4/4/06

ANNA

Nancy,
Enjoy the book. Thank
you for all you have
done and continue to
do for Nephrology Nursing.
and for your very
special friendship.

Best Regards,
Evelyn

Contemporary Nephrology Nursing:
Principles and Practice

Contemporary Nephrology Nursing: Principles and Practice

Second Edition

Anita E. Molzahn, PhD, RN
Editor

Evelyn Butera, MS, RN, CNN
Assistant Editor

Copyright © 2006
American Nephrology Nurses' Association

Publication Management by
Anthony J. Jannetti, Inc.; East Holly Avenue/Box 56; Pitman, New Jersey 08071-0056

ISBN No. 0-9768125-4-1

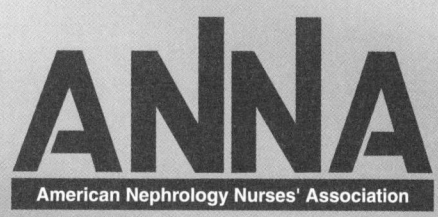

ANNA
American Nephrology Nurses' Association

Preface

Janel Parker left a wonderful legacy with the publication of the first edition of *Contemporary Nephrology Nursing*. Evelyn and I were looking forward to working with her as Associate Editors on this second edition, but Janel's unexpected and tragic death in 2003 left a huge vacuum. I have often reflected on how we would have enjoyed working with her on this publication (she was such fun to work with), but we know that Janel would have wanted us to continue on and build on the strong foundation of the first edition.

This edition of *Contemporary Nephrology Nursing: Principles and Practice* is directed to a North American audience of front-line nephrology nurses. We recognize that there are many practice patterns and cultural perspectives that will be different in other regions of the world. Nevertheless, there has been interest in the book from many areas of the world and from other health professionals working in nephrology settings. We hope that graduate and undergraduate students in nursing also find it to be a useful reference book.

Knowledge in nephrology nursing continues to grow at a rapid rate. We have integrated current research findings and best current practices into the various chapters of this text. As ANNA continues to strive towards the goal of research-based practice, we expect that this book will move us forward in attaining that goal.

In this edition, there is a new opportunity for nurses to earn CE credits for each chapter that they read. Not only can you increase your knowledge base, but now you can also obtain CE credit!

This is an exciting and dynamic specialty in nursing. It blends rich opportunities to come to know individuals and their families with opportunities to integrate complex knowledge and skills in a wide range of care settings. There are few more rewarding or challenging opportunities in nursing. We hope that this book will prove to be a valuable resource to you as you deal with the many challenges in nephrology nursing practice.

Knowledge in our specialty will continue to grow, as will nursing knowledge and medical knowledge. Please offer your suggestions of areas that you would like to see addressed in future editions, by contacting either of the editors or ANNA, the publisher.

Anita Molzahn, PhD, RN
Editor

Evelyn Butera, MS, RN, CNN
Assistant Editor

Foreword

A decade, a century and a millennium have all passed since the first edition of *Contemporary Nephrology Nursing* was published in 1998. In the past 8 years, many events have transformed the healthcare landscape of our country and the world. Many of these have influenced the manner in which professional nurses deliver care to patients with kidney disease. With policy focus on value-based reimbursement; concern for the exponential increase in chronic conditions such as diabetes, hypertension, and obesity; the demands of a mobile, aging population; the emphasis on quality of life and end of life options; and the decrease in the number of nurses available to provide care, our nursing specialty has many opportunities to become preoccupied. However, the second edition of the *Contemporary Nephrology Nursing: Principles and Practice* Textbook brings nephrology nursing back to the basics of our practice regardless of the setting and supports ANNA's mission to advance nephrology nursing practice and positively influence outcomes for patients with kidney or other disease processes requiring replacement therapies through advocacy, scholarship, and excellence.

The new edition builds upon the foundation set forth in the first edition as nephrology nurses faced a new millennium. The ANNA Board of Directors and I are grateful to Editor Dr. Anita Molzahn and Assistant Editor Evelyn Butera for assembling expert contributors and reviewers to deliver a publication that I would recommend be available for frequent reference in resource libraries of individuals as well as educational and work settings. Few can comprehend the time, dedication and commitment that a project of this magnitude involves, but all who benefit will appreciate the product.

Finally, it is fitting to remember Janel Parker, Editor of the first edition of *Contemporary Nephrology Nursing,* whose untimely death in 2003 brought great sadness to many whose personal and professional lives were touched by the contributions she made to nephrology nursing. Few nephrology nurses have played such a significant role in the professional growth and development of nephrology nursing as Janel. She would be proud of the second edition of this textbook if she were here today!

Suzann VanBuskirk, BSN, RN, CNN
ANNA President, 2005-2006

Dedication to Janel Parker

On August 26, 2003, nephrology nursing and the American Nephrology Nurses' Association (ANNA) lost one of our best and brightest colleagues when Janel Parker passed away following injuries sustained in an automobile accident in Philadelphia. Janel, who had served as the first Editor of *Contemporary Nephrology Nursing* in 1998, had just been appointed Editor for the second edition of this publication at the time of her sudden and unexpected death.

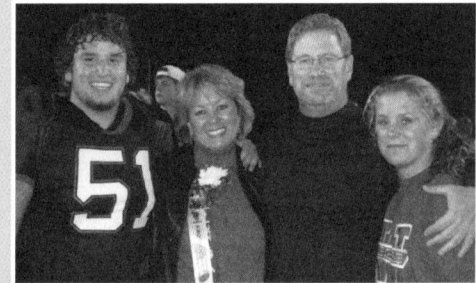

Not only did Janel leave behind her wonderful family – daughter Ellen, son J.D., and husband David – but she left behind a professional legacy that was brilliant and lengthy to say the least. Where do we begin when speaking of Janel's many professional accomplishments? During her career, she:

Janel Parker (2nd from L), with her son J.D., husband David, and daughter Ellen, was a dedicated mother and wife as well as a devoted colleague and friend to nephrology nurses around the country.

- Served as President of ANNA in 1986-87;
- Helped to form the Nephrology Nursing Certification Board (NNCB) and develop the first Nephrology Nursing Certification Examination;
- Served as Charter President of NNCB, now known as the Nephrology Nursing Certification Commission (NNCC);
- Served as NNCC's first full-time Executive Director;
- Served as the first Editor of the *Contemporary Nephrology Nursing* textbook; and
- Helped to organize the American Board of Nursing Specialties (ABNS), serving a term as its first President.

Janel was honored for her many accomplishments in 1992 when she was awarded the Outstanding Contribution to ANNA Award, the association's highest honor! She received additional honors as well from other organizations for her ongoing role in patient advocacy.

Those of us who were close to her, of course, knew Janel for her bright, caring, and energizing personality! She took many of her colleagues and friends under her wing, and helped all of us fulfill accomplishments and goals we thought beyond our reach.

Ironically, it was primarily Janel's outgoing and caring personality that have led us to bestow upon her one more honor. The Editors, staff, and members of the ANNA Board of Directors would like to dedicate this Second Edition of *Contemporary Nephrology Nursing: Principles and Practice* to Janel Parker, for whom this project was close to her heart.

Thank you Janel for your wonderful legacy. We have missed you!

Anita E. Molzahn, PhD, RN
Editor

Evelyn Butera, MSN, RN, CNN
Assistant Editor

Table of Contents

Contemporary Nephrology Nursing: Principles and Practice
Second Edition

Table of Contents and Contributors

Unit One
Nature and Scope of Nephrology Nursing

Unit Two
The Kidney

Table of Contents

Table of Contents

Table of Contents

Table of Contents

Contributors

Editor
Anita E. Molzahn, PhD, RN
University of Victoria
Vancouver, British Columbia, Canada

Assistant Editor
Evelyn Butera, MS, RN, CNN
Mills-Peninsula Health Services
A Sutter Health Affiliate
Burlingame, CA

Contributors

Cynthia Baker, PhD, MN, RN
University of New Brunswick
Fredericton, New Brunswick, Canada

Marilyn Bartucci, MSN, RN, CS, CCTC
Fujisawa Healthcare, Inc.
Euclid, OH

Patricia Brennan, MSN, RN
Fresenius Medical Care
Lexington, MA

LaVonne M. Burrows, M-SCNS, BC, RN, CNN
Springfield Nephrology Associates
Springfield, MO

Lori Candela, EdD, RN, APRN, BC, FNP
University of Nevada, Las Vegas
Las Vegas, NV

Laurie Carlson, RN, MSN
UCSF Transplant Service
San Francisco, CA

Ann Cashion, PhD, RN
University of Tennessee Health
Science Center
Memphis, TN

Christine Chmielewski, MS, CRNP, CNN, CS
Edward Filippone MD, PC
Philadelphia, PA

Elaine R. Colvin, BSN, RN, MEPD
Gundersen Lutheran
La Crosse, WI

Caroline S. Counts, MSN, RN, CNN
Medical University of South Carolina
Charleston, SC

Leanne Dekker, MBA, MN, RN
University of Alberta Hospitals
Edmonton, Alberta, Canada

Lesley C. Dinwiddie, MSN, RN, FNP, CNN
Nephrology Nurse Consultant
Cary, NC

Carolyn J. Driscoll, MSN, RN, FNP-C
University of Tennessee Health
Sciences Center
Memphis, TN

Annette Frauman, PhD, RN, FAAN
Atlanta, GA

Cyrena Gilman, MN, RN, CNN
Riley Hospital for Children
Indianapolis, IN

Jordi Goldstein-Fuchs, DSc, RD
DaVita, Inc.
Sparks Dialysis
Sparks, NV

David Guthrie, MN, ARNP
University of Florida
Gainesville, FL

Lori Harwood, MSc, RN, CNeph(C)
London Health Science Centre
London, Ontario, Canada

Maryse Pelletier Hibbert, MN, RN
University of New Brunswick
Fredericton, Canada

Mary Jo Holechek, MS, CRNP, CNN
Johns Hopkins Hospital
Baltimore, MD

Elizabeth Kelman, MEd, RN, CNeph(C)
University Health Network/Toronto GH
Toronto, Ontario, Canada

Carolyn E. Latham, MSN, MBA, RN, CNN
Renal Care Group
Nashville, TN

Francis Lau, PhD
University of Victoria
Victoria, British Columbia, Canada

Rosemary Leitch, RN, CNeph(C)
London Health Science Centre
London, Ontario, Canada

Marlys Ludlow, MS, RN
Stanford University Hospital
Palo Alto, CA

Terran Mathers, DNS, RN
Spring Hill College
Mobile, AL

Patricia McCarley, MSN, RN, ACNPc, CNN
Diablo Nephrology Group
Walnut Creek, CA

Janice McCormick, PhD, RN
University of Victoria
Lower Mainland Campus
Vancouver, British Columbia, Canada

Anita E. Molzahn, PhD, RN
University of Victoria
Vancouver, British Columbia, Canada

Christine Mudge, RN, MS, PNPc/CNS, CNN, FAAN
University of California
San Francisco, CA

Janice A. Neil, PhD, RN
East Carolina University
Greenville, NC

Kathy P. Parker, PhD, RN, FAAN
Emory University
Atlanta, GA

Eileen J. Peacock, MSN, RN, CNN, CIC, CPHQ
DaVita, Inc.
Berwyn, PA

Barbara F. Prowant, MS, RN, CNN
University of Missouri
Columbia, MO

David Quan, PharmD
UCSF
San Francisco, CA

Christy Price Rabetoy, NP
Nephrology Associates, Inc.
Salt Lake City, UT

Mary Rau-Foster, MBA, BS, JD, RN
Foster Seminars and Communication
Brentwood, TN

Karen C. Robbins, MS, RN, CNN
Hartford Hospital
Hartford, CT

Patricia Baltz Salai, MSN, RN, CNN, CRNP
VA Pittsburgh Healthcare System
Pittsburgh, PA

Contributors

Kristine Schonder, PharmD
University of Pittsburgh School of Pharmacy
Pittsburgh, PA

Kathleen Smith, BS, RN, CNN
Fresenius Medical Care
Washington, DC

Rosalie Starzomski, PhD, RN
University of Victoria
Vancouver, British Columbia, Canada

Nicola Thomas, MA, BSc (Hons), RN
St. Helier Hospital
Carshalton, Surrey, England

Charlotte Thomas-Hawkins, PhD, RN
Rutgers University
Newark, NJ

Isabelle Toupin, MN, RN
University of Laval
Laval, Quebec, Canada

Beth Tamplet Ulrich, EdD, RN, CHE
Nephrology Nursing Journal
Pearland, TX

Diane M. Watson, RN, MSc, CNeph(C)
Toronto General Hospital, University Health Network
Toronto, Ontario, Canada

Janet L. Welch, DNS, RN, CNS
Indiana University
Indianapolis, IN

Randee Breiterman White, MS, RN, CNN
Vanderbilt Medical Center
Nashville, FL

Gail S. Wick, BSN, RN, CNN
Consultant
Atlanta, GA

Carolyn B. Yucha, PhD, RN, FAAN
University of Nevada
Las Vegas, NV

Reviewers

The Editors of *Contemporary Nephrology Nursing* wish to thank the following professionals, who reviewed and commented on the content of the chapters in this publication.

Kim M. Alleman, MS, RN, FNP, CNN
Hartford Hospital
Hartford, CT

Joan Arslanian, MSN, RN, CNN, FNP, CS
New York Hospital Medical Center of Queens
Fresh Meadows, NY

Lynda Ball, BS, BSN, RN, CNN
Northwest Renal Network
Seattle, WA

Donna Bednarski, MSN, APRN, BC, CNN, CNP
Harper University Hospital
Detroit, MI

Judy Bernardini, BSN, RN
University of Pittsburgh
Pittsburgh, PA

Geri Biddle, RN, CNN, CPHQ
Nephrology Nurse Consultants
Loudonville, NY

Joan Brookhyser, RD, CSR, CD
St. Joseph Medical Center
Tacoma, WA

Laura Broome, RN, CPN
Children's Hospital of Alabama
Birmingham, AL

Deborah J. Brouwer, RN, CNN
Renal Solutions, Inc.
Warrendale, PA

Gillian Brunier, MScN, RN
Sunnybrook & Womens Hospitals
Toronto, Canada

Sally Burrows-Hudson, MS, RN, CNN
Nephrology Management Group, Inc.
Sunnyvale, CA

Anita Catlin, DNSc, FNP, FAAN
Sonoma State University
Rohnert Park, CA

Christine M. Ceccerelli, MS, MBA, RN, CNN
Hartford Hospital
Hartford, CT

Christine Chmielewski, MS, CRNP, CNN, CS
Edward J. Filippone, MD, PC
Philadelphia, PA

Jean Colaneri, MS, RN, CNN
Albany Medical Center Hospital
Albany, NY

Caroline S. Counts, MSN, RN, CNN
Medical University of South Carolina
Charleston, SC

Nancy Fleming Courts, PhD, RN, NCC
University of North Carolina
Greensboro, NC

Patricia A. Cowan, PhD, RN
University of Tennessee Health Science Center
Memphis, TN

Kennith Culp, PhD, RN
University of Iowa
Iowa City, IA

Roberta Braun Curtin, PhD
Medical Education Institute
Madison, WI

Peggy Devney, RN, CNS, ACNP
University of California
San Francisco, CA

Sheila J. Doss, RN, CNN
Satellite Healthcare, Inc.
Mountain View, CA

Claudia M. Douglas, MA, RN, CNN
Hackensack University Medical Center
Hackensack, NJ

Andrea Easom, MA, MNSc, APN, BC, CNN
University of Arkansas for Medical Science Kidney Center
Little Rock, AR

Reviewers

The Editors of *Contemporary Nephrology Nursing* wish to thank the following professionals, who reviewed and commented on the content of the chapters in this publication.

Pamela R. Frederick, MSB
Centers for Medicare & Medicaid
Baltimore, MD

Nancy M. Gallagher, BSN, RN, CNN
St. Joseph Medical Center
Tacoma, WA

Karen K. Guiliano, MSN, CCRN, NP
Phillips Medical Systems
Andover, MA

Nancy Hoffart, PhD, RN
Northeastern University
Boston, MA

Mary Jo Holchek, MS, CRNP, CNN
Johns Hopkins Hospital
Baltimore, MD

Dawn T. Holcombe, MSN, RN, CDE
Eli Lilly & Company
Indianapolis, IN

Jean A. Jacko, PhD, RN
Capital University
Columbus, OH

Tamara M. Kear, MSN, RN, CNN
Physicians Dialysis, Inc.
Philadelphia, PA

Karen Kelley, BSN, RN, CNN
Baxter Healthcare Corporation, Renal
Division
McGaw Park, IL

Maria Luongo, MSN, BA, RN
Massachusetts General Hospital
Boston, MA

Jean A. S. MacMullen, RN, CNA
Health Care Consultant
Inverness, FL

Harold Manley, PharmD, BCPS, FASN
Albany College of Pharmacy
Albany, NY

Judith C. Meraw, BHScN, RN, CNeph(C)
London Health Sciences Centre
London, Ontario, Canada

Sheila G. Mitchell, MSN, ACNP, CNN
Network 8, Inc.
Jackson, MS

Amy Barton Pai, PharmD, BCPS, FASN
University of New Mexico Health Sciences
Center
College of Pharmacy
Albuquerque, NM

Eileen J. Peacock, MSN, RN, CNN, CIC, CPHQ
DaVita, Inc.
Berwyn, PA

Daisy Perry, BScN, RN
Retired, University of Alberta Hospitals
Edmonton, Alberta, Canada

Marcia Phillips, DNSc, RN
St. Luke's Medical Center
Chicago, IL

Mary A. Pipkin, BA, RN, CNN
Lynchburg Nephrology, Inc.
Lynchburg, VA

Linda M. Plush, MSN, RN, CNS/FNP, CNN
Plush Systems, Inc.
Palmdale, CA

Christy A. Price Rabetoy, NP
Nephrology Associates, Inc.
Salt Lake City, UT

Fannie Rankin-Vinci, RN, CDE
Mills-Peninsula Health Services
Burlingame, CA

Kitty Richardson
Falls Church, VA

Sue Dickey Roberts
Abbott Laboratories
Oakland, CA

Joan H. Ruppert, MSN, RN, CNN
St. Louis Community College
Kirkwood, MO

Patricia Baltz Salai, MSN, RN, CNN, CRNP
VA Pittsburgh Healthcare System
Pittsburgh, PA

Mary Scott, PhD, RN
UCSF Department of Psychological Nursing
San Francisco, CA

Nancy J. Sharp, MSN, RN, FAAN
Sharp & Associates
Bethesda, MD

Rosalie C. Starzomski, PhD, RN
University of Victoria
Vancouver, British Columbia, Canada

Donna J. Swartzendruber, MSN, RN, CNN
DaVita, Inc.
Denver, CO

Charlotte Szromba, MSN, APRN, NP, CNN
University of Chicago
Chicago, IL

Charlotte Thomas-Hawkins, PhD, RN
Rutgers University
Newark, NJ

Annie W. Tu, MSN, ARNP, CNN, RN
University of Washington Medical Center
Seattle, WA

Diane M. Watson, MSc, RN, CNeph(C)
Toronto General Hospital, University Health
Network
Toronto, Ontario, Canada

Patricia D. Weiskittel, MSN, RN, APRN, BC, CNN
VA Hospital Medical Center
Cincinnati, OH

Joan K. Werner, BSN, CNN, MBA
Fresenius Medical Care
Lexington, MA

Beth Witten, MSW
Medical Education Institute
Madison, WI

Gail S. Wick, BSN, RN, CNN
Consultant
Atlanta, GA

Barbara Wilson, MScN, RN, CNeph(C)
London Health Sciences Centre
London, Ontario, Canada

Rebecca P. Winsett, PhD
University of Tennessee
Memphis, TN

Karen C. Wiseman, MSN, RN, CNN
Renal America, Inc.
Brentwood, TN

Cynthia Yam, BScN, RN
University of Alberta Hospital
Edmonton, Alberta, Canada

Acknowledgments

There are many people who contribute to the publication of a comprehensive textbook like *Contemporary Nephrology Nursing: Principles and Practice.* We would like to express our sincere gratitude to the many people who made this book possible. In particular, we would like to extend our appreciation to:

Gus Ostrum, for his wonderful organizational ability, expert advice, good judgment, and invaluable support,

Mike Cunningham and the **Board of Directors of ANNA,** for their confidence in our abilities and ongoing support of the project,

Katie Brownlow and **Lauren McClintock,** for their administrative, organizational, and editorial skills,

To the authors, for their creativity, persistence and cooperation in meeting deadlines, despite many personal and family responsibilities and challenges.

Anita Molzahn, PhD, RN
Editor

Evelyn Butera, MS, RN, CNN
Assistant Editor

Sponsorships
ANNA would like to thank the following companies for their sponsorships of this textbook.

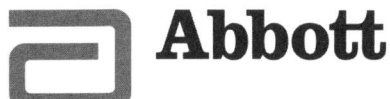
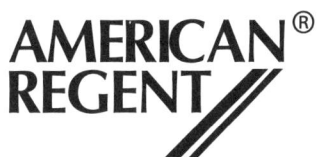
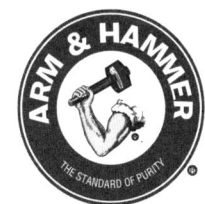

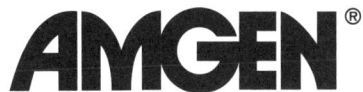
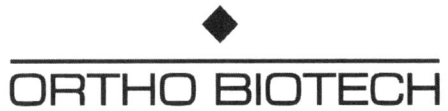
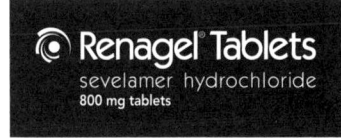

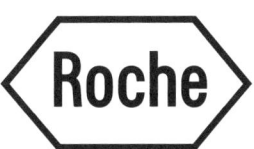
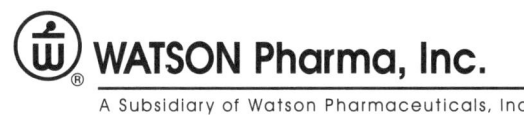

Nature and Scope of Nephrology Nursing

UNIT 1

Unit 1 Contents

Professional Nephrology Nursing

Beth Tamplet Ulrich, EdD, RN, CHE

Chapter Contents

Professional Nephrology Nursing

Chapter 1

Beth Tamplet Ulrich, EdD, RN, CHE

Professional nursing has evolved from the most basic caring behaviors to the complex knowledge and expertise of today's advanced practice nurses. Nursing theories range from Nightingale's first theory that the goal of nursing is to "put the patient in the best condition for nature to act upon him," (Nightingale, 1859, p. 75) which stressed manipulating the patient's environment to theories that emphasize self-care, adaptation, systems, caring, goal attainment, etc.

Contemporary nephrology nursing is exciting and fulfilling. Few other nursing specialties offer the wide range of opportunities in nursing roles, practice settings, in-depth and long-term relationships with patients, and collaboration with other health care professionals. Professional nephrology nursing is, however, complex and requires an understanding of both the role of the professional nurse and the practice of nephrology nursing.

The Development of Professional Nursing Practice

Contemporary nursing practice traces its roots back to 1860 when the Nightingale School for Nurses at St. Thomas Hospital in London opened its doors. Created from donations collected by the English people to honor the work of Florence Nightingale in the Crimea, the Nightingale School was the first formal program to educate and train nurses. At its foundation were principles established by Florence Nightingale including: classes taught by both nurses and physicians, an apprentice model that required many hours in the clinical setting, and 360° evaluations between students and teachers. Florence Nightingale herself was a great role model for nurses of the future. Everything she set out to do was aimed at improving the health or health care of individuals, whether it was caring for the soldiers in the Crimea, improving the health care of the British Military, reforming sanitation practices in India, creating a statistical system to determine which hospitals delivered better care, or designing hospitals.

The Civil War created the first major demand for nurses in the United States (U.S.). During and after the war, members of the U.S. Sanitary Commission consulted with Florence Nightingale about nursing and the education of nurses (Flanagan, 1976). In 1873, three schools of nursing were established in the U.S. based on the Nightingale model – the Bellevue Training School for Nurses in New York City; the Connecticut Training School for Nurses in New Haven, Connecticut; and the Boston Training School for Nurses at Massachusetts General Hospital (Dock, 1907). At about the same time, significant advances were being made in the areas of anesthesia, germ theory, antisepsis, and diagnostic tools. Hospitals moved from being almshouses for the poor to becoming institutions for the care and curing of the sick and injured (Starr, 1982). Nursing also advanced. As a result of the efforts of the nurses who volunteered to serve in the Spanish-American war in 1898, Congress determined that nurses should be a part of the defense forces of the U.S. The Army Nurse Corps was established in 1901 and the Navy Nurse Corps in 1908.

Hospitals and physicians quickly discovered the benefits of having a labor force of nursing students and a staff of graduate nurses. By 1900, the number of nursing schools in the U.S. had grown rapidly to 432 and increased to 1,129 by 1910 (Ashley, 1976). However, as the number of schools of nursing and hospitals grew, conflicts often arose between the educational needs of the students and the hospitals' needs for students to care for the hospitals' patients. In what was perhaps the beginning of the quality and quantity discussions surrounding nursing, nursing educators attempted to improve the quality of nursing education, while hospitals wanted the nursing schools to provide a larger quantity of nursing students. Hospitals grew rapidly in the early 1900s, but often preferred to use nursing students rather than hiring graduate nurses.

The need for nurses in World War I birthed several new nursing programs. During the depression years, as the number of paying patients declined significantly, many hospitals closed their nursing programs in an effort to save money and replaced nursing students with untrained staff. It quickly became apparent, however, that patient care was suffering and hospitals began to hire graduate nurses. An available work pool of unemployed graduate nurses willing to work for minimum wages, the new Blue Cross health insurance program, and the passage of national legislation to fund health and medical care for indigent Americans resulted in an increase in the number of graduate nurse positions in hospitals from 4,000 in 1929, to 28,000 in 1937, and over 100,000 by 1941 (Cannings & Lazonick, 1975). The shortage of nurses in World War II lead to the creation of the Cadet Nurse Corps in 1943, which provided funds for nursing education to students who agreed to serve in military or civilian agencies until the war was over as well as funds for the nursing schools who participated. The Cadet Nurse Corps program added over 100,000 new nurses to the work force. After World War II, many nurse veterans used the G.I. Bill of Rights benefits to expand their nursing education, and as a result, the number of undergraduate nursing programs expanded significantly. In addition, community college programs were created in the late 1950s and early 1960s to provide associate degree programs in nursing.

The 1950s and 1960s were also a time of dramatic technological and scientific advances in medicine and surgery, a huge population explosion as the Baby Boomer generation was born, and an increased consumer demand for health services. Clinical subspecialties were developed and coronary care units and intensive care units proliferated. To keep pace and to function in these new specialties, nurses needed to acquire additional knowledge and more complex clinical competencies. Masters' and doctoral programs in nursing were created to meet the growing need for advanced practice nurses.

Nursing went through many phases as it moved into the latter part of the 20th century and the beginning of the 21st century. Issues such as defining the role of the nurse, determining what differentiated the practice of nurses educated at the various levels of nursing education, defining what level of education should constitute entry into nursing practice,

Table 1-1

Staff Nurse Self-Assessment to Determine Readiness to Pursue Magnet Recognition

- Do the nursing services of this health care organization have excellent patient outcomes?
- Is there a high level of staff job satisfaction?
- Does the health care organization have a low turnover rate among nurses who provide direct patient care?
- Are grievances heard and responded to in a timely and appropriate manner?
- Are nurses actively involved in matters that impact the provision of patient care?
- Are the contributions of nurses who provide direct patient care valued by nurses serving in leadership positions?
- Are nurses involved in the collection of data that affects patient outcomes or care or that affects the delivery of nursing care within the organization?
- Are nurses provided time, compensation, and involvement in the data collection, data analysis, and decision-making activities that impact nursing practice and the delivery of patient care?
- Are policies, procedures, and guidelines for nursing practice based on research and/or data collection findings?
- Is there open communication between nurses and members of other disciplines?
- Are personnel utilized appropriately to attain the highest levels of patient outcomes and to optimize the staff work environment? Are nurses encouraged to advance nursing practice within the work environment?
- Is the advancement of the individual nurse encouraged and rewarded?
- Am I proud of the organization that I work for?
- Would I recommend to my nurse friends that they work for this organization?

Note: From American Nurses' Credentialing Center (ANCC). (2004b). *Staff nurse self-assessment to determine readiness to pursue magnet recognition.* Washington, DC: Author. Retrieved July 18, 2004, from www.nursingworld.org/ancc/magnet/selfassess.pdf.

Table 1-2

Hallmarks of the Professional Nursing Practice Environment

- Manifests a philosophy of clinical care emphasizing quality, safety, interdisciplinary collaboration, continuity of care, and professional accountability.
- Recognizes contributions of nurses' knowledge and expertise to clinical care quality and patient outcomes.
- Promotes executive level nursing leadership.
- Empowers nurses' participation in clinical decision-making and organization of clinical care systems.
- Maintains clinical advancement programs based on education, certification, and advanced preparation.
- Demonstrates professional development support for nurses.
- Creates collaborative relationships among members of the health care provider team.
- Utilizes technological advances in clinical care and information systems.

Note: From American Association of Colleges of Nursing (AACN). (2002). *Hallmarks of the professional nursing practice environment.* Washington, DC: Author. Retrieved July 9, 2004, from www.aacn.nche.edu/Publications/Positions/Hallmarks.htm

ine characteristics of systems that impeded or facilitated the professional practice of nursing in hospitals (McClure, Poulin, Sovie, & Wandelt, 1983). As a result, 41 hospitals were identified that were known for patient care excellence and for their ability to attract and retain registered nurses (thus, the title of "magnet" hospitals). In 1994, the American Nurses' Association (ANA), through its subsidiary the American Nurses' Credentialing Center (ANCC), established a magnet hospital designation process. In order to achieve Magnet Recognition status, organizations must perform a self-appraisal and undergo a site visit to demonstrate that they meet the criteria for Magnet Recognition.

Subsequent research has continued to support the characteristics identified in the original Magnet research as being beneficial to both patients and registered nurses. As a result, the Magnet Recognition Program has now expanded beyond hospitals and broadened its activities beyond recognition. Its current goals are to recognize nursing services that build programs of excellence for the delivery of nursing care to patients, promote a work environment that supports professional nursing practice, provide a vehicle to disseminate successful nursing practices and strategies, and promote positive patient outcomes (ANCC, 2004a). Registered Nurses are encouraged to use the Magnet criteria to evaluate current and potential work environments (see Table 1-1) (ANCC, 2004b).

In 2002, the American Association of Colleges of Nursing (AACN) identified the environmental characteristics that best support professional nursing practice and also allow nurses to practice to their full potential (AACN, 2002). These hallmarks of a professional nursing practice environment are summarized in Table 1-2.

The science of nursing began to expand significantly in latter part of the 20th century and the beginning of the 21st

and determining whether or not it was beneficial for nurses to unionize both brought some nurses together but, at the same time, caused much dissension. As more women entered the work force and career options for women expanded, nursing school enrollments declined and did not begin to pick back up until 2001. Extensive national, regional, and local efforts to recruit more people into nursing were so effective that by 2003, many schools of nursing were experiencing a number of qualified applicants far exceeding the number of student slots available.

Nursing shortages have come and gone in an almost cyclic nature – sometimes as the result of changes in reimbursement for care (such as when Medicare was enacted in 1965 or when managed care became the norm in the late 1990s) and sometimes as a result of the attention or lack of attention paid to the environments within which nurses practiced and the compensation they received. In 1983, the American Academy of Nursing launched a project to exam-

century. Traditional practices were investigated to determine what really worked and what didn't. In 1985, the National Center for Nursing Research was established within the National Institutes of Health (NIH), thereby moving nursing research into the mainstream. Research on the outcomes of nursing care is increasingly resulting in an evidence base for the practice of nursing in the care of patients and in the way care is delivered.

In care delivery, for example, nurse staffing levels have been found to be related to quality of care. Needleman, Buerhaus, Mattke, Stewart, and Zelevinsky (2002) found that higher proportions of registered nurses as well as a greater amount of care by registered nurses were both associated with better patient care outcomes. Aiken, Clarke, Sloane, Sochalski, and Silber (2002) studied the care of surgical patients in hospitals and concluded that surgical patients had higher risk-adjusted 30-day mortality and failure-to-rescue rates and nurses were more likely to experience burnout and job dissatisfaction in hospitals with higher patient-to-nurse ratios. The effect of the educational level of nurses has also been studied in relation to patient outcomes. Aiken, Clarke, Cheung, Sloane, and Silber (2003) found that a 10% increase in the proportion of nurses holding a bachelor's degree was associated with a 5% decrease in 30-day mortality and the odds of failure to rescue. These kinds of studies have provided a solid evidence base for changing practices in the delivery of patient care.

The roles of advanced practice nurses have continued to expand. Prescriptive authority and independent practice have been authorized in many states, and the ability for advanced practice nurses to be reimbursed for their services has increased.

Organized Nursing

The first organized meeting of nurses in America occurred in 1893 at the Chicago World's Fair – the same meeting at which a paper written by Florence Nightingale was presented that laid the foundation for modern holistic nursing by discussing prevention as well as sick care as a part of the role of nursing. Superintendents from 18 U.S. nursing schools met to discuss nursing education problems. As a result, the American Society of Superintendents of Training Schools for Nurses of the U.S. and Canada (renamed the National League for Nursing Education in 1912 and along with two other nursing organizations formed the National League for Nursing in 1952) was created in 1894 to establish and maintain a universal standard of training, promote the fellowship of its members, and to further the best interests of the nursing profession (Canavan, 1996). In 1886, this society established the Committee for the Organization of a National Association for Nurses to prepare a constitution and bylaws for a new organization that would meet the needs of nurses. That organization, the Nurses' Associated Alumnae of the U.S. and Canada, was formed in 1896 and, in 1911, was renamed the American Nurses' Association (Canavan, 1996). Its first initiative was to obtain legal registration for nurses. With the number of untrained "nurses" growing steadily, nursing leaders felt that the only way to protect the public was to enact state licensure. In addition, they believed that licensure based on educational credentials and an examina-

Figure 1-1
Model for Nephrology Nursing Practice Base

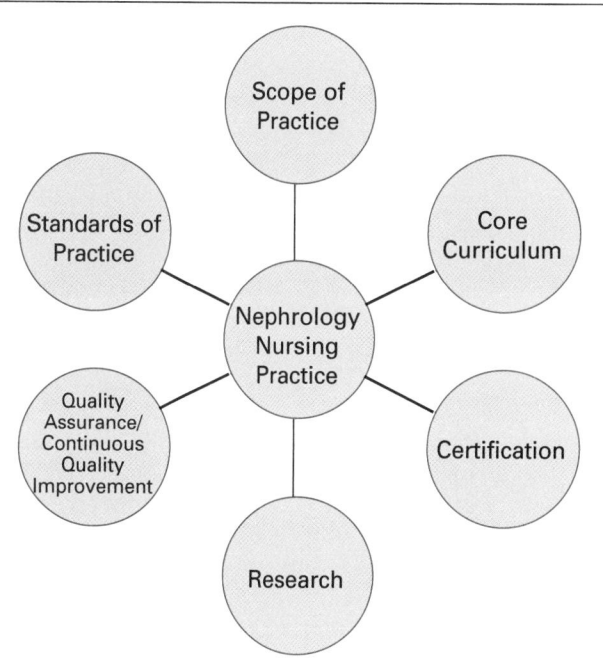

Note: Revised from Jordan, P.J. (1993). *Professional development guide* (p. 8). Pitman, NJ: American Nephrology Nurses' Association. Reprinted with permission.

tion would encourage higher educational standards and would also enhance the public's view of nursing as a profession (Brodie & Keeling, 2001). State associations of the Nurses' Associated Alumnae were formed to lobby for state licensure laws. In March 1903, North Carolina became the first state to enact a nurse registration act, and all states had nurse registration laws by 1923.

Professional Nursing Today

Nursing is defined as "the protection, promotion, and optimization of health and abilities, prevention of illness and injury, alleviation of suffering through the diagnosis and treatment of human response, and advocacy in the care of individuals, families, communities, and populations" (ANA, 2003). The authority for the practice of nursing, according to the *ANA Nursing: Scope and Standards of Practice* (2004), "is based on a social contract that acknowledges the professional rights and responsibilities of nursing and includes mechanisms for public accountability" (p. vi).

Nursing has evolved over the years into a profession that has a distinct body of knowledge, a social contract, and an ethical code. Professional nursing practice is complex and multifaceted (see Figure 1-1). As noted by Koerner and Burgess (1997), "The new health care paradigm demands extraordinary expertise, phenomenal creativity, a command of finance and information systems, mastery of managed care principles, and a great sense of humor" (p. 2).

Standards of Nursing Practice

Standards, as defined by the ANA (2004), are "authoritative statements by which the nursing profession describes the responsibilities for which its practitioners are accountable. Consequently, standards reflect the values and priorities of the profession. Standards provide direction for professional nursing practice and a framework for the evaluation of this practice. Written in measurable terms, standards also define the nursing profession's accountability to the public and outcomes for which registered nurses are responsible" (p. 1).

ANA published the first *Standards of Nursing Practice* in 1973. The standards were generic and focused on the basic nursing process (ANA, 2004). The current standards, published in 2004, include standards of practice, which describe a competent level of nursing care, and standards of professional practice, which describe a competent level of behavior in the professional role (ANA, 2004). All of the standards have basic measurement criteria as well as additional measurement criteria for advanced practice RNs and nursing role specialties. Leadership has been added to the standards of professional practice in this revision reflecting the belief that all RNs are expected to act in a leadership role appropriate to their education and position. Several themes have been identified that span all areas of nursing practice, are fundamental to many of the standards, and are consistently and significantly influential in nursing practice. These themes are: providing age-appropriate and culturally and ethnically sensitive care, maintaining a safe environment, educating patients about healthy practices and treatment modalities, assuring continuity of care, coordinating the care across settings and among caregivers, managing information, communicating effectively, and utilizing technology (ANA, 2004).

Code of Ethics

The ANA Code of Ethics for Nurses is a succinct statement of the ethical obligations and duties of every individual who enters the nursing profession, is the profession's nonnegotiable ethical standard, and is an expression of nursing's own understanding of its commitment to society (ANA, 2001). The nine provisions in the Code of Ethics describe the fundamental values and commitment of the RN, the boundaries of duty and loyalty, and the duties beyond individual patient encounters (see Table 1-3) (ANA, 2001).

Public Trust

Another important aspect of professional nursing today is the public's view of the nursing profession. Beginning in 1999, the Gallup organization included nurses in their annual survey on the honesty and ethics of various professions. Nurses have ranked higher than any other profession every year since, with the exception of 2001. That year, firefighters were included and ranked just above nurses in the wake of the September 11 attacks. In the November, 2004 survey, 79% of the public surveyed ranked the honesty and ethics of nurses as high or very high (Gallup Poll News Services, 2004).

Specialty Nursing Practice

The proliferation of medical and nursing knowledge and the necessary competencies that must accompany that knowledge have made it virtually impossible for any one practitioner to acquire all the knowledge and competencies required to care for the health and illness needs of all indi-

Table 1-3
ANA Code of Ethics

Provision 1. The nurse, in all professional relationships, practices with compassion and respect for the inherent dignity, worth, and uniqueness of every individual, unrestricted by considerations of social or economic status, personal attributes, or the nature of health problems.

Provision 2. The nurse's primary commitment is to the patient, whether an individual, family, group, or community.

Provision 3. The nurse promotes, advocates for, and strives to protect the health, safety, and rights of the patient.

Provision 4. The nurse is responsible and accountable for individual nursing practice and determines the appropriate delegation of tasks consistent with the nurse's obligation to promote optimum patient care.

Provision 5. The nurse owes the same duties to self as to others, including the responsibility to preserve integrity and safety, to maintain competence, and to continue personal and professional growth.

Provision 6. The nurse participates in establishing, maintaining, and improving health care environments and conditions of employment conducive to the provision of quality health care and consistent with the values of the profession through individual and collective action.

Provision 7. The nurse participates in the advancement of the profession through contributions to practice, education, administration, and knowledge development.

Provision 8. The nurse collaborates with other health professionals and the public in promoting community, national, and international efforts to meet health care needs.

Provision 9. The profession of nursing, as represented by associations and their members, is responsible for articulating nursing values, for maintaining the integrity of the profession and its practice, and for shaping social policy.

Note: From American Nurses' Association (ANA). (2001). *Code of ethics for nurses with interpretive statements.* Washington, DC: Author. Retrieved March 21, 2004, from www.nursingworld.org/ethics/code/ethicscode 150.htm.

viduals. Specialization provides the opportunity for individual practitioners to focus on one area of care and, as a result, to provide the best possible care those in need (Parker, 1998).

Though the nation's first clinical specialty organization, the National Organization for Public Health Nursing, was formed in 1912, organized specialty nursing practice really began in earnest in 1966 when the ANA established divisions of practice. These divisions were based on evidence that a substantial number of nurses were practicing in a field of nursing with a well-defined and unique body of nursing knowledge and skills and/or upon evidence that a significant health problem existed in which nursing was involved. The divisions established were community health nursing, geriatric nursing, maternal and child nursing, and psychiatric and mental health nursing. The purpose of each division of practice was to establish standards for nursing practice, conduct clinical and scientific sessions at ANA conventions, stimulate research, disseminate relevant information in areas of practice, provide recognition for professional achieve-

Table 1-4
Benefits of Achieving Certification

- Quality Care
- Patient Satisfaction
- Professional Recognition
- Financial Compensation
- Career Advancement
- Staff Retention
- Personal Growth & Self Confidence
- Professional Autonomy

Note: From Cary, A. (2001). Certified registered nurses: Results of the study of the certified workforce. *American Journal of Nursing, 101*(1), 44-52.

ment, and establish certification boards (Flanagan, 1976). Although ANA represented all professional RNs and made an effort with the divisions of practice to represent nurses in various specialties, one organization was unable to meet the needs of nurses in all specialties. Specialty organizations rapidly began to emerge to meet the demands of nurses requiring distinctive knowledge and skills for practice (Parker, 1998).

Certification

Certification and credentialing in nursing have benefits for both nurses and patients. In 1979, when credentialing in nursing was in its infancy, the main objective of certification in nursing, according to the ANA (1979), was to assure that the public received quality nursing care and was safe from incompetent caregivers. Expanding on that, Cary (2001) described the purposes of certification in nursing as protecting the public from unsafe and incompetent providers, giving consumers more choices in selecting health care providers, distinguishing among levels of care, and giving better-trained providers a competitive advantage.

The ANCC and the Nursing Credentialing Research Coalition have conducted the largest international study of the certified nurse workforce (ANCC, 2004c). In the third phase of research, Cary (2001) surveyed a random sample of 40,426 certified nurses in the U.S. and Canada, and found that "certification may give nurses the means or opportunity to practice in a manner likely to improve outcomes" and that "certification may afford nurses professional growth and financial rewards, such as recognition, reimbursement, salary increases, and career opportunities, as well as opportunity for personal growth" (p. 49). Certified nurses in the study also reported increased confidence, competence, credibility, and control (see Table 1-4). Many nurses in the study who were certified within 5 years prior to the study believed that the certification process and the knowledge gained from preparing for the certification examination improved their confidence in detecting signs and symptoms of complications and initiating prompt intervention and also was responsible for them having fewer adverse incidents in patient care.

In 1991, the American Board of Nursing Specialties

(ABNS) was established. The ABNS is a national peer review program that promotes the highest quality of specialty nursing practice through the recognition of approved national certification bodies and their programs. The goal of ABNS is to serve as an advocate for consumer protection by establishing and maintaining standards of professional specialty nursing certification and to increase consumers' awareness of the meaning and value of specialty nursing certification (Parker, 1994). Janel Parker, President of ANNA in 1986-87, served as the first President of ABNS.

The Development of Nephrology Nursing As A Specialty

The specialty of nephrology nursing traces its beginnings to the arrival of the artificial kidney developed by Willem Kolff in 1947. Initially, nurses collected research data, prepared dialysis equipment, provided nursing care to patients receiving dialysis, and acted as patient advocates (Hoffart, 1989a, 1989b). Transplantation became a part of the nephrology nursing specialty in 1954 with the first successful kidney transplants performed at Peter Bent Brigham (Merrill, Murray, Harrison, & Guild, 1956). Although many dialysis and transplant nurses had experience with peritoneal dialysis, it wasn't until the 1970s, when continuous modes were developed, that peritoneal dialysis programs were developed in renal centers (Hoffart, 1989a, 1989b).

American Nephrology Nurses' Association

The specialty of nephrology nursing is represented by the American Nephrology Nurses' Association (ANNA). In 1969, the American Association for Nephrology Nurses (AANN) was created, becoming one of the nation's earliest specialty nursing organizations. Its purpose was "to promote knowledge about the care of patients with renal disease" (AANN, 1969, p. 1).

At the time, there were relatively few dialysis and transplants units. Treatment alternatives were costly, demand exceeded supply, and selection committees were used to determine who received treatment and who did not. The technology in use today was only in its most basic design, and many of the drugs we currently rely on to care for patients with chronic kidney disease (CKD) were unheard of.

Nephrology nursing, however, was on the cutting edge of specialty nursing and interdisciplinary care teams. In 1970, AANN changed its name to the American Association of Nephrology Nurses and Technicians (AANNT) and held its first national symposium. In 1974, AANNT launched its official journal, then known as the *AANNT Journal* and now named the *Nephrology Nursing Journal*. AANNT returned to its roots as purely a professional nursing organization in 1984 and became the American Nephrology Nurses' Association (ANNA).

Today, ANNA is a vibrant specialty nursing organization, composed of over 10,000 members and more than 100 local chapters. Its mission is to advance nephrology nursing practice and positively influence outcomes for patients with kidney or other disease processes requiring replacement therapies through advocacy, scholarship, and excellence (see Table 1-5) (ANNA, 2003a).

ANNA achieves its mission through establishing standards of care, providing education and information for

Table 1-5
ANNA Mission, Philosophy, Purpose, Values, Objectives

Mission
ANNA will advance nephrology nursing practice and positively influence outcomes for patients with kidney or other disease processes requiring replacement therapies through advocacy, scholarship, and excellence.

Philosophy
The American Nephrology Nurses' Association (ANNA) believes that the role of nephrology nursing is to assess the real or threatened impact of renal disease on the individual as well as to diagnose and treat his or her responses to this problem. Within this context, we also believe in the commitment of nursing to assist each individual to achieve an optimum level of functioning, whether it be in preventing renal disease, arresting further dysfunction, or rehabilitating the individual throughout the life cycle. In order to achieve these goals, we believe that practitioners within the field of nephrology nursing should set forth high standards of patient care that are continually updated. We believe that through the continued education of nurses in the field of nephrology, we can assure high quality patient care. We further believe that a sound educational program is necessary to develop, maintain, and augment competence in practice. Because research is essential for the advancement of nursing science, new concepts must be developed and tested to sustain the continued growth and maturation of nephrology nursing. We believe in the team approach to patient care and embrace interdisciplinary communication and collaboration as being essential to the achievement of the highest attainable level of cost-effective, quality patient care. As members of the nephrology team, it is our duty to respond to issues affecting our practice in both private and public sectors.

Purpose
The American Nephrology Nurses' Association as a professional organization has the obligation to set forth and update high standards of patient care, educate its practitioners, stimulate research, disseminate new ideas throughout the field, promote interdisciplinary communication and cooperation, and address issues encompassing the practice of nephrology nursing. ANNA fulfills its mission through the strategies that address clinical practice, education, research, representation, and operations.

Values
Advocacy, Scholarship, Excellence

Objectives
To foster the highest attainable level of patient care, the American Nephrology Nurse's Association endeavors to:
1. Develop and continually update standards for the practice of nephrology nursing.
2. Provide the mechanisms and stimuli to promote individual professional growth.
3. Assist practitioners within the nephrology field to utilize the standards of practice for the purpose of professional audit and peer review.
4. Enhance the competence of the membership through education programs at the local, regional, and national levels.
5. Promote members' awareness of issues affecting both the professional and sociological spheres of their practice.
6. Encourage the individual member to participate in the growth and development of the organization.
7. Promote research, development, and demonstration of advances in nephrology nursing and provide the opportunity to disseminate these new ideas.
8. Maintain a functional rapport and serve as a resource body to professional groups, government agencies, and lay organizations.
9. Respond to the issues encompassing the practice of nephrology nursing.

Note: From American Nephrology Nurses' Association (ANNA). (2003b). *Constitutions and bylaws.* Pitman, NJ: Author.

Table 1-6
ANNA Position Statements

Advanced Practice in Nephrology Nursing (*Revised April 2005*)

Autonomy of the Nephrology Nursing Certification Commission (NNCC) (*Reaffirmed April 2005*)

Certification in Nephrology Nursing (*Revised April 2005*)

Concerns Regarding Inclusion of End Stage Renal Disease Patients in Managed Care Plans (*Revised April 2005*)

Daily Hemodialysis (DHD)/Nocturnal Hemodialysis (NHD) (*Revised April 2005*)

Delegation of Nursing Care Activities (*Revised October 2003*)

Financial Incentives for Organ Donation (*Reaffirmed April 2005*)

ANNA Health Policy Agenda (*Revised April 2005*)

ANNA Health Policy Statement (*Revised April 2005*)

Impact of the National Nursing Shortage on Quality Nephrology Nursing Care (*Reaffirmed April 2005*)

Joint Position Statement of the American Nephrology Nurses' Association (ANNA) and the National Association of Nephrology Technicians/Technologists (NANT) on Unlicensed Personnel in Dialysis (*Reaffirmed April 2005*)

Minimum Preparation for Entry Into Nursing Practice (*Reaffirmed April 2005*)

Nondiscrimination in Educational Programs (*Revised April 2005*)

Role of Nephrology Nursing in ESRD Disease Management (*Reaffirmed April 2005*)

Role of Unlicensed Assistive Personnel in Dialysis Therapy (*Revised April 2005*)

RPA/ASN and ANNA Joint Position Paper on Collaboration Between Nephrologists and Advanced Practice Nurses (*Revised April 2005*)

Self-Care, Rehabilitation, and Optimal Functioning (*Adopted September 2005*)

Vascular Access for Hemodialysis (*Revised April 2005*)

nephrology nurses, enunciating positions on issues relevant to nephrology nursing practice and patients requiring the care of nephrology nurses, educating and lobbying legislators and other relevant regulatory agencies on behalf of nephrology nurses and patients, encouraging and sponsoring research, etc.

Position statements. ANNA advocates for nephrology nurses and patients through the issuance of position statements. Position statements address a broad range of issues, such as the use of unlicensed personnel in dialysis therapy, mandatory HIV testing, reuse of dialysis disposables, and solicitation of organs and tissues. A list of ANNA position statements as of 2006 is found in Table 1-6. The complete set of updated ANNA positions statements is available on the ANNA Web site (www.annanurse.org).

Educational activities. ANNA's educational activities include national, regional, and local educational meetings, publication of the *Nephrology Nursing Journal* and books such as *Contemporary Nephrology Nursing*, and the *Core Curriculum;* audio conferences, etc.

Legislative and regulatory activities. Very few specialty nursing organizations have as long a history of legislative involvement as does ANNA. Dating back to the early 1970s,

ANNA's extensive involvement has been driven by the presence of the federal government in the reimbursement and regulation of nephrology care and the commitment and perseverance of ANNA leaders.

As the professional association for nephrology nursing, ANNA takes a leadership role in legislative and regulatory activities relevant to the practice of nephrology nursing and the care of nephrology patients. The ANNA Health Policy Statement (2004a) states the association's positions on various issues regarding nursing and patient care and serves as the basis for association decisions. It is reviewed and revised annually. ANNA also develops a Health Policy Agenda for congressional sessions to establish the legislative priorities of the association (see Appendix F).

Through a network of ANNA members serving as legislative representatives at local, state, regional, and national levels, ANNA educates individuals involved in legislative and regulatory activities and advocates for nephrology patients and nurses. In 2003, ANNA instituted an ESRD Education Day for legislators and their staffs. As a part of that project, an ESRD Briefing Book for State and Federal Policymakers was developed and distributed and legislators, their staffs, and others associated with ESRD policymaking and regulation were invited to visit dialysis units across the country. As in many other endeavors, ANNA collaborated with other members of the ESRD community to assure the success of the program. ESRD Education Day has now become an annual event.

Sponsorship of nephrology nursing education and research. ANNA provides grants for nephrology nurses to pursue their educational advancement and to perform research related to nephrology nursing and patient care.

Scope of Practice

The scope of practice for nephrology nursing was first delineated by ANNA in 1986 (ANNA, 1986) and has been revised over the years as the scope of nephrology nursing has expanded. The current version is based on the scope of nursing practice as defined by the ANA (2004) and describes the scope of nephrology nursing practice (ANNA, 2004b).

"The practice of nephrology nursing encompasses the roles of direct caregiver, educator, coordinator, consultant, administrator, and researcher; it extends to all care delivery settings in which patients experiencing or at risk for developing chronic kidney disease (CKD), stages 1 through 5, receive health care, education, and counseling for kidney disease prevention, diagnosis, and treatment. Optimal individual and family functioning throughout all phases of disease management are the primary goals of nephrology nursing.

The nephrology nurse achieves these primary goals by diagnosing and treating human responses exhibited by individuals and families with CKD diagnoses or at risk for developing CKD. These human responses include, but are not limited to, physical symptoms, functional limitations, psychosocial disruptions, and knowledge needs. Treatment of these responses involves the delivery of replacement therapies including transplantation, restorative physical care to manage disease and treatment-related symptoms;

health promotion and disease prevention counseling; health maintenance education; psychosocial support to build or sustain coping capacity; and education to encourage active participation in decision-making and self-care. The focus of the nephrology nurse is the patient, which can include individuals, families, groups, and communities.

Nephrology nursing practice occurs throughout the lifespan, along a continuum of care, and across delivery settings. Care requirements extend beyond CKD to address chronic causative disease processes as well as subsequent co-morbid complications. The nature of this nursing care spans the spectrum from preventive and acute through replacement therapies and rehabilitation as well as palliative supportive care as necessary. Nephrology nursing may be provided in a variety of settings: inpatient, outpatient, freestanding clinics, and home care" (p. 1).

Advanced practice. In 1997, ANNA adopted a Position Statement on Advanced Practice in Nephrology Nursing. That statement has been revised and reaffirmed a number of times since its adoption.

ANNA defines advanced practice in nephrology nursing as "expert competency and leadership in the provision of care to individuals with an actual or potential diagnosis of kidney disease" (ANNA, 2005a). It is the position of ANNA that advanced practice requires "substantial theoretical knowledge in nephrology nursing and proficient use of the knowledge in providing expert care to individuals diagnosed with CKD and the families as well as the community at large" (2005a). Advanced practice roles in nephrology include "direct caregiver, coordinator, consultant, educator, researcher, and administrator" (2005a).

The scope of practice for advanced practice in nephrology nursing is described as follows (ANNA, 2005a).

"The advanced practice nurse in nephrology, transplantation, and related therapies, by virtue of education, training, and certification, as well as documented competencies, is able to provide safe, competent, high-quality care in a cost-effective manner. In addition, the advanced practice nurse focuses on promoting the health and well being of patients and on preventing disease or its subsequent complications along the entire continuum of renal dysfunction. The advanced practice nurse may provide and coordinate the care of renal patients in both the acute and chronic settings and across all treatment modalities. The advanced practice nephrology nurse is an integral member of the healthcare team and works collaboratively with other healthcare professionals to assure the highest standard of quality care."

Nephrology Nursing Certification

In 1986, the ANNA Board of Directors voted to pursue the development of a process that would certify proficiency in nephrology nursing practice. A criterion-referenced examination designed to identify the proficient nephrology nurse practitioner was initially developed by an ANNA Certification Ad Hoc Committee with the assistance of the National League of Nursing Testing Service. In 1987, after

Table 1-7
Certified Nephrology Nurse (CNN)

- Designed to test proficiency in nephrology nursing practice.
- Administered by the Center for Nursing Education and Testing (C-NET), which specializes in test development and test administration.
- Credential: Certified Nephrology Nurse (CNN)
- Certification is effective for 3 years.

Eligibility Requirements:
1. A current license as a registered nurse in the United States or its territories.
2. Within 3 years prior to application, a minimum of 2 years of nephrology experience as a registered nurse.
3. In meeting the above criteria, at least 50% of employment hours spent in nephrology nursing.
4. Candidates for certification must possess a minimum of a Baccalaureate Degree in Nursing.
5. Candidates for certification must have completed 30 hours of approved continuing education in nephrology nursing within 3 years prior to submission of application for certification.

Examination Content:
Concepts of renal failure – 35%
Hemodialysis – 30%
Peritoneal dialysis – 20%
Transplant – 15%

Note: From Nephrology Nursing Certification Commission (NNCC). (2005b). *About Becoming a CNN*. Pitman, NJ: Author. Retrieved October 22, 2005, from www.nncc-exam.org.

Table 1-8
Certified Dialysis Nurse (CDN)

- A competency-level examination for nephrology nurses working in a dialysis setting.
- Administered by the Center for Nursing Education and Testing (C-NET).
- Credential: Certified Dialysis Nurse (CDN)
- Certification is effective for 3 years.

Eligibility Requirements:
1. The applicant must hold a full and unrestricted license as a registered nurse in the United States or its territories.
2. The applicant must have completed a minimum of 2,000 hours experience in nephrology nursing as a registered nurse during the last 2 years.
3. The applicant must have completed 15 contact hours of approved continuing education credit in nephrology nursing within 2 years prior to submitting the CDN examination application.

International Eligibility Criteria
1. Hold a current, full, and unrestricted license as a first-level general nurse in the country in which one's general nursing education was completed and meet the eligibility criteria for licensure as a registered nurse (RN) in the United States in accordance with requirements of the Commission on Graduates of Foreign Nursing Schools (CFGNS).
2. A minimum of 2,000 hours experience (1 year full-time employment) in nephrology nursing in the last 2 years.
3. Documentation of 15 hours of education in nephrology nursing within 2 years prior to submission of application.

Examination Content:
Hemodialysis – 50%
Concepts of renal failure – 30%
Peritoneal dialysis – 16%
Transplant – 4%

Note: From Nephrology Nursing Certification Commission (NNCC). (2005c). *About Becoming a CDN*. Pitman, NJ: Author. Retrieved October 22, 2005, from www.nncc-exam.org.

administration of the pilot examination, the Certification Ad Hoc Committee incorporated to form the Nephrology Nursing Certification Board (NNCB) (Parker, 1998). To assure independence and autonomy related to the certification process, the NNCB was established as a separate corporation from ANNA, with its own by-laws, officers, and Board of Directors. The first examination was given in September 1987. In 2000, the NNCB changed its name to the Nephrology Nursing Certification Commission (NNCC) to reflect a broader scope of certification and recertification activities.

Nephrology nursing certification. Janel Parker (1991), President of ANNA when the Board of Directors voted to pursue the development of a nephrology nursing certification examination and the first President of the NNCB, described the purposes of certification for nephrology nursing to be to "reflect attainment of special knowledge beyond the basic nursing credential and documentation of that achievement, promote a high quality of nephrology nursing care by providing a mechanism for nurses to demonstrate their proficiency in the nursing specialty area, enhance the standards of nephrology nursing practice, and provide for expanded career opportunities and advancement within the specialty of nephrology nursing" (p. 543).

The NNCC believes that "the attainment of a common knowledge base, utilization of the nursing process, and a predetermined level of skill in the practice setting are required for practice in nephrology nursing" (NNCC, 2005a). The NNCC further believes that certification exists primarily to benefit the public and that all caregivers providing care to renal patients should demonstrate a minimum level of knowledge, skills, and abilities (NNCC, 2005a). Two nephrology nurse certifications are offered by NNCC: the certified nephrology nurse (CNN), designed to test proficiency in nephrology nursing practice; and the certified dialysis nurse (CDN), an examination for entry level nephrology nurses practicing at a competent level in the dialysis setting (NNCC, 2005a). Details on the CNN certification can be found in Table 1-7 and on the CDN certification in Table 1-8.

Professional Nephrology Nursing Practice

Nephrology nursing practice occurs in primary, secondary, and tertiary health care settings as well as in the community and in the homes of individuals with CKD. The specialty of nephrology nursing offers a wide variety of roles for nephrology nurses and an even wider variety of settings in which to practice in the selected roles. Professional nephrol-

Table 1-9
Nephrology Nursing Standards of Nursing Practice

Standards of Practice	Standards of Professional Performance
Standard 1. Assessment The nephrology registered nurse collects comprehensive data pertinent to the patient's health or the situation.	**Standard 7. Quality of Practice** The nephrology registered nurse systematically enhances the quality and effectiveness of nursing practice.
Standard 2. Diagnosis The nephrology registered nurse analyzes the assessment data to determine the diagnosis or issues.	**Standard 8. Education** The nephrology registered nurse attains knowledge and competency that reflects current nursing practice.
Standard 3. Outcomes Identification The nephrology registered nurse identifies expected outcomes for a plan individualized to the patient or the situation.	**Standard 9. Professional Practice Evaluation** The nephrology registered nurse evaluates one's own nursing practice in relation to professional practice standards and guidelines, relevant statutes, rules, and regulations.
Standard 4. Planning The nephrology registered nurse develops a plan that prescribes strategies and alternatives to attain expected outcomes.	**Standard 10. Collegiality** The nephrology registered nurse interacts with and contributes to the professional development of peers and colleagues.

Standard 5. Implementation
The nephrology registered nurse implements the identified plan.
  Standard 5A. Coordination of Care
  The nephrology registered nurse coordinates care delivery.
  Standard 5B. Health Teaching and Health Promotion
  The nephrology registered nurse employs strategies to promote health and a safe environment.
  Standard 5C. Consultation
  The advanced practice nephrology registered nurse and the nursing role specialist provide consultation to influence the identified plan, enhance the abilities of others, and affect change.
  Standard 5D. Prescriptive Authority and Treatment
  The advanced practice nephrology registered nurse uses prescriptive authority, procedures, referrals, treatments, and therapies in accordance with state and federal laws and regulations.
	Standard 11. Collaboration
	The nephrology registered nurse collaborates with patient, family, and others in the conduct of nursing practice.
	
	Standard 12. Ethics
	The nephrology registered nurse integrates ethical provisions into all areas of practice.
	
	Standard 13. Research
	The nephrology registered nurse integrates research findings into practice.
	
	Standard 14. Resource Utilization
	The nephrology registered nurse considers factors related to safety, effectiveness, cost, and impact on practice in the planning and delivery of nursing services.

Standard 6. Evaluation The nephrology registered nurse evaluates progress towards the attainment of outcomes.	**Standard 15. Leadership** The nephrology registered nurse provides leadership in the professional practice setting and the profession.

Note: Burrows-Hudson, S., & Prowant, B.F. (Eds.). (2005). *Nephrology nursing standards of practice and guidelines for care.* Pitman, NJ: American Nephrology Nurses' Association (ANNA).

ogy nursing practice, like professional nursing practice, is complex and multidimensional.

Standards of Practice

The first standards of practice in nephrology nursing were in the form of standards of clinical practice for the nephrology patient and covered the care of patients receiving hemodialysis, peritoneal dialysis, and transplantation as well as patients experiencing acute renal failure, by nurses and other health care practitioners (AANNT, 1977). In 1982, these standards were redone using the nursing process and expanded to include conservative management, hemoperfusion, and pediatrics (AANNT, 1982). Over the years, the standards have been revised to include updated information, structure standards, patient teaching, patient outcomes, and new therapeutic modalities. The 1993 revision of the standards incorporated the revised ANA format for standards of practice and care including standards of professional performance (Burrows-Hudson, 1993). In 2002, the *Advanced Practice Nurse Standards of Care* and the *Advanced Practice Nurse Standards of Professional Performance* were published (ANNA, 2002). These standards were modeled after the ANA *Scope and Standards of Advanced Practice Registered Nursing.*

The *Nephrology Nursing Standards of Practice*, revised in 2005, are based on the *2004 ANA Standards of Nursing Practice* (see Table 1-9) (Burrows-Hudson & Prowant, 2005). They include Standards of Practice (assessment, diagnosis, outcomes identification, planning, implementation, and evaluation) and Standards of Professional Performance (quality of practice, education, professional practice evaluation, collegiality, collaboration, ethics, research, resource utilization, and leadership). Each standard includes measurement criteria for the nephrology RN as well as for the nephrology advanced practice RN.

In order to meet the standards of nursing practice and professional performance, nephrology nurses must possess certain knowledge and skills. To meet the standards of nursing practice (Burrows-Hudson & Prowant, 2005), nephrology nurses must have the knowledge and experience to:

- collect comprehensive data pertinent to the patient's health or the situation.
- analyze the data collected.
- determine diagnoses or issues.
- identify expected outcomes.
- develop a plan to achieve outcomes.
- implement the plan.
- coordinate care.
- provide health teaching and health promotion.

Table 1-10
ANNA Advanced Practice Nurse Standards

Standards of Care
Standard I. Assessment
The nephrology advanced practice nurse (APN) collects and integrates comprehensive health data about the patient from a holistic approach using resources that include the patient and his or her family, as well as their community and environment, and other health care team members.

Standard II. Diagnosis
The nephrology APN synthesizes and critically analyzes the data collected from all sources to identify normal and abnormal findings to diagnose actual/potential problems.

Standard III. Outcome Identification
The nephrology APN identifies expected outcomes based upon assessment data and diagnoses and individualizes the expected outcomes with the patient, the family, and other health care team members in accordance with nationally accepted clinical practice guidelines.

Standard IV. Planning
The nephrology APN develops a holistic and individualized plan of care that is derived from the assessment data and diagnoses, includes interventions and treatments to attain the expected outcomes, and is in accordance with nationally accepted clinical practice guidelines.

Standard V. Implementation
The nephrology APN prescribes and/or recommends and implements interventions and therapies consistent with the plan of care to achieve expected outcomes.

    Standard V-A. Case Management/Coordination of Care
    The nephrology APN provides holistic care coordinating clinical interventions and case management.

    Standard V-B. Consultation
    The nephrology APN provides consultation to influence the comprehensive plan of care for the patient, family, community, and environment to enhance the abilities of others and to effect change in the health care system.

    Standard V-C. Health Promotion, Health Maintenance, and Health Teaching
    The nephrology APN promotes, maintains, and improves health, as well as prevents illness and injury in the nephrology patient.

Standard V-D. Prescriptive Authority and Treatment
The nephrology APN utilizes prescriptive authority, procedures, and therapeutic interventions in accordance with institutional, state, and federal regulations to treat illness, improve health status, and/or provide preventative care for the nephrology patient.

Standard V-E. Referral
The nephrology APN identifies the need for adjunct care and makes referrals as appropriate.

Standard VI. Evaluation
The nephrology APN continuously evaluates the patient's changing condition, response to therapy, functional status, and progress toward attaining expected outcomes.

Standards of Professional Performance
Standard I. Quality of Care
The nephrology APN develops criteria for and evaluates the quality and effectiveness of nephrology APN nursing care.

Standard II. Self-Evaluation.
The nephrology APN continuously evaluates own nursing practice in relation to professional practice standards and relevant statutes and regulations, and is accountable to the public and to the profession for providing competent clinical care.

Standard III. Education
The nephrology APN acquires and maintains knowledge related to current scientific findings and advanced practice in nephrology nursing.

Standard IV. Leadership
The nephrology APN serves as a leader and role model for the professional development of peers, colleagues, and others.

Standard V. Ethics
The nephrology APN demonstrates clinical thinking and discriminating judgment integrating ethical principles into practice.

Standard VI. Interdisciplinary Process
The nephrology APN promotes the interdisciplinary approach to providing advanced nephrology nursing care to the patient, family, and community.

Standard VII. Research
The nephrology APN provides evidence-based care to achieve and improve outcomes for the patient, family, and community.

Note: From American Nephrology Nurses' Association (ANNA). (2002). *Scope and standards of advanced practice in nephrology nursing.* Pitman, NJ: Author.

- evaluate progress.

To meet the standards of professional performance, nephrology nurses must have the knowledge and expertise to:

- systematically enhance the quality and effectiveness of nursing practice.
- attain knowledge and competency that reflects current practice.
- evaluate one's own practice.
- interact with and contribute to the professional development of peers and colleagues.
- collaborate.
- integrate ethical provisions into all areas of practice.
- integrate research findings into practice.
- utilize resources effectively and efficiently.
- provide leadership.

Advanced practice. The *Advanced Practice Standards of Care and Standards of Professional Performance* reflect the increased expectations of advanced practice nurses in knowledge, clinical expertise, autonomy, and leadership (see Table 1-10) (ANNA, 2002).

Clinical Practice Guidelines

Guidelines convert scientific knowledge into clinical action and have the potential for decreasing variability in practice (Dean-Barr, 2001). Studies have shown that following best practice guidelines results in decreased patient suffering, decreased mortality, improved quality of life, and improved clinical outcomes (Agency for Healthcare Research and Quality [AHRQ], 2004a).

The goals of clinical practice guidelines, as defined by Bednar and Peacock (1998) are to:

- provide guidance to clinicians based on the best

Table 1-11
Nephrology Nursing Guidelines for Care

Chronic Kidney Disease, Stages	Acute Peritoneal Dialysis
Hypertension	Dialysis Prescription and Adequacy
Glycemic Control	Prevention and Treatment of Complications
Nutrition and Metabolic Control	**Self-Care and Home Dialysis**
Fluid Balance and Congestive Heart Failure	Evaluation and Education
Anemia	Dialysis Training
Bone Metabolism and Disease	Ongoing Monitoring
Dyslipidemia and Reduction of	**Apheresis and Therapeutic Plasma Exchange**
Cardiovascular Disease Risk Factors	Pretreatment Patient Education
Preparation for Replacement Therapy	Patient Assessment
Universal Guidelines for Nephrology Nursing Care	Equipment Assessment
Anemia	Initiation of Treatment
Bone Metabolism and Disease	Anticoagulation
Fluid Balance and Congestive Heart Failure	Intratherapy Monitoring
Nutrition and Metabolic Control	Fluid Management
Dyslipidemia and Reduction of	Acid/Base and Electrolyte Balance
Cardiovascular Disease Risk Factors	Complications
Residual Kidney Function	Termination of Treatment
Integrity of Skin and Mucous Membranes	**Continuous Renal Replacement Therapy**
Bowel Function	Pretreatment Assessment
Sleep	Prior to Initiation of Therapy
Coping	Initiation of Therapy
Family Process	Intratherapy Monitoring
Sexuality – Adult	Anticoagulation
Sexuality – Adolescent	Fluid Management
Self-Concept and Self-Management	Acid/Base and Electrolyte Balance
Rehabilitation	Metabolic Stability
Infection Control	Nutrition
Bacterial Infection	Complications
Hepatitis B	Termination of Therapy
Hepatitis C	Elements of a CRRT Monitoring Tool
Tuberculosis	**Kidney and Pancreas Transplantation**
Hemodialysis	Deceased Donor
Vascular Access	Living Donor
Adequacy	Recipient
Treatment and Equipment-related Complications	Universal Postoperative Guidelines for Care of
Patient Management	Donor and Recipient
Peritoneal Dialysis	Allograft Dysfunction
Catheter Implantation	**Palliative Care and End-of-Life Care**

Note: From Burrows-Hudson, S., & Prowant, B.F. (Eds.). (2005). *Nephrology nursing standards of practice and guidelines for care.* Pitman, NJ: American Nephrology Nurses' Association (ANNA).

available scientific information and clinical judgment
- enhance the quality of care.
- combine the science and art of nursing practice to provide a structure for nursing judgment.
- reduce the incidence of inappropriate care.
- reduce the wide variation in practice patterns.

The guidelines for nephrology nursing care grew out of the standards of clinical practice, which originated in 1977. Guidelines for clinical practice were published in 1999 (Burrows-Hudson, 1999) and revised and expanded in 2005 (Burrows-Hudson & Prowant, 2005) (see Table 1-11).

Education, Clinical Competence, and Professional Development

Nephrology nurses are individually responsible for obtaining basic nursing education, education in the specialty of nephrology nursing, and life-long learning to assure that their education is always up-to-date. Education involves theoretical as well as clinical and hands-on knowledge and experience.

Educational preparation. It is the position of ANNA that "the minimum preparation for beginning technical nursing practice is the associate degree in nursing" and "the minimum preparation for beginning professional nursing practice is to be the baccalaureate degree in nursing" (ANNA, 2005b). This position is in agreement with and re-affirms the positions of the ANA and the majority of professional nursing organizations.

Clinical competence. Clinical competence involves theoretical and clinical competence. While theoretical nursing knowledge can be acquired in the classroom, much of the knowledge required to attain and maintain clinical competence is obtained in the clinical setting and through experience. Patricia Benner's *Novice to Expert Model* (Benner, 1984) provides an excellent framework for developing clinical competence in both general nursing and in the specialty of nephrology nursing.

Benner based her model on the Dreyfus Model of Skill Acquisition, which describes the process of acquiring and developing skills as including movement from relying on abstract principles to using past concrete experiences as paradigms, from seeing situations less as a compilation of equally relevant pieces to seeing situations as a whole with only certain parts being relevant, and from being a detached observer to being an involved performer (Dreyfus & Dreyfus, 1980). Benner's model, like that of Dreyfus and Dreyfus, includes five levels of proficiency: novice, advanced beginner, competent, proficient, and expert (see Table 1-12).

It is important to remember that the novice-to-expert concept is situational; you can be an expert in one aspect of nursing and a novice in another. This occurs, for example, when experienced nurses come into nephrology nursing. Even the most expert medical-surgical nurse is initially a novice in the dialysis unit. Nurses with knowledge and experience, however, can transfer learning and concepts from previous experience and, so, tend to progress through the stages of skill acquisition at a quicker pace.

Professional development. Continued professional development is the responsibility of every nurse. Maslow's Hierarchy of Needs continues to be a sound basis for a model of professional development. Maslow's original Hierarchy of Needs contained five levels of need: biological and physiological needs, safety needs, belongingness and love, esteem, and self-actualization (Maslow, 1954). These needs were based on the belief that an individual is ready to act upon growth needs only if the deficiency needs are met. In the initial conceptualization, Maslow only identified one growth need – self-actualization. In subsequent work (Maslow, 1971; Maslow, 1998), additional growth needs were identified – two below self-actualization (the cognitive need to know, understand, and explore and the aesthetic need for symmetry, order, and beauty) and one above (self-transcendence, the need to connect with something beyond one's ego and to help others find self-fulfillment and realize their potential (see Figure 1-2). Maslow's concept of becoming more self-actualized and self-transcendent aligns with Benner's expert level of practice in that Maslow believes that at this stage, one develops wisdom and automatically or intuitively knows what to do in a wide variety of situations.

Maslow also points out that even though individuals are striving toward higher goals, they can enjoy experiences along the way. "Achieving basic-need gratifications," Maslow said, "gives us many peak experiences, each of which are absolute delights, perfect in themselves, and needing no more than themselves to validate life" (Maslow, 1998, pp. 169-170).

In nursing, when someone starts a new job, we often refer to "survival needs," meaning those things you have to know to get the basic job done. First, we need to learn the basics, and only when we feel secure with the basics are we inclined to move to the next level. Similarly, in developing professionally, we are only motivated to expand our horizons when we feel secure in what we have already done.

Problem-Solving, Critical Thinking, Critical Judgment, and Critical Synthesis

A crucial part of developing expert practice is expanding one's thought processing abilities. The abilities of problem-solving, critical thinking, clinical judgment, and critical synthesis are all vital to the practice of professional nursing and,

Table 1-12

Stages of Professional Development: From Novice to Expert

Novice
No experience of situations
Practice based on theoretical knowledge
Rule-governed behavior
Little understanding of contextual meaning of information

Advanced Beginner
Minimal experience
Marginally acceptable performance
Task oriented
Operates on general guidelines
Beginning to see contextual meaning of information
Need assistance in setting priorities

Competent
2 to 3 years experience
Consciously aware of long-range plan and goals
Beginning to see actions in terms of long-range plan and goals
Begins to feel mastery of specific situations
Copes with and manages contingencies

Proficient
Perceives and understands situations as a whole
Performance is guided by maxims but driven by experience
Learns from experience what typical events to expect
Modifies plans in response to typical events
Recognizes when expected does not occur
Hones in quickly on problem
Prioritizes information and occurrences as well as responses

Expert
Large amount of experience
Relies on an intuitive grasp of each situation
Quickly identifies problems and causes
Deep understanding of total situation

Note: Adapted from Benner, P. (1984). From novice to expert: *Excellence and power in clinical nursing practice.* Menlo Park, CA: Addison-Wesley Publishing Company.

Figure 1-2

Maslow's Hierarchy of Needs

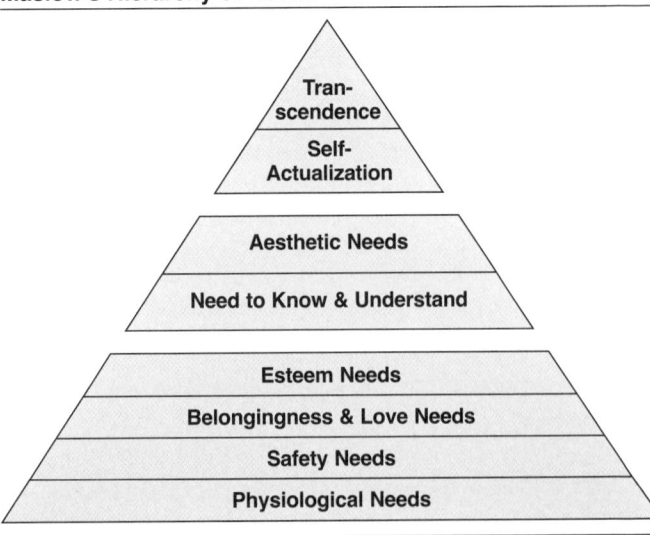

Note: Adapted from Maslow, A.H. (1998). *Toward a psychology of being* (3rd ed.). New York: John Wiley & Sons.

Table 1-13
Characteristics of Critical Thinkers

- Active thinkers
- Fair-minded
- Persistent
- Good communicators
- Open-minded
- Empathetic
- Independent thinkers
- Curious and insightful
- Humble
- Honest with themselves and others
- Proactive
- Organized and systematic in approach
- Flexible
- Cognizant of rules of logic
- Realistic
- Team players
- Creative and committed to excellence

Note: From Alfaro-Lefevre, R. (1999). *Critical thinking in nursing: A practical approach* (2nd ed.). Philadelphia: W.B. Saunders.

like Benner's Novice to Expert Model or Maslow's Hierarchy of Needs, are hierarchical in nature.

Problem-solving is a basic nursing skill and is taught in nursing through the use of the nursing process, which involves five steps: assessment, problem identification (diagnosis), planning, implementation, and evaluation. The process is sequential in theory, but since patients rarely present with only one single-faceted problem, in reality, the process is dynamic and requires parallel thinking, critical thinking, clinical judgment, and critical synthesis.

Critical thinking is "careful, deliberate, outcome-focused (results-oriented) thinking" (Alfaro-LeFevre, 2002, p. 23). It involves clearly and quickly focusing one's thinking, using well-reasoned strategies, to achieve desired results. The key differences between thinking and critical thinking are control and purpose (Alfaro-LeFevre, 1999). The characteristics of critical thinkers are detailed in Table 1-13.

Clinical judgment refers to "the ways in which nurses come to understand the problems, issues, or concerns of clients/patients, to attend to salient information, and to respond in concerned and involved ways" (Benner, Tanner, & Chesla, 1996, p. 2). Clinical grasp and clinical forethought are two components of thought and action that describe clinical judgment (Benner, 2000). Clinical grasp, according to Benner (2000), includes "making qualitative distinctions, engaging in detective work, recognizing changing clinical relevance, and developing clinical knowledge in specific populations," while clinical forethought includes "future think, clinical forethought about specific diagnoses and injuries, anticipation of risks for particular patients, and seeing the unexpected" (p. 317). Nurses develop clinical judgment as they gain more knowledge and experience.

Tim Porter-O'Grady has suggested that the next step beyond critical thinking is critical synthesis (Ulrich, 2003). Critical synthesis involves being able to combine and unite many pieces of data, knowledge, and experience together to form a more complex whole.

Accountability

The *ANA Scope of Practice* makes it clear that RNs are "accountable for judgments made and actions taken in the course of their nursing practice" (ANA, 2004, p.10). The interpretive statements that accompany the ANA Code of Ethics (2001) detail the accountability of the nursing profession ("Nursing is responsible and accountable for assuring that only those individuals who have demonstrated knowledge, skill, practice experiences, commitment, and integrity essential to professional practice are allowed to enter into and continue to practice within the profession.") as well as the accountability of individual nurses ("In order to be accountable, nurses act under a code of ethical conduct that is grounded in the moral principles of fidelity and respect for the dignity, worth, and self-determination if patients. Nurses are accountable for judgments made and actions taken in the course of nursing practice, irrespective of health care organizations' policies or providers' directives.")

Accountability includes, at a minimum, accountability to self, to other health care professionals, to the nursing profession, to one's employer, to the patient, and to the public. The nursing profession and nursing specialties describe the responsibilities for which nurses are accountable through standards of care, clinical practice, and performance.

Delegation. Delegation is an aspect of accountability. Delegation is both a legal and a professional responsibility. What can and cannot be delegated and to whom is determined by individual state nursing practice acts, state and federal regulations, and by professional associations. It is the responsibility of nurses to know the limits of delegation for the states in which they practice and for the applicable limits of delegation from state and federal regulations and from both general and specialty professional nursing associations. It is also nurses' responsibility to know the scope of legal and professional practice for the profession of any individual to whom they are delegating.

In nephrology nursing, ANNA has defined the delegation of nursing care activities. It is the position of ANNA (2003a) that the RN must never delegate a nursing care activity that requires

- the knowledge and expertise derived from completion of a nursing education program and the specialized skill, judgment, and decision-making of a RN or
- an understanding of the core nephrology nursing principles necessary to recognize and manage real or potential complications that may result in an adverse outcome to the health and safety of the patient.

ANNA has also determined specific criteria for delegation to LPNs/LVNs and to unlicensed assistive personnel (ANNA, 2003a).

The RN retains the legal accountability and clinical responsibility for the delegated activities, and the RN is legally accountable and clinically responsible for the complete documentation of the entire nursing process (ANNA, 2003a). It is also important to note that nurses are individually accountable for what they delegate regardless of organizational policies or directives. The ANA Code of Ethics (2001) states that "Employer policies or directives do not relieve the nurse of the responsibility for making judgments about the delegation and assignment of nursing tasks."

Leadership

Leadership was added to the ANA and the ANNA *Standards of Professional Practice* in 2004. Part of being a professional nurse is being a leader. Few RNs practice in isolation. By having LVNs/LPNs and unlicensed personnel working with them, they become de facto leaders. RNs also assume a leadership role with patients and families as professionals experienced in not only care of patients but also as people knowledgeable in navigating the health care system. Whether it is leading a patient care team in a dialysis unit or being the charge nurse on the night shift, all RNs takes on the mantle of leadership when they sign their first nursing license.

In accord with the ANA Standard, the ANNA Standard on leadership is: "The nephrology registered nurse provides leadership in the professional practice setting and the profession." Both ANA and ANNA measurement criteria for the leadership standard state that it is the responsibility of **every** RN to:

- engage in teamwork as a team player and a team builder.
- work to create and maintain healthy work environments in local, regional, national, or international communities.
- display the ability to define a clear vision, the associated goals, and a plan to implement and measure progress.
- demonstrate a commitment to continuous, life-long learning for self and others.
- teach others to succeed by mentoring and other strategies.
- Exhibit creativity and flexibility through times of change.
- demonstrate energy, excitement, and passion for quality work.
- willingly accept mistakes by self and others, thereby creating a culture in which risk-taking is not only safe, but expected.
- inspire loyalty through valuing of people as the most precious asset in an organization.
- direct the coordination of care across settings and among caregivers, including oversight of licensed and unlicensed personnel in any assigned or delegated tasks.
- serve in key roles in the work setting by participating on committees, councils, and administrative teams.
- promote advancement of the profession through participation in professional organizations.
- work to influence decision-making bodies to improve patient care, health services, and policies.
- promote communication of information and advancement of the profession through writing, publishing, and presentations for professional or lay audiences.
- design innovations to effect change in practice and outcomes.
- provide direction to enhance the effectiveness of the multidisciplinary or interdisciplinary team.

Obviously, you learn more about leadership and expand your leadership skills as you grow as a nurse, but the leadership responsibility starts on day one. Fay Bower (2000) says that every nurse "must develop the attitudes, the motivation, and the skills to become a leader at any time" (p. 2) and she describes twelve principles for developing leadership: knowing self, looking forward: being and becoming a futurist, seeing the big picture (having a vision), building self-directed work teams, taking a risk, recognizing the right time for action, seeing change as an opportunity, being proactive and not reactive, communicating effectively, mentoring others, letting go and taking on, and keeping informed.

It is also important to remember that leadership is not always about the big things. Sometimes it is about how to connect with a patient or a family member or help them find their way through the health care maze. Sometimes it is as simple as a new idea for an old problem that a new set of eyes sees differently. Sometimes it is having the courage to say the obvious.

Collegiality and Collaboration

RNs serve as one member of an extensive health care team. Nowhere is this more evident than in the nephrology specialty, one of the first clinical specialty areas to stress the necessity and advantage of multidisciplinary care and interdisciplinary collaboration. Within the nephrology community, the health care team is composed of nurses, physicians, patients, significant others, dietitians, social workers, technicians, manufacturers, professional and lay organizations, and others. According to the ANNA *Standards of Nursing Practice* (Burrows-Hudson & Prowant, 2005), nephrology nurses are responsible for interacting with and contributing to the professional development of peers and colleagues and for collaborating with patients, families, and others in the conduct of nursing practice.

Collaboration goes beyond cooperation. It is the "concerted efforts of individuals and groups to attain a shared goal" and requires "mutual trust, recognition, and respect among the health care ream, shared decision-making about patient care, and open dialogue among all parties who have and interest in and a concern for health outcomes" (ANA, 2001).

There are many examples of collaboration in nephrology beyond the collaboration that occurs at the bedside or in the dialysis unit. ANNA and the National Association of Nephrology Technicians/Technologists (NANT) worked together in 1997 to create a joint position statement on the role of unlicensed personnel in nephrology. The National Kidney Foundation's Dialysis Outcomes Quality Initiative and the subsequent Kidney Disease Outcomes Quality Initiative (KDOQI) are both examples of multidisciplinary collaboration. In 2000, a variety of nephrology professionals worked together on end-of-life care (Robert Woods Johnson Foundation, 2003). Kidney Care Partners is an alliance of patient advocates, dialysis professionals, providers, and suppliers that collaborates to assure quality, accessible care for individuals with end stage renal disease (ESRD). The list goes on and on. The nephrology community is large and continues to grow. A list of the major nephrology-related organizations and their contact information can be found in Table 1-14.

Table 1-14
Nephrology-Related Organizations and Contact Information

American Association of Kidney Patients (AAKP)	**National Association of Nephrology Technicians Technologists / (NANT)**
3505 E. Frontage Road, Suite 315	PO Box 2307
Tampa, FL 33607	Dayton, OH 45401-2307
Executive Office (800) 749-2257	Office (937) 586-3705
Fax (813) 636-8122	Fax (937) 586-3699
www.aakp.org	www.dialysistech.org
American Diabetes Association (ADA)	**National Kidney Foundation Inc. (NKF)**
1701 North Beauregard Street	30 East 33rd Street
Alexandria, VA 22311	New York, NY 10016
National Office (800) 342-2383	Office (212) 889-2210
www.diabetes.org	Fax (212) 689-9261
	www.kidney.org
American Kidney Fund (AKF)	**National Renal Administrators Association (NRAA)**
6110 Executive Boulevard, Suite 1010	1904 Naomi Place
Rockville, MD 20852	Prescott, AZ 86303-5061
Office (800) 638-8299	Office (928) 717-2772
Fax (301) 881-0898	Fax (928) 441-3857
www.kidneyfund.org	www.nraa.org
American Nephrology Nurses' Association (ANNA)	**North American Transplant Coordinators' Organization (NATCO)**
East Holly Avenue/Box 56	PO Box 15384
Pitman, NJ 08071	Lenexa, KS 66285-5384
Office (856) 256-2320	Office (913) 492-3600
Fax (856) 589-7463	Fax (913) 599-5340
www.annanurse.org	www.natco1.org
American Society of Nephrology (ASN)	**Renal Physicians Association (RPA)**
1725 I Street NW, Suite 510	1700 Rockdale Pike, Suite 220
Washington, DC 20006	Rockdale, MD 20852
Office (202) 659-0599	Office (301) 468-3515
Fax (202) 659-0709	Fax (301) 468-3511
www.asn-online.org	www.renalmd.org
Association for the Advancement of Medical Instrumentation (AAMI)	**United Network For Organ Sharing (UNOS)**
1110 North Glebe Road, Suite 220	PO Box 2484
Arlington, VA 22201-4795	Richmond, VA 23218
Office (703) 525-4890	Office (804) 782-4800
Fax (703) 276-0793	Fax (804) 782-4817
www.aami.org	www.unos.org
ESRD Network Organizations	
www.cms.hhs.gov/esrd/default.asp	
Kidney Care Partners (KCP)	
2550 M Street NW	
Washington, DC 20037-1350	
Office (202) 457-6620	
Fax (202) 457-6313	
www.kidneycarepartners.org	

Quality

There are several levels of nursing responsibilities with regard to quality, but ultimately, all center on assuring the best care for the patient. As noted in the ANA Code of Ethics (2001), "The nurse's primary commitment is to the healthy well-being and safety of the patient across the life span and in all settings in which health care needs are addressed"

It is the responsibility of every nephrology RN to enhance the quality and effectiveness of nursing practice (Burrows-Hudson & Prowant, 2005). In order to achieve this, nephrology nurses must understand the minimum standards of care for nephrology patients, the expected patient outcomes, and the basics of processes used to evaluate quality.

The search for quality goes by many names like quality assurance, continuous quality improvement, evidence-based practice, and outcomes research. It has often been said that quality is in the eyes of the beholder and that is part of the problem – quality can not be aimed for, reached, or evaluated until it can be defined. The Institute of Medicine (IOM) defines quality of care as "the degree to which health services for individuals and populations increase the likelihood of desired health outcomes and are consistent with current professional knowledge" (IOM, 2003a).

Outcomes. The systematic use of patient outcomes to evaluate care began with Florence Nightingale's work in the Crimea and, later, her attempts to create a uniform hospital data system to compare the quality of care in hospitals. Donabedian (1966) created a model to assess the quality of physician practice that emphasized structure, process, and outcomes. The model was adopted by many health care disciplines; however, for many years, standards and process, not outcomes, dominated quality programs. The national medical outcomes study of physician practice in the late 1980s changed the scope of past quality work by broadening the outcomes to include functional status, general well-being, and patient satisfaction (Tarlov et al., 1989).

In addition, several government groups began taking an active role in outcomes evaluation and research. In 1989, Congress created the Agency for Health Care Policy and Research, later renamed the Agency for Healthcare Research and Quality. Its mission is to improve the quality, safety, efficiency, and effectiveness of health care for all Americans (AHRQ, 2004b). AHRQ notes that outcomes research provides evidence about benefits, risks, and results so clinicians and patients can make informed decisions and identifies potentially effective strategies to improve the quality and value of care (AHRQ, 2000).

Research and Evidence-Based Practice

All nursing practice should be based on solid research. According to Stevens (1999), "the *raison d'etre* for research in a practice discipline is to provide scientific guidelines for effective and efficient practice" (p. 2). In order to use research in the practice setting, however, nephrology nurses must have at least a basic understanding of the research process and the criteria for acceptable research.

Evidence-based practice. Evidence-based practice involves using research and clinical expertise in patient care. The concept of evidence-based practice began in medical practice in England in the early 1990s. Sackett et al. (1996) define evidence-based medicine as "the conscientious, explicit and judicious use of current best evidence in making decisions about the care of individual patients" and say that the practice of evidence-based medicine "means integrating individual clinical expertise with the best available external clinical evidence from systematic research" (p. 71). Following the concept of evidence-based medicine, evidence-based nursing practice and multidisciplinary evidence-based practice have also developed. Some, but not all, evidence-based practice concepts also include patient preferences as a critical component. Mulhall (1998) defines evidence-based practice as the "incorporation of evidence from research, clinical expertise, and patient preferences into decisions about the health care of individual patients" (p. 5).

All agree that basing decisions on valid evidence is the key. According to Stetler et al. (1998), evidence-based nursing practice "de-emphasizes ritual, isolated and unsystematic clinical experiences, ungrounded opinions, and traditions as a basis for nursing practices and stresses instead the use of research findings and, as appropriate, quality improvement

data or other operational and evaluation data, the consensus of recognized experts, and affirmed experience to substantial practice" (p. 49). The concept of evidence-based practice is being expanded in all nursing settings – clinical, education, research, and management. Stevens (2002) has developed a five-step model for evidence-based practice: knowledge discovery, evidence synthesis, translation into practice recommendations, implementation into practice, and evaluation.

In nephrology, one of the best examples of evidence-based practice is the KDOQI of the NKF. In 1995, NKF launched the Dialysis Outcomes Quality Initiative (DOQI) to develop clinical practice guidelines for dialysis patients and health care providers. Guiding principles in the development of DOQI guidelines included scientific rigor that critically appraised available evidence, the involvement of multiple disciplines with a part in nephrology care, vesting decision authority in the multidisciplinary work groups appointed to create the guidelines, and an open development process to encourage peer review and debate (NKF, 2005). The first guidelines were published in 1997 and began immediately to have an impact on the care and outcomes for patients requiring dialysis. It soon became clear, however, that the emphasis of the guidelines on dialysis needed to be expanded to include all stages of kidney disease, from early to end stage. In 1999, NKF expanded the scope of DOQI, changing the name to the KDOQI. Using the same guiding principles that successfully developed the DOQI guidelines, the KDOQI initiative has created clinical practice guidelines addressing the evaluation, classification, and stratification of CKD.

Legal Aspects of Professional Nursing Practice

Two key concepts of the legal aspects of professional nursing practice that should be known by every nurse are that each nurse is legally responsible and individually liable for his or her own actions and that the nurse-patient relationship is not a derivative of any other relationship. The case establishing the nurse-patient relationship precedent occurred in Texas in 1983 when the court held that there is a nurse-patient relationship separate and apart from other relationships and that a nurse has a duty to the patient which cannot be superseded by hospital policy or physician's order (*Lunsford v. Board of Nurse Examiners*, 1983).

Part of a nurse's responsibility to a patient is keeping the patient safe. The extent of this role was highlighted in the IOM report, *Keeping Patients Safe: Transforming the Work Environment of Nurses,* which recognized the importance of nurses in creating a safe environment for patients through the care they give and the defense they provide against errors by others (IOM, 2003b). Not only must nurses adhere to the principle of nonmaleficence (first, do no harm), but also they are also responsible for assuring that no one else – health care professional, family member, etc. – harms the patient. Provision 3 of the ANA Code of Ethics (2001) states that "the nurse promotes, advocates for, and strives to protect the health, safety, and rights of the patient" Further, the Code of Ethics states that "As an advocate for the patient, the nurse must be alert to and take appropriate action regarding instances of incompetent, unethical, illegal, or impaired practice by any member of the health care team or the health care system or any action on the part of others that places the rights or best interests of the patient in jeopardy."

Malpractice in nursing is the "failure of one rendering professional services to exercise that degree of skill and learning commonly applied in the community by the average prudent reputable member of the nursing" (Hall & Hall, 2001, p. 136). Most lawsuits result from the failure to maintain a standard of practice. Examples of such failures are found in Table 1-15.

Ethics

Ethical principles and the ethical dilemmas faced by nurses and other health care professionals are important aspects of professional nursing practice. They are discussed in detail in Chapter 33.

Nephrology Nursing Roles

Nephrology nurses have many options in the roles they chose and often occupy more than one role at a time (see Table 1-16). The role options multiply exponentially when one considers the various practice settings available to the nephrology nurse (Table 1-17).

Caregiver. The most fundamental and, arguably, most important role of nephrology nurses is that of caregiver. In nephrology nursing, nurses have opportunities to work with adults and with children and with people who are chronically ill as well as those experiencing acute episodes of illness. Nephrology nursing care is provided in a range of settings ranging from patient homes to the most tertiary hospitals. Major benefits of nephrology nursing also include the opportunity to get to know the patient's family and significant others, as well as the patient, and the time to form long-term relationships.

Teacher. The role of teacher may involve teaching patients, families, other health care professionals, or students. Teaching is an art and a science that requires additional knowledge and expertise. Teaching, like nursing care, requires assessment, planning, intervention, and evaluation.

In most cases, teaching will also require knowledge of adult learning theory. Adult learners are characterized by being independent, often resistant to the learner role, possessing a background of experience and knowledge, a variety of motivations, and definite expectations about the teaching, the system, and the need to learn what is being taught (Knowles, 1990).

Advocate. Advocacy can occur at many levels – nurses may advocate for individual patients, groups of patients, health and illness issues, nursing as a profession, etc. Key aspects of the patient advocacy role are mutuality, facilitation, protection, and coordination (Leddy & Pepper, 1998). Mutuality involves respect and sharing. Both the nurse and the patient respect each other's knowledge, experiences, and feelings. Neither is more powerful than the other in the relationship. Facilitation requires assuring that the patient has whatever knowledge and support needed to make necessary decisions and the support for whatever decision the patient makes. Sometimes, the advocacy role involves protection – either from treatments or a lack of treatments or from potentially dangerous situations or people. Coordination is a part of the advocacy role and includes assuring that the patient

Table 1-15
Malpractice – Recurring Causes of Nurse Liability

- Failure to assess
- Failure to plan
- Failure to follow organization policy and procedure
- Failure to implement a plan of care
- Failure to advocate for the patient through the organization hierarchy
- Medication errors – failure to follow the five rights – right drug, right dose, right patient, right route, right time
- Failure to implement specific actions – failure to respond, failure to educate the patient, failure to perform according to the standards of care, failure to adequately supervise care
- Failure to evaluate – observe, monitor, communicate, follow up
- Failure to follow-up or to document follow-up

Note: From Hall, J.K., & Hall, D. (2001). Negligence specific to nursing. In M.E. O'Keefe (Ed.), *Nursing practice and the law: Avoiding malpractice and other legal risks* (pp. 132-149). Philadelphia: F.A. Davis.

Table 1-16
Nephrology Nursing Roles – A Sample

• Staff nurse – hospital	• Quality assurance coordinator
• Staff nurse – outpatient	• Manager
• Patient educator	• Administrator
• Staff educator	• Executive
• Nursing faculty	• Surveyor
• Clinical nurse specialist	• Consultant
• Nurse practitioner	• Leader
• Transplant coordinator	• Volunteer
• Organ recovery coordinator	• Mentor
• Researcher	

Table 1-17
Nephrology Nurse Practice Settings – A Sample

Hospitals	Government
Dialysis units	Schools of nursing
Corporate settings	Physicians' offices
Pharmaceutical companies	Organ procurement organizations
	Professional associations

has access to whatever is needed in the health care delivery systems and that the responses to the patient's needs are coordinated in a manner that is most in line with the patient's needs and desires.

Advocating for groups of patients, for nephrology nursing, and for nursing in general often involves volunteer work like that done by many ANNA members. This aspect of advocacy works best when people with the same goals join together to pool their expertise and resources for a common good.

Manager/executive. Every nurse manages just as every nurse leads whether management involves oneself, a group of patients, or a group of staff. Some nursing roles, such as assistant nurse manager or charge nurse, include both direct care and management components. Management is a learned set of knowledge and expertise. The more complex the management role, the more complex is the required knowledge and expertise to adequately perform the role. Numerous studies have shown that the performance of the frontline manager is a primary reason that nurses and many other health care professional stay in their jobs or leave.

Case manager/care coordinator. There are many names for the role of case manager or care coordinator. This role has arisen primarily due to the increased complexity of the health care system combined with the scarcity of resources. The goals of case management are to ensure access to needed care, continuity of care, optimal use of resources, the achievement of desired patient outcomes.

Researcher. In order for nursing to improve and advance, nurse researchers must study the work of nurses and the resulting outcomes. There are many levels of research involvement: using research findings in practice, data collection, identification of research topics, collaboration on a research project, and being the principal investigator of a research project. While leading research generally requires an advanced degree, participating in it does not.

Mentor. In the mid-1980s, ANNA had a slogan, "Protecting the Future of Quality Care," that guided many of the association's efforts and is at the heart of the concept of mentoring. Mentoring has many valuable outcomes, not the least of which is assuring the future of nephrology nursing and the care of patients with kidney disease.

Mentoring can occur in a formal mentoring relationship and in informal ways. Bell (2002) describes the mentoring process through the SAGE model - surrendering, accepting, gifting, and extending. Surrendering involves understanding that a mentor-mentee relationship is designed to be mutually beneficial with power, authority, and control either eliminated or shared. Accepting means creating a safe environment in which each person can be open and where honest constructive feedback is encouraged and welcomed. Gifting is giving of oneself. In Maslow's hierarchy, it is the self-transcendence level in which we help others find fulfillment and reach their potential. Extending is helping, encouraging, and challenging mentees to move forward – often further than they think they can go, but never farther than the mentor knows they can be successful.

Being a mentor requires a number of skills including listening, communicating, facilitating, guiding, counseling, coaching, relationship building, setting goals, developing and implementing a plan, managing conflict, etc. The rewards, however, can be enormous to both the mentor and mentee.

Summary

Nursing is one of life's most rewarding professions. Obtaining that reward requires extensive study, life-long learning, care and compassion, a commitment to nursing's professional standards and ethics, and a true dedication to the people who entrust us with their care. The opportunities in nursing and the joy that can be derived from it are immense.

Nephrology nursing is an especially exciting specialty. As one of the first nursing specialties, it has a long history of excellent care and active participation in achieving the best outcomes for patients with kidney disease – whether through actions at the bedside or in the legislative and regulatory arenas. Nephrology nurses have always been on the cutting edge as the intricacies of the specialty have developed and have stood side-by-side with other members of the healthcare team in improving care for patients with kidney disease. The past has been full of success and pride and the opportunities for the future are almost endless.

References

Agency for Healthcare Research and Quality (AHRQ). (2000). *Outcomes research fact sheet. AHRQ Publication No. 00-P011.* Rockville, MD: Author. Retrieved July 19, 2004, from www.ahrq.gov/clinic/outfact.htm

Agency for Healthcare Research and Quality (AHRQ) (2004a). *Closing the quality gap: A critical analysis of quality improvement strategies. Fact sheet.* Rockville, MD: Author. Retrieved July 19, 2004 from www.ahrq.gov/clinic/epc/qgapfact.htm

Agency for Healthcare Research and Quality (AHRQ). (2004b). *About AHRQ.* Rockville, MD: Author. Retrieved July 19, 2004, from www.ahrq.gov/about/

Aiken, L.H., Clarke, S.P., Sloane, D.M., Sochalski, J., & Silber, J.H. (2002). Hospital nurse staffing and patient mortality, nurse burnout, and job dissatisfaction. *Journal of the American Medical Association, 288,* 1987-1993.

Aiken, L.H., Clarke, S.P., Cheung, R.B., Sloane, D.M., & Silber, J.H. (2003). Educational levels of hospital nurses and surgical patient mortality. *Journal of the American Medical Association, 290,* 1617-1623.

Alfaro-Lefevre, R. (1999). *Critical thinking in nursing: A practical approach* (2nd ed.). Philadelphia: W.B. Saunders.

Alfaro-LeFevre, R. (2002). *Applying nursing process: Promoting collaborative care* (5th ed.). Philadelphia: Lippincott.

American Association of Colleges of Nursing (AACN). (2002). *Hallmarks of the professional nursing practice environment.* Washington, DC: Author. Retrieved July 9, 2004, from www.aacn.nche.edu/Publications/Positions/Hallmarks.htm

American Association for Nephrology Nurses (AANN). (1969). *Constitutions and bylaws.* Pitman, NJ: Author.

American Association of Nephrology Nurses and Technicians (AANNT). (1977). *Standards of clinical practice for the nephrology patient.* Pitman, NJ: Author.

American Association of Nephrology Nurses and Technicians (AANNT). (1982). *Nephrology nursing standards of clinical practice.* Pitman, NJ: Author.

American Nephrology Nurses' Association (ANNA). (1986). *Scope of practice for nephrology nursing.* Pitman, NJ: Author.

American Nephrology Nurses' Association (ANNA). (2002). *Scope and standards of advanced practice in nephrology nursing.* Pitman, NJ: Author.

American Nephrology Nurses' Association (ANNA). (2003a). *Delegation of nursing care activities.* Pitman, NJ: Author.

American Nephrology Nurses' Association (ANNA). (2003b). *Constitutions and bylaws.* Pitman, NJ: Author.

American Nephrology Nurses' Association (ANNA). (2004a). *Health policy statement.* Pitman, NJ: Author.

American Nephrology Nurses' Association (ANNA). (2004b). *Scope of practice for nephrology nursing.* Pitman, NJ: Author.

American Nephrology Nurses' Association (ANNA). (2005a). *Advanced practice in nephrology nursing.* Pitman, NJ: Author. Retrieved October 22, 2005, from www.annanurse.org

American Nephrology Nurses' Association (ANNA). (2005b). *Minimum preparation for entry into nursing practice.* Pitman, NJ: Author.

American Nephrology Nurses' Association (ANNA) & National Association of Nephrology Technicians/Technologist (NANTT). (1997). *Joint position statement of the American Nephrology Nurses' Association and the National Association of Nephrology Technicians/Technologists on unlicensed personnel in dialysis.* Pitman, NJ: Author.

American Nurses' Association (ANA). (1979). *The study of credentialing in nursing: A new approach.* Kansas City, MO: Author.

American Nurses' Association (ANA). (2001). *Code of ethics for nurses with interpretive statements.* Washington, DC: Author. Retrieved March 21, 2004, from www.nursingworld.org/ethics/code/ethicscode150.htm

American Nurses' Association (ANA). (2003). *Nursing's social policy statement.* Washington, DC: Author.

American Nurses' Association (ANA). (2004). *Nursing: Scope and standards of practice.* Washington, DC: Author.

American Nurses' Credentialing Center (ANCC). (2004a). *ANCC magnet program.* Washington, DC: Author. Retrieved July 18, 2004, from www.nursingworld.org/ancc/magnet/html

American Nurses' Credentialing Center (ANCC). (2004b). *Staff nurse self-assessment to determine readiness to pursue magnet recognition.* Washington, DC: Author. Retrieved July 18, 2004, from www.nursingworld.org/ancc/magnet/selfassess.pdf

American Nurses' Credentialing Center (ANCC). (2004c). *Expanding through research the frontiers of nurse credentialing: A program of the Institute for Research, Education, and Consultation.* Washington, DC: Author. Retrieved May 2, 2004, from www.nursingworld.org/ancc/education/research.html

Ashley, J.A. (1976). *Hospitals, paternalism, and the role of the nurse.* New York: Teachers College Press.

Bednar, B., & Peacock, E. (1998) Maintaining and documenting standards of care: Use of the nursing process. In J. Parker (Ed.), *Contemporary nephrology nursing* (pp. 3-42). Pitman, NJ: American Nephrology Nurses' Association.

Bell, C.R. (2002). *Managers as mentors: Building partnerships for learning.* San Francisco: Berrett-Koehler Publishers, Inc.

Benner, P. (1984). *From novice to expert: Excellence and power in clinical nursing practice.* Menlo Park, CA: Addison-Wesley Publishing Company.

Benner, P. (2000). Claiming the wisdom and worth of clinical practice. *Nursing and Health Care Perspectives, 20*(6), 312-319.

Benner, P.A., Tanner, C.A., & Chesla, C.A. (1996). *Expertise in practice: Caring, clinical judgment, and ethics.* New York: Springer.

Bower, F.L. (2000). *Nurses taking the lead: Personal qualities of effective leadership.* Philadelphia: W.B. Saunders.

Brodie, B., & Keeling, A.W. (2001). Historical highlights: The foundations of professional nursing in the United States. In J.L. Creasia & B. Parker (Eds.), *Conceptual foundations: The bridge to professional nursing practice* (3rd ed.) (pp. 3-25). St. Louis: Mosby.

Burrows-Hudson, S. (Ed.). (1993). *Standards of clinical practice for nephrology nursing.* Pitman, NJ: American Nephrology Nurses' Association (ANNA).

Burrows-Hudson, S. (Ed.). (1999). *ANNA standards and guidelines of clinical practice for nephrology nursing.* Pitman, NJ: American Nephrology Nurses' Association (ANNA).

Burrows-Hudson, S., & Prowant, B.F. (Eds.). (2005). *Nephrology nursing standards of practice and guidelines for care.* Pitman, NJ: American Nephrology Nurses' Association (ANNA).

Canavan, K. (1996). ANA's centennial: The birth of a professional organization. *American Nurse, 28*(6), 28.

Cannings, K., & Lazonick, W. (1975). The development of the nursing labor force in the United States: A brief analysis. *International Journal of Health Sciences, 5,* 185-217.

Cary, A. (2001). Certified registered nurses: Results of the study of the certified workforce. *American Journal of Nursing, 101*(1), 44-52.

Dean-Barr, S.L. (2001). Standards and guidelines: Have they made any difference? In J.M. Dochterman & H.K. Grace (Eds.), *Current issues in nursing* (6th ed.) (pp. 234-240). St. Louis: Mosby.

Dock, L. (1907). *A history of nursing* (Vol. 2). New York: G.P. Putnam's Sons.

Donabedian, A. (1966). Evaluating the quality of medical care. *Millbank Memorial Fund Quarterly, 44*(3), 166-206.

Dreyfus, S.E., & Dreyfus, H. L. (1980). *A five-stage model of the mental activities involved in directed skill acquisition.* Unpublished report supported by the Air Force Office of Scientific Research (AFSC), USAF, University of California at Berkeley.

Flanagan, L. (1976). *One strong voice: The story of the American Nurses' Association.* Kansas City, MO: American Nurses' Association.

Gallup Poll News Service. (2004). *Honesty/Ethics in Professions.* Retrieved October 22, 2005, from http://brain.gallup.com/content//?ci=1654

Goode, C.J., & Krugman, M. (2001). Evidence-based practice: A tool for clinical and managerial decision making. In Dochterman, J.M. & Grace, H.K. (Eds.). *Current issues in nursing* (6th ed.) (pp. 60-68). St. Louis: Mosby.

Hall, J.K., & Hall, D. (2001). Negligence specific to nursing. In M.E. O'Keefe (Ed.), *Nursing practice and the law: Avoiding malpractice and other legal risks* (pp. 132-149). Philadelphia: F.A. Davis.

Hoffart, N. (1989a). A professional organization for nephrology nurses. *ANNA Journal, 16*(3), 197-199.

Hoffart, N. (1989b). Nephrology nursing 1915-1970: A historical study of the integration of technology and care. *ANNA Journal, 16*(3), 169-178.

Institute of Medicine (IOM). (2003a). *Crossing the quality chasm: The IOM health care quality initiative.* Washington, DC: Author. Retrieved October 22, 2005, from http://www.iom.edu/focuson.asp?id=8089

Institute of Medicine (IOM). (2003b). *Keeping patients safe: Transforming the work environment of nurses.* Washington, DC: Author.

Knowles, M. (1990). *The adult learner* (4th ed.). Houston: Gulf Printing.

Koerner, J., & Burgess, C.S. (1997). Nursing's role and functions in a seamless continuum of care. In S. Morrhead & D.G. Huber (Eds.), *Nursing roles: Evolving or recycled?* (pp. 1-14). Thousand Oaks, CA: Sage Publications.

Leddy, S., & Pepper, J.M. (1998). *Conceptual basics of professional nursing.* Philadelphia: J.B. Lippincott.

Lunsford v. Board of Nurse Examiners, 648 S.W. 2d 391 (Tex. Civ App 3 Dist, 1983).

Maslow, A.H. (1954). *Motivation and personality.* New York: Harper.

Maslow, A.H. (1971). *The farther reaches of human nature.* New York: Viking Press.

Maslow, A.H. (1998). *Toward a psychology of being* (3rd ed.). New York: John Wiley & Sons.

McClure, M.L., Poulin, M.A., Sovie, M.D., & Wandelt, M.A. (1983). *Task force on nursing practice in hospitals.* Kansas City: American Nurses' Association.

Merrill, J.P., Murray, J.E., Harrison, J.H., & Guild, W.R. (1956). Successful homotransplantations of the human kidney between identical twins. *Journal of the American Medical Association, 160,* 277-281.

Mulhall, A. (1998). Nursing research and the evidence. *Evidence-Based Nursing, 1,* 4-6.

National Kidney Foundation (NKF). (2005). KDOQI History. Retrieved October 22, 2005, from www.kidney.org/professionals/KDOQI/abouthistory.cfm

Needleman, J., Buerhaus, P., Mattke, S., Stewart, M., & Zelevinsky, K. (2002). Nurse-staffing levels and the quality of care in hospitals. *New England Journal of Medicine, 346*(22), 1715-1766.

Nephrology Nursing Certification Commission (NNCC). (2005a). *About NNCC.* Pitman, NJ: Author. Retrieved October 22, 2005, from www.nncc-exam.org

Nephrology Nursing Certification Commission (NNCC). (2005b). *About Becoming a CNN.* Pitman, NJ: Author. Retrieved October 22, 2005, from www.nncc-exam.org

Nephrology Nursing Certification Commission (NNCC). (2005c). *About Becoming a CDN.* Pitman, NJ: Author. Retrieved October 22, 2005, from www.nncc-exam.org

Nightingale, F. (1859). *Notes on Nursing: What it is and What it is Not.* London: Harrison & Sons.

Parker, J. (1991). The development of the nephrology nursing certification program. *ANNA Journal, 18*(6), 543-547, 571.

Parker, J. (1994). The development of the American Board of Nursing Specialties. *Nursing Management, 25*(1), 33-35.

Parker, J. (1998). Nephrology nursing as a specialty. In J. Parker (Ed.), *Contemporary nephrology nursing* (pp. 3-42). Pitman, NJ: American Nephrology Nurses' Association.

Robert Woods Johnson Foundation. (2003). ESRD workgroup final report summary on end-of-life care: Recommendations to the field. *Nephrology Nursing Journal, 30*(1), 59-63.

Sackett, D.L., Rosenberg, W.M, Gray, J.A., Haynes, R.B., & Richardson, W.S. (1996). Evidence-based medicine: What it is and what it isn't. *British Medical Journal, 312,* 71-72.

Starr, P. (1982). *The social transformation of American medicine.* New York: Basic Books, Inc.

Stetler, C.B., Brunell, M., Guiliano, K.K., Morsi, D., Prince, L., & Newell-Stokes, V. (1998). Evidence-based practice and the role of nursing leadership. *Journal of Nursing Administration, 28,* 45-53.

Stevens, K.R. (1999). Advancing evidence-based teaching. In K.R. Steven & V.R. Cassidy (Eds.), *Evidence-based teaching: Current research in nursing education* (pp. 1-22). Boston: Jones and Bartlett Publishers.

Stevens, K.R. (2002). *ACE star model of EBP: The cycle of knowledge transformation.* Academic Center for Evidence-Based Practice. Retrieved June 12, 2004, from www.acestar.uthscsa,edu

Tarlov, A.R., Ware, J.E. Jr., Greenfield, S., Nelson, E.C., Perrin, E., & Zubkoff, M. (1989). The Medical Outcomes Study. An application of methods for monitoring the results of medical care. *Journal of the American Medical Association, 262*(7), 925-930.

Ulrich, B.T. (2003). Leader to watch: Tim Porter O'Grady. *Nurse Leader, 1*(5), 20-25.

Zachary, L.J. (2002). *The mentor's guide.* San Francisco: Jossey-Bass.

- Contemporary nursing practice traces its roots back to 1860 when the Nightingale School for Nurses at St. Thomas Hospital in London opened its doors.

- The first organized meeting of nurses in America occurred in 1893 at the Chicago World's Fair – the same meeting at which a paper written by Florence Nightingale was presented that laid the foundation for modern holistic nursing by discussing prevention as well as sick care as a part of the role of nursing.

- Nursing has evolved over the years into a profession that has a distinct body of knowledge, a social contract, and an ethical code. Professional nursing practice is complex and multifaceted.

- Standards reflect the values and priorities of the profession.

- The ANA Code of Ethics for Nurses is a succinct statement of the ethical obligations and duties of every individual who enters the nursing profession, is the profession's non-negotiable ethical standard, and is an expression of nursing's own understanding of its commitment to society (ANA, 2001).

- An important aspect of professional nursing today is the public's view of the nursing profession.

- Specialization provides the opportunity for individual practitioners to focus on one area of care and to provide the best possible care those in need (Parker, 1998). The specialty of nephrology nursing traces its beginnings to the arrival of the artificial kidney developed by Willem Kolff in 1947.

- Certification and credentialing in nursing have benefits for both nurses and patients.

- In 1969, the American Association for Nephrology Nurses (AANN) was created, becoming one of the nation's earliest specialty nursing organizations. In 1970, AANN changed its name to the American Association of Nephrology Nurses and Technicians (AANNT), and in 1984 and became the American Nephrology Nurses' Association (ANNA).

- ANNA's mission is to advance nephrology nursing practice and positively influence outcomes for patients with kidney or other disease processes requiring replacement therapies through advocacy, scholarship, and excellence.

- ANNA achieves its mission through establishing standards of care, providing education and information for nephrology nurses, enunciating positions on issues relevant to nephrology nursing practice and patients requiring the care of nephrology nurses, educating and lobbying legislators and other relevant regulatory agencies on behalf of nephrology nurses and patients, and encouraging and sponsoring research.

- The Nephrology Nursing Certification Board (NNCB) was formed in 1987. In 2000, the NNCB changed its name to the Nephrology Nursing Certification Commission.

- Two nephrology nurse certifications are offered by NNCC: the certified nephrology nurse (CNN), designed to test proficiency in nephrology nursing practice; and the certified dialysis nurse (CDN).

- Nephrology nurses are individually responsible for obtaining basic nursing education, education in the specialty of nephrology nursing, and life-long learning to assure that their education is always up-to-date. Education involves theoretical as well as clinical and hands-on knowledge and experience.

- The Standards of Nursing Practice include Standards of Practice (assessment, diagnosis, outcomes identification, planning, implementation, and evaluation) and Standards of Professional Performance (quality of practice, education, professional practice evaluation, collegiality, collaboration, ethics, research, resource utilization, and leadership).

- Nephrology nurses have many options in the roles they chose and often occupy more than one role at a time.

ANNP601

Professional Nephrology Nursing

Beth Tamplet Ulrich, EdD, RN, CHE

Contemporary Nephrology Nursing: Principles and Practice contains 39 chapters of educational content. Individual learners may apply for continuing nursing education credit by reading a chapter and completing the Continuing Education Evaluation Form for that chapter. Learners may apply for continuing education credit for any or all chapters.

Please photocopy this page and return to ANNA.
COMPLETE THE FOLLOWING:

Name: _____

Address:_____

City:_____ State: _____ Zip: _____

E-mail: _____

Preferred telephone: ☐ Home   ☐ Work: _____

State where licensed and license number (optional): _____

CE application fees are based upon the number of contact hours provided by the individual chapter. CE fees per contact hour for ANNA members are as follows: 1.0-1.9 - $15; 2.0-2.9 - $20; 3.0-3.9 - $25; 4.0 and higher - $30. Fees for nonmembers are $10 higher.

ANNA Member: ☐ Yes   ☐ No   Member # (if available) _____

☐ Checked Enclosed   ☐ American Express   ☐ Visa   ☐ MasterCard

Total Amount Submitted: _____

Credit Card Number: _____ Exp. Date: _____

Name as it appears on the card: _____

CE Evaluation Form
To receive continuing education credit for individual study after reading the chapter
1. Photocopy this form. (You may also download this form from ANNA's Web site, **www.annanurse.org**.)
2. Mail the completed form with payment (check) or credit card information to American Nephrology Nurses' Association, East Holly Avenue, Box 56, Pitman, NJ 08071-0056.
3. You will receive your CE certificate from ANNA in 4 to 6 weeks.

Test returns must be postmarked by **December 31, 2010.**

CE Application Fee
ANNA Member $20.00
Nonmember $30.00

EVALUATION FORM

1. I verify that I have read this chapter and completed this education activity. Date: _____

   _____
   Signature

2. What would be different in your practice if you applied what you learned from this activity? *(Please use additional sheet of paper if necessary.)*

   _____
   _____
   _____
   _____
   _____
   _____
   _____
   _____
   _____
   _____
   _____
   _____
   _____

Evaluation	Strongly disagree				Strongly agree
3. The activity met the stated objectives.					
a. Outline the development of professional nursing practice from the late 1800's through today.	1	2	3	4	5
b. Describe the attributes of professional nursing practice.	1	2	3	4	5
c. Compare and contrast the development of nephrology nursing as a specialty to the development of professional nursing practice.	1	2	3	4	5
4. The content was current and relevant.	1	2	3	4	5
5. The content was presented clearly.	1	2	3	4	5
6. The content was covered adequately.	1	2	3	4	5
7. Rate your ability to apply the learning obtained from this activity to practice.	1	2	3	4	5

Comments _____
_____

8. Time required to read the chapter and complete this form: _____ minutes.

This educational activity has been provided by the American Nephrology Nurses' Association (ANNA) for 2.6 contact hours. ANNA is accredited as a provider of continuing nursing education (CNE) by the American Nurses Credentialing Center's Commission on Accreditation (ANCC-COA). ANNA is an approved provider of continuing education by the California Board of Registered Nursing, CEP 0910.

The Evolution of Nephrology and Nephrology Nursing

Caroline S. Counts, MSN, RN, CNN

Chapter Contents

Caroline S. Counts, MSN, RN, CNN

It is not without reason that this textbook contains a chapter that reviews the history of nephrology and nephrology nursing. History offers contextual perspective as well as enlightenment. Nephrology nursing has been shaped by social pressures that persist today only under new forms. Insight into the past may help face the challenges of present times.

Classic reasons to look at the past are either to avoid repeating it or to learn from previous experience. Today's nephrology nurse will understand the tremendous work that was accomplished by nurses who led the crusade for improved health care for persons with kidney disease. They will gain a sense of professional identity. Exposing nephrology nurses to their heritage is a part of proper orientation (American Association for History of Nursing [AAHN], 2001).

Reconstructing the History of Nephrology

Hippocrates is described by some as the father of clinical nephrology, not just the father of medicine. Hippocratic medicine looked for natural causes for diseases, not divine intervention, as was the prevailing belief at the time. He and his colleagues at the medical school at Kos focused on the common elements of various disease processes, accurate descriptions of signs and symptoms, and prognosis.

Also at the time, under the leadership of Euryphon at the medical school of Knidos, interest focused on the systematic classification of diseases according to the body systems involved. Galen, a member of the Knidian school, mentions that his colleagues were familiar with four renal diseases.

In the book, *About Inner Sufferings,* four renal diseases are described. It is not known with certainty who the author is; some experts say Hippocrates, some say Galen. It may have even been a collaborative effort since the two were familiar with each other. The first renal disease described is nephrolithiasis with renal colic. And, for the first time a differential diagnosis between renal and urinary bladder stones is made. The second disease is renal tuberculosis and is mentioned as renal phthisis. The third renal disease resembles either renal vein thrombosis or bilateral papillary necrosis. The fourth disease is described in greatest detail and is acute suppurative renal condition or a sexually transmitted urethritis. Hippocrates states that sexual abuse can be harmful to the kidney (Dardioti et al., 1997). As far as treatment goes, it remained empirical. In the words of Galen, "All who drink of this remedy recover in a short time, except those whom it does not help, who all die. Therefore it is obvious that it fails only in 'incurable cases'" (Eknoyan, 2002).

During the Byzantine period (330 – 1453), medical science was both original and innovative. Many diseases of the time were widespread and had a high mortality rate. New diagnostic tests were introduced to examine urine, feces, spittle, sperm, and blood. The dissection of dead bodies was seen as a necessity to study anatomy and improve medical science. Oribasius correctly described blood circulation and discerned the micro histology of the kidneys, including the capillary vessels in the renal bodies. Hypertension as a plentitude of blood was noted by Alexander of Tralles, who forbid salt in food.

Important elements of nephrology began to surface – acute and chronic renal failure, acute and chronic nephritis, pyelonephritis, necrotic renal disease, crush syndrome, and ulcer of the kidney or tuberculosis. Diabetes was considered a disease of the kidneys (Eftychiadis, 1997).

During the Renaissance, the anatomy of the kidney continued to be studied and described. This was a period of scientific inquiry. Men such as Andreas Vesalius (1514 – 1564) and Bartholomeo Eustachio (about 1510 – 1574) described in excellent fashion the normal organs. This led the way for others to be able to describe pathological states (George, 2002). In his writings, Vesalius described the location of the kidneys in the abdominal cavity with the right kidney being higher than the left. He described his own ideas concerning kidney architecture and function. And, he dwelt on the misconceptions and misinterpretations of his contemporaries concerning the kidneys (DeBroe, Sacre, Snelders, & De Weerdt, 1997).

Hieronymus Fabrici, who graduated in medicine in 1556, also gave much to the study of anatomy. He was the first to describe venous valves. In addition, his initial description of the bursa led to recognizing the immune response and B- and T-dependent lymphocytes (Antonello et al., 1997).

Marcello Malpighi (1628 – 1694) is credited to be the founder of functional microscopic anatomy. He pioneered the development of medicine as a science as he observed nature and searched for the truth. During the early 1600s, a very strong opposition to traditional science emerged. The passive descriptive culture was no longer acceptable. A new era began that involved experimentations based on new methodological and analytical approaches. The focus switched to how phenomena take place. Galilei's microscope introduced new questions into morphological science.

By the end of his career Malpighi had: defined the direction of blood flow, discovered glomerular and tubular structures in the renal parenchyma, and resolved the relationship between renal glomerules and excretory outlets. The basis for the beginning of modern nephrology had been laid (Mezzogiorno & Mezzogiorno, 1997).

The Era of Correlating Pathology to Clinical Manifestations

Giovanni Battista Morgagni (1682 – 1771) took the crucial step of linking specific anatomical pathology to a clinical syndrome – chronic renal failure. Upon performing an autopsy, Morgagni described a pair of small, hard and irregular kidneys. The symptoms this person had experienced included nausea, vomiting, headache, and episodic coma (Eknoyan, 2002).

Morgagni is the acknowledged father of pathological anatomy. He first proposed a classification of ischuria into four categories: ischuria vesicalis, ischuria ureterica, ischuria urethralis, and ischuria renalis. The latter class was essential for the kidney to become a taxon around which the causes of ischuria due to kidney injury or disease could be grouped, studied, and described (Eknoyan, 2002, p. 226).

Others followed in Morgagni's footsteps (George, 2002). William Heberden (1710 – 1801) gave what can be considered a classic description of the clinical course of acute renal failure. "A total suppression has lasted seven days, and yet the patient has recovered. It has been fatal as early as the fourth day. But in general those patients, who could not be cured, have sunk to their malady on the sixth or seventh day" (Eknoyan, 2002). William Charles Wells (1757 – 1815) provided descriptions of persons who suffered from nephritic or nephrotic syndromes. In 1827, Richard Bright (1789 – 1858) addressed the same topic but in much greater detail. He presented case histories on 24 patients who had had proteinuria and edema during their lives. Bright speculated that there were three types of kidney disease based on microscopic appearances. And, he described secondary consequences that could cost the patients lives; these were inflammation of serous membranes (pericarditis or pleuritis) and cerebral hemorrhage. He considered the cause of the renal disease to be either intemperate consumption of alcohol or exposure to a wet and cold environment, or possibly a combination of the two.

Bright enlisted the help of two chemists, William Prout (1785 – 1850) and John Bostock (1773 – 1846). One recognized that the level of urea in the blood was high while the other recognized that the level in the urine was very low. Thus raised the possibility of gross chemical abnormalities in kidney disease (George, 2002).

John Abercrombie (1780 – 1828) taught in Edinburgh at the same time Richard Bright was studying medicine there. Abercrombie provided a description of acute renal failure with more detail than did Heberden. "The disease seems, in general to come suddenly. The peculiar symptom is a sudden diminution of secretion of urine, which soon amounts to a complete suspension of it. The affliction is probably first considered a retention; but the catheter being employed, the bladder is found to be empty…after several days, the patient begins to talk incoherently, and shows a tendency to stupor. This increases gradually to perfect coma, which in a few days is fatal. The occurrence of coma may be expected about the fourth or fifth day from the time when urine becomes suspended" (Eknoyan, 2002, p. 227)

In 1827 in Berlin, Friedrich Wohler (1800 – 1882) succeeded in synthesizing urea. This was the same year that Bright published his clinico-pathological observations about renal disease. Attention focused upon this chemical substance that occurred naturally in both blood and urine, but accumulated in the blood in some cases of renal damage.

In 1829 in Edinburgh, Robert Christison (1797 – 1882) was the first to draw a clear linkage between a rising urea level in the blood to a falling urea level in the urine and connected this occurrence with subsequent symptoms. He visualized renal disease as being a single variety that progressed through three anatomical distinct stages. He distinguished the immediate changes in the urine and blood from secondary complications – edema, dyspnea, vomiting, diarrhea, pleurisy, peritonitis, coma, apoplexy, pneumonia, heart disease, liver disease, and 'general infirmity.' Christison's emphasis on the rising level of urea in the blood led Pierre

Piorry (1794 – 1879) to coin the term 'uremie' to describe patients with elevated blood urea levels. The year was 1847 (George, 2002).

Another key figure of the time was William Bowman (1816 – 1892). Bowman's description of the glomerular capsule was a fundamental step in understanding kidney function and pathophysiology. He was the first to use the microscope to study the diseased kidney and described the microscopic features of Bright's disease. With Richard B. Todd (1809 – 1860), he edited one of the first textbooks on pathophysiology in which he wrote and illustrated the section on the kidneys (Eknoyan, 2002).

By 1877, the enigma of renal disease was resolved. Fatal outcomes were dependent upon toxic levels of urea. By 1900, the idea of uremia was well established, yet it was more qualitative than quantitative. Efforts were put into developing tests of renal function. The earliest methods left a lot to be desired. They relied upon the smell of urine after consumption of turpentine or asparagus. Other tests that researchers developed over the years depended on the concentrating, diluting, and acidifying abilities of the kidneys (George, 2002).

It was in 1917 that a report in the *Lancet* described "War Nephritis." Captains Davies and Weldon presented the morphologic and clinical features of 53 cases of kidney disease in observations made in 173 autopsies performed in connection with World War I. Today these would be classified as acute renal failure.

Between World War I and World War II there was emphasis placed on experimental medicine and in understanding vascular hemodynamics, kidney function, and tubular epithelial cell regeneration. Colonel W.B. Cannon (1871 – 1945) elaborated on the role of sympathetic and adrenal mechanisms of homeostasis. Alfred N. Richards (1876 – 1946) began a series of studies on urine formation. He used micro puncture while manipulating glomerular function with vasoconstrictors and tubular function with nephrotoxins. About the same, time Jean Oliver (1889 – 1976) was using micro dissection to clarify epithelial cell regeneration following exposure of micro dissected tubules to the same nephrotoxins Richards was using. Yet despite the flurry of clinical, structural, and functional studies many terms were used to describe the entity of acute renal failure. For example, in 1941, E.G.L. Bywaters and D. Beall reported on four cases of 'crush injuries with impairment of renal function' that were observed during the bombing of London in World War II (Eknoyan, 2002).

The preferential use of the term acute renal failure (ARF) is credited to Homer W. Smith (1895 – 1962). Smith is known as the founding father of the study of kidney function. Adoption of the term acute renal failure led to the term being used in making a diagnosis. It is relevant that at the same time William Kolff was introducing the artificial kidney, thus providing a supportive therapy for the person with acute renal failure (Eknoyan, 2002).

Hemodialysis

Thomas Graham (1805 – 1869) was a Scotsman who is considered to be the father of modern dialysis. He discovered the laws that govern the diffusion of gases, now known as Graham's law. He investigated osmotic force and the fractionation of biologic or chemical fluids by dialysis. He provided the original distinction between colloids and crystalloids. Colloids were described as a fixed class of chemical substances that are unable or are very slow to crystallize or diffuse (i.e., starch, gum, albumin, gelatin, and animal extractive matters). He named a variety of inorganic salts, sugars, and alcohols that are more volatile and are able to diffuse more easily as crystalloids. And, he introduced the concept of the semipermeable membrane (Gottschalk & Fellner, 1997).

Over 50 years later, John J. Abel, Leonard Rowntree, and B.B. Turner were the first to apply the principle of diffusion to actually remove substances from the blood of living animals. In 1914, they published two papers that gave more details about their apparatus that they called an artificial kidney. Their artificial kidney was made of celloidin tubes immersed in dialysate fluid housed in a glass jacket. In anesthetized animals, usually dogs, an arterial cannula carried the blood to the apparatus; another cannula returned the blood to the animal. Arterial pressure drove the system; no additional pump was used. Anticoagulation was achieved by using hirudin obtained from leeches as heparin had yet to be discovered. Abel, Rowntree, and Turner were forced to abandon their work when World War I began. They were unable to obtain the expensive anticoagulant.

George Haas (1886 – 1971) is credited with performing dialysis on a human being for the first time in October 1924 in Germany. This first dialysis lasted 15 minutes. Under local anesthesia, cannulae were inserted into the patient's left radial artery and antecubital vein. While the patient suffered no complications from the surgery or the procedure, the dialysis treatment lacked therapeutic effect. Haas calculated that only 150 cc of blood had been cleansed. Because of lack of support from the medical community, Haas did not pursue his work in this area (Gottschalk & Fellner, 1997).

Technological advancements continued. Heparin replaced the toxic and expensive hirudin; cellophane tubing replaced the celloidin tubes (Gottschalk & Fellner, 1997). A Dutch physician, Willem Johan Kolff, may be considered the major contributor to convince others that uremic patients could be managed by the use of an artificial kidney (Gottschalk & Fellner, 1997; McBride, 1989).

In the spring of 1940 in Groningen, Kolff became distressed over not being able to help a young patient dying of uremia. He performed some simple experiments with cellophane tubing to study the dialyzability of urea. He and his colleagues worked under the pressure of World War II as Germany was invading the Netherlands. Because of the most difficult surroundings, Kolff decided to move to the small town of Kampen, where he remained during the war. There he convinced the Berk Enamel Company that he needed their assistance. With the help of engineer Hendrik Berk, the first device was designed and built – the rotating artificial kidney. It was a mechanically sound piece of equipment and demonstrated that a dialysis machine could overcome the problems of renal failure. A rotating drum that was covered with cellophane tubing and partially submerged in a tank of dialysis fluid was the original design (Gottschalk & Fellner, 1997; McBride, 1989).

By 1944, 15 patients had been dialyzed. Unfortunately none had survived, but most underwent autopsy, allowing Kolff to discuss the causes of their deaths. Then on September 3, 1945, a 67-year-old woman was admitted to the surgical service with acute cholecystitis, jaundice, and near anuria. Ironically, this woman was a Nazi collaborator during the war. She was treated with sulfathiazide for $2^1/_2$ days. Her blood urea nitrogen (BUN) rose to 185 mg/dl and her potassium was an unbelievable 13.7 mEq/l. On September 11th she was dialyzed for 11.5 hours at which time her BUN fell to 56 mg/dl and her potassium to 4.7 mEq/l. Her clinical condition as well as her sensorium improved, she entered the polyuric phase of acute renal failure, and went on to recover completely.

Kolff later wrote in 1946 that chronic nephritis was no indication for treatment with the artificial kidney. His enthusiasm lay with the treatment of acute renal failure (Gottschalk & Fellner, 1997). Nonetheless, the development of successful dialysis by Kolff brought a fresh focus to ideas about uremia. Previously an aura of imprecision prevailed. This, however, was to change (George, 2002).

Unfortunately, the events of World War II limited communication among scientists in different countries. While Kolff was working in Kampen, another group was working in Toronto, Canada developing a clinical useable artificial kidney. Neither group knew of the other. Gordan Murray, Edmund Delorme, both surgeons, and Newell Thomas, an undergraduate chemistry student, built an artificial kidney in the basement of Murray's home. The cost of this project was 8,000 United States dollars. Murray had previously worked with transplanting kidneys into nephrectomized, heparinized animals to clear their blood of toxic substances. He was a pioneer in the clinical use of heparin and he developed several new surgical techniques, including vein grafting. He performed the first heart valve transplant using a cadaveric aortic valve. The patient was suffering from aortic insufficiency and was dying (Gottschalk & Fellner, 1997).

Murray performed the first dialysis in North America on December 6, 1946 on a comatose young woman. She was in acute renal failure following an attempted abortion 9 days earlier. The treatment was terminated after 1 hour because of severe chills. The dialysate fluid had not been warmed nor was the sterility of the system ensured. Her next treatment was 36 hours later when she underwent an 8-hour treatment; 3 days later she underwent another 6-hour dialysis. She eventually recovered completely. And, for whatever reason, the use of this artificial kidney stopped.

But, by this time some of Kolff's machines had been shipped to Canada, New York, and England. Kolff himself came to the United States and helped to initiate the first dialysis at Mount Sinai Hospital in New York City in 1947. Dr. George Thorne and Dr. John Merrill were present and decided to start a program in Boston that would support the transplant unit they were going to start (McBride, 1989).

Dr. Kolff guided the Boston group in modifying the original design of his artificial kidney. Edward Olsen, a machinist, and Dr. Carl Walters at the Peter Bent Brigham Hospital began building the Kolff-Brigham artificial kidney. This would be the machine that was used in the 1950s and by the military physicians of the United States Army during the

Korean War. The system was effective, but cumbersome, and treatments were time consuming.

Because of these limitations and the expense of the rotating drum system, Kolff abandoned the concept. He accepted a position at the Cleveland Clinic and continued his work in designing a more practical system. Dr. Bruno Wattschinger helped Kolff modify a coil dialyzer that was originally designed by Inouye and Ingelberg. Their modifications included two blood paths to lower the internal resistance and sterilization of the coil. While they had a prepackaged, presterilized, ready-to-use artificial kidney, they lacked a way to manufacture them.

Kolff was finally able to team with William Graham, President of Baxter Laboratories. At the time, Baxter was a relatively small company that focused on manufacturing disposable products using plastic components and intravenous devices. Their collaboration led to an artificial kidney system that went on sale October 30, 1956. The price of the machine was $1,000; the disposable kidneys were $53 each. Several limiting factors precluded the immediate success of the venture. First was the cost. Then there was the fact that it could only be used in acute renal failure. And, there were few medical groups who were trained in the use of the equipment. Yet the single most prohibitive factor was access to the bloodstream (McBride, 1989).

Access to the Bloodstream

Originally hemodialysis required venous and arterial cut downs with each treatment to gain access to the bloodstream. Obviously, the patient was quickly depleted of viable access sites. In 1960, Belding Scribner designed the revolutionary Scribner shunt while at the University of Washington (Schwab & Butterly, 2001; University of Washington, 1996). The impetus for Scribner was a very ill young man named Joe Sanders from Spokane, Washington. He had been treated for acute renal failure that turned out to be chronic renal failure. He and his family had to be told that there could be no further treatment and he was sent home to die, much to the dismay of Scribner and his staff (Blagg, 2004).

This externalized silastic shunt, connected by a short Teflon bridge, was usable right after it had been placed. The shunt was designed in a U-shape so that when not in use the tubing served as an extension of the circulatory system. On the arterial side the radial artery was usually used; on the venous side the cephalic vein was used. However, the shunts could be placed in the lower extremity if the need existed.

On March 9, 1960, the first Scribner shunt was implanted in the arm of a Boeing machinist, Clyde Shields (Schwab & Butterly, 2001; University of Washington, 1996). David Dillard, a pediatric heart surgeon, performed the surgery (Blagg, 2004). Shields lived for 11 years with hemodialysis and died in 1971 from a heart attack (Fresenius, 2001).

The disadvantages of the shunts included the fact that they clotted fairly regularly and then had to undergo embolectomy. They were also prone to infection. The lifespan of a shunt was about 6 months secondary to intimal hyperplasia. Once a shunt had been inserted into a vessel, the site was often not usable for future vascular access (Schwab & Butterly, 2001; University of Washington, 1996).

In 1966, Brescia and Cimino described the radio cephalic fistula. Either a side to side or end to side surgical technique created the anastomosis of the radial artery to the cephalic vein. The fistula continues to be the access of choice (Schwab & Butterly, 2001).

Home Hemodialysis

With the improvements in technology and a means for permanent access, the medical community's interest in chronic hemodialysis developed rapidly in the 1960s. Chronic renal care became an actuality (McBride, 1989). In 1963, the Veteran's Administration announced that it was going to open approximately 30 dialysis treatment centers around the country (Rettig, 1991). For others, treatments would be performed in the home.

Worldwide, credit for doing the first home hemodialysis goes to Yuke Nosé in Japan, in 1960 (Blagg, 2003). In the United States, Scribner demonstrated that indeed patients could be treated on hemodialysis equipment safely and effectively. However, available financial resources were not enough to meet the needs (McBride, 1989). Scribner became the leading advocate for treating patients by dialysis in the United States. His efforts resulted in Seattle receiving the first dialysis center grant from the Public Health Service in 1964. Seattle continued to pioneer the home dialysis treatment in the following years (Rettig, 1991).

Over the next 5 years, more than 50 patients from all over the United States and abroad came to the University of Washington in Seattle to be trained for home hemodialysis (Blagg, 2003). The number of treatment centers steadily increased, and patients trained for home dialysis to get the most out of the limited funding (Rettig, 1991).

By 1972, when Congress passed the Social Security Amendment of 1972 (H.R.1), there were approximately 10,000 patients being treated for renal failure. This law allowed for a source of funding from the federal government to pay for the treatment of end stage renal disease (Rettig, 1991). The number of home patients dropped dramatically after this legislation passed and more patients went to outpatient dialysis facilities (McBride, 1989).

Peritoneal Dialysis

The initial concept of peritoneal dialysis may date back to the early 1740s in England, Christopher Warrick treated a 50-year-old woman with severe ascites. He instilled Bristol water and claret wine into the patient's peritoneum through a leather pipe. The wine was to have an antibacterial effect. After three treatments, therapy was stopped because the patient reacted so violently. Despite her treatment, the patient recovered in a period of weeks and reportedly was able to walk 7 miles in a day without difficulty.

Early investigators were more interested in the peritoneal membrane and its ability to remove toxins than they were in its ability to remove fluid. In a period of several years ,these investigators were able to discover the membrane's ability to do both (International Society of Peritoneal Dialysis [ISPD], n.d.):

- 1877 Germany – G. Wegner determines the absorption rate of various solutions from the peritoneum.
- 1894 – E.H.Starling and A.H.Tubby describe the fluid removal characteristics of the peritoneum.

- 1895 – W.N. Orlow points out that fluid absorption also occurs from the peritoneal cavity.
- 1918 Prague and China – Desider Engel demonstrates that protein can pass through the peritoneal membrane.
- 1919 – M. Rosenberg notes that the fluid in the peritoneum contained the same amount of urea as the blood.
- 1923 John Hopkins – Tracy Putnam suggests that the peritoneum might be used to correct physiological problems (ISPD, n.d.).

The physiologic milestones had been laid that were necessary for the development and understanding of peritoneal dialysis (Diaz-Buxo, 1995).

In 1923 in Germany, Georg Ganter took this knowledge and put it into clinical practice. Under his care was a woman who suffered from renal failure following the birth of her child. Ganter prepared a sterile physiological solution that contained the correct amounts of electrolytes along with dextrose for fluid removal. The solution was placed in large bottles that were then boiled to insure sterilization. This solution was then infused into the woman's peritoneum through a rubber tubing connected to a hollow needle. Ganter instilled 1 to 3 liters of solution and let it dwell for 30 minutes to 3 hours each time. He continued to do the exchanges until the blood chemistries were more acceptable. He then discharged the patient to home, where she died. Ganter noted that he did not realize that he would have to continue the treatments for the patient to live.

From this very first patient, Ganter made several important observations. He noted the importance of the access, especially in relation to maintaining adequate outflows. He was very much aware of the possibility of infection and saw it as the most common complication of the treatment. Ganter knew that fluid removal depended on dextrose. And, he recognized the fact that dwell time and fluid volume affect solute clearance. These principles remain important today (ISPD, n.d.).

In 1936 at the Wisconsin General Hospital, a group led by J.B. Wear, R. Sisk, and A.J. Tinkle treated a patient with urinary obstructive disease with peritoneal dialysis. They maintained the patient on continuous dialysis until the obstruction was resolved. For the first time, it was shown that a patient could be treated with continued peritoneal dialysis.

In the mid 1940s, P.S.M. Kop, an associate of Willem Kolff's, created an integrated system that used gravity to instill the dialysate solution into the patient. The components of the system – porcelain containers, latex tubing, and a large glass catheter – could be easily sterilized. His group treated 21 patients; 10 were successful (ISPD, n.d.).

During World War II, researchers at Beth Israel Hospital in Boston were directed to devise a method of treating renal failure in battlefield conditions. Arnold Seligman, Jacob Fine, and Howard Frank developed a system for peritoneal dialysis that was similar to Kop's. In designing their system they addressed optimal flow rates and modification of the solution to meet the individual needs of the patient. Large bottles of solution that were sterilized were used to prevent infection. And, two catheters were used to minimize potential outflow obstruction.

In 1945, Seligman and his coworkers used their system to successfully treat a patient who had acute renal failure secondary to an overdose of sulfa drugs. This was a milestone in the development of peritoneal dialysis (ISPD, n.d.).

In 1952, Arthur Grollman at the Southwestern Medical School in Dallas, described intermittent peritoneal dialysis in a book he published. Grollman wrote about a 1 liter container with a cap that connected to a piece of plastic tubing. The tubing connected to the catheter. The catheter was made out of polyethylene; it was flexible, it had very small holes in the distal end to prevent outflow obstruction, and it was revolutionary. It resulted in better inflow and outflow. Grollman recommended that the fluid be instilled by gravity, that it be allowed to dwell for 30 minutes and then drained out into the same container. The technique was to be repeated hourly until the patient's chemistries were again normal (ISPD, n.d.).

Morton Maxwell, at the Wadsworth Veteran's Administration Hospital in Los Angeles, thought that hemodialysis was too difficult for most practitioners to use to treat acute renal failure. In 1959, he published a procedure that would become known as the "Maxwell Technique." Maxwell first convinced a local manufacturer of intravenous solutions, Don Baxter, to develop a peritoneal solution in a custom-designed container with a plastic tubing set and a polyethylene catheter. This allowed peritoneal dialysis to be performed in any hospital where the supplies were available and the procedure was understood (ISPD, n.d.; McBride, 1989).

It was during the Korean War that Paul Doolan, with the help of William Murphy, developed a catheter for long-term use. They worked at the Naval Hospital in San Francisco. The polyethylene catheter was flexible and contained a number of grooved segments to prevent the blockage of drain holes and maximize drainage. The consideration of using peritoneal dialysis in a chronic situation emerged.

Dr. Richard Reuben, who was finishing his tour of duty with the Navy in 1956, was consulted about a woman in renal failure. Reuben decided to use Doolan's techniques and implanted the catheter into the patient's abdomen. Once treatment began, the patient's condition improved dramatically only to deteriorate again once the treatment was finished. Eventually, the patient was allowed to go home during the week and received chronic peritoneal dialysis on the weekends in the hospital. The catheter was replaced once in a 7-month period (ISPD, n.d.).

The technical difficulties associated with having an adequate access, with maintaining sterility, and with providing large volumes of dialysate in a practical and economic manner, had thwarted the evolution of peritoneal dialysis (Diaz-Buxo, 1995). But, the lack of funding and resources for dialysis in the 1960's, led to Belding Scribner proposing that peritoneal dialysis be used as an alternative treatment to hemodialysis (ISPD, n.d.).

Automated peritoneal dialysis became a term used to describe all modalities of peritoneal dialysis that used a mechanical device to perform the dialysis (Diaz-Buxo, 2001). Automated peritoneal dialysis dates back to the 1960s, when Scribner invited Fred Boen to come to Seattle to set up a chronic home peritoneal dialysis program. Boen led a team that developed an automated unit that could be operated unattended at night. However, the logistical support required prevented the widespread use of this system. The system used 40-liter "carboy" containers that were filled and sterilized at the University of Washington and delivered to the patient's home. After the treatment, the containers were returned to the University. An automatic solenoid device opened and closed a switch to regulate the fluid into and out of the peritoneum. A physician would go to the patient's home to insert the catheter and initiate the exchange. After insuring that the treatment had begun, the physician would leave and the treatment would continue for approximately 24 hours. At this time the patient's caregiver would help the patient remove the catheter and cover the wound with a bandage. The patient would lead a normal life until the following weekend when the whole scenario was repeated (ISPD, n.d.).

In 1963, Henry Tenckoff accepted a position at the University of Washington to continue and improve the work of Boen. He first focused on improving the equipment being used. He got rid of the 40-liter bottles and replaced them by installing a water still in the patient's home to provide a supply of sterile water that could be mixed with the peritoneal concentrate. This too was time consuming and cumbersome.

In 1969, Tenckoff replaced the still with a reverse osmosis water purification system (ISPD, n.d.). The dialysate solution flowed in by gravity; clocks controlled the duration of the cycle phase; and, mechanical occluders directed the flow of solution (Diaz-Buxo, 2001). A simplified automated peritoneal dialysis system evolved that served as the prototype for all the reverse osmosis peritoneal machines that were later developed.

Next, Tenckoff modified a catheter that had been developed by Wayne Quinton. The catheter sealed properly at the exit site and prevented bacteria from migrating into the peritoneal cavity. But, Tenckoff wanted the catheter to be easier to insert and use. He added Dacron felt cuffs to help seal the openings through the peritoneum; he shortened the catheter; and, he suggested two designs – straight and curled. He developed an insertion tool called a trocar designed to make the placement of the catheter easier (ISPD, n.d.).

It was then that long-term access for peritoneal dialysis became a reality. Methods of accessing the peritoneum had changed over the years. Not only had the peritoneal catheter changed, but also the placement techniques. These changes led to the reduction in peritonitis and elongated the life of the catheter. In addition to the improvements in the catheters and placement techniques, came improvements in various types of cycler machines, assistive devices, and solution containers (Warren, 1989).

As early as 1970, Norman Lasker, at the Thomas Jefferson School of Medicine in Philadelphia, sent patients home on his "cycler." This system was able to measure the volume of fluid to be instilled and was able to warm the fluid prior to instillation. Whereas most of the medical community did not accept Lasker's device, Dimitrios Oreopoulos was very much interested. Oreopoulos was in charge of a four-bed intermittent peritoneal dialysis unit at Toronto Western Hospital. Because of the space limitations, he began sending patients home on intermittent peritoneal dialysis using the Lasker cycler. By 1974, he managed more than 74 patients at home (ISPD, n.d.).

In 1975, Jack Moncrief was practicing medicine in Austin, Texas. He had a patient, Peter Pilcher, who required dialysis but whose fistula had failed. He had no access through which to dialyze. The patient refused to relocate to a city where peritoneal dialysis was available; the only solution was peritoneal dialysis in Austin until a transplant could be done. Moncrief worked with a biomedical engineer, Robert Popovich, to determine the kinetics of long dwell equilibrated peritoneal dialysis. They discovered that Pilcher needed five exchanges of 2 liters per day to achieve appropriate chemistries and removal of 12 liters of equilibrated solution each day. They used 2-liter bottles, a simple piece of tubing, and a Tenckoff catheter. Fluid was instilled for 4 hours then drained out. Continuous ambulatory peritoneal dialysis was the outcome.

Moncrief noted several important facts. The patient's diet needed to be supplemented with protein, and other dietary restrictions could be relaxed. And, the solution could be left in the peritoneum overnight (ISPD, n.d.). Technological advances in biomaterials and kinetics have revived interest in this mode of therapy (Diaz-Buxo, 1995).

Renal Transplant

Throughout history the possibility of transplanting organs and tissues from one body to another has been intriguing. There are references dating back to the 15th century in historical medical literature regarding attempted blood transfusions and the transplantation of teeth. As far back as 1880, there were attempts at corneal and skin transplants. These early efforts were usually unsuccessful. It was not until the 20th century that transplantation offered real hope for renewed health and life (Transplant Network, n.d.).

The kidney became the pilot organ for transplantation research since it could be removed fairly easily and transplanted quickly. The assessment of the transplant's success could be evaluated by observing serial renal function. In the early 1900s, animal kidneys were transplanted into humans but without success (Novartis, n.d.). When dialysis became available, it offered only temporary improvement for patients with renal failure. It was logical to continue to seek a more permanent therapy (Murray, 1990).

In 1933, the first recorded human cadaveric transplant took place in Russia. In 1936, the first human kidney transplant from an allograft was performed by U. Voronoy. Like all transplants performed before the rejection process was understood, they failed (Renal Unit, 2001).

It was Peter Medawar, a young immunologist in England, who helped to discover why transplants failed. During World War II, Medawar studied the problems with skin grafts in soldiers who had been severely burned. He noted that initial skin grafts transplanted from one animal to another survived 7 days. If a second skin graft was performed between the same two animals, the graft survived a much shorter time. This became known as the second set response and formed the basis of the rejection process (Novartis, n.d.). It also implied that the rejection process was an allergic or immunologic process and meant it could be manipulated (Murray, 1990).

Planned programs for human organ transplantation started in the late 1940s in Paris, London, Edinburgh, and Boston. This was in spite of warnings and the pessimistic predictions of many scientists and clinicians (Murray, 1990).

By the late 1940s, there were two surgical prerequisites in place in order for renal transplant to be successful. The first of these was the perfected techniques to ensure the vascular anastomosis and the second was the suture techniques to establish the continuity of the urinary tract (Richet, 1997).

In Boston, at the Peter Bent Brigham Hospital, all elements for a sound renal transplant program were in place. There was experienced knowledge in renal disease. There was availability of dialysis. There were skilled and imaginative surgeons. Dr. David Hume was one such surgeon.

In the first allografts, the kidneys were added as a third kidney and placed in the thigh by Dr. Hume. The renal vessels were anastomosed to the femoral vessels, and urine was collected in a bag from a skin ureterostomy. Several of these grafts worked better than expected. This may have been due to the immunosuppressive effect of uremia or the acute tubular necrosis often seen in inadequately preserved donor kidneys. One thigh transplant functioned for almost 6 months (Murray, 1990).

By 1947 in Paris, Jean Hamburger had mapped out a course of action to transplant kidneys successfully. He emphasized four points. First, graft ischemia could cause functional deterioration to the kidney so it should be perfused extracorporally. Second, vascular coagulation within the kidney could be avoided by using heparin, which caused no harm to the kidney. Third, immune tolerance for organ grafts was probably like immune tolerance for blood transfusions. And fourth, the variable length of graft survival meant that it should be possible to overcome rejection (Richet, 1997).

On December 18, 1952, Dr. Hamburger performed a right nephrectomy on Marius Renard, a 15-year-old roofer. Marius had fallen off of a roof and ruptured the kidney. After surgery, anuria followed secondary to a congenitally absent left kidney. His mother proposed and insisted that she donate one of her kidneys to her son. On December 25th, the surgery took place. Upon removing the clamps, urine began to flow freely and the blood urea nitrogen returned to normal. Despite the hope of recovery, on the 22nd day the kidney became hard, thick, and ceased to function. Marius died 10 days later.

Marius' death had a global impact and affected the scientific community as well. J.P. Merrill, who was from the Boston group and on sabbatical in London with Medawar, immediately flew to Hospital Necker. The friendships that formed would have important bearings on the future of renal transplantation (Richet, 1997).

In the fall of 1954, Dr. Merrill was referred a patient in renal failure. What was particularly interesting about this man was that he had a healthy, identical twin brother. There was an opportunity for transplantation and the transplantation team of Joseph Murray and David Hume was very interested in transplanting a genetically compatible kidney. Cross skin grafting established genetic identity.

However, an ethical question remained. Should a normal healthy person be subjected to a major surgical operation if it was not for his own benefit? Physicians both within and outside of Peter Bent Brigham Hospital were consulted. Clergy of all denominations were consulted. Both patients and their families were consulted. The patients and the team decided to proceed.

The transplanted kidney began to function immediately and brought a dramatic improvement to the patient's renal and cardiopulmonary status. It was a clear demonstration that organ transplantation could be life saving (Murray, 1990). The recipient had a normal functioning kidney for 8 years. And, Dr. Joseph Murray won a Nobel Prize for Medicine in 1990 for his efforts in this field (Transplant Network, n.d.).

By transplanting identical twins, the issue of biological incompatibility had been bypassed, not solved, as no immunosuppression was required. Despite the success of this and other transplants between identical twins, the problem of transplanting tissues and organs between nongenetically identical persons still needed to be overcome. Widespread research into potential immunological barriers was stimulated (Murray, 1990; Renal Unit, 2001; Novartis, n.d.). An additional seven successful transplants between identical twins confirmed that rejection was an immunological event (Richet, 1997).

Important observations emerged in the laboratory that shed light on the role of the immune system in transplant rejection. Rupert Billingham, Leslie Brent, and Peter Medawar reported the use of lymphoid cells to transfer immunity to skin grafts in the mouse. Others demonstrated that the lymphocytes could attack the transplant without the presence of antibodies. Jean Dausset was able to describe the histocompatability complex in humans. From his work, tissue typing came into being and he received a Nobel Prize for his pioneering work (Richet, 1997; Novartis, n.d.).

As knowledge about the immune system emerged, attempts were made to alter it to prevent or control rejection episodes. Some of the first attempts included total body irradiation. While the treatment did prevent rejection, it could cause aplasia and could lead to destruction of the nervous system, fluid loss, and/or bacterial invasion. Total body irradiation had a high mortality rate. Death could occur within a few hours to a few days (Novartis, n.d.; Renal Unit, 2001). In Boston, total body X-ray was followed by marrow infusion and a renal allograft. In most patients the transplant worked immediately and continued to work for several weeks. However, only 1 of 12 patients, still had a functioning transplant after 3 months (Murray, 1990).

Real breakthroughs began to happen as the immunosuppressive drugs were introduced (Murray, 1990). Antineoplastic drugs, like methotrexate and cyclophosphamide, proved to be too toxic. Research continued (Novartis, n.d.).

In 1960, Sir Peter Medawar advised Roy Caine to go to Boston to work with Dr. Murray. In 1962, the pair reported the successful use of azathioprine, a derivative of 6-mercaptopurine, in a transplant patient who had received a kidney from a cadaver. This was the world's first successful unrelated renal allograft and it survived over a year. The second half of this first batch of azathioprine was used with success in a renal transplant patient in Edinburgh that same year (Murray, 1990; Renal Unit, n.d.; Novartis, n.d.).

At the same time, Dr. Willard Goodwin at the University of California in Los Angeles introduced the use of corticosteroids to immunosuppressive therapy. Worldwide, several transplant groups began their own successful programs. By 1965, the 1-year survival rate from living related donors was about 80%; from cadavers the rate was 65% (Murray, 1990).

Optimism and enthusiasm ran high. New drugs and other methods of immunosuppression were tested. Anti-lymphocyte serum and globulin prepared in sheep, horse, and rabbit was tested. Lymphocyte drainage via the thoracic duct was utilized. The role of human leukocyte antigens (HLA) became clearer. The relationship between HLA typing and clinical outcomes was established. The criteria for brain death were created and the Uniform Anatomical Gift Act was passed. This legislation allowed organs to be given as gifts to others. The Uniform Organ Donor Card followed as a legal document. Folkert O. Belzer improved preservation of tissues and cadaver organs as he developed cold hypothermic solution applied by a perfusion machine (Murray, 1990; Novartis, n.d.; Transplant Network, n.d.).

In 1972, Jean-Francois Borel, through chance, discovered the selective action of cyclosporine on helper t lymphocytes. Testing began in 1978 and the Federal Drug Administration gave approval in 1983. The use of cyclosporine improved graft survival but high doses were nephrotoxic and carried a high incidence of lymphoma. Lowering the dose of cyclosporine and combining it with corticosteroids could control the nephrotoxicity. This combination quickly became the standard regimen following transplant (Novartis, n.d.; Transplant Network, n.d.).

In 1984, the National Organ Transplant Act was passed. This law established a nationwide computer registry operated by the United Network for Organ Sharing (UNOS). It authorized financial support for organ procurement organizations, and it outlawed the purchase or sales of organs.

Shortly thereafter, in 1986, the Consolidated Omnibus Budget Reconciliation Act passed. This law requires that all potential donors be approached. It supersedes state laws and adds that hospitals must comply if they are to receive Medicare benefits. In 1988, the Joint Commission on Accreditation of Health Care Organizations added donor identification and notification standards. The Joint Commission requires hospitals to have policies and procedures in place for the identification, referral, and procurement of organs and tissues (Transplant Network, n.d.).

It has been over 50 years since that first successful transplant performed by Murray and Hume in Boston. Increased experience, advances in surgical technique, tissue preservation, post-transplantation care, and immunosuppression have led to improved success rates (Norvatis, n.d.). Yet serious complications still occur. The ultimate goal is to achieve an immunological tolerance between the donor and recipient and eliminate the need for drugs (Murray, 1990).

Pediatric Nephrology

Pediatric nephrology arose out of the clinical research that had been conducted from 1820 to 1950. Pediatric scientists were interested in the definition of glomerular disorders, fluid and electrolytes, the maintenance of normal volume, tonicity, acid-base balance, and the pathophysiology of conditions such as rickets and diarrhea. Pediatric kidney disease was initially viewed from a descriptive perspective rather than a quantitative one.

During the late 19th and early 20th centuries, most textbooks described renal tuberculosis, Bright's disease, post-scarlet fever renal disease, and albuminuria. German and Viennese pediatrics dominated this phase of pediatric nephrology.

The term nephrosis was used frequently in the first half of the 20th century to denote pale, enlarged, swollen kidneys that resulted from hypoproteinemia. The term was mostly gone by the 1960s and replaced by the more descriptive term nephrotic syndrome. This latter term indicates hypoproteinuria, edema, and hypercholesterolemia. Another term that vanished was Bright's disease. This denoted chronic renal failure, proteinuria, edema, and hypertension. Bright's disease carried with it a fatal prognosis (Chesney, 2002).

In this same time period, other investigators in Germany and in the United States, studied normal and pathophysiologic processes in the kidneys of neonates. They examined the composition of urine, urine volume excretion, and the disorder urate nephropathy. Improvements in laboratory methods allowed the field to develop. The field of study became known as metabolism and encompassed studies of rickets, the acidosis of the dehydration resulting from diarrhea, nephrosis, and factors related to growth. From the broad field of metabolism emerged several specialties – one of them was pediatric nephrology.

In 1912, John Howland founded the first department of pediatrics at a medical school. As chair at John Hopkins, Howland focused on pediatric research. He emphasized quantitative data collection, physiologic principles, and biochemical techniques (Chesney, 2002).

The early scholars tended to place all nephritis into limited forms. They largely based their views on the fact that some children recovered with bed rest and various diets; other views were based on the findings at autopsy. Their descriptions of disease progression were sometimes on target and sometimes were not. However, this changed once there were enough scientific advancements, including the development of the percutaneous renal biopsy (Chesney, 2002).

Chesney (2002) described the evolution of pediatric nephrology as having gone through six fundamental scientific and/or technologic discoveries regarding the kidney. These findings ensured that pediatric nephrology could never again be considered a part of another discipline. First, it was discovered that ACTH or glucocorticoids could induce remission in childhood idiopathic nephrotic syndrome. Second, a percutaneous renal biopsy could help define the underlying renal disease and the histological variants of the nephrotic syndrome, thus permitting the classification of glomerular disease. Third, the emerging immunologic techniques could be used to help define the type and mechanism of glomerular injury. Fourth, children can be treated with peritoneal dialysis or hemodialysis to prolong their lives when faced with end stage renal disease. Fifth, children can be considered as candidates for renal transplant whether it is from a cadaver or living donor. And sixth, approximately 80% of the children with hypertension have an underlying renal disease.

The treatment of childhood renal disease moved to focusing on the structure and function of the kidney. The renal biopsy, dialysis, and transplantation became essential components of care. By 1970, the uremic child was becoming a focus for study and clinical care. Pediatric nephrology continues to expand its knowledge base and still supports strong improvements in care (Chesney, 2002).

Nephrology Nursing

In 1944 as Willem Kolff worked in Kampen, Holland, three nurses worked along with him. The nurses were involved in all aspects of care except setting up the dialyzer. M. ter Welle was the head nurse of the medical department at the Kampen Hospital and was also a coauthor of Kolff's first report to the medical community. In 1950, Barbara Coleman, RN, worked along side John P. Merrill at the Peter Bent Brigham Hospital. Together they wrote an article for the *American Journal of Nursing*, "The Artificial Kidney" – it was the first article published in nursing literature to describe the role of the nurse in dialysis. In 1952, Anna Smyth, of the Army Nurse Corps, worked alongside Dr. Paul Teschan in the Renal Insufficiency Center at the 11th Evacuation Hospital in Wonju, Korea. The early home training programs relied heavily on registered nurses, as did transplant and peritoneal dialysis programs (Coleman & Merrill, 1952; Hoffart, 1989a).

As reported by Hoffart (1989a), nursing care of the patient with renal failure was presented in the literature as early as 1915. Nursing responsibilities included recording intake and output, controlling the diet, stimulating elimination of waste through the gastrointestinal tract, providing rest, preventing infection, providing comfort measures, and decreasing muscle activity to reduce the production of metabolic wastes. Nephrology nursing as a specialty did not come into being until dialysis and transplant programs had been established.

While nephrology nursing was evolving, nursing in general was changing in response to social pressures and changes within medicine and health care. The nurse's relationship with the physician changed from one of being a handmaiden to one of being an assistant to the physician. The level of knowledge the nurse needed was expanding. And, the medical care the patient was receiving was more complex and there was more concern for the patient as a person (Hoffart, 1989a).

One of the first practice areas to reflect these changing roles of nurses was in the dialysis units (Albers, 1989). In 1962 in Boston, a dialysis nurse was a professional nurse who had a physician in attendance at all times. The nurse provided care to the patient with acute renal failure during hemodialysis. The physician was responsible for setting up the $80 coil, performing the cut down, and weighing out the chemicals for the bath and then changing the bath every 2 hours (Fulton & Cameron, 1989). Very soon thereafter, nurses initiated technical procedures and were responsible for independent assessments of the patient (Albers, 1989). The descriptions of the nurses in dialysis units demonstrate that they were assisting the physician and were using scientific knowledge as well as expanding knowledge (Hoffart, 1989a).

The early dialysis nurse faced challenges in several

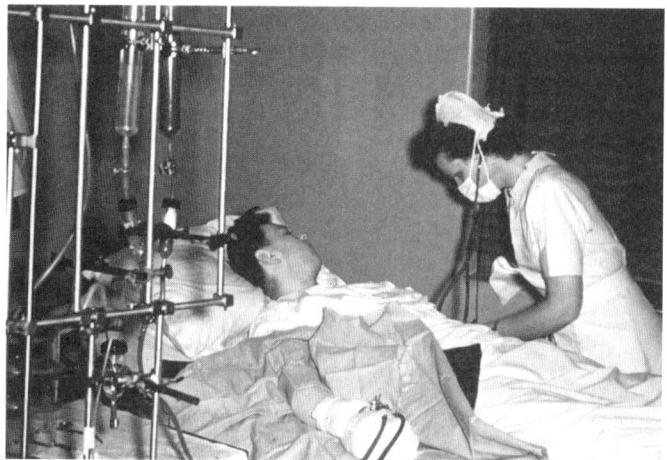

Photo courtesy of Bill Murphy, Miami, FL

Barbara Coleman-Wysocki, RN, provides nursing care for a patient on the artificial kidney at Peter Bent Brigham Hospital in Boston in 1949. The Brigham team worked on the first dialysis program in the United States.

areas, including making the patient comfortable. The equipment itself was large, cumbersome, and frightening. There were no safety features. The first dialysis patients ran in a room that had little else in it other than the plumbing. Nursing tasks included back rubs, repositioning, explaining the procedure, offering reassurance, and easing the patient's last hours or days in cases where death was immanent. There were often a lot of staff, teachers, medical students, and so forth coming to see the equipment in action. The nurse was also responsible for trying to protect the patient from all of this activity (Hoffart, 1989a).

With the development of the arteriovenous shunt, nephrology nursing continued to evolve. The shunt provided a means for chronic dialysis to become a reality. This in turn meant that it was no longer feasible to have the physician present at all times. Additional technical tasks were delegated to the nurse – initiating and terminating the treatment, declotting the shunt, administering blood; yet, the nurse did not lose sight of the patient's personal needs amidst the tubing and equipment (Hoffart, 1989a).

By 1963 home dialysis was begun and again the role of the nephrology nurse expanded. Patient education became a top priority as patients and their partners trained to go home with a complicated treatment regimen. Keep in mind that textbooks focusing on patient education did not appear until 1968; patient teaching was a new concept in nursing. Providing interpersonal care was another challenge. Patients and their families were under the stress of being dependent on the dialysis machine, of following a strict medical regimen, of changes in lifestyle, of changes in roles within the family, and of financial concerns (Hoffart, 1989a). Without federal funding, home dialysis was only available to those patients who had either personal or community funds. There were a few patients whose employers provided extended benefits (Fulton & Cameron, 1989). Nurses made home visits to assess the medical, technical, socioeconomic, and psychological problems (Hoffart, 1989a).

In less than a decade the dialysis treatment went from being a procedure done by the doctors, to one done by registered nurses, to one done by the patient in the home. The nurse's role went from assistant, to provider, to educator and supporter (Hoffart, 1989a).

Like dialysis nurses, transplant nurses faced many challenges in delivering patient care and were required to expand their knowledge base. During the early years, transplantation was full of risks and complications. The nurse was there to help the patient and the family with the uncertainty of the treatment. In the 1960s, some hospitals established transplant units. Patients underwent total body irradiation and were in isolation for weeks. Strict infection control techniques were required (Hoffart, 1989a).

Postoperative care made it necessary for the nurse to know about the transplant procedure, renal system physiology, immunosuppression, and the rejection process. Providing psychological care was paramount. The patient's fears and emotions were intense. And, patient and family education was extremely important. They had to know about blood pressure, weight, medications, laboratory values, and signs of infection and rejection.

The nurse was able to assist the patient and family through the physiological and psychological rigors of transplant. It necessitated attention to the physical, emotional, and learning needs (Hoffart, 1989a).

Nurses who worked in peritoneal dialysis, like the nurses working in hemodialysis and transplant, learned new technical skills. They had to maintain and monitor the procedure recording the intake and output, handling drainage problems, and keeping the patient safe. Infection control and the prevention of peritonitis were concerns. In addition, they were required to fulfill supportive and educational roles (Fulton & Cameron, 1989; Hoffart, 1989a).

These were the beginnings of the specialty of nephrology nursing. It evolved out of the needs of a growing population of persons with renal disease. These patients required care that was not only specific to their needs, but also cost-effective (Fulton & Cameron, 1989). Early registered nurse (RN) advocates for the end stage renal disease (ESRD) program can be seen in Table 2-1 (Sharp, 2004).

The American Nephrology Nurses' Association

The pioneers in nephrology nursing had few opportunities to meet each other or to come together. In the 1960s there were few units and those that existed employed only one or two registered nurses who typically reported to the physician rather than nursing administration (Hoffart, 1989b).

In 1955, the American Society for Artificial Internal Organs, better known as ASAIO, was founded. Their meetings focused on topics related to machines and equipment that simulated the functions of human organs and provided a venue for learning, discussions, and networking. Those in attendance included physicians, researchers, engineers, and eventually those RNs working in dialysis (Hoffart, 1989b).

In October 1966, at the Peter Bent Brigham Hospital in Boston, a nurse named Barbara Fulton planned the first nephrology nursing educational program. Over 150 nurses attended. Based on the success of this program, the nurses who came to the ASAIO meeting in 1967 in Chicago decided to plan a second meeting.

Table 2-1
Early RN Advocates for ESRD Program

Bernice Hinckley, RN	Washington, DC
Barbara Fulton, RN	Boston, MA
Barbara Wysocki, RN	Rexford, NY
Barbara Fellows, RN	Seattle, WA
Margery Fearing, RN	Iowa City, IA
JoAnn Albers, RN	Seattle, WA
Elizabeth Cameron, RN	Philadelphia, PA
Lo Schlotter Binkley, RN	Indianapolis, IN
Mary O'Neil, RN	Philadelphia, PA
Betty Preston Oates, RN	Jackson, MS
Mary Mallison, RN	Atlanta, GA
Martha Leonard Orr, RN	Yonkers, NY
Marcia Keen, RN	San Francisco, CA
Donna Mapes, RN	San Francisco, CA
Marcia Clark, RN	Seattle, WA
Lynn Poole, RN	Charlottesville, VA
Nancy Sharp, RN	Chicago, IL & Washington, DC

Bernice Hinckley, a nurse consultant with the Kidney Disease Control Program (KDCP) of the United States Public Health Service, arranged for a 1-day meeting for nurses during the 1968 ASAIO meeting held in Philadelphia. KDCP, ASAIO, the Milton Roy Company, and Travenol Laboratories sponsored the meeting. Hinckley, Elizabeth Cameron, and Mary O'Neill planned the meeting and focused its contents on nephrology nursing, not simply dialysis. Over 200 nurses attended (Hoffart, 1989b).

Following the 1969 ASAIO meeting in Atlantic City, a core group of about 50 nurses came together and formed the American Association for Nephrology Nurses (AANN). This core group had seen the need to ensure the continuation of nephrology nursing conferences. The organization's purpose was to promote knowledge in this field. The first officers were Bernice Hinckley, president; Barbara Fulton, vice president; and, JoAnn Albers, secretary. Full membership was open only to RNs (Hoffart, 1989b).

The following year the name of the organization changed to the American Association of Nephrology Nurses and Technicians (AANNT). The bylaws were changed and full membership was opened to technicians as well as RNs (Hoffart, 1989b). In 1983, the decision was made to focus the association's efforts and resources on the RN. The name of the association was once again changed; it now became the American Nephrology Nurses' Association (ANNA) and full membership was limited to registered nurses. Highlights of the many accomplishments of the association from its inception can be found in Figure 2-1.

Summary

The evolution of nephrology began centuries ago. A deeper wide-spreading understanding of kidney function, technological advances, improvements in surgical techniques, and discovery of new medications, have changed kidney disease from a potentially life-threatening disease to a treatable one. Life-saving renal replacement therapy now exists for the hundreds of thousands of persons who reach the end stage of kidney disease.

continued on page 48

Figure 2-1

The History of the American Nephrology Nurses' Association (ANNA) at a Glance

---

ANNA

Looking Back: 1969-1970
Bernice Hinckley
President

The Year in Review

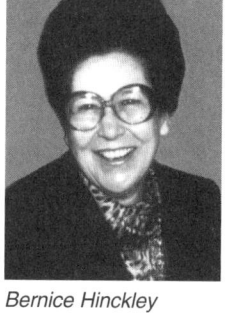

- The success of a 1968 dialysis symposium for physicians and nurses in Philadelphia led to the announcement of a formal educational program for nurses the following year.
- In Atlantic City in April 1969, a formal educational meeting, "A Dialysis Symposium for Nurses," was sponsored by the Kidney Disease Control Program under the Department of Health, Education, and Welfare.
- During this historic meeting in Atlantic City, a small group of nephrology nurses met to formally begin a new organization.

Bernice Hinckley

- During the Atlantic City Meeting, the name American Association for Nephrology Nurses (AANN) was formally adopted for the new nursing organization.
- In Atlantic City, AANN held its first elections, developed its charter and bylaws, and established its membership fee of $2.50.
- Bernice I. Hinckley was elected as the Association's first President.
- The new organization spent the following year promoting networking with other dialysis professionals and industry sponsors as well as implementing plans to increase its membership.
- The First Annual AANN National Symposium, held in Washington, DC in April 1970 in conjunction with ASAIO, attracted 450 registrants. Proceedings from the symposium were published.

Looking Back: 1970-1971
Beth Cameron
President

The Year in Review

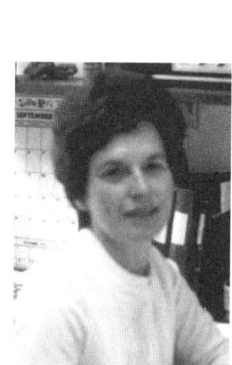

- Recognizing the important contributions of the technicians, a vote was taken to include technicians as full members in the Association.
- AANN subsequently changed its name to the American Association of Nephrology Nurses and Technicians (AANNT), allowing LPNs and technicians full membership.
- In an effort to allow all members to participate in the organization, members received the first mailed ballot, including a CV. Membership dues of $5.00 were barely enough to pay for one mailing.

Beth Cameron

- Arrangements were made to continue to meet concurrently with ASAIO for the next 3 years, including the desire to meet in split sessions.
- The Second Annual National Meeting in Chicago in Spring 1971 drew 574 attendees.
- Papers were presented at the Annual Meeting by nationally known speakers who could pay their own way! Meeting expenses were defrayed by the controversial registration fee and the continued help of corporate sponsors and ASAIO.
- Total membership in AANNT reached 800 under Beth Cameron, the young organization's second president.

Looking Back: 1971-1973
Mary O'Neill
President

The Years in Review

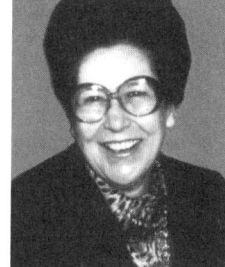

- The original AANNT Bylaws were significantly changed to allow for growth development and expansion of the organization's services.
- The AANNT Newsletter (volume 1, number 1) began national publication on a quarterly basis in 1972.
- Standards of Hemodialysis, the first ones throughout the world for this field, were developed.

Mary O' Neill

- President Mary O'Neill and President-Elect Betty Preston attended the first meeting of NFSNO, held at the Western White House in San Clemente, CA.
- Communication to the membership was through AANNT general information sheet, newsletters, bylaws, standards, and membership card.
- AANNT's first official organization logo was approved by the Board of Directors.
- First President Bernice Hinckley was appointed liaison to the European Dialysis and Transplant Nurses' Association (EDTNA).
- Membership increased to over 900 while five regions (Northeast, Southeast, North Central, Middle Mountain, and Western) were developed.
- The Third National Symposium (1972) in Seattle attracted 423 attendees while the Fourth National Symposium (1973) in Boston had more than 500 registrants in attendance.

Looking Back: 1973-1975
Betty Preston Oates (1973)
Lois Bernbeck (1973-1975)
Presidents

The Years in Review

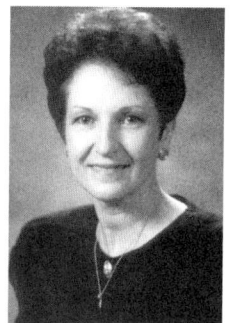

- AANNT representatives attended the Chronic Renal Disease Conference to discuss the chronic renal disease provision of the Social Security Amendments of 1972 (HR-1).
- The Continuing Education Board was established under the Standards of Education Committee.
- Publication of Standards for Hemodialysis, Transplantation, and Peritoneal Dialysis was complete.

Betty Preston Oates

- The first issue of the *Journal of AANNT* was published in Fall 1974 with Margery Fearing serving as the first Editor.
- In collaboration with another organization, AANNT took part in the formation of BONENT, and work on certification progressed.
- Seminars-at-Sea were offered to the membership as a means of vacationing and learning at the same time.
- To keep up with increasing activity, Human Resources, Inc. was hired as the association's management firm.
- Membership increased to over 1,600 under Lois Bernbeck during her second year as president in 1974-1975.
- Attendance at the Fifth National Symposium (1974) in Chicago reached 800 while attendance at the Sixth National Symposium (1975) in Washington also reached 800.

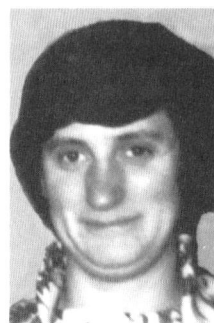
Lois Bernbeck

Looking Back: 1975-1976
Martha Leonard Orr
President

The Year in Review

- Membership under President Martha Leonard Orr reached about 2000.
- A successful National Symposium was held in San Francisco, CA.
- The National Association of Patients on Hemodialysis and Transplantation (NAPHT) presented its annual award for Outstanding Contributions to Patient Welfare to AANNT.
- The Peritoneal Dialysis section of the Standards of Clinical Practice (Section III) was published and distributed to Association members.
- The Association continued its work on the development and promotion of its new journal, which today is known as *Nephrology Nursing Journal.*
- AANNT planned and implemented a new organizational framework for the Executive Committee and Executive Council.
- The Association moved in the direction of a centralized administrative office by consolidating the convention management functions under the Executive Director.
- AANNT helped to sponsor the first summer camp for children on hemodialysis at Frost Valley in upstate New York.
- The Association co-sponsored its first management seminar, the "Laboratory for Leadership," geared toward nurses in nephrology management positions.

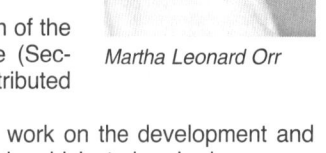
Martha Leonard Orr

Looking Back: 1976-1977
Marcia Clark
President

The Year in Review

- Membership under President Marcia Clark numbered approximately 2,200.
- The Eighth National Symposium, held in Montreal, attracted 800 registrants.
- The position paper "The Role of the Dialysis Technician" was published.
- Standards of Clinical Practice for Hemodialysis, Transplantation, and Peritoneal Dialysis were revised, and an additional set addressing acute renal failure was developed.
- The Continuing Education Approval Board published "Guidelines for Continuing Education Approval" to assist members with this process.
- A booklet on anticoagulation, sponsored by Abbott Laboratories, was prepared and presented under the AANNT name and distributed to the members.
- Twenty-five position descriptions were written to facilitate members' understanding of the roles and duties of the various officers and committees.
- Efforts were begun to develop a nephrology core curriculum, which resulted in the first draft of a content outline.
- The concept of Basic Learning Institutes was formulated with two pilot programs in 1977.

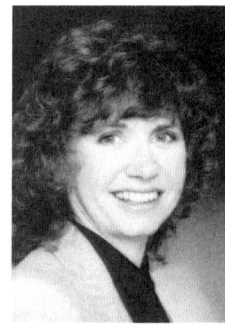
Marcia Clark

Looking Back: 1977-1978
Susan Hopper
President

The Year in Review

- Ten Basic Learning Institutes were presented to the AANNT membership.
- AANNT received accreditation from the American Nurses' Association as a provider and approval body for continuing education in nursing.
- Recruitment began for an Educational Director for AANNT.
- Work began on the second position paper, "The Role of the LPN in Dialysis."
- The monograph series was initiated with the publication of the Monograph on Self-Dialysis.
- Ten National Newsletters and four issues of the *Journal of AANNT* were published and sent to the membership.
- Through correspondence with European colleagues, AANNT participated in initial plans to form an international organization of nephrology nurses.
- A membership recruitment and retention campaign resulted in a 52% membership increase under President Susan Hopper.
- A successful 9th Annual National Symposium was held in Chicago.

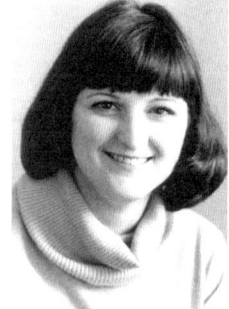
Susan Hopper

Looking Back: 1978-1979
Lois Foxen
President

The Year in Review

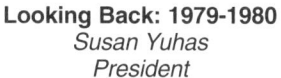
Lois Foxen

- AANNT membership reached 4000 by April 1979, with chapters totaling 40.
- The milestone 10th Anniversary National Symposium was held in New York City.
- Plans were initiated for the publication of a Skills Resource Book, intended to serve as a resource for those seeking potential speakers or advisors for programs or projects.
- AANNT's second position paper, "The Role of the Licensed Practical Nurse in Dialysis," was published.
- Francine Hekelman was employed by AANNT to fill the position of full-time Education Director.
- Nine Learning Institutes/Workshops were conducted, with over 700 people in attendance.
- The Continuing Education Approval Board reviewed and processed over 100 applications for national, regional, and chapter programs.
- Publications included 10 informative newsletters, the quarterly publication of JAANNT, and initial work on the monograph "Transplantation."
- President Lois Foxen journeyed to the Republic of South Africa to be the guest speaker at the Renal Care Society of Southern Africa's Annual Congress.

Looking Back: 1979-1980
Susan Yuhas
President

The Year in Review

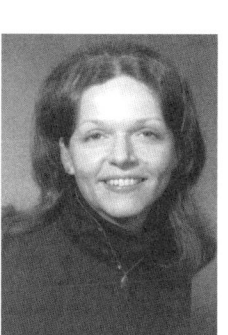
Susan Yuhas

- Under President Susan Yuhas, the Association experienced a year of critical decision making that ultimately affected the future of AANNT.
- A Long Range Planning Retreat was held in which several major short and long-term objectives were addressed.
- The Association's Executive Committee approved a decision to change association management firms.
- A monograph on hepatitis was published in the *AANNT Journal*.
- A written Policy and Procedure Manual, providing continuity in function, was initiated.
- The Executive Committee approved the concept of the AANNT Foundation, the first step prior to formation of the Foundation the following year.
- The 11th National Symposium, "The Realities of Nephrology Patient Care in the New Decade," was held at the Hyatt Regency Hotel/Louisiana Superdome in New Orleans.
- Membership in AANNT held steady at approximately 2,200 members while the number of chapters continued to increase.

Looking Back: 1980-1981
Carmella Bocchino
President

The Year in Review

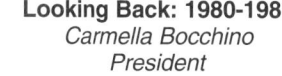
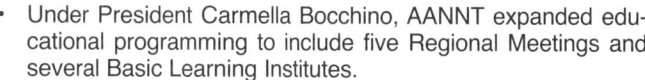
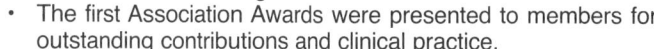
Carmella Bocchino

- In a transition year, the Association's management firm changed twice. Anthony J. Jannetti, Inc. was hired in 1980 and still serves as the association's management firm today.
- The strength and dedication of the volunteer members held the Association intact through a difficult transition year.
- The 12th National Symposium was held with about 800 registrants attending a successful meeting in Anaheim, CA.
- Under President Carmella Bocchino, AANNT expanded educational programming to include five Regional Meetings and several Basic Learning Institutes.
- The first Association Awards were presented to members for outstanding contributions and clinical practice.
- The position paper, "Role of the Registered Nurse in Dialysis," was published.
- The *AANNT Journal* began publishing bimonthly instead of quarterly.
- Monographs on renal osteodystrophy and transplantation were published.
- The AANNT Foundation was established by a vote of the Board of Directors.
- The Board of Directors voted to host independent national meetings, beginning in 1983.

Looking Back: 1981-1982
Nancy Sharp
President

The Year in Review

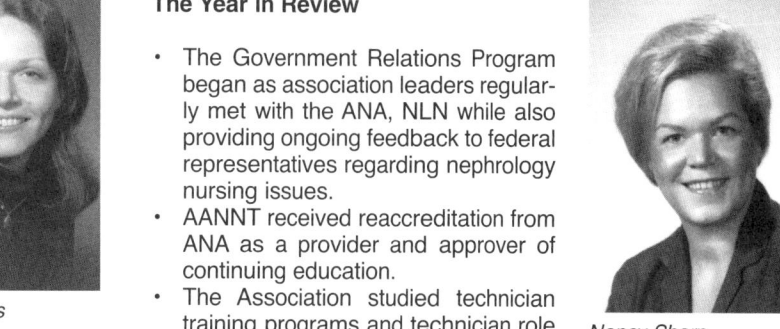
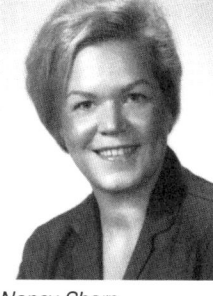
Nancy Sharp

- The Government Relations Program began as association leaders regularly met with the ANA, NLN while also providing ongoing feedback to federal representatives regarding nephrology nursing issues.
- AANNT received reaccreditation from ANA as a provider and approver of continuing education.
- The Association studied technician training programs and technician role descriptions through a national Ad Hoc Committee.
- AANNT hosted the NFSNO Annual Meeting.
- AANNT formed the Long Range Planning Committee, the Professional Relations Committee, and the Corporate Liaison Committee.
- The entire AANNT Awards Program was expanded as awards in nephrology education and research were instituted.
- The Standards of Clinical Practice were revised to conform to the nursing process format.
- The Association held five regional meetings in Monterey, Denver, Milwaukee, Atlanta, and Philadelphia while also holding an "Advances in Dialytic Therapy Seminar."
- The 13th National Symposium in Chicago attracted 1,000 registrants.
- Membership grew to 3,237 under President Nancy Sharp.

Looking Back: 1982-1983
Dawn Brennan
President

The Year in Review

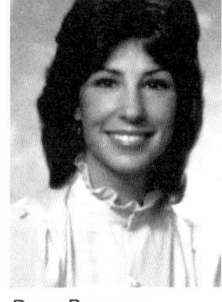

- The association bylaws changed to limit full membership to registered nurses only, an important step toward development of a professional nursing organization.
- The Independent First National Meeting separate from ASAIO was held in Philadelphia in June 1983 and attracted 1,000 registrants and 300 industrial representatives.
- The First Congress of Chapters was held at the 14th National Symposium in Philadelphia.

Dawn Brennan

- An International Workshop on Nephrology Nursing followed the 14th National Symposium.
- A 5-year contract was signed with Anthony J. Jannetti, Inc. to provide central office management, exhibit management, and conference management.
- A brochure, "Careers in Nephrology Nursing," was published while a slide/tape presentation about AANNT was developed to foster membership growth.
- The association sent a delegation to the White House for National Nurses' Day and presented a sculpture to Vice President George Bush.
- The Special Interest Group (SIG) concept was accepted for implementation at the 1983 National Symposium.
- Despite the bylaws change, membership held steady at nearly 3,000 under President Dawn Brennan.

Looking Back: 1983-1984
Mary Baker
President

The Year in Review

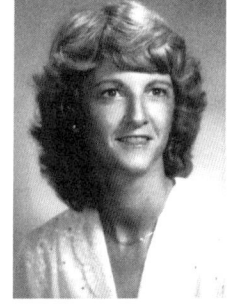

- The organization approved a new name —The American Nephrology Nurses Association (ANNA).
- Special Interest Groups (SIGs) became an official subcommittee of the Clinical Practice Committee. The identified groups were Administration, Education, Hemodialysis, Pediatrics, Peritoneal Dialysis, Research, and Transplantation.
- 54 chapters were in place representing all areas of the United States.

Mary Baker

- A high visibility theme was encouraged among the leaders to educate members who chose to be inactive and promote AANNT among those people who were not members.
- Government Relations became more evident for AANNT with the adoption of the AANNT Legislative Policy Statement/ Platform. Input was provided to Senator Albert Gore for proposed legislation relating to transplantation.
- Mary Baker was appointed by President Reagan to serve on a National Health Steering Committee that met in November in Washington DC. As chairperson of the Public Relations Committee of the National Federation for Specialty Nursing Organizations, Ms. Baker was the only nurse appointed to the committee, representing 15 associations.
- The *ANNA Journal* published a Monograph on Renal Rehabilitation.

- The 15th National Symposium was held in Hollywood, FL with attendance reaching 1,000. Donna Mapes served as the keynote speaker.
- Betty Irwin Crandall was the recipient of the Outstanding Contribution to Nephrology Nursing.
- During the opening ceremonies of the 15th National Symposium, 11 past presidents and 16 of the original founding members of the organization were recognized.

Looking Back: 1984-1985
Beth Ulrich
President

The Year in Review

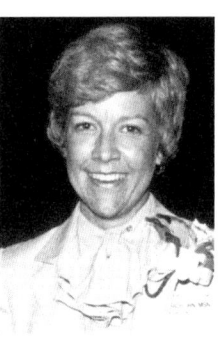

- The organization enjoyed a successful first full year with its new identity of the American Nephrology Nurses' Association (ANNA).
- Educational opportunities were provided this year at the four regional meetings, the National Symposium, and through printed media.
- The *ANNA Journal* monograph, Protecting the Future of Quality Care through an Understanding of Hemodialysis Principles, was distributed.

Beth Ulrich

- Special Interest Groups (SIGs) began to function effectively in 1984. A ninth SIG for Renal Staff Nurses was formed in 1985 for nurses who work on inpatient renal units.
- ANNA contributed significantly to the passage of the organ procurement legislation and maintained an ongoing dialogue with members of Congress and HCFA.
- In an attempt to promote collaboration among nephrology associations and their members, ANNA organized and hosted the first Assembly of Nephrology Organizations.
- Membership exceeded 3,000 and the number of chapters increased to 55 under President Beth Ulrich.
- A successful 16th National Symposium was held at the Sheraton Harbor Island Hotel in San Diego, CA.

Looking Back: 1985-1986
Geri Biddle
President

The Year in Review

- ANNA continues to become financially stable and membership increased 12% between March and December 1985.
- The position of education director was reinstituted for ANNA after being vacant since 1981.
- Planning took place to publish the Scope of Practice for Nephrology Nursing.
- The development of the Core Curriculum for Nephrology Nursing was established as a major priority.

Geri Biddle

- Regional educational programming was redefined with the First Clinical Concerns in Nephrology Meetings planned for Fall 1986, while the final Regional Meetings were held in Fall 1985.
- ANNA reevaluated and established new directions for nephrology nursing certification with actions that eventually led to the

development of a new certification examination.
• Membership surpassed 3,000 under President Geri Biddle.
• A successful 17th Annual National Symposium was held at the Hyatt Regency Hotel in New Orleans, LA.

Looking Back: 1986-1987
Janel Parker
President

The Year in Review

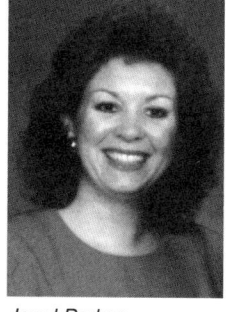

• The 18th National Symposium in New York City attracted 1,335 participants.
• Membership reached an all-time high of 3,690 while chapters increased to 65 under President Janel Parker.
• The Nephrology Nursing Certification Board (NNCB) was incorporated.
• The Nephrology Nursing Certification Examination was developed and a pilot examination was administered at the 18th Annual National Symposium in New York City.

Janel Parker

• The definition of nephrology nursing and the components of a practice base for nephrology nursing were identified.
• The Scope of Practice for Nephrology Nursing was published.
• The Core Curriculum for Nephrology Nursing, First Edition, was published.
• The position of ANNA Education Director was established.
• The First Clinical Concerns in Nephrology Meetings were held in Chicago and San Diego.
• The Third International Nephrology Nursing Workshop and the first hosted in the United States was held in conjunction with the 18th National Symposium in New York City.
• The American Society for Artificial and Internal Organs (ASAIO) met in conjunction with the 18th National Symposium in New York City.
• The Renal Coalition was formed consisting of ANNA, the National Association of Patients on Hemodialysis and Transplantation (NAPHT), the Renal Physicians Association (RPA), the National Dialysis Association (NDA), and the National Renal Administrators' Association (NRAA).

Looking Back: 1987-1988
Gail Wick
President

The Year in Review

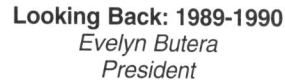

• In December 1987, ANNA officially became a $1 million organization!
• The Standards of Clinical Practice for Nephrology Nursing were revised by the Clinical Practice Committee and were available for purchase.
• The ANNA Career Guide was revised to promote the specialty practice and address the increasing shortage of nephrology nurses.
• Two major projects were launched: a head nurse survey and a pilot research project addressing nephrology care in the United States.

Gail Wick

• The Long Range Planning Committee began the important, challenging, and timely task of evaluating the direction, structure, and future priorities of ANNA.

• A guide to help chapters develop and implement certification review courses was produced, while two national certification review courses were conducted.
• The association also promoted the newly developed certification exam offered by the NNCB. The exam was offered three times during the year and twice at the 18th National Symposium.
• The Association, under President Gail Wick, reached a long sought-after goal of surpassing the 4,000-membership mark!
• A highly successful 18th National Symposium was held in Reno, Nevada.

Looking Back: 1989-1990
Patricia Jordan
President

The Year in Review

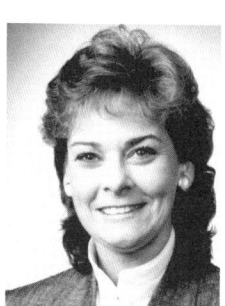

• A nursing shortage survey was conducted and published in the *ANNA Journal*.
• The ANNA staffing survey was distributed to ESRD facilities with the HCFA Facility Report.
• The Quality Assurance Manual for Nephrology Nurses was developed.
• The association established a legislative office in Washington, DC.
• A bylaws change extended the term of office for regional vice presidents from 1 to 2 years, eliminated the regional secretary position, and estab-

Patricia Jordan

lished the positions of chapters coordinator and chapters coordinator-elect.
• ANNA laid the groundwork for a research-based nephrology nursing practice by establishing a standing Research Committee.
• The Association continued to support certification in nephrology nursing as the number of nurses earning the CNN credential grew to more than 600.
• Membership surpassed 5,000 and chapters grew to 70 under President Patricia S. Jordan.
• The association celebrated its 20th anniversary with a successful National Symposium in Dallas that attracted 1,355 registrants.

Looking Back: 1989-1990
Evelyn Butera
President

The Year in Review

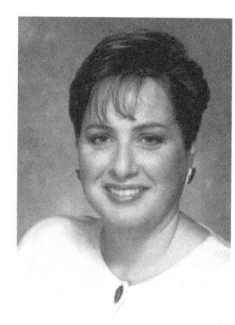

• A 5-year strategic plan for the association was developed by the Strategic Planning Task Force in Philadelphia.
• The ANNA Staffing Mix Survey was distributed nationally by the ESRD Networks.
• The ANNA Board of Directors approved the development of a Patient Classification System.
• A study was approved to validate ANNA's Standards of Clinical Practice.
• The Nephrology Nursing Clinical Ladder Program was published.

Evelyn Butera

• ANNA President Evelyn Butera was appointed chairperson of the National Federation For Specialty Nursing Organization's

(NFSNO) Health Policy Committee.
- The association's membership increased 12% to 5,745 while chapters grew to an all-time high of 70!
- ANNA received 6-year reaccreditation as a provider and approver of Continuing Education by the American Nurses' Association Board of Accreditation.
- ANNA participated as a member of HCFA's Medical Review Indicators Committee.
- The first ANNA-sponsored research grants were awarded at the 21st National Symposium in Washington, DC.

Looking Back: 1990-1991
Sally Burrows-Hudson
President

The Year in Review

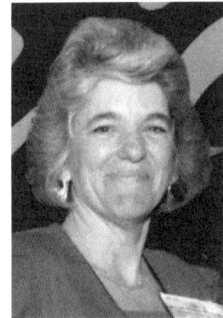

- The Association's membership grew to 6,400 members under President Sally Burrows-Hudson.
- ANNA initiated and sought Congressional approval for the Nephrology Nursing Demonstration Project.
- ANNA chaired the NFSNO Health Policy Committee.
- The Association approved development of a Conceptual Model for Nephrology Nursing.

Sally Burrows-Hudson

- The first ANNA audio-teleconference educational programs were conducted.
- The "For Chapters Only" leadership development program was created.
- ANNA established positions on HIV, the world-wide nursing shortage, substance abuse, transplant of living related organs, staff-assisted home hemodialysis, and use of EPO.
- A standardized analysis of State Nurse Practice Acts was begun.
- The successful 22nd National Symposium was held in San Francisco in April 1991 with more than 1,000 members in attendance.

Looking Back: 1991-1992
Marilyn Neff
President

The Year in Review

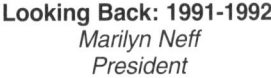

- The Board of Directors approved bylaws changes for the NNCB to allow for improved continuity of leadership on the Board, and to require that all directors hold a minimum of a BSN degree.
- Two new research grants were approved to encourage collaboration between experienced and novice investigators.
- The Conceptual Model Task Force met twice and conducted a survey to begin identifying a study model for nephrology nursing.

Marilyn Neff

- A first time, 3-day national Legislative Workshop was held in February 1992 to increase chapter leaders' knowledge about the legislative and regulatory processes.

- ANNA maintained an active role in multiple organizations, including the Renal Coalition, the NFSNO, AAMI, and NOLF.
- ANNA endorsed position statements developed by other nursing organizations on the management of analgesia by catheter techniques and the management of patients receiving IV conscious sedation for short-term therapeutic, diagnostic, or surgical procedures.
- Three successful workshops for chapter leaders were held in conjunction with the Fall 1991 Clinical Concerns Meetings and the January 1992 Management/Education Seminar.
- Membership grew to more than 7,500 under President Marilyn Neff.
- American Nurses Association President Lucille Joel served as the keynote speaker for ANNA's 23rd National Symposium in Chicago.

Looking Back: 1992-1993
Barbara Bednar
President

The Year in Review

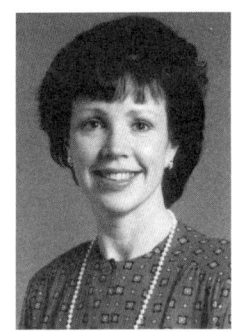

- ANNA finalized an agreement with Mecon Associates to design and develop a Patient Classification System (PCS) for chronic hemodialysis patients.
- The Board formally endorsed the clinical practice guideline developed by AHCPR, "Urinary Incontinence in the Adult."
- In October, the Board approved the revision of the Standards of Clinical Practice for Nephrology Nursing to reflect current technology.

Barbara Bednar

- The Board approved the formation of a task force to investigate the feasibility of ANNA developing a clinical practice guideline with funding from AHCPR or another agency.
- In November 1992, written testimony from the ANNA and NNCB Joint Task Force on Advanced Practice was presented at federal hearings on credentialing in advance nursing practice.
- The Board approved the formation of the Nephrology Nursing Needs Assessment Task Force in July 1992.
- "For Leaders Only" Workshops were held in conjunction with the Fall 1992 Clinical Concerns Meetings.
- Recognizing the importance of certification for nephrology nurses, the Board approved a task force to assess the feasibility of a chapter-sharing Certification Review Course.
- Membership reached 8,200 under President Barbara Bednar, and attendance at the 24th Annual Symposium in Orlando reached nearly 2,000!

Looking Back: 1993-1994
Terran Warren Sims
President

The Year in Review

- The association celebrated its 25th anniversary of service to the nephrology nursing community.
- Involvement in the national health care reform movement was very strong, including representation at the National Nursing Summit on Health Care Reform.
- ANNA released a Patient Classification System.
- The association provided representation for the First UNOS/DOT Public Forum on Transplantation.
- ANNA initiated revisions and expansions of the Quality Assurance Guide for Nephrology Nursing and the Core Curriculum for Nephrology Nursing.
- The association conducted a 2-day Strategic Planning Think Tank in Philadelphia and a 2-day "Team Think" session with ANNA committees in Dallas.
- The association's 25th Anniversary National Symposium was held in Dallas.
- Membership grew to an all-time high of over 9,000 under President Terran Warren Sims while chapters expanded to more than 100!

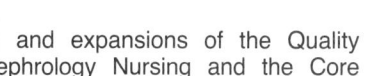
Terran Warren Sims

Looking Back: 1994-1995
Karen E. Schardin
President

The Year in Review

- The ground breaking Consensus Development Conference focused on the role of the nephrology nurse. ANNA was invited to share the results of this conference with NFSNO.
- The first formal 3-year ANNA educational plan was created.
- Several key publications – Continuous Quality Improvement: From Concept to Reality; ANNA's Scope of Practice; and The Core Curriculum for Nephrology Nursing – contributed to the cornerstone of nephrology nursing practice.
- In collaboration with AADE, a Diabetes Monograph was completed.
- Facing potential cuts in the entitlement program, ANNA met with AAKP to discuss the future health care for ESRD patients and later testified before the House Ways and Means Committee regarding the impact of possible cuts.
- ANNA was represented on the HCFA Core Indicators Workgroup and the Renal Quality Census Committee.
- The 26th National Symposium was held in Philadelphia, the site of ANNA's first independent meeting, and marked the first year that the ANNA meeting was held in a convention center.
- Membership reached 9727, an all-time high under President Karen E. Schardin.

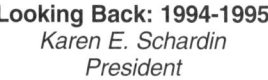
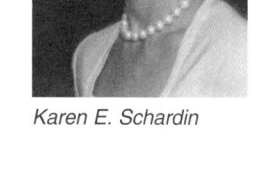
Karen E. Schardin

Looking Back: 1995-1996
Nancy Gallagher
President

The Year in Review

- A national 800 number for association leaders was established to strengthen and enhance the lines of communication.
- The position of ANNA Research Consultant was created, in part, to further develop a plan toward research-based nursing practice and to assist in integrating research and clinical practice in the workplace.
- A Task Force completed the groundwork of taking the scope of legislative activities into state government to promote and support the role of the registered nurse in the delivery of patient care.
- An ANNA-sponsored preconference workshop was presented at the Clinical Concerns Meetings, where participants linked their professional issues to association goals.
- An Advanced Practice SIG, chaired by Christine Chmielewski, was formed to address the needs of that group and provide a forum for dialogue.
- The Administrative SIG participated in the program development for the Management/Education Seminar to address the educational needs of both the new and experienced manager.
- ANNA membership grew to more than 10,500 members under President Nancy Gallagher.
- A successful 27th National Symposium, with more than 1,000 registrants, was held in Anaheim, CA.

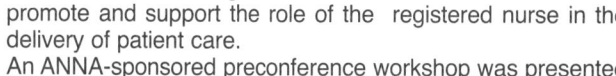
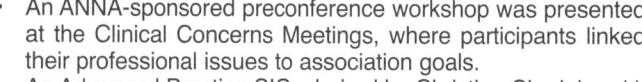
Nancy Gallagher

Looking Back: 1996-1997
Christy Price
President

The Year in Review

- ANNA reviewed and commented on the DOQI guidelines with nephrology nurses' input clearly heard by the committees.
- The Association responded to the PEW Health Professions Commission report on regulation and licensure of all health professionals.
- A work group met with the RPA to explore consensus and a possible position statement on collaborative practice arrangements between nephrologists and nephrology advanced practice nurses.
- ANNA developed and endorsed a joint position statement with NANT on the use of unlicensed assistive personnel in dialysis.
- The Association responded to ANA's survey on standards for specialty nursing practice and sent a representative to participate in ANA's work group for nursing standards.
- Chris Chmielewski was appointed as Project Director to develop a curriculum for Orientation to the Specialty.
- The ANNA Advance Practice Nursing Conference was held.
- ANNA secured a joint research award from Sigma Theta Tau for investigation of clinical practice outcomes related to treating chronic illness.

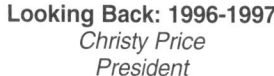
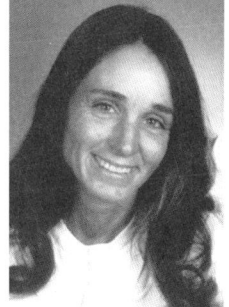
Christy Price

- Jeannette Chambers was appointed as ANNA's representative to the ANA/AACN Creative Solutions Initiatives.
- More than 1,200 nephrology nurses attended the 28th National Symposium in Minneapolis while ANNA membership reached an all-time high of 10,500.

Looking Back: 1997-1998
Karen C. Robbins
President

The Year in Review

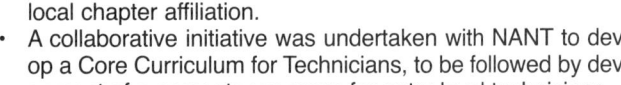

- Contemporary Nephrology Nursing, ANNA's comprehensive textbook for nephrology nursing, was published.
- The Management/Education Seminar and Advanced Practice Seminar were combined for a very successful meeting.
- A consultant for Distance Learning/ On-Line Services was appointed.
- Chapter choice was implemented to allow individual members to select local chapter affiliation.

Karen C. Robbins

- A collaborative initiative was undertaken with NANT to develop a Core Curriculum for Technicians, to be followed by development of a competency exam for entry level technicians.
- Collaborative efforts were undertaken with the RPA and the ASN for a position statement, "The RPA/ASN/ANNA Joint Position Statement on Collaboration Between Nephrologists and Advanced Practice Nurses."
- ANNA participated in the ANA/AACN Best Practices Network as a charter member.
- ANNA mourned the passing of long-time Executive Director Ron Brady.
- Membership exceeded 11,000 under President Karen C. Robbins while a successful 29th National Symposium was held in San Antonio, TX.

Looking Back: 1998-1999
Carolyn E. Latham
President

The Year in Review

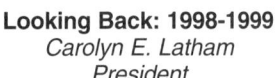

- The Standards and Guidelines of Clinical Practice for Nephrology Nursing were revised.
- The Scope of Advanced Practice in Nephrology Nursing was developed.
- ANNA collaborated with other renal-related organizations (RPA, ASN, NKF, HCFA, Renal Coalition) on numerous projects.
- The Leadership '99 Meeting was held for incoming volunteer leaders on local, regional, and national levels.

Carolyn E. Latham

- A comprehensive Association Assessment was conducted, including operational, business and financial evaluations and recommendations.
- The following positions were approved: A full-time Executive Director, combined Clinical Practice and Research Consultant, Assistant Director of Professional Development, and Leadership Development Consultant.
- The Association renewed its successful relationship with Jannetti, Inc.

- The following project directors were named: Dr. Nancy Hoffart for ANNA's 1999 Research Project; Dr. Larry Lancaster for the revision of the Core Curriculum for Nephrology Nursing; and Leanne Dekker for Essentials for Nephrology Nursing Practice.
- Eileen Meier was appointed Legislative Consultant while ANNA's Legislative Services were restructured.
- The Clinical Practice Committee formed two subcommittees: Disaster Management and Ethics.
- The *ANNA Journal* published a monograph on end-of-life issues.
- A successful 30th Anniversary National Symposium was celebrated in Baltimore.

Looking Back: 1999-2000
Pat Weiskittel
President

The Year in Review

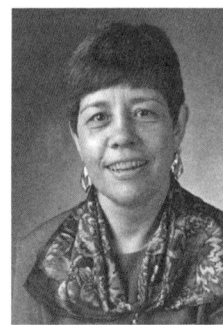

- The newly published Standards and Guidelines of Clinical Practice for Nephrology Nursing, edited by Sally Burrows-Hudson, were distributed to all ANNA chapters to promote their use.
- The Professional Practice Committee and the ANNA Board of Directors reviewed and endorsed the RPA/ASN Clinical Practice Guideline on shared decision-making in the initiation and withdrawal of renal replacement therapies.

Pat Weiskittel

- ANNA and the National Association of Nephrology Technicians and Technologists (NANT) Task Force completed the second phase toward administering a pilot competency test for patient care technicians.
- Dr. Charlotte Thomas-Hawkins joined ANNA as the clinical practice/research consultant and was instrumental in coordinating project development in the areas of research and clinical practice.
- Together with colleagues in the Renal Coalition, ANNA supported an increase in the composite rate and provided testimony at a HCFA town hall meeting regarding current issues and problems with the ESRD Networks.
- The Awards Committee, chaired by Kitty Thomas, received and processed 118 applications from 49 applicants for scholarship/fellowship awards and achievement awards. Over $100,000 in grants and awards were made available to ANNA members.
- Membership exceeded 11,500 under President Pat Weiskittel.
- The 31st National Symposium, held at the Opryland Hotel in Nashville, attracted nearly 1,500 registrants as well as more than 200 exhibitors from around the country.

Looking Back: 2000-2001
Jean Nardini
President

The Year in Review

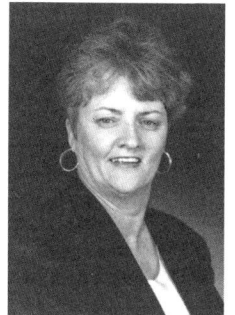

- Twenty two (22) ANNA leaders, executive staff, and industry and professional organization representatives helped to develop the Association's 2000-2001 Strategic Plan during a think tank session in Philadelphia.
- Dr. Nancy Hoffart completed the ANNA research project entitled "An Exploration of Nephrology Nursing Practice and Dialysis Patient Outcomes" and presented her findings at the National Symposium in Las Vegas.

Jean Nardini

- The Awards Committee, chaired by Cynthia Frazier, saw a 24% increase in applications for scholarship/fellowship awards and achievement awards. Once again, over $100,000 in grants and awards were made available to ANNA members.
- The Core Curriculum for Nephrology Nursing, Fourth Edition, edited by Dr. Larry E. Lancaster, was published in April 2001.
- The Advanced Practice SIG task force developed the first draft of the ANNA APN Standards of Care and Professional Performance.
- ANNA membership exceeded 12,000 under President Jean Nardini.
- The 32nd National Symposium, held at the MGM Grand Hotel in Las Vegas, attracted a record attendance of about 2,300 paid registrants and more than 250 exhibit booths.

Looking Back: 2001-2002
Mary Ann Gould
President

The Year in Review

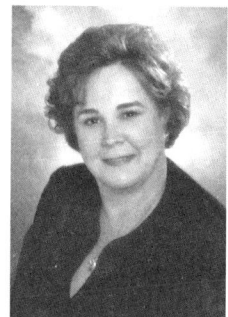

- ANNA worked with the Renal Physicians Association to develop a Practice Guideline for Chronic Renal Insufficiency.
- ANNA received a significant educational grant for development of a three-part series, Delaying and Preparing for Renal Disease Progression, edited by Charlotte Szromba.
- Mike Cunningham was appointed ANNA's Executive Director while all association functions were consolidated at the National Office in Pitman, NJ.

Mary Ann Gould

- *Nephrology Nursing Journal* began its own Web site at nephrologynursingjournal.net, and featured complete abstracts of articles and full text of all departments.
- The Advanced Practice SIG task force published the ANNA APN Standards of Care and Professional Performance.
- ANNA collaborated with the National Kidney Foundation Singapore to successfully participate in NephroAsia 2001, an international renal health care congress.
- ANNA membership exceeded 12,000 members under President Mary Ann Gould while there were a total of 108 chapters.
- The 33rd National Symposium, held at the Walt Disney World Dolphin Hotel in Orlando, attracted an attendance of about 1,600 paid registrants and more than 250 exhibit booths.

Looking Back: 2002-2003
Gail Wick
President

The Year in Review

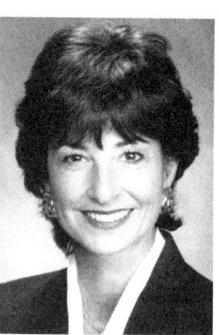

- Beth Ulrich, EdD, RN, CHE, was appointed as the fifth Editor of *Nephrology Nursing Journal* in June 2002.
- ANNA hosted a landmark meeting of the renal community, "Nephrology Nursing Shortage and Solutions: An Invitational Summit," in March 2003 in Baltimore.
- Sally Russell, MN, RN, was appointed as ANNA's Director of Educational Services in late 2002.

Gail Wick

- Under the authorship of Nancy Syzmanski, Nancy Sharp, and Kathleen Smith, ANNA published the well-received ESRD Briefing Book for State and Federal Policymakers.
- The Hemodialysis, Peritoneal Dialysis and Pediatrics SIGs developed and distributed a series of fact sheets that provided essential information on the care of adults and children.
- The Work Environment Survey (WES), a first of its kind survey of staff nurses in outpatient dialysis settings, was published and will allow ANNA to more accurately advocate for nephrology nurses in that setting.
- The ANNA Strategic Plan was revised, simplified and operationalized at all levels of the organization. Strategic actions for 2003-2005 were reached by consensus of the 2002-2003 and 2003-2004 ANNA boards.
- Four new position papers were added and all remaining statements were revised, allowing ANNA to communicate the position of nephrology nursing on a number of important issues while facilitating our role in the public policy arena.
- The 34th National Symposium, held in Chicago, proved to be another highly successful educational and networking event!

Looking Back: 2003-2004
Caroline Counts
President

The Year in Review

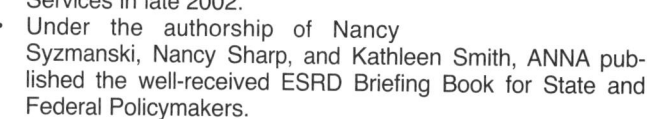
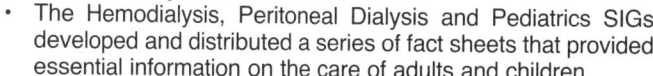

- ANNA produced the Discover Nephrology Nursing brochure, which was designed to attract both student nurses and registered nurses to nephrology, and to attract nephrology nurses who are not members of ANNA to join the Association.
- The Association joined Kidney Care Partners (KCP), a coalition of kidney disease organizations representing professionals, providers, pharmaceutical manufacturers, and patient support organizations.

Caroline Counts

- ANNA chose to honor Janel Parker, one of its greatest leaders and visionaries following her untimely and accidental death on August 26, 2003. A Career Mobility Scholarship was renamed the Janel Parker Career Mobility Scholarship.
- ANNA held its first ESRD Education Day on August 15, 2003, under the leadership and guidance of ANNA Legislative Consultant Nancy Sharp.
- ANNA's Fall Meeting in Savannah, GA broke attendance records for a Fall program with 425 registrants and 35

exhibitors. The Fall 2003 and Winter 2004 Audio-Confererences also set new records with chapters hosting a combined 193 sites and 1550 participants!

- The Association subscribed to a Web-based political communications service called CapWiz that allowed ANNA members to gain more political information and to easily write letters to their legislators with just a few clicks of the mouse!
- ANNA delivered its biweekly "RenalWEB E-News" and monthly "ANNA E-News" to members via email. Member contacts throughout the past 12 months through mail and email totaled more than 500,000!
- With Suzann VanBuskirk at the helm, ANNA continued the work of the Nephrology Nursing Shortage and Solutions: An Invitational Summit as four task forces worked on the outcomes of the Summit.
- ANNA was awarded a $13,000 Nurse Competence in Aging Grant by the American Nurses Association (ANA). The funds will be used over 2 years to enhance the education of nurses in caring for older adults.
- The 35th National Symposium, held in Washington, DC, proved to be another highly successful educational and networking event!

Looking Back: 2004-2005
Lesley C. Dinwiddie
President

The Year in Review

- ANNA prepared written responses to CMS to the long-awaited Conditions for Coverage (CfC), the notice on proposed rule making for the Medicare Modernization Act, and the rule on erythropoeitin reimbursement.
- The Association continued to monitor legislative and regulatory activities and published in *Nephrology Nursing Journal* a state-specific table detailing state laws affecting the practice of nephrology nursing complete with state Boards of Nursing Web site addresses.

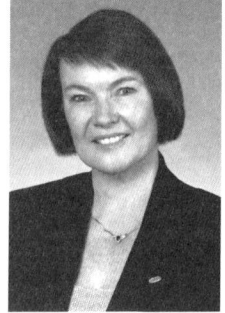
Lesley C. Dinwiddie

- The Nephrology Nursing Standards of Practice and Guidelines for Care were revised and published along with the revised Scope of Practice.
- ANNA unveiled an all-new Association Web site on October 1, 2004 that was much more efficient and comprehensive with the content presented to members. Included on the new site were archived past issues of ANNA's efficient communication tool, E-News.
- A new clinical SIG was approved for those members whose special interest is CKD.
- ANNA successfully nominated a representative to the ESRD Demonstration Project Advisory Board.
- ANNA held its very successful Second Annual ESRD Education Day on August 13, 2004, and voted to expand the activity to a full week beginning in 2005.
- The *Nephrology Nursing Journal* published A Monograph on Peritoneal Dialysis Topics in its September-October 2004 issue with copies mailed to the 500 largest PD units in the country.
- The Association continued its partnership with Kidney Care Partners (KCP) and secured a seat on the Operations Committee.
- ANNA's All Region Executive Committee created a program for chapters called CE on Wheels.
- The Association joined ANA as an organizational affiliate member.
- ANNA's Fall Meeting in New Orleans broke attendance records for a Fall program with 500 registrants and 40 exhibitors.
- The 36th National Symposium, held in Las Vegas, proved to be another highly successful educational and networking event with more than 1800 registrants in attendance!
- Collaboration and Outreach were the hallmarks of ANNA's 2004-2005!

Summary
continued from page 38

The history of nephrology nursing is not as old as nephrology itself; but nephrology nursing has been closely intertwined with the more recent developments and improvements in renal care. Nurses have played key roles in every aspect of nephrology. While the evolutionary process continues as new discoveries continue, the specialty of nephrology nursing continues to grow and develop.

References

Albers, J. (1989). Reflections on the first dialysis nurse training program. *ANNA Journal, 16*, 3, 230-231.

American Association for the History of Nursing, Inc. (2001). *Position paper nursing history in the curriculum: Preparing nurses for the 21st century.* On-line:Author. Available: http://www.aahn.org/position.html

Antonello, A., Bonfante, L., Bordin, V., Calò, L., Favaro, S., Rippa-Bonati, M., & D'Angelo, A. (1997). The bursa of Hieronymus Fabrici d'Acquapendente: Past and present of an anatomical structure. *American Journal of Nephrology, 17*, 248-251.

Blagg, C.R. (2003). The Northwest Kidney Centers has carried the ban-ner for home hemodialysis for four decades. *Contemporary Dialysis & Nephrology, 24*(2), 22-23.

Blagg, C.R. (2004). Tribute to Belding Scribner, MD: The Scribner shunt. *Hemodialysis International, 8*(1), 4-5.

Chesney, R.W. (2002). The development of pediatric nephrology. *Pediatric Research 52*(5), 770–777.

Coleman, B.K., & Merrill, J.P. (1952). The artificial kidney. *American Journal of Nursing, 52*, 327–329.

Dardioti, V., Angelopoulos, N., & Hadjiconstantinou, V. (1997). Renal diseases in the Hippocratic era. *American Journal of Nephrology, 17*, 214-216.

DeBroe, M.E., Sacrè, D., Snelders, E.D., & De Weerdt, D.L. (1997). The Flemish anatomist Andreas Vesalius (1514–1564) and the kidney. *American Journal of Nephrology, 17*, 252-260.

Diaz-Buxo, J.A. (1995). Technology of peritoneal dialysis. In H.R. Jacobson, G.E. Striker, & S. Klahr (Eds.), *The principles and practice of nephrology* (p. 690). St. Louis: Mosby.

Diaz-Buxo, J.A. (2001). Automated peritoneal dialysis. In S.G. Massry & R.J. Glassock (Eds.), *Massry & Glassock's textbook of nephrology* (4th ed, p. 1549). Philadelphia: Lippincott Williams & Wilkins.

Eftychiadis, A.C. (1997). Diseases in the Byzantine world with special emphasis on the nephropathies. *American Journal of Nephrology, 17*, 217-221.

Eknoyan, G. (2002). Emergence of the concept of acute renal failure. *American Journal of Nephrology, 22*, 225-230.

Fresenius. (2001). *Dialysis – History of dialysis.* Author: On-line. Available: http://www.fresenius.de/e/5/e_05_1_3.html

Fulton, B.J., & Cameron, E. (1989). Perspectives on our beginnings: 1962 – 1979. *ANNA Journal, 16*(3), 201–203.

George, C.R.P. (2002). Development of the idea of chronic renal failure. *American Journal of Nephrology, 22,* 231-239.

Gottschalk, C.W., & Fellner, S.K. (1997). History of the science of dialysis. *American Journal of Nephrology, 17,* 289-298.

Hoffart, N. (1989a). Nephrology nursing 1915-1970: A historical study of the integration of technology and care. *ANNA Journal, 16*(3), 169-178.

Hoffart, N. (1989b). A professional organization for nephrology nurses. *ANNA Journal, 16*(3), 197-199.

International Society for Peritoneal Dialysis. (n.d.). *The emergence of peritoneal dialysis.* On-Line: Author. Available: http://www.ispd.org/history/genesis.php3

McBride, P. (1989). Industry's contribution to the development of renal care. *ANNA Journal, 16*(3), 217-226.

Mezzogiorno, A. & Mezzogiorno, V. (1997). Marcello Malpighi (1628 – 1694). *American Journal of Nephrology, 17,* 269-273.

Murray, J.E. (1990). *Nobel lecture.* Available: http://www.nobel.se/medicine/laureates/1900/murray-lecture.html

Novartis Transplant. (n.d.). *Milestones in transplantation.* On-Line: Author. Available: http://www.novartis-transplant.com/medpro/symposia/milestones_in_TX.html

Renal Unit of the Royal Infirmary of Edinburgh. (2001). On-Line: Author. Available: http://renux.dmed.ed.ac.uk/EdREN/Unitbits/historyweb/transplant.html

Rettig, R.A. (1991). *Origins of the Medicare kidney disease entitlement: The Social Security amendments of 1972.* Available: http://books.nap.edu/books/0309044863/html/index.html (pp. 176-214).

Richet, G. (1997). Hamburger's achievement with early renal transplants. *American Journal of Nephrology, 17,* 315-317.

Schwab, S.J., & Butterly, D.W. (2001). Vascular access for hemodialysis. In S.G. Massry & R.J. Glassock (Eds.), *Massry & Glassock's textbook of nephrology* (4th ed., p. 1482). Philadelphia: Lippincott Williams & Wilkins.

Sharp, N. (2004). *Nephrology nurses: Pioneers then, futurists now.* Paper presented at the ANNA 35th National Symposium. Washington, DC.

The Transplant Network. (n.d.). *The history of transplantation.* On-line. Available: http://www.thetransplantnetwork.com/history_of_transplantation.htm

University of Washington. (1996). *Pioneers in kidney dialysis: From the Scribner shunt and the Mini-II to the "One-Button Machine."* On-line. Available: http://www.washington.edu/research/pathbreakers/1960c.html

Warren, H. (1989). Changes in peritoneal dialysis nursing. *ANNA Journal, 16*(3), 237-241.

- Classic reasons to look at the past are either to avoid repeating it or to learn from previous experience. Today's nephrology nurse will understand the tremendous work that was accomplished by nurses who led the crusade for improved health care for persons with kidney disease.

- Hippocrates is described by some as the father of clinical nephrology, not just the father of medicine. Hippocratic medicine looked for natural causes for diseases, not divine intervention, as was the prevailing belief at the time.

- The Renaissance was a period of scientific inquiry as the anatomy of the kidney continued to be studied and described. Men such as Andreas Vesalius (1514 – 1564) and Bartholomeo Eustachio (about 1510 – 1574) described in excellent fashion the normal organs. This led the way for others to be able to describe pathological states (George, 2002).

- Giovanni Battista Morgagni (1682 – 1771) is the acknowledged father of pathological anatomy. He first proposed a classification of ischuria into four categories: ischuria vesicalis, ischuria ureterica, ischuria urethralis, and ischuria renalis. The latter class was essential for the kidney to become a taxon around which the causes of ischuria due to kidney injury or disease could be grouped, studied, and described (Eknoyan, 2002).

- By 1877, the enigma of renal disease was resolved. Fatal outcomes were dependent upon toxic levels of urea. By 1900, the idea of uremia was well established, yet it was more qualitative than quantitative. Efforts were put into developing tests of renal function. The earliest methods left a lot to be desired

- Thomas Graham (1805 – 1869) was a Scotsman who is considered to be the father of modern dialysis. He discovered the laws that govern the diffusion of gases, now known as Graham's law... Over 50 years later, John J. Abel, Leonard Rowntree, and B.B. Turner were the first to apply the principle of diffusion to actually remove substances from the blood of living animals. In 1914, they published two papers that gave more details about their apparatus that they called an artificial kidney.

- In the small town of Kampen, Kolff convinced the Berk Enamel Company that he needed their assistance. With the help of engineer Hendrik Berk, the first rotating artificial kidney was designed and built. It was a mechanically sound piece of equipment and demonstrated that a dialysis machine could overcome the problems of renal failure. A rotating drum that was covered with cellophane tubing and partially submerged in a tank of dialysis fluid was the original design (Gottschalk & Fellner, 1997; McBride, 1989).

- On March 9, 1960, the first Scribner shunt was implanted in the arm of a Boeing machinist, Clyde Shields (Schwab & Butterfly, 2001; University of Washington, 1996). David Dillard, a pediatric heart surgeon, performed the surgery (Blagg, 2004). Shields lived for 11 years with hemodialysis and died in 1971 from a heart attack (Fresenius, 2001).

- It was during the Korean War that Paul Doolan, with the help of William Murphy, developed a catheter for long-term use. They worked at the Naval Hospital in San Francisco. The polyethylene catheter was flexible and contained a number of grooved segments to prevent the blockage of drain holes and maximize drainage. The consideration of using peritoneal dialysis in a chronic situation emerged.

- Automated peritoneal dialysis became a term used to describe all modalities of peritoneal dialysis that used a mechanical device to perform the dialysis (Diaz-Buxo, 2001). Automated peritoneal dialysis dates back to the 1960s, when Scribner invited Fred Boen to come to Seattle to set up a chronic home peritoneal dialysis program.

- Throughout history the possibility of transplanting organs and tissues from one body to another has been intriguing. There are references dating back to the 15th century in historical medical literature regarding attempted blood transfusions and the transplantation of teeth. As far back as 1880, there were attempts at corneal and skin transplants. These early efforts were usually unsuccessful. It was not until the 20th century that transplantation offered real hope for renewed health and life (Transplant Network, n.d.).

- The early dialysis nurse faced challenges in several areas, including making the patient comfortable. The equipment itself was large, cumbersome, and frightening... Nursing tasks included back rubs, repositioning, explaining the procedure, offering reassurance, and easing the patient's last hours or days in cases of death... The nurse was also responsible for trying to protect the patient from all of this activity (Hoffart, 1989a).

- Following the 1969 ASAIO meeting in Atlantic City, a core group of about 50 nurses came together and formed the American Association for Nephrology Nurses (AANN). This core group had seen the need to ensure the continuation of nephrology nursing conferences. The organization's purpose was to promote knowledge in this field. The first officers were Bernice Hinckley, president; Barbara Fulton, vice president; and, JoAnn Albers, secretary. Full membership was open only to RNs (Hoffart, 1989b).

ANNP602

The Evolution of Nephrology and Nephrology Nursing

Caroline S. Counts, MSN, RN, CNN

Contemporary Nephrology Nursing: Principles and Practice contains 39 chapters of educational content. Individual learners may apply for continuing nursing education credit by reading a chapter and completing the Continuing Education Evaluation Form for that chapter. Learners may apply for continuing education credit for any or all chapters.

Please photocopy this page and return to ANNA.
COMPLETE THE FOLLOWING:

Name: _____

Address:_____

City:_____ State: _____ Zip: _____

E-mail: _____

Preferred telephone: ☐ Home   ☐ Work: _____

State where licensed and license number (optional): _____

CE application fees are based upon the number of contact hours provided by the individual chapter. CE fees per contact hour for ANNA members are as follows: 1.0-1.9 - $15; 2.0-2.9 - $20; 3.0-3.9 - $25; 4.0 and higher - $30. Fees for nonmembers are $10 higher.

ANNA Member: ☐ Yes   ☐ No   Member # (if available) _____

☐ Checked Enclosed   ☐ American Express   ☐ Visa   ☐ MasterCard

Total Amount Submitted: _____

Credit Card Number: _____ Exp. Date: _____

Name as it appears on the card: _____

CE Evaluation Form
To receive continuing education credit for individual study after reading the chapter
1. Photocopy this form. (You may also download this form from ANNA's Web site, **www.annanurse.org.**)
2. Mail the completed form with payment (check) or credit card information to American Nephrology Nurses' Association, East Holly Avenue, Box 56, Pitman, NJ 08071-0056.
3. You will receive your CE certificate from ANNA in 4 to 6 weeks.

Test returns must be postmarked by **December 31, 2010.**

CE Application Fee
ANNA Member $20.00
Nonmember $30.00

EVALUATION FORM

1. I verify that I have read this chapter and completed this education activity. Date: _____

   _____
   Signature

2. What would be different in your practice if you applied what you learned from this activity? *(Please use additional sheet of paper if necessary.)*

   _____
   _____
   _____
   _____
   _____
   _____
   _____
   _____
   _____
   _____
   _____
   _____

Evaluation	Strongly disagree				Strongly agree
3. The activity met the stated objectives.					
a. Outline the history of nephrology.	1	2	3	4	5
b. Briefly describe the progression of treatments available for renal failure.	1	2	3	4	5
c. Summarize the development of nephrology nursing as a specialty practice.	1	2	3	4	5
4. The content was current and relevant.	1	2	3	4	5
5. The content was presented clearly.	1	2	3	4	5
6. The content was covered adequately.	1	2	3	4	5
7. Rate your ability to apply the learning obtained from this activity to practice.	1	2	3	4	5

Comments _____

_____

8. Time required to read the chapter and complete this form: _____ minutes.

This educational activity has been provided by the American Nephrology Nurses' Association (ANNA) for 2.5 contact hours. ANNA is accredited as a provider of continuing nursing education (CNE) by the American Nurses Credentialing Center's Commission on Accreditation (ANCC-COA). ANNA is an approved provider of continuing education by the California Board of Registered Nursing, CEP 0910.

Chronic Illness Management and Outcomes: A Theory-Based Approach

Charlotte Thomas-Hawkins, PhD, RN

Chapter Contents

Chronic Illness Management and Outcomes: A Theory-Based Approach

Chapter 3

Charlotte Thomas-Hawkins, PhD, RN

End-stage renal disease (ESRD) is a condition that requires individuals who are affected by this illness to manage a complex treatment regimen. Historically, a dialysis double bind has been described for the majority of individuals with ESRD who receive chronic dialysis treatments (Alexander, 1976). These individuals are expected to be self-directed and independent in managing their illness while at the same time acknowledging dependence on dialysis. On the other hand, while transplantation removes many of the problems associated with dialysis, individuals who have received a kidney transplant are expected to manage and adhere to complex and lifelong regimens of immunosuppressant therapy with the possibility of unpleasant side effects; these individuals also are faced with the ubiquitous threat of rejection. The management of a complex chronic illness like ESRD is a challenge for individuals and families affected by this condition. The purpose of this chapter is to present a theoretical framework for understanding and managing chronic illness from the perspective of the individual with ESRD. This chapter will use the Common-Sense Model of Self-Regulation of Health and Illness (CSM) as a guiding theoretical framework for chronic illness self-management.

Chronic Illness: An Overview

Chronic illness in the United States (U.S.) is a common problem. More than 90 million Americans live with chronic illnesses, and 25 million have major limitations in activities of daily living due to their chronic conditions (Centers for Disease Control and Prevention [CDC], 2003). Approximately 80% of all persons over 65 years of age have at least one chronic condition, and 50% of older individuals have at least two chronic illnesses (CDC, 2004). Chronic diseases account for 70% of all deaths in the U.S., and the medical care costs for chronically ill individuals comprise more than 75% of U.S. health care costs (CDC, 2003). The prevalence of chronic conditions in individuals with ESRD is very similar to the occurrence of chronic conditions in the general U.S. population. For example, data from the United States Renal Data Systems (USRDS) (2003) indicate that 57% of individuals who begin a renal replacement therapy have diabetes, and 50% have cardiovascular disease. USRDS data also reveal that an increasing number of individuals are initiating treatment for ESRD with a cancer diagnosis. These data emphasize the complexity of the population receiving treatment for ESRD and underscore the need for nurses to effectively help these individuals understand and manage their illness and its treatment.

A generally accepted definition of chronic illness is not available. However, Verbrugge and Patrick (1995) provide a definition of chronic illness that appears broad enough to encompass most descriptions of the concept. They define chronic conditions as "long-term diseases, injuries with long sequelae, and enduring structural, sensory, and communication abnormalities. They are physical and mental (cognitive or emotional) in nature, their onset time ranges from before birth to late in life. Their defining aspect is duration. Once they are past certain symptomatic or diagnostic thresholds, chronic conditions are essentially features for the rest of life. Medical and personal regimens can sometimes control but can rarely cure them" (p. 173). Characteristics of most chronic illnesses are consistent with this definition and include (1) symptoms that interfere with normal activities and routines; (2) a need for palliation rather than cure; (3) stable phases that are often punctuated with episodic flares or complications; and (4) treatment interventions that alleviate the symptoms and long-term effects of the disease but also contribute substantially to the disruption of routine daily activities and patterns of living (Reif, 1975).

For the individual, being chronically ill entails ongoing involvement with health professionals in a health care system. However, this involvement is limited for most chronically ill individuals. Research findings have indicated that a majority of persons with chronic illnesses spend approximately an hour a year in face-to-face encounters with their health care provider (Kaptein, Scharloo, Helder, Kleijn, van Korlaar, & Woertman, 2003). Similarly, for individuals with ESRD who are receiving chronic hemodialysis, research findings have shown that the amount of time physicians spend with each patient in U.S. dialysis centers averages only 32 minutes per month, or 6.4 hours per year (Pifer, Satayathum, Dykstra, Mapes, Goodkin, Canaud et al., 2002). This fairly simple arithmetic demonstrates quite clearly that individuals with chronic illnesses have no choice but to self-manage and incorporate their chronic illness into their daily lives. These individuals must find ways to make sense of what is happening to them, to manage their illness and its symptoms, and to make adjustments in their daily living in order to maintain some sense of balance and quality in their lives. Health care providers have an important role in trying to keep the medical condition stable and under control, but for the chronically ill individual, his or her self-management skills are equally as important (Lorig, 2002). It is important, then, for nurses to understand chronic illness and its management from the individual's perspective in order to assist persons with ESRD to manage their illness effectively.

Use of Theory for Chronic Illness Management

An individual's beliefs about a particular chronic illness can have important influences on his or her behavioral responses to the illness; that is, what an individual does in response to the illness. A theory-based approach to chronic illness management can help nurses and other health care providers understand and identify relevant personal, sociocultural, and health-related characteristics of individuals that may affect how they self-manage their chronic illness (Sidani, Doran, & Mitchell, 2004). The use of theory in clinical practice also helps health care providers understand the potential effect of individual characteristics on the health outcomes of chronically ill individuals. In addition, a theory-based approach to chronic illness management offers both a target for intervention efforts and markers for the effectiveness of treatment. Finally, theory helps nurses recognize the unique needs of individuals and tailor care to specific personal needs, values, and preferences (Fawcett, Watson, Neuman, Walker, & Fitzpatrick, 2001; Lauver, Ward, Heidrich, Keller, Bowers, Brennan et al., 2002).

For the purposes of this chapter, it is important to make a conceptual distinction between disease and illness. Disease is often conceptualized as a malfunctioning or maladaptation of biologic and psychophysiologic processes in the individual (Horne & Weinman, 1994). The traditional biomedical framework, which underlies many aspects of disease management in Western medical practice, places an emphasis on diagnosing and treating diseases and understanding the biological processes that cause disease (Engel, 1977). Diseases are seen as entities with specific signs and symptoms, and in many cases, specific treatments. The biomedical orientation for chronic illness management typically considers the diagnosis, identification, and description of disease-related physiological, structural, and mechanical changes as critical steps in chronic illness management. The biomedical framework also considers timely and appropriate treatment as critical for the control, and in some cases, the reversal or delay of physiological changes and the reduction in the physical and psychological dysfunctions that they create (Leventhal, Halm, Horowitz, Leventhal, & Ozakince, in-press).

Conversely, Kleinman (1980) distinguishes illness as an individual's subjective response to the disease. Subjective responses are frequently referred to as *illness experiences* and entail one's personal, interpersonal, and cultural reactions to disease or discomfort. An individual's experience of illness, including its management, is shaped by the processes of perception, labeling, explanation, and coping (Horne & Weinman, 1994). While the expressions "disease management" and "chronic illness management" are often used interchangeably, the nature and meaning of chronic illness and its management may differ in important ways for the health care provider and the individual who is chronically ill, and these differences in perceptions and beliefs can have important effects on health outcomes (Kleinman, 1980; Cameron & Leventhal, 2003). For example, studies have demonstrated that nonadherence to treatment regimens for hypertension frequently occurs when the patient and health care provider have different explanations and beliefs about an illness and its treatment. In what is considered a seminal study of illness representations in chronic illness, 230 individuals were interviewed about their hypertension beliefs (Meyer, Leventhal, & Gutmann, 1985). Many of the participants with hypertension viewed their illness as a symptomatic disease; physicians did not. For the study participants, the goal of hypertension treatment was the amelioration of symptoms. For physicians, the treatment goal was a lowering of blood pressure. The implication of these disparate views of hypertension and treatment goals was that physicians were asking their patients to begin and sustain a treatment that basically made no sense from patients' point of view. Patients were told they were "ill" but asymptomatic, and needed to take medicine that would have no effect on the way they felt. On the other hand, the patients believed that they only needed to take their medications when they experienced symp-

toms. The participants' illness beliefs influenced the action they took in dealing with their illness. They were significantly more likely to drop out of treatment or tended to use their medications intermittently in response to perceived symptoms. The findings from this study also illustrate the theoretical supposition that the way in which individuals self-manage their chronic condition is strongly influenced by what they think about their illness (Horne & Weinman, 1998). Thus, for nurses and other health care providers to be successful in helping individuals successfully manage their chronic kidney disease, it is important to understand what people think about their illness and how their cognitive interpretations of illness influence their self-management behaviors.

The Common-Sense Model of Self-Regulation of Health and Illness

The study of individual beliefs about illness and the relationship of these beliefs to illness-related behavior, including illness self-management, have been referred to as the illness perceptions approach to illness self-management (Horne, 2000). This approach has been used extensively in studies of individuals' adjustment to and management of a wide range of illnesses, including chronic illnesses (Weinman & Petrie, 1997a). The illness perceptions approach to chronic illness management is based on the Common Sense Model of Self-Regulation of Health and Illness (CSM) (Leventhal, Brissette, & Leventhal, 2003). The CSM is an information-processing model built on the proposition that individuals construct their own "common-sense" representations or interpretations of illnesses and symptoms. A basic assumption of the CSM is that individuals are viewed as active problem solvers when faced with an illness or health threat. According to the CSM, the individual is actively involved in (a) interpreting the meaning of somatic experiences; (b) deciding how best to respond to these experiences and then taking action; and (c) evaluating the effectiveness of the response for achieving a desired outcome (for example, the relief of bothersome symptoms). This problem solving depends heavily on the individual's interpretation or representation of the illness. According to the CSM, an individual's response to an illness threat follows three broad stages that are listed below and illustrated in Figure 3-1.

- The cognitive and emotional representation of the illness by which the individual makes sense of a health threat or illness.
- The development and implementation of an action plan or coping procedures to deal with the health threat or illness
- Appraisal of the outcome of the action plan.

Key features of the CSM are that the three stages of processing occur in parallel at a cognitive and emotional level. One level of processing creates a psychologically "objective" cognitive representation of the threat with its coping procedures and evaluative processes; the other is a psychologically "subjective" or emotional processing system that creates feeling states, and coping procedures and appraisal for the management of emotion. There is a dynamic interaction between the processes of representation, coping, and

Figure 3-1

Common Sense Model of Self-Regulation of Health and Illness

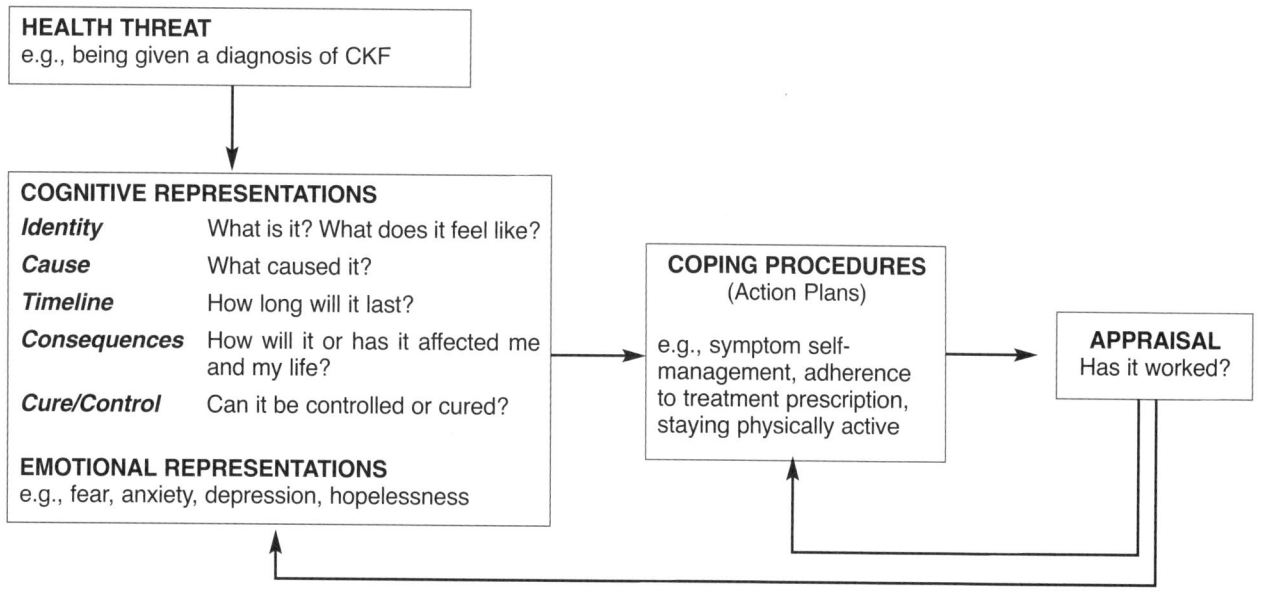

appraisal. Figure 3-1 shows that the interaction proceeds in both directions. The individual's coping procedures and appraisal may arise from a particular representation. But equally, the appraisal of the outcome of coping procedures may feed back to influence either the representation or coping procedure, or both. For example, in the hypertension study discussed previously (Meyer et al., 1985), individuals who perceived that hypertension was a symptomatic illness (cognitive representation) took their medications to relieve symptoms (coping procedure in response to representation). The relief of symptoms (appraisal of outcome) supported their beliefs that hypertension is a symptomatic disease, and that taking medications to relieve symptoms was appropriate and made sense to them (feedback to representations and coping procedures). In this case, if symptoms were not relieved, the CSM postulates that individuals would either change their representation ("Maybe hypertension does not have symptoms") or their coping procedures ("I will double the dose of my medication the next time I have symptoms"). This example illustrates how misrepresentations about illness can arise and how people may manage their illnesses based on misrepresentations in ways that could potentially afford less than optimal outcomes. The CSM offers a framework for understanding and improving an individual's management of chronic illness.

Cognitive Representations of Illness

Research findings have consistently shown that when faced with a health threat, such as a chronic illness, people try to make sense of it (define the problem) by forming a mental image or model of the problem. The illness representations domain of the CSM is a stage in which people analyze information about health threats and give meaning to them. Cognitive representation of illness refers to the individual's efforts to organize, analyze, and interpret diverse types of information about an illness or its symptoms. Research has consistently shown that the beliefs that comprise an individual's cognitive representation of a particular illness fall into five domains: illness identity, cause, timeline, consequences, and cure/control. A description of each of these domains follows.

Illness identity. *Illness identity* refers to the way in which an individual identifies an illness by both its abstract label and by the physical symptoms that one experiences. For example, at diagnosis, individuals are given an abstract label "ESRD" for their illness. The CSM postulates that these individuals will then seek to define or give meaning to this label in concrete terms by looking for or attaching physical symptoms to the label. In other words, the individual will attempt to discern what ESRD "feels" like. On the other hand, when symptoms occur before a label is identified, the individual will make meaning of the symptoms and give them a label that makes common sense to him. For example, an individual who may not know or has not been informed that she or he has kidney problems, and has no personal experience with this illness may not link the experience of uremic symptoms (such as loss of appetite and weight loss) to kidney failure. This individual may interpret these symptoms differently and give them a label (for example, gastrointestinal problems or even cancer) that makes common sense to him. In a qualitative study that explored the illness representations of 24 elderly hemodialysis patients (Thomas-Hawkins, 2004), content analysis of the data revealed that many participants did not link their uremic symptoms (such as loss of appetite and weight loss) to kidney failure. These individuals received no information regarding their diagnosis or the symptoms of ESRD, and many interpreted their uremic symptoms as gastrointestinal problems. This illness label made "common sense" to them based on their past experiences with gastrointestinal symptoms and their lack of experience with uremic symptoms or ESRD.

Cause. *Cause* representations relate to an individual's beliefs about the likely cause or causes of an illness or its physical symptoms. At the individual level, most chronic conditions are perceived to have complex causes (Taylor, Repetti, & Seeman, 1997). The individual's age and experience with treatment and whether or not it is successful will also affect causal beliefs. For example, research has consistently shown that older individuals are likely to attribute the cause of many of their symptoms to aging (Leventhal & Crouch, 1997). One consequence of this type of "aging attribution" by older individuals is that they may fail to report their symptoms to family, friends, or health professionals, and they will attempt to manage the symptoms by themselves. A second example relates to one's belief that treatment for an illness may cause a particular symptom. In Thomas-Hawkins' study (2004), several dialysis patients attributed the cause of many of their symptoms to the dialysis treatment. As a result, many felt that they had no personal control over the management of their symptoms since they could not control their dialysis treatments. This is a single study of illness representations in elderly dialysis patients, and the findings are not generalizable. However, the study findings should suggest to nurses and other health professionals that it is important to understand how patients are interpreting the cause of their illness and symptoms. Often, patients' causal representations will differ in important ways from the typical "medical" causes held by health professionals, and the procedures or strategies these individuals select to manage their illness or symptoms based on their causal representations may not be consistent with what may be deemed appropriate by the nurse or physician.

Timeline. *Timeline* representations focus on one's perceptions of the likely duration or course of the illness or its symptoms. The initiation of chronic renal replacement therapy often signals to the individual that the duration of kidney failure is permanent. On the other hand, research has shown that individuals receiving chronic hemodialysis treatments perceive many of the symptoms of ESRD (such as fatigue) as variable and cyclic (Thomas-Hawkins, 1998). Illness and symptom timeline representations have important implications for nurses who care for individuals with ESRD. Nursing interventions can be designed and tailored to this knowledge to assist patients to self-manage their illness and symptoms appropriately. For example, nurses can encourage increased participation in daily activities during times when a patient is not fatigued with a goal of expanding the individual's asymptomatic periods and encouraging appropriate energy conservation techniques during times when patients are fatigued.

Consequences. *Consequence representations* are the perceptions one has of the seriousness of an illness or its symptoms, and its short- and long-term consequences for the individual's life. Research that has explored ESRD patients' perceptions of the consequences of their illness have revealed that these individuals believe there are many negative and some positive illness effects on their daily lives. In one study (Lindqvist, Carlsson, & Sjoden, 2000), hemodialysis and peritoneal dialysis patients perceived many negative consequences of dialysis treatments (such as a lack of freedom to do things, a lack of control over their lives, significant losses (for example, having to give up work and social activities), dependence on others, and changes in physical appearance). On the other hand, transplant patients appeared to perceive some positive consequences of transplantation (such as a feeling of freedom and control over one's life, and fulfilled dreams of leading a normal life). Every chronic illness has a set of expected and perceived consequences of the impact of the illness on the individual and their lives. For example, anemia is an expected medical consequence of ESRD. On the other hand, an example of a perceived consequence of ESRD at the individual level is that a person may believe his health status will get worse with participation in exercise or regular daily physical activity. An individual's perceptions of the consequences of ESRD are certainly non-trivial and may have important implications for the selection of self-management procedures or strategies. For example, if one perceives that participation in regular physical activity will result in increased levels of fatigue or a worsening of the illness, then that individual will likely not engage in regular exercise despite the advice of health professionals. Assessment of an individual's consequence representations can provide information for health professionals to reshape consequence misrepresentations and assist patients to adopt illness management strategies that are adaptive and likely to result in positive health outcomes.

Control/Cure. *Cure/control representations* are concerned with the extent to which the individual believes the illness or its symptoms is amenable to cure or control. Chronic conditions differ with respect to expectations of *control* and *actual control*. Some are more controllable than others, but few are curable with current technology. While some studies in ESRD populations have shown that dialysis patients, in particular, perceive little to no control over their illness and its symptoms (Lindqvist et al., 2000; Thomas-Hawkins, 2004), other studies have indicated that ESRD patients' desire to control their health led to positive illness response behaviors such as maintaining independence, monitoring responses to treatment, and seeking disease-related information (Rittman, Northsea, Hausauer, Green, & Swanson, 1993). While more research is needed in this area, these findings do indicate a need for health professionals to explore the control representations of individuals with ESRD. This information can assist nurses to distinguish aspects of ESRD perceived by individuals as subject to personal control. If nurses can gain an understanding of their patients' control representations, this knowledge can support nursing interventions to help these individuals recognize and manage controllable aspects of their illness.

To illustrate the cognitive representations stage of the CSM, findings from the hypertension study (Meyer et al., 1985) will be discussed again. Medical clinicians assert that hypertension is an asymptomatic disease. On the other hand, Meyer's study demonstrated that many individuals with this condition think otherwise. The investigation revealed that many individuals with hypertension develop representations of the illness that differ from the medical view of hypertension. In Meyer's study, a majority of participants identified symptoms (for example, flushed face, headache, shakiness) for detecting and self-monitoring elevated blood pressure soon after diagnosis, and symptom monitoring increased over time. Moreover, a higher percentage of individuals in treatment for a long time (92%) reported monitoring symptoms for detecting elevated blood pressure compared to those with newly-diagnosed hypertension (71%). These findings support the premises of the CSM. That is, when given an illness diagnosis, individuals with hypertension will likely seek to define what the illness means for them in concrete terms; that is, they will seek to determine what hypertension *feels like* by discerning somatic symptoms that give meaning to the illness label of hypertension. Meyer's study also revealed that many participants' personal *identity* representation of hypertension consisted of a combination of symptoms and a label that differed from the medical view of hypertension as an asymptomatic illness. Study participants' beliefs about the duration and cause of hypertension also were not consistent with health care providers' views. Participants indicated that hypertension was limited in its duration and that it was caused by a variety of environmental conditions such as work, family, stress, and diet. In addition, participants indicated that they used their medication as prescribed if they perceived it controlled their symptoms; they did not adhere to their prescribed medication regimen if they felt that the medication did *not* control their symptoms. The important implication of these findings is that cognitive representations influence illness self-management behaviors. When individuals misinterpret somatic symptoms or an illness label, the procedures that they adopt to manage the illness or its symptoms, while sensible to the individual, may be misguided and could result in less than optimal outcomes.

For individuals with ESRD, there has been little research aimed at exploring illness representations of those persons affected by this condition. In Thomas-Hawkins' study (2004), the content of participants' representations for ESRD differed somewhat from the content of their representations for symptoms commonly associated with this condition. Many participants were not able to link their uremic symptoms with the label "ESRD." In addition, a majority of these individuals did not know the reason why their kidneys had failed. While many of these individuals had either diabetes or hypertension, most did not seem to understand that these conditions were major causes of kidney failure. Many participants viewed their illness as chronic and long-term. In addition, all participants indicated that the consequences of their illness, if not treated, were serious. While a few individuals expressed "hope" for a cure, most of the individuals did not feel that they had any control over their illness. Similarly, a majority of the participants did not seem to understand the cause of many symptoms that they were experiencing after starting dialysis, and many felt that they had little control over their symptoms. However, while many identified multiple symptoms that they were experiencing, most did not view their symptoms as serious or cause for concern. While more research is needed in this area, these findings suggest that many individuals with ESRD may not have clear or coherent representations of their illness, and educational interventions that are tailored to individual representations can help to reshape misrepresentations so that these individuals gain a clearer understanding of their illness and its symptoms.

Emotional Representations of Illness

Emotional representations are one's emotional responses to a health threat; these include feeling states such as anxiety, fear, worry, denial, and depression (Leventhal et al., 2003). Similar to cognitive representations, emotional representations also influence the procedures that one adopts to deal with emotional responses to illness. For the individual, chronic illness can represent a fundamental threat to survival and well being, and quite often, chronic illnesses can generate high and long-lasting levels of emotional distress. Individuals receiving dialysis cannot ignore the significant level of morbidity and mortality associated with the illness. Many of these individuals experience complications soon after the start of dialysis, and most have described similar experiences of distress and even depression when learning of the death of another patient in the dialysis facility (Harris & Brown, 1998). In a qualitative study by Curtin, Mapes, Petillo, & Oberly (2002), processes that were involved in ESRD patients' ability to survive on dialysis were explored, and all participants alluded to the "nearness of death and/or insecurity of their lives" (p. 618). Several participants described the anxiety associated with living with a risk of death and uncertain future. Similarly, individuals who have received a kidney transplant also experience distress and anxiety about an uncertain future, the constant threat of allograft rejection and return to dialysis, and the experience of medication side effects (Wainwright, Fallon, & Gould, 1999).

There is a growing body of research that addresses the stressors associated with ESRD and its treatment, and many of these stressors are listed in Table 3-1. Many studies have revealed that for patients receiving hemodialysis and continuous ambulatory peritoneal dialysis (CAPD), the most frequent stressors reported by these individuals include dietary and fluid restrictions, time constraints, risk of vascular access infection and loss, itchiness, fatigue, physical weakness, frequent hospitalizations, loss of employment, alterations in sexual function, decrease in social contacts, dependence on others, lack of control and freedom to do things, changes in physical appearance, worry and uncertainty about the future, and fear of death (Gurklis & Menke, 1995; Lindqvist, et al., 2000; Welch & Austin, 1999).

After transplantation, research has indicated that the most frequent stressors that these individuals experience include the cost of health care and related financial strains, long-term side effects of medications, anxiety and depression related to illness-related physical limitations, worry about physical appearance (for example, swelling of the face from medications), fear of repeated hospitalizations and transplant rejection, risk of infection, and uncertainty about the future (Fallon, Gould, & Wainwright, 1997; Lindqvist et al., 2000; Starzomski & Hilton, 2000).

ESRD stressors can generate an array of emotional responses, and emotional reactions to ESRD stressors such as fear, anxiety, depression, and pain-related distress are commonly reported in the literature (Kimmel, 2001; Watnick, Kirwin, Mahnensmith, & Concato, 2003). It is important to recognize that emotional representations of health threats (such as depression) may differ from the nurse's and other health care providers' understanding of emotional reactions to illness. For example, many chronically ill individuals may

Table 3-1
Common Stressors in ESRD by Treatment Modality

Hemodialysis	Peritoneal Dialysis	Transplant
Alterations in sexual function	Alterations in sexual function	Chages in bodily appearance
Changes in bodily appearance	Changes in bodily appearance	Cost of health care and related financial strains
Fatigue	Decrease in income and financial consequences of illness	Fear of repeated hospitalizations
Fear of death	Decrease in sex drive	Fear of transplant rejection
Fear of vascular access infection and/or failure	Dependence on others	Illness-related physical limitations
Financial consequences of illness	Fatigue	Risk of infection
Functional limitations	Fear of death	Side effects of medication
Loss of income and financial constraints	Fear of access failure	Worry and uncertainty about the future
Powerlessness and lack of control	Fear of infection/peritonitis	
Role reversal with children	Limited physical activity	
Sleep disturbances	Loss of income and financial constraints	
Social isolation	Treatment regimen complexities and intrusiveness	
Time constraints for work and leisure activities	Worry and uncertainty about the future	
Treatment regimen complexities and intrusiveness		
Worry and uncertainty about the future		

reject psychological labels like depression and depressed mood, because these labels may be perceived as stigmatizing (Leventhal, Diefenback, & Leventhal, 1992). Often, individuals may interpret symptoms of depression in physical rather than psychological terms (for example, feeling tired rather than sad), generate causal explanations that are physical rather than psychological (such as thinking this is due to my illness rather than interpersonal stress), and seek treatments that are physiological rather than psychological (for example, taking drugs rather than undergoing psychological therapy). Of the wide range of emotional responses in ESRD, depression is regarded as the most common psychological problem in patients treated with dialysis (Finkelstein & Finkelstein, 2000; Kimmel, 2001). Since many of the symptoms of depression are similar to symptoms associated with ESRD (such as fatigue, sleep difficulties, and loss of appetite) it can be easy for individuals to misrepresent these as physical symptoms rather than psychological manifestations. Emotional responses such as depression can have a negative effect on patient outcomes and need to be actively managed. For example, in the *Dialysis Outcomes and Practice Patterns Study* (DOPPS), a well-designed, multi-national, prospective observational study that examined dialysis practice patterns and patient outcomes, hemodialysis patients' self-reports of depression were associated with increased risks of mortality and hospitalizations for hemodialysis patients (Lopes, Bragg, Young, Goodkin, Mapes, Combe et al., 2002). These findings point to the need for nurses and other health professionals to assess emotional representations so that negative emotional responses to ESRD can be detected and addressed. It is important to note that the depression data in the DOPPS study were analyzed from two simple questions that were independently predictive of outcomes: (1) Have you felt so down in the dumps that nothing could cheer you up? and (2) Have you felt downhearted and blue? Nurses and other health professionals can easily incorporate these questions into their patient assessment forms. This would facilitate routine screening for depression as well as early detection and treatment.

Social Context of Illness Representations

Past illness experiences, social observation, information from others, and culture can help to shape an individual's representation of their health condition or somatic experiences (Brownlee, Leventhal, & Leventhal, 2000; Leventhal, Leventhal, & Contrada, 1998). In Thomas-Hawkins' study of older adult dialysis patients (2004), participants' lack of experience with ESRD appeared to shape their representation of uremic symptoms as "non-uremic" in nature. Moreover, many of the participants indicated that they compared their symptom experiences with other dialysis patients. This process of social comparison helped these individuals give meaning to their symptoms, and they frequently concluded that the symptoms they were experiencing were normal and should be expected for individuals with ESRD because other dialysis patients had experienced similar symptoms. Social contacts and social comparison, however, often fail to lead to appropriate illness representations or self-management behaviors. Other individuals may encourage each individual's preference to manage a particular problem or symptom alone or to delay seeking medical advice. The participants in Thomas-Hawkins' study who compared new symptoms with other patients' symptom experiences did not report their symptoms to the nurse or physician, but sought advice about symptom management from other dialysis patients. Similarly, in another qualitative study that examined the self-management strategies of long-term dialysis patients (Curtin & Mapes, 2001), many participants revealed a self-management strategy of selective symptom reporting and self-management.

Family Context of Illness Representations

It is also important to understand that illness takes place within the context of the family. Most chronic illnesses are managed within the home environment and inevitably involve other family members. Thus, for the chronically ill individual, the family provides the central context for chronic illness management. Every aspect of chronic illness self-management from the representation of illness through the development and execution of coping procedures to appraisal is heavily influenced by interactions with the family and by its impact on the family unit (Leventhal, Leventhal, & van Nguyen, 1986). Although spouses and other family members are the most important sources of emotional and instrumental support for patients, patients and their spouses or significant others may have divergent ideas about an illness. For example, the spouse may feel that the consequences of an illness are far more serious than the patient claims.

While no research related to family members' representations of ESRD has been done, nephrology professionals can learn from the few studies conducted in other chronically ill populations that have explored representations of significant others and compared them to their chronically ill family member. Researchers have conducted a number of studies in which they have explored the illness perceptions of significant others as a factor influencing illness representations and adaptive outcomes in their ill family member. For example, two studies have explored the illness representations of 49 individuals suffering from chronic fatigue syndrome (CFS) and 52 individuals with Addison's disease (AD) and their spouses (Fukuda, Straus, Hickie, Sharpe, Dobbins, & Komaroff, 1994; Heijmans, de Ridder, & Bensing, 1999). The results of these studies showed considerable differences in the illness representations of patients and their spouses. In the study of CFS patients and their spouses, partners tended to minimize the seriousness of the illness; they were less convinced that CFS had a biological basis or serious consequences. On the other hand, partners of AD patients tended to maximize the seriousness of the illness; they perceived more negative consequences, were less optimistic about the possibilities for cure, and believed more in a chronic timeline than did the patients. The perceptions of spouses influenced the illness representations and coping procedures of the patients. The spouses of AD patients tended to curb the enthusiasm of their sick partners for undertaking activities whereas the spouses of CFS patients tried to motivate their partners to fight the illness and become more active. The perceptions of spouses also appeared to have important influences on the outcomes of the patients. In general, the partner's minimization of the patient's illness appeared to be detrimental to the patient's well being. Those AD patients with minimizing spouses reported more problems, especially in mental and social functioning.

While there are no empirical comparisons of the illness representations of caregivers, partners, and individuals with ESRD, there is an emerging body of literature that under-scores the importance of dyadic and social relationships for the health of individuals with ESRD (Christenson, Wiebe, Smith, & Turner, 1994; Kimmel, Peterson, Weihs, Shidler, Simmens, Alleyne et al., 2000). It is likely that empirical approaches to chronic illness management for the individual with ESRD could be enhanced by assessing the degree of consonance of illness representations between individuals with ESRD and their significant others. The findings from Fukuda et al. (1994) and Heijmans et al. (1999) studies suggest the degree of illness representation congruence between patients and spouses is likely to have important, independent effects on the patients' well-being and other health outcomes. While the samples were small in these studies and the findings are not generalizable to individuals with ESRD and their families, these studies should raise the consciousness of nurses and other professionals that patient and family congruence or incongruence in illness representations is likely to be particularly influential for ESRD health outcomes. Understanding the illness representations of chronically individuals can only assist in providing a fundamental and theoretically based starting point for developing nursing interventions to facilitate effective illness self-management and outcomes in individuals with ESRD.

Health Care Provider Context of Illness Representations

Another important social dyad in the health care process is that between the patient and health care provider. Research has demonstrated that there is frequently a mismatch between a patient and his or her health care provider's perceptions of illness. One study compared the illness representations of individuals with diabetes and those of their general practitioners (Heijmans, Foets, Rijken, Schreurs, de Ridder, & Bensin, 2001). The findings from this investigation revealed that, compared to their doctor, persons with diabetes viewed their illness as more changeable, less controllable by medical care, more painful, and less life-threatening but more progressive. The general practitioners' perceptions were linked more to medical factors, as they seemed to attach more weight to the medical severity of the illness. In addition, differences in patient and health care provider perceptions were associated with patients' poor health status and an increase in their use of non-prescription drugs, and more paid visits to paramedical and alternative healers.

For many health care professionals, medical knowledge is the main source of information on which their representations and ideas about disease are based (Weinman, Heijmans, & Figueiras, 2003). These perceptions are grounded in the medical model, and they typically guide the actions and advice of health professionals. However, individuals who are chronically ill live with their illness for a very long time, and their interactions with health care providers are only one of many social situations that shape the content of their illness representations. Their day-to-day experiences with diseases and their symptoms are the main sources of information on which their representations are based (Leventhal et al., 2003). In health care encounters, health care providers should elicit their patient's illness representations as a basis for effective communication and care. A potential danger of this approach is that instead of using this information as a way of understanding the patient's views and needs, the provider may rush to replace the patient's beliefs with his or her own "medically correct" version (Weinman et al., 2003). Nurses and other health care providers should understand that it is unlikely that their patients will readily accept the provider's explanations of symptoms and diseases as replacements for their own ideas or perceptions (Leventhal et al., 1997). This is discussed in further detail later in this chapter.

Cultural Context of Illness Representations

A basic assumption of the CSM is that the individual is an active problem solver. Since the active problem solver is hypothesized to be actively involved in interpreting the meanings of somatic experiences, there seems to be a logical connection between illness representations and culture. The culture and the experiences of individuals are enmeshed in their interpretations of their illness experiences and health practices as they process internal and external information (Baumann, 2003). Culture can play a significant role in how an individual interprets, clarifies, and categorizes body symptoms, and it provides the context of normative beliefs. For example, diabetes has reached almost epidemic proportions among Native Indian groups in regions of the US. Leventhal and colleagues (1992) provide a cultural context for illness representations for this group of chronically ill individuals. Leventhal, Diefenbach, and Leventhal (1992) reported that Native Indian communal leaders sought advice from nonphysician professionals because of a lack of fit between their traditional models of illness and the disease models of their physicians; physicians were avoided because they were viewed as hostile to traditional medicine. According to Leventhal, some Indian tribes classified diabetes as a "white man's disease" that they felt had been thrust upon their community. They also attributed the cause of diabetes to contamination of food by electricity. This attribution was grounded in the culture of this group and recognized the link between the adoption of Western practices and the movement away from traditional diet and work. The anxiety and suspicion evident in this cultural interpretation of diabetes described by Leventhal appeared to be associated with dissatisfaction with treatment by physicians and decisions to seek alternative sources of care. This example serves as an illustration of the influence of culture on illness representations and the potential effect of cultural interpretations on procedures adopted to manage illness.

There has been little research related to the cultural aspects of illness representations, and much of the research in ESRD populations has not addressed culture as a variable. Nurses must recognize that culture affects illness beliefs. It is important that nurses, in their work with patients from different cultural groups, attempt to gain an understanding of that culture and work with individuals and their families in culturally relevant ways.

Assessment of Illness Representations

Nurses and other health care professionals should recognize that illness representations are, by their nature, private. In encounters between chronically ill individuals and their health care providers, these individuals are often reluctant to discuss their beliefs about their illness because they fear conflict or the risk of being thought of as misinformed or even unintelligent (Kleinman, Eisenberg, & Good, 1978; Weinman & Petrie, 1997b). As discussed, illness representations also vary between patients and health care providers (Leventhal et al., 2003), and health care providers generally do not explore the illness representations of their patients (Weinman & Petrie, 1997b).

When people think about their illnesses, the CSM suggests that they appear to organize their thoughts around five key questions: What is it and what does it feel like (illness identity)? What caused it (cause)? How long will it last (timeline)? How will it or has it affected me (consequences)? Can it be controlled or cured (cure/control)? An individual's representation or lay model of a particular illness is comprised of his or her answers to these questions. In order to help individuals manage their illness appropriately, it is important that nurses and other health care providers gain an understanding of how patients are interpreting their illness and its symptoms. Using the CSM as a guide, nurses can elicit their patients' illness representations using closed and open-ended assessment questions that are listed in Table 3-2. The information gleaned from assessment of illness representations can help nurses and other health professionals gain an understanding of their patients' interpretations of ESRD and its symptoms, and help improve patients' illness management. Assessment questions can be incorporated into nursing admission assessment and routine screening tools in the clinical setting. In that way, illness representations could be assessed on an ongoing basis, and nurses could use this information to tailor interventions, in collaboration with the patients and families. Interventions that are tailored to individual beliefs and perceptions could help to support coherent representations and reshape or alter misrepresentations.

Coping Procedures (Illness Self-Management Strategies)

The CSM postulates that illness representations guide coping procedures, the second stage in the CSM. This stage reflects the illness self-regulation strategies that individuals select and execute in response to their beliefs about the illness. There are a multitude of procedures selected by patients for managing chronic illnesses that range from the use of dietary products, alternative healers, and over-the-counter medications to meditation, exercise, energy conservation, and treatments prescribed by health professionals, family, friends, and/or acquaintances. The particular attributes of an individual's illness representations guide the coping procedures or strategies that the individual adopts for coping with or managing the illness. For example, an individual who represents colon cancer as chronic and due to a weakened immune system may execute coping procedures (actions) to deal with the cancer that might include exercise to strengthen body resistance, ingestion of a high-bran diet to remove carcinogenic poisons from the gut, and positive thinking to invigorate immune defenses. Given this common-sense representation of colon cancer, the specific procedures or actions selected to cope with the disease are perceived by the individual as necessary and appropriate; that is, they are correct psychologically for the individual, though they may be viewed by the health professional as irrelevant to the control and cure of colon cancer.

Table 3-2
Illness Representation Assessment Questions

Cognitive Representations	Assessment Questions
Illness identity	What do you think your illness (or symptom) is? What does it do to you? What do you call it?
Cause	What do you think caused your illness? What do you think caused your symptom?
Timeline/Duration	How long do you think your illness will last? When does your symptom occur? How long does your symptom last?
Consequences	How severe do you think your illness (symptom) is? What are the chief problems your illness (symptom) has caused you?
Cure/control	What control do you think you have over your illness (symptom)? What are the results you hope to receive from your treatment?

Emotional Representations Assessment Questions
How do you feel about your kidney disease?   Does your illness make you angry?   Do you worry about your illness?   Are you afraid of anything? If so, what?   Do you feel anxious? If so, what is making you feel this way?   Have you felt so down in the dumps that nothing could cheer you up?   Have you felt downhearted and blue?

The CSM is in many ways well-suited for nurses and other health professionals to use as a framework for understanding and improving patients' management of chronic illness. There are a number of strategies that an individual may choose to select, but nurses must understand that the coping procedures selected and executed by patients are based on common-sense representations of illness, and they may be inconsistent with nurses' ideas about the what the patient should be doing. The CSM provides a theory-based approach to assist nurses to understand the bases for individual patient approaches for managing ESRD and its symptoms, and it can guide nurses to shape or change particular aspects of a patient's illness beliefs or self-management behaviors.

Adherence to Treatment in Chronic Illness

In the CSM, adherence to treatment is viewed as one of a number of coping procedures that an individual has available to deal with the illness threat. Since adherence to treatment is a problem in most chronic illnesses including ESRD, this particular aspect of chronic illness self-management will be discussed.

Until relatively recently, compliance was the most common term used for following treatment regimen instructions. However, this term suggests a relationship in which the individual has a passive role and is expected to follow the health care provider's orders (Horne, 2000). In this regard, non-compliance may be seen as the individual's fault. Many have adopted the term adherence as an acceptable alternative to compliance. The term adherence emphasizes a person's freedom to decide whether to follow the health care provider's recommendations and implies that failure to do so may not

be a reason to blame the patient. This reasoning also implies that health care providers have a responsibility to facilitate adherence to treatment regimens rather than assume that it is the patient's responsibility to comply with instructions. Recently, the term concordance has been used to denote the degree to which the patient and health practitioner agree about the nature of the illness and need for treatment (Horne, 2000).

Poor adherence to treatment in chronic conditions is well documented, and research has shown that non-adherence contributes significantly to treatment failures and poor health outcomes. Although the level of non-adherence in the general population varies depending on the patient population, medical condition, form of treatment, and the definition of adherence, estimates of non-adherence have ranged from 15 to 93% with an average estimate of approximately 50% of individuals who fail to adhere to their treatment regimens (Horne & Weinman, 1998).

Adherence to Treatment in ESRD

The concept of adherence in ESRD involves a variety of health-related behaviors, and adherence with the prescribed treatment regimen is a challenge for most individuals. For dialysis patients, the prescribed treatment regimen is complex and includes regularly scheduled and relatively time-consuming dialysis treatments, strict dietary and fluid restrictions, multiple prescribed medications, participation in regular physical activity, and frequent medical appointments. Nonadherence to particular aspects of this complex regimen may result in acute health crises, such as acute volume overload or hyperkalemia, or may have long-term negative consequences on health outcomes, such as crippling metabolic bone disease. Individuals who have received a kidney transplant also are expected to adhere to complex, lifelong immunosuppressant medications and to adjust to the side effects that accompany these medications (Siegel & Greenstein, 1999). Non-adherence to immunosuppressant medications can lead to rejection episodes, allograft loss, and resumption of dialysis. Non-adherence to treatment regimens is a pervasive problem among individuals with ESRD. Research that examined the prevalence of non-adherence in individuals receiving dialysis has indicated that 30 to 60% of individuals do not adhere to fluid intake, dietary, and medication regimens (Christensen, Benotsch, & Smith, 1997). Curtin and her colleagues (1999) examined compliance with antihypertensive and phosphate binding medications in a sample of 135 individuals receiving chronic hemodialysis treatments. The findings of this study revealed that more than 70% of the participants missed 20% or more of their phosphate binding medications over a 6-week period, and 43% of the patients missed 20% or more of their antihypertensive doses of medication. Similarly, investigations of adherence to immunosuppressive medications in transplant patients reveal nonadherence rates that range from 5% to more than 45% (DeGeest, Abraham, & Dunbar-Jacob, 1996).

Adherence and Outcomes in ESRD

Adherence to treatment in ESRD is an important self-management issue because of the relationship of adherence to health outcomes in individuals with this condition. Several studies have revealed that individuals who make decisions, either intentionally or non-intentionally, to not adhere to particular aspects of treatment are at higher risk for adverse health outcomes. Saran, Bragg-Gresham, Rayner, Goodkin, Keen, van Dijk et al. (2003) reviewed data from the *Dialysis Outcomes and Practice Patterns Study* to assess nonadherence and outcomes in an international sample of 7,676 hemodialysis patients. In this study, nonadherence was operationalized as: (1) skipping one or more dialysis treatments in a month, (2) shortening the dialysis session by > 10 minutes in one month, (3) serum potassium level of > 6.0 mEq/l, (4) serum phosphate level of > 7.5 mg/dl, and (5) an interdialytic weight gain of > 7% of dry weight. The major findings of this study revealed that hemodialysis patients who skipped dialysis treatments had excessive interdialytic weight gains and high phosphate levels, and had significantly increased mortality rates compared to those who were adherent in these areas. In addition, patients who skipped treatments and had high serum phosphate levels also had higher rates of hospitalization compared to patients who were more adherent in these areas. Similar associations between adherence and outcomes have been demonstrated in research with individuals who had received a kidney transplant. In one prospective study that examined the cause of allograft loss in 58 transplant patients, 27% of the losses were attributed to nonadherence (Dunn, 1990). Similarly, in another study that examined graft loss in kidney transplant patients, 13% of allograft losses were attributed to medication non-adherence (Hong, Sumrani, Delaney, Dibenedetto, & Butt, 1992). These research findings underscore the importance of individual behaviors for health outcomes. Equally as important, these findings seem to indicate that despite the advice of health care professionals to adhere to prescribed treatment regimens, many individuals with ESRD are non-adherent. There is clearly a need for research that examines ESRD patients' beliefs about their illness and treatment to understand the influence of these beliefs on adherence coping procedures. Moreover, the CSM offers a framework for nurses and other health professionals in clinical practice to understand why individuals may not adhere and to assist patients to improve their adherence self-management behaviors.

Common Sense Model and Treatment Beliefs

From the health care provider perspective, an individual's adherence to treatment plans is considered an appropriate coping procedure. Health professionals believe that adherence to prescribed treatment regimens will result in optimal outcomes, the prevention of complications, and the success of therapeutic treatment plans. Unfortunately, most interventions and treatment plans designed and executed by health care professionals to assist patients to manage their illnesses are rarely theoretically based (Petrie, Broadbent, & Meechan, 2003). Individuals who are chronically ill rarely blindly follow health advice. People tend to interpret advice about treatment and make a decision about whether or not they need it (Horne, 2003).

Horne (2003) hypothesizes that individuals must be convinced that a condition warrants treatment. It is logical that perceptions of treatment necessity are ultimately intertwined with illness representations as the individual attempts to achieve common-sense coherence. For example, symptoms experiences and perception (illness identity) may stimulate medication use by reinforcing beliefs about its necessity. On the other hand, research has shown that the absence of severe symptoms might cause one to interpret one's condition as more benign that it actually is (Horne, Cooper, Fischer, & Buick, 2001; Siegel & Gorey, 1997). A study by Horne and colleagues (2001) revealed a relationship between hemodialysis patients' belief about treatment and adherence to treatment regimens. In a study of 47 hemodialysis patients that assessed their beliefs about medication, fluid and diet restrictions, Horne et al. (2001) found that 90% of the participants agreed that their medications were necessary for maintaining their health, but 32% had concerns about becoming too dependent on their medications or about the long-term effects of medication. These beliefs had important implications for adherence. Participants who had concerns about their medications were more likely to report intentionally missing doses of medication. Forty-three percent of the study participants also believed their fluid and diet restrictions were too strict, and these participants were less likely to adhere to their fluid and dietary restrictions. This study had several limitations including the small sample size and the use of self-report measures for medication adherence that did not detail the exact number of medications doses taken. Patients may have underestimated the extent of their non-adherence in this study. While the findings are not generalizable to all hemodialysis patients, they can be considered preliminary. Study findings identify potential targets for intervention; that is, concerns about medications, and diet and fluid restrictions. For example, particular concerns about medications might be misplaced, and these concerns could be addressed by appropriate educational interventions. The decision to adhere or not to adhere to treatment is the prerogative of the patient. However, nurses should help patients ensure that their decisions about treatment are informed by fact rather than by misguided beliefs about the relative risks and benefits of treatment. The findings from this study, while preliminary, reinforce the need for a negotiated approach to adherence decisions that take into account patients' beliefs about illness and its treatment.

Assessment of Adherence in ESRD

The assessment of adherence is a complex task, and adherence to the ESRD treatment regimen is difficult to quantify. There are no standard criteria that have been developed to measure adherence or non-adherence. In research investigations, interdialytic weight gain and laboratory values (such as serum potassium and phosphate levels) have been used as objective measures of adherence to dietary and fluid treatment prescriptions, and missed or shortened dialysis treatments have been used as objective measures of adherence to dialysis treatment schedules. Researchers have used various methods for assessing medication adherence in dialysis and transplant patients including self-report (Curtin, Svarstad, & Keller, 1999; Siegel & Greenstein, 1999), pill count (Curtin et al., 1999; Hillbrands, Hoitsma, & Koene, 1995; Long, Kee, Graham. Saethang, & Dames, 1998), electronic monitoring devices (Curtin et al., 1999), and serum drug levels (Kiley, Lan, & Pollack, 1993).

Objective criteria (such as laboratory values and body weight) are useful in clinical practice, but the lack of standardization for these measures may make it difficult to compare adherence outcomes across patient settings. For example, scales to measure body weight vary in their accuracy from treatment center to treatment center, and scale precision may even vary from day-to-day within a single dialysis center. Moreover, the use of self-report, pill counts, and microelectronic monitor devices for the assessment of medication adherence have particular advantages and disadvantages for clinical practice.

Pill count. The pill count is a commonly used method of assessing medication adherence. This method entails counting the number of pills that remain in a medication container and comparing this number to the number that would have been left if the individual took the medication as prescribed. This method has the advantage of being easy to do in a clinical setting and is inexpensive. However, there is no guarantee that a tablet that has been removed from a container has actually been ingested. Patients may remove medications from pill containers for many reasons. They might give medications to someone else or transfer it to another container. In some cases, patients may deliberately discard doses prior to assessment to create an impression of high adherence, a practice commonly known as "dose-dumping." Another source of inaccuracy in the pill counting method arises with needing to know when the individual started taking pills from the container. Relying on the date that the drug was dispensed, which is included on the medication label, may be misleading. Frequently, individuals receiving medications for a chronic illness will obtain a supply of their

medication in advance to avoid running out, and they may start their medication after it was dispensed. An individual's recall of when they started taking medications from the pill container may also be inaccurate.

Electronic monitoring devices. Electronic monitoring of adherence to medications entails the use of microelectronic devices that are inserted into medication containers to record the date and time that the pill container was opened. Each time the pill container is opened, the device records this as a medication event that can be regarded as a presumptive ingestion of the medication dose. However, one limitation of this method of assessment is that removal of the cap does not necessarily mean that a dose of the medication was taken. A major advantage of this method is that it may capture a profile or pattern of medication taking rather than simply detailing how much was taken (Horne, 2000). This method is frequently used in research but may be impractical for the assessment of medication adherence in clinical practice because the monitors are expensive, multiple devices are required for individuals who take multiple medications, and the devices change the appearance of the pill container and may alert the patient that their medication usage is being monitored. Consequently, this may affect pill-taking behavior during the assessment period.

Self-Report. Patient self-report is a commonly used method of assessing adherence to treatment recommendations. When self-reports have been compared to other objective measures of medication taking in individuals, research findings have shown that patients are accurate when they say that they have not taken their medication (Fletcher, 1989). However, for individuals who say they have taken their medications as prescribed, their verbal reports have not been confirmed by objective measures (Curtin et al., 1999; Spector, Kinsman, Mawhinney, Siegel, Radhelesfsky, Katz et al., 1986). One problem with self-reported adherence to medication regimens is that questions are usually asked at a time and place which is distant from the actual event, which produces problems with recall. People are often unable to recall exactly what they did and tend to remember the good rather than the bad, frequently referred to as the halo effect. The reliability and validity of self-report medication adherence assessment methods in clinical practice can be enhanced in a number of ways (Horne, 2000). When asking individuals about adherence to medications, it may help to pose these questions in a non-threatening manner that might increase an individual's tendency to report medication-taking behaviors more accurately. The following is an example of a question that one might ask about adherence to medications: "Some patients say that they may forget to take some of their medication doses. In the past week, how often would you say that this happened to you?" Another method for improving the quality of information that is obtained from patients about medication adherence is to offer a range of responses rather than relying on simple yes or answers. The following is an example: "How often do you miss a dose of your medicines: never, rarely, sometimes, often, very often?"

In the clinical setting, assessment of adherence to medication regimens may be difficult to quantify, and there are no standard criteria for this assessment. In a study by Curtin et al. (1999) of medication compliance in hemodialysis patients, microelectronic monitoring, pill count, and self-report methods of adherence were used and compared. In this study, microelectronic monitoring was considered to have the greatest potential for providing the most reliable estimates of compliance, and pill count and self-report findings were compared against this measure. The estimates of noncompliance acquired through pill count in this study were similar to the electronic monitoring assessments. Electronic monitoring revealed that 52% of patients monitored for antihypertensive use were repeatedly noncompliant, and 42% were repeatedly non-compliant on pill count. For phosphate binders, 70% of patients were assessed to be repeatedly non-compliant by both electronic monitoring devices and pill counts. On the other hand, noticeable differences were observed in rates of noncompliance when comparing electronic monitoring assessments and self-reports. For example, only 12% of patients monitored for antihypertensive use were assessed by self-report to be repeatedly non-compliant compared to 52% who were monitored electronically. Similarly, only 8% of patients were assessed by self-report to be repeatedly noncompliant with phosphate binder use compared to 70% who were repeatedly noncompliant as assessed with electronic monitor devices. While findings by Curtin et al. (1999) should be validated with replication studies, they suggest that pill count may be a reasonable and cost-effective method for the assessment of medication adherence in ESRD patients in the clinical setting.

Appraisal of Coping Procedures

The coping procedure stage is followed by an appraisal stage in which the individual evaluates the effectiveness of his or her coping procedures. An individual's illness representations help to establish questions and set criteria for appraisal of coping procedures. To illustrate this point, findings from the Meyer et al. (1986) study of hypertension will be used. Many participants in this study viewed hypertension as a symptomatic, believed that the timeline for the disease was limited (for example, not chronic), and perceived the causes to be related to the environment, work, or stress. Many individuals used somatic symptoms (headache, shakiness, flushed face) to monitor and treat their hypertension. For these individuals, the goal for treatment was the amelioration of symptoms. Thus, the implicit question these individuals likely established for appraisal of their coping procedures (taking medication for symptomatic relief) was "Are my symptoms gone?" (after taking medication), and the criterion for appraisal was "absence of symptoms."

The appraisal domain of the CSM has received little empirical attention. Research that has examined this stage of the CSM is sparse. One pilot intervention study that examined the effect of an energy conservation intervention for cancer treatment-related fatigue included appraisal as a variable (Barsevick, Whitmer, Sweeney, & Nail, 2002). The outcome variable (appraisal criterion) in this study was fatigue intensity, and the 5-item fatigue scale of the *Profile of Mood States* was the instrument used to measure this variable. The researchers noted that the nurse and the participant performed the outcome appraisal.

While research in this area is clearly needed, the tenets

of the CSM indicate that it is essential to address all three stages of information processing to bring about necessary changes in illness representations and self-management behaviors. Equally as important is the fact that chronically ill individuals may set unrealistic criteria for evaluating coping procedures or treatment outcomes (such as amelioration of symptoms as a goal for hypertension treatment). Nurses should recognize that in many instances, they must assist in helping patients establish appropriate goals and criteria for appraisal of self-management efforts. This should only be done in collaboration with the patient and with a clear understanding and knowledge of his or her illness beliefs, personal goals for the illness, and coping procedures. Otherwise, the therapeutic goals that nurses and other health professionals set for patients may not make common sense to them. In this situation, a plausible outcome is that the patient and nurse will not agree with the goals that are set, and patients will continue to execute self-management strategies that make sense to them.

Improving the Management of Chronic Illness

Tenets of the CSM indicate that representations and coping procedures are alterable (Leventhal, Brisette, & Leventhal, 2003). Research in non-ESRD populations has demonstrated that illness misrepresentations and misguided coping procedures can change with theory-guided interventions. One study will be discussed to illustrate this supposition. A randomized controlled educational intervention trial was conducted to investigate whether a brief, hospital-based intervention designed to change inaccurate and negative illness representations of myocardial infarction (MI) would result in an earlier return to work, less long-term disability, and improved cardiac rehabilitation attendance (Petrie, Cameron, Ellis, Buick, & Weinman, 2002). Previous work by the researchers revealed that many individuals who had an MI believed that this event would have serious and long-lasting consequences, and some believed that they had little or no control over their heart condition. These representations were associated with a slower return to work after the MI (coping procedure). In the randomized controlled trial, participants who were hospitalized after suffering a MI for the first time were randomized to an education intervention group or a control group. The educational intervention included four sessions that were conducted during participants' hospital stay. The intervention was specifically structured and tailored to each participant's representations in order to change highly negative representations of MI and to alter their views of the timeline and consequences of MI. The results of the study revealed that the intervention significantly altered individuals' beliefs about their MI. Compared to participants in the control group, those individuals who received the educational intervention were significantly less likely to perceive that their heart condition would cause serious consequences and last a long time or indefinitely. Intervention group participants were significantly more likely to perceive that their heart condition could be controlled. The intervention group participants also had lower levels of distress about symptoms as compared to the control group. Moreover, the intervention group participants returned to work at significantly faster rates compared to the control group, and their rates of cardiac rehabilitation attendance were higher than control group attendance rates. This study suggests that illness representations may be successfully altered by brief cognitive-based educational interventions and provides further evidence that interventions based on the CSM have considerable potential to improve adjustment to and management of chronic illness.

Summary

The CSM provides nurses and other health professionals who care for individuals with ESRD with a practical blueprint to guide these individuals in the management of their illnesses. The view of the patient as an active problem solver is in stark contrast with the passive role to which patients are often relegated in the medical treatment process. There is an emerging chronic illness paradigm that favors a less paternalistic model of care and greater involvement of patients in decisions and management (Holman & Lorig, 2000).

The central role that a theory-based approach to chronic illness management affords in ESRD care is that an understanding of the patient's view of his or her illness provides nurses and other health care providers with several advantages. Most importantly, CSM theory-guided practice will assist health professionals to gain an understanding of patients' interpretations and views of their illness and the particular strategies that individuals have adopted to manage the illness. Secondly, the CSM provides both a target for intervention efforts and a marker for the effectiveness of therapy. The importance of this advantage should not be understated as many interventions designed to improve illness management behaviors (such as cardiac rehabilitation, pain management programs, and exercise interventions) are not theoretically based and are unclear about the types of perceptions and behaviors they are designed to change (Petrie et al., 2003). The CSM provides a sound theoretical basis for the improvement of chronic illness management behaviors and outcomes in ESRD.

References

Alexander, L. (1976). The double-bind theory and hemodialysis. *Archives of General Psychiatry, 33,* 1353-1356.

Barsevik, A.M., Whitmer, K., Sweeney, C., & Nail, L.M. (2002). A pilot study examining energy conservation for cancer treatment-related fatigue. *Cancer Nursing, 25,* 333-341.

Baumann, L.C. (2003). Culture and illness representation. In L.D. Cameron & H. Leventhal (Eds.), *The self-regulation of health and illness behavior* (pp. 242-253). London: Routledge.

Brownlee, S., Leventhal, H., & Leventhal, E.A. (2000). Regulation, self-regulation, and regulation of the self in maintaining physical health. In M. Boekarts, P.R. Pintrich, & M. Ziedner (Eds.). *Handbook of self-regulation* (pp. 369-416). San Diego, CA: Academic Press.

Cameron, L. & Leventhal, H. (2003). Self-regulation, health, and illness: an overview. In L.D. Cameron & H. Leventhal (Eds.). *The self-regulation of health and illness behavior* (pp. 42-65). London: Routledge.

Centers for Disease Control and Prevention. (2003). *Chronic disease overview.* Retrieved March 3, 2004, from http://www.cdc.gov/nccdphp/overview.htm

Christensen, A.J., Benotsch, E.G., & Smith, T.W. (1997). Determinants of regimen adherence in renal dialysis. In Gochman, D.S. (Ed.). *Handbook of health behavior research: Vol. 2* (pp. 231-244). New York: Plenum.

Christenson, A.J., Wiebe, J.S., Smith, T.W., & Turner, C.W. (1994). Predictors of survival among hemodialysis patients: Effects of per-

ceived family support. *Health Psychology, 13,* 521-525.

Curtin, R.B. & Mapes, D.L. (2001). Health care management strategies of long-term dialysis survivors. *Nephrology Nursing Journal, 27,* 385-392, 394.

Curtin, R.B., Mapes, D., Petillo, M., & Oberly, E. (2002). Long-term dialysis survivors: A transformational experience. *Qualitative Health Research, 12,* 609-624.

Curtin, R.B., Svarstad, B.L., & Keller, T.H. (1999). Hemodialysis patients' noncompliance with oral medications. *ANNA Journal, 26,* 307-316.

DeGeest, S., Abraham, L., & Dunbar-Jacob, J. (1996). Measuring transplant patients' compliance with immunosuppressant therapy. *Western Journal of Nursing Research, 18,* 595-599.

Dunn, J. (1990). Causes of graft loss beyond two years in the cyclosporin era. *Transplantation, 49,* 49-53.

Engel, G.L. (1977). The need for a new medical model: A challenge for biomedicine. *Science, 196,* 129-136.

Fallon, M., Gould, D., & Wainwright, S.P. (1997). Stress and quality of life in the renal transplant patient: A preliminary investigation. *Journal of Advanced Nursing, 25,* 562-570.

Fawcett, J., Watson, J., Neuman, B., Walker, P.H., & Fitzpatrick, J.J. (2001). On nursing theories and evidence. *Journal of Nursing Scholarship, 33,* 115-119.

Finkelstein, F.O. & Finkelstein, S.H. (2000). Depression in chronic dialysis patients: Assessment and treatment. *Nephrology, Dialysis, and Transplantation, 15,* 1911-1913.

Fletcher, R.H. (1989). Patient compliance with therapeutic advice: Modern view. *The Mount Sinai Journal of Medicine, 56,* 453-458.

Fukuda, K., Straus, S.E., Hickie, I., Sharpe, M.C., Dobbins, J.G., & Komaroff, A. (1994). The chronic fatigue syndrome: A comprehensive approach to its definition and study. *Annals of Internal Medicine, 121,* 953-959.

Gurklis, J.A., & Menke, E.M. (1995). Chronic hemodialysis patients' perceptions of stress, coping, and social support. *ANNA Journal, 22,* 381-389.

Harris, S. & Brown, E. (1998). Patients surviving more than 10 years on dialysis. The natural history of complications of treatment. *Nephrology, Dialysis, and Transplantation, 13,* 1226-1233.

Heijmans, M., de Ridder, D., & Bensing, J. (1999). Dissimilarity in patients' and spouses' representations of chronic illness: Exploration and relations to patient adaptation. *Psychology and Health, 14,* 451-466.

Heijmans, M., Foets, M., Rijken, M., Schreurs, K., de Ridder, D., & Bensing, J. (2001). Stress in chronic disease: Do the perceptions of patients and their general practitioners match? *British Journal of Health Psychology, 6,* 229-242.

Hillbrands, L.B., Hoitsma, A.J., & Koene, R.A. (1995). Medication and compliance after renal transplantation. *Transplantation, 60,* 914-920.

Hong, J.H., Sumrani, N., Delaney, V., Dibenedetto, V., & Butt, K.M. (1992). Cases of late allograft loss in the cyclosporin era. *Nephron, 62,* 272-279.

Holman, H., & Lorig, K.R. (2000). Patients as partners in managing chronic illness. *British Medical Journal, 320,* 526-527.

Horne, R. (2000). Nonadherence to medication: Causes and implications for care. In P.R. Gard (Ed.). *A behavioural approach to pharmacy practice* (pp. 111-130). Oxford: Blackwell Sciences, Inc.

Horne, R. (2003). Treatment perceptions and self-regulation. In L.D. Cameron & H.Leventhal (Eds.). *The self-regulation of health and illness behavior* (pp. 138-153). London: Routledge.

Horne, R., Cooper, V., Fisher, M., & Buick, D. (2001). Beliefs about HIV and HAART and the decision to accept or reject HAART. *HIV Medicine, 2,* 195-200.

Horne, R., Sumner, S., Jubraj, B., Weinman, J., & Frost, S. (2001). Haemodialysis patients' beliefs about treatment: implications for adherence to medication and fluid-diet restrictions. *International Journal of Pharmacy Practice, 9,* 169-175.

Horne, R. & Weinman, J. (1998). Predicting treatment adherence: An overview of theoretical models. In L.B. Myers & K. Midence (Eds.). *Adherence to treatment in medical conditions* (pp. 25- 50). London: Harwood Academic.

Horne, R., & Weinman, J. (1994). Illness cognitions: Implications for the treatment of renal disease. In H.M. McGee & C. Bradley (Eds.).

Quality of life following renal failure (pp. 113-132). Switzerland: Harwood Academic.

Kaptein, A.A., Scharloo, M., Helder, D.I., Kleijn, W.C., van Korlaar, I.M., & Woertman, M. (2003). Representations of chronic illnesses. In L.D. Cameron & H. Leventhal (Eds.). *The self-regulation of health and illness behavior* (pp. 97-118). New York: Routledge.

Kiley, D.J., Lan, C.S., & Pollak, R. (1993). A study of treatment compliance following kidney transplantation. *Transplantation, 55,* 51-56.

Kimmel, P.L. (2001). Psychosocial factors in dialysis patients. *Kidney International, 59,* 1599-1613.

Kimmel, P.L., Peterson, R.A., Weihs, K.L., Shidler, N.R., Simmens, S.J., & Alleyne, S., et al. (2000). Marital conflict, gender and survival in urban hemodialysis patients. *Journal of the American Society of Nephrology, 11,* 1518-1525.

Kleinman, A. (1980). *Patients and healers in the context of culture.* Berkeley, CA: University of California Press.

Kleinman, A., Eisenberg, I., & Good, B. (1978). Clinical lessons learned from anthropologic and cross-cultural research. *Annals of Internal Medicine, 88,* 251-258.

Lauver, D.R., Ward, S.E., Heidrich, S.M., Keller, M.L., Bowers, B.J., Brennan, P.F., et al. (2002). Patient-centered nursing interventions. *Research in Nursing & Health, 25,* 246-255.

Leventhal, H., Benyamini, Y., Brownlee, S., Diefenbach, M., Leventhal, E.A., Patrick-Miller, L., & Robitalle, C. (1997). Illness representations: Theoretical foundations. In. K.J. Petrie & J.A. Weinman (Eds.). *Perceptions of health & illness* (pp. 19-45). Amsterdam, The Netherlands: Harwood Academic.

Leventhal, H., Brissette, I., & Leventhal, E.A. (2003). The common-sense model of self-regulation of health and illness. In L.D. Cameron & H. Leventhal (Eds.), *The self-regulation of health and illness behavior,* (pp. 42-65), London: Routledge.

Leventhal, E.A., & Crouch, M. (1997). Are there differences in perceptions of illness across the lifespan? In K.J. Petrie & J. Weinman (Eds.), *Perceptions of health and illness: Current research and applications* (pp. 77-102). London: Harwood Academic Press.

Leventhal, H., Diefenbach, M., & Leventhal, E.A. (1992). Illness cognitions: Using common sense to understand treatment adherence and affect cognition interactions. *Cognitive Therapy and Research, 16,* 143-163.

Leventhal, H., Halm, E., Horowitz, C., Leventhal, E.A. & Ozakince, G. (in-press). Living with chronic illness: A contextualized self-regulation approach. In M. Johnston, S.R. Sutton, & A. Baum (Eds.), *Handbook of health psychology.* Thousand Oaks: Sage.

Leventhal, H., Leventhal, E.A., & Contrada, R.J. (1998). Self-regulation, health, and behavior: A perceptual-cognitive approach. *Psychology & Health, 13,* 717-733.

Leventhal, H., Leventhal, E.A., & van Nguyen. (1986). Reactions of families to illness: Theoretical models and perspectives. In D. Turk & R. Kerns (Eds.), *Health, illness, and families: A life-span perspective* (pp. 108-147). New York: Wiley.

Lindqvist, R., Carlsson, M., & Sjoden, P-O. (2000). Perceived consequences of being a renal failure patient. *Nephrology Nursing Journal, 27,* 291-298.

Lopes, A.A., Bragg, J., Young, E., Goodkin, D., Mapes, D., Combe, C., et al. (2002). Depression as a predictor of mortality and hospitalization among hemodialysis patients in the United States and Europe. *Kidney International, 62,* 199-207.

Lorig, K. (2002). Partnerships between expert patients and physicians. *Lancet, 359,* 814-815.

Meyer, D., Leventhal, H., & Guttman, M. (1985). Common-sense models of illness: the example of hypertension. *Health Psychology, 4,* 115-135.

Petrie, K.J., Broadbent, E., & Meechan, G. (2003). Self-regulatory interventions for improving the management of chronic illness. In L.D. Cameron & H. Leventhal (Eds.), *The self-regulation of health and illness behavior* (pp. 257-277). London: Routledge.

Petrie, K.J., Cameron, L.D., Ellis, C.J., Buick, D., & Weinman, J. (2002). Changing illness perceptions after myocardial infarction: An early intervention randomized controlled trial. *Psychosomatic Medicine, 64,* 580-586.

Pifer, T.B., Satayathum, S., Dykstra, D.M., Mapes, D.L., Goodkin, D.A., Canaud, B., et al. (2002). Hemodialysis (HD) staffing and patient outcomes in the Dialysis Outcomes Practice Patterns Study (DOPPS). *Journal of the American Society of Nephrology Abstracts, 13,* 425A.

Reif, L. (1975). Beyond medical intervention strategies for managing life in face of chronic illness. In. M. Davis, M. Kramer, & M. Strauss (Eds.), *Nurses in practice: A perspective on work environments* (pp. 261-273). St. Louis: Mosby.

Rittman, M., Northsea, C., Hausauer, N., Green, C., & Swanson, L. (1993). Living with renal failure. *ANNA Journal, 20,* 327-331.

Saran, R., Bragg-Gresham, J.L., Rayner, H.C., Goodkin, D.A., Keen. M.L., van Dijk, P.C. et al. (2003). Nonadherence in hemodialysis: Associations with mortality, hospitalizations, and practice patterns in the DOPPS. *Kidney International, 64,* 254-262.

Sidani, S., Doran, D.M., & Mitchell, P.H. (2004). A theory-driven approach to evaluating quality of nursing care. *Journal of Nursing Scholarship, 36,* 60-65.

Siegel, B., & Greenstein, S. (1999). Compliance and noncompliance in kidney transplant patients: Cues for transplant coordinators. *Journal of Transplant Coordinators, 9,* 104-108.

Siegel, K., & Gorey, E. (1997). HIV infected women: Barriers to AZT use. *Social Science Medicine, 45,* 15-22.

Spector, S.L., Kinsman, R., Mawhinney, H., Siegel, S.C., Radhelesfsky, G.S., Katz, R.M., et al. (1986). Compliance of patients with asthma with an experimental aerolized medication: Implications for controlled clinical trials. *Journal of Allergy and Clinical Immunology, 77,* 65-70.

Starzomski, R., & Hilton, A. (2000). Patient and family adjustment to kidney transplantation with and without an interim period of dialysis. *Nephrology Nursing Journal, 27,* 17-32.

Taylor, S.E., Repetti, R.L., & Seeman, T. (1997). Health psychology: What is an unhealthy environment and how does it get under the skin? *Annual Review of Psychology, 48,* 411-447.

Thomas-Hawkins, C. (2004). Illness representations and activity self-regulation of elders with ESRD. *Nephrology Nursing Journal, 139.*

Thomas-Hawkins, C. (1998). Correlates of changes in functional status in chronic in-center hemodialysis patients. *Unpublished dissertation data,* University of Pennsylvania, Philadelphia.

United States Renal Data Systems. (2003). *USRDS 2003 Annual Data Report.* [Online].Available: http://www.usrds.org

Verbrugge, L.M., & Patrick, D.I. (1995). Seven chronic conditions and their impact on U.S. adults' activity levels and use of medical services. *American Journal of Public Health, 85,* 173-182.

Wainwright, S.P., Fallon, M., & Gould, D. (1999). Psychosocial recovery from adult kidney transplantation: A literature review. *Journal of Clinical Nursing, 8,* 233-245.

Watnick, S., Kirwin, P., Mahnensmith, R., & Concato, J. (2003). The prevalence and treatment of depression among patients starting dialysis. *American Journal of Kidney Diseases, 41,* 105-110.

Weinman, J., Heijmans, M., & Figueiras, M.J. (2003). Carer perceptions of chronic illness. In L.D. Cameron & H. Leventhal (Eds.), *The self-regulation of health and illness behavior* (pp. 207-219). London: Routledge.

Weinman, J., & Petrie, K.J. (1997a). Illness perceptions: A new paradigm for psychosomatics. *Journal of Psychosomatic Research, 42,* 113-116.

Weinman, J.A., & Petrie, K.J. (1997b). Perceptions of health and illness. In K.J Petrie & J.A. Weinman (Eds.), *Perceptions of Health and Illness* (pp. 1-17). The Netherlands:Harwood Academic.

Welch, J.L., & Austin, J.K. (1999). Factors associated with treatment-related stressors in hemodialysis patients. *Nephrology Nursing Journal, 26,* 318-325.

Additional Readings

Centers for Disease Control and Prevention. (2004). Public health and aging: Trends in aging – United States and worldwide. *MMWR, 52,* 101-106 [Electronic version].

Long, J.M., Kee, C.C., Graham, M.V., Saethang, T.B., & Dames, F.D. (1998). Medication compliance and the older hemodialysis patient. *ANNA Journal, 25,* 43-49.

- More than 90 million Americans live with chronic illnesses, and 25 million have major limitations in activities of daily living due to their chronic conditions.

- Approximately 80% of all persons over 65 years of age have at least one chronic condition, and 50% of older individuals have at least two chronic illnesses.

- A theory-based approach to chronic illness management can help nurses and other health care providers understand and identify relevant personal, sociocultural, and health-related characteristics of individuals that may affect how they self-manage their chronic illness.

- The study of individual beliefs about illness and the relationship of these beliefs to illness-related behavior, including illness self-management, have been referred to as the illness perceptions approach to illness self-management.

- The illness representations domain of the CSM is a stage in which people analyze information about health threats and give meaning to them. Cognitive representation of illness refers to the individual's efforts to organize, analyze, and interpret diverse types of information about an illness or its symptoms.

- Emotional representations are one's emotional responses to a health threat; these include feeling states such as anxiety, fear, worry, denial, and depression. Similar to cognitive representations, emotional representations also influence the procedures that one adopts to deal with emotional responses to illness.

- Past illness experiences, social observation, information from others, and culture can help to shape an individual's representation of their health condition or somatic experiences.

- For the chronically ill individual, the family provides the central context for chronic illness management. Every aspect of chronic illness self-management from the representation of illness through the development and execution of coping procedures to appraisal is heavily influenced by interactions with the family and by its impact on the family unit.

- The culture and the experiences of individuals are enmeshed in their interpretations of their illness experiences and health practices as they process internal and external information. Culture can play a significant role in how an individual interprets, clarifies, and categorizes body symptoms, and it provides the context of normative beliefs.

- The CSM provides a theory-based approach to assist nurses to understand the bases for individual patient approaches for managing ESRD and its symptoms, and it can guide nurses to shape or change particular aspects of a patient's illness beliefs or self-management behaviors.

- Adherence to treatment in ESRD is an important self-management issue because of the relationship of adherence to health outcomes in individuals with this condition. Several studies have revealed that individuals who make decisions, either intentionally or non-intentionally, to not adhere to particular aspects of treatment are at higher risk for adverse health outcomes.

- Objective criteria (such as laboratory values and body weight) are useful in clinical practice, but the lack of standardization for these measures may make it difficult to compare adherence outcomes across patient settings.

- Tenets of the CSM indicate that representations and coping procedures are alterable. Research in non-ESRD populations has demonstrated that illness misrepresentations and misguided coping procedures can change with theory-guided interventions. One study will be discussed to illustrate this supposition.

- The CSM provides nurses and other health professionals who care for individuals with ESRD with a practical blueprint to guide these individuals in the management of their illnesses. The view of the patient as an active problem solver is in stark contrast with the passive role to which patients are often relegated in the medical treatment process.

ANNP603

Chronic Illness Management and Outcomes:
A Theory-Based Approach

Charlotte Thomas-Hawkins, PhD, RN

Contemporary Nephrology Nursing: Principles and Practice contains 39 chapters of educational content. Individual learners may apply for continuing nursing education credit by reading a chapter and completing the Continuing Education Evaluation Form for that chapter. Learners may apply for continuing education credit for any or all chapters.

Please photocopy this page and return to ANNA.
COMPLETE THE FOLLOWING:

Name: _____

Address: _____

City: _____ State: _____ Zip: _____

E-mail: _____

Preferred telephone: ☐ Home ☐ Work: _____

State where licensed and license number (optional): _____

CE application fees are based upon the number of contact hours provided by the individual chapter. CE fees per contact hour for ANNA members are as follows: 1.0-1.9 - $15; 2.0-2.9 - $20; 3.0-3.9 - $25; 4.0 and higher - $30. Fees for nonmembers are $10 higher.

ANNA Member: ☐ Yes ☐ No Member # (if available) _____

☐ Checked Enclosed ☐ American Express ☐ Visa ☐ MasterCard

Total Amount Submitted: _____

Credit Card Number: _____ Exp. Date: _____

Name as it appears on the card: _____

CE Evaluation Form
To receive continuing education credit for individual study after reading the chapter
1. Photocopy this form. (You may also download this form from ANNA's Web site, **www.annanurse.org.**)
2. Mail the completed form with payment (check) or credit card information to American Nephrology Nurses' Association, East Holly Avenue, Box 56, Pitman, NJ 08071-0056.
3. You will receive your CE certificate from ANNA in 4 to 6 weeks.

Test returns must be postmarked by **December 31, 2010.**

CE Application Fee
ANNA Member $20.00
Nonmember $30.00

EVALUATION FORM

1. I verify that I have read this chapter and completed this education activity. Date: _____

_____
Signature

2. What would be different in your practice if you applied what you learned from this activity? *(Please use additional sheet of paper if necessary.)*

_____
_____
_____
_____
_____
_____
_____
_____
_____
_____

Evaluation	Strongly disagree				Strongly agree
3. The activity met the stated objectives.					
a. Explain the cognitive representations of illness.	1	2	3	4	5
b. Describe the Common Sense Model (CSM) of Self-Regulation of Health and Illness and the components of it.	1	2	3	4	5
c. Discuss ways the CSM theory-guided practice can be of use to nephrology nurses.	1	2	3	4	5
4. The content was current and relevant.	1	2	3	4	5
5. The content was presented clearly.	1	2	3	4	5
6. The content was covered adequately.	1	2	3	4	5
7. Rate your ability to apply the learning obtained from this activity to practice.	1	2	3	4	5

Comments _____
_____

8. Time required to read the chapter and complete this form: _____ minutes.

This educational activity has been provided by the American Nephrology Nurses' Association (ANNA) for 2.1 contact hours. ANNA is accredited as a provider of continuing nursing education (CNE) by the American Nurses Credentialing Center's Commission on Accreditation (ANCC-COA). ANNA is an approved provider of continuing education by the California Board of Registered Nursing, CEP 0910.

The Kidney

UNIT

2

Unit 2 Contents

Renal Physiology

Christine Chmielewski, MS, CRNP, CNN, CS
Mary Jo Holechek, MS, CRNP, CNN
Marlys Ludlow, MS, RN
Carolyn B. Yucha, PhD, RN, FAAN

David Guthrie, MN, ARNP
Jennifer Dungan, MSN, RN, ARNP
Lori Candela, EdD, RN, APRN, BC, FNP

Chapter Contents

Renal Physiology

Chapter 4

Christine Chmielewski, MS, CRNP, CNN, CS
Mary Jo Holechek, MS, CRNP, CNN
Marlys Ludlow, MS, RN
Carolyn B. Yucha, PhD, RN, FAAN

David Guthrie, MN, ARNP
Jennifer Dungan, MSN, RN, ARNP
Lori Candela, EdD, RN, APRN, BC, FNP

Chapter Editor's Note: This chapter is a compilation of the renal physiology series published in the Nephrology Nursing Journal between April 2003 and August 2004. The individual articles have only been modified as needed to enhance the continuity of the chapter or for formatting consistency. The basic content of each article is unchanged from that published in the series and reflects the opinions and understanding of the individual authors. Textbook Editors Anita Molzahn and Evelyn Butera are indebted to the authors who wrote the individual articles for their contributions to this book. They are Christine Chmielewski ("Renal Anatomy and Overview of Nephron Function," April 2003 issue; Vol. 30, pp. 185-190); Mary Jo Holechek ("Glomerular Filtration: An Overview," June 2003 issue; Vol. 30, pp. 285-290; and "Renal Hemodynamics: An Overview," August 2003 issue; Vol. 30, pp. 441-446); Marlys Ludlow ("Renal Handling of Potassium," October 2003 Issue; Vol. 30, pp. 493-497); Carolyn Yucha and David Guthrie ("Renal Homeostasis of Calcium," December 2003 issue, Vol. 30, pp. 621-626); Carolyn Yucha and Jennifer Dungan ("Renal Handling of Phosphorus and Magnesium," January-February 2004 issue, Vol. 31, pp. 33-37); Carolyn Yucha ("Renal Regulation of Acid-Base Balance," March-April 2004 issue, Vol. 31, pp. 201-206); David Guthrie and Carolyn Yucha ("Urinary Concentration and Dilution," May-June 2004 issue, Vol. 31, pp. 297-301); and Lori Candela and Carolyn Yucha ("Renal Regulation of Extracellular Fluid Volume and Osmolality," July-August 2004 issue, Vol. 31).

Chapter 4 provides an overview of the normal anatomy and physiology of the renal system to serve as a foundation for understanding renal assessment and renal abnormalities. The chapter is divided into 9 sections, which are briefly described below.

Section 1: Renal Anatomy and Overview of Nephron Function

The kidneys are highly vascularized organs that are responsible for maintaining the body's internal environment. The nephron is the basic structural and functional unit of the kidney involved in the complex interplay between tubular and vascular components resulting in the excretion of fluid and solutes. The regulation of body fluid and solutes is governed by the processes of filtration, reabsorption, and secretion. Unwanted fluid and substances are excreted from the body as urine.

This section (a) identifies the anatomic components of the renal system; (b) describes the functional components of the nephron; and (c) explains the various processes involved in urine formation.

Section 2: Glomerular Filtration: An Overview

This section examines the unique characteristics of the renal circulation, describes the physiology of glomerular filtration and reviews the extrinsic and intrinsic factors that can alter renal hemodynamics. Nephrology nurses will be able to (a) define and explain the process of glomerular filtration, (b) identify factors that can influence the glomerular filtration process, and (c) list methods to measure or estimate glomerular filtration rate (GFR).

Section 3: Renal Hemodynamics: An Overview

This section also examines the unique characteristics of the renal circulation, describes the physiology of glomerular filtration and reviews the extrinsic and intrinsic factors that can alter renal hemodynamics. Nephrology nurses will be able to: (a) discuss the intrinsic and extrinsic factors that alter renal hemodynamics, (b) describe the renin-angiotensin mechanism and its role when renal ischemia occurs, and (c) explain the multiple integrated factors that work in concert to maintain a consistent renal blood flow and glomerular filtration despite systemic pressure changes.

Section 4: Renal Handling of Potassium

Under normal physiologic conditions, the kidney is the organ chiefly responsible for the maintenance of potassium balance. Knowledge of the physiologic properties of the distal nephron that affect potassium secretion allows for a better understanding of how potassium excretion can be modulated. This section will review the normal renal handling of potassium and the factors responsible for maintaining potassium balance.

Section 5: Renal Homeostasis of Calcium

Calcium is critical for many metabolic functions. While 99% of body calcium is found as part of the structure of bone and teeth, 1% found in plasma and body cells is crucial for such functions as blood clotting, nerve impulse conduction, and muscle contraction. The homeostasis of calcium is complex because the gastrointestinal tract, the bones, and the kidneys all affect calcium balance. This section reviews the functions, homeostasis, and renal handling and regulation of calcium. The major sites of renal tubular reabsorption and the related cellular mechanisms are described.

Section 6: Renal Handling of Phosphorus and Magnesium

Phosphorus and magnesium are important components of many organic molecules and serve as intermediates of metabolic pathways. As such, their concentration in the body must be maintained within narrow limits. Phosphorus and magnesium balance is maintained by the kidney, the bone, and the gastrointestinal system. Accordingly, the roles and interactions of all three sites must be considered. This section focuses on the renal regulation of phosphorus and magnesium.

Section 7: Renal Regulation of Acid-Base Balance

Because maintaining a normal body pH is essential to the efficient functioning of many physiologic processes, the body has a number of mechanisms that prevent pH fluctuations. Some of these prevent minute-to-minute pH fluctuations over the course of the day, whereas others maintain pH balance from day to day. The kidney plays a key role in both processes. The renal process of bicarbonate reclamation prevents the loss of bicarbonate in the urine and, thus, maintains plasma levels of one substrate that is instrumental to preventing minute-to-minute pH fluctuations. The other renal process, bicarbonate regeneration, replenishes the body's supply of bicarbonate and, thus, maintains pH balance on a day-to-day basis. This section will discuss basic principles of acid-base physiology, the mechanisms that prevent fluctuations in body pH, and the renal processes involved in maintaining a homeostatic pH environment.

Section 8: Urinary Concentration and Dilution

Water constitutes approximately 60% of the healthy adult human body. Water balance in the body is regulated by the kidneys, which excrete either concentrated or dilute urine in accordance with physiological needs. This section describes the mechanisms by which the kidneys vary water excretion independent of excretion of other physiological important substrates such as sodium, potassium, hydrogen, and urea. These mechanisms involve the loops of Henle, the distal tubules, the collecting ducts, and the vasa recta, and are under the control of vasopressin (antidiuretic hormone).

Section 9: Renal Regulation of Extracellular Fluid Volume and Osmolality

In order for our body cells to function properly, they must be surrounded in extracellular fluid that is relatively constant with regard to osmolality. This section describes the mechanisms by which sodium and water input and output are controlled; outlines the neurological and endocrine effects on sodium and water homeostasis; and compares and contrasts the mechanisms for sodium, chloride and water transport in the proximal tubule, the thick ascending limb, and the collecting duct.

Section 1: Renal Anatomy and Overview of Nephron Function

The kidneys are paired vascular organs that perform excretory, regulatory, and secretory functions. In order to understand how these complex organs work, it is necessary to review renal anatomy and understand the renal processes involved in maintaining the body's internal milieu.

The renal system is comprised of the kidneys, ureters, bladder, and urethra (see Figure 4-1). Urine is formed by

Figure 4-1
General Organization of the Kidneys and the Urinary System

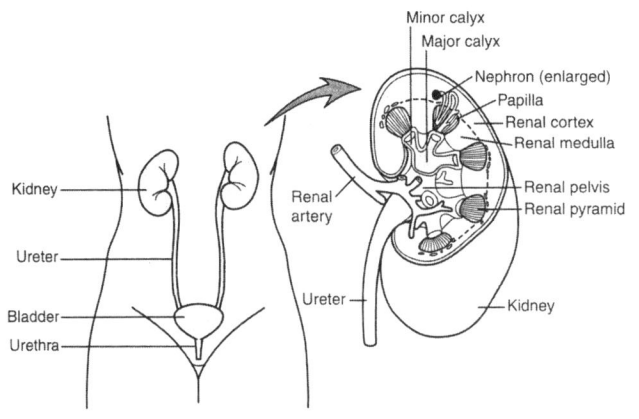

the kidneys and then flows through the other structures to be excreted from the body. The kidneys are located bilaterally in the retroperitoneal space at the level of T-12 to L-3. The organs are bean-shaped, measure approximately 12 cm in length, 6 cm in width, and 2.5 cm in thickness, and weigh 120 to 170 grams in the normal adult. The right kidney is slightly lower than the left because of the liver. The kidneys are protected, not only by their anatomical position within the rib cage, but also by the perinephric structures. A tough fibrous capsule covers each kidney. The renal fascia provides support and perirenal fat acts as a cushion.

The ureters are hollow fibromuscular tubes that begin at the renal pelvis, extend downward retroperitoneally, and join the bladder. Urine flows away from the kidneys by peristalsis. The urinary bladder, located in the pelvic region, is a spherical, muscular sac with a capacity of 300 to 500 ml in the normal adult. Urine enters via the ureteral orifices and is excreted through the urethra.

Vascular Supply

The kidneys are highly vascularized organs and receive approximately 20% of the resting cardiac output. Thus, renal blood flow is about 1,200 ml/min. Two characteristics of the renal vasculature make it different from most other vascular beds in the body. First, there are two capillary beds in series, the glomerular capillary bed and peritubular capillary bed. These capillary beds are separated by the efferent arteriole. This arrangement, a capillary bed surrounded by arterial vasculature, is referred to as a portal system. Second, the capillary bed is more porous. For example, it has a higher rate of fluid exudation than do the systemic

Figure 4-2

Section of the Human Kidney Showing the Major Vessels that Supply the Blood Flow to the Kidney and Schematic of the Microcirculation of Each Nephron

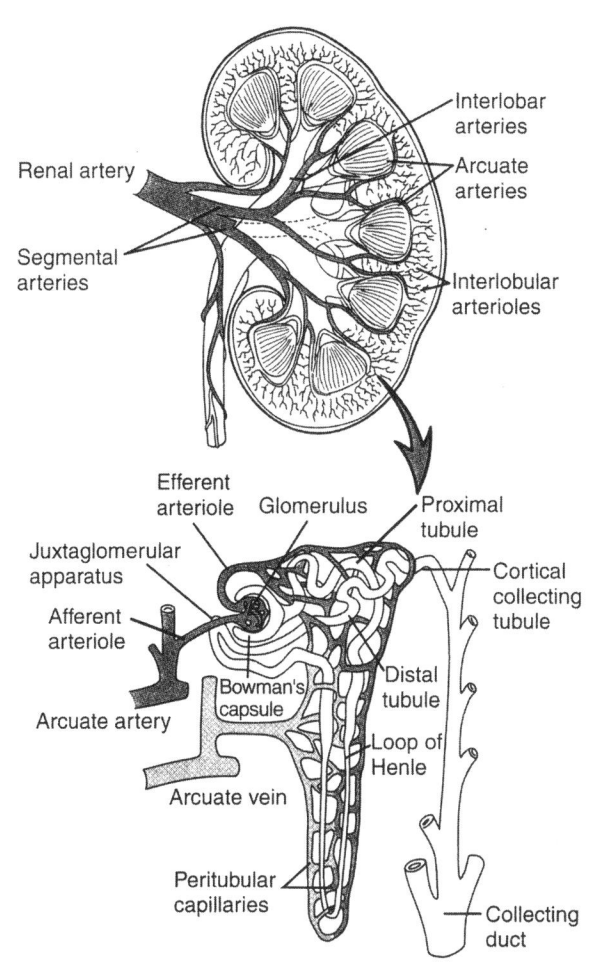

water and solutes reabsorbed from the nephron structures. Blood flow in the remainder of the venous system follows the same pattern as the arterial vessels and returns to the inferior vena cava.

Macroscopic Anatomy

The renal parenchyma consists of two distinct regions, the cortex and medulla (see Figures 4-3 and 4-4). The cortex has a granular appearance because of the structures contained in this layer, namely, the glomeruli, proximal and distal tubules, cortical collecting tubules, and adjacent peritubular capillaries. The medulla contains triangular wedges that have a striped appearance. These wedges are the renal pyramids formed by the long loops of Henle, medullary collecting tubules, and vasa recta. The tapered end of the pyramid, the papilla, directs urine toward the minor and major calyces. Urine then enters the hollow, funnel-shaped renal pelvis, which has a volume of 5 to 10 ml, before flowing into the ureters.

Microscopic Anatomy

The nephron is the basic functional unit of the kidney. There are approximately 1 million nephrons in each kidney. There are two types of nephrons, cortical and juxtamedullary, named according to the location of their glomeruli within the renal parenchyma (see Figures 4-3 and 4-4). The cortical nephrons, which comprise about 85% of the total nephrons, are subdivided into superficial and midcortical nephrons. The superficial cortical nephrons have their glomeruli in the outer cortex and have short loops of Henle. The midcortical nephrons, as their name suggests, have their glomeruli in the midcortex region. Their loops vary in length and may be either short (contained within the cortex) or long (extending partially into the outer medulla). The cortical nephrons perform excretory and regulatory functions. The juxtamedullary nephrons make up the remaining 15% of the nephrons. Their glomeruli are located deep in the cortex near the corticomedullary border. They have long loops of Henle that descend into the medulla often to the tips of the pyramids. These nephrons play an important role in the concentration and dilution of urine by generating a steep interstitial fluid osmotic gradient between the cortex and deep medulla. The vasa recta are responsible for maintaining this gradient.

Glomerulus. This specialized capillary bed is a network of interconnected loops surrounded by Bowman's capsule. As described above, the glomerular capillaries have unique characteristics that contribute to its filtering capabilities. The porosity of the endothelial layer increases capillary permeability, the meshlike structure of the basement membrane provides a barrier to large molecules, and the portal structure allows maintenance of an intracapillary pressure that favors filtration.

The glomerular membrane has three layers: (a) endothelial, (b) basement membrane, and (c) epithelial. The endothelium lines the capillary lumen and contains many pores, or fenestrae, that favor the filtration of fluid and small solutes. The glomerular basement membrane (GBM) is a matrix of collagen and similar proteins as well as glycosaminoglycans that provides a size and charge bar-

capillaries and provides a size and charge barrier to large molecules such as albumin, unlike the systemic capillaries.

The aorta gives rise to the renal artery, which enters the kidney at the hilar region. This, in turn, branches to increasingly smaller vessels, that is, the interlobar, arcuate, and interlobular arteries. The interlobular arteries extend into the cortex and become the afferent arterioles that branch to form the glomerular capillary tufts (see Figure 4-2). The efferent arterioles receive blood from the glomerular capillaries. The presence of arteriolar structures on either end of the glomerular capillaries allows maintenance of an intracapillary pressure favoring the movement of fluid out of the capillary lumen. The efferent arterioles give rise to the second capillary bed, the peritubular network. These capillaries are a low pressure system that favors fluid movement into the capillary lumen. In the medulla, these capillaries, called the vasa recta, form long straight loops that run parallel to the loops of Henle of the juxtamedullary nephrons and play an important role in the concentration and dilution of urine. In the cortex, the peritubular capillaries form a network surrounding nephron segments located within the cortex. This meshwork is designed to efficiently pick up

rier to the movement of large particles out of the capillary lumen. The visceral epithelial cells of Bowman's capsule, or the podocytes, have cytoplasmic foot processes that extend over the basement membrane. Spaces between these foot processes are called slit-pores and allow the filtrate into Bowman's space. Mesangial cells are located between the capillary loops of the glomerulus and form a support network within the tuft. Some of these cells have phagocytic properties.

The glomerular membrane allows filtration of fluid and small molecules. Large molecules are prevented from entering the filtrate in two ways. First the size of the spaces in the glomerular epithelium and basement membrane limits the passage of these larger molecules and cells such as the white and red blood cells and albumin. Second, the podocytes and, to some extent the GBM, have a net negative charge that repels large negatively charged molecules, particularly the plasma proteins. Small anions that easily filter through the pores are not influenced by the negative electrical charge.

Bowman's capsule. Bowman's capsule is made up of two cell layers: the visceral layer that forms the epithelial layer (podocytes) of the filtration barrier and the parietal cell layer that forms the outer layer of the capsule. The space between the two cell layers, referred to as Bowman's space, collects the filtered fluid and solutes and directs this filtrate toward the proximal tubule.

Tubular system. The tubular system has four components: (a) proximal tubule (PT), (b) loop of Henle, (c) distal tubule (DT), and (d) collecting tubule. These components are divided further into subsegments each with specific cellular structures and functions. The kidneys filter about 180 liters of fluid per day with an electrolyte composition similar to that of plasma. Clearly, if all of this filtrate were excreted, total body water and electrolytes would be excreted in a few hours. Thus, the nephrons have the responsibility of handling this large volume of filtrate and separating out that which must be conserved and that which needs to be excreted. The advantage of filtering such a large volume of fluid is that plasma clearance of waste products can occur rapidly. The disadvantage, however, is that the majority of the filtrate must be recycled back to the plasma, with little room for error.

In order to accomplish this tenuous task, the nephron is physically divided into subsegments with "assigned" specific tasks. In general, the proximal tubule can be thought of as the "bulk-phase" segment of the nephron as it transports water and solutes in bulk. It reabsorbs, and thus, returns to the plasma, up to 100% of the filtered solutes that the body does not routinely wish to discard, such as glucose, amino acids, and bicarbonate and reabsorbs a large percentage of solutes, such as sodium, potassium, chloride, calcium, and magnesium, and water whose amounts of excretion will vary throughout the day. This is not to say that regulation of transport of any of these solutes does not occur in the proximal tubule. In fact, transport of most of these solutes is tightly regulated, but the regulation involves a gross versus fine-tune regulation.

The distal nephron, including all subsegments between the thin descending limb of the loop of Henle and

Figure 4-3
Basic Tubular Segments of the Nephron

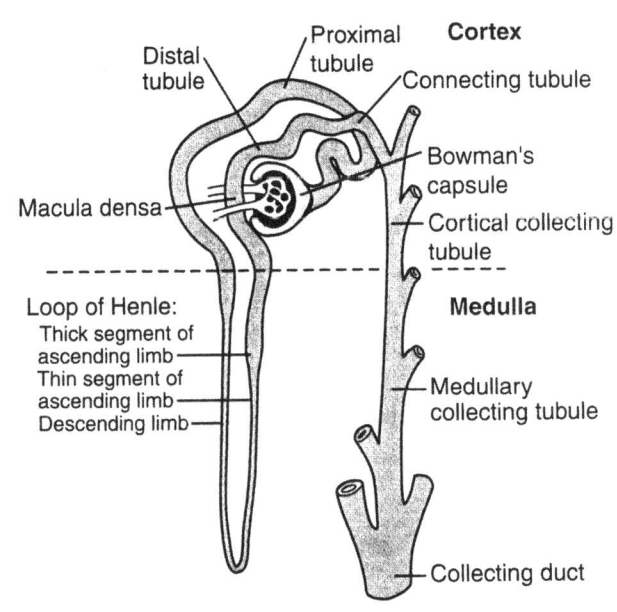

Note: The relative lengths of the different tubular segments are not drawn to scale.
From Guyton & Hall (2000), page 282. Reprinted with permission.

the inner-medullary collecting tubule, is the site of fine-tune regulation of all solutes and water that leave the proximal tubule. In the sections that follow in this series, the nephron segments specifically handling these solutes and water will be discussed in detail, along with discussions of the regulation of solute and water excretion. In total, these processes govern maintenance of a systemic homeostatic milieu with regards to volume regulation, acid-base balance, and electrolyte balance. The next section introduces the nephron subsegments, describing their anatomic differences, and summarizing their roles in water and solute regulation.

Proximal tubule. The PT, which drains the glomerular filtrate from Bowman's space, is located in the renal cortex. The pars convoluta is the convoluted section of the PT and the pars recta is the straight section that descends toward the medulla. The cellular structures of the PT give evidence of its high transport capacity. The flattened epithelial cells have microvilli on the luminal border, which create a brush border and increase surface area available to solute and fluid transport. The cells contain a large number of mitochondria, which are necessary for active transport.

The PT is the major site of reabsorption in the nephron. Sixty-five percent of the filtered water and sodium is reabsorbed here. Other substances reabsorbed include all of the filtered glucose and amino acids, some of the water soluble vitamins, 50% of the filtered chloride, potassium, and urea, 80%-90% of the filtered bicarbonate, 75% of the filtered phosphate, 60% of the filtered calcium, and one-third of the filtered magnesium and remaining solutes. The PT also secretes substances into the tubular fluid. Secretion occurs primarily in the pars recta and includes many endogenous

Figure 4-4
Schematic of Relations Between Blood Vessels and Tubular Structures and Differences Between Cortical and Juxtamedullary Nephrons

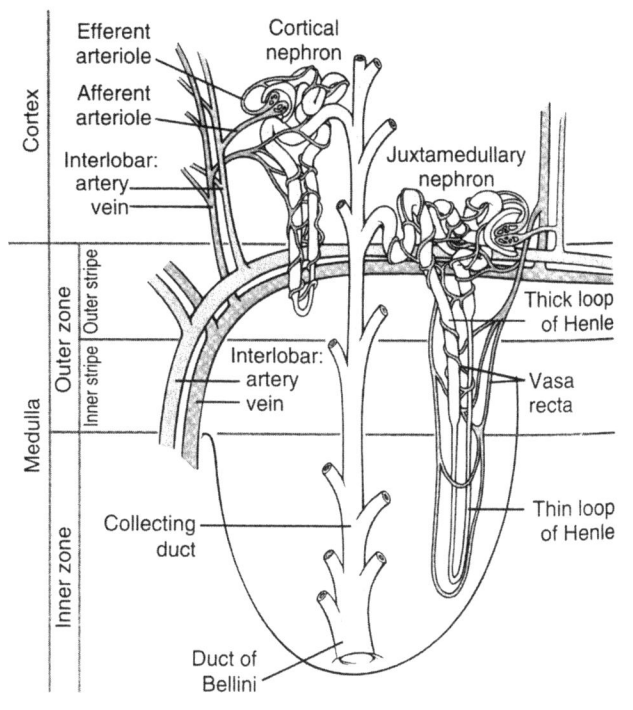

and exogenous organic anions and cations. As a result of these reabsorptive and secretory processes, the osmolarity of the tubular fluid at the end of the PT is isosmotic, that is, essentially equivalent to plasma, or approximately 300 mOsm/L.

Loop of Henle. The loop of Henle is the next component of the tubular system and consists of the thin descending limb, thin ascending limb, and thick ascending limb. Of note, these segments differ between the cortical and juxtamedullary nephrons. Superficial cortical nephrons, with their short loops, do not have a thin ascending segment. This is also true of the midcortical nephrons with short loops. However, the juxtamedullary nephrons and those midcortical nephrons with loops extending into the inner medulla do have a thin ascending limb. In the juxtamedullary nephrons, the long loops of Henle together with the vasa recta are components of the countercurrent mechanism responsible for urine concentration and dilution.

In the thin descending limb and thin ascending segment, the cells are flat with few microvilli and mitochondria. Movement of solutes is by diffusion rather than by active transport. There are functional differences between the two thin segments. The thin descending limb is highly permeable to water but much less permeable to urea, sodium, and most of the other solutes. The thin ascending limb is virtually impermeable to water but transports sodium, chloride, and urea.

The epithelial cells of the thick ascending limb become thick and are similar to those in the PT but with fewer microvilli. The thick ascending limb, like the thin ascending limb, is impermeable to water. Although sodium and chloride are the major solutes reabsorbed, other ions including potassium, bicarbonate, magnesium, and calcium are also reabsorbed. Because of the high solute but low water reabsorption in this segment, the tubular fluid becomes hypo-osmotic.

Distal tubule. The DT is located in the cortical region of the kidney. The initial section of the DT immediately after the thick ascending limb of the loop of Henle contains specialized cells, the macula densa cells, which are a component of the juxtaglomerular apparatus. Following this specialized region, there are two sections of the DT, the distal convoluted segment or early distal tubule and the late distal segment. The tubular epithelial cells of these subsegments are thick and have both microvilli and mitochondria.

The early DT transports a number of solutes including sodium, chloride, bicarbonate, potassium, calcium, and magnesium. However, it is quite impermeable to water. With reabsorption of solutes but virtually no reabsorption of water, the tubular fluid remains hypo-osmotic.

The late DT is a site for regulation of sodium, chloride, bicarbonate, potassium, and calcium transport. These processes are regulated in a variety of manners, including hormonal, physical factors, and/or systemic acid-base or electrolyte balance.

Water-permeability of the late distal tubule is influenced by antidiuretic hormone (ADH), which is produced by the hypothalamus and released in response to input by systemic baroreceptors, osmoreceptors, and angiotensin II. In the presence of ADH, the late DT is impermeable to water, and the tubular fluid remains hypo-osmotic, as solutes, not water, are reabsorbed.

Collecting tubule. A number of DTs join together to form the collecting tubules, which extend from the cortex through the medulla and empty into the papilla. The collecting tubule has three subsegments: the cortical collecting tubule, the outer medullary collecting tubule, and the inner medullary collecting tubule. For the first two subsegments, there are two predominant cell types, the principal cells and intercalated cells. The principal, or light cells, is the predominant cell in the cortical collecting tubule, comprising approximately 90% of the epithelial cells. These cells are involved in the transport of sodium and potassium. The intercalated, or dark cells, are the predominant cell type in the outer medullary collecting tubules, and account for about 10% of the epithelial cells in the cortical collecting tubule. These cells are involved in the transport of hydrogen and bicarbonate and play an important role in the acidification of urine.

In the inner medullary collecting tubules, some intercalated cells are still present, but a different cell type, called the inner medullary collecting duct cells, appears. The exact role of this latter cell type is not fully known, but since sodium, chloride, potassium, and ammonia transport all occur in this segment, this cell may be involved in these processes.

All along the collecting tubule, water permeability is ADH dependent. In the absence of ADH, water absorption along the collecting tubule is minimal and a dilute urine is excreted. In the presence of ADH, water absorption occurs. When ADH secretion is maximal, osmotic equilibration can occur between the collecting tubule fluid and the surrounding interstitium, which can lead to a maximally concentrated urine of > 1000 mOsm/L depending on the interstitial osmolality. Urine osmolalities between these extremes occur with submaximal ADH secretion.

Juxtaglomerular Apparatus

This autoregulatory structure participates in maintaining systemic blood pressure and, consequently, intraglomerular pressure and glomerular filtration. It involves the interplay between vascular and tubular components in the nephron. As the ascending limb of the loop of Henle moves upward, the initial portion of the DT passes between the afferent and efferent arterioles that proceed or form from, respectively, the glomerulus of that nephron. Specialized cells, the macula densa cells, are found in the walls of the tubule juxtapositioned to the glomerular hilus (see Figure 4-3). This region of the distal tubule "touches" the cells of the afferent arteriole, feeding the glomerular capillary associated with that nephron. At this point, the afferent arteriole basement membrane is absent so that the macula densa cells and the afferent arteriole cells "touch," forming a synsitium that allows communication between these specialized cells. These granular smooth muscle cells of the afferent arteriole are called juxtaglomerular cells, which synthesize and store renin, a proteolytic enzyme.

Renal Processes

As blood flows through the kidneys, approximately 20% of the plasma passes from the glomerulus into Bowman's space, forming the glomerular filtrate. This fluid contains no red blood cells, has approximately 0.03% small molecular weight proteins (primarily albumin), and has essentially the same concentration of electrolytes and other small molecules as the plasma. This filtrate undergoes many changes in the tubular system before it is excreted as urine.

Glomerular filtration is the initial process in the formation of urine. The glomerular membrane is highly permeable and allows fluid and small molecular weight solutes to pass into Bowman's space. The glomerular capillary tuft with its interconnected loops increases available surface area. Finally, arterioles at both ends of the glomerulus modulate intraglomerular pressure.

Tubular reabsorption is the movement of fluid and solutes from the tubular system into the peritubular capillaries. This process allows the body to retain fluid and desired solutes. At a glomerular filtration rate of 125 ml/min., the kidneys produce 180 liters of filtrate daily. Yet the average urine output is only 1000 to 1500 ml. Through reabsorption, 99% of the glomerular filtrate is returned to the bloodstream.

The proximal tubule is the major site of reabsorption in the tubular system although reabsorption occurs throughout the nephron. Reabsorption involves both passive and active transport mechanisms. Passive transport includes osmosis and diffusion while active transport mechanisms, such as primary and secondary transport and endocytosis,

require the use of energy to move substances against an electrochemical gradient. Reabsorption of fluid and solutes is regulated to meet the body's physiological needs, through a number of hormonal and neural systems including ADH, aldosterone, angiotensin II, parathyroid hormone, prostaglandins, and alpha and beta adrenergics.

Tubular secretion is the movement of solutes from the peritubular capillaries into the tubular system. It is the process by which the body secretes unwanted or excess substances. Like reabsorption, secretion occurs by both passive and active transport mechanisms. As with reabsorption, secretion of substances is regulated by a number of factors, many of them hormonal in nature.

With regard to active transport mechanisms in both tubular reabsorption and secretion, reference is made to the maximal transport capacity (Tm). Specific carriers exist in the tubular epithelium that are responsible for the movement of substances in and out of the tubular system. However, there is a maximum rate at which substances can be transported in this way. This is known as the maximal transport capacity, or Tm, of the substance. Once the threshold or maximal solute transport rate has been reached, the presentation of larger amounts of solute results in the substance remaining in the tubular fluid (not reabsorbed) or in the plasma (not secreted). All substances actively transported have a Tm. As with all physiological processes, the Tm is subject to regulatory factors, most notably physiological, pathological, and pharmacological.

Excretion is the process by which unwanted substances are eliminated from the body through the passage of urine. These substances include the end products of metabolism such as urea, creatinine, uric acid, drugs, and foreign chemicals and unwanted ingested substances such as sodium, potassium, and phosphate.

Conclusion

The kidneys are responsible for performing various roles in the maintenance of the body's internal environment. A thorough understanding of the renal system with its components and specialized functions is necessary to grasp not only its role in the healthy individual but also in the individual with renal disease.

This section is the basis for the physiology series. Subsequent sections will deal with renal functions in more detail. Topics include renal hemodynamics and glomerular filtration, urine concentration and dilution, renal acidification, renal regulation of extracellular volume, osmolality and electrolytes, and the effect of aging on the kidney.

Section 2: Glomerular Filtration

Glomerular filtration is the first step in the complex process of urine formation. For filtration to occur, a rapid renal blood flow (RBF) at a consistent pressure is essential. There are many factors that can alter RBF and, thus, the rate of glomerular filtrate generation. At any given time, especially under the condition of stress, multiple factors act and counteract to maintain a normal glomerular filtration rate (GFR) despite changes in RBF. This section will examine the unique characteristics of the renal circulation, describe the

Figure 4-5
Renal Circulatory Anatomy: The renal artery branches into the segmental artery, interlobar artery, arcuate artery, interlobular artery, afferent artery, and finally, the glomerulus.

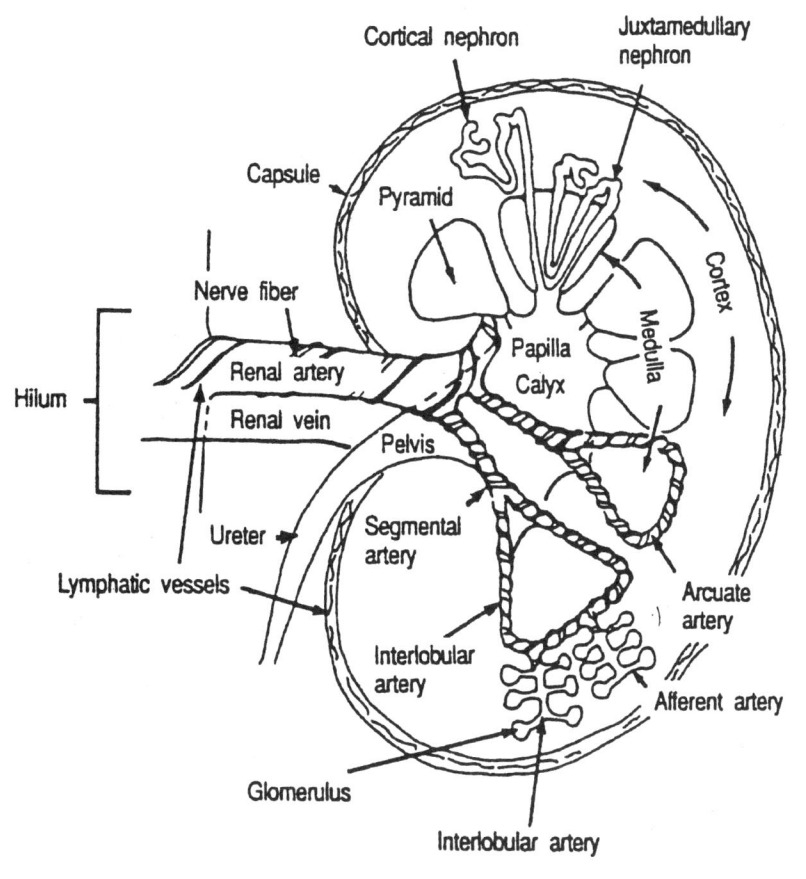

Note: From Richard, C.J. (1986). *Comprehensive nephrology nursing* (p. 12). Boston: Little, Brown & Co. Copyright 1986 by C.J. Richard. Reprinted by permission.

physiology of glomerular filtration, review the extrinsic and intrinsic factors that can alter renal hemodynamics, and discuss a clinical situation in which multiple factors are interacting in an effort to maintain the RBF and GFR despite systemic pressure changes.

Renal Circulation

Blood flows into the kidneys at a rate of about 1,000-1,200 ml per minute, representing approximately 20%-25% of the cardiac output. This rapid blood flow rate exceeds the metabolic and oxygen needs of the kidneys but facilitates efficient clearance of metabolic waste products.

To understand glomerular filtration, it is essential to consider the special characteristics of the renal circulation. Figure 4-5 illustrates the gross renal circulatory anatomy.

The renal artery pressure is approximately 100 mmHg. This high pressure is maintained up to the afferent arteriole, the location of the first major point of vascular resistance. Across the afferent arteriole, the arterial pressure falls to about 40-60 mmHg. Although this is a significantly lower pressure than present in the systemic circulation, this pressure is higher than that in the glomerular capillary bed. This

pressure is referred to as hydrostatic pressure. Maintaining a hydrostatic pressure of about 50 mmHg is the key to glomerular filtration, as it is needed to overcome other opposing pressures present in the glomerular capillaries and Bowman's space.

The glomerulus is a bundle of capillaries that are highly porous compared to systemic capillaries. The portion of the blood that is not filtered across the filtration barriers in the glomerular capillaries returns to the central circulation via the peritubular capillary (PTC) network. (See the first section in the physiology series for a discussion of the PTC network.)

Glomerular Filtration

Glomerular anatomy. The porous glomerular capillaries rest between the afferent and efferent arterioles (see Figure 4-6). Their function is to filter large quantities of water and solutes from the plasma. As blood flows through the glomerulus a portion is sieved through the filtering layers of the glomerular capillaries into the Bowman's space. The filtration barrier is composed of three layers that allow for the filtration of solutes (eg., blood urea nitrogen, creati-

Figure 4-6
Glomerular Anatomy

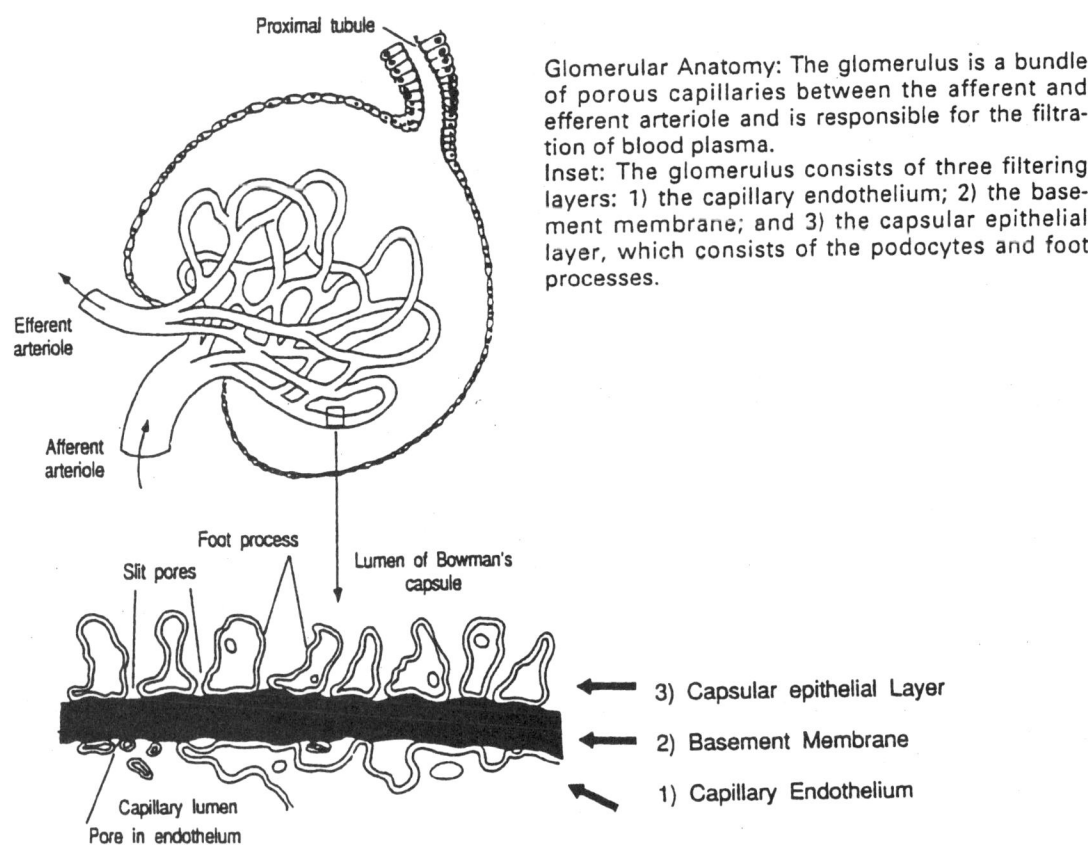

Glomerular Anatomy: The glomerulus is a bundle of porous capillaries between the afferent and efferent arteriole and is responsible for the filtration of blood plasma.
Inset: The glomerulus consists of three filtering layers: 1) the capillary endothelium; 2) the basement membrane; and 3) the capsular epithelial layer, which consists of the podocytes and foot processes.

Note: From Marsh, D.J. (1983). *Renal physiology* (p. 41). New York: Raven Press. Copyright 1983 by Raven Press. Reprinted by permission.

nine, electrolytes) and water, but prevent the loss of blood components such as red and white blood cells and plasma proteins. The three layers are the glomerular capillary endothelium, glomerular basement membrane, and visceral layer of Bowman's capsule (epithelial cell layer) (see Figure 4-6).

The first layer of the filtration barrier is the capillary endothelium, which has large fenestrations that allow the free filtration of substances with diameters up to 100 nm, thus excluding blood cells and large plasma proteins. The surface of the endothelial cells has a negative charge that inhibits the movement of negatively charged substances such as plasma proteins, as like-charges repel each other.

The second layer, the glomerular basement membrane, represents the major barrier to the filtration of macromolecules. The glomerular basement membrane is made of fibrous proteins such as collagen, fibrin, and laminin, which intertwine to form a meshwork. As the fibers cross each other, small openings are created through which selective filtration occurs. The crossed fibers act as a size barrier and restrict the filtration of large molecules. This layer also contains anionic sialoproteins that further inhibit filtration by repelling other negatively charged ions.

The third layer, composed of epithelial cells, is the visceral layer of the Bowman's capsule. These epithelial cells, called podocytes, are attached directly to the exterior surface of the basement membrane. The podocytes branch into multiple finger-like projections called foot processes. These foot processes, which cover the outer surface of the basement membrane, are in close proximity to each other forming narrow elongated, slit-type openings about 25-60 nm wide. These openings, called slit pores, are covered by thin diaphragms. The foot processes have anionic sialoproteins on their borders that form the slit pores, generating a highly negatively charged region through which the filtrate must pass. These negative charges assist in preventing plasma proteins from entering the tubular fluid since plasma proteins carry negative charges. These narrow slits combined with the negative charges of the podocytes provide the final barrier to molecule movement through the glomerular membrane.

The glomerulus is a selective filtration membrane. The factors that determine which molecules are filtered are molecular size, electrical charge, protein binding, configuration, and rigidity. Small molecules with molecular weights (MW) less than 7,000 Daltons (eg., water, MW 18; and all ions including sodium, potassium, chloride, phosphate, magnesium, and calcium) are filtered without restriction. Larger molecules, such as myoglobin with a MW of 17,000 Daltons, are filtered to a lesser degree. Very large molecules, such as plasma proteins with molecular weights approaching 70,000 Daltons, are restricted from passing through the normal glomerulus.

As the filtration barrier has a net negative electrical charge, the movement of large negatively charged molecules is restricted more than molecules with a positive or neutral charge. As a result, proteins, which are negatively charged, are not freely filtered by the glomerulus. Likewise, drugs, ions, or small molecules bound to protein are not filtered. Round molecules do not filter as easily as ellipsoid molecules. The more rigid a molecule, the less easily it filters. Normal glomerular filtrate is essentially protein free but contains crystalloids (eg., sodium, chloride, creatinine, urea, uric acid, and phosphate) in the same concentration as plasma.

A final anatomical aspect of the glomerulus is the mesangial cells, which are located between the capillary loops. They support the capillary structures and carry out some phagocytic activities. They also demonstrate contractile properties and can alter the total filtration surface area. Mesangial cells contract when exposed to vasoconstrictive substances, such as angiotensin II, thus decreasing the effective filtration surface area and glomerular filtration rate. The special filtering characteristics of the glomerulus coupled with the unique renal circulation allow for effective glomerular filtration to occur.

Glomerular Filtration Rate and Filtration Fraction

Glomerular filtrate moves into the Bowman's space and then into the tubular component of the nephron. In the average 70 kg adult, glomerular filtration rate (GFR) is approximately 125 ml/minute. This means that about 180 L of glomerular filtrate is produced in a 24-hour period, which is more than 30 times the average total blood volume. All but one to two liters are reabsorbed from the nephron into the peritubular capillary and vasa recta network. The formation of such a large amount of filtrate assures adequate filtration of plasma, but requires very efficient reabsorptive processes to prevent volume and electrolyte depletion.

GFR, which indicates the volume of filtrate moving from the glomerular capillaries into Bowman's space per unit of time, is calculated by determining the renal clearance of a marker substance. Clearance (CL) is defined as the volume of plasma from which a substance is completely removed or cleared by the kidneys per unit of time. The ideal marker for measuring CL does not bind to proteins, is freely filtered at the glomerulus, and is neither reabsorbed, secreted, synthesized, nor metabolized by the tubules. Substances that do not meet these requirements can result in falsely elevated or decreased values of GFR. As there is no naturally occurring ideal marker, endogenous creatinine (Cr) often is used to measure clearance; however, since a small amount of creatinine is secreted into the tubule, GFR measured with creatinine clearance (CrCL) will be overestimated. Since individual GFRs vary widely, a change in GFR over time is more important than the absolute value of the GFR. Thus, if the CrCL method is used, it should be used for all measurements of GFR to allow for comparison of values over time.

Inulin is a marker that meets all the requirements of an ideal marker for measuring GFR, but is not often used because it is an exogenous substance that must be infused for several hours at a constant rate making it both impractical and costly.

A more practical method to determine the CrCL involves the collection of a 24-hour urine and midpoint plasma Cr (PCr). CrCL is calculated using Equation 1 where UCr is the urine creatinine concentration, mg/dl; Uv is the average urine flow rate, ml/min; and PCr is the plasma creatinine concentration, mg/dl.

Equation 1

$$CrCL = \frac{UCr\ Uv}{PCr}$$

Another method for determining CrCL involves the intravenous injection of a radioactive marker. Clearance of the radioactive marker is assessed by serial scans. The results using this method correlate closely with inulin clearance. The CrCL estimates the GFR and gives a gross indication of how well the kidneys are functioning based on their ability to remove a marker substance.

As using inulin is impractical, urine collections are often inaccurate, and renal scans are costly and require special equipment, the use of alternative methods to estimate GFR have been proposed. The National Kidney Foundation, in its Kidney Disease Outcome Initiative Guidelines, recommends the use of the Cockcroft-Gault formula (see Equation 2) or the more complicated Modification of Diet in Renal Disease (MDRD) study formula (available at www.kidney.org).

Equation 2: Cockcroft-Gault Formula

$$GFR = \frac{(140 - Age) \times Body\ weight\ (kg)}{72 \times Serum\ creatinine}$$

(X 0.85 for females)

Both consider the effects of age, gender, and body weight on creatinine, but no special lab or diagnostic tests are required. The MDRD formula also factors in the effects of race, albumin, and serum urea nitrogen. There are hand-held personal data assistant programs and Web-based calculators with these formulas that easily complete the calculations after the raw data has been entered. Use of one of these standardized formulas with a programmed calculator ensures accurate, consistent results when tracking a GFR over time.

The glomerular filtrate is derived from the plasma portion of whole blood. The term filtration fraction (FF) describes the percentage of the plasma that becomes glomerular filtrate. Since plasma volume is about 55% of total blood volume, normal renal plasma flow (RPF) is approximately 660 ml/min (1200 ml/min x 0.55 = 660 ml/min). The FF can then be determined using Equation 3.

Figure 4-7
Pressures Influencing Normal Glomerular Filtration

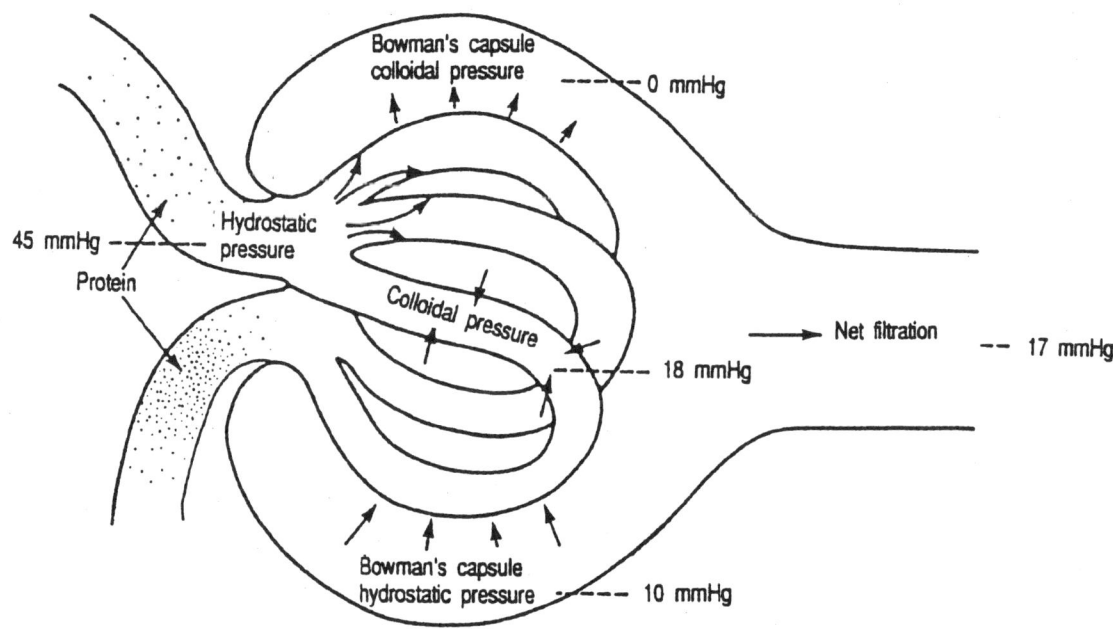

Pressures Influencing Normal Glomerular Filtration. The factor favoring filtration is capillary hydrostatic pressure (45 mmHg). The factors opposing filtration are Bowman's capsule hydrostatic pressure (10 mmHg) and capillary colloidal osmotic pressure (18 mmHg). As Bowman's capsule colloidal pressure is usually 0 mmHg it has no effect. The net filtration pressure produced by these opposing pressures is 17 mmHg.

Note: Adapted from Richard, C. (1986). *Comprehensive nephrology nursing* (p. 23). Boston: Little, Brown & Co. Copyright 1986 by C.J. Richard. Reprinted by permission.

Equation 3

$$FF = \frac{GFR}{RPF} = \frac{125 \text{ ml/min}}{660 \text{ ml/min}} \sim= 19\%$$

Thus, almost 20% of the plasma passing through the glomerulus becomes glomerular filtrate in the average adult.

Pressures influencing normal glomerular filtration. Glomerular filtration is controlled by four pressures, the algebraic sum of which defines the net filtration pressure. These pressures are:

1. Glomerular capillary hydrostatic pressure (PGC), which is the pressure exerted against the capillary wall by fluid within the capillary lumen. This pressure is generated by the blood pressure. This value ranges from 40-60 mmHg and favors the movement of fluid from the capillary lumen to the Bowman's space (see Figure 4-7).

2. Glomerular capillary colloid osmotic pressure (PGC), which is about 18 mmHg. This force, generated by plasma proteins within the capillaries, retards the movement of fluid out of the capillary lumen.

3. Bowman's space hydrostatic pressure (PBS), which is the pressure exerted against the outer layer of the capillary walls by fluids within Bowman's space. This value is about 10 mmHg and also retards the movement of fluid out of the capillary lumen.

4. Bowman's space colloid osmotic pressure (PBS), which is normally 0 mmHg because normal filtrate is void of protein.

Net filtration pressure (NFP), which is the sum of these negative and positive pressures, can be calculated with the following formula (see Equation 4). An average PGC of 45 mmHg is used.

Equation 4

$$\begin{aligned} NFP &= (PGC - PBS) - (PGC - PBS) \\ &= (45 \text{ mmHg} - 10 \text{ mmHg}) \\ &\quad - (18 \text{ mmHg} - 0 \text{ mmHg}) \\ &= 17 \text{ mmHg} \end{aligned}$$

These pressures are based on animal models but are thought to be similar to those in humans. Therefore, for adequate filtration to occur, an NFP of approximately 17 mmHg is required to produce approximately 125 ml/min of glomerular filtrate.

As blood progresses through the glomerulus toward the efferent arteriole, the PGC increases from 18 to approximately 35 mmHg, reflecting the removal of protein free fluid from the glomerular capillary. PGC, PBS, and PBS remain essentially unchanged along the capillary loop. As a result, NFP decreases along the length of the capillary and in some species is zero before or at the end of the capillary. The point at which NFP falls to zero is called filtration equilibrium and is the point at which glomerular filtration ceases.

Conditions altering glomerular filtration rate. The GFR can be altered by changes in any of the above four pressures or the ultrafiltration coefficient. Theoretically, there is a direct relationship between the renal plasma flow rate (the primary determinant of PGC) and the GFR. If RPF increases due to volume expansion or other causes, GFR should also rise. However, a change in RBF rarely occurs in isolation and is usually accompanied by changes in afferent or efferent arteriolar resistance designed to maintain a consistent PGC and, therefore, GFR at normal levels. Through a process called autoregulation, the kidney is adept at maintaining a normal GFR over a wide range of vascular pressures.

Changes in the glomerular colloid osmotic pressure (PGC) can also alter GFR. Serum protein is the major determinant in colloid osmotic pressure. If PGC increases due to increased protein concentration, as in hypovolemic states, NFP and, thus, GFR will fall in an effort to prevent further intravascular volume loss. If the PGC decreases due to protein losses, as in severe malnutrition or hypoalbuminemic states, GFR can increase.

When PBS increases, as in urinary tract obstruction, GFR falls. GFR decreases as glomerular filtrate outflow from the tubule is obstructed and the pressure of the increased filtrate volume in the Bowman's space opposes the forces favoring filtration.

If PBS rises above 0 mmHg, as it does in nephrotic conditions where protein is filtered into the Bowman's space because of changes in the filtering membrane, GFR can increase. The presence of plasma proteins in Bowman's space favors increased filtration due to the increased colloid osmotic pressure within that compartment.

A final factor that can alter GFR is a change in the ultrafiltration coefficient (Kf) of the glomerular capillary membrane. The Kf is the product of the surface area and hydraulic permeability of the glomerular membrane. Vasoactive substances such as angiotensin II can cause the mesangial cells to contract thereby decreasing the available surface area for filtration resulting in a decreased GFR.

Glomerular filtration is the critical initial step in urine formation. In order for adequate solute and water removal to occur, glomerular filtrate must be generated at a constant rate. Changes in RPF, hydrostatic and osmotic pressures, available filtering surface area, and glomerular membrane permeability can upset the internal environment by increasing or decreasing GFR. Fortunately, there exists a complicated system where factors both extrinsic and intrinsic to the kidneys act simultaneously to minimize the effects of these changes.

Summary

Glomerular filtration is a complex process that is impacted by numerous intrinsic and extrinsic factors that can alter renal hemodynamics and RBF. These factors interact in an attempt to maintain a consistent glomerular filtration rate under a wide variety of normal and pathologic conditions. If these integrated systems fail, serious problems can develop with renal function and urine production and excretion.

Understanding the physiology of glomerular filtration and the interactions of factors altering renal hemodynamics will help the nephrology nurse in predicting, identifying, and assisting in the treatment of clinical conditions that alter glomerular filtration and renal hemodynamics.

Section 3:
Renal Hemodynamics

Renal blood flow (RBF), which defines renal plasma flow (RPF), is controlled by a number of physical and humoral factors. These factors are both intrinsic and extrinsic to the kidney. Some of the intrinsic factors include an autoregulatory mechanism, intrarenal renin-angiotensin mechanism, eicosanoids, and kinins. Critical extrinsic factors include the Sympathetic Nervous System (SNS), angiotensin II, antidiuretic hormone, dopamine, and histamine. Endothelin, nitric oxide (NO), and atrial natriuretic peptide (ANP) also play important roles in altering renal hemodynamics. These multiple factors work in concert to sustain glomerular filtration despite wide variations in systemic pressures.

Intrinsic Factors

Autoregulation. The autoregulatory mechanism (ARM), an intrarenal system, maintains a consistent RBF despite mean arterial pressure (MAP) fluctuations from about 80-180 mmHg, but becomes dysfunctional when the MAP is outside this range. The ARM maintains renal perfusion at a constant level during exercise, postural changes, sleep, and physiological crises, even though these conditions lead to systemic pressure changes.

There are two mechanisms believed to be involved in this autoregulatory phenomena: the myogenic and the tubuloglomerular feedback (TGF) mechanisms. The myogenic mechanism is based on the function of baroreceptors (stretch receptors) in the afferent arterioles. When the MAP increases, these receptors respond to the increased vascular wall tension or stretch and cause afferent arteriolar constriction. This constriction prevents transmission of the elevated arterial pressure to the glomerulus, thus maintaining a normal PGC and GFR. There appears to be no effect on the efferent arteriole. Conversely, if the MAP falls, afferent arteriolar dilation occurs to allow for increased blood flow and maintenance of a normal PGC and GFR. This mechanism may also be stimulated by increases and decreases in the delivery of oxygen and other nutrients to the tissues. This mechanism provides a rapid response to changes that can alter GFR and is thought to be most important during episodes where the blood pressure rises rapidly.

The TGF mechanism relates to the function of the macula densa and juxtaglomerular cells. In conditions that increase RBF and, thus, GFR, there is an increased delivery of sodium chloride (NaCl) to the macula densa cells in the distal nephron. When these cells detect this increased NaCl load, they mediate vasoconstriction of the afferent arteriole via an unknown messenger substance, resulting in a decrease in the glomerular blood flow, a decrease in PGC, and a return of the GFR toward normal. Conversely, when there is a decrease in glomerular blood flow, there is a decrease in NaCl delivered to the macula densa cells. This leads to afferent arteriolar dilatation, increased glomerular blood flow, increased PGC, and return of GFR toward normal. Adenosine has been identified as the possible mediator for TGF. This mechanism works more slowly than the myogenic mechanism, but is critical to GFR maintenance in conditions that cause changes in intra-arteriolar pressure.

Neither of these mechanisms alone or together fully explains the ARM, and in all likelihood numerous other factors contribute to this phenomena. There are several essential facts to be noted about the ARM. The ARM cannot completely override changes in the MAP, but it can limit the degree of change transmitted to the glomerulus and the degree to which GFR changes. The ARM will fail to function when there is severe hypotension (MAP < 70-80).

Renin-Angiotensin Mechanism (RAM). The RAM is a critical regulator of intrarenal blood flow that is triggered by internal and external stimuli (see Figure 4-8). It is more important than any other regulatory mechanism during episodes of hypotension. When renal ischemia occurs due to hypovolemia, decreased cardiac contractility, or renal artery stenosis, among other conditions, the kidney produces the proteolytic enzyme, renin, from the granular cells of the juxtaglomerular apparatus (JGA).

Renin release is regulated by two intrarenal mechanisms, the afferent arteriole baroreceptors and the macula densa cells, and one extra-renal mechanism, the SNS. Local renal baroreceptors located in the afferent arterioles constrict in the face of decreased volume, which leads to renin release. The macula densa cells stimulate renin release when they detect a decreased NaCl load being delivered to the distal tubule because of decreased RBF.

Renin cleaves angiotensin I (AI) from angiotensinogen that is produced mainly by the liver. A converting enzyme in the lungs and other tissues splits angiotensin II (AII), a potent vasoconstrictor, from angiotensin I. Angiotensin II is a biologically active compound and causes vasoconstriction of both the afferent and efferent arterioles, but affects the efferent arteriole to a greater degree. Through afferent arteriole constriction, angiotensin II decreases RBF. However, concurrent efferent arteriolar constriction creates a resistance to fluid leaving the glomerular

Figure 4-8
Renin-Angiotensin Mechanism: Local and Systemic Effects

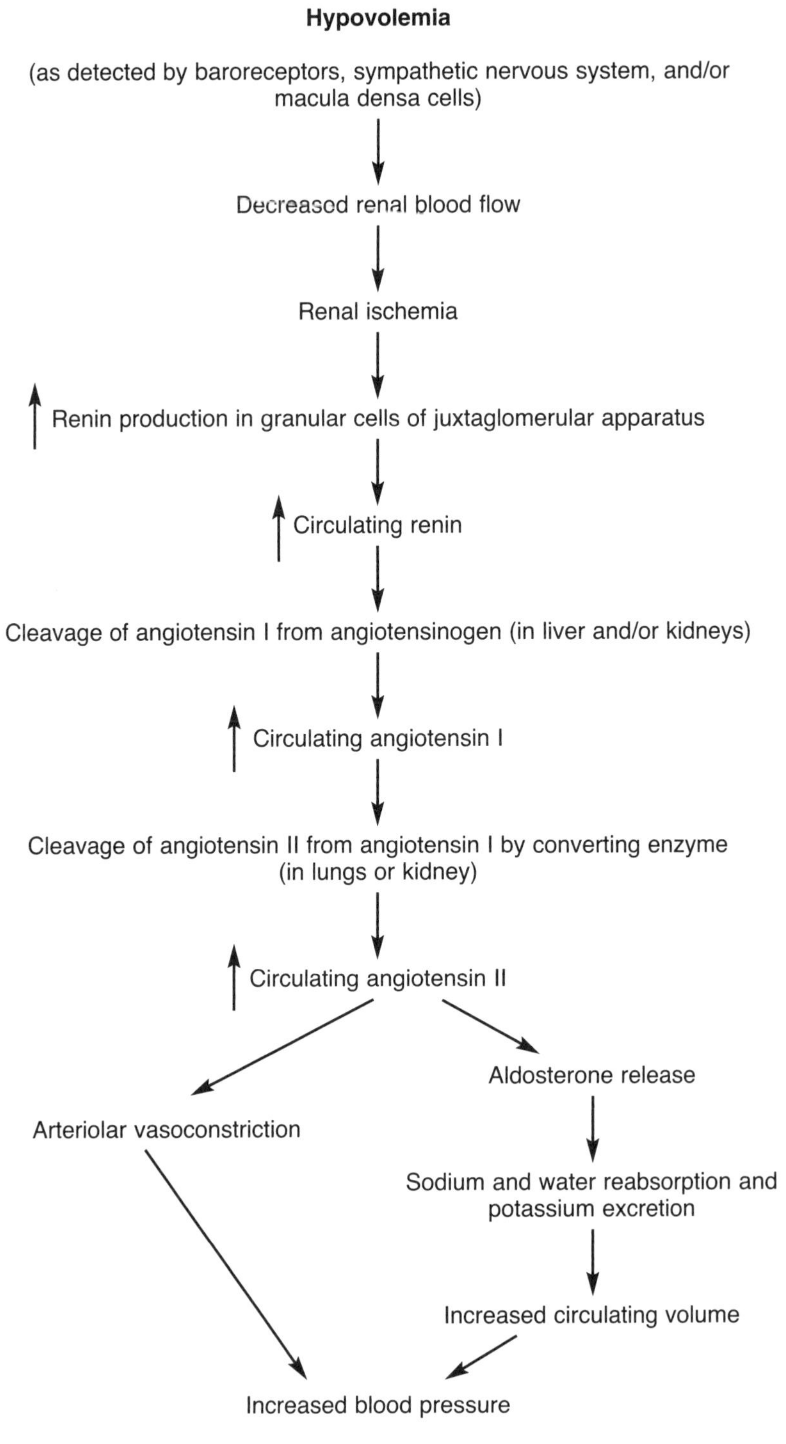

Hypovolemia

(as detected by baroreceptors, sympathetic nervous system, and/or macula densa cells)

↓

Decreased renal blood flow

↓

Renal ischemia

↓

↑ Renin production in granular cells of juxtaglomerular apparatus

↓

↑ Circulating renin

↓

Cleavage of angiotensin I from angiotensinogen (in liver and/or kidneys)

↓

↑ Circulating angiotensin I

↓

Cleavage of angiotensin II from angiotensin I by converting enzyme (in lungs or kidney)

↓

↑ Circulating angiotensin II

↙ ↘

Arteriolar vasoconstriction   Aldosterone release

↓

Sodium and water reabsorption and potassium excretion

↓

Increased circulating volume

↘ ↙

Increased blood pressure

capillaries, which maintains glomerular hydrostatic pressure and GFR at normal values despite the fall in RBF.

The RAM is an intrinsic system that is triggered by local and systemic stimuli. One purpose of this system is to maintain perfusion of vital organs (heart and brain) in the face of hypovolemia, an effect mediated by peripheral and intrarenal vasoconstriction. Unfortunately for the kidney, this system does not spare the kidneys, and RBF is compromised in such situations. However, the decreased RBF will, to some degree, be compensated for by increased efferent arteriolar resistance, preventing a proportional decrease in GFR. When the RBF returns to normal, renin production returns to normal.

Eicosanoid synthesis. Eicosanoids are vasoactive substances produced locally in the kidney by the glomerular and vascular endothelium, nephrons, and interstitial cells. Eicosanoids include prostaglandins, thromboxanes, leukotrienes, and monooxygenase products. Some prostaglandins such as PGE_1, PGE_2, and PG_{I2} (prostacyclin) are vasodilators. Thromboxane, leukotrienes, and some monooxygenase products are vasoconstrictors. The physiologic role of the vasoconstrictor substances is unclear, but the vasodilatory prostaglandins play a major role in maintaining RBF in individuals with impaired renal function.

Prostaglandins are produced in response to increased levels of angiotensin II and norepinephrine and attenuate the vasoconstrictive effects of these agents. The vasodilatory prostaglandins act primarily on the afferent arterioles, counteracting the vasoconstrictive effects of angiotensin II and SNS stimulation, and maintaining RBF despite systemic arteriolar vasoconstriction. The prostaglandins also offset the angiotensin II mediated mesangial constriction preserving adequate surface area for filtration. The vasodilatory prostaglandins protect the kidneys by preventing extreme vasoconstriction in response to AII or norepinephrine. PGE_2 is also a renin agonist. They have little systemic effect as they are rapidly metabolized in the pulmonary circulation. The production of vasodilatory prostaglandins is blocked by non-selective cyclooxygenase inhibitors such as indomethacin, ibuprofen, or other non-steroidal anti-inflammatory drugs. These drugs should not be administered to individuals with renal insufficiency to prevent the loss of this crucial protective mechanism. Only limited data is available on the effects of selective COX-2 inhibitors (eg., celecoxib, raloxifene) on vasodilatory prostaglandins. Preliminary data indicates that COX-2 inhibitors also negatively impact renal function in those with impaired kidneys.

Kallikrein-Kinin synthesis. The kinins are inflammatory mediators produced locally in the kidney. The distal nephron cells secrete the enzyme kallikrein that initiates the process, whereby bradykinin is eventually formed. Bradykinin is a vasodilator, but its physiologic role in the control of renal hemodynamics is not fully understood. It stimulates the release of nitric oxide that leads to vasodilation. It also attenuates the renal ischemic effects of AII and norepinephrine. Although overall bradykinin appears to reverse the effects of AII on RBF, it is ineffective in increasing GFR because of the simultaneous decrease in Kf induced by angiotensin AII. It is important to note that kinins are broken down by the angiotensin converting enzyme (ACE). For individuals on ACE inhibitors, kinins accumulate leading to decreased bradykinin breakdown. This phenomena is responsible for the dry cough and angioedema seen in persons on ACE inhibitors.

Extrinsic Factors

There are multiple extrarenal factors that influence renal hemodynamics. These substances or systems are based outside of the kidneys, but can directly or indirectly initiate changes in RBF and the GFR.

SNS. As noted earlier the SNS plays a role in the RAM (see Figure 4-8). The SNS detects systemic volume changes via cardiac and arterial baroreceptors and can increase or decrease renin secretion and levels of circulating catecholamines accordingly. Catecholamines (eg., epinephrine, norepinephrine) act on the adrenergic receptor sites of the arterioles causing vasoconstriction. In hypovolemic states, the SNS mediates arterial vasoconstriction including vasoconstriction of the renal vasculature. In addition, the decreased volume detected by the stretch receptors in the afferent arteriole leads to the release of renin into the systemic circulation resulting in the extrarenal production of AII.

The sympathetic nerves enter the kidney at the hilum and parallel the arterial system. The nerve endings terminate in the smooth muscle cells of the afferent and efferent arterioles. Direct stimulation of the adrenergic receptors at these locations will result in afferent and efferent arteriolar vasoconstriction. This leads to a decreased RBF, but the concurrent efferent arteriolar vasoconstriction helps to maintain glomerular hydrostatic pressure so that GFR is maintained.

Angiotensin II (AII). In addition to the afferent and efferent arteriolar vasoconstriction described earlier, AII mediates peripheral vasoconstriction. AII also stimulates the release of aldosterone that allows for sodium and water reabsorption thus increasing circulating volume. These two effects combined allow for maintenance of systemic pressure and perfusion of critical body organs. As noted earlier, AII also stimulates the release of vasodilatory prostaglandins attenuating the vasoconstrictive effects of AII on the kidneys allowing for preservation of RBF and GFR.

Antidiuretic hormone (ADH). ADH (vasopressin) in high plasma concentrations also results in renal vessel vasoconstriction, as well as mesangial cell contraction. In the presence of ADH, the RBF and GFR decrease. ADH will also trigger the production of prostaglandins that attenuate its own vasoconstrictive effects. ADH is produced in hypovolemic states, and production decreases when the serum osmolality and/or extracellular volume returns to normal.

Endothelins. Endothelins are potent vasoconstrictors. Three endothelins have been identified (ET-1, ET-2, ET-3), with ET-1 being the most active in the group. Endothelins are synthesized in the endothelial cells of the kidneys, lungs, cerebellum, and major arteries. They are produced in response to increased vessel wall tension, vasoconstrictive agents (AII, vasopressin, thrombin), and inflammatory cytokines (TNF, interleukin). Endothelin works locally within the organ or vessel in which it is produced. It is thought that there are endothelin receptors in the renal vessels and that endothelin causes increased vascular resistance in both the afferent and efferent arterioles leading to decreased RBF and GFR. The endothelins main mechanism of action is through potent vasoconstriction of the smooth muscle cells. ET-1 is inhibited by PG_{I2}, PGE_2, bradykinin, atrial natriuretic peptide, and nitric oxide. In contrast to many other vasoactive agents, ET-1 has a long half-life.

Nitric oxide (NO). NO, formerly known as endothelium-derived relaxing factor, is a substance released from the vascular endothelium. NO triggers the generation of a vasodilatory messenger that causes the relaxation of vascular smooth muscle. It is also thought to block the production of arachidonic acid metabolites that cause vasoconstriction. NO is believed to work in conjunction with other vasoactive substances to maintain normal physiologic tone in the glomerular vessels 24 hours a day. NO is released in response to several vasodilators including histamine, bradykinin, serotonin, and acetylcholine. It is speculated that NO may be a mediator of the vasorelaxation produced by these substances. It also seems to be an AII antagonist at baseline. When precursors of NO are blocked, systolic blood pressure (BP) increases resulting in decreased RPF and variable changes in the GFR.

Atrial natriuretic peptide (ANP). ANP is a hormone secreted by specialized granular cardiac cells primarily in the right atrium in response to right atrial distention and increased right atrial pressure. ANP induces vasodilation of the afferent arteriole and vasoconstriction of the efferent arteriole resulting in an increased GFR. Natriuresis and diuresis are enhanced because of the rise in the GFR. ANP directly blocks ADH release and interferes with aldosterone release directly at the adrenal gland and indirectly by blocking the RAM, thus increasing sodium and water loss from the kidney. The cumulative effects are reduced peripheral and renal vasoconstriction and decreased circulating volume. In conditions of volume overload, as in congestive failure and vasoconstrictive states such as hypertension, ANP attempts to reduce the circulating volume and induce vascular relaxation.

Dopamine. Dopamine receptors within the renal vasculature respond to low-dose dopamine by increasing the renal plasma flow and the GFR through vasodilation. How much of a role dopamine plays in normal renal hemodynamics, however, is not clear.

In this section some of the important intrinsic and extrinsic factors that regulate the hemodynamics of the kidney are examined. All of these factors react and interact simultaneously in the normal individual with intact kidneys. The net result of the interplay of these factors is the maintenance of RBF and glomerular filtration. To close this section, a clinical situation will be examined demonstrating the interaction of these factors.

Integration of Renal Hemodynamic Control Factors

Hemorrhage. In low volume states, such as hemorrhage, multiple alterations occur in both systemic and intrarenal hemodynamics (see Figure 4-9). Uncontrolled hemorrhage ultimately leads to hypovolemia and hypotension. At the extrarenal level, there is increased SNS activity

and catecholamine production as a result of decreased stretch detected by the cardiac and arterial baroreceptors. These extrinsic forces result in generalized vasoconstriction including the renal arterial system. The ARM, particularly the myogenic component, attempts to compensate by dilating the afferent arteriole, but this becomes dysfunctional when the MAP falls below about 70-80 mmHg.

As a result of direct sympathetic stimulation of the juxtaglomerular cells and ischemia initiating the renin-angiotensin cascade, renin and eventually AII are produced. AII causes further systemic and intrarenal vasoconstriction. All of these efforts are directed towards maintaining the MAP at the sacrifice of non-priority organs and structures. Although the RBF falls in response to AII, the fall in GFR is not of equal magnitude because AII maintains pressure within the glomerular capillary by causing greater vasoconstriction of the efferent than of the afferent arteriole.

Another protective mechanism demonstrated by AII is that it stimulates the release of vasodilatory prostaglandins, which will attenuate to a degree the intrarenal vasoconstriction induced by the RAM and SNS. NO may also limit the vasoconstrictive effects of AII. Bradykinin probably also plays a minor role in attenuating the vasoconstriction. ADH will also be produced, contributing to the vasoconstriction. ADH also stimulates prostaglandins release in an effort to diminish its intrarenal vasoconstrictive effects.

The cumulative result of all these forces, in an individual with normal renal function, would be increased vascular resistance with a fall in RBF and GFR. The decrease in GFR will not be nearly as great as it would be without the protective effects of efferent arteriolar vasoconstriction, prostaglandins, nitric oxide, and bradykinin. These mechanisms allow for the maintenance of a reasonable MAP and at the same time protection of the kidney from severe ischemia. If the hemorrhage is not controlled, eventually these protective mechanisms will be exhausted, GFR will decline, and renal failure will ensue.

Summary

Glomerular filtration is a complex process that is impacted by numerous intrinsic and extrinsic factors that can alter renal hemodynamics and RBF. These factors interact in an attempt to maintain a consistent glomerular filtration rate under a wide variety of normal and pathologic conditions. If these integrated systems fail, serious problems can develop with renal function and urine production and excretion. Understanding the physiology of glomerular filtration and the interactions of factors altering renal hemodynamics will help the nephrology nurse in predicting, identifying, and assisting in the treatment of clinical conditions that alter glomerular filtration and renal hemodynamics.

Section 4:
Renal Handling of Potassium

Potassium (K) is the most abundant cation in the human body. The total body K stores in an adult are approximately 50-55 milliequivalents (mEq)/Kilogram (Kg) body weight with 98% of the K located intracellularly. Skeletal muscle has the highest K content per unit dry weight and, therefore, contains the bulk of total body K, while fat and

Figure 4-9
Integration of Major Renal Hemodynamic Control Factors in Hemorrhage

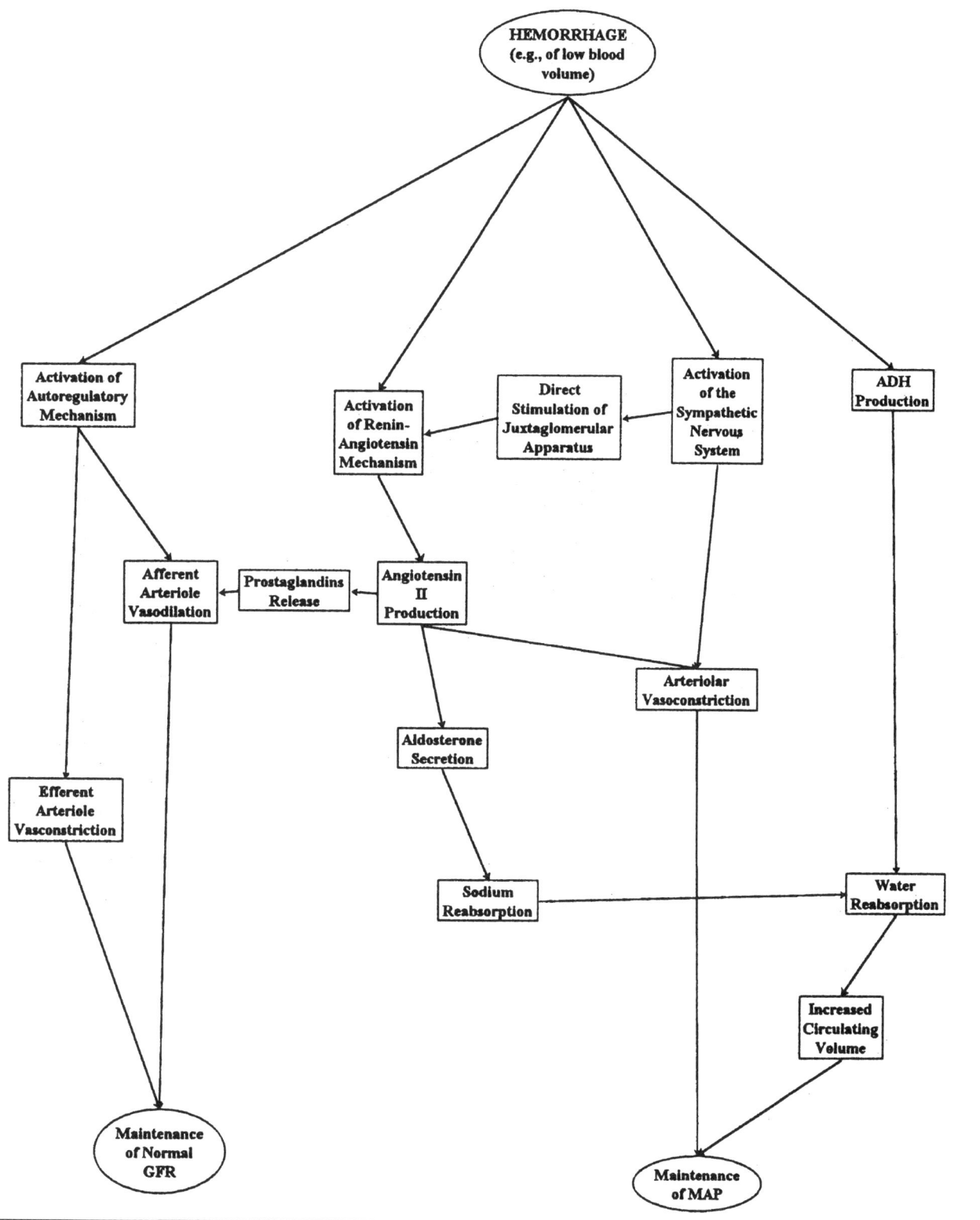

Figure 4-10
Body Cell

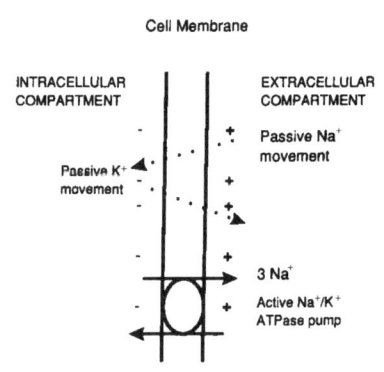

Figure 4-11
Segmental Handling of Potassium

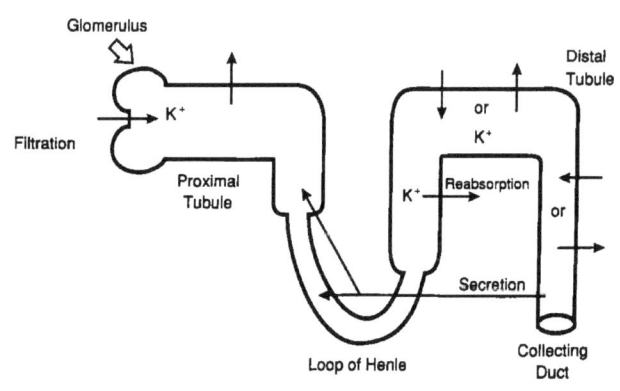

bone have relatively low K content. The high intracellular concentration of K (150 mEq/L) versus the low extracellular concentration (4-5 mEq/L) is a delicate balance critical for normal cell functions. Before reviewing how renal cells control body K content, it is important to understand how individual cells regulate K content. The following discussion addresses the mechanisms responsible for maintaining the K balance in the intracellular and extracellular fluid compartment of individual body cells.

Potassium Functions

Each body cell must regulate its internal K content and concentration in order to regulate cell growth and division, metabolic reactions, acid-base balance, and cell volume. It is also important that appropriate K concentration gradients be maintained across nerve and muscle cells so that appropriate electrical polarization of these cells is maintained for normal neuromuscular and cardiac activity. The movement of as little as 1.5%-2% of the cell K into the extracellular fluid (ECF) can result in a potentially fatal increase in the plasma K concentration.

Sodium-Potassium ATPase Pump

The most important mechanism in maintaining the critical balance of K between the extracellular and intracellular compartments is the sodium-potassium (Na/K) ATPase pump located in the cell membrane. The Na/K ATPase pump actively transports Na out and K into the cell in a 3:2 ratio (3 Na out for every 2K in, thus a net loss of cations). In addition to the active transport system for Na and K, the cells have tiny channels that allow for the passive movement of Na and K through the cell membrane. Because the cell membrane is 50-100 times more permeable to K than to Na, K continually diffuses down its concentration gradient from the intracellular to the extracellular compartment. Na diffuses back into the intracellular compartment but at a much slower rate than the outward movement of K, resulting in a net cation (+ charge) loss from the cell. The consequence of both the Na/K ATPase pump and the cation diffusion process both carrying net positive charges out of the cell is that the cell interior has a negative electrical potential relative to the extracellular compartment (see Figure 4-10).

Extrarenal Regulation of Internal Potassium

An average American diet includes 60-100 mEq of K per day, which requires that 60-100 mEq of K must be excreted daily in order to maintain a homeostatic balance. After a meal, the K absorbed from the gastrointestinal tract rapidly enters the extra cellular fluid. This rise in plasma K is attenuated by the rapid uptake of K into cells in order to prevent life-threatening hyper-kalemia. K absorption by the gastrointestinal tract stimulates insulin secretion from the pancreas, aldosterone release from the adrenal cortex, and epinephrine secretion from the adrenal medulla. These hormones promote the uptake of K into muscle, liver, bone, and red blood cells by stimulating the Na/K pumps on these cell membranes.

Renal Handling of Potassium

Although small amounts of K are lost each day in stool and sweat, the kidney plays the major role in maintenance of K balance. The kidney is able to alter the excretory rate of K in response to the quantity of K ingested. The following discussion will address the renal segmental handling of K and factors that normally regulate K transport in these segments (see Figure 4-11).

Segmental Handling of Potassium

The kidney must excrete >90% of daily K intake in order for the body to remain in K balance. Because potassium is freely filtered at the glomerulus, the K concentration of the fluid entering the proximal tubule is essentially equal to that of plasma (3.5-5.0 mEq/L). Along the proximal tubule, potassium is generally reabsorbed in proportion to solute and water reabsorption. Accordingly, ~60% of filtered K is reabsorbed in the proximal tubule. Entering the descending limb of Henle's loop, a small amount of K is secreted into the luminal fluid, and along the ascending limb, particularly the thick ascending limb of Henle's loop, K is avidly reabsorbed. Consequently, the K concentration of the fluid entering the distal convoluted tubule is lower than plasma, about 2 mEq/L. The connecting tubule and cortical connecting tubule actively secrete K into the tubule lumen. Potassium is passively reabsorbed in the medullary segment with the remainder excreted in the urine. The K

Figure 4-12
Cellular Model for Potassium Handling by the Distal Nephron

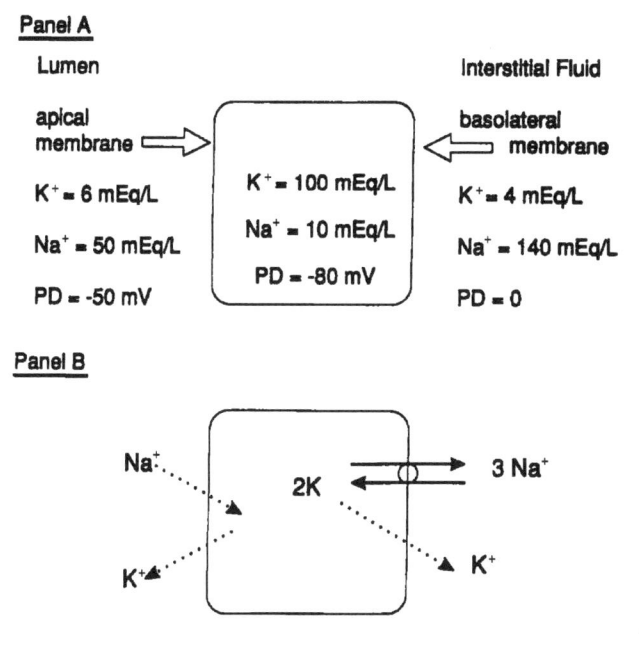

difference or PD) across the basolateral membrane of the cell, such that the cell interior is electrically negative by about 80 mV in reference to the exterior of the cell (see Figure 4-12A).

Across the apical membrane, Na is the primary cation (positively charged ion) reabsorbed under normal conditions. Since the cell interior is negative (280mV) and the Na concentration inside the cell (~10 mEq/L) is less than that in the tubular fluid (~50 mEq/L) (see Figure 4-12A), both the electrical and chemical driving forces for Na favor Na reabsorption from the luminal fluid into the cell. Since the anion most frequently accompanying Na is Cl, which is reabsorbed at a much slower rate than Na, the luminal compartment develops a negative PD as a consequence of Na diffusing into the cell.

As shown in Figure 4-12A, both the cell interior and the luminal compartment are negative in reference to the interstitial fluid. Because the cell is more negative than the luminal compartment, the electrical driving force between the lumen and cell interior opposes the movement of K (a positively charged ion) out of the cell, that is K is 'held' within the cell. However, due to the high intracellular K concentration (100 mEq/L) and the low luminal fluid K concentration (mean luminal ~6 mEq/L), the chemical driving force for K favors K secretion from the cell to the luminal compartment. These are opposing forces. However, the chemical driving force is larger than the electrical driving force, therefore, the net driving force favors K secretion.

In summary, the net movement of K from the extracellular fluid into the tubule lumen occurs by K first being actively transported from the interstitial fluid, which is in equilibrium with plasma, into the cell across the basolateral membrane on the Na/K ATPase pump, and then passively diffusing from the cell into the tubule fluid through the K channels in the apical membrane, driven by the electrochemical gradient. Changes in the rate of K secretion are secondary to changing (a) the rate of K accumulation within the cell, that is, the activity of the Na/K ATPase pump on the basolateral membrane; or (b) the magnitude and direction of the driving force for K secretion across the apical membrane. The latter involves the intracellular K concentration, luminal K concentration, and electrical gradient across the apical membrane. The influence of various factors on net K secretion will be discussed below in relationship to altering one or more of these determinants of K secretion.

reabsorbed in the medullary segment of the tubule is the source of the K secreted into the proximal straight tubule and descending loop of Henle.

The major site for regulating net K excretion occurs in the late distal tubule and cortical collecting tubule. The cellular mechanisms for regulating K transport are essentially the same in the 2 nephron segments, and therefore, will be discussed together using 1 cellular model (see Figures 4-12A and 4-12B). Depending on the K balance of the body, these nephron segments will either reabsorb or secrete K. In conditions of K deficiency, reabsorption will occur, and when the body is in a positive K balance, secretion will occur. The latter is the normally occurring situation. In order to discuss regulation of K transport in these segments, it is necessary to characterize the cell responsible for K transport. The discussion below will focus on K secretion, since that is the more frequent direction of net transport.

Cellular model for potassium transport. In the late distal tubule, the cell type responsible for K transport is the late distal tubule cell, and in the cortical collecting tubule, the cell type is the principal cell. The late distal tubule cell is similar in many ways to the principal cell, but is so named because of its location. In these cells (see Figure 4-12B), the basolateral membrane (side of the cell facing the peritubular capillaries) contains the Na/K ATPase pump and a K channel. The apical membrane (side of the cell facing the tubule lumen) contains both Na and K channels.

The activity of the Na/K pump transporter is exquisitely sensitive to the K concentration of blood. When extracellular K concentration increases, the pump increases its activity and more K is taken up by the cell. When plasma K concentration is decreased, the reverse is true. Due to the imbalance of charge generated by exchanging 3 Na ions for 2 K ions, there is an electrical gradient (called a potential

Regulation of potassium secretion. Major factors that influence net K secretion include: (a) dietary K intake, (b) distal tubule flow rate, (c) distal delivery of non-reabsorbable anions, (d) aldosterone levels, and (e) acid-base balance.

Dietary potassium intake. When K intake increases, the K absorbed from the GI tract first appears in the extracellular pool (plasma and interstitial fluid). The Na/K ATPase pump on the baso-lateral membrane is exquisitely sensitive to the extracellular K concentration, and the uptake of K from the extracellular to the intracellular pool is a mechanism of defense against an increase in extracellular K concentration. Although this uptake of K occurs in almost all cells of the body, its occurrence in the late distal

Figure 4-13
Effect of Luminal Flow Rate on Potassium Secretion

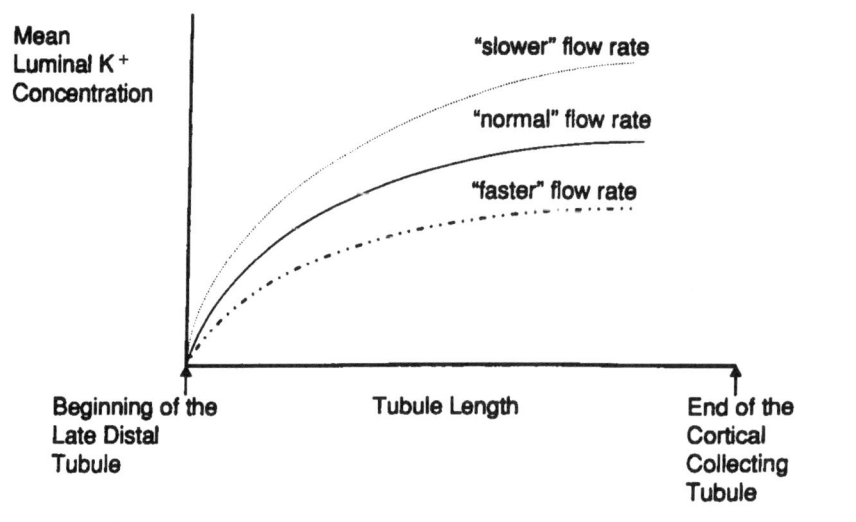

tubule and principal cells facilitate K secretion by increasing the intracellular K concentration, and therefore, the chemical gradient for K secretion into the luminal fluid (see Figure 4-12A). The increase in K secretion leads to an increase in K excretion. Increases in plasma K concentration also stimulate aldosterone secretion, which contributes to enhancing K secretion as described below.

Distal tubule flow rate. K is secreted into the luminal fluid as the fluid flows along the distal and cortical collecting tubules. Consequently, the K concentration rises along the length of the tubule (see Figure 4-13, solid line). If luminal fluid flow rate increases, that is, transverses the distal and cortical collecting tubules in a shorter time period, the mean luminal K concentration will be less than "normal" due to less time available for K to be secreted into the luminal fluid (see Figure 4-13, dashed line). The reverse is true for a decrease in luminal fluid flow rate (see Figure 4-13, dotted line). When luminal flow rate is slower than normal, the mean K concentration will be higher than "normal," due to the longer time available for K to enter the luminal compartment. At theoretical extremes of flow rate, luminal K concentration would remain at 2 mEq/L (infinitely fast flow rate) or become equal to intracellular K concentration (100 mEq/L) at infinitely slow flow rates.

Since the K concentration of the luminal fluid is one determinant of the net driving force governing K secretion across the apical membrane, it follows that when distal tubule fluid flow rate increases, the rate of K secretion, and therefore, excretion will increase. When distal tubule flow rate decreases, the rate of K secretion and excretion will decrease.

Although changes in extracellular fluid volume lead to changes in distal tubule flow rate, K secretion is relatively unaffected because of the offsetting effects of aldosterone. In the presence of loop diuretics, such as furosemide, or thiazide diuretics, which inhibit NaCl and secondarily water reabsorption prior to the late distal tubule, luminal

flow rates increase substantially in the late distal and cortical collecting tubules. This leads to an increase in K secretion, and thus K excretion. This is the mechanism by which K depletion occurs in patients on these diuretics.

Distal delivery of nonreabsorbable anions. The anion accompanying the majority of Na delivered to the distal tubule is chloride. Although Cl is reabsorbed in these segments, the rate of reabsorption is slower than that of Na, which explains the luminal negativity of these nephron segments. If the anion accompanying Na is not Cl, then the magnitude of the luminal negativity will depend on the rate at which the anion is reabsorbed. If the anion is reabsorbed more easily than Cl, the lumen will become less negative, and if the anion is less readily reabsorbed the luminal negativity will increase. The latter situation occurs when bicarbonate or organic anions, such as penicillin, are the anions accompanying Na. These anions are less readily reabsorbed than Cl. Subsequently, luminal negativity increases and K secretion and excretion are enhanced.

Aldosterone. Aldosterone is a hormone synthesized and secreted from the adrenal cortex. Aldosterone secretion is influenced by many factors, two of which are pertinent to the regulation of K balance. These are plasma K concentration and extracellular volume. Increases in aldosterone secretion are associated with increases in plasma K concentration and decreases in extracellular volume.

Aldosterone has three major effects on the cells in the distal nephron involved in regulating K excretion. The first is to increase Na/K ATPase pump activity. This results in an increase in cellular K uptake, intracellular K content, and the magnitude of the K concentration gradient across the apical membrane. These results cause an increase in the rate of K secretion into the luminal fluid. The second effect is the increase in the K permeability of the apical membrane. K transverses the apical membrane through channels. Because aldosterone increases the ease with which K can pass through the channels, more K can be secreted in a given period of time. The third effect is to increase the rate of Na uptake across the apical membrane. The consequence is an increase in the luminal negativity, an effect that enhances K secretion by the same mechanism described above for increased delivery of nonreabsorbable anions.

Increases in dietary intake of K lead to enhanced secretion secondary to raising intracellular K concentrations. In addition, intake-induced increases in plasma K concentration stimulate aldosterone secretion, which will facilitate K secretion by the three mechanisms described above.

The effects of aldosterone associated with changes in extracellular volume are more complex. When extracellular volume is low, GFR decreases, distal delivery of solutes and water decreases, and luminal flow rate is reduced. If this were the sole effect of extracellular volume, then K secretion should be significantly impaired as previously discussed (see Figure 4-13). However, decreases in extracellular volume stimulate aldosterone secretion, which enhances K secretion. When extracellular volume is increased, the opposite occurs, that is that distal flow rate increases and aldosterone secretion is suppressed. The net effect of these two opposing factors is that changes in extracellular volume, although associated with dramatic changes in distal tubular flow rate, are not associated with dramatic effects on net K secretion. Therefore, K balance remains relatively independent of extracellular volume status.

Acid-base balance. The acid-base balance of the body is another factor that affects K secretion in the distal tubule. In acidemic states, some of the excess hydrogen (H) is buffered intracellularly. To maintain electroneutrality, K moves into the extracellular fluid, raising the plasma K concentration. The result is a decrease in the amount of K available for secretion into the luminal fluid. In addition, a decrease in cell pH (acidosis) decreases the K permeability of the apical membrane. Accordingly, at any given driving force for K secretion, less K will be secreted because of the enhanced difficulty of K passing through the K channels.

The cation shifts are reversed in alkalemia, and the plasma K+ concentration tends to fall and the intracellular K content increases. In addition, alkalosis is associated with an increase in the K permeability of the apical membrane. Therefore, during metabolic alkalosis, there is an increase in K secretion into the lumen. These changes are usually transient and of minor significance.

In general, metabolic acidosis results in a decrease in K excretion and an increase in plasma K. Conversely, metabolic alkalosis enhances K excretion and decreases plasma K. The changes in plasma K concentration associated with respiratory acid-base disturbances are described as minor. The reason for this is not know.

Conclusion

The maintenance of a normal plasma K concentration depends upon extrarenal and renal control mechanisms. The extrarenal mechanisms (insulin, epinephrine, aldosterone) are effective in the transitory movement of K into the intracellular compartment. The renal mechanism is responsible for the chronic maintenance of "normal" body K content. When these transient and chronic regulatory mechanisms are functioning in concert, large variations in K intake have relatively minor effects on plasma K concentration.

Section 5:
Renal Homeostasis of Calcium

The homeostasis of calcium is complex because the gastrointestinal tract, the bone, and the kidney all affect calcium balance. Earlier sections in this chapter have been concerned almost entirely with the *renal* handling of ions and water homeostasis. This approach is not possible when dealing with calcium because two other major organ systems are also involved in controlling its concentration – the skeletal system and the gastrointestinal system. The fact that redundant regulatory processes have evolved that enable calcium concentration to be maintained underscores the importance of calcium for optimal physiological functioning. Accordingly, the roles and interactions of all three sites must be considered.

Functions and Forms of Calcium

Calcium is a necessary ion for many metabolic processes. Due to its structural features, which make it well suited for its diverse biological roles, calcium can be rapidly bound and released from many different proteins. This enhances calcium's ability to regulate ion channels and promote activation of enzymes. It is the major cation within the structure of bone and teeth. The following processes depend on calcium:

Neuromuscular excitability. Normal membrane excitability depends on a consistent calcium level. When extracellular calcium falls, membrane permeability increases nonselectively. This increase in permeability increases neuromuscular excitability. If left unchecked, a decreasing serum calcium level will result in spontaneous muscle contractions (tetany). On the other hand, hypercalcemia has the opposite effect and may lead to decreased neuromuscular activity, cardiac arrhythmias, lethargy, muscle weakness, and disorientation.

Secretion. Calcium is essential for secretion of many hormones and neurotransmitters. When serum calcium levels drop, both hormone and neurotransmitter secretion is impaired. Enzymes activated by calcium binding regulate critical intracellular functions such as DNA formation, glycogen metabolism, actin/myosin muscular filament contraction, and mitosis.

Alveolar surfactant. In the setting of reduced calcium, surfactant spreads so slowly that its role in reducing alveolar surface tension is impaired.

Coagulation. Calcium is required for blood clotting to occur. It promotes several reactions along the coagulation cascade, most notably the conversion of prothrombin to thrombin and the conversion of fibrinogen to fibrin. Fortunately, calcium ion concentration rarely falls low enough to significantly affect clotting. However, with severe blood loss requiring multiple red blood cell (RBC) transfusions, calcium ion concentration is lowered because the citrate ion (present in transfusion preparations) reacts with and lowers the total body calcium ion concentration.

Figure 4-14
Calcium Homeostasis: Daily Calcium Metabolism

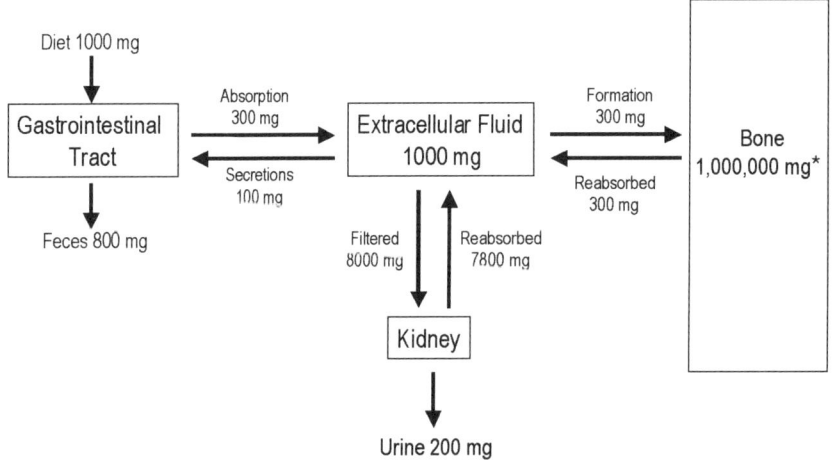

The regulation of extracellular calcium concentration is a complex phenomena affected by the rates of formation and absorption of bone, by the rates of secretion and absorption in the GI tract, and by the rates of filtration and reabsorption by the kidney.

*Total amount stored in the bone

The total body calcium is about 1,200 g, 99% of which is located within bone as hydroxyapatite. The remainder is in the plasma and body cells. The total plasma calcium reflects the extracellular calcium level, which is less than the intracellular calcium level. The phosphate level is normally higher intracellularly (due to its role in ATP); keeping a low intracellular calcium level prevents precipitation of calcium phosphate within the cell. The total plasma calcium (normally 4.5-5.5 mEq/L or 8.6-10.5 mg/dl) exists in three general forms.

Ionized. Approximately 45% (4.5 mg/dl) is in the free or ionized form (Ca^{++}). This is the only biologically active form in nerve, muscle, and other target organs and is the form that is regulated. This form of calcium is diffusible across cell membranes and can be filtered at the glomerulus of the nephron.

Bound. About 40% (4.0 mg/dl) is reversibly bound to plasma proteins, with albumin accounting for 90% of this. When the serum protein level is reduced, more calcium is in the ionized state; when serum proteins are elevated, more calcium is in the bound form. Protein binding is also influenced by plasma pH. During alkalosis, hydrogen ions are released from protein exposing more negatively charged binding sites. This increases the sites available for calcium binding and reduces the amount of free calcium in the plasma. Thus, a patient with alkalosis is susceptible to tetany. In contrast, under acidotic conditions, proteins are saturated with hydrogen. Therefore, there are fewer sites on proteins available for calcium binding and more calcium remains in the plasma in its ionized form. Thus, an acidotic patient may not show tetany at calcium levels low enough to produce symptoms in other people. Bound calcium is not diffusible across cell membranes and is not filtered at the glomerulus.

Complexed. Approximately 15% of the calcium in plasma (1.5 mg/dl) is complexed to anions such as chloride, citrate, and phosphate. This form of calcium is diffusible and available for filtration at the glomerulus.

Calcium Imbalances

The importance of the control of calcium concentration can be illustrated by considering the consequences of abnormal concentrations of calcium. Hypercalcemia decreases the permeability of the cell membranes to sodium ions, preventing normal depolarization of nerve and muscle cells. This can lead to cardiac arrhythmias, fatigue, weakness, lethargy, anorexia, nausea, and constipation. Hypercalcemia also leads to the deposition of calcium carbonate salts in soft tissues, resulting in irritation and inflammation or in the development of kidney stones. In contrast, hypocalcemia increases the permeability of cell membranes to sodium ions such that nerve and muscle tissues undergo spontaneous action potential generation. This may lead to confusion, muscle spasms, hyperreflexia, intestinal cramping, and may progress to convulsions, tetany, and respiratory failure.

Calcium Homeostasis

Calcium is regulated at three different sites, the bone, the intestine, and the kidney, as shown in Figure 4-14. Of the 1,000 mg ingested each day, approximately 300 mg is absorbed from the GI tract and enters the extracellular fluid. From here it may be stored in bone or excreted by the kidney, depending on the presence of parathyroid hormone, Vitamin D3, and calcitonin.

Control of calcium concentration may be divided into daily control and long-term control. The calcium ion concentration in the extracellular fluid (ECF) remains within a few percent of 2.4 mEq/l and on a day-to-day basis is controlled principally by the effect of parathyroid hormone on

Table 4-1
Calculating the Amount of Calcium Filtered

Amount filtered per minute	= GFR	x	[Ca]
	120 ml/min	x	5.0 mg/dl
	120 ml/min	x	0.05 mg/ml
	6 mg/min		
Amount filtered per day	= 6 mg/min x 60 min x 24 hours = 8,640 mg.		

bone absorption. Bone is not a fixed, dead tissue; rather, it is cellular and well supplied with blood. Bone is constantly broken down (absorbed) and simultaneously reformed under the influence of the bone cells, osteoclasts and osteoblasts, respectively. Thus, bone provides a huge source or storage area for the withdrawal or deposit of calcium. Typically 300 mg of calcium is used to build new bone and 300 mg is reabsorbed from bone each day.

The long-term control of calcium results from the reabsorption of calcium from the kidney tubules and from the gut through the intestinal mucosa. Under normal conditions, only part of the ingested calcium (approximately 300 mg) is absorbed from the intestine. Gastric secretions contain about 100 mg of calcium; thus, 800 mg is excreted in the feces. Accordingly, control of the active transport system that moves calcium from the intestinal lumen to the blood can result in large increases or decreases in net calcium absorption, thereby assisting in the regulation of total body calcium.

Renal Handling of Calcium

The kidneys control calcium by filtration and reabsorption. Only about 60% of the plasma calcium is filterable, the free calcium and that bound to anions. Protein-bound calcium is not filterable and remains in the plasma. Since calcium is both filtered at the glomerulus and reabsorbed by the tubules but is not secreted, the amount of calcium excreted can be described by the following equation:

Calcium Excreted = Calcium Filtered – Calcium Reabsorbed

The amount of calcium filtered can be calculated by multiplying the glomerular filtration rate (GFR) by the serum concentration of filterable calcium. To illustrate, if the GFR is 120 ml/min and the serum filterable calcium concentration is 5.0 mg/dl, the daily filtered load would be approximately 8,640 mg (see Table 4-1).

The filtered load may be altered by changes in the GFR or the serum calcium concentration. For example, the filtered load is reduced by a decreased GFR, such as occurs in chronic renal failure, or by a fall in the serum calcium concentration. Such alterations would lead to a reduction in the renal excretion of calcium if the amount reabsorbed were unchanged.

Changing the amount that is reabsorbed can also alter the amount of calcium excreted. In many situations, both the amount filtered and the amount reabsorbed change. For example, when calcium intake rises, the plasma calcium concentration increases. This increases the amount of calcium that is filtered. In addition, the rise in plasma calcium

triggers hormonal changes that cause a diminished reabsorption. The net result is an increase in calcium excretion. Of the amount of calcium filtered, 98%-99% is reabsorbed. Approximately 60%-70% of the filtered load is reabsorbed in the proximal tubule, 20% in the thick ascending limb of Henle's loop, and 5%-10% in the distal tubule.

Proximal tubule. The majority of the calcium filtered by the glomerulus is recovered by the proximal tubule along with sodium and chloride. Sodium is actively reabsorbed in the proximal tubule. It is followed passively by chloride and water. The ratio of the calcium concentration [Ca] in tubule fluid (TF) relative to the plasma ultrafiltrate (UF) is represented by the expression $[TF/UF]_{Ca}$. This ratio remains near one along the proximal tubule, indicating that calcium reabsorption is paralleling sodium and fluid reabsorption. Changes in the rate of fluid reabsorption are accompanied by changes in calcium reabsorption. This suggests that calcium reabsorption in the proximal tubule occurs primarily through passive diffusion, probably by moving between the cells (i.e., a paracellular route), rather than through the cells (i.e., a transcellular route). A small amount of calcium is also absorbed via an active-transport pathway (requiring expenditure of energy in the form of ATP). This route requires transport proteins capable of moving calcium from the tubular cells across the basolateral membrane against its electrochemical gradient. Two such transporters are the plasma membrane Ca^{2+}-ATPase, which is an ATP-dependent pump, and the Na^+-Ca^{2+}-exchanger, a carrier protein that derives its energy from the inwardly directed Na^+ gradient that is generated by the continuous activity of the Na^+-K^+-ATPase. By the end of the proximal tubule, 60% to 70% of the filtered calcium has been absorbed.

Loop of Henle. Calcium transport by thin descending and thin ascending limbs is minimal because of the low calcium permeability of these segments. In the thick ascending limb (where 20%-25% of filtered calcium is reabsorbed), calcium is reabsorbed by both passive and active mechanisms. In this segment, chloride is actively reabsorbed. Movement of a negatively charged ion out of the tubular fluid leaves behind a positive voltage in the lumen. Calcium reabsorption is driven passively, paracellularly, as the lumen-positive voltage repels the positively charged calcium ions. When the transepithelial voltage is manipulated experimentally, the direction and rate of calcium movement is changed. That is, when the voltage is zero, there is no net calcium movement, and when the voltage is negative, calcium secretion occurs. An active transport mechanism may also exist in this nephron segment, transcellularly, since under certain conditions calcium reabsorption occurs, even when the electrochemical driving forces are eliminated.

Distal tubule. Since more calcium than water is reabsorbed in the thick ascending limb, the calcium concentration in the fluid entering the distal tubule is less than that of plasma ultrafiltrate. The $[TF/UF]_{Ca}$ ratio is about 0.6 at the beginning of the distal tubule and falls along the length of it to 0.3 or less. This information, taken together with the lumen-negative transepithelial voltage, provides evidence for an active calcium reabsorptive mechanism that pro-

Figure 4-15
Calcium Transport in the Distal Tubule

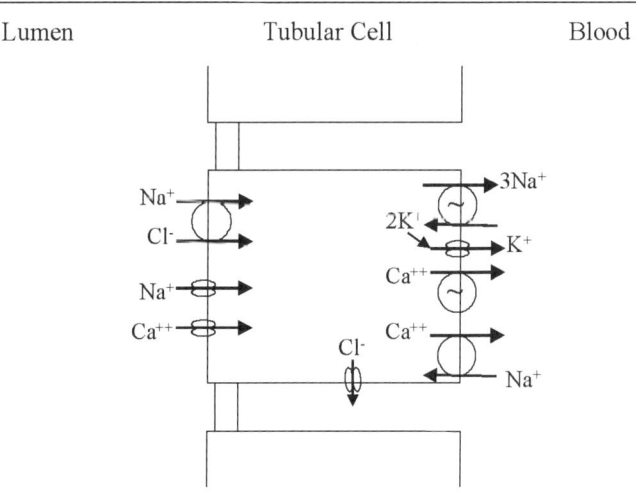

In the distal tubule, calcium crosses the luminal membrane, driven by the chemical gradient. Transport across the basolateral membrane involves an ATP-driven calcium pump and a Ca^{2+}-Na^+ exchanger. The latter is powered by the Na+ gradient established by the extrusion of Na+ from the cell. (Double ovals represent ion channels, circles with arrows adjacent represent transporters, ~ represents ATPase driven transport.)

ceeds against both electrical and chemical gradients. This is in contrast from proximal tubule calcium absorption, which is primarily passive and paracellular in nature.

A simplified model illustrating the mechanisms of transfer of calcium across the membranes of the distal tubule is shown in Figure 4-15. Calcium enters the distal tubule cell from the tubular lumen through a calcium channel. Its exit from the cell into the blood is mediated by a combination of Na^+ - Ca^{2+} exchange and Ca^{2+} ATPase. The first of these is driven by sodium gradients established by sodium entry across the luminal membrane and its extrusion from the cell across the basolateral membrane by the $3Na^+$ - $2K^+$ ATPase. Calcium reabsorption in the distal tubule is regulated by PTH, calcitonin, and vitamin D $(1,25(OH)_2D_3)$.

Collecting tubule. The contribution of the cortical collecting tubule to overall calcium reabsorption is small because the calcium permeability in the cortical collecting tubule is lower than in the thick ascending limb and proximal tubule. Calcium reabsorption in this segment varies with the magnitude and direction of the transepithelial voltage. In summary, calcium is reabsorbed passively via the paracellular pathways, driven by a chemical gradient in the proximal tubule and by the lumen-positive transepithelial voltage in the thick ascending limb. In the distal tubule, calcium is actively reabsorbed. Calcium activity within the renal cells is about four times lower than that of the ECF. Calcium moves passively from the lumen into the renal epithelial cells driven by the chemical gradient. Calcium extrusion from the cell across the basolateral membrane occurs against an electrochemical gradient. This transport involves both an ATP-driven calcium transport pump and Ca^{2+}-Na^+ exchange.

Regulation of Calcium Excretion

The renal excretion of calcium may vary considerably. In normal subjects, an average of 200 mg/day is excreted, but may reach up to 300 mg/day for men and 250 mg/day for women. In severe states of calcium depletion, it may be reduced to 50 mg/day.

Tubular calcium reabsorption may be altered by many factors. In general, those maneuvers that alter sodium transport in the proximal tubule or chloride transport in the thick ascending limb cause parallel alterations in calcium transport by interfering with the passive driving forces (concentration gradient in the proximal tubule and lumen-positive voltage in the thick ascending limb). For example, as ECF volume expansion inhibits salt and water reabsorption, calcium reabsorption in the proximal tubule is diminished. Loop diuretics, such as furosemide, decrease the lumen-positive transepithelial voltage in the thick ascending limb. The usual passive driving force for calcium reabsorption is thereby eliminated, and sodium excretion is accompanied by calcium excretion.

The reabsorption that occurs in the distal tubule and collecting duct is very selective, depending upon the calcium ion concentration in the blood. In these segments of the nephron, sodium and calcium reabsorption can be dissociated from one another, suggesting that the reabsorptive mechanisms differ. This is supported by the observation that parathyroid hormone (PTH) reduces urinary excretion of calcium while enhancing urinary excretion of sodium. In addition, thiazide diuretics, acting in the early portion of the distal tubule induce a natriuresis, but cause urinary retention of calcium when administered on a chronic basis.

Phosphorus levels also affect calcium excretion. An increase in phosphorus may decrease urinary excretion of calcium. Presumably, this is due to deposition of calcium phosphate in the bone, thereby decreasing serum calcium levels and the filtered load. Although the mechanism has not been defined, phosphate depletion leads to an increased urinary excretion of calcium.

Acid-base disturbances, most notably metabolic in nature, also affect calcium excretion. Hydrogen ions, increased in acidosis, displace protein bound calcium resulting in more ionized calcium without affecting the total calcium concentration. This leads to a reduced distal tubule calcium reabsorption and increased calcium excretion. Conversely, metabolic alkalosis reduces ionized calcium levels through the mechanism of increased protein binding. Thus, an increased distal tubule reabsorption of calcium occurs and calcium excretion is reduced.

Parathormone (parathyroid hormone, PTH). Movement of calcium into and out of the bone, gastrointestinal tract and kidney is under the control of a hormone called PTH. PTH is a single chain polypeptide, composed of 84 amino acids, produced by the chief cells of the parathyroid glands. Its production is controlled directly by the calcium concentration of the fluid bathing the cells of these glands. When the extracellular calcium concentration falls too low, the parathyroid glands are directly stimulated to increase their secretion of PTH. As shown in Figure 4-16, PTH increases the ECF concentration of calcium through effects on the bone, GI system, and the kidney.

Figure 4-16
PTH Regulation of Calcium

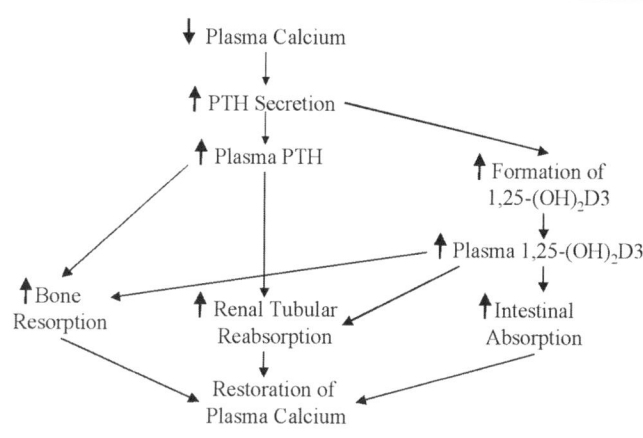

PTH increases the extracellular calcium concentration by stimulating the absorption of bone salts and by increasing the intestinal absorption and renal reabsorption of calcium.

1. PTH stimulates the absorption of bone salts (by increasing bone osteoclastic activity), thereby releasing large amounts of calcium into the ECF. (Related to this is the fact that PTH decreases renal bicarbonate reabsorption. Since renal bicarbonate reabsorption and renal chloride reabsorption are inversely related, this causes a rise in serum chloride concentrations. This, in turn, produces hyperchloremic acidosis, which aids in bone demineralization).

2. PTH stimulates the renal mediated conversion of vitamin D_3 to calcitriol. Calcitriol increases calcium and phosphate absorption in the intestine.

3. Since PTH increases serum calcium through its effects on the bone and GI system, a greater load of calcium passes through the glomerulus. This increases the reabsorption in the proximal tubule. However, PTH has also been reported to decrease or not to change proximal tubule calcium reabsorption. In fact, the primary action of PTH on proximal tubule transport is to inhibit phosphate reabsorption. This decreased reabsorption is so pronounced that it offsets the increase in GI phosphate absorption, thus resulting in a net decrease in serum phosphate concentrations. This is important because it decreases the likelihood of calcium-phosphate precipitates in the setting of rising serum calcium levels.

PTH increases calcium reabsorption in the thick ascending limbs, the distal tubules, and the collecting ducts through activation of renal adenylate cyclase and generation of cyclic adenosine monophosphate (AMP) within the tubular cells. All of the effects of PTH on the bone, intestine, and kidney result in a higher ECF calcium concentration. Ninety percent of circulating PTH is degraded in the liver and kidney, and the circulating half-life is short.

In contrast, when the calcium level becomes too great, PTH secretion falls and almost no bone absorption occurs. Since new bone continues to be formed by the osteoblastic system, calcium is removed from the ECF. In addition, without PTH, fecal and urinary calcium losses are increased and the ECF calcium level returns toward normal.

Vitamin D3 (calcitriol). A second hormone that affects calcium homeostasis is 1,25 dihydroxyvitamin D3 (also known as calcitriol). This hormone is metabolized from ingested vitamin D and from Vitamin D3 (cholecalciferol) formed by the action of ultraviolet radiation on 7-dehydrocholesterol in the skin. These precursors enter the blood and a hydroxyl group (OH^-) is added in the 25 position by the liver. This chemical reaction is called hydroxylation and, in this case, involves the addition of a hydroxy group to the 25th carbon atom of Vitamin D3. When PTH is present, 25, hydroxyvitamin D3 is further hydroxylated in the 1 position within the proximal tubules of the kidney. The mitochondria of the proximal tubules contain the enzyme 1-alpha-hydroxylase, which is responsible for this conversion. The end result is the formation of 1,25 dihydroxyvitamin D3, the active form of vitamin D. One-alpha-hydroxylase activity is directly regulated by PTH (which stimulates renal synthesis of the enzyme) and serum phosphate levels (a decrease in serum phosphate stimulates enzymatic activity).

Calcitriol stimulates active absorption of calcium (and phosphate) by the intestine, enhances bone absorption, and stimulates the renal-tubular reabsorption of calcium. Throughout the cells of the body calcitriol regulates the synthesis of several proteins, most notably a family of proteins known as calbindin D. These proteins bind calcium with a high affinity and are widely found in the intestine, kidney, and bone, as well as other organs. In the presence of calbindin D, there is an increase in transmembrane calcium pump activity within the membranes of the intestine and the distal tubule of the nephron. This increased pump activity combined with calbindin's greater affinity for calcium facilitates an influx of calcium into the ECF and the plasma.

Osteoclastic activity and bone turnover is increased when calcitriol works together with PTH. However, due to increases in intestinal and renal absorption of calcium, calcitriol ultimately provides the high ECF calcium levels necessary for bone mineralization. Finally, calcitriol decreases the synthesis of collagen and PTH, which also favors bone mineralization. In summary, calcitriol's actions on the bone, intestines, and kidney serve to increase the ECF calcium concentration.

Calcitonin. Calcitonin is a 24 amino acid polypeptide secreted by the parafollicular cells of the thyroid gland. It is secreted in response to hypercalcemia and tends to lower plasma calcium primarily by inhibiting osteoclastic bone absorption. Both osteoclast differentiation from precursor cells and activity of existing osteoclasts are reduced in the presence of calcitonin. Calcitonin also increases urinary excretion of calcium, but the mechanism for this is undefined. Its role is thought to be of minor significance in comparison to that of PTH and 1,25 dihydroxyvitamin D3.

Conclusion

New information about the renal regulation of calcium is being discovered on a regular basis. Numerous genetic mutations have been identified that are associated with calcium imbalances. A calcium-sensing receptor located in the membranes of cells involved in regulating calcium homeostasis has been identified. Such receptors in the

Figure 4-17
Reabsorption of Phosphate and Magnesium

Phosphate is primarily reabsorbed in the proximal tubule, and magnesium is primarily reabsorbed in the thick ascending limb.

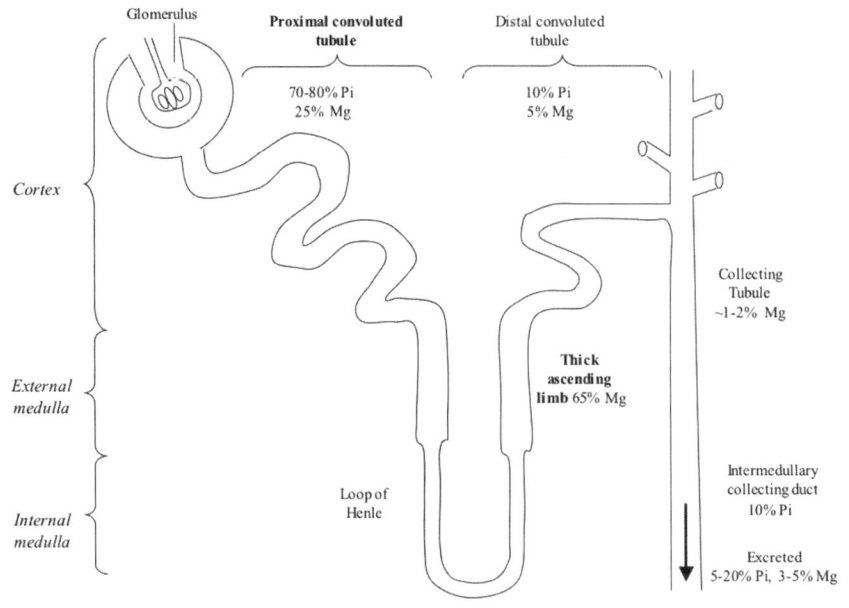

Note: Pi=phosphate

thick ascending limb and distal tubule respond directly to changes in plasma calcium and regulate calcium absorption by these nephron segments. Mutations in the gene coding for the calcium-sensing receptors cause disorders in calcium homeostasis. A PTH-related peptide (PTHrP) has been identified in proximal and distal convoluted tubules and cortical collecting ducts. While its actions have not been well delineated yet, its effects on renal calcium absorption appear to be significant in the hypercalcemia that occurs on some patients with cancer. Thus, we continue to enhance our understanding of the kidney's role in homeostasis.

This section has reviewed the roles, homeostasis, and renal handling of calcium. The homeostasis of calcium is complex and involves the gastrointestinal tract, the bone, the kidney as well as interaction among these sites. The major sites of tubular reabsorption (the proximal tubule, thick ascending limb of Henle and the distal tubule) and the presumed cellular mechanisms involved have been described. In addition, the regulation of calcium by PTH, calcitonin, and vitamin D has been described.

Section 6:
Renal Handling of Phosphorus and Magnesium

Phosphorus and magnesium are important components of many organic molecules and serve as intermediates of metabolic pathways. As such, their concentration in the body must be maintained within narrow limits. Phosphorus and magnesium balance is maintained by the kidney, the bone, and the gastrointestinal system. Accordingly, the roles and interactions of all three sites

must be considered. This chapter focuses on the renal regulation of phosphorus and magnesium.

Phosphorus and its Functions

Phosphorus is located primarily within body cells in combination with hydrogen and oxygen, as a major intracellular anion. It is found in the plasma and interstitial fluid in two forms at pH 7.4: the divalent or alkaline form, known as sodium monohydrogen phosphate ($NaHPO_4^{2-}$), and the monovalent or acid form, sodium dihydrogen phosphate ($NaH_2PO_4^{1-}$), in a ratio of 4:1. Because of their ability to pick up and release hydrogen, both of these forms play important roles as acid- base buffers. In acidosis, $NaH_2PO_4^{1-}$ shows a relative increase, while $NaHPO_4^{2-}$ decreases. The opposite occurs when the extracellular fluid becomes alkaline.

The total quantity of phosphate in the body includes both forms and is expressed in milligrams per deciliter of blood. In the plasma, phosphate ranges from 2.0 - 4.5 mg/dl in adults, with concentrations slightly higher in children. Approximately 5%-10% of plasma phosphate is protein-bound and is, therefore, not filterable at the renal glomerulus. Within the cells, phosphates are also found combined with lipids (phospholipids) as part of the lipid bilayer of the cell membrane, with nucleic acids in DNA and RNA, and as part of adenosine triphosphate (ATP), adenosine diphosphate (ADP), and cyclic adenosine monophosphate (cAMP), providing the energy currency of the cell. Lastly, the major crystalline salt found in bone, hydroxyapatite, is composed of phosphate and calcium.

The effects of hypophosphatemia and hyperphosphatemia illustrate the importance of phosphate homeostasis. Hypophosphatemia produces consequences secondary to the red blood cells' reduced capacity for oxygen transport and to disturbed energy metabolism. Reduced levels of 2,3-diphosphoglycerate and ATP may lead to hypoxia, while the derangement in energy metabolism may lead to nerve and muscle dysfunction, as manifested by irritability, confusion, numbness, coma, convulsions, muscle weakness, and respiratory and cardiac failure. Alternatively, hyperphosphatemia may lower calcium levels because increased amounts of phosphate and calcium are deposited in bone and soft tissues. Thus, symptoms of hyperphosphatemia are primarily those of hypocalcemia, such as confusion, muscle spasms, hyperreflexia, intestinal cramping, and may progress to convulsions, tetany, and respiratory failure.

Phosphorus Homeostasis

Phosphates are found in meats, cereals, and dairy products. When these foods are ingested, they are hydrolyzed in the gastrointestinal tract to form inorganic phosphate and are readily absorbed through the intestinal mucosa. Under normal conditions, the intestinal absorption of phosphate is unregulated in that the net absorption is directly proportional to the amount ingested.

The amount of phosphate released during bone resorption and taken up during bone formation depends primarily on the same mechanisms that govern calcium homeostasis. That is, when serum calcium level drops, bone is absorbed, releasing both phosphate and calcium into the extracellular fluids. When serum calcium level rises, bone is formed, withdrawing both phosphate and calcium from body fluids. Thus, neither the intestines nor the bone have a specific way to control phosphorus levels that are based on the body's needs. This is the role of the kidneys.

Renal Handling of Phosphorus

Phosphate is regulated within the normal range primarily by renal excretion. More than 90% of plasma phosphate is filterable at the glomerulus, and 70%-80% of this is reabsorbed by the proximal tubule, as shown in Figure 4-17. Under normal conditions, the renal tubules reabsorb phosphate at a maximum rate of about 0.1 mmol/min. When less phosphate is present in the glomerular filtrate, all of it is reabsorbed. When more is present, the excess is excreted. Because phosphate is not secreted by the tubules, its renal excretion may be described by the following equation:

Phosphate excreted = Phosphate filtered - Phosphate reabsorbed.

Accordingly, phosphate excretion may be altered by changing the amount filtered and/or the amount reabsorbed. Because the maximum amount of phosphorus that can be reabsorbed is close to the normal filtered amount, even relatively small increases in plasma phosphate concentration can produce relatively large increases in phosphate excretion. Thus, when plasma phosphate concentration increases due to an increase in phosphate intake, the amount filtered increases and the amount excreted increases.

Most of the filtered phosphate is actively reabsorbed in

Figure 4-18
Phosphate Transport in the Proximal Tubule

In the proximal tubule, phosphate transport across the luminal membrane depends on the Sodium gradient via type I and II co-transporters. Most of the phosphate enters the cell as NaHPO$_4^{--}$ along with two Na$^+$ via the Type II co-transporters. Phosphate exits the cell by simple diffusion along its electrochemical gradient (as indicated by the dashed arrow) and perhaps by an anion exchange mechanism.

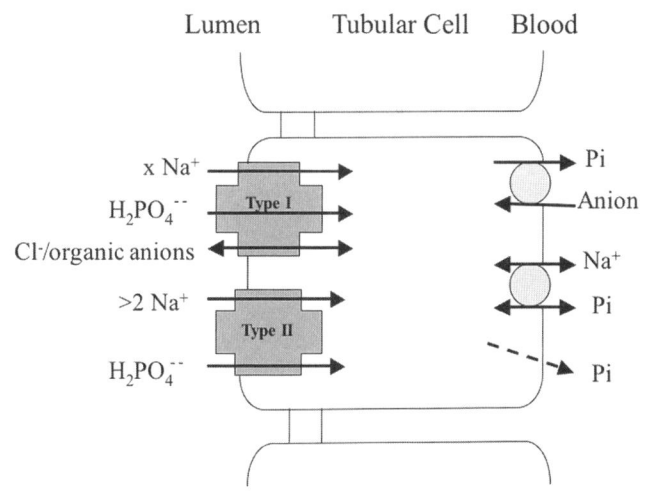

Note: Pi=phosphate

the proximal tubule in co-transport with sodium. Distal nephron segments have shown some capacity for reabsorbing additional phosphate, but that capacity is very limited and has been demonstrated only in the acute absence of parathyroid hormone (PTH) (such as post parathyroidectomy) or with severe dietary phosphate restriction.

The cellular mechanisms for phosphate reabsorption in the proximal tubule are shown in Figure 4-18. Phosphate enters the cells across the luminal membrane by way of type I and II sodium/phosphate (Na$^+$/Pi) co-transporters. Type II co-transporters facilitate the majority of tubular phosphate reabsorption and are the main target for regulating phosphate by PTH and dietary phosphate content. Most of the phosphate enters the proximal tubule cell as divalent phosphate (NaHPO$_4^{2-}$) along with two sodium ions and is, therefore, electroneutral. In contrast, the smaller transport volume of monovalent phosphate (NaH$_2$PO$_4^{1-}$) is electrogenic. A hallmark of these Na$^+$/Pi co-transporter mechanisms is dependency on pH in that HPO$_4^{2-}$ (divalent) is reabsorbed at physiologic pH, while H$_2$PO$_4^{1-}$ (monovalent) is only reabsorbed at low pH. Hydrogen in the luminal fluid alters this transport by inhibiting the sodium site and decreasing the availability of divalent phosphate. It is thought that basolateral phosphate exit is controlled so that intracellular phosphate concentration remains high enough to sustain cellular metabolism. Phosphate exit probably occurs via Na$^+$ co-transport and an anion-exchange mechanism, in addition to passive diffusion along its electrochemical gradient. The rate-limiting event in phosphate reabsorption appears to be phosphate entry at the luminal membrane, which is determined by the number of phosphate co-transporters located in the luminal membrane and the intensity of the inward-directed sodium gradient. Mechanisms that modify existing transporters insert new co-transporters into the luminal membrane or delete existing co-transporters, change the number and velocity of phosphate co-transporters, and are thought to provide the physiological basis by which phosphate excretion is regulated.

Regulation of Phosphate Excretion

Two major factors regulate urinary phosphate excretion: dietary adaptation and PTH. Over time, a diet low in phosphates increases the amount of phosphate reabsorbed in the tubules; whereas a diet high in phosphate reduces the amount reabsorbed. Because dietary adaptation changes the velocity of phosphate transport, dietary-induced changes in reabsorption are likely to remove existing co-transporters or insert new co-transporters into the luminal membrane. For example, if co-transporters are removed due to a high phosphate diet, phosphate reabsorption decreases and excretion increases.

PTH also affects phosphate excretion. Increases or decreases in PTH due to changes in calcium concentration inhibit or stimulate tubular phosphate reabsorption, respectively. This phenomenon is explained if one remembers that in hypocalcemia, the parathyroid gland releases PTH, which induces bone resorption, thereby increasing blood levels of both calcium and phosphate. Similarly, hypocalcemia stimulates activation of Vitamin D_3, which enhances the intestinal absorption of both calcium and phosphate. Therefore, through its adaptive mechanisms, low calcium produces a rise in plasma phosphate. The ability of PTH to inhibit phosphate reabsorption in the kidney prevents this rise, thus increasing phosphate excretion. The mechanism by which PTH does this is, however, unclear. It may stimulate a rapid endocytosis of type II Na^+/Pi co-transporters on the luminal membrane, thereby decreasing reabsorption.

Urinary phosphate excretion is also affected by other hormonal and nonhormonal factors. Vitamin D increases excretion of phosphate, perhaps by enhancing the effects of PTH. The thyroid hormone thyroxine also increases phosphate reabsorption, probably by inserting new phosphate co-transporters into the luminal membrane. Other hormones that increase phosphate reabsorption and, thus, decrease excretion include: somatotropin (human growth hormone), serotonin, insulin, and norepinephrine. Dopamine inhibits reabsorption of phosphate, and controversy remains over whether or not glucocorticoids are similarly phosphaturic. Nonhormonal factors such as metabolic acidosis, respiratory acidosis, hypercapnia, and extracellular volume expansion also decrease reabsorption, thereby increasing excretion of phosphate. In contrast, phosphate excretion is decreased in respiratory alkalosis.

Magnesium and its Functions

Magnesium is the second most abundant and important intracellular cation. It is found mostly within bone (55%) and other intracellular fluids (44%). Only about 1% of the body's magnesium is found in plasma and other extracellular fluids. Plasma concentration is 1.8-2.5 mEq/L or 1.8-2.4 mg/dl, with about 20% of this bound to proteins.

Magnesium functions as a cofactor in many intracellular enzymatic reactions. It helps to regulate potassium and calcium cell membrane channels, is vital for protein synthesis, and also helps to fuel energy production in the mitochondria. While rare, hypomagnesemia increases neuromuscular excitability, producing symptoms such as behavioral changes, irritability, hyperreflexia, ventricular arrhythmias, muscle weakness, tetany, and convulsions. Excess magnesium depresses skeletal muscle contraction and nerve function producing nausea and vomiting, muscle weakness, hypotension, bradycardia, and respiratory depression.

Magnesium Homeostasis

Magnesium is ubiquitous in our diet, being abundant in green vegetables, seafood, grains, nuts, and meats. About 30%-40% of our dietary intake of magnesium is absorbed in the small intestine via saturable and passive transport processes. This absorption varies inversely with dietary intake and does not seem to be affected by Vitamin D or PTH. Magnesium concentrations in the intracellular and extracellular fluid are primarily regulated by the gastrointestinal tract, the kidney, and the bone, although these processes are not well understood.

Renal Handling of Magnesium

With a normal dietary intake of magnesium, urinary excretion averages 100-150 mg per day. This may decrease to 10 mg per day with dietary restriction or may increase to 600 mg per day in patients receiving magnesium-containing antacids. Thus, the kidney is very adept at conserving or excreting magnesium as necessary. Control of magnesium occurs primarily by filtration and tubular reabsorption, although the mechanisms involved are not yet well defined.

Seventy to 80% of the plasma magnesium is filterable; the remainder is bound to protein and is not filterable. As shown in Figure 4-17, 10%-25% of the filtered magnesium is reabsorbed along the length of the proximal tubule. In contrast to sodium and calcium, which are reabsorbed along the proximal tubule in equivalent concentrations to plasma, the ratio of the magnesium concentration [Mg] in tubule fluid relative to the plasma ultrafiltrate ($[TF/UF]_{Mg}$) rises as a function of water absorption along the length of the proximal tubule to a value as high as 2.0. This indicates that the proximal tubule is comparatively impermeable to magnesium. Although the orientation of the electrochemical gradient along most of the proximal tubule favors diffusion of magnesium from the lumen to blood through the paracellular pathway, this has not been demonstrated.

The thick ascending limb of the loop of Henle is the principle site of magnesium reabsorption, where 50%-65% of the filtered load is reabsorbed. Here, as depicted in Figure 4-19, sodium chloride transport is coupled to potassium, probably via an electroneutral $Na^+/2Cl^-/K^+$ co-transport. The selective movement of potassium back across the luminal membrane and the preferential transfer of chloride across the basolateral membrane accounts for the lumen-

Figure 4-19
Magnesium Transport in the Thick Ascending Limb

In the thick ascending limb, sodium chloride transport is coupled to potassium, probably via an electroneutral $Na^+/2Cl^-/K^+$ co-transport. This is an active transport process, indicated by the multi-arrow symbol. Selective diffusion (as indicated by the dashed arrows) of potassium back across the luminal membrane and chloride across the basolateral membrane creates a lumen positive voltage that allows for magnesium to move passively through the paracellular pathway (indicated by the hatched arrows).

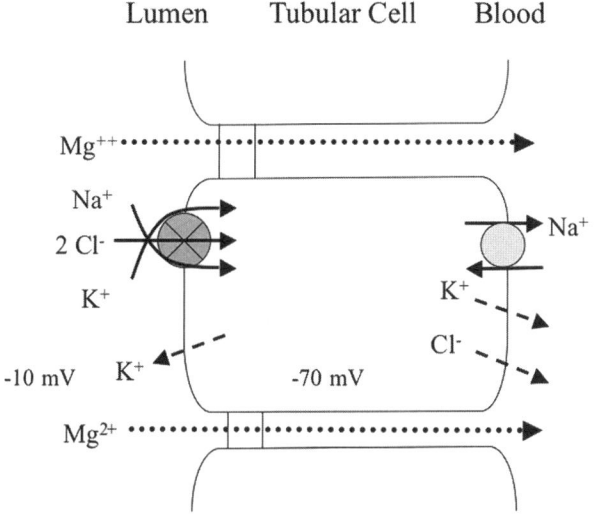

positive voltage in the thick ascending limb. The lumen-positive voltage allows for magnesium to move passively between the cells (through the paracellular pathway).

The distal tubule and collecting duct have a very limited role in renal magnesium conservation, reabsorbing only about 5%-10% of the filtered load. This reabsorption appears to be load dependent, but again the cellular mechanisms involved are not well understood. There is some evidence that magnesium moves passively into the cell across the luminal membrane, driven by the transmembrane voltage difference (i.e., -10mV in the lumen vs. –70 mV in the cell). Magnesium then leaves the cell against both electrical and concentration gradients, perhaps via Na^+/Mg^+ exchange.

Regulation of Magnesium Excretion

The amount of magnesium excreted is primarily dependent on the amount reabsorbed. No single hormone appears to regulate urinary magnesium reabsorption directly. Rather, excretion varies according to many factors, such as those affecting reabsorption in the thick ascending limb, dietary magnesium intake, calcium concentration, pH balance, and certain hormones. Since transport in the thick ascending limb depends on sodium chloride transport and on the electrical potential, factors that alter these (e.g., loop diuretics such as furosemide) also alter magnesium reabsorption.

Excretion also varies with dietary magnesium intake. A high dietary intake decreases reabsorption in the proximal tubule and ascending limb markedly. In contrast, hypo-

magnesemia reduces reabsorption in the proximal tubule corresponding to the reduction in filtered load. At the same time, the reabsorption in the thick ascending limb is enhanced leading to excellent conservation of magnesium.

Hypercalcemia markedly increases magnesium excretion by reducing both magnesium and calcium reabsorption in the thick ascending limb. In contrast, hypocalcemia decreases magnesium excretion. These effects of calcium are thought to be due to a Ca^{+2}/Mg^{+2}-sensing receptor located in glomeruli, proximal tubules, thick ascending limbs, and distal tubules. Binding of Ca^{+2} or Mg^{+2} to this sensor initiates intracellular signals that alter reabsorption.

Metabolic acidosis is associated with increased magnesium excretion, and metabolic alkalosis is associated with decreased excretion, probably through changes in transport in the loop of Henle and distal tubule. In addition, a number of hormones, including PTH, calcitonin, and vasopressin, enhance magnesium reabsorption in the thick ascending limb and distal tubule, thereby decreasing excretion.

Conclusion

In contrast to renal homeostasis of calcium, much less is known about renal homeostasis of phosphate and especially of magnesium. New information about renal regulation of these elements is being discovered on a regular basis. Many genetic products associated with phosphorus reabsorption have been identified. Mutational alterations of these and other proteins are associated with familial hypo- and hyper-phosphatemias. Scientists are beginning to describe age-related reductions of co-transporter molecules that, coupled with new information on age-related changes in cholesterol (and concomitantly the membrane fluidity), may lead to better understanding of the changes in renal function that occur with age.

Section 7:
Renal Regulation of Acid-Base Balance

This section covers renal acidification and is divided into two major sections. The first section reviews principles of acid-base physiology, describing pH and hydrogen ions, buffer systems, and intracellular and extracellular buffering mechanisms. The second section discusses the renal contribution to maintaining pH balance and describes: (a) the reabsorption of filtered bicarbonate, (b) the regeneration of bicarbonate, (c) how hydrogen ion balance is maintained over a 24-hour period, and (d) adaptations that occur in response to changes in the daily acid load.

Principles and Definitions: Acid-Base Physiology

The normal free hydrogen ion concentration in the plasma is 0.000035 – 0.000045 mEq/L. Because this concentration is so low, pH is used to describe it. pH is the negative logarithm of the free hydrogen ion concentration, shown as pH = -log [H^+]. Thus, hydrogen ion (H^+) concentration defines the pH of a solution. Only free hydrogen ions, also called protons, contribute to the measured pH. If hydrogen ions are bound to other ions (such as phosphate or bicarbonate) or proteins, they are not free and do not contribute to the measured pH. Solutes and proteins that

Table 4-2
Physiological Buffer Systems

Buffer Pair	H$^+$ Acceptor	H$^+$ Donor	Reaction	pKa
Bicarbonate	HCO_3^-	H_2CO_3	$HCO_3^- + H^+ \leftrightarrow H_2CO_3 \leftrightarrow CO_2 + H_2O$	6.1
Phosphate	HPO_4^{2-}	$H_2PO_4^-$	$HPO_4^{2-} + H^+ \leftrightarrow H_2PO_4^-$	6.8
Ammonia	NH_3	NH_4^+	$NH_3 + H^+ \leftrightarrow NH_4^+$	9.2
Protein	Protein	Protein	Protein + H$^+$ $\leftrightarrow$ Protein - H$^+$	Depends on the amino acids in the protein

can donate or release hydrogen ions are referred to as acids, and those that can absorb or bind hydrogen ions are referred to as bases.

The normal plasma pH is about 7.30 – 7.45 and must be maintained within this narrow range for optimal physiological function. A number of physiologic processes such as (a) the metabolic enzymes that maintain adenosine triphosphate (ATP) or energy stores within cells; (b) transport proteins that move substances across cell membranes; and (c) signaling systems that transmit messages between cells or intracellular compartments, are pH-dependent, meaning they are most efficient when pH is normal. If pH levels change significantly in either the acid (lower pH, higher free H$^+$ concentration) or alkaline (higher pH, lower free H$^+$ concentration) direction, a number of physiologic processes required for life become altered, and the homeostatic milieu begins to deteriorate.

The chemical systems that maintain a normal pH are called buffer systems, because they buffer the pH and prevent it from drifting far from normal. Each buffer system is made up of two compounds, together referred to as a buffer pair. One of the members of the pair is an acid because it is capable of donating a proton, thus lowering pH. The second member of the pair is a base, because it is capable of accepting a proton, thus raising pH.

Table 4-2 shows four buffer pairs. All the buffer systems listed, except for ammonia, whose primary buffering role is in the kidney and is discussed below, exist both inside and outside of cells and contribute to the intracellular and extracellular buffering, respectively, of the two fluid compartments. Note that each buffer system is in equilibrium, meaning that there is continual adjustment in the ratio of the acid (proton donor) to base (proton acceptor) members of the buffer pair. If the pH drops (becomes more acidic) in the environment in which the buffer exists, then the base member of the pair will accept protons, the ratio of acid to base members will increase, and the pH will increase back towards normal. Conversely, if the pH increases (becomes more alkaline) in the environment in which the buffer exists, then the acid members of the pair will donate protons, the ratio of acid to base members will decrease, and the pH will decrease back toward normal.

Each buffer system has an equilibrium point (pKa), defined as the pH at which 50% of the buffer members are in the acid form (capable of donating protons), and 50% are in the base form (capable of accepting protons). At this

pH, the buffer system has the highest buffering potential because it has equal amounts of substrate in each form and, thus, can readily respond to either an acid or alkali load.

The right column of Table 4-2 shows the pKa for each buffer system. Of the systems listed, phosphate has a pKa closest to normal plasma pH and, thus, has the greatest buffering potential for plasma. Since pH is a logarithmic function of [H$^+$], at a pH of 7.32 (normal plasma pH) less than 10% of phosphate's members are in the acid form, and more than 90% are in the base form. From the standpoint of balance, then, phosphate is not the ideal system to defend body pH, especially in response to an alkali (hydroxyl ion) load. However, since the body is presented daily with a net acid load from metabolic processes, a buffer system with 90% of its members in the base form (capable of accepting a proton) is useful. In addition, the extracellular bicarbonate concentration is 25 mM and the phosphate concentration is around 5 mM; thus, there is much more bicarbonate than phosphate around to contribute to the buffer pool.

Some proteins carry a large number of negative charges, some of which can readily bind hydrogen ions at physiologic pH (7.30 – 7.45). Hemoglobin is one such protein. It is instrumental in carrying acids (CO$_2$ that has been converted to a hydrogen ion and bicarbonate ion) from the peripheral tissues to the lungs, where the reaction reverses and CO$_2$ is expired. Other cellular and plasma proteins can also accept and donate protons and contribute significantly to defending body pH. In addition, other buffer systems are also at work in the body. For example, the sulfate system is present but does not contribute much to maintaining a homeostatic environment because its pKa (1.9) is too distant from physiological pH.

Intracellular and extracellular buffering systems. Since adding free hydrogen (acid) or hydroxyl (alkali) ions to either the intra- or extracellular fluid will immediately change the pH, a number of buffer mechanisms (see Table 4-3) are ready to respond, ranging from ones that respond immediately to those that respond over a period of hours-to-days. The buffer mechanisms in the extracellular fluid respond immediately to prevent minute-to-minute pH fluctuations. The processes that take longer to respond regulate the excretion rate of hydrogen ions from the body, thereby replenishing the buffering systems.

Thus, as seen in Table 4-3, extracellular buffering (predominantly by the bicarbonate buffering system) occurs

 Contemporary Nephrology Nursing: Principles and Practice, Second Edition © — American Nephrology Nurses' Association 2006

Table 4-3

Mechanisms that Buffer an Acid Load

Mechanisms	Site	Time Frame
Buffer systems (primarily bicarbonate)	Extracellular fluid	Immediate
Increased rate and depth of breathing to decrease CO_2	Lungs	Minutes to hours
Buffer systems (phosphate, bicarbonate, protein)	Intracellular fluid	2-4 hours
Hydrogen ion excretion, bicarbonate reabsorption, and bicarbonate generation	Kidneys	Hours to days

Figure 4-20

Segmental Reabsorption of Bicarbonate

Normally the entire load of filtered HCO_3^- is reabsorbed, primarily in the proximal tubule.

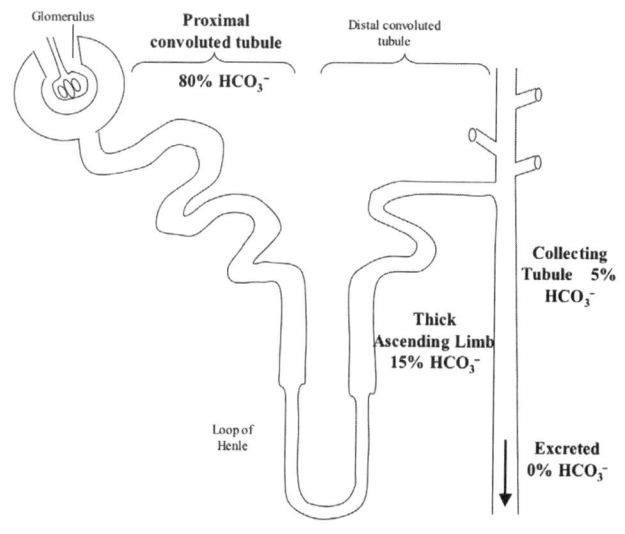

almost instantaneously as H^+ is added to the plasma. Next, neurons in the medullary respiratory center respond to the change in plasma pH by altering the rate and depth of respiration, which increases the excretion of carbon dioxide (CO_2), thus decreasing plasma CO_2, which is part of the bicarbonate buffer system (see Table 4-2). Since the members of the bicarbonate buffering system are in equilibrium with one other, the decrease in plasma CO_2 drives the reaction to the right, lowering the free H^+ concentration and increasing plasma pH. Although the respiratory response is identified as a separate responding mechanism, it uses the bicarbonate buffer system to provide the regulated substrate (CO_2).

Third in line of defense are the intracellular buffering systems such as the bicarbonate and phosphate systems and the intracellular proteins. These sometimes take a little longer to respond because of the time required for protons to enter the various cellular compartments.

Finally, the renal system regulates H^+ excretion on a time scale of hours-to-days. Since it takes the kidneys longer to respond to changes in acid load, body pH would fluctuate widely during a 24-hour period if the fast-responding extra-and intracellular buffering mechanisms and respiratory system described above were not operating to protect plasma pH until the kidneys were able to alter the rate of H^+ excretion. Although not responsible for the minute-to-minute buffering of plasma pH, the kidneys play a very important part because they are the final step in excreting H^+ from the body and thereby returning the net balance of H^+ to the body. In the steady state, in order for plasma pH to be maintained within a normal range over a long period of time, the rate of H^+ addition to the body must equal its rate of exit from the body. The renal mechanisms that contribute to pH balance are complex and allow for adjustment of H^+ excretion in accordance with acid production in the body. This is the focus of the remainder of this section.

The daily maintenance of acid-base balance. In a typical diet, food metabolism generates 60 - 100 mEq of protons per day for a 70 kg person. If these protons were not

buffered, a person would become increasingly acidotic in response to normal metabolic processes. Thus, each day the body must buffer the acids produced from normal metabolic processes to maintain a normal pH. Similarly, if the body faced a daily alkali load, the base compounds would have to be buffered to prevent the individual from becoming increasingly alkalotic. Since acid addition is the typical daily metabolic "insult" to the body, however, we will discuss the renal contribution to maintaining acid-base homeostasis in this context.

Renal Mechanisms Involved in the Maintenance of Acid-Base Homeostasis

The kidney has two major responsibilities in maintaining acid-base balance. The first is to reabsorb any bicarbonate that is filtered at the glomerulus and to return it to the plasma, so that it is not excreted in the urine. Since bicarbonate is a small ion, it is freely filtered at the glomerulus; therefore, the bicarbonate concentration in the filtrate entering the proximal tubule is essentially equal to that in the plasma. If all of this filtered bicarbonate were excreted in the urine, the body would lose one of its predominant extracellular and intracellular defenses against acid or alkaline loads. In fact, if all of the filtered bicarbonate were excreted, total body bicarbonate would be depleted in a matter of hours.

Bicarbonate reabsorption. Bicarbonate reabsorption is the process of returning filtered bicarbonate to the plasma. Figure 4-20 shows the segmental reabsorption of bicarbonate in the nephron. Approximately 80% of the filtered bicarbonate is reabsorbed in the proximal tubule, 15% in the thick ascending limb, and 5% in the collecting duct.

Figure 4-21 depicts the mechanism of bicarbonate reabsorption in the proximal tubules. On the left side of the cell is the tubular fluid; on the right side are the interstitial

Figure 4-21
Bicarbonate Reabsorption in the Proximal Tubule

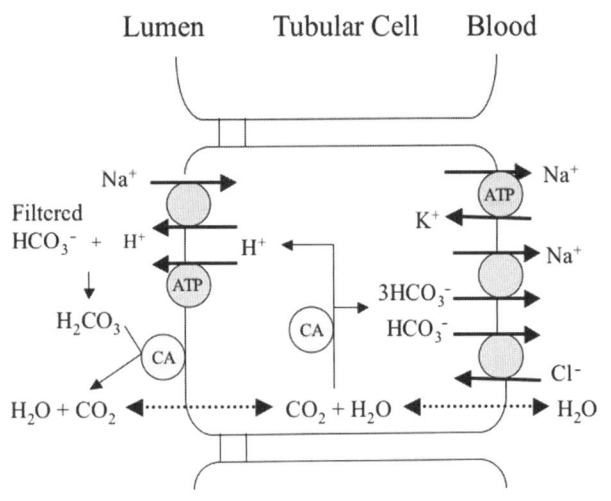

Figure 4-22
Bicarbonate Generation: H+ Excretion with Nonbicarbonate Buffers

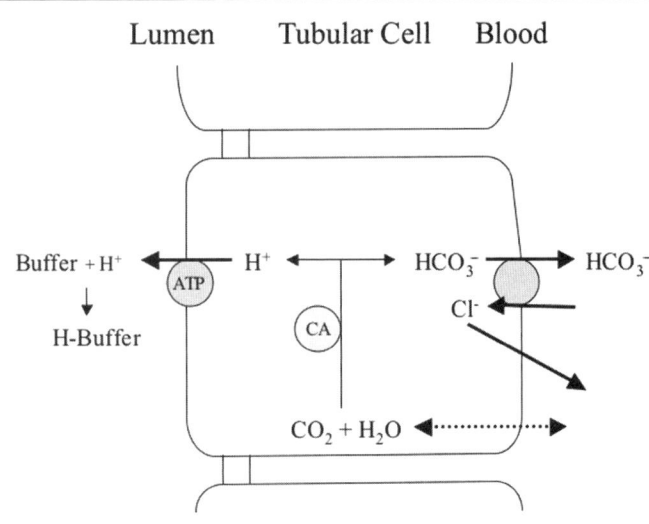

and peritubular capillary fluids. Because bicarbonate ions are too large to be transported across the paracellular pathway (between the cells), and there are no transport mechanisms on the apical membrane capable of transporting bicarbonate ions, the ions must be converted to some other form for transport. In the proximal tubule, H^+ is secreted across the apical membrane (from the cell into the tubular fluid) in counter-transport with Na^+. In the tubular lumen, H^+ combines with HCO_3^- and is converted into CO_2 and H_2O by the enzyme carbonic anhydrase (CA), which is located on the luminal membrane. The CO_2 readily diffuses across the apical cell membrane to the intracellular compartment. Once inside the cell, the reaction reverses and CO_2 combines with H_2O, catalyzed again by CA, to be converted back to H^+ and HCO_3^-. The bicarbonate ion is then transported across the basolateral membrane in co-transport with sodium on the $Na^+/3HCO_3^-$ transporter or in counter-transport with chloride (Cl^-). Bicarbonate then diffuses across the interstitial space to be returned to the systemic plasma. The H^+ generated in the cell is free to be secreted into the lumen again, and the process is repeated.

A similar mechanism occurs in the thick ascending limb and the collecting duct with a few minor deviations. First, CA is not present on the luminal membrane. Second, in the collecting duct, HCO_3^- reabsorption occurs in a specialized type of cell known as an intercalated cell and is not dependent on sodium movement.

In summary, HCO_3^- reabsorption completely removes HCO_3^- from the tubular fluid and adds it into the plasma, although the HCO_3^- added to the plasma is not the "same" ion that was originally filtered at the glomerulus. While the process uses free H^+, there is no net consumption or production of H^+; the H^+ ions merely circulate between the intracellular and tubular fluid compartments to facilitate the conversion of HCO_3^- to CO_2 and H_2O, and then back to HCO_3^-.

The pH of the glomerular filtrate is about 7.3, essentially the same as plasma pH; thus, the free H^+ concentration is 0.000050 mEq/L. At the limiting pH of 4.0, free H^+

concentration will be 0.1 mEq/L. The difference between these two values is 0.09995 mEq/L. Thus, if secreted protons were not buffered within the tubular fluid, the maximum number of protons that could be excreted per day would be 0.09995 mEq, assuming a daily urine output of 1 liter. Clearly, this rate is insufficient to balance the daily addition of H^+ at least 60 mEq/day.

Bicarbonate generation. Bicarbonate reabsorption alone does not replenish the HCO_3^- that is lost when the nonvolatile acids produced by metabolism are titrated. To maintain acid-base balance, the kidneys must replace the lost HCO_3^- with new HCO_3^-. This process is known as bicarbonate generation and couples the excretion of H^+ from the body with HCO_3^- generation within the kidney. As discussed previously, when the bicarbonate buffer system responds to an acid load, HCO_3^- is consumed. When an acid is added or produced, plasma HCO_3^- concentration declines as the HCO_3^- molecules combine with the added H^+, form carbonic acid, convert to CO_2 and H_2O, and exit from the body via the respiratory system.

The kidney generates bicarbonate through non-bicarbonate buffer systems and by metabolizing glutamine. Let us first describe buffer systems. Bicarbonate generation occurs predominantly in the collecting tubule, although some occurs in earlier nephron segments. Bicarbonate generation is similar in many ways to bicarbonate reabsorption, but involves nonbicarbonate buffers such as phosphate and protein. As shown in Figure 4-22, the process again involves the movement of H^+ from the intracellular to the tubular fluid compartments by way of an H^+ ATPase. The proton is generated in the cell when CO_2 and H_2O join to form H_2CO_3 (catalyzed by CA), which then dissociates to form H^+ and HCO_3^-. This process of generating intracellular protons for secretion into the luminal fluid is the same as that used in the HCO_3^- reabsorption process.

The HCO_3^- formed in the cell is transported across the basolateral membrane in counter-transport with Cl^-, ulti-

Figure 4-23
Ammonia Production in the Proximal Tubule

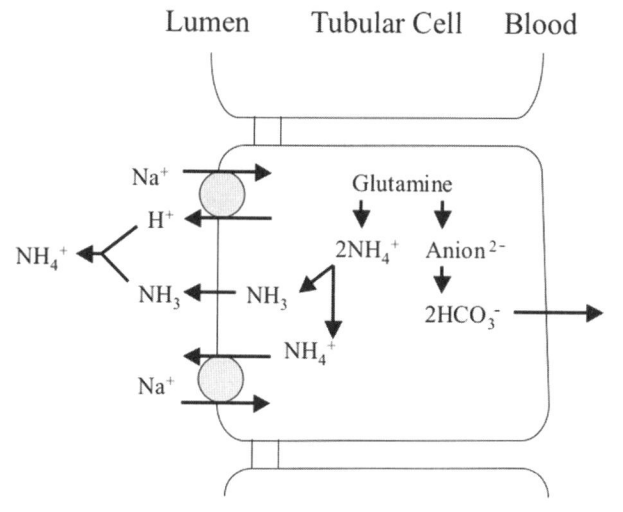

mately to be returned to the peritubular fluid and systemic circulation. The proton that is secreted into the tubular fluid combines with a base molecule, predominantly a protein or dibasic phosphate (HPO_4^{-2}) to form monobasic phosphate ($H_2PO_4^{-1}$). These acid forms of their respective buffer systems are then excreted in the urine. Thus, the major difference between HCO_3^- reabsorption and generation is that the secreted H^+ is not excreted in the reabsorption process, but is excreted in the regeneration process.

To be excreted, secreted protons must be coupled with another ion because protons that remain free in the tubular fluid have the same effect on tubular fluid pH as protons that remain free in the systemic plasma: the higher the free H^+ concentration, the lower the pH. Tubular fluid pH affects the ability of nephron segments to secrete protons; therefore, net proton secretion does not occur when tubular fluid pH is lower than about pH 4.0. At this point, the rate of proton secretion into the luminal fluid is balanced by the rate of proton reabsorption, so that net proton movement is zero.

The kidney also generates bicarbonate by metabolizing glutamine in the proximal tubule, as shown in Figure 4-23. The cells of the proximal tubule break down each glutamine molecule into 2 molecules of ammonium (NH_4^+) and a divalent anion. The metabolism of this ion provides 2 molecules of HCO_3^-, which exits the cell across the basolateral membrane and enters the blood as new HCO_3^-. NH_4^+ may enter the lumen in counter-transport with sodium or may dissociate into H^+ and NH_3, both of which may also cross the luminal membrane. Once in the lumen, H^+ and NH_3 join to reform NH_4^+, which gets trapped as the luminal fluid flows through the proximal tubule. NH4+ may be reabsorbed when it reaches the thick ascending limb because it substitutes for potassium (K^+) on a transporter located in this segment that transports Na^+, K^+, and 2 Cl^- from the lumen into the cell. In addition, this segment has a lumen-positive voltage, which drives NH_4^+ through the paracellular pathway into the peritubular fluid. The reab-

sorbed NH_4^+ accumulates in the interstitial fluid, where it exists in chemical equilibrium with NH_3. While NH_4^+ remains trapped in the interstitial fluid, NH_3 is able to diffuse into the tubular fluid of the collecting duct. As described above, when H^+ is secreted by the intercalated cell of the collecting duct, the luminal fluid acidifies (pH as low as 4.0). H^+ combines with NH_3 to form NH_4^+, which is less able to diffuse out of the collecting duct than is NH_3. NH_4^+ is therefore trapped in the tubular lumen and excreted in the urine.

Unlike the other bicarbonate handling systems, the NH_4^+ system can be regulated. During systemic acidosis, the proximal tubular cells are stimulated to synthesize more enzymes that metabolize glutamine: phosphate-dependent glutaminase and glutamate dehydrogenase. This synthesis requires several days for complete adaptation. With increased levels of enzymes, NH_4^+ production is increased, thus allowing more H^+ excretion and enhanced production of new HCO_3^-. Conversely, NH_4^+ production is reduced in alkalosis. Plasma potassium concentration also alters NH_4^+ production: hyperkalemia inhibits NH_4^+ production and hypokalemia stimulates NH_4^+ production.

Maintenance of systemic acid-base balance. Systemic acid-base homeostasis will be maintained only when the net balance of protons is zero, which can be accomplished only when all protons added to the body are removed. Remember that when a proton is picked up by one of the buffer systems, the pH is protected. From a homeostatic standpoint, however, the system is not the same because a buffer system has been disturbed. Thus, acid-base homeostasis is not solely defined by the pH, but also by the balance between the acid and base forms of each buffer system. The renal bicarbonate generation process is the primary mechanism responsible for maintaining the balance between the acid and base forms of the bicarbonate buffer system. When this system buffers a proton, a HCO_3^- is consumed and is effectively lost from the body (since the CO_2 molecule that is generated is excreted from the body by the respiratory system). Then when the kidney regenerates a HCO_3^-, the base molecule of the buffer system is replenished and homeostasis reestablished.

Adaptations to changes in the magnitude of daily acid load. Although the typical daily acid-base insult to the body is a metabolic acid load, the magnitude of this acid load can vary widely depending on the composition of the diet and will, thus, consume varying amounts of the buffer systems' base members and place varying demands on the kidney for the amount of bicarbonate that must be generated daily.

As described above, bicarbonate generation is coupled with and dependent on proton excretion, and predominantly uses both phosphate and ammonia to entrap the protons and ensure their excretion. In an average American diet, of the 60 mEq of hydrogen that are excreted each day, 20 mEq are entrapped by phosphate and 40 mEq are entrapped by ammonia. In a severe acidosis, these values can increase to about 80 mEq/day for phosphate and 500 mEq/day for ammonia. Thus, our ability to respond to widely different acid excretion needs resides predominantly in the kidneys' ability to provide varying amounts of ammonia on demand. Note in Table 4-2 that the pKa of the ammonia system is 9.2. At a tubular fluid pH of 7.3, 99% of the synthesized and secreted ammonia (NH_3) molecules will exist as ammonium (NH_4^+). At a lower tubular fluid pH, essentially all synthesized and secreted ammonia has picked up a proton. Thus, this system is especially well poised to trap secreted protons within the tubular fluid.

Ammonia is produced by the proximal tubule cells, and its generation is regulated by enzymes whose activities are modified by the pH in the surrounding environment. Thus, in the case of a large acid load, more ammonia is produced, more secreted H^+ is entrapped by ammonia, and more HCO_3^- is generated to replenish the extracellular and intracellular stores that were consumed in protecting plasma pH. And visa versa, in the case of an alkaline load, less ammonia is produced, fewer secreted H^+ are entrapped by ammonia, and less HCO_3^- is generated. The continual monitoring of body pH allows renal ammonia production to be tightly regulated and a homeostatic pH environment maintained.

Conclusion

Maintaining a homeostatic pH environment is essential for normal functioning of most physiologic processes. To achieve this goal, the body has rapid-response, short-term approaches as well as slower-response, long-term mechanisms that play critical roles in maintaining pH within a narrow range.

Section 8: Urinary Concentration and Dilution

This section covers urinary concentration and dilution and is adapted from an article published in the August 1992 issue of *ANNA Journal*, volume 19, number 4.

Since water is the major component of all living cells, the ability to absorb and release water is a fundamental aspect of life. In humans, 60%-70% of body weight is water, which equilibrates across the lipid bilayer in cell membranes throughout the body. Because we live on land, the human body is exposed to constant, daily unregulated losses of water through the feces, sweat, and lungs. Without fluid replacement, these losses would ultimately dehydrate the body. Water balance is tightly regulated by the kidneys, because they are the only organ capable of regulating total body water balance based on their ability to concentrate urine (thus saving body water) or dilute it (thus ridding the body of excess water). This paper reviews the mechanisms involved in urinary concentration and dilution.

An Evolutionary Perspective

It is theorized that the kidneys evolved from early excretory structures in primitive multicellular sea organisms. As these organisms developed increasingly complex cellular structures, simple diffusion of solutes and water through the skin became impossible. Thus, a single tubular structure evolved that secreted or reabsorbed solutes (primarily sodium chloride [NaCl]) and water and opened at one end to the sea, enabling the organism to maintain an internal osmotically favorable environment. This earliest form of kidney, analogous to the tubule structures present in human kidneys, provides the basis for the additional structures and processes present in the human kidneys.

When early vertebrates were exposed to freshwater, the kidney evolved further. The simple tubular kidney was no longer adequate to maintain the internal osmotic environment – it could not eliminate enough water, and too much solute was lost, so the organism succumbed to extreme hypo-osmolality. Thus, the glomerulus evolved. This structure rapidly dumped the contents of the extracellular fluid into the tubule, thus solving the problem of water elimination. However, since a significant amount of valuable solute was also discarded at the glomerulus, a mechanism for recapturing solutes and some water evolved along the tubular structures.

The kidneys' ability to regulate solute and water balance probably did not achieve present day potential until animals emerged permanently onto dry land. Then, within the tubular structure, mechanisms continued to evolve that recaptured solutes, allowing for the excretion of dilute urine. Hormonal regulation and the collecting duct system evolved, allowing the kidneys to produce urine that was more concentrated than body fluids. This conservation of body water was refined in the mammalian kidneys with the loop of Henle, which is a countercurrent mechanism to further concentrate urine and conserve body water. With these water conservation mechanisms, mammals could leave pools of water for extended periods.

Anatomy of the Mammalian Kidney

Tubular structure and orientation. The ability of the kidney to concentrate or dilute urine is structurally based on the orientation of the nephron within the three layers of the kidney. These layers are (a) the cortical layer, the most superficial layer; (b) the outer medullary layer, medial to the cortical layer; and (c) the inner medullary layer, the deepest layer. As shown on the left side of Figure 4-24, each layer has a higher osmotic gradient than the one external to it. The osmolality rises from 300 mOsm/kg H_2O in the cortical layer (similar to that of plasma) to 1200 mOsm/kg H_2O in the inner medullary layer. These different gradients are important in establishing the various solute and water properties present in different segments of the tubule and collecting ducts.

The tubules of the nephron extend perpendicularly through all three layers of the kidney; however, each layer houses different tubule segments (see Figure 4-24). The proximal convoluted tubule, receiving tubular fluid from the Bowman's capsule, resides in the cortical layer. It connects to the proximal straight tubule, which begins in the cortical layer and joins the descending limb of the loop of Henle in the outer medullary layer.

Two different types of nephrons receive output from the proximal tubule, conduct it through the medullary layer via the loop of Henle, and pass it on to the distal convoluted tubule. Superficial nephrons have short loops of Henle that extend only to the outer medullary layer, and their efferent arterioles branch into peritubular capillaries that surround the nephron segments. Juxtamedullary nephrons (see Figure 4-24) have longer loops of Henle that extend to the deep layers of the inner medulla, and their efferent arteri-

Figure 4-24
The orientation of different tubular segments as they pass through the layers of the kidneys. The numbers on the left are typical osmolalities of the different layers in mOsm/kg H$_2$O. The bold numbers within the lumen shown the urine osmolality during diuresis. The italicized numbers within the lumen shown the urine osmolality when vasopressin is present.

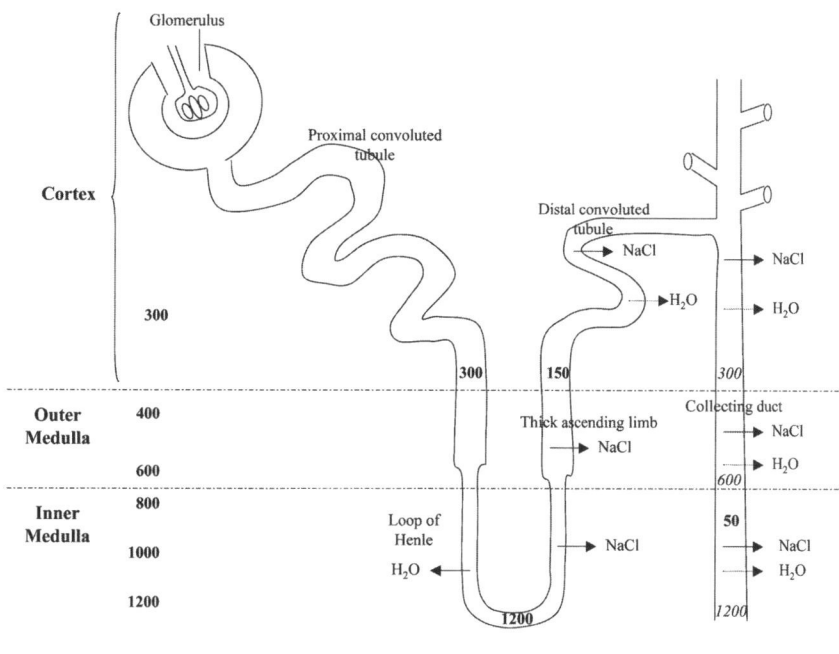

oles form both a network of peritubular capillaries and a series of vascular loops called the vasa recta.

Upon exit from the loop of Henle, tubule fluid enters the distal convoluted tubule (DCT) in the cortical layer. Several DCTs merge to form a connecting tubule, which in turn, joins other collecting tubules to conduct tubule fluid to a cortical collecting duct. Arranged parallel to the loops of Henle, the collecting ducts extend from the superficial layer of the cortical layer to the deepest inner medullary layer. Similar to the loop of Henle, the passage of the collecting duct through different layers of the kidney permits differentiation in water and solute transport.

Tubule vasculature. The blood vessels that carry blood in and out of the renal medulla, collectively called the vasa recta, lie in close proximity to the loops of Henle and collecting ducts. A dense capillary bed projects within the medulla between the afferent (descending) and efferent (ascending) vasa recta. More capillary beds exist in the outer medullary layer than in the inner medullary layer.

The arrangement of the tubule vasculature helps the nephrons concentrate or dilute fluid by creating a countercurrent exchange between the solute- and water-rich fluid within the tubule (coming from the Bowman's capsule) and the solute- and water-poor descending vasa recta (and proximal capillaries) coming from the glomerulus. There is a reverse relationship in the osmolality between the tubule fluid and the interstitium and vasa recta plasma. That is, as the tubular fluid becomes more concentrated, the sur-

rounding interstitium and plasma within the vasa recta become more dilute. The arrangement of the tubule vasculature in the medulla creates a low flow/high perfusion state (by having dense capillary beds) that facilitates efficient countercurrent exchange and maintains the differentiation of solute concentrations within the interstitium of the medulla. High flow rates would wash out this difference. In contrast to the medulla, the cortical layer has a high flow rate of blood through its capillaries, which facilitates the rapid return of solutes and water from the nephron to the blood.

Water Regulation Along the Tubule Segments

The key factors that allow the kidneys to produce either a concentrated urine or a dilute urine, depending on our body's fluid needs are: (a) tubular segments with different permeability to water, NaCl, and urine (see Table 4-4); (b) an increase in the osmolality of the interstitial space from the cortical to the inner medullary layer (see Figure 4-24); and (c) the presence of vasopressin, which alters the water permeability of the distal tubule and collecting ducts. Thus, water transport in each of the nephron segments differs markedly.

Proximal tubule. The proximal tubule wall reabsorbs approximately 67% of tubular fluid water as well as sodium, potassium, and other ions. These components move through the cortical layer interstitium where high vasa recta flow rates cause rapid reabsorption into the plasma. Solute

Table 4-4
Permeability of the Nephron Segments

Segment	Water	NaCl	Urea
Proximal tubule	Yes	Yes	No
Loop of Henle - Descending limb	Yes	Slight	Slight
Loop of Henle – Thin ascending limb	No	Yes	Slight
Loop of Henle - Thick ascending limb	No	Slight	No
Distal tubule and cortical collecting duct*	No	Slight	No
Medullary collecting duct*	Slight	Slight	Slight**

Note: * When vasopressin is present, these segments become highly permeable to water
allowing a concentrated urine to be excreted.
** When vasopressin is present, urea permeability in the medullary collecting duct
rises. The concentration of urea increases due to water reabsorption and diffuses
into the medullary interstitium.

movement (mainly sodium) into the interstitial space occurs through active and facilitative transport mechanisms, creating an osmotic gradient that is higher in the interstitium than in the tubular fluid. Water diffuses through the tubular wall to dilute the higher interstitial concentration, so that the tubular fluid that ultimately exits the proximal tubule (and enters the descending loop of Henle) is relatively isosmotic with respect to the vasa recta plasma. Because simple diffusion across or between tubular wall cells is too slow to account for the rapidity of water movement across the tubule wall, specialized water channels in the cells of the tubular walls allow for the rapid movement of water. At the end of the proximal tubule, the tubular fluid is isosmotic to that of plasma (300 mOsm/kg H_2O).

Loop of Henle

In the loop of Henle, 25% of the filtered NaCl is rapidly absorbed by active transport into the medullary interstitium and, ultimately, into the vasa recta plasma. The descending limb is highly permeable to water and much less so to solutes such as NaCl and urea. Consequently, as the fluid descends into the medulla, water is reabsorbed because of the osmotic gradient between the tubular and interstitial fluid. Thus, at the tip of the loop, the tubular fluid has an osmolality equal to that of the surrounding interstitial fluid. However, the NaCl concentration is greater than the surrounding interstitial fluid, while the urea concentration is less than that of the surrounding interstitial fluid. The thin ascending limb is impermeable to water, but permeable to NaCl and urea. Consequently, as tubular fluid moves up the ascending limb, NaCl is passively reabsorbed because the tubular fluid NaCl concentration is greater than that of the surrounding interstitial fluid. In contrast, urea passively diffuses into the lumen because the tubular fluid urea concentration is less than that of the surrounding interstitial fluid. The net movement of urea is less than that of NaCl, and the tubular fluid becomes hypo-osmolar. The net effect is that while the volume of fluid remains unchanged along the thin ascending limb, the NaCl concentration decreases and the urea concentration increases. The fluid becomes more dilute as it moves into the

thick ascending limb, which is impermeable to water and urea, but actively reabsorbs NaCl. Fluid leaving this segment is hypo-osmotic with respect to plasma (approximately 150 mOsm/kg H_2O).

The processes by which the kidney makes concentrated or dilute urine are the same up to this point. The major distinguishing factor occurs with the presence of vasopressin (antidiuretic hormone [ADH]). Vasopressin is made in the cell bodies of the hypothalamus. When plasma osmolality rises, it stimulates osmoreceptors located in the hypothalamus, which, in turn, sends signals to the vasopressin synthesizing cells located in the supraoptic and paraventricular nuclei of the hypothalamus. Vasopressin is transported along the axons for release in the posterior pituitary gland.

Distal tubule and collecting duct. The same processes that regulate water and solute movement in the distal tubule also do so in the cortical portion of the collecting duct. At the beginning of the distal tubule, the tubular fluid is hypo-osmotic to that of plasma. In the absence of vasopressin, this hypotonicity is maintained throughout the distal tubule and collecting duct system, as these segments are impermeable to water. The distal tubule and the cortical portion of the collecting duct actively reabsorb NaCl but are impermeable to urea. Thus, the urine is made more dilute and hypo-osmotic with respect to plasma. The sodium concentration in the cortex remains close to the plasma concentration due to the high flow rate of blood within the vasa recta in this area. As the collecting duct extends into the medullary layers, NaCl is still actively reabsorbed, increasing the osmolality of the medullary interstitium. In the medullary layer, the collecting duct becomes slightly permeable to water and urea, thereby allowing a small amount of urea into the collecting duct and a small amount of water into the medullary interstitium. Under diuretic conditions, the volume of urine excreted can be as much as 18 L/day or approximately 10% of the glomerular filtration rate (GFR).

In contrast, a rise in the vasopressin level increases water permeability in the distal tubule and collecting ducts. Water flows towards the higher concentration in the inter-

Table 4-5
Aquaporin Expression Disorders

Water Losing Disorders (Overexpression of aquaporins)	Water Retaining Disorders (Underexpression of aquaporins)
Hereditary nephrogenic diabetes insipidus	SIADH
Acquired nephrogenic diabetes insipidus	Vasopressin escape
Lithium	Congestive heart failure
Primary polydipsia	Cirrhosis
Hypokalemia	Pregnancy
Hypercalcemia	Glucocorticoid deficiency
Urinary tract obstruction	
Acute and chronic renal failure	
Nephrotic syndrome	
Hypothyroidism	
Low protein diet	

stitium and plasma; the high flow rate within the vasa recta in the cortex maintains the cortical osmolality close to the plasma osmolality. The cortical collecting duct, however, can only concentrate urine to an osmolality that is no higher than the plasma osmolality (approximately 300 mOsm/kg H_2O). Urine becomes more concentrated as it passes down the collecting duct from the cortical layer through the medullary layers. Due to the hyperosmolality of the interstitium in these layers (up to 1200 mOsm/kg H_2O in the inner medullary layer), water is reabsorbed into the interstitium. The resulting urine is concentrated more than the plasma and the primary remaining solute is urea. Urine volume under this condition can be as low as .5 L/day.

Mechanism of Water Movement Across the Walls of the Tubules

Aquaporins. Now that we have reviewed the fundamentals of urinary concentration and dilution in the kidneys, let us take a closer look at the mechanisms underlying water movement through the tubule walls. Over the past decade, experiments have demonstrated that the velocity of water traveling from inside the tubular lumen to the surrounding interstitium cannot be explained by simple diffusion through the cells' lipid bilayers or between cell junctions in the tubule wall. It was theorized that specialized water channels existed within the cells that allowed the rapid movement of water from the lumen into the interstitium.

This water channel theory was supported by the discovery of Aquaporin-1 in the proximal tubule, which is highly permeable to water. Aquaporin-1 is a channel composed of protein that spans the cell membrane and is specific for water only. Water passes more rapidly through this channel than through the lipid bilayer or between cell junctions. There are many Aquaporin-1 channels on the tubular lumen side and the interstitial side of the tubule wall cells.

In healthy individuals, the Aquaporin-1 channels remain an ever-present structure in the luminal wall cells of the proximal tubule and the descending limb of the loop of Henle. Therefore, these two segments are always permeable to water. Aquaporin-1 is not located in the distal tubule or the collecting duct, other sites with well-known water movement. This makes sense, since the "always open" nature of the Aquaporin-1 channels would make them unsuitable for regulation. Indeed, a second aquaporin channel, Aquaporin-2, was discovered. These water channels are removed from the membrane of the distal tubules and the collecting ducts and are stored within vesicles within the cells during urinary dilution. As a result, the water is kept in the collecting duct lumen. Once activated by an increase in vasopressin, these vesicles move towards and integrate themselves within the cell membranes of the distal tubules and collecting ducts. This movement leads to greater water permeability and, therefore, greater water absorption. Surprisingly, while short bursts of vasopressin liberate Aquaporin-2 channels from storage vesicles, chronic exposure to vasopressin produces new Aquaporin-2 channels that have never been stored.

While Aquaporin-2 are integrated into the luminal side of the cells in the distal tubule and collecting duct, Aquaporin-3 and Aquaporin-4 are integrated into the interstitial side of the cell. These water channels have the same function as Aquaporin-2; that is, as water flows through the channels at one side of the cell, they conduct it out of the cell at the other side. As always, the direction of water movement still depends on the solute concentration gradient on either side of the tubule lumen. Although the list of known aquaporins has grown to 10, many of them have unclear roles; however, experimental studies have discovered a correlation between expression and integration of aquaporin channels (mostly type 2) and human disorders (see Table 4-5).

Role of vasopressin. Vasopressin affects the expression

of aquaporin channels, mainly the Aquaporin-2 channels. When vasopressin activity is low, water permeability is low in the collecting ducts, and relatively little water is absorbed in this segment. The dilute fluid exiting the loop of Henle remains hypotonic all the way to the final urine. With high vasopressin, more water channels exist; water exits the tubular lumen and urine becomes more hypertonic. Only the distal tubules and the collecting ducts exhibit vasopressin regulated water transport.

During water diuresis, when vasopressin levels are low, a small amount of water is still reabsorbed, primarily at the inner medullary layer where the medullary osmotic gradient is highest and the basal water permeability is also highest. This results in a reduction of the inner medullary osmolality. Vasopressin also increases urea permeability in the collecting duct within the inner medullary layer and increases the rate of active NaCl absorption from the loop of Henle. Urea and NaCl absorption contribute to increasing the hypertonicity of the inner medullary layer. In the cortical layer section of the collecting duct, vasopressin increases water absorption where rapid blood flow can return it to the circulation.

Summary

The mammalian kidneys have evolved into a structure capable of regulating several complex mechanisms simultaneously. The link between structure and function is exemplified by the perpendicular orientation of the tubule structures within the layers of the kidney. The nephrons could not produce both a concentrated or dilute urine without traveling through these layers of differing osmolality. The anatomical structure of the kidney serves one important function: to maintain total body water balance.

Section 9: Renal Regulation of Extracellular Fluid Volume and Osmolality

Proper functioning of the cells of the body requires that their environment, the extracellular fluid (ECF), contain the fluid and electrolyte balance within narrow limits. All body systems, principally the cardiovascular, nervous and endocrine systems, contribute to maintaining fluid and electrolyte homeostasis. This section describes the mechanisms by which the kidneys integrate signals from other body systems to control the ECF volume and osmolality.

Paramount in the control of the ECF volume and osmolality is the regulation of sodium and water. The osmolality is set by the ratio of solute to water so that controlling either the amount of solute or water can set the extracellular osmolality to the optimal level. The osmolality and ionic composition of ECF are controlled within very narrow limits, as illustrated by the observation that a rise in body osmolality of as little as 1% to 2% results in a conscious desire to drink and near maximal renal water conservation.

Body Requirements for Sodium and Water

Table 4-6 shows the typical routes of water gain and loss in adults in steady state. The majority of water gain comes from fluid and food intake. In addition, oxidation of food produces a small amount of water, primarily as a

Table 4-6
Normal Routes for Water and NaCl Gain and Loss

Intake	Water (ml/day)	NaCl (g/day)
Fluid	1200	10.50
Food	1000	
Metabolism	350	
Total	2550	10.50
Output		
Insensible (skin & lungs)	900	
Sweat	50	0.25
Feces	100	0.25
Urine	1500	10.00
Total	2550	10.50

result of carbohydrate metabolism. While water loss is primarily in the form of urine, a sizable, insensible component of fluid loss occurs through evaporation from the skin and respiratory tract. This can be significantly augmented by evaporative loss from the skin in environments that induce sweating for thermal regulation. There is also a small fecal water loss. The major ways that fluid balance is controlled and maintained are through fluid intake (stimulated by thirst) and urine output.

Table 4-6 also shows the normal routes for the intake and output of sodium chloride (NaCl). The majority of sodium (Na^+) and chloride (Cl^-) intake, which averages 10.5 grams per day, is through food ingestion. Sodium balance is controlled primarily by renal excretion of Na^+ and Cl^-. The small amount of fluid lost through sweating is normally hypotonic. Sodium chloride loss via this route is modest except in situations that produce prolonged, copious sweating.

Homeostatic Control of Sodium and Water

Renal control and excretion of sodium, chloride, and water (H_2O) is the most important contributor to the control of ECF volume and osmolality. There is no minimum requirement for sodium intake to maintain extracellular fluid homeostasis unless there are significant changes in body water osmolality due to Na^+ losses. In contrast, there is an obligatory water loss, and thus an obligatory water intake, to allow excretion of daily waste products (e.g., urea, sulfates, and phosphates). The typical daily production of these waste products requires a urine volume of at least 400-500 ml/day with a maximal osmolality of 1400 mOsm/L to allow for excretion.

The renal regulation of total body sodium simultaneously achieves regulation of the ECF. This is because sodium is essentially an extracellular solute so that changes in total body sodium are accompanied by virtually identical changes in the extracellular sodium. Since sodium and its associated anions account for more than 90% of all osmotically active ECF solutes, the amount of sodium in the ECF is the major determinant of the ECF volume. Thus ECF and

Figure 4-25

The major determinants of sodium and water excretion. Neural and hormonal signals are integrated by the kidneys, which alter filtration and reabsorption. This results in changes in sodium and water excretion.

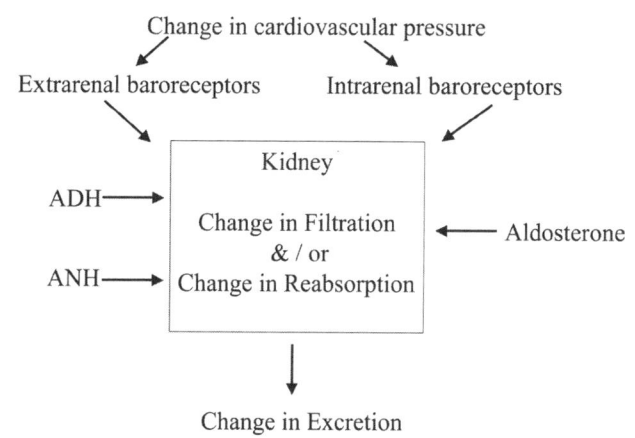

plasma volume normally change in the same direction as total body sodium. Plasma volume, in turn, is a major determinant of cardiovascular pressures, which control total body sodium by acting directly on the kidneys and by stimulating reflexes that alter sodium and water excretion. The term effective circulating volume (ECV) is used to describe the vascular space of the ECF that perfuses tissues throughout the body. In normal states, the volume of the ECF and ECV, blood pressure, and cardiac output will increase as sodium levels rise and decrease as sodium levels fall. The kidneys respond to these changes through adjustment of sodium chloride excretion. In certain disease states (for example, congestive heart failure), blood pressure, cardiac output, and ECF and ECV volumes may not function as in normal states. In any case, the kidneys will adjust sodium excretion according to the ECV. The overall regulation of sodium and water excretion is highly complex with many interactions among neurological and hormonal stimuli. The major determinants of sodium and water excretion are depicted in Figure 4-25 and outlined in Table 4-7, but are described more fully in the text.

Control of sodium filtration. The kidneys play the major role in the maintenance of body sodium and water content. Because they are small and not bound to protein, sodium, chloride, and water are all freely filtered at the glomerulus and are reabsorbed throughout most of the nephron. Since sodium is not also secreted, the amount that is finally excreted depends on filtration and reabsorption alone:

Amount Na⁺ excreted = amount Na⁺ filtered - amount Na⁺ reabsorbed

The amount of Na⁺ that is filtered is equal to the glomerular filtration rate (GFR) times the plasma concentration of sodium (P_{Na^+}). It is theoretically possible then to alter sodium excretion by altering GFR, P_{Na^+}, and/or sodium reabsorption. Under normal conditions the plasma concentration of sodium does not vary greatly and there-

fore contributes little to the regulation of sodium excretion. GFR, on the other hand, is influenced by volume sensors, osmoreceptors, and arterial oncotic pressure.

Antidiuretic hormone (ADH), also known as vasopressin, is the primary regulator of the volume and osmolality of the urine. It is a small peptide (9 amino acids long) that is made in the hypothalamus. From there it is transported down the axon and stored in the nerve terminals located in the posterior pituitary gland. Hypothalamic synthesis and pituitary secretion of ADH occurs rapidly in response to hemodynamic and osmolality changes.

Volume sensors. Sodium reabsorption and GFR are controlled by extrarenal and intrarenal sensors. Extrarenal sensors located in the vascular system respond to changes in volume (stretch). High pressure sensors are located in the aortic arch and carotid sinus. A rise in vascular pressures (secondary to increased plasma volume, for example) stimulates these extrarenal baroreceptors to transmit signals to the brainstem via the vagus and glossopharyngeal afferent nerve fibers. Ultimately, the signal is transmitted to the ADH-producing cells of the hypothalamus to decrease ADH production and secretion. Low pressure sensors are located in the walls of the cardiac atria and pulmonary vessels. Signals from the low volume sensors are transmitted to the ADH-producing cells of the hypothalamus to increase ADH production and secretion. Generally, a 5%-10% decrease in blood volume is necessary to stimulate ADH secretion.

Intrarenal solute sensors in the juxtaglomerular apparatus (JGA) sense changes in GFR via NaCl concentration in the tubular fluid of the macula densa. Increased NaCl concentration is associated with increased GFR, whereas decreased NaCl concentration is associated with decreased GFR. Signals from the JGA are transmitted to either dilate or constrict renal arterioles; this process is known as tubuloglomerular feedback. Dilation of the renal arterioles allows renal blood flow to increase, leading to a reduction in the normal rise of osmotic pressure along the glomerular capillary. The decreased osmotic pressure contributes to a higher net filtration pressure and consequently an increase in GFR. At the same time, increased vascular pressure within the kidneys stimulates intrarenal baroreceptors, decreasing renin secretion and angiotensin II. This also contributes to the vasodilation of the afferent and efferent arterioles, supporting the rise in GFR (and consequently, a rise in the amount of sodium filtered). In contrast, reduced stimulation of extrarenal and intrarenal baroreceptors leads to constriction of afferent and efferent arterioles and a reduction in renal blood flow. This results in a faster rise of osmotic pressure, which leads to filtration pressure equilibrium prior to the efferent end of the glomerular capillary bed. The consequence of this is that glomerular filtration stops earlier in the capillary bed, resulting in a reduction in GFR (and consequently, a fall in the amount of sodium filtered).

Osmoreceptors. Within the hypothalamus, osmoreceptor cells sense changes in ECF osmolality. The receptors selectively sense changes in the concentration of effective osmoles. These are solutes able to exert an osmotic pressure sufficient to balance the pressure exerted by intracellular solutes, thus resisting permeation of the cell mem-

Table 4-7
Major Determinants of Sodium and Water Excretion

Stimulus	Signaling Pathway	Renal Response	Net Effect
↓ plasma volume	↓ stimulation of extrarenal baroreceptors → ↑ renal sympathetic nerve activity → afferent & efferent arteriole constriction	↓ RBF & GFR	↓ Na⁺ & H₂0 excretion
	↓ stimulation of intrarenal baroreceptors → ↑ renin → ↑ angiotensin II → ↑ aldosterone	↑ Na⁺ & H₂0 reabsorption	
	↓ stimulation of intrarenal baroreceptors ↑ renin → ↑ angiotensin II → vasoconstriction	↓ GFR	
	↓ atrial distention → ↓ release of ANH	↓ GFR ↑ Na⁺ & H₂0 reabsorption	
↓ plasma volume & ↑ plasma osmolality	↑ ADH	↑ H₂0 reabsorption	
↑ plasma osmolality	stimulation of extrarenal baroreceptors → ↓ renal sympathetic nerve activity → afferent & efferent arteriole dilation	↑ RBF & GFR	↑ Na⁺ & H₂0 excretion
	stimulation of intrarenal baroreceptors → ↓ renin → ↓ angiotensin II → ↓ aldosterone	↓ Na⁺ & H₂0 reabsorption	
	stimulation of intrarenal baroreceptors → ↓ renin → ↓ angiotensin II → vasodilation	↑ GFR	
	atrial distention → release of ANH	↑ GFR ↓ Na⁺ & H₂0 reabsorption	
↑ plasma volume & ↓ plasma osmolality	↓ ADH	↓ H₂0 reabsorption	

brane. Increases in effective ECF osmolality stimulate osmoreceptors to send signals to the hypothalamus to stimulate ADH synthesis and secretion. Conversely, decreases in effective ECF osmolality result in ADH inhibition. The osmoreceptors are highly sensitive, responding to osmolality changes in the ECF of as little as 1%.

Arterial oncotic pressure. A last contributor to GFR is arterial oncotic pressure (the pressure due to plasma protein concentration). As plasma protein concentration rises (secondary to severe sweating for example), GFR decreases; as the protein concentration falls, GFR increases. These changes have the effect of decreasing or increasing sodium and water excretion respectively, thereby correcting the initial change in oncotic pressure.

Control of sodium reabsorption. Changes in tubular sodium reabsorption have a greater effect on sodium excretion than do changes in the amount of sodium filtered. This is because the changes in GFR are small and these changes automatically induce proportional changes in sodium reabsorption by the proximal tubule, a phenomenon known as glomerulotubular balance. That is, if GFR decreases by 25%, the rate of sodium reabsorption also decreases by close to 25% in the proximal tubule. Glomerulotubular balance is maintained because sodium reabsorption in the proximal tubule is by cotransport with glucose, amino acids, and other substances. The higher the GFR filtered

load of these substances, the higher the sodium reabsorption. Glomerulotubular balance is also influenced by oncotic and hydrostatic pressures between renal capillaries (Starling forces).

Homeostatic control of sodium excretion is achieved via changes in sodium reabsorption in the late distal and collecting tubules. This requires some explanation since more than 90% of the filtered sodium is reabsorbed before the filtrate even reaches these nephron segments. Aldosterone is the single most important controller of sodium excretion, despite the fact that only 2% of the total filtered sodium is dependent on it for reabsorption. Although this seems small, it is actually quite large because of the large amount of sodium that is filtered. Each day the total filtered sodium is equal to the GFR times the concentration of sodium in the plasma. This equals approximately 180 L/day times 145 mmol/L, or 26,100 mmol of sodium each day. Aldosterone controls the reabsorption of 2% of this or 522 mmol/day. This sums to approximately 30 g NaCl per day or 3 times more than the average NaCl intake (see Table 4-6).

Aldosterone is secreted by the adrenal cortex in response to adrenocorticotropic hormone (ACTH) released from the anterior pituitary gland, high levels of potassium, and angiotensin II. The latter stimulator of aldosterone is the most important in regard to sodium-regulating reflexes and is mediated by the renin angiotensin system. The factors that regulate renin secretion (intrarenal baroreceptors, the macula densa, and the renal sympathetic nerves) also regulate aldosterone secretion. In response to low plasma volume (due to low sodium intake or hemorrhage, for example), the kidney releases renin. Renin is a proteolytic enzyme that catalyzes the splitting of angiotensin I from a plasma protein known as angiotensinogen, which is produced mainly by the liver and is present in the plasma in high concentration. Next, the terminal two amino acids are split from the relatively inactive angiotensin I to yield the highly active octapeptide angiotensin II. This is catalyzed by angiotensin converting enzyme (ACE), found primarily within the pulmonary capillaries.

Although angiotensin II acts directly on the tubular cells to stimulate sodium reabsorption, it has two major additional effects: (a) it causes vasoconstriction, thereby raising blood pressure; and, (b) it stimulates the release of aldosterone from the adrenal cortex. Aldosterone travels via the blood stream to the late distal tubule and collecting ducts. Being a fat-soluble steroid, aldosterone enters the cells where it combines with intracellular receptors and stimulates the synthesis of mRNA within the cell nucleus. The mRNA mediates translation of specific proteins that increase the activity and/or number of the luminal membrane sodium channels and basolateral membrane Na^+/K^+ ATPase pumps. These proteins cause more Na^+ to be reabsorbed and more K^+ to be secreted. In contrast, ingestion of a high sodium diet results in a reduction of renin secretion, plasma angiotensin II, and aldosterone secretion. Ultimately sodium and water excretion increase.

In addition to stimulating renin secretion, the renal sympathetic nerves stimulate sodium reabsorption by directly acting on proximal tubular cells. When impulses traveling through these nerves are very high, afferent and efferent arteriolar constriction occurs, resulting in a decrease in renal blood flow and GFR. Ultimately, proximal sodium reabsorption rises. The resulting decrease in fluid delivered to the macula densa is accompanied by decreased sodium and chloride concentrations in the macula densa lumen and decreased NaCl reabsorption by the macula densa cells. While the pathway by which this occurs is unclear, the decreased reabsorption by the macula densa stimulates renin secretion. The rise in renin ultimately results in vasoconstriction (due to angiotensin II) and increased sodium reabsorption (due to aldosterone). Conversely, when flow, and hence, NaCl concentration in the macula densa are high, renin secretion is inhibited.

Another hormone affecting sodium reabsorption is atrial natriuretic hormone (ANH), also known as atrial natriuretic peptide, atrial natriuretic factor, or atriopeptin. ANH is secreted from the cells in the cardiac atria in response to distention of the atria, secondary to plasma volume expansion. Its ultimate effects are opposite to those of aldosterone, inhibiting sodium, and therefore water, reabsorption. ANH acts directly on the medullary collecting ducts and indirectly on other tubular segments (by inhibiting several steps in the renin-angiotensin-aldosterone pathway) to inhibit sodium reabsorption. It inhibits renin and aldosterone secretion, and causes an increase in GFR (via its

effects on the renal arterioles), all of which increase sodium and water excretion.

Other hormones also influence sodium reabsorption, but are not reflexly controlled specifically for the homeostatic regulation of sodium balance. Cortisol, estrogen, growth hormone, thyroid hormone, and insulin all increase sodium reabsorption. In contrast, glucagon, progesterone, and parathyroid hormone decrease sodium reabsorption.

Control of water excretion. Like sodium, water excretion is the difference between the amount filtered and the amount reabsorbed. Similarly, the baroreceptor-initiated reflexes controlling GFR have the same effects on water filtration as on sodium filtration described earlier so that the major regulated determinant of water excretion is the rate of water reabsorption. Changes in ECF volume simultaneously elicit reflex changes in the excretion of both sodium and water. This works well since alterations in ECF volume are normally associated with loss or gain of sodium and water in approximately proportional amounts.

In situations whereby total body water increases without a proportional rise in total body sodium, the kidneys must be able to increase water excretion without increasing sodium excretion. The action of ADH is very important in managing such situations. As noted earlier, the ADH secreting hypothalamic cells receive two inputs, from baroreceptors and from osmoreceptors. An increase in plasma volume accompanied by a decrease in osmolality inhibits ADH secretion, while a decrease in plasma volume accompanied by an increase in osmolality increase ADH secretion (see Table 4-7). In other cases, baroreceptor and osmoreceptor inputs oppose each other, if, for example, volume and osmolality are both decreased. Such situations wherein water and sodium balance are dissociated from one another occur in rare clinical conditions (for example, diabetes insipidus).

ADH acts on principal cells within the late distal tubule and the cortical and medullary collecting ducts and markedly increases the water permeability of the luminal membrane. Receptors located in the basolateral membrane of these tubular segments bind ADH, eliciting a second messenger that leads to the insertion of protein channels into the luminal membrane through which water can move. ADH also increases sodium reabsorption by the cortical collecting duct, appearing to synergize the effect of aldosterone in this segment. If high enough concentrations of ADH result, ADH exerts direct vasoconstrictor effects on arteriolar smooth muscle, resulting in a rise in blood pressure. Concurrent constriction of renal arterioles and mesangial cells in the glomerular membrane lowers GFR, also promoting sodium and water retention.

Taken together, the interactions of various hormones and changes in renal vessel diameter allow the kidneys to maintain the ECF within very narrow limits conducive to optimal cell functioning. These effects are summarized in Table 4-7. In addition, homeostatic balance of salt and water may also be affected by altering the intake of these substances, as shown in Table 4-6. The centers that mediate thirst are located in the hypothalamus and are stimulated by reduced plasma volume and increased body fluid osmolality (the same stimuli that increase ADH secretion).

Although salt craving does occur in humans who are severely salt depleted, its contribution to sodium homeostasis is probably minimal since, on a daily basis, we ingest 20 times the amount of salt needed.

General Renal Reabsorptive Mechanisms

As described earlier, alterations in reabsorption are the primary renal mechanism for regulation of sodium and water. The magnitude of sodium and water reabsorption can be appreciated in that approximately 180 liters of water and 630 grams of sodium are filtered every day by the kidney. In spite of this impressive filtered load, only about 0.5% to 1.0% of the filtered amounts are normally excreted in the urine.

Several pathways exist for the movement of ions and water between the tubule and the peritubular capillaries. One route is the transcellular pathway in which a solute traverses through the epithelial cells lining the tubules, moving through both the luminal and basolateral membranes. Transcellular ionic movement generally requires the expenditure of energy. Another transport route is the paracellular pathway, between or around cells through cellular junctional complexes and lateral intercellular spaces. Ionic movement via the paracellular pathway occurs passively by diffusion along chemical and/or electrical gradients and does not require energy expenditure directly. The permeability of the junctional complexes varies among nephron segments. In those nephron sites where the permeability of the junctional complexes is high, the paracellular movement of solute may dissipate the concentration gradients between the tubular lumen and the interstitium. In contrast, in tubule segments with low permeability of the junctional complexes, large solute concentration differences may be generated between the lumen, tubular cells, and the capillaries.

In general, primary active transport of sodium provides the energy for subsequent reabsorption of chloride and water. The Na^+/K^+ ATPase pumps found on the basolateral membrane of all tubular segments are the primary active transport mechanism. Using ATP, they work diligently to exclude Na^+ from the cell while bringing K^+ into the cell. The low intracellular sodium provides the driving force for Na^+ movement across the luminal membrane. Depending on the tubular segment, the movement of Na^+ down this concentration gradient into the cell may be as a sodium ion alone, in cotransport with other organic substances such as amino acids and glucose or ions such as chloride, or in a countertransport mechanism with ions such as hydrogen. Transporters that do not require ATP directly, but are driven by the extracellular to intracellular sodium concentration gradient are called secondary active transporters.

The mechanisms by which Na^+ reabsorption drives reabsorption of other substances are varied. The loss of Na^+ from the tubular lumen decreases the osmolality of the tubular fluid while increasing the intracellular osmolality. Depending on the water permeability, water crosses the luminal membrane to restore osmotic equilibrium between these two compartments. Movement of water out of the lumen concentrates other intraluminal substances such as urea, allowing these substances to diffuse out of the lumen

Figure 4-26
Segmental reabsorption of sodium. Percent of sodium reabsorbed in each segment is shown for three different conditions: euvolemia (bold), after ECF expansion (italics), & in ECF contraction (regular).

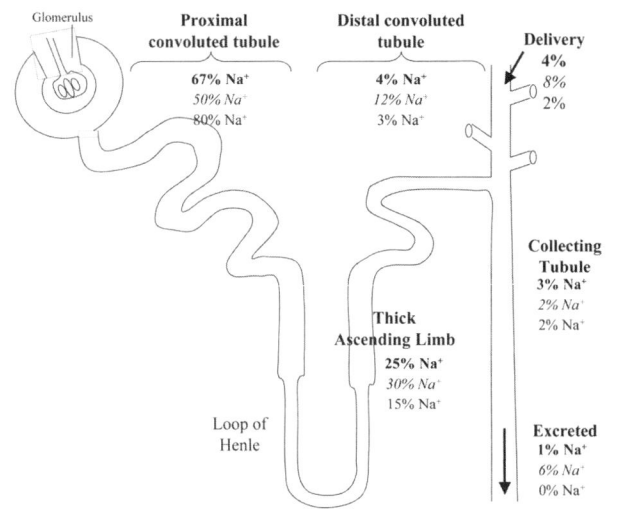

along their concentration gradients. In some nephron segments, such as the collecting duct, water permeability is under hormonal control and varies according to the body's osmolality. This reabsorption of water into the peritubular capillaries is dependent upon the presence of ADH and the hypertonic medullary interstitium, as described in an earlier article of this series.

Similarly, Cl^- reabsorption occurs passively as a consequence of chemical and/or electrical concentration gradients between the tubular lumen, tubular cells, and the peritubular capillaries. The movement of sodium from the tubular lumen to the cell leads to the development of a lumen-negative transtubular potential difference that drives Cl^- movement. In addition, water reabsorption from the tubular lumen increases the luminal Cl^- concentration, which establishes a chemical gradient favoring Cl^- movement. In many segments Cl^- diffuses passively via the paracellular pathway driven by both chemical and electrical gradients established secondary to the active reabsorption of Na^+.

Specific Tubular Reabsorptive Mechanisms

The actual transport mechanisms differ among the various nephron segments. The segments of primary interest in sodium, chloride, and water reabsorption are the proximal tubule, the loop of Henle, the late distal tubule, and the collecting ducts, as shown in Figure 4-26.

Proximal tubule. Over the course of the convoluted and straight portions of the proximal tubules, approximately 67% of filtered Na^+, Cl^-, and water is reabsorbed. The large reabsorptive capacity is facilitated by the high permeability of the junctional complexes. As shown in Figure 4-27, the active movement of 3 Na^+ and 2 K^+ across the basolateral membrane by the Na^+/K^+ ATPase pump creates both a chemical gradient and an electrical gradient that provide

Figure 4-27

Sodium and chloride reabsorption in the early proximal tubule. In this segment, the lumen is negative with respect to the interstitium and the paracellular pathway is highly permeable to Cl- and H₂O. CA = carbonic anhydrase.

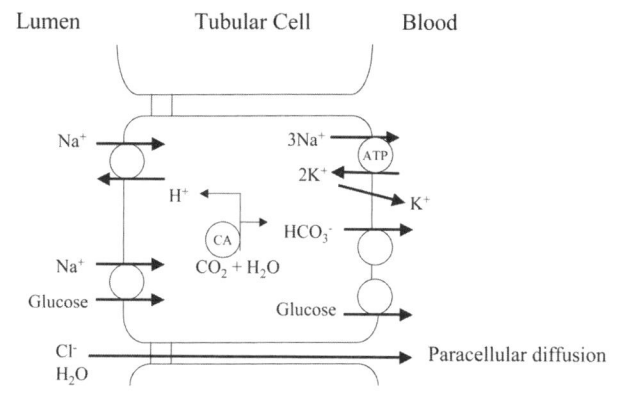

the energy needed to move Na⁺ across the luminal membrane. The luminal entry of sodium requires various carriers that transport sodium coupled or in countertransport with other solutes across the luminal membrane.

In the early proximal tubule, Na⁺ leaves the lumen in cotransport with phosphate or organic solutes such as amino acids and glucose. As a result, the luminal concentration of these solutes decreases and the intracellular concentration increases. These solutes then diffuse passively across the basolateral membrane into the peritubular capillaries. In this segment, the transcellular transport rates of sodium and chloride are quite high, but because the paracellular pathway is highly permeable to water, high sodium and chloride concentration gradients between the lumen and the interstitium are not generated.

Although there is some transport of Cl⁻ that occurs via anion countertransport in the luminal membrane and cotransport with potassium across the basolateral membrane (not depicted in Figure 4-27), most Cl⁻ is passively reabsorbed via the paracellular pathway secondary to the chemical and electrical gradients established by Na⁺ movement. Luminal Cl⁻ concentration increases because water is reabsorbed along the proximal tubule. The loss of Na⁺ from the luminal fluid leads to a lumen negative potential difference. The chemical and electrical gradients allow Cl⁻ to diffuse out of the lumen and into the interstitial space.

In the proximal tubule, Na⁺ also crosses the luminal membrane in countertransport with hydrogen ion (H⁺), thereby exchanging electropositive ions. The dissociation of H_2CO_3 within the proximal cells and subsequent movement of H⁺ into the lumen enhances the secondary active reabsorption of bicarbonate in cotransport with sodium across the basolateral membrane. Thus bicarbonate reabsorption is mostly sodium-coupled. Further information regarding renal acidification is described in an earlier article of this series.

As a result of the tightly coupled reabsorption of sodium, chloride, and water over the course of the proximal

tubule, tubular fluid undergoes little change in Na⁺ concentration or osmolality. Luminal fluid bicarbonate concentration decreases to about 20% of filtered concentration and glucose falls to zero. In the presence of osmotic agents such as mannitol or high glucose concentration in the tubular fluid (often seen in patients with diabetes mellitus), water reabsorption may be sharply reduced, which leads to an osmotic diuresis. This situation can also lead to renal excretion of large quantities of Na⁺ and Cl⁻ because the retardation of water reabsorption leads to a drop in luminal Na⁺ concentration, creating a concentration gradient favoring net diffusion of sodium into the tubular lumen and subsequent excretion.

Loop of Henle. The loop of Henle consists of several segments including the thin descending limb, the thin ascending limb of Henle, and the thick ascending limb. Together these segments reabsorb approximately 25% of filtered Na⁺ and Cl⁻ and about 15% of filtered water. The individual segments have important differences in Na⁺ and water reabsorption. At the beginning of the thin descending limb where the tubular fluid has an osmolality of 300 mOsm/L, the interstitial osmolality is maintained at approximately 400 mOsm/L. At the tip of the loop, the interstitial osmolality may be as high as 1200 mOsm/L. The interstitial gradient is established by Na⁺ and Cl⁻ reabsorption in the ascending limb of the loop and by urea reabsorption in the collecting ducts. Because the thin descending limb is highly permeable to water and relatively impermeable to Na⁺ and Cl⁻, water moves out of the lumen into the hypertonic medullary interstitium. As a consequence, there is an increase in tubular fluid Na⁺ and Cl⁻ and urea concentrations as the tubular fluid travels through the descending limb.

In contrast, the thin and thick ascending limbs are highly permeable to Na⁺ and Cl⁻ while being impermeable to water. Na⁺ and Cl⁻ are reabsorbed, contributing to the hypertonic medullary interstitium, and the tubular fluid becomes more dilute because water is not able to follow.

As tubular fluid moves into the thick ascending limb, more Na⁺ and Cl⁻ than water has been reabsorbed leading to a relatively lower ion concentration and osmolality compared to plasma. As shown in Figure 4-28, Na⁺ is moved across the basolateral membrane by the Na⁺ / K⁺ ATPase pump. Chloride moves out of the tubular cells into the interstitium in cotransport with potassium and via diffusion. The resulting low intracellular concentrations of sodium and chloride drive a luminal membrane carrier, known as a Na⁺ / K⁺ /2 Cl⁻ cotransporter. Diffusion of potassium back across the luminal membrane (driven by the concentration gradient between the cell and the lumen) creates a lumen-positive voltage. The positive voltage favors passive sodium movement through paracellular pathways. In addition, this segment contains luminal Na⁺/H⁺ countertransport as previously described in the proximal tubule.

By the end of the ascending limb of the loop of Henle, more than 90% of filtered Na⁺ and Cl⁻ and 80% of filtered water have been reabsorbed. Under normal homeostatic conditions, Na⁺ and Cl⁻ reabsorption continues until the final urine contains less than 1% of the filtered Na⁺ and Cl⁻. However, the actual Na⁺ and Cl⁻ reabsorption is under the

Figure 4-28
Sodium and chloride reabsorption in the thick ascending limb of Henle. In this segment, the lumen is positive with respect to the interstitium. This is because potassium rapidly diffuses back into the lumen driven by the chemical gradient. CA = carbonic anhydrase.

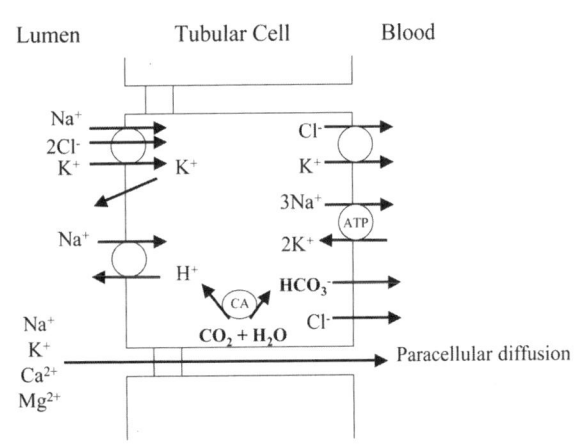

Figure 4-29
Sodium and chloride reabsorption in the late distal tubules and collecting ducts. In these segments, the lumen is negative with respect to the interstitium.

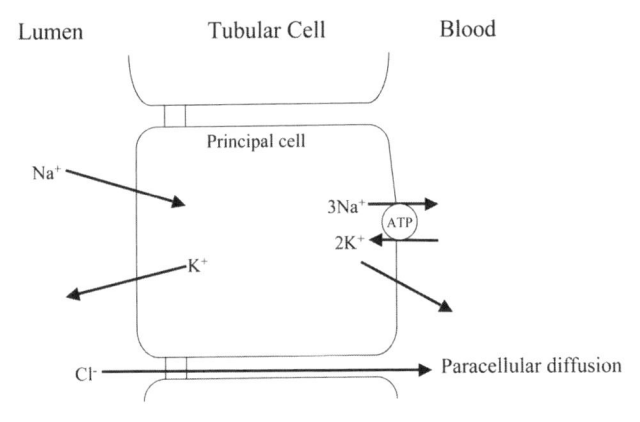

physiologic control of aldosterone and varies as a function of the body's salt balance.

Early distal tubule. Although the early distal convoluted tubule also serves as a diluting segment, some of the transporters differ from those in the thick ascending limb. Na^+/K^+ ATPase pumps are again located on the basolateral membrane, maintaining a low concentration of sodium intracellularly. Sodium crosses the luminal membrane in cotransport with Cl^- and by simple diffusion driven by the low intracellular sodium, and leaving behind a negative potential. Cl^- reabsorption occurs via secondary active cotransport with Na^+ across the luminal membrane and passive diffusion across the basolateral membrane. Since the water permeability of the distal convoluted tubule is quite low, little or no water is reabsorbed in this nephron segment and the luminal fluid osmolality continues to decrease.

Late distal tubule and collecting duct. The late distal tubule is similar in function to the collecting duct. Two different cell types are involved in Na^+ and Cl^- reabsorption in these segments, principal cells and intercalated cells. As shown in Figure 4-29, Na^+ enters the principal cells through sodium channels and leaves the cells via the Na^+/K^+ ATPase pump. Intercalated cells (not shown) reabsorb chloride. The luminal membrane contains Cl^-/HCO_3^- countertransporters; once inside the intercalated cell, Cl^- diffuses passively across the basolateral membrane. In addition, some Cl^- reabsorption occurs by paracellular diffusion, driven by the lumen-negative PD.

The final regulation of NaCl and water reabsorption occurs by the late distal tubule and the collecting ducts under hormonal control. In the presence of aldosterone, the principal cells synthesize proteins that increase the activity and/or number of the luminal membrane sodium channels and the basolateral Na^+/K^+ ATPase pumps, ultimately increasing sodium reabsorption. In response to plas-

ma volume expansion, ANH inhibits sodium reabsorption in the medullary collecting duct, resulting in natriuresis. The water permeability of these segments is under control of ADH secretion. Without ADH, the late distal tubule and collecting ducts are impermeable to water, and the water that is within the tubular fluid is excreted, resulting in a dilute urine. In contrast, in the presence of ADH, the late distal tubule and collecting ducts are permeable to water and water is reabsorbed in proportion to the interstitial fluid osmolality. A description of the mechanisms whereby the kidney is able to produce either a dilute or concentrated urine as needed is described in an earlier article of this series.

Summary

In summary, regulation of sodium, chloride, and extracellular fluid volume and osmolality is complex, but very efficient. The excretion of sodium and water is altered through changes in GFR and reabsorption. As summarized in Figure 4-25, these changes are stimulated by alterations in cardiovascular pressure and are mediated by the nervous system (signals passing through extrarenal and intrarenal baroreceptors) and the endocrine system (ADH, ANH, and aldosterone). Integration of the neural and hormonal signals by the kidney results in changes in filtration and reabsorption and, therefore, changes in sodium, chloride, and water excretion.

Ninety percent of the filtered sodium, chloride, and water is reabsorbed by the proximal tubule, loop of Henle, and early distal tubule. Aldosterone, ADH, and ANH work primarily on the late distal tubule and collecting duct system to fine tune sodium reabsorption in accordance with our body's needs. In normal persons, the mechanisms for regulating sodium excretion are so precise that sodium balance does not vary by more than a small percentage despite marked changes in dietary intake or losses caused by sweating, vomiting, diarrhea, hemorrhage, or burns.

Bibliography

Agre, P. (2000). Aquaporin water channels in kidney: Homer W. Smith award lecture. *Journal of the American Society of Nephrology, 11*(4), 764-777.

Alpern, R.J. (2000). Renal acidification mechanisms. In B.M. Brenner (Ed.), *Brenner & Rector's, the kidney* (6th ed., Vol 1). Philadelphia: W.B. Saunders Company.

Brenner, B.M., & Rector, F.C. (2000). *The kidney* (6th edition), Volume I. Philadelphia: W.B. Saunders Company.

Cook, N.E., & Haddad, J.G. (1997). Vitamin D protein binding. In D.W. Feldman, F.H. Glorieux, & J.W. Pike (Eds.), *Vitamin D*. San Diego: Academic Press.

Dolan, J.T. (1991). Anatomy and physiology of the renal/urinary system. In J.T. Dolan, *Critical care nursing: Clinical management through the nursing process* (pp. 399-416). Philadelphia: F.A. Davis.

Drüeke, T., & Lacour, B. (2000). Disorders of calcium, phosphate, and magnesium metabolism. In R.J. Johnson & J. Freehally (Eds.), *Comprehensive clinical nephrology* (pp. 3.11.1-3.11.16). London: Mosby.

Dworkin, L.D., Sun, A.M., & Brenner, B.M. (2000). The renal circulations. In B.M. Brenner (Ed.), *The kidney: Volume I* (pp. 277-311). Philadelphia: W.B. Saunders Co.

Friedman, P.A. (2000). Renal calcium metabolism. In D.W. Seldin & G. Giebisch (Eds.), *The kidney: Physiology and pathophysiology* (3rd ed.). Philadelphia: Lippincott, Williams & Wilkins.

Gabbai, F.B., & Blantz, R.C. (2001). Glomerular filtration. In S.G. Massry & R.J. Glassock (Eds.), *Textbook of nephrology: Volume I* (4th ed.) (pp. 56-60). Philadelphia: Lippincott, Williams & Wilkins.

Giebisch, G., Mainic, G., & Berliner, W. (1991). Renal transport and control of potassium excretion. In B.M. Brenner & F.C. Rector (Eds.), *The kidney*, Vol. 1 (6th edition) (pp. 419-446). Philadelphia: W.B. Saunders Company.

Goraca, A. (2002). New views on the role of endothelin. Endocrine Regulations, 36, 161-167.

Grantham, J.J., & Wallace, D.P. (2002). Return of the secretory kidney. *American Journal of Physiology: Renal Physiology, 282,* F1-F9.

Guthrie, D., & Yucha, C. (2004). Urinary concentration and dilution. *Nephrology Nursing Journal, 31*(3), 297-301.

Guyton, A.C. & Hall, J.E. (2000). *Textbook of medical physiology* (10th ed.). Philadelphia: W. B. Saunders Company.

Guyton, A.C., & Hall, J.E. (2000). Unit V: The kidneys and body fluids. In A.C. Guyton & J.E. Hall, *Textbook of medical physiology* (10th ed.) (pp. 264-379). Philadelphia: W.B. Saunders.

Hladsky, S.B., & Rink, T.J. (1986). *Physiological principles in medicine series: Body fluid and kidney physiology*. London: Edward Arnold Publishers Ltd.

Horio, M., Orita, Y., & Fukunaga, M. (2001). Assessment of renal function. In R.J. Johnson & J. Feehally (Eds.), *Comprehensive clinical nephrology* (pp. 3.1-3.6). London: Mosby.

Inoue, T., Nonoguchi, H., & Tomita, K. (2001). Physiological effects of vasopressin and atrial natriuretic peptide in the collecting duct. *Cardiovascular Research, 59,* 470-480.

Jackson, B.A., & Ott, C.E. (1999). Renal system. Madison, CT: Fence Creek Publishing.

Kishore, B.K., Krane, C.M., Reif, M., & Menon, A.G. (2001). Molecular physiology of urinary concentration defect in elderly population. *International Urology and Nephrology, 33,* 235-248.

Koeppen, B.M., & Stanton, B.A. (2001). *Renal physiology* (3rd ed.). St. Louis: Mosby.

Koeppen, B.M., & Stanton, B.A. (2003). *Renal physiology* (3rd ed.) (pp. 75-92). St. Louis: Mosby, Inc.

Levey, A., Bosch, J., Lewis, J., Greene, T., Rogers, N., & Roth, D. (1999). A more accurate method to estimate glomerular filtration rate from serum creatinine: A new prediction equation. *Annals of Internal Medicine, 130,* 461-470.

Levin, E.R. (1995). Endothelins. *New England Journal of Medicine, 333,* 356-363.

Lote, C.J. (2000). *Principles of renal physiology* (4th ed.). Boston, MA: Klewer Academic Publishers.

Maddox, D.A., & Brenner, B.M. (2000). Glomerular ultrafiltration. In B.M. Brenner (Ed.), *The kidney: Volume I* (pp. 319-359). Philadelphia: W.B. Saunders.

Marsh, D.J. (1983). *Renal physiology* (p. 41). New York: Raven Press. Copyright 1983 by Raven Press. Reprinted by permission.

Masilamani, S., Knepper, M.A., & Burg, M.B. (2000). Urine concentration and dilution. In B.M. Brenner (Ed.), *Brenner and Rector's the kidney* (6th ed.) (pp. 595-635). Philadelphia: Saunders.

McCance, K.L., & Huether, S.E. (2001). *Pathophysiology: The biologic basis for disease in adults and children* (4th ed.). St Louis: Mosby, Inc.

Meyers, B.D. (2001). Determinants of the glomerular filtration of macromolecules. In S.G. Massry & R.J. Glassock (Eds.), *Textbook of nephrology: Volume I* (4th ed.) (pp 61-64). Philadelphia: Lippincott, Williams & Wilkins.

Miyataka, M., Rich, K.A., Ingram, M., Yamamoto, T., & Bing, R.J. (2002). Nitric oxide, antiinflammatory drug on renal protoglandin and cyclooxygenase2. *Hypertension, 39,* 785-789.

Murer, H., Kaissling, B., Forster, I., & Biber, J. (2000). Cellular mechanisms in proximal tubular handling of phosphate. In, D.W. Seldin & G. Giebisch (Eds.), *The kidney: Physiology and pathophysiology* (pp. 1869-1884) (3rd ed.) (Vol. 2). Philadelphia: Lippincott.

Osborn, J.L., Greenberg, S., & Plato, C.F. (2001). The neural control of renal function and extracellular fluid volume. In S.G. Massry & R.J. Glassock (Eds.), *Textbook of nephrology: Volume I* (4th ed.) (pp. 65-69). Philadelphia: Lippincott, Williams & Wilkins.

Pallone, T.L., & Mattson, D.L. (2002). Role of nitric oxide in the regulation of the renal medulla in normal and hypertensive kidneys. *Current Opinion in Nephrology and Hypertension, 11,* 93-98.

Paul, R.V., & Ploth, D.W. (2001). Renal circulation. In S.G. Massry & R.J. Glassock (Eds.), *Textbook of nephrology: Volume I* (4th ed.) (pp. 43-55). Philadelphia: Lippincott, Williams & Wilkins.

Porterfield, S.P. (2001). *Endocrine physiology* (2nd ed.). St. Louis: Mosby.

Preisig, P., Chmielewski, C., Keen, M., Holechek, M.J., Ludlow, M.K., & Yucha, C.B. (1998). Renal physiology. In J. Parker (Ed.), Contemporary nephrology nursing (pp. 127-176). Pitman, NJ: American Nephrology Nurses' Association.

Quamme, G.A., & Rouffignac, C. (2000). Renal magnesium handling. In D.W. Seldin & G. Giebisch (Eds.), *The kidney: Physiology and pathophysiology* (pp. 1711-1729) (3rd ed.) (Vol. 2). Philadelphia: Lippincott.

Rose, B.D., & Rennke, H. (1994). *Renal pathophysiology*. Baltimore: Williams & Wilkins.

Rose, B.D. (1994). Potassium homeostasis. In B.D. Rose (Ed.), *Clinical physiology of acid-base and electrolyte disorders* (4th edition) (pp. 323-349). New York: McGraw-Hill Book Company.

Sansom, S.C. & Giebisch, G.H. (1989). Potassium homeostasis. In S.G. Massry & R.J. Glassock (Eds.), *Textbook of nephrology*, Vol. 1 (4th ed.) (pp. 276-293). Baltimore: Williams & Wilkins.

Schrier, R.W., & Cadnapaphornchai, M.A. (2002). Renal aquaporin channels: From molecules to human disease. *Progress in Biophysics and Molecular Biology, 81,* 117-131.

Seeley, R.R., Stephens, T.D., & Tate, P. (2002). *Anatomy and physiology* (6th ed.). New York: McGraw-Hill.

Silve, C., & Friedlander, G. (2000). Renal regulation of phosphate excretion. In D.W. Seldin & G. Giebisch (Eds.), *The kidney: Physiology and pathophysiology* (pp.) (3rd ed.) (Vol. 2). Philadelphia: Lippincott.

Stanton, B.A., & Koeppen, B.M. (1998). Control of body fluid osmolality and volume. In R.M. Berne & M.N. Levy (Eds.), *Physiology* (4th ed.) (pp. 715-743). St. Louis: Mosby, Inc.

Thomson, S. (2002). Adenosine and puringenic mediators of tubuloglomerular feedback. *Current opinions in nephrology and hypertension, 11,* 81-86.

Unwin, R.J., & Capasso, G. (2000). *Renal physiology*. In R.J. Johnson & J. Feehally (Eds.), *Comprehensive clinical nephrology* (pp. 2.1-2.12). London: Mosby.

Veenstra, D.A., & Kumar, R. (2000). Hormonal regulation of calcium metabolism. In D.W. Seldin & G. Giebisch (Eds.), *The kidney: Physiology and pathophysiology* (3rd ed.). Philadelphia: Lippincott, Williams, and Wilkins.

Vander, A.J. (1994). Renal regulation of potassium balance. In A.J. Vander (Ed.), *Renal Physiology* (5th edition) (pp. 139-154). New York: McGraw-Hill.

Vander, A.J. (1995). *Renal physiology* (5th ed.) New York: McGraw-Hill Inc

Vander, A.J. (1994). *Renal physiology* (5th ed.) New York: McGraw-Hill, Inc.

Verkman, A.S. (1999). Lessons on renal physiology from transgenic mice lacking aquaporin channels. *Journal of the American Society of Nephrology, 10,* 1126-1135.

Yucha, C. (2004). Renal regulation of acid-base balance. *Nephrology Nursing Journal, 31*(2), 201-208.

- The kidneys are paired vascular organs that perform excretory, regulatory, and secretory functions. In order to understand how these complex organs work, it is necessary to review renal anatomy and understand the renal processes involved in maintaining the body's internal milieu.

- Glomerular filtration is the first step in the complex process of urine formation. For filtration to occur, a rapid renal blood flow (RBF) at a consistent pressure is essential. There are many factors that can alter RBF and, thus, the rate of glomerular filtrate generation. At any given time, especially under the condition of stress, multiple factors act and counteract to maintain a normal glomerular filtration rate (GFR) despite changes in RBF.

- Renal blood flow (RBF), which defines renal plasma flow (RPF), is controlled by a number of physical and humoral factors. These factors are both intrinsic and extrinsic to the kidney. Some of the intrinsic factors include an autoregulatory mechanism, intrarenal renin-angiotensin mechanism, eicosanoids, and kinins. Critical extrinsic factors include the Sympathetic Nervous System (SNS), angiotensin II, antidiuretic hormone, dopamine, and histamine. Endothelin, nitric oxide (NO), and atrial natriuretic peptide (ANP) also play important roles in altering renal hemodynamics.

- Potassium (K) is the most abundant cation in the human body. The total body K stores in an adult are approximately 50-55 milliequivalents (mEq)/Kilogram (Kg) body weight with 98% of the K located intracellularly. Skeletal muscle has the highest K content per unit dry weight and, therefore, contains the bulk of total body K, while fat and bone have relatively low K content. The high intracellular concentration of K (150 mEq/L) [L] versus the low extracellular concentration (4-5 mEq/L) is a delicate balance critical for normal cell functions.

- The homeostasis of calcium is complex because the gastrointestinal tract, the bone, and the kidney all affect calcium balance... Two other major organ systems are also involved in controlling calcium concentration – the skeletal system and the gastrointestinal system. The fact that redundant regulatory processes have evolved that enable calcium concentration to be maintained underscores the importance of calcium for optimal physiological functioning. Accordingly, the roles and interactions of all three sites must be considered.

- Phosphorus and magnesium are important components of many organic molecules and serve as intermediates of metabolic pathways. As such, their concentration in the body must be maintained within narrow limits. Phosphorus and magnesium balance is maintained by the kidney, the bone, and the gastrointestinal system. Accordingly, the roles and interactions of all three sites must be considered.

- Since water is the major component of all living cells, the ability to absorb and release water is a fundamental aspect of life. In humans 60%-70% of body weight is water, which equilibrates across the lipid bilayer in cell membranes throughout the body. Because we live on land, the human body is exposed to constant, daily unregulated losses of water through the feces, sweat, and lungs. Without fluid replacement, these losses would ultimately dehydrate the body.

- Proper functioning of the cells of the body requires that their environment, the extracellular fluid (ECF), contain the fluid and electrolyte balance within narrow limits. All body systems, principally the cardiovascular, nervous, and endocrine systems, contribute to maintaining fluid and electrolyte homeostasis. Thus, it is important to understand the mechanisms by which the kidneys integrate signals from other body systems to control the ECF volume and osmolality.

ANNP604

Renal Physiology

Christine Chmielewski, MS, CRNP, CNN, CS; Mary Jo Holechek, MS, CRNP, CNN; Marlys Ludlow, MS, RN; Carolyn B. Yucha, PhD, RN, FAAN; David Guthrie, MN, ARNP; and Lori Candela, EdD, RN, APRN, BC, FNP

Contemporary Nephrology Nursing: Principles and Practice contains 39 chapters of educational content. Individual learners may apply for continuing nursing education credit by reading a chapter and completing the Continuing Education Evaluation Form for that chapter. Learners may apply for continuing education credit for any or all chapters.

Please photocopy this page and return to ANNA.
COMPLETE THE FOLLOWING:

Name: _____

Address:_____

City:_____ State: _____ Zip: _____

E-mail: _____

Preferred telephone: ☐ Home   ☐ Work: _____

State where licensed and license number (optional): _____

CE application fees are based upon the number of contact hours provided by the individual chapter. CE fees per contact hour for ANNA members are as follows: 1.0-1.9 - $15; 2.0-2.9 - $20; 3.0-3.9 - $25; 4.0 and higher - $30. Fees for nonmembers are $10 higher.

ANNA Member: ☐ Yes   ☐ No   Member # (if available) _____

☐ Checked Enclosed   ☐ American Express   ☐ Visa   ☐ MasterCard

Total Amount Submitted: _____

Credit Card Number: _____ Exp. Date: _____

Name as it appears on the card: _____

CE Evaluation Form
To receive continuing education credit for individual study after reading the chapter
1. Photocopy this form. (You may also download this form from ANNA's Web site, **www.annanurse.org.**)
2. Mail the completed form with payment (check) or credit card information to American Nephrology Nurses' Association, East Holly Avenue, Box 56, Pitman, NJ 08071-0056.
3. You will receive your CE certificate from ANNA in 4 to 6 weeks.

Test returns must be postmarked by **December 31, 2010.**

CE Application Fee
ANNA Member $30.00
Nonmember $40.00

EVALUATION FORM

1. I verify that I have read this chapter and completed this education activity. Date: _____

_____
Signature

2. What would be different in your practice if you applied what you learned from this activity? *(Please use additional sheet of paper if necessary.)*

_____
_____
_____
_____
_____
_____
_____
_____
_____
_____
_____
_____

Evaluation	Strongly disagree				Strongly agree
3. The activity met the stated objectives.					
a. Explain glomerular filtration.	1	2	3	4	5
b. Outline renal hemodynamics.	1	2	3	4	5
c. Describe renal management of electrolytes and acid base balance.	1	2	3	4	5
d. Relate urinary concentration and dilution to regulation of extracellular fluid volume and osmolality.	1	2	3	4	5
4. The content was current and relevant.	1	2	3	4	5
5. The content was presented clearly.	1	2	3	4	5
6. The content was covered adequately.	1	2	3	4	5
7. Rate your ability to apply the learning obtained from this activity to practice.	1	2	3	4	5

Comments _____

_____

8. Time required to read the chapter and complete this form: _____ minutes.

This educational activity has been provided by the American Nephrology Nurses' Association (ANNA) for 5.5 contact hours. ANNA is accredited as a provider of continuing nursing education (CNE) by the American Nurses Credentialing Center's Commission on Accreditation (ANCC-COA). ANNA is an approved provider of continuing education by the California Board of Registered Nursing, CEP 0910.

C
H
A
P
T
E
R

5

Alterations in Fluid, Electrolyte, and Acid-Base Balance

Kathy P. Parker, PhD, RN, FAAN

Chapter Contents

Kathy P. Parker, PhD, RN, FAAN

Normal renal function is essential for the optimal regulation of the volume and ionic composition of body fluids (see Chapter 4). When renal function is compromised, alterations in fluid, electrolytes, and acid-base balance occur. Hypervolemia often becomes a problem; however, in certain circumstances, the diseased kidney is unable to conserve water leading to hypovolemia. Sodium excess and depletion may also develop, depending on the free water load. Imbalances of other electrolytes including potassium, phosphate, calcium, and magnesium are common. Although metabolic acidosis related to retention of fixed acids is more likely, metabolic alkalosis can develop in selected situations if the kidneys become unable to excrete bicarbonate loads. Thus, in caring for patients with both acute and chronic kidney disease, the nurse should be knowledgeable regarding these potential abnormalities, their clinical presentation, and appropriate medical and nursing interventions.

Alterations in Fluid Balance

Body water represents approximately 55% to 60% of the total body weight in young, lean adults. As the water content of fat is less than that of lean body mass, the percentage of total body weight that is water is lower in obese individuals and in women (who typically have a higher body fat content than men). In a newborn, water may account for as much as 75% of the total body weight. In contrast, total body water decreases with age and may compose as little as 50% of the body weight in the elderly.

Body water is divided into two major compartments: extracellular fluid and intracellular fluid. Fluids outside the cells are in the extracellular fluid compartment (ECF) and account for approximately one-third of the total body water. This compartment can be further divided into interstitial fluids (fluid in between cells), intravascular fluid (plasma water), lymph, and transcellular fluid (fluid in joints, peritoneal and pleural cavities, etc). Conceptually, fluid (along with blood

components) that is available to fill the arterial vascular system and perfuse tissues and organs is specifically referred to as the effective arterial blood volume (EABV). Intracellular fluid (ICF), which makes up the remaining two-thirds of total body water, is that volume inside the cells (see Table 5-1). Fluid shifts between the fluid compartments through the semipermeable membranes that separate them often occurs, depending on both fluid and electrolyte status.

Although the plasma and interstitial fluids are very similar, the composition of the intracellular fluid compartment differs significantly (see Figure 5-1). In fact, all fluid compartments are characterized by a selected pattern of cations (positively charged ions) and anions (negatively charged ions). According to the principle of electrical neutrality, the number of positively and negatively charged substances in each compartment should be equal. Although maintenance of this balance is clinically important, it is impractical to routinely measure all of the relevant substances. Typically, only sodium (Na^+), potassium (K^+), chloride (Cl^-), and bicarbonate (HCO_3^-) are readily available. When these major ions are summed (as below), there is a gap (anion gap; AG).

Anion gap $= Na^+ - (Cl^- + HCO_3^-)$
$= 145$ mEq/L $- (101$ mEq/L $+ 35$ mEq/L$) = 9$ mEq/L

The normal AG is 9 ± 3 mEq/L; it represents the unmeasured anions and other negatively charged substances that are present in plasma (albumin, globulins, phosphates, sulfates, and other organic anions). An increase in AG can result from an increase in unmeasured anions (lactate - high anion gap acidosis). A decrease in AG can result from a decrease in unmeasured anions (i.e. low albumin as in nephritic syndrome, protein malnutrition). The assessment of acid-base disorders usually includes a calculation of the AG as it helps infer the underlying pathophysiology, (i.e., whether the disturbance is organic or inorganic in nature).

Fluid balance is determined by daily gains and losses. Most of the daily intake of water is oral. The remainder is water in food and a small amount produced by metabolic

Table 5-1
Classification of Body Fluid

Compartment	Volume of Fluids in Liters	Percentage of Body Fluid	Percentage of Body Weight
Total body fluid	42	100%	60%
Intracellular fluid (ICF)	28	67	40
Extracellular fluid (ECF)	14	33	20
• Interstitial fluid	2.8	6.6 (20% in ECF)	4
• Plasma	11.2	26.4 (80% in ECF)	16
• Lymph	negligible	negligible	negligible
• Transcellular fluid	negligible	negligible	negligible

Note: Reprinted with permission from Sherwood,L. (2004). *Human physiology: From cells to systems* (5th edition), page 561 (Table 15-1). Belmont, CA: Brooks/Cole-Thomas Learning.

Figure 5-1
Ionic Composition of Major Body-Fluid Compartments

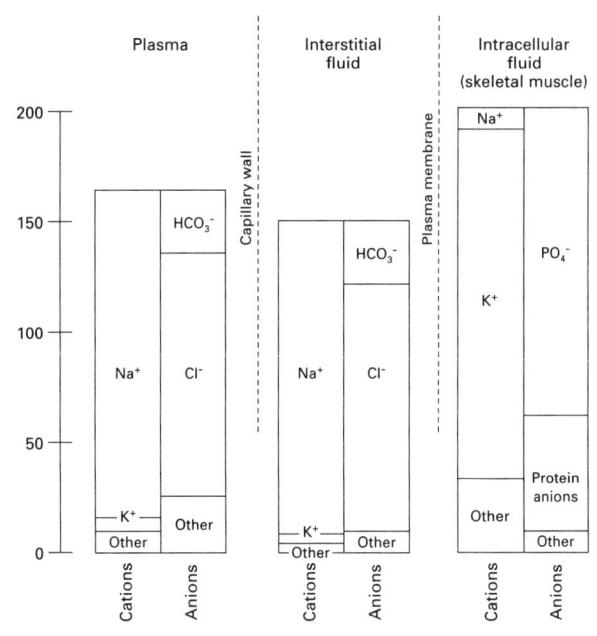

Note: From Sherwood, L. (2004). *Human physiology: From cells to systems, 5th edition.* Belmont, CA: Brooks/Cole – Thomas Learning. Reprinted with permission.

oxidation processes. A majority of body fluid losses occur in the form of urine (sensible fluid loss). Gastrointestinal losses are typically small but may become important when renal function is disturbed. Hidden water losses through the skin and respiratory tract (insensible water loss) also occur but vary significantly with dress, humidity, temperature, and exercise. Under sedentary and temperature-controlled conditions, daily insensible water loss is approximately 10 mL/kg of body weight (700 cc in a 70 kg individual). However, this amount can increase considerably and, under extremes of temperature and other abnormal physiological states, may approximate the amount of fluid excreted by the kidney. Thus, insensible loss can be just as important to body fluid regulation as urine output.

Hypervolemia, or volume excess (see Table 5-2), is a serious complication of acute renal failure and may develop insidiously or abruptly. Control of volume intake may be especially difficult to manage if the patient is receiving hyperalimentation, blood products, multiple intravenous medications, and continuous intravenous infusions. Therefore, medications should be given in the smallest volume possible, and this may necessitate the use of double-, triple-, or quadruple-strength solutions. Although intravenous medications are frequently given in 5% dextrose solution (D_5W), large amounts of this fluid can precipitate hyponatremia, and, therefore, normal saline may be more appropriate. Treatment of volume overload in acute renal failure usually includes an attempt to induce diuresis using high does loop diuretics (such as furosemide; bolus doses of

up to 200 mg or up to 20 mg/hour as an intravenous infusion) or sequential thiazide and loop diuretics if there is no response to conventional doses. Although patients may not respond to this treatment with increased urine output, some may show some resolution of pulmonary edema, if present, as furosemide increases large vein capacitance and shunts blood away from the pulmonary circulation. Dialysis with ultrafiltration may be required if attempts to induce diuresis are not successful. When the patient is hemodynamically unstable, a slow continuous renal replacement therapy may be the treatment of choice (see Chapter 9).

Fluid management in the patient with end-stage renal disease on dialysis is often a challenge for both the patient and the nurse. The daily fluid allowance is usually 1 liter plus the volume of urine produced. Sodium is also restricted to 2 g/day. Thirst can cause significant distress, particularly following dialysis, due to fluid removal and increases in serum osmolality. Patients can be advised to chew gum and suck on hard candy to help relieve this symptom. Ice chips can also be used to moisten the mucous membranes of the mouth and throat. However, the volume of fluid given with ice must be included in that volume permitted per day (the water volume of ice chips is approximately one-half of the measured volume). Good oral hygiene is also crucial.

Although volume overload is more common in patients with renal abnormalities, hypovolemia (see Table 5-2) may also occur. Fluid losses can develop from hemorrhage, burns, vomiting/diarrhea, diaphoresis, or excessive fluid removal during hemodialysis or peritoneal dialysis. Fluid losses should be replaced as soon as possible with solutions similar in composition to the lost fluid. Chronic kidney and end-stage renal disease patients can develop volume deficits for many of the same reasons. In addition, these patients may have increased insensible losses during elevations in ambient temperature and increased activity. In most cases, fluid losses can be replaced orally or during dialysis.

Although fluid intake and output are valuable guides, weight remains the most important indicator of overall fluid status. However, the information obtained from frequent measurements of weight does have its limitations. It is important to remember that patients with renal disease may become catabolic and develop protein wasting; dry body weight can be insidiously lost and replaced with fluid weight. Thus, it is important to complete a thorough assessment of the patient's fluid status on a regular basis (see Chapter 8). A summary of the signs and symptoms of alterations in fluid balance appears in Table 5-2.

Alterations in Sodium Balance

Sodium (Na+) is a major determinant of serum osmolality. It also plays an essential role in nerve conduction, acid-base balance, and numerous chemical reactions. Because water is freely permeable across cell membranes, changes in the extracellular sodium concentration result in shifts in water distribution in ECF and ICF compartments. (This process by which this occurs is referred to as osmosis, the passive movement of water through a membrane from an area of lower concentration of solutes to an area of greater concentration of solutes.) For example, a decrease in the sodium concentration of the intravascular compartment

Table 5-2
Alterations in Water Balance

Major Causes	Signs and Symptoms
Hypervolemia	
Renal insufficiency Renal failure Congestive heart failure Cirrhosis Nephrotic syndrome	Weight gain Edema Headache Visual blurring Hypertension Tachycardia Engorged neck veins Cough, dyspnea S3 gallop Pulmonary rales
Hypovolemia	
Renal losses of salt and water • Diuretics • Post-obstructive diuresis • Renal tubular defects GI losses • Vomiting • Diarrhea Skin losses • Diaphoresis • Burns • Insensible Losses Third-spacing of fluid • Ascites Blood loss	Weight loss Reduced skin turgor Dry, cracked mucous membranes Dizziness, syncope Orthostatic hypotension Hypotension Tachycardia Postural hypotension and tachycardia Thirst

Note: Adapted from Berl & Schrier (2003); Berl & Verbalis (2004); Huether (2002); Nielsen, Knepper, Kwon, & Frokiaer (2004); Schrier, Gurevich & Abraham (2003); Sherwood (2004).

results in a shift of water into the cells, causing an increase in cell volume. On the other hand, an increase in intravascular sodium concentration produces a shift of water from the intracellular to the extracellular compartment, and cells shrink.

In kidney disease, the ability to excrete sodium often becomes limited. In contrast, however, the ability to conserve sodium may be decreased, resulting in "salt wasting." Therefore, although sodium restriction is commonly necessary in the treatment of patients with acute or chronic kidney disease, the dietary prescription of sodium should be individualized and based on urinary sodium losses.

Hypernatremia, defined as a plasma sodium concentration above 146 mEq/L, is extremely dangerous. The condition is rare, but when it occurs is associated with a 10% to 60% mortality rate. Hypernatremia results from an excess in sodium relative to free water and always reflects a hyperosmolar state. It can occur with decreased, normal, or increased total body water (see Table 5-3) and with low, normal, or high total body sodium. This condition is most commonly seen in patients with restricted access to fluid, such as

the elderly or critically ill, or those with impaired thirst regulation. In the patient with renal failure, hypernatremia may also occur during peritoneal dialysis when high-dextrose, short-dwell exchanges are used to remove fluid quickly.

The symptoms associated with hypernatremia vary with the speed of onset and result from a loss in intracellular fluid stores. Manifestations include dry mucous membranes, intense thirst, flushed skin, fever, and oliguria. Central nervous systems symptoms include lethargy, altered mentation, and seizures (see Table 5-3). Physical examination may be unremarkable.

The treatment of hypernatremia depends on two very important factors - the ECF volume status of the patient and the rate of development of the hypernatremia. The overall goal of treatment is to restore normal osmolality. If the imbalance is caused by water deficits, it is important to replace volume with free water, hypotonic sodium chloride, or D_5W. If it is associated with volume expansion, diuretics may be used to enhance sodium excretion if renal function permits.

Severe neurologic signs and symptoms are associated with the rapid correction of hypernatremia and may result in

Table 5-3
Alterations in Sodium Balance
Normal rage – 135 to 145 mEq/L

Major Causes	Signs and Symptoms
Hypernatremia - Serum Na+ > 146 mEq/L	
Hypovolemic • GI losses of water • Renal losses of water • Skin losses of water Euvolemic • Renal losses of water • Skin and respiratory water losses • Inability to gain access to fluids Hypervolemic • Hypertonic saline administration • Infants given hypertonic feedings • Hyperaldosterism Sodium chloride intake	Depression of sensorium Seizures Irritability Focal neurologic deficits Muscle spasticity Fever Nausea, vomiting Labored respiration Intense thirst Flushed skin Dry mucous membranes
Hyponatremia - Serum Na+ < 135 mEq/L	
Hypovolemic • Vomiting • Diarrhea • Diuretics • Salt-losing nephritis • Third spacing Euvolemic • Drugs • Pain • Emotional distress • Syndrome of inappropriate ADH secretion Hypervolemic • Congestive heart failure • Acute renal failure • Chronic renal failure • Cirrhosis • Nephrotic syndrome	Headache Abnormal sensorium Depressed deep tendon reflexes Cheyne-Stokes respiration Hypothermia Pathologic reflexes Pseudobulbar palsy Seizures Lethargy Disorientation Muscle cramps Anorexia, nausea Agitation

Note: Adapted from Berl & Schrier (2003); Berl & Verbalis (2004); Huether (2002); Nielsen et al. (2004); Schrier et al. (2003); Sherwood (2004).

cerebral edema, seizures, and death. In general, the serum sodium level should be reduced no faster than 2 mEq/L/hour during the first 48 hours. If dialysis is being used, the safest approach is to dialyze a patient with a dialysis solution sodium level close to that of the plasma and then correct the hypernatremia by slow administration of isotonic saline. (When comparing the concentration of fluids to the blood or plasma, isotonic refers to those fluids with the same concentration of solutes; hypertonic refers to those having a greater concentration; and hypotonic refers to those with a lower concentration.)

Hyponatremia, defined as a plasma sodium concentration less than 135 mEq/L, is a state in which there is a decrease in sodium relative to water. It is among the most common electrolyte disorders seen in clinical practice.

Depending on the etiology of the hyponatremia, this condition may be associated with hypervolemia, hypovolemia, and euvolemia (see Table 5-3). Hyponatremia may also be associated with decreased, increased, or near-normal amounts of total body sodium. Pseudohyponatremia is sometimes seen with hyperlipidemia (a rise of plasma lipids of 4.6 g/L leads to a decrease in sodium of 1 mEq/L), hyperproteinemia (plasma concentration > 10g/dl lead to a comparable effect), and hyperglycemia (decrease in plasma sodium is approximately 1.6 mEq/L for every 100 mg/dl increase in plasma glucose) as these conditions are osmotically active and pull water into the intravascular space. In these cases, correction of the underlying problem also corrects the hyponatremia.

The signs and symptoms that may be associated with hyponatremia (see Table 5-3) are caused by the decreased

Table 5-4
Alterations in Potassium Balance
Normal range – 3.5 to 5.5 mEq/L

Major Causes	Signs and Symptoms
Hyperkalemia - Serum K⁺ > 5.5 mEq/L	
Increased dietary intake • Rapid IV K⁺ infusion • Transfusion of stored blood • Salt substitutes Decreased renal excretion • Acute renal failure • Chronic renal failure • Adrenal insufficiency • Potassium sparing diuretics • Angiotensin converting/enzyme inhibitors • Nonsteroidal anti-inflammatory drugs Release of intracellular K⁺ • Hemolysis • Catabolism • Burns • Rhabdomyolysis Shift of K⁺ from cells to ECF • Insulin deficiency • Acidosis • Beta blockers	Skeletal muscle weakness and paralysis Tingling of lips and fingers Restlessness Intestinal cramping Diarrhea Cardiac arrythmias – bradycardia, sinus arrest, ventricular tachycardia, ventricular fibrillation, asystole Cardiac changes – tall peaked T waves, prolonged PR intervals, progressive widening of the QRS complex
Hypokalemia - Serum K⁺ < 3.5 mEq/L	
Decreased dietary intake • Anorexia • Alcoholism Renal losses • Diuretics • Steroids GI losses • Vomiting • Diarrhea • Laxative abuse Shift of K⁺ from ECF to cells • Alkalosis • Insulin • Hypothermia	Muscle weakness and paralysis Generalized malaise Fatigue Restless legs syndrome Myalgias Rhabdomyolysis Cardiac arrythmias (atrial and ventricular) Cardiac changes – flattening of the T wave, ST depression, QT prolongation (often accompanied by hypomagnesemia) Possible increase in blood pressure Carbohydrate intolerance Polydipsia Polyuria Renal abnormalities Constipation Intestinal distention Anorexia Nausea, vomiting Paralytic ileus

Note: Adapted from Huether (2002); Ludlow (2003); Mount & Zandi-Nejad (2004); Peterson & Levi (2003); Sherwood (2004); Velazquez & Wright (2001).

Table 5-5
Treatment of Hyperkalemia

Mechanism	Onset of action
Antagonism of membrane actions • Calcium	Several minutes and then rapidly waves
Increased potassium entry into cells • Insulin and glucose • β-2 adrenergic agonists • Sodium bicarbonate	Each of these modalities works within 30-60 minutes, lowers the serum potassium concentration by 0.5 – 1.5 mEq/L, and lasts for several hours
Potassium removal from the body • Diuretics	Several hours but many patients with advance renal failure show little response
• Cation exchange resin • Dialysis	2-3 hours Several hours

Note: Reprinted with permission from Rose, B.D. & Rennke, H.G. (1994). *Renal pathophysiology - The essentials* pg. 183. Baltimore: Williams & Wilkins.

osmolality of the extracellular fluid and generally correlate with the rate of development of the abnormality. Although the majority of patients with hyponatremia are asymptomatic, early manifestations include gastrointestinal symptoms such as anorexia, nausea, vomiting, generalized weakness, and muscle cramps. The later and more severe signs and symptoms relate to the central nervous system (cerebral edema) and include malaise, headache, confusion, lethargy, seizures, and coma. These problems usually develop when the sodium decreases rapidly to 120 to 125 mEq/L.

The medical management of hyponatremia is determined by the degree of symptoms exhibited as well as by the onset and duration of the abnormality. Treatment may include water restriction, administration of intravenous sodium chloride solutions, or discontinuation of diuretic therapy. In the renal failure patient, the sodium content of the dialysate bath in hemodialysis can be increased. Overly rapid or a large change in serum sodium in those with the condition for > 48 hours may cause shrinkage of the brain tissue, resulting in severe neurologic signs and symptoms and even death (central pontine myelinolysis). Rapid correction (1 to 2 mEq/L/hour) may be indicated in those patients with acute (< 48 hours) and symptomatic hyponatremia.

Alterations of Potassium Balance

Potassium (K$^+$) is one of the most abundant cations in the body, with total body potassium stores in adults approximating 50-55/mEq per kilogram of body weight. Approximately 150 mEq of potassium are present in each liter of intracellular fluid while only 4.0 mEq are present in each liter of extracellular fluid. Thus, more than 98% of total body potassium is present inside the cells. As the major intracellular cation, potassium helps maintain intracellular osmolality, regulates skeletal, cardiac, and smooth muscle activity, influences acid-base balance, and is crucial for many intracellular enzyme reactions.

Changes in the plasma potassium concentration have important effects on neuronal membrane excitability. A fall in extracellular potassium concentration (hypokalemia) lowers the resting membrane potential (E_m) of the cell, leading to hyperpolarization and decreased neuronal excitability. A rise in potassium concentration (hyperkalemia) increases the resting membrane potential, bringing it closer to the threshold potential (E_t) for neuronal firing (see Figure 5-2). Hyperkalemia, therefore, causes increased neuronal excitability. The effects of alterations in potassium levels on neuromuscular transmission are clinically important, because they are largely responsible for the most serious symptoms associated with disturbances in potassium balance: muscle weakness, potentially fatal cardiac arrhythmias, and disturbances in cardiac conduction.

Hyperkalemia, defined as a serum potassium > 5.5 mEq/L, is caused by factors such as increased potassium intake, decreased renal excretion, increased release of intracellular potassium, or a shift of potassium from the cells into the extracellular fluid (see Table 5-4). In the acute setting, hyperkalemia is a serious complication and may be aggravated by release of intracellular stores with hypercatabolism or hemolysis. In the chronic setting, hyperkalemia occurs most often in individuals who have failed to report for dialysis for several days or follow the prescribed dietary regimen. Diabetes may aggravate hyperkalemia because of insulin deficiency or resistance. Medications that can impair potassium entry into cells such as alpha-adrenergic receptor agonists (nasal sprays), nonselective beta-blockers, or agents that interfere with potassium secretion such as nonsteroidal anti-inflammatory drugs, angiotensin-converting enzyme inhibitors, and potassium-sparing diuretics can also increase potassium levels. Pseudohyperkalemia may be seen when blood is hemolyzed or an excessively tight tourniquet is used during the blood collection procedures.

As hyperkalemia develops, the smooth and skeletal muscles become hypopolarized and more reactive to stimuli (see

Figure 5-3). Early hyperkalemia is associated with mild intestinal cramping and diarrhea, nausea, and vomiting. Later, muscle weakness and flaccid paralysis are common. Ultimately, hyperkalemia decreases the duration and rate of rise of the cardiac action potential, and decreases conduction velocity. Acute hyperkalemia is potentially life threatening because of the risk of cardiac arrest. In some patients, treatment with diuretics may be helpful. The various treatments for acute hyperkalemia are outlined in Table 5-5. When hyperkalemia is mild and chronic, therapeutic measures should address the specific cause. In the patient with kidney disease, adherence to the diet is often the problem.

Hypokalemia is defined as a serum potassium level less than 3.5 mEq/L. Generally, this condition occurs in one of four major situations: decreased dietary intake, increased urinary losses, excessive GI losses, or increased entry of potassium into the cells (see Table 5-4). This electrolyte disturbance is commonly seen in the acute renal failure patient with nonoliguric renal failure caused by diuretics, cisplatin , or amphotericin B. In those with chronic kidney disease, hypokalemia typically occurs when food intake is poor or the patient has diarrhea. Pseudohypokalemia is caused by the movement of K^+ inside metabolically-active cells after the blood has been removed from the patient. This is more likely to happen if the patient has a high white blood count or if the blood has stood for a prolonged period of time at room temperature; this problem can be avoided by refrigeration of the sample.

As previously mentioned, the clinical manifestations of hypokalemia result from hyperpolarization of cellular membranes of nerve and muscle cells which decrease neuromuscular excitability (see Figure 5-3). The most significant effect of hypokalemia is on cardiac function. Manifestations include alterations in the electrocardiogram (ECG) (see Table 5-4), predisposition to digitalis toxicity, and atrial and ventricular arrhythmias. Hypomotility of the gastrointestinal tract leading to constipation also occurs. Patients may experience malaise, weakness, fatigue, and myalgia. Paralysis of the extremities and respiratory muscles has been described with a serum K < 2.0.

Treatment for hypokalemia usually involves replacement of the deficit with potassium salts either orally or intravenously. The oral route is preferable if tolerated by the patient (particularly with foods high in potassium such as orange juice). However, a common complication of oral potassium chloride supplementation is gastrointestinal bleeding. Phlebitis may occur with intravenous administration of potassium chloride, especially when the concentration exceeds 40 mEq/L. The major risk of potassium replacement in patients with renal impairment is the development of hyperkalemia. If the patient is receiving dialysis, the potassium content of the dialysate should be increased, particularly if the patient is on digitalis.

Alterations in Calcium and Phosphorous Balance

There is a close link between the regulation of calcium and phosphate in the body. A change in the concentration of one is often associated with a change in the concentration of the other; when one substance is elevated, the other tends to drop and visa versa. Thus, both calcium and phosphate are discussed together in this section.

Calcium (Ca^{2+}) plays a major role in many important metabolic and physiologic processes. In addition to being a major constituent of bone, calcium ions are important in intracellular and enzymatic reactions, and in blood coagulation. Calcium is also critical for neuromuscular transmission. About 99% of the calcium in the body is found in the skeleton and teeth. Of the remaining 1%, about 0.9% is found intracellularly with less than 0.1% being present in the ECF. Approximately half of the plasma calcium is bound to plasma proteins. The other half of the plasma calcium is ionized and, therefore, can freely diffuse through cell membranes. Only the free, or ionized, calcium is biologically active. Natural cheeses, milk, and dairy products are major sources of dietary calcium.

Phosphorous (PO_4^{2-}) is the sixth most abundant element in the human body. Approximately 80% of phosphorous is also found in the bones. Only a small amount is found in the ECF, the normal level being 2.5 to 4.5 mg/dL. Phosphorous is the major anion in the ICF where it functions primarily as a cofactor in many metabolic processes, including the formation of high-energy phosphate bonds such as those in ATP. It is also an important component of nucleic acids. In the ECF, phosphorus plays an important role in acid-base buffering and calcium homeostasis. Milk and its products are the richest source of phosphorus. However, both are found in other foods, such a meat, fish, poultry, whole grains, eggs, and peanuts.

Serum calcium and phosphorous are maintained within their normal ranges via regulatory mechanisms involving the gastrointestinal tract, the skeleton, and the kidneys under the influence of parathyroid hormone (PTH), vitamin D, and calcitonin. PTH, a substance produced by the parathyroid glands, is sensitive to the level of serum calcium. When serum calcium levels drop, PTH is released, causing enhanced renal absorption of calcium and increased activity of bone osteoclasts (bone breakdown cells) that liberate ionized calcium. The result is an increase in serum calcium.

PTH also activates the production of the most active form of vitamin D (1,25-$(OH)_2D_3$; 1, 25-dihydroxycholecalciferol; or calcitriol) by the kidney. This substance facilitates the absorption of calcium from the GI tract that also increases the serum calcium level. However, a series of metabolic changes must occur before calcitriol is produced. Initially, Vitamin D_3 (cholecalciferol, a fat-soluble steroid ingested in food or synthesized in the skin in the presence of ultraviolet light) is converted by the liver into 25-$(OH)D_3$ (calcifediol). This substance is subsequently converted into calcitriol [1,25-$(OH)_2D_3$] by the kidney. Thus, both normal liver and kidney function are required for these processes to occur.

Calcitonin, produced by the C cells in the thyroid, also play a role in calcium balance. Hypercalcemia stimulates release of calcitonin, which lowers serum calcium through inhibition bone osteoclastic activity and increased renal excretion of calcium (see Figure 5-4).

Although PTH also increases the absorption of phosphorous from the GI tract, it enhances renal phosphate excretion. This action is very important in calcium-phosphate regulation. Significantly elevated phosphate levels actually lower ionized calcium because phosphate binds

Figure 5-2
Effects of Potassium and Calcium on Membrane Excitability

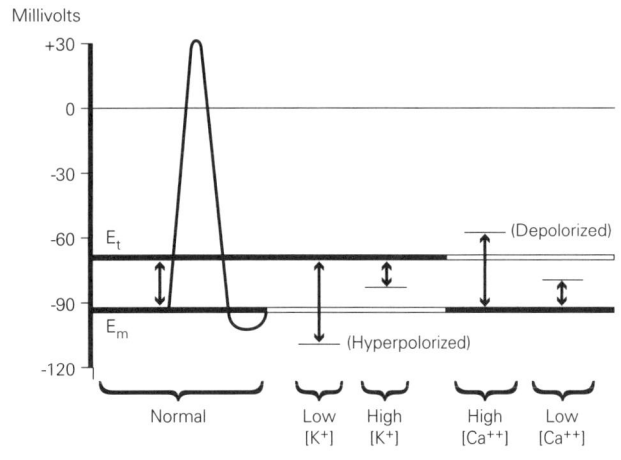

Note: From McCance, K.L., & Huether, S.E. (1994). *Pathophysiology: The biologic basis for disease in adults and children* (p. 105). St. Louis, MO: Mosby Yearbook. Reprinted with permission.

with calcium, forming a complex which precipitates out of solution. These "calcium-phosphate complexes" can deposit in the soft tissues and blood vessels, a process called calciphylaxis or metastatic calcification. Thus, maintenance of normal calcium and phosphate levels is important in preventing calcium-phosphate deposition. Under normal circumstances, the calcium phosphate product (calcium in mg/dl X phosphate in mg/dl) is approximately 40. If the product exceeds 70, complex deposition may occur.

In summary, three principal mechanisms involving the bone, the kidney, and the GI tract, all controlled by PTH, vitamin D, and calcitonin (see Figure 5-4), bring a low calcium level back to within its normal range. The processes reverse in the presence of high calcium levels. Alterations in the levels of calcium, phosphate, and their products occurs frequently in renal failure and are related to abnormalities in the excretion, absorption, and metabolism of the electrolytes. In patients with chronic kidney disease, these alterations may lead to metastatic calcifications, secondary hyperparathyroidism, and renal bone disease. A thorough discussion of these abnormalities appears in Chapter 13.

Hypercalcemia

Hypercalcemia is defined as a total plasma calcium greater than 10.0 mg/dl. Hypercalcemia causes the neuronal threshold potential to become more positive and depresses neuromuscular excitability (see Figure 5-2). The major causes of hypercalcemia include increased GI absorption, increased calcium release from bone, and increased physiologically available calcium (see Table 5-6). Hypercalcemia may be seen in the acute renal failure patient with a malignancy, such as multiple myeloma or a solid tumor, because of bone destruction and release of intracellular stores. Hypercalcemia often occurs in patients with chronic kidney disease and is usually attributable to secondary hyperparathyroidism or aluminum toxicity. Medications associated

with hypercalcemia include lithium, thiazides, and excessive vitamin A and D ingestion.

The neuropsychiatric manifestations of hypercalcemia range from subtle personality changes to acute psychosis. There may also be weakness, lethargy, confusion, and coma. Vomiting and constipation may occur (see Table 5-6). Hypercalcemia shortens the QT interval on electrocardiogram (see Figure 5-5), potentiates the action of cardiac glycosides, and may cause arrhythmias. When hyperphosphatemia is also present, calcium will bind with the phosphate, precipitate, and deposit in soft tissues.

Although treatment of chronic hypercalcemia depends on the underlying cause, immediate therapy is required for patients with acute, severe hypercalcemia; symptomatic patients usually have a calcium greater than 12 mg/dl and require prompt treatment. If renal function permits, the administration of saline (hydration) and diuretics can assist in increasing calcium excretion in the urine. To maintain normocalcemia, pamidronate may be used to inhibit osteoclastic bone resorption. Calcitonin may also be used as it inhibits bone resorption and increases urinary calcium excretion. In addition, therapy for renal failure patients includes reducing calcium in dialysis bath and withdrawing vitamin D therapy and calcium containing binders.

Hypocalcemia

Hypocalcemia is defined as a plasma calcium level below 8.5 mg/dL. Calcium deficits cause partial depolarization of neuronal cells resulting in an increase in neuromuscular irritability (see Figure 5-2). The major causes of hypocalcemia include decreased intake or gastrointestinal absorption of calcium, increased urinary excretion of calcium, disturbances of the parathyroid gland, and decreased physiologically-available calcium (see Table 5-5). Selected medications may also alter levels. As mentioned previously, hypocalcemia in renal failure occurs predominantly because of abnormalities in the absorption and metabolism of calcium.

The clinical features of hypocalcemia depend on the rapidity of onset and duration of the abnormality. Circumoral and acral (fingers and toes) paresthesias and tingling around the mouth and lips are frequently the initial manifestations of hypocalcemia-induced increased neuromuscular excitability. Latent tetany may be detected by tapping over the facial nerve to produce a facial twitch (Chvostek's sign) or by inflation of a blood pressure cuff to a level between systolic and diastolic pressure for more than 5 minutes to produce carpopedal spasm (Trousseau's sign; see Figure 5-6). In more severe cases, laryngeal stridor/spasm and convulsions can occur. Neuropsychiatric manifestations range from emotional lability to depression or frank psychosis. Weakness and fatigue may also be present. The characteristic electrocardiographic finding is a prolonged QT interval (see Figure 5-5). In chronic cases, papilledema, cataracts, dental caries, rickets, and osteomalacia may be present. The skin may also become dry and scaly, the nails brittle, and the hair coarse (see Table 5-6).

Decreased calcium levels are frequently seen in association with hypoalbuminemia, a condition common in renal failure patients. This decrease occurs in the protein-bound

Table 5-6
Alterations in Calcium Balance
Normal Range – 8 to 10 mg/dL

Major Causes	Signs and Symptoms
Hypercalcemia - Serum Ca⁺⁺ > 10.0 mg/dL	
Increased GI absorption of Ca^{++} • Milk-alkali syndrome • Vitamin A or D intoxication • Sarcoidosis Increased release of Ca^{++} from bone • Hyperparathyroidism • Malignancies • Immobilization Decreased physiologic availability of Ca^{++} • Acidosis Medications • Thiazide diuretics • Lithium carbonate • Estrogens	Altered mental status Fatigue Weakness Lethargy Anorexia Nausea, vomiting Constipation Impaired renal function Shortened QT segment and depressed T waves Polyuria Polydipsia
Hypocalcemia - Serum Ca⁺⁺ < 8.5 mg/dL	
Decreased intake or poor GI absorption of Ca^{++} • Poor diet • Malabsorption • Renal failure Increased urinary losses of Ca^{++} • Renal defects Decreased physiologic availability of Ca^{++} • Alkalosis • Massive transfusion with citrated blood • Hypoalbuminemia Disturbances of parathyroid system • Hypoparathyroidism • Pseudohypoparathyroidism Medications • Biphosphates • Mithramycin • Calcitonin • Citrated blood	Anxiety, depression Paresthesias Laryngospasm Chvostek's sign Trousseau's sign Convulsions Tetany Prolonged QT interval Intestinal cramping Hyperactive bowel sounds Longstanding hypocalcemia • Dry skin • Coarse hair • Alopeci • Brittle nails

Note: Adapted from Huether, 2002; Pollak & Yu 2004; Popovtzer, 2003.

fraction of the calcium, with a negligible change in the ionized component. A decrease in albumin of 1 g/dL is associated with an increase in plasma calcium of approximately 0.8 mg/dL. One way of "correcting" the measured serum calcium level when the concentration of albumin is low is to add 0.8 mg/dL to the patient's calcium for every 1.0 g/dL that the serum albumin is below 4.0 g/dL. Acid-base disturbances also affect the ionized fraction of calcium. A drop in pH of 0.1 units results in a reciprocal rise in ionized calcium of approximately 0.1 mEq/L. Therefore, renal failure patients who have acidosis may be asymptomatic from hypocalcemia because metabolic acidosis increases the level of ionized calcium and counterbalances its effect on the neuromuscular system. In critically ill patients, total calcium levels may be a poor indicator of the ionized calcium as a number of factors in this setting may change calcium/protein binding (intravenous contrast, albumin infusion, citrate, intravenous fluids, acid/base disturbances, dialysis therapy). Thus, it is important to measure ionized calcium in these situations.

Therapy for acute hypocalcemia is replacement with intravenous calcium salts such as calcium chloride, calcium citrate, and calcium gluconate, for example, 1 to 3 g of intra-

Figure 5-3
Electrocardiogram Abnormalities Associated with Potassium Changes

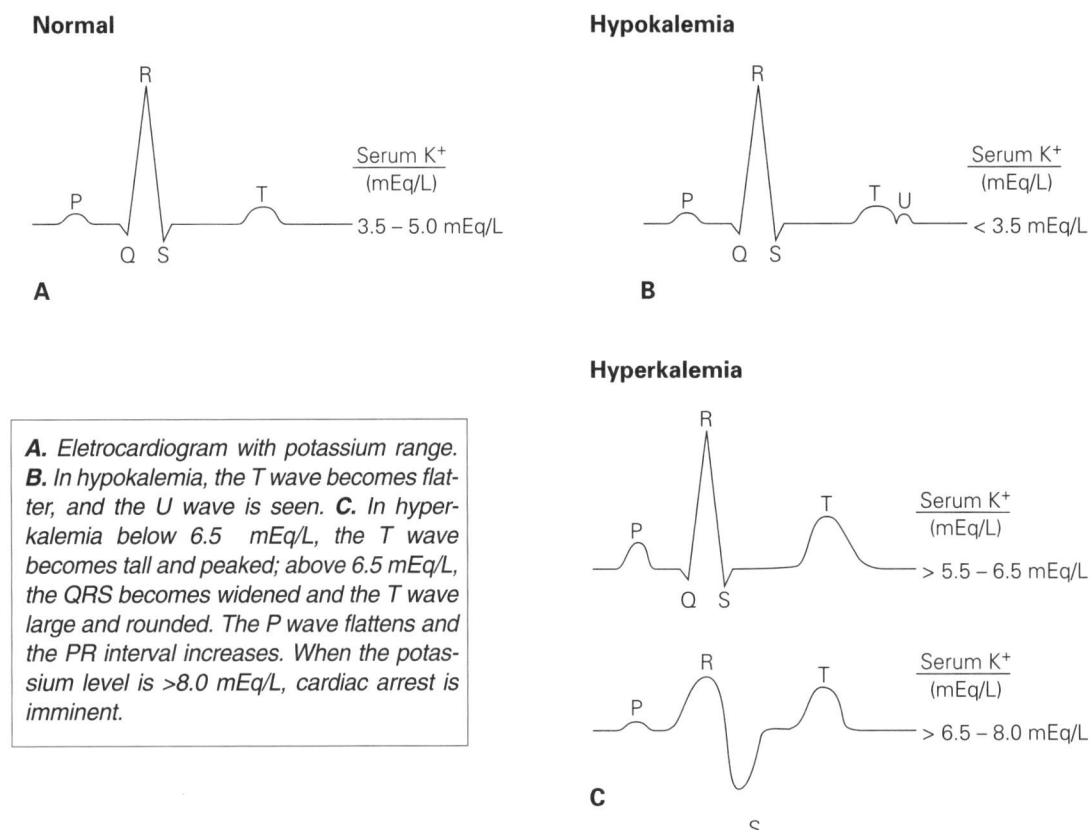

Normal

Serum K⁺ (mEq/L)
3.5 – 5.0 mEq/L

A

Hypokalemia

Serum K⁺ (mEq/L)
< 3.5 mEq/L

B

A. Eletrocardiogram with potassium range. B. In hypokalemia, the T wave becomes flatter, and the U wave is seen. C. In hyperkalemia below 6.5 mEq/L, the T wave becomes tall and peaked; above 6.5 mEq/L, the QRS becomes widened and the T wave large and rounded. The P wave flattens and the PR interval increases. When the potassium level is >8.0 mEq/L, cardiac arrest is imminent.

Hyperkalemia

Serum K⁺ (mEq/L)
> 5.5 – 6.5 mEq/L

Serum K⁺ (mEq/L)
> 6.5 – 8.0 mEq/L

C

Note: From Bullock, B.L. (1996). *Pathophysiology: Adaptations and alterations in function* (p. 201). Philadelphia: J.B. Lippincott Company. Reprinted with permission.

venous calcium gluconate given over a period of 10 to 20 minutes. Replacement should also be done slowly and carefully if the patient is on digitalis or hypokalemia is present. Treatment of chronic hypocalcemia includes oral calcium, vitamin D supplementation, and control of hyperphosphatemia. Correction of hypomagnesemia and hyperphosphatemia should also be done.

Hyperphosphatemia

Hyperphosphatemia is defined as a plasma phosphate concentration above 4.5 mg/dl. A decrease in the glomerular filtration rate (usually < 25 mL/min) accounts for more than 90% of the cases of hyperphosphatemia and is a common complication of both acute and chronic renal failure. In acute renal failure, levels rarely rise above 7 mg/dL, but very high levels may be seen with severe tissue breakdown as in rhabdomyolysis and tumor lysis syndrome. The most important short-term consequence of hyperphosphatemia is hypocalcemia. Calcium phosphate crystals form and deposit in soft tissues including the joints, myocardium, brain, lungs, skin, and blood vessels. Clinical symptoms of hyperphosphatemia are primarily related to low serum calcium levels and are comparable to symptoms of hypocalcemia (see Tables 5-6 & 5-7).

Treatment for hyperphosphatemia in the renal failure

patient includes dietary restriction of phosphorus (600 to 1000 mg/day). Intestinal absorption is frequently blocked with an aluminum antacid. However, aluminum-containing agents are rarely used to manage hyperphosphatemia as they have been shown to be toxic to bone, brain, and the myocardium of patients and are not ideal for long-term use. Constipation is also a major complication. Calcium salts, in the form of calcium carbonate or calcium acetate, are the preferred maintenance binders. Maximal binding occurs when these binders are taken with meals. Dialysis also assists in removing phosphorous.

A plasma phosphate concentration of 2.5 mg/dl or less indicates hypophosphatemia. This condition can be caused by decreased intestinal absorption of phosphorous, increased urinary losses, or a shift of phosphorus from extracellular to intracellular compartments (such as during nutritional repletion or in alkalosis (see Table 5-7). Hypophosphatemia may be seen in some patients with acute renal failure, particularly those with burns, on hyperalimentation, or alcoholics. In the chronic renal failure patient, this abnormality can be seen in association with poor nutritional intake or excessive phosphorous-binder therapy.

Mild or moderate hypophosphatemia frequently has no clinical manifestations. Symptoms usually do not occur until serum phosphate levels approach or fall below 1 mg/dl. The

Table 5-7
Alterations in Phosphorous Balance
Normal range - 2.5 mg/dL to 4.5 mg/dL

Major Causes	Signs and Symptoms
Hyperphosphatemia - Serum $PO_4^=$ > 4.5 mg/dL	
Decreased renal excretion • Renal failure • Hypoparathyroidism • Acromegaly Increased $PO_4^=$ loads or GI absorption • IV, oral, or rectal administration of $PO_4^=$ • Vitamin D administration Release of intracellular $PO_4^=$ into ECF • Catabolism • Infections • Crush injuries • Cytotoxic therapy Respiratory Acidosis	Symptoms are primarily related to low serum calcium levels and thus are comparable to symptoms of hypocalcemia
Hypophosphatemia - Serum $PO_4^=$ < 2.5 mg/dL	
Decreased intake or poor GI absorption of $PO_4^=$ • Alcoholism • Malabsorption • Vitamin D deficiency • Starvation • Chronic diarrhea • Phosphate binding antacids Increased urinary losses • Hyperparathyroidism • Acidosis • Renal tubular defects • Drugs - diuretics, calcitonin Shift of $PO_4^=$ from ECF into cells • Nutritional repletion • Alkalosis • Salicylate poisoning • Insulin • "Hungry bone syndrome (post-parathyroidectomy)	Hypoxia Bradycardia Leukocyte and platelet dysfunctions; greater risk of infection and blood-clotting impairment Rhabdomyolysis Irritability Confusion Numbness Coma Convulsions Respiratory failure Cardiomyopathies

Note: Adapted from Huether, 2002; Pollak & Yu, 2004; Popovtzer, 2003.

mechanisms believed to be responsible for the clinical manifestations include diminished ATP production, decreased concentrations of 2,3 diphophoglycerate in erythrocytes (causing a decreased binding affinity for oxygen), and stimulation of other electrolyte imbalances.

Neurologic manifestations of hypophosphatemia include encephalopathy, paresthesias, and hyperreflexia (see Table 5-7). Skeletal muscles become weak, possibly leading to respiratory failure. Hematologic abnormalities include decreased platelet aggregation, loss of erythrocyte oxygen binding capacity, hemolysis, and immunosuppression. Acute hypophosphatemia can also result in impaired leukocyte function and increase the risk of infections.

The appropriate treatment of hypophosphatemia requires identification and correction of the underlying cause. When supplementation is necessary, it can be done with milk (if the patient can tolerate lactose), an excellent source of phosphorus. Neutraphos tablets can also be used. Intravenous supplementation may be necessary for severe cases. Intravenous supplementation is usually safe and effective. Complications of repletion therapy include diarrhea, hyperphosphatemia, and hypocalcemia with metastatic calcifications.

Alterations in Magnesium Balance

Magnesium (Mg^{2+}) is the fourth most abundant cation in the body (normal range 1.8 to 2.4 mg/dL) and is involved in enzymatic reactions and the maintenance of cellular permeability and neuromuscular excitability. In addition, it is important in the production and use of energy essential in

Figure 5-4
Hormonal Regulation of Calcium Balance

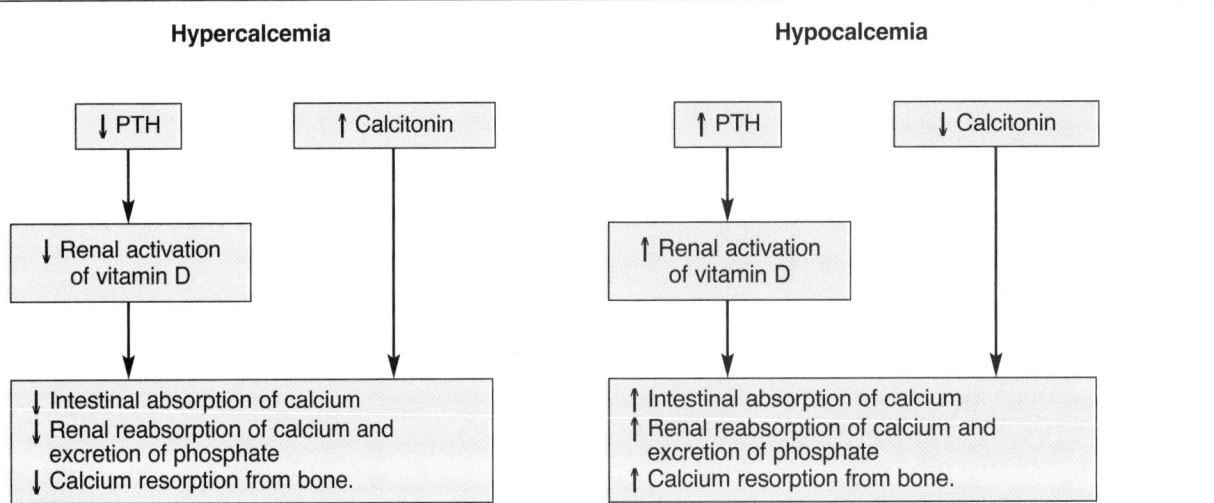

aNote: From McCance, K.L. & Huether, S.E. (2002). *Pathophysiology: The Biological Basis for Disease in Adults and Children*, pg. 99 (Figure 3-7). St. Louis: Mosby

Figure 5-5
EKG Abnormalities Associated with Alterations in Calcium Levels

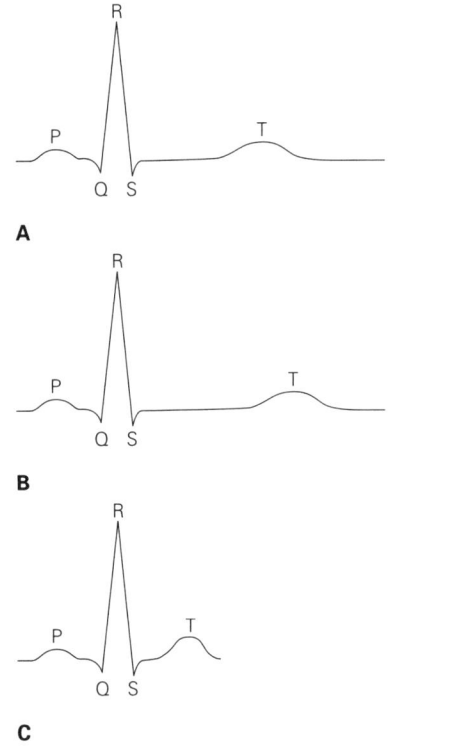

*A. Normal electrocardiogram tracing. **B.** Prolongation of the QT interval in hypocalcemia may increase risk of dysrhythmias or heart block and may be associated with poor contractility. **C.** Shortening of QT in hypercalcemia may cause severe dysrhythmias that may result from increased cardiac irritability.*

Note: From Bullock, B.L. (1996). *Pathophysiology: Adaptations and alterations in function* (p. 203). Philadelphia: J.B. Lippincott Company. Reprinted with permission.

Figure 5-6
Position of the Hand in Hypocalcemic Tetany (Trousseau's Sign)

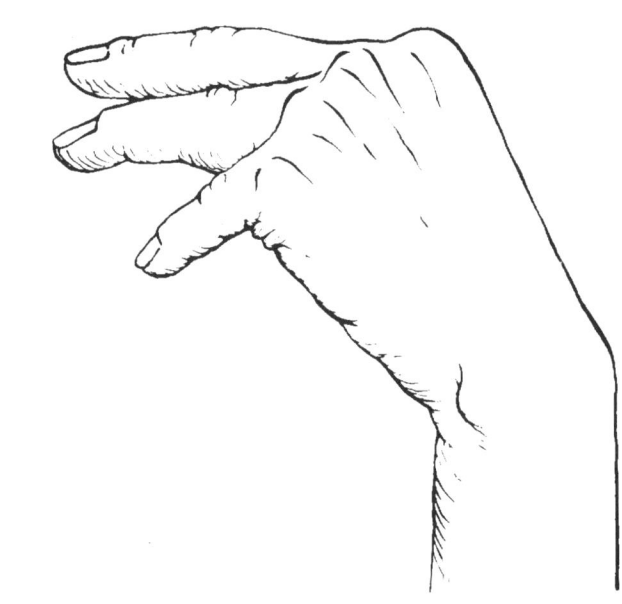

Note: From Ganong, W.F. (1993). *Review of medical physiology* (p. 357). Norwalk, CT: Appleton & Lange. Reprinted with permission.

the maintenance of normal intracellular electrolyte composition. Approximately 40 to 60% is stored in muscles and bone with 30% in the cells. Regulation of magnesium is a function of both gastrointestinal absorption and renal excretion.

Hypermagnesemia is defined as a serum magnesium greater than 2.5 mg/dL and can result from increased magnesium absorption, decreased renal excretion, and certain medications (see Table 5-8). Symptoms of hypermagnesemia

Table 5-8
Alterations in Magnesium Balance
Normal range – 1.8 to 2.4 mg/dL

Major Causes	Signs and Symptoms
Hypermagnesemia - Serum Mg^{++} > 2.5 mg/dL	
Increased intake • Oral or parenteral Mg^{++} administration Decreased renal excretion • Renal failure Miscellaneous • Lithium • Bone metastasis • Hypothyroidism • Addison's disease	Lethargy Dilated pupils Nausea Vomiting Muscle weakness Depression of deep tendon reflexes Paralytic illeus Hypotension Bradycardia, complete heart block, cardiac arrest Respiratory depression Coma
Hypomagnesemia - Serum Mg^{++} < 1.5 mg/dL	
Increased GI loss of Mg^{++} • Steatorrhea • Diarrhea • Hereditary absorption defect Increased renal excretion • Renal tubular defects • Diuretics • Aminoglycosides • Cisplatin • Amphotericin B • Volume expansion Miscellaneous • Alcoholism • Thyrotoxicosis • Burns • Prolonged, intense physical exertion	Depression Confusion Irritability Increased reflexes Tetany Positive Trousseau's and Chvostek's signs Muscle weakness Ataxia Nystagmus Convulsions ECG abnormalities • Nonspecific T save changes • U waves • Prolonged QT and QU intervals • Ventricular ectopy/fibrillation • Torsades de pointes Hypocalcemia Hypokalemia

Note: Adapted from Alfry, 2003; Huether, 2002; Pollak & Yu, 2004.

are related to diminished neuromuscular transmission and cardiac conduction. Therefore, patients have nausea, vomiting, lethargy, confusion, respiratory depression, and absent tendon reflexes. Cardiovascular effects include hypotension, bradycardia, heart block, and cardiac arrest.

Mild degrees of asymptomatic hypermagnesemia are common in patients with renal failure, though higher levels may be seen with the injudicious use of magnesium-containing antacids, enemas, or laxatives. Treatment is to stop ingestion of magnesium-containing compounds. In symptomatic patients, urgent treatment with intravenous calcium gluconate as a magnesium antagonist, and insulin and glucose to promote entry of magnesium into cells, is required. Calcium acts as a direct antagonist to magnesium; the injection of as little as 10 mEq of calcium can reverse potentially lethal respiratory depression or cardiac arrhythmia. Thus, intravenous calcium is often used as an initial therapy when life-threatening complications of hypermagnesium are present. Dialysis quickly improves the condition. In patients with renal failure, the only way to clear the excess magnesium may be by dialysis.

Hypomagnesemia is defined as a serum magnesium less than 1.5 mg/dl, but symptoms are unusual unless the level is < 1 mg/dL. The major causes of hypomagnesemia are increased GI and urinary losses (see Table 5-8). Elevated serum ionized Ca^{2+} levels directly induce renal magnesium wasting and hypomagnesemia, an observation often noted in the setting of hypercalcemia caused by malignant bone metastases. The clinical manifestations depend on the total body deficit and the rate of the development of the deficiency. Tetany is a common finding, Chvostek's sign more frequently positive than Trousseau's sign. Other neuromuscular and psychiatric manifestations include tremors, asterixis, myoclonus, and seizures (see Table 5-8). Cardiac dysrythmias, including ventricular tachycardia, fibrillation, and asystolic arrest, can occur. By causing intracellular potassium loss, a magnesium deficiency will increase the risk of digitalis toxicity. Hypomagnesemia may occasionally be seen in patients with renal tubular injury from nephrotoxic agents such as cisplatin, amphotericin B, and aminoglycoside antibiotics and in malnourished dialysis patients, including those receiving TPN.

Table 5-9
Alterations in Acid-Base Balance

Major Causes	Signs and Symptoms
Metabolic Acidosis - systemic pH < 7.35	
Decreased renal excretion of H⁺ • Renal failure • Renal tubular acidosis Increased production of H⁺ • Lactic acidosis • Ketoacidosis • Starvation Bicarbonate loss • Renal defects • Diarrhea Ingestions • Salicylate • Ethylene glycol • Methanol	Headache Lethargy Deep, rapid respiration (Kussmaul respirations) Anorexia Nausea Vomiting Diarrhea Abdominal discomfort Life-threatening cardiac dysrhythmias
Metabolic Alkalosis - systemic pH > 7.45	
Increased intake of alkali • Sodium bicarbonate administration Gastric losses of H⁺ • Vomiting • Gastric suction Renal losses of H⁺ • Diuretics • Renal tubular defects • Mineralocorticoid excess Movement of H⁺ from ECF into cells • Hypokalemia	Weakness Muscle cramps Hyperactive reflexes Slow, shallow respirations Confusion Convulsions Artial tachycardia
Respiratory Acidosis – systemic pH < 7.35	
Depression of the respiratory center • Brain stem trauma • Oversedation Respiratory muscle paralysis Disorders of the chest wall • Kyposcoliosis • Picwickian syndrome • Flail chest Disorders of the lung parenchyma • Pneumonia • Pulmonary edema • Emphysema • Asthma • Bronchitis	Lethargy Muscle twitching Tremors Convulsions Coma

continued on next page

Table 5-9 (continued)
Alterations in Acid-Base Balance

Major Causes	Signs and Symptoms
Respiratory Alkalosis – systemic pH > 7.45	
Stimulation of ventilation • Pulmonary disease • Congestive heart failure • High altitudes Hypermetabolic states • Fever • Anemia • Thyrotoxicosis • Salicylate intoxication Hysteria Cirrhosis Gram negative sepsis	Dizziness Confusion Tingling of extremities or around mouth and lips Convulsions Coma Carpopedel spasm and other symptoms of hypocalcemia

Note: Adapted from Huether, 2002.

Treatment involves oral or intravenous supplementation with magnesium sulfate. When a patient has compromised renal function, magnesium should be administered carefully with close monitoring of plasma levels. Magnesium repletion may be useful in treating a variety of tachyarrhythmias and is recommended in all patients with a significant underlying cardiac or seizure disorder, and patients with concurrent severe hypocalcemia or hypokalemia.

Alterations in Acid-Base Balance

The pH of a solution is a measurement of its hydrogen ion concentration and is expressed as the logarithm (log) to the base 10 of the reciprocal of the hydrogen ion concentration [H+]:

$$pH = \log 1/[H+]$$

Under normal circumstances, systemic acid-base balance is well regulated within a relatively narrow range (7.36 to 7.44) by buffering systems in the blood and renal and respiratory mechanisms. The maintenance of this narrow range is very important because small changes in [H+] have dramatic effects on normal cell function. The effects of changes in pH include changes in the excitability of nerve and muscle cells, alterations in the rate and direction of enzymatic reactions, and changes in the potassium levels in the ICF and ECF.

Acidosis is present when the blood pH falls below 7.35, while alkalosis occurs when the blood pH is above 7.45. Acidosis and alkalosis can both be caused by metabolic and respiratory abnormalities (see Table 5-9). Each of the acid-base disorders can potentially occur in the renal failure patient. However, because metabolic derangements in acid-base balance are more common, a brief discussion of metabolic acidosis and alkalosis will be presented here.

Metabolic acidosis results from an excess of hydrogen ions in the body fluids. Three major defects cause this con-

dition including renal abnormalities in hydrogen ion excretion, an increase in acid burden, or a loss of bicarbonate; ingestion of selected substances can also trigger acidosis (see Table 5-9). The most striking clinical manifestation of metabolic acidosis is an increase in the rate and depth of respiration. This change in the pattern of breathing is termed "Kussmaul's respirations" and assists in compensating for the acidosis by lowering the PCO_2. In severe acidosis, the respiratory rate may increase so much as to cause extreme fatigue. Hyperkalemia may develop or worsen as potassium ions move from the ICF to the ECF in exchange for hydrogen ions, also in an attempt to compensate.

In acute renal failure, acidosis may be severe and occur in conjunction with diabetic ketoacidosis, lactic acidosis, or septic catabolism. In addition to displaying Kussmaul's respirations, the patient may develop myocardial depression and hypotension, insulin resistance, impaired carbohydrate utilization, and increased protein degradation. In contrast, the patient with chronic renal failure may exhibit a slow progressive retention of acid that can also become severe. Chronic metabolic acidosis, even if mild, causes loss of calcium from the bone as calcium acts as a buffer.

Decreasing acid production by reducing dietary protein is frequently the first line of treatment in the renal failure patient. Depending on the severity of the acidosis, oral or IV sodium bicarbonate can also be administered. Dialysis is an effective treatment and may be used on an emergent basis for the patient in acute renal failure with severe acidosis.

Metabolic alkalosis is an acid-base disorder characterized by an elevated bicarbonate concentration, an alkaline blood pH, and an increase in PCO2. The major causes of metabolic alkalosis include increased loads of alkali such as bicarbonate, gastric or renal losses of hydrogen ions, and potassium depletion (see Table 5-9). No specific signs or symptoms are associated with metabolic alkalosis. However, patients can experience muscle cramps, weakness, arrhythmias, or seizures. Some of these problems may be related to alterations in ionized calcium because increases in pH cause increased binding of calcium to proteins.

In acute renal failure, the most common cause is administered lactate or acetate, especially with TPN. Dialysis usually assists in correcting this abnormality. A custom dialysate bath with a lower acetate or bicarbonate level can be used depending on the degree of the alkalosis. Metabolic alkalosis rarely occurs in the chronic renal failure patient but may occur in several of the situations listed in Table 5-9.

The most important part of treatment is to address the underlying cause. Administration of HCL is sometimes used in selected cases. Treatment of associated electrolyte disturbances, such as hypochloremia and hypokalemia, is also important.

Summary

Fluid, electrolyte, and acid-base balance are essential for normal physiologic function. Patients with renal disease are prone to a wide variety of problems in these areas. Hypervolemia often becomes a problem, but hypovolemia may also occur. Sodium excess and depletion may develop, depending on the free water load. Imbalances of other electrolytes including potassium phosphate, calcium, and magnesium are common. Although metabolic acidosis is more likely to occur, metabolic alkalosis may develop in selected situations. Thus, the nurse should be knowledgeable regarding these potential abnormalities, their clinical presentation, and appropriate nursing interventions.

References/Readings

Agraharkar, M., Guba, S. C., & Safirstein, R. L. (2001). Acute renal failure associated with cancer chemotherapy. In B. A. Molitoris & W. F. Finn (Eds.), *Acute renal failure: A companion the Brenner & Rector's the kidney* (pp. 365-375). Philadelphia: W.B. Saunders Company.

Alfry, A.C. (2003). Normal and abnormal magnesium metabolism. In R. W. Schrier (Ed.), *Renal and electrolyte disorders* (pp. 278-302). Philadelphia: Lippincott Williams & Wilkins.

Berl, T., & Schrier, R.W. (2003). Disorders of water metabolism. In R.W. Schrier (Ed.), *Renal and electrolyte disorders* (6th ed.) (pp. 1 - 63). Philadelphia: Lippincott Williams & Wilkins.

Berl, T., & Verbalis, J. (2004). Pathophysiology of water metabolism. In B.M. Brenner (Ed.), *Brenner and Rector's the kidney* (7th ed.) (Vol. 1) (pp. 857-920). Philadelphia: W.B. Saunders Company.

Bliss, D.E. (2002). Calciphylaxis: What nurses need to know. *Nephrology Nursing Journal, 29*(5), 433-438, 443-434; quiz 435-436.

Daugirdas, J.T., Ross, E.A., & Nissenson, A.R. (2001). Acute hemodialysis prescription. In J.T. Daugirdas, P.G. Blake & T.S. Ing (Eds.), *Handbook of dialysis* (3rd ed.) (pp. 102-120). Philadelphia: Lippincott Williams & Wilkins.

Dillon, J.J. (2001). Nephrotoxicity from antibacterial, antifungal, and antiviral drugs. In B.A. Molitoris & W.F. Finn (Eds.), *Acute renal failure: A companion to Brenner & Rector's the kidney* (pp. 349-364). Philadelphia: W.B. Saunders Company.

DuBose, T.D., Jr. (2004). Acid-base disorders. In B.M. Brenner (Ed.), *Brenner & Rector's the kidney* (7th ed.) (Vol. 1) (pp. 921-1041). Philadelphia: W.B. Saunders Company.

Edelstein, C.L., & Schrier, R.W. (2004). Acute renal failure (7th, Trans.). In B.M. Brenner (Ed.), *Brenner and Rector's the kidney* (Vol. 2) (pp. 1041-1071). Philadelphia: W.B. Saunders Company.

Huether. (2002). The cellular environment: Fluids and electrolytes, acids, and bases. In K.L. McCance & S.E. Huether (Eds.), *Pathophysiology: The biologic basis for disease in adults & children* (pp. 85-113). St. Louis, MO: Mosby.

Korbet, S.M., & Kronfol, N.O. (2001). Acute peritoneal dialysis prescription. In J.T. Daugirdas, P.G. Blake & T.S. Ing (Eds.), *Handbook of dialysis* (3rd ed.) (pp. 333-342). Philadelphia: Lippincott Williams & Wilkins.

Ludlow, M. (2003). Renal handling of potassium. *Nephrology Nursing Journal, 30*(5), 493-497; quiz 498-499.

Michael, M., & Garcia, D. (2004). Secondary hyperparathyroidism in chronic kidney disease: Clinical consequences and challenges. *Nephrology Nursing Journal, 31*(2), 185-194; quiz 195-186.

Mount, D.B., & Zandi-Nejad, K. (2004). Disorders of potassium balance. In B.M.Brenner (Ed.), *Brenner & Rector's the kidney* (7th ed.) (Vol. 1) (pp. 997-1041). Philadelphia: W.B. Saunders Company.

Nielsen, S., Knepper, M.A., Kwon, T.H., & Frokiaer, J. (2004). Regulation of water balance. In B. M. Brenner (Ed.), *Brenner and Rector's the kidney* (7th ed.) (Vol. 1) (pp. 109-134). Philadelphia: W.B. Saunders Company.

Peterson, L.N., & Levi, M. (2003). Disorders of potassium metabolism. In RW. Schrier (Ed.), *Renal and electrolyte disorders* (6th ed.) (pp. 171-215). Philadelphia: Lippincott Williams & Wilkins.

Pollak, M.R., & Yu, A.S.L. (2004). Clinical disturbances of calcium, magnesium, and phosphate metabolism. In B. M. Brenner (Ed.), *Brenner & Rector's the kidney* (Vol. 1) (pp. 1041-1078). Philadelphia: W.B. Saunders Company.

Popovtzer, M.M. (2003). Disorders of calcium, phosphorous, vitamin D, and parathyroid hormone activity. In R. W. Schrier (Ed.), *Renal and electrolyte disorders* (pp. 216-277). Philadelphia: Lippincott Williams & Wilkins.

Schrier, R.W., Gurevich, A.K., & Abraham, W.T. (2003). Renal sodium excretion, edematous disorders, and diuretic use. In R.W. Schrier (Ed.), *Renal and electrolyte disorders* (6th ed.) (pp. 64-114). Philadelphia: Lippincott Williams & Wilkins.

Shapiro, J.I., & Kaehny, W.D. (2003). Pathogenesis and management of metabolic acidosis and alkalosis. In R.W. Schrier (Ed.), *Renal and electrolyte disorders* (6th ed.) (pp. 115-153). Philadelphia: Lippincott Williams & Wilkins.

Sherwood, L. (2004). *Human physiology: From cells to systems.* Belmont, CA: Brooks/Cole – Thomson Learning.

Velazquez, H.E., & Wright, F.S. (2001). Tubular potassium transport. In R.W. Schrier (Ed.), *Diseases of the kidney and urinary tract* (Vol. 1) (pp. 177-201). Philadelphia: Lippincott Williams & Wilkins.

Welch, J.L., & Davis, J. (2000). Self-care strategies to reduce fluid intake and control thirst in hemodialysis patients. *Nephrology Nursing Journal, 27*(4), 393-395.

Yu, A.S.L. (2004). Renal transport of calcium, magnesium, and phosphate. In B.M. Brenner (Ed.), *Brenner & Rector's the kidney* (7th ed.) (Vol. 1) (pp. 535-573). Philadelphia: W.B. Saunders Company.

Yucha, C., & Guthrie, D. (2003). Renal homeostasis of calcium. *Nephrology Nursing Journal, 30*(6), 621-626; quiz 627-628.

- In a newborn, water may account for as much as 75% of the total body weight. In contrast, total body water decreases with age and may compose as little as 50% of the body weight in the elderly.

- Although fluid intake and output are valuable guides, weight remains the most important indicator of overall fluid status. However, the information obtained from frequent measurements of weight does have its limitations... thus, it is important to complete a thorough assessment of the patient's fluid status on a regular basis.

- Sodium (Na+) is a major determinant of serum osmolality. It also plays an essential role in nerve conduction, acid-base balance, and numerous chemical reactions. Because water is freely permeable across cell membranes, changes in the extracellular sodium concentration result in shifts in water distribution in ECF and ICF compartments.

- Hypernatremia, defined as a plasma sodium concentration above 146 mEq/L, is extremely dangerous. The condition is rare, but when it occurs is associated with a 10% to 60% mortality rate.

- Hyponatremia, defined as a plasma sodium concentration less than 135 mEq/L, is a state in which there is a decrease in sodium relative to water. It is among the most common electrolyte disorders seen in clinical practice.

- As the major intracellular cation, potassium helps maintain intracellular osmolality, regulates skeletal, cardiac, and smooth muscle activity, influences acid-base balance, and is crucial for many intracellular enzyme reactions.

- There is a close link between the regulation of calcium and phosphate in the body. A change in the concentration of one is often associated with a change in the concentration of the other; when one substance is elevated, the other tends to drop and vice versa.

- Magnesium (Mg^{2+}) is the fourth most abundant cation in the body (normal range 1.8 to 2.4 mg/dL) and is involved in enzymatic reactions and the maintenance of cellular permeability and neuromuscular excitability. In addition, it is important in the production and use of energy essential in the maintenance of normal intracellular electrolyte composition.

- Under normal circumstances, systemic acid-base balance is well regulated within a relatively narrow range (7.36 to 7.44) by buffering systems in the blood and renal and respiratory mechanisms. The maintenance of this narrow range is very important because small changes in [H^+] have dramatic effects on normal cell function.

- Metabolic alkalosis is an acid-base disorder characterized by an elevated bicarbonate concentration, an alkaline blood pH, and an increase in PCO_2. The major causes of metabolic alkalosis include increased loads of alkali such as bicarbonate, gastric or renal losses of hydrogen ions, and potassium depletion.

ANNP605

Alterations in Fluid, Electrolyte, and Acid-Base Balance

Kathy P. Parker, PhD, RN, FAAN

Contemporary Nephrology Nursing: Principles and Practice contains 39 chapters of educational content. Individual learners may apply for continuing nursing education credit by reading a chapter and completing the Continuing Education Evaluation Form for that chapter. Learners may apply for continuing education credit for any or all chapters.

Please photocopy this page and return to ANNA.
COMPLETE THE FOLLOWING:

Name: _____

Address:_____

City:_____ State: _____ Zip: _____

E-mail: _____

Preferred telephone: ☐ Home   ☐ Work: _____

State where licensed and license number (optional): _____

CE application fees are based upon the number of contact hours provided by the individual chapter. CE fees per contact hour for ANNA members are as follows: 1.0-1.9 - $15; 2.0-2.9 - $20; 3.0-3.9 - $25; 4.0 and higher - $30. Fees for nonmembers are $10 higher.

ANNA Member: ☐ Yes   ☐ No   Member # (if available) _____

☐ Checked Enclosed   ☐ American Express   ☐ Visa   ☐ MasterCard

Total Amount Submitted: _____

Credit Card Number: _____ Exp. Date: _____

Name as it appears on the card: _____

CE Evaluation Form
To receive continuing education credit for individual study after reading the chapter
1. Photocopy this form. (You may also download this form from ANNA's Web site, **www.annanurse.org.**)

2. Mail the completed form with payment (check) or credit card information to American Nephrology Nurses' Association, East Holly Avenue, Box 56, Pitman, NJ 08071-0056.

3. You will receive your CE certificate from ANNA in 4 to 6 weeks.

Test returns must be postmarked by **December 31, 2010.**

CE Application Fee
ANNA Member $15.00
Nonmember $25.00

EVALUATION FORM

1. I verify that I have read this chapter and completed this education activity. Date: _____

_____
Signature

2. What would be different in your practice if you applied what you learned from this activity? *(Please use additional sheet of paper if necessary.)*

_____

_____

_____

_____

_____

_____

_____

_____

_____

_____

_____

_____

Evaluation	Strongly disagree				Strongly agree
3. The activity met the stated objectives.					
a. State reasons that observing more than one parameter for fluid change is necessary.	1	2	3	4	5
b. Describe physiological consequences of electrolytes being elevated or decreased.	1	2	3	4	5
c. Compare and contrast metabolic acidosis and metabolic alkalosis as to causes and effects.	1	2	3	4	5
4. The content was current and relevant.	1	2	3	4	5
5. The content was presented clearly.	1	2	3	4	5
6. The content was covered adequately.	1	2	3	4	5
7. Rate your ability to apply the learning obtained from this activity to practice.	1	2	3	4	5

Comments _____

_____

8. Time required to read the chapter and complete this form: _____ minutes.

This educational activity has been provided by the American Nephrology Nurses' Association (ANNA) for 1.3 contact hours. ANNA is accredited as a provider of continuing nursing education (CNE) by the American Nurses Credentialing Center's Commission on Accreditation (ANCC-COA). ANNA is an approved provider of continuing education by the California Board of Registered Nursing, CEP 0910.

Diseases of the Kidney

LaVonne M. Burrows, M-SCNS, BC, RN, CNN

Chapter Contents

Diseases of the Kidney

LaVonne M. Burrows, M-SCNS, BC, RN, CNN

Understanding diseases of the kidney will assist nephrology nurses in the management of patients entrusted to our care. Increasing our knowledge base related to disease process, prognosis, and therapy will facilitate delivery of high quality care. The purpose of this chapter is to provide a framework for understanding disease processes affecting the kidney; it is beyond the scope of this overview to detail pathophysiology of every disease. An anatomical approach is used to organize the content, with diseases discussed as glomerular, tubulointerstitial, vascular, cystic, infectious, obstructive, or neoplastic. Issues associated with the kidney in pregnancy are briefly reviewed. Diabetic nephropathy is addressed elsewhere in this text. Figure 6-1 illustrates trends of disease incidence over the last decade (1990-2000), based on United States Renal Data System (USRDS) statistics (USRDS, 2002). The rising overall incidence of kidney disease is clearly evident.

Glomerular Diseases

Glomerulonephritis (GN) refers to a complex group of disease processes affecting the glomerulus. It is beyond the scope of this text to address all these individual disease processes, but a discussion of general principles will facilitate assessment and nursing management. Although the term GN implies inflammation or infection, some lesions are not associated with inflammatory cells. Primary glomerular diseases affect the kidney nearly exclusively, while secondary diseases are the result of systemic disease processes that include glomerular pathology. In the U.S. and Europe, GN is the third most common cause of ESRD, accounting for 10%-15% of U.S. cases with only diabetes mellitus and hypertension more prevalent (Couser, 1999). Some diseases may have a primary (idiopathic) and a secondary variant (e.g., focal segmental glomerulosclerosis).

Glomerular diseases present with abnormalities in the urine, most notably proteinuria, due to damage to the filtering membrane. Although patient history, clinical presentation, and blood and urine tests may provide a presumptive diagnosis, renal biopsy is required for a definitive diagnosis. In systemic diseases with renal manifestations, the systemic signs and symptoms provide additional information helpful in establishing the likely cause. Indications for biopsy include establishing or confirming the diagnosis to determine therapy or establishing activity, chronicity, and potential reversibility of the disease process. When treatment would require the use of potentially toxic drugs, the risks of therapy may outweigh the potential benefit in cases where significant scarring has already occurred. The best predictors of reversibility are level of renal function and kidney size (Couser, 1999). Size can be easily assessed by renal ultrasound, which can also evaluate for cortical thickness and evidence of obstruction.

Renal biopsy samples are evaluated via a variety of techniques. Abnormalities seen in fewer than 50% of glomeruli are termed focal, with diffuse being the term used for findings seen in over 50% of glomeruli. Cellular or fibrous crescents in Bowman's capsule are generally indicative of more aggressive disease. Presence or absence of immune deposits and degree of cellular proliferation in various areas of the renal tissue help distinguish disease processes. Figure 6-2 shows normal renal tissue, Figure 6-3 a normal glomerulus, Figure 6-4 a glomerulus with a cellular crescent.

Acute GN

Early detection and therapeutic intervention in acute GN is critical since prompt treatment may reverse renal damage with return to near-normal function. Even if recovery is not achieved, progression of renal disease may be slowed (Mookerjee, Lohr, Jenis, & Heffner, 2001). The classic presentations of acute GN are nephritic and/or nephrotic syndrome (see Table 6-1), with many underlying causes of GN capable of either nephrosis or nephritis (Madaio &

Figure 6-1
Trends in Incident Rates by Primary Diagnosis

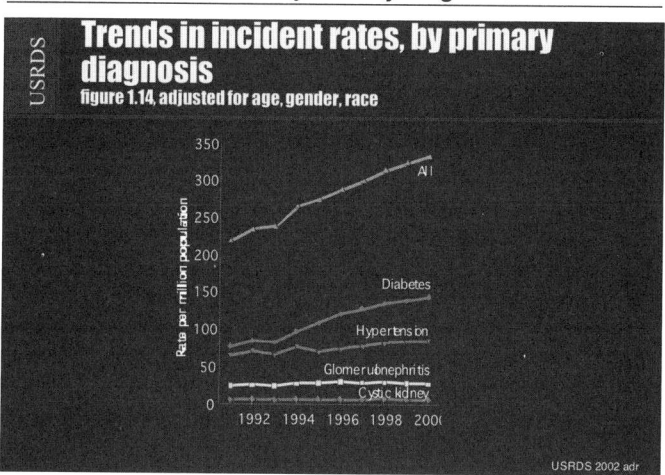

Note: From USRDS. (2002). USRDS Annual Data Report. Bethesda, MD: Author.

Figure 6-2
Normal Kidney

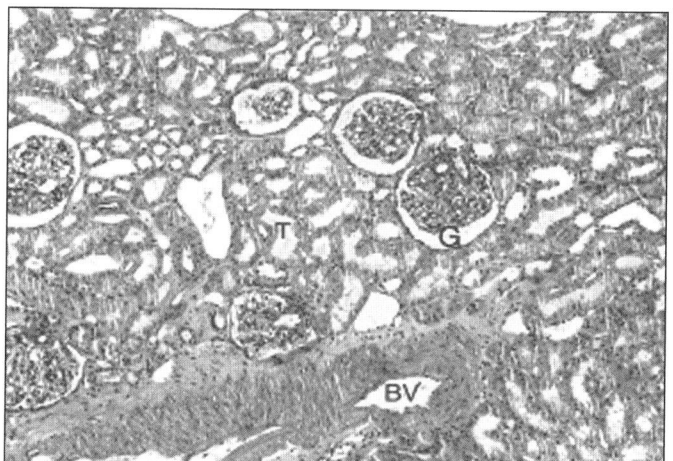

Note: G = glomerulus; T = tubule; BV = blood vessel. PAS, original magnification 100x

Figure 6-3
Normal Glomerulus

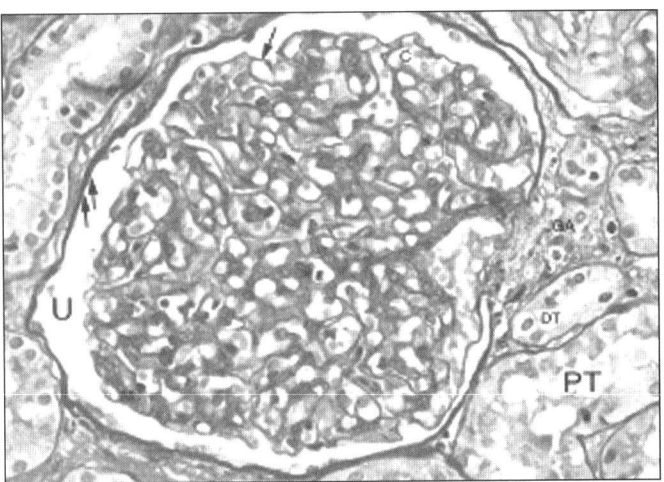

Note: U = urinary space; C = capillary space; M = mesangium; PT = proximal tubule; DT = distal tubule; JGA = juxtaglomerular apparatus; single arrow = glomerular basement membrane; double arrow = Bowman's capsule. PAS, original magnification 400x.

Figure 6-4
Glomerulus with a Circumferential Crescent (arrow).
PAS Original Magnification 400x.

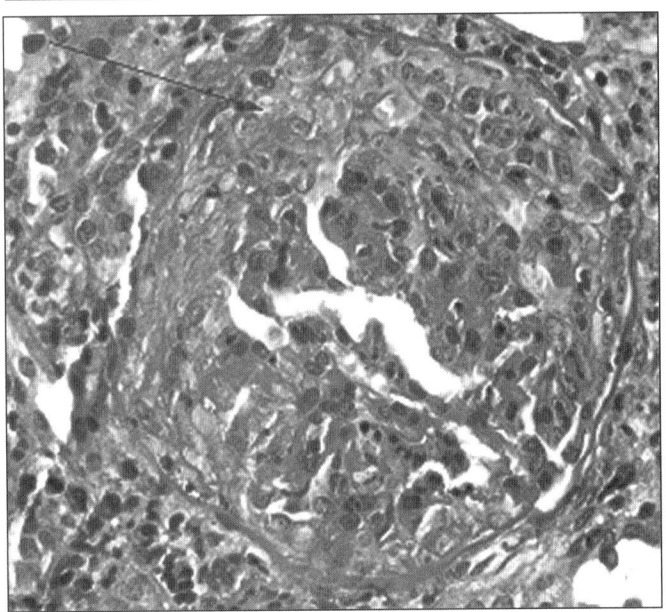

Table 6-1
Characteristics of Nephrotic and Nephritic Syndromes

Nephrotic Syndrome
*Proteinuria >3.5 grams per 24 hours per 1.73 m^2
Lipiduria
Bland urine sediment (may have oval fat bodies)
*Hypoalbuminemia
*Hyperlipidemia
Hypercoagulability
Edema
          *"Classic triad"

Nephritic Syndrome
Hematuria (microscopic or gross)
Mild or no proteinuria
Active urine sediment (especially cellular casts)
Azotemia
Hypertension

Figure 6-5
Wegener's Granulomatosis. Medium sized artery showing necrotizing destruction of the vessel (arrow) surrounded by inflammatory cells. PAS original magnification 200x.

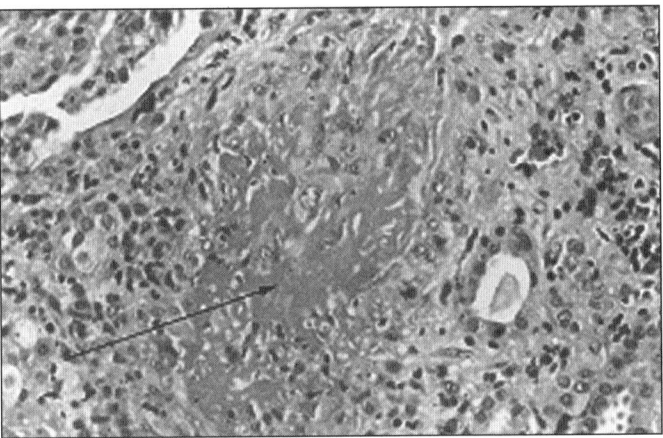

Harrington, 2001). Clinically, most patients exhibit hematuria, proteinuria, and impaired renal function that occur over days to weeks (Vinen & Oliveira, 2003). Edema, fluid retention, hypertension, and oliguria are frequent. Urine is often dark in color with an "active" urine sediment, a term referring to the presence of red or white blood cells, debris, and/or cellular casts.

Immune reactions within the glomerulus may activate mediators of tissue injury and consume complement, with resulting low serum complement levels. Other disease processes do not consume complement, and serum levels remain normal (see Table 6-2). Besides complement, other serologic markers can be helpful in the diagnosis of glomerular diseases. Table 6-3 lists blood tests used and its associated diagnosis. Pulmonary renal syndromes involving both lung and glomerular tissue include Goodpasture's syndrome and Wegener's granulomatosis. Figure 6-5 shows blood vessel destruction seen in Wegener's granulomatosis.

Treatment regimens are aimed at arresting the inflammatory process. Pharmacologic agents that may be used include glucocorticoids, azathioprine, mycophenolate mofetil, cyclophosphamide, cyclosporine, and omega-3 fatty acids (Glassock, 2001). Combinations of these agents, either oral or intravenous, may be indicated; oral prednisone and either intravenous or oral cyclophosphamide is commonly effective. Other interventions, such as therapeutic plasma exchange, may be useful in certain disease processes. Supportive care including fluid and electrolyte management, renal replacement therapies, and control of hypertension are important adjuncts to treatment of the underlying disease process. Use of ACE inhibitors and angiotensin receptor

Table 6-2
Acute Glomerulonephritis

Systemic Diseases with Renal Involvement	
Low Serum Complement	*Normal Serum Complement*
SLE (focal, 75%; diffuse, 90%)	Polyarteritis nodosa
Subacute bacterial endocarditis (90%)	Hypersensitivity vasculitis
Visceral abscess	Wegener's granulomatosis
"Shunt" nephritis (90%)	Henoch-Schönlein purpura
Cryoglobulinemia (85%)	Goodpasture's syndrome

Primary Renal Diseases	
Low Serum Complement	*Normal Serum Complement*
Acute post-infectious GN	IgA nephropathy
Membranoproliferative GN	Idiopathic rapidly progressive GN
Type I (50%-80%)	Anti-GBM disease
Type II (80%-90%)	Immune complex disease

Notes: Adapted from Yoshizawa, 2000.
*Percentages indicate the approximate frequencies of low C3 or hemolytic complement

Table 6-3
Serologic Markers Associated with Glomerular Diseases

Primary Glomerular Disease	Serologic Markers
Post-infectious GN	Antibodies to streptococcus Low complement
Anti-GBM nephritis	Anti-GBM antibody
Idiopathic crescentic GN	ANCA (vasculitis)

Systemic Disease	Serologic Markers
SLE	ANA Low complement Double-stranded DNA antibody
Wegener's granulomatosis	ANCA
Hepatitis C	Cryoglobulins Rheumatoid factor Low complement (C3) Hepatitis C antibody Hepatitis C RNA in serum

Note: Adapted from Couser (1999).

blockers has been shown to be especially beneficial in these individuals (Glassock, 2001).

Chronic GN

Similarly to acute GN, chronic GN generally manifests with proteinuria, often in the nephrotic range. Nephrotic syndrome consists of the triad of proteinuria, hypoalbuminemia, and hyperlipidemia (see Table 6-1). Urine sediment is usually "bland," with few cellular elements or casts, and edema is commonly seen along with hypertension. Although nephrotic syndrome is common, chronic GN can occur in virtually any glomerular disease, even those where proteiniuria is not generally seen or when hematuria is present. As implied by the term chronic, progression of disease is indolent, and some disease processes are unlikely to result in renal failure (e.g., thin basement membrane disease), while others tend to progress despite current interventions (e.g., diabetic nephropathy).

The glomerulonephritides are complex, with a broad spectrum of presentations and clinical courses even within the same disease entity. For example, membranous glomerulonephropathy (MN) is the most common form of nephrotic syndrome and idiopathic GN in the adults (Mookerjee et al., 2001). This disease can be idiopathic or secondary to malignancy, infections, auto-immune disease, or hepatitis B. Approximately one third of affected individuals slowly

Figure 6-6
Post-Infectious Glomerulonephritis with a Markedly Hypercellular Glomerulus

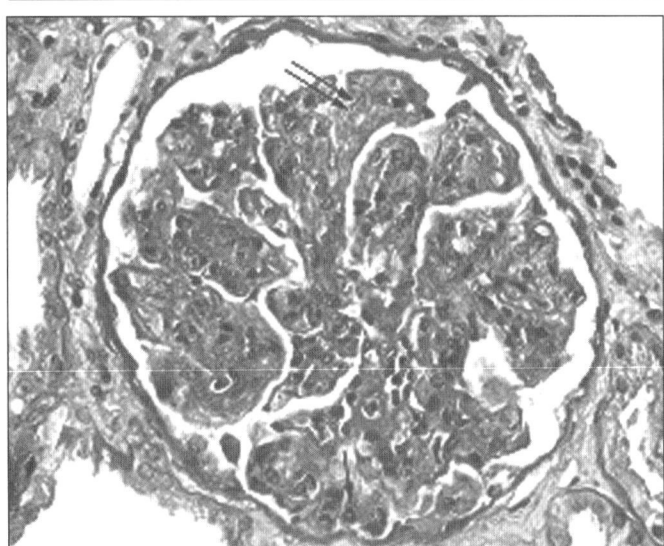

Arrow = neutrophil; double arrow = endocapillary proliferation. PAS, original magnification 400x.

progress to end-stage disease over a 15- to 20-year course (Kunis & Teng, 2000), one third have persistent proteinuria without disease progression, and one third undergo spontaneous remission with resolution of symptoms (Mookerjee et al., 2001). Some diseases are more common in specific age groups (amyloidosis in the elderly, IgA nephropathy in adults, and minimal change disease in children), some are associated with systemic diseases (lupus nephritis), and others have associations with antecedent infections (post-streptococcal GN) (Kunis & Teng, 2000; Mookerjee et al., 2001). An example of glomerular changes in post-infectious GN is shown in Figure 6-6. Note the increased number of cells compared to the normal glomerulus in Figure 6-3.

Patients who initially present with impaired renal function or significant proteinuria tend to have more progression of disease. In the chronic progressive phase of GN, damage continues mediated by non-immune mechanisms associated with increases in glomerular pressure, sclerosis, and interstitial fibrosis. Cellular mechanisms such as cytokines, ischemic changes, and toxic effects of excess filtered protein have all been implicated in causing the damage and subsequent loss of filtration (Couser, 1999). The goals of treatment are "protection of renal structure and function: control of blood pressure, action on renal hemodynamics and proteinuria via pharmacological inhibition of the renin-angiotensin system, control of hyperlipidemia and limitation of fibrosis" (Kiperova, 2003, p. v31). In secondary GN, treatment of the underlying systemic disease is generally beneficial for preservation of renal function.

Tubulointerstitial Diseases

Acute Interstitial Nephritis

Acute interstitial nephritis (AIN) describes injury to the interstitium of the kidney resulting in abrupt deterioration of

Table 6-4
Drugs Associated with Acute Interstitial Nephritis

Antibiotics	NSAIDS	MISCELLANEOUS
Cephalosporins	Fenoprofen	Allopurinol
Ciprofloxacin		Azathioprine
Macrolides	**DIURETICS**	Cocaine
Penicillins	Furosemide	Mesalazine
Rifampin	Bumetanide	Omeprazole
Sulfonamides	Thiazides	Phenytoin
		Triamterene

renal function. The etiology of AIN is most often secondary to drug therapy but may also be from infections, certain immune diseases, or idiopathic causes. A list of drugs associated with AIN is shown in Table 6-4. This is not an exhaustive list since many drugs have been implicated. Disease development is not related to drug dose, and symptoms generally become clinically evident approximately 2 weeks after the drug is initiated (Kodner & Kudrimott, 2003). Bacterial or viral infections may result in AIN, particularly infections of the kidney itself, including renal tuberculosis, fungal nephritis, and acute bacterial pyelonephritis. Local or systemic autoimmune diseases such as Sjögren's syndrome, SLE, and Wegener's granulomatosis may cause immune complex-mediated AIN.

The symptoms of AIN are those of acute renal failure: oliguria, nausea, vomiting, anorexia, and malaise along with biochemical abnormalities including elevated blood urea nitrogen (BUN) and creatinine levels. Low-grade fever, skin rash, and arthralgias have been called the "classic triad" of AIN but are present in only 5% of cases overall (Kodner & Kudrimott, 2003). Eosinophilia with or without eosinophiluria can add to the body of evidence for a presumptive diagnosis of AIN but do not reliably confirm or exclude AIN. Urinary findings of proteinuria may be present, generally less than 1 gram per 24 hours, and leukocytes or leukocyte casts may be found. Red cell casts are rare. Although renal biopsy is the gold standard for diagnosis of AIN, it is not always necessary in mild cases or where improvement is rapid. Biopsy findings show inflammatory infiltrates in the peritubular spaces of the interstitium, typically by mononuclear cells and T lymphocytes, along with edema. Granuloma formation with epithelioid giant cells may be found, particularly in AIN from tuberculosis, sarcoidosis, or Wegener's granulomatosis (Kodner & Kudrimott, 2003). Interstitial fibrosis may be seen and is a poor prognostic indicator for ultimate recovery of function, especially if it is diffuse. Renal ultrasound demonstrates normal to large kidneys, likely from edema associated with the inflammatory process.

In individuals who present with acute or subacute decline in renal function, a careful history should be taken to evaluate for drugs implicated in AIN or a history of a recent infection associated with AIN. Withdrawal of any and all potentially offending agents should be done, with substitution of medications not associated with AIN when clinically indicated. The majority of patients with AIN improve after withdrawal of the offending agent(s), with recovery of near baseline renal function most likely when the agent is withdrawn within 2 weeks of creatinine elevation (Kodner &

Table 6-5
Relative Risk of Analgesic Nephropathy with ESRD

Phenacetin	2.66 – 19.05
Aspirin	1.0 – 2.5
Acetaminophen	2.1 – 4.06
NSAIDs	1.0

Note: Data from studies between 1969-1992.
Adapted from Guo & Nzerue (2002).

Kudrimott, 2003). In cases where recovery of function is delayed or not seen, supportive care measures including fluid and electrolyte management, volume management, and symptomatic relief are indicated. Renal replacement therapy indications are the same as for other forms of acute renal failure (ARF) (hyperkalemia, uremia, or fluid control). Corticosteroids have been used empirically, with case reports of improved function, but controlled clinical trial data is lacking.

Chronic Tubulointerstitial Nephritis

Tubulointerstitial nephritis (TIN) can be a primary disease or can occur in the setting of glomerular injury. Prolonged exposure to therapeutic and environmental agents as well as systemic illnesses may result in chronic TIN. Antibody-mediated TIN in humans is rare, with the anti-tubular basement membrane antibody being found in the renal tubules as well as the intestinal mucosa (Yoshioka, Takemura, & Hattori, 2002). The clinical course in chronic TIN is more indolent than in AIN. Urinary findings mirror those of AIN. Fluid and electrolyte disturbances are varied and may reflect the area of the tubular involvement.

Severe glomerular pathology rarely exists without tubulointerstitial inflammation and damage (Meyers, 1999). The excessive filtered protein seen in severe glomerular disease has been postulated as one link to the development of tubulointerstitial disease (Harris, 2001). Tubular epithelial cell damage is likely mediated by multiple pathways in chronic progressive kidney disease with cytokines, growth factors, hormones, complement, and immune mechanisms all implicated (Cao & Cooper, 2001; Hsu & Couser, 2003). Since indices of tubular damage correlate best with ultimate renal function (Hsu & Couser, 2003), the potential to intervene in the processes leading to this damage is intriguing.

Analgesic Nephropathy

Chronic ingestion of analgesics was noted to be associated with chronic renal failure as early as the 1950s. Initially, the combination analgesics, including phenacetin, were implicated, and phenacetin was removed from the market in the U.S. and many other countries. Still, analgesic nephropathy (AN) continues to cause chronic renal failure, likely through the accumulation of metabolites of analgesics within the kidney. Table 6-5 lists the relative risk of AN associated renal failure. It was initially hoped newer NSAIDs called COX-2 inhibitors would not lead to renal failure, but there are recent reports of cases, so the relative risk of ESRD will likely increase in the future. (Guo & Nzerue, 2002). Although ARF occurs in less than 10% of cases of severe acetamino-

phen poisoning, patients with glutathione-depletion (alcoholism, starvation) are at increased risk (Guo & Nzerue, 2002). Combinations of analgesics are more nephrotoxic than single agents, as is prolonged or excessive intake of these drugs. There is no clear contribution of caffeine to AN (Fox & Siebers, 2003).

Pathogenesis of AN involves microangiopathy of the renal papilla, papillary necrosis, and chronic TIN (see above). Clinical presentation is one of slowly progressive declining renal function; episodes of worsening function may be related to passage of sloughed papillae and subsequent obstruction (Guo & Nzerue, 2002). Patient history usually includes chronic pain (i.e., headaches or back pain) with associated intake of analgesics. The majority of patients are women between the ages of 30 and 70 years. Renal ultrasound may show small kidneys. Non-contrast computed tomography (CT) is recommended as the diagnostic modality of choice for AN (DeBroe & Elseviers, 1998), being more sensitive than ultrasound, but without requiring contrast.

Treatment consists of cessation of the offending agent; otherwise, the disease process will continue to progress. Mild improvement or stabilization of renal function is seen in most cases of AN, though in some cases renal function continues to deteriorate even after stopping the analgesic. "Acetaminophen taken alone is probably safe for episodic use. If patients have chronic pain, tramadol (Ultram®), a centrally acting analgesic with weak opiod activity, can be tried, as it has not yet been found to be nephrotoxic." (Guo & Nzerue, 2002, p.305).

NSAIDs, both non-selective and selective COX-2 inhibitors, appear to be equally nephrotoxic (Gambara & Perazella, 2003). Mechanisms of injury may be via an allergic AIN or by the changes resulting in renal hemodynamics from inhibition of renal prostaglandins. These prostaglandins contribute to control of renal blood flow by vasodilatory effects on the afferent arteriole. Individuals who are dependent on these effects to maintain glomerular filtration are more susceptible to adverse effects from these drugs. In states of volume depletion, congestive heart failure, or in combination with ACE inhibitors or angiotension receptor blockers, ARF can result. These drugs have also been shown to blunt antihypertensive effects of diuretics, ACE inhibitors, and β adrenergic blockers (Gambara & Perazella, 2003), and thus may contribute to hypertensive nephrosclerosis.

Contrast-Induced Nephropathy

Of unselected populations undergoing intravascular radiocontrast administration, about 15% develop contrast-induced nephropathy (CIN), with higher incidence seen in diabetics with pre-existing renal insufficiency (Isenbarger, Kent, & O'Malley, 2003). CIN, defined as a sudden decline of renal function after contrast administration, is the third leading cause of hospital acquired acute renal failure (Asif, Preston, & Roth, 2003). Clinically, serum creatinine begins to rise within 24 to 72 hours following administration, peaks at 3 to 5 days, and returns to baseline in another 3 to 5 days. Definitions of CIN generally include a rise in serum creatinine of 25% - 50% above baseline or an absolute increase of 0.5 mg/dL. Risk factors for CIN include diabetes with renal insufficiency or pre-existing renal insufficiency from any cause, intravascular volume depletion, older age, and increased total dose of contrast.

Pathophysiologic mechanisms of renal injury include medullary hypoxia and direct tubular toxicity. Impairment of vasodilatory prostaglandin production, similar to that which occurs with use of NSAIDs, can contribute to intrarenal vasoconstriction and hypoxia. Tubular injury is via direct damage by generation of reactive oxygen species and tubular obstruction from increased urate excretion and aggregation and precipitation of Tamm-Horsfall proteins (Asif et al., 2003).

Interventions to minimize incidence of CIN in high-risk groups include hydration with IV fluids prior to contrast administration, use of the lowest possible volume of contrast, and preferential use of low-osmolar contrast media that is less nephrotoxic. Avoidance of NSAIDs concomitantly with contrast is preferred. Likewise, due to the risk of renal impairment immediately following contrast administration, metformin use should be discontinued for 48 hours prior to the procedure and held until creatinine is stable at baseline. Use of fenoldopam, a vasodilator that increases renal blood flow, has had mixed results, but a recent study by Kini et al. (2002) found an incidence of CIN of 4.7% in the fenoldopam group compared to 18.8% in the control group. N-acetylcysteine, a scavenger of reactive oxygen species and a potent vasodilator, has also demonstrated significant benefit with low cost and is easily administered via oral dosing (Isenbarger et al., 2003).

Other Nephrotoxic Agents

Chemotherapeutic agents such as mitomycin C, bleomycin, and cisplatin can result in ARF from thrombotic thrombocytopenic purpura (TTP) (see section on TTP for further discussion). The potent antifungal agent Amphotericin B has been associated with ARF with urinary magnesium and potassium wasting, renal tubular acidosis, and polyuria from nephrogenic diabetes insipidus (Guo & Nzerue, 2002). So-called Chinese herb nephropathy is characterized by renal interstitial fibrosis, thought to be from the aristolochic acid found in these preparations. About 50% of individuals with ESRD from this disease process develop urothelial cancers. Valvular heart disease is also common (Guo & Nzerue, 2002). Cocaine abuse is associated with rhabdomyolysis and ARF as well as AIN and hypertension. Heavy metals, including lead, cadmium, gold, and mercury, can also cause renal toxicity. It is beyond the scope of this discussion to provide an exhaustive list of nephrotoxins. Be aware that many therapeutic, diagnostic, and environmental agents have potential for toxicity.

Vascular Diseases

Renal Artery Stenosis

Renal artery stenosis (RAS) is defined as narrowing of the renal artery lumen by 50% or more (Martin et al., 2003). Renovascular disease is present in 10%-40% of patients with ESRD and is the fastest growing group of ESRD patients (Radermacher, Weinkove, & Haller, 2001). Despite this, not all patients with RAS have concomitant impairment of renal function or hypertension (Vagaonescu & Dangas, 2002). This

Table 6-6
Percutaneous Renal Revascularizations Major Complications

Complication	Reported Rate (%)
30-day mortality	1
Secondary nephrectomy	<1
Surgical salvage operation	1
Main or branch renal artery occlusion	2
Acute renal failure	2
Worsening chronic renal failure	2
Symptomatic embolization	3
Access site hematoma requiring surgery, transfusion, or prolonged hospital stay	5

Note: Adapted from Martin et al. (2003).

is best understood by reviewing the pathophysiologic mechanisms by which RAS can result in renovascular hypertension and impaired renal function.

RAS results in a decrease in renal blood flow when the stenosis is functionally significant. Decreased renal blood flow triggers the renin-angiotensin-aldosterone system with resulting vasoconstriction, retention of fluid with volume expansion, and hypertension. Unilateral RAS with two functioning kidneys leads to increased renin and hypertension. This process may ultimately result in damage to the kidney not affected by RAS (Vashist, Heller, Brown, & Alhaddad, 2002). If the RAS is bilateral or unilateral affecting a solitary functioning kidney, renal clearance can be affected to the point where serum creatinine rises. RAS is caused by atherosclerosis in over 90% of cases, with the remainder caused by fibromuscular dysplasia (Haller & Keim, 2003). Not surprisingly, individuals with RAS generally have atherosclerosis in other vessels, including coronary arteries, carotid vessels, and the abdominal aorta.

Diagnosis of RAS requires a high degree of suspicion. In individuals with hypertension that cannot be controlled with at least triple drug therapy at near maximum doses and who have other known vascular disease and reduced renal function, RAS should be considered. An abdominal bruit supports the diagnosis, but may not always be heard. Imaging studies including ultrasound (conventional or duplex), magnetic resonance imaging, and angiography have been used. Catheter directed imaging should only be undertaken in patients where RAS would be treated if found (Martin et al., 2003). Not all patients with RAS require revascularization; many can be managed conservatively. Revascularization can be done surgically, but recent success with endovascular intervention in combination with stent placement is gaining in popularity. Not all patients with RAS benefit from treatment, and risks of intervention must be weighed against potential benefit. In general, intervention is considered with refractory hypertension (on $\geq$ 3 medications), progressive azotemia, recurrent flash pulmonary edema, bilateral RAS, or RAS in a single functioning kidney. Major complications are rare (see Table 6-6).

Table 6-7

Events Secondarily Associated with TTP/HUS

Escherichia coli 0157:H7 infection (especially in children)
Pregnancy (most common in third trimester)
Hormone contraceptive therapy (progestogen only)
Bone marrow or solid organ transplantation
Use of chemotherapeutic agents (especially cisplatin and
   mitomycin-C)
HIV infection
Use of ticlopidine

Hypertensive Nephrosclerosis

Hypertension and large vessel disease is listed as the cause of renal failure in 26.3% of cases requiring renal replacement therapy in the U.S. according to the 1990-2000 USRDS statistics (USRDS, 2002). Despite this seemingly large incidence, it represents less than 2% of the total hypertensive population in western society (Tylicki, Rutkowski, & Hörl, 2002). The low incidence of ESRD relative to the large number of individuals with hypertension led to research to identify additional factors that might predict hypertensive individuals at risk for ESRD. The risk factors identified include African-American race, advancing age, male gender, smoking, lipid abnormalities, insulin resistance, hyperuricemia, and hyperhomocysteinemia (Tylicki et al., 2002).

Pathogenesis of vascular injury within the kidney is similar to that sustained elsewhere in the body. The mechanical forces of stretch and shear stress are thought to contribute. Biochemical pathways of injury include growth factors such as angiotensin II and transforming growth factor-1, as well as oxidative stress from reactive oxygen species. Progressive nephron loss occurs at least in part via ischemic changes from narrowed preglomerular vessels with resultant limited supply of oxygenated blood. Loss of autoregulation in preglomerular vessels allows for the direct transmission of the elevated systemic pressure to the delicate glomerular capillaries, causing scarring and sclerosis (Tylicki et al., 2002). Further damage may occur due to inflammation in the tubulointerstitial compartment.

Hypertensive nephrosclerosis (HN) is generally a clinical diagnosis, and often no renal biopsy is done. Clinical presentation is typically long-term essential hypertension and progressive renal insufficiency with a urinalysis showing absent or mild proteinuria. Extra-renal signs such as retinal changes and left ventricular hypertrophy are frequently seen (Bleyer & Appel, 1999). There is a correlation between elevated blood pressure and increasing serum creatinine, though it is sometimes unclear whether the chronic kidney disease is the result of hypertension or its cause. This is illustrated by the finding that renal damage occurs in some individuals despite blood pressure controlled to target. Patients with diabetes mellitus or with evidence of renal damage, such as proteinuria, should have their blood pressure controlled to less than 130/80 mmHg according to recently published guidelines (Chobanian, Bakris, Black, & Cushman, 2003).

Although there is a wide range of pharmacologic agents available for blood pressure control, agents such as ACE inhibitors that block the renin-angiotensin system are considered more renoprotective than other antihypertensive agents, independent of blood pressure control achieved (Segura, Campo, Rodicio, & Ruilope, 2001). Lifestyle modifications to augment pharmacotherapy and achieve blood pressure control include weight reduction, regular exercise, smoking cessation, and dietary restriction of sodium intake (JNC VII). Tylicki, Rutkowski, and Hörl (2002) cite strong evidence that urinary sodium excretion (an index of salt intake) is a determinant of microalbuminuria. Increases in dietary sodium intake are associated with reduced renal plasma flow; associated increase in blood volume contributes to shear stress and glomerular injury.

Microangiopathic Diseases

Thombotic thrombocytopenic purpura (TTP)/hemolytic uremic syndrome (HUS). The multisystem syndromes of TTP and HUS were initially thought to be two separate entities but are now considered to be different presentations of the same syndrome. Although rare, with an incidence of 3.7 cases per 1,000,000 U.S. residents (Rock, 2000), it was an almost universally fatal disorder with a mortality rate in excess of 95% if left untreated (Lara et al., 1999). Initial treatments with plasma infusion showed some benefit, but therapeutic plasma exchange has an approximately 80% response rate, with survival rates greater than 90% (Lara et al., 1999).

Classically, TTP consists of a pentad of symptoms: microangiopathic hemolytic anemia, thrombocytopenia, central nervous system abnormalities, fever, and renal impairment. In individuals where neurologic deficits dominate, the disease is termed TTP; in those where renal impairment is predominant, HUS is used. Clinical presentation varies since there are several causative factors. The most common episode is a single acute event that resolves with appropriate therapy, generally within weeks, but chronic relapsing forms are also seen. Kidney biopsy in HUS patients shows severe cortical injury, with platelet thrombi obstructing glomerular blood vessels and the tubular lumen (Baker & Moake, 2000).

Although the majority of TTP/HUS seen in adults is idiopathic, Table 6-7 lists disorders secondarily associated with TTP/HUS. A deficiency in a cleaving metalloproteinase results in unusually large von Willebrand factor multimers in the blood. These appear to adhere to platelets, leading to platelet aggregation and deposition in the microvasculature. This leads to the purpura and thrombocytopenia. Red blood cell fragments including schistocytes, helmet cells, and triangle forms are seen on peripheral blood smears. This red blood cell destruction results in anemia, a universal finding. Elevation of lactate dehydrogenase (LDH) levels results from ischemic tissue. Despite the low platelet counts, significant bleeding is rare, and platelet transfusion should be avoided since it may exacerbate the underlying disease process.

Treatment is with plasma exchange, with plasma being separated from the cellular portion of blood by a cell separation device. If renal failure occurs, renal replacement therapy is also indicated. In patients who do not respond to plasma exchange or who have rapid disease recurrence, splenectomy may be beneficial.

Scleroderma. Scleroderma is a mixed connective tissue

Figure 6-7
Autosomal Dominant Polycystic Kidney Disease (ADPKD)

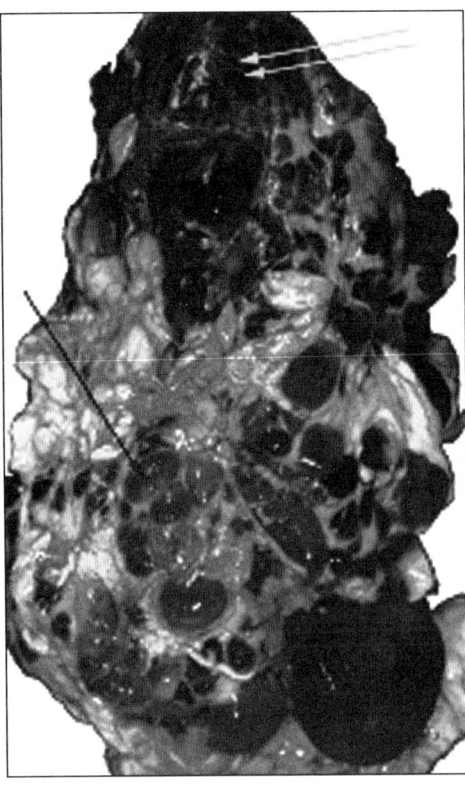

Nephrectomy specimen showing complete replacement of the usual renal architecture by cysts (arrows) of varying sizes. Some are hemorrhagic (double arrow).

parenchyma was historically thought to be progressively compressed and destroyed by multiple epithelial lined cysts, with renal function deteriorating as a result. However, there is little evidence of similar destruction in other organs with cystic involvement, such as the liver. Progressive renal failure correlates most closely with interstitial fibrosis and vascular sclerosis. The relationship to cyst formation is unclear, but normal renal architecture is replaced by cysts as shown in Figure 6-7. ADPKD is inherited in both men and women and affects all ethnic groups. The underlying inherited mutation affecting all body cells requires a somatic "second hit" to the tubular epithelial cells which begins the cyst formation process (Somlo & Markowitz, 2000).

There are two subtypes of ADPKD, with PKD1 progressing more rapidly than PKD2 but otherwise sharing nearly identical disease courses. Harris (2002) notes the average age at onset of kidney failure is 53 years for PKD1 compared with 69 years for PKD2. PKD1 is more common, accounting for nearly 85% of affected individuals (Chapman, 2003).

Hypertension is common and accompanied by severe sclerosis of the preglomerular vessels (Qian, Harris, & Torres, 2001). There is evidence of involvement of the renin-angiotensin system, raising the possibility of benefit by treatment regimens including ACE inhibitors or angiotensin receptor blockers. Other common renal complications include rupture of cysts with associated pain, hemorrhagic cysts (seen in Figure 6-7), gross hematuria, urinary tract infections, and nephrolithiasis. Extra-renal manifestations include cysts in other organs (such as liver, ovaries, spleen, and pancreas), diverticulosis, and intracranial aneurysms.

Autosomal recessive polycystic kidney disease (ARPKD) has an incidence of 1 in 20,000 live births (Guay-Woodford & Desmond, 2003), with the majority of cases being identified either in utero or at birth. A recent breakthrough demonstrated the defect to be a mutation at a single locus, PKHD1 (polycystic kidney and hepatic disease 1). Renal manifestations include hypertension, urinary tract infections, and renal failure. Extrarenal manifestations include pulmonary hypoplasia (potentially fatal in the perinatal period), hepatic fibrosis, and biliary dysgenesis (Harris, 2002). The highest mortality is generally in the first month of life, with the Guay-Woodford and Desmond (2003) study reporting survival rates in 85.5% at 1 month, but only declining to 74.6% at 5 years.

Medullary Cystic Kidney Disease

Medullary cystic kidney disease is a relatively rare inherited disorder characterized by structural defects in the tubules at the corticomedullary junction. Historically, medullary cysts were a predominant feature, but not all patients have cysts. The initial clinical indications are inability to concentrate urine with resultant polyuria and salt wasting. Disease progression results in declining glomerular filtration rate and chronic kidney disease with associated anemia, metabolic acidosis, and uremia (Scolari et al., 2001). Tubular atrophy and interstitial fibrosis are the most frequent lesions seen, and medullary cysts develop late in the disease, if at all. Kidney failure generally occurs in the fourth or fifth decade of life. The disease does not recur in a transplanted kidney.

disease characterized by connective tissue proliferation and vascular lesions. In patients with renal involvement, the disease results in narrowing of the lumen of the small interlobular and arcuate arteries (Shor & Halabe, 2002). In approximately 10% of individuals with scleroderma, an abrupt onset of severe hypertension and rapidly progressive oliguric renal failure is seen, termed scleroderma renal crisis (Prisant, Loebl, & Mulloy, 2003). Though not predictive of scleroderma renal crisis, increased plasma renin levels are felt to mediate the accelerated or malignant hypertension and rapidly deteriorating renal function. Survival of individuals with scleroderma renal crisis was dismal prior to use of ACEI's, with one series of 68 patients studied between 1955 and 1981 having an 84% mortality rate (Prisant et al., 2003). Survival has improved with ACE inhibitors, with 76% survival at 1 year after crisis compared to 15% survival rate in untreated individuals (Prisant et al., 2003).

Cystic Diseases

Polycystic Kidney Disease

Autosomal dominant polycystic kidney disease (ADPKD) is a common genetic cause of kidney failure, accounting for approximately 5% of hemodialysis patients worldwide (Sutters & Germino, 2003). Functional renal

Acquired Cystic Kidney Disease

Acquired cysts are found in individuals with chronic kidney disease, usually after beginning renal replacement therapy, and are thought to develop from sustained uremia. Cysts are more common in males than in females but progress in both sexes and are associated with duration of dialysis. Ishikawa et al. (2003) found cysts in 44% of patients with less than 3 years on dialysis, increasing to 97.2% of patients on dialysis for more than 20 years. Between 2%-7% of patients with acquired cysts ultimately develop renal cancers, a risk 41-100 times that of the general population (Choyke, 2000). Following transplant cysts regress, but pre-existing tumors may become more aggressive with immunosuppression. Patients who have been on dialysis prior to transplant may benefit from screening for acquired cysts.

Simple Renal Cysts

Simple renal cysts are a common finding in adult populations. These cysts are discrete, fluid filled, usually oval or round, and benign. Terada et al. (2002) found that of 1,700 individuals, approximately 12% had at least one renal cyst on ultrasound. Their origin is currently believed to be from diverticula of the tubules. Prevalence increases with age, and cysts occur twice as often in men as in women. Simple renal cysts progress in size and number but have not been associated with carcinoma or loss of renal function.

Infectious Diseases

Urinary Tract Infections/Pyelonephritis

Infections of the urinary tract are common in women, affecting more than half of all women at least once in their lifetime (Fihn, 2003). Infections of the lower urinary tract are termed cystitis, while upper urinary tract infections are described as pyelonephritis. Urinary tract infections (UTIs) are generally classified as uncomplicated or complicated. Uncomplicated UTIs occur in an otherwise healthy, non-pregnant female and are community acquired. Complicated UTIs include infections in any other setting, such as with structural abnormalities of the urinary tract, in males, or with resistant or multiple organisms (Rubenstein & Schaeffer, 2003). Symptoms of cystitis include dysuria, urinary frequency, and occasionally gross hematuria. If fever, chills, nausea, vomiting, costovertebral angle tenderness, or flank pain is present, pyelonephritis is likely. These patients are at higher risk for bacteremia, sepsis, perinephric abscess, emphysematous pyelonephritis, and renal insufficiency (Rubenstein & Schaeffer, 2003).

Uncomplicated UTIs are most often caused by *Escherichia coli*, a short course of oral antibiotics is generally effective, and renal function is rarely impaired. Recurrent UTIs are associated with sexual activity and use of spermicidal contraceptives (Krieger, 2002). In complicated UTIs or pyelonephritis, the spectrum of causative organisms is broader, with diabetics five times more likely to have upper urinary tract involvement (Melekos & Naber, 2000). Hospitalization and intravenous antibiotic therapy may be required. Impaired renal function and even renal failure can result from scarring, especially if there is obstruction or a perinephric abscess.

Viral Diseases

Hepatitis B virus. Viral infections can cause several types of glomerular diseases. Hepatitis B virus (HBV) is a known cause of membranous glomerulonephritis (MGN). Clinical presentation in children from endemic areas is an initial flu-like illness followed by hematuria, proteinuria often in the nephrotic range, and mildly elevated liver transaminases. Renal function is normal, spontaneous remission occurs in about 60% of patients, and chronic renal failure or end stage disease is rare (Lhotta, 2002). In adults, liver transaminases at presentation tend to be normal, but disease progression is more likely, occurring in approximately one third of patients regardless of treatment, and spontaneous remission is rare (Pyrsopoulos & Reddy, 2001). Ten percent of patients will require renal replacement therapy within 5 years (Lhotta, 2002). Histologically, immune deposits are seen in the subepithelial space. Treatment is directed toward eradicating the virus, with interferon alfa used most often. In patients who do not tolerate interferon, lamivudine may be tried. Steroid therapy is not effective and may even be detrimental (Lhotta, 2002). Less frequently, HBV may cause membranoproliferative glomerulonephritis (MPGN) or IgA nephropathy (IgAN) (di Belgiojoso, Ferrario, & Landriani, 2002). MPGN is discussed with Hepatitis C virus (HCV).

HCV. The most common renal manifestation of HCV is MPGN (Giannico, Manno, & Schena, 2000), frequently associated with essential mixed cryoglobulinemia (EMC). Cryoglobulinemia refers to serum immunoglobulins (Ig) that reversibly precipitate when cooled to ≤ 37° C. Between 10% and 50% of HCV patients develop EMC, with renal involvement occurring in approximately half of patients with EMC (Pyrsopoulos & Reddy, 2001). Immune complexes are deposited in the glomerulus, resulting in microscopic proteinuria, overt proteinuria, or even a nephrotic syndrome type presentation in approximately 20% of cases (Lhotta, 2002). In the past, acute flares of EMC glomerulonephritis were treated with steroids, cyclophosphamide, and plasmapheresis (Giannico et al., 2000). Although often effective, side effects and recurrent disease were frequent problems. Current treatment is usually targeted at the virus, often with interferon alfa. Response to treatment may lead to clinical improvement, but relapses after discontinuation of therapy are frequent. Ribavirin may be used in combination with interferon alfa for treatment of HCV liver disease but must be used with caution if renal impairment is present due to risk of profound hemolytic anemia (Pyrsopoulos & Reddy, 2001). Despite the chronic kidney disease seen in about half of HCV patients with EMC, only a minority requires renal replacement therapy (Lhotta, 2002).

Less commonly, HCV is associated with MGN, IgAN, rapidly progressive GN, exudative-proliferative GN, fibrillary and immunotactoid GN, and lupus nephritis (di Belgiojoso et al., 2002). Human immunodeficiency virus-HCV co-infection has been related to immune complex GN.

Human immunodeficiency virus. The human immunodeficiency virus (HIV) has been linked with several types of renal disease. Initial cases were an aggressive, collapsing form of focal segmental glomerulosclerosis (FSGS) termed HIV-associated nephropathy (HIVAN) (Herman & Klotman, 2003). The spectrum of kidney disease among HIV infected

Figure 6-8
Viral Tubulitis

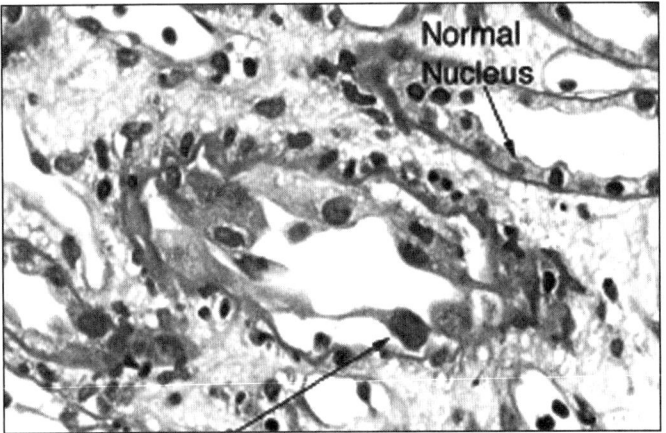

Polyoma viral infection in a renal transplant patient. A tubular injury with viral inclusions. PAS original magnification 200x.

patients is now known to be broader, consisting of at least three syndromes: FSGS, immune complex GN, and thrombotic microangiopathies (Weiner, Goodman, & Kimmel, 2003). FSGS in HIV affects predominantly black males, currently the third leading cause of ESRD in black males between the ages of 20 and 64 based on USRDS data. Presentation is with nephrotic range proteinuria (often greater than 10 g/day), hypoalbuminemia, but generally without hypertension. Approximately half of these cases are in individuals with a history of IV drug use, raising a question about the role of heroin nephropathy (Moroni & Antinori, 2003). Ultrasound shows large, echogenic kidneys, hypothesized to be from interstitial expansion and dilated tubules. Progression to renal failure is rapid, with a median of 2 months (Moroni & Antinori, 2003).

HIV associated immune complex GN is more common among Caucasians and includes a proliferative GN, a mixed sclerotic-immune complex GN, and IgAN (Weiner et al., 2003). These patients may present with hematuria and proteinuria, usually in the range of 1-3 g/day. The disease tends to follow a more indolent course that is less likely to progress to renal failure. The thrombotic microangiopathies TTP/HUS in HIV have a similar presentation to their idiopathic forms, but the prognosis is considerably worse, with mortality rates of 66% to 100% (Weiner et al., 2003) (see the section on TTP/HUS).

Treatment of HIVAN is based on observational evidence. Highly active antiretroviral therapy (HAART) to reduce viral replication has been shown to be associated with improved outcomes. Use of ACE inhibitors has also been shown to improve renal survival. The use of steroids is controversial, since although it may result in decreased proteinuria, complications such as gastrointestinal bleeding, new opportunistic infections, and psychosis were observed (Weiner et al., 2003). Szczech (2001) recommends considering prednisone use only when HAART and ACE inhibitors fail to stabilize renal function.

Miscellaneous virus-related glomerular disease. Recent reports implicate parvovirus B19 in "idiopathic" collapsing FSGS, immune complex GN, and Coxsackie B virus may be associated with IgAN. Polyoma virus BK affects renal transplants and can lead to loss of function (di Belgiojoso et al., 2002). Figure 6-8 shows viral tubulitis in a transplanted kidney; tubular injury includes a sloughed cell that contains the viral nucleus. Fulminant hepatitis A has been associated with acute renal failure.

Obstructive Diseases

Obstruction of the urinary tract is classified by degree (partial or complete), duration (acute or chronic), and site (location within the urinary tract). Obstructive uropathy is the term used to describe the change in structure or function resulting in alteration of the normal flow of urine. Obstructive nephropathy refers to the kidney disease that occurs as a result of the obstruction, including a decrease in renal blood flow, decreased glomerular filtration rate, and tubular dysfunction (Klahr, 2000). Obstruction is relatively common and can occur at any age. Anatomical abnormalities are more common in childhood, renal calculi in middle-aged males, pelvic tumors in middle-aged females, and prostatic hypertrophy or malignancy in older males (Rose & Black, 1988).

Acute Obstructive Nephropathy

Though urinary tract obstruction is frequently asymptomatic, pain can be a typical presenting symptom with acute obstruction, particularly if the obstruction is complete. This is from distention of the bladder, collecting system, or renal capsule. Unrelieved obstructive uropathy can lead to nephropathy with clinical and laboratory findings consistent with impaired renal function. Early diagnosis and intervention to relieve the obstruction enhances the chances of recovery of function. Bladder catheterization can relieve obstruction of the urethra or bladder neck. Radiologic studies such as ultrasound may be used to diagnose obstruction at the level of the ureters or above, though hydronephrosis (dilatation of the urinary tract) may not be present initially due to limited compliance of the collecting system. Intravenous pyelogram can be used to identify the site of obstruction and has few false positives but has the disadvantage of requiring radiocontrast, which can be nephrotoxic. After relief of the obstruction, the kidney may initially be unable to appropriately concentrate the urine, leading to a post-obstructive diuresis (Palmieri, 2002). The majority of the functional recovery is seen in the first 7 to 10 days.

Chronic Obstructive Nephropathy

An incomplete obstruction may be present for weeks, months, or even years prior to diagnosis since it is often asymptomatic. Because of the variability in degree and duration, its course is harder to predict and may be influenced by comorbid factors such as hypertension, infection, or underlying renal disease. The mechanism of kidney injury is thought to be multifactorial, with increased pressures within the kidney leading to decreased renal blood flow and decreased glomerular filtration. Interstitial fibrosis is also common in chronic obstruction, likely from ischemia and inflammatory factors (Klahr, 2000). Renal failure can be acute or chronic and may require temporary or permanent renal replacement therapy.

Neoplasms of the Kidney

Renal Cell Carcinoma

Kidney cancers are relatively rare, accounting for 3% of adult malignancies (Zweizig, 2002). These cancers present a diagnostic and therapeutic challenge, since symptoms can be myriad or absent until the tumor has invaded surrounding structures. Males are nearly twice as likely to develop the disease as females, commonly during the fifth through seventh decades of life, though cases have been reported in younger individuals. Risk factors include cigarette smoking, obesity, hypertension, high protein diets, and chronic dialysis-acquired renal cystic disease (Figlin, 1999; Zweizig, 2002).

The incidence of renal cell carcinoma (RCC) has increased by 43% since 1973, thought to be at least in part due to increasing frequency of abdominal imaging. In the early 1970s, only 10% of tumors were discovered incidentally, compared to 61% found incidentally in 1998 (Zweizig, 2002). Ultrasound is highly sensitive in distinguishing solid lesions from cystic lesions; magnetic resonance imaging (MRI) can also assess lesions using gadolinium contrast, which is not nephrotoxic. Due to its sensitivity, MRI can assess tumor extension into the vasculature and may be useful in preparation for surgery. Computed tomography (CT) with contrast is the imaging modality of choice, but should be avoided in individuals with significant renal insufficiency due to the need for potentially nephrotoxic contrast (Herts, 2003).

RCC is often clinically occult in its early stages. Symptoms at presentation may include hematuria, abdominal pain, palpable mass, weight loss, fever, night sweats, or hypertension. "The classic triad of pain, hematuria, and a flank mass is found in less than 10% or patients with kidney cancer, and usually indicates advanced disease" (Zweizig, 2002, pp. 885-886). One third of patients have evidence of metastatic disease at the time of diagnosis (Leibovich et al., 2003), with hematogenous spread common to lung, bone, adrenal gland, liver, or brain. Tumor staging represents the anatomic spread and disease involvement. All RCC is classified as adenocarcinoma, with four main histologic subtypes. Each subtype has distinguishing characteristics and disease patterns that may influence prognosis (Leibovich et al., 2003). Von Hippel-Lindau disease is an inherited disease that may be associated with multiple malignancies including clear cell carcinoma of the kidney (Figlin, 1999). Table 6-8 shows relative frequency of the main subtypes based on data from Leibovich et al. (2003). Sarcomatoid histology is no longer considered a distinct subtype of RCC, but represents an aggressive variant that can be found with any histologic subtype.

Surgical excision is the only primary treatment, since RCC tumors are poorly responsive to chemotherapy or radiation therapy. Figure 6-9 shows a nephrectomized kidney with RCC. Total nephrectomy is indicated unless the mass is small, 4 cm or less. In these cases, a subtotal nephrectomy has shown outcomes of equal efficacy to radical surgery while sparing nephron mass (Zweizig, 2002). Needle biopsy is not generally recommended. Recent research in the treatment of advanced disease shows some benefit to immunotherapy with interferon α and interleukin-2 (Figlin, 1999). Nephrectomy in metastatic disease has been shown to have a positive impact on survival (Mejean, Oudard, & Thiounn, 2003). The 5-year survival rate for individuals diagnosed between 1983 and 1989 is 58% overall, but varies widely based on tumor stage and grade at time of diagnosis (Zweizig, 2002). Incidentally discovered tumors tend to be smaller and of lower stage and grade, with 5-year survival rates of 85.3% compared to 62.5% for symptomatic tumors in the same series (Leibovich et al., 2003).

Wilm's tumor (nephroblastoma), although rare, is the most common malignant neoplasm of the urinary tract in children (Ozcan & Bahado-Singh, 2001). Ninety percent of these tumors are found by age 7. The tumor is usually an encapsulated solitary tumor that can occur in any part of the kidney. These may be asymptomatic, found by a parent or clinician as an abdominal mass on physical exam, or may present with hematuria or obstruction if the renal pelvis is involved. Fatigue, weight loss, and malaise are late symptoms of the condition. Treatment generally consists of nephrectomy with adjuvant chemotherapy or radiotherapy, with prognosis dependent upon the size, grade, and stage of the tumor. Early stage disease has a good prognosis, and the

Table 6-8
Relative Frequency of Histologic Types of RCC

Histologic Type	Frequency
Clear cell carcinoma	70% - 80%
Papillary RCC	10% - 20%
Chromophobe RCC	5%
Collecting duct carcinoma	< 1%

Figure 6-9
Renal Cell Carcinoma

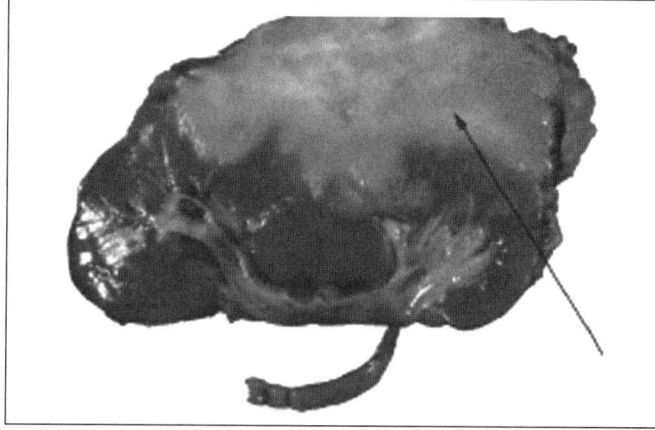

Whitish tumor mass infiltrating renal parenchyma (arrow).

Acknowledgment: Photographs and captions courtesy of Dr. Patrick D. Walker, Nephropathologist, Little Rock, AR.

Table 6-9
Potential Causes of ARF in Pregnancy

Hypoperfusion
    Sepsis
    Volume contraction (i.e., hyperemesis graviderum)
    Hemorrhage (placenta previa, abruptio placentae, postpartum)
    UTI/pyelonephritis
Urinary obstruction
    Uterine leiomyomata
    Urolithiasis
    Polyhydramnios
Pre-eclampsia / Eclampsia
HELLP Syndrome
TTP/HUS
Idiopathic postpartum renal failure

recurrence rate is lower for children diagnosed prior to 2 years of age (Ozcan & Bahado-Singh, 2001).

Renal Disease in Pregnancy

Physiologic Changes in Renal Function During Pregnancy

During normal pregnancy, extensive changes occur in kidney function. The kidney actually increases in size by approximately 1 cm, with increased glomerular size and dilatation of the urinary tract (Thorsen & Poole, 2002). This physiologic ureteral dilatation is primarily from smooth muscle relaxing effects of progesterone (Sanders & Lucas, 2001) and may result in urinary stasis.

Increased sodium and water retention leads to increased vascular volume and a slight fall in serum sodium concentration ($\approx$ 5 mEq/L). Serum sodium levels above 140 mEq/L are considered hypernatremia (Thorsen & Poole, 2002). Cardiac output increases 30%-50% above normal, and GFR increases within the first month, peaking at nearly 50% above baseline by the end of the first trimester. Concomitantly, plasma creatinine concentration is reduced ($\approx$ 0.5 mg/dL), so values in the "normal" range may actually reflect impaired renal function. Increased filtration fraction combined with changes in tubular reabsorption of glucose and protein is altered; mild glycosuria and proteinuria up to 300 mg/ 24 hours is considered normal (Thorsen & Poole, 2002). GFR declines slightly during the third trimester and returns to prepregnancy levels within 3 months after delivery.

Types of Renal Diseases in Pregnancy

UTI is the most common renal disease in pregnancy. The urinary stasis seen during pregnancy predisposes to UTI. Both symptomatic and asymptomatic bacteriuria should be treated, with antibiotic selection made considering potential maternal and fetal toxicity (Melekos & Naber, 2000). Untreated bacteriuria can lead to pyelonephritis, which in turn can lead to high rates of premature infants and perinatal mortality if untreated (Melekos & Naber, 2000).

ARF in pregnancy is rare, with an incidence of only $\approx$ 1 in 10,000 due to improved medical and prenatal care for women (Thorsen & Poole, 2002). Table 6-9 lists potential causes of ARF in pregnancy. Several of these have been previously discussed since these conditions are also seen in non-pregnant states.

Pre-eclampsia/eclampsia, HELLP syndrome (hemolysis, elevated liver enzymes, low platelets), and idiopathic postpartum renal failure will be briefly discussed.

Pre-eclampsia is defined as hypertension and proteinuria in excess of 300 mg/day. Incidence is approximately 3%-5% of pregnancies. Neurologic abnormalities such as headache and visual disturbances are seen with severe pre-eclampsia, though renal failure with elevated serum creatinine and oliguria (< 500 ml urine/day) are rare. Fetal growth retardation may be seen (McMinn & George, 2001). Eclampsia is defined by the occurrence of generalized seizures with no other apparent neurologic etiology. HELLP syndrome is closely associated with pre-eclampsia or eclampsia, with the additional features of microangiopathic hemolysis, thrombocytopenia, and liver function abnormalities. Pre-eclampsia and HELLP syndrome typically resolve spontaneously after delivery, so once the fetus is felt to be viable, delivery is generally the "treatment" of choice (McMinn & George, 2001). TTP/HUS is clinically very similar to pre-eclampsia and HELLP syndrome, but requires urgent intervention with plasma exchange (McMinn & George, 2001). See TTP/HUS for discussion of this disease process.

A rare but often fatal syndrome, idiopathic postpartum renal failure typically presents following an uneventful pregnancy. Severe hypertension, microangiopathic hemolytic anemia, and oliguric renal failure are hallmarks. Congestive heart failure and central nervous system involvement may also be seen. The cause is unknown, and treatment is not well established (Thorsen & Poole, 2002).

Pregnancy and Preexisting Renal Disease

Mild renal impairment (serum creatinine less than 1.5 mg/dL) at the onset of pregnancy is associated with a low risk of decline in renal function. Serum creatinine of greater than 2.0 mg/dL poses an increased risk (nearly 50%) for progression to renal failure requiring renal replacement therapy (Sanders & Lucas, 2001). Chronic kidney disease in pregnancy increases the risk of fetal loss, preterm birth, and low birth weight. Maternal hypertension is the most common risk factor for unfavorable perinatal outcomes (Thorsen & Poole, 2002), with the degree of hypertension directly related to the prognosis. Sanders and Lucas (2001) conclude that women with mild renal impairment should expect a good maternal and fetal outcome, but for individuals with moderate to severe renal impairment, risk of preterm delivery, low birth weight, and still birth increases proportionately to the degree of renal dysfunction.

Pregnancy following renal transplant is not uncommon, but should be avoided for the first year (living donor) or two (cadaveric donor) to allow for stabilization of immunosuppression (Thorsen & Poole, 2001). While control of hypertension is important, certain antihypertensives, such as ACE inhibitors, should be avoided in all women of childbearing age who may conceive due to predictable toxicity to the fetal kidney (Sanders & Lucas, 2001).

Women receiving dialysis rarely become pregnant, with estimated conception rates in the U.S. of 0.5% (Hou, 2001). Incidence of pregnancy in women on peritoneal dialysis is two to three times lower than for women on hemodialysis (Hou, 2001). Increasing the dialysis dose prolongs gestation and improves infant survival chances (Holley & Reddy, 2003). More frequent hemodialysis sessions are generally recommended, with a goal pre-dialysis BUN of ≤ 50 mg/dL. This is also felt to minimize fluid shifts and helps control maternal intravascular volume, reducing chances of hypotension. Low birth weight is common, and the fetus is rarely carried to term, but survival rates are improving from only ≈ 20% in the 1980s to ≈ 50% now. Adjustment of estimated dry weight must be done frequently to account for fetal growth as well as amniotic fluid and maternal weight gain. A successful pregnancy in a dialysis patient requires collaboration of the entire renal team as well as the obstetric team. Nurses and physicians should discuss fertility and contraception issues with premenopausal women on dialysis.

Summary

Kidney disease continues to be a major health problem in the U.S. Disease states can involve any part of the kidney, be acute or chronic, potentially reversible, chronically progressive, or even fatal. Early detection and intervention has the potential to improve outcomes and lessen the medical, psychosocial, and financial impact of these diseases on millions of individuals. Participation by nephrology nurses in educational efforts, research, and treatment delivery is enhanced by improving the knowledge base of kidney disease. Nephrology nurses are important members of the multidisciplinary team, with the potential to have a positive impact on the course of kidney disease and its sequelae. Understanding disease processes can guide the nurses' assessments and interventions, as well as facilitate meeting the educational needs of patients and family members.

References

Asif, A., Preston, R.A., & Roth, D. (2003). Radiocontrast-induced nephropathy. *American Journal of Therapeutics, 10,* 137-147.

Baker, K.R., & Moake, J.L. (2000). Thrombocytopenic purpura and the hemolytic-uremic syndrome. *Current Opinion in Pediatrics, 12*(1), 23-28.

Bleyer, A.J., & Appel, R.G. (1999). Risk factors associated with hypertensive nephrosclerosis. *Nephron, 82,* 193-198.

Cao, Z., & Cooper, M. (2001). Role of angiotensin II in tubulointerstitial injury. *Seminars in Nephrology, 21,* 554-562.

Chapman, A.B. (2003). Cystic disease in women: Clinical characteristics and medical management. *Advances in Renal Replacement Therapies, 10*(1), 24-30.

Chobanian, A.V., Bakris, G.L., Black, H.R., & Cushman, W.C. (2003). The seventh report of the joint national committee on prevention, detection, evaluation, and treatment of high blood pressure: The JNC 7 report. *Journal of the American Medical Association, 289,* 2560.

Choyke, P.L. (2000). Acquired cystic kidney disease. *European Radiology, 10,* 1716-1721.

Couser, W.G. (1999). Glomerulonephritis. *Lancet, 353,* 1509-1515.

DeBroe, M.E., & Elseviers, M.M. (1998). Analgesic nephropathy. *New England Journal of Medicine, 338,* 446.

di Belgiojoso, G.B., Ferrario, F., & Landriani, N. (2002). Virus-related glomerular diseases: Histological and clinical aspects. *Journal of Nephrology, 15,* 469-479.

Figlin, R.A. (1999). Renal cell carcinoma: Management of advanced disease. *The Journal of Urology, 161,* 381-387.

Fihn, S.D. (2003). Acute uncomplicated urinary tract infection in women. *The New England Journal of Medicine, 349,* 259-266.

Fox, J.M., & Siebers, U. (2003). Caffeine as a promoter of analgesic-associated nephropathy – where is the evidence? *Fundamental & Clinical Pharmacology, 17,* 377-392.

Gambara, G., & Perazella, M.A. (2003). Adverse renal effects of anti-inflammatory agents: evaluation of selective and nonselective cyclooxygenase inhibitors. *Journal of Internal Medicine, 253,* 643-652.

Giannico, G., Manno, C., & Schena, F.P. (2000). Treatment of glomerulonephritides associated with hepatitis C virus infection. *Nephrology Dialysis Transplantation, 15*(Suppl. 8), 34-38.

Glassock, R.J. (2001). Glomerular therapeutics: Looking back, looking forward. *Heart Disease, 3,* 276-281.

Guay-Woodford, L.M., & Desmond, R.A. (2003). Autosomal recessive polycystic kidney disease: The clinical experience in North America. *Pediatrics, 111,* 1072-1080.

Guo, X., & Nzerue, C. (2002). How to prevent, recognize, and treat drug-induced nephrotoxicity. *Cleveland Clinic Journal of Medicine, 69,* 289-312.

Haller, C., & Keim, M. (2003). Current issues in the diagnosis and management of patients with renal artery stenosis: A cardiologic perspective. *Progress in Cardiovascular Diseases, 46*(3), 271-286.

Harris, D.C.H. (2001). Tubulointerstitial renal disease. *Current Opinion in Nephrology & Hypertension, 10*(3), 303-313.

Harris, P.C. (2002). Molecular basis of polycystic kidney disease: PKD1, PKD2 and PKHD1. *Current Opinion in Nephrology and Hypertension, 11,* 309-314.

Herman, E.S., & Klotman, P.E. (2003). HIV-Associated nephropathy: Epidemiology, pathogenesis, and treatment. *Seminars in Nephrology, 23,* 200-208.

Herts, B.R., (2003). Imaging for renal tumors. *Current Opinion in Urology, 13,* 181-186.

Holley, J.L., & Reddy, S.S. (2003). Pregnancy in dialysis patients: A review of outcomes, complications, and management. *Seminars in Dialysis, 16,* 384-387.

Hou, S. (2001). Conception and pregnancy in peritoneal dialysis patients. *Peritoneal Dialysis International, 21*(Suppl. 3), S290-S294.

Hsu, S.I., & Couser, W.G. (2003). Chronic progression of tubulointerstitial damage in proteinuric renal disease is mediated by complement activation: A therapeutic role for complement inhibitors? *Journal of the American Society of Nephrology, 14*(7 Suppl. 2), S186-S191).

Isenbarger, D.W., Kent, S.M., & O'Malley, P.G. (2003). Meta-Analysis of randomized clinical trials on the usefulness of acetylcysteine for prevention of contrast nephropathy. *The American Journal of Cardiology, 92,* 1454-1458.

Ishikawa, I., Saito, Y., Asaka, M., Tomosugi, N., Yuri, T., Watanbe, M., & Honda, R. (2003). Twenty-year follow-up of acquired renal cystic disease. *Clinical Nephrology, 59*(3), 153-159.

Kini, A.S., Mitre, C.A., Kamran, M., Suleman, J., Kim, M., Duffy, M.E., Marmur, J.D., & Sharma, S.K. (2002). Changing trends in incidence and predictors of radiographic contrast nephropathy after percutaneous coronary intervention with use of fenoldopam. *The American Journal of Cardiology, 89,* 999-1002.

Kiperova, B. (2003). The treatment of glomerular disease – a compromise between the standard and the individual approach. *Nephrology Dialysis Transplantation, 18*(Suppl. 5), v31-v33.

Klahr, S. (2000). Obstructive nephropathy. *Internal Medicine, 39*(5), 355-361.

Kodner, C.M., & Kudrimoti, A. (2003). Diagnosis and management of acute interstitial nephritis. *American Family Physician, 67,* 2527-2534.

Krieger, J.N. (2002). Urinary tract infections: What's new? *The Journal of Urology, 168,* 2351-2358.

Kunis, C.L., & Teng, S.N. (2000). Treatment of glomerulonephritis in the elderly. *Seminars in Nephrology, 20,* 256-264.

Lara, P.N., Coe, T.L., Shou, H., Fernando, L., Holland, P.V., & Wun, T. (1999). Improved survival with plasma exchange in patients with thrombotic thrombocytopenic purpura-hemolytic uremic syndrome. *The American Journal of Medicine, 107,* 573-579.

Leibovich, B.C., Pantuck, A.J., Bui, M.H.T., Ryu-Han, K., Zisman, A., Figlin, R., & Belldegrun, A. (2003). Current staging of renal cell carcinoma. *Urologic Clinics of North America, 30,* 481-497.

Lhotta, K. (2002). Beyond hepatorenal syndrome: Glomerulonephritis in patients with liver disease. *Seminars in Nephrology, 22,* 302-308.

Madaio, M.P., & Harrington, J.T. (2001). The diagnosis of glomerular diseases. *Archives of Internal Medicine, 161,* 25-34.

Martin, L.G., Rundbacj, J.H., Sacks, D., Cardella, J.F., Rees, C.R., Matsumoto, A.H., Meranze, S.G., Schwartzberg, M.S., Silverstein, M.I., & Lewis, C.A. (2003). Quality improvement guidelines for angiography, angioplasty, and stent placement in the diagnosis and treatment of renal artery stenosis in adults. *Journal of Vascular Interventional Radiology, 14,* S297-S310.

McMinn, J.R., & George, J.N. (2001). Evaluation of women with clinically suspected thrombotic thrombocytopenic purpura-hemolytic uremic syndrome during pregnancy. *Journal of Clinical Apheresis, 16,* 202-209.

Mejean, A., Oudard, S., & Thiounn, N. (2003). Prognostic factors of renal cell carcinoma. *The Journal of Urology, 169,* 821-827.

Melekos, M.D., & Naber, K.G. (2000). Complicated urinary tract infections. *International Journal of Antimicrobial Agents, 15,* 247-256.

Meyers, C.M. (1999). New insights into the pathogenesis of interstitial nephritis. *Current Opinion in Nephrology & Hypertension, 8*(3), 287-292.

Mookerjee, B.K., Lohr, J.W., Jenis, E.H., & Heffner, H.M. (2001). Glomerulonephritis for the generalist. *Journal of Medicine, 32*(3-4), 115-134.

Moroni, M., & Antinori, S. (2003). HIV and direct damage of organs: disease spectrum before and during the highly active antiretroviral therapy era. *AIDS, 17*(Suppl. 1), S51-S64.

Ozcan, T., & Bahado-Singh, R. (2001, August 7). Prenatal diagnosis of fetal renal masses. *UpToDate® in Medicine.*

Palmieri, P.A. (2002). Obstructive nephropathy: Pathophysiology, diagnosis, and collaborative management. *Nephrology Nursing Journal, 29,* 15-21, 96.

Prisant, L.M., Loebl, D.H., & Mulloy, L.L. (2003). Scleroderma renal crisis. *The Journal of Clinical Hypertension, 5,* 168-170, 176.

Pyrsopoulos, N.T., & Reddy, K.R. (2001). Extrahepatic manifestations of chronic viral hepatitis. *Current Gastroenterology Reports, 3,* 71-78.

Qian, Q., Harris, P.C., & Torres, V.E. (2001). Treatment prospects for autosomal-dominant polycystic kidney disease. *Kidney International, 59,* 2005-2022.

Radermacher, J., Weinkove, R., & Haller, H. (2001). Techniques for predicting a favorable response to renal angioplasty in patients with renovascular disease. *Current Opinion in Nephrology and Hypertension, 10,* 799-805.

Rock, G.A. (2000). Management of thrombotic thrombocytopenic purpura. *British Journal of Haematology, 109*(3-l), 496-507.

Rose, B.D., & Black, R.M. (1988). In *Manual of clinical problems in nephrology* (pp. 337-343). Boston: Little, Brown.

Rubenstein, J.N., & Schaeffer, A.J. (2003). Managing uncomplicated urinary tract infections: The urologic view. *Infectious Disease Clinics of North America, 17,* 333-351.

Sanders, C.L., & Lucas, M.J. (2001). Renal disease in pregnancy. *Obstetrics and Gynecology Clinics, 28,* 593-600.

Scolari, F., Viola, B.F., Prati, E., Ghiggeri, G.M., Caridi, G., Amoroso, A., Casari, G., & Maiorca, R. (2001). Medullary cystic kidney disease: Past and present. *Contributions to Nephrology, 136,* 68-78.

Segura, J., Campo, C., Rodicio, J.L., & Ruilope, L.M. (2001). ACE Inhibitors and appearance of renal events in hypertensive nephrosclerosis. *Hypertension, 38*(Part 2), 645-649.

Shor, R., & Halabe, A. (2002). New trends in the treatment of scleroderma renal crisis. *Nephron, 92,* 716-718.

Somlo, S., & Markowitz, G.S. (2000). The pathogenesis of autosomal dominant polycystic kidney disease: An update. *Current Opinion in Nephrology and Hypertension, 9,* 385-394.

Sutters, M., & Germino, G.G. (2003). Autosomal dominant polycystic kidney disease: Molecular genetics and pathophysiology. *Journal of Laboratory Clinical Medicine, 141,* 91-101.

Szczech, L.A. (2001). Renal diseases associated with human immunodeficiency virus infection: Epidemiology, clinical course, and management. *Clinical Infectious Diseases, 33,* 115-119.

Terada, N., Ichioka, K., Matsuta, Y., Okubo, K., Yoshimura, K., & Arai, Y. (2002). The natural history of simple renal cysts. *The Journal of Urology, 167,* 21-23.

Thorsen, M.S., & Poole, J.H. (2002). Renal disease in pregnancy. *Journal of Perinatal & Neonatal Nursing, 15*(4), 13-26.

Tylicki, L., Rutkowski, B., & Hörl, W.H. (2002). Multifactorial determination of hypertensive nephroangiosclerosis. *Kidney & Blood Pressure Research, 25,* 341-353.

U.S. Renal Data System (USRDS). (2002). USRDS Annual Data Report: Atlas of end stage renal disease in the United States. Bethesda, MD: National Institutes of Health, National Institute of Diabetes and Digestive and Kidney Diseases.

Vagaonescu, T.D., & Dangas, G. (2002). Renal artery stenosis: Diagnosis and management. *The Journal of Clinical Hypertension, 5,* 363-370.

Vashist, A., Heller, E.N., Brown, Jr., E.J., & Alhaddad, I.A. (2002). Renal artery stenosis: A cardiovascular perspective. *American Heart Journal, 143,* 559-564.

Vinen, C.S., & Oliveira, D.B.G. (2003). Acute glomerulonephritis. *Postgraduate Medical Journal, 79,* 206-213.

Weiner, N.J., Goodman, J.W., & Kimmel, P.L. (2003). The HIV-associated renal diseases: Current insight into pathogenesis and treatment. *Kidney International, 63,* 1618-1631.

Yoshioka, K., Takemura, T., & Hattori, S. (2002). Tubulointerstitial nephritis antigen: Primary structure, expression and role in health and disease. *Nephron, 90,* 1-7.

Zweizig, S.L. (2002). Cancer of the kidney. *Clinical Obstetrics and Gynecology, 45*(3), 884-891.

- Although the term GN implies inflammation or infection, some lesions are not associated with inflammatory cells. Primary glomerular diseases affect the kidney nearly exclusively, while secondary diseases are the result of systemic disease processes that include glomerular pathology.

- Early detection and therapeutic intervention in acute GN is critical since prompt treatment may reverse renal damage with return to near-normal function. Even if recovery is not achieved, progression of renal disease may be slowed (Mookerjee, Lohr, Jenis, & Heffner, 2001).

- Patients who initially present with impaired renal function or significant proteinuria tend to have more progression of disease. In the chronic progressive phase of GN, damage continues mediated by non-immune mechanisms associated with increases in glomerular pressure, sclerosis, and interstitial fibrosis.

- Acute interstitial nephritis (AIN) describes injury to the interstitium of the kidney resulting in abrupt deterioration of renal function. The etiology of AIN is most often secondary to drug therapy but may also be from infections, certain immune diseases, or idiopathic causes.

- In individuals who present with acute or subacute decline in renal function, a careful history should be taken to evaluate for drugs implicated in AIN or a history of a recent infection associated with AIN. Withdrawal of any and all potentially offending agents should be done, with substitution of medications not associated with AIN when clinically indicated.

- Of unselected populations undergoing intravascular radiocontrast administration, about 15% develop contrast-induced nephropathy (CIN), with higher incidence seen in diabetics with pre-existing renal insufficiency (Isenbarger, Kent, & O'Malley, 2003).

- Renal artery stenosis (RAS) is defined as narrowing of the renal artery lumen by 50% or more (Martin et al., 2003). Renovascular disease is present in 10%-40% of patients with ESRD and is the fastest growing group of ESRD patients (Radermacher, Weinkove, & Haller, 2001).

- Hypertension and large vessel disease is listed as the cause of renal failure in 26.3% of cases requiring renal replacement therapy in the U.S. according to the 1990-2000 USRDS statistics (USRDS, 2002). Despite this seemingly large incidence, it represents less than 2% of the total hypertensive population in western society (Tylicki, Rutkowski, & Hörl, 2002).

- The multisystem syndromes of TTP and HUS were initially thought to be two separate entities but are now considered to be different presentations of the same syndrome. Although rare, with an incidence of 3.7 cases per 1 million U.S. residents (Rock, 2000), it was an almost universally fatal disorder with a mortality rate in excess of 95% if left untreated (Lara et al., 1999).

- Infections of the urinary tract are common in women, affecting more than half of all women at least once in their lifetime (Fihn, 2003). Infections of the lower urinary tract are termed cystitis, while upper urinary tract infections are described as pyelonephritis.

- During normal pregnancy, extensive changes occur in kidney function. The kidney actually increases in size by approximately 1 cm, with increased glomerular size and dilatation of the urinary tract (Thorsen & Poole, 2002). This physiologic ureteral dilatation is primarily from smooth muscle relaxing effects of progesterone (Sanders & Lucas, 2001) and may result in urinary stasis.

- UTI is the most common renal disease in pregnancy. The urinary stasis seen during pregnancy predisposes to UTI. Both symptomatic and asymptomatic bacteriuria should be treated, with antibiotic selection made considering potential maternal and fetal toxicity (Melekos & Naber, 2000).

- Kidney disease continues to be a major health problem in the U.S. Disease states can involve any part of the kidney, be acute or chronic, potentially reversible, chronically progressive, or even fatal. Early detection and intervention has the potential to improve outcomes and lessen the medical, psychosocial, and financial impact of these diseases on millions of individuals.

ANNP606

Diseases of the Kidney

LaVonne M. Burrows, M-SCNS, BC, RN, CNN

Contemporary Nephrology Nursing: Principles and Practice contains 39 chapters of educational content. Individual learners may apply for continuing nursing education credit by reading a chapter and completing the Continuing Education Evaluation Form for that chapter. Learners may apply for continuing education credit for any or all chapters.

Please photocopy this page and return to ANNA.
COMPLETE THE FOLLOWING:

Name: _____

Address:_____

City:_____State: _____Zip: _____

E-mail: _____

Preferred telephone: ☐ Home   ☐ Work: _____

State where licensed and license number (optional): _____

CE application fees are based upon the number of contact hours provided by the individual chapter. CE fees per contact hour for ANNA members are as follows: 1.0-1.9 - $15; 2.0-2.9 - $20; 3.0-3.9 - $25; 4.0 and higher - $30. Fees for nonmembers are $10 higher.

ANNA Member: ☐ Yes   ☐ No   Member # (if available) _____

☐ Checked Enclosed   ☐ American Express   ☐ Visa   ☐ MasterCard

Total Amount Submitted: _____

Credit Card Number: _____ Exp. Date: _____

Name as it appears on the card: _____

CE Evaluation Form
To receive continuing education credit for individual study after reading the chapter
1. Photocopy this form. (You may also download this form from ANNA's Web site, **www.annanurse.org.**)
2. Mail the completed form with payment (check) or credit card information to American Nephrology Nurses' Association, East Holly Avenue, Box 56, Pitman, NJ 08071-0056.
3. You will receive your CE certificate from ANNA in 4 to 6 weeks.

Test returns must be postmarked by **December 31, 2010.**

CE Application Fee
ANNA Member $15.00
Nonmember $25.00

EVALUATION FORM

1. I verify that I have read this chapter and completed this education activity. Date: _____

_____
Signature

2. What would be different in your practice if you applied what you learned from this activity? *(Please use additional sheet of paper if necessary.)*

_____
_____
_____
_____
_____
_____
_____
_____
_____
_____
_____
_____
_____

Evaluation	Strongly disagree				Strongly agree
3. The activity met the stated objectives.					
a. Identify various diseases of the kidney by nursing assessment findings.	1	2	3	4	5
b. Relate treatment of a specific renal disease to the pathophysiologic basis of the disease.	1	2	3	4	5
c. Outline a nursing plan of care for a patient with a specified renal disease.	1	2	3	4	5
4. The content was current and relevant.	1	2	3	4	5
5. The content was presented clearly.	1	2	3	4	5
6. The content was covered adequately.	1	2	3	4	5
7. Rate your ability to apply the learning obtained from this activity to practice.	1	2	3	4	5

Comments _____

_____

8. Time required to read the chapter and complete this form: _____ minutes.

This educational activity has been provided by the American Nephrology Nurses' Association (ANNA) for 1.9 contact hours. ANNA is accredited as a provider of continuing nursing education (CNE) by the American Nurses Credentialing Center's Commission on Accreditation (ANCC-COA). ANNA is an approved provider of continuing education by the California Board of Registered Nursing, CEP 0910.

Genetics and Kidney Disease

Ann Cashion, PhD, RN
Carolyn J. Driscoll, MSN, RN, FNP-C

C
H
A
P
T
E
R
7

Chapter Contents

Genetics and Kidney Disease

Chapter 7

Ann Cashion, PhD, RN
Carolyn J. Driscoll, MSN, RN, FNP-C

With the inception of the International Human Genome Project begun in 1990, health care and the diagnosis, treatment, and monitoring of diseases has been transformed. Nurses are increasingly incorporating genetic concepts into their practice and answering questions related to genetic issues ranging from genetic testing to pharmacogenomics. Genetics has always played a key role in nephrology, particularly in determining the genetic origins of single gene disorders including polycystic kidney disease, cystinuria, Alport syndrome, Bartter syndrome, and various renal neoplasms (George & Neilson, 2000). More recently, it has been recognized that multifactorial genetic disorders, which have both gene and environmental interaction, also lead to chronic renal dysfunction. Research on multifactorial diseases such as diabetes mellitus, systemic lupus erythematosis, and hypertension focuses on identifying the multiple genes involved and addressing the environmental components that can be modified with intervention. Results of these clinical and laboratory studies will change nursing practice. However, to understand and apply these findings, nurses need to know the basics of genetics.

This explosion in genetic technologies and methodologies to identify disease-related genes has led to an increase in the number of genetic tests and genetic-based therapies available to identify, monitor, and treat kidney diseases. The role of the clinical practitioner includes interpreting clinical reports, applying evidenced-based research to patient care, and communicating this information to patients, all of which require a basic understanding of how genetic principles apply to kidney disease. This chapter provides a genetic foundation of the structure and function of deoxyribonucleic acid (DNA) and patterns of inheritance that will enable nephrology nurses to integrate genetics knowledge into their clinical practice. The focus is on defining and understanding key genetic terminology, identifying genetic mutations associated with kidney disease, and summarizing new genetic technologies and therapies needed to understand and apply genetic information to the care of nephrology

patients. For a more in-depth exploration of genetics, it is suggested that the reader refer to the Web sites listed at the end of this chapter and to genetics textbooks (Lewin, 2000; Nussbaum, McInnes, & Willard, 2001).

ACTG: The Basics of Genetics

Nephrology nurses have become increasingly aware of a new genetic language, and although most are familiar with terms such as *DNA*, other terms (such as *allele*) are less familiar (see Table 7-1). This section will provide a foundation in basic genetics.

Genes are DNA organized into linear structural units called *chromosomes*. Genes are found in the nucleus of almost all human cells, with a notable exception being red blood cells, which have no nucleus. Small subsets of genes are also found in the

Table 7-1
Common Genetic Terms

Genetic Term	Definition
Allele	Alternative form of a gene
Autosome	Any chromosome except sex chromosomes
Centromere	A constriction in the chromosome
Chromosome	The linear arrangement of genes
Concordance	Similarities among phenotypes of individuals
DNA	Deoxyribonucleic acid
Dizygous	Derived from two eggs
Exon	Region of a gene containing code for the gene's protein
Expressivity	The degree to which a person with a genotype is affected
Gene	Unit of genetic material located on a chromosome
Gene expression	Activity of the gene as measured by the amount of mRNA produced
Gene therapy	Introduction of a gene into a cell as a treatment modality to improve the patient's health by correction of the mutant phenotype
Genome	All the DNA in an organism
Genotype	Genetic identity of an individual
Heterozygous	A gene pair having different alleles at the same locus
Homozygous	A gene pair having the same alleles at the same locus
Intron	Non-coding region in a gene
Karyotype	The entire chromosome complement of a cell
Locus	A position on a chromosome where a gene is located

Table 7-1 (continued)
Common Genetic Terms

Genetic Term	Definition
mRNA	Messenger ribonucleic acid
Mitochondrial DNA	Tiny cell organelles that make energy for the body's cells and have their own DNA separate from chromosomal DNA
Monogenic	Controlled by or associated with a single gene
Monozygous	Derived from a single egg
Multifactorial	Traits determined by numerous factors both genetic and environmental
Mutation	A change in the normal gene sequence in < 1% of the population
Penetrance	The proportion of individuals with the genotype who are affected
Phenotype	Observable traits of an individual, not necessarily genetic
Polygenic	Controlled by or associated with a number of genes
Polymorphism	A common variation in the gene sequence seen in > 1% of the population
Sex Chromosomes	The X and Y chromosomes that determine the sex of an individual
Somatic cell	Any cell in the body except sex (germ) cells
Sporadic	Occurring occasionally; a new mutation
Telomere	The tip or end of the chromosome
Transcription	Formation of mRNA by using DNA as a template
Translation	Formation of a protein directed by mRNA
Wild-type	The genotype considered to be normal

Note: Information for this table was modified from the *Talking Glossary* at the National Human Genome Research Institute at http://www.genome.gov/glossary.cfm

cytoplasm in the *mitochondria*. Mitochondrial genes exclusively exhibit maternal inheritance, which means an individual can only inherit these genes from his/her mother. Several nephrology disorders, such as renal tubular defects and Toni- Fanconi-Debre syndrome, are inherited through the mother in mitochondrial DNA (Nussbaum, McInnes, & Willard, 2001).

The building blocks of DNA are the four nucleotide bases, adenine (A), cytosine (C), guanine (G), and thymine (T), with the addition of sugar (deoxyribose) and phosphate (see Figure 7-1).

The bases align into two complementary DNA chains to create the double-helix form identified by James Watson and Francis Crick in 1953 (Watson & Crick, 1953). Together, they compose approximately 25,000 genes that are contained in 46 chromosomes that are organized into 23 pairs of chromosomes. Of those 23 pairs, 22 are the same in both males and females, and are known as *autosomes*. The remaining pair is known as the *sex chromosomes*, which are XX in females and XY in males. Each chromosome carries a different subset of genes; however, pairs of

chromosomes carry matching genetic information in the same sequence. An individual's chromosomes can be arranged and displayed in a standard format showing the number, size, and shape of each chromosome. This is known as a karotype (see Figure 7-2).

Because one chromosome of each pair is inherited from each parent, individuals have two alleles, or alternative copies of each gene, one on each chromosome. The most common version of an allele is considered "normal" and is called the *wild-type*, while alleles that differ from the wild-type are known as *polymorphisms* or *mutations*. Polymorphisms vary from mutations in that they are observed more frequently in the general population. This will be discussed in more detail later in the chapter. Chromosomes are divided into two arms by the *centromere*, a constriction in the chromosome (see Figure 7-3). The short or petite arm is designated p and the long arm is q. To identify a specific location, or *locus*, on a chromosome, both the number of the chromosome and the arm is identified. For example, the gene involved with IgA Nephropathy is located at 6q22-q23, which means on the long arm (q) of chromosome 6 at locus 22-23. Each end of the chromosome is called the *telomere* and has been associated with the aging process.

The genome is an individual's complete genetic makeup containing the entire genetic information for that individual. An individual's genetic sequence is known as his *genotype*, while *phenotype* is an individual's observable traits.

Each gene has coding regions known as *exons*, which make up less than 10% of the human genome, and noncoding regions called *introns*. A primary function of exons is to code for about 60,000 to 80,000 proteins. This is accomplished by two processes known as *transcription* and *translation* (see Figure 7-4). Transcription occurs when *messenger ribonucleic acid (mRNA)* is formed using DNA as a template. The mRNA undergoes some changes within the nucleus and is then transported through the nuclear membrane into the cytoplasm. Once in the cytoplasm, mRNA is decoded, or translated, to produce the protein that has been designated by the gene. Physiologically, when genes increase transcription of mRNA (sometimes known as upregulation), their expression, or activity,

Figure 7-1
The Building Blocks of DNA, the Double Helix

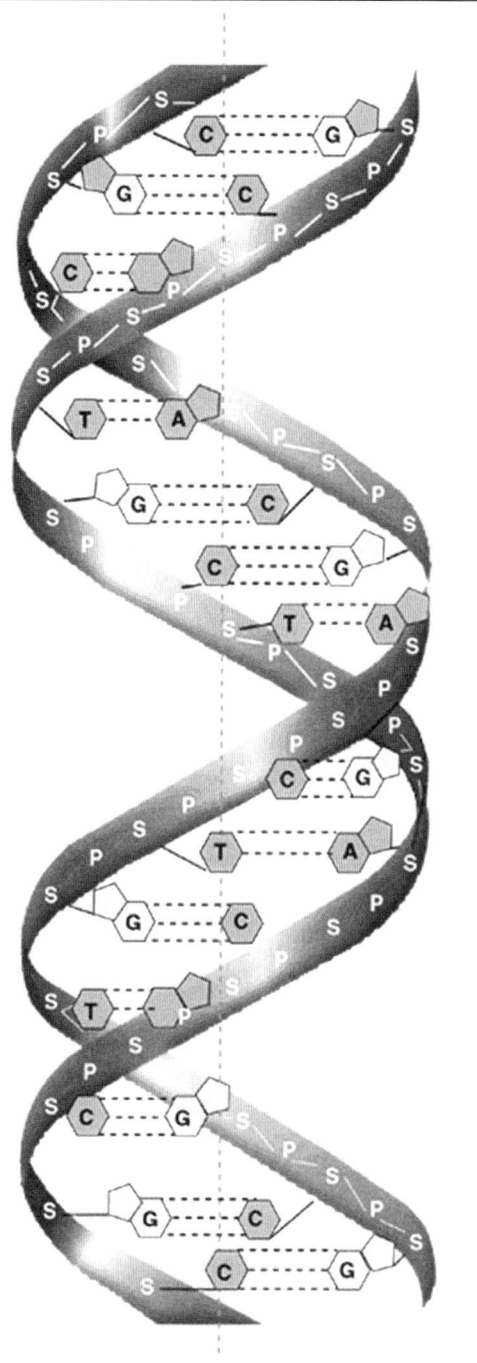

DNA is composed of 4 nucleotide bases: adenine (A), cytosine (C), guanine (G), and thymine (T), with the addition of deoxyribose sugar (S) and phosphate (P). The bases align into two complementary DNA chains with C always aligning with G, and A always aligning with T. This creates the double-helix form.

increases resulting in the production of more proteins. *Gene expression* is the activity of the gene at the time of measurement. Currently, clinical and research endeavors are targeted toward quantifying gene activity. Although an individual's entire genome is in each cell, each gene does not actively express the entire genome at one time. In fact, most cells only express about 30% of the genes in the genome

(Nussbaum, McInnes, & Willard, 2001). For example, neural cells only express the genes needed for normal neural function, and kidney cells express genes related to renal function. To determine expression levels of a gene, the mRNA produced by the gene is measured using genetic technologies such as polymerase chain reaction, (PCR), real time PCR, and microarray analysis. These genetic technologies will be further explained in a later section.

Another key concept in genetics involves *polymorphisms* and *mutations*, which are variations in the DNA sequence of a gene from the normal gene. They are key determinants of an individual's observable traits, or phenotype, and clinical status (see Figure 7-5). Whether the gene variation is identified as a mutation or polymorphism has more to do with how often the allele is seen versus whether the allele is harmful or beneficial. A polymorphism is a change in the DNA sequence that is more common and has been identified in >1% of the population. Conversely, a mutation has been identified in <1% of the population. For example, in more than 1% of the population, a polymorphism in the PIGR gene has been identified that increases genetic susceptibility to IgA nephropathy. This polymorphism results in the substitution of one protein for another (Obara , Iida, Suzuki, Tanaka, Akiyama, Maeda et al., 2003). Also, in less than 1% of the population, a genetic sequence change occurs creating a mutation in the PKD1 gene, and this has been associated with the development of autosomal dominant polycystic kidney disease (Rizk & Chapman, 2003).

There are associations between an individual's genotype and phenotype. Knowledge of which mutation the patient has (genotype) and how that influences the clinical presentation (phenotype) affects nursing management of the patient. Nurses can collect and organize family histories known as pedigrees to trace the disease allele (variation of the gene) as it is inherited through family members. Genotyping, a method used to identify an individual's genetic sequence at a particular locus, may also be conducted. This is generally a non-invasive, relatively easy test to conduct using blood, buccal (cheek) or skin cells as specimens. However, feasibility issues related to this analysis remain. These issues are dependent on the number of known mutations associated with the phenotype. For diseases where the mutation has not been identified, genotyping is not an appropriate diagnostic method.

In conclusion, when considering genetic variation and its association with disease, it is important to differentiate between a gene and a mutation of a gene. Many individuals believe that if you have the gene associated with a disease, then you are predisposed to the disease. This is not the case. All humans have essentially the same 25,000 genes; therefore, it is a mutation or polymorphism in a gene that predisposes some of us for disease – not just having the gene itself. For example, each individual has a gene named the polycystic kidney disease (PKD1) gene and the Wilms tumor gene (WT1). Only those who develop the diseases have a mutation in that gene. Mutations in a gene may be *sporadic* (a new mutation) or inherited. Determining genetic patterns of inheritance can assist in differentiating between sporadic and inherited mutations.

Patterns of Inheritance

In 1865, Gregor Mendel reported on the fundamental patterns of inheritance of specific traits based on his experi-

Figure 7-2
Karyotype

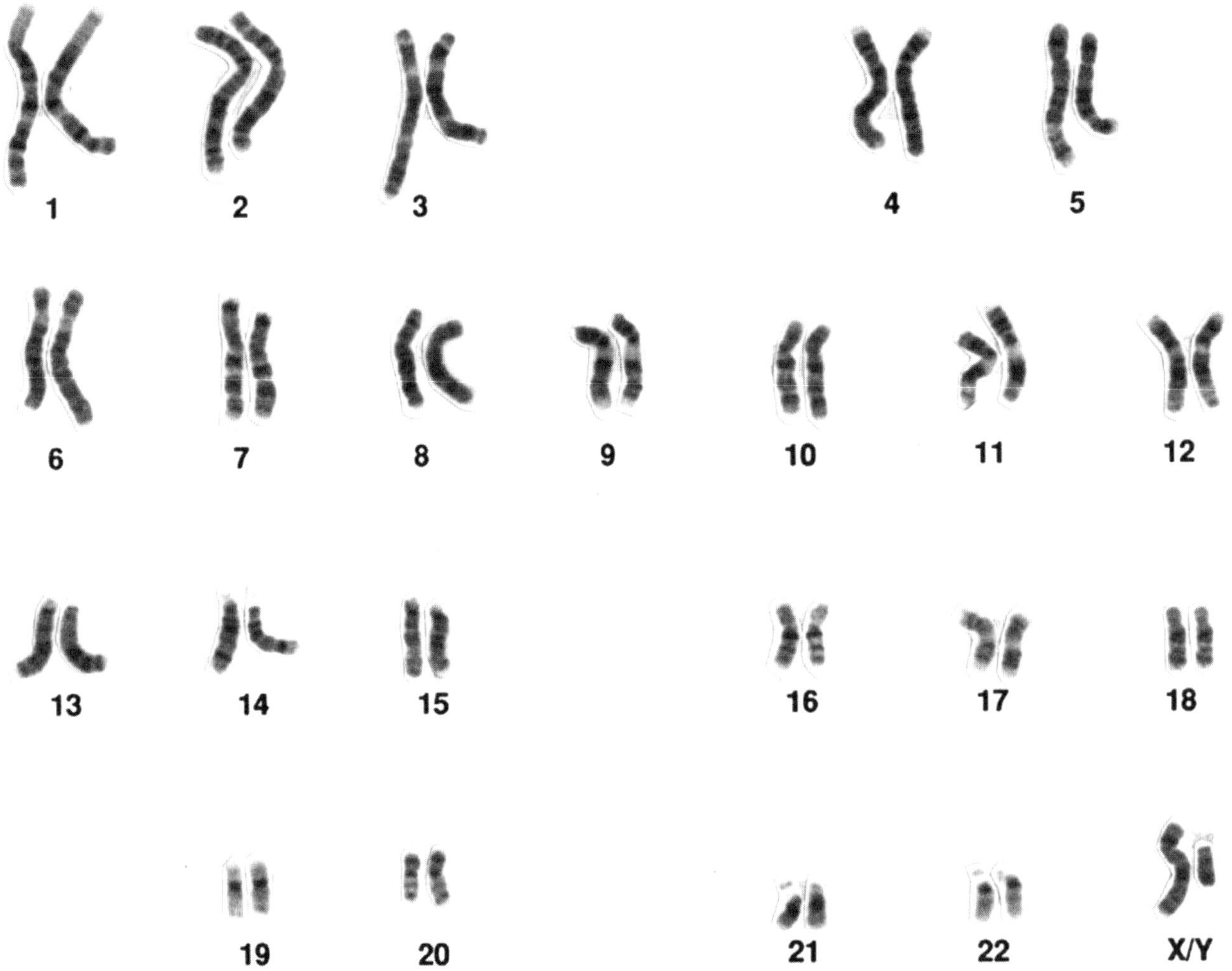

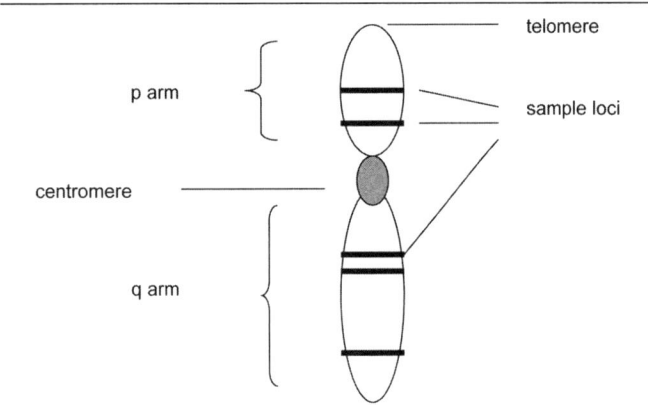

The human karyotype of a human male showing the size and shape of each chromosome. They are arranged in order of size from largest to smallest.

Figure 7-3
Chromosome

There are 24 different chromosomes: 22 autosomes and 2 sex chromosomes (X and Y). This diagram is an example of a generic chromosome. Each chromosome has a short (p) and long (q) arm, which are formed by the placement of the centromere. The ends of the chromosome are known as the telomeres. A position on the chromosome is known as the locus.

ments using pea plants. From his reports, three typical patterns of inheritance emerged: autosomal recessive, autosomal dominant, and sex influenced (X-linked). Examples of three generational pedigrees illustrating these different patterns of inheritance are seen in Figure 7-6.

Autosomal Recessive

Autosomal recessive diseases, such as Bartter syndrome, occur when two mutant alleles are present and no normal alleles are present. The mutation may be *homozygous*, where both alleles carry the same mutation, or compound *heterozygous*, where each allele has a mutation but they are not the same mutation. Individuals with only one mutated gene are carriers of the disease and are usually not affected by the disease because the normal allele is able to compensate for the mutant allele, thus preventing the disease from occurring. Characteristics of autosomal recessive diseases include an equal distribution of disease frequency in males and females, absence of the disease in successive generations, and a 25% chance of inheriting the disease if both parents are carriers of the mutant allele.

Figure 7-4
Overview of Transcription and Translation Processes in Protein Synthesis

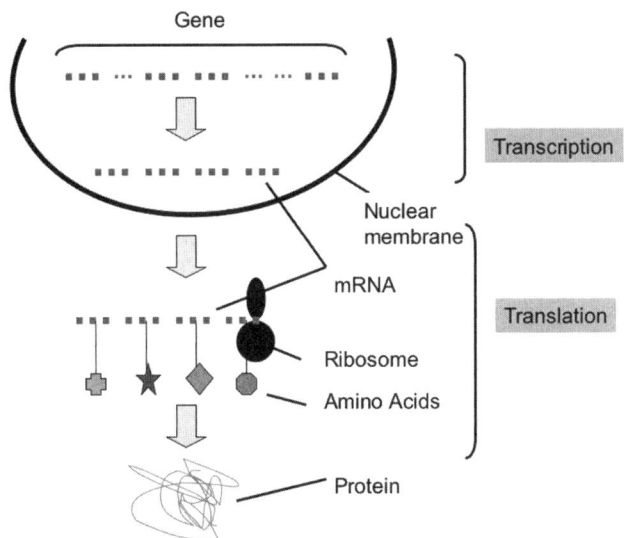

Note: ••• = introns; ■ ■ ■ = exons. The process of transcription forms RNA, which is complementary to its DNA template. Within the nucleus, RNA processing occurs so that the introns or noncoding regions are excised, leaving only the coding regions, exons, in the mRNA. mRNA is transported through the nuclear membrane into the cytoplasm where it binds to ribosomes, which are cellular organelles, where protein synthesis occurs. While mRNA is bound, each triplet (3 successive bases) is translated into one amino acid and a polypeptide sequence is formed.

Figure 7-5
Mutations and Polymorphisms

Individual	DNA Sequence	Product
Person 1	GT**A**ACG	Normal Protein
Person 2	GT**T**ACG	Low or Nonfunctioning Protein

Genetic variation originates from mutations and polymorphisms, which are defined as a change in genetic sequence. In this example, Person 1 has the normal DNA sequence resulting in a normal protein product. Person 2 has a change in one base; T replaces A, and this results in either a low or nonfunctioning protein. The frequency with which this change is observed determines whether it is considered a mutation or polymorphism.

X-linked

X-linked diseases, such as Alport syndrome, occur when there is a mutation in a gene on the X chromosome. Females have two X chromosomes, while males have one X and one Y chromosome. Therefore, if a male has a mutation in a gene on the X chromosome, he is much more likely to have the disease than a female who has another X-linked gene that could potentially compensate for the mutated X-linked gene. X-linked diseases may have recessive or dominant patterns of inheritance.

Pedigrees

Patterns of inheritance can be determined based on a thorough family history. This family history information would be organized into a family tree, or pedigree, to visualize how diseases and characteristics are clustered within a family and through generations. Obtaining a complete and accurate family history is becoming increasingly important as we discover that genes are associated with common chronic diseases, such as diabetes and hypertension, as well as single gene disorders, such as Alport syndrome. In addition, as more becomes known about the great variety of genetic mutations leading to diseases, we discover that a disease such as Alport syndrome can be classified as X-linked, autosomal recessive, or autosomal dominant. In order to determine which form of Alport syndrome the patient has, a detailed family history is needed. The most informative family history includes information on three generations of relatives.

Identification of the pattern of inheritance affects clinical management, patient education, and prognosis. Tools have been developed to assist health care providers in documenting a pedigree (see www.ama-assn.org/go/genetics). For each family member, the most important information to record is the current age (or age at death), ethnicity, and relevant medical conditions including onset or duration. Pedigrees can be used to identify disease risk and to develop a personalized prevention program for chronic conditions as well as single gene diseases.

For some diseases, the cluster patterns do not appear to follow an autosomal dominant, recessive, or X-linked pattern of inheritance. Occasionally, this is due to either incomplete pene-

Autosomal Dominant

In contrast, autosomal dominant inheritance occurs when only one mutated allele is needed for the disease to occur, and the individual would be considered heterozygous for the mutation. Each affected individual would have an affected parent. Examples of diseases transmitted through autosomal dominant inheritance patterns include polycystic kidney disease and IgA nephropathy. Characteristics of autosomal dominant diseases include an equal distribution of the disease in males and females, the appearance of the phenotype in each generation, and a 50% chance of inheriting the disease for children of an affected parent.

Figure 7-6
Three Generational Pedigrees

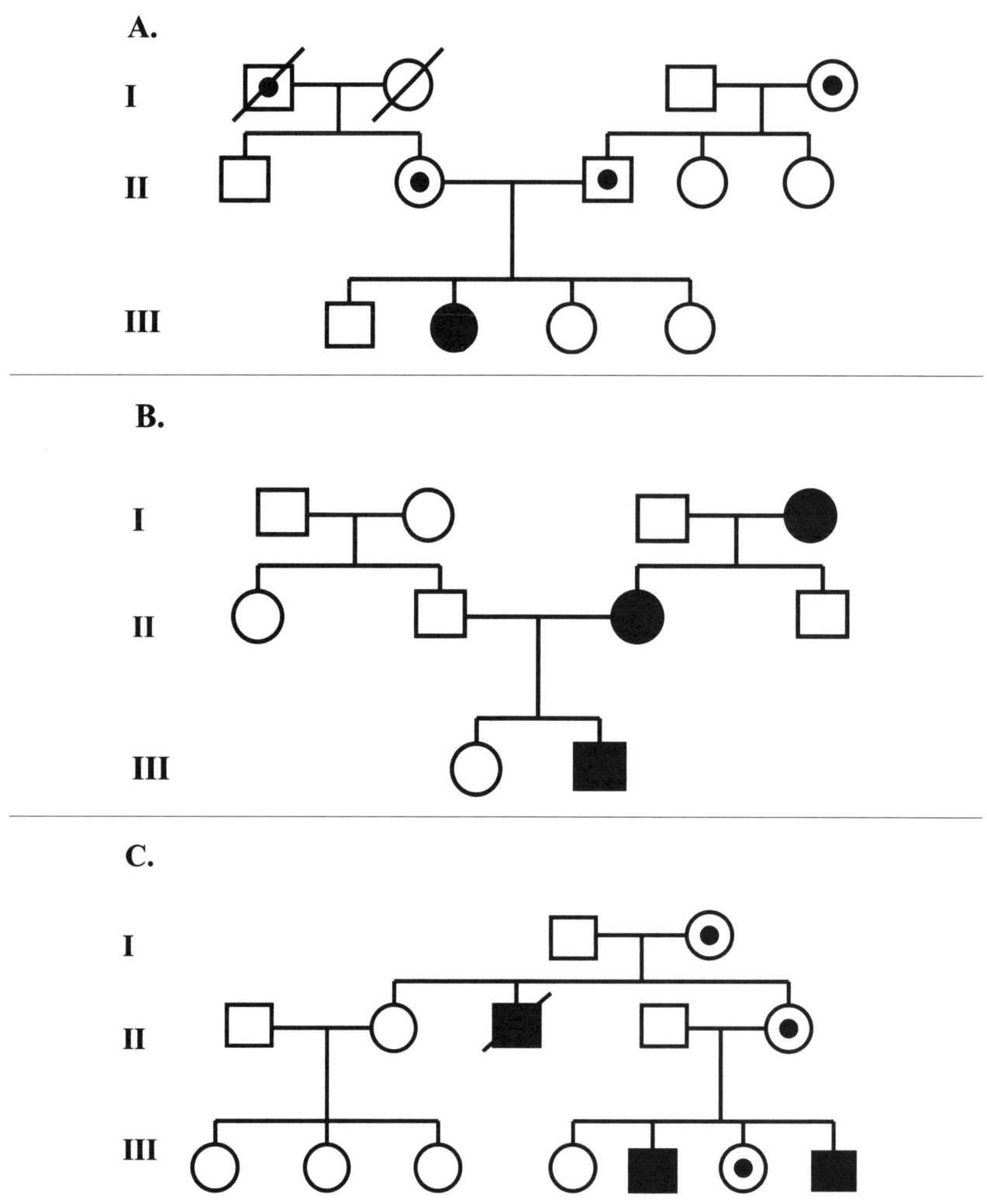

To visualize patterns of inheritance, 3 generational family histories are arranged into diagrams known as pedigrees. Pedigree symbols are commonly used in genetic counseling. It is customary to show females as circles and males as squares. A horizontal line represents mating, a vertical line shows offspring, and a diagonal line through a circle or square indicates that the person is deceased. Individuals who are affected with a disease or condition are shaded. A dot within a figure illustrates carriers of the trait. Roman numerals indicate generations. Figure 7-6A – autosomal recessive, shows an affected individual is the offspring of carriers of the trait. Figure 7-6B – autosomal dominant, shows affected individuals in each generation. Figure 7-6C – sex-influenced, shows female carriers and males who are affected.

trance or varied expressivity. *Penetrance* is the proportion of individuals with the genotype who actually manifest the disease at all. It is considered an all-or-none concept. This means that an individual with a specific genotype either will or will not be affected with the disease. Some diseases have incomplete or reduced penetrance where some individuals with the genotype are affected and some are not. *Expressivity* is the degree to which a person with a specific genotype is affected. For example, two individuals may have the same genotype; one may have all the symptoms of the disease, while the other has relatively few symptoms. This is known as variable expressivity.

Types of Genetic Disorders

Genetic disorders are generally categorized into one of three groups: single gene (*monogenic*), chromosomal, or multifactorial. In this section, these three groups will be discussed, and examples of nephrology patients with these diseases will be provided.

Single Gene Disorders

Single gene disorders are caused by a mutation within a single gene. Examples of single gene disorders that lead to renal failure include polycystic kidney disease and Alport syndrome. For each of these diseases, mutations may be on one or both alleles of the gene of the chromosome pair. Whether or not the individual is affected by the disease depends on if the disease is inherited in a recessive or dominant pattern.

Chromosomal Disorders

Chromosomal disorders occur when there is an abnormal number or structure of chromosomes. We normally have 22-paired autosomal chromosomes and 2 sex chromosomes (XX or XY) for a total of 46 chromosomes. Traditionally, this is written as 46XX (females) or 46XY (males). Two examples of chromosomal disorders that are associated with renal failure are Down syndrome and Turner syndrome. Down syndrome is the most common chromosomal condition in humans and results from an extra chromosome 21. The karyotype of a female with Down syndrome would be written as 47,XX,+21. This means that there are 47 chromosomes, two X chromosomes, and one extra chromosome (+21). In contrast, Turner syndrome occurs when one of the X chromosomes is missing in a female. The karyotype of an individual with Turner syndrome would be written as 45,X indicating that there are a total of 45 chromosomes and only one X chromosome. The missing chromosome is the other X chromosome. Chromosomal disorders can lead to kidney disease when genes on the extra or missing chromosome are responsible for protein products that are functionally important to the renal system. Chromosomal disorders can also result when there are extra or missing pieces of chromosomes.

Multifactorial Disorders

Multifactorial disorders are caused by gene-environment interaction. These disorders occur when a mutation in a gene predisposes an individual to a disease, and the environment also influences the onset of the disease. Mutations in several interacting genes, which is known as *polygenic* inheritance, are often needed for the development of multifactorial disor-

ders. Certain environmental factors combined with these genetic mutations can predispose an individual to disease. Diabetes mellitus type 1 is a multifactorial disorder that can lead to complications, which include renal failure. Surgical treatments for diabetes and its complications include pancreas, islet cell, and kidney transplantation. Because many chronic diseases (such as diabetes mellitus, cardiovascular disease, and cancer), are multifactorial disorders, they are the focus of intense clinical and basic science research. Most kidney complications arise from single-gene or multifactorial disorders.

Genetic Variations That Lead To Kidney Failure

Clinical genetics has traditionally focused on single-gene disorders that are transmitted through families as recessive, dominant, or X-linked traits. Examples of single-gene disorders include polycystic kidney disease and Alport Syndrome. We are now expanding our knowledge to include multifactorial disorders as well. Table 7-2 lists several of the genetic conditions that have renal involvement, the gene symbol, name, location (locus) on the chromosome, and the pattern of inheritance. These conditions have a broad range of symptoms and outcomes ranging from potentially mild (such as hypertension) to life-threatening (such as end-organ failure). In addition, some of these disorders, such as Congenital Nephrotic Syndrome, manifest immediately following birth and are followed in pediatric genetic clinics. While others, such as type 2 diabetes mellitus, are not apparent until adulthood and are followed primarily in family practice settings.

The following diseases have a genetic component that can lead to renal failure. Some diseases and syndromes were originally thought to be single-gene disorders. However, with improved genetic methodologies and technologies, it is becoming apparent that one phenotype, such as Alport syndrome, can result from a variety of inheritance patterns. This knowledge is still in its infancy and will expand as we discover more associations between specific diseases and specific genes, in addition to knowledge on how mutations in modifier genes affect the disease phenotype.

Alport Syndrome

Alport syndrome, a progressive hereditary nephritis associated with hearing loss and eye abnormalities in up to 40% of patients, is caused by the production of a defective type IV collagen. Alport syndrome accounts for 1 to 2% of end stage renal disease (ESRD) cases (Rizk & Chapman, 2003) and encompasses four different diseases. The majority of cases (85%) are X-linked and due to mutations in the COL4A5 gene that codes for the 5-chain of type IV collagen. The autosomal recessive form of Alport syndrome accounts for about 15% of the cases and involves mutations of the COL4A3 and COL4A4 genes coding for the 3 and 4 chains of type IV collagen. The autosomal dominant form, which is rare, also results from mutations in the COL4A3 ad COL4A4 genes. A very rare variant of this disease results from deletions on two contiguous genes (COL4A5 and COL4A6) on the long arm of the X-chromosome (Torres & Scheinman, 2004). There is a wide range of symptoms in Alport syndrome, and the severity of symptoms depends on the gene mutation. Thin basement membrane disease has also been associated with mutations in the COL4A3 and COL4A4 genes (Rizk & Chapman,

Table 7-2
Single Gene and Multifactorial Genetic Diseases that Can Lead to Kidney Dysfunction

Disease	Gene Symbol	Inheritance	Locus	Gene Name
Alport syndrome	COL4A5, ATS	X-linked	Xq22.3	Collagen IV, alpha-5 polypeptide
	COL4A5&COL4A6	X-linked	Xq22.3	Collagen IV, alpha-5 and 6 polypeptides
	COL4A3	AR	2q36-q37	Collagen IV, alpha-3 polypeptide
	COL4A4	AR	2q36-q37	Collagen IV, alpha-4 polypeptide
IgA nephropathy	IGAN	AD	6q22-q23	IgA nephropathy
	PIGR	Susceptibility	1q31-q42	Polymeric immunoglobulin receptor
	ACE	Susceptibility	17q23	Angiotensin I converting enzyme
Polycystic kidney disease	PKD1	AD	16p13.3-p13.12	Polycystin-1
	PKD2	AD	4q21-q23	Polycystin-2
	PKHD1	AR	6p21.1-p12	Fibrocystin
Wilms tumor	WT1	Sporadic, AD	11p13	Wilms tumor-1
	WT2, MTACR1	Sporadic	11p15.5	Multiple tumor associated chromosome region-1
	WT3	AD	16q	Wilms tumor-3
	GPC3	Sporadic	Xq26	Glypican-3
	FWT1, WT4	Susceptibility	17q12-q21	Wilms tumor-4
	FWT2	Susceptibility	19q13.4	Familial Wilms tumor-2
von Hippel-Lindau syndrome	VHL	AD	3p26-p25	von Hippel Lindau syndrome
Bartter syndrome	CLCNKB	AR	1p36	Chloride channel, kidney, B
	SLC12A1	AR	15q15-q21.1	Solute carrier family 12 (sodium/potassium/ chloride transporters), member-1
	KCNJ1	AR	11q24	Potassium inwardly-rectifying channel, subfamily J, member-1
Focal segmental glomerulosclerosis	ACTN4, FSGS1	AD, Susceptibility	19q13	Actinin, alpha-4
	FSGS2	Susceptibility	11q21-q22	Focal segmental glomerulosclerosis-2
	CD2AP, CMS	Susceptibility	6p12	CD 2 Associated protein
Congenital nephrotic syndrome	NPHS1	AR	19q13.1	Nephrin
Steroid resistant nephrotic syndrome	NPHS2	AR	1q25-q31	Podocin
Systemic lupus erythematosis	SLEB1, SLE1	Susceptibility	1q41-q42	Systemic lupus erythematosus susceptibility to, 1
	SLEN1	Susceptibility	10q22.3	Systemic lupus erythematosus with nephritis, susceptibility to, 1
	SLEN2	Susceptibility	2q34-q35	Systemic lupus erythematosus with nephritis, susceptibility to, 2
	SLEN3	Susceptibility	11p15.5	Systemic lupus erythematosus with nephritis, susceptibility to, 3
	FCGR2A	Susceptibility	1q21-q23	Fc fragment of IgG, low affinity IIa, receptor for (CD32)
	SLEB3	Susceptibility	4p16-p15.2	Systemic lupus erythematosus susceptibility to, 3
	PDCD1, SLEB2	Susceptibility	2q37.3	Programmed cell death-1

Table 7-2 (continued)
Single Gene and Multifactorial Genetic Diseases that Can Lead to Kidney Dysfunction

Disease	Gene Symbol	Inheritance	Locus	Gene Name
Hypertension				
Liddle syndrome	SCNN1B	AD	16p13-p12	Sodium channel, nonvoltage-gated 1, beta
Liddle syndrome	SCNN1G	AD	16p13-p12	Sodium channel, nonvoltage-gated 1, gamma
Gordon syndrome	WNK1, PHA2C, PRKWNK1	AD	12p13	Pseudohypoaldosteronism, type IIC
	WNK4, PHA2B, PRKWNK4	AD	17q21-q22	Pseudohypoaldosteronism type II
	ACE	Susceptibility	17q23	Angiotensin I converting enzyme
	AGT	Susceptibility	1q42-q43	Angiotensinogen
	HYT1	Susceptibility	17q	Hypertension, essential, susceptibility to, 1
	HYT2	Susceptibility	15q	Hypertension, essential, susceptibility to, 2
	HYT3	Susceptibility	2p25-p24	Hypertension, essential, susceptibility to, 3
Diabetes mellitus				
Type 1 DM	IDDM1*	Susceptibility	6p21.3	Insulin-dependent diabetes mellitus-1
	IDDM2*	Susceptibility	11p15.5	Insulin-dependent diabetes mellitus-2
	CTLA4	Susceptibility	2q33	Cytotoxic T-lymphocyte-associated serine esterase-4
Type 2 DM	ZNF236	Susceptibility	18q22-q23	Zinc finger protein-236
	CAPN10	Susceptibility	2q37.3	Calpain-10
	LPL	Susceptibility	8p22	Lipoprotein lipase
	BDKRB2	Susceptibility	14q32.1-q32.2	Bradykinin receptor B2
	ACE	Susceptibility	17q23	Angiotensin I converting enzyme
	GCGR	Susceptibility	17q25	Glucagon receptor
	GCK	Susceptibility	7p15-p13	Glucokinase (hexokinase-4)
	PPARG	Susceptibility	3p25	Peroxisome proliferator activated receptor, gamma
	HNF4A	Susceptibility	20q12-q13.1	Hepatocyte nuclear factor 4, alpha (transcription factor-14)
	INS	Susceptibility	11p15.5	Insulin
MODY1	HNF4A	AD	20q12-q13.1	Hepatocyte nuclear factor 4, alpha (transcription factor-14)
MODY2	GCK	AD	7p15-p13	Glucokinase (hexokinase-4)
MODY3	TCF1, HNF1A	AD	12q24.2	Interferon production regulator factor (HNF1), albumin proximal factor
MODY4	IPF1	AD	13q12.1	Insulin promoter factor 1, homeodomain transcription factor
MODY5	TCF2, HNF1B	AD	17cen-q21.3	Transcription factor-2, hepatic; LF-B3; variant hepatic nuclear factor
MODY6	NEUROD1	AD	2q32	Neurogenic differentiation-1

Note: AR = autosomal recessive; AD=autosomal dominant. Information for this table was obtained on August 17, 2004, from *Online Mendelian Inheritance in Man (OMIM)*, Genome, LocusLink, Gene available online from the National Center for Biotechnology Information (www.ncbi.nlm.nih.gov).

* IDDM1 and IDDM2 are loci that contain more than one gene. The IDDM1 locus contains many diabetes susceptibility genes, including the HLA genes. The genes encoding class II MHC proteins are most strongly linked with diabetes; these genes are HLA-DR, HLA-DQ, and HLA-DP. The IDDM2 locus contains the insulin gene (INS).

2003). It has been hypothesized that these cases represent the heterozygous state of autosomal recessive Alport syndrome (Torres & Scheinman, 2004).

IgA Nephropathy

This disorder is one of the most common kidney diseases causing glomerulonephritis, and it affects up to 1% of the population worldwide. The cause of IgA nephropathy is unknown (Donadio & Grande, 2002). However, there may be genetic factors that predispose families or individuals to IgA nephropathy. Mutations in several genes have been associated with this disease, most of which represent *sporadic mutations* (McKusick, 1986a). One location on chromosome 6 (6q22-q23) has been found to have an autosomal dominant mode of transmission with incomplete penetrance (Torres & Scheinman, 2004) in a study of 30 families. These findings support the suggestion that IgA nephropathy is a multifactorial disease with gene-environment interaction (Donadio & Grande, 2002).

Polycystic Kidney Disease

Autosomal dominant polycystic kidney disease (ADPKD), which is characterized by massive enlargement of the kidneys secondary to cyst growth and development, is the most common hereditary kidney disease. Extrarenal complications (such as hepatic cysts, intracranial aneurysms, cardiac disease, diverticular disease, vascular abnormalities, and hernias) may also occur. ADPKD affects 1 in 400 to 1,000 live births, is equally distributed in all races, and accounts for 5% of ESRD cases in the U.S. and Europe (Rizk & Chapman, 2003). Most cases of ADPKD (85%) result from a mutation in the PKD1 gene located on chromosome 16, while the remaining 15% of cases are associated with a mutation in the PKD2 gene located on chromosome 4. Prognostic implications vary depending on which mutation is present. Individuals with PKD2 mutations develop renal cysts, hypertension, and ESRD at a later age than individuals with mutations in PKD1 (Rizk & Chapman, 2003).

Autosomal recessive polycystic kidney disease (ARPKD), which is characterized by various combinations of bilateral renal cystic disease and congenital hepatic fibrosis (Torres & Scheinman, 2004), is much less common than ADPKD and affects 1 in 10,000 to 40,000 individuals. ARPKD results from mutations in the PKHD1 gene located on chromosome 6 (Rizk & Chapman, 2003).

Wilms Tumor

Wilms tumor, which is the most common childhood tumor (Kalapurakal, Dome, Perlman, Malogolowkin, Haase, Grundy et al., 2004), is associated with several syndromes, including (but not limited to) WAGR, Denys-Drash, and Wiedemann-Beckwith syndromes. All three of these syndromes have mutations located on Chromosome 11. Both WAGR and Denys-Drash are associated with the WT1 gene, located at 11p13. Mutations associated with Wiedemann-Beckwith syndrome are found at 11p15, which is sometimes called WT2, even though the precise gene at this location has not yet been defined. Familial Wilms tumor is rare, affecting only 1.5% of individuals with this condition. Two genes are associated with this familial type, FWT1 and FWT2, located on chromosomes 17 and 19 respectively. It is thought that other genes must be implicated in Wilms tumor as well.

Von Hippel-Lindau Syndrome

Von Hippel-Lindau syndrome, which results from a mutation in the VHL gene, is an autosomal dominant disease characterized by a variety of benign and malignant tumors. The most commonly seen tumors are retinal, cerebellar, spinal hemangioblastoma, renal cell, pheochromocytoma, and pancreatic (McKusick, 1986b). Von Hippel-Lindau syndrome has several subtypes: Type 1, which does not include pheochromocytoma, and Type 2, which includes pheochromocytoma (Torres & Scheinman, 2004).

Focal Segmental Glomerulosclerosis

Focal segmental glomerulosclerosis (FSGS) is a histopathologic diagnosis seen in approximately 5% of adult and 20% of pediatric ESRD (Winn, 2003). Several subtypes of FSGS exist including primary, secondary, familial, and FSGS associated with congenital syndromes. Some forms of FSGS are thought to be multifactorial in nature. Primary FSGS, which is sporadic in nature and has no known cause, is the most common subtype. Secondary FSGS is associated with another disease process (such as sickle cell disease) or human immunodeficiency virus. Familial FSGS, which has virtually the identical histopathologic and clinical characteristics as primary FSGS, is seen in families and has both autosomal dominant and recessive patterns of heritability. Congenital syndromes associated with FSGS include Charcot-Marie-Tooth and Laurence-Moon-Biedl syndromes (Winn, 2003).

Broad spectrums of renal diseases associated with a histopathologic diagnosis of FSGS exist. Congenital nephrotic syndrome and steroid resistant nephrotic syndrome are two disorders that are similar to FSGS. However, these disorders have an autosomal recessive pattern of inheritance and are linked with different mutations than that identified for FSGS (Pollak, 2003).

Multifactorial Diseases Associated with Renal Failure

In addition to genetic mutations that have a direct effect on the kidney, there are other diseases that have particular impact on the kidney. Examples of such systemic diseases include systemic lupus erythematosis, hypertension, and diabetes. Each of these diseases is considered a multifactorial disorder and is associated with a variety of genetic mutations or polymorphisms. The focus of this section is to highlight the genetic mutations or polymorphisms associated with the expression of renal disease in these patients.

Systemic Lupus Erythematosis

Systemic lupus erythematosis (SLE) is an inflammatory autoimmune disease that affects many organ systems, including the kidney, joints, and skin (Pullen, Cannon, & Rushing, 2003). It occurs predominantly in women (>90%), and the incidence in African-Americans is four times greater than in Caucasians (Pullen, Cannon, & Rushing, 2003). African-Americans may also have an earlier onset and more severe presentation of the disease (Lindqvist & Alarcon-Riquelme, 1999). Renal disease is one of the most common causes of morbidity and mortality associated with SLE, occurring in at least 50% of patients within one year of diagnosis. Renal replacement therapy is eventually needed in 15 to 20% of those with renal involvement (Pullen, Cannon, & Rushing, 2003).

Evidence supports a strong genetic basis for the development of SLE. The *concordance* rate (similarities between phenotypes) for the clinical expression of SLE in *monozygotic* twins is 25-69% and the presence of autoantibodies may be as high as 92% (Lindqvist & Alarcon-Riquelme, 1999). In siblings and *dizygotic* twins, the concordance rate for the clinical expression of SLE is only 1-2%.

Many genes have been identified either as potential candidate genes for SLE or as contributing factors to the development of SLE. Mutations or polymorphisms have been identified and some have been associated with a specific phenotypic expression of SLE, such as photosensitivity (C4A deficiency), hemolytic anemia (SLEH1), or nephritis.

Table 7-3
Genetic Educational Web Sites

Web Site	Address
GeneTests	http://www.geneclinics.org/
Online Mendelian Inheritance in Man	http://www.ncbi.nlm.nih.gov/
Genetic Science Learning Center at the University of Utah	http://gslc.genetics.utah.edu/
Dolan DNA Learning Center	http://www.dnalc.org/
Genetics Educational Center, University of Kansas Medical Center	http://www.kumc.edu/gec/
National Human Genome Research Institutes: Talking Glossary of Genetic Terms	http://www.genome.gov/glossary.cfm
American Medical Association	http://www.ama-assn.org/ama/pub/category/2380.html
National Newborn Screening and Genetic Resource Center	http://genes-r-us.uthscsa.edu/

Susceptibility to lupus nephritis has also been linked to genes on three different chromosomes (see Table 7-3). Two of these genes, SLEN2 (2q34-q35) (McKusick, 2003a) and SLEN3 (11p15.6), (McKusick, 2003.) are associated with increased susceptibility to nephritis in African Americans. The third gene, SLEN1 (10q22.3), (McKusick, 2003c) is associated with increased susceptibility in European Americans.

Hypertension

Hypertensive nephrosclerosis is one of the leading causes of ESRD in the U.S. (Hayden, Iyengar, Schelling, & Sedor, 2003). Although some single gene mutations are responsible for hypertension, these causes are rare (see Table 7-2). It is generally accepted that for most individuals a combination of up to five or six genes contributes to arterial pressure (O'Shaughnessy & Karet, 2004). This indicates that a complex network of gene-gene as well as gene-environment interactions contributes to the development of hypertension. However, the underlying pathophysiology leading to renal disease in the setting of hypertension is not well described (Hayden, Iyengar, Schelling, & Sedor, 2003).

Some data suggest that hypertension alone does not result in ESRD (Hayden, Iyengar, Schelling, & Sedor, 2003). Rather, for some patients, the development of renal nephrosclerosis is associated with the development of small and large vessel vasculopathy. This is consistent with the idea that hypertension is a multifactorial disorder that involves multiple gene-gene and gene-environment interactions. In this setting, one specific mutation may not be solely responsible for the development of hypertensive nephrosclerosis. Instead, mutations in a variety of genes may increase an individual's predisposition to develop ESRD in the setting of hypertension. Another hypothesis implicates an alteration in sodium handling as an underlying etiology for the development of renal disease in hypertension (O'Shaughnessy & Karet, 2004). Some examples of genes that have been associated with the development of renal complications in the setting of hypertension can be found in Table 7-2. It is important to note that these genes may play a role in other diseases or symptoms.

Diabetes Mellitus

The phenotype of diabetes is characterized by abnormally high blood glucose levels (Dean & McEntyre, 2004). Typically, the body releases insulin from the pancreas to remove the glucose from the blood and return the serum glucose levels to normal. In patients with diabetes, however, this response does not occur. Reasons for this lack of response include an inability to produce sufficient amounts of insulin or a poor response to the circulating insulin. Several subtypes of diabetes have been identified. Type 1 diabetes, which accounts for 5% of all cases of diabetes, is an autoimmune disorder in which the pancreas does not produce sufficient insulin. Approximately 95% of all cases of diabetes fall into the category of type 2 diabetes that is associated with a relative deficiency of insulin, either from insulin resistance or a defect in insulin secretion. Type 2 diabetes commonly occurs in obese individuals. Other forms of diabetes include maturity onset diabetes of the young and gestational diabetes (Dean & McEntyre, 2004).

Type 1 diabetes mellitus. The onset of type 1 diabetes is associated with both genetic and environmental risk factors (Dean & McEntyre, 2004). Although there is an increased prevalence of type 1 diabetes in relatives, identical twin studies demonstrate less than 50% concordance for the disorder. Eighteen regions of the genome, each of which may contain more than one gene, have been associated with increased risk for the development of type 1 diabetes. These regions have been labeled IDDM1 to IDDM18. IDDM1 is the best studied of these regions and contains the HLA genes that encode immune response proteins. IDDM2 contains the insulin gene. Although many genes have been associated with increased susceptibility to the development of type 1 diabetes, few genes have been linked with the development of diabetic kidney disease. One such gene, ZNF236, is located at the IDDM6 locus.

Type 2 diabetes mellitus. Type 2 diabetes is associated with relative insulin deficiency and/or insulin resistance (Dean & McEntyre, 2004). It is more common in obese individuals, and until recently, it has been linked with adults. Now it is increasingly common in children as well. There is an increased prevalence of type 2 diabetes among relatives and a high concordance rate (>70%) among monozygotic twins.

Environmental factors such as weight, food intake, and physical activity level play an important role in the development of type 2 diabetes (Dean & McEntyre, 2004). Many genes have been associated with type 2 diabetes, yet most are poorly defined. Few genes have been associated specifically with diabetic nephropathy (see Table 7-2). One such gene, LPL, has been associated with microalbuminuria (Mattu, Trevelyan, Needham, Khan, Adiseshiah, Richter et al., 2002). This gene produces an enzyme, lipoprotein lipase, which breaks down triglycerides. The LPL gene is found on chromosome 8. Genetic variants of LPL correlated with the presence and severity of microalbuminuria. Higher concentrations of LDL constituents have been linked with the development of microalbuminuria.

Maturity onset diabetes in the young. Maturity onset diabetes in the young (MODY) is an uncommon cause of diabetes and is triggered by a single gene mutation (Dean & McEntyre, 2004). MODY is inherited in an autosomal dominant fashion and has several subtypes (see Table 7-2). Just as the majority of mutations associated with type 1 and type 2 diabetes are not associated specifically with the development of renal disease, neither are the mutations that cause MODY particularly linked to this complication. This suggests that the development of renal disease in the setting of diabetes may result from other pathophysiologic mechanisms or may be associated with genetic susceptibility in genes other than diabetes associated genes.

Genetic Testing

The last 10 years has seen an explosion in genetic knowledge and in technologies used to examine the genetic components of diseases. Much of this information is being broadly disseminated in newspapers and television as soon as it is reported in major journals and at conferences. Because of public access to cutting-edge research, patients are requesting genetic testing for conditions ranging from breast cancer to colon cancer from their primary health care provider. Traditionally, genetic counselors have provided guidance and counseling for genetic testing. However, there are not enough genetic counselors to meet the needs of patients referred for genetic testing. In addition, while it is still appropriate to obtain genetic counseling for inherited genetic conditions (such as polycystic kidney disease), it is not always possible for patients with chronic conditions of adulthood (for example, diabetes) to receive this type of counseling. This means a nurse is frequently the one responsible for patient education related to genetic testing. This section will briefly describe the purpose of several types of genetic tests, and discuss legal and ethical issues related to genetic testing.

Prenatal Genetic Testing and Newborn Screening

Prenatal genetic testing is usually offered when there is increased risk determined by information such as maternal age, family history, ethnicity, multiple marker screen, or fetal ultrasound. Biochemical, chromosomal, or molecular-based approaches are used to identify individuals with a variety of genetic disorders. As an example, biochemical testing of alphafetoprotein levels may be done to assess for neural tube defects, chromosomal testing for Down syndrome, and molecular-based approaches can detect single gene disorders such as cystic fibrosis. Informed consent is required prior to conducting prenatal testing because of risks to the fetus.

Each year, newborn screening tests are conducted on over 4 million newborns in the United States. These screening tests were begun in an effort to prevent death or life-long debilitating conditions. Newborn screening tests commonly screen for a minimum of 9 disorders including metabolic, hematological, and endocrine disorders. State laws require newborn screening unless parents decline testing. States vary on the number and type of genetic screening tests required. Recently, some states have expanded their newborn screening program by using tandem mass spectrometry, a new laboratory testing technology, to substantially increase the number of metabolic disorders that can be detected. To view up-to-date information on what tests are required in each state, visit the National Newborn Screening and Genetic Resource Center at http://genes-r-us.uthscsa.edu/

Carrier Genetic Tests

Carrier genetic tests are conducted to determine if an unaffected individual has *one* copy of a gene that has a mutation. This can be valuable information in common recessive disorders such as cystic fibrosis and sickle cell anemia. It is important information to use in family planning. If both parents are carriers of a recessive gene, there is a 25% risk that each child will have the disease and a 50% chance that the child will be a carrier.

Diagnostic Genetic Tests

Diagnostic genetic tests are conducted on symptomatic individuals to identify the genetic disease and assist with specific treatment and prognosis. For example, when the clinician knows there is a mutation in the p53 tumor-suppressor gene, the decision can be made to treat the cancer more aggressively because it is more likely to grow aggressively. As more and more treatments and prognostic indicators are associated with the specific mutation (such as BRCA1 vs. BRCA2) instead of the disease (such as breast cancer), molecular approaches have been used. In general, age is not a factor when determining whether or not to conduct a diagnostic genetic test.

Predictive Genetic Tests

Predictive genetic tests are gaining in usefulness, and much of the current excitement in genetic testing revolves around these tests. These tests are offered to asymptomatic individuals with a family history of a genetic disorder. There are two types of predictive tests; presymptomatic and susceptibility. *Presymptomatic genetic testing* is conducted on individuals who will eventually develop symptoms if the gene mutation is present. An example of this is an individual who has the mutation for Huntington disease, a fatal neurologic genetic disease. *Susceptibility genetic testing* is conducted on individuals who are at-risk for developing symptoms associated with the disorder. An example of this is someone who has a mutation in the APOE gene, which has been associated with Alzheimer's disease. Many laboratories conducting predictive genetic testing require patient informed consent and counseling.

There are many sources from which to obtain samples appropriate for predictive genetic testing because the mutation will be in the DNA of any cells in the body. DNA analysis is usually conducted using blood specimens, buccal cells, or skin cells because they are relatively non-invasive and easy to obtain. Only a limited number of predictive genetic tests are available at this time, one of which is the genetic test for Wilms tumor.

Benefits and Limitations of Genetic Tests

Genetic tests differ from other medical tests because they provide genetic information about the health of the individual *and his or her family*. In addition, they test for potential diseases for which the individual may be at risk. Genetic testing is controversial because of the fear of discrimination against the individual and family members based on genetic test results, and individuals may be discriminated against at work or in obtaining insurance. Health care providers should offer pretest counseling and obtain informed consent prior to most genetic tests. After the results are obtained, adequate time should be allowed to explain the genetic results to the patient and to plan adequate follow-up when needed.

Whether or not the genetic test will be covered by insurance is dependent on the type of insurance and the indication for the test. Genetic tests can be costly, and many are only conducted in research laboratories, which have a much slower return time. Many patients do not want to inform their insurance companies that genetic tests are being conducted for fear of discrimination, so they pay for the genetic tests themselves. However, if the insurance company pays for the test, it is entitled to the results. Currently, there is pending state and federal legislation to protect the patient from employment or insurance discrimination. In addition, Health Information Portability Accountability and Accessibility (HIPAA) is addressing these issues by affording genetic information increased confidentiality.

Limitations of genetic testing depend on the type of genetic test conducted. For example, a predictive test does not give a diagnosis; instead, it identifies if the patient is "at-risk" for a genetic condition. In addition, many molecular genetic tests check for a specific mutation and will not identify mutations in other areas of the genome. For example, cystic fibrosis is diagnosed by a mutation in the cystic fibrosis gene. However, over 900 different mutations have been identified in that one gene, and the assay panel only tests for the 25 most common mutations. The other 875 mutations would be missed, and the disease would go undiagnosed by genetic testing.

One of the primary risks of genetic testing is the emotional response of the individual or family to the test result. The nurse can be actively involved in preparing the individual and family to receive those results. For example, the nurse may need to prepare the patient for possible lifestyle changes, changes in family dynamics, and decisions related to medical treatment (for example, breast removal). It is also possible for test results to inadvertently uncover a paternity or adoption issue.

Genetic testing may be important to the health care of the individual and his or her family. Benefits can include an opportunity for counseling and health promotion activities to reduce risk for the disease. Results can be important for future decision making in terms of children, financial planning, career choices, and lifestyle. In addition, for some individuals, knowing the test results may decrease stress and anxiety by eliminating uncertainty – even if the test is positive.

Increasingly, DNA testing is being directly marketed to consumers and is available over the Internet. Predictive genetic tests are being marketed through the Internet for conditions ranging from breast cancer to cardiovascular disease; however, because of the complexity of the interpretation and patient education issues related to the results of genetic tests, there are emerging concerns about these marketing techniques. For example, a woman can discover she has a mutation associated with breast cancer by sending a specimen directly to a laboratory located through the Internet. Ethical issues related to how that woman will obtain appropriate psychological and medical counseling to follow-up on the results are not resolved. Because of the role that nurses play in patient education, it is increasingly important that nurses become familiar with these emerging genetic technologies.

Emerging Genetic Technologies

Emerging genetic technological and methodological advances, such as polymerase chain reaction (PCR), real-time PCR, and microarrays, allow us to identify disease susceptibility genes and monitor gene activity, bringing applied genetics to the clinical practitioner (Cashion & Driscoll, 2004). These genetic technologies are based on gene expression (the activity of the gene as measured by the amount of mRNA produced) and the complimentary binding nature (A binds to T, and C binds to G) of DNA bases. If you take two individuals and sequence their DNA, you will find that 99.9% of the DNA is identical. Clinical studies that have been conducted to examine the association between genetic variation and disease susceptibility focus on this remaining 0.1% where genetic variation occurs.

Polymerase Chain Reaction

Kary Mullis developed PCR in 1983, and its use has revolutionized the field of molecular biology. PCR is used to replicate, or amplify, as few as one copy of a gene into billions of copies of that gene using a special heat tolerant polymerase known as *Taq* DNA. Why do we need so many copies of a gene? Because one gene is too small to measure using current technology. The many exact copies of a gene made by PCR enable researchers and clinicians to identify and study that gene. PCR has become a valuable tool in nephrology, with uses ranging from identifying human leukocyte antigens (HLA) in kidney transplant patients (Gallon, Leventhal, & Kaufman, 2002) to examining genetic determinants in various renal diseases such as Alport syndrome (Coll, Campos, Gonzalez-Nunez, Botey, & Poch, 2003).

Real-time Polymerase Chain Reaction

Real-time PCR allows for the detection and quantification of a small fragment of replicating DNA during the amplification process. It is an improvement over PCR because it offers more rapid and sensitive quantification of the gene of interest. Clinically, real-time PCR is used to obtain viral load levels of many different viruses including cytomegalovirus, hepatitis B, hepatitis C, and others. Recently, real-time PCR has also been used in research studies to detect and monitor for rejection episodes in kidney transplant patients.

Microarray Analysis

Although primarily still in the research setting, microarray analysis is one of the newest emerging genetic technologies. However, it is increasingly clear that microarrays will have a clinical application. When conducting a microarray analysis, specialized equipment using sophisticated computer programs simultaneously evaluate up to 33,000 genes that have been placed on a small, one-inch solid support (usually glass) chip. During this analysis, a pattern emerges that demonstrates the genes that are most active. Clinicians and researchers may use gene expression patterns that emerge to obtain a more specific diagnosis and to better manage patient care (Cashion & Driscoll, 2004). In some conditions, a more accurate prognosis is possible following microarray analysis. For example, one study used microarray analysis to identify a subset of genes that predicted survival in metastatic renal cell cancers (Vasselli, Shih, Iyengar, Maranchie, Riss, Worrell et al., 2003).

As genomic health care expands into the clinical setting, nurses will be required to understand the concepts and principles that underpin emerging genetic technologies. Having a basic understanding of these technologies allows the nurse to recognize the benefits, limitations, and applications of each technology and to translate this knowledge to the patient, thereby improving patient care (Cashion, Driscoll, & Sabek, 2004).

Emerging Genetic Therapies

Genetics has played a key role in nephrology and in particular, kidney transplantation. Since the 2001 publication of the sequencing of the human genome (Venter, Adams, Myers, Li, Mural, Sutton et al., 2001), the research focus has shifted appropriately from sequencing the genome to applying this knowledge to treat diseases. This continues to build on a long history of success using genetic therapies in the care of renal patients, such as the use of human leukocyte antigen (HLA) genes to accurately match organs for transplantation.

The explosion in bioinformatics and molecular technology is bringing about new options using gene therapy and stem cell transplantation that may prove to deter the progression of disease. Gene therapy is the correction of a genetic mutation by the introduction of DNA into a cell as a treatment modality to improve the patient's health. Kidney transplantation can be considered gene therapy because the transplanted organ retains the genotype of the donor and therefore modifies the recipients' *somatic* genome (Nussbaum, McInnes, & Willard, 2001).

Stem cells research offers opportunities for developing new medical therapies. Stem cells are unspecialized cells that have the potential to divide without limit and to develop into specialized cells, such as kidney or muscle cells. Because there is a worldwide shortage of organs for transplantation, stem cells have been suggested as a potential source of tissues for transplantation. At this time, it appears that whole organs may be too complex to grow in vitro. While in theory, embryonic stem cell research remains promising; in reality, many political and ethical issues must be resolved.

Summary

With the increase in genetic knowledge and advances in genetic technologies and therapies, genetics is emerging in a key role in the diagnosis, monitoring, and treatment of patients with kidney diseases. In addition to providing a foundation in basic genetics, this chapter provides an overview of the genetic variations that potentially lead to kidney disease. To provide education, support, and care to patients with renal disease, nephrology nurses need to be knowledgeable in basic genetics and in the new methodologies used to identify and modify the genetic components that place the patient at risk for disease. Nurses are on the front line of care and will be asked to provide information and comfort to individuals and their families while they undergo genetic testing or therapy. There are excellent Web sites available to help clinical nurses understand the molecular mechanisms underlying specific diseases and their clinical implications.

References

Cashion, A.K., & Driscoll, C.J. (2004). Genetics and kidney dysfunction. *Nephrology Nursing Journal, 31*(1), 14-18, 29.

Cashion, A.K., Driscoll, C.J., & Sabek, O. (2004). Emerging genetic technologies in clinical and research settings. *Biological Research for Nursing, 5*(3), 159-167.

Coll, E., Campos, B., Gonzalez-Nunez, D., Botey, A., & Poch, E. (2003). Association between the A1166C polymorphism of the angiotensin II receptor type 1 and progression of chronic renal insufficiency. *Journal of Nephrology, 16*(3), 357-364.

Dean, L., & McEntyre, J. (2004). *The genetic landscape of diabetes*: [Internet]. Bethesda (MD): National Library of Medicine (U.S.), NCBI.

Donadio, J.V., & Grande, J.P. (2002). IgA nephropathy. *New England Journal of Medicine, 347*(10), 738-748.

Gallon, L.G., Leventhal, J.R., & Kaufman, D.B. (2002). Pretransplant evaluation of renal transplant candidates. *Seminars in Nephrology, 22*(6), 515-525.

George, A.L., Jr., & Neilson, E.G. (2000). Genetics of kidney disease. *American Journal of Kidney Diseases, 35*(4, Suppl. 1), S160-S169.

Hayden, P.S., Iyengar, S.K., Schelling, J.R., & Sedor, J.R. (2003). Kidney disease, genotype and the pathogenesis of vasculopathy. *Current Opinion in Nephrology and Hypertension, 12*(1), 71-78.

Kalapurakal, J.A., Dome, J.S., Perlman, E.J., Malogolowkin, M., Haase, G.M., Grundy, P., et al. (2004). Management of Wilms' tumor: Current practice and future goals. *Lancet Oncology, 5*(1), 37-46.

Lewin, B. (2000). *Genes VII*. New York City: Oxford University Press.

Lindqvist, A.K., & Alarcon-Riquelme, M.E. (1999). The genetics of systemic lupus erythematosus. *Scandinavian Journal of Immunology, 50*(6), 562-571.

Mattu, R.K., Trevelyan, J., Needham, E.W., Khan, M., Adiseshiah, M.A., Richter, D., et al. (2002). Lipoprotein lipase gene variants relate to presence and degree of microalbuminuria in Type II diabetes. *Diabetologia, 45*(6), 905-913.

McKusick, V.A. (1986a). IgA nephropathy. *Online Mendelian Inheritance in Man (OMIM™)*. MIM no. 161950. Baltimore, MD: Johns Hopkins University. Retrieved August 17, 2004, from http://www.ncbi.nlm.nih.gov/entrez/dispomim.cgi?id=161950

McKusick, V.A. (1986b). Von Hippel-Lindau syndrome (VHL). *Online Mendelian Inheritance in Man (OMIM™)*. MIM no. 193300. Baltimore, MD: Johns Hopkins University. Retrieved August 17, 2004, from http://www.ncbi.nlm.nih.gov/entrez/dispomim.cgi?id=193300

McKusick, V.A. (2003a). Susceptibility to Systemic Lupus Erythematosus with Nephritis 2 (SLEN2). *Online Mendelian Inheritance in Man, OMIM™*. MIM no. 607966. Baltimore, MD: Johns Hopkins University. Retrieved August 17, 2004, from http://www.ncbi.nlm.nih.gov/entrez/dispomim.cgi?id=607966

McKusick, V.A. (2003b). Susceptibility to Systemic Lupus Erythematosus with Nephritis 3 (SLEN3). *Online Mendelian Inheritance in Man, OMIM™*. MIM no. 607967. Baltimore, MD: Johns Hopkins University. Retrieved August 17, 2004, from http://www.ncbi.nlm.nih.gov/entrez/dispomim.cgi?id=607967

McKusick, V.A. (2003c). Susceptibility to Systemic Lupus Erythematosus with Nephritis 1 (SLEN1). *Online Mendelian Inheritance in Man, OMIM™*. MIM no. 607965. Baltimore, MD: Johns Hopkins University. Retrieved August 17, 2004, from http://www.ncbi.nlm.nih.gov/entrez/dispomim.cgi?id=607965

Nussbaum, R.L., McInnes, R.R., & Willard, H.F. (2001). *Thompson & Thompson genetics in medicine* (6th ed.). Philadelphia: W.B. Saunders Company.

Obara, W., Iida, A., Suzuki, Y., Tanaka, T., Akiyama, F., Maeda, S., et al. (2003). Association of single-nucleotide polymorphisms in the polymeric immunoglobulin receptor gene with immunoglobulin A nephropathy (IgAN) in Japanese patients. *Journal of Human Genetics, 48*(6), 293-299.

O'Shaughnessy, K.M., & Karet, F.E. (2004). Salt handling and hypertension. *Journal of Clinical Investigation, 113*(8), 1075-1081.

Pollak, M.R. (2003). The genetic basis of FSGS and steroid-resistant nephrosis. *Seminars in Nephrology, 23*(2), 141-146.

Pullen, R.L. Jr., Cannon, J.D., & Rushing, J.D. (2003). Managing organ-threatening systemic lupus erythematosus. *MEDSURG Nursing, 12*(6), 368-379.

Rizk, D., & Chapman, A.B. (2003). Cystic and inherited kidney diseases. *American Journal of Kidney Diseases, 42*(6), 1305-1317.

Torres, V., & Scheinman, S. (2004). Genetic Diseases of the Kidney, *NephSAP* (Vol. 3, pp. 1-76): Lippincott Williams & Wilkins.

Vasselli, J.R., Shih, J.H., Iyengar, S.R., Maranchie, J., Riss, J., Worrell, R., et al. (2003). Predicting survival in patients with metastatic kidney cancer by gene-expression profiling in the primary tumor. *Proceedings of the National Academy of Sciences of the United States of America., 100*(12), 6958- 6963.

Venter, J.C., Adams, M.D., Myers, E.W., Li, P.W., Mural, R.J., Sutton, G.G., et al. (2001). The sequence of the human genome. *Science, 291*(5507), 1304-1351.

Watson, J.D., & Crick, F.H. (1953). Molecular structure of nucleic acids: A structure for deoxyribose nucleic acid. *Nature, 171*(4356), 737-738.

Winn, M.P. (2003). Approach to the evaluation of heritable diseases and update on familial focal segmental glomerulosclerosis. *Nephrology, Dialysis, Transplantation, 18*(Suppl. 6), vi, 14-20.

- The explosion in genetic technologies and methodologies to identify disease-related genes has led to an increase in the number of genetic tests and genetic-based therapies available to identify, monitor, and treat kidney diseases. The role of the clinical practitioner includes interpreting clinical reports, applying evidenced-based research to patient care, and communicating this information to patients, all of which require a basic understanding of how genetic principles apply to kidney disease.

- The genome is an individual's complete genetic makeup containing the entire genetic information for that individual. An individual's genetic sequence is known as his *genotype*, while *phenotype* is an individual's observable traits.

- Another key concept in genetics involves *polymorphisms* and *mutations*, which are variations in the DNA sequence of a gene from the normal gene. They are key determinants of an individual's observable traits, or phenotype, and clinical status.

- In 1865, Gregor Mendel reported on the fundamental patterns of inheritance of specific traits based on his experiments using pea plants. From his reports, three typical patterns of inheritance emerged: autosomal recessive, autosomal dominant, and sex influenced (X-linked).

- Genetic disorders are generally categorized into one of three groups: single gene (*monogenic*), chromosomal, or multifactorial... Single gene disorders are caused by a mutation within a single gene... Chromosomal disorders occur when there is an abnormal number or structure of chromosomes... Multifactorial disorders are caused by gene-environment interaction.

- Clinical genetics has traditionally focused on single-gene disorders that are transmitted through families as recessive, dominant, or X-linked traits. Examples of single-gene disorders include polycystic kidney disease and Alport Syndrome. We are now expanding our knowledge to include multifactorial disorders as well.

- In addition to genetic mutations that have a direct effect on the kidney, there are other diseases that have particular impact on the kidney. Examples of such systemic diseases include systemic lupus erythematosis, hypertension, and diabetes.

- While it is still appropriate to obtain genetic counseling for inherited genetic conditions (such as polycystic kidney disease), it is not always possible for patients with chronic conditions of adulthood (for example, diabetes) to receive this type of counseling. This means a nurse is frequently the one responsible for patient education related to genetic testing.

- Many patients do not want to inform their insurance companies that genetic tests are being conducted for fear of discrimination, so they pay for the genetic tests themselves. However, if the insurance company pays for the test, it is entitled to the results. Currently, there is pending state and federal legislation to protect the patient from employment or insurance discrimination.

- Limitations of genetic testing depend on the type of genetic test conducted. For example, a predictive test does not give a diagnosis; instead, it identifies if the patient is "at-risk" for a genetic condition. In addition, many molecular genetic tests check for a specific mutation and will not identify mutations in other areas of the genome.

- Emerging genetic technological and methodological advances, such as polymerase chain reaction (PCR), real-time PCR, and microarrays, allow us to identify disease susceptibility genes and monitor gene activity, bringing applied genetics to the clinical practitioner (Cashion & Driscoll, 2004).

Genetics and Kidney Disease

Ann Cashion, PhD, RN
Carolyn J. Driscoll, MSN, RN, FNP-C

Contemporary Nephrology Nursing: Principles and Practice contains 39 chapters of educational content. Individual learners may apply for continuing nursing education credit by reading a chapter and completing the Continuing Education Evaluation Form for that chapter. Learners may apply for continuing education credit for any or all chapters.

Please photocopy this page and return to ANNA.
COMPLETE THE FOLLOWING:

Name: _____

Address: _____

City: _____ State: _____ Zip: _____

E-mail: _____

Preferred telephone: ☐ Home ☐ Work: _____

State where licensed and license number (optional): _____

CE application fees are based upon the number of contact hours provided by the individual chapter. CE fees per contact hour for ANNA members are as follows: 1.0-1.9 - $15; 2.0-2.9 - $20; 3.0-3.9 - $25; 4.0 and higher - $30. Fees for nonmembers are $10 higher.

ANNA Member: ☐ Yes ☐ No Member # (if available) _____

☐ Checked Enclosed ☐ American Express ☐ Visa ☐ MasterCard

Total Amount Submitted: _____

Credit Card Number: _____ Exp. Date: _____

Name as it appears on the card: _____

CE Evaluation Form
To receive continuing education credit for individual study after reading the chapter
1. Photocopy this form. (You may also download this form from ANNA's Web site, **www.annanurse.org.**)
2. Mail the completed form with payment (check) or credit card information to American Nephrology Nurses' Association, East Holly Avenue, Box 56, Pitman, NJ 08071-0056.
3. You will receive your CE certificate from ANNA in 4 to 6 weeks.

Test returns must be postmarked by **December 31, 2010.**

CE Application Fee
ANNA Member $15.00
Nonmember $25.00

EVALUATION FORM

1. I verify that I have read this chapter and completed this education activity. Date: _____

   _____
   Signature

2. What would be different in your practice if you applied what you learned from this activity? *(Please use additional sheet of paper if necessary.)*

   _____
   _____
   _____
   _____
   _____
   _____
   _____
   _____
   _____
   _____
   _____
   _____

Evaluation	Strongly disagree				Strongly agree
3. The activity met the stated objectives.					
a. Relate the basics of genetics to genetic variations that lead to kidney disease.	1	2	3	4	5
b. Describe the pathophysiologic basis of a chosen multifactorial disease associated with renal failure.	1	2	3	4	5
c. Discuss new avenues of medical treatment that may occur in the future because of gene therapy research.	1	2	3	4	5
4. The content was current and relevant.	1	2	3	4	5
5. The content was presented clearly.	1	2	3	4	5
6. The content was covered adequately.	1	2	3	4	5
7. Rate your ability to apply the learning obtained from this activity to practice.	1	2	3	4	5

Comments _____

_____

8. Time required to read the chapter and complete this form: _____ minutes.

This educational activity has been provided by the American Nephrology Nurses' Association (ANNA) for 1.9 contact hours. ANNA is accredited as a provider of continuing nursing education (CNE) by the American Nurses Credentialing Center's Commission on Accreditation (ANCC-COA). ANNA is an approved provider of continuing education by the California Board of Registered Nursing, CEP 0910.

Assessment of the Renal System

Kathy P. Parker, PhD, RN, FAAN

Chapter Contents

Chapter 8

Assessment of the Renal System

Kathy P. Parker, PhD, RN, FAAN

Individuals with kidney disease may present in a variety of ways. Some have symptoms that are directly related to the kidney, such as flank pain and hematuria, while others may present with associated extrarenal abnormalities such as edema, hypertension, and signs of uremia. Some may be critically ill. Others, such as persons with mild renal insufficiency, may be completely asymptomatic and only incidentally found to have abnormal renal function on routine screening tests (Anderson & Schrier, 2001; Toto, 2004). Clinical management, prevention of complications, and patient prognosis differ depending on the clinical presentation.

Once the renal abnormality is discovered, the primary goals are to establish the correct diagnosis; to assess and monitor the severity of the renal dysfunction; to reverse or slow the progression of renal dysfunction, if possible (Anderson & Schrier, 2001; National Kidney Foundation [NKF], 2000a; Toto, 2004); and to address the associated nursing concerns (Thomas, 2002). As part of this process, it is important to determine whether the renal failure is acute or chronic and to assess the systemic impact of the renal abnormality. This may not be simple, especially if previous data are not readily available. Thus, it is important to know how to collect and process the appropriate information.

The initial approach to the evaluation of a person with renal failure begins with the history, physical examination, and appropriate diagnostic tests (Anderson & Schrier, 2001; Toto, 2004). This information is crucial not only in identifying the problem, but also in designing an effective nursing care plan, setting appropriate clinical goals, and assessing treatment outcomes. Because the clinical presentation of renal failure may vary substantially, nurses who work in settings ranging from walk-in clinics and emergency rooms to hospitals and critical care units are likely to be involved in the evaluation, education, follow-up, and emotional support of persons with renal function abnormalities and their families. Therefore, nurses should be knowledgeable regarding the components of the history and physical examination that are specifically related to the renal system as well as the most frequently used diagnostic tests.

History

The purpose of the history is to collect subjective data, or what persons say about themselves. A history can be divided into six components including the chief complaint, history of present illness, past medical and surgical history, family history, personal and social history, and a review of body systems (Bickley & Szilagyi, 2003). Although a general discussion of the overall health history is beyond the scope of this text, it is important to be aware that each element of the history can contain information that is relevant to the renal system.

The *chief complaint* is the individual's description of the symptom or symptoms that precipitated the decision to seek medical attention (Bickley & Szilagyi, 2003). Thus, the presentation of renal-related symptoms can provide important clues that will assist the nurse in assessing the patient. A list of these symptoms and potential associated conditions are summarized in Table 8-1. The *history of present illness* flows from the chief complaint and is a detailed "story" of the cur-

Table 8-1

Renal-Related Symptoms and Potential Associated Pathological Conditions

Symptoms	Potential Condition
Anuria	Obstruction Renal failure
Dysuria	Infection
Dribbling	Prostatic enlargement Strictures
Edema	Renal failure Nephrotic syndrome
Frequency	Infection Diabetes
Hematuria	Trauma Glomerular disease Neoplasia Infection
Hesitancy	Prostatic enlargement Strictures
Incontinence	Infection Neoplasia Diabetes
Flank pain	Infection Trauma Neoplasms Ischemia Calculi Papillary necrosis Infection
Nocturia	Renal insufficiency Renal failure
Oliguria	Renal insufficiency
Polyuria	Diabetes insipidus Glomerular diseases Diabetes
Frothy urine (proteinuria)	Nephrotic syndrome
Cloudy urine	Infection, crystalluria
Bloody urine	Glomerular disease
Renal colic	Calculi Papillary necrosis
Urgency	Infection Prostatic disease

Note: From Bickley & Szilagyi (2003); Parker (1998); Swartz (2002); Toto (2004).

rent problems from the person's perspective. If present, each of the symptoms listed should be evaluated for the onset and temporal sequence of events, the quality and quantity of the symptoms, aggravating and alleviating factors, and associated symptoms (Bickley & Szilagyi, 2003). In addition, it is also appropriate to inquire concurrently about other ongoing medical problems.

The *past medical and surgical history* is a catalog of significant past health problems including childhood diseases, congenital abnormalities (especially urologic abnormalities), previous medical examinations, hospitalizations, surgeries, radiation exposure, dental work, pregnancies, malignancies, and genitourinary disorders (Anderson & Schrier, 2001; Bickley & Szilagyi, 2003; Swartz, 2002; Toto, 2004). They should also be asked about any recent illness or trauma, including those associated with a history of fever or sore throat, fluid losses (vomiting, diarrhea, excessive sweating, burns) or gains (dyspnea and peripheral edema), hypotension (syncope, dizziness), hypertension (headache or epistaxis), trauma (with or without blood loss), or immunological abnormalities (HIV infection) (Toto, 2004). Because of the risk of nephrotoxicity, information should also be collected regarding the use of medications to diagnose or treat these conditions such as dyes for vascular studies, antibiotics, antihypertensive agents, cancer chemotherapy, herbal remedies, or other medications such as nonsteroidal antiinflammatory drugs (NSAIDs) (Anderson & Schrier, 2001; Toto, 2004). (Additional information regarding these and other potential nephrotoxins appears in Chapter 9, Acute Renal Failure.) It is especially important to obtain information related to systemic diseases that might have a direct impact on renal function such as immunological diseases, infection, hypertension, and diabetes. A careful review of past or current medical records, if available, should also be conducted (Anderson & Schrier, 2001; Toto, 2004).

The *family history* is an important component of the health history (Bickley & Szilagyi, 2003; Swartz, 2002). The presence of hereditary renal diseases in the family can alert the nurse to the potential of a preexisting chronic disorder. Examples of familial renal disorders include Alport's syndrome, Fanconi's syndrome, Barter's syndrome, cystinuria, and polycystic kidney disease (autosomal dominant), Fabry's disease (sex-linked), and medullary cystic disease (autosomal recessive). A family history of other common diseases such a diabetes, hypertension, and sickle cell disease should also be elicited. The construction of a family pedigree that includes parents, grandparents, great-grandparents, siblings, and offspring is often helpful in determining the diagnosis and the need for genetic tests and counseling (Toto, 2004). Ethnic background is also important. Although the reasons are unclear and likely multifactorial, ethnic minorities (African, Asian, and Native Americans) have a higher incidence of chronic kidney disease in comparison to Whites (Toto, 2004).

The *personal and social history*, often called the patient profile, is an inventory of medically relevant aspects of lifestyle (Bickley & Szilagyi, 2003; Swartz, 2002). It is intended to obtain information about the person as a member of society and family including educational level, employment history, current living situation, family structure and support systems, hobbies, sexual activity, general health habits, and daily routine. There are several renal-related factors important to explore in this section of the health history, including:

1. History of exposure to environmental agents at home or work that could precipitate acute or chronic renal dysfunction.
2. Travel to particular areas of the world, which could place individuals at risk for exposure to infectious agents and subsequent renal abnormalities.
3. Illegal drug or over-the-counter medication use, as these substances are potential sources of nephrotoxicity.
4. Weight changes, which might reflect fluid gains or losses or changes in appetite.
5. Changes in activity and exercise tolerance, which could be related to the anemia associated with renal failure.
6. Allergies, as these have the potential to precipitate renal dysfunction.
7. Diet, including history of dietary (sodium, protein) or fluid restriction that may have been prescribed for a pre-existing renal condition.

General health habits should also be explored, as this information can be used to plan health promotion and disease prevention activities (Bickley & Szilagyi, 2003; Swartz, 2002).

Finally, individuals may present with extrarenal symptoms associated with kidney disease. Therefore, it is important to seek specific information that will reflect the impact of renal dysfunction in relation to each body system *(review of body systems)* (Bickley & Szilagyi, 2003). A summary of these symptoms according to body system appears in Table 8-2. As in the renal-related symptoms previously highlighted, many of these symptoms can be seen in both acute and chronic renal failure. However, history does not always serve to distinguish these two problems due to variability in patient recall and the sudden onset of symptoms that sometimes occurs in chronic kidney disease (Toto, 2004).

Physical Examination

The physical examination consists of the process by which the clinician observes, palpates, percusses, and auscultates the body of an individual and describes the findings (signs) elicited by these processes. Inspection is the informed and critical use of the examiner's eyes. Palpation is a form of touching and feeling used to assess the skin and both superficial and deep structures. Percussion is the use of sound to define structure density and content. The classical percussion method is to create vibration by tapping against the body surface and listening for differences in sound wave conduction. Auscultation is the use of the stethoscope to judge the sounds made by the movement of gases, fluid, or internal organs. Each of these modes is used to varying degrees, depending on the body region being examined (Bickley & Szilagyi, 2003; Swartz, 2002).

The physical examination begins with a general survey or inspection of the whole person covering the general health state and significant physical characteristics, such as level of consciousness, signs of distress, skin color, grooming and personal hygiene, facial expression, odors of the body and breath, and posture, gait, and motor activity (Bickley & Szilagyi, 2003; Swartz, 2002). Overall appearance can provide tremendous help in determining the health status of the individual as well as functional ability. For example, pallor, cachexia, and weariness are frequently associated with chronic illnesses. Other the other hand, cyanosis and immobility related to pain are associated with acute processes.

The vital signs, including blood pressure, pulse, respira-

Table 8-2

Renal-Related Information to Be Documented in a General Systems Review

Body System	Information to be Elicited	Clinical Significance
General	Fatigue, weakness	Uremia, anemia
Integumentary	Dryness	Fluid volume deficit Uremia
	Pruritus	Hyperphosphatemia secondary to uremia
	Ecchymosis	Platelet dysfunction secondary to uremia
	Petechiae	Platelet dysfunction secondary to uremia
	Delayed healing	Uremia
	Pallor	Anemia secondary to renal failure
	Yellowness	Uremia
	Reduced skin turgor	Volume depletion
Neurological	Headaches	Hypertension Fluid volume excess Uremia
	Syncope	Uremia
	Seizures	Metabolic imbalances Uremia
	Paresthesias	Hypocalcemia Uremia
	Footdrop	Uremia
	Decreased cognitive ability	Uremia Electrolyte imbalance
	Memory loss	Uremia
	Sleep disturbances	Uremia
	Confusion, somnolence	Uremia
Psychological	Apathy	Uremia
	Depression	Uremia
	Anxiety	Uremia
Visual	Blurring	Fluid volume excess Electrolytes imbalances Hypotension Malignant hypertension
	Ocular muscle paralysis	Ethylene glycol poisoning Necrotizing vasculitis
	Conjunctivitis	Vasculitis, drug toxicity, chronic kidney disease
Auditory	Decrease acuity	Alport's syndrome, medications
Cardiovascular	Dizziness	Volume depletion
	Syncope	Heart failure Cardiac tamponade
Respiratory	Cough	Volume overload, pneumonia
	Dyspnea Hemoptysis	Goodpasteur's syndrome, Wegener granulomatosis, Churg-Strauss vasculitis, pulmonary edema
Gastrointestinal	Stomatitis	Uremia
	Ageusia	Uremia
	Dysgeusia	Uremia
	Anorexia	Uremia
	Nausea and vomiting	Uremia Electrolyte imbalances
	Constipation or diarrhea	Fluid volume changes Electrolytes imbalances
	Bloody stools	Uremia
	Abdominal tenderness	Uremia Ureteral obstruction Renal infarction
	Abdominal swelling	Nephrotic syndrome
	Pain	Liver disease Obstructive uropathies, acute inflammation of the kidney, renal infarction

Table 8-2 (continued)
Renal-Related Information to Be Documented in a General Systems Review

Body System	Information to be Elicited	Clinical Significance
Renal	(see Table 8-1)	(See Table 8-1)
Reproductive	Impotence Decreased libido Amenorrhea	Uremia Uremia Uremia
Musculoskeletal	Cramps Muscle weakness Less movement at night Muscle tenderness	Uremia Uremia Uremia Tissue ischemia Rhabdomyolysis
Endocrine	Tetany Thirst	Hypocalcemia Volume deficits
Hematopoietic	Fatigue Malaise Bleeding	Uremia Uremia Uremia

Note: From Headley & Wall (2002); Parker (1998); Toto (2004).

tion, and temperature are important parts of the physical exam and may reflect alterations in the renal system. The blood pressure and pulse, both lying and standing, should be taken approximately 2-3 minutes apart in order to check for orthostasis. If the patient is unable to stand, simply raising and lowering the head of the bed during blood pressure and pulse measurements can be helpful. An increase in pulse (> 30 beats/minute) and a decrease in arterial pressure (> 20 mm/Hg) following change from a supine to either a sitting or standing position is often seen with extracellular fluid volume depletion (Anderson, 2001; Anderson & Schrier, 2001; Bickley & Szilagyi, 2003). An increase in pulse rate is frequently noted before any changes in blood pressure occur (Anderson & Schrier, 2001; McGee, Abernethy, & Simel, 1999). Hypertension and tachycardia frequently occur in states of volume excess.

Respiratory rate can increase with air hunger, pulmonary edema related to volume retention, pulmonary-renal syndromes, or in compensation for the metabolic acidosis that develops in renal failure (Bickley & Szilagyi, 2003; Swartz, 2002; Toto, 2004). Therefore, careful assessment of the rate and quality of respirations, in addition to auscultation of the lungs, is important.

For reasons poorly understood, uremia is associated with hypothermia, and several studies have reported body temperatures averaging 96.8° (F) in persons with chronic kidney disease (Schneditz, 2001). In fact, body temperature may show an inverse relationship with the degree of uremia (Lewis, 1992). Therefore, infection should be suspected with even small increases in temperature (98° to 99° F). All persons with renal abnormalities should also be assessed for fever, chills, and other signs of both local and systemic infection.

Height and weight should be measured, as these variables are useful in assessing fluid status and in calculating ideal body weight and nutritional requirements. A weight change of greater than 0.25 to 0.50 kg/day indicates gain or loss of salt and/or water (Anderson & Schrier, 2001).

Following the collection of the preliminary data described above, a complete physical examination is performed. As the effects of renal dysfunction are often multi-systemic, it is important that nurses familiarize themselves with the basic approach and techniques involved. Numerous textbooks thoroughly describe the physical examination process (Bickley & Szilagyi, 2003; Swartz, 2002). Renal-related signs that might be identified during the examination and associated pathological conditions appear in Table 8-3.

The kidneys, which are usually assessed during the abdominal examination, are located in the right and left upper quadrants at the midclavicular line. Because of their location, only limited information about the kidneys can be obtained by physical examination. This area should be inspected from both a standing and supine position for raised masses and unusual pulsations. During auscultation, a renal bruit may be heard slightly above the umbilicus using the diaphragm of the stethoscope held lightly against the abdomen. A bruit, which can have both systolic and diastolic components, sounds like a low-pitched murmur and indicates a renal arterial stenosis (RAS) (Bickley & Szilagyi, 2003; Swartz, 2002).

Renal palpation is usually attempted by elevating the flank with the nondominant hand and pressing the dominant hand deep and upward under the rib cage. The kidneys, as retroperitoneal organs, are rarely felt unless they are enlarged as in polycystic kidney disease or ptotic kidneys. However, the right kidney lies 1-2 cm lower than the left and is occasionally palpable in the adult, even when normal in size (Bickley & Szilagyi, 2003; Swartz, 2002). Using the technique described previously, anterior percussion may be done to assist in assessing kidney size.

In addition, the individual should be checked for renal tenderness. This is usually done at the costovertebral angle (CVA), the area where the twelfth rib and vertebral column intersect. The palm is placed over this area and hit with the ulnar surface of the other hand that has been curled into a fist. The patient should feel a "thud." If pain occurs, renal

Table 8-3

Systems Oriented Physical Examination, Renal-Related Signs, and Associated Pathological Conditions

Body System	Sign	Clinical Significance
HEENT	Dry, thin hair	Chronic kidney disease
	Periorbital edema	Nephrotic syndrome
	Optic fundi - hemorrhages, exudates	Hypertension/diabetes
	Uveitis	Interstitial nephritis, necrotizing vasculitis
	Ocular muscle paralysis	Ethylene glycol poisoning, necrotizing vasculitis
	Conjunctivitis	Vasculitis, drug toxicity, uremia
	Hearing loss	Drug reaction, Wegener's granulomatosis, Alport syndrome
	Epistaxis	Uremia, Wegener's granulomatosis
	Halitosis	Uremia
	Dry, cracked mucous membranes	Volume depletion
	Nasal/oropharyngeal ulcers	Active lupus nephritis
	Perforated nasal septum	Wegener granulomatosis
	Engorged neck veins	Volume excess
	Carotid bruits	Vascular disease
Integumentary	Decreased tissue turgor (forehead and sternum most reliable)	Volume depletion
	Dry, scaly skin	Uremia
	Pallor	Uremia
	Yellowness	Uremia
	Cyanosis	Cardiac failure
	Maculopapular rash	Drug reaction
	Petechiae, purpura, echymoses	Uremia, vasculitis, disseminated intravascular coagulation, septic shock, thrombotic purpura
	Livedo reticularis	Vasculitis
	Pallor of nail beds	Uremia
	Excoriation	Uremia
	Vitiligto/periungual fibromas	Tuberous sclerosis
	Neurofibromas	Neurofibromatosis (renal artery stenosis)
	Butterfly rash	Lupus erythematosus
	Half-and-half nails (Lindsay's nails)	Chronic kidney disease
Cardiac	Murmurs	Valvular disease
	Pericardial friction rub	Uremia
	S3, S4	Congestive heart failure
Lungs	Pleural rub	Uremia
	Rales	Volume excess
	Decreased breath sounds	Uremia
	Hemoptysis	Pulmonary-renal syndromes
Abdomen	Bruits	Vascular disease
	Enlarged liver	Congestive heart failure
	Enlarged kidneys	Polycystic kidney disease, hydronephrosis
	Ascites	Liver failure, acute renal failure
Rectal	Enlarged prostate	Obstruction
	Tender prostate	Infection
	Occult blood	Uremia
Genitourinary	Distended bladder	Obstruction
	Prostate enlargement	Prostatic hypertrophy
	Flank masses	Polycystic kidney disease
	Pelvic masses	Obstruction

Table 8-3 (continued)
Systems Oriented Physical Examination, Renal-Related Signs, and Associated Pathological Conditions

Body System	Sign	Clinical Significance
Extremities	Peripheral edema Ischemia, muscle tenderness	Volume excess Rhabdomyolysis
Musculoskeletal	Joint pain Bone pain Proximal muscle weakness	Immunologic disorders, uremia Uremia Uremia
Neurological	Altered levels of consciousness Seizures, coma Tetany (Chvostek's/Trousseau's) Depressed reflexes	Uremia Uremia Electrolyte disturbances Electrolyte disturbances, uremia

Note: From Anderson (2001); Headley & Wall (2002); Parker (1998); Toto (2004).

tenderness may be present. This physical finding is commonly seen in pyelonephritis. However, positive results may also occur in tense persons and in some musculoskeletal strains and inflammations of the midback (Bickley & Szilagyi, 2003; Swartz, 2002).

The bladder should be examined for distention. As the bladder fills, it ascends into the abdomen. When containing more than approximately 500 cc of urine, it can be seen as an ovoid mass in the lower abdomen. A full bladder also elicits a dull sound to percussion and can be felt as a slightly tense suprapubic mass on palpation. A distended bladder suggests obstruction, while tenderness over the area (suprapubic tenderness) upon palpation is associated with infection. An assessment of post-void residual urine to assess bladder emptying may also be done as part of the physical examination. The patient is first asked to void. Then a straight catheterization is done to determine how much urine remains in the bladder after voiding. Although an ultrasound provides more reliable information, a post-void residual volume of more than 50 to 100 cc suggests a bladder outlet obstruction or neurological abnormality (uropathy) (Stern, Hsieh, & Schaeffer, 2004). A disadvantage of this procedure is the possibility of introducing infection.

Diagnostic Tests

Diagnostic tests are crucial in evaluating patients with renal function abnormalities. In addition to the complete history and physical, the information obtained from these tests helps to describe the degree of renal dysfunction present and associated systemic effects. Directly or indirectly, these tests measure both kidney structure and function, help establish the diagnosis, and suggest the appropriate treatment (Silkensen & Kasiske, 2004). Nurses frequently review the reports and, therefore, should know which results suggest renal abnormalities. The diagnostic tests most commonly used include analyses of the blood and urine, measures of renal clearance and glomerular filtration rate (GFR), selected radiologic procedures, and renal biopsy.

Blood Analyses

As discussed in Chapter 5, the kidneys play a major role in electrolyte balance, acid-base homeostasis, and in the reg-

ulation of the serum concentration of non-electrolyte substances such as blood urea nitrogen (BUN) and creatinine. In addition, the kidneys normally produce the hormone erythropoietin, which stimulates red blood cell production. When renal dysfunction occurs, marked changes in the amount of substances normally found in the blood change. The laboratory measures that are most commonly used in the evaluation of the patient with renal failure are outlined in Table 8-4. The normal ranges of these values and changes indicating possible renal dysfunction are also listed.

Levels of serum creatinine and BUN, both by-products of metabolism, are commonly used to help estimate renal function. Creatinine is a waste product of muscle metabolism that originates from creatine and phosphocreatine. It is continuously produced in amounts that depend on muscle mass (Silkensen & Kasiske, 2004); its production can change over long periods of time if there is a change in muscle mass. Although approximately 5% to 15% of urinary creatinine is secreted by the tubules, it is predominately filtered at the glomerular level and then excreted (Silkensen & Kasiske, 2004). Because of this characteristic, measurements of serum creatinine are typically inversely correlated with GFR. However, several factors other than GFR can affect serum creatinine levels. Age, gender, and race-associated differences in creatinine production have been observed and are largely related to differences in muscle mass (mean creatinine generation is higher in men than women, in younger than older individuals, and in Blacks than in Whites) (NKF, 2000a, 2002). Because the conversion of creatine to creatinine can occur during cooking, intake of cooked meat can also lead to an increase in serum levels. In contrast, serum creatinine is typically lower than expected in patients following a low protein diet. Certain medications and laboratory techniques may interfere with the measurement of serum creatinine and cause elevations without an actual decrease in GFR. Although, extra-renal (bowel) excretion of creatinine is minimal in those with normal kidney function, it may be significantly increased in persons with chronic kidney disease. In fact, as much as two thirds of total daily creatinine excretion can occur via this route in the face of severe kidney disease, and 40% of individuals with a significantly decreased GFR can have a serum creatinine level within nor-

Table 8-4
Blood and Serum Laboratory Values and Changes in Renal Dysfunction

Substance	Normal Range	Renal Dysfunction
Sodium	135 - 145 mEq/L	Varies with free water load
Potassium	3.5 - 5.3 mEq/L	Increases, but may also change with acid-base balance
Chloride	98 - 106 mEq/L	Varies
CO_2 combining power	23 - 30 mEq/L	Decreases
BUN	10 - 20 mg/dl	Increases
Creatinine	0.5 - 1.5 mg/dl	Increases
Phosphorus	2.5 to 4.5 mg/dl	Increases
Calcium	8.4 - 10.2 mg/dl	Decreases
Magnesium	1.6 - 2.6 mg/dl	Increases
Hematocrit	35 - 55%	Decreases
Hemoglobin	12 - 16 g/dl	Decreases

Note: From Fischback (2004); Parker (1998).

mal range. In summary, serum creatinine is affected, not only by GFR, but also age, gender, race, body size, diet, drugs, laboratory analytical techniques, and extrarenal creatinine excretion (NKF, 2000a, 2002; Silkensen & Kasiske, 2004) (see Table 8-5).

BUN is formed from the hepatic metabolism of amino acids (Fischback, 2004; Silkensen & Kasiske, 2004). When dietary protein is digested, the ammonia formed is absorbed from the intestinal tract and routed to the liver through the portal vein. The liver combines the ammonia with carbon dioxide to form urea, a much less toxic substance. Like creatinine, BUN is excreted by glomerular filtration and tends to increase as the GFR decreases. However, the tubule reabsorbs up to 50% of the filtered urea. This amount can increase in physiologic states characterized by decreased tubular flow (i.e. volume depletion) causing elevations in BUN. Levels of BUN may also increase due to large protein loads, gastrointestinal bleeding, corticosteroid intake, increased catabolic states (muscle breakdown) (Silkensen & Kasiske, 2004). Conversely, BUN decreases in liver dysfunction and protein restriction. In addition, numerous substances can interfere with the laboratory measurement of urea. For example, bilirubin, chloral hydrate, dextran, free hemoglobin, lipids, tetracycline, and uric acid can cause elevations, while ascorbic acid, levodopa, and streptomycin can cause falsely low values (Silkensen & Kasiske, 2004)(see Table 8-5).

The normal range of BUN is 10 to 20 mg/dl while the normal value of creatinine is 0.5 to 1.5 mg/dl (Fischback, 2004). The ratio of BUN: creatinine is usually 15:1 (Anderson, 2001). In most cases of renal failure, both the BUN and serum creatinine increase while maintaining this ratio. As previously discussed, however, in certain renal abnormalities characterized by low tubular flow, the BUN may increase more than the creatinine yielding an increased BUN: creatinine ratio. Thus, it is important to note not only the absolute levels of BUN and serum creatinine, but also their ratio.

Measures of GFR and Renal Clearance

GFR provides an excellent measure of renal function. A low or decreasing GFR precedes kidney failure, and monitoring changes can help determine the progression of the disease. The GFR of normal kidneys is approximately 125 ml/minute/1.73m^2 (the body surface area of an average 70 kg adult) (Holechek, 2003; NKF, 2002; Silkensen & Kasiske, 2004). However, kidney damage with clinical manifestations (nephritic syndrome, urinary tract symptoms, tubular syndromes) can be present even with a normal GFR (GFR $\geq$ 90 ml/minute; Stage 1). A mild reduction in GFR (60–89 ml/minute; Stage 2) is usually associated with hypertension and laboratory abnormalities indicative of dysfunction in other organ systems. Persons with a GFR of 30–59 ml/minute (moderately reduced GFR, Stage 3) also have laboratory abnormalities, but few symptoms. Those with severely reduced GFR (15–29 ml/minute; Stage 4) have laboratory abnormalities in several organ systems and mild symptoms. A GFR of less than 15 ml/minute (Stage 5) is classified as renal failure, a state in which the kidneys are unable to maintain a homeostatic internal environment and a level at which patients usually have many symptoms and laboratory abnormalities in several organ systems (NKF, 2000a).

Unfortunately, although GFR cannot be measured directly, it can be estimated via measures of renal clearance. Renal clearance is that amount of blood that is cleared of a substance in a given unit of time. If it is assumed that there is no extrarenal elimination, tubular reabsorption, or secretion of the substance, then an estimate of the GFR can be calculated as follows:

$$UV/P$$

where U is the urine concentration of that substance, V is the urine volume per unit time, and P is the plasma concentration of the marker (Silkensen & Kasiske, 2004). The substance measured must have several properties including constant production, no tubular reabsorption or secretion, and no extrarenal elimination. Inulin, a fructose polysaccharide, is such a substance, and inulin clearance is widely regarded as the gold standard for measuring GFR. However, its calcula-

Table 8-5

Conditions Causing an Increase in Creatinine and Urea in Blood Without a Decrease in Glomerular Filtration Rate (GFR)

Interference with creatinine assays
  Cefoxitin
  Cephalothin
  Cephaloridine
  Other cephalosporins
  Ketoacidosis

Decreased tubule secretion of creatinine
  Cimetidine
  Trimethoprim

Increased creatinine production
  Intake of cooked meat
  Muscle disorders (rare)

Decreased creatinine production
  Malnutrition
  Women and older patients

Abnormal renal handling of urea
  Familial azotemia

Increased production of urea
  Excessive protein intake
  Amino acid infusion
  Increased catabolism
  Tetracycline
  Corticosteroids
  Acute illness
  Accelerated catabolism
  Gastrointestinal bleeding

Increased renal absorption of urea
  Dehydration
  Reduced renal perfusion (congestive heart failure)

Reduced renal reabsorption of urea
  Overhydration
  Increased renal perfusion (pregnancy, syndrome of inappropriate ADH secretion)

Interference with BUN assays
  Bilirubin
  Chloral hydrate
  Dextran
  Free hemoglobin
  Lipids
  Tetracycline
  Uric Acid

Note: Adapted with permission from Brezis, M., Rosen, S. & Epstein, F.H. (1993). Acute renal failure due to ischemia. In J.M. Lazarus & B.M. Brenner (Eds.), *Acute renal failure* (3rd ed.) (pg. 222). New York: Churchill Livingstone; NKF (2000a); Lafayette, Perrone, & Levey (2001); Parker (1998); Silkensen & Kasiske (2004).

tion requires an intravenous infusion and timed urine collections over several hours making it both time consuming and expensive (NKF, 2000a).

The most widely used estimate of GFR in clinical practice is based on the 24-hour creatinine clearance. Creatinine clearance is usually measured by obtaining a 24-hour urine specimen for the urine volume and urine creatinine concentration and a venous blood specimen, ideally drawn at the midpoint (12 hours) of the urine collection, for the plasma creatinine concentration. The normal values for creatinine clearance in adults are 95 ± 20 ml/min in women and 120 ± 25 ml/min in men (Fischback, 2004). After the age of 30, there is a gradual reduction in renal mass and a subsequent decrease in creatinine clearance.

The formula for creatinine clearance (CC) is:
$$CC = Ucr \times V/Pcr$$
Ucr = urine creatinine in mg/dl
V = urine volume in cc/min
Pcr = serum creatinine in mg/dl

Small changes in serum creatinine can reflect marked decreases in creatinine clearance. For example, an increase in serum creatinine from 1 to 2 mg reflects a 50% decrease in creatinine clearance.

The most common error in calculating creatinine clearance results from an incomplete urine collection leading to an underestimation of creatinine clearance. (The relative consistent rate of creatinine production and excretion can be helpful in assessing completeness of collection. In adults, daily creatinine excretion is approximately 25 mg/kg of lean body mass for men and 20 mg/kg for women. If total creatinine excretion is less than these normal values, then an incomplete collection is likely.) Prolonged storage of urine can also alter results. High ambient temperature and low urine pH can increase the conversion of creatine to creatinine in the urine. Refrigeration of the specimen and prompt measurement reduces these effects (Fischback, 2004; Silkensen & Kasiske, 2004).

When used as an estimate of GFR, creatinine clearance has limitations. First, as previously discussed, serum creatinine (the variable in the denominator of the equation used to calculate creatinine clearance) can be affected by a number of variables. In severe kidney disease, because of enhanced tubular secretion and extra-renal elimination, the serum creatinine can remain quite low. In fact, only 60% of patients with a decreased GFR have an increased serum creatinine (NKF, 2000a). Second, enhanced tubular excretion of creatinine in renal disease also affects urine creatinine (a variable in the numerator of the equation used to calculate creatinine clearance). Thus, creatinine clearance will systematically overestimate GFR. This overestimation is approximately 10% to 40% in normal individuals (due to the normal tubular secretion of creatinine) but is greater and more unpredictable in patients with chronic kidney disease. Because tubular secretion of creatinine is a major limitation of creatinine clearance, some have tried to enhance its accuracy by blocking this action with the histamine receptor blocker antagonist cimetidine with varied success (Silkensen & Kasiske, 2004).

Recently, several studies have shown that equations used to estimate GFR based on serum creatinine and some or all of the following variables (age, gender, race, and body size) provide better estimates of GFR (NKF, 2000a). The most widely used formula, originally developed by Cockroft and Gault to better estimate creatinine clearance, reduces the

Table 8-6
Formulas for Estimating Glomerular Filtration Rate (GFR)

Cockcroft-Gault Equation
Creatinine clearance (ml/min) = $\dfrac{(140 - Age) \; X \; (0.85 \; if \; female)}{72 \; X \; serum \; creatinine}$

MDRD Formula (adults)
GFR =   170 X serum creatinine concentration $^{-0.999}$
               X age $^{-0.176}$
               X 0.762 (if female)
               X 1.18 (if race is black)
               X blood urea nitrogen concentration $^{-0.17}$
               X serum albumin concentration $^{-0.318}$

Schwartz Formula (children)
Creatinine clearance (ml/min) = $\dfrac{0.55 \; X \; length}{Serum \; creatinine}$

Note: From www.nkdep.nih.gov/GFR-cal.htm; NKF (2000a).

variability of serum creatinine estimates in men and women but may overestimate it in those who are obese or edematous. Nonetheless, the Cockcroft and Gault equation can be used to estimate creatinine clearance if only the serum creatinine is known (see Table 8-6). In the large adult population studied in the Modification of Diet in Renal Disease (MDRD) Study, an equation was developed to estimate GFR based on multiple serum values (creatinine, urea, and albumin) and patient characteristics (age, gender, and race) (Coresh et al., 1998; Silkensen & Kasiske, 2004). The Schwartz equation was developed for use in children. GFR calculators are readily available on the Internet (www.nkdep.nih.gov/GFR-cal.htm). Estimates of GFR are the best overall indices of the level of kidney function (NKF, 2000a)(see Table 8-6).

Urinalysis

The urine is a very complex body fluid, containing filtrates from blood and other elements from the kidneys, ureters, and bladder. Therefore, the urinalysis is a major diagnostic tool for evaluating the patient with renal abnormalities (Silkensen & Kasiske, 2004). In order to yield optimal information, the specimen must be appropriately collected and stored. A morning, first voided urine specimen obtained by a midstream, clean catch technique is preferred (Fischback, 2004); random urine specimens are also acceptable if first morning specimens are not available (Toto, 2004). If urine cannot be delivered to the laboratory immediately, it should be refrigerated. After urine stands at room temperature for 1 hour, red blood cells (RBCs) hemolyze, tubercle bacilli die, and bacteria grow. In addition, bacterial action decomposes urea to ammonia and the urine becomes alkalotic causing casts that may be present to disintegrate. The analysis should ideally be conducted within 1 to 2 hours after voiding and typically includes visual inspection, dipstick testing, and examination of urine sediment.

Inspection. A urinalysis begins with inspection of the specimen for its odor, clarity, and color. Normal urine has a faint, ammonia odor. Foul-smelling urine usually indicates infection. The sweet smell of acetone can be recognized in diabetic ketosis, while some foods, such as asparagus, can produce characteristic odors. After urine stands for a long time, ammonia is formed by bacterial activity causing the decomposition of urea and producing a very pungent odor

(Kim & Corwin, 2001).

Normal urine is usually clear. However, certain types of crystals may appear or disappear in the urine and change its turbidity depending on the pH. The presence of RBCs, white blood cells (WBCs), bacteria, spermatozoa, prostatic fluid, and mucus can also cause cloudiness. Foamy urine usually indicates the presence of protein. Normal urine ranges from almost colorless to deep yellow, depending on its chemical content (Silkensen & Kasiske, 2004). The color intensity varies with the concentration of these substances. An unusually intense color might imply a normal solute load contained in a small urine volume (as in dehydration) or abnormal substances in a normal quantity (Fischback, 2004). Abnormal urine colors may be a sign of disease or indicate the presence of a pigmented drug, dye, or food (see Table 8-7).

Dipstick testing. The urine is assessed chemically with the "dipstick," a plastic strip impregnated with various reagents that detect selected substances. These variables include specific gravity, urinary pH, protein, blood, bilirubin and urobilinogen, glucose, ketones, leukocytes, and nitrates (see Table 8-8).

Specific gravity reflects the size, weight, and number of substances in the urine in comparison to distilled water at 4∞ C (Kim & Corwin, 2001; Silkensen & Kasiske, 2004). The specific gravity of water is 1.000, while normal urine specific gravity ranges from 1.001 to 1.030. The first voided specimen of the morning should be approximately 1.020, indicating normal concentrating ability. When the kidneys lose their ability to concentrate, the first voided morning specimen is often around 1.010, the specific gravity of plasma. Specific gravity as measured by reagent strip is not affected by the presence of albumin, glucose, or radiographic contrast media in the urine (Kim & Corwin, 2001). However, these substances will raise the reading of specific gravity if it is measured by a hydrometer or urometer (Fischback, 2004; Kim & Corwin, 2001).

Although the measurement of specific gravity is a useful screening tool, the kidney's ability to concentrate or dilute urine is reflected in the number of particles present and not their size or weight. Thus, urine osmolality, which measures the number of dissolved solutes per unit of volume (mosm/kg), is often more clinically useful (Silkensen &

Table 8-7
Urinary Color Variations

Color	Etiology
Orange	Pyridium Bilirubin Azulfidine Carrots or vitamin A (in large amounts)
Red	Hemoglobin Red blood cells Myoglobin Porphyrin Beets
Brown to black	Hemoglobin Mercury poisoning Lead poisoning Methyldopa Levodopa Phenylpyruvic acid
Blue, blue green	Methylene blue Amitriptyline Pseudomonas
White	Phosphates Chyle Lipiduria

Note: From Fischback (2004).

Kasiske, 2004). Urine osmolality requires a 24-hour urine collection, is measured by an osmometer, and normally ranges from approximately 50 to 1200 mosm/kg H_2O. When the kidneys lose their ability to concentrate, as in chronic kidney disease and some types of acute renal failure, both the urine specific gravity and osmolality are low and do not change appropriately with changes in volume status (Fischback, 2004).

The symbol pH is used to denote the amount of the free hydrogen ion (H^+) present in a solution; 7.0 is the neutral point (pH of water) (Fischback, 2004). The lower the pH, the greater the acidity; the higher the pH, the greater the alkalinity. The pH of urine can range between 4.5 and 8.0. Normal urine typically has an acidic pH (between 5.0 and 6.0) because of the excretion of acids from metabolism. Urine pH can be helpful in diagnosing acid-base disorders when used with other laboratory tests (Kim & Corwin, 2001) (see Table 8-8).

Under normal circumstances, individuals excrete a very small amount of protein in the urine with a 24-hour total protein excretion of less than 300 mg/day (30 mg/dL) (see Table 8-9). In normal urine, 60% of the proteins present are plasma proteins from the GFR and 40% are from the kidney and the urogenital tract (Kim & Corwin, 2001). Although there are over 32 different plasma proteins, albumin is the most abundant (normal excretion is < 30 mg/day). Increased albumin excretion is a sensitive marker for chronic kidney disease due to diabetes, glomerular disease, and hypertension. Increased excretion of other low molecular weight proteins is a sensitive marker for some types of tubulointerstitial dis-

ease. "Total protein" refers to urinary excretion of albumin and other proteins. "Albuminuria" refers to increased urinary excretion of albumin. "Microalbuminuria" refers to albumin excretion above the normal range but below the level of detections by tests for total protein (NKF, 2000a) (see Table 8-8).

An untimed (spot) urine sample should be used to detect and monitor proteinuria in children and adults (NKF, 2000b). A 24-hour collection is not routinely recommended because variability in hydration, effects of postural changes and exercise, and collection errors can affect test results (NKF, 2000b). The urine is screened for total protein by dipstick with results, based on color change, being graded from negative to trace to 4+. The urine dipstick is sensitive to negatively charged proteins such as albumin but often insensitive to positively charged immunoglobulin light chains such as those found in multiple myeloma (Kim & Corwin, 2001). The lower limit of protein that a dipstick will detect is 10 to 20 mg/dL, a trace positive indicates approximately 15 to 30 mg/dL, and 4+ indicates greater than 2,000 mg/dL. Persistently increased protein excretion usually indicates renal damage. Albumin-specific dipsticks detect albumin above a concentration of 3 to 4 mg/dl and are useful for detection of microalbuminuria. When results are positive, a quantification of the urinary protein-to-creatinine or albumin-to-creatinine ratio is recommended; this ratio correlates well with the 24-hour protein excretion and is both a convenient and inexpensive method of monitoring proteinuria over time.

For information regarding other substances measured via dipstick, see Table 8-8.

Urinary sediment. A microscopic examination of the urine may reveal the presence of urinary sediment, cells, casts, and crystals (see Table 8-10), substances that cannot be detected by urine dipsticks (NKF, 2000c). Squamous, transitional, and renal tubular epithelial cells can be found in the urine. Squamous epithelial cells originate from the lower urinary tract and usually represent normal cell turnover. Transitional cells come from the renal pelvis, ureter, and bladder and, when found in the urine, indicate disorders in those areas. Renal tubular epithelial cells are found in the urine when abnormalities in the kidney occur. Oval fat bodies are a special type of renal tubular epithelial cells that have undergone fatty degeneration and indicate heavy proteinuria.

Casts are precipitated proteins (Tamm-Horsfall mucoprotein) and cells that form within the tubular lumen and, thus, have a cylindrical shape. When the lumen is free of cells, the casts are composed almost entirely of this protein, called hyaline casts, and are of little clinical significance. However, cellular casts form if there are cells in the lumen. This is a clinically important finding as it identifies the kidney as the source of the cells. Casts generally form in the collecting tubules, the site at which the urine is most concentrated and most acidic. Urinary stasis, as in poorly functioning nephrons with low flow, also promotes cast formation (Kim & Corwin, 2001).

Crystals are composed of salts and can be seen in the urine sediment depending on the urine composition, concentration, and pH. Uric acid and calcium crystals are found in an acid urine. Calcium phosphate and triphosphate crystals are found in alkaline urine. Urine crystals can be seen in normal subjects but may also indicate renal disease.

Table 8-8

Variables Measured by Dipstick in a Urinalysis, Normal, and Abnormal Findings

Variable	Normals	Abnormals
Specific gravity	1.001 to 1.030	Low in chronic kidney disease and some types of ARF. High in dehydration and prerenal states. Can be pH dependent with falsely elevated values at urine pH less than 6 and falsely lower values at urine pH greater than 7.
pH	4.5 to 8.0	Alkaline in certain urinary tact infections (ureasplitting organisms such as Proteus and Klebsiella), metabolic alkalosis, potassium depletion, drugs (sodium bicarbonate), or if the specimen has sat around for a long time. Acidic in metabolic or uncompensated respiratory acidosis, fever, drugs (calcium chloride), ingestion of large amounts of meat. False-positive changes may be seen if the urine is very alkaline or if there is contamination with bacteria, blood, or chlorhexidine (a skin cleanser)
Protein	Negative	The standard dipstick is sensitive to 10 to 20 mg/dl of total protein but is insensitive for low concentrations of albumin that may occur in patients with microalbuminuria (i.e. diabetics). It is also insensitive to immunoglobulin light changes. Albumin-specific dipsticks detect albumin above a concentration of 3 to 4 mg/dl and are useful for detection of microalbuminuria. False positive results may be seen with dehydration, hematuria, exercise, infection, or alkaline urine. False negative results may be seen with excessive hydration or the presence of proteins that do not react with the reagent on the dipstick.
RBCs	Negative	The dipstick will detect RBCs, hemoglobin, and myoglobin (0.3 mg/dl or 10/HPF).
WBCs	Negative	The dipstick will detect neutrophils and eosinophils (10/HPF).
Bilirubin	Negative	The dipstick detects conjugated (water soluble) bilirubin. Will show up positive in obstructive liver disease (obstructive jaundice or jaundice due to hepatocellular injury). Will be negative in patients with jaundice due to hemolysis. False positive results can occur if urine is contaminated with stool. Prolonged storage and exposure to light can lead to false-negative results.
Urobilinogen	Negative to trace	A by-product of bilirubin breakdown in the gut and can be elevated in liver disease.
Glucose	Negative	May be positive in some renal diseases that are characterized by proximal tubular defects and, of course, in diabetes when serum glucose levels exceed the renal transport maximum. Indicates a high serum glucose level. Dipsticks detect glycosuria in concentrations ranging from 50 mg/dl to over 1,000 mg/dl. False negative results can be seen if ascorbic acid or aspirin is present in the urine. False positive results can be seen with hydrogen peroxide.
Ketones	Negative	Positive when fats are being used for energy (fasting or starvation) and in insulin deficiency.
Nitrate	Negative	Nitrate is changed to nitrite by bacteria. When positive, suggests urinary tract infection. However, the urine must be in the bladder for about 4 hours for this to be positive. Will be negative in the presence of enterococcus (anaerobic streptococci in the bowel, such a Streptococcus faecalis). False positive results can occur with vaginal contamination. False negative results can occur with high levels of glucose, albumin, ascorbic acid, tetracycline, cephalexin, or cephalothin.

HPF = high powered field

Note: From Fischback (2004); Kim & Corwin (2001); Silkensen & Kasiske (2004).

Table 8-9
Definitions of Proteinuria and Albuminuria *

	Urine Collection Method	Normal	Microalbuminuria
Total Protein	24-hour urine	< 300 mg/day	N/A
	Spot urine dipstick	< 30 mg/dl	N/A
	Spot urine	< 200 mg/g	
	Protein: creatinine ratio		
Albumin	24-hour urine	< 30 mg/day	> 30 to 300 mg/day
	Spot urine **	< 3 mg/dl	> 3 mg/dl
	Spot urine	< 17 mg/g (men)	17-250 mg/g (men)
	Albumin: creatinine ratio	< 25 mg/g (women)	25-355 mg/g (women)

Notes: * = Adults; values for children are not well established but appear to be similar to those observed in adults;
** = Albumin-specific dipstick.
Note: From NKF (2000a).

However, an exception is the presence of cystine crystals, which are seen only in patients with cystinuria, a hereditary disorder. Sulfa crystals may be found in patients on sulfa drugs. Large numbers of calcium oxalate crystals are associated with ethylene glycol overdose (Kim & Corwin, 2001)

Urinary Electrolytes

The kidneys regulate electrolytes via several complex processes. When renal abnormalities occur, the amount of these substances found in the urine changes. To measure urinary electrolyte levels, a 24-hour sample is usually required. However, electrolytes are frequently measured using an aliquot of urine when an estimate is needed or a 24-hour collection is not practical. The results vary greatly and depend on a variety of dietary and hormonal influences. In addition, diuretics can alter test results, regardless of their site of action. The normal ranges of urinary electrolytes appear in Table 8-11.

The urine sodium is of particular clinical importance in evaluating the patient with renal function abnormalities. A urine sodium concentration less that 20 mEq/L is usually associated with volume depletion or decreased blood flow to the kidneys and suggests that renal tubular mechanisms are intact, actively conserving sodium, and able to concentrate urine. A urine sodium in excess of 40 mEq/L may indicate that the kidneys are loosing their ability to concentrate as seen in some type of acute renal failure and chronic renal disease.

The fractional excretion of sodium (FENa) is an additional parameter used to assess renal tubular function. The FENa is the ratio of the amount of sodium excreted in the urine to the amount of sodium filtered by the kidney. Normally, the amount of sodium actually excreted is less that 1% because a functioning kidney reabsorbs 99% of filtered sodium. The FENa is greater than 1% when tubular dysfunction with the inability to absorb normal amounts of sodium is present; this may also be seen with diuretic use (Anderson & Schrier, 2001; Toto, 2004). To measure the FENa, a spot urine sample for sodium and creatinine is obtained simultaneously with a serum sample for sodium (Na) and creatinine (cr) (Anderson & Schrier, 2001). The FENa is calculated as follows:

$$FENa = \frac{U_{Na} \times P_{cr}}{U_{cr} \times P_{Na}} \times 100$$

Urine Volume

The normal adult produces approximately 600 to 2500 mL in 24 hours, an amount that is directly related to fluid intake, the temperature and climate, and the amount of perspiration. Children void smaller quantities in proportion to their body weight. The volume of urine produced at night is < 700 mL, making the day-to-night ratio approximately 2:1 to 4:1(Fischback, 2004). The urine volume, however, is generally of little diagnostic value. Even patients with advanced renal disease may maintain an adequate urine volume, as total output is determined not by the GFR alone but by the difference between the GFR and tubular reabsorption. Thus, a patient whose GFR has fallen from the normal of 180 L/day down to near end stage renal failure of 10 L/day will still have a urine output of 2 liters if only 8 liters of the filtrate are reabsorbed. In early renal failure, urine volume may actually increase as tubular function decreases and patients complain of polyuria and nocturia.

Anuria, oliguria, and polyuria are terms used to denote the volume of urine produced. Anuria is defined as the excretion of 100 ml or less of urine a day and suggests urinary tract obstruction or other more rare conditions such as rapidly progressive glomerulonephritis, mechanical occlusion of renal blood flow, and diffuse renal cortical necrosis (Anderson & Schrier, 2001; Toto, 2004). Oliguria is defined as the production of less than 400 ml of urine a day and is often seen in volume depletion and both acute and chronic renal failure (Anderson & Schrier, 2001). Nonoliguria is used to describe renal failure states accompanied by the production of significant volumes of urine; in acute renal failure, a nonoliguric clinical picture is associated with lower morbidity and mortality and better long-term outcome than an oliguric state (Allgren et al., 1997; Lewis et al., 2000). Polyuria refers to excessive urine production and can occur with both normal BUN and creatinine levels (diabetes mellitus, diabetes insipidus, compulsive water drinking, and certain tumors of the brain and spinal cored) and in the face of elevated BUN and creatinine (acute renal failure and partial urinary tract obstruction) (Fischback, 2004).

Table 8-10
Urinary Sediment and Clinical Significance

Finding	Normal	Clinical Significance
Cells		
RBC	0-5/HPF	2 to 3 RBCs/HPF may be very significant. Present in urinary calculi, UTIs, urinary tract inflammation, malignancies, bleeding from trauma, glomerulopathies, tubulointerstitial nephrities, vascular disease, urologic disorders renal vein thrombosis, coagulopathies, and anticoagulant drugs. Dysmorphic (malformed) cells indicate glomerular disease.
WBC	0-5/HPF	UTIs, urinary tract inflammation, tubulointerstitial nephritis. Eosinophils are associated with drug induced interstitial nephritis.
Epithelial cells		
Transitional	None	Inflammatory conditions of the renal pelvis, ureters or bladder; malignancies
Squamous	None	Female and terminal male urethra
Renal tubular	None	Acute tubular necrosis, nephrotoxicity, transplant rejection
Casts		
RBC	None	Glomerulopathies, vasculitis
WBC	None	Interstitial nephritis, pyelonephritis, acute tubular necrosis
Granular	Occasional	Seen in small numbers in normal urine, but common in disease states. May have fine granules that are small and regular. Coarse granular cats may represent early degeneration of cellular casts. Muddy brown granular cast is characteristic of acute tubular necrosis
Waxy	None	Advanced renal failure
Fatty	None	Heavy proteinuria
Hyaline	Occasional	Appear in small numbers in normal urine or in stress, exercise, fever, diuretics, and dehydration. Appear in large number in disease states. Casts may be much wider (broad casts) when formed in damaged, dilated, or hypertrophied nephrons.
Epithelial cell	None	Tubular injury, glomerulonephritis, drug effects
Crystals		
Uric acid	Occasional	Acid urine, acute uric acid nephropathy, hyperuricosuria
Ca phosphate	Occasional	Alkaline urine
Ca oxalate	Occasional	Acid urine, hyperoxaluria, ethylene glycol poisoning
Sulfur	None	Sulfadiazine antibiotics
Cystine	None	Cystinuria, a hereditary disorder

HPF = high powered field

Note: From Kim & Corwin (2001); NKF (2000c); Parker (1998).

Radiologic Studies in Renal Disease

Several radiologic studies are used to provide data in the evaluation of a patient with renal failure. A list of these procedures and the information they provide are outlined in Table 8-12.

The following nursing interventions are important for any individual who is undergoing these procedures.
1. Explain the procedure to the individual, emphasizing the individual's responsibilities during the procedure.
2. Reinforce the explanations that have been previously provided by other health care team personnel concerning the procedure.
3. Complete any preparatory activities required for the procedure; inquire regarding any allergies to IV contrast material.
4. Provide appropriate fluids to assist the individual in maintaining an adequate hydration state before and after the procedure.
5. Assist with the procedure whenever possible or necessary.

6. Document the individual's response to the procedure (Parker, 1998; Thomas, 2002).

Renal Biopsy

A renal biopsy is performed in patients with renal parenchymal disease when other tests have been unable to identify the correct diagnosis or in order to prescribe the most appropriate therapy. This is especially important in patients with glomerular disease or vasculitis when the urinalysis, serum creatinine, and serologic studies have not provided sufficient information. Indications for renal biopsy include hematuria of renal origin; proteinuria; rapidly progressing, unexplained renal failure; and acute renal failure of undetermined etiology or with a prolonged course. Contraindications to a renal biopsy include bleeding, solitary or horseshoe kidney, urinary tract infection, uncontrolled hypertension, and an uncooperative patient. Kidney biopsy is not indicated for patients with chronic, end stage kidney disease and, in this setting, may be associated with a higher risk of complications (Croker & Tisher, 2001; Silkensen & Kasiske, 2004).

A percutaneous renal biopsy is a procedure during which a biopsy needle is inserted through the skin of the flank area under local anesthesia and directed by ultrasonography or computed tomography (CT) (Silkensen & Kasiske, 2004). Open surgical biopsy under local or general anesthesia may be performed if a biopsy is needed and the patient has a bleeding abnormality or has some technical contraindication to the percutaneous procedure. Following the biopsy, the small piece of renal cortical tissue that was obtained is submitted to histological examination by light, electronmicroscopy, and immunoflouresence. This examination provides specific information about the glomerular basement membrane and surrounding renal tissues and greatly assists in determining the diagnosis and appropriate medical therapy.

The nurse's responsibilities in preparing the patient for a renal biopsy include:

1. explaining the procedure, postprocedural care, and client responsibilities and ensuring that salicylates and nonsteroidal anti-inflammatory drugs have been discon-

Table 8-11
Normal Urinary Electrolytes

Electrolyte	Normal Range
Sodium	40 – 220 mEq/24 hours
Potassium	25 – 125 mEq/24 hours
Chloride	140 – 250 mE/24 hours
Calcium	100 – 300 mg/24 hours
Magnesium	12 – 199 mg/24 hours

Note: From Fischback (2004).

Table 8-12
Radiologic Procedures Used in the Evaluation of the Patient with Renal Failure

Test	Use
KUB	Kidney number, size, shape, and placement Diagnosis and monitoring of radiopaque stones
IVP	Kidney number, size, shape, and calyceal anatomy Detection of site and cause of obstruction (ultrasound preferable for screening) Bladder
Ultrasound & CT	General appearance, size, and scarring Evaluation for possible urinary tract obstruction Evaluation for renal mass (cyst versus tumor) Early diagnosis of polycystic kidney disease Detection of radiolucent kidney stones
Radionuclide studies	Screening for renovascular hypertension Screening for renal thrombo-emboli Screening for tumors and cysts Assess symmetry of blood flow
Renal arteriography	Direct visualization of renal arterial system for renovascular hypertension, thrombo-emboli, or diagnosis of renal mass that seems noncystic on other studies
Voiding cystourethrogram	Detection of vesicoureteral reflux
Retrograde or antegrade pyelography	Determination of site of obstruction Relief of obstruction (catheters inserted)
Magnetic resonance imaging (MRI)	More specific than ultrasonography and CT. Helpful in detection of renal masses and malformations of vessels and tubules

Note: From Chang & Hricak (2001); Croker & Tisher (2001); Hricak, Meux, & Reddy (2004); Morris & Rimmer (2001); NKF (2000c); Parker (1998); Webb & Britton (2001).

tinued 1 to 2 weeks before the procedure (to help prevent bleeding).

2. demonstrating position during the test and breathing techniques, and having the patient return the demonstration.
3. verifying that informed consent has been obtained.
4. verifying that hematologic evaluation such as CBC, prothrombin, partial thromboplastin time, bleeding and clotting time, and type and crossmatching for possible transfusion have been completed.
5. verifying that evaluation of renal function by urinalysis and determination of kidney position and depth by ultrasonography or KUB has been done.
6. providing sedation, depending on the patient.

Following biopsy, the major potential complications are hemorrhage and gross hematuria. These complications occur in less than 10% of patients and frequently subside after 24 hours of bed rest. Perirenal hematomas radiologically develop in 50% to 80% but are rarely clinically significant. Other possible complications include laceration of the spleen, liver, gallbladder, and bowel; arteriovenous fistulae formation; and infection. The overall risk of kidney loss following biopsy is less than 0.1 percent (Croker & Tisher, 2001; Korbel, 2002).

The nurse should monitor the patient frequently during the post-procedure period checking the vital signs every 15 minutes for the first hour, every 30 minutes for the second hour, every hour for the next 4 hours, and every 4 hours for the next 24 hours. The nurse should also inspect all urine produced for blood. This can be done by saving specimens in clear plastic cups from one voiding to the next in order to observe the color changes closely. The biopsy site should be inspected frequently for signs of bleeding, and the patient should be assessed and treated for flank pain. In addition, fluids should be given either orally or parenterally in order to dilute the urine and prevent intrarenal clot formation (Parker, 1998).

Summary

The assessment of the renal system includes the history, physical examination, and diagnostic tests. The history includes an evaluation of the persons' chief complaint and history of present illness, past medical and surgical history, family history, personal and social history, and a review of body systems. The physical examination consists of the general survey, vital signs, height and weight, and examination. Diagnostic tests include analyses of the blood and urine, measures of renal clearance and GFR, radiologic procedures, and renal biopsy. Nurses have an important role in the evaluation of individuals with renal problems and should be well versed in the findings that indicate abnormalities and clinical change.

References

Allgren, R.L., Marbury, T.C., Rahman, S.N., Weisberg, L.S., Fenves, A.Z., Lafayette, R.A., et al. (1997). Anaritide in acute tubular necrosis. Auriculin anaritide acute renal failure study group. *New England Journal of Medicine, 336*(12), 828-834.

Anderson, R.J. (2001). Clinical and laboratory diagnosis of acute renal failure. In B.A. Molitoris & W.F. Finn (Eds.), *Acute renal failure: A companion to Brenner & Rector's the kidney* (pp. 157-168). Philadelphia: W.B. Saunders Company.

Anderson, R.J., & Schrier, R.W. (2001). Acute renal failure. In R.W. Schrier (Ed.), *Diseases of the kidney and urinary tract* (7th ed.) (Vol.

2). Philadelphia: Lippincott Wilkins & Williams.

Bickley, L.S., & Szilagyi, P.G. (2003). *Bates' guide to physical examination and history taking* (8th ed.). Philadelphia: Lippincott Williams & Wilkins.

Chang, S.D., & Hricak. (2001). Computed tomography and magnetic resonance imaging. In R.W. Schrier (Ed.), *Diseases of the kidney and urinary tract* (7th ed.) (Vol. 1) (pp. 411-430). Philadelphia: Lippincott Williams & Wilkins.

Coresh, J., Toto, R.D., Kirk, K.A., Whelton, P.K., Massry, S., Jones, C., et al. (1998). Creatinine clearance as a measure of GFR in screening for the African-American study of kidney disease and hypertension pilot study. *American Journal of Kidney Disease, 32*(1), 32-42.

Croker, B.P., & Tisher, C.C. (2001). Indications for and interpretation of the renal biopsy. In R.W. Schrier (Ed.), *Diseases of the kidney and urinary tract* (7th ed.) (Vol. 1) (pp. 457-487). Philadelphia: Lippincott Williams & Wilkins.

Fischback, F.T. (2004). *Manual of laboratory and diagnostic tests* (7th ed.). Philadelphia: Lippincott Williams & Williams.

Headley, C.M., & Wall, B. (2002). ESRD-associated cutaneous manifestations in a hemodialysis population. *Nephrology Nursing Journal, 29*(6), 525-539.

Holechek, M.J. (2003). Glomerular filtration: An overview. *Nephrology Nursing Journal, 30*(3), 285-290.

Hricak, H., Meux, M., & Reddy, G. (2004). Radiologic assessment of the kidney. In B.M. Brenner (Ed.), *Brenner & Rector's the kidney* (7th ed., Vol. 1, pp. 1183-1214). Philadelphia: Saunders.

Kim, M.S., & Corwin, H.L. (2001). Urinalysis. In R.W. Schrier (Ed.), *Diseases of the kidney and urinary tract* (7th ed.) (Vol. 1) (pp. 317-331). Philadelphia: Lippincott Wilkins & Williams.

Korbel, S.M. (2002). Percutaneous renal biopsy. *Seminars in Nephrology, 22*, 254-267.

Lafayette, R.A., Perrone, R.D., & Levey, A.S. (2001). Laboratory evaluation of renal function. In R.W. Schrier (Ed.), *Disease of the kidney and urinary tract* (7th ed.) (Vol. 1) (pp. 333-369). Philadelphia: Lippincott Williams & Wilkins.

Lewis, J., Salem, M.M., Chertow, G.M., Weisberg, L.S., McGrew, F., Marbury, T.C., et al. (2000). Atrial natriuretic factor in oliguric acute renal failure. Anaritide acute renal failure study group. *American Journal of Kidney Disease, 36*(4), 767-774.

Lewis, S.L. (1992). Fever: Thermal regulation and alterations in end stage renal disease patients. *ANNA Journal, 19*(1), 13-18.

McGee, S., Abernethy, W.B., 3rd, & Simel, D.L. (1999). The rational clinical examination. Is this patient hypovolemic? *Journal of the American Medical Association, 281*(11), 1022-1029.

Morris, C.S., & Rimmer, J.M. (2001). Diagnostic and therapeutic angiography of the renal circulation. In R.W. Schrier (Ed.), *Diseases of the kidney and urinary tract* (7th ed.) (Vol. 1) (pp. 431-456). Philadelphia: Lippincott Williams & Wilkins.

National Kidney Foundation (NKF). (2000a). *K/DOQI clinical practice guidelines for chronic kidney disease evaluation. Part 4. Definition and classification of stages of chronic kidney disease. Guideline 1. Definition and stages of chronic kidney disease.* www.kidney.org/professionals/doqi/kdoqi/p4_classg2.htm

National Kidney Foundation (NKF). (2000b). *K/DOQI clinical practice guidelines for chronic kidney disease: Evaluation, classification, and stratification. Part 5. Evaluation of laboratory measurements for clinical assessment of kidney disease. Guideline 5. Assessment of proteinuria.* Retrieved from www.kidney.org/professionals/doqi/kdoqi/p5_lab_g5.htm

National Kidney Foundation (NKF). (2000c). *K/DOQI clinical practice guidelines for chronic kidney disease: Evaluation, classification, and stratification. Part 5. Evaluation of laboratory measurements for clinical assessment of kidney disease. Guideline 6. Markers of chronic kidney disease other than proteinuria*. Retrieved from www.kidney.org/professionals/doqi/kdoqi/p5_lab_g6.htm

National Kidney Foundation (NKF). (2002). K/DOQI clinical practice guidelines for chronic kidney disease: Evaluation, classification, and stratification. *American Journal of Kidney Disease, 39*(2 Suppl. 1), S1-266.

Parker, K.P. (1998). Renal patient assessment. In M.R. Kinney, S.B. Dunbar, J. Brooks-Brunn, N. Molter, & J.M. Vitello-Cicciu (Eds.), *AACN's clinical reference for critical care nursing* (4th ed., pp. 785-796). St. Louis, MO: Mosby.

Schneditz, D. (2001). Temperature and thermal balance in hemodialysis. *Seminars in Dialysis, 14*(5), 357-364.

Silkensen, J.R., & Kasiske, B.L. (2004). Laboratory assessment of kidney disease: Clearance, urinalysis, and kidney biopsy. In B.M. Brenner (Ed.), *Brenner and Rector's the kidney* (7th ed.) (Vol. 1) (pp. 1107-1150). Philadelphia: Saunders.

Stern, J.A., Hsieh, Y.C., & Schaeffer, A.J. (2004). Residual urine in an elderly female population: Novel implications for oral estrogen replacement and impact on recurrent urinary tract infection. *Journal of Urology, 171*(2 Pt. 1), 768-770.

Swartz, M.H. (2002). *Textbook of physical diagnosis history and examination* (4th ed.). Philadelphia: W.B. Saunders.

Thomas, N. (2002). *Renal nursing* (2nd ed.). London: Bailliere Tindall.

Toto, R.D. (2004). Approach to the patient with kidney disease. In B.M. Brenner (Ed.), *Brenner & Rector's the kidney* (Vol. 7) (pp. 1070-1106). Philadelphia: Saunders.

Webb, J.A.W., & Britton, K.E. (2001). Intravenous urography, ultrasonography, and radionuclide studies. In R.W. Schrier (Ed.), *Disease of the kidney and urinary tract* (7th ed.) (Vol. 1) (pp. 371-410). Philadelphia: Lippincott Williams & Wilkins.

- If renal abnormality is identified, the primary goals are to establish the correct diagnosis; to assess and monitor the severity of the renal dysfunction; to reverse or slow the progression of renal dysfunction, if possible (Anderson & Schrier, 2001; National Kidney Foundation [NKF], 2000a; Toto, 2004); and to address the associated nursing concerns (Thomas, 2002).

- A history can be divided into six components including the chief complaint, history of present illness, past medical and surgical history, family history, personal and social history, and a review of body systems (Bickley & Szilagyi, 2003).

- The physical examination consists of the process by which the clinician observes, palpates, percusses, and auscultates the body of an individual and describes the findings (signs) elicited by these processes.

- Diagnostic tests are crucial in evaluating patients with renal function abnormalities. In addition to the complete history and physical, the information obtained from these tests helps to describe the degree of renal dysfunction present and associated systemic effects.

- The most commonly used tests include blood analyses, measures of glomerular filtration rate (GFR) and renal clearance, urinalysis, urinary electrolytes, urine volume, radiologic studies in renal disease, and renal biopsy.

- Serum creatinine is affected, not only by GFR, but also age, gender, race, body size, diet, drugs, laboratory analytical techniques, and extrarenal creatinine excretion.

- GFR provides an excellent measure of renal function. A low or decreasing GFR precedes kidney failure, and monitoring changes can help determine the progression of the disease.

- The urine is a very complex body fluid, containing filtrates from blood and other elements from the kidneys, ureters, and bladder. As a result the urinalysis is a major diagnostic tool for evaluating the patient with renal abnormalities. The analysis should ideally be conducted within 1 to 2 hours after voiding and typically includes visual inspection, dipstick testing, and examination of urine sediment.

- Anuria, oliguria, and polyuria are terms used to denote the volume of urine produced.

- Radiologic studies are used to provide data in the evaluation of a patient with renal failure.

- A renal biopsy is performed in patients with renal parenchymal disease when other tests have been unable to identify the correct diagnosis or in order to prescribe the most appropriate therapy.

- Nurses have an important role in the evaluation of individuals with renal problems and should be well versed in the findings that indicate abnormalities and clinical change.

Assessment of the Renal System

Name of Resource	Brief Description	Where to Obtain Resource
Calculation of Glomerular Filtration Rate	Provides a GFR calculator using the Cockcroft and Gault, Modified Diet in Renal Disease, and Schwartz equations.	www.nkdep.nih.gov/GFR-cal.htm
K/DOQI Clinical Practice Guidelines for Chronic Kidney Disease: Evaluation, Classification, and Stratification	Part 5. Evaluation of Laboratory Measurements for Clinical Assessment of Kidney Disease Guideline 4. Estimation of GFR. Provides background and information regarding measures of renal clearance and glomerular filtration rate.	www.kidney.org/professionals/doqi/kdoqi/p5_lab_g4.htm
K/DOQI Clinical Practice Guidelines for Chronic Kidney Disease: Evaluation, Classification, and Stratification	Part 5. Evaluation of Laboratory Measurements for Clinical Assessment of Kidney Disease Guideline 5. Assessment of Proteinuria. Provide guidelines for the assessment of proteinuria and appropriate clinical follow-up.	www.kidney.org/professionals/doqi/kdoqi/p5_lab_g5.htm
K/DOQI Clinical Practice Guidelines for Chronic Kidney Disease: Evaluation, Classification, and Stratification	Part 5. Evaluation of Laboratory Measurements for Clinical Assessment of Kidney Disease. Guideline 6. Markers of Chronic Kidney Disease Other Than Proteinuria. Provides information regarding urine sediment and imaging studies often performed in persons with chronic kidney disease.	www.kidney.org/professionals/doqi/kdoqi/p5_lab_g6.htm

ANNP608

Assessment of the Renal System

Kathy P. Parker, PhD, RN, FAAN

Contemporary Nephrology Nursing: Principles and Practice contains 39 chapters of educational content. Individual learners may apply for continuing nursing education credit by reading a chapter and completing the Continuing Education Evaluation Form for that chapter. Learners may apply for continuing education credit for any or all chapters.

Please photocopy this page and return to ANNA.
COMPLETE THE FOLLOWING:

Name: _____

Address:_____

City:_____ State: _____ Zip: _____

E-mail: _____

Preferred telephone: ☐ Home   ☐ Work: _____

State where licensed and license number (optional): _____

CE application fees are based upon the number of contact hours provided by the individual chapter. CE fees per contact hour for ANNA members are as follows: 1.0-1.9 - $15; 2.0-2.9 - $20; 3.0-3.9 - $25; 4.0 and higher - $30. Fees for nonmembers are $10 higher.

ANNA Member: ☐ Yes   ☐ No   Member # (if available) _____

☐ Checked Enclosed   ☐ American Express   ☐ Visa   ☐ MasterCard

Total Amount Submitted: _____

Credit Card Number: _____ Exp. Date: _____

Name as it appears on the card: _____

CE Evaluation Form
To receive continuing education credit for individual study after reading the chapter
1. Photocopy this form. (You may also download this form from ANNA's Web site, **www.annanurse.org.**)
2. Mail the completed form with payment (check) or credit card information to American Nephrology Nurses' Association, East Holly Avenue, Box 56, Pitman, NJ 08071-0056.
3. You will receive your CE certificate from ANNA in 4 to 6 weeks.

Test returns must be postmarked by **December 31, 2010.**

CE Application Fee
ANNA Member $15.00
Nonmember $25.00

EVALUATION FORM

1. I verify that I have read this chapter and completed this education activity. Date: _____

_____
Signature

2. What would be different in your practice if you applied what you learned from this activity? *(Please use additional sheet of paper if necessary.)*

Evaluation	Strongly disagree				Strongly agree
3. The activity met the stated objectives.					
a. Summarize the important information to be collected in the patient history portion of a nursing assessment.	1	2	3	4	5
b. Describe an ideal physical assessment of a patient with renal abnormalities.	1	2	3	4	5
c. Analyze diagnostic test results for suggestions of renal abnormalities.	1	2	3	4	5
4. The content was current and relevant.	1	2	3	4	5
5. The content was presented clearly.	1	2	3	4	5
6. The content was covered adequately.	1	2	3	4	5
7. Rate your ability to apply the learning obtained from this activity to practice.	1	2	3	4	5

Comments _____

8. Time required to read the chapter and complete this form: _____ minutes.

This educational activity has been provided by the American Nephrology Nurses' Association (ANNA) for 1.7 contact hours. ANNA is accredited as a provider of continuing nursing education (CNE) by the American Nurses Credentialing Center's Commission on Accreditation (ANCC-COA). ANNA is an approved provider of continuing education by the California Board of Registered Nursing, CEP 0910.

Acute Renal Failure

Christy Price Rabetoy, NP

Chapter Contents

Christy Price Rabetoy, NP

Acute renal failure (ARF) may be defined as a rapid decline in glomerular filtration rate (GFR) (greater than 50% reduction), usually causing oliguria or anuria and resulting in the accumulation of metabolic wastes in the blood (azotemia). This condition is a potentially fatal complication of critical illness, traumatic injury, and certain therapeutic regimens. The term ARF is generic and refers to this sudden renal impairment without regard to a specific cause or mechanism. ARF happens most often in acute care facilities, reaching an overall incidence of 2%-5% of hospitalized patients (Kellerman, 1994). The incidence increases to 10%-30% in the critically ill (Mehta et al., 2004; Schrier & Wang, 2004). Although ARF is frequently a reversible process (often self-limiting), it may also be irreversible and lead to chronic kidney disease (CKD) or failure. ARF may occur in a patient with pre-existing CKD, and in this situation, it is often reversible but only to the previous baseline of renal function. However, quite often ARF in the setting of CKD leads to severe chronic renal failure (CRF) because the additional insult to already marginal renal function cannot be overcome.

Although renal replacement therapies have been available for over 30 years, the mortality associated with ARF continues to be approximately 50% (Siegel & Shah, 2003; Swartz, Perry, & Daley, 2004). For those with ARF requiring dialysis, the mortality is often higher (Kjellstrand & Solez, 1993; Siegel & Shah, 2003). Thus, the outcome of ARF is not exclusively related to the sequelae associated with failure of the kidneys. Rather, numerous studies have demonstrated that the outcome of ARF is dependent on age, intercurrent sepsis, hypoalbuminemia, and factors that determine failure of other organs (Kellerman, 1994; Siegel & Shah, 2003; Spurney, Fulkerson, & Schwab, 1991). There is a general belief that dialysis significantly influences mortality outcomes of patients with these comorbid conditions (Alexopoulos et al., 1994; Mehta et al., 2004; Siegel & Shah, 2003).

The treatment of ARF in the U.S. has military roots coinciding with the treatment of war casualties during World War II, Korean police action, and the Vietnam conflict. The clinical experience gained from these difficult periods in history has led to changes, which in current practice allow nephrology and critical care professionals to effectively manage the fluid, electrolyte, and acid/base abnormalities that occur secondary to acute kidney dysfunction. The mortality and morbidity associated with ARF was extremely high during the two world wars. The multisystem sequelae and sepsis that often accompany ARF secondary to traumatic injuries and/or gunshot wounds led to the triage of many soldiers to the "expectant" category. In 1948, the first successful use of hemodialysis (HD) in the U.S. was reported as a treatment for ARF related to self-administration of vaginal mercury to induce a spontaneous abortion (McBride, 1987). During the Korean police action, military nephrologists were able to use HD successfully, which led to saving many young lives. Upon returning to civilian practice, these military physicians provided valuable experience for the training of future

nephrologists. Shortly thereafter, nurses became involved in the delivery of HD and the care of patients with ARF. After the passage in 1972 of PL 92-603, which assured Medicare coverage for patients with CKD at Stage 5, more physicians and nurses were needed to provide dialytic therapy to the growing patient population. It is this expanded coverage and availability for the treatment of CKD that led to an increase in the number of professionals with the knowledge and experience to safely and effectively treat ARF. However, the best treatment for ARF is prevention by close monitoring of hemodynamic parameters, avoidance of known nephrotoxic exposures, and early intervention for vascular volume deficit.

Definitions and Types of Acute Renal Failure

The continuum of renal function (see Table 9-1) is historical and has been defined in terms of GFR. Normal renal function is at one end of this continuum and is a state in which the kidneys can easily meet the metabolic demands of the body. The GFR of normal kidneys is approximately 100-125 ml/minute/1.73m^2 (the body surface area of an average 70 kg adult). Diminished renal reserve (DRR), defined as a GFR of 50-70 ml/minute, is a state in which the patient is asymptomatic and the small but significant decrease in renal function can be detected only by specific laboratory tests. Loss of additional function leads to renal insufficiency with a GFR of 15-50 ml/min, a condition that can be identified easily with routine laboratory tests and that may produce symptoms as the kidneys become increasingly unable to meet metabolic and dietary stresses. A GFR of less than 10-15 ml/minute is classified as end stage renal disease (ESRD), a state in which the kidneys are unable to maintain a homeostatic internal environment. The current classification of chronic renal dysfunction is introduced in Chapter 10.

Renal failure is broadly classified as acute and chronic. In ARF, renal function deteriorates rapidly, whereas CKD develops slowly, sometimes over a period of years or decades. ARF may also be superimposed on preexisting CKD. In all situations, the associated pathophysiology triggers multisystemic abnormalities that predispose the patient to several serious problems requiring complex medical and nursing care. The needs of ARF patients are complex, and the nurse must possess a knowledge base characterized by breadth as well as depth. The purpose of this chapter is to provide the nurse with an overview of the processes, manifestations, and implications of ARF. The material covered will include assessment and diagnostic parameters; etiology and pathophysiologic bases; and clinical presentation, treatment, and nursing management.

The clinical assessment of renal failure may be very comprehensive. Patients with ARF may present in a variety of ways. Some have symptoms that are directly related to the kidney, such as flank pain and gross hematuria, while others may present with associated extrarenal abnormalities such as edema; hypertension; and signs and symptoms of uremia, for example nausea, vomiting, or pruritus (Rose & Rennke, 1994). Patients with mild renal insufficiency may be completely asymptomatic and only incidentally found to have

Table 9-1
Continuum of Renal Function from Normal to Renal Failure

Stage	Clinical Symptoms	GFR (ml/minute/1.73m²)/Signs
Normal		GFR: 125 ml/min
Diminished Renal Reserve	Asymptomatic	GFR: 50 to 70 ml/min Small elevations in serum creatinine Possibly proteinuria
Renal Insufficiency	Early symptoms may include nocturia. Later, signs and symptoms of uremia develop, including nausea, edema, fatigue, and hypertension	GFR: 10 to 50 ml/min Azotemia, acidosis, hyperkalemia, hypocalcemia, hyperphosphatemia, anemia
Renal Failure	Manifestations of uremic syndrome	GFR: less than 10 ml/min Azotemia, acidosis, hyperkalemia, hypocalcemia, hyperphosphatemia, anemia

Note: Adapted from Dubrow & Levin (1995); Price (1992a); Ulrich (1989).

abnormal renal function during the course of their hospitalization. Patients may experience ARF in a community setting and never know it, as it resolves before laboratory data are collected. Clinical management, prevention of complications, and patient prognosis differ depending on the etiology and clinical presentation.

Once the renal abnormality is discovered, the primary goals are to establish the correct diagnosis, to assess and monitor the severity of the renal dysfunction (Rose & Rennke, 1994), to reverse or slow the progression of renal dysfunction, if possible, and to address the associated nursing concerns. As part of this process, it is important to determine whether the renal failure is acute or chronic and to assess the systemic impact of the renal abnormality. This may not be simple, especially if previous data are not readily available. Thus, it is important to know how to collect and process the appropriate information.

The initial approach to the evaluation of patients with renal failure begins with the history, physical examination, and appropriate diagnostic tests. Not only is this information crucial in diagnosing the problem, but also it is important in designing an effective medical and nursing treatment plan with appropriate expected patient outcomes. The clinical presentation of renal failure may vary, and nurses who work in settings ranging from walk-in clinics and emergency rooms to hospitals and critical care units are likely to be involved in the evaluation, education, follow-up, and emotional support of patients and their families. Therefore, nurses should be knowledgeable regarding the evaluation process, including the components of the history and physical exam that are specifically related to the renal system as well as the most frequently used diagnostic tests (Baer, 1993a). It is critical that a detailed present patient history, the presenting patient symptoms and complaints, and the patient past medical history and the family history of illness are thoroughly documented. As with any disease process, there are several factors of particular importance to explore with the patient and family (see Table 9-2).

Renal function begins with ultrafiltration of blood, proceeds with the intrarenal processing of the filtrate, and ends with excretion of urine via the ureters, bladder, and urethra. It follows, then, that the syndrome of ARF may develop from reduced renal blood flow (RBF), prerenal ARF; from a sudden, severe renal parenchymal insult, intrarenal ARF; or from obstruction to urine flow, postrenal ARF. Although all three disturbances ultimately reduce the GFR, each disorder causes a different physiological response. These differences form the basis of the tests used to identify the specific disorder and, subsequently, to determine the appropriate treatment and nursing care (Faber, Kupin, Krishna, & Narins, 1993).

Prerenal Failure

Etiology and pathophysiology. The kidneys receive approximately 20% of the cardiac output. This blood flow provides the large GFR that is necessary for efficient clearance of metabolic waste products and exceeds the metabolic needs of the kidney tissue (Holechek, 1992). A reduction in RBF diminishes the fundamental driving force for glomerular filtration. It also decreases the nutrients and oxygen for basic renal cellular metabolism and tubular transport systems (Baer & Lancaster, 1992; Lancaster, 2001). Thus, prerenal failure (also referred to as prerenal azotemia) results when the blood fails to reach the kidneys, causing renal hypoperfusion and a subsequent reduction in glomerular perfusion and filtration. This state is immediately reversed upon restoration of RBF and is not associated with structural damage in the kidney. However, prerenal failure frequently precedes or contributes to the development of acute intrarenal failure.

The causes of prerenal failure can be divided into four

Table 9-2

Factors to Explore with the Patient and Family that are Potentially Related to

History of exposure to environmental agents

Travel to areas of the world where exposure to infectious agents is high

Illegal drug use, over-the-counter (OTC) use, and use of prescription medication

Weight changes reflective of fluid gains or loss of appetite

Changes in routine activities and exercise tolerance

Allergies related to potential precipitation of renal dysfunction

Diet patterns, including use of supplements and weight reduction aids

Any underlying chronic diseases or conditions

Table 9-3

Causes of Prerenal Failure (Azotemia)

Decreased Cardiac Output

Myocardial infarction
Cardiac failure
Cardiac dysrhythmias
Cardiac tamponade

Volume Depletion

Skin losses (excessive sweating or burns)
Gastrointestinal losses (vomiting and diarrhea)
Urinary losses (diuretics)
Hemorrhage
Third spacing of fluid (ascites, nephrotic syndrome, burns, acute pancreatitis)

Vasodilation

Shock
Sepsis
Anaphylaxis
Extreme acidosis
Treatment with antihypertensive agents

Renovascular Obstruction

Renal artery thrombosis (usually accompanied by renal parenchymal damage)
Renal vein thrombosis (usually accompanied by renal parenchymal damage)
Renal artery stenosis

Note: Adapted from Agmon & Brezis (1993); Faber et al. (1993); Rose & Rennke (1994); Toto (1990).

major categories: decreased cardiac output, volume depletion, vasodilation, and obstruction of renal vessels (see Table 9-3). A decrease in effective arterial blood volume (EABV) characterizes the first three of these situations. The EABV is an unmeasurable parameter that refers to that part of the extracellular fluid in the arterial system actually available for perfusion of the tissues (Rose & Rennke, 1994). The EABV can be decreased as a result of true intravascular volume depletion from hemorrhage, diarrhea, over diuresis, isotonic fluid losses, or from a redistribution of plasma volume to a third space. However, reductions in EABV can also occur in volume expanded states that are characterized by decreased renal perfusion, such as congestive heart failure (decreased cardiac output), advanced liver disease (pooling of blood in the portal circulation), and vasodilation from sepsis (Faber et al., 1993). Occasionally, prerenal failure can result from a vessel obstruction, such as renal artery stenosis or thrombosis, or damage to small vessels and glomerular capillaries, as in atherosclerosis and diabetes mellitus.

Under normal circumstances, the GFR is maintained despite changes in renal perfusion by several intrinsic and extrinsic factors. Autoregulation is an intrinsic mechanism that preserves renal perfusion and GFR through dilation of the afferent and constriction of the efferent arterioles in the face of reductions in renal perfusion pressure. This process serves as an important defense mechanism against intrarenal failure in kidneys that are underperfused. However, the autoregulation process is effective until the systolic blood pressure decreases below approximately 70 mm/Hg, at which point maximal afferent vasodilation occurs (Burnett, 1993). Below this level, renal autoregulation is severely altered by the associated intense sympathetic and renin-angiotensin activity. In response, the afferent arteriole constricts and glomerular blood flow and GFR decrease (Baer & Lancaster, 1992).

Reduced renal perfusion also stimulates the renin-angiotensin mechanism (RAM). Renin is released and subsequently converted to angiotensin I and angiotensin II (a powerful vasoconstrictor), which also stimulates the production of aldosterone. Aldosterone increases renal absorption of sodium. The resulting increase in serum osmolality stimulates the release of antidiuretic hormone (ADH) and enhances tubular absorption of water (Holechek, 1992). The net result is renal and systemic vasoconstriction, and sodium and water retention (see Figure 9-1).

It is the ability of the kidney to successfully retain salt

Figure 9-1
Intrarenal Responses to Decreased Renal Perfusion

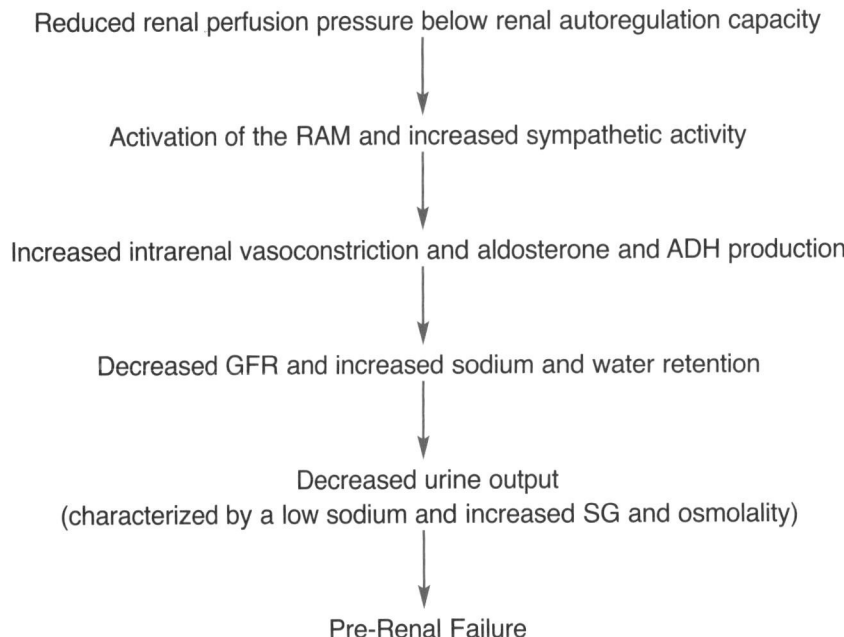

Reduced renal perfusion pressure below renal autoregulation capacity

Activation of the RAM and increased sympathetic activity

Increased intrarenal vasoconstriction and aldosterone and ADH production

Decreased GFR and increased sodium and water retention

Decreased urine output
(characterized by a low sodium and increased SG and osmolality)

Pre-Renal Failure

Note: Adapted from Burnett, J.C. (1993). Acute renal failure associated with cardiac failure and hypo-volemia. In J.M. Lazarus & B.M. Brenner (Eds.), *Acute renal failure* (3rd edition) (p. 200). New York: Churchill Livingstone.

and water that distinguishes prerenal failure from intrarenal and the early stages of postrenal failure (Faber et al., 1993). This increased absorption causes a decrease in urine flow, a drop in urea clearance, and an increase in serum blood urea nitrogen (BUN). Because early prerenal failure depresses the urea clearance more than it depresses the creatinine clearance (because filtered urea is avidly absorbed by the tubules while creatinine is not), BUN increases proportionately more than serum creatinine concentration (Faber et al., 1993). Therefore, the hallmark of prerenal failure is an increase in the BUN to creatinine ratio (> 15:1).

Clinical and laboratory features. Nurses should complete a thorough history and physical assessment on all patients at risk for developing prerenal failure. Risk factors include use of diuretics and antihypertensive agents, exposure to hot weather, fever, diarrhea and vomiting, wounds, burns, recent surgery, cardiac arrest, and other situations listed in Table 9-3. The presence of true volume depletion is usually evident from the history. In addition, fluid loss severe enough to decrease renal perfusion usually causes some of the physical findings associated with volume depletion, such as decreased skin turgor (best assessed on the forehead and sternum) (Faber et al., 1993), dry mucous membranes, postural tachycardia with or without hypotension, and weight loss. Those patients in hypovolemic shock may also have signs of hypoperfusion (due in part to intense peripheral vasoconstriction), such as cold, clammy extremities; cyanosis; agitation; and confusion. Those with decreased EABV from cardiac or hepatic failure may present with signs

and symptoms of volume overload, such as peripheral and pulmonary edema, ascites, jugular vein distention, liver congestion, and an S3 gallop. A decrease in urinary output characterizes prerenal failure. Anuria is rare and is more commonly seen in some types of postrenal failure. Table 9-4 summarizes a systems approach to the physical examination and renal-related signs and symptoms.

Laboratory studies for the assessment of prerenal failure include blood and urine analyses. As previously mentioned, the hallmark of prerenal failure is an elevation in the BUN to creatinine ratio (may be as high as 40:1). Due to hemoconcentration, plasma albumin and hematocrit may increase. If volume overload is present, decreases in hematocrit and albumin may be noted. Because of the increased renal absorption of sodium and water, urinary sodium levels are characteristically less than 20 mEq/L with elevated urinary specific gravity and osmolality. A summary of the serum and urinary laboratory values found in prerenal failure in comparison to other types of renal failure are summarized in Table 9-5.

Prerenal failure may also be associated with other abnormalities in electrolyte and acid-base balance. For example, elderly patients with diminished mental or physical capabilities may become hypovolemic from the inability to obtain fluid and replace insensible losses. Because of the free water deficit, hypernatremia may develop. On the other hand, the sodium level may be normal if sodium and water have been lost in proportion, as with diuretic therapy. Metabolic alkalosis may be seen with diuretic therapy or

Table 9-4

Systems Oriented Physical Examination, Renal-Related Signs, and Their Correlated Pathological Conditions

Body System	Sign	Clinical Significance
HEENT	Dry, thin hair	Chronic renal disease
	Periorbital edema	Nephrotic syndrome
	Optic fundi - hemorrhages, exudates	Hypertension/diabetes
	Hearing loss	Drug reaction, Wegener's granulomatosis
	Epistaxis	Uremia, Wegener's granulomatosis
	Halitosis	Uremia
	Dry, cracked mucous membranes	Volume depletion
	Engorged neck veins	Volume excess
	Carotid bruits	Vascular disease
Skin	Decreased tissue turgor (forehead and sternum most reliable)	Volume depletion
	Dry, scaly skin	Uremia
	Pallor	Uremia
	Yellowness	Uremia
	Cyanosis	Cardiac failure
	Maculopapular rash	Drug reaction
	Purpura	Uremia, vasculitis
	Livedo reticularis	Vasculitis
	Pallor of nail beds	Uremia
	Butterfly rash	Lupus erythematosus
Heart	Murmurs	Valvular disease
	Pericardial friction rub	Uremia
	S_3, S_4	Congestive heart failure
Lungs	Pleural rub	Uremia
	Rales	Volume excess
	Decreased breath sounds	Uremia
	Hemoptysis	Pulmonary-renal syndromes
Abdomen	Bruits	Vascular disease
	Enlarged liver	Congestive heart failure
	Enlarged kidneys	Polycystic kidney disease, Hydronephrosis
Rectum	Enlarged prostate	Obstruction
	Tender prostate	Infection
	Occult blood	Uremia
Genitourinary Tract	Distended bladder	Obstruction
	Prostate enlargement	Prostatic hypertrophy
	Flank masses	Polycystic kidney disease
	Pelvic masses	Obstruction
Extremities	Peripheral edema	Volume excess
Musculoskeletal System	Joint pain	Immunologic disorders, uremia
	Bone pain	Uremia
	Proximal muscle weakness	Uremia
Neurologic System	Altered levels of consciousness	Uremia
	Tetany (Chvostek's/Trousseau's)	Electrolyte disturbances
	Depressed reflexes	Electrolyte disturbances, uremia
	Depressed reflexes	Electrolyte disturbances, uremia

Note: Adapted from Baer (1993a); Richard (1986b).

Table 9-5
Significant Laboratory Findings in Acute Renal Failure

Laboratory Test	Pre-Renal	ATN	Post-Renal
Urine volume	Oliguria	Oliguria, nonolguria	Anuria, oliguria, polyuria
Urine osmolality	Concentrated	Isosmotic	Isosmotic
Urine specific gravity	High	Low, fixed	Variable
Urine Na$^+$	< 20	> 20	Variable
FeNa	< 1	> 1	> 1
RFI	< 1	> 1	> 1
BUN	Increased	Increased	Increased
Serum creatinine	May be normal	Increased	Increased
BUN: creatinine	> 15:1	10:1	Normal to increased
Urine creatinine: Plasma creatinine	> 15:1	< 15:1	< 15:1
Urine sediment	Normal (hyaline casts and rare granular casts)	Granular casts Epithelial casts RBC casts Cellular debris	Normal or RBCs, WBCs, and crystals

Note: Adapted from Bonaventre et al. (1995); Rose & Black (1988); Schrier (1995).

Table 9-6
Nursing Interventions Appropriate for Patients with Renal Failure

Identify patients at risk.

Provide patients with adequate amounts of fluids, unless volume restricted.

Monitor volume status, intake and output, daily weight, and assessment of edema.

Monitor vital signs, especially observe for orthostasis with decreased blood pressure and increased heart rate.

Monitor urine output; outputs of < 30 ml/hr should be reported to the physician.

Review appropriate urine and serum analyses routinely.

vomiting. In contrast, metabolic acidosis may be seen with diarrhea, diabetic ketoacidosis, or shock-induced lactic acidosis. A therapeutic fluid challenge is frequently given (usually 250 to 500 ml of 5% dextrose in water or normal saline over a 30-minute period) to ascertain if the renal abnormality is a result of prerenal failure from volume depletion. An attempt may also be made to increase the response of the kidney by the concurrent administration of a diuretic such as mannitol or furosemide. The nurse should carefully assess the patient during this procedure for side effects of the diuretics and acute changes in volume status.

Treatment and prevention. Management of the patient with prerenal failure seeks to restore normal hemodynamic status and varies depending on the cause of the renal hypoperfusion. Volume-depleted patients should have their volume replaced with appropriate fluids. In patients with cardiac failure, treatment may include those interventions aimed at increasing cardiac output and normalizing fluid balance, including positive inotropic agents and/or vasodilating agents and sodium restriction. In patients with prerenal fail-

ure from vasodilation, volume replacement and the use of vasoconstrictors may be successful in restoring renal perfusion. When these therapies are unsuccessful, ventricular assist devices or aortic balloon counterpulsation may be of benefit. For renal artery disease, surgery may be required to eliminate the cause (Burnett, 1993).

Appropriate treatment frequently reverses the pathophysiologic processes of prerenal failure. However, if therapy is not instituted promptly or is not effective, prerenal failure can lead to acute intrarenal failure (Bonventre, Shah, Walker, & Humphreys, 1995). The most effective treatment for prerenal failure, therefore, is prevention, and the nurse can play a major role in implementing prevention strategies. Appropriate nursing interventions are outlined in Table 9-6.

Postrenal Failure

Etiology and pathophysiology. Postrenal failure results from an obstruction to urine flow that can occur anywhere within the urinary tract (Hagland, 1993) (see Figure 9-2). The most common causes of postrenal failure in adults are

Table 9-7

Radiologic Procedures Used in the Evaluation of the Patient with Renal Failure

Test	Use
Kidney-ureter-bladder x-ray (KUB)	Kidney number, size, shape, and placement Diagnosis and monitoring of radiopaque stones
Intravenous pyelography (IVP)	Kidney number, size, shape, and calyceal anatomy Detection of site and cause of obstruction (ultrasound preferable for screening)
Ultrasound and CT	Evaluation for possible urinary tract obstruction Evaluation for renal mass (cyst versus tumor) Early diagnosis of polycystic kidney disease Detection of radiolucent kidney stones
Radionuclide studies	Screening for renovascular hypertension Screening for renal thromboemboli Screening for tumors and cysts Assess symmetry of blood flow
Renal arteriography	Direct visualization of renal arterial system for renovascular hypertension, thromboemboli, or diagnosis of renal mass that seems noncystic on other studies
Voiding cystourethrogram	Detection of vesicoureteral reflux
Retrograde or antegrade pyelography	Determination of site of obstruction Relief of obstruction (catheters inserted)
Magnetic resonance imaging (MRI)	More specific than ultrasonography and CT Helpful in detection of renal masses and malformations of vessels and tubules

Note: Adapted from Baer (1993b); Borkowski (1995); Doherty (1995); Geisinger & Pohl (1995); Nally & Pohl (1995); Occhipinti & Hricak (1995); Parker, Older, Wertman, Crane, & Hidalgo (1995); Richard (1986b); Rose & Rennke (1994); Sarno (1995).

benign prostate hypertrophy and nephrolithiasis, while obstruction secondary to congenital abnormalities occurs frequently in children (Llach, 1993; Yarger, 1991). The obstruction may have little permanent effect on renal function, may cause progressive kidney damage over a period of months or years, or may cause rapid destruction of the kidneys (Llach, 1993). The exact nature and site of the occlusion and its speed of onset determine the pathophysiology as well as the clinical presentation (Faber et al., 1993). Urinary tract obstruction causes an increase in pressure proximal to the obstruction due to continued glomerular filtration. Depending on the site of the obstruction, this leads to dilation of the proximal collecting system such as the ureter (hydroureter) and the renal pelvis (hydronephrosis). These anatomic changes are important clinically because ultrasonography or computed tomography (CT) scanning can detect them. The elevation in pressure is transmitted back to the proximal tubule. If the obstruction is complete, the increase in intratubular pressure eventually exceeds the hydrostatic pressure of the glomerulus, stopping glomerular filtration. With partial obstruction, the rise in tubular pressure may lower filtration, but it will not completely stop (Yarger, 1993). Intrarenal vasoconstriction mediated by renin, angiotensin II, and thromboxan helps reduce GFR.

In the first 1 to 2 hours following acute obstruction, the decrease in GFR is associated with an increase in tubular absorption of sodium and water. Thus, the urine produced in this setting is decreased in volume, hypertonic, and has a low sodium concentration. The reduced GFR also results in increased urea absorption by functional tubules leading to an elevated BUN. Following several hours of obstruction, sodium and water reabsorption decline because of tubular injury, and an isotonic urine is produced. Distal potassium and hydrogen ion secretion and water reabsorption are also diminished and frequently cause hyperkalemia, hyperchloremia, and a metabolic acidosis (see Figure 9-2). The extent of the subsequent renal damage depends on the degree, duration, and location of the obstruction as well as the presence and severity of infection (Llach, 1993). Acute obstruction is a urological emergency. In most cases, if the obstruction is not relieved, permanent renal damage occurs.

Clinical and laboratory features. Although it may develop acutely, postrenal failure is frequently a chronic condition that has gone unnoticed or unreported by the patient (Price, 1994). However, a thorough assessment of all patients who present with renal abnormalities can frequently help identify those with postrenal abnormalities. The history may be positive for either obstructive and/or irritation symptoms of the bladder. Obstructive symptoms include hesitancy, decreased size and force of the urine stream, and postvoid dribbling. Irritation symptoms include dysuria, frequency, and urgency. A history positive for irritation symptoms is especially significant, as urinary tract infection remains a leading cause of death in patients with ARF (Yarger, 1993). Pain is a common

Figure 9-2
Renal Responses to Bilateral Urinary Tract Obstruction

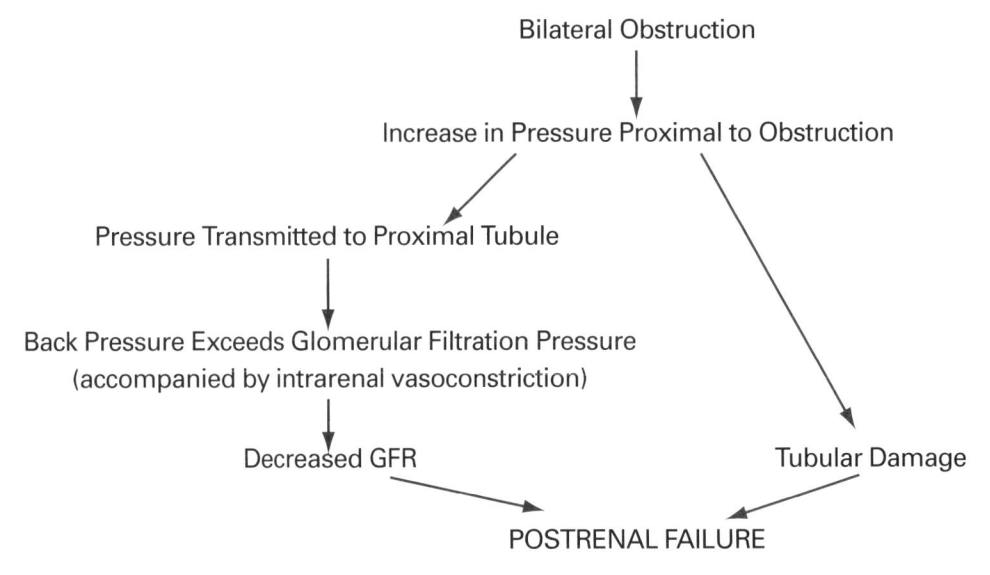

Note: Adapted from Yarger (1991, 1993); Richard (1986a).

symptom if the obstruction has occurred suddenly. The pain generally begins in the flank and radiates toward the labia in women or the scrotum in men (Yarger, 1991).

The symptoms may be followed by the sudden onset of anuria or oliguria. However, some patients may present with no changes in urine flow, and it is important to note that urine volume does not necessarily reflect renal function. Depending on the type of obstruction, urine volume may vary from zero to several thousand milliliters daily. Thus, in the azotemic patient, the presence of large volumes of urine is consistent with partial but severe urinary tract obstruction (Yarger, 1993).

Physical examination may reveal a distended abdomen or dullness to percussion over the bladder as a result of a distention. Costovertebral (CVA) tenderness may be present if hydronephrosis or infection has developed. A large, postvoid residual urine noted after straight catheterization indicates a lower urinary tract obstruction.

The urine and serum laboratory findings seen in postrenal failure are summarized in Table 9-5. Microscopic hematuria and proteinuria are common. In addition, some patients may develop a salt-losing state accompanied by hyponatremia and extracellular volume contraction. Others develop hyperkalemia due to decreased levels of aldosterone and increased tubular resistance to the hormone. Patients may also have a hyperchloremic, hyperkalemic metabolic acidosis due to diminished ability of the nephron to excrete hydrogen ions (Yarger, 1993).

A plain film of the abdomen may reveal kidney enlargement and often provides clues about the cause of the obstruction. Ultrasonography, CT, and magnetic resonance imaging (MRI) can be done safely to screen an azotemic patient, as contrast media is not required. An anterograde or retrograde pyelogram may also help visualize the site of obstruction (Faber et al., 1993; Yarger, 1993). Table 9-7 summaries the radiologic and angiographic procedures used in evaluation of a patient with renal failure.

Treatment and prevention. Postrenal failure is treated by relieving the obstruction, preserving renal function, and preventing and treating any complications. An acute obstruction lasting less than 24 hours is generally accompanied by complete recovery. In the absence of complicating infection, decompression of the urinary tract after 1 to 2 weeks of even total obstruction may still allow for complete functional recovery. However, it may take days or weeks to return to baseline renal functioning (Faber et al., 1993). The nurse plays a key role in the assessment, management, education, and support of these patients before and during relief of the obstruction.

After the obstruction has been relieved, renal concentrating abnormalities may persist, such that large amount of solutes and water are excreted (generally from 5 to 8 L/day). This condition is referred to as postobstructive diuresis (Yarger, 1991, 1993). Three factors are thought to contribute to its development. First, fluid taken orally or administered intravenously before removal of the obstruction can cause volume expansion, which is later excreted. Second, solutes such as urea and electrolytes that were also retained can act as osmotic diuretics and facilitate the diuresis. Third, tubular damage may have occurred during the obstruction that inhibits the normal concentrating abilities of the kidney. The polyuria is usually associated with the excretion of large amounts of sodium, potassium, magnesium, and other electrolytes. Although the condition is self-limiting, the fluid and electrolyte losses that occur can be life-threatening (Yarger, 1991).

The nurse should carefully monitor the patient with postobstructive diuresis. Intake and output should be measured hourly and fluid replaced if needed. Daily or more frequent weights provide information regarding net fluid balance. Vital signs, including checks for orthostasis, should be taken every 1 to 2 hours. Electrolytes, including sodium, potassium, and magnesium, should be measured daily. Urine specific gravity and osmolality provide information regarding the ability of the kidneys to concentrate urine. The condition usually resolves in several days to a week (Yarger, 1991). Activities for the prevention of postrenal failure include careful assessment of patients at risk and education of those individuals regarding symptoms, including both irritation and obstructive symptoms, which require further medical evaluation. Early intervention is paramount to avoid permanent kidney damage.

Intrarenal Failure

Etiology and pathophysiology. Injury to the renal tissues causes intrarenal failure and leads to the rapid decline of GFR; elevation of BUN and serum creatinine; and frequently, progressively diminishing urine output. The condition most commonly occurs in high-risk clinical settings (see Table 9-8) and in those patients with acute risk factors and pre-existing renal disease (see Table 9-9). The severe insults that cause this abnormality result from damage or inflammation of the glomerulus and/or other renal vessels, the interstitial tissues, or the tubule system.

Glomerulonephritis and vasculitis result from inflammatory or immunologic disorders, such as poststreptococcal glomerulonephritis, systemic lupus erythematosus, and Goodpasture's Syndrome. In these diseases, the GFR is reduced from the hemodynamic changes that result from acute immune injury as well as structural damage. Occlusion of the renal vessels from conditions such as renal thrombosis, sickle cell disease, and thrombotic thrombocytopenic purpura also cause intrarenal failure by inducing ischemia and necrosis (Bonventre et al., 1995; Levine, Lieberthal, Bernard, & Salant, 1993). In contrast, interstitial nephritis, an abnormality characterized by inflammatory cell infiltrates within the renal interstitium without glomerular or tubular damage, results from certain infections, infiltrative diseases (such as lymphoma, leukemia, and sarcoidosis), and drugs (antibiotics, diuretics, analgesics) (Bonventre et al., 1995; Faber et al., 1993). Approximately 5% to 20% of acute intrarenal failure is from these types of abnormalities (Anderson, 1993; Faber et al., 1993; Llach 1993).

More commonly, intrarenal failure results from acute tubular necrosis (ATN). Although in most cases of ATN the pathology involves the renal tubules, other renal tissues may also become damaged. The major causes of ATN are ischemia and nephrotoxicity. The pathophysiology of each disorder will be discussed in the following sections; however, it is important to note that these two conditions may act in combination to produce renal damage (refer to Figure 9-3). For example, some patients with underlying renal ischemia may develop ATN after only a brief exposure to a nephrotoxic agent (Anderson, 1993; Brezis, Rosen, & Epstein, 1993).

Ischemic ATN. Renal ischemia is the most common cause of ATN. This may seem like a paradox given that the kidney is one of the best oxygenated organs of the body and

Table 9-8

Clinical Settings Associated with a High Risk of Acute Renal Failure

Patients Undergoing Surgery
  Open heart surgery
  Abdominal aortic surgery
  Surgery in a jaundiced patient

Cadaveric Renal Transplantation
  Warm and cold ischemia
  Cyclosporine nephrotoxicity

Nephrotoxic agents (see Table 9-10)

Inflammatory Processes
  Bacterial
  Viral
  Septicemia

Trauma
  Penetrating
  Nonpenetrating
  Burns

Systemic and Vascular Disorders
  Renal vein, artery, arteriolar thrombosis
  Sickle cell disease
  Systemic Lupus Erythematosus

Pigment Induced
  Disseminated intravascular hemolysis (hemoglobin)
  Transfusion reactions (hemoglobin)
  Rhabdomyolysis (myoglobin)

Multiorgan Failure

Note: Adapted from Leiberthal & Levinsky (1990); Richard (1986a); Wardle (1994).

Table 9-9

Acute and Chronic Risk Factors Associated with the Development of Acute Renal Failure

Acute Risk Factors

  Volume depletion
  Aminoglycoside use
  Radiocontrast exposure
  NSAID exposure
  Septic shock
  Dehydration
  Hypotension
  Pigmenturia

Chronic Risk Factors

  Preexisting renal disease
  Hypertension
  Congestive heart failure
  Diabetes mellitus
  Age
  Liver cirrhosis

Note: From Brezis, M., Rosen S., & Epstein, F.H. (1993). Acute renal failure due to ischemia (acute tubular necrosis). In J.M. Lazarus & B.M. Brenner (Eds.), *Acute renal failure* (3rd edition) (pp. 210). New York: Churchill Livingstone.

Figure 9-3
Ischemic and Nephrotoxic ATN

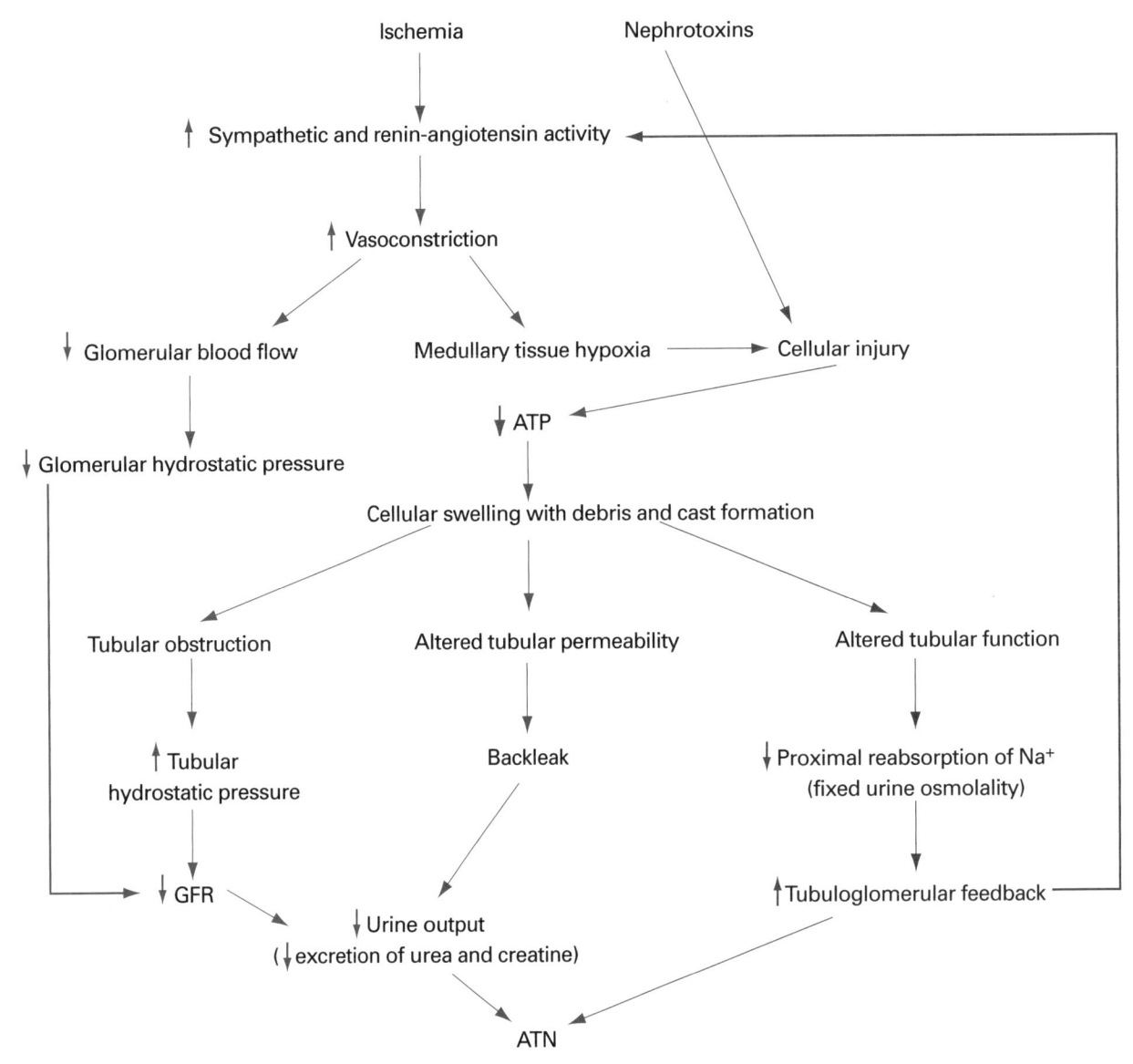

Note: Adapted from Baer & Lancaster (1992); Hays (1992); Iaina & Schwartz (1994); Stark (1994); Richard (1986a).

receives approximately 25% of the cardiac output each minute. However, most of the RBF goes to the cortex (which houses the glomeruli) for the formation of filtrate and the clearance of wastes. Only about 1/10 goes to the medulla, the minimal amount necessary for oxygen delivery while at the same time permitting urine concentration. A higher blood flow would disrupt the osmotic gradient generated in the medulla by the countercurrent system (Brezis et al., 1993). Therefore, when RBF is reduced, the medulla (along with the tubules) is the area most severely compromised. According to Brezis et al. (1993), this susceptibility of the medulla to hypoxia and subsequent tubule damage "may be considered the price paid for an efficient urinary concentrating mechanism" (p. 214).

The cell damage that actually occurs during periods of reduced renal perfusion depends on the extent and duration of the ischemia. When the mean arterial pressure (MAP) falls below 50 to 70 mm/Hg, RBF and perfusion pressure decrease and ischemia begins. If this ischemia is less than 25 minutes, the damage is often mild and reversible. Ischemia of 40 to 60 minutes results in more severe damage, which may recover in 2 to 3 weeks. However, periods of ischemia of up to 60 to 90 minutes usually result in permanent kidney damage (Kjellstrand & Solez, 1993).

The initial pathophysiologic event in ischemic ATN is intrarenal vasoconstriction. As discussed previously, reduced RBF causes activation of the sympathetic and renin-angiotensin systems (see Figure 9-3). In response, the afferent arteriole of the glomerulus constricts and reduces glomerular blood flow. This response may also be mediated by other vasoconstrictors such as endothelin and thromboxane (Wardle, 1994). The reduced glomerular blood flow causes a decrease in hydrostatic pressure and a subsequent decrease in GFR. These events are in part responsible for the reduced urinary output frequently seen in ATN. A variety of factors contribute to the development of tubular injury in ischemic ATN. These factors include cellular adenosine triphosphate (ATP) depletion, alteration in normal polarity of the epithelial layer of the tubular walls, disruption of the basement membrane, and generation of oxygen-free radicals. The damage causes both functional impairment and cell necrosis (Rose & Rennke, 1994; Weinberg, 1995).

The presence of ATP is essential for cell homeostasis, maintenance of cellular volume and ionic concentration, and integrity of the cell membrane (Stark, 1994). Within 30 seconds of an ischemic episode, the tubular cells experience ATP depletion. This occurs because of conversion from aerobic to anaerobic metabolism, a state in which less ATP is produced (Baer, 1993b). The intracellular energy depletion associated with low levels of ATP causes inactivation of the Na^+-K^+ pump, a system that helps regulate tubular cell volume. Sodium and chloride accumulate in the cell, and the cells take up water and swell. The cellular swelling contributes to tubular obstruction and medullary ischemia and injury (Baer & Lancaster, 1992; Stark, 1994; Weinberg, 1995). Other cellular pumps also fail, causing a decrease in intrarenal cell potassium, magnesium, and inorganic phosphates and an increase in calcium, all of which may also enhance cell injury (Stark, 1994). Sloughed necrotic cells and casts that form obstruct the tubular lumen. This obstruction to tubular flow causes an increase in Bowman's capsule hydrostatic pressure, which opposes the glomerular hydrostatic pressure. The changes cause a reduction of GFR and a decreased excretion of urea and creatinine and urinary output.

The lesion of ischemic ATN is characterized by patchy necrosis and is commonly associated with disruption of the basement membrane (Llach, 1993). Injury to the basement membrane increases tubular permeability and allows tubular filtrate to leak back into the interstitium and peritubular capillaries. This backleak of tubular filtrate also contributes to the reduced urine output (Baer & Lancaster, 1992). Production of oxygen-free radicals is also believed to play a major role in the development of cellular injury (Weinberg, 1995). Cells that are experiencing aerobic metabolism (with oxygen) produce oxygen-free radicals as part of the normal process. However, these substances are highly reactive and can cause disruption of cellular functioning. Usually, the cell defends itself against these normal elements by utilizing intracellular mechanisms to destroy the free radicals. However, during ischemia and anaerobic metabolism, the cell is unable to protect itself and damage occurs (Stark, 1994). Oxygen-free radicals may be particularly important in the cellular injury known to continue after reperfusion of the ischemic kidney (ischemic-reperfusion injury) (Iaina & Schwartz, 1994; Stark, 1994).

Nephrotoxic ATN. Nephrotoxic ATN is defined as the deterioration of renal function over a matter of days to weeks following toxin exposure (see Table 9-10). This type of ATN accounts for 30% to 40% of the cases of ATN and may cause

Table 9-10
Nephrotoxic Agents

Classification	Example
Drugs	Antibacterial Antiviral Antifungal Antiprotozoal Nonsteroidal antiinflammatory Antineoplastic Angiotensin-converting enzyme inhibitors Diuretics Anti-ulcer
Anesthetics	Methoxyflurane Enflurane
Contrast Media	Diatrizoate Iothalamate Bunamiodyl
Organic Solvents	Glycols Halogenated hydrocarbons Aromatic hydrocarbons Gasoline, kerosene, turpentine
Heavy Metals	Arsenic Bismuth Barium Copper Lead Gold Mercury Lithium
Heme Pigments	Hemoglobin Myoglobin
Intrarenal Crystal Deposition	Uric acid Calcium Oxalate
Products from Multiorgan Failure	Endotoxins Tumor necrosis factor (TNF) Interleukin-1

Note: Adapted from Baer & Lancaster (1992); Brezis et al. (1991); Llach (1993a); Swan & Bennett (1993); Richard (1986a).

renal damage ranging from mild renal insufficiency to frank renal failure. Nephrotoxic ATN is commonly seen in hospitalized patients receiving certain antibiotics, particularly aminoglycosides. In fact, it has been estimated that an elevation in the serum creatinine concentration of 0.5 to 4.0 mg/dl occurs in 10% to 20% of patients who receive a full 7- to 10-day course of aminoglycosides (Anderson, 1993; Rose & Rennke, 1994). The kidney is very vulnerable to toxic damage for several reasons. First, the blood circulates through the kidneys many times per hour. Thus, the renal tissue is repeatedly exposed to substances that are carried in the blood. Second, the kidneys play a major role in the concentration and excretion of toxic substances and are, therefore, exposed to high concentrations of these substances. Finally, the renal tubular cells are very susceptible to direct toxic effects of a wide variety of drugs, solvents, heavy metals, and other products (Brezis et al., 1993). Thus, the nurse should carefully monitor the renal function of any patient who has been exposed to or is receiving a potentially nephrotoxic substance. In toxic ATN, the initial event is injury to the tubular cell from the toxic substance. Thereafter, the pathophysiology is basically the same as with ischemic ATN (see Figure 9-3). There is tubular damage, followed by necrosis and cast formation, tubular obstruction, and decreased GFR (Baer & Lancaster, 1992).

In contrast to that of ischemic ATN, the lesion of nephrotoxic ATN is uniform and may be localized to the proximal and distal tubule (Llach, 1993). The basement membrane of the renal tubular cells is usually not injured and remains intact. This type of lesion frequently causes a renal-concentrating defect rather than the impairment of the urinary flow seen with tubular backleak and obstruction as in ischemic ATN. As a result, dilute urine flows freely through intact, unobstructed tubules. This condition is referred to as nonoliguric ATN. The urine volume may vary from normal to as much as 2 L/h. Nonoliguric ATN is associated with a shortened clinical course (ranging from as little as 5 to 8 days in comparison to weeks or months in the case of ischemic ATN) and a 50% to 60% reduction in mortality (Douglas, 1992; Stark, 1992a). The severity and time course of the renal failure depends on the nature and dose of the toxin as well as a variety of host factors. Thus, individual nephrotoxic insults that are tolerated by healthy persons may produce severe and prolonged injury in elderly patients or those with dehydration, vascular insufficiency, or circulatory failure. Nephrotoxic ATN is reversible if it is identified early and if exposure to the offending agent is removed.

Clinical and laboratory features. Before the diagnosis of ATN is made, it is crucial to rule out prerenal and postrenal causes of renal failure. This can be done by obtaining an in-depth health history, performing a complete physical examination, and reviewing the results of appropriate urine and blood analyses. The laboratory analyses used to assist in distinguishing pre-, intra-, and postrenal failure are summarized in Table 9-5.

The clinical course of ATN is divided into four stages, including onset, oliguric-anuric phase, diuretic phase, and recovery. The onset begins with the precipitating event and lasts hours or days until renal cell injury occurs along with oliguria or anuria. The onset is usually a period of hours when caused by ischemia but may last 2 to 7 days when caused by a nephrotoxin (Lancaster, 1992; Rose & Rennke, 1994). If the conditions that trigger the onset of ATN are not reversed, the oliguric-anuric phase begins. This stage is characterized by a urine output of less than 400 ml per 24 hours. Although this period usually lasts from 7 to 14 days, it can persist for weeks or months depending on the extent of the renal injury (Stark, 1992a). The longer an individual remains in the oliguric-anuric phase, the poorer the prognosis for recovery because of the increased risk of complications (Baer & Lancaster, 1992; Baer, 1993b). Renal dysfunction persists throughout the duration of this stage, although the healing of renal tissue begins within 25 to 48 hours after the insult. During the oliguric-anuric phase, the BUN and serum creatinine are elevated in a ratio of approximately 10:1. In

addition, there are increases in the levels of potassium, phosphorus, and magnesium, and decreases in the levels of pH, bicarbonate, calcium, hematocrit, and hemoglobin (see Table 9-11). As previously mentioned, the urine volume is usually less than 400 cc/24 hours. However, if the patient has nonoliguric ATN, urine volumes may be considerably greater. The urine that is produced has a low specific gravity and osmolality, a sodium level greater than 20 mEq/L, and contains granular and epithelial casts.

Because the kidney has lost most or all of its regulatory and excretory functions, the patient may develop many of the signs and symptoms of acute uremia within as few as 72 hours. The clinical problems that can occur during this phase are summarized in Table 9-11. The diuretic phase usually lasts about 7 to 14 days and begins when the daily urinary output is greater than 400 ml per 24 hours (Baer & Lancaster, 1992; Llach, 1993). Although renal healing occurs during this stage, the tubule system is frequently unable to concentrate urine effectively. In addition, retained fluid and the diuretic affect of urea may facilitate the diuresis. Thus, patients may ultimately excrete large volumes of urine (in excess of 10 L/day) and lose substantial amounts of important electrolytes (Llach, 1993). Hypokalemia and metabolic alkalosis may develop. Initially the urine is comparable to plasma filtrate, but then urea excretion gradually increases and urinary sodium decreases. The BUN and serum creatinine usually slowly decrease but rapid correction may also occur. The onset of the diuretic phase does not signify a halt to all the clinical problems associated with ARF. For several days after diuresis begins, renal function remains poor, the BUN may continue to rise, infection may occur, and the uremic syndrome may become worse. In fact, 20% to 25% of the deaths occur during the diuretic phase (Llach, 1993). Thus, the nurse must carefully monitor the patient for fluid and electrolyte deficits, acid-base disorders, and the other systemic complications of uremia.

The convalescent phase begins when the BUN is stable and lasts until the patient is able to return to normal activity. Complete recovery may require several months to a year. For many patients, renal function never returns to baseline and some are left with significant renal impairment, requiring dialysis and renal transplantation.

Treatment and prevention. The goals of treatment for the patient with ATN include the following: (a) prevention or correction of the primary disorder, if possible; (b) correction of fluid, electrolyte, and acid-base disorders; (c) prevention of infection; (d) maintenance of an optimal nutrition state; (e) treatment of the systemic effects of uremia; and (f) provision of patient and family support (Baer & Lancaster, 1992; Kjellstrand & Barsoum, 1995; Stark, 1994). The nurse should carefully monitor the volume status of all patients at risk for the development of ATN. Blood pressure, body weight, urinary output, central venous pressure, and pulmonary capillary wedge pressure are all valuable parameters that can help determine if a patient is volume depleted. Prompt correction of volume deficits and maintenance of cardiac output can help prevent ATN. Even when this intervention is not successful in preventing ATN, it can still contribute to the formation of a nonoliguric state by reducing renal tubular damage and, thus, reducing both morbidity and mortality (Stark,

Table 9-11

Acute Bremia: Pathophysiology and Related Clinical Findings

Body System	Pathophysiology	Clinical Findings
Fluid, electrolyte, and acid-base status	Kidneys have decreased ability or are unable to regulate fluid, electrolyte, and acid-base balance.	Fluid retention, hypertension, edema, hyperkalemia, hypocalcemia, hyperphosphatemia, hypermagnesemia, and metabolic acidosis.
General metabolic status	Kidneys have decreased ability or are unable to excrete metabolic wastes. There is an increase in the peripheral resistance to insulin and decreased renal excretion of insulin.	Increased BUN and creatinine, and glucose intolerance.
Urinary system	Kidney damage is reflected in decreased output and presence of abnormal sediment in urine that is produced. Foley catheters are frequently in place to facilitate urine output measurement; therefore, the risk of infection is high.	Anuria or oliguria; urine sediment—red and white cells, casts, proteinuria; potential for urinary tract infection.
Gastrointestinal system	Uremic wastes are retained and exert effects on mucous membranes along GI tract. Hyper- or hypomotility can occur with electrolyte imbalances.	Anorexia, nausea and vomiting, stomatitis, constipation/diarrhea, GI bleeding, abdominal distention.
Cardiovascular system	Fluid is retained, electrolyte abnormalities (particularly hyperkalemia) are present, and uremia causes increased permeability of the pericardial membrane.	Hypertension or hypotension, congestive heart failure, pericarditis, dysrhythmias, pericardial effusion, cardiac tamponade, edema.
Respiratory system	Hyperventilation is a compensatory mechanism for metabolic acidosis. Pulmonary edema may develop with volume overload. Decreased lung expansion in patients on bed rest, along with the decreased immunologic response seen in acute renal failure, facilitates development of pneumonia.	Kussmaul respirations, pulmonary edema, pneumonia, pneumonitis,. pleural effusions.
Hematologic system	Anemia is related to depressed erythropoietin secretion. Uremia decreases platelet adhesiveness and immunologic responses.	Anemia, potential for bleeding and infections.
Neurologic system	Accumulation of metabolic wastes may result in alteration of mental status.	Drowsiness, coma, convulsions, myoclonus, psychosis.
Dermatologic system	Skin changes result from accumulation of metabolic wastes, calcium and phosphate imbalances, and platelet abnormalities associated with uremia.	Dryness, pruritus, purpura, potential for infection as a result of cracking of the skin.
Skeletal system	Decreased GI absorption of calcium and decreased renal excretion of phosphate causes electrolyte imbalances.	Hypocalcemia, hyperphosphatemia, metastatic calcifications.

Note: From Parker, K.P. (1992). Disorders of the kidney. In L. Burrell (Ed.), *Adult health nursing in hospital and community settings* (p. 1249). Norwalk, CT: Appleton Lange.

1992a). The nurse should also carefully monitor patients receiving potentially nephrotoxic agents, particularly those who are elderly, diabetic, volume depleted, or receiving multiple nephrotoxic drugs. Dosages of these medications should be calculated and given according to renal function and drug levels checked when appropriate.

Several pharmacologic agents are available to help prevent and treat ATN. These agents can also be used create a nonoliguric ATN (Stark, 1994). Although the exact physiologic effects of many of these medications are poorly understood, potential mechanisms of action in the prevention and treatment of ARF include:

1. improvement of renal hemodynamics by increasing blood flow, glomerular hydrostatic pressure, and GFR;
2. decrease of tubular obstruction by reducing the formation of casts and enhancing their removal;
3. decrease of tubular cell injury and backleak; and
4. enhancement of tubular epithelial regeneration and

Table 9-12
Pharmacologic Agents Potentially Useful in the Treatment of Acute Renal Failure

Drugs	Possible Action	Nursing Considerations

Diuretics
  Lasix
  Mannitol
	• Increases GFR and helps create non-oliguric ATN.
	• Increases tubular flow and prevents cast formation and obstruction.
	• Lasix produces a resting state due to blockage of Na$^+$-K$^+$ pump in ascending loop of Henle. May help preserve ATP levels.
	• Mannitol may help prevent cellular swelling and/or destroy oxygen-free radicals.
		• There is no evidence whether diuretics influence the clinical course of ARF, they do increase urine flow rate.
		• Lasix is ototoxic.
		• Lasix may enhance the ototoxicity of aminoglycosides and nephrotoxicity of cephalosporins.
		• Mannitol may cause volume expansion. Lasix should be considered if the patient is volume overloaded.
		• Urine chemistries should be obtained prior to diuretic administration.
		• May prevent ATN if administered before or during the onset phase of ATN.

Dopamine	• Acts on the dopaminergic receptors of the renal vasculature to cause vasodilation. • Increases renal blood flow by decreasing renal vascular resistance.	• Effect decreases as the dosage requirements increase to maintain BP. • Restoration of intravascular volume is essential when using dopamine. • May be more effective if used in conjunction with Lasix. • May alter the course of ATN by increasing GFR and/or urinary output.
Atrial natriuretic peptide (ANP)	• Animal studies have shown that IV infusion can reverse experimental ATN. The mechanism is thought to be due to the vasodilatory action of ANP.	• A series of studies is currently being conducted at multiple sites to test its effectiveness in humans. • Causes hypotension in large doses. • ANP is rapidly degraded and quickly becomes ineffective. • May prevent ATN if administered during onset phase.
Calcium channel blockers	• Dilate afferent arteriole and increase GFR. • Prevent influx of calcium into the cell and thereby decrease cellular damage.	• May cause hypotension. • May prevent ATN if administered during onset phase. • May alter course of ATN by increasing GFR and urine output. • Not extensively studied in humans.
Prostaglandins	• Mechanism of action unclear but may be related to increase in renal blood flow, increased solute excretion, inhibition of platelet aggregation, and/or a direct cytoprotective effect.	• Insufficient studies in humans.

Adenine nucleotides (ATP, ADP, or AMP complexed to MgCl$_2$)	• In animals:
	  -decreases cell damage.
	  -enhances GFR.
	• Provides ATP at cellular level and preserves cell function
		• Causes of the fall in systemic resistance and an increase in cardiac output.
		• Further research in humans needed.

Amino acids
  Glycine
  Alanine
	• May be beneficial by both preventing or reducing cell injury and by enhancing regeneration and repair of tubular cells.
	• The mechanism of protective effect has not been established.
		• Effects not well studied in humans.
		• Amino acids can be nephrotoxic in selected situations.

Antioxidants
  Allopurinol
  Deferoxamine
	• Inhibits production of oxygen-free radicals.	• Effectiveness remains controversial.

Growth factors
  Insulin-like Growth Factor (IGF-1)
  Epidermal Growth Factor (EGF)
  Hepatocyte Growth Factor
	In animal models:
	• Accelerates recovery of renal tubular cells.
	• May also enhance GFR and RBF.
		• Further study will be required in humans.

Note: Adapted from Dolleris (1992); Fischereder et al. (1994); Hammerman & Miller (1994); Hays (1992); Lieberthal & Levinsky (1990); Nouwen, Verstrepen, & DeBroe (1994); Shilliday & Allison (1994); Stark (1994); Strupp (1988).

repair. A summary of these medications, their mechanism of actions, and nursing considerations appear in Table 9-12.

Infection is one of the most frequent complications of ATN and occurs in as many as 70% of patients (Kjellstrand & Barsoum, 1995; Stark, 1994). More importantly, infections have been implicated in the deaths of 29% to 72% of patients with ARF (Finn, 1993). The most common infections seen in patients with ARF include septicemia, pulmonary infections, urinary tract infections, peritonitis, and intraabdominal abscess formation (Finn, 1993; Schrier & Wang, 2004). Thus, nurses should continually assess the patient for signs of infection. Interventions should include the use of aseptic technique, maintenance of skin integrity, avoidance of indwelling catheters, pulmonary toilet, and the prophylactic use of antibiotic therapy when indicated (Kjellstrand & Barsoum, 1995; Stark, 1994).

Nutrition. ATN frequently occurs in conjunction with other pathologic processes and is characterized by increased caloric needs and a susceptibility to catabolism. Metabolic changes caused by renal failure and the metabolic effects of the primary illness both contribute to these alterations. Therefore, patients with ARF frequently display the signs and symptoms of protein catabolism, such as negative nitrogen balance, loss of lean body mass, and enhanced production of urea with severe hyperkalemia and acidosis (Schaefer, Schaefer, & Horl, 1994). In addition, the effects of protein and calorie malnutrition are delayed wound healing and impaired immune function (Wolfson & Kopple, 1993).

Although not conclusive, the results of numerous studies suggest that a considerable amount of the morbidity and mortality associated with ARF may result from a failure to take into account these increased nutritional requirements (Kjellstrand & Barsoum, 1995; Wolfson & Kopple, 1993). Thus, adequate nutrition is essential. However, the metabolic disturbances and alterations in fluid and electrolyte excretion mandate careful planning of nutritional support. The goals of dietary management are to minimize uremic toxicity, to minimize fluid and electrolyte imbalances, and to maintain adequate nutrition (Baer & Lancaster, 1992; Kjellstrand & Barsoum, 1995).

Appropriate nutrition is paramount in the management of ARF. Adequate calories should be given to meet energy needs (35 to 45 kcal/kg of IBW/day) (Druml, 1995). Protein requirements vary from 0.6 to 1.5 g/kg/day, and the protein given should be of high biological value and, thus, contain all essential amino acids (Rodriquez & Lewis, 1997; Wolfson & Kopple, 1993). Sodium, potassium, and phosphorous are usually restricted because the tubules are not able to secrete them. However, electrolyte replacement should be individualized based on blood levels of these substances. Fluid is restricted to output plus 500 to 1000 cc for insensible losses. Water-soluble vitamin supplementation is required, but care must be taken in the administration of fat-soluble vitamins because of the risk of vitamin toxicity (Wolfson & Kopple, 1993). Whenever feasible, the gastrointestinal (GI) tract should be used for nutrition. If the patient is unable to eat, administration of nutrition via enteral tubes is frequently preferred to intravenous administration. Early dialysis may be required secondary to volume overload if intravenous nutri-

tional therapy is necessary. The systemic effects of uremia frequently appear when the BUN level rises above 70 to 100 mg/dl (Stark, 1994) (see Table 9-11). The nurse should carefully assess the patient for the development of these symptoms. Careful dietary management is helpful in preventing uremic manifestations. However, renal replacement therapy may be required. Treatment used may include HD, peritoneal dialysis (PD), or continuous renal replacement therapies (CRRTs). The advantages and disadvantages of each type of therapy are listed in Table 9-13.

Treatment and Symptom Management

Patients with ARF and their families must cope with the sudden loss of health in the face of a very serious illness. The loss of renal function may require prolonged hospitalization, complex dietary and medication management, and dialysis. The nurse should continually assess the educational and emotional needs of both the patient and family, providing them with appropriate explanations of the disease process, its prognosis, and all procedures and components of treatment (Baer & Lancaster, 1992). Permitting the patient and family members to express their needs and concerns is essential. Allowing frequent family visits helps support the entire family, decreases anxiety, and provides the patient with a source of comfort (Stark, 1994).

The patient in renal failure is at risk for developing a wide variety of systemic abnormalities. Although existing medical treatments, including dialysis, correct many of these problems, they cannot reverse several of the maladaptive physiologic changes induced by renal failure. In addition, the psychosocial responses to the disease are profound. Thus, patients with renal failure and their families require complex nursing care. Patients and families need information about the many pathological conditions that result from ARF as well as the possible planned interventions. A patient with ARF requires a variety of pharmacological supports. Along with pharmacological agents, some patients will require HD, PD, CRRT, and/or therapeutic plasma exchange (TPE). All of these therapies have an appropriate place in the treatment of ARF, but in this chapter only CRRT and TPE will be discussed.

In general, the manifestations of renal failure can be divided into four areas including:
1. manifestations specifically related to disorders of fluid and electrolyte excretion and acid-base disturbances;
2. manifestations related to disordered metabolic and regulatory functions;
3. alterations related to the effects of uremia (uremic syndrome); and
4. psychosocial responses of the patient and family to acute/chronic illness.

Cardiovascular manifestations. The cardiovascular system is greatly affected by renal failure and dialysis. Salt and water retention, anemia, hypertension, and numerous metabolic abnormalities are contributing factors. These complications occur in ARF patients and are a leading cause of morbidity and mortality in those with CRF (Suki & Eknoyan, 1995) (see Figure 9-4).

Hypertension. Hypertension occurs in approximately 10% to 30% of patients with ARF (O'Meara & Bernard,

Table 9-13

Renal Replacement Therapies Used in the Treatment of Acute Renal Failure

Renal Replacement Therapy Option	Indications	Contraindications	Advantages	Disadvantages
Hemodialysis (HD) - removal of soluble substances and water from the blood into a dialysate bath across a semipermeable membrane by diffusion, filtration, and use of a transmembrane pressure gradient.	• uremia and related symptoms • electrolyte imbalances • volume overload • symptomatic acidosis • contraindications to other forms of dialysis • availability of highly trained staff and equipment	• hemodynamic instability • lack of access to circulation • inability to anticoagulate • lack of highly trained staff and/or equipment	• rapid and efficient • intermittent treatment usually sufficient	• hemodynamic instability • rapid fluid and solute shifts • membrane incompatibility • blood loss • anticoagulation needed • access to circulation • equipment/personnel
Peritoneal dialysis (PD) - removal of soluble substances and water from the body by transfer across the peritoneum through diffusion, filtration, and osmosis using a dialysate solution that is intermittently introduced into and removed from the peritoneal cavity.	• uremia • electrolyte imbalance • volume overload • blood access failure • hemodynamic instability • inability to anticoagulate • contradiction to hemodialysis	• need for rapid removal of fluid or solute • presence of abdominal adhesions • traumatized abdomen • consider postoperative abdomen • consider peritonitis • history of ineffective clearances	• slow, gradual dialysis • indicated for unstable or bleeding patients • requires less technical support and equipment • no anticoagulation needed	• slow fluid and solute removal • less predictable • infection • drainage failure • respiratory compromise • hyperglycemia
Continuous renal replacement therapies (CRRT) - an extracorporeal process for removing fluid, electrolytes, and small to medium-sized molecules from the blood by ultrafiltration or combinations of ultrafiltration, fluid replacement, and dialysis. (Ultrafiltration is the removal of soluble substances and water from the blood across a semipermeable membrane.)	• hypervolemia • need to remove large volumes of fluid in hemodynamically unstable patients • oliguric patients requiring large quantities of volume replacement • contraindication to HD/PD dialysis • lack of hemodialysis staff	• hematocrit over 45% • inability to anticoagulate	• maintains consistent homeostasis • avoids hypotensive episodes • permits continuous control of fluid balance	• nursing time involved • technical problems

Note: Adapted from Daugirdas & Ing (1994); Mehta (1994); Price (1992b); Stark (1992b, pp. 40-44).

1995), and it is usually volume dependent (related to the retention of salt and water). However, it may be complicated by decreased renal perfusion and activation of the renin-angiotensin system, excess aldosterone secretion, increased sympathetic tone, diminished production of vasodepressor hormones, and excess release of vasoconstrictor natriuretic factors (Suki & Eknoyan, 1995). Blood pressure medications are, therefore, an important component of treatment. However, most antihypertensive agents may increase vascular instability and can cause profound hypotension during HD.

Congestive heart failure. Congestive heart failure is often present in varying degrees, depending on volume status, and may be aggravated by other problems such as hypertension, anemia, electrolyte abnormalities, and acidosis (Suki & Eknoyan, 1995). Reduction of blood pressure and correction of acidosis and hyperkalemia often have marked effects on

the stabilization of cardiac function (O'Meara & Bernard, 1995). Serious disturbances in cardiac rhythm may develop secondary to hyperkalemia, hypermagnesemia, hypocalcemia, and severe acidosis. In the ARF patient, hypomagnesemia and hypokalemia frequently occur after diuretic administration, predisposing the individual to digitalis intoxication (O'Meara & Bernard, 1995; Suki & Eknoyan, 1995).

Uremic pericarditis. Uremic pericarditis, an inflammation of the membrane surrounding the heart, is a condition often accompanied by the collection of varying amounts of fluid and/or blood in the pericardial sac (Suki & Eknoyan, 1995). In most cases, the inflammation is aseptic, although some cases of bacterial and viral pericarditis have been reported (Suki & Eknoyan, 1995). Clinical manifestations include pain, fever, and a pericardial friction rub (a harsh leathery sound heard over the precordium). The friction rub may precede the pain, often persists when the pain has sub-

Figure 9-4
Etiologic Factors of the Cardiovascular Manifestations

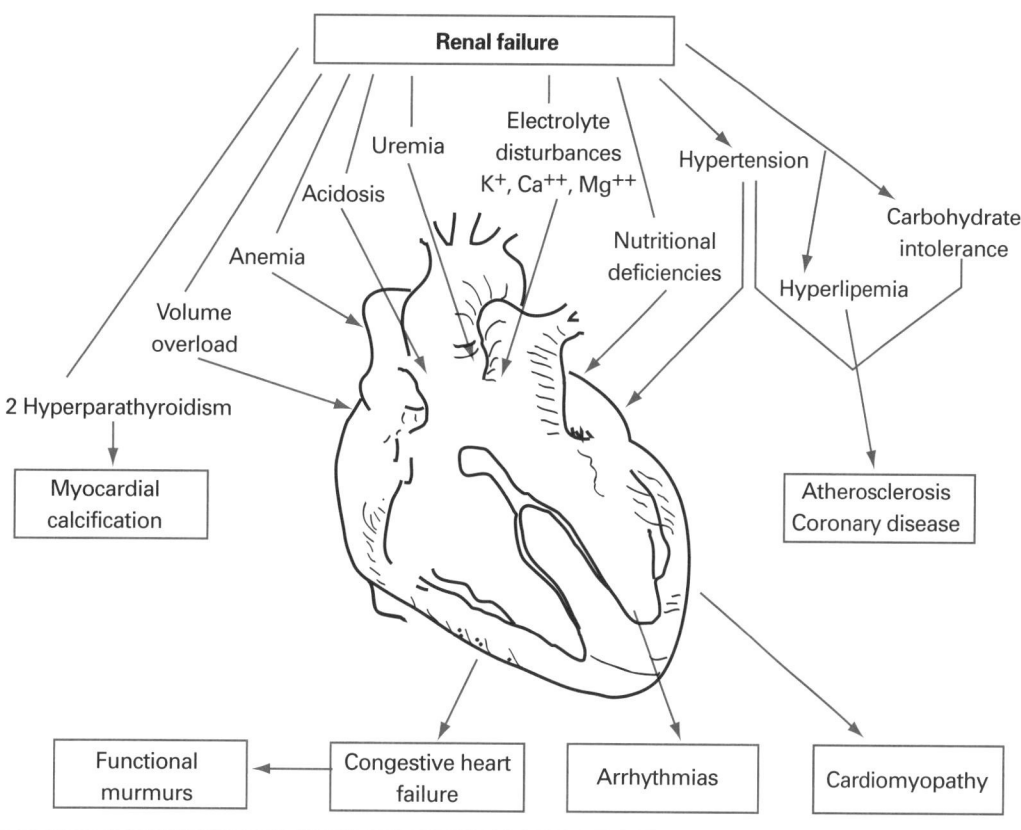

Note: From Eknoyan, G. (1977). Chronic renal failure and uremic syndrome. In N.A. Kurtzman & M. Martinez-Maldonado (Eds.), *Pathophysiology of the kidney* (p. 856). Springfield, IL: Charles C. Thomas Publishers. Reprinted with permission.

sided, and may disappear when fluid begins collecting. Other symptoms include tachycardia, low-grade fever, hypotension, narrowing pulse pressure, and a paradoxical pulse (see Table 9-14). About 50% of patients will have the EKG changes. Tamponade may also occur with the development of severe right ventricular failure, requiring pericardiocentesis or tube pericardiostomy. Treatment usually includes daily HD or CRRT. No or minimal doses of heparin or regional anticoagulation should be used during dialysis to minimize the risk of pericardial bleeding and tamponade (O'Meara & Bernard, 1995). Normal saline flushes every half hour may be attempted to maintain the extracorporeal circulation. Anti-inflammatory agents such as indomethacin and corticosteroids may also be effective in relieving the pericardial inflammation. Appropriate nursing management includes a careful assessment of the cardiovascular status of the patient and careful monitoring of fluid, electrolyte, and acid-base balance. Many cardiac medications require dosage adjustments in renal failure, and patients' responses to these agents may vary with electrolyte levels.

Respiratory manifestations. A variety of pulmonary complications are associated with the uremic syndrome. These complications include pulmonary edema, pleuritis with or without pleural effusion, and increased susceptibility to pulmonary infection. In addition, Kussmaul respirations secondary to metabolic acidosis are frequently encountered. Thus,

Table 9-14
Checking for a Paradoxical Pulse by Sphygmomanometer

A paradox is often cited as specific for pericardial effusion. Normally, on inspiration, increased venous return to the right heart and increased pulmonary vascular capacity results in less blood in the left heart and a small decrease in cardiac output. This change in cardiac output is evidenced as the arterial blood pressure falls as much as 10 mm/Hg during inspiration. A paradoxical pulse is an exaggeration of this normal event. On inspiration, the arterial blood pressure falls more than 10 mm/Hg. The pericardial effusion limits or restricts cardiac filling and decreases cardiac output. The result is a marked fall in blood pressure on inspiration (paradoxical pulse) (Lancaster, 1983, p. 44).

1. Ask the patient to breathe as easily and normally as possible.
2. Apply sphygmomanometer and inflate it until no sounds are audible.
3. Deflate the cuff gradually until sounds are audible only during expiration. Note the pressure.
4. Deflate the cuff further until sounds are also audible during inspiration. Note the pressure.

The difference in systolic pressure between expiration and inspiration should be 5 mm/Hg. If it is greater than 10 mm/Hg, the paradoxical pulse is exaggerated. Associated findings include low blood pressure and weak and rapid pulse (Seidel et al., 1991, p. 343).

Figure 9-5
Factors Contributing to Uremic Pneumonitis

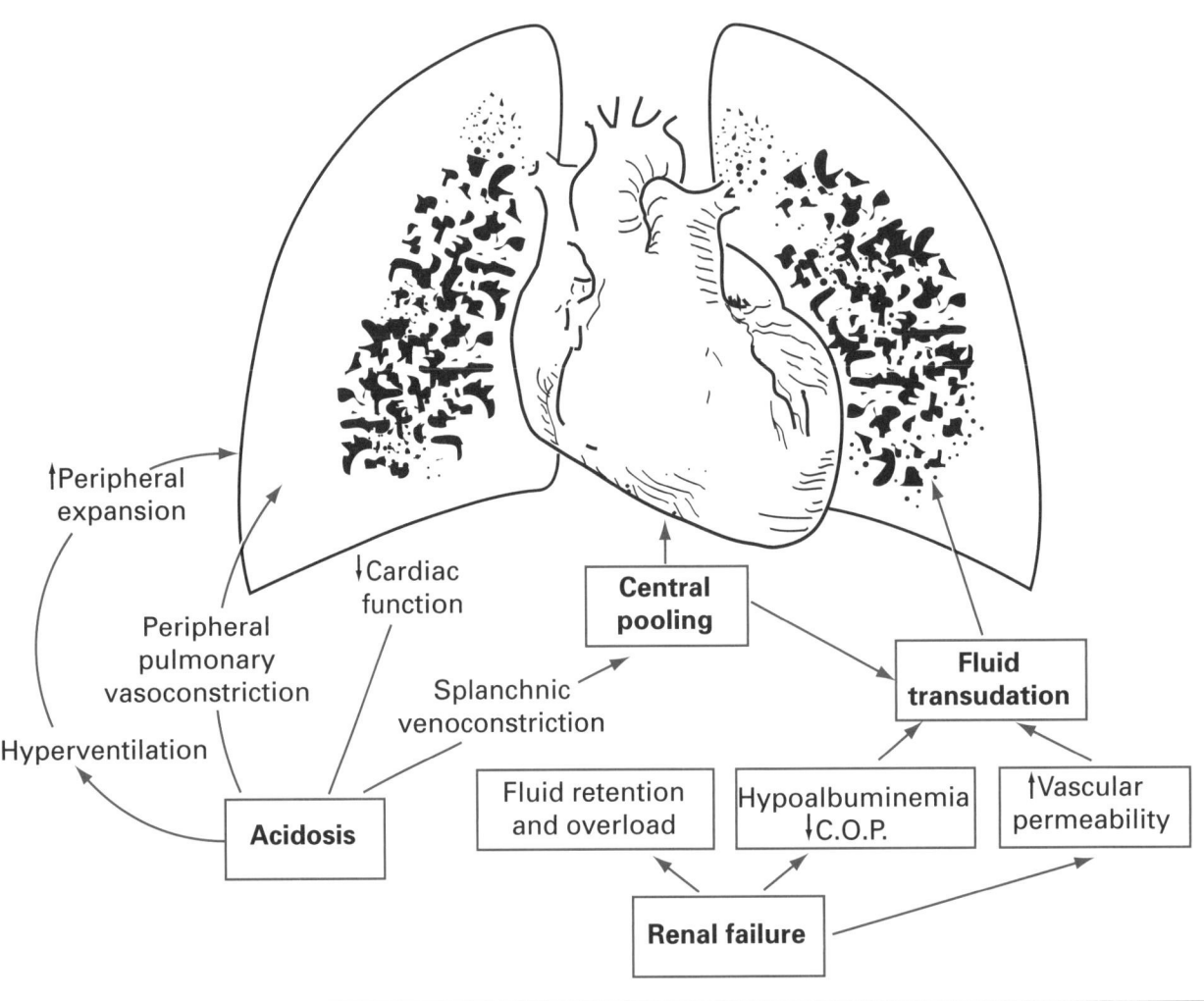

↑Peripheral expansion

Peripheral pulmonary vasoconstriction

↓Cardiac function

Central pooling

Hyperventilation

Splanchnic venoconstriction

Fluid transudation

Acidosis

Fluid retention and overload

Hypoalbuminemia ↓C.O.P.

↑Vascular permeability

Renal failure

Note: From Eknoyan, G. (1977). Chronic renal failure and uremic syndrome. In N.A. Kurtzman & M. Martinez-Maldonado (Eds.), *Pathophysiology of the kidney* (p. 859). Springfield, IL: Charles C. Thomas Publishers. Reprinted with permission.

a careful assessment of the pulmonary system is crucial in the management of these patients as prompt treatment with HD is often required.

Pulmonary edema. Pulmonary edema occurs frequently in patients with renal failure and is generally related to congestive heart failure and volume overload. Associated symptoms include shortness of breath, frothy sputum, and rales and rhonchi over lung fields. Although invasive monitoring is of great help in assessing volume status, pulmonary edema may occur in some patients with normal central venous or pulmonary artery pressures as acute uremia may damage capillaries, causing the leakage of fluid (Kjellstrand & Barsoum, 1995). In addition, a low serum albumin level resulting in decreased colloidal osmotic pressure (COP) of the blood may favor the formation of pulmonary edema in some patients. Central fluid collection, a phenomenon associated with metabolic acidosis, may also contribute to the problem (Suki & Eknoyan, 1995) (see Figure 9-5). X-rays often reveal a characteristic pattern in which opacities of the

central peripheral areas of the chest give a bat wing appearance (uremic pneumonitis). Pulmonary edema usually resolves after treatment with diuretics and/or dialysis (Suki & Eknoyan, 1995).

Pleuritis. Pleuritis, an inflammation of the pleura, can occur in ARF patients and may be accompanied by effusion. The etiology is believed to be similar to that of pericarditis and the two conditions frequently coexist. Symptoms include chest pain on inspiration and dyspnea. Decreased breath sounds over the area and a pleural friction rub are common physical findings (Suki & Eknoyan, 1995). Treatment with intensive dialysis is frequently helpful. Diagnostic thoracentesis may be necessary to exclude other causes of effusion, such as malignancy (Daugirdas & Ing, 1994).

Infection. Uremic patients exhibit an increased susceptibility to infection, including pneumonia and pulmonary tuberculosis. When infection is present, the sputum is often thick and tenacious. The cough reflex may also be depressed. Prompt treatment with antibiotics is required.

Table 9-15

Protocols for Pharmacologic Reduction of the Bleeding Time in Uremia

Agent	Usual dosage	Onset of action	Peak action	Duration of effect	Comments
Cryoprecipitate (IV)	10 units over 30 min	1 h	4-12 h	24-36 h	Effective on repeat dosing; hepatitis or HIV risk equivalent to transfusion of 10 units of blood.
DDAVP	0.3 mg/kg IV or SC	1 h	2-4 h	6-8 h	May not be effective on repeated dosing.
Intranasal DDAVP[a]	3.0 mg/kg	Same	Same	Same	Convenient, but only limited clinical experience.
IV estrogen[b]	0.6 mg/kg/day for 5 days (days 1-5)	6 h (day 1)	day 5-7	21-30 days	No reported adverse effects.

Notes: [a] Desmopressin (DDAVP) is available from Armour Pharmaceutical Co., Kankakee, IL; [b] Conjugated estrogen (Emopreparin) is available from Ayerst Pharmaceutical Co., New York, NY.

From Daugirdas, J.T., & Ing, T.S. (1994). *Handbook of dialysis* (p. 465). Boston: Little, Brown and Company. Reprinted with permission.

Hematologic manifestations. Anemia is a well-known complication of renal failure, generally worsens as renal function deteriorates, and is related to a decreased production of erythropoietin. In ARF, anemia can occur as early as 10 days after the onset. The hematocrit gradually falls, stabilizing in the 20% to 30% range (O'Meara & Bernard, 1995). Other factors that may contribute to the anemia of renal failure include bone marrow suppression, bleeding, hemodilution, decreased red blood cell survival, gastrointestinal hemorrhage, perioperative blood loss, and intravascular hemolysis (Eschbach & Adamson, 1993; O'Meara & Bernard, 1995). The anemia is usually normocytic (normal red blood cell [RBC] size) and normochromic (normal RBC color) unless it is complicated by iron deficiency, folate deficiency, or aluminum overload secondary to the administration of aluminum-containing phosphate binders (Daugirdas & Ing, 1994; Suki & Eknoyan, 1995). Associated symptoms include fatigue, reduced exercise tolerance, depression, decreased appetite, increased angina, cold intolerance, and hypotension.

Administration of recombinant human erythropoietin (r-HuEPO) has dramatically improved most patients by correcting anemia, increasing exercise tolerance, and improving subjective well-being, appetite, cognitive functioning, and overall quality of life. Because of the length of time required for full effects, transfusions may be used instead of r-HuEPO to treat the anemia of ARF. Adequate assessment of iron stores through measurements of ferritin, iron saturation, and transferrin are important, and iron adequate replacement (oral and IV) is essential (Daugirdas & Ing, 1994). In addition, supplementation of folic acid, iron, and amino acids is often given to patients with renal failure to replace suspected dietary deficiencies or extra losses due to dialysis (Eschbach & Adamson, 1993). Androgens can increase the red cell mass in some anemic dialysis patients. However, because of the high incidence of side effects, r-HuEPO should be the primary therapy.

A bleeding tendency related to platelet dysfunction also develops in uremia manifested by easy bruising, GI bleeds, epistaxis, bleeding gums, and spontaneous ecchymosis. Uremic platelets display defective aggregation and adhesiveness related to a decreased availability of platelet factor 3 and an altered platelet response to clotting factor VIII (von Willebrand's factor) (Suki & Eknoyan, 1995). The platelet count is usually only slightly reduced but may be very low in patients with hemolytic uremic syndrome or disseminated intravascular coagulation (DIC) (O'Meara & Bernard, 1995). The most reliable test to evaluate this bleeding tendency and its response to therapeutic interventions is the bleeding time (Suki & Eknoyan, 1995). Interventions that can improve the bleeding time include intensive dialysis (especially in the acute setting); increasing the hematocrit; and treatment with cryoprecipitate, desmopressin, and estrogen (Daugirdas & Ing, 1994; Eschbach & Adamson, 1993) (see Table 9-15). Cryoprecipitate and desmopressin are believed to improve the bleeding time by supplying or inducing other forms of factor VIII. The action of estrogen is not known (Daugirdas & Ing, 1994).

Uremia also induces impairment of several aspects of lymphocyte and granulocyte function (Daugirdas & Ing, 1994; Eschbach & Adamson, 1993). Although the leukocyte count is normal and increases appropriately in response to infection, the phagocytic capacity of the cell is compromised. In addition, the absolute number of circulating T cells is reduced, and suppressor cell activity seems to be increased while helper cell activity is decreased (Suki & Eknoyan, 1995). These factors increase the susceptibility of the patients to infections.

In summary, the hematologic manifestations of uremic syndrome have the potential to profoundly affect the health outcomes of patients with ARF. Nursing management should begin with a careful assessment of hematologic parameters and evaluation of related signs and symptoms. Evaluation of the patient's status and response to treatment is an ongoing process.

Figure 9-6
Factors Contributing to the Development of Gastrointestinal Bleeding in Renal Failure

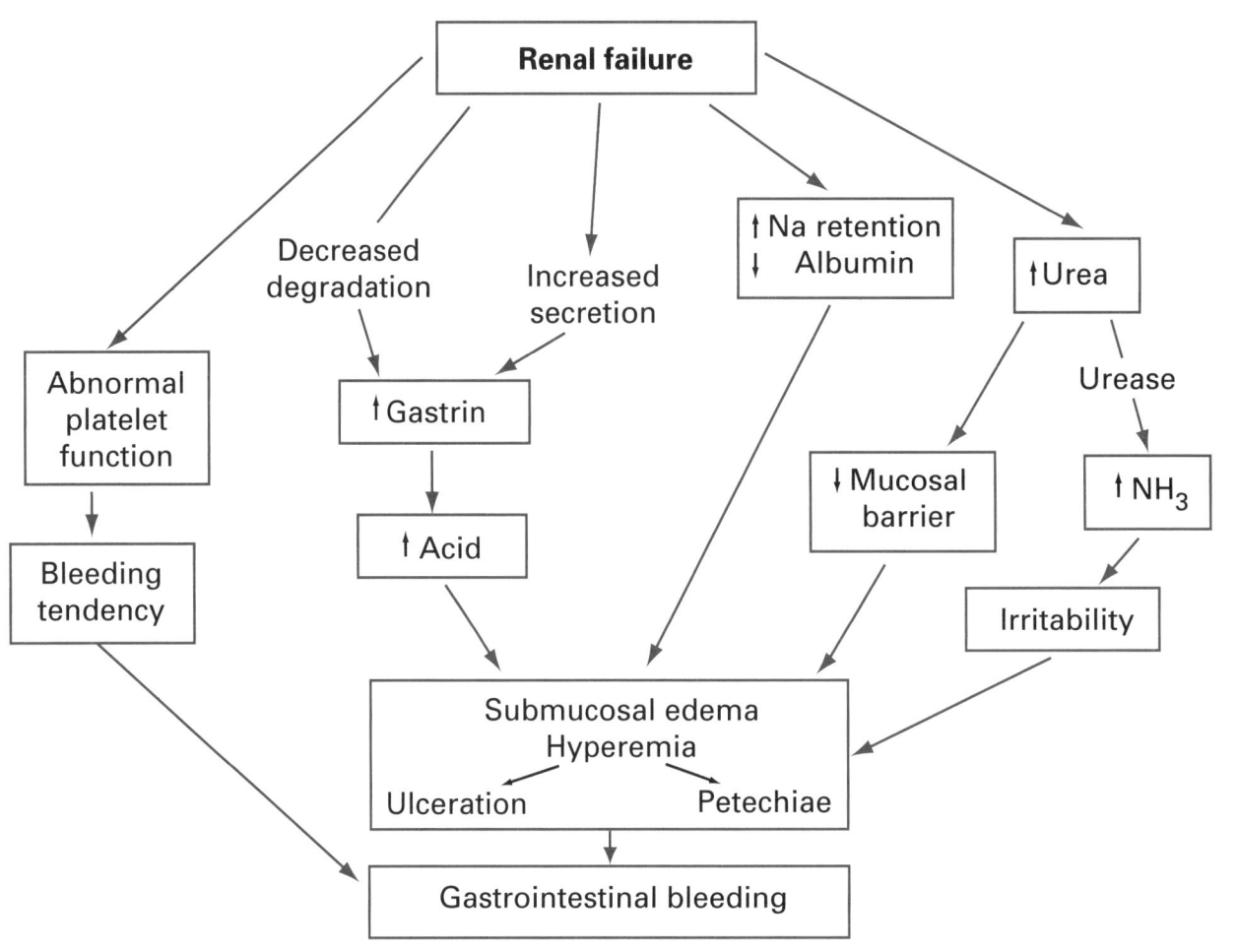

Note: Adapted with permission from Eknoyan, G. (1977). Chronic renal failure and uremic syndrome. In N.A. Kurtzman & M. Martinez-Maldonado (Eds.), *Pathophysiology of the kidney* (p. 854). Springfield, IL: Charles C. Thomas.

Gastrointestinal manifestations. Patients with ARF commonly manifest a variety of gastrointestinal symptoms related to mucosal alterations from uremia such as anorexia, nausea, dyspepsia, and vomiting. Hiccups also occur but are usually a late sign occurring in patients with advanced uremia (O'Meara & Bernard, 1995). Although diarrhea may be severe (especially if secondary to diabetic autonomic neuropathy), constipation is very common and a side effect of the aluminum binders patients often take with meals to decrease serum phosphate levels (Daugirdas & Ing, 1994). Patients may also complain of a metallic or salty taste in the mouth that is probably related to the high concentration of urea in the saliva. Halitosis and stomatitis are common. Spontaneous gingival bleeding often occurs and may be related to abnormalities in clotting mechanisms and high circulating levels of gastrin (Suki & Eknoyan, 1995). High amylase levels occur in ARF that are related to reduced renal excretion of the enzyme, but levels rarely exceed twice the upper limit of normal (O'Meara & Bernard, 1995; Suki & Eknoyan, 1995).

As renal failure progresses, patients may develop gastritis, duodenitis, ileitis, colitis, or proctatitis. Pathologic examination of the gastrointestinal system frequently reveals mucosal abnormalities such as edema, capillary hyperemia, angiodysplasia, multiple superficial shallow areas of ulceration, and necrotic lesions (Suki & Eknoyan, 1995). Although the pathophysiological basis is not fully understood, the formation of these alterations seems to be related to elevated levels of serum urea nitrogen. Urea diffuses into the bowel lumen and is converted by bacterial enzymes into ammonia and carbon dioxide (Suki & Eknoyan, 1995) (see Figure 9-6). Mucosal and submucosal edema may also contribute to decreased gastric peristalsis with prolonged emptying time.

ARF is associated with gastrointestinal bleeding in up to 25% of the cases (O'Meara & Bernard, 1995). The acute erosive ulcerations may affect any part of the upper or lower GI tract. Gastrointestinal blood loss may be exacerbated by the bleeding tendency or uremia and the use of heparin during HD. HD or CRRT will need to be offered without heparin or the use of trisodium sodium citrate anticoagulation. Early institution of dialysis and prophylactic antacids and H$_2$ blockers may prevent problems. Treatment with a medication such as metoclopramide can control nausea and enhance gastric emptying. Because of the increased tendency to bleed, medications such as steroids and NSAIDs should be avoided. Diets high in fiber and laxatives free of magnesium or phosphate can be safely used for patients with constipation. Diarrhea is often successfully treated with diphenoxylate hydrochloride (Lomotil®). Nursing care should begin with a thorough assessment of the oral cavity, abdomen, and bowel patterns. All vomitus and stool should be checked for occult blood, the presence of which can potentially increase the BUN. Good oral hygiene not only makes the patient more comfortable, but may also help enhance the appetite. Tables 9-4 and 9-11 summarize the systemic manifestations that occur with ARF.

Summary

Developments in the field of nephrology have presented the nursing profession with great challenges. Not only is the scientific and theoretical basis of the discipline exceedingly complicated, but also the nursing management required by patients with ARF continues to grow in complexity with further scientific developments. A thorough understanding of the physiologic basis and human responses, both systemic and psychosocial, is essential in order to effectively plan appropriate nursing interventions and evaluate patient outcomes. Equally as imperative, the nephrology nurses must understand the complexities of all of the potential extracorporeal therapies that may be necessary in the management of patients with ARF.

Continuous Renal Replacement Therapy

Whether on a battle ground or in a hospital intensive care unit (ICU), since 1982 nephrology professionals have not had to rely on hemodialysis (HD) or peritoneal dialysis (PD) for the treatment of ARF. Continuous renal replacement therapy (CRRT) has received popular acceptance in Europe and the United States, particularly for hemodynamically unstable patients who are unresponsive to conservative management with pharmacologic and dietary interventions. In the simplest form, CRRT is an arterial to venous extracorporeal whole blood circuit that uses the patient's mean arterial pressure (MAP) as a driving force to propel blood through the circuit and create an ultrafiltration of plasma water. Many nephrologists and nephrology nurses have embraced CRRT because it is recognized as meeting the total 24-hour needs of the patient for hourly fluid and electrolyte balance, adjustment of acid/base status, and continuous removal of uremic toxins. Furthermore, correction of the patient's clinical profile can be accomplished while maintaining hemodynamic stability and providing essential nutritional and pharmacokinetic support. The development of CRRT therapy has permitted an expansion of critically ill patients who can benefit from dialytic therapies (Baldwin, 2002; Teechan, Liangos & Jaber, 2003).

CRRT Technologies, Hemofilters, and Equipment

The early literature describing CRRT highlighted the benefits of continuous fluid removal for patients with renal dysfunction (Kramer et al., 1980). The extracorporeal circuit required arterial and venous vascular access and a hemofilter as a highly porous device for removal fluid and small molecular weight plasma contents. A continuous heparin infusion was used to maintain anticoagulation of the system. Replacement fluids were administered continuously or intermittently to balance the hourly fluid removal. Figure 9-7 provides a pictorial view of basic CRRT components.

The first acronyms for these treatments were CAVH (continuous arteriovenous hemofiltration), CAVU (continuous arteriovenous ultrafiltration), and SCUF (slow continuous ultrafiltration), respectively (Price, 1989a). A basic definition of these procedures is: an arteriovenous extracorporeal circuit with the patient's whole blood flowing through a hemofilter to create an ultrafiltrate of plasma. A hemofilter is a medical device of either hollow fiber or parallel plate membrane geometric design that allows plasma water and dissolved contents to freely move across the membrane and out of the patient's blood. Ultrafiltrate is plasma water free of formed cells and protein, and it is isotonic with plasma for small molecules, for example, electrolytes, creatinine, and urea. The system is blood pressure-dependent as the driving force for the blood flow rate (BFR), and it uses a gravity drain for ultrafiltration into a fluid collection container. Ideally the patient's systolic blood pressure (SBP) is constantly > 90 mmHg and the MAP is > 70 mmHg. The plasma ultrafiltrate is collected and measured hourly to calculate the ultrafiltration rate (UFR). Although historically important, this basic approach to CRRT is rarely practiced today. Automated, pump-assisted, volumetric equipment is the standard of care. There are a number of machines on the market available for hospital use. The therapy is now referred to as continuous venovenous hemofiltration (CVVH) or continuous venovenous hemodialysis/diafiltration (CVVHD).

The use of CRRT is limited to an ICU setting where close hourly monitoring and fluid adjustments are possible. The original intent of CRRT was to augment existing renal dysfunction. The most conservative of the CRRT therapies for fluid removal is SCUF. Generally, the patient is not anuric, but requires ultrafiltration of an extra 100-300 ml of fluid/hour for a short period of time, possibly 12-48 hours. Replacement fluid for the ultrafiltrate is usually not necessary. A typical patient profile might be an individual with renal insufficiency post-myocardial infarction, or a patient with moderate oliguria who is resistant to diuretics.

When the patient's clinical status is more critical or involves multisystem failure, both solute and fluid must be effectively managed. With CVVH the hourly UFR can range from 200-800 ml of fluid, which is poorly tolerated by most hemodynamically unstable patients. The patient may be oliguric or anuric. If replacement fluid is not delivered intravenously (IV) every hour, the patient may experience significant hypotension and other cardiac abnormalities. Physicians will prescribe an hourly net loss of fluid as their goal for the patient, for example 100 - 300 ml/hr. The orders will also prescribe the type of replacement fluid to be infused, for example, normal saline with potassium, 5% dextrose and .45% normal saline, or 5% albumin solution. The replacement is customized to meet the patient's unique needs. The CRRT machine is programmed to deliver the prescribed therapy, including fluid replacement. With the equipment of today being computerized, all parameters can be set at the initiation of the treatment, and only need adjust-

Figure 9-7
Arterial Bloodline, Ultrafiltrate Line, Venous Bloodline, Hemofilter, and CAVHD Port

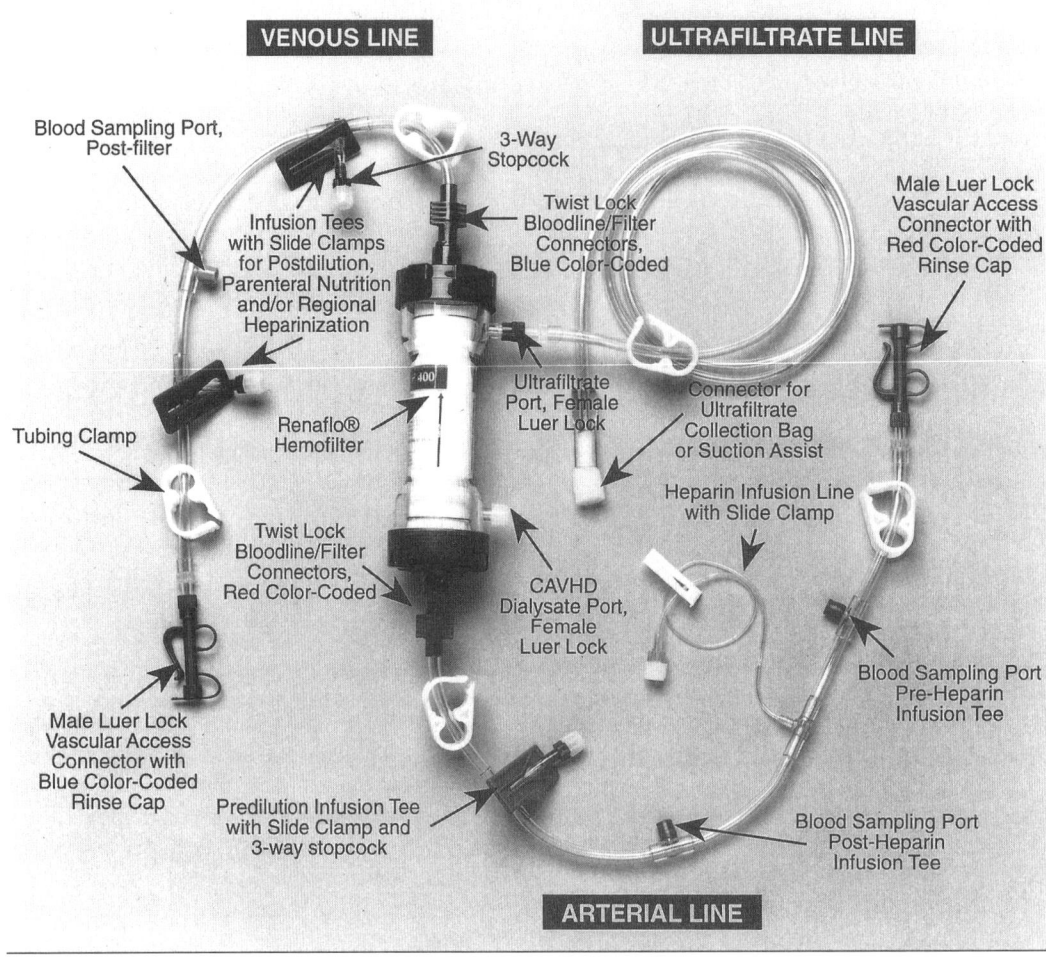

Note: Printed with permission from Renal Systems.

ing if the physician changes the orders or the patient does not respond well to the therapy.

The replacement fluid is infused either predilution in the arterial blood tubing, before the hemofilter, or postdilution in the venous blood tubing, after the hemofilter, as labeled in Figure 9-7. Predilution will dictate the use of more solution, but it may decrease the anticoagulation requirements and increase clearance of plasma contents because of the hemodilution effect of expanding the blood volume. Postdilution is simpler to monitor because none of the fluid is lost in the ultrafiltrate and less expensive because generally less replacement fluid is needed.

In addition to maintaining the BFR (range 150-300 ml/min), UFR (range 0-500+ml/hour) and fluid requirements, the CRRT circuit requires an ongoing method of anticoagulation to maintain the long-term patency. A patient clinical presentation may require the application of CRRT for a short period, that is 24- 8 hours, or a prolonged period of > 2 weeks. Heparin therapy is the standard means of assuring patency of the extracorporeal circuit. Heparin administration is prescribed usually as a bolus dose to be given prehemofilter at the initiation of CRRT. Depending on the patient's

injuries or wounds, postsurgical status, and risk for hemorrhage, the heparin dose may range from 0 - 2000 units IV bolus. During the course of therapy, an hourly heparin infusion may be prescribed that may range from 0 to 5 - 10 u/kg. The heparin administration may be regulated by the platelet count, partial prothrombin time (PTT), prothrombin time (PT), or activated clotting time (ACT). Problems related to heparin therapy include bleeding and heparin associated antibodies, which leads to thrombocytopenia and clotting of the hemofilter (Davenport, 1998). The experience of health care professionals, available hospital equipment, and established ICU protocols will dictate the use of heparin therapy.

In lieu of heparin anticoagulation, some centers have a protocol for the use of trisodium citrate anticoagulation (Ashton, Mehta, Ward, McDonald & Aguilar, 1991). With this system, the trisodium citrate is infused prehemofilter and a 10% calcium chloride replacement solution is infused posthemofilter (Kutsogiannis, Mayers, Chin, & Gibney, 2000. The nurse must monitor for cardiac dysarhythmias and neurological deficits related to hypocalcemia. Serum ionized calcium and total calcium levels must be monitored every 4-8 hours. An additional problem related to citrate anticoagulation is acid/base disturbance, which may lead to severe alkalosis.

For several years, CVVH and SCUF served the nephrology and critical care communities well for the treatment of ARF. Fluid and some solute removal can be achieved with CVVH or SCUF, but for patients who had no kidney function, the removal of uremic toxins and electrolytes was inadequate. Continuous arteriovenous hemodiafiltration or hemodialysis (CAVHD) was introduced for the treatment of patients who required considerable adjustment for serum electrolyte abnormalities, intervention for severe acid/base disturbance, and correction of moderate to severe uremia (Geronemus, 1988). As with CVVH, the current standard of practice is the venovenous approach, or CVVHD. However, we now have better technology that allows the health care providers to customize CRRT to match the needs of the patient (Luyckx & Bonventre, 2004; Mehta, 1993).

In the ARF setting, therapy for correction of fluid overload is of paramount importance. Equally important is the removal of toxins that under normal conditions would be excreted through the kidneys. Clearance of metabolic waste products is a goal of renal replacement therapy. Clearance of plasma substances is achieved by convection during CVVH. Adequate clearance can be achieved if the patient is not extremely catabolic and/or nephrology service is consulted early in the ARF setting. There is only minimal clearance achieved using SCUF because of the low hourly UFR. Convective clearance is the removal of a substance along with fluid, that is, the ultrafiltrate. The plasma contents are essentially carried across the hemofilter membrane. In this situation, clearance is reflective of the sieving coefficient (see Table 9-16). The more ultrafiltrate generated, the higher will be the clearance of molecules. The measurement is based on every 100 ml of fluid ultrafiltrated.

With CVVHD, the CRRT system is not dependent on convective clearance alone. Adding a dialysate solution to run countercurrent to the patient's blood flow in the extracorporeal circuit permits diffusion of substances across the hemofilter membrane. Plasma contents will move in the direction of higher concentration to lower concentration. The dialysate solution will customarily be prescribed for concentration of sodium, potassium, calcium, bicarbonate, and possibly glucose. Solutions similar to PD solutions may be used, that is, Na: 134 mEq/L; K: 0-4 mEq/L; Ca: 2.5-3.5 mEq/L; HCO_3: 25-35 mEq/L; Mg: 0.5-1.5 mEq/L; and glucose: 0-1500 mg dextrose/L. If the patient's serum level is higher than the dialysate level, then that particular substance will diffuse across the membrane with the ultrafiltrate. During CVVHD, the dialysate flow rate (DFR) may range from 1-3 L/hr, or 16.7-50 ml/min. CVVHD rapidly replaced CVVH for critically ill patients whose health care needs necessitated more intense management. The clearance of plasma water contents is improved by having convection and diffusion principles operational. However, this complicates a rather simple procedure and adds to the expense of providing the therapy (Henrich, 1993). Patients who might benefit from CVVHD are patients who have sustained severe traumatic injuries or burns, patients with extremely compromised cardiac function, and/or patients who are status post-extensive vascular repair surgery.

Table 9-16
Formulae and Calculations for Monitoring CRRT

A. Blood flow rate

QBi = (Qf x Hct outlet) / (Hct outlet - Hct inlet)
QBi = blood flow rate in ml/min
Qf = ultrafiltation rate in ml/min
Hct inlet = hematocrit prehemofilter in percent
Hct outlet = hematocrit posthemofilter in percent

B. Ultrafiltration rate

UFR = TV / 60 min
UFR = ultrafiltration rate in ml/min
TV = total volume of ultrafiltrate in 1 hour

C. Sieving coefficient for solute removal

Sieving coefficient = ultrafiltrate level/ plasma level
Sieving coefficient = ratio of the ultrafiltrate concentration of a solute to the plasma concentration of the solute

D. Fluid replacement using net loss concept

Total fluid output - total fluid intake = volume of fluid loss
Volume of fluid loss - prescribed net loss = fluid replacement
Total fluid output = urine, gastric tubes, chest tubes, stool, UF, insensible loss, etc.
Total fluid intake = IVs, blood products, oral, nutritional support, etc.
Net loss must be in physician's orders
Replacement fluid will be infused over following hour

CVVH and CVVHD further complicate the simple CRRT system, but they have definite advantages and they have allowed for a greater number of patients to be treated (Mehta, 1993; Paganini, 1993). The patient's MAP does not influence the BFR with CVVH or CVVHD, but in lieu of the MAP, a blood pump is set from 50 - 350 ml/min. Problems can arise during periods of hypotension because the BFR is not altered, nor is the UFR lowered to compensate for the decreased MAP. The patient may continue to lose intravascular fluid volume and quickly develop a fluid deficit. However, during the venovenous approach to CRRT the infusion of heparin is more consistent, therefore, clotting of the hemofilter may be less problematic. The venovenous system equipment requirements add to the expense of providing CRRT and to the nurse's time and attention for monitoring patient care. Continuous venovenous therapy equipment has a blood pump, dialysate pump, fluid replacement pumps, air alert detector, and arterial and venous pressure alarms, in addition, to various monitoring systems that are specific to the equipment manufacturer. CVVHD may require the use of one or more dialysate delivery pumps to maximize the therapy for achieving diffusive clearance (Bonnardeaux et al.,

1992). Patients who would be candidates for these therapies include diabetics, patients with advanced cardiovascular disease, elderly patients with significant arteriolosclerosis or atherosclerosis, and/or neonatal or pediatric patients.

The treatment of ARF has changed considerably over the years. Likewise, the practice of CRRT has changed. The advantage of CRRT over standard acute HD is that there are several different approaches in the health care professionals' armamentarium of therapies (Abdeen & Mehta, 2002). Treatment can be provided on a continuous basis, rather than attempting to fit the patient's needs into a time-prescribed therapy, like 3 or 4-hour treatment with HD. The approach to CRRT most often is based on the knowledge and skill of the nephrology and critical care professionals, the availability of necessary equipment, and the patient's clinical status. Treatment with planned patient outcomes and expected goals guides the use of CRRT. CRRT is often considered the treatment of choice for ARF (Vanholder, VanBieson & Lameire, 2001)

Responsibilities of Health Care Professionals

In a collaborative effort, the American Nephrology Nurses' Association (ANNA) developed *Standards of Clinical Practice for Continuous Renal Replacement Therapy,* and these standards were reviewed and subsequently endorsed by the American Association of Critical Care Nurses (AACN). Nursing professionals recognize collaboration and communication should exist for successful management of patients receiving CRRT (Politosk, Mayer, Davy, & Swartz, 1998). Unlike the nursing care for patients receiving HD, where the lines of responsibility are fairly well defined, there is a blending of nursing roles and care, when CRRT is the treatment of choice (Price, 1992; Martin, 1997). The continuous nature of CRRT over hours or days requires a delineation of who will provide the care and when the necessary nursing interventions will occur. Of equal importance is the delineation of physicians' responsibilities for the nephrologists and intensivists. However, this chapter will only address the nursing care from the perspective of pre-CRRT assessment, intra-CRRT monitoring and interventions, and post-CRRT evaluation.

Unfortunately, as CRRT has matured in its clinical application and allowed for treatment of more patients, the implementation of CRRT programs remains somewhat controversial. Many nephrologists, as do many nephrology nurses, view CRRT as one of several dialytic therapies that are within the realm of their practice (Price, 1993,1994; Yagi & Paganini, 1997). On the other hand, many intensivists and critical care nurses consider interventions provided in an ICU within their realm of expertise (Bellomo, Cole, Reeves, & Silvester, 1997; Giuliano & Pysznik, 1998). From a nursing viewpoint, Martin (2002) points out the benefits of a joint nephrology and critical care nursing model that promotes collaboration between the two distinct nursing specialties with opportunities for setting joint standards and promoting research. It is the opinion of this author that striving towards collaborative practice should be the goal of all involved professionals for the enhancement of their clinical knowledge, but moreover, because this approach will best serve the needs of critically ill patients who suffer the injuries related to ARF.

Nursing Care Before CRRT

When critically ill patients present to the hospital emergency room or develop ARF while hospitalized, intensive monitoring and intervention are often required. Critical care nurses are always responsible for the total nursing management of ICU patients. This includes following the nursing process of systematic data collection, setting expected patient outcomes, planning nursing interventions accordingly, and evaluating the patient's response to the nursing care provided. A total body systems physical assessment is completed upon admission to the ICU and then at the beginning of each nursing shift. Using the cephalocaudal approach, the nurse incorporates any findings that are caused by ARF, or may be exacerbated by the ARF, for example, fluid imbalance and cardiac dysrhythmias. Additionally, the critical care nurse assesses findings of available pertinent laboratory analyses and diagnostic tests. This might include serum chemistries, arterial blood gases, urine analysis, and blood and/or urine cultures. Diagnostic procedures might include renal biopsy, radiography, ultrasound, flow scans, computed tomography (CT), and/or magnetic resonance imaging (MRI) studies.

Ideally, after the nephrologist has been consulted regarding the patient's medical problems, nephrology nurses are alerted to the possibility of providing dialysis. Often the nephrologist, a nephrology clinical nurse specialist (CNS), or a nephrology nurse practitioner (NP) will collaborate on the type of dialysis that would best meet the patient's needs. Alternatively, an intensivist or nephrologist and a critical care nurse may collaborate on a plan of care. If CRRT is the selected renal replacement modality, the physician, CNS, or NP will review the patient's clinical presentation, the need for fluid and/or solute removal, and the availability of venous vascular access. Most often the vascular access used will be a standard dual lumen HD catheter placed in the intrajuglar, subclavian, or femoral vein. Based on these considerations, SCUF, CVVH, or CVVHD will be prescribed. Figure 9-8 provides a pictorial view of all CRRT therapies.

A nephrology nurse will prepare the CRRT system to assure removal of all air, sterilant, and packing agents. This is necessary to avoid an adverse reaction upon initiation of the therapy. After priming the system with heparinized normal saline (5000 u/L), the nephrology nurse usually takes the CRRT system to the patient's ICU bedside. Before proceeding with the initiation of CRRT, the nephrology nurse completes an assessment of the patient's condition. Additionally, she or he completes, or consults with the critical care nurse regarding the total patient physical assessment. The nephrology nurse reviews the nursing documentation and the physician's orders and progress notes. Collaboratively, the nurses perform an assessment of the vascular access that has been placed either by the nephrologist, the intensivist, or the surgeon. The nephrology nurse and the responsible critical care nurse discuss the intended interventions and assure that all appropriate supplies are readily available, which include replacement fluids, dialysate, heparin infusion, and CRRT machine.

Ideally, nurses work together to initiate the treatment. The venovenous vascular access is flushed per protocol, the blood tubing is connected using strict sterile technique, and the extracorporeal blood circuit is established. If prescribed, a heparin bolus will be administered into the arterial blood line. The heparin or citrate infusion will be started and gradually

Figure 9-8
Diagrams of Continuous Renal Replacement Therapies

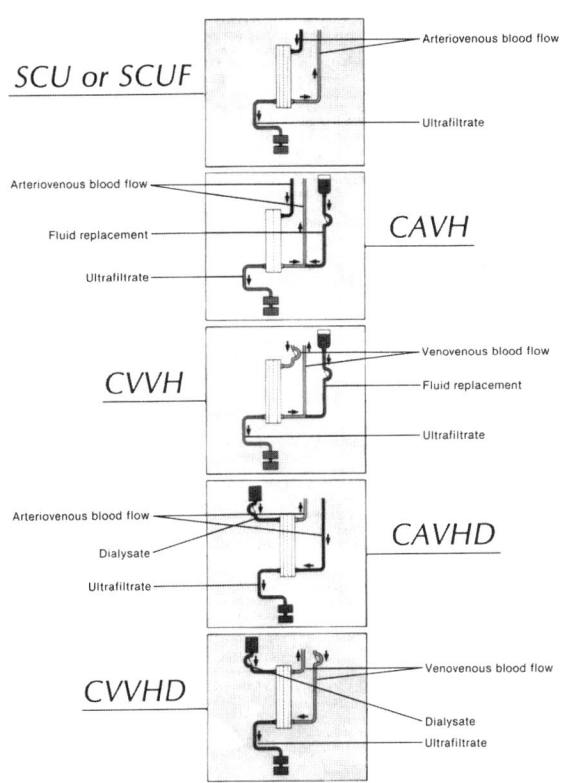

SCU or SCUF
- Arteriovenous blood flow
- Ultrafiltrate

CAVH
- Arteriovenous blood flow
- Fluid replacement
- Ultrafiltrate

CVVH
- Venovenous blood flow
- Fluid replacement
- Ultrafiltrate

CAVHD
- Arteriovenous blood flow
- Dialysate
- Ultrafiltrate

CVVHD
- Venovenous blood flow
- Dialysate
- Ultrafiltrate

Note: Printed with permission from Cobe Gambro-Hospital Medical, Inc.

increased based on the ICU protocol, which generally requires monitoring the patient's activated clotting time (ACT), partial prothrombin time (PTT), or prothrombin time (PT), and titrating the infusion for delivery of the correct dose. There is no universal or standard approach for anticoagulation therapy related to CRRT, but rather hospital-specific guidelines.

The nurses monitor the patient's response to the initiation of the treatment. Particularly the patient's blood pressure and pulse are observed to avoid sudden changes that indicate cardiac distress. During the first 30 minutes of treatment, the nurses observe the ultrafiltrate for color and amount. The BFR is slowly increased as ordered, usually from 50 to 350 ml/min. The UFR is set along with the fluid replacement rate. Finally, if prescribed, a dialysate solution is prepared on a fluid administration pump to be delivered countercurrent to the BFR. This dialysate solution is delivered to the space on the outside of the hollow fiber or parallel plate membrane to promote clearance of small molecular weight solutes across the membrane by diffusion. The nurses share the responsibility for assuring correct solution and delivery rate as prescribed in the physician's orders.

Nursing Care During CRRT

Once the therapy is ongoing and the patient remains stable, critical care nurses assume primary responsibility for the CRRT treatment (Bosworth, 1992; Martin, 1997). However, a nephrology nurse, NP, or CNS is expected to visit the patient daily or more often, if necessary, and complete a physical assessment of

the patient and an equipment assessment of the CRRT system. After consulting with the nephrologist, if patency of the system is suspect, a nephrology nurse arranges for discontinuation of the present CRRT circuit and reinitiation of CRRT with a new hemofilter and tubing. A nephrology nurse checks daily laboratory analyses to assess adequacy of clearances and ultrafiltration, which might also necessitate a new hemofilter and tubing if the therapy is not meeting expected goals. The nephrology and critical care personnel usually collaborate on making adjustments in the CRRT system depending on the patient's response to therapy. A nephrology nurse should be available by telephone or pager to assist critical care nurses with nursing care related to CRRT.

In performing routine intensive care, the critical care nurse consults with the intensivist or nephrologist and relates the nursing assessment and any changes in the patient's clinical course. The skill and expertise of the critical care nurses will enhance the probability of successful management of patients with ARF. Appropriate nursing policies, procedures, and standards of practice are developed and communicated to all nurses. Particularly important during the intratherapy period, all nurses must comprehend and follow protocols for intervening to resolve problems related to CRRT or make adjustments based on evaluation of the patient's response to therapy. Some of the most frequent patient complications that may occur are hypotension, cardiac dysrhythmias, excessive fluid loss, electrolyte imbalance, acid/base abnormalities, neuromuscular changes, local and/or systemic infection, and blood loss. Some of the most frequent CRRT circuit problems that may occur are disconnection of blood lines at the vascular access site, clotting of the hemofilter, blood leak in the hemofilter, physical damage to the hemofilter plastic case, and malfunctioning of the CRRT equipment. The patient-related problems often with regards to the patient's underlying diagnosis, comorbid factors, and/or need to make changes in the CRRT circuit, for example, advancing CVVH to CVVHD or changing the replacement or dialysate fluid prescription. The equipment-related problems mandate changing the sterile set-up, increasing attention to all tubing connections, having the hemofilter clearly visible at all times (that is, not covered with bed linens), increasing anticoagulation delivery, monitoring for positional or kinked catheters, and securing biomedical assistance for equipment support. If the system should clot, the critical care nurse must disconnect the tubing from the vascular access and focus on maintaining patency of the access until a new system is available.

Nursing Care After CRRT

With resolution of the patient's ARF or with a decision to withdraw therapy, the CRRT circuit is discontinued. Often this task is a joint responsibility shared by the nurses. If the ARF has resolved, the critical care nurse assumes total responsibility for managing the patient's nursing care. After a day or 2, if the vascular access is no longer needed, either the nephrology or critical care nurse will remove the catheter. Often shortly afterwards, the patient is transferred out of the ICU. If the patient's condition has deteriorated and the prognosis is poor, the nurses, physicians, and family discuss the decision to withdraw care and prepare for comfort measures only. A written advance directive, living will, and/or durable power of attorney become extremely important to assure that the patient's wishes are followed.

Nursing Literature and Research Related to CRRT

The medical professional literature covering CRRT dates back to the 1970s and is vast. The introduction of CRRT into clinical practice involved nephrology and critical care nurses from the very beginning, but often the nurses' contributions were only acknowledged as a note of appreciation from manuscript authors. The earliest nursing publication appeared in the *AANNT Journal* in 1981 (Rainone & Littman). Nursing involvement with CRRT during the early 1980s was primarily the work of two critical care nurses, Gayle Whitman and Susan Dirkes, and this author, Christy Price. The Cleveland Clinic in Ohio, under the physician direction of Emil Paganini, MD, has been heavily involved in research related to CRRT, and nursing assistance has been recognized in joint physician and nurse publications. Paganini, Fisque, Whitman, and Nakamoto (1982) published the first studies using SCUF in the treatment of ARF. Several years later Cindy Bosworth, RN, was the primary author of a paper published from data collected on using pump-assisted ultrafiltration and dialysate delivery during CAVHD (Bosworth, Swann, & Paganini, 1990). An early reference guide for CRRT was coauthored by physicians and a nurse from the University of Michigan in 1984, but the 1989 edition specifically listed the contributing professionals (Mault, Dirkes, Swartz, & Bartlett, 1989). Rabetoy, Mosley, Duke, and Price (1989) collaboratively presented a review of the literature and summarized their early experience with CRRT being practiced in a military teaching hospital.

After the above initial nurse-coauthored publications, nurses independently published in nursing journals. The nursing literature addressed the principles and procedures related to CRRT, but several articles appeared that outlined nursing interventions, continuous critical care monitoring, potential patient and system complications, and expected patient outcomes (Williams & Perkins, 1984; Kiely, 1984; Cant, 1984; Locke, Groth, & Lees, 1985; Winkelman, 1985; Whittaker, Brown, Grabenbauer, & Cauble, 1986; Palmer, Koorejian, London, Dechert, & Bartlett; 1986; Lawyer, 1987; Bell, 1988, Wedel, 1988; Dirkes, 1989; Kaplow & Bendo, 1989; Paradiso, 1989; Price, 1989a, 1989b,1991a, b). These authors represent a mix of nephrology and critical care nurses in professional positions as inservice coordinator, clinical nurse specialist, clinical staff nurse, and/or nursing director of a particular ICU or renal unit.

The nursing literature after the 1980s became less descriptive of the principles and supplies and began to focus on specific areas of concern and on patient presentations. The first comprehensive nursing care plan using nursing diagnoses was published in 1990 by four critical care nurses (Coloski, Mastrianni, Dube, & Brown, 1990). An experienced nephrology nurse investigated the cost comparisons between HD, PD, and CRRT (Lees, 1991). The treatment of ARF using CRRT was recommended as the treatment of choice and as collaborative practice between intensive care physicians and nurses, and nephrology physicians and nurses (Price, 1991b). Nephrology nurses reported an alternative to standard heparin anticoagulation using trisodium citrate (Ashton et al., 1991). Butler (1991) presented nutritional considerations for patients with ARF requiring renal replacement therapy. Successful medical and nursing management of a patient with hepatorenal syndrome using CAVH has been reported (Chmielewski, Zellers, & Eyer, 1990). The experience of Canadian nurses with CAVH and CAVHD has appeared

in the literature (Graham & Urquhart, 1990). The clinical application of CAVH for treating neonates and pediatric patients has demonstrated the increasing popularity of CRRT over conventional HD and PD (Stapleton & Wright, 1992; Hendrix, 1992). Several nurse authors focused on preventing complications, nursing management, and the advantages of CRRT (Bosworth, Paganini, Consentino, & Heyka, 1991; Lievaart & Voerman, 1991; Pinson, 1992; Stark, 1992b; Price, 1992). Others have suggested establishing a CRRT program as a unilateral critical care nursing practice is possible (Giuliano & Pysznik, 1998). Martin (1997, 2002) has explored the roles of all nurses in the management of CRRT.

Researchers continue to investigate the optimal means of managing patients with continuous therapies. Adequate nutrition remains a primary concern, and it is being addressed by nurses (Chima et al., 1993; Hagland, 1993). A case presentation involving a severely injured trauma patient using CVVHD has been reported (Strohshein, Caruso, & Greene, 1994). The application of dialysis therapies for treatment of ARF as a sequelae of sepsis highlighted nursing challenges (Price, 1994). ANNA added content related to CRRT in the 2nd edition of the *Core Curriculum for Nephrology Nursing* (Price, 1991b). AACN included discussion of CRRT in the Fourth edition of the *Core Curriculum for Critical Care Nursing* (Stark, 1991). Nursing professionals have worked closely in providing the necessary knowledge and clinical skills to the practice environment.

Summary

The treatment of ARF continues to evolve as pharmacologic agents and medical devices improve. All technological advances present new opportunities and challenges for professionals. Possibly nowhere else in health care has a diagnosis and treatment had more of an impact on collaborative practice than with ARF and CRRT. Nurses and the physicians have benefited, but the true beneficiaries have been critically ill patients.

Therapeutic Plasma Exchange (TPE)

Historical Review of Therapeutic Apheresis

Apheresis simply means to separate a part from its whole. It is the umbrella term used to describe all blood separation techniques. TPE and cytapheresis are the two primary categories of apheresis. TPE was introduced for medicinal purposes in the early 1900s. It was described as a process for removing blood factors and relief of toxaemia (Abel, Rowntree, & Turner, 1914). As with other beginning approaches for improving an individual's health status, physicians were not always certain if a benefit would be realized from their prescriptions.

A bloodletting procedure, or technique of cannulating a vein for the removal of whole blood, was a rather aggressive approach for removal of plasma. If the patient did receive a beneficial response from this intervention, there was an uncertainty as to why it occurred. The simple explanation provided the patient may have been a description of a process for removing toxins, poisons, or "bad" substances that were the cause of their illness. The short- and long-term adverse effects were unknown. Possible complications were anemia, electrolyte imbalance, vascular collapse, immune suppression, and infection. After this crude beginning, plasmapheresis, plasma exchange, or TPE as it is currently identified, became a therapy

Figure 9-9
Advances in Therapeutic Apheresis Time Line

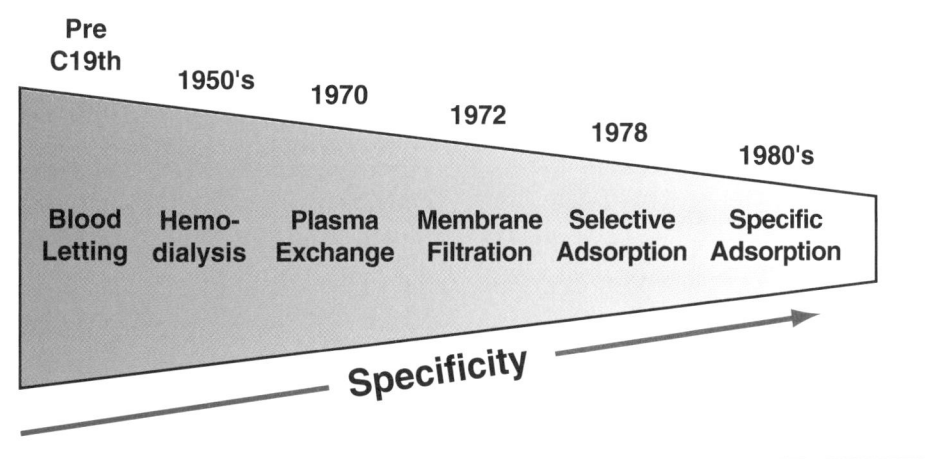

of more widespread application. With refinement of the technology and procedures, it became a frequent practice of blood banking facilities for plasma donations and for therapeutic applications. To summarize, as the medical indications for prescribing plasma exchange increased, intermittent therapies advanced to continuous flow techniques and eventually plasma membrane separators. Plasma exchange therapy gained acceptance when the patient's disease or syndrome was characterized as antibody or immune complex mediated, monoclonopathy, or for replacement of certain plasma factors (Dau, 1983; Kaplan, 1995; Ward, 1984).

To a limited extent, nephrology practices are involved in collection and processing of cellular components of whole blood. As an example, stem cell transplants may be a treatment of amyloidosis, which may present as acute or chronic renal failure. Cytapheresis is the collection of one particular formed cell by means of centrifuge apheresis equipment. The procedure could be performed for the removal of white cells, red cells, or platelets. Cytapheresis is clinically indicated for the reduction of a particular cell in an individual patient, or for donation of a particular cell to another individual or self in the future. An example for these procedures would include routine red cell reduction, which is a treatment for a patient who has hemochromatosis, a disease characterized by an inborn error in iron metabolism leading to very elevated iron levels that result in excessive pathological iron deposits throughout the body. The treatment plan may include cytapheresis for the removal of stored iron through red cell reduction. Plateletapheresis is an example of a procedure performed with the intention of collecting platelets from a healthy individual. The purpose of platelet collection is for transfusion of platelets to achieve hemostasis, such as for a severely injured trauma patient, intraoperatively to control blood loss or to treat severe thrombocytopenia. Presently, peripheral stem cell collection with preservation of these cells until the patient completes a course of chemotherapy is becoming a widespread practice. Stem cells are immature cells that can become normal blood cells. The healthy stem cells are retransfused back to the patient where they can differentiate into white cells.

With the introduction of HD in the early 1950s,

researchers, engineers, and physicians recognized that whole blood could be processed extracorporeally using membrane technology for the correction of metabolic, electrolyte, and fluid imbalances. The dialyzer membrane has a particular molecular weight (MW) above which substances cannot be removed. Uremic toxins, specifically urea (MW 69 daltons) and creatinine (MW 113 daltons) could be removed along with other small molecular weight substances typically less than 10,000 daltons. High-flux or synthetic dialyzer membranes have the ability to remove molecules up to 50,000 daltons. An example is beta 2 microglobulin, which has a MW of 11,800 daltons. The clearance capacity of the human kidney is controlled by several factors, one of which is that substances over 69,000 daltons are poorly removed. Proteins, immunoglobulins and antibodies have molecular weights of 69,000 to over 1 million daltons. Therefore, they require a much more porous membrane to effectively use TPE to treat immune complex or antibody mediated diseases or syndromes, or to remove large plasma factors.

It is this development of a membrane technology approach to TPE that has lead to nephrology nurses' roles in the care of patients for whom TPE is prescribed. The similarity in the equipment and procedural considerations between HD and TPE is the primary reason for establishing a TPE program in a dialysis unit. (Gerhardt, Ntoso, Koethe, Lodge & Wolf, 1992; Price, 1987). However, the expertise of nephrology nurses in patient assessment and treatment monitoring is essential to providing safe and effective therapy. Nephrologists and nephrology nurses are becoming more interested and involved in research related to the numerous applications of TPE in treating acute and chronic illnesses. Additionally, the newer therapies of secondary cascade filtration and immunoadsorption therapy are gaining widespread acceptance for certain identified patient populations. Figure 9-9 provides a pictorial view of the advancement of extracorporeal therapies.

Intermittent flow centrifugation. The early equipment for TPE used centrifugal forces to separate whole blood into its formed elements and plasma. The original machines relied on anticoagulating and pumping blood into a bowl that rotates and thereby separates the blood components by their density (Gardner & Gilcher, 1990; Hakim & Siami, 1994). The red

Figure 9-10
Continuous Centrifuge Apheresis
A. Extracorporeal blood and plasma circuit
B. Therapeutic plasma exchange channel

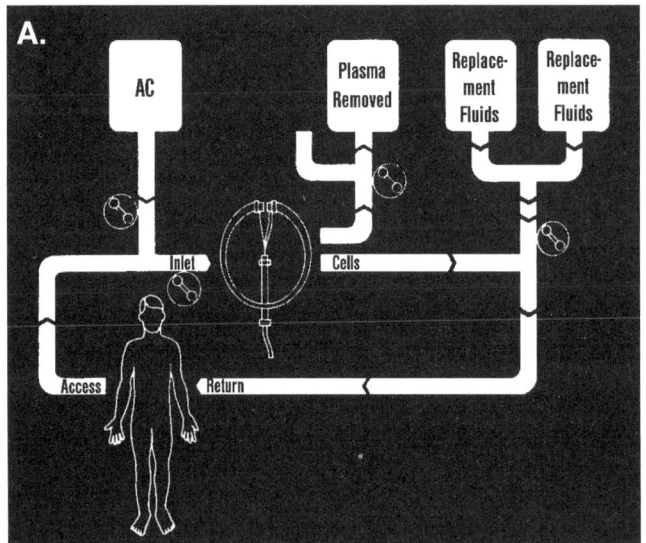

B.

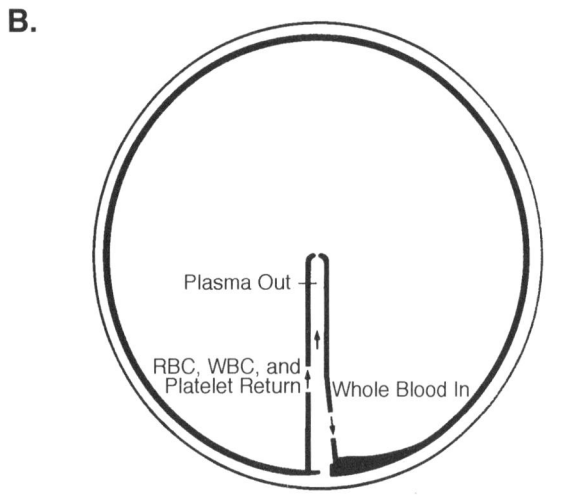

Note: Printed with permission from Cobe BCT, Lakewood, CO.

cells, having the highest density, move toward the center, and the plasma, being the lightest component, moves out to the periphery of the bowl. The white cells and platelets align themselves between the red cells and the plasma according to their respective density. Any of the components can be discarded, collected, or reinfused depending on the indication and goals of performing the procedure. The intermittent nature of the blood flow and removal of a blood component or plasma generally results in a longer procedure time and some intravascular fluid imbalance being experienced by patients. For intermittent flow centrifuge TPE procedures, the standard anticoagulant is acid-citrate dextrose (ACD).

Vascular access is achieved by cannulating usually only one antecubital vein with a 17-gauge needle. Although these machines continue to be used in clinical practice, they are being replaced by continuous flow centrifuge machines. A centrifugal process for separating blood components is necessary for removing or collecting one particular component, for example, platelets, but centrifugation is not necessary for simple separation of plasma.

Continuous flow centrifugation. As the name implies, continuous flow machines use an uninterrupted blood flow path. The whole blood enters into a rotating channel, or space, that generates a centrifugal force. The spinning blood into the channel separates into cellular elements and plasma (Hakim & Siami, 1994; Senack, 1990). The red cells move to the outside of the channel and the plasma moves toward the inside, and similar to an intermittent system the white cells and platelets divide the remaining space. Any blood component can be collected, discarded, or reinfused. The continuous nature of these procedures helps to avoid intravascular fluid shifts once the treatment is ongoing, but this also requires two sites for vascular access – blood flow out to the machine and blood return to the patient. The anticoagulation method is called acid-citrate dextrose (ACD) (see Figure 9-10).

Continuous flow centrifugal therapies are preferred because of increased patient comfort and, usually, decreased treatment time. Cytapheresis procedures are performed in blood banks or donor collection centers. Relatively few nephrology nurses are involved with cytapheresis and, therefore, continuous flow centrifuge equipment.

Membrane plasma separators. In 1983, the first medical devices for membrane TPE were introduced in the United States. A plasma membrane separator device is similar to a hemodialyzer in appearance, that is, either hollow fiber or parallel device, but the membrane properties are significantly different. Whereas, conventional dialyzers remove blood components up to 10,000 daltons, and high-flux, high permeable dialyzers remove elements up to 50,000 daltons, plasma separators are capable of removing plasma and all dissolved components up to 3 million daltons in size (Asaba, Rekola, Bergstrand, Wasserman, & Bergstrom, 1980). Although this extracorporeal circuit for TPE looks quite similar to an HD circuit (see Figure 9-11), there are major differences in the ways of priming, monitoring, and performing TPE (Price & McCarley, 1993). Membrane plasma separation has been proven to be as effective as the centrifuge techniques for the removal of plasma, plasma proteins, and other plasma components (Samtleben et al., 1984; Wood, Bond & Jacobs, 1984). The continuous flow extracorporeal circuit requires use of a central line dual lumen catheter or permanent vascular access, such as an arteriovenous fistula or synthetic graft. The anticoagulation of choice is heparin.

TPE has been recognized as part of the core curriculum content for clinical nephrology nurses (Price, 1995). Clinical practice standards have been written to guide patient care (McCarley, Wingard, & White, 1993). Nephrology nurses are recognized for their expertise with extracorporeal therapies, systematic anticoagulation, and sophisticated technology and equipment. The total body systems nursing assessment required for a patient receiving TPE and/or HD is the identical first step of the nursing process (Price & McCarley, 1994). TPE has been a natural transition and incorporation of membrane technology into nephrology nursing's scope of prac-

Figure 9-11
Membrane Plasma Exchange Circuit

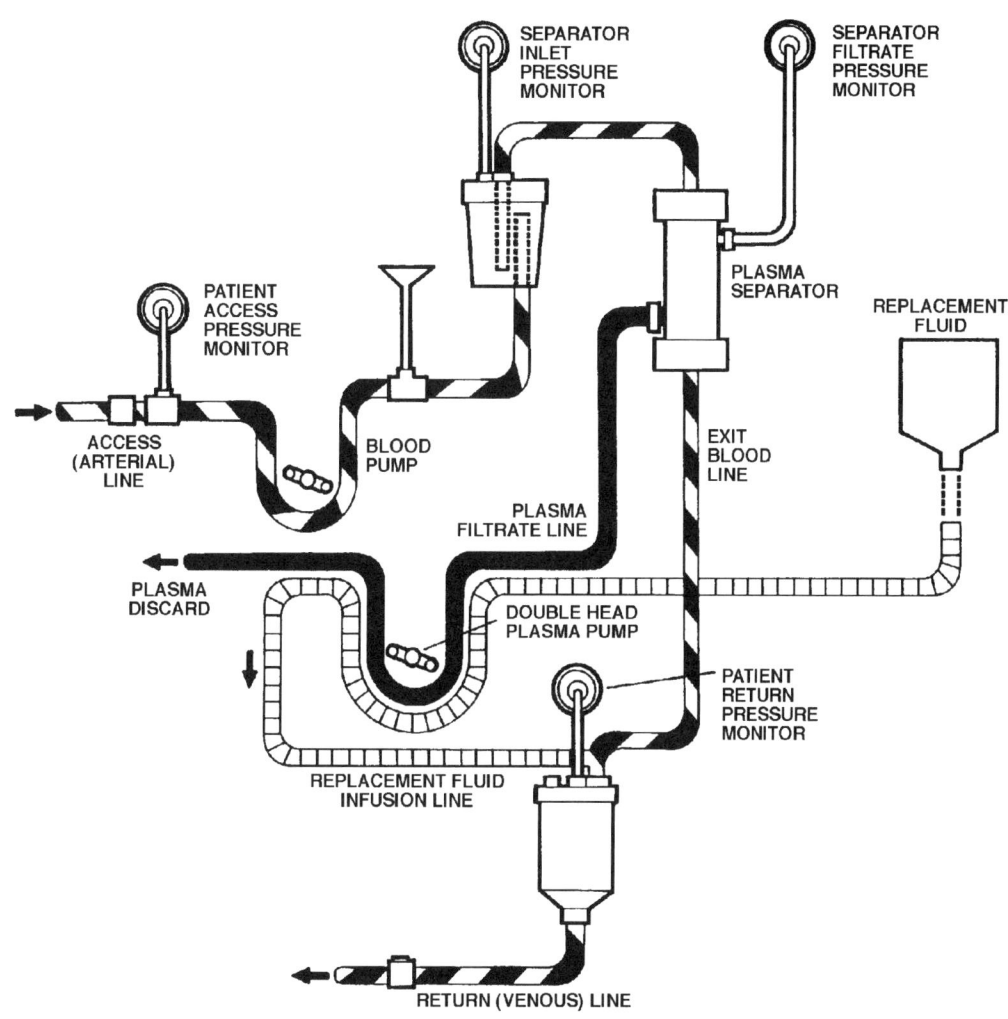

Note: Printed with permission from Apheresis Technologies Inc., Palm Harbor, FL.

tice. However, cytapheresis and related procedures have not become a major component in nephrology clinical practice.

Cascade or secondary plasma filtration. As illustrated in Figure 9-9, the wave of the future is incorporating plasma filtration therapies under the parent heading of apheresis. Selective adsorption of a particular plasma component by perfusing the separated plasma through a secondary column may become the therapy of choice as these techniques are further researched (see Figure 9-12). Currently in the United States, there is only one secondary column available, and it is limited to the treatment of idiopathic thrombocytopenia purpura (ITP) (Guthrie & Oral, 1989). Cascade plasma filtration requires a dual lumen catheter or a permanent arteriovenous vascular access. Anticoagulation therapy is prescribed cautiously because of the patient's underlying thrombocytopenia. The significant increase in TPE being performed by nephrology nurses has lead to their involvement with secondary filtration therapy. It is again a natural extension of procedural skills and nursing assessment required.

Figure 9-12
Cascade, or Secondary, Plasma Filtration Circuit

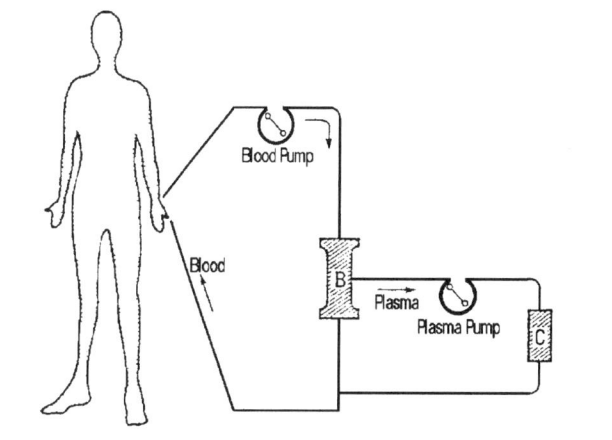

Note: Printed with permission from Apheresis Technologies Inc., Palm Harbor, FL.

Table 9-17
Comparison of HD and TPE

	HD	TPE
.9% NaCl priming	1000 ml	1000 to 3000 ml
vascular access	dual lumen catheter dialysis needles	dual lumen catheter dialysis needles
equipment	dialysis machine	dialysis machine & plasma pump TPE machine
tubing	arterial & venous	arterial & venous plasma discard fluid replacement
initial heparin	zero to > 8000 u	zero to 100 u/kg
heparin infusion	zero to > 2000 u/hr	1000 to 2000 u/hr
systemic ACTs	125 to 250 sec	200 to > 400 sec
ACTs obtained	postdialyzer	preplasma filter
heparin administered	predialyzer	postplasma filter
treatment time	3 to 4 hours	1.5 to 3 hours
fluid replacement	normal saline	normal saline 2.5% - 5% albumin FFP
staffing (acute care)	one nurse	one nurse
patient diagnosis	ARF or CRF drug overdose	every organ system drug overdose

Notes:
ARF = acute renal failure   HD = hemodialysis
CRF = chronic renal failure TPE = therapeutic plasma exchange
FFP = fresh frozen plasma

Similarities and Differences Between TPE and HD

HD and TPE share many of the same equipment and supplies, although the indications are quite different. The performance of TPE by membrane technology involves an extension of preexisting HD skills, principles, protocols, and nursing assessment.

Table 9-17 provides a comparison between the two procedures. HD is prescribed when a patient has acute renal failure, chronic renal insufficiency in the setting of fluid or electrolyte imbalance, or chronic renal failure. TPE is prescribed when a patient is diagnosed with a disease or syndrome involving autoantibodies, alloantibodies, monoclonal proteins, immune complexes, unidentified plasma factors, or for the replacement of certain plasma factors (Dau, 1983;

Hakim & Siami, 1994; Ward, 1984). TPE may be recommended for certain drug overdoses or ingestion of poisonous substances (Chu, Mantin, Shen, Baskett, & Sussman, 1993; Kale, Thomson, Provenzano, & Higgins, 1993; Rabetoy, Price, Findlay, & Sailstad, 1990). The goal for HD may be to reduce the patient's intravascular blood volume, but the expectation for TPE is that the patient will remain euvolemic. TPE involves replacing the discarded plasma with an equal volume of a replacement fluid.

Pretreatment Nursing Assessment

A total body systems assessment is identical for HD and TPE. As the initial step in the nursing process, a complete patient assessment is an expectation before proceeding with any nursing intervention. The physical assessment for a patient receiving TPE may focus on a certain body system, depending on the medical diagnosis (Price & McCarley, 1994). Unlike a patient being treated with HD for renal failure, a patient receiving TPE may not have renal dysfunction. The etiology for the primary condition may involve hematology/oncology, neurology, cardiology, dermatology, nephrology, gastroenterology, obstetrics/gynecology, and/or transplantation. Although serial monitoring of serum electrolytes and complete blood count (CBC) is standard operating procedure, laboratory analyses may also include the following titers for antibodies, identified markers of disease activity, drug levels, circulating immune complexes, and immunoglobulins. Pulmonary function tests, nerve conduction tests, and cardiac stress tests are a few of the invasive and noninvasive diagnostic examinations that may be required depending on the patient's diagnosis. It is important that the nephrology nurse is aware of the need for such testing and the findings to appropriately plan the nursing component for total patient care. Finally, prior to initiating TPE, it may be the responsibility of the nephrology nurse to calculate the patient's plasma volume. This may be estimated at 40 ml/kg, using a formula for estimated plasma volume (EPV) (Kaplan, 1992) or by using a nomogram for plasma volume (Buffaloe & Heineken, 1983; Price, 1995). Generally, 1 to 1 1/2 plasma volumes are exchanged every treatment.

Vascular Accesses

HD may be performed using two single lumen catheters, a dual lumen catheter, or a permanent arteriovenous fistula or graft. For TPE any of these vascular accesses are acceptable. The placement, monitoring, use, and nursing care of the vascular accesses are described elsewhere in this book. The primary difference is that unlike HD where the standard blood rate is 200 to 450 ml/min, the usual blood flow rate for membrane plasma exchange is 100 to 150 ml/min. TPE performed by intermittent or continuous flow centrifuge technique may range from 30 to 90 ml/min.

Equipment and Supplies

Standard HD requires the use of a HD machine with the appropriate blood pump, dialysate delivery system, ultrafiltration controls, pressure monitors, and an air alert detector. The disposable supplies include a dialyzer, arterial and venous blood tubing, and dialysate concentrate solutions. Heparin (1000 u/ml) is available to be given by the nurse as prescribed. Normal saline (.9% NaCl) is used as necessary for priming the system, fluid replacement during the treatment, and returning the patient's blood at termination of the treatment. Centrifuge TPE will require the use of a dedicated machine, as previously described. Membrane TPE may involve a dedicated machine or the use of a standard dialysis machine, but the essential equipment needs include a blood pump, pressure monitoring devices, an air alert detector, and a plasma pump that is ideally a dual track pump. Dialysate is never used when performing TPE. The disposable supplies include a plasma membrane separator, TPE arterial and venous blood tubing, a plasma discard line, and a fluid replacement line. Heparin is the standard anticoagulant, but a physician may elect to use citrate anticoagulation from a protocol adapted for performing HD. Heparinized .9% NaCl is used as the priming solution for preparing the extracorporeal circuit. However, the replacement fluids will vary depending on the patient's diagnosis and anticoagulation parameters; that is, platelet count, PT, PPT, or fibrinogen level. Plasma replacement fluids may involve a combination of crystalloids, colloids, and/or fresh frozen plasma (FFP).

Intraprocedural Monitoring for TPE

Like HD, TPE requires continuous monitoring of the patient's hemodynamic status. Vital signs, that is, blood pressure and pulse, are recorded every 15 to 20 minutes. If blood products are being administered, the patient's temperature must also be checked before and after each unit. It is imperative when monitoring the patient's vital signs that the underlying diagnosis is taken into consideration, as often patients with neurologic disorders will be hypotensive. During TPE the patient should remain euvolemic; therefore, hypotension generally is not related to a fluid imbalance. However, as with HD, normal saline must be available for immediate bolus infusion, and the patient is placed in Trendelenburg to treat hypotension.

During TPE, the nurse is continuously monitoring the plasma discard volume and plasma replacement fluid. It is the nurse's responsibility to make certain the output and intake are balanced. The plasma replacement fluid may be .9% NaCl, Lactate Ringers, a 2.5% to 5% albumin solution, or FFP. It is a nursing responsibility to assure that the correct solution and amount is administered by following the physician's prescription. A typical prescription may instruct the nurse to remove 3 liters of plasma and replace the plasma with 1 liter of .9% NaCl and 2 liters of 5.0% albumin solution.

Standard initial heparin prescriptions for HD range from 0 to 8000 units IV, followed by hourly doses of 0 to 2000 units. Patients who are being treated for acute renal failure tend to receive less heparin than chronic renal failure patients. Similarly, patients receiving TPE may have a range of heparin doses depending on the patient's diagnosis. A heparin bolus of 0, or 50 to 100 units/kg of body weight is administered at the initiation of the treatment. If the patient has significant thrombocytopenia, heparin may be contraindicated. The nurse will monitor activated clotting times (ACTs) every 20 to 30 minutes and administer a heparin bolus of 1000 to 2000 units, if indicated. Anticoagulation therapy during TPE is prescribed in consideration of the

patient's diagnosis, platelet count, hematocrit, PT, and fibrinogen level. It may vary from no heparin to systemic range anticoagulation, generally with ACTs maintained higher than during an HD treatment, that is, greater than 300 seconds. Depending on the patient's pretreatment PT or fibrinogen level, FFP may be used as part of the plasma replacement fluid.

Potential complications that require continuous monitoring during TPE are hypotension, fluid imbalance, electrolyte imbalance, air embolism, blood leak, and hemolysis. Hypotension and fluid imbalance have been addressed. The first intervention would be fluid recessitation with follow-up assessment for possible etiologies.

All small molecules, including electrolytes, are removed along with the plasma. The nurse checks the pretreatment sodium, potassium, calcium, and magnesium serum levels, and if they are not within normal to possibly high normal ranges, the physician is consulted for appropriate intervention. Often, patients are prescribed routine oral calcium supplementation to avoid hypocalcemia. Generally, if other electrolyte replacement is necessary it can be provided through dietary or nutritional changes. Intravenous replacement may be indicated if the patient is not eating well or the levels are critically low and need a faster replacement route for correction. If during TPE, the patient complains of tingling over fingers or face, numbness around the mouth, nausea or feeling "washed out," or develops muscle flaccidity or tetany, the physician is consulted and along with serum labs for calcium, potassium and magnesium, an electrocardiogram is obtained.

If the air alert detector is not armed or if the equipment is faulty, the patient is at risk for receiving an air embolism. Monitoring of the situation is an expected nephrology nurse responsibility. Should an air embolism be suspected, the treatment is immediately stopped, the patient is placed in Trendelenburg on her or his left side, and oxygen is administered. The rationale for these actions is to trap any air in the right atrium of the heart and prevent it from escaping into the carotid arteries causing a cerebral embolism. The patient is likely to become hypotensive and possibly hypoxic. Preparations for possible cardiac resuscitation are made.

Occasionally, a product fault may occur, and it may result in a broken hollow fiber or parallel plate that allows a small amount of blood to leak into the plasma discard. This is not a medical emergency, but the treatment should be discontinued. Unlike HD, the patient can safely have the blood returned because there is no possibility of contamination with nonsterile dialysate. A new TPE system is prepared if the treatment is to be continued.

During HD, hemolysis may occur secondary to a contaminant in the dialysate, like chloramine, or secondary to the dialysate being too warm, that is, greater than 40.5° C. During TPE, hemolysis may also occur. However, the causes are different, and the situation is not a medical emergency, as with HD. Unlike HD, the patient's blood may be returned during TPE. Hemolysis may occur because the transmembrane pressure for TPE has been exceeded or because the plasma filter is significantly clotted. There is no nonsterile dialysate as a possible etiology for the hemolysis as in HD. Monitoring for hemolysis is an ongoing procedural concern, and it is usually avoided. Under normal circumstances, plasma is light to moderately dark yellow. When hemolysis occurs, the discarded plasma changes to an orange color. If hemolysis should occur, the intervention is to simply stop the plasma exchange and flush the filter with normal saline to reestablish pressure equilibrium within the system. Generally only a very small amount of whole blood is actually hemolyzed, and the red cell fragments and free hemoglobulin are discarded with the plasma.

Postprocedural Nursing Care

After the appropriate plasma volume has been exchanged, the plasma pump is turned off, and the patient's whole blood is returned via the venous line. The TPE circuit is disposed of as contaminated waste, as the plasma filters are not reused as in HD. The vascular access is given appropriate attention that will vary depending on the access used.

The nephrology nurse completes a posttreatment assessment and evaluation. Vital signs, subjective responses, and laboratory analyses are obtained. The patient is allowed 15 to 30 minutes to adjust and stabilize her or his blood pressure and pulse back to baseline parameters. Most patients will be transferred back to their hospital room, although other patients will return home. Patients and/or other hospital personnel are instructed on the two most frequent postprocedural complications, that is bleeding and infection.

During TPE, heparin therapy may be provided, but also unlike HD, clotting factors, particularly fibrinogen, are removed. This increases the patient's risk for postprocedural bleeding. Precautions must include allowing no invasive procedures for the next 24 hours. This includes surgery, and/or intraarterial and spinal punctures. Likewise, intravenous catheters should not be attempted unless absolutely necessary for several hours. Patients are cautioned about protecting themselves against blunt trauma, falling against a hard surface, shaving cuts, or vigorous teeth brushing. Protocols should be in place that prohibit discontinuing central line catheters until possibly 24 hours after TPE and a fibrinogen or PT level has been recorded. Hospital staff should be prepared to hold direct pressure against the site for 15 to 20 minutes.

Patients receiving TPE are at high risk for secondary or opportunistic infections. Many will be receiving steroids or cytotoxic agents as part of their treatment regimen. Any patient with an indwelling central line catheter and undergoing intermittent invasive procedures is considered at high-risk for infection. Patients are to be instructed to report to the nurses any ill feeling, sweating, chills, or fever. Hospital staff monitor for signs and symptoms of systemic infection, including hemodynamic instability, hyperthermia, and elevated white cell count with an abnormal differential. Signs of local infection include observing for induration, erythema, drainage, and warmth. Appropriate interventions are taken immediately because a patient receiving TPE can become septic quickly.

The long-term care, monitoring, and clinical outcomes of patients receiving TPE will vary greatly and will be directly related to the patient's primary diagnosis. Depending on the patient's presentation and disease course, the patient's illness may be resolved or cured, placed in a state of remission, or require long-term chronic treatments. Health care professionals must tailor their therapeutic interventions, patient education, and psychosocial support in consideration of the immediate circumstances and clinical situation.

Nursing Literature and Research Related to TPE

Over the past decade, there have been more published reports of the nursing care provided for patients treated with TPE. TPE has become recognized as a safe and effective therapy. The involvement of various nursing specialties demonstrates some of the clinical applications.

Neuroscience nurses have recognized the therapeutic value of TPE and the related nursing concerns for patients diagnosed with Guillain-Barre Syndrome, myasthenia gravis, and neuromuscular respiratory failure (George, 1988; Hinkle, Albanese, & McGinty, 1993; Hood, 1990; Parobeck, Burnham, & Laukhuf, 1992; Sulton, 2002; Weeks, 1991). The primary nursing concern with these neurologic disorders is respiratory depression or arrest. Function of the cranial nerves, gag reflex, and ability to swallow are monitored closely to assure the patient has a protected airway. These patients may have a self-limited condition that will resolve over a period of weeks to months, or they may have a chronic condition that could require repeated courses of TPE over their lifetime.

Professional nurses who specialize in perinatology neonatal nursing have been confronted with pregnant women needing TPE for the treatment of myasthenia gravis and Guillain-Barre Syndrome (Burke, 1993; Graves & Oates, 1994). This may be a frightening situation for all because the goal of therapy is to sustain normal fetal growth and development without complications, while treating the mother's disorder.

A patient who developed Stevens-Johnson Syndrome secondary to medication reaction has been reported in the nursing literature (Sherry, 1993). The florid and painful rash that occurs may resolve with conventional prescription of steroids and antihistamines, skin lotions, and hygiene care.

Critical care nurses have experienced an increased use of TPE for critically ill patients with a variety of clinical presentations, including those already mentioned plus thrombotic thrombocytopenic purpura (TTP), idiopathic thrombocytopenic purpura (ITP), cardiac transplantation, cardiac surgery, and familial hypercholesterolemia (Bell, 1989; Cohen, 1989; Eggenberger, Coker, & Menezes, 1993; Ellenberger, Haas, & Cundiff, 1993; Ellis, 1994; Folkes, 1990; Krnsak, 1994; Pfister & Bullas, 1990; White-Williams, 1993). ITP is a hematological syndrome resulting from the presence of antiplatelet antibodies. Patients may present with neurologic deficits, renal failure, and/or gastrointestinal or cerebral hemorrhage. TTP is believed to be a nonimmunological syndrome that mimics ITP with either a fulminant or subacute presentation.

All transplant patients develop antibodies against the donor organ, and occasionally TPE is prescribed in conjunction with pharmacologic management. TPE protocols have been developed for patients with high panel reactive antibodies (PRA) to receive TPE prior to, and occasionally after, kidney transplant (Gloor, 2005). Familial hypercholesterolemia is a genetic disorder characterized by elevated levels of serum cholesterol that are not amenable to the standard therapy of diet, exercise, and cholesterol lowering agents.

With the changes in technology, nephrology nursing literature has increased content related to its scope of practice for the treatment of rapidly progressive glomerulonephritis (RPGN), Goodpasture's Syndrome, hemolytic uremia syndrome (HUS), hyperviscosity syndrome, cryoglobulinemia, as well as all diseases previously listed (Duff & Dugas, 1991; Graves & Oates, 1994; Isaacs, 1994; Klee, McAfee, & Greenleaf, 1993; Neumann & Urizar, 1994; Price, 1987; Price & McCarley, 1994; Wingard, 1993; Wiseman, 1993). Antibody mediated renal diseases are often treated with TPE. Likewise, sepsis and kidney failure may be amenable to TPE (Klenzak & Himelfarb, 2005). Paraproteinemias are disorders of the blood in which a particular protein becomes elevated, resulting in changes of the pressures in the vascular space and disruption of normal clotting processes.

Along with the professional health care community becoming increasingly aware of the value of TPE, the general public has been informed of this wonder of modern medicine through lay public journals, like *Woman's Day* and *Saturday Evening Post* (Coudert, 1993; Martin, 1993).

Summary

As the science and technology related to TPE and cascade or immunoadsorption therapy are advanced, the role of nephrology nurses will parallel these developments. As evidenced by the several specialty nurses involved, collaborative practice will continue to be of great importance for the sharing of education and support for patients and professionals. Reinforced by their expertise with HD, nephrology nurses will be called upon to develop specific TPE protocols and practices related to vascular accesses, anticoagulation prescriptions, treatment regimens, and expected patient outcomes. Experience with the Medicare ESRD program will assist nephrology nurses in designing appropriate checks and balances as society debates the long-term treatment of chronic disease. Similarly, the evolution of the treatment of ARF as a component of multisystem failure should serve nephrology nurses as a guide for end-of-life patient care considerations. Nephrology nurses have been at the forefront of aggressive, invasive health care practices for the treatment of acute illness and chronic disease. This past experience is an asset as their scope of practice expands to encompass caring for patients and families when TPE is the treatment of choice.

References

Abdeen, O., & Mehta, R. (2002). Dialysis modalities in the intensive care unit. *Critical Care Clinics, 18*(2), 223-247.

Abel, S., Rowntree, L., & Turner, B. (1914). Plasma removal with return of corpuscles (plasmapheresis). *Journal of Pharmacologic Experiment Therapy, 5,* 625-641.

Alexopoulos, E., Vakianis, P., Kokolina, E., Koukoudis, P., Sakellariou, G., Memmos, D., et al. (1994). Acute renal failure in the medical setting: Changing patterns and prognostic factors. *Renal Failure, 16*(2), 273-284.

Anderson, R.J. (1993). Prevention and management of acute renal failure. *Hospital Practice, 28*(8), 61-75.

Asaba, H., Rekola, S., Bergstrand, A., Wasserman, H., & Bergstrom, J. (1980). Clinical trial of plasma exchange with a membrane filter in the treatment of crescentic glomerulonephritis. *Clinical Nephrology, 14*(2), 60-65.

Ashton, D., Mehta, R., Ward, D., McDonald, B., & Aguilar, M. (1991). Recent advances in continuous renal replacement therapy: Citrate anticoagulated continuous arteriovenous hemodialysis. *ANNA Journal, 18*(3), 269-267, 329.

Baer, C. (1993a). Renal data acquisition. In M. Kinney, D. Packa, & S. Dunbar (Eds.), *AACN's clinical reference of critical care nursing* (pp. 873-883). St. Louis: Mosby Year Book.

Baer, C. (1993b). Acute renal failure. In M. Kinney, D. Packa, & S. Dunbar (Eds.), *AACN's clinical reference of critical care nursing* (pp. 885-901). St. Louis: Mosby Year Book.

Baer, C.L., & Lancaster, L.E. (1992). Acute renal failure. *Critical Care Nursing Quarterly, 14*(4), 1-21.

Baldwin, I. (2002). Continuous renal replacement therapy. Keeping pace with changes in technology and technique. *Blood Purification, 20*(3), 269-274.

Bell, J. (1989). Understanding and managing myasthenia gravis. *Focus on Critical Care, 16*(1), 57-65.

Bell, S. (1988). CAVH in pediatrics: Meeting the challenge...continuous arteriovenous hemofiltration. *ANNA Journal, 15*(1), 25-26.

Bellomo, R., Cole, L., Reeves, J., & Silvester, W. (1997). Who should manage CRRT in the ICU? The intensivist's viewpoint. *American Journal of Kidney Diseases, 30*(5 Suppl. 4), S109-S111.

Bonnardeaux, A., Pichette, V., Quimet, D., Geadah, D., Habel, F., & Cardinal, J. (1992). Solute clearances with high dialysate flow rates and glucose absorption from the dialysate in continuous arteriovenous hemodialysis. *American Journal of Kidney Diseases, 19*(1), 31-38.

Bonventre, J.V., Shah, S.V., Walker, P.D., & Humphreys, M.H. (1995). Acute renal failure: Ischemic, toxic, other. In H.R. Jacobson, G.E Striker, & S. Klahr (Eds.), *The principles and practice of nephrology* (2nd ed.) (pp. 564-576). St. Louis: Mosby Year Book.

Bosworth, C. (1992). SCUF/CAVH/CAVHD: Critical differences. *Critical Care Nursing Quarterly, 14*(4), 45-55.

Bosworth, C., Paganini, E., Consentino, F., & Heyka, R. (1991). Long-term experience with continuous renal replacement therapy in intensive care unit acute renal failure. *Contributions in Nephrology, 93,* 13-16.

Bosworth, C., Swann, S., & Paganini, E. (1990). Evaluation of the IMED infusion pumps in extracorporeal continuous therapy circuits. *Dialysis & Transplantation, 19*(1), 26-28.

Brezis, M., Rosen, S., & Epstein, F.H. (1993). Acute renal failure due to ischemia (acute tubular necrosis). In J.M. Lazarus & B.M. Brenner (Eds.), *Acute renal failure* (3rd ed.) (pp. 207-229). New York: Churchill Livingstone.

Buffaloe, G., & Heineken, F. (1983). Plasma volume nomograms for use in therapeutic plasma exchange. *Transfusion, 23*(4), 355-358.

Burke, M. (1993). Myasthenia gravis and pregnancy. *Journal of Perinatology Neonatal Nursing, 7*(1), 11-21.

Burnett, J.C. (1993). Acute renal failure associated with cardiac failure and hypovolemia. In J.M. Lazarus & B.M. Brenner (Eds.), *Acute renal failure* (3rd ed.) (pp.193-206). New York: Churchill Livingstone.

Butler, B. (1991). Nutritional management of catabolic acute renal failure requiring renal replacement therapy. *ANNA Journal, 18*(3), 247-259.

Cant, J. (1984, January). Haemofiltration. *Nursing Mirror*, pp. 3-6.

Chima, C., Meyer, L., Hummell, A., Bosworth, C., Heyka, R., Paganini, E., & Werynski, A. (1993). Protein catabolic rate in patients with acute renal failure on continuous arteriovenous hemofiltraton and total parenteral nutrition. *Journal of American Society of Nephrology, 3*(8), 1516-1521.

Chmielewski, C., Zellers, L., & Eyer, J. (1990). Continuous arteriovenous hemofiltration in the patient with hepatorenal syndrome: A case study. *Critical Care Nursing Clinics of North American, 2*(1), 115-122.

Chu, G., Mantin, R., Shen, Y., Baskett, G., & Sussman, H. (1993). Massive cisplatin overdose by accidental substitution of carboplatin. *Cancer, 72*(12), 3707-3714.

Cohen, J. (1989). Reducing cholesterol: Strategies for increasing patient awareness. *Critical Care Nurse, 9*(3), 25-28.

Coloski, D., Mastrianni, J., Dube, R., & Brown, L. (1990). Continuous arteriovenous hemofiltration patient: Nursing care plan. *Dimensions of Critical Care Nursing, 9*(3), 130-142.

Coudert, J. (1993). I was trapped in a useless body (pregnant woman suffers from Guillian-Barre syndrome). *Woman's Day, 57*, 56-60.

Dau, P. (1983). *Therapeutic plasma exchange disease compendium.* Lakewood, CO: Cobe Laboratories, Inc.

Daugirdas, J.T., & Ing, T.S. (1994). *Handbook of dialysis* (2nd ed.) Boston: Little, Brown and Company.

Davenport, A. (1998). Management of heparin-induced thrombocytopenia during continuous renal replacement therapy. *American Journal of Kidney Diseases, 32*(4), E3.

Dirkes, S. (1989). Making a critical difference with CAVH...continuous arteriovenous hemofiltration. *Nursing 1989, 19*(11), 57-60.

Douglas, S. (1992). Acute tubular necrosis: Diagnosis, treatment, and nursing implication. *ACCN Clinical Issues, 3*(3), 688-697.

Druml, W. (1995). Nutritional management of acute renal failure. In H.R. Jacobson, G.E. Striker, & S. Klahr (Eds.), *The principles and practice of nephrology* (2nd ed.) (pp. 745- 753). St. Louis: Mosby Year Book.

Duff, B., & Dugas, A. (1991). A clinical picture of a patient with thrombotic thrombocytopenia purpura. *CANNT Journal, 1*(4), 23-24.

Eggenberger, E., Coker, S., & Menezes, M. (1993). Pediatric Miller Fisher syndrome requiring intubation: A case report. *Clinical Pediatrics, 32*(6), 373-376.

Ellenberger, B., Haas, L., & Cundiff, L. (1993). Thrombotic thrombocytopenia purpura: Nursing during the acute phase. *Dimensions of Critical Care Nursing, 12*(2), 58-65.

Eschbach, J.W., & Adamson, J.W. (1993). Anemia in renal disease. In R.W. Schrier & C.W. Gottschalk (Eds.), *Diseases of the kidney* (5th ed.) (pp. 2743-2758). Boston: Little, Brown and Company.

Faber, M.D., Kupin, W.L., Krishna, G.G., & Narins, R.G. (1993). The differential diagnosis of acute renal failure. In J.M. Lazarus & B.M. Brenner (Eds.), *Acute renal failure* (3rd ed.) (pp. 133-192). New York: Churchill Livingstone.

Finn, W.F. (1993). Recovery from acute renal failure. In J.M. Lazarus & B.M. Brenner (Eds.), *Acute renal failure* (3rd ed.) (pp. 553-596). New York: Churchill Livingstone.

Folkes, M. (1990). Transfusion therapy in critical care nursing. *Critical Care Nursing Quarterly, 13*(2), 15-28.

Gardner, J., & Gilcher, R. (1990) Haemonetics V-50 and plasma collection system: Common concerns and troubleshooting. *Journal of Clinical Apheresis, 5*, 106-109.

George, M. (1988) Neuromuscular respiratory failure: What the nurse knows may make the difference. *Journal of Neuroscience Nursing, 20*(2), 110-117.

Gerhardt, R., Ntoso, A., Koethe, J., Lodge, S., & Wolf, C. (1992). Acute plasma separation with hemodialysis equipment. *Journal of American Society of Nephrology, 2*, 1455-1458.

Geronemus, R. (1988). Slow continuous hemodialysis. *Transactions of ASAIO, 34*, 59-60.

Giuliano, K., & Pysznik, E. (1998). Renal replacement therapy in critical care: Implementation of a a unit-based continuous venovenous hemodialysis program. *Critical Care Nurse, 18*(1), 40-51.

Gloor, J. (2005). Kidney transplantation in the hyperimmunized patient. *Contribution in Nephrology, 146*, 11-21.

Graham, K., & Urquhart, G. (1990). Continuous arteriovenous hemofiltration/dialysis. *Canadian Critical Care Nursing Journal, 7*(1), 18-24.

Graves, G., & Oates, M. (1994). Therapeutic plasma exchange for Guillian-Barre syndrome during pregnancy. *ANNA Journal, 21*(4), 277-278.

Guthrie, T., & Oral, A. (1989). Immune thrombocytopenia purpura: A pilot study of staphylococcal protein A immunomodulation in refractory patients. *Seminars in Hematology, 26*(2), 3-9.

Hagland, M. (1993). The management of acute renal failure in the intensive therapy unit. *Intensive & Critical Care Nursing, 9*(4), 237-241.

Hakim, R., & Siami, G. (1994). Plasmapheresis. In Daugirdas & Ing (Eds.), *Handbook of dialysis* (2nd ed.) (pp. 218-241). Boston: Little, Brown & Company.

Hendrix, W. (1992). Dialysis therapies in critically ill children. *AACN Clinical Issues in Critical Care Nursing, 3*(3), 605-613.

Henrich, W. (1993). Arteriovenous of venovenous continuous therapies are not superior to standard hemodialysis in all patients with acute renal failure. *Seminars in Dialysis, 6*(3), 174-176.

Hinkle, J., Albanese, M., & McGinty. (1993). Development of printed teaching materials for neuroscience patients. *Journal of Neuroscience Nursing, 25*(2), 125-129.

Holechek, M.J. (1992). Glomerular filtration and renal hemodynamics. *ANNA Journal, 19*(3), 237-248.

Hood, L. (1990). Myasthenia gravis: Regimens and regimen-associated problems in adults. *Journal of Neuroscience Nursing, 22*(6), 358-364.

Iaina, A., & Schwartz, D. (1994). Renal tubular cellular and molecular events in acute renal failure. *Nephron, 68*, 413-418.

Isaacs, P. (1994). Combined therapy management for patients with thrombolytic thrombocytopenic purpura. *ANNA Journal, 21*(4), 196-197, 199.

Kale, P., Thomson, P., Provenzano, R., & Higgins, M. (1993). Evaluation of plasmapheresis in the treatment of an acute overdose of carbamazepine. *Annals of Pharmacotherapy, 27*(7-8), 866-870.

Kaplan, A. (1992).Toward the rational prescription of therapeutic plasma exchange: The kinetics of immunoglobulin removal. *Seminars in Dialysis, 5*(3), 227-229.

Kaplan, A. (1995). General principles of therapeutic plasma exchange. *Seminars in Dialysis, 8*(5), 294-298.

Kaplow, R., & Bendo, K. (1989). QA in continuous arteriovenous hemofiltration. *Dimensions of Critical Care Nursing, 8*(3), 170-174.

Kellerman, P. (1994). Perioperative care of the renal patient. *Archives of Internal Medicine, 154*(15), 1674-1688.

Kiely, M. (1984). Continuous arteriovenous hemofiltration. *Critical Care Nurse, 4*(4), 39-43.

Kjellstrand, C.M., & Barsoum, R. (1995). Management of acute renal failure. In H.R. Jacobson, G.E. Striker, & S. Klahr (Eds.), *The principles and practice of nephrology* (pp. 584-594). St. Louis: Mosby Year Book.

Kjellstrand, C.M., & Solez, K. (1993). Treatment of acute renal failure. In R. Schrier & C. Gottschalk (Eds.), *Diseases of the kidney* (5th ed.) (pp. 1371-1404). Boston: Little Brown and Company.

Klee, K., McAfee, N., & Greenleaf, K. (1993). Pediatric case study: Hemolytic uremic syndrome. *ANNA Journal, 20*(4), 505-506.

Klenzak, J., & Himmelfarb, J. (2005). Sepsis and the kidney. *Critical Care Clinics, 21*(2), 211-222.

Kramer, P., Kaufhold, G., Grone, H., Wigger, J., Rieger, D., Matthaei, D., Stokke, T., Burchardi, H., & Scheler, F. (1980). Management of anuric intensive care patients with arteriovenous hemofiltration. *International Journal of Artificial Organs, 3*(4), 225-230.

Krsnak, J. (1994). Immunoadsorption column treatment for refractory ITP. *ANNA Journal, 21*(4), 198-199.

Kutsogiannis, D., Mayers, I., Chin, W., & Gibney, R. (2000) Regional citrate anticoagulation in continuous venovenous hemofiltration. *American Journal of Kidney Diseases, 35*(5), 802-811.

Lancaster, L.E. (1992). Acute renal failure. In V.B. Huddleston (Ed.), *Multisystem organ failure: Pathophysiology and clinical implications* (pp. 222-235). St. Louis: Mosby Year Book.

Lancaster, L. (2001). Systemic manifestations of renal failure. In L. Lancaster (Ed.), *ANNA's core curriculum for nephrology nursing* (4th edition) (pp. 117-158). Pitman, NJ: American Nephrology Nurses' Association.

Lawyer, L. (1987). *Clinical experience and application of continuous arteriovenous hemodialysis in the intensive care unit.* Reprint from the Third International Symposium on Acute Continuous Renal Replacement Therapy.

Lees, P. (1990, April). Acute renal replacement treatment alternatives. *Contemporary Dialysis & Nephrology*, pp. 22-27.

Levine, J.S., Lieberthal, W., Bernard, D.B., & Salant, D.J. (1993). Acute renal failure associated with renal vascular disease, vasculitis, glomerulonephritis, and nephrotic syndrome. In J.M. Lazarus & B.M. Brenner (Eds.), *Acute renal failure* (3rd ed.) (pp. 247- 355). New York: Churchill Livingstone.

Lievaart, A., & Voerman, H. (1991). Nursing management of continuous arteriovenous hemodialysis. *Heart & Lung, 29*(2), 152-160.

Llach, F. (1993). Acute renal failure. In F. Llach (Ed.), *Papper's clinical nephrology* (3rd ed., pp. 109-134). Boston: Little, Brown and Company.

Locke, S., Groth, N., & Lees, P. (1985). Continuous arteriovenous hemofiltration: An alternative to standard hemodialysis in unstable patients. *ANNA Journal, 12*(2), 127-131.

Luyckx, V., & Bonventre, J. (2004). Dose of dialysis in acute renal failure. *Seminars in Dialysis, 17*(1), 30-36.

Martin, L. (1993, July-August). Mommy, why don't you hug me? (women suffers from Guillian-Barre syndrome). *Saturday Evening Post, 265,* 60-67.

Martin, R. (1997). Who should manage CRRT ? The nursing perspective. *American Journal of Kidney Disease, 30*(5) Suppl. 4, 3105-3108.

Martin, R. (2002). Who should manage continuous renal replacement in the intensive care setting? A nursing viewpoint. *EDTNA/ERCA Journal,* (Suppl. 2), 43-45, 53.

Mault, J., Dirkes, S., Swartz, R., & Bartlett, R. (1989). *Continuous hemofiltration: A reference guide for SCUF, CAVH, and CAVHD.* Ann Arbor, MI: University of Michigan Medical Center.

McBride, P. (1987). *Genesis of the artificial kidney.* Deerfield, IL: Baxter Health Care Corporation.

McCarley, P., Wingard, R., & White, R. (1993). Therapeutic plasma exchange. In S. Burrows-Hudson (Ed.), *ANNA standards of clinical practice for nephrology nursing* (2nd ed.) (115-135), Pitman, NJ: American Nephrology Nurses' Association.

Mehta, R. (1993). Renal replacement therapy for acute renal failure: Matching the method to the patient. *Seminars in Dialysis, 6*(4), 253-259.

Mehta, R., Pascual, M., Soroto, S., Savage, B., Himmerfarb, J., Jkizler, T., et al. (2004). Spectrum of acute renal failure in the intensive care unit: The PICARD experience. *Kidney International, 66*(4), 1613-1621.

O'Meara, Y. M., & Bernard, D.B. (1995). Clinical presentation, complications, and prognosis of acute renal failure. In H.R. Jacobson, G.E. Striker, & S. Klahr (Eds.), *The principles and practice of nephrology* (2nd ed.) (pp. 577-584). St. Louis: Mosby Year Book.

Neumann, M., & Urizar, R. (1994). Hemolytic uremic syndrome: Current pathophysiology and management. *ANNA Journal, 21*(2), 137-143.

Paganini, E. (1993). Continuous renal replacement is the preferred treatment for all acute renal failure patients receiving intensive care. *Seminars in Dialysis, 6*(3), 176-179.

Paganini, E., Fisque, J., Whitman, G., & Nakamoto, S. (1982). Amino acid balance in patients with oliguric acute renal failure undergoing slow continuous ultrafiltration (SCUF). *Transactions of ASAIO, 28,* 615-620.

Palmer, J., Koorejian, K., London, J., Dechert, R., & Bartlett, R. (1986). Nursing management of continuous arteriovenous hemofiltration for acute renal failure. *Focus on Critical Care, 13*(5), 21-30.

Paradiso, C. (1989). Hemofiltration: An alternative to dialysis. *Heart & Lung, 18*(3), 282-290.

Parobeck, V., Burnham, S., & Laukhuf, G. (1992). An unusual nursing challenge: Guillian-Barre syndrome following cranial surgery. *Journal of Neuroscience Nursing, 24*(5), 251-255.

Pfister, S., & Bullas, J. (1990). Acute Guillian-Barre syndrome. *Critical Care Nurse, 10*(10), 68-73.

Pinson, J. (1992). Preventing complications in the CAVH patient. *Dimensions of Critical Care Nursing, 11*(5), 242-248.

Politosk, G., Mayer, B., Davy, T., & Swartz, M. (1998). Continuous renal replacement therapy: A national perspective AACN/NKF. *Critical Care Nursing Clinics of North America, 10*(2), 171-177.

Price, C. (1987). Therapeutic plasma exchange in a dialysis unit. *ANNA Journal, 14*(2), 103-108.

Price, C. (1989a). Continuous arteriovenous ultrafiltration: A monitoring guide for ICU nurses. *Critical Care Nurse, 9*(1), 12-19.

Price, C. (1989b). Continuous renal replacement therapy from a professional nursing perspective. *Nephrology News & Issues, 3*(7), 31-34.

Price, C. (1991a). Continuous renal replacement therapy. In L. Lancaster (Ed.), *Core curriculum for nephrology nursing* (2nd ed.) (pp. 323-340). Pitman, NJ: American Nephrology Nurses' Association.

Price, C. (1991b). Continuous renal replacement therapy: The treatment of choice for acute renal failure. *ANNA Journal, 18*(3), 239-244.

Price, C. (1992). An update on continuous renal replacement therapies. *AACN Clinical Issues in Critical Care Nursing, 3*(3), 597-604.

Price, C. (1993). Standards of clinical practice for continuous renal replacement therapy. In S. Burrows-Hudson (Ed.), *Standards of clinical practice for nephrology nursing.* Pitman, NJ: American Nephrology Nurses' Association.

Price, C. (1994). Acute renal failure - A sequelae of sepsis. *Critical Care Nursing Clinics of North America, 6*(2), 359-372.

Price, C. (1995). Therapeutic plasma exchange. In L. Lancaster (Ed.), *Core curriculum for nephrology nursing* (3rd ed.) (pp. 347-365). Pitman, NJ: American Nephrology Nurses' Association.

Price, C., & McCarley, P. (1993). Technical considerations of therapeutic plasma exchange as a nephrology nursing procedure. *ANNA Journal, 20*(1), 41-46.

Price, C., & McCarley, P. (1994). Physical assessment for patients receiving therapeutic plasma exchange. *ANNA Journal, 21*(4), 149-154, 201.

Rabetoy, G., Mosley, C., Duke, M., & Price, C. (1989). Continuous arteriovenous hemofiltration (CAVH). *Dialysis & Transplantation, 18*(3), 120-125, 128.

Rabetoy, G., Price, C., Findlay, J., & Sailstad, J. (1990). Treatment of digoxin intoxication in a renal failure patient with digoxin-specific antibody fragments and plasmapheresis. *American Journal of Nephrology, 10,* 510-521.

Rainone, A., & Littman, E. (1981). The use of the Amicon filter in dialysis related complications. *AANNT Journal, 8*(3), 32-33.

Rodriquez, D., & Lewis, S. (1997). Nutritional management of patients with acute renal failure. *ANNA Journal, 24*(2), 232-234, 238-243.

Rose, B.D., & Rennke, H.G. (1994). *Renal pathophysiology – The essentials.* Baltimore: Williams & Wilkins.

Samtleben, W., Randerson, D., Blumenstein, M., Habersetzer, R., Schmidt, B., & Gurland, H. (1984). Membrane plasma exchange: Principles and application techniques. *Journal of Clinical Apheresis, 2*(2), 163-169.

Schaefer, R.M., Schaefer, L., & Horl, W.H. (1994). Mechanisms for protein catabolism in acute renal failure. *Nephrology Dialysis Transplantation,* (Suppl. 3), 44-47.

Schrier, R., & Wang, W. (2004). Acute renal failure and sepsis. *New England Journal of Medicine, 351*(2), 159-169.

Senack, E. (1990). Cobe: 2997 TPE Spectra, troubleshooting and common concerns. *Journal of Clinical Apheresis, 5,* 110-114.

Sherry, M. (1993). Wound care. A rash cure. Stevens-Johnson syndrome. *Nursing Times, 89*(25), 68, 71.

Siegel, N., & Shah, S. (2003). Acute renal failure direction for the next decade. *Journal of the American Society of Nephrology, 14*(8), 2176-2177.

Spurney, R.F., Fulkerson, W.J., & Schwab, S.J. (1991). Acute renal failure in critically ill patients: Prognosis for recovery of kidney function after prolonged dialysis support. *Critical Care Medicine, 19*(1), 8-11.

Stapleton, S., & Wright, J. (1992). Continuous arteriovenous hemofiltration: An alternative dialysis therapy in neonates. *Journal of Neonatal Nursing, 11*(4), 17-29.

Stark, J. (1991). The renal system. In J. Alspach (Ed.), *Core curriculum of critical care nursing* (4th edition) (pp. 472-608). Philadelphia: W.B. Saunders Company.

Stark, J. (1992a). Acute tubular necrosis: Differences between oliguria and nonoliguria. *Critical Care Nursing Quarterly, 14*(4), 22-27.

Stark, J. (1992b). Dialysis options in the critically ill patient: Hemodialysis, peritoneal dialysis, and continuous renal replacement therapy. *Critical Care Nursing Quarterly, 14*(4), 40-44.

Stark, J. (1994). Acute renal failure in trauma: Current perspectives. *Critical Care Nursing Quarterly, 16*(4), 49-60.

Strohshein, B., Caruso, D., & Greene, K. (1994). Continuous venovenous hemodialysis. *American Journal of Critical Care, 3*(2), 92-100.

Suki, W.N., & Eknoyan, G. (1995). Pathophysiology and clinical manifestations of chronic renal failure and the uremic syndrome. In H.R. Jacobson, G.E. Striker, & S. Klahr (Eds.), *The principles and practice of nephrology* (2nd ed.) (pp. 603-614). St. Louis: Mosby Year Book.

Sulton, L. (2002). Meeting the challenge of Guillain-Barre syndrome. *Nursing Management, 33*(7), 25-30.

Swartz, R., Perry, E., & Daley, J. (2004). The frequency of withdrawal from acute care is impacted by severe renal failure. *Journal of Palliative Medicine, 7*(5), 676-682.

Teechan, G., Liangos, O., & Jaber, B. (2003). Update on dialytic management of acute renal failure. *Journal of Intensive Care Medicine, 18*(3), 130-138.

Vanholder, R., VanBieson, W., & Lameire, N. (2001). What is the renal replacement method of first choice for intensive care patients. *Journal of American Society of Nephrology. 12* (Suppl. 17), 540-543.

Ward, D. (1984). Therapeutic plasmapheresis and related apheresis techniques. In *Update to Harrison's principles of internal medicine* (volume 5, pp. 67-95). New York: McGraw-Hill.

Wardle, E.N. (1994). Acute renal failure and multiorgan failure. *Nephron, 66*(4), 380-385.

Wedel, S. (1988). Continuous arteriovenous hemofiltration. *Current Reviews in Respiratory and Critical Care, 11*(5), 34-40.

Weeks, D. (1991). Washing the blood, *RN, 54*(5), 60-64.

Weinberg, J.M. (1995). Pathogenetic mechanisms of ischemic acute renal failure. In H.R. Jacobson, G.E. Striker, & S. Klahr (Eds.), *The principles and practice of nephrology* (2nd ed.) (pp. 544-555). St. Louis: Mosby Year Book.

White-Williams, C. (1993). Immunosuppressive therapy following cardiac transplantation. *Critical Care Nursing Quarterly, 16*(2), 1-10.

Whittaker, A., Brown, C., Grabenbauer, K., & Cauble, L. (1986). Preventing complications in continuous arteriovenous hemofiltration. *Dimensions of Critical Care Nursing, 5*(2), 72-79.

Williams, V., & Perkins, L. (1984). Continuous ultrafiltration. *Critical Care Nurse, 4,* 44-49.

Wingard, R. (1993). Familial hypercholesterolemia treated by plasma exchange and immunoadsorption. *ANNA Journal, 20*(1), 84-85.

Winkelman, C. (1985). Hemofiltration: A new technique in critical care nursing. *Heart & Lung, 14*(3), 265-271.

Wiseman, K. (1993). New insights on Goodpasture's syndrome. *ANNA Journal, 20*(1), 17-26.

Wolfson, M., & Kopple, J.D. (1993). Nutritional management of acute renal failure. In J.M. Lazarus & B.M. Brenner (Eds.), *Acute renal failure* (3rd ed.) (pp. 467-485). New York: Churchill Livingstone.

Wood, L., Bond, R., & Jacobs, P. (1984). Comparison of filtration to continuous-flow centrifugation for plasma exchange. *Journal of Clinical Apheresis, 2*(2), 155-162.

Yagi, N., & Paganini, E. (1997). Acute dialysis and continuous renal replacement: The emergence of new technology involving the nephrologists in the intensive care setting. *Seminars in Nephrology, 17*(4), 306-320.

Yarger, W.E. (1991). Urinary tract obstruction. In B.M. Brenner & F.C. Rector (Eds.), *The kidney* (4th ed.) (pp. 1768-1808). Philadelphia: W.B. Saunders Company.

Yarger, W.E. (1993). Obstructive urinary tract disease as a cause of acute renal failure. In J.M. Lazarus & B.M. Brenner (Eds.), *Acute renal failure* (3rd ed.) (pp. 393-415). New York: Churchill Livingstone.

- Acute renal failure (ARF) may be defined as a rapid decline in glomerular filtration rate (GFR) (greater than 50% reduction), usually causing oliguria or anuria and resulting in the accumulation of metabolic wastes in the blood (azotemia).

- Although renal replacement therapies have been available for over 30 years, the mortality associated with ARF continues to be approximately 50%.

- The best treatment for ARF is prevention by close monitoring of hemodynamic parameters, avoidance of known nephrotoxic exposures, and early intervention for vascular volume deficit.

- Management of the patient with prerenal failure seeks to restore normal hemodynamic status and varies depending on the cause of the renal hypoperfusion.

- Postrenal failure results from an obstruction to urine flow that can occur anywhere within the urinary tract. The most common causes of postrenal failure in adults are benign prostate hypertrophy and nephrolithiasis, while obstruction secondary to congenital abnormalities occurs frequently in children.

- Postrenal failure is treated by relieving the obstruction, preserving renal function, and preventing and treating any complications.

- Injury to the renal tissues causes intrarenal failure and leads to the rapid decline of GFR; elevation of BUN and serum creatinine; and frequently, progressively diminishing urine output.

- Patients with ARF and their families must cope with the sudden loss of health in the face of a very serious illness. The loss of renal function may require prolonged hospitalization, complex dietary and medication management, and dialysis. The nurse should continually assess the educational and emotional needs of both the patient and family, providing them with appropriate explanations of the disease process, its prognosis, and all procedures and components of treatment.

- Many nephrologists and nephrology nurses have embraced CRRT because it is recognized as meeting the total 24-hour needs of the patient for hourly fluid and electrolyte balance, adjustment of acid/base status, and continuous removal of uremic toxins.

- The advantage of CRRT over standard acute HD is that there are several different approaches in the health care professionals' armamentarium of therapies. Treatment can be provided on a continuous basis, rather than attempting to fit the patient's needs into a time-prescribed therapy, like 3 or 4-hour treatment with HD.

- The treatment of ARF continues to evolve as pharmacologic agents and medical devices improve. All technological advances present new opportunities and challenges for professionals. Possibly nowhere else in health care has a diagnosis and treatment had more of an impact on collaborative practice than with ARF and CRRT.

- The similarity in the equipment and procedural considerations between HD and TPE is the primary reason for establishing a TPE program in a dialysis unit. However, the expertise of nephrology nurses in patient assessment and treatment monitoring is essential to providing safe and effective therapy.

- Patients receiving TPE are at high risk for secondary or opportunistic infections. Many will be receiving steroids or cytotoxic agents as part of their treatment regimen. Any patient with an indwelling central line catheter and undergoing intermittent invasive procedures is considered at high-risk for infection.

- Over the past decade, there have been more published reports of the nursing care provided for patients treated with TPE. TPE has become recognized as a safe and effective therapy. The involvement of various nursing specialties demonstrates some of the clinical applications.

ANNP609

Acute Renal Failure

Christy Price Rabetoy, NP

Contemporary Nephrology Nursing: Principles and Practice contains 39 chapters of educational content. Individual learners may apply for continuing nursing education credit by reading a chapter and completing the Continuing Education Evaluation Form for that chapter. Learners may apply for continuing education credit for any or all chapters.

Please photocopy this page and return to ANNA.
COMPLETE THE FOLLOWING:

Name: _____

Address: _____

City: _____ State: _____ Zip: _____

E-mail: _____

Preferred telephone: ☐ Home   ☐ Work: _____

State where licensed and license number (optional): _____

CE application fees are based upon the number of contact hours provided by the individual chapter. CE fees per contact hour for ANNA members are as follows: 1.0-1.9 - $15; 2.0-2.9 - $20; 3.0-3.9 - $25; 4.0 and higher - $30. Fees for nonmembers are $10 higher.

ANNA Member: ☐ Yes   ☐ No   Member # (if available) _____

☐ Checked Enclosed   ☐ American Express   ☐ Visa   ☐ MasterCard

Total Amount Submitted: _____

Credit Card Number: _____ Exp. Date: _____

Name as it appears on the card: _____

CE Evaluation Form
To receive continuing education credit for individual study after reading the chapter
1. Photocopy this form. (You may also download this form from ANNA's Web site, **www.annanurse.org.**)
2. Mail the completed form with payment (check) or credit card information to American Nephrology Nurses' Association, East Holly Avenue, Box 56, Pitman, NJ 08071-0056.
3. You will receive your CE certificate from ANNA in 4 to 6 weeks.

Test returns must be postmarked by **December 31, 2010.**

CE Application Fee
ANNA Member $30.00
Nonmember $40.00

EVALUATION FORM

1. I verify that I have read this chapter and completed this education activity. Date: _____

_____
Signature

2. What would be different in your practice if you applied what you learned from this activity? *(Please use additional sheet of paper if necessary.)*

_____
_____
_____
_____
_____
_____
_____
_____
_____
_____

Evaluation	Strongly disagree				Strongly agree
3. The activity met the stated objectives.					
a. Compare and contrast the three types of acute renal failure as to definitions, treatment, and symptom management.	1	2	3	4	5
b. Describe the nursing responsibilities related to CRRT.	1	2	3	4	5
c. Discuss the nursing care needed by patients having a therapeutic plasma exchange.	1	2	3	4	5
4. The content was current and relevant.	1	2	3	4	5
5. The content was presented clearly.	1	2	3	4	5
6. The content was covered adequately.	1	2	3	4	5
7. Rate your ability to apply the learning obtained from this activity to practice.	1	2	3	4	5

Comments _____

_____

8. Time required to read the chapter and complete this form: _____ minutes.

This educational activity has been provided by the American Nephrology Nurses' Association (ANNA) for 4.4 contact hours. ANNA is accredited as a provider of continuing nursing education (CNE) by the American Nurses Credentialing Center's Commission on Accreditation (ANCC-COA). ANNA is an approved provider of continuing education by the California Board of Registered Nursing, CEP 0910.

Chronic Kidney Disease

Unit 3 Contents

Chronic Kidney Disease

Unit 3 Contents

UNIT
3

Diagnosis, Classification and Management of Chronic Kidney Disease

Patricia Bargo McCarley, MSN, RN, ACNPc, CNN

Chapter Contents

Diagnosis, Classification and Management of Chronic Kidney Disease

Chapter 10

Patricia Bargo McCarley, MSN, RN, ACNPc, CNN

Chronic kidney disease (CKD) is a growing public health problem. Projections indicate that the number of patients with end stage renal disease (ESRD), dialyzing at home or incenter, or with functioning renal transplant, is expected to increase from a prevalence of 406,081 as of December 31, 2001 to an estimated 651,000 patients in 2010 (USRDS, 2003; Xue, Ma. Louis, & Collins, 2001). The number of patients with ESRD, however, appears to represent only the "tip of the iceberg," as data show there are many more "undiagnosed and untreated" patients with CKD (National Kidney Foundation [NKF], 2002).

The Third National Health and Nutrition Examination Survey (NHANES III), a survey conducted between 1988 and 1994, examined 15,624 participants, age 20 years or older, to provide data on the health and nutritional status of the U.S. population. Renal dysfunction was measured as serum creatinine (SCr) and albuminuria. Results from the study, when extrapolated to the U.S. population of adults over 20 years old, revealed the following findings: (a) 6.2 million individuals had a serum creatinine (SCr) $\geq$ 1.5 mg/dl, (b) 2.5 million had a SCr $\geq$ 1.7 mg/dl, and (c) 0.8 million patients had a SCr $\geq$ 2.0 mg/dl (Jones et al., 1998). In further analysis of the NHANES III data, calculating glomerular filtration rate (GFR) from serum creatinine based on the Modified Diet in Renal Disease (MDRD) equation, the prevalence of CKD, Stage 1 – 4, was 19.2 million persons (see Table 10-1), or 11% of the U.S. population (Coresh, Astor, Greene, Eknoyan, & Levey, 2003).

The NHANES III study also measured the presence of CKD based on the presence of albuminuria. Albuminuria was measured on a random spot urine sample along with the urine creatinine to allow for determination of the albu-

min-to-creatinine ratio. Albuminuria was defined as two spot albumin-to-creatinine ratios (mg/g) of greater than 17 mg/g in men and greater than 25 mg/g for women. Persistent albuminuria was present in 6.3 % or 11.2 million of the U.S. population with GFR > 60 ml/min/1.73 m² (Coresh et al., 2003). Nissenson, Pereria, Collins, and Steinberg (2001) also predicted the CKD prevalence in the U.S. Based on a large analysis of over 150,000 patients in an HMO data base, the number of patients in the U.S. with a Cr $\geq$ 2.0 mg/dl was estimated to be 4.2 million, higher than the NHANES III findings. Mortality rates of patients on dialysis remain in excess of 20% per year despite improved dialytic technology, and expenditures are greater than $260 billion dollars per year as of 2002 (USRDS, 2004). Clearly, the rising incidence and prevalence of CKD, along with the poor outcomes and high cost, create a growing health care concern.

This chapter is focused on CKD and delaying its progression, and will address: (a) definition and classification of the stages of CKD, (b) diagnosis and early detection of CKD, (c) risk factor identification and strategies to delay progression, (d) identification and treatment of co-morbid conditions, and (e) prevention and treatment of complications of CKD. This chapter will also discuss the efforts by the nephrology community to improve outcomes and the quality of care of persons with CKD. Treatment of ESRD is discussed in detail later in this book.

Defining and Classifying Chronic Kidney Disease

In an effort to address this growing public health care concern, the National Kidney Foundation (NKF) Kidney Disease Outcome Quality Initiative (K/DOQI) Advisory

Table 10-1

Stages and Prevalence of Chronic Kidney Disease in the Adult U.S. Population

Stage	Description	GFR ml/min/1.73 m²	Prevalence* N (1000s)	%
1	Kidney damage with normal or ↑ GFR	$\geq$90	5,900	3.3
2	Kidney damage with mild or ↓ GFR	60-89	5,300	3.0
3	Moderate ↓ GFR	30-59	7,600	4.3
4	Severe ↓ GFR	15-29	400	0.2
5	Kidney Failure	<15 or dialysis	300	0.1

*Data for Stages 1-4 from NHANES III (1988-1994). Population 177 million adults age $\geq$20 years. Data for Stage 5 from USRDS (1998) include approximately 230,000 patients treated by dialysis and assuming 70,000 additional patient not on dialysis. GFR estimated from serum creatinine using MDRD Study equation based on age, gender, race and calibration for serum creatinine. For Stages 1 and 2, kidney damage estimated by spot albumin-to creatinine ratio > 17 g/g in men or >25 mg/g in women on two measurements.

Note: From K/DOQI Clinical practice guidelines for chronic kidney disease: Evaluation, classification, and stratification (2002).

Table 10-2
Definition of Chronic Kidney Disease

1. Kidney damage for ≥ 3 months as defined by structural or functional abnormalities of the kidney, with or without decreased GFR, manifested by *either*:
   - Pathological abnormalities; or
   - Markers of kidney damage, including abnormalities in the composition of the blood and urine, or abnormalities in imaging tests.

2. GFR < 60 mL/min/1.73 m² for ≥ 3 months, with or without kidney damage.

Note: From K/DOQI Clinical practice guidelines for chronic kidney disease: evaluation, classification, and stratification (2002).

Table 10-3
Screening for CKD

Laboratory and Radiologic Markers of CKD
- Serum creatinine to estimate GFR from prediction equation
- Protein-to-creatinine ratio or albumin-to-creatinine ratio in a first-morning or random untimed "spot" urine specimen
- Urine sediment evaluation
- Urinalysis or dipstick for red blood cells and white blood cells
- Imaging studies of the kidneys (e.g., ultrasound)
- Serum electrolytes (e.g., sodium, potassium, chloride and bicarbonate)

Note: From K/DOQI Clinical practice guidelines for chronic kidney disease: evaluation, classification, and stratification (2002).

Board approved development of clinical practice guidelines for CKD in 2001, and a K/DOQI work group was identified. The CKD work group goals were to define CKD and to develop a classification system for the stages of chronic kidney disease. Additionally the work group provided an evaluation of lab measurements for clinical assessment of CKD and association of level of CKD with development of complications. Finally the group was challenged to stratify risk for loss of kidney function and development of cardiovascular disease. The guidelines were published in February 2002 and provide a foundation for the identification, evaluation and treatment of patients with CKD (NKF, 2002).

Definition of CKD

The K/DOQI workgroup (see Table 10-2) defined CKD as either kidney damage or glomerular filtration rate (GFR) < 60 ml/min/1.73 m² for ≥ 3 months. Kidney damage is defined irrespective of the specific pathology. Markers of damage include abnormalities in the blood or urine tests or imaging studies. The level of GFR, accepted as the best measure of the kidney's ability to filter blood, allows for the expression of kidney function on a continuous scale (NKF, 2002).

Classification System

The K/DOQI work group also developed a classification system of the stages of chronic kidney disease based on level of kidney function measured by GFR (see Table 10-1). The classification system is meant to provide a common language for patients and practitioners to improve communication, enhance education, and promote the conduct of clinical research. Adverse outcomes of CKD can be based on the level of kidney function, thus the classification system provides a framework for the evaluation and development of a clinical action plan for patients with CKD (NKF, 2002).

The classification system is based on the calculated GFR, which is widely accepted as the best measure of kidney function in health and disease. Stage 1 includes persons with normal function, GFR > 90 ml/min/1.73 m², but with kidney damage. This would include a patient with polycystic kidney disease, as detected by ultrasound, or a diabetic patient with microalbuminuria, but with normal GFRs.

Stage 2 CKD includes persons with kidney damage and a mild decrease in the kidney function as defined by GFR between 60 – 89 ml/min/1.73 m². Examples of persons with Stage 2 kidney disease would be a patient with hypertension or diabetes with albuminuria or proteinuiria and a GFR between 60 - 89 ml/min/1.73 m². Persons with a GFR between 60 – 89 ml/min/1.73 m², and no known marker of kidney damage (e.g., abnormality in urine or imaging test), are not considered to have CKD. An example would be an elderly patient with mild decrease in function but no marker of kidney damage. Other causes of decreased GFR without kidney damage include unilateral nephrectomy or extracellular fluid volume depletion with reduced kidney perfusion.

Stage 3 kidney disease is defined as a GFR between 30 and 59 ml/min/1.73 m² and is based on the level of GFR regardless of the presence of kidney damage. An example of a patient with Stage 3 kidney function might be an older person with no kidney damage but a moderate decrease in kidney function or a person with hypertension, albuminuria, and a GFR between 30 and 59 ml/min/1.73 m².

Stage 4 is defined as a GFR between 15 and 29 ml/min/1.73 m² and represents severe loss of kidney function. Persons are often diagnosed at this stage as they usually become symptomatic (e.g., weakness, low energy, appetite loss). Stage 5, GFR < 15 ml/min/1.73 m², is defined as kidney failure and is usually accompanied by signs and symptoms of uremia such as nausea and vomiting, malaise, or mental lassitude. Persons at this level usually need to initiate renal replacement therapy (RRT) for treatment of the complication of decreased GFR. Although not all patients at this stage are treated with RRT, these persons nonetheless are considered to have kidney failure (NKF, 2002).

Etiology and Pathophysiology

Historically the classification of the type of kidney disease has been based on pathology and etiology. The new classification system focuses on the GFR, but is not meant to minimize the need to diagnose the cause of CKD. Patients with CKD should be evaluated to determine the etiology or type of kidney disease, as early treatment may prevent or slow progression.

Table 10-4

Simplified Classification of Chronic Kidney Disease by Diagnoses

Disease	Major types (Examples)
Diabetic Kidney Disease	Type 1 and Type 2 diabetes
Nondiabetic Kidney Disease	Glomerular diseases (autoimmune diseases, systemic infections, drugs, neoplasia) Vascular diseases (large vessel disease, hypertension, microangiopathy) Tubulointerstitial diseases (urinary tract infection, stones, obstruction, drug toxicity) Cystic diseases (polycystic diseases)
Diseases in the Transplant	Chronic rejection Drug toxicity (cyclosporin or tacrolimus) Recurrent diseases (FSGS) Transplant glomerulopathy

Note: From K/DOQI Clinical practice guidelines for chronic kidney disease: Evaluation, classification, and stratification (2002).

In many patients, clinical history, physical examination, and presentation provide sufficient information to determine the etiology of CKD. Critical to establishment of the diagnosis in other patients are other diagnostic findings, including imaging of the kidney, evaluation of urine sediment, kidney biopsy, and measurement of serum electrolytes and other markers of CKD listed in Table 10-3 (NKF, 2002).

A simplified classification of CKD based on diagnosis is presented in Table 10-4. The leading cause of CKD is diabetes mellitus. A second group of diseases can be grouped under the label of nondiabetic kidney disease. This includes glomerular diseases (primary and secondary), vascular diseases, tubulointerstitial diseases, and cystic diseases. Included among these nondiabetic kidney diseases are hypertensive nephrolosclerosis and glomerular diseases, the second and third leading causes of CKD. Finally, kidney disease in the renal transplant is the fourth leading cause of CKD (NKF, 2002). Details of diseases causing CKD can be found in Chapter 6.

Mechanisms for Disease Progression

Although there are many diseases that can cause CKD, there appear to be common pathways for disease progression. Prominent morphologic features are fibrosis, loss of native renal cells, and infiltration by monocytes and macrophages, the result of the constant interplay between vasoactive substances. Mediators of the process are many and include abnormal glomerular hemodynamics, proteinuria, hypoxia, and angiotensin II (Yu, 2003).

Briefly, adaptive effects by the glomerulus to maintain GFR, leads to elevated glomerular pressures and hyperfiltration. This hyperfiltration causes endothelial injury, stimulation of profibrotic cytokines by mesangiam, infiltration by monocytes and macrophages, and detachment of glomerular epithelial cells. Glomerular growth, another adaptive change, leads to increased wall stress and even more increased glomerular pressure and injury. Proteinuria results from the increased glomerular permeability and increased capillary pressure (Remuzzi & Bertani, 1998).

Accompanying all forms of glomerular injury is disease of the tubulointerstitium. The pathophysiology involved in tubulointerstitial disease begins with abnormal glomerular permeability with resultant proteinura (Remuzzi & Bertani, 1998). The filtered protein is reabsorbed by the proximal tubular cells and accumulates within the cells, causing abnormal production of cytokines. The release of these proinflammatory factors leads to injury and ultimately fibrosis and scarring of the tubulointerstitium (Yu, 2003).

Hypoxia is also regarded as a potential cause for progression of kidney disease. Loss of the peritubular capillaries by various causes diminishes capillary perfusion of the tubules. Hypoxia favors release of proinflammatory and profibrotic cytokines, leading to injury and fibrosis (Nangaku, 2004). Angiotensin II increases glomerular hypertension. Besides its hemodynamic effect on the glomerulus, angiotensin II also stimulates cytokines and growth factor that favor fibrogenesis (Yu, 2003; Remuzzi, Ruggenent, & Perico, 2002).

The cause and location of the initial renal injury may vary, however, and as discussed the mechanisms of renal injury share common pathways. Although the rate of progression may vary substantially, the level of proteinuria is one of the strongest predictor of progression of kidney disease (Keane, 2000).

Treatment of CKD Based on Diagnoses

Specific treatment to delay progression should be based initially on treating the primary disease. Table 10-4 provides a simplified classification system based on diagnosis. Diabetic kidney disease follows a characteristic course, presenting with microalbuminuria or proteinuria,

Table 10-5
Equations to Estimate GFR based on Serum Creatinine

Cockroft-Gault equation:

$$\text{CrCl (ml/min)} = \frac{(140 - \text{age})(\text{weight in kg})}{(\text{serum Cr})(72)} \times 0.85 \text{ if female}$$

From: Cockcroft, D.W. & Gault, M.H.. (1976). Prediction of creatinine clearance from serum creatinine. *Nephron, 16*, 31-41.

Abbreviated MDRD equation:

$$\text{GFR(ml/min per 1.73 m}^2) = 186 \times (\text{SCr})^{-1.154} \times (\text{age})^{-0.203}$$
$$\times \quad (0.742 \text{ if female}) \text{ and} \quad \times \quad (1.210 \text{ if African-American})$$

Note: From Levey, A.S., Bosch, J., Lewis, J. B., Greene, T., Rogers, N. & Roth, D. (1999). A more accurate method to estimate glomerular filtration rate from a serum creatinine: A new prediction equation. *Annals of Internal Medicine, 130*, 461-470.

and developing nephropathy if left untreated. Effective treatment includes strict glycemic control, effective hypertension management, and reduction of proteinuria with angiotensin converting enzyme (ACE) inhibitors and angiotensin receptor blockers (ARB) (American Diabetes Association [ADA], 2004a, b, and c; Bakris et al., 2000; Wolf & Ritz, 2003). Treatment of nondiabetic kidney disease is based on specific cause, usually identified by biopsy. Specific therapies are directed to reverse abnormalities in structure or function. For example, treatment of chronic urinary tract infection with antibiotics or cessation of nephrotoxic drugs such as nonsteriodal anti-inflammatory drugs (NSAIDS). Treatment also includes effective hypertensive management and reduction in proteinuria (Levey, 2002).

Finally, treatment of diseases of the transplant kidney again is biopsy guided and focuses on reversing the cause. Patients with a kidney transplant should be considered at high risk for development of CKD as GFR is lower in patients with a solitary kidney. There is a low threshold for biopsy in kidney transplant patients in order to provide the differential diagnosis for treatment. The most common cause of CKD in the transplanted kidney is chronic rejection and toxicity due to cyclosporin or tacrolimus. The predominant challenge for clinicians is to provide a level of immunosuppression that increases long-term patient and allograft survival while preventing or reducing rejection episodes. The differential diagnosis also includes all the diseases of the native kidney (Kirk, Mannon, Swanson, & Hale, 2005). Treatment of specific diseases of the kidney are discussed in Chapter 6 and diseases of the transplanted kidney are discussed in Chapter 31. Slowing the progression of CKD, regardless of diagnosis, is discussed in detail later in this chapter.

Assessment of Severity of CKD

Using Glomerular Filtration Rate (GFR)

In addition to the establishment of a diagnosis, it is important to assess the severity of kidney dysfunction and establish the stage of CKD. Serum creatinine and proteinuria are key markers for determining the degree of kidney dysfunction. Serum creatinine, still widely used by many practitioners as a marker of the level of kidney function, is not an accurate index of kidney dysfunction. It is affected by age, gender, race, body mass, muscle mass, body fat, metabolic states, pharmacological agents, and lab analytical methods. Glomerular filtration rate (GFR) is now accepted as the best overall measure of kidney function and as previously discussed is used to define the stages of CKD. GFR represents the best measure of the kidney's ability to filter blood (NKF, 2002).

The most accurate method to measure GFR involves substances that are cleared 100% by the kidney, such as inulin or inthalamide. Normal GFR, based on inulin clearance and adjusted to standard body surface area of 1.73 m², is 127 ml/min/1.73 m² for men and 118 ml/min/1.73 m² for women (standard deviation is approximately 20 ml/min/1.73 m²). The use of inulin or inthalamide, however, is expensive and impractical for screening purposes (NKF, 2002). A number of equations, estimating GFR based on serum creatinine, have been developed and studied. These equations provide a more accurate prediction of GFR than measurement of serum creatinine alone. Most widely used are the Cockcroft-Gault equation (Cockcroft & Gault, 1976), which takes into account age, weight and gender, and the abbreviated Modified Diet in Renal Disease (MDRD) equation, which factors in age, gender, and race (Levey et al., 1999) (see Table 10-5). The level of kidney function should be determined based on a prediction equation using the serum creatinine and some or all of the following variables: age, gender, race, and body size (NKF, 2002).

Albuminuria and Proteinuria

A measurement of the level of albumin or protein in the urine helps to establish the diagnosis and also the severity of kidney disease. It is a sensitive marker for many types of kidney disease from very early to advanced stages. It is also a prognostic finding, as increasing levels of albumin-

Table 10-6
JNC VII Classification of Blood pressure for Adults Aged 18 Years or Older

BP Classification	Systolic BP (mmHg)		Diastolic BP (mmHg)
Normal	<120	and	<80
Prehypertension	120 – 139	or	80 - 89
Stage 1 Hypertension	140 – 159	or	90 - 99
Stage 2 Hypertension	≥180	or	≥100

Note: From Chobanian, A.V., Bakis, G.L., Black, H.R., Cushman, W.C., Green, L.A., Izzo, J.L., Jones, D.W., Materson, B.J., Oparil, S., Wright, J.T., Rocella, E.J., & the National High Blood Pressure Education Programming Coordinating Committee (2003). The Seventh Report of the Joint National Committee on Prevention, Detection, Evaluation, and Treatment of High Blood Pressure. *JAMA, 289*, 2560-2562

uria or proteinuria are associated with higher-rates of loss of kidney function. Albuminuria or proteinuria are also targets of treatment in slowing progression. Early identification of albuminuria or proteinuria permits a timely introduction of therapy that can slow the course of kidney disease (Keane, 2000; Rugenenti, Gaspari, Perna, & Remuzzi, 1998).

Proteinuria refers to increased secretion of albumin and other specific proteins in the urine. Albuminuria refers to increased excretion of only albumin in the urine and is preferred over measuring proteinuria unless protein in the urine is substantially elevated (e.g., > 500–1000 mg/g) (NKF, 2002).

Albuminuria or proteinuria can be measured in a 24-hour urine or from an untimed spot urine sample. In a 24-hour urine, microalbuminuria is defined as 30–300 mg/day and albuminuria as levels > 300 mg/day. Although the 24-hour urine collection has been the standard for quantitative evaluation of albuminuria or proteinuria, the random-spot urine measurement of the albumin or protein-to-creatinine ratio is now more widely used due to the difficulty in collecting an accurate 24-hour specimen. In the measurement of a spot urine albumin-to-creatinine ratio, microalbuminuria is defined as a ratio between 17–250 mg/g in males and 25–355 mg/g in females, and albuminuria as a ratio greater than 250 mg/g in men and 355 mg/g in women. When albumin excretion exceeds > 500-1000 mg/g as measured in a spot albumin-to-creatinine ratio, it is acceptable to measure protein-to-creatinine ratio due to cost and technical difficulty in measuring albumin. Measurement of urine protein concentrations by standard dipsticks are not sufficiently sensitive to pick up microalbuminuria. However, albumin-specific dipsticks are available that can detect albumin above a concentration of 3 to 4 mg/dl, and are useful in detecting microalbuminuria (NKF, 2002).

Signs and symptoms of CKD

Interventions during the early stages of CKD are critical in slowing disease progression. However, CKD often goes undetected because patients are frequently asymptomatic. The GFR provides an indication of what signs and symptoms may be seen based on the degree of decline. As GFR declines, patients begin to show hypertension, a wide

range of lab abnormalities, and symptoms due to disorders in other organ systems, including anemia, dyslipidemia, disorders of bone metabolism, protein energy malnutrition, neuropathy, and alterations in health status (NKF, 2002). Specific discussion of each of the complications of kidney disease will follow a brief discussion of the association of levels of GFR with complications of CKD.

Stage 1 patients have normal GFR, but some structural or functional abnormality in the kidney. Usually they have normal blood pressure, no lab abnormalities, and no symptoms. Stage 2 patients (GFR 60- 89 ml/min/1.73 m²) generally are asymptomatic, however, hypertension usually develops during this stage. Lab abnormalities, indicative of dysfunction in other organ systems, may or may not be present. Stage 3 patients (GFR 30–59 ml/min/1.73 m²) usually have lab abnormalities in several organ systems (e.g., anemia, disorders of bone metabolism), but again are usually asymptomatic, although hypertension is almost always present. Stage 4 patients (GFR 15–29 ml/min/1.73 m²) usually have lab abnormalities in several organ systems and begin to experience mild symptoms associated with CKD (e.g., fatigue, poor appetite). Stage 5 patients (GFR <15 ml/min/1.73 m²) usually have lab abnormalities in several systems and symptoms of renal failure (e.g., malnutrition, malaise, neuropathy) (NKF, 2002). A thorough discussion of symptom and symptom management is provided in Chapter 9. As CKD is often asymptomatic until late stages, establishment of GFR and early identification of complications through lab testing is critical to improve outcomes and delay progression.

Complications of CKD

The complications of CKD and the stage at which they are usually observed will be discussed, including: (a) hypertension, (b) anemia, (c) protein-energy malnutrition, (d) metabolic acidosis, (e) disorders of bone metabolism, (f) neuropathy, and (g) dyslipidemias. Treatment of these complications will be discussed later in the chapter.

Hypertension

Hypertension, the second leading cause of CKD, is also a complication of CKD. It is well recognized as a public health care problem and is a significant contributor to cardiovascular morbidity and mortality. The higher the blood pressure the greater the risk of myocardial infarction, heart failure, and kidney damage (Chobanian et al., 2003). For each 20 mmHg increase in systolic blood pressure or 10 mmHg increase in diastolic blood pressure in persons 40–70 years old, there is a doubling of the risk of cardiovascular disease across the entire blood pressure range from 115/75 to 185/115 mmHg (Lewington et al., 2002). Antihypertensive therapy has been associated with more than 50% mean reduction in heart failure, 20% to 25% mean reduction in myocardial infarction, and 35%-40% mean reduction in stroke (Neal, MacMahon, & Chapman, 2000).

Hypertension in CKD increases the risk of loss of kidney function (Bakris, 1998; Bakris & Weir, 2000; Jafar et al., 2001; Hovind, Rossing, Tarnow, Smidt, & Parving, 2001). JNC VII defines Stage 1 hypertension as systolic BP between 140 to 159 mmHg and diastolic BP between 90-99 mmHg. Stage 2 hypertension is systolic BP $\geq$ 160 or diastolic BP $\geq$ 100. JNC VII establishes a prehypertension category. Patients with prehypertension, systolic BP between 120–139 mmHg or diastolic BP between 80–89 mmHg, are at increased risk of progression to hypertension (see Table 10-6) (Chobanian et al., 2003).

Hypertension occurs with mild decreases in the GFR. Data from the NHANES II study showed 40% of individuals with GFR < 90 ml/min/m² had hypertension (Coresh, 2001). Buckalew and colleagues (1996), in the MDRD study (1795 patients), showed that hypertension was present in persons with a GFR of 60–90 ml/min/1.73m², 65%–75% of the time. Numerous studies have shown that improved BP control decreases progression (Brenner et al., 2001; Hovind et al., 2001). The high prevalence of hypertension among persons with mildly decreased GFR, emphasizes the importance of early monitoring and treatment of hypertension in patients with CKD.

Anemia

Anemia, as defined by the World Health Organization (WHO), is hemoglobin (Hgb) < 13 g/dl for males and Hgb < 12 g/dl for women (WHO, 1998). Its prevalence is common in CKD. Although there are many contributing factors, the major cause is a decline in the erythropoietin synthesis by the kidneys. Other causes include iron deficiency, blood loss, presence of uremic inhibitors, reduced half-life of blood cells, vitamin B1 or B12 deficiency, or a combination of factors. In the majority of studies examining anemia of CKD, there is an association between the level of Hgb and the level of kidney disease (Astor, Munter, Levin, Eustace, & Coresh, 2002; Hsu, McCulloch, & Curhan, 2002). Astor and colleagues (2002), in the NHANES III study, showed an increase in the presence of anemia in stage 3 patients (GFR less than 60 ml/min/1.75 m²). Results from the Prevalence of Anemia in Early Renal Insufficiency (PAERI) Study showed there was an increase in the percentage of patients with anemia (Hgb <12 g/dl) and the severity of anemia (Hgb <10 g/dl) as creatinine clearance decreased from 60–90 ml/min/1.73 m² to less than 15 ml/min/1.73 m² (McClellan, Tran, & The PAERI Study Group, 2002). Anemia is associated with higher hospitalization rates, increased

cardiovascular diseases, and increased mortality (Collins et al., 2001; Levin, 2002). Patients with CKD should be routinely assessed and treated for anemia.

Protein-Energy Malnutrition

Many factors in CKD contribute to protein-energy malnutrition (PEM). Usually multifactorial, the causes of PEM include the following: (a) poor nutritional intake due to uremic-induced anorexia, (b) increased protein catabolism caused by metabolic acidosis, (c) negative effect of inflammation and infection on decreasing visceral protein synthesis, and (d) endocrine disorders in uremia, including derangements of insulin and parathyroid hormone. Comorbid conditions, frequently common in CKD, including diabetes mellitus, older age, and cardiovascular disease, also contribute to PEM in patients with CKD (Mehrotra & Kopple, 2004). Evidence of nutritional decline begins long before patients reach end stage renal disease. In the Modification of Diet in Renal Disease (MDRD) Study (1785 patients), patients with Stage III (mean $\pm$ S.D.GFR: 39.8 $\pm$ 21.1 mL/min/1/73 m²) demonstrated a decline in nutritional status as measured by dietary protein intake, serum albumin and transferrin, and body weight and body mass index (Kopple et al., 2000).

Hypoalbumin is associated with increased morbidity and mortality. Many studies show there is a high prevalence of PEM in patients undergoing maintenance dialysis and a strong association between increased morbidity and mortality in this population (Pupim, Calgar, Hakim, Shyr, & Ikizler, 2004; Combe et al., 2004). The patient with CKD should be evaluated early and frequently for the nutritional status and the adequacy of the diet in order to prevent PEM. Patients with severe hypoalbuminuria should be given special attention.

Metabolic Acidosis

Metabolic acidosis occurs as the number of functioning nephrons declines. Decreased ammonia and phosphate excretion lead to the development of acidosis in CKD. A decrease in the serum bicarbonate level occurs when the patient reaches Stage III and the GFR falls below 60 mL/min/1.73 m². It is associated with many adverse consequences, including protein catabolism, fatigue, and demineralization of bone (Franch & Mitch, 2004). It should be identified and treated in patients with CKD.

Disturbances in Mineral and Bone Metabolism

Disturbances in mineral and bone metabolism develop as the GFR declines. Abnormal calcium and phosphorous metabolism and elevated PTH can lead to pruritis; bone disease; proximal myopathy; and soft tissue calcification, including vascular, visceral, periauricular, and cutaneous calcifications (NKF, 2003a). Briefly, the major features of the disturbances in mineral and bone metabolism include the following: (a) hyperphosphatemia develops due to impaired urinary excretion; (b) phosphate retention suppresses calcitriol [dihydroxyvitamin D3] production; (c) reduced calcitriol production leads to defective intestinal absorption of calcium leading to hypocalcemia; (d) hyperphosphatemia, hypocalcemia, and reduced calcitriol synthesis combine to stimulate the production of PTH; (e) continuous PTH stimulation leads to hyperplasia and proliferation of the parathryroid cells, resulting in hyperparathyroidism; (f) high PTH levels stimulate osteoblasts, resulting in high-turnover bone disease with significant bone demineralization; and (g) high PTH, along with hyperphosphatemia, hypercalcemia, and elevated calcium-phosphorus product, leads to soft tissue calcification (Lach & Bover, 2000).

Phosphate retention first occurs in Stage 2 but becomes more evident in patients at Stage 4 when GFR falls below 30 mL/min/1.73 m^2. Patients with Stage 2 and Stage 3 CKD may have a calcitriol-resistant state, but as GFR falls below 30 mL/min/1.73 m^2 an absolute calcitriol deficiency develops (Martinez, Saracho, Montengro, & Llach, 1997). There is no consistent data that shows a relationship exists between the level of serum calcium and the level of kidney function (NKF, 2003a). Elevated PTH, the earliest and most sensitive marker of abnormal bone metabolism, develops when the GFR level falls below 80 ml/min/1.73 m^2 (Martinez et al., 1997).

The consequences of secondary hyperparathyroid (SHPT) disease include metabolic bone disease with reduction in bone mass and changes in microarchitecture (Goodman, 2004). In a study by Balon, Hoss, and Zavrantnik (2002), abnormal bone histology was present in most patients with CKD before the initiation of dialysis.

Extraskeletal calcification has also become the recent focus of practitioners due to the burden of cardiovascular disease in patients with ESRD and has been associated with increased morbidity and mortality (Block, Julbert-Shearon, Levin, & Port, 1998; Ganesh, Stach, Levin, Hylbert-Shearon, & Port, 2001). Cardiovascular mortality in the United States is 10-30 times higher in individuals receiving dialysis than in age-matched controls (Foley et al., 1998). A number of studies have shown the increased risk of cardiovascular disease with elevations in calcium, phosphorous and PTH (Block et al., 1998; Ganesh et al., 2001; Goodman et al., 2004). Indeed, SHPT disease has received considerable attention as a nontraditional risk factor in cardiovascular morbidity and mortality. Clearly, early identification and treatment of the disturbances in metabolism of bone and minerals can reduce the associated increased morbidity and mortality observed in patients with CKD.

Neurological Disturbance

Neuropathy is a common feature of CKD. Although its pathophysiology is not well understood, increased levels of uremic toxins have correlated with reduction of nerve conduction velocity and peripheral manifestations of neuropathy. Peripheral neuropathy develops during the course of CKD and is present in up to 65% of patients at the initiation of dialysis (Burns & Bates, 1998). Generally, uremic polyneuropathy is a symmetrical, mixed sensory and motor polyneuropathy and affects distal nerves more severely. Symptoms usually do not present until the patient (Stage 4 and 5) has a GFR < 12 to 20 mL/min/1.73 m^2. Patients may complain of puritis, burning, muscle irritability, cramps, and weakness (Burns & Bates, 1998).

Uremic toxins may also affect the autonomic and central nervous systems. Autonomic dysfunction also occurs frequently both in patients with CKD, caused by diabetes, and in patients with severely impaired kidney function (GFR < 15 ml/min/1.73 m^2. Symptoms include impaired heart rate and blood pressure variability in response to respiratory cycle, postural change, and Valsalva maneuver (K/DOQI, 2002). Central nervous system symptoms associated with uremia include fatigue, apathy, clumsiness, impaired concentration and/or memory, and sleep disturbances. A patient who presents with altered mental status may progress to uremic encephalopathy, if CKD goes untreated. The patient may become delirious, disoriented, and agitated, which may evolve to preterminal coma and convulsions (Burns & Bates, 1998).

Treatment with renal replacement therapy improves the more severe symptoms and signs of CNS involvement and can also improve peripheral neuropathy. There is limited research associating the level of kidney function and markers of neuropathy as most of the information regarding neuropathy is from studies of patients with ESRD (NKF, 2002). Patients with CKD should be periodically assessed for neurologic involvement in order to develop a treatment plan that may include the initiation of renal replacement therapy if symptoms continue to progress. In fact, altered mental status related to uremia is a key indicator that renal replacement therapy should be initiated.

Dyslipidemias

Hyperlipidemia is common in patients with CKD. The typical pattern consists of elevated triglycerides and low high-density lipoprotein (HDL) cholesterol. Low-density lipoprotein is usually variable. Proteinuria, prevalent in many diseases causing CKD, also contributes to dyslipidemia. Nephrotic range proteinuria is usually associated with increases in total and LDL cholesterol and triglycerides. Although the cause of the accumulation of cholesterol and triglycerides is not fully known, it may result from delayed lipoprotein catabolism (Sahadevan & Kasiske, 2002). Other factors affecting lipoprotein levels in patients with CKD include level of GFR, although there is no correlation to the stage of CKD, and development of dyslipidemias (K/DOQI, 2003).

Atherosclerotic cardiovascular disease (ACVD) is higher in patients with CKD than the general population (Tonelli et al., 2001; Jungers et al., 1997). In the MDRD Study of patients without diabetes who initiated dialysis, 25% of the first hospitalizations were related to cardiovascular disease. Go, Chertow, Fan, McCulloch, and Hsu (2004), who followed more then 1 million patients in a large health care system for a median of 2.84 years, found an independent graded association between lower levels of kidney function and the risks of death, cardiovascular events, and hospitalizations. Although there are no randomized, controlled intervention trials testing the hypothesis that dyslipidemias cause ACVD in CKD patient, there are no compelling reasons to assume that dyslipidemias do not contribute to ACVD in patients with CKD. In addition to detecting abnormalities that may contribute to ACVD, evaluation and treatment of dyslipidemias may preserve kidney function (Fried, Orchard, & Kasisko, 2001). Dyslipidemias should be evaluated early, and treated and followed closely in order to reduce the incidence of ACVD (NKF, 2003a).

Quality of Life

There is good evidence that declining GFR is associated with abnormalities in health status, functioning, and well being (e.g., weakness, poor appetite, anxiety, decreased sense of well-being). In the MDRD study, it was found that reduced kidney function was associated with an array of symptoms, including weakness and low energy, affecting quality of life and well-being (Rocco et al., 1997). In the NHANES III study, declining GFR was associated with impaired walking and lifting ability (NKF, 2002). Decreased GFR is also associated with poorer psychosocial functioning, including higher depression, reduced social activity, and interaction (Rocco et al., 1997). Functional status and well being should be assessed in order to establish baseline data and early intervention to improve quality of life of patients with CKD.

Comorbid Conditions

Patients with CKD usually have comorbid conditions in addition to CKD. Management of unrelated diseases is important to the health of the patient but does not affect the course of CKD (e.g., chronic obstructive pulmonary disease, degenerative joint disease). Treatment of other diseases, such as diabetes and hypertension, which cause CKD, does affect the course of CKD. Diabetes is singled out for this discussion, as it is the leading cause of CKD. Cardiovascular disease, the leading cause of death in patients with kidney disease, will also be discussed because of its importance as a preventable cause of morbidity and mortality in patients with CKD (NKF, 2002).

Diabetes

Diabetes, a leading cause of morbidity and death in the United States, is the leading cause of CKD. Patients with diabetes on hemodialysis consume more financial resources and have worse outcomes than those without diabetes (Wolf & Ritz, 2003). Microalbuminuria (> 30 mg/day) is the first sign of renal disease. Most adverse outcomes of diabetes are associated with vascular complications. The complications may be microvascular, including retinopathy, neuropathy or nephropathy, or macrovascular, including coronary artery disease, cerebrovascular disease, or peripheral vascular disease. Without action to manage, nearly one-third of patients with diabetes will develop CKD. Evidence indicates that the course of microalbuminuria can be altered with early intervention (Snow, Weiss, & Mottar-Pilson, 2003). Albuminuria and proteinuria are also associated with high risk for non-kidney complications, including cardiovascular disease, retinopathy, and neuropathy. Early detection and treatment of diabetic nephropathy cannot only minimize the loss of renal function, but also improve long-term survival (NKF, 2002). Effective management strategies in preventing vascular complications include good glycemic control, tight hypertensive control, and lifestyle modifications when appropriate (Bakris et al., 2000; Snow et al., 2003). In Chapter 11 diabetic kidney disease is discussed in detail.

Cardiac Disease

Cardiac disease is the leading cause of death in patients with ESRD, accounting for half of all deaths. Dialysis patients have a 10 to 30 times greater CVD mortality compared to age-matched individuals in the general population (Foley, Parfrey, & Sarnak, 1998). CKD appears to be a risk factor for cardiac disease. Several large prospective studies have reported that cardiovascular disease is a risk independently associated with elevated serum creatinine, low GFR, and microalbumunuria (Fried et al., 2003; Manjunath et al., 2003).

Patients with CKD have many of the traditional risk factors for CVD, including older age, hypertension, dyslipidemias, diabetes mellitus, and physical inactivity. In addition, patients with CKD have other unique renal-related risk factors for the development of CVD, including anemia, disturbances of mineral metabolism, proteinuria, extracellular volume overload, malnutrition, inflammation, elevated homocysteine, and decreased GFR (Sarnak et al., 2003).

In the Framingham Heart study, males with mild kidney disease (SCr level between 1.5 and 3.0 mg/dl) had 2 ? times more episodes of congestive heart failure (CHF) and 3 times higher incidence of left ventricular hypertrophy (LVH) when compared with males with normal SCr (Culleton et al., 1999). Anavekar and colleagues (2004) found a decreased calculated GFR was associated with increased mortality in over 14,000 patients with myocardial infarction complicated by heart failure, left ventricular dysfunction, or both. It is clear that patients with CKD should be considered at highest risk for CVD and its associated mortality. Risk factor reduction for CVD should be initiated early to reduce the morbidity and mortality associated with CKD and ESRD (Coresh, Astor, & Sarnak, 2004; Sarnak et al., 2003).

Although CKD is estimated to afflict 20 million adults in the United States; in contrast, the estimated prevalence of ESRD in the U.S. population is 400,000. Only a small percentage of patients progress to kidney failure and renal replacement therapy, the most visible outcome of CKD. In a study by Keith, Nichols, Guillion, Brown, and Smith (2002), 27,998 patients with CKD were followed for up to 66 months over a 5-year period. Only 3.1% of patients with Stage 2 through 4 CKD progressed to renal replacement therapy, while 24.9% died. Indeed patients are more likely to die than to progress to kidney failure, emphasizing the need to recognize patients at risk and identify and treat CKD early in order to delay and prevent adverse outcomes.

Identification of Individuals at Risk for CKD

Epidemiological studies show that individuals with certain clinical and socio-demographic characteristics are at increased risk for CKD, suggesting that there are identifiable risk factors for CKD. Knowing these risk factors allows for early identification of those likely to develop CKD and initiation of treatment to slow progression. Risk factors for CKD can be divided into susceptibility factors and initiation factors (see Table 10-7).

Susceptibility factors would include those that increase a patient's susceptibility to kidney damage, including older age, family history, ethnic status (African American, American Indian, Hispanic, Asian or Pacific Islander), exposure to

Table 10-7
Potential Risk Factors for Susceptibility to and Initiation of CKD

Susceptibility Factors	Initiating Factors
Older age	Diabetes
US ethnic minority status: African American, American Indian, Hispanic, Asian, or Pacific Islander	Hypertension
	Autoimmune disease
	Systemic infections
Exposure to certain chemical and environmental conditions (e.g. lead)	Chronic urinary tract infections
	Urinary stones
Low income	Lower urinary tract obstruction
Limited education	Neoplasia
Family history of CKD	History of acute kidney failure
Reduction in kidney mass	Exposure to certain drugs (e.g. NSAIDS, aminoglycosides)
Low birth weight	

Note: From K/DOQI Clinical practice guidelines for chronic kidney disease: Evaluation, classification, and stratification (2002).

chemical and environmental conditions, low income/education levels, reduction in kidney mass, and low birth weight. Initiation factors are those that directly initiate kidney damage, including diabetes and hypertension, the leading causes of kidney damage. Other initiating factors are autoimmune disease, chronic urinary tract infections, urinary stones, lower urinary tract obstruction, neoplasia, drug toxicity, and history of acute renal failure. Individuals at risk of developing CKD should undergo routine screening for the markers of kidney disease (NKF, 2002).

Screening

Patients at risk for CKD should be screened. SCr should be assessed on a routine basis and used in a prediction equation to estimate the level of GFR. Serum electrolytes should also be checked routinely. Blood pressure and glycemic control should be measured as they are early potential risks for development of CKD. Urinalysis may uncover evidence of kidney damage such as pyuria, proteinuria, hematuria, and abnormal sediment. Patients with diabetes should have the presence of microalbuminuria measured annually (NKF, 2002). Those found to have CKD should be evaluated, as previously discussed (see Table 10-3), and treated. Those found not to have CKD should be advised to follow a program of risk factor reduction, where appropriate, with repeat periodic evaluations (NKF, 2002).

Clinical Action Plan to Treat CKD

The ultimate goal of therapy is to slow the progression of CKD. The care of patients with CKD is a complex process involving diagnosis and treatment, delaying progression, preventing and treating complications, treating comorbidities, and preparing for RRT. Table 10-8 outlines a clinical action plan based on the stage of CKD (NKF, 2002).

Regardless of the stage at which the patient presents, the cause of CKD should be diagnosed and treated, rate of progression should be delineated, and all efforts to slow progression should be initiated. Risk factors for progression should be identified and reduced. Comorbid conditions should be addressed and treated at each stage, and specifically cardiac risk factor reduction should begin with diagnosis of CKD. Evaluation for the presence of complications of CKD should begin in Stage 2 in order to initiate treatment. Finally, preparation for renal replacement should begin in Stage 3 with education concerning treatment options. Optimal preparation for RRT should include the placement of a vascular access for dialysis in Stage 4 and referral for renal transplant evaluation. RRT is usually initiated in Stage 5 when GFR is < 10 – 15 ml/min/1.73 m^2 (NKF, 2002).

Risk Factors for Progression

Many patients are unaware of the fact that they have kidney disease until the later stages. Without treatment, kidney function progressively declines in most patients with CKD after sufficient damage has occurred. For this reason it is essential that health care providers be vigilant in assessing patients at risk and identifying factors that can be modified. A variety of factors have been associated with more rapid progression. Factors may be nonmodifiable or modifiable (NKF, 2002).

Nonmodifiable Risk Factors

Among the nonmodifiable risk factors is the underlying cause of the kidney disease. Diabetic, glomerular, and polycystic kidney disease, and kidney disease in transplant patients are associated with faster GFR decline than hypertensive and tubulointerstitial kidney disease, although few studies specifically relate the rate of GFR decline to the type of disease (NKF, 2002). Other nonmodifiable risk factors that affect GFR are race, level of kidney function, gender, and age. African-American race, lower baseline kidney function, male gender, and older age are associated with more rapid rates of decline (Hunsicker et al., 1997; Krop et al., 1999; Nakano et al., 1999).

Table 10-8
Clinical Action Plan for CKD

Stage	Description	GFR ml/min/ 1.73 m²	Frequency of Visit (minimum)	Focus of Care	Lab and Frequency* (located at bottom unless specified otherwise)	Referrals	Education
Stage 0	Increased risk	Normal	Annual	• Screen and control risk factors	• CMP • CBC • Urinalysis • Urine albumin-to-creatinine ratio *Annual		• Reduce risk factors
Stage 1	Kidney damage with normal GFR	>90	Diagnosis dependent (q 3 – 6 months)	• Diagnose and treat • Slow progression • Screen and control risk factors • Treat comorbid conditions • Cardiovascular risk reduction	• CMP • CBC • Lipid Panel • Urinalysis • Urine albumin-to-creatinine ratio *Q 3 – 6 months	• Dietary • Diagnosis dependent	• CKD • Reduce risk factors • Comorbid conditions • Cardiovascular risk reduction
Stage 2	Mild decrease in GFR	60 - 89	Diagnosis dependent (q 3 – 6 months)	• Treat CKD • Slow progression • Screen and control risk factors • Treat comorbid conditions • Cardiovascular risk reduction • Treat complications	• CMP-annual • CBC-annual • PTH-annual • Lipid panel-annual • BMP • Hgb/Hct • Urinalysis • Urine albumin-to-creatinine ratio *Q 3 – 6 months	• Dietary • Diagnosis dependent	• CKD • Reduce risk factors • Comorbid conditions • Cardiovascular risk reduction • CKD complications
Stage 3	Moderate decrease in GFR	30 - 59	Every 2 – 3months	• Treat CKD • Slow progression • Screen and control risk factors • Treat comorbid conditions • Cardiovascular risk reduction • Treat complications	• CMP-annual • CBC-annual • PTH-annual/QTR/tx • Lipid Panel-annual/QTR/tx • BMP • Hgb/Hct • Urine albumin-to-creatinine ratio *Q 2 – 3 months	• Dietary • Diagnosis dependent	• CKD • Reduce risk factors • Comorbid conditions • Cardiovascular risk reduction • CKD Complications • CKD Treatment Options
Stage 4	Severe decrease in GFR	15 - 29	Monthly	• Treat CKD • Slow progression • Screen and control risk factors • Treat comorbid conditions • Cardiovascular risk reduction • Treat complications • Prepare for RRT	• CMP-annual • CBC-annual • PTH-annual/QTR/tx • Lipid Panel-annual/QTR/tx • BMP • Hgb/Hct • Urine albumin-to-creatinine ratio *Monthly	• Dietary • Transplant • Access	• CKD • Reduce risk factors • Comorbid conditions • Cardiovascular risk reduction • CKD Complications • CKD Treatment Options • Individual treatment options
Stage 5	Kidney Failure	<15 or dialysis dependent	Monthly	• Treat comorbid conditions • Treat complications • Cardiovascular risk reduction • Prepare for RRT	• CMP-annual • CBC-annual • PTH-annual/QTR/tx • Lipid Panel-annual/QTR/tx • BMP • Hgb/Hct *Monthly	• Dietary • Transplant • Access	• ESRD • Comorbid conditions • Cardiovascular risk reduction • CKD Complications • CKD – Individual treatment options

Abbreviations: CMP-comprehensive metabolic profile (BUN, Cr, electrolytes, albumin, Ca, PO4, LFT)
CBC-complete blood count; PTH-parathyroid hormone, BMP- basic metabolic profile, (BUN,Cr, NA, K, CO2, Cl, CA, PO4, Alb)
Hgb-hemoglobin, HCT-hematocrit,; GFR-glomerular filtration rate; RRT-renal replacement therap, Q – every
QTR/TX-quarterly if treating

Note: Adapted from: K/DOQI Clinical Practice Guidelines for CKD, *American Journal of Kidney Diseases*, February, Suppl, 1, 2002.

Modifiable Risk Factors

Modifiable patient characteristics that are associated with faster GFR decline include proteinuria, high blood pressure, poor glycemic control, and smoking. There is inconclusive evidence concerning the effect of anemia and dyslipidemia on GFR, but both may be associated with faster GFR decline (Keane et al., 2003; Massy, 1999; NKF, 2002; NKF, 2003a, b). Each of these modifiable risk factors will be briefly discussed.

Proteinuria. The quantity of protein excreted in the urine is one of the strongest predictors of renal disease progression (Keane, 2000). A simple spot urine measuring the albumin or protein-to-creatinine ratio can help to predict the progression of renal disease. In a study by Ruggenenti et al. (1998), patients with a urinary protein to SCr ratio < 1g/g creatinine had no decline in GFR compared to a progressive decrease in GFR in those patients with a urinary protein ratio > or g/g creatinine. Results from the RENAAL (Reduction in End Point in Noninsulin-Dependent Diabetes Mellitus with the Angiotensin II Antagonist Losartan) Study showed patients with high baseline albuminuria (≥ 3g/g creatinine) had an 8.1-fold increased risk for progressing to ESRD compared to the low albuminuria group (< 1.5 g/g creatinine) (DeZeeuw et al., 2004). Increasing evidence suggests that reduction and normalizing proteinuria may confer renal protection independent of blood pressure reduction (Parving et al., 2001; Viberti & Wheeldon, 2002). Proteinuria is a risk marker for progressive loss of kidney function and should be a target for treatment.

High blood pressure (BP). Hypertension is a risk factor for accelerated progression of renal disease and is the second leading cause of ESRD. Numerous trials have shown the effect of elevated BP on progression of renal disease. Higher blood pressures in patients with renal insufficiency correlate linearly with decreases in GFR (Klahr et al., 1994; Bakris, 1998; Sheinfield & Bakris, 1999). The RENAAL Study showed that patients with type 2 diabetes with BP treated to < 140/90 with losartan had a reduced incidence of doubling of the serum creatinine (25%) and reduced progression to ESRD (28%) (Brenner et al., 2001). The MDRD study showed strict blood pressure control decreased the rate of decline of GFR by 28% in nondiabetic kidney disease and showed that a slower rate of decline was seen in patients with stricter BP control (Hunsicker et al., 1997). Hovind and colleagues (2001) showed that aggressive antihypertensive treatment in type 1 diabetics achieved regression in the decline of GFR to < or = 1 ml/min/yr - 22% of the time. Hypertension also plays a role as a major cardiovascular risk factor. Based on numerous studies, the recommendation of the JNC VII (7th Report of the Joint National Committee on Prevention, Detection, Evaluation, and Treatment of Hypertension) and NKF-K/DOQI is to aggressively treat hypertension to slow progression of CKD and reduce cardiovascular disease risk (Chobanian et al., 2003; NKF, 2004).

Poor glycemic control. The Diabetes Control and Complications Trial (DCCT), a prospective study, compared conventional (average HbA1c - 9%) with intensive treatment (average HbA1c < 7.2%) of 1,441 patients with insulin-dependent diabetes mellitus (IDDM). Patients were followed for 6.5 years. The DCCT firmly established the benefit of tight glycemic control in reducing the occurrence of nephropathy in patients with IDDM (DCCT Research Group, 1993). The United Kingdom Prospective Diabetes Study (UKPDS) compared intensive glycemic control (sulfonylureas, metformin or insulin) to standard therapy (diet only) in newly diagnosed patients with Type 2 diabetes. The study showed a lower mean HbA1c level (HbA1c 7.0% in intensive control compared with HbA1c 7.9% in conventional control) was associated with a reduction (25%) in microvascular events, including kidney disease with a decreased incidence of reduced GFR (UKPDS Study Group, 1998).

Smoking. The mechanisms of the effect of smoking on renal disease progression are unclear, but studies have shown an association between smoking and worsening renal function in certain diseases. An early study by Shulman and colleagues (1989) of 10,940 patients showed tobacco use was a predictor of progression of renal disease. A recent study by Chuahirun et al. (2004) showed smoking is associated with the progression of diabetic nephropathy. Halimi, Giraideau, and Vol (2000) showed smoking to be a risk factor for proteinuria, and, thus may contribute to progression. Smoking has been shown to increase the risk of developing Type 2 diabetes and microalbuminuria and further progression of diabetic nephropathy (Wolf & Ritz, 2003). Finally, Fox and colleagues (2004) found smoking was related to the development of kidney disease (odds ratio 1.42; confidence interval 95%, 1.06-1.91) in a community-based longitudinal cohort study of 2585 individuals with a mean follow-up of 18.5 years in persons with no previous history of kidney disease.

Anemia

Although there is not sufficient evidence to associate rate of decline of GFR with anemia (NKF, 2002), one study by Kuriyama et al. (1997) revealed that progression of renal failure could be slowed with treatment of anemia. More recently a study by Jungers and colleagues (2001) showed that treatment of anemia with epoietin alfa therapy resulted in significant slowing of the progression of CKD in 10 of the 20 patients followed. Several randomized controlled clinical trials are underway to answer the question of whether treatment of anemia has renoprotective action.

Dyslipidemias

Studies of the impact of dyslipidemias on the rate of progression of kidney disease are inconclusive (NKF, 2002). Experimentally hypercholesterolemia and hypertriglyceridemia can promote proteinuria and tubulointerstitial injury (Yu, 2003). Although there are no randomized controlled trials testing the hypothesis that treatment of dyslipidemia preserves kidney function, meta-analysis of several small studies, totaling 362 patients with CKD, suggested that there was a lower rate of decline in GFR (0.156 ml/min/month; 95% CI, 0.026 to 0.285 ml/min/month, P = 0.008) with treatment with a cholesterol-lowering agent compared to placebo (Fried et al., 2001).

As discussed there is growing evidence that certain factors are associated with more rapid progression of CKD and

Table 10-9
Strategies to Slow Progression

Risk Factor	Target/Treatment Recommendations	Nursing Considerations
Hypertension	• Target: 130/80 mmHg • ACE inhibitor/ARB preferred in diabetics and patients with protein-to-creatinine ratio >200 mg/g. • All antihypertensive agents effective in nondiabetic and protein-to-creatinine ratio <200 mg/gl. Follow recommendations of JNC VII for drug selection in other comorbidities. • Diuretics are ideal second drug (thiazides not effective GFR < 30 ml/min/1.73m^2	• Initiate TLC(weight reduction, DASH diet, ↓ dietary Na, ↑ physical activity, alcohol moderation). • Side effects of ACE inhibitor or ARB include hyperkalemia and ↓ GFR (↑ Scr). • ACE inhibitors can cause angioedema and cough. • Monitor for hypotension with all agents. • Monitor for electrolyte abnormalities with diuretics.
Proteinuria	• Target: <500 mg - 1g/24 hour • ACE inhibitor and ARB effective in reducing proteinuria. Combination may have increased effect. • In stage 3 & 4 limiting protein intake to 0.6 g/kg/day –0.8 g/kg/day may be effective in reducing uremic manifestations; controversial concerning reduction in proteinuria.	• Monitor protein-to-creatinine ratio for improvements. • Side-effects of ACE inhibitor/ARB listed above. • Monitor for PEM.
Hyperglycemia	• Targets: HbA1c <7.0 % Preprandial glucose - 90-130 mg/dl Peak postprandial glucose <180 mg/dl • Avoid Metformin due to development of lactic acidosis.	• Diabetic self-management education essential. • Monitor patients for side effects: hypoglycemia, weight gain and edema.
Hyperlipidemia	• Targets: LDL <100 mg/dl Non-HDL <130 mg/dl Trig. <150 mg/dl HDL >40 mg/dl (varies by gender) • TLC + Statin recommended. • Fibrate and Niacin as needed.	• Monitor patients for rhabdomyolysis and increased LFTs with statin. • Fibrate renally excreted, use lower doses.
Smoking	• Target: Cessation of smoking	• Counseling, Nicotine replacement, bupropion.
Nephrotoxic Drugs	• Target: Avoid exposure to nephrotoxic drugs (NSAIDS, Cox-2 inhibitors, cephalosporins, contrast media, amphotericin, cyclosporin)	• Teach patient about over-the-counter medications to avoid, particularly NSAIDS. • Teach patient GFR level and communication of this level to other prescribing providers. Call if questions about a new drug.
Nephrology Referral	• Target: Refer early for diagnosis and recommendations. • Stage 3 for treatment and follow-up.	• Community outreach and education. • Promote and calculate GFR to be shown on labs when creatinine drawn.

Abbreviations: TLC-therapeutic lifestyle changes; ACE-angiotensin converting enzyme; ARB-angiotensin receptor blocker; GFR-glomerularfiltration rate; Scr-serum creatinine; JNC VII-Joint national committee on treatment of hypertension; PEM-protein energy malnutrition; LDL-low density lipoprotein; HDL high density lipoprotein; LFT-liver function test; NSAIDS-nonsteroidal anti-inflammatory drugs; Cox-2- cyclooxygenase-2

Note: From K/DOQI Guidelines 2000-2004. ATP III, 2001; JNC VII (2003).

Figure 10-1
Algorithm for Blood Pressure Management and Use of Antihypertensive Agents in CKD

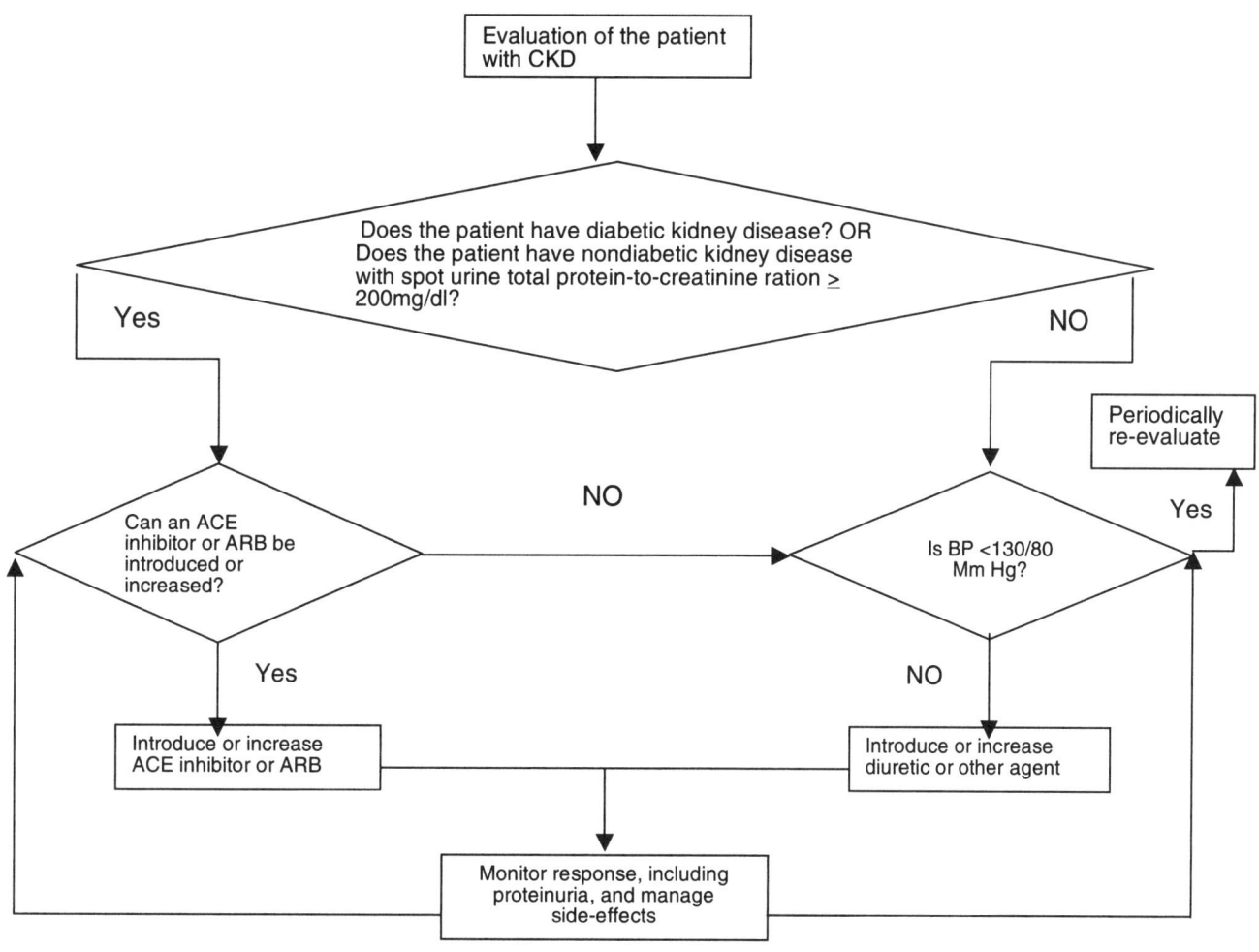

Note: From National Kidney Foundation. (2004). K/DOQI clinical practice guidelines on blood pressure management and use of antihypertensive agents in chronic kidney disease, *American Journal of Kidney Diseases, 43*(suppl 1), S1-S268.

that interventions can slow the decline of GFR and prevent the development of ESRD. Given the high mortality rates of patients with ESRD, it is critical that we treat modifiable risk factors during the earlier stages of CKD.

Strategies to Slow Progression

Certain treatment strategies are proven to slow the progression of CKD. This section will discuss these interventions, including: antihypertensive therapy, reduction of proteinuria, strict glycemic control, treatment of dyslipidemias, diet and lifestyle modifications, avoidance of nephrotoxic drugs, and referral to a nephrologist. These strategies are summarized in Table 10-9.

Antihypertensive Therapy

The NKF-K/DOQI Clinical Practice Guidelines on Blood Pressure Management and Use of Antihypertensive Agents in Chronic Kidney Disease (2004) state the goals of antihypertensive therapy in CKD are to lower BP, slow the progression of kidney disease, and reduce the risk of CVD. Additionally, the guidelines recommend that proteinuira should be moni-

tored as it is known to increase risk of progression and is a CVD risk factor. Target of therapy based on the NKF-K/DOQI (2004) report are listed in Table 10-10. Patients with CKD should have a BP < 130/80 mmHg. The NKF-K/DOQI recommends a lower target BP, if moderate proteinuria is present (spot urine protein-to-creatinine ratio > 500-1000 mg/g). Antihypertensive therapy includes lifestyle modifications and pharmacological therapy (NKF, 2004).

Lifestyle modifications are critical in the treatment of hypertension. Table 10-11 presents the JNC VII recommendations for therapeutic lifestyle changes (TLC), that have shown to lower BP including: (a) weight reduction in overweight individuals, (b) DASH (Dietary Approached to Stop Hypertension) eating plan, (c) dietary sodium reduction (2,400 mg sodium/day), (d) physical activity (30 minutes of aerobic exercise on most days), and (e) moderation of alcohol consumption (2 drinks/day-men and 1 drink/day-women (Chobanian et al., 2003). The K/DOQI recommendations differ only in the area of diet. The DASH diet is recommended for patients with CKD in stages 1 and 2. In stages 3-5, however, modifications in the diet are necessary

Table 10-10

Summary of Recommendations on Hypertension and Antihypertensive agents in CKD

Population	BP Goal (mmHg)	Preferred Agents for CKD with (or without) Hypertension	Other Agents to Reduce CVD Risk and Reach Blood Pressure Targets
Diabetic Kidney Disease	<130/80	ACE inhibitor or ARB	Diuretics preferred, then BB or CCB
Nondiabetic kidney disease with spot urine total protein-to-creatinine ratio ≥ 200 mg/g	<130/80	ACE inhibitor or ARB	Diuretics preferred, then BB or CCB
Nondiabetic kidney disease with spot urine total protein-to-creatinine ratio ≥ 200 mg/g	<130/80	None preferred	Diuretic preferred, then ACE inhibitor, ARB, BB, or CCB
Kidney Disease in the Transplant Recipient	<130/80	None preferred	CCB, diuretic, BB, ACE inhibitor, ARB

Abbreviations: ACE-angiotensin converting enzyme, ARB-angiotensin receptor blocker, BB-beta blocker, CCB-calcium channel blocker

From: K/DOQI Clinical practice guidelines on blood pressure management and use of antihypertensive agents in CKD (2004).

due to the possibility of hyperkalemia with a diet rich in fruit and vegetables and hyperphosphatemia with low fat dairy products (see Table 10-12). A dietary consult will be helpful in assisting the patients to meet the dietary recommendations and modifications required by CKD.

In spite of lifestyle modifications, most patients with CKD will require pharmacological intervention with two or more drugs (NKF, 2004). According to JNC VII recommendations, angiotensin converting enzyme (ACE) inhibitor and angiotensin receptor blockers (ARB) should be used in patients with diabetic or nondiabetic renal disease as the initial drug of choice (see Table 10-13). Both drugs have proven to lower BP, reduce proteinuria, and slow the progression of kidney disease (Chobanian et al., 2003). The Clinical Practice Guidelines on Blood Pressure Management and Use of Antihypertensive Agents in Chronic Kidney Disease (2004) divide hypertension treatment for diabetic patients and nondiabetic patients with kidney disease (see Table 10-10). For patients with diabetic kidney disease and a protein-to-creatinine ratio > 200 mg/gm, the guidelines recommend an ACE inhibitor or ARB initially. ACE inhibitors are preferred in patients with type 1 diabetes and ARBs are preferred in patients with type 2 diabetes. For patients with kidney disease and a protein-to-creatinine ratio < 200 mg/gm, the guidelines do not recommend a preferred drug (NKF, 2004). Figure 10-1 presents an algorithm for blood pressure management and use of antihypertensive agents in patients with CKD.

Precautions with initiation of an ACE inhibitor and/or ARB include a decrease in GFR. An increase in serum creatinine (SCr) of 20% - 30%, which then stabilizes, is acceptable. In fact, increases of SCr up to 30% from baseline (up to 3 mg/dl) within the first 4 months of initiation of any ACE inhibitor are correlated with slower rate of decline in renal function after 3 or more years (Bakris & Weir, 2000). If there is greater than 30% increase or repeated measures of serum creatinine show a progressive increase, the drug should be discontinued and the patient evaluated for other causes of renal failure. Conditions in which an

ACE inhibitor or ARB may exaggerate decline of renal function include: renal artery stenosis, polycystic kidney disease, decreased arterial blood volume, use of nonsteroidal anti-inflammatory drugs, use of cyclosporine or tacrolimus, and sepsis. Renal function should be checked 1-2 weeks after initiation of an ACE inhibitor or ARB (Palmer, 2003).

Hyperkalemia is also associated with the use of an ACE inhibitor or ARB. To minimize the likelihood of hyperkalemia, first discontinue drugs known to interfere with renal potassium secretion. Low potassium diet and use of thiazide or loop diuretics can be effective in minimizing hyperkalemia. Patients with metabolic acidosis should be treated with alkali salts. Serum potassium should be monitored closely after initiating the drugs and with dose increases (Palmer, 2003).

ACE inhibitors may cause angioedema or cough. Patients should be warned of angio-edema so they can seek emergency treatment. Cough is resolved with discontinuing the ACE inhibitor and substituting an ARB, which usually does not cause a cough (Palmer, 2003).

In addition to monitoring the patient's BP response to therapy, patients with proteinuria > 500 – 1000 mg/g (protein-to-creatinine ratio) should have proteinuria monitored so that antihypertensive agents known to reduce proteinuria, including ACE, ARBs, and beta blockers can be initiated or increased. Studies have shown a combination of ACE inhibitor and ARB significantly improves BP control and further reduces albuminuria (Campbell et al., 2003; Mogensen et al., 2000). Patients with proteinuria should be treated with antihypertensive agents known to reduce proteinuria even if they are not hypertensive (K/DOQI, 2004).

As monotherapy rarely achieves BP goals in hypertensive patients with CKD, a second or third agent is often required. Diuretics are an ideal second drug and potentiate the BP-lowering effects of an ACE inhibitor and/or ARB. In addition to treating hypertension, diuretics reduce edema and correct metabolic acidosis and hyperkalemia. Although thiazide diuretics have been the basis of antihypertensive therapy in most outcome trials, they are ineffective in

Table 10-11

Lifestyle Modifications to Manage Hypertension

Modification	Recommendation	Approximate systolic BP Reduction Range
Weight reduction	Maintain normal body weight (BMI, 18.5 – 24.9)	5-20 mmHg/10-kg weight loss
Adopt DASH eating plan (CKD Stage 1 – 2 only)	Consume a diet rich in fruits, vegetables, and low-fat dairy products with a reduced content of saturated and total fat	8-14 mmHg
Dietary sodium reduction	Reduce dietary sodium intake to no more than 100 mEq/L (2.4 g sodium or 6 g sodium chloride)	2-8 mmHg
Physical activity	Engage in regular aerobic physical activity such as brisk walking (at least 30 minutes per day, most days of the week)	4-9 mmHg
Moderation of alcohol consumption	Limit consumption to no more than 2 drinks per day (1 oz or 30 mL ethanol in most men and no more than 1 drink per day in women and lighter-weight persons	2-4 mmHg

Abbreviations: BMI-body mass index calculated as Weight in kilograms divided by the square of the height in meters; BP-blood pressure; DASH-Dietary Approaches to Stop Hypertension

Note: From Chobnian, A.V., Bakis, G.L., Black, H.R., Cushman, W.C., Green, L.A., Izzo, J.L., Jones, D.W., Materson, B.J., Oparil, S., Wright, J.T., Rocella, E.J., & the National High Blood Pressure Education Programming Coordinating Committee (2003). The seventh report of the joint national committee on prevention, detection, evaluation, and treatment of high blood pressure. *JAMA, 289*, 2560-2562.

Table 10-12

Macronutrient Composition and Mineral Content of the Dietary Approaches to Stop Hypertension (DASH) Diet Recommended by JNC VII, With Modification for Stages 3 – 4 of CKD

Nutrient	Stage of CKD	
	Stages 1-2	Stages 3-4
Sodium (g/dl)	<2.4	<2.4
Total Fat (% of calories)	<30	<30
Saturated Fat (% of calories)	<10	<10
Cholesterol (mg/dl)	<200	<200
Carbohydrates (% of calories)	50-60	50-60
Protein (g/kg/d, % of calories)	1.4 (~18)	0.6-08 (~10)
Phosphorus (g/dl)	1.7	0.8-1.0
Potassium (g/dl)	>4	2-4

Note: From *K/DOQI Clinical practice guidelines on blood pressure management and use of antihypertensive agents in CKD* (2004).

patients with GFR < 30 ml/min/1.73m^2. Loop diuretics are then the diuretic of choice. Dose-related hypokalemia is the most common metabolic side effect of diuretics. Other electrolyte abnormalities include hypomagnesemia and hyponatremia. Supplements can be added if indicated. Patients should also be monitored for volume depletion, which can cause acute renal dysfunction (Wilcox, 2002).

Additional antihypertensive medications should be added until target BP is achieved. The JNC VII provides recommendations (see Table 10-13) for the addition of drugs based on comorbid conditions, including ischemic heart disease, heart failure, diastolic hypertension, and CVD. Other special situations addressed in the JNC VII recommendations for drug selection include minority popula-

Table 10-13
JNC VII Guideline Bases for Compelling Indicator for Individual Drug Classes

High-Risk Conditions with compelling Indication*	Diuretic	Beta-Blocker	ACE Inhibitor	ARB	CCB	Aldosterone Antagonist
Heart failure	•	•	•	•		•
Post-myocardial infarction		•	•			•
High coronary disease risk	•	•	•		•	
Diabetes	•	•	•	•	•	
Chronic kidney disease			•	•		
Recurrent stroke prevention	•		•			

Abbreviations: ACE-angiotensin converting enzyme; ARB-angiotensin receptor blocker; CCB-calcium channel blocker

*Compelling indications for antihypertensive drugs are based on benefits from outcome studies or existing clinical guidelines; the compelling indication is managed in parallel with the blood pressure

Note: From Chobanian, A.V., Bakis, G.L., Black, H.R., Cushman, W.C., Green, L.A., Izzo, J.L., Jones, D.W., Materson, B.J., Oparil, S., Wright, J.T., Rocella, E.J., & the National high blood pressure Education Programming Coordinating Committee (2003). The seventh report of the joint national committee on prevention, detection, evaluation, and treatment of high blood pressure. *JAMA, 289*, 2560-2562.

tions, obesity, left ventricular hypertrophy, peripheral arterial disease, older individuals, and others. The drug selection is based on favorable outcomes from clinical trials (Chobanian et al., 2003).

Because of the increased risk of complications from pharmacologic therapy in persons with CKD, there should be frequent monitoring. The NKF-K/DOQI Clinical Practice Guidelines on Blood Pressure Management and Use of Antihypertensive Agents in Chronic Kidney (2004) recommend that the blood pressure, GFR, and serum potassium be checked before initiation and within 12 weeks of initiation or a change in dose of an ACE inhibitor, ARB, and/or diuretic. Monitoring should be every 4 weeks or more frequent in patients with systolic BP <120 or $\geq$ 140 mm Hg, GFR < 60 ml/min/1.73 m^2, or if there is a change in GFR greater than 15% in 2 months. If an ACE inhibitor or ARB is used in CKD patients with serum potassium > 4.5 mEq/L or a diuretic is used in patient with serum potassium $\leq$ 4.0 mEq/L, then monitoring of serum potassium should be every 4 weeks or more often (NKF, 2004).

Tight Glycemic Control

The American Diabetes Association (ADA), through its Clinical Practice Recommendations (2004, 2005), provides goals for treatment of patients with diabetes. The target for key parameters are: glycosolated hemoglobin (HbA1c) < 7.0%, a preprandial plasma glucose of 90 – 130 mg/dl, and a peak postprandial plasma glucose of < 180 mg/dl (ADA, 2004, 2005). The cornerstone of glycemic control is lifestyle modification, including dietary control, weight loss, and exercise. Diabetes self-management education is an integral component of care with frequent monitoring of blood glucoses and medical nutrition therapy. Co-management with a diabetes team, change in pharmacological therapy, initiation of or increase in self-monitoring of blood glucose, more frequent

contact with the patient, and referral to an endocrinologist may assist in achieving treatment goals (ADA, 2004a, b, and c).

Potential problems in the treatment of patients with diabetes and kidney disease can occur with drugs used to treat hyperglycemia. Sulfonylureas accumulate in renal failure with the exception of gliquidone and glimepiride. Prolonged hypoglycemia is possible as drug excretion is delayed. Metformin, one of the most widely prescribed oral antidiabetic agents in the country, must be used with caution in patients with CKD and should be discontinued when a patient has a GFR < 40 ml/min/1.73 m^2 due to the risk of life-threatening lactic acidosis. Glitizones may aggravate edema and congestive heart failure (CHF). Insulin degradation by the kidney is decreased and dose reduction is necessitated by reduced renal function. As patients reach stage 5, oral hyperglycemic agents and insulin may often be discontinued (Wolf & Ritz, 2003). Patients with diabetes and CKD must be followed closely to achieve optimal HbA1c target while avoiding hypoglycemic risks.

Treating Dyslipidemias

Treatment of dyslipidemias has been shown to slow the progression of CKD. Because of the burden of cardiac disease in patients with CKD, and the association of dyslipidemias with ACVD, dyslipidemias should be treated aggressively. The K/DOQI Clinical Practice Guidelines for Managing Dyslipidemias in CKD (NKF, 2003b) recommends assessment of all patients with CKD for dyslipidemias. This should include a complete fasting lipid profile with total cholesterol, LDL, HDL, and triglycerides. Changes in proteinuria and GFR affect lipoprotein levels, so it is recommended that patients with CKD be evaluated more frequently than the general population. The NKF-K/DOQI Guidelines recommend that patients with CKD be considered to be in the highest risk cat-

Table 10-14
The Management of Dyslipidemias in Adults with CKD

Dyslipidemia	Goal	Initiate	Increase	Alternative
TG ≥150 mg/dl	TG <150 mg/dl	TLC	TLC + Fibrate or Niacin	Fibrate or Niacin
LDL 100-129mg/dl	LDL <100 mg/dl	TLC	TLC + low dose Statin	Bile acid seq. or Niacin
LDL ≥130 mg/dl	LDL <100 mg/dl	TLC + low dose Statin	TLC + max dose Statin	Bile acid seq. or Niacin
TG ≥200 mg/dl and non-HDL ≥130 mg/dl	Non-HDL <130 mg/dl	TLC + low dose Statin	TLC + max dose Statin	Fibrate or Niacin

Abbreviations: TG-triglycerides; LDL-low-density lipoprotein cholesterol; HDL-high-density lipoprotein cholesterol; TLC-therapeutic lifestyle changes

Note: From Clinical practice guidelines for managing dyslipidemias in CKD (2003).

egory, the same as coronary heart disease (CHD) risk equivalent. With this in mind, the NKF-K/DOQI Guidelines recommend that clinicians treating CKD patients in Stages 1-4 should follow the recently updated Adult Treatment Panel (ATP III) Guidelines as adopted in the Table 10-14 for CKD patients.

The K/DOQI guidelines define the goal for LDL as < 100 mg/dl for patients at highest risk. If levels of LDL are greater than 100 but < 130 mg/dl, then therapeutic lifestyle changes (TLC) can be initiated. This includes lowering of saturated fats; increasing fiber intake, especially viscous fiber; glycemic control; weight management; and increased physical activity. In addition, moderation in alcohol consumption is advised and smoking cessation is recommended. If LDL exceeds 130 mg/dl initially or does not reach target after 3 months of TLC, then drug therapy should be initiated (see Table 10-14). HMG CoA reductase inhibitors, nicotinic acid, bile acid sequestants, fibric acids, and combinations can be used to lower LDL (NKF, 2003b).

Treatment goal for triglycerides is less than 150 mg/dl (ATP III). If triglycerides are between 150 - 499 mg/dl after the LDL goal is reached, then set the secondary goal for non-HDL cholesterol (total – HDL) to 130 mg/dl. Drugs should be added to reach the non-HDL goal along with intensifying weight management and physical activity. If triglycerides are ≥ 150 mg/dl, the first treatment should include low fat diet, weight management, physical activity, and drugs, including nicotinic acid or fibrate. Finally, the goal for HDL cholesterol is > 40 mg/dl (ATP, III). Although the first target for lipid therapy is LDL, if HDL is low, then intensify weight management and physical activity. If HDL remains low or there is isolated low HDL cholesterol, consider nicotinic acid or fibrate (Expert Panel, 2001).

Therapeutic Lifestyle Changes

Lifestyle modifications include changes in diet, exercise and other habits that may affect the progression of CKD. Analysis of data from the NHANES II study showed there was increased risk of CKD associated with morbid obesity (BMI > 35), physical inactivity, and smoking (Tarver-Carr, Powe, Eberhardt, & Brancati, 2003). The JNC VII rec-

ommendations form the cornerstone of the lifestyle modifications recommended by the K/DOQI Clinical Practice Guideline for Patients With CKD (see Table 10-11).

Diet. Diet recommendations for adults with CKD are often complex as patients must limit certain foods based on diagnosis (e.g., diabetes) and stage of kidney disease. Table 10-11 makes recommendations for modification of macronutrient composition and mineral content of the DASH diet recommended by JNC VII. Restrictions are recommended for protein, total fat and saturated fats, cholesterol, phosphorous, potassium, and sodium. The lack of clear evidence supporting the impact of low protein diet on the rate of GFR decline and the logistics of providing intensive nutritional intervention preclude recommendation for a low protein diet (0.6 g/kg/d) in all patients with CKD. K/DOQI currently recommends protein restriction for patients in Stage 3-4, which may help to avoid generation of nitrogenous metabolites and reduce uremic manifestations (NKF, 2004). Patients who do not meet the recommended body weight (BMI 18.5-25.9) should be encouraged to begin a weight-loss program that promotes healthy behaviors to lose weight and maintain the loss over time. Referral to a dietitian should be made to help patients achieve the many dietary recommendations.

A special note is in order concerning sodium and fluid restriction in patients with CKD. Sodium restriction is critical as renal failure progresses, as there is evidence that sodium retention plays a major role in hypertension in CKD. The mechanism appears to be expansion of extracellular fluid volume (Vasavada & Agarwal, 2003). Patients should be taught to limit their sodium intake to less than 2.4 g/day and limit fluid intake to 500 cc above their previous day's output. Strategies to reduce both salt intake and fluid intake may also be useful in reducing CVD morbidity and mortality.

Exercise. The health benefits of exercise are many, including reducing blood pressure, lowering cholesterol and triglycerides, reducing body weight and fat, and lowering the risk of cardiovascular disease (Fletcher et al., 1996). Patients should be encouraged to begin an exercise program that includes aerobic physical activity such as brisk walking (at least 30 minutes per day, most days of the week) (Chobanian et al., 2003). If patients do not usually engage in regular physical activity, then they should be counseled and encouraged to begin regular exercises slowly and only after consulting with their primary health care provider. CKD patients with cardiovascular risk factors should be evaluated for CVD prior to the initiation of any exercise program. Patients with musculo-skeletal problems might benefit from a physical therapy referral.

Smoking cessation. According to the American Heart Association (AHA), as many as 30% of all coronary heart disease deaths in the United States are attributable to cigarette smoking, and smoking nearly doubles the risk of ischemic stroke (Ockene & Miller, 1997). Cigarette smoking also exacerbates renal injury, and its cessation in those with microalbuminuria ameliorates the progressive renal injury caused by continued smoking (Chuahirun et al., 2004; Orth, 2004). Clinicians have a powerful impact in motivating patients to try to quit smoking. As little as 3 minutes of clinician time can double the rate of smoking cessation among the clinician's smoking patients. Smoking cessation treatments that have been found to be safe and effective include counseling and medications or a combination of both. Effective counseling and behavior therapies with patients attempting tobacco cessation include provision of practical counseling (problem solving/skill building) and helping secure social support as part of the treatment and outside of treatment. Pharmacotherapies for smoking cessation that reliably increase long-term smoking abstinence rates include: nicotine gum, inhaler, nasal spray, patch, and lozenge and bupropion SR (Fiore, 2000).

Avoidance of nephrotoxic drugs. Because the kidneys are a major route of excretion for a variety of drugs, they are a frequent target for toxic injury. Injury is due to the concentration of the drug within the renal tubular cells during the excretory process. Additionally, the high blood flow through the kidney results in exaggerated exposure of renal endothelial cells and glomeruli (Coffman, 2002).

Drug toxicity is manifested through the same clinical syndromes that are associated with kidney disease of other causes, including acute and chronic renal dysfunction and nephritic syndrome. Some common agents include contrast media; heavy metals including lead, barium, and copper; and drugs, including antibiotics, antineoplastic, and antiviral medications (Coffman, 2002). In Chapter 11, there is further discussion of the nephrotoxic agents that should be avoided and the renal syndromes caused by these therapeutic agents.

Large number of Americans are exposed to over-the-counter and prescription analgesics, and this class of drugs will be addressed. Moderate to severe pain often accompanies chronic disease. Patients with CKD are at risk for reduction of renal blood flow and GFR with use of nonsteroidal anti-inflammatory drugs (NSAIDS). NSAIDS can also exaggerate hypertension and lead to edema formation and hyponatremia. Selective cyclooxygenase-2 (COX-2) inhibitors appear to exert similar effects on the kidney. Both drugs should be avoided. In patients with known risk of CKD and use of NSAIDS, renal function should be checked routinely (Kurella, Bennett, & Chertow, 2003).

Referral to Nephrologist

Many patients begin renal replacement therapy (RRT) less than 6 months after they are referred to a nephrologist, and thus may not benefit from renoprotection measures, halting or slowing the rate of progression of GFR (Obrador, Ruthazer, Pradeep, Kausz, & Pereria, 1999). Studies of the effect of timely nephrology referral show increased morbidity associated with later referral (Roubicek et al., 2000; Jungers et al., 2001). Although the effect of late referral on mortality has yielded conflicting results, a study by Stack (2003) evaluating early nephrology referral and pre-ESRD care on mortality risk in a national cohort of patient starting dialysis in 1996 and 1997 (n=2264), showed late referral was associated with greater risk of death in patients with ESRD. More frequent pre-ESRD care confirmed increased survival benefits. Studies in France have suggested longer nephrology care is associated with better CV outcomes and lower CV mortality (Jungers et al., 2001). It appears clear that late referral patients may not benefit from optimal CKD therapy.

Early consultation with a nephrologist is important in establishing an accurate diagnosis, allowing for the opportunity to prevent, slow, or reverse the development of CKD. Immediate diagnosis of potential and reversible kidney disease is critical to avoid RRT (e.g., obstructive nephropathy, glomerulonephritis). Intervention in the early stages of other diseases is aimed at slowing progression (e.g., diabetes, polycystic kidney disease). Additionally, because cardiovascular risk factors appear to develop early in CKD, cardioprotection has emerged as another early target of treatment for patients with CKD. Indeed studies have shown that patients referred late to a nephrologist may not receive optimal treatment of hypertension and anemia and exhibit high prevalence of CVD (Jungers et al., 2001; Obrador et al. 1999).

Management of CKD also involves identification and treatment of complications and adequate preparation for dialysis, including informed choice regarding RRT and referral for transplantation. Placement of dialysis access may not occur in a timely manner with late referral, and this puts the patient at increased risk of hospitalization and emotional distress when starting RRT. While awaiting placement and utilization of a permanent access, the patient may require a dialysis catheter for hemodialysis, which is associated with a 39% annual increased risk of death. Transplant referral is also often delayed, and most eligible recipients in the United States have not been placed on a transplant waiting list 6 months after beginning dialysis (Owen, 2003). Communication within the referring health care community about the importance of early referral and collaborative care of the patients with CKD is critical to improving outcomes.

Prevention and Treatment of Complication of CKD

Many of the complications of CKD can be prevented or delayed by earlier detection and appropriate evaluation and management. The following complications will be discussed: hypertension, anemia, malnutrition, disorders of calcium and phosphorus metabolism, metabolic acidosis, nephropathy, and dyslipidemias. Table 10-15 summarizes

Table 10-15

CKD Complication Treatment Targets with Suggested Strategies to Achieve Target

ANEMIA: (K/DOQI) *Target*: Hgb 11 – 12 g/dl • Anemia workup: Assess RBC indices, stool for occult blood, retic ct, iron parameters, B12 & folate levels • Epoetin alfa • Darbopoietin	**HYPERTENSION:** (JNC VII, KDOQI) *Target*: BP <130/80 for all patients • Proteinuria >200 mg/g – Use ACE inhibitor or ARB initially • Diabetic Kidney Disease Type 1 – ACE inhibitor Type 2 – ARB

HYPERLIPIDEMIA: (ATP III, K/DOQI) *Targets:* *Treatment:* • LDL-C <100 mg/dl - > initiate TLC then add statin • Non-HDL-C <130 mg/dl > initiate TLC then add statin • Triglyceride <150 mg/dl > initiate TLC then add fibrate or niacin • HDL >40 mg/dl < then TLC then add fibrate or niacin • TLC - low saturated fats, increase fiber intake emphasizing viscous fiber, glycemic control, weight management, increase physical activity, moderation in alcohol consumption, smoking cessation.	**BONE METABOLISM:** (K/DOQI) *Stage 3* Phos. 2.7 – 4.6 mg/dl *Targets:* iPTH 35-70 pg/ml Ca – normal for lab *Stage 4* Phos. 2.7 – 4.6 mg/dl *Targets:* iPTH 70 – 110 pg.ml Ca – normal for lab *Stage 3 & 4* ↑ Phos. – low phos diet/phos binders *Treatment:* ↓ Ca – Ca supplements ↑ Ca – dc supplemental Ca, Vitamin D ↑ PTH – Measure serum 25 – hydroxyvitamin D <30ng/ml - oral ergocaciferolol (D2) ** >30 ng/ml- active oral Vitamin D

NUTRITION: (K/DOQI) *Targets*: **HCO$_3$** >22 mg/dl **BMI** - 18.5 - 25.9 **Albumin** >3.5 g/dl **K$^+$** 3.5-5.5mg/dl • Protein - 1.2 – 1.4 mg/kg/day Stage 3 & 4 - 0.6 – 0.8 mg/kg/day • Calorie – 35 kcal/kg/day <60yo 30 – 35 kcal/kg/day >60yo • Potassium <2000 mg/day(based on serum K$^+$ level) • Sodium <2400 mg/day • Calcium <2000 mg/day • Phosphorous <1000 mg/day (Stage 3 & 4) • Fluid - 500 cc + 24-hour urine output/day • HCO3$^-$ <22 mg/dl - alkali salts 0.5-1.0 meq/kg/day	*Stage 5* Phos 3.5 – 5.5 mg/dl *Targets:* iPTH – 150 – 300 pg/ml Ca – lower end of normal (8.4- 9.5) *Stage 5* *Treatment:* ↑ PTH – active oral Vitamin D ↑ Phos. – low phos diet/phos binders ↓ Ca – Ca supplements ↑ Ca – dc supplemental Ca, Vitamin D ** *Ergocalciferol (D2) Dosing in Stage 3 & 4* <5 ng/ml – 50,000 IU x 12 wks then monthly x 3 5 – 15 ng/ml – 50,000 IU x 4 wks then monthly x 3 16 –30 ng/ml – 50,000 IU q month x 6 After 6 months re-measure level of PTH

Glycemic Control: (ADA) *Targets:* HBA1$_c$ <7 % Preprandial 90-130 mg/dl Peak postprandial <180 mg/dl • Avoid Metformin • Blood glucose monitoring, medications	**Cardiac Risk Reduction:** (K/DOQI, JNC VII) • TLC–weight reduction, DASH diet, sodium, physical activity, moderation in alcohol • Treat ↑ BP, ↑ Lipids, anemia, & bone metab. • Smoking cessation • Fluid restriction/diuretics • Treat hyperhomocytenemia –B$_{12}$, Folate, B$_6$

Abbreviations: Hgb – hemaglobin, RBC – red blood cell, retic ct – reticulocyte count, LDL – low density lipoprotein, HDL – high density lipoprotein, TLC – therapeutic lifestyle changes, BMI – body mass index, K$^+$– potassium, HCO3$^-$ – bicarbonate, BP – blood pressure, ACE – angiotensin converting enzyme, ARB – angiotensin receptor blocker, Phos – phosphorous, Ca – calcium, iPTH – intact parathyroid hormone

Note: From K/DOQI Guidelines 2000-2004. ATP III, 2001; JNC VII, 2003, ADA (2004).

treatment of CKD complications.

Hypertension

As previously discussed, hypertension is both a cause of CKD and a complication. It occurs with mild decreases in GFR and should be treated early. Data from the NHANES III shows that hypertension in patients with CKD is not adequately controlled. In this study of patients with an elevated serum creatinine, only 75% received treatment for hypertension. Additionally only 11% of all patients with CKD and hypertension had blood pressure reduced to 130/85 mmHg (Coresh et al., 2001). Recommendations concerning treatment of hypertension were previously discussed in relationship to delaying progression of CKD.

Anemia

Anemia is a common and important complication of CKD. It most commonly presents in Stage 3 of CKD but can be present in earlier stages. The major physiologic consequence of anemia is reduced oxygen-carrying capacity of the blood. Patients with anemia attempt to offset tissue hypoxia by compensating with increased cardiac output. The heart must increase in mass and contractile strength to respond to the increased workload (NKF, 2000a). Anemia, in fact, is a risk factor for left ventricular hypertrophy (LVH) and increased cardiovascular mortality. In a study by Levin and colleagues (1999), decreased Hgb (decreases of 0.5 g/dl) was associated with a 32% increase in the odds of having LVH. LVH is an independent risk factor for morbidity and mortality in dialysis patients (Levin et al., 1999).

Treatment of anemia in CKD has been inadequate. In a study by Obrador et al. (1999) of patients beginning dialysis between April 1, 1995 and June 30, 1997 (n= 155,051), only 23% of patients received epoetin alfa prior to ESRD. Anemia (Hct < 33%) in patients with ESRD is associated with increased risk of hospitalization and death (Collins et al., 2001). Fink, Blahut, Reddy, and Light (2001) showed that patients on dialysis who had been treated with epoetin alfa prior to dialysis had a 20% lower relative risk of death. Anemia is associated with many symptoms, including low energy, fatigue, sleep disturbances, alterations in cognitive function and ability to concentrate, sexual dysfunction, gastrointestinal symptoms, and decreased quality of life (NKF, 2000a).

An anemia work-up should be initiated in patients with CKD when the Hgb is less than 11 g/dl in premenopausal females and prepubertal patients and less than 12 g/dl in adult males and postmenopausal females. Parameters to be assessed include red blood cell (RBC) indices, reticulocyte count, and iron parameters. The workup should also include checking stools for occult blood and evaluating the patient for vitamin deficiencies. After deficiencies have been treated, and if no cause for anemia is detected, then anemia is most likely due to erythropoietin deficiency, and treatment with human erythropoietin (r-HuEPO) or darbopoetin alfa should begin. K/DOQI Guidelines recommend a target hematocrit level of 33% to 36% for patients with CKD. An anemia management protocol is useful in providing for consistent treatment and follow-up of patients with anemia of CKD (NKF, 2000a).

Vitamins should also be administered prior to and during therapy to prevent deficiencies. Iron parameters should be checked quarterly. Targeted levels for iron supplementation are as follows: ferritin - 100 mg/dl and and iron saturation - 20%. Provision of 200 mg elemental iron orally may be sufficient to replace losses and support erythopoiesis. Intravenous iron therapy may be indicated if iron stores fall below targeted levels and the patient is unable to achieve the targeted Hgb and Hct with oral iron supplementation.

Blood pressure should be controlled before initiation of an erythropoietin agent and should be monitored closely during initiation. Initiation of or an increase in antihypertensive therapy is indicated if there is a rise in blood pressure above the K/DOQI target of 130/80 mmHg (NKF, 2000a).

Malnutrition

Protein-energy malnutrition commonly develops during the course of CKD and contributes to morbidity and mortality (Obrador et al., 1999). K/DOQI Clinical Practice Guidelines for Chronic Kidney Disease Failure (NKF, 2002) recommend that patients should be assessed for dietary protein and energy intake and nutritional status at Stage 3 (GFR < 60 ml/min per 1.73 m^2). Protein nutritional status should be evaluated by the following: (a) serial measurements of a panel of markers, including serum albumin; (b) edema-free body weight, % standard NHANES III body weight, or subjective global assessment; and (c) normalized protein nitrogen appearance (nPNA) or dietary interview and food consumption diaries. Assessments should occur every 6-12 months beginning at Stage 3 and increase in frequency to every 1-3 months in patients as CKD progresses toward ESRD. Patients with decreased dietary intake or malnutrition should be referred for dietary consult (NKF, 2000b).

The recommendations for dietary protein and other nutrients are listed in Table 10-15. Recommended dietary energy intake for individuals in stage 4 with GFR < 25 ml/min per 1.73 m^2 is 35 kcal/kg per day for those < 60 years old and 30–35 kcal/kg per day for those > 60 years old. If patients with GFR < 20 ml/min per 1.73 m2 develop signs of protein-calorie malnutrition, that does not respond to nutritional intervention, then initiation of renal replacement therapy should be considered (NKF, 2000b).

Disorders of Calcium and Phosphorus Metabolism

Disorders of calcium, phosphorus metabolism and the resulting secondary hyperparathyroid (SPTH) disease are evident early in CKD. Assessment and treatment of SPTH is inadequate in this population. Kauz and colleagues (2001) found screening for SHPT was low. In a retrospective cohort of 602 patients with CKD, serum parathyroid hormone levels were obtained in only 15% of the sample.

Metabolic bone disease presents with a spectrum of bone lesions, including osteitis fibrosa, adynamic bone disease, and mixed forms. It is the end result of a protracted and severe derangement and may put patients at increased risk of fracture. Patients with SHPT disease also frequently complain about bone pain and tenderness. Excess PTH is linked not only to bone disease but also to nonskeletal tissue deposition in the heart, cardiovascular system, brain, peripheral nerves, pancreas, and lungs (Goodman et al., 2004). Goals of treatment of SPTH include prevention of hyperphosphatemia, maintenance of normal serum calcium levels, treatment of vitamin D deficiency, and suppression of PTH (NKF, 2002).

The NKF/KDOQI Clinical Practice Guidelines for Bone Mineral Metabolism and Disease in CKD (NKF, 2003a) recommend annual measurement of serum calcium, phosphorus, and PTH levels beginning at Stage 3 (GFR < 60 ml/min per 1.73 m^2). The measurements should be made more frequently, if the patient is receiving therapy for abnormal levels.

The K/DOQI guidelines (NKF, 2003a) state that the target range for phosphorus is 2.7 mg/dl to 4.6 mg/dl. in stages 3, 4 and 5 prior to dialysis. Dietary restriction of phosphate and phosphate binders, that prevent its absorption, are the first steps in preventing hyperphosphatemia. Dietary phosphorus restriction is a challenge as eating enough protein to prevent malnutrition can result in an overload of phosphorus. Calcium-based phosphate binders and noncalcium-based phosphate binders are effective in lowering serum phosphorous levels in patient with GFR < 60 ml/min/ 1.73 m^2 (NKF, 2003a).

Target levels for corrected total calcium should be maintained in the normal range, preferably toward the lower end of normal (8.4 to 9.5 mg/dl) for the laboratory used. Total elemental calcium intake should not exceed 2000 mg/day. If calcium exceeds 10.2 mg/dl, then therapies that cause hypercalcemia should be adjusted, including calcium supplementation and/or vitamin D supplementation (NKF, 2003a).

Intact PTH (iPTH) is an assay used to measure the biologically active level of PTH in assessment, monitoring, and treatment of disorders of bone and mineral metabolism. The target for intact PTH (iPTH) for patients in Stage 3 is 35–70 pg/ml. and for patients with Stage 4 the level is 70–110 pg/ml. If PTH levels exceed these target levels, then vitamin D (serum 25 hydroxyvitamin D) should be measured. In stage 3 and 4, supplementation with oral vitamin D2 (ergocalciferol) is initiated if levels are less than 30 nmol/L. The dose of oral Vitamin D supplementation is based on the level of deficiency. If the level of Vitamin D2 is > 30 nmol/L, then treatment with active oral Vitamin D sterol is indicated. Calcium, phosphorus and PTH levels should be monitored closely during therapy with Vitamin D sterols. Doses should be adjusted or held if PTH falls below the target range, if corrected serum calcium exceeds 9.5 mg/dl, or if serum phosphorus levels rise > 4.6 mg/d (NKF, 2003a).

Research concerning the calcium-sensing receptor (CaR) located in the parathyroid gland has led to development of new therapeutic agents that might lead to improved control of SPTH disease. Calcimemetics are small organic compounds that increase CaR sensitivity to extracellular calcium. Cincalcet HCl, a second-generation calcimemetic, specifically binds and modulates the calcium-sensing receptor, resulting in a rapid decrease in PTH secretion. It was approved by the FDA in March 2004 and has shown to be safe and efficacious in reducing PTH in patients with ESRD (Block et al., 2004). Although most of the studies of this drug have been with patients on dialysis, Coburn and associates (2003) used the drug in patients not yet on dialysis and found it effective in lowing iPTH by 30%. The drug was generally well tolerated.

Metabolic Acidosis

Metabolic acidosis develops in Stage 3 and is associated with protein catabolism and demineralization of bones, due to the body's mechanism to buffer and excrete excess hydrogen ions (Franch & Mitch, 2004). The Clinical Practice Guideline for Nutrition in Chronic Renal Failure recommends a target serum bicarbonate level of > 22 mEq/L. Supplementation with alkali salts (sodium bicarbonate) should start at 0.5 to 1.0 mEq/kg per day (NKF, 2000b).

Neurologic Disorders

Neurologic disorders are present in up to 60% of patients starting dialysis. These disorders may include peripheral polyneuropathy, encephalopathy, autonomic dysfunction, and sleep disorders. Patients with CKD should be assessed for signs and symptoms during routine office visits. The lower the GFR the more likely that neurologic problems will be seen. If, however, the severity of neurologic problems appears out of proportion to the level of function, other co-existing causes should be evaluated (Burns & Bates, 1998). Tricyclic antidepressants, anticonvulsants, capsaicin, and lidoderm patches may be efficacious in reducing the pain of peripheral polyneuropathy (Newton, Collins, & Fotino, 2004). Treatment with dialysis usually improves the more severe symptoms in central nervous system involvement.

Dyslipidemias

As previously discussed hyperlipidemia, which may contribute to the progression of renal disease, is a complication of CKD, and contributes to the increased occurrence of artherosclerotic cardiovascular disease (ACVD) in CKD. It is estimated that 36% of all outpatients in the U.S. have cholesterol levels high enough for treatment, but only 12%–20% actually receive treatment. Among those outpatients receiving therapy, cholesterol goals were reached in not more than 39% of patients treated by cardiologists (Allison, Squires. Johnson, & Gau, 1999). Aggressive assessment and treatment of dyslipidemias is critical to morbidity and mortality associated with CKD.

Complications of CKD contribute to morbidity and mortality. Reports suggest that current treatment is suboptimal (Nissenson et al., 2001; Obrador et al., 1999). Patient outcomes should benefit form early identification and treatment of complications.

Modification of Co-Morbid Conditions

Cardiac Disease

CVD mortality rates in CKD are 10–30 times higher than the general population. At the start of renal replacement therapy, 40% of the patients have coronary heart disease and 75% of the patients have abnormal left ventricular size and function (Foley et al., 1998). Although no prospective studies have been performed that show risk factor reduction reduces the risk of cardiovascular disease in patients with CKD, most clinicians recommend aggressive therapy to reduce risks (NKF, 2002). This includes management of hypertension and dyslipidemias, as previously discussed. Disturbances of mineral metabolism and development of SPTH and anemia play an important role in the development of cardiac disease and should also be treated vigorously. Other cardioprotective strategies include treatment of elevated homocysteinemia and prevention of fluid overload (Sarnak et al., 2003).

Hyperhomocysteinemia, plasma homocysteine (Hcy) levels > 15 mol/L, is an independent risk factor for atherosclerosis. Hyperhomocystenemia is observed in 85% of patients with ESRD. The cause of consistently elevated Hcy levels in ESRD patients is not known. Vitamin deficiencies (B_{12}, Folate, and B_6), a common cause of hyperhomocystenemia, are frequently found in patients with CKD. Uremic-induced anorexia, dietary restrictions, and poor nutritional intake, along with increased diuretic use with losses of water-soluble vitamins, can lead to vitamin deficiencies (Bostom & Culleton, 1999).

The American Heart Association (AHA) recommends those patient with increased risk of heart disease should have a Hcy level < 10 mol/L. Folic acid and B_{12} work to reduce Hcy levels by metabolizing it back to the amino acid, methionine. Vitamin B_6 facilitates the breakdown of Hcy to cystene and other waste products. Supplementation with folic acid, B_{12}, and B_6 should be considered and has shown to reduce Hcy levels (Shemin, Bostom, & Sellhub, 2001). It may also lower the incidence of atherosclerotic CVD outcomes.

Extracellular volume overload appears early in CKD. Patients with CKD may have a 10%–30% increase in extracellular and blood volume in the absence of peripheral edema (Wilcox, 2002). Fluid overload is a major contributor to hypertension in patients with CKD. Additionally, extracellular fluid volume overload leads to left ventricular hypertrophy (Foley et al., 1998). Strategies to reduce volume overload appears important in reducing cardiovascular morbidity and mortality. Patients should be instructed to monitor fluid intake and limit it to 500 cc plus their previous day's 24-hour urine output.

Diabetes Mellitus

Patients with diabetes mellitus, type 1 and type 2, have the lowest overall age adjusted survival of all patients with ESRD. Patients should have intensified glycemic control with target HgbA1c < 7.0 %. Tight antihypertensive control (BP < 130/80 mm Hg) with a regimen that includes an ACE inhibitor or ARB. Albuminuria and proteinuria should be targeted and reduced to the lowest possible levels.

Dyslipidemia should be controlled to reduce cardiovascular risk. Lifestyle modification, including weight reduction and cessation of smoking, should be initiated. Nephrotoxic drugs should be avoided, including light use of minor analgesics (e.g., NSAIDS, salicylates) (Bakris et al., 2000; Wolf & Ritz, 2003). A multidisciplinary integrated structured treatment in diabetics has shown significantly less loss of GFR as compared to private physician-managed care (Wolf & Ritz, 2003). Chapter 11 discusses in more detail the treatment of diabetes and kidney disease.

Preparation for Renal Replacement Therapy

In stage 4 when the GFR is < 30 ml/min/1.73 m² discussions of RRT should begin. The focus should be on selection of the treatment modality with establishment of a plan for access placement. Patients should be referred to the transplant center when the GFR is < 30 ml/min/1.73 m². Plans can be made for a preemptive transplant if a suitable donor is available.

Indications for initiation of RRT are based on the level of kidney function and presence of signs and symptoms of uremia. Most individuals begin dialysis or receive a transplant when GFR is < 10 – 15 ml/min/1.73 m². Preparation for RRT and treatment of ESRD is discussed in detail in Chapter 12.

Summary

It is clear that early identification of patients with CKD is important to not only delay disease progression and treat complications, but to reduce related morbidity and mortality. Identification of patients with a disease that is mainly asymptomatic until the later stages poses a challenge. Nurses are in a unique position to identify patients with risk factors and initiate appropriate screening for early referral, evaluation, and treatment of patients with CKD.

References

American Diabetes Association. (2005a). Standards of medical care. *Diabetes Care, 28,* S4-S36.

American Diabetes Association. (2005b). Nephropathy in diabetes. *Diabetes Care, 27,* S79-S83.

Anavekar, N.S., McMurray, J.J., Velazquez, E.J., Solomon, S.D., Kober, L., Rouleau, J.L., et al. (2004). Relation between renal dysfunction and cardiovascular outcomes after myocardial infarction, *New England Journal of Medicine, 351*(13), 1344-1346.

Astor, B.C., Munter, P., Levin, A., Eustace, J.A., & Coresh, J. (2002). Association of kidney function with anemia: The Third National Health and Nutrition Examination Survey (1988-1994). *Archives of Internal Medicine, 162*(12), 1401-1408.

Bakris, G.L. (1998). Progression of diabetic nephropathy. A focus on arterial pressure level and methods of reduction. *Diabetes Research and Clinical Practice, 39*(Suppl), S35-42.

Bakris, G.L. Williams, M., Dworkin, L., Elliott, W.J. Epstein, M. Toto, R., et al. (2000). Preserving renal function in adults with hypertension and diabetes: A consensus approach. National Kidney Foundations Hypertension and Diabetes Executive Committees Working Group. *American Journal of Kidney Diseases, 36*(3), 646-661.

Bakris, G.L., & Weir, M.R. (2000). ACE inhibitor-associated elevations in serum creatinine: Is this a cause for concern? *Archives of Internal Medicine, 160*(5), 685-693.

Balon, P.B., Hojs, R., Zavratnik, A., & Kos, M. (2002). Bone mineral density in patients beginning hemodialysis treatment. *American Journal of Nephrology, 22*(1), 14-17.

Block, G.A., Julbert-Shearon, T.E., Levin, N.W. & Port, F.K. (1998). Association of serum phosphorus and calcium x phosphate product with mortality risk in chronic hemodialysis patients: a national study. *American Journal of Kidney Diseases, 31*(4), 607-617.

Block, G.A., Martin, K.J., de Francisco, A.L., Turner, S.A., Avram, M.M., Suranyi, M.G., et al. (2004). Cinacalcet for secondary hyperparathyroidism in patients receiving hemodialysis. *New England Journal of Medicine, 350*(15), 1516-1525.

Bostom, A.G., & Culleton, B.F. (1999) Hyperhomocysteinemia in chronic renal disease. *Journal of the American Society of Nephrology, 10*(4), 891-900.

Brenner, B.M., Cooper, M.E., de Zeeuw, D., Keane, W.F., Mitch, W.E., Parving, H.H., et al. & RENAAL Study Investigators. (2001). Effects of losartan on renal and cardiovascular outcomes in patients with type 2 diabetes and nephropathy. *New England Journal of Medicine, 345*, 861-869.

Buckalew, V.M., Berg, R.I., Wang, S.R., Porush, J.G., Rauch, S., & Schulman, G. (1996). Prevalence of hypertension in 1,790 subjects with chronic renal disease: The modification of diet in renal disease study baseline cohort. Modification of Diet in Renal Disease Study Group. *American Journal of Kidney Diseases, 28*, 811-821.

Burn, D.J., & Bates, D. (1998). Neurology and the kidney. *Journal of Neurological Neurosurgic Psychiatry, 65*, 810-821.

Campbell, R., Sangalli, F., Perticucci, E., Aros, C., Viscarra,C. Perna, A., et al. (2003). Effects of combined ACE inhibitor and angiotensin II antagonist treatment in human chronic nephropathies. *Kidney International, 63*, 1094-1103.

Chobanian, A.V., Bakis, G.L., Black, H.R., Cushman, W.C., Green, L.A., Izzo, J.L., et al. & the National high blood pressure Education Programming Coordinating Committee. (2003). The seventh report of the joint national committee on prevention, detection, evaluation, and treatment of high blood pressure. *Journal of the American Medical Association, 289*, 2560-2562.

Chuahirun, T., Simoni, J., Hudson, C., Seipel, T., Khanna, A., Harrist, R.B. et al. (2004). Cigarette smoking exacerbates and its cessation ameliorates renal injury in type 2 diabetes. *American Journal of Medical Science., 327*(2), 57-67.

Coburn, J.W., Charytan, C., Chonchol, M., Herman, J., Lien, Y.H., Liu, W., et al. (2003). *Cinacalcet HCL is an effective treatment for secondary hyperparathyroidism in patients with chronic kidney disease not yet receiving dialysis.* Abstract presented at the ASN meeting. Abstract SA-P0740.

Cockcroft, D.W., & Gault, M.H. (1976). Prediction of creatinine clearance from serum creatinine. *Nephron, 16*, 31-41.

Coffman, T.M. (2002). Renal failure caused by therapeutic agents. In Greenberg, A., Cheung, A.K., Coffman, T.M., Folk, R.J., Jeanette, J.C. (Eds). *Primer on kidney diseases* (pp. 260-265). New York: Academic Press.

Collins, A.J., Li, S., St. Peter, W., Ebben, J., Roberts, T., Ma, J.Z., et al. (2001). Death, hospitalization, and economic associations among incident hemodialysis patients with hematocrit values of 36% to 39%. *Journal of the American Society of Nephrology, 12*, 2465-2473.

Combe, C., McCullough, K.P., Asano, Y., Ginsberg, N., Maroni, B.J., & Pifer, T.B. (2004). Kidney Disease Outcomes Quality Initiative (K/DOQI) and the Dialysis Outcomes and Practice Patterns Study (DOPPS): Nutrition guidelines, indicators, and practices. *American Journal of Kidney Diseases, 44*(5Suppl3), 39-3346.

Coresh, J., Wei, G.L., McQuillan, G., Branccati, F.L., Levey, A.S., Jones, C., et al. (2001). Prevalence of high blood pressure and elevated serum creatinine level in the United States: Findings from the Third National Health and Nutrition Examination Survey (1988-1994). *Archives of Internal Medicine, 161*, 1207-1216.

Coresh J., Astor, B.C., Greene, T., Eknoyan, G., & Levey, A.S. (2003). Prevalence of chronic kidney disease and decreased kidney function in the adult US population: Third National Health Nutrition Examination Survey. *American Journal of Kidney Diseases, 41*(1), 1-12.

Coresh, J., Astor, B., & Sarnak, M.J. (2004). Evidence for increased cardiovascular disease risk in patients with chronic kidney disease. *Current Opinions in Nephrology Hypertension, 13*, 73-81.

Culleton, B.F., Larson, M.G., Wilson, P.W., Evans, J.C., Parfrey, P.S., & Ievy, D. (1999). Cardiovascular disease and mortality in a community-based cohort with mild renal insufficiency. *Kidney International, 56*(6), 2214-2219.

De Zeeuw, D., Remmuzzi, G., Parving, H.H., Keane, W.F., Zhang, A., Shahinfar, S., et al. (2004). Proteinuria, a target for renoprotection in patients with type 2 diabetic nephropathy: Lessons form RENAAL. *Kidney International, 65*(6), 2309-2320.

Diabetes Control and Complications Trial Research Group. (1993). The effect of intensive treatment of diabetes on the development and progression of long-term complications in insulin-dependent diabetes mellitus. *New England Journal of Medicine, 329*, 977-986.

Expert Panel on Detection, Evaluation and Treatment of High Blood Cholesterol in Adults (ATP III Guidelines). (2001). Executive summary of the third report of the national cholesterol education program (NCEP) expert panel on detection, evaluation, and treatment of high blood cholesterol in adults (Adult Treatment Panel III). *Journal of the American Medical Association, 285*, 2486-2497.

Fink, J.C., Blahut, S.A., Reddy, M., & Light, P. (2001). Use pf erythropoietin before the initiation of dialysis and its impact on mortality. *American Journal of Kidney Diseases, 37*(2), 348-355.

Fiore, M.C. (2000). U.S. public health service clinical practice guideline: Treating tobacco use and dependence. *Respiratory Care, 45*, 1200-1262.

Fletcher, G.F, Balady, G., Blair, S.N., Blumenthal, J., Caspersen, C., Chaitman, B., Epstein, S., Sivarajan Froelicher, E.S., Froelicher, V.F., Pina, I.L., & Pollock, M.L. (1996).Statement on exercise: benefits and recommendations for physical activity programs for all Americans. A Statement for Health Professionals by the Committee on Exercise and Cardiac Rehabilitation of the Council on Clinical Cardiology, American Heart Association. *Circulation, 94*, 857-862,

Foley, R.N., Parfrey, P.S., & Sarnak, M.J. (1998). Clinical epidemiology of cardiovascular disease in chronic renal disease. *American Journal of Kidney Diseases, 32*, 112-119.

Fox, C.S., Larson, M.G., Leip, E.P., Culleton, B., Wilson, P.W., & Levy, D. (2004). Predictors of new-onset kidney disease in a community-based population. *Journal of the American Medical Association, 291*(7), 844-850.

Franch, H.A., & Mitch,W.E. (2004). Metabolic and nutritional responses to academia. In J.D. Kopple & S.G. Massry (Eds). *Nutritional management of renal disease* (pp. 151-165). Philadelphia: Lippincott, Williams & Wilkins.

Fried, L.F., Orchard, T.J., & Kasiske, B.L. (2001). The effect of lipid reduction on renal disease progression: A meta analysis. *Kidney International, 59*, 260-269.

Fried L.F., Shlipak, M.G., Crump, C., Bleyer, A.J., Gottdiener, J.S., Kronmal, R.A., Kuller, L.H., & Newman, A.B. (2003). Renal insufficiency as a predictor of cardiovascular outcomes and mortality in elderly individuals. *Journal of the American College of Cardiology, 41*(8), 1364-1372.

Ganesh, S.K., Stach, A.G., Levin, N.W., Hylbert-Shearon, R., & Port, F.K. (2001). Association of level serum phosphorous, Calcium x phosphorous predict and parathyroid hormone with cardiac mortality risk in chronic hemodialysis patient. *Journal of the American Society of Nephrology, 12*, 2131 – 2138.

Goodman, W.G., London, G., Amann, K., Block, G.A., Giachelli, C., Hruska, K.A., Ketteler, M., Levin, A., Massy, Z., McCarron, D.A., Raggi, P., Shanahan, C.M., Yorioka, N.; & Vascular Calcification Work Group. (2004). Vascular calcification in chronic kidney disease. *American Journal of Kidney Diseases, 43*, 572-529.

Goodman, W.G. (2004). The consequences of uncontrolled secondary hyperparathyroidism and its treatment in chronic kidney disease. *Seminars in Dialysis, 17*(3), 209-216.

Go, A.S., Chertow, G.M., Fan, D., McCulloch, C.E., & Hsu, C.Y. (2004). Chronic kidney disease and the risks of death, cardiovascular events, and hospitalization. *New England Journal of Medicine, 351*(13),1296-1305..

Halimi, J., Giraideau, B. & Vol, S. (2000). Effect of current smoking and smoking discontinuation on renal function, proteinuria in the general population. *Kidney International, 58*, 1285-1292.

Hovind, P., Rossing, P., Tarnow, L., Smidt, U.M. & Parving, H.H. (2001). Progression of diabetic nephropathy. *Kidney International, 59,* 702-709.

Hsu, C.Y., McCulloch, C.E.. & Curhan, G.C. (2002). Epidemiology of anemia associated with chronic renal insufficiency among adults in the United States: results from the Third National Health and Nutrition Examination Survey. *Journal of the American Society of Nephrology, 13*(2), 504-510.

Hunsicker, L.G., Adler, S., Caggiula, A., England, B.K., Greene, T., Kusek, J.W., Rogers, N.L., & Teschan, P.E. (1997). Predictors of the progression of renal disease in the Modification of Diet in Renal Disease Study. *Kidney International, 51*(6), 1908-1919.

Jarfar, T.H., Schmid, C.H., Landa, M., Fiatras, I., Toto, R., & Remizzo. G., Maschio, G., Brenner, B.M., Kamper, A., Zucchelli, P., Becker, G., Himmelmann, A., Bannister, K., Landais, P., Shahinfar, S., de Jong, P.E., de Zeeuw, D., Lau, J. & Levey, A.S. (2001). Angiotensin-converting enzyme inhibitors and progression of nondiabetic renal disease. A meta-analysis of patient-level data. *Annals of Internal Medicine, 35,* 73-87.

Jones, C.A., McQuillan, G.M., Kusek, J.W., Eberhardt, M.S., Herman, W.H., Coresh, J., Salive, M., Jones, C.P., & Agodoa, L.Y. (1998). Serum creatinine levels in the U.S. population: Third National Health and Nutrition Examination Survey. *American Journal of Kidney Diseases, 32,* 992-999.

Jungers, P., Massy, Z.A., Khoa, T.N., Fumeron, C., Labrunie, M., Lacour, B., Descamps-Latscha, B., & Man, N.K. (1997). Incidence and risk factors of atherosclerotic cardiovascular accidents in predialysis chronic renal failure patients: A prospective. *Nephrology Dialysis and Transplantation, 12*(12), 2597-2600.

Jungers, P., Massy, Z.A., Nguyen-Khoa, T., Choukroun, G., Robino, C., Fakhouri, F., Touam, M., Nguyen, A.T., & Grunfeld, J.P. (2001). Long duration of pre-dialysis nephrological care is associated with improved long-term survival of dialysis patients. *Nephrology Dialysis and Transplantation, 12,* 2357-2364.

Kausz, A.T., Khan, S.S., Abichandani, R., Kazmi, W.H., Obrador, G.T., Ruthazer, R., & Pereira, B.J. (2001). Management of patients with chronic renal insufficiency in the Northeastern United States. *Journal of the American Society of Nephrology, 12*(7), 1501-1507.

Keane, WF. (2000). Proteinuria: its clinical importance and role in progressive renal disease. *American Journal of Kidney Diseases, 35*(4suppl1), S97-S105.

Keane, W.F., Brenner, B.M., de Zeeuw, D., Grunfeld, J.P., McGill, J., Mitch, W.E., Ribeiro, A.B., Shahinfar, S., Simpson, R.L., Snapinn, S.M., & Toto, R.; & RENAAL Study Investigators. (2003). The risk of developing end-stage renal disease in patients with type 2 diabetes and nephropathy: The RENAAL study. *Kidney International, 63*(4), 1499-1507.

Keith, D., Nichols, G., Gullion, C., Brown, J., & Smith, D. (2002). Mortality of chronic kidney disease (CKD) in a large HMO population. (2002). *Journal of the American Society of Nephrology, 13,* 620A. Abstract SU-PO740.

Kirk, A.D, Mannon, R.G., Swanson, S.J., & Hale, D.A. (2005). Strategies for minimizing immunosuppression in kidney transplantation. *Transplant International, 18*(1), 2-14.

Klahr, S., Levey A.S., Beck G.J., Caggiula A.W., Hunsicker L., Kusek J.W., & Striker G. (1994). The effects of dietary protein restriction and blood pressure control on the progression of chronic renal disease Modification of Diet in Renal Disease Study Group. *New England Journal of Medicine, 330,* 877-84

Kopple, J.D., Greene, T., Chumlea, W.C. Hollinger, D., Maroni, B.J., Merrill, D., Scherch, L.K., Schulman, G., Wang, S.R., & Zimmer, G.S. (2000). Relationship between nutritional status and the glomerular filtration rate. Results from the MDRD study. *Kidney International, 55,* 1688-1703.

Krop, J.S., Coresh, J., Chambless, L.E., Shahar, E., Watson, R.L., Szklo M. & Brancati, F.L. (1999). A community-based study of explanatory factors for the excess risk for early renal function decline in blacks vs. whites with diabetes: The Atherosclerosis Risk in Communities study. *Archives of Internal Medicine, 159*(15), 1777-1783.

Kurella, M., Bennett, W.M., & Chertow, G.M. (2003). Analgesia in patients with ESRD. A review of available evidence. *American Journal of Kidney Diseases, 42,* 217-228.

Kuriyama, S., Tomonari, H. Yoshida. H., Hashimoto, T., Kawagauchi, Y., & Sakai, O. (1997). Reversal of anemia by erythropoietin therapy retards the progression of chronic renal failure, especially in nondiabetic patients. *Nephron, 77,* 176-185.

Lach, F., & Bover, J. (2000). Renal osteodystrophies. In B.M. Brenner (Ed.)., Brenner & Rector *The Kidney* (6th edition) (pp. 2103-2186). Philadelphia: W.B. Saunders, Company.

Levey, A.S., Bosch, J., Lewis, J. B., Greene, T., Rogers, N. & Roth, D. (1999). A more accurate method to estimate glomerular filtration rate from a serum creatinine: A new prediction equation. *Annals of Internal Medicine, 130,* 461-470.

Levey, A.S. (2002). Non-diabetic kidney disease. *New England Journal of Medicine, 347*(19), 1505-1511.

Levin, A., Thompson, C.R., Ethier, J., Carlisle, E.J., Tobe, S., Mendelssoh, D., Burgess, D., Jindal, K., Barrett, B., Singer, J & & Djidjev, O. (1999). Left ventricular mass index increase in early renal disease: impact of decline in hemoglobin. *American Journal of Kidney Diseases, 34,* 125-134.

Levin, A. (2002). The role of anemia in the genesis of cardiac abnormalities in patients with chronic kidney disease. *Nephrology, Dialysis and Transplantation, 17,* 207-210.

Lewington S., Clarke R., Qizilbash N., Peto R., Collins R., & Prospective Studies Collaboration. (2002). Age-specific relevance of usual blood pressure to vascular mortality: a meta-analysis of individual data for one million adults in 61 prospective studies. *Lancet, 360*(9349), 1903-1913.

Manjunath, G., Tighiouar,t H., Ibrahim, H., MacLeod, B., Salem, D.N., Griffith, J.L., Coresh, J., Levey, A.S., & Sarnak, M.J. (2003). Level of kidney function as a risk factor for atherosclerotic cardiovascular outcomes in the community. *Journal of the American College of Cardiology, 41*(1), 47-55).

Martinez, I., Saracho, R., Montenegro, J., & Llach, F. (1997). The importance of dietary calcium and phosphorous in the secondary hyperparathyroidism of patients with early renal failure. *American Journal of Kidney Diseases, 29,* 496-502.

Massy, Z.A., Khoa, T.N., Lacour, B., Descamps-Latscha, B., Man, N.K., & Jungers, P. (1999). Dyslipidaemia and the progression of renal disease in chronic renal failure patients. *Nephrology, Dialysis and Transplantation, 14*(10), 2392-7.

McClellan, W., Tran, L.L., & the PAERI Study Group. (2003). *The prevalence of anemia in patients with chronic kidney disease. The final results of the PAERI Study.* Poster presented at the 35th Annual Meeting and Scientific Exposition of the American Society of Nephrology, Philadelphia, PA, Abstract 955.

Mehrotra, R., & Koppel, J. (2004). Causes of protein-energy malnutrition in chronic renal failure. In J.D. Kopple & S.G. Massry (Eds). *Nutritional management of renal disease* (pp. 161-182). Philadelphia: Lippincott, Williams & Wilkins.

Mogensen, C.E., Neldan, S., Tikkanen, I., Oren, S., Viskoper, R., Watts, R.W. & Cooper, M.E.. (2000). Randomized controlled trail of dual blockage of renin-angiotensin system in patients with hypertension, microalbuminuria, and non-insulin dependent diabetes: the candesartan and lisinopril microalbuminuria (CALM) study. *British Medical Journal, 321,*1440-1444.

Nakano, S., Ogihara, M., Tamura, C., Kitazawa, M., Nishizawa, M., Kigoshi, T., & Uchida K. (1999). Reversed circadian blood pressure rhythm independently predicts end stage renal failure in non-insulin-dependent diabetes mellitus subjects. *Journal of Diabetes Complications, 13*(4), 224-231.

Nangaku, M. (2004). Hypoxia and tubulointerstitial injury: A final common pathway to end-stage renal disease. *Experimental Nephrology, 98*(1), e8-12.

National Kidney Foundation. (2000a). K/DOQI Clinical practice guidelines for anemia of chronic kidney disease update. *American Journal of Kidney Diseases, 37*(1 Suppl 1), S182-238.

National Kidney Foundation. (2000b). K/DOQI Clinical practice guidelines for nutrition in chronic renal failure. *American Journal Kidney Diseases, 35*(6 Suppl 2), S1-S140.

National Kidney Foundation. (2002). K/DOQI clinical practice guidelines for chronic kidney disease: Evaluation, classification and stratification. *American Journal of Kidney Diseases, 39*(suppl1), S1-S266.

National Kidney Foundation. (2003a). K/DOQI clinical practice guidelines for bone metabolism and disease in chronic kidney disease. *American Journal of Kidney Diseases. 42*(suppl 3), S1-S201.

National Kidney Foundation. (2003b). K/DOQI clinical practice guidelines for managing dyslipidemias in chronic kidney disease. *American Journal of Kidney Diseases, 41*(suppl 3), S1-S91.

National Kidney Foundation. (2004). K/DOQI clinical practice guidelines on blood pressure management and use of antihypertensive agents in chronic kidney disease. *American Journal of Kidney Diseases, 43*(suppl 1), S1-S268.

Neal, B., MacMahon, S., Chapman, N., & Blood Pressure Lowering Treatment Trialists' Collaboration. (2000). Effects of ACE inhibitors, calcium antagonists, and other blood-pressure-lowering drugs: results of prospectively designed overviews of randomized trials. Blood Pressure Lowering Treatment Trialists' Collaboration. *Lancet, 356*(9246), 1955-1964.

Newton, W.P., Collins, L., & Fotino, C. (2004). What is the best treatment for diabetic neuropathy. *Journal of Family Practice. 53*, 403-408.

Nissenson, A.R., Pereria, B.J., Collins, A.J., & Steinberg, E.P. (2001). Prevalence and characteristics of individuals with chronic kidney disease in a large health maintenance organization. *American Journal of Kidney Diseases, 37*, 1177-1183.

Nissenson, A.R., Collins, A.J., Hurley, J., Petersen, H., Pereira, B.J. & Steinberg, E.P. (2001). Opportunities for improving the care of patients with chronic renal insufficiency: Current practice patterns. *Journal of the American Society of Nephrology, 12*(8), 1713-1720.

Obrador, G.T., Ruthazer, R., Pradeep, A., Kausz, A., & Pereria, B.J. (1999). Prevalence of factors associated with suboptimal care before initiation of dialysis in the United States. *Journal of the American Society of Nephrology, 10*, 1793-1800.

Ockene, I.S., & Miller, N.H. For the American Heart Association Task Force on Risk Reduction. (1997). Cigarette smoking, cardiovascular disease, and stroke. *Circulation, 96*, 3243-3247.

Orth, S.R. (2004). Effects of smoking on systemic and intrarenal hemodynamics: influence on renal function. *Journal of the American Society of Nephrology, 15*(Suppl 1), S58-S63.

Owen, W.F. Jr. (2003). Patterns of care for patients with chronic kidney disease in the United States: Dying for improvement. *Journal of the American Society of Nephrology, .14*(7 Suppl 2), S76-80.

Palmer, B.F. (2003). Renal dysfunction complicating the treatment of hypertension. *New England Journal of Medicine, 337*(6), 1256-1261.

Parving, H-H, Lehnert, H., Brochner-Mortensen, J., Gormis, R., Anderson, S. & Arner, P., for the Irbesartan in Patients with Type 2 Diabetes and Microalbuminuria Study Group. (2001). The effect of irbesartan on the development of diabetic nephropathy in patients with type 2 diabetes. *New England Journal of Medicine, 345*, 870-888.

Pupim, L.B., Caglar, K., Hakim, R.M., Shyr, Y., & Ikizler, T.A. (2004). Uremic malnutrition is a predictor of death independent of inflammatory status. *Kidney International, 66*(5), 2054-2060.

Remuzzi, G., & Bertani, T. (1998). Pathophysiology of progressive nephropathies. *New England Journal of Medicine, 339*, 1448-1556.

Remuzzi, G., Ruggenent, P., & Perico, N. (2002). Chronic renal diseases: renoprotective benefits of renin-angiotensin system inhibition. *Annals of Internal Medicine, 136*, 604-615.

Rocco, M.V., Gassman, J.J., Wang, S.R., & Kaplan, R.M. (1997). Cross-sectional study of quality of life and symptoms in chronic renal disease patients: The Modification of Diet in Renal Disease Study. *American Journal of Kidney Diseases, 29*, 888-896.

Roubicek, C., Brunet, P., Huiart, L., Thiron, X., Leonetti, F., Dussol, B., Jaber, K., Andrieu, D., Rarmananarivo, P., & Berland, Y. (2000). Timing of nephrology referral: Influence on mortality and morbidity. *American Journal of Kidney Diseases, 36*, 35-41.

Ruggenenti, P., Gaspari, F., Perna, A., & Remuzzi, G. (1998). Cross sectional longitudinal study of spot morning urine protein:creatine ratio, 24 hour urine protein excretion rate, glomerular filtrations rate and end stage renal failure in chronic renal disease in patients without diabetes. *British Medical Journal, 316*, 504-509.

Sahadavan, M., & Kasiske, B.L. (2002). Hyperlipidemia in kidney disease: Causes and consequences. *Current Opinions in Nephrology and Hypertension, 11*(3), 323-329.

Sarnak, M.J., Levey, A.S., Schoolwerth, A.C., Coresh, J., Culleton, B., Hamm, L.L., McCullough, P.A., Dasiske, B.L, Kelepouris, E., Klag, M.J., Parfrey, P., Pfeffer, M., Raij, L, Spinosa, D.J., & Wilson, P.W. (2003). Kidney disease as a risk factor for development of cardiovascular disease: A statement from the American Heart Association Councils on Kidney in cardiovascular disease, high blood pressure research, clinical cardiology, and epidemiology and prevention. *Circulation, 1008*, 2154-2169.

Sheinfeld, G.R., & Bakris, G.L. (1999). Benefits of combination angiotensin-converting enzyme inhibitor and calcium antagonist therapy for diabetic patients. *American Journal of Hypertension, 12*, 80S-85S.

Shemin, D., Bostom, A.G., & Selhub, J. (2001). Treatment of hyperhomocystenemia in ESRD. *American Journal of Kidney Diseases, 38*(4 suppl), 591-595.

Shulman, N.B., Ford, C.E., Hall, W.D., Blaufox, M.D., Simon, D., Langford, H.G. & Schneider, K.A. (1989). Prognostic value of serum creatinine and effect of treatment of hypertension on renal function. Results from the hypertension detection and Follow-up program. The Hypertension Detection and Follow-up Program Cooperative Group.*Hypertension, 13*(Suppl 5), I80-I93.

Snow, V., Weiss, K.B., Mottur-Pilson, C., for the Clinical Efficacy Assessment Subcommittee of the American College of Physicians. (2003). The evidence base for tight blood pressure control in management of type 2 diabetes mellitus. *Annals of Internal Medicine, 138*, 593-602.

Stack, A.G. (2003). Impact of timing of nephrology referral and pre-ESRD care on mortality risk among new ESRD patients in the U.S. *American Journal of Kidney Diseases, 41*, 310-318.

Tarver-Carr, M.E., Powe, N.R., Eberhardt, M.S., & Brancati, F.L. (2003). Lifestyle factors, obesity and the risk of chronic kidney disease. *Epidemiology, 14*, 479-487.

Tonelli, M., Bohm, C., Pandeya, S., Gill, J., Levin, A., & Kiberd, B.A. (2001). Cardiac risk factors and the use of cardioprotective medications in patients with chronic renal insufficiency. *American Journal of Kidney Diseases, 37*(3), 484-489.

United Kingdom Prospective Diabetes Study Group (UKPDS). (1998). Tight blood pressure control and risk of macrovascular and microvascular complications in type 2 diabetes. *British Medical Journal, 317*, 703-713.

U.S. Renal Data System. (2003). *USRDS 2003 annual data report. Atlas of end-stage renal disease in the United States.* Bethesda MD, National Institutes of Health, NIDDK.

U.S. Renal Data System. (2004). *USRDS 2004 annual data report: Atlas of end-stage renal disease in the United States.* Bethesda MD, National Institutes of Health, NIDDK.

Vasavada, N., & Agarwal, R. (2003). Role of excess volume in the pathophysiology of hypertension in chronic kidney disease. *Kidney International, 64*(5), 1772-1779.

Viberti, G., & Wheeldon, N.M., for the MARVAL Study Investigators. (2002). Microalbuminuria reduction with valsartan patients with type 2 diabetes mellitus: A blood pressure-independent effect. *Circulation, 106*, 672-678.

Wilcox, C.S. (2002). New insights into diuretic use in patients with chronic renal disease. *Journal of the American Society of Nephrology, 13*, 798-805.

Wolf, G., & Ritz, E. (2003). Diabetic nephropathy in type 2 diabetes prevention and patient management. *Journal of the American Society of Nephrology, 14*, 1396-1405.

World Health Organization. (1998). *Nutritional anemia.* Report of a WHO Scientific Group in Geneva, Switzerland, WHO.

Xue, J.L., Ma, J.Z., Louis, T.A. & Collins, A.J. (2001). Forecast of the number of patients with end-stage renal disease in the United States to the year 2020. *Journal of the American Society of Nephrology, 12*, 2753-2758.

Yu, H.T. (2003). Progression of chronic kidney disease. *Archives of Internal Medicine, 163*, 1417-1429.

Readings

Jungers, P., Choukrousn, G., Oualim, Z., Nguyen, A.T., & Man, N.K. (2002). Beneficial influence of recombinant human erythropoietin therapy on the rate of progression of chronic renal failure in predialysis patients. *Nephrology, Dialysis and Transplantation, 16*, 175-176.

Pearson , T.A., Blair, S.N., Daniels, S.R., Eckel, R.H., Fair, J.M., Fortman, S.P., Franklin, B.A., Goldstein, L.B., Greenland, P., Grundy, S.M., Hong, Y., Miller, N.H., Lauer, R.M., Ockene, I.S, Sacco, R.L., Sallis, J.F. Jr, Smith, S.C. Jr, Stone, N.J., & Taubert, K.A. (2002). AHA Guidelines for Primary Prevention of Cardiovascular Disease and Stroke: 2002 Update: Consensus Panel Guide to Comprehensive Risk Reduction for Adult Patients Without Coronary or Other Atherosclerotic Vascular Diseases. American Heart Association Science Advisory and Coordinating Committee, Circulation. *Circulation, 106*(3), 388-391.

Rigotti, N.A., & Pasternak, R.C. (1996). Cigarette smoking and coronary heart disease: Risks and management. *Cardiology Clinics, 14*(1), 51-68.

- In an effort to address this growing public health care concern, the National Kidney Foundation (NKF) Kidney Disease Outcome Quality Initiative (K/DOQI) Advisory Board approved development of clinical practice guidelines for CKD in 2001, and a K/DOQI work group was identified.

- Although there are many diseases that can initiate and cause CKD, there appear to be common pathways for disease progression. Prominent morphologic features are fibrosis, loss of native renal cells, and infiltration by monocytes and macrophages, the result of the constant interplay between vasoactive substances.

- In addition to the establishment of a diagnosis, it is important to assess the severity of kidney dysfunction and establish the stage of CKD. Serum creatinine and proteinuria are key markers for determining the degree of kidney dysfunction.

- Interventions during the early stages of CKD are critical in slowing disease progression, however, CKD often goes undetected because patients are frequently asymptomatic. The GFR provides an indication of what signs and symptoms may be seen based on the degree of decline.

- The complications of CKD include: (a) hypertension, (b) anemia, (c) protein-energy malnutrition, (d) metabolic acidosis, (e) disorders of bone metabolism, (f) neuropathy, and (g) dyslipidemias.

- Patients with CKD usually have comorbid conditions in addition to CKD. Management of unrelated diseases is important to the health of the patient but does not affect the course of CKD (e.g., chronic obstructive pulmonary disease, degenerative joint disease). Treatment of other diseases, such as diabetes and hypertension, which cause CKD, does affect the course of CKD.

- Epidemiological studies show that individuals with certain clinical and socio-demographic characteristics are at increased risk for CKD... Knowing these risk factors allows for early identification of those likely to develop CKD and initiation of treatment to slow progression.

- Certain treatment strategies are proven to slow the progression of CKD, including: antihypertensive therapy, reduction of proteinuria, strict glycemic control, treatment of dyslipidemias, diet and lifestyle modifications, avoidance of nephrotoxic drugs, and referral to a nephrologist.

Diagnosis, Classification, and Management of CKD

Name of Resource	Brief Description	Where to Obtain Resource
K/DOQI Clinical Practice Guidelines for: 1. **Nutrition in Chronic Renal Failure** (AJKD, 35, no. 6, suppl. 2). 2. **Anemia of Chronic Kidney Disease Update** (AJKD, 37, no. 1, suppl. 1). 3. **Clinical Practice Guidelines for Chronic Kidney Disease: Evaluation, Classification and Stratification** (AJKD, 39, no. 2, suppl. 1). 4. **Bone Metabolism and Disease in Chronic Kidney Disease** (AJKD 42, no. 4, suppl. 3). 5. **Managing Dyslipidemias in Chronic Kidney Disease** (AJKD, 41, no. 4, suppl. 3). 6. **Hypertension and Antihypertensive Agents in Chronic Kidney Disease** (AJKD, 43, suppl. 1).	Content includes guidelines for the identification, management and treatment of patients with CKD.	*American Journal of Kidney Disease* (AJKD) – Medical Library * Free, full-text Guidelines available on line at www.kidney.org/professionals/ kdoqi/index.cfm
The Seventh Report of the Joint National Committee on Prevention, Detection, Evaluation and Treatment of High Blood Pressure (JNC 7 Report) (JAMA, 289, no. 19, 2560-2572.	Content provides guidelines for hypertension prevention, detection, evaluation, and treatment.	*Journal of American Medical Association* (JAMA) – Medical Library * Full-text available online at www.nhlbi.nih.gov/guidelines/ hypertension/
United States Renal Data System Annual Report	The United States Renal Data System (USRDS) is a national data system that collects, analyzes, and distributes information about end-stage renal disease in the United States.	Report available from: USRDS Coordinating Center 914 South 8th Street Suite D-206 Minneapolis, MN 55404 (612) 347-7776 1-888-99USRDS USRDS Coordinating * Full-text report available online at www.usrds.org/
Online resources Web sites for professional and patients concerning the latest in treatment and care of patients with CKD.	Up-to-date information to guide both the protessionals and patients.	**Professionals:** www.kidney.org www.niddk.nih.gov/ www.kidneydirections.com **Patients:** www.kidney.org www.aakp.org www.lifeoptions.org www.kidneyschool.org www.kidneydirections.com www.kidneypatientguide.org.uk

ANNP610 ## Diagnosis, Classification and Management of Chronic Kidney Disease

Patricia Bargo McCarley, MSN, RN, ACNPc, CNN

Contemporary Nephrology Nursing: Principles and Practice contains 39 chapters of educational content. Individual learners may apply for continuing nursing education credit by reading a chapter and completing the Continuing Education Evaluation Form for that chapter. Learners may apply for continuing education credit for any or all chapters.

Please photocopy this page and return to ANNA.
COMPLETE THE FOLLOWING:

Name: _____

Address: _____

City: _____ State: _____ Zip: _____

E-mail: _____

Preferred telephone: ☐ Home   ☐ Work: _____

State where licensed and license number (optional): _____

CE application fees are based upon the number of contact hours provided by the individual chapter. CE fees per contact hour for ANNA members are as follows: 1.0-1.9 - $15; 2.0-2.9 - $20; 3.0-3.9 - $25; 4.0 and higher - $30. Fees for nonmembers are $10 higher.

ANNA Member: ☐ Yes   ☐ No   Member # (if available) _____

☐ Checked Enclosed   ☐ American Express   ☐ Visa   ☐ MasterCard

Total Amount Submitted: _____

Credit Card Number: _____ Exp. Date: _____

Name as it appears on the card: _____

CE Evaluation Form
To receive continuing education credit for individual study after reading the chapter
1. Photocopy this form. (You may also download this form from ANNA's Web site, **www.annanurse.org**.)
2. Mail the completed form with payment (check) or credit card information to American Nephrology Nurses' Association, East Holly Avenue, Box 56, Pitman, NJ 08071-0056.
3. You will receive your CE certificate from ANNA in 4 to 6 weeks.

Test returns must be postmarked by **December 31, 2010.**

CE Application Fee
ANNA Member $25.00
Nonmember $35.00

EVALUATION FORM

1. I verify that I have read this chapter and completed this education activity. Date: _____

_____
Signature

2. What would be different in your practice if you applied what you learned from this activity? *(Please use additional sheet of paper if necessary.)*

_____

_____

_____

_____

_____

_____

_____

_____

_____

_____

Evaluation	Strongly disagree				Strongly agree
3. The activity met the stated objectives.					
a. Outline methods used to determine the severity of CKD.	1	2	3	4	5
b. Discuss the prevention and treatment of the complications of CKD.	1	2	3	4	5
c. Describe strategies to slow progression of CKD.	1	2	3	4	5
d. Summarize ways to modify co-morbid conditions of CKD.	1	2	3	4	5
4. The content was current and relevant.	1	2	3	4	5
5. The content was presented clearly.	1	2	3	4	5
6. The content was covered adequately.	1	2	3	4	5
7. Rate your ability to apply the learning obtained from this activity to practice.	1	2	3	4	5

Comments _____

_____

8. Time required to read the chapter and complete this form: _____ minutes.

This educational activity has been provided by the American Nephrology Nurses' Association (ANNA) for 3.2 contact hours. ANNA is accredited as a provider of continuing nursing education (CNE) by the American Nurses Credentialing Center's Commission on Accreditation (ANCC-COA). ANNA is an approved provider of continuing education by the California Board of Registered Nursing, CEP 0910.

Contemporary Nephrology Nursing: Principles and Practice, Second Edition © — American Nephrology Nurses' Association 2006

Symptom Management
Janet L. Welch, DNS, RN, CNS

Chapter Contents

Symptom Management

Chapter 11

Janet L. Welch, DNS, RN, CNS

Symptoms have variously been described as (a) experiences reflecting changes in biopsychosocial function, sensation, or cognition (Lenz, Pugh, Milligan, Gift, & Suppe, 1997); (b) indicators of change in normal functioning (University of California, San Francisco, School of Nursing Symptom Management Faculty Group [UCSF], 1994); and (c) cognitive-perceptual stimuli subject to complex psychosocial processes (Cioffi, 1991). Symptoms are subjective in nature, are experienced by the individual, and cannot be detected by another person such as a health care worker (UCSF, 1994). In contrast, signs are objective in nature, may or may not be subjectively experienced, and can be detected by another person such as a health care worker (UCSF, 1994). The focus of this chapter is on symptoms occurring in patients with kidney failure.

Individuals diagnosed with kidney failure commonly face a variety of concurrent symptoms such as fatigue, thirst, or trouble falling asleep. The causes of and the individual responses to these symptoms, however, may vary. In many acute and chronic illnesses, symptoms provide the patient with a signal indicating that some change in functioning has occurred; the signal prompts the individual to seek health care (Dodd et al., 2001; UCSF, 1994). The symptom experience of the individual with kidney failure, however, is somewhat different. Similar to other chronic illnesses, some symptoms, such as dyspnea, provide information to the patient that a physical change has occurred, thus prompting the patient to seek immediate health care. Unlike some other chronic illnesses, however, other symptoms, such as fatigue, occur not only at the onset of chronic kidney disease, but they also persist throughout the course of renal replacement therapy. Patients must learn to distinguish between immediately reportable symptoms and those they can treat themselves. Most patients self-manage these latter symptoms at home. It is not clear what self-care strategies are used to treat these symptoms or how patients respond to the chronicity of the symptoms. Furthermore, symptoms experienced in kidney failure, unfortunately, are often unpredictable and may contribute to feelings of powerlessness (Stapleton, 1992).

Assisting patients with symptom management is an essential component of nursing practice. The effective management of symptoms is a high priority both for patients afflicted with kidney failure and for the nurse caring for these patients. Patients state, however, that they selectively report the symptoms that they experience (Curtin & Mapes, 2001). An accurate and comprehensive assessment must be done, therefore, in order for nurses to begin effective symptom management. Once the presence and probable etiology of the symptom has been identified, appropriate interventions to prevent, reduce, or relieve the symptom are mutually selected and often implemented by the patient in the home setting.

Complicating effective symptom management in the patient with kidney failure are the patterns of symptoms that may occur. For example, Sklar and colleagues (1996, 1999) differentiate postdialysis fatigue from the persistent fatigue experienced by hemodialysis (HD) patients. In addition, the intensity of thirst varies between the interdialytic and intradialytic period (Giovannetti et al., 1994). The best times to assess, intervene, and vary management techniques are unknown. Also unknown are whether management techniques should be different in the intradialytic and interdialytic periods.

Symptom management goals are to delay or prevent negative outcomes (Dodd et al., 2001). Evaluation of symptoms should include not only an evaluation of the effectiveness of the interventions used in preventing, reducing, or relieving the symptom, but also of the patient outcomes that result from experience with the symptom. Symptoms experienced by patients with kidney failure affect not only physical functioning, but also psychological and social functioning. Moreover, when patients avoid addressing the symptoms they experience, physical and mental functioning is often negatively affected (Curtin, Bultman, Thomas-Hawkins, Walters, & Schatell, 2002; Curtin, Sitter, Schatell, & Chewning, 2004; Welch & Austin, 2001). The best time to evaluate nursing interventions to prevent, reduce, or relieve a symptom and the outcomes that result from the symptom is unknown. Functioning among HD patients fluctuates and depends upon the number of days between treatments or whether it's the first, second, or third treatment in a given week. For example, functioning is lower on the day before the first HD session of a week compared to the previous day. Moreover, functioning is lower on the second dialysis day of the week compared to previous and subsequent nondialysis days (Thomas-Hawkins, 2000). These findings suggest that nurses should pay careful attention to when they evaluate the outcomes of symptom management interventions.

This chapter presents an overview of symptom management models that have been formulated to promote more accurate and effective symptom management. Instruments for assessing general symptoms are reviewed; these instruments contain lists of symptoms experienced by individuals with kidney failure and can be used to conduct comprehensive symptom assessment. Finally, the definition, assessment, etiologies, and interventions for three symptoms are discussed: fatigue, pruritus, and thirst. These three symptoms are included because there is existing empirical evidence applicable to the patient with kidney failure. Although other symptoms such as anorexia, constipation, dyspnea, nausea, and pain are frequently reported in patients with kidney failure, no reported studies have evaluated these symptoms in patients with kidney failure. Most of this chapter focuses on patients receiving traditional, three-times-a-week HD because literature was available about these patients. Patients receiving other renal replacement therapies were included when literature was available.

Symptom Management Models

Five symptom management models have been proposed to assist nurses when helping patients manage their symptoms. These models include the Symptom Self-Care Response Model (Sorofman, Tripp-Reimer, Lauer, & Martin, 1990), the Model of Somatic Interpretation (Cioffi, 1991), the

Symptom Interpretation Model (Teel, Meek, McNamara, & Watson, 1997), the Middle-Range Theory of Unpleasant Symptoms (Lenz et al., 1997), and the Symptom Management Model (UCSF, 1994; Dodd et al., 2001). A brief description of each model follows.

The Symptom Self-Care Response Model

The Symptom Self-Care Response Model (Sorofman et al., 1990) focuses on the individual and his or her response to the symptom experience. In this model, patients examine changes in health status that they perceive as abnormal in six stages. In the first stage, symptom recognition, an individual recognizes a change in physical, psychological, or social functioning. During symptom evaluation, the second stage, individuals attach labels to explain an unexpected or unexplainable symptom. During this stage, individuals determine the impact of the symptom on social roles. In the third stage, consultation, individuals decide whether or not to treat the symptom. During this stage, information or skills needed to manage the symptom are requested from professional and nonprofessional sources. During the fourth stage, treatment consideration, specific interventions are selected and ways to avoid related symptoms are considered. The fifth stage, treatment implementation, occurs when individuals select and use an intervention or interventions. The final stage, symptom outcome, occurs when the effectiveness of an intervention is evaluated and/or a new intervention is selected.

When nephrology nurses use the Symptom Self-Care Response Model, the dynamic nature of symptom recognition and treatment is assessed. The model prompts the nurse to assess for symptoms the patient may be experiencing, the interventions that have been selected for use, and how effective these interventions were in treating the symptom.

Model of Somatic Interpretation

The Model of Somatic Interpretation (Cioffi, 1991) is a cognitive-perceptual model focusing on the awareness of physical sensations, what is felt, and how individuals feel about the sensation. Physical sensations are labeled, interpreted, and responded to when an individual becomes aware of them. Attributions, goals, coping behaviors, previous hypotheses, and consequences affect how much attention is given to a physical sensation and the extent to which the individual perceives the sensation as a threatening event. Perception of somatic information may also be influenced by the situation and by the behavior of others.

When using the Model of Somatic Interpretation in clinical practice, the nephrology nurse would assess for a specific symptom. In particular, the nurse would focus on explaining what the symptom means to the patient, how it feels, and whether it is perceived as a threat to his or her well-being.

Symptom Interpretation Model

The Symptom Interpretation Model (Teel et al., 1997) also focuses on the meaning attached to a symptom. The underlying meaning is thought to be crucial to understanding decisions in response to the symptom. An assumption in this model is that patients have control over their behavioral, cognitive/intellectual, and emotional responses to a symp-

tom experience. There are three major constructs in the model: input, interpretation, and outcome. Input refers to a recognition of a symptom, interpretation involves naming and attaching meaning to a sensation, and outcome refers to the decision an individual makes to do something or do nothing about the symptom. In this model, the consequences of the responses to a symptom experience provide information for future symptom interpretations.

The nephrology nurse would assess for a specific symptom when using the symptom interpretation model. Similar to the Model of Somatic Interpretation, the meaning of the symptom is assessed. In addition, the self-care behaviors a patient uses in response to the symptom are assessed.

The Middle-Range Theory of Unpleasant Symptoms

The Middle-Range Theory of Unpleasant Symptoms (Lenz et al., 1997) also has three major components: symptoms, influencing factors, and consequences. This model asserts that, although symptoms may occur alone, more often individuals experience multiple, concurrent symptoms and that similar interventions may relieve more than one symptom. In this model, the symptom experience is a multidimensional phenomenon that can be described in terms of intensity, distress, timing, and quality. Antecedents to a symptom include physiologic factors such as existing pathology or nutritional status, psychological factors such as mental state or mood, and situational factors such as marital status or social support. In this model, the antecedent factors affect each other as well as the symptom experience. Consequences of the symptom experience include functional status, cognitive functioning, and physical performance. In this feedback model, consequences affect both the symptom experience and antecedents.

The nephrology nurse would use the Middle-Range Theory of Unpleasant Symptoms to help explain a symptom. In addition, the nurse would explore how the symptom affects functioning.

The Symptom Management Model

The Symptom Management Model (UCSF, 1994; Dodd et al., 2001) focuses on three interrelated dimensions common to a variety of symptoms: (a) the symptom experience, (b) symptom management strategies, and (c) symptom outcomes. The major premise of the theory is that all three dimensions must be considered to manage a symptom effectively. The symptom experience has two important components, symptom evaluation and response. Symptom evaluation refers to how people describe their symptoms, for example, in terms of distress, duration, frequency, and intensity. Evaluation of each dimension of a symptom is important in the model. For example, some patients may experience a symptom as less intense, but so frequent as to cause considerable distress. Conversely, some patients may experience a symptom less often, but when it occurs it is very intense and distressing. The inherent threat of a symptom, such as whether or not it is dangerous or disabling, is also evaluated in this dimension. Symptom response includes physiological, emotional, and/or behavioral reactions to a particular symptom, such as physical, cognitive, or affective alterations. The symptom experience in this model influences both symptom management and symptom outcomes. The second dimension of the symptom management model, symptom management strategies, follows assessment of the symptom experience. Successful management of the symptom usually requires a partnership of the patient, family, health care provider, and health care system to identify possible management strategies and, in turn, whether the patient is willing and/or able to implement these strategies. Symptom outcomes are the third dimension of the symptom management model and include costs, emotional status, functional status, self-care ability, comorbidity, quality of life, morbidity, and mortality. Symptom outcomes influence both the symptom experience and self-management strategies.

Nephrology nurses using the Symptom Management Model would assess multiple components of a particular symptom to gain understanding. The nurse would design or develop self-management strategies and may seek to involve the family members of the individual. A comprehensive evaluation of outcomes would occur.

Summary of Symptom Management Models

The five symptom management models are not inconsistent with one another. Each model provides a valuable perspective and can be used according to one's purpose, whether it is a research or practice goal. However, the decision to use one model or another to guide practice will affect subsequent decisions of the nurse in the assessment, intervention, and evaluation of a patient's symptom. For example, it would not be appropriate to use a symptom checklist to assess symptoms or the dimensions of a symptom if the Model of Somatic Interpretation (Cioffi, 1991) was guiding clinical practice because the model focuses on the process of awareness and how the individual feels about a particular sensation.

General Symptom Measures

Many tools have been used to assess symptoms in patients with kidney failure. When deciding whether or not to use a tool in clinical practice, the nurse needs to pay attention to its reliability and validity. Reliability, often defined as consistency or stability, is often reported in one or two different ways. Internal consistency reliability tells the nurse how well the items in a tool relate to one another, a characteristic that is desirable if the items are supposed to measure the same concept. Internal consistency reliability is often reported using Cronbach's alpha. In general, an acceptable level of Cronbach's alpha is greater than .70 (Nunnally & Bernstein, 1994). The second measure of reliability, test-retest, refers to how stable scores on a tool are over short periods of time. Generally, a satisfactory level for test-retest reliability is .70 or above (Polit & Beck, 2004). Validity is concerned with whether the items in a tool are assessing what is intended. There are three methods that are often used to determine validity: content, criterion, and construct (DeVellis, 2003). Content validity is usually assessed by having content experts review the items in a tool. Criterion-related validity simply refers to whether the instrument or assessment tool is related to a "gold standard" or, in other words, if another established tool were used to assess the same thing, would scores on the two different assessment tools be

statistically related to one another? Construct validity is theory driven and often assessed by determining whether proposed theoretical relationships are consistently and statistically demonstrated.

Another term that is often used when discussing assessment tools is sensitivity or responsiveness to change (Puhan, Brant, Guyatt, Heels-Ansdell, & Schunemann, 2005). This simply means, for example, that if we expect a change to occur following an intervention, we want the assessment tool to be able to capture that change. For more detail on reliability and validity, there are several texts written on these properties (Carmines & Zeller, 1979; DeVellis, 2003; Nunnally, 1978; Nunnally & Bernstein, 1994).

The nurse should carefully select the tool or tools to be used in clinical practice. Reliable and valid tools that are sensitive to changes in the patient will assist the nurse in symptom management.

Symptoms experienced by patients with kidney failure have been assessed in a number of ways. Often investigators develop their own tools to assess symptoms in dialysis patients. For example, Virga and colleagues (1998) assessed the frequency of occurrence of 14 symptoms in HD patients, Friedrich (1980) assessed the distress associated with 20 symptoms in HD patients, and Merkus and colleagues (1999) assessed 9 symptoms in HD and peritoneal dialysis (PD) patients. In addition, many instruments to evaluate health-related quality of life (Hays, Kallich, Mapes, Coons, & Carter, 1994; Laupacis, Muirhead, Keown, & Wong, 1992; Rao et al., 2000), and stressors of dialysis patients (Baldree, Murphy, & Powers, 1982) have embedded items that pertain to symptoms.

Two published instruments assessing overall symptoms in dialysis patients have been reported: the Symptom Assessment Index (Parfrey et al., 1987; Parfrey et al., 1989; Parfrey, Vavasour, & Gault, 1988) and the Dialysis Symptom Index (Weisbord et al., 2004). The Symptom Assessment Index measures 12 symptoms including fatigue, muscle weakness, headaches, cramps, pruritus, dyspnea, angina, lack of sleep, joint pain, nausea/vomiting, stomach pain, and an "other" category. Patients rate the intensity of the symptoms on a 5-point response scale from absent to very severe. Content validity has not been reported. Evidence of construct validity was supported by differences in symptoms between dialysis and transplant patients. Although there were no changes in symptom scores among HD or transplant patients who did not change kidney failure therapy over the course of 1 year, symptom scores improved in newly transplanted patients, indicating that the instrument was sensitive to change.

The Dialysis Symptom Index (DSI) (Weisbord et al., 2004) assesses 30 symptoms including, for example, appetite, constipation, nausea, muscle cramps, and shortness of breath. The degree to which the symptoms are perceived as "bothersome" is measured on 5-point response scales from not at all to very much. Content validity was assessed by experts in health-related quality of life, kidney failure, and clinical nephrologists. Test-retest reliability was reported as .48. No data are available about sensitivity to change.

In summary, a list of symptoms is presented to patients

in each of these two instruments. Each instrument measures only one symptom dimension, either intensity or distress. The instruments show initial evidence of reliability and validity, but there is little evidence about sensitivity to change. Assessing the overall symptom experience of a patient with kidney failure may be useful in clinical practice. Nurses could use these entire instruments to help establish priorities of care.

Fatigue

Fatigue has been variously defined as a "decreased capacity for physical and mental work" (Potempa, Lopez, Reid, & Lawson, 1986, p. 165) and as a "subjective, unpleasant symptom which incorporates total body feelings ranging from tiredness to exhaustion creating an unrelenting overall condition which interferes with individuals' ability to function in their normal capacity" (Ream & Richardson, 1996, p. 527). Estimates of fatigue are from 61%-82% for patients receiving HD (Merkus et al., 1999; Parfrey et al., 1989), 87% for patients receiving PD (Merkus et al., 1999), and 23% for patients with a functioning transplant (Parfrey et al., 1989). Moderate to severe levels of fatigue distress are experienced by 50% of patients with kidney failure (Friedrich, 1980).

Postdialysis fatigue is described as an intermittent fatigue experienced soon after HD treatment (Sklar, Riensenberg, Silber, Ahmed, & Ali, 1996; Sklar, Newman, Scott, Semenyuk, & Fiacco, 1999), but a precise conceptual definition of postdialysis fatigue is not available. Approximately 50% of patients experience postdialysis fatigue, and in those patients this fatigue occurs following 80% of their HD treatments, with 65% reporting that postdialysis fatigue began with the first HD treatment (Sklar et al., 1996).

Assessment

Various instruments have been used to measure fatigue in research studies with patients with kidney failure. The instruments are grouped into four categories: single-item measures, multiple-item scales measuring one dimension of fatigue, multiple-item instruments measuring more than one dimension of fatigue, and instruments used to assess postdialysis fatigue.

Single-item measure. A visual analogue scale has been used to assess fatigue intensity. Patients are asked to rate their fatigue on a scale from no tiredness at all to complete exhaustion (Brunier & Graydon, 1996; McCann & Boore, 2000; Tsay, 2004). Criterion-related validity for this scale was supported by high correlations with the fatigue-inertia subscale contained within the Profile of Mood States (Brunier & Graydon, 1996) and with the Piper Fatigue Scale (Piper, 1997). One major advantage of single-item measures is that they are short and easily applied to a busy clinical practice area.

Unidimensional subscales. Unidimensional scales or subscales are often short assessment tools that measure one thing, such as fatigue intensity. Several unidimensional subscales are embedded in general instruments. Those used in patients with kidney failure include the vitality subscale of the SF-36 developed by Ware, Kosinski, and Gandek (2000) and the fatigue-inertia subscale contained within the Profile of Mood States (McNair, Lorr, & Droppleman, 1981).

The vitality subscale of the SF-36 contains four items measuring frequency of fatigue. Frequency is measured on 6-point response scales from none of the time to all of the time (Ware, Kosinski, & Gandek, 2000). A Cronbach's alpha of .89 was reported in a sample of HD patients (McCann & Boore, 2000).

The fatigue-inertia subscale assesses fatigue intensity. Fatigue is assessed on 5-point response scales from not at all to extremely. A Cronbach's alpha of .95 was reported in dialysis patients (Brunier & Graydon, 1996). Test-retest reliability has been reported as .74 in cancer patients (Meek et al., 2000), but there is no evidence about stability in patients with kidney failure. Criterion-related validity was supported by high correlations with a visual analogue scale measuring fatigue intensity (Brunier & Graydon, 1996). Construct validity has been supported by high correlations with mood, pain, and performance status in patients with cancer (Cassileth et al., 1985; Glover, Dibble, Dodd, & Miaskowski, 1995; Jamar, 1989; Meek et al., 2000), but has not been determined for patients with kidney failure. In addition, there are no data about sensitivity to change among patients with kidney failure.

The fatigue subscale of the Kidney Disease Questionnaire (KDQ) (Laupacis et al., 1992) assesses how much of a problem the fatigue is on 7-point response scales from no problem to severe problem. No reliability or validity information has been reported. In one study, scores changed over a 24-week period of intravenous carnitine therapy (Brass et al., 2001), indicating the scale's sensitivity to change.

Multiple-item, multidimensional scales. Several multiple-item, multidimensional scales are available to assess fatigue. Those used in patients with kidney failure include the Multidimensional Fatigue Inventory (MFI-20) developed by Smets and colleagues (1995) and the Piper Fatigue Scale developed by Piper and colleagues (1989).

The MFI-20 is a 20-item scale with subscales measuring general fatigue, physical fatigue, reduced activity, mental fatigue, and reduced motivation subscales. Cronbach's alphas for the subscales ranged from .52 to .82 in samples of dialysis patients (McCann & Boore, 2000) and from .60 to .87 in caregivers of dialysis patients (Schneider, 2001). Although there is no evidence about construct validity in patients with kidney failure, the scale correlated with measures of mood, activities of daily living, and emotional distress in cancer patients (Meek et al., 2000; Smets, Garssen, Cull, & de Haes, 1996).

The Piper Fatigue Scale is a 41-item scale that assesses the temporal, affective, sensory, and intensity domains of fatigue. The perceived cause, relief measures, and associated symptoms are assessed using three open-ended items. A visual analogue scale is embedded in the instrument (Piper, 1997). The Cronbach's alpha for the total scale was reported to be .92 in a sample of dialysis patients (Tsay, 2004), with subscales ranging from .69 to .95 in patients with cancer (Berger & Walker, 2001; Piper, Dodd, Paul, Welcer, 1989). Content validity was supported. Evidence of construct validity in cancer patients was supported by high correlations between the Profile of Mood States subscales and the Fatigue Symptom Checklist (Piper et al., 1989). A significant change in fatigue following an acupuncture intervention (Tsay, 2004) provided evidence that it is sensitive to change.

Scales to assess postdialysis fatigue. Three different ways to assess postdialysis fatigue have been reported. First, a Fatigue Index Questionnaire developed by Sklar and colleagues (1996) has been used (Dreisbach, Hendrickson, Beezhold, Riesenberg, & Sklar, 1998; Sklar et al., 1996), but no description of the scale is available. Second, a summed score calculated from the hours of sleep and the hours of fatigue for up to 6 hours after each dialysis (Sklar, Beezhold, Newman, Hendrickson, & Dreisbach, 1998) was reported, but no other data are available. Finally, a single item on a 5-point intensity scale was developed, with response options of *none, mild* (noticeable but without effect), *moderate* (felt sluggish), *severe* (required rest), and *overwhelming* (slept) (Sklar et al., 1999). There is no evidence about reliability or validity for these measures.

The decision about which fatigue instrument to use depends on the purpose of the clinical assessment and the instrument's psychometric properties. Single-item and unidimensional scales can be used to assess the severity of fatigue and evaluate the effectiveness of interventions to relieve this symptom. Single-item measures provide a global measure of fatigue severity and do not tire patients, but they do not provide information about which dimensions of the fatigue experience are affected. Unidimensional scales offer different descriptors of fatigue so respondents can choose the one best describing their experience. Multidimensional scales are useful by providing a comprehensive assessment of the patients' experience with fatigue, which may be more helpful for planning care and evaluating its effectiveness. In general, nurses working in the clinical setting can evaluate items in any given scale to determine which scale best captures the patient's symptom experience. A complete and appropriate assessment will help the nurse select or design intervention strategies.

Etiologies of Fatigue

There are many possible etiologies for fatigue in dialysis patients. These include the side effects of medications, poor nutrition, physiological alterations, psychological factors, sleep disorders, and factors relating to HD treatment itself.

Medications. Fatigue is a side effect of many antihypertensive medications. Antihypertensive medication may contribute to the fatigue experience of patients with kidney failure (Sklar et al., 1996).

Nutrition. L-carnitine insufficiency (Brass et al., 2001; Wanner & Horl, 1988) and protein and energy malnutrition (Ikizler & Hakim, 1996; Lindsay, Heidenheim, Spanner, Kortas, & Blake, 1994) are thought to contribute to fatigue in patients with kidney failure. L-carnitine helps oxidize fatty acids, which are used by skeletal and cardiac muscles as a major source of energy, and carnitine administration has been successful in reducing fatigue in dialysis patients (Brass et al., 2001). In malnutrition, a reduction in essential metabolites and loss of muscle mass may result in abnormal muscle function (Smets, Garssen, Schuster-Uitterhoeve, & de Haes, 1993).

Physiological. Physiological variables that may contribute to fatigue include anemia, uremia, and peripheral neuropathy (Blank, Gonen, Zilberman, & Magora, 1986). Reduced erythropoietin production (National Kidney Foundation [NKF], 2000a) causes anemia, reducing oxygen supply to tissues, and is thought to be a major contributor to fatigue in patients with kidney failure; however, not all patients with kidney failure who are anemic have fatigue (Srivastava, 1986). Uremia is also thought to influence fatigue in patients requiring dialysis and fatigue decreases following a kidney transplant (Parfrey et al., 1988).

Psychological factors. Depression may cause fatigue in patients on dialysis, especially for those who experience fatigue upon rising (Cardenas & Kutner, 1982). Flat affect, often considered a symptom of depression, may also contribute to fatigue in patients with kidney failure (Barrett, Vasavour, Major, & Parfrey, 1990).

Sleep disorders. Poor sleep patterns may contribute to the fatigue experienced by patients with kidney failure (Brunier & Graydon, 1993). Disturbances of sleep are extremely common in dialysis patients (Hui et al., 2002; Parker, 2003), and daytime sleepiness is also common even on nondialysis days (Parker, Bliwise, Bailey, & Rye, 2003).

HD treatment. There is some evidence to suggest that exponential, linear, or step sodium modeling may be preferable to constant dialysate sodium. Patients who receive a constant dialysate sodium of 138 mEq/L were shown to have more fatigue than those receiving sodium modeling beginning at 148 mEq/L and decreased by exponential, linear, or a step program to 138 mEq/L (Sadowski, Allred, & Jabs, 1993).

Etiologies of Postdialysis Fatigue

Several etiologies of postdialysis fatigue have also been proposed. These include excessive ultrafiltration, decreased osmolality during dialysis (Driesbach et al., 1998), and an increase in tumor necrosis factor (Driesbach et al., 1998; Sklar et al., 1998; Sklar et al., 1999). Use of a high sodium dialysate may reduce postdialysis fatigue (Sklar et al., 1999).

Interventions

Several independent nursing interventions have been suggested to reduce fatigue in dialysis patients. These include nutritional, sleep, and alternative therapy interventions.

Medications. Nurses may want to review the medications a patient is receiving to determine if any have the side effect of fatigue. Advocating for a potential change in medication may help decrease the fatigue experienced by the patient who has kidney failure.

Nutrition. An adequate intake of protein and calories should be encouraged. The K/DOQI guidelines recommend a protein intake of 1.2 gm per kg body weight per day and suggest a dietary energy intake of 35 kcal per kg body weight per day in individuals under 60 years of age and 30 to 35 kcal per kg body weight for those over 60 (NKF, 2000). Psychoeducational strategies to increase protein and caloric intake may include tailoring messages to reduce the perceived barriers and to increase the perceived benefits of implementing dietary recommendations, teaching patients how to self-monitor intake, or suggesting ways to improve the taste of food.

Physiological. Anemia management is a priority when

caring for patients with kidney failure. Administering prescribed medications is imperative. Careful monitoring of monthly laboratory work for the patient's response to medical therapy is essential.

Equally important is assessing the dialysis prescription to determine that patients are receiving the total dose of dialysis that is prescribed (NKF, 2001). Approximately 20% of patients shorten HD treatments and 7% skip treatments (Gordon, Leon, & Sehgal, 2003). Identifying the reasons why patients shorten or skip treatment may help nurses develop interventions to reduce barriers and improve the receipt of an adequate dialysis dose (Gordon et al., 2003).

Psychological. Depression symptoms occur frequently in patients with kidney failure (Lopes et al., 2004), and nurses may need to consider routine depression screening for patients who are experiencing fatigue. Instruments that are commonly used to screen for depression symptoms in dialysis patients are the Beck Depression Inventory (Beck & Beamesderfer, 1974) and the Center for Epidemiologic Studies Depression Scale (CES-D) (Comstock & Helsing, 1976; Radloff, 1977). A positive depression screen may indicate the need for referral to a mental health care provider.

Sleep and waking patterns. The nurse should conduct a complete assessment of sleep patterns and/or disturbances (Hopkins, 2005; Locking-Cusolito, Huyge, & Strangio, 2001; Parker, 1997). Rogers (1997a) suggests that the assessment should include a sleep history with the patient and his/her bed partner, including a description of the sleep problem and a 24-hour evaluation of sleep/wake patterns.

This intervention category also may include interventions that encourage better sleep. Sleep hygiene, wake-promoting diversional activities during HD, and limits placed on daytime naps may promote better sleep patterns (Parker, Bliwise, & Rye, 2000). There are numerous sleep hygiene interventions suggested by Rogers (1997b) and Locking-Cusolito et al. (2001). These sleep hygiene interventions include: avoidance of caffeine after noon, no alcohol in the evening, no smoking just before bedtime, regular exercise, maintenance of a regular time for bedtime and awakening, no napping during the day, dark and quiet bedroom, comfortable bedroom temperature, a sleep preparation routine, and the use of the bedroom for sleep or sexual activity only (Rogers, 1997b).

Alternative therapies. Alternative therapies such as acupuncture (Tsay, 2004) have been empirically tested, and acupuncture is the only intervention that has been investigated for its efficacy in reducing fatigue in patients with kidney failure. In a randomized controlled study of 106 patients with kidney failure, fatigue was significantly reduced in those patients receiving an acupuncture intervention (Tsay, 2004). Similar findings were obtained by Cho and Tsay (2004) in a pretest-posttest design with 62 HD patients.

In summary, most of the interventions to reduce or alleviate fatigue are based on clinical experience or trial and error; few have been systematically investigated by research. Future research is needed to determine whether fatigue is responsive to nursing interventions in the dialysis population.

Outcomes

Patients with kidney failure may experience many negative consequences associated with fatigue. Fatigue negatively affects physical and emotional functioning (Curtin et al., 2002). Fatigue may exacerbate depression, reduce quality of life, and alter role performance (McCann & Boore, 2000; Sklar et al., 1996). Nurses working with these patients should consider intervening to reduce the negative consequences of fatigue.

Pruritus

Pruritus, defined as generalized itching and often referred to as uremic pruritus or renal itch, is a common symptom experienced by dialysis patients. Uremic pruritus has been additionally defined as pruritus that occurs shortly before beginning dialysis therapy or any time after dialysis begins, with no other active disease to explain the symptom (Zucker, Yosipovitch, David, Gafter, & Boner, 2003). Pruritus is estimated to occur in 45% to 90% of HD patients (Goicoechea, de Sequera, Ochando, Andrea, & Caramelo, 1999; Kato, Hamada, Maruyama, Maruyama, & Hishida, 2000; Merkus et al., 1999; Parfrey et al., 1989; Subach & Marx, 2002; Vergili-Nelson, 2003; Virga et al., 1998; Virga, Visentin, La Milia, & Bonadonna, 2002; Zakrzewska-Pneiwska & Jedras, 2001; Zucker et al., 2003) and in 68% of patients receiving PD (Merkus et al., 1999). Approximately 40%-50% describe moderate to severe levels of distress (Friedrich, 1980). The most frequently reported sites of itching are the back, legs, abdomen, arms, face, chest, buttocks, and head (Subach & Marx, 2002; Yosipovitch & Boner, 1997; Zucker et al., 2003). Uremic pruritus often occurs daily, gets worse at night, and does not worsen during HD (Zucker et al., 2003).

Assessment

Numerous instruments have been used to measure pruritus in research studies with patients with kidney failure. The instruments are grouped into two categories: single-item measures and a multidimensional instrument measuring more than one dimension of pruritus. Pruritus has been assessed most often using single-item scales.

Single-item measures. Single-item measures have been used to measure pruritus in a number of ways. In some studies, patients were asked to rate pruritus on a visual analogue scale from no itch to severe itch (Kato et al., 2000) or from no itch to worst possible itch (Subach & Marx, 2002). A 3-point response scale with options of absent, moderate, and severe was used by Virga and colleagues (2002). In another study, pruritus intensity was measured on a 4-point response scale with responses of absent to every day, severe, or major problem (Zakrzewska-Pneiwska & Jedras, 2001). Patients have also rated intensity of pruritus on 5-point scales from absent to severe and constant, disturbing work and sleep (Kato et al., 2000) or from rarely to most of the time and interferes with rest and activity (Yoshimoto-Futuro et al., 1999). A graded 5-point response scale from slight itch without scratching to pruritus with total restlessness (Pauli-Magnus et al., 2000) was used in another study. Finally, an open-ended question was used in which patients were asked to indicate the intensity and discomfort of their pruritus experience using one or more sentences (Jimenez, Monte, El-Mir, Pascual, & Marin, 2002).

Several measures have been used to assess duration, location, and frequency of pruritus. A visual analogue scale was used to assess pruritus duration from no feeling to full time feeling for one day (Kato et al., 2000). Location was assessed by Pauli-Magnus and colleagues (2000) using a 3-point response scale: less than 2 locations, more than 2 locations, and generalized. Finally, frequency was assessed on a 3-point scale with responses of never, occasionally, and every day (Virga et al., 2002).

Four different visual analogue scales were used by Zucker and colleagues (2003). These scales assessed the intensity of pruritus during four different situations: at the time of data collection, pruritus at its worst, pruritus at its best, and after a mosquito bite.

Multiple-item, multidimensional scale. One multidimensional instrument was found that assesses pruritus in patients with kidney failure (Yosipovitch et al., 2001). This instrument, adapted from the short form of the McGill Pain Questionnaire, was tested in 145 patients with pruritus. The instrument contains open-ended questions on frequency, duration, concurrent circumstances, and accompanying symptoms. In addition, verbal descriptors of the itch are elicited and affective sensations are assessed. The instrument also includes a visual analogue scale for intensity. There was no significant difference in scores 2 weeks apart for verbal descriptors, affective sensations, or site of the itch. In addition, 2-week test-retest reliability of the visual analogue scale was high (r = .72).

The nurses' decision about which pruritus instrument to use in clinical practice should depend upon the purpose of the assessment and the instrument's psychometric properties. Unfortunately, the reliability and validity of the single, global items measuring pruritus were not evaluated or reported in any of the sources included in this review. Single-item measures provide valuable information about the intensity of a symptom; assessing test-retest reliability and construct validity, however, is important in order to determine whether the single item (Youngblut & Casper, 1993) accurately assesses pruritus. The major advantage of a single item to measure pruritus is less burden on the patient. In addition, single-item measures provide a quick and easy way to measure pruritus in clinical practice. The multidimensional scale provides useful and comprehensive information about patients' experience with pruritus, which may help in planning and delivering care and evaluating its effectiveness.

Etiologies of Pruritus

The exact mechanism inducing pruritus in patients with kidney failure is unknown, although many potential causes have been proposed. These include medications, environmental conditions, nutritional alterations, physiological changes, reactions to products used during dialysis, and changes in the integument.

Medications. In one study (Zucker et al., 2003), pruritus occurred more commonly in patients who received ACE inhibitors. This same study found that those who had received furosemide did not experience pruritus while taking the medication.

Environmental conditions. One environmental condition may contribute to pruritus. High levels of air temperature have been reported to exacerbate pruritus (Zucker et al., 2003).

Nutritional alterations. Elevated Vitamin A has been proposed as a potential etiology for pruritus in patients with kidney failure (Berne, Vahlquist, Fisher, Danielson, & Berne, 1984). However, although increased epidermal levels of retinol, or pre-formed vitamin A, were shown in kidney failure, no relationship was found with pruritus (Stahle-Backdahl, 1995).

Physiological alterations. The role of metabolic alterations as the origin of pruritus is still unknown (Vanholder & De Smet, 1999), although many possibilities have been proposed. These include hypercalcemia, hypermagnesemia, hyperphosphatemia, uremia, accumulation of bile acids, amplified mast cell production, high calcium-phosphate product, inadequate dialysis, middle molecule accumulation, neuron-specific enolase, and secondary hyperparathyroidism (Crawford, Sands, & Neiwirth, 2000; Goicoechea et al., 1999; Jimenez et al., 2002; Klein, Klein, Hanno, & Callen, 1988; Kyriazis & Glotsos, 2000). Some studies suggest that persons who receive more adequate HD have less pruritus (Goicoechea et al., 1999), but others do not (Zucker et al., 2003). Some have found evidence that a high calcium-phosphate product is associated with more pruritus (Chou, Ho, Huang, & Sheen-Chen, 2000), but others have not (Stahle-Backdahl, 1995). In addition, although mast cells multiply in renal failure and play an important roll in the release of histamines (Cohen, Russell, & Garancis, 1992), an increase in mast cells has not been shown to increase pruritus (Klein et al., 1988). Finally, Goicoechea and colleagues (1999) found no significant difference in serum phosphorus levels in patients with and without pruritus.

Reactions to products used during dialysis. Contact with substances used in dialysis treatment has also been proposed as contributing to pruritus. These may include particular dialyzing membranes or the use of porcine heparin.

Changes in the integument. Dry skin and sweat have been reported to make pruritus worse in HD patients (Zucker et al., 2003). A decrease in the function of sweat and oil glands in patients with kidney failure is often thought to contribute to pruritus as is the presence of dry skin. Kato and colleagues (2000) reported that, although the water content of skin was less in dialysis patients, there was no relationship between water content and pruritus intensity.

Interventions

A variety of independent nursing interventions have been suggested to reduce pruritus. These include a review of medications, nutritional interventions, skin care regimens, changes in the environment, alternative therapies, and those related to the dialysis procedure.

Medications. Nurses may want to review the medication list to determine if the patient is receiving an ACE inhibitor. Although only one study reported that ACE inhibitors were associated with pruritus, a reported side effect of ACE inhibitors is pruritus without the presence of a skin rash (Zucker et al., 2003).

Nutritional. Nutritional dietary supplements, such as

fish oil, have been proposed as a possible intervention for pruritus (Vergili-Nelson, 2003). In one study of 25 patients, there was a nonsignificant reduction in pruritus intensity and distribution in participants receiving fish oil compared to those receiving olive or safflower oil (Peck, Monsen, & Ahmad, 1996). Further work in this area is recommended (Vergili-Nelson, 2003). In addition, clinicians are advised to promote adherence to both dietary phosphorus restriction and the prescribed phosphate binders by recommending various visual or auditory cues (Crawford et al., 2000). Changing dietary behavior and promoting medication adherence, however, have not been studied in the kidney failure patient population.

Skin care. A variety of skin care recommendations have been given to patients in an effort to reduce pruritus. For example, patients are often advised to cleanse daily; use cornstarch, baking soda, or oatmeal baths; avoid very hot bath water; use calamine lotion and daily emollients; and wear cotton clothing (Crawford et al., 2000). Goicoechea and colleagues (1999) found no differences between the efficacy of emollients and antihistamines in reducing pruritus in 73 HD patients. However, when emollients and antihistamines were used together, pruritus was totally resolved in 38%, partially resolved in 48%, and not resolved in 14% of the patients. Hot and cold showers have also been reported to reduce pruritus (Zucker et al., 2003). Whether or not these showers need to alternate hot and cold or be either hot or cold is not clear.

Environmental. Particular changes in the home environment are also recommended for patients with pruritus and kidney failure. Patients are often encouraged to install and use home humidifiers. In addition, for those patients doing their own laundry, laundry detergents without perfume are recommended (Crawford et al., 2000). Encouraging patients to avoid extreme temperature may also be helpful.

Alternative therapies. Alternative therapies have been suggested that include aromatherapy (Ro, Ha, Kim, & Yeom, 2002), phototherapy (ultraviolet light) (Cohen et al., 1992; Hindson, Taylor, Martin, & Downey, 1981), or the use of a TENS unit (Robertson & Mueller, 1996). Ro and colleagues (2002) found significant reduction in pruritus scores in a sample of 29 HD patients who received aromatherapy three times per week for 4 weeks. Hindson and colleagues reported a reduction in pruritus for patients receiving phototherapy, although Cohen et al. (1992) did not.

Dialysis procedure. Adherence to the prescribed dose of dialysis is often poor in the United States. As mentioned, some patients shorten treatments and others skip treatments altogether (Bleyer et al., 1999; Gordon et al., 2003; Saran et al., 2003). Efforts to promote adherence to the prescribed dose of dialysis are often recommended to reduce pruritus (Daugirdas, Blake, & Todd, 2001). Medical problems during HD, such as cramping; technical problems during treatment, such as clotting of the extracorporeal circuit; and transportation problems have all been reported as possible explanations for reduced or skipped treatment. Assessing why patients skip treatment may help nurses develop effective interventions to reduce these problems, promote greater adherence to the HD procedure, and reduce pruritus (Gordon et al., 2003).

In summary, most of the interventions to reduce or alleviate pruritus are based on clinical experience or trial and error; few have been systematically investigated by research. Future research is needed to determine whether pruritus is responsive to nursing care in the dialysis population.

Outcomes

Nurses should deliberately assess and evaluate the negative outcomes patients experience as a result of pruritus. Changes in mood (Zucker et al., 2003), interference with daytime activity (Goicoechea et al., 1999; Zucker et al., 2003), sleep disturbances (Goicoechea et al., 1999; Ro, Ha, Kim, & Yeom, 2002; Yosipovitch & Boner, 1997; Zucker et al., 2003), nervousness, depression (Yosipovitch & Boner, 1997), and physical functioning (Curtin et al., 2002) have been reported. In addition, reduced quality of life, skin excoriation as a result of scratching, and even suicide are potential outcomes (Headley & Wall, 2002).

Thirst

Thirst has been defined as a conscious desire for water (Guyton & Hall, 1996), a desire to drink caused by a deficit in fluid (Greenleaf, 1992), a drive to drink water (Thompson & Baylis, 1988), a desire for fluid that is not ignorable and causes a behavioral drive to drink (Toto, 1994), a conscious need to obtain and drink water (Porth & Erickson, 1992), and a conscious and subjective sensation of desiring fluids (Welch, 2002). In contrast, a nonregulatory thirst has been described that is based on social cues and personal habits (Woodtli, 1990). Some research indicates that exaggerated thirst begins 4 to 6 hours after a dialysis treatment ends, persists during the interdialytic period, and disappears during the next dialysis (Giovannetti et al., 1994). Others have found that thirst increases during dialysis treatment (Shepherd, Farleigh, Atkinson, & Pryor, 1987).

Thirst is a common problem for individuals receiving HD therapy. Thirst has been reported to occur daily in over 85% of HD patients (Virga et al., 1998), and 30%-86% experience moderate to high levels of thirst intensity (Dominic, Ramachandran, Somiah, Mani, & Dominic, 1996; Giovannetti et al., 1994; Virga et al., 1998).

Assessment

There are few instruments to assess thirst among patients with kidney failure. The instruments are grouped into two separate categories: single-item measures and a unidimensional scale measuring one dimension of thirst.

Single-item measures. Single-item measures have been used to assess thirst intensity in two ways. First, a 100 mm visual analogue scale has been used to assess thirst intensity (Dominic et al., 1996; Martinez-Vea, Garcia, Gaya, Rivera, & Oliver, 1992; Welch, 2002; Welch, Perkins, Evans, & Bajpai, 2003; Wirth & Folstein, 1982) ranging from not at all to extremely thirsty. A 125 mm visual analogue scale was also used to assess thirst intensity from no thirst to maximal thirst (Argent, Burrell, Goodship, Wilkinson, & Baylis, 1991). Construct validity was supported by positive relationships with thirst distress (Welch, 2002) and by changes in thirst intensity as serum osmolality changed (Baylis & Thompson, 1988). Another single-item measure used a 4-point response scale to measure intensity of thirst from 0 (no abnormal thirst) to 3 (almost always present and disturbing sleeping and working) (Giovannetti et al., 1994).

Unidimensional scale. A unidimensional scale measuring thirst distress had a Cronbach's alpha of .78 in HD patients (Welch, 2002). A panel of experts in instrument development, symptom management, and nephrology nursing assessed content validity. Construct validity was supported by confirmatory and exploratory factor analysis and by positive relationships between thirst distress and, respectively, thirst intensity and interdialytic weight gain.

Overall, there are few instruments to choose from when assessing thirst in clinical practice. All are brief and do not overly burden the patient with kidney failure. More data are needed to determine their effectiveness for use in clinical practice.

Etiologies of Thirst

Several factors have been suggested as influencing thirst. These include demographic factors, environmental conditions, physiological alterations, psychological/social variables, and factors related to HD treatment.

Demographic factors. The age of an individual has been proposed as a factor that may influence the experience of thirst although findings have been conflicting. In some studies, healthy older adults often rated themselves as less thirsty than younger persons (Miescher & Fortney, 1989; O'Neill & McLean, 1992), although other studies have found no difference (de Castro, 1992). Moreover, when healthy elderly men received hypertonic saline, they reported less thirst intensity than younger men (Phillips, Bretherton, Johnston, & Gray, 1991).

Environmental conditions. Two potentially important environmental variables may contribute to thirst. High levels of humidity and the season of year, particularly when outside temperatures are elevated, may cause more thirst (Tozawa et al., 1999).

Physiological alterations. Several metabolic alterations as the etiology of thirst have been proposed. These include lowered plasma osmolarity, hypovolemia without a corresponding loss of sodium, osmotic shift of water from cells to extracellular fluid induced by excessive intake of sodium, increased levels of arginine vasopressin, hyperglycemia, increased levels of urea, and a decrease in saliva (Andersson, 1987; Argent et al., 1991; Brunstrom, Macrae, & Roberts, 1997; Giovannetti et al., 1994; Kimura, 1989; Rogers & Kurtzman, 1973; Yamamoto et al., 1986).

HD treatment. Many factors associated with dialysis treatment have been investigated as etiologies of thirst. The role of sodium modeling has received the most attention. There are some data indicating that individuals who receive low sodium dialysate during treatment experience less thirst intensity (Dominic et al., 1996) and that exponential sodium modeling is associated with higher interdialytic weight gain (Daugirdas, Al-Kudsi, Ing, & Norusis, 1985; Sang, Kovithavongs, Ulan, & Kjellstrand, 1997).

Medications. The side effect of some medications may also need to be considered as a potential etiology for thirst. Patients may have antihypertensive medications or antihistamines prescribed affecting thirst intensity.

Interventions

A variety of independent nursing interventions have been suggested to reduce or alleviate thirst in dialysis patients. These include nutritional interventions, environmental modifications, moisturizing interventions, and psychological recommendations.

Nutritional. Decreased amounts of dietary sodium are often prescribed to patients with kidney failure. Psycho-educational interventions to help patients reduce salt intake are often implemented, although these strategies have not been empirically tested (Welch & Thomas-Hawkins, 2005). For example, patients report many barriers to implementing a sodium restriction (Welch, Bennett, Delp, & Agarwal, in press). These barriers include the poor taste of food and difficulty in eating in restaurants or away from home. Ways to improve the taste of foods without adding salt or salt substitute and ways to eat at restaurants while following a salt restriction may need to be incorporated into psycho-educational interventions. New and creative cooking interventions may need to be developed to improve the taste of foods for these patients to reduce the experience of thirst. In addition, the ways foods are prepared by African Americans may increase salt intake, for example, when salted meats or bacon fats are added to vegetables (Jones, 1989). Assessing for sodium content that is hidden presents a unique challenge. Moreover, there is some evidence that HD patients have less ability to detect the salty taste of food (Fernstrom, Hylander, & Rossner, 1996), creating a challenging situation for both the patient and care providers when discussing diet alternatives.

Environmental. A variety of environmental recommendations are given to patients to help reduce thirst. For example, patients are often advised to avoid prolonged exposure to outside heat, keep home temperatures moderate, and to use home humidifiers.

Moisturizing. Many strategies to moisturize the mouth are recommended because decreases in saliva are associated with increases in thirst (Brunstrom et al., 1997). For example, recommendations include ice cubes or ice chips, chewing gum, and oral lubricants. Drinking cold water (3°C) may also increase saliva flow and make the mouth feel wetter (Brunstrom et al., 1997).

Psychological. Distraction is often proposed as a strategy to reduce the perception of thirst. Distracting activities include watching television, reading, or engaging in other pleasurable activities.

Unfortunately, most of the foregoing strategies have not been systematically investigated for their efficacy in relieving thirst. In one study (Welch & Davis, 2000), the investigators examined strategies used to limit fluid intake and/or relieve thirst. The use, perceived effectiveness, and plans for future use of 40 self-management strategies were examined. Most patients reported they regularly avoided the sun, took medications with mealtime fluid, limited salt on the foods, avoided salty foods, stayed busy, stayed away from fast food restaurants, drank ice-cold drinks, and drank only when thirsty to reduce fluid intake and relieve thirst. They also planned to use these strategies in the future. The strategies perceived as most effective, however, such as measuring daily allotted fluids in a pitcher to drink from all day, spacing liquids over the entire day, and measuring the fluid they drank, were not the same as those they used the most. A more recent study (Welch, Evans, Juliar, & Agarwal, 2004) found that an increase in the number and perceived effectiveness of fluid management strategies, including those for thirst, were associated with less interdialytic weight gain.

Outcomes

The effects of thirst are multiple. Thirst becomes a significant problem in HD patients when it interferes with adherence to a prescribed fluid limit (Welch et al., in press). In addition, thirst may indirectly affect physical and emotional functioning and also affect social relationships because usual activities may be hindered. Finally, thirst may indirectly increase morbidity and mortality by leading to medical complications such as pulmonary edema. Thirst may also indirectly increase the incidence of pulmonary edema or exaggerated hypertension because of its effect on interdialytic weight gain (Bots et al., 2004).

Summary

Symptom management in patients with kidney failure includes an assessment of symptoms patients are experiencing, the interventions used to treat the symptoms, and evaluation of outcomes. The literature reviewed in this chapter can be summarized by seven key points. First, most of the symptom literature in the kidney failure population focuses on the patient receiving HD. Few studies have focused on individuals who receive PD or transplantation. In addition, the symptom experience of people with chronic kidney disease who do not require a renal replacement therapy has not been reported. Second, individuals diagnosed with kidney failure experience a variety of symptoms. We have not studied the concurrent nature of symptoms experienced by the patient with kidney failure. Third, many instruments were reviewed in this chapter and have initial evidence of reliability and validity. Before widespread use in clinical practice, many need further testing in research studies. Fourth, most nursing interventions are based on conventional wisdom. Few nursing interventions have been empirically evaluated for their effectiveness in managing the various symptoms experienced by the patients with kidney failure. When you consider that the etiologies for the three symptoms that were reviewed were often similar, it's entirely possible that an intervention for the etiology of one symptom may have effects on another, less dominant symptom. Fifth, educational or psychoeducational interventions have not been tested to provide patients with the knowledge and skills needed to recognize and manage the symptoms they experience. Nor have we explored psycho-educational interventions that may be needed to help patients distinguish between the acute and chronic symptoms they experience. Knowledge is a prerequisite to any behavior (Maibach & Cotton, 1995), and empirically tested interventions that include education, self-care skills, and support are needed. Sixth, symptoms interfere with physical, psychological, and social functioning. Inclusion of these outcomes in evaluating the symptom experience will help us improve these quality of life outcomes. Finally, assessing symptoms as an outcome of nursing care is necessary to determine the effectiveness of care in

daily practice. The same instrument used for initial assessment could be used to evaluate effectiveness. Because of the possible patterns in symptoms in HD patients, symptoms should be assessed and evaluated on the same day of the week at approximately the same time, during or after treatment.

The patient with chronic kidney failure has an extremely difficult condition to live with. Nurses must be vigilant in their search for new ways to help patients deal with their symptoms. Preventing, relieving, or reducing the symptoms patients experience will help improve the quality of life in these patients.

Acknowledgments — The author would like to thank Roberta Delp, MSN, RN, NP, for conducting the literature searches and retrieving all literature. The author also wishes to thank Dr. Phyllis Dexter and the anonymous reviewers for their thoughtful reviews, helpful comments, and editorial recommendations.

References

Andersson, B. (1987). Thirst mechanism and its inhibition. *Bibliotheca Nutritio et Dieta, 40,* 122-129.

Argent, N.B., Burrell, L.M., Goodship, T.H., Wilkinson, R., & Baylis, P.H. (1991). Osmoregulation of thirst and vasopressin release in severe chronic renal failure. *Kidney International, 39,* 295-300.

Baldree, K.S., Murphy, S.P., & Powers, M.J. (1982). Stress identification and coping patterns in patients on hemodialysis. *Nursing Research, 31,* 107-112.

Barrett, B.J., Vasasour, H.M., Major, A., & Parfrey, P.S. (1990). Clinical and psychological correlates of somatic symptoms in patients on dialysis. *Nephron, 55,* 10-15.

Baylis, P.H., & Thompson, C.J. (1988). Osmoregulation of vasopressin secretion and thirst in health and disease. *Clinical Endocrinology, 29,* 549-576.

Beck, A.T., & Beamesderfer, A. (1974). Assessment of depression: The depression inventory. *In Modern problems in pharmacopsychiatry* (Vol. 7). Basel: Basel & Karger.

Berger, A.M., & Walker, S.N. (2001). An explanatory model of fatigue in women receiving adjuvant breast cancer chemotherapy. *Nursing Research, 50,* 42-52.

Berne, B., Vahlquist, A., Fisher, T., Danielson, B.G., & Berne, C. (1984). UV treatment of uraemic pruritus reduces the vitamin A content of the skin. *European Journal of Clinical Investigation, 14,* 203-206.

Blank, A., Gonen, B., Zilberman, S., & Magora, A. (1986). Electrophysiological pattern of development of muscle fatigue in patients undergoing dialysis. *Electromyography & Clinical Neurophysiology, 26,* 489-497.

Bleyer, A.J., Hylander, B., Sudo, H., Nomoto, Y., de la Torre, E., Chen, R.A., et al. (1999). An international study of patient compliance with hemodialysis. *JAMA, 281,* 1211-1213.

Bots, C.P., Brand, H.S., Veerman, E.C., Valentijn-Benz, M., van Amerongen, B.M., Valentijn, R.M., et al. (2004). Interdialytic weight gain in patients on hemodialysis is associated with dry mouth and thirst. *Kidney International, 66,* 1662-1668.

Brass, E.P., Adler, S., Sietsema, K.E., Hiatt, W.R., Orlando, A.M., & Amato, A. (2001). Intravenous L-carnitine increases plasma carnitine, reduces fatigue, and may preserve exercise capacity in hemodialysis patients. *American Journal of Kidney Diseases, 37,* 1018-1028.

Brunier, G., & Graydon, J. (1993). The influence of physical activity on fatigue in patients with ESRD on haemodialysis. *ANNA Journal, 20,* 457-461.

Brunier, G., & Graydon, J. (1996). A comparison of two methods of measuring fatigue in patients on chronic haemodialysis: Visual analogue versus Likert scale. *International Journal of Nursing Studies, 11,* 338-347.

Brunstrom, J.M., Macrae, A.W., & Roberts, B. (1997). Mouth-state dependent changes in the judged pleasantness of water at different temperatures. *Physiology & Behavior, 61,* 667-669.

Cardenas, D.D., & Kutner, N.G. (1982). The problem of fatigue in dialysis patients. *Nephron, 30,* 336-340.

Carmines, E.G., & Zeller, R.A. (1979). *Reliability and validity assessment.* Newbury Park: Sage.

Cassileth, B.R., Lusk, E.J., Bodenheimer, B.J., Farber, J.M., Jochimsen, P., & Morrin-Taylor, B. (1985). Chemotherapeutic toxicity: The relationship between patients' pretreatment expectations and post-treatment results. *American Journal of Clinical Oncology, 8,* 419-425.

Cho, Y.C., & Tsay, S.L. (2004). The effect of acupressure with massage on fatigue and depression in patients with end stage renal disease. *Journal of Nursing Research, 12,* 51-59.

Chou, F.F., Ho, J.C., Huang, S.C., & Sheen-Chen, S.M. (2000). A study on pruritus after parathyroidectomy for secondary hyperparathyroidism. *Journal of the American College of Surgeons, 190,* 65-70.

Cioffi, D. (1991). Beyond attentional strategies: A cognitive-perceptual model of somatic interpretation. *Psychological Bulletin, 109,* 25-41.

Cohen, E.P., Russell, T.J., & Garancis, J.C. (1992). Mast cells and calcium in severe uremic itching. *American Journal of the Medical Sciences, 303,* 360-365.

Comstock, G.W., & Helsing, K. (1976). Symptoms of depression in two communities. *Psychological Medicine, 6,* 551-563.

Crawford, S., Sands, L., & Neiwirth, J. (2000). Dialysis and skin care. *Journal of Renal Nutrition, 10,* 105-109.

Curtin, R.B., Bultman, D.C., Thomas-Hawkins, C., Walters, B.A., & Schatell, D. (2002). Hemodialysis patients' symptom experiences: Effects on physical and mental functioning. *Nephrology Nursing Journal, 29,* 562, 567-574.

Curtin, R.B., & Mapes, D.L. (2001). Health care management strategies of long-term dialysis survivors. *Nephrology Nursing Journal, 28,* 385-392.

Curtin, R.B., Sitter, D.C., Schatell, D., & Chewning, B.A. (2004). Self-management, knowledge, and functioning and well-being of patients on hemodialysis. *Nephrology Nursing Journal, 31,* 378-386, 396.

Daugirdas, J.T., Al-Kudsi, R.R., Ing, T.S., & Norusis, M.J. (1985). A double-blind evaluation of sodium gradient hemodialysis. *American Journal of Nephrology, 5,* 163-168.

Daugirdas, J.T., Blake, P.G., & Todd, S.I. (2001). Special problems in the dialysis patient. In J.T. Daugirdas, P.G. Blake, & T.S. Ing (Eds.), *Handbook of dialysis* (pp. 413-579). New York: Lippincott.

de Castro, J.M. (1992). Age-related changes in natural spontaneous fluid ingestion and thirst in humans. *Journal of Gerontology, 47,* P321-P330.

DeVellis, R.F. (2003). *Scale development: Theory and applications* (2nd ed.), Thousand Oaks: Sage.

Dodd, M., Janson, S., Facione, N., Faucett, J., Froelicher, E.S., Humphreys, J., Lee, K., et al. (2001). Advancing the science of symptom management. *Journal of Advanced Nursing, 33,* 668-676.

Dominic, S.C., Ramachandran, S., Somiah, S., Mani, K., & Dominic, S.S. (1996). Quenching the thirst in dialysis patients. *Nephron, 73,* 597-600.

Dreisbach, A.W., Hendrickson, T., Beezhold, D., Riesenberg, L.A., & Sklar, A.H. (1998). Elevated levels of tumor necrosis factor alpha in postdialysis fatigue. *International Journal of Artificial Organs, 21,* 83-86.

Fernstrom, A., Hylander, B., & Rossner, S. (1996). Taste acuity in patients with chronic renal failure. *Clinical Nephrology, 45,* 169-174.

Friedrich, RM. (1980). Patient perception of distress associated with hemodialysis: A state survey. *Journal of the American Association of Nephrology Nurses & Technicians, 7,* 252-258.

Giovannetti, S., Barsotti, G., Cupisti, A., Morelli, E., Agostini, B., Posella, L., et al. (1994). Dipsogenic factors operating in chronic uremics on maintenance hemodialysis. *Neprhon, 66,* 413-420.

Glover, J., Dibble, S.L., Dodd, M.J., & Miaskowski, C. (1995). Mood states of oncology out-patients: Does pain make a difference? *Journal of Pain and Symptom Management, 10,* 120-128.

Goicoechea, M., de Sequera, P., Ochando, A., Andrea, C., & Caramelo,

C. (1999). Uremic pruritus: An unresolved problem in hemodialysis patients. *Nephron, 82,* 73-74.

Gordon, E.J., Leon, J.B., & Sehgal, A.R. (2003). Why are hemodialysis treatments shortened and skipped? Development of a taxonomy and relationship to patient subgroups. *Nephrology Nursing Journal, 30,* 209-217.

Greenleaf, J.E. (1992). Problem: Thirst, drinking behavior, and involuntary dehydration. *Medicine & Science in Sports & Exercise, 24,* 645-656.

Guyton, A.C., & Hall, J.E. (1996). *Textbook of medical physiology* (9th ed.). Philadelphia: Saunders.

Hays, R.D., Kallich, J.D., Mapes, D.L., Coons, S.J., & Carter, W.B. (1994). Development of the kidney disease quality of life (KDQOL) instrument. *Quality of Life Research, 3,* 329-338.

Headley, C.M., & Wall, B. (2002). ESRD-associated cutaneous manifestations in a hemodialysis population. *Nephrology Nursing Journal, 29,* 525-527, 531-539.

Hindson, C., Taylor, A., Martin A., & Downey, A. (1981). UVA light for relief of uraemic pruritus. *Lancet, 1* (8213), 215.

Hopkins, K. (2005). Facilitating sleep for patients with end stage renal disease. *Nephrology Nursing Journal, 32,* 189-195.

Hui, D.S., Wong, T.Y., Li, T.S., Ko, F.W., Choy, D.K., Szeto, C.C., et al. (2002). Prevalence of sleep disturbances in Chinese patients with end stage renal failure on maintenance hemodialysis. *Medical Science Monitor, 8,* CR331-CR336.

Ikizler, T.A., & Hakim, R.M. (1996). Nutrition in end stage renal disease. *Kidney International, 50,* 343-357.

Jamar, S.C. (1989). Fatigue in women receiving chemotherapy for ovarian cancer. In S.G. Funk, E.M. Tornquist, M.T. Champagne, L.A. Copp, & R.A. Wiese (Eds.), *Key aspects of comfort: Management of pain, fatigue, and nausea* (pp. 224-228). New York: Springer.

Jimenez, F., Monte, M.J., El-Mir, M.Y., Pascual, M.J., & Marin, J.J. (2002). Chronic renal failure-induced changes in serum and urine bile acid profiles. *Digestive Diseases and Sciences, 47,* 2398-2406.

Jones, W.O. (1989). Bridging the gap between black food preferences and the renal diet. *Transplantation Proceedings, 21,* 3990-3992.

Kato, A., Hamada, M., Maruyama, T., Maruyama, Y., & Hishida, A. (2000). Pruritus and hydration state of stratum corneum in hemodialysis patients. *American Journal of Nephrology, 20,* 437-442.

Kimura, G. (1989). Quantitative assessment of sodium and water metabolism in hemodialyzed patients. *International Journal of Artificial Organs, 12,* 744-748.

Klein, L.R., Klein, J.B., Hanno, R., & Callen, J.P. (1988). Cutaneous mast cell quantity in pruritic and nonpruritic hemodialysis patients. *International Journal of Dermatology, 27,* 557-559.

Kyriazis, J., & Glotsos, J. (2000). Dialysate calcium concentration of ≤ 1.25 mmol/l: Is it effective in suppressing uremic pruritus? *Nephron, 84,* 85-86.

Laupacis, A., Muirhead, N., Keown, P., & Wong, C. (1992). A disease-specific questionnaire for assessing quality of life in patients on hemodialysis. *Nephron, 60,* 302-306.

Lenz, E.R., Pugh, L.C., Milligan, R.A., Gift, A., & Suppe, F. (1997). The middle-range theory of unpleasant symptoms: An update. *Advances in Nursing Science, 19,* 14-27.

Lindsay, R.M., Heidenheim, A.P., Spanner, E., Kortas, C., & Blake, P.G. (1994). Adequacy of hemodialysis and nutrition: Important determinants of morbidity and mortality. *Kidney International, 44,* S85-S91.

Locking-Cusolito, H., Huyge, L., & Strangio, D. (2001). Sleep pattern disturbance in hemodialysis and peritoneal dialysis patients. *Nephrology Nursing Journal, 28,* 40-44.

Lopes, A.A., Albert, J.M., Young, E.W., Satayathum, S., Pisoni, R.L., Andreucci, V.E. et al. (2004). Screening for depression in hemodialysis patients: Associations with diagnosis, treatment, and outcomes in the DOPPS. *Kidney International, 66,* 2047-2053.

Maibach, E.W., & Cotton, D. (1995). Moving people to behavior change: A staged social cognitive approach to message design. In E. Maibach & R.L. (Eds.), *Designing health messages: Approaches from communication theory and public health practice.* Thousand Oaks, CA: Sage.

Martinez-Vea, A., Garcia, C., Gaya, J., Rivera, F., & Oliver, J.A. (1992). Abnormalities of thirst regulation in patients with chronic renal failure on hemodialysis. *American Journal of Nephrology, 12,* 73-79.

McCann, K., & Boore, J.R. (2000). Fatigue in persons with renal failure who require maintenance haemodialysis. *Journal of Advanced Nursing, 32,* 1132-1142.

McNair, D.M., Lorr, M., & Droppleman, E.F. (1981). *Profile of mood states.* San Diego: Educational and Industrial Testing Service.

Meek, P.M., Nail, L.M., Barsevick, A., Schwartz, A.L., Stephen, S., Whitmer, K. et al. (2000). Psychometric testing of fatigue instruments for use with cancer patients. *Nursing Research, 49,* 181-190.

Merkus, M.P., Jager, K.J., Dekker, F.W., de Haan, R.J., Boeschoten, E.W., & Krediet, R.T. (1999). Physical symptoms and quality of life in patients on chronic dialysis: Results of The Netherlands Cooperative Study on Adequacy of Dialysis. *Nephrology Dialysis Transplantation, 14,* 1163-1170.

Miescher, E., & Fortney, S.M. (1989). Responses to dehydration and rehydration during heat exposure in young and older men. *American Journal of Physiology, 257,* R1050-R1056.

National Kidney Foundation (NKF). (2000). Kidney disease outcomes quality initiative (KDOQI) clinical practice guidelines for anemia of chronic kidney disease [Online]. Retrieved August 9, 2004, from www.kidney.org/professionals/kdoqi/guidelines_updates/doqi

Nunnally, J.C. (1978). *Psychometric theory* (2nd ed.). New York: McGraw-Hill.

Nunnally, J.C., & Bernstein, I.H. (1994). *Psychometric theory* (3rd ed.). New York: McGraw-Hill.

O'Neill, P.A., & McLean, K.A. (1992). Water homeostasis and aging. *Medical Laboratory Sciences, 49,* 291-298.

Parfrey, P.S., Vavasour, H., Bullock, M., Henry, S., Harnett, J.D. & Gault, M.H. (1987). Symptoms in end stage renal disease: Dialysis versus transplantation. *Transplantation Proceedings, 19,* 3407-3409.

Parfrey, P.S., Vavasour, H., Bullock, M., Henry, S., Harnett, J.D., Gault, M.H. (1989). Development of a health questionnaire specific for end stage renal disease. *Nephron, 52,* 20-28.

Parfrey, P.S., Vavasour, H.M., & Gault, M.H. (1988). A prospective study of health status in dialysis and transplant patients. *Transplantation Proceedings, 20,* 1231-1232.

Parker, K.P. (1997). Sleep and dialysis: A research-based review of the literature. *ANNA Journal, 24,* 626-639.

Parker, K.P. (2003). Sleep disturbances in dialysis patients. *Sleep Medicine Reviews, 7,* 131-143.

Parker, K.P., Bliwise, D.L., Bailey, J.L, & Rye, D.B. (2003). Daytime sleepiness in stable hemodialysis patients. *American Journal of Kidney Diseases, 41,* 394-402.

Parker, K.P., Bliwise, D.L., & Rye, D.B. (2000). Hemodialysis disrupts basic sleep regulatory mechanisms: Building hypotheses. *Nursing Research, 49,* 327-332.

Pauli-Magnus, C., Mikus, G., Alscher, D.M., Kirschner, T., Nagel, W., Gugeler, N., et al. (2000). Naltrexone does not relieve uremic pruritus: Results of a randomized double-blind, placebo-controlled crossover study. *Journal of the American Society of Nephrology, 11,* 514-519.

Peck, L., Monsen, E., & Ahmad, S. (1996). Effect of three sources of long-chain fatty acids on the plasma fatty acid profile, plasma prostaglandin E2 concentration and pruritus symptoms in hemodialysis patients. *American Journal of Clinical Nutrition, 64,* 210-214.

Phillips, P.A., Bretherton, M., Johnston, C.I., Gray, L. (1991). Reduced osmotic thirst in healthy elderly men. *American Journal of Physiology, 261,* R166-R171.

Piper, B.F. (1997). Measuring fatigue. In M. Frank-Stromborg & S.J. Olsen (Eds.), *Instruments for clinical health care research* (pp. 482-496). Boston: Jones & Bartlett.

Piper, B.F., Dodd, M.L., Paul, S.M., & Welcer, S. (1989). The development of an instrument to measure the subjective dimension of fatigue. In S.G. Funk, E.M. Tornquist, M.T. Champagne, L.A. Copp, & R.A. Wiese (Eds.), *Key aspects of comfort management of pain, fatigue, and nausea* (pp. 199-208). New York: Springer.

Polit, D.F., & Beck, C.T. (2004). *Nursing research: Principles and methods* (7th ed.). Philadelphia: Lippincott Williams & Wilkins.

Porth, C.M., & Erickson, M. (1992). Physiology of thirst and drinking:

Implications for nursing practice. *Heart & Lung, 21,* 273-282.

Potempa, K., Lopez, M., Reid, C., & Lawson, L. (1986). Chronic fatigue. *Image: The Journal of Nursing Scholarship, 18,* 165-169.

Puhan, M.A., Bryant, D., Guyatt, G.H., Heels-Ansdell, D., & Schunemann, H.J. (2005). Internal consistency reliability is a poor predictor of responsiveness. *Health and Quality of Life Outcomes.* Retrieved from www.hqlo.com/content/3/1/33.

Radloff, L.S. (1977). The CES-D scale: A self-report depression scale for research in the general population. *Applied Psychological Measurement, 1,* 385-401.

Rao, S., Carter, W.B., Mapes, D.L., Kallich, J.D., Kamberg, C.J., Spritzer, K.L., & Hays, R.D. (2000). Development of subscales from the symptoms/problems and effects of kidney disease scales of the kidney disease quality of life instrument. *Clinical Therapeutics, 22,* 1099-1111.

Ream, E., & Richardson, A. (1996). Fatigue: A concept analysis. *International Journal of Nursing Studies, 33,* 519-529.

Ro, Y.J., Ha, H.G., Kim, C.G., & Yeom, H.A. (2002). The effects of aromatherapy on pruritus in patients undergoing hemodialysis. *Dermatology Nursing, 14,* 231-238, 256.

Robertson, K.E., & Mueller, B.A. (1996). Uremic pruritus. *American Journal of Health-System Pharmacy, 53,* 2159-2170.

Rogers, A.E. (1997a). Nursing management of sleep disorders: Part 1 – Assessment. *ANNA Journal, 24,* 666-671.

Rogers, A.E. (1997b). Nursing management of sleep disorders: Part 2 – Behavioral interventions. *ANNA Journal, 24,* 672-675.

Rogers, P.W., & Kurtzman, N.A. (1973). Renal failure, uncontrollable thirst, and hyperreninemia: Cessation of thirst with bilateral nephrectomy. *JAMA, 225,* 1236-1238.

Sadowski, R.H., Allred, E.N., & Jabs, K. (1993). Sodium modeling ameliorates intradialytic and interdialytic symptoms in young hemodialysis patients. *Journal of the American Society of Nephrology, 4,* 1192-1198.

Sang, G.L., Kovithavongs, C., Ulan, R., & Kjellstrand, C.M. (1997). Sodium ramping in hemodialysis: A study of beneficial and adverse effects. *American Journal of Kidney Diseases, 29,* 669-677.

Saran, R., Bragg-Gresham, J.L., Rayner, H.C., Goodkin, D.A., Keen, M.L., Van Dijk, P.C., et al. (2003). Nonadherence in hemodialysis: Associations with mortality, hospitalization, and practice patterns in DOPPS. *Kidney International, 64,* 254-262.

Schneider, R.A. (2001). Preliminary data on the Multidimensional Fatigue Inventory-20 from female caregivers of male hemodialysis patients. *Psychological Reports, 88,* 699-700.

Shepherd, R., Farleigh, C.A., Atkinson, C., & Pryor, J.S. (1987). Effects of haemodialysis on taste and thirst. *Appetite, 9,* 79-88.

Sklar, A.H., Beezhold, D.H., Newman, N., Hendrickson, T., & Dreisbach, A.W. (1998). Postdialysis fatigue: Lack of effect of a biocompatible membrane. *American Journal of Kidney Diseases, 31,* 1007-1010.

Sklar, A.H., Newman, N., Scott, R., Semenyuk, J., & Fiacco, V. (1999). Identification of factors responsible for postdialysis fatigue. *American Journal of Kidney Diseases, 34,* 464-470.

Sklar, A.H., Riensenberg, L.A., Silber, A.K., Ahmed, W., & Ali, A. (1996). Postdialysis fatigue. *American Journal of Kidney Diseases, 28,* 732-736.

Smets, E.M., Garssen, B., Bonke, B., & de Haes, J.C. (1995). The multidimensional fatigue inventory: Psychometric qualities of an instrument to assess fatigue. *Journal of Psychosomatic Research, 39,* 31-325.

Smets, E.M., Garssen, B., Schuster-Uitterhoeve, A., & de Haes, J.C. (1993). Fatigue in cancer patients. *British Journal of Cancer, 68,* 220-224.

Smets, E.M., Garssen, B., Cull, A., & de Haes, J.C. (1996). Application of the multidimensional fatigue inventory (MFI-20) in cancer patients receiving radiotherapy. *British Journal of Cancer, 73,* 241-245.

Sorofman, B., Tripp-Reimer, T., Lauer, G.M., & Martin, M.E. (1990). Symptom self-care. *Holistic Nursing Practice, 4,* 45-55.

Srivastava, R.H. (1986). Fatigue in the renal patient. *ANNA Journal, 13,* 246-249.

Stahle-Backdahl, M. (1995). Uremic pruritus. *Seminars in Dermatology, 14,* 297-301.

Stapleton, S (1992). Etiologies and indicators of powerlessness in persons with end stage renal disease. In J.F. Miller (Ed.), *Coping with chronic illness: Overcoming powerlessness* (pp. 163-178). Philadelphia: F.A. Davis.

Subach, R.A., & Marx, M.A. (2002). Evaluation of uremic pruritus at an outpatient hemodialysis unit. *Renal Failure, 24,* 609-614.

Teel, C.S., Meek, P., McNamara, A.M., & Watson, L. (1997). Perspectives unifying symptom interpretation. *Image: The Journal of Nursing Scholarship, 29,* 175-181.

Thomas-Hawkins, C. (2000). Symptom distress and day-to-day changes in functional status in chronic hemodialysis patients. *Nephrology Nursing Journal, 27,* 369-380, 428.

Thompson, C.J., & Baylis, P.H. (1988). Osmoregulation of thirst. *Journal of Endrocrinology, 117,* 155-157.

Toto, K.H. (1994). Regulation of plasma osmolality: Thirst and vasopressin. *Critical Care Nursing Clinics of North America, 6,* 661-674.

Tozawa, M., Iseki, K., Iseki, C., Morita, O., Yoshi, S., & Fukiyama, K. (1999). Seasonal blood pressure and body weight variation in patients on chronic hemodialysis. *American Journal of Nephrology, 19,* 660-667.

Tsay, S.L. (2004). Acupressure and fatigue in patients with end stage renal disease: A randomized controlled trial. *International Journal of Nursing Studies, 41,* 99-106.

University of California, San Francisco, School of Nursing Symptom Management Faculty Group (UCSF). (1994). A model for symptom management. *Image: Journal of Nursing Scholarship, 26,* 272-276.

Vanholder, R., & De Smet, R. (1999). Pathophysiologic effects of uremic retention solutes. *Journal of the American Society of Nephrology, 10,* 1815-1823.

Vergili-Nelson, J.M. (2003). Benefits of fish oil supplementation for hemodialysis patients. *Journal of the American Dietetic Association, 103,* 1174-1177.

Virga, G., Mastrosimone, S., Amici, G., Munaretto, G., Gastaldon, F., & Bennadonna, A. (1998). Symptoms in hemodialysis patients and their relationship with biochemical and demographic parameters. *International Journal of Artificial Organs, 21,* 788-793.

Virga, G., Visentin, I., La Milia, V., Bonadonna, A. (2002). Inflammation and pruritus in haemodialysis patients. *Nephrology Dialysis Transplantation, 17,* 2164-2169.

Wanner, C., & Horl, W. (1988). Carnitine abnormalities in patients with renal insufficiency: Pathophysiological and therapeutic aspects. *Nephron, 50,* 89-102.

Ware, J.E., Kosinski, M., & Gandek, B. (2000). *SF-36 health survey: Manual and interpretation guide.* Lincoln, RI: Quality Metric Inc.

Weisbord, S.D., Fried, L.F., Arnold, R.M., Rotondi, A.J., Fine, M.J., Levenson, D.J., Switzer, G. E. (2004). Development of a symptom assessment instrument for chronic hemodialysis patients. *Journal of Pain and Symptom Management, 27,* 226-240.

Welch, J.L. (2002). Development of the thirst distress scale. *Nephrology Nursing Journal, 29,* 337-342.

Welch, J.L., & Austin, J.K. (2001). Stressors, coping, and depression in hemodialysis patients. *Journal of Advanced Nursing, 33,* 200-207.

Welch, J.L., Bennett, S.J., & Delp, R.L., Agarwal, R. (in press). Benefits and barriers to dietary sodium adherence. *Western Journal of Nursing Research.*

Welch, J.L., & Davis, J. (2000). Self-care strategies to reduce fluid intake and control thirst in hemodialysis patients. *Nephrology Nursing Journal, 27,* 393-395.

Welch, J.L., Evans, J.D., Juliar, B., & Agarwal, R. (2004). Abstracts from the 2nd Scientific Conference on Compliance in Health Care and Research: Predictors of fluid adherence in adult hemodialysis patients. *Circulation, 109,* 8.

Welch, J.L., Perkins, S.M., Evans, J.D., Bajpai, S. (2003). Differences in perceptions by stage of fluid adherence. *Journal of Renal Nutrition, 13,* 275-281.

Welch, J.L., & Thomas-Hawkins, C. (2005). Psycho-educational strategies to promote fluid adherence in adult hemodialysis patients: A review of intervention studies. *International Journal of Nursing Studies, 42,* 597-608

Wirth, J.B., & Folstein, M.F. (1982). Thirst and weight gain during maintenance hemodialysis. *Psychosomatics, 23,* 1125-1127, 1130-1131, 1134.

Woodtli, A.O. (1990). Thirst: A critical care nursing challenge. *Dimensions of Critical Care Nursing, 9,* 6-15.

Yamamoto, T., Shimizu, M., Morioka, M., Kitano, M., Wakabayashi, H., & Aizawa, N. (1986). Role of angiotensin II in the pathogenesis of hyperdipsia in chronic renal failure. *JAMA, 256,* 604-608.

Yoshimoto-Futuro, K., Yoshimoto, K., Tanaka, T., Saima, S., Kikuchi, Y., Shay, J., et al. (1999). Effects of oral supplementation with evening primrose oil for 6 weeks on plasma essential fatty acids and uremic skin symptoms in hemodialysis patients. *Nephron, 81,* 151-159.

Yosipovitch, G., & Boner, G. (1997). Pruritus and skin hydration during dialysis. *Nephrology Dialysis Transplantation, 12,* 1769-1770.

Yosipovitch, G., Zucker, I., Boner, G., Gafter, U., Shapira, Y., & David, M. (2001). A questionnaire for the assessment of pruritus: Validation in uremic patients. *Acta Derm Venereol, 81,* 108-111.

Youngblut, J.M., & Casper, G.R. (1993). Single-item indicators in nursing research. *Research in Nursing and Health, 16,* 459-465.

Zakrzewska-Pneiwska, B., & Jedras, M. (2001). Is pruritus in chronic hemodialysis patients related to peripheral somatic and autonomic neuropathy? *Neurophysiologic Clinics, 31,* 181-193.

Zucker, I., Yosipovitch, G., David, M., Gafter, U., & Boner, G. (2003). Prevalence and characterization of uremic pruritus in patients undergoing hemodialysis: Uremic pruritus is still a major problem for patients with end stage renal disease. *American Academy of Dermatology, 49,* 842-846.

- Individuals diagnosed with kidney failure commonly face a variety of concurrent symptoms, the most common of which are fatigue, pruritus, and thirst. The causes of and the individual responses to these symptoms vary.

- Five symptom management models are available to assist nurses when helping patients manage their symptoms. These models include the Symptom Self-Care Response Model, the Model of Somatic Interpretation, the Symptom Interpretation Model, the Middle-Range Theory of Unpleasant Symptoms, and the Symptom Management Model.

- Many tools have been used to assess symptoms in patients with kidney failure. When deciding which tool to use in clinical practice, the nurse needs to pay attention to its reliability and validity.

- There are many possible etiologies for fatigue in dialysis patients. These include the side effects of medications, poor nutrition, physiological alterations, psychological factors, sleep disorders, and factors relating to HD treatment itself.

- Several independent nursing interventions have been suggested to reduce fatigue in dialysis patients. These include nutritional, sleep, and alternative therapy interventions.

- Pruritus, defined as generalized itching and often referred to as uremic pruritus or renal itch, is a common symptom experienced by dialysis patients.

- The exact mechanism inducing pruritus in patients with kidney failure is unknown, although many potential causes have been proposed. These include medications, environmental conditions, nutritional alterations, physiological changes, reactions to products used during dialysis, and changes in the integument.

- Most of the interventions to reduce or alleviate pruritus are based on clinical experience or trial and error; few have been systematically investigated by research. Future research is needed to determine whether pruritus is responsive to nursing care in the dialysis population.

- Thirst is a common problem for individuals receiving HD therapy. Thirst has been reported to occur daily in over 85% of HD patients with 30%-86% experiencing moderate to high levels of thirst intensity.

- Several factors have been suggested as influencing thirst. These include demographic factors, environmental conditions, physiological alterations, psychological/social variables, and factors related to HD treatment.

- Thirst becomes a significant problem in HD patients when it interferes with adherence to a prescribed treatment. In addition, thirst may indirectly affect physical and emotional functioning and also affect social relationships because usual activities may be hindered. Finally, thirst may indirectly increase morbidity and mortality by leading to medical complications such as pulmonary edema.

- Symptom management in patients with kidney failure includes an assessment of symptoms patients are experiencing, the interventions used to treat the symptoms, and evaluation of outcomes.

ANNP611

Symptom Management

Janet L. Welch, DNS, RN, CNS

Contemporary Nephrology Nursing: Principles and Practice contains 39 chapters of educational content. Individual learners may apply for continuing nursing education credit by reading a chapter and completing the Continuing Education Evaluation Form for that chapter. Learners may apply for continuing education credit for any or all chapters.

Please photocopy this page and return to ANNA.
COMPLETE THE FOLLOWING:

Name: _____

Address:_____

City:_____State:_____Zip:_____

E-mail: _____

Preferred telephone: ☐ Home   ☐ Work: _____

State where licensed and license number (optional): _____

CE application fees are based upon the number of contact hours provided by the individual chapter. CE fees per contact hour for ANNA members are as follows: 1.0-1.9 - $15; 2.0-2.9 - $20; 3.0-3.9 - $25; 4.0 and higher - $30. Fees for nonmembers are $10 higher.

ANNA Member: ☐ Yes   ☐ No   Member # (if available) _____

☐ Checked Enclosed   ☐ American Express   ☐ Visa   ☐ MasterCard

Total Amount Submitted: _____

Credit Card Number: _____ Exp. Date: _____

Name as it appears on the card: _____

CE Evaluation Form
To receive continuing education credit for individual study after reading the chapter
1. Photocopy this form. (You may also download this form from ANNA's Web site, **www.annanurse.org.**)
2. Mail the completed form with payment (check) or credit card information to American Nephrology Nurses' Association, East Holly Avenue, Box 56, Pitman, NJ 08071-0056.
3. You will receive your CE certificate from ANNA in 4 to 6 weeks.

Test returns must be postmarked by **December 31, 2010.**

CE Application Fee
ANNA Member $20.00
Nonmember $30.00

EVALUATION FORM

1. I verify that I have read this chapter and completed this education activity. Date: _____

   _____
   Signature

2. What would be different in your practice if you applied what you learned from this activity? *(Please use additional sheet of paper if necessary.)*

   _____
   _____
   _____
   _____
   _____
   _____
   _____
   _____
   _____
   _____
   _____
   _____
   _____

Evaluation	Strongly disagree				Strongly agree
3. The activity met the stated objectives.					
a. Provide an overview of at least 3 symptom management models.	1	2	3	4	5
b. Describe the use of a symptom management model with patients experiencing chronic kidney disease.	1	2	3	4	5
c. Using a symptom management model, describe the plan of care for a patient with chronic kidney disease who has either thirst, pruritus, or fatigue.	1	2	3	4	5
4. The content was current and relevant.	1	2	3	4	5
5. The content was presented clearly.	1	2	3	4	5
6. The content was covered adequately.	1	2	3	4	5
7. Rate your ability to apply the learning obtained from this activity to practice.	1	2	3	4	5

Comments _____

_____

8. Time required to read the chapter and complete this form: _____ minutes.

This educational activity has been provided by the American Nephrology Nurses' Association (ANNA) for 2.0 contact hours. ANNA is accredited as a provider of continuing nursing education (CNE) by the American Nurses Credentialing Center's Commission on Accreditation (ANCC-COA). ANNA is an approved provider of continuing education by the California Board of Registered Nursing, CEP 0910.

Diabetes and Kidney Disease: A Challenge in Chronic Disease Management

Janice A. Neil, PhD, RN

Chapter Contents

Diabetes and Kidney Disease: A Challenge in Chronic Disease Management

Chapter 12

Janice A. Neil, PhD, RN

Diabetes is defined as an alteration in the metabolism of carbohydrates, proteins, and fats. It is a multisystem disease related to a decrease in insulin production, insulin utilization, or both defects. Insulin is responsible for the active transport of glucose into the cell where it is utilized to make ATP and, thus, provide energy (Kumar & Young, 1999). Insulin is released from the beta cells of the pancreas. A basal rate of insulin is produced at a steady state to maintain blood glucose and a bolus of insulin is released in response to the fed state, that is, the intake of food and nutrients. Diabetes is the leading cause of renal disease in the U.S. It causes blood vessel and nerve damage leading to the involvement of many organs including the kidneys.

There are an estimated 18 million people in the U.S. with diabetes and an estimated 20 million with "pre-diabetes," an altered fasting glucose state. Diabetes is also the 5th leading cause of death in the U.S., and nearly 20% of people over 65 years old have diabetes. The incidence continues to rise worldwide with younger people developing diabetes related to obesity. Diabetes is the leading cause of heart disease, blindness, and lower limb amputations (American Diabetes Association [ADA], 2004a). The cost of caring for diabetes in the U.S. now exceeds $137 billion per year, including 30% of the Medicare budget. Diabetes now accounts for 40% of patients entering dialysis or requiring transplantation, making it the leading cause of end stage renal disease (ESRD) (Skyler, 2001).

Diabetes affects 1%-1.5% of the general population. The incidence is highest in the Native American population, followed by the Latino population. African Americans and Pacific Islanders are affected more than Caucasians (ADA, 2004b). It is estimated that 10% of diabetics have type 1 diabetes and 90% have type 2. Both types of diabetes are characterized by polydipsia, polyphagia, and polyuria when glucose levels are elevated. All are the result of a hyperosmolar state that occurs in the vascular compartment (ADA, 2004d). Clinical diabetes is diagnosed by fasting blood glucose levels greater than 126 mg/dL on two occasions or a random blood glucose greater than 200 mg with acute symptoms (Diagnosis and Classification of Diabetes Mellitus, 2005).

Types of Diabetes Mellitus

Type 1 Diabetes

Type 1 diabetes, formerly known as insulin dependent diabetes or juvenile diabetes, occurs most often in people under the age of 30. It results from a destruction of the pancreatic beta cells due to an autoimmune process. Although not inherited, genetic predisposition has been linked to the human leukocyte antigens (HLAs). In theory, when a genetically susceptible person is exposed to a virus or other environmental antigen with a certain HLA-DR3 or HLA-DR4, the autoimmune process begins. Also, cold weather has been shown to have some effect on the development of the autoimmune process, with more people developing the dis-

ease in the winter and in colder climates. Caucasians have the highest incidence of type 1 diabetes (ADA, 2004e).

Type 2 Diabetes

Type 2 diabetes is the most prevalent and usually occurs in people over age 40. The prevalence of type 2 increases with age and generally has an insidious onset. Some people are not diagnosed for years because of multiple vague symptoms that occur over time. The chronic complications of diabetes may be the first sign of disease. The pancreas continues to make some insulin; however, the amount may be insufficient or is poorly utilized. There are multiple genes responsible, and type 2 does have some hereditary factors, especially in families where both parents have type 2 diabetes. Type 2 diabetes is characterized by a decrease in insulin production, increased insulin resistance (decreased number of insulin receptor site), and increased hepatic glucagon output. Obesity is a factor in the development of type 2 (ADA, 2004b).

Gestational Diabetes

Gestational diabetes manifests in pregnancy with over 135,000 women in the U.S. affected a year. Hormones produced by the placenta block the action of insulin in the mother's body that leads to insulin resistance and results in hyperglycemia. Since the baby is subject to higher glucose levels, excess glucose is stored by the fetus, which may result in macrosomia, an infant with a birth weight over 4,500 g. There is a 40% incidence of the development of type 2 diabetes later in life in women who have had gestational diabetes. Gestational diabetes is treated with diet and exercise primarily. Insulin may be necessary if medication is needed to control blood glucose levels (ADA, 2004c).

Secondary Diabetes

Diabetes develops in some people secondary to other medical conditions that cause blood glucose to rise. These include Cushing syndrome, hyperthyroidism, and the use of parenteral nutrition. Some medications can also cause blood glucose to rise such as prednisone, phenytoin, and antipsychotics such as clozapine. Secondary diabetes often disappears when the underlying cause is removed (Semb, 2004).

Pre-Diabetes

The ADA has identified a state of "pre-diabetes." This is a state of impaired glucose tolerance or impaired fasting glucose with a fasting blood glucose between 100 and 125 mg/dL. (Normal fasting plasma glucose should be less than 100 mg/dl and less than 140 mg/dl 2 hours after eating.) These people are at high risk for developing type 2 diabetes and are also at risk for developing cardiovascular disease. At this point, diabetes may be avoided with lifestyle changes such as weight loss and exercise. Even a 10%-15% weight loss may delay the onset of diabetes.

Guidelines for Diabetic Nephropathy Screening

Current Screening Procedures

Screening for diabetic nephropathy should include (Taylor, 1998):

- Clinical history and physical examination:
  - ✓ Family history of diabetes.
  - ✓ Onset of symptoms: changes in the kidney usually happen within 10-15 years after the onset of diabetes. In patients with type 2, diagnosis may not be made until the chronic complications occur.
  - ✓ Current therapeutic management including insulin and hypoglycemic oral agents.
  - ✓ Other organ involvement (i.e., retinopathy- another serious complication of diabetes that leads to blindness, cardiac disease, and peripheral vascular disease).
  - ✓ Test for peripheral neuropathy – Semmes Weinstein test to determine the sensory status of the foot.
  - ✓ Hypertension and how it is being treated. ACE inhibitors are now used even in normotensive individuals to protect the kidneys.

Laboratory Tests

Laboratory tests include:

- Urine tests.
  - ✓ Urinalysis – a dipstick method may be used for macroalbuminuria. Urine may also be microscopically examined for red blood cells (RBCs) and crystals.
  - ✓ Creatinine clearance: 24-hour urine test – measures kidney function. Creatinine is formed by the breakdown of muscle creatinine and is proportional to muscle mass. Changes in creatinine reflect changes in the glomerular filtration rate (GFR). Abrupt cessation of GFR causes a rise of 1-3 mg/dL/day. Blood urea nitrogen (BUN) is affected by protein intake, catabolism, and gastrointestinal (GI) bleeding. BUN is often a late sign of kidney dysfunction because the GFR may be 75% down before the creatinine starts to rise. Non-renal variables affect BUN. BUN and creatinine are in a 20:1 ratio.
- Blood tests.
  - ✓ Fasting blood glucose – normal fasting glucose should be 70-100 mg/dl; pre-diabetes 101-125 mg/dl; and a diagnosis of diabetes greater then 126mg/dl (ADA, 2004). The fasting glucose test should be done every 3 years after the age of 45.
  - ✓ Random plasma glucose measurements greater than 200mg/dl, plus the manifestations of diabetes as polydipsia, polyphagia, and polyuria indicates diabetes (Semb, 2004).
  - ✓ 2-hour oral glucose tolerance test – a value over 200 mg/dl that began with a loading dose of 75 g of glucose indicates diabetes (Semb, 2004).
  - ✓ Glycemic control – the hemoglobin A1C (HbA1C) is useful in evaluating blood glucose control over the past 3 months.
  - ✓ Proinsulin – the measurement of proinsulin is a very sensitive marker of beta cell destruction, therefore it may be a helpful tool in medication decision making by health care providers in patients with type 2 diabetes. It is useful in selecting what type of medication would be the most effective; secretagogues, sensitizers, and/or insulin therapy (Pfutzner et al., 2004)

Structural and Functional Abnormalities in Nephropathy as a Result of Diabetes

The clinical course leading to nephropathy differs in the two types of diabetes. For patients with type 1, their diabetes occurs usually at a much younger age. Nephropathy usually occurs 15-25 years after the onset of diabetes and almost inevitably results in ESRD. Type 2 diabetes is more insidious in its onset. It also usually occurs at a more advanced age. Often, early renal involvement is missed. Since the comorbid conditions such as coronary artery disease and hypertension exist, it is not always clear that diabetes is the cause of renal failure. Hypertension and diabetes are comorbid conditions that independently increase the risk of developing and accelerating both cardiovascular and renal disease (Rabkin, 2003).

Diabetes is responsible for 35% of renal failure. In fact, diabetes is the most common cause of renal failure. Thirty percent of patients with type 1 diabetes, and 10-40 % of those with type 2 diabetes will eventually require dialysis or transplantation (Diabetes and Kidney Disease, 2005). Both types have similar effects on the kidneys. If a person with diabetes develops renal failure the mortality rises dramatically in comparison to those with diabetes alone. The rate of renal disease in patients with diabetes is increasing related to the increase in type 2 diabetes, the extended lifespan of those with diabetes, and the improved management of comorbid conditions.

Diabetes alters the flow of blood to the glomeruli causing numerous complex biochemical changes in their function. These changes lead to severe scarring or "leaks" in the filtering mechanism manifested by excessive loss of proteins like albumin into the urine. The leakage itself may be toxic leading to further damage. In the diabetic kidney, there is overproduction and impaired degradation of the extracellular matrix components that lead to accumulations in the basement membranes of the mesangial regions of the glomerulus. In the now expanded mesangium, diffuse glomerulosclerosis occurs. This leads to a reduction in the density of the capillaries and the glomerular filtration area is decreased. Now, decreased permeability exists and, thus, albumin leakage. Extracellular matrix also accumulates in the tubular basement membranes and the interstitial compartment. Tubulointerstitial fibrosis leads to nephron destruction and resulting renal failure (Rabkin, 2003).

The key to development of nephropathy is the hyperglycemic state; therefore, blood glucose should be tightly controlled. Glucose in high concentrations leads to renal impairment for several reasons. High glucose concentrations are toxic, altering cellular growth and gene and protein expression. There is also an increase in extracellular matrix and growth factor production causing hypertrophy. Glucose may indirectly affect the kidneys by production of metabolic derivatives, such as oxidants, that modify extracellular proteins.

Table 12-1

Prevalence of Total Diabetes by Race/Ethnicity Among People Aged 20 Years or Older – United States, 2002

Ethnic Group	Numbers with Diabetes	Percentage of Ethnic Group with Diabetes
Non-Hispanic Whites	12,500,000	8.4%
Non-Hispanic Blacks	2,700,000	11.4%
Hispanic/Latino Americans	2,000,000	8.2%
American Indians and Alaska Natives	107,775	14.5%
Asian Americans and Native Hawaiian or other Pacific Islanders – Chinese (24%), Filipino (18%), Asian Indian (16%), Vietnamese (11%), Korean (11%), Japanese (8%), and other Asian (13%) ancestry	Unavailable – diverse group	Estimated 10%

Note: From American Diabetes Association (2004).

These products may induce continuous activation and signaling pathways involving kinases that elevate blood pressure. Kinase also alters renal blood flow and vascular permeability, and increases growth factor release that can again result in increased extracellular matrix formation (Rabkin, 2003). Diabetic kidney disease occurs in four stages that eventually lead to end stage renal failure (Kumar & Young, 1999).

Stage 1: Microalbuminuria

Microalbuminuria is the initial stage of kidney damage related to diabetes. Soon after the onset of diabetes, the kidneys hypertrophy, and renal blood flow and glomerular blood flow increases. Over the next 5-15 years the GFR remains elevated but falls within normal limits, and there is no elevation in systemic blood pressure. Small amounts of albumin, microalbuminuria, leak through the glomeruli. The leakage of this protein may be evident by using sensitive antibody based assays with a 24-hour urine collection. This small amount of protein is predictive of renal damage over the next 10-15 years, especially in patients with type 1. If microalbuminuria is detected, then it is important to begin treatment so that renal failure can be prevented or retarded. Therefore, it is important to screen for microalbumin 5 years after the onset of type 1 and immediately after the diagnosis of type 2. After 1-5 years of microalbuminuria, larger amounts appear in the urine that can be detected by dipstick. However, by now, blood pressure is elevated and renal function has deteriorated.

Stage 2: Macroproteinuria

At this stage, protein can be detected in a routine urinalysis. The urine often appears frothy. As protein leakage becomes massive, a nephrotic syndrome occurs with a loss of albumin, peripheral edema, and an increase in serum cholesterol. Usually hypertension also co-exists, which exacerbates renal damage. Once macroproteinuria exists, kidney damage is inevitable, but further deterioration can be slowed with treatment.

Stage 3: Chronic Kidney Disease

At this stage, early signs of nephropathy appear. GFR is reduced and mild symptoms of renal failure are possible. Because the kidneys metabolize insulin, insulin may remain in the body longer and predispose them to hypoglycemia. Patients taking insulin may need an adjustment in their insulin dose.

Stage 4: ESRD

GFR is less than 15 mL/min/1.73 m^2. The patient is uremic and may experience symptoms such as nausea, vomiting, anorexia, itching, hiccups, irritability, and confusion. At this point the patient will require dialytic therapy or renal transplantation. Proteinuria greater than 300 mg/day will be present.

Diagnosis of Nephropathy in Patients with Diabetes

Of those with type 1 diabetes, 20%-40% will develop renal disease and another 20%-30% will develop microalbuminuria (Kumar & Young, 2004). The peak onset occurs 10-15 years after the onset of type 1, and if after 25 years microalbuminuria does not develop, they are at low risk for developing renal disease. There is also a genetic susceptibility if one or both parents have diabetes and renal disease. Researchers are now in the process of isolating genes that may predispose people with diabetes to renal disease. Ethnic background seems to be an important determinant (see Table 12-1). It is extremely important that blood glucose be kept as close to normal as possible to avoid developing renal disease with a target average blood glucose of 100-110 mg/dl.

In addition to nephropathy, diabetes can affect other parts of the urinary track. Patients with diabetes are prone to urinary track infections and papillary necrosis. Autonomic nervous system damage results in neuropathy that leads to bladder dysfunction with obstruction and can lead to impaired kidney function. Renal artery stenosis may also be accelerated due to atherosclerosis. Atherosclerosis is accelerated with high glucose levels (Rabkin, 2003).

Table 12-2
Hyperglycemic Medications and Their Use With Renal Patients

Drug	Advantages	Precautions	Use with Renal Patients
Insulin	• Must be used in persons with type 1 diabetes • May be added to PD fluid • Some types may be given intravenously	• Hypoglycemia • Amount may need to be decreased as renal failure progresses	• Rate of catabolism decreased • Half-life of insulin in the circulation prolonged • Use with caution
Sulfonylureas Acetohexamide (Dymelor), Chlorpropamide (Diabinese), Tolazamide (Tolinase), Tolbutamide (Orinase). Glimepiride (Amaryl), Glipizide (Glucotro, Glucotrol XL, and Glyburide (Diabeta, Glynase, Micronase)	• Oral agent • Lower serum glucose • Least expensive	• Hypoglycemia: stimulate the beta cells to produce insulin • Acetohexamide, chlor-propamide, tolazamide excreted in the urine: not used with dialysis patients	• Use shorter half-life agents metabolized in the liver • Glipizide and tolbutamide are almost completely hepatically metabolized: drugs of choice
Biguanides Metformin (Glucophage)	• Oral agents • Weight loss, insulin sensiti-zation, positive lipid effects, mild hypotensive effect • Low or no incidence of hypoglycemia	• Metformin: may cause lac-tic acidosis • Must discontinue use before studies using con-trast	• Metformin should not be used in renal failure
Thiazolidinediones Rosiglitazone (Avandia), Pioglitazone (Actos)	• Improved peripheral utiliza-tion, increases insulin sen-sitivity increased glucose uptake • Rosiglitazone (Avandia) and pioglitazone (Actos) can be taken once daily	• May cause fluid retention and edema	• Hepatically metabolized can be used safely
Meglitinides Repaglinide (Prandin)	• Repaglinide acts like an extremely short-acting sul-fonylurea • Ultra-short half-life (1 hour)	• Should be taken right before meals	• Safe: metabolized in the liver
Alpha-Glucosidase Inhibitors Miglitol (Glyset), acarbose (Precose)	• Non-systemic oral agents • Delay absorption of carbo-hydrates	• Excess flatulence, bloating, diarrhea in some patients	• Use with caution with gastroparesis • Acarbose may cause liver toxicity

Management of Patients with Diabetes and Renal Disease

Medication Management

Insulin. The maintenance of normal blood glucose lev-els is always the goal of drug therapy in patients with dia-betes (see Table 12-2). For patients with type 1 diabetes, insulin is used because the pancreatic beta cells have been destroyed by an autoimmune process. However, as renal fail-ure progresses, insulin treated patients may need to reduce their dose because real disease decreases the rate of insulin clearance. About 10%-20% of insulin is metabolized in the kidneys, and as function deteriorates, less insulin is cleared. Uremia also affects glucose tolerance by increasing insulin

resistance both peripherally and in the liver. Therefore, it is important the blood glucose levels be checked frequently and appropriate dosage changes made (Bilous, 2003).

Oral hypoglycemic agents. Before 1994, the treatment for type 2 diabetes was limited to the sulfonylurea class of oral hypoglycemic agents, insulin, and diet and exercise. Today, there are an additional four new classes of oral agents and several new types of insulin (Quillen, 2004). Management of type 2 diabetes with all the available agents is now much more complex, and patients with renal failure pose a larger problem. A common problem for all oral hypo-glycemic agents is that there are few appropriate studies of their use in dialysis patients (Daugirdis, Blake, & Ing 2001). Below are listed the classes of hypoglycemic agents, their action, and precautions for renal patients.

Sulfonylureas. The sulfonylurea class of oral hypoglycemic agents (insulin secretagogues) has been in existence since 1956 and was the mainstay of noninsulin treatment. The older first-generation sulfonylureas are acetohexamide *(Dymelor),* chlorpropamide *(Diabinese),* tolazamide *(Tolinase),* and tolbutamide *(Orinase).* The second-generation sulfonylureas are glimepiride *(Amaryl),* glipizide *(Glucotrol and Glucotrol XL),* and glyburide *(Diabeta, Glynase, Micronase).* The major adverse effects of these first- and second-generation drugs are hypoglycemia because they stimulate the beta cells to produce insulin. The main difference between the between first and second generation agents is cost. All are equally effective in lowering serum glucose. The safety of this group in renal patients depends on their mode of metabolism and their half-life. Using those with a shorter half-life that are metabolized in the liver is safer for renal patients. Acetohexamide, chlorpropamide, and tolazamide are excreted in the urine and are usually not used with dialysis patients because their half-life will be prolonged in the absence of renal function. This may cause severe hypoglycemia. Glipizide and tolbutamide are almost completely hepatically metabolized and are the drugs of choice in patients with renal failure (Daugirdis et al., 2001).

Biguanides. Metformin *(Glucophage)* has been available in the U.S. since 1994. Metformin has many characteristics that are ideal for treating type 2 diabetes, including weight loss, insulin sensitization, positive lipid effect, mild hypotensive effect, and low or no incidence of hypoglycemia. Many experts believe that because metformin addresses so many of the key effects of type 2 diabetes, it should be considered the first-line medication. The major complication of metformin is a low, but significant, risk for fatal lactic acidosis. Because the kidneys excrete metformin, it can accumulate in renal failure patients, with the risk of severe lactic acidosis. Diabetic patients undergoing contrast dye studies and taking metformin should have the drug stopped at least 24 hours prior to the procedure. Patients receiving metformin should have their serum creatinine monitored periodically. Patients with serum creatinine above 1.4 (women) and 1.5 (men) should not take metformin (Quillen, 2004).

Thiazolidinediones (TZDs). The TZD class of oral hypoglycemics is a recent addition to the oral hypoglycemic agents. The first, troglitazone *(Rezulin),* was taken off the market in 1999 because of its association with hepatic toxicity. Rosiglitazone *(Avandia)* and pioglitazone *(Actos)* have been available since 1999. The primary effect of TZDs is peripheral, with increasing insulin sensitivity and increased glucose uptake. TZDs are hepatically metabolized and, thus, can be used safely in patients with renal dysfunction. They can be dosed once daily, although rosiglitazone works better with twice-daily dosing (Quillen, 2004).

Meglitinides. Repaglinide *(Prandin),* from the meglitinide drug class, is another recent class of oral hyperglycemic agents on the market. Repaglinide acts like an extremely short-acting sulfonylurea (an insulin secretagogue). The effect of repaglinide on the pancreas is very similar to that of the sulfonylureas, stimulating the secretion of insulin. What makes repaglinide clinically different from the sulfonylureas is its ultra-short half-life (1 hour). Repaglinide is

taken just before or with meals, and the stimulation of the pancreas is limited only to a brief time around meals. Because of the short duration, the patient does not have continuous high levels of insulin and the resulting adverse effects. It allows for meals to be more flexibly timed. It is metabolized in the liver so it is safe for renal patients (Quillen, 2004).

Alpha-glucosidase inhibitors (AGIs). The AGIs are unique nonsystemic oral agents that can help manage type 2 diabetes. The AGIs target the alpha-glucosidase enzyme of the proximal small intestine. Physiologically, the alpha-glucosidase enzyme is used to breakdown disaccharide-polysaccharides (starch) and sucrose (glucose + fructose). These medications delay the absorption of carbohydrates. However, there are GI effects such as bloating, flatulence, and diarrhea. There are currently two alpha-glucosidase inhibitors available in the U.S., miglitol *(Glyset)* and acarbose *(Precose).* Acarbose has occasionally been associated with liver toxicity and requires liver monitoring, whereas miglitol does not (Quillen, 2004). These drugs are safe for renal patients except for those with gastroparesis or gastric enteropathies that further delay or accelerate the absorption of food.

Blood pressure management. Careful screening of blood pressure should be done at each visit. Several medications are useful in treating hypertension in patients with renal disease and diabetes. Angiotensin converting enzymes (ACE inhibitors) and angiotension receptor blockers (ARBs) can modify the progress of kidney disease even in normotensive people. In a study using Captopril in patients with type 1 diabetes, the ACE inhibitor significantly reduced the progression of diabetic nephropathy as well as decreased proteinuria (Lewis, Hunsicker, Bain & Roche, 1993). In a study with ARBs in patients with type 2 diabetes, the drugs reduced the progression from microalbuminuria to macroalbuminuria in 37% of the patients. Because these two drug categories have an effect on nephropathy over and above their blood pressure lowering effects, their usage is now the mainstay of hypertension and renal protection in patients with diabetes (Taal & Brenner, 2002). It is also suggested that if one agent is ineffective in treating hypertension and proteinuria, then they should be used in combination. Hypertension treatment must be especially aggressive in the client with diabetes, not only for kidney protection but also to prevent the high rate of cardiovascular complications. Keeping the blood pressure under control is also important in avoiding or slowing renal disease. A target of less than 130/80 should be the goal (K/DOQI Guidelines, 2005). ACE inhibitors are especially renal protective because they decrease the pressure in the glomeruli that subsequently decrease protein leakage and scarring. Current therapy includes giving patients with diabetes ACE inhibitors before any renal changes start as a regular medication, even those without hypertension. However, there are side effects that include an annoying cough in 25% of the patients, and there can also be an increase in serum potassium. The new ARBs are a useful alternative for those who do not tolerate ACE inhibitors.

For patients with macroalbuminuria, blood pressure and blood glucose control is essential. These patients may also need dietary protein restriction and diuretics. When the third stage or renal failure develops, chronic renal failure patients need to be under the care of a nephrologist as well as an endocrinologist. At this point, dialysis may need to be instituted along with the medications mentioned above. Patients also need to see a renal social worker to help prepare for dialysis emotionally. The final stage, ESRD, will require complex management including medications and dialysis. At this point, patients with diabetes and ESRD may benefit from a renal and pancreatic transplant to help both diseases.

Blood Glucose Testing in Patients with Renal Disease

Patients with diabetes need intensive glycemic control to avoid the chronic complications of the disease including renal failure. Treatment guidelines have been established. Glycemic control is set forth by the ADA and others. Results of glucose monitoring are used to assess the effectiveness of therapy and to make adjustments in nutrition therapy, exercise, and medications to achieve optimum blood glucose control. Blood glucose control is important to prevent or delay diabetic nephropathy. Currently, the recommendations suggest a hemoglobin A1c of less than 6, which depending on the laboratory assay used, translates into an average daily blood glucose of less than 135 mg/dL (Goldstein et al., 2003). The Diabetes Control and Complications Trial (DCCT) revealed the health benefits of normal or near-normal blood glucose levels. Self-management by patients has revolutionized the management of diabetes. The ADA recommends that patients with diabetes attempt to keep blood glucose levels as close to normal as possible. Frequency and timing of self-monitoring should be centered on the needs and goals of the individual, but for patients with type 1, three times a day or more is recommended. The frequency of monitoring with type 2 is not specifically prescribed, but regular surveillance should be done, especially those who are taking insulin. Hypoglycemic and hyperglycemic states should be avoided. At a minimum, those taking sulfonylureas or insulin should monitor their blood glucose once a day. However, data indicates that only a minority of patients perform self-monitoring. Barriers to self-testing were identified as cost, inadequate understanding by patients and health care providers about the health benefits and usage of self-monitored glucose results, patient psychological and physical discomfort associated with finger stick sampling, inconvenience in terms of time requirements, physical settings, and complexity of technique. It is important that health care providers evaluate the patient's monitoring technique initially and at regular intervals. Also, proper interpretation is needed to adjust dietary intake, exercise, and pharmacological therapy.

Urine glucose testing has been replaced by self-monitored blood glucose; however, urine ketone measurement is important in patients with type 1 diabetes and in women with gestational diabetes. Ketoacidosis requires immediate attention. During times of stress of illness or when symptoms such as nausea and vomiting or abdominal pain exist, it is important to measure urine ketones by the use of a dipstick method (Goldstein et al., 2003).

Glycated protein testing. Measurement of glycated proteins, especially hemoglobin, has added a new dimension to monitoring glycemic control. These tests quantify glucose over weeks to months, complementing daily testing.

Glycated hemoglobin testing (HbA1c) measures hemoglobin components that form slowly from hemoglobin and glucose. The rate of formation is directly proportional to the glucose concentration. Since erythrocytes are freely permeable to glucose, the HbA1c in the blood sample provides a glycemic history of the past 120 days, the average life span of an erythrocyte. The A1C test should be performed routinely on patients, first to document glycemic control at an initial assessment and then as a part of ongoing care. The current recommended A1C is less than 6%, which translates into a mean plasma glucose of 135 mg/dL (Goldstein et al., 2003).

HbA1c values may not be accurate in patients with chronic renal failure. HbA1c levels have been reported to be elevated in this population. The laboratory values often do not correlate with the actual daily blood glucose levels due to changes in hematocrit, especially in dialysis patients. Acidosis also may increase HbA1c in uremic patients on hemodialysis (HD) (DeMarchi et al., 1983). Erythropoietin (EPO) treatment may also significantly influence HbA1c levels, and the more erythropoiesis fluctuates, the more HbA1c levels change even though there may not be changes in the blood glucose levels (Nakao et al., 1998).

Dietary Guidelines

A nutritional assessment is a necessary component of the ESRD patient treatment regimen. The dietary management of a person with diabetes and renal failure is complex. Qualified dietitians should complete a nutritional assessment within the first month of treatment. To prevent further or worsening diabetic complications, acceptable glucose control is essential. Hyperglycemia also causes thirst due to the hyperosmolar state of the vascular compartment drawing in cellular water causing dehydration at the cellular level. Managing fluid intake is an important step in preventing serious complications such as hypertension and congestive heart failure. Patients with ESRD can exhibit anorexia and nausea and vomiting. They may show evidence of malnutrition and wasting due to contributing factors such as poor intake, gastroparesis, enteropathy, and the catabolic stress associated with frequent illness (Daugirdis, Blake, & Ing, 2001). Patients with renal failure should have their diet closely monitored at regular intervals.

General dietary guidelines for patients with renal disease and diabetes include:

- Keep weight at a healthy level by eating a well-balanced diet and avoiding concentrated sweets
- Eat three meals a day about the same time each day
- Eat a bedtime snack
- Use sugar substitute
- Use fresh fruits and vegetables instead of canned (Fresenius Medical Care - Nutrition Education, 2003)

Protein restriction is often ordered for patients with renal failure. The recommended levels of protein intake must balance protein anabolism and amino acid losses with phosphorus restrictions that limit protein intake, especially in dialysis patients (Daugirdis et al., 2001).

Dialysis and the Renal Client with Diabetes Mellitus

Provisions for the maintenance of dialysis for patients with diabetes can be challenging. Morbidity and mortality is

Table 12-3
Dialysis Modalities for Persons with Diabetes

Modality	Advantages	Disadvantages
Hemodialysis (HD)	• Very efficient • No protein loss to dialysate • Frequent monitoring of renal failure	• Frequent medical follow-up • Higher risk for those with cardiovascular disease • More hypotensive episodes related to autonomic neuropathy • More prone to hypoglycemia • Survival rate of vascular access may be reduced • High risk for infection of vascular access
Peritoneal dialysis (PD)	• Better cardiovascular tolerance • No need for vascular access • Better control of serum potassium • Possible better glycemic control with intraperitoneal insulin • Less hypoglycemia	• Protein loss to dialysate • Glucose solutions used in PD fluid-glucose metabolism more stressed • Challenging control of glycemia • Increased hernias, fluid leaks, abdominal wall stress • Retinopathy may hinder sterile technique • More home assistance needed • Decreased appetite-increased glucose absorption through abdominal wall

Note: From Daugirdas, J.T., Blake, P.G., & Ing, T.I. (2001).

higher for diabetics with renal failure than non-diabetics. The most common co-morbidities responsible for mortality rates of approximately 25% per year are cardiovascular (Agarwal & Levi, 1994). The hypertension that accelerates atherosclerosis and retinopathy can be difficult to control when creatinine clearance falls below 15 mL/min. (Daugirdis et al., 2001). Table 12-3 describes the advantages and disadvantages of HD versus peritoneal dialysis (PD).

HD. One of the major challenges is the establishment and maintenance of a vascular access. The high incidence of peripheral vascular disease in diabetic patients can make placement of native fistulae difficult. However, changes in surgical techniques have made upper arm arteriovenous fistulas possible for more diabetic patients. The use of synthetic grafts may be necessary. (See Chapter 24, Hemodialysis Access for more information). Regulating blood glucose levels during dialysis may be challenging for some diabetic patients. Blood glucose monitoring during dialysis can avoid hypoglycemia and subsequent intradialytic complications. Fluid management is important in the control of hypertension. Sodium restriction and control of fluid by the patient is the first line of prevention. During HD treatments, regular observation of blood pressures and fluid removal rates to avoid hypotensive episodes is essential. Regular patient medication reviews by the nurse can help improve compliance with anithypertensive medications. (See chapter 13 End Stage Renal Disease and chapter 25 Preventing and Managing Complications Associated with Hemodialysis for more information.)

PD. PD produces less strain on the cardiovascular system and should be considered as a dialytic therapy for patients with these conditions. Patients with lung function or lumbar sacral problems may find it difficult to tolerate the volume of fluid in the abdomen. Advantages of PD may include better control of serum potassium and fluid retention. Patients may achieve better glycemic control with the use of intraperitoneal insulin. Disadvantages include peritonitis, catheter exit site infections, hernias, and fluid leaks. PD involves the use of glucose solutions that may be absorbed, causing anorexia with subsequent malnutrition. Protein losses across the peritoneal membrane can impact serum albumins and contribute to infection, malnutrition, and morbidity and mortality. Diabetic patients may need assistance from family members to perform their exchanges due to retinopathy. (See chapter 29 Preventing and Managing Complications Associated with Peritoneal Dialysis; Chapter 28 Peritoneal Dialysis Access for more information.)

Renal transplantation. Patients with diabetes account for over 30% of patients with ESRD. In choosing transplantation, the indications and contraindications must be considered as applying to the general ESRD population. The Diabetes Control and Complications Trial Group reported the risks for long-term complications from type 1 diabetes can be significantly minimized with the maintenance of normoglycemia (Implications of the Diabetes Control and Complications Trial, 2003). Pancreas transplantation for type 1 diabetics with simultaneous kidney/pancreas transplantation has a 3-year graft survival at an estimated 80%. Posttransplant, type

1 and type 2 diabetics require intensive glucose monitoring and management. Generally, they are controlled with a continuous intravenous insulin infusion. Assessment of insulin needs is required because of alteration in glucose metabolism caused by prednisone and other medications patients may be taking (see Chapter 31 on Transplantation for more information.)

Complications of Diabetes Mellitus and Renal Disease

The chronic complications of diabetes are entities that lead to morbidity and mortality in patients with diabetes. Renal disease itself is often a complication of diabetes. In addition, the following are diabetic complications with emphasis on the client with renal failure.

Diabetic Ketoacidosis (DKA)

Ketoacidosis is the result of a rapid fat breakdown leading to metabolic acidosis. It results from an absolute or relative deficiency of insulin and is characterized by a hyperglycemic state. It is a severe, sometimes fatal complication characterized by ketosis, acidosis, hyperglycemia, and dehydration (Funnell, Hunt, & Kulkarni, 1998). This condition is often a result of illness with counter regulatory hormones such as cortisol being released, stimulating gluconeogenesis (the process of making glucose from the breakdown products of lipids or proteins). Hyperglycemia results from inadequate insulin needed to transport glucose into the cell. DKA is much more common in patients with type 1 diabetes because people with type 2 usually have some endogenous insulin that prevents the breakdown of lipids that leads to DKA. In a person with renal failure and heart failure, DKA has a higher mortality rate because it may be concurrent with cardiac disease or infection. DKA leads to severe dehydration because the hyperosmolar state of the blood draws in water from the cellular compartment, dehydrating the cells. When correcting DKA, care must be taken to closely monitor the replacement of fluids and electrolytes, especially potassium. If heart failure also exists with DKA, intensive hemodynamic monitoring should occur in an intensive care setting. Sodium bicarbonate is not recommended due to its accompanying sodium burden in renal patients (Bloomgarden, 2002).

Hyperosmolar non-ketotic syndrome. Prolonged hyperglycemia can also lead to an acute metabolic crisis known as hyperosmoloar hyperglycemic state (HHS). This life-threatening condition is usually seen in elderly patients with type 2 diabetes. Signs and symptoms include severe hyperglycemia (blood glucose greater than 600 mg/dL), absence of ketoacidosis, profound dehydration, and mild to severe neurologic signs. Precipitating factors for HHS in the elderly include HD and PD treatments that lead to dehydration, infections, stress, and uremia. Treatment of HHS is rehydration, as appropriate, to restore plasma volume and correct electrolyte disturbances. Additional treatments are similar to those for DKA (Sagarin & McAfee, 2005).

GI Complications of Diabetes Mellitus

GI disorders in patients with diabetes include esophageal reflux, gastroparesis, diarrhea, constipation, and biliary tract abnormalities (Montgomery, 1999). These problems are common and can be debilitating. The common element in GI problems is dysmotility. Normal GI function requires coordinated contractions of the muscular layer of the gastrointestinal organs coordinated by the myenteric plexus, a network of nerves that run the length of the GI tract. In patients who have had diabetes for many years, especially those who have had prolonged periods of hyperglycemia, autonomic neuropathy develops, which leads to dysfunction of the nervous innervation to the GI tract.

Gastropathy

Gastropathy, or gastroparesis, is a chronic condition that can have significant consequences of glycemic and metabolic control leading to a poor quality of life. It occurs as a result of the stomach not functioning in an efficient or timely manner often rendering medication regimens ineffective. The stomach normally empties within 20 minutes to 6 hours after eating. The digestive process is controlled by the smooth muscles coordinated by the autonomic nervous system. Autonomic neuropathy can cause this process to go awry. The nervous innervation of the GI tract is altered, which changes the muscular activity of the stomach. There can be erratic absorption of oral medications and/or the formation of gastric bezoars causing obstruction or vomiting that leads to dehydration, electrolyte imbalance, weight loss, and nutritional compromise. The "diabetic stomach" is rarely a client's primary complaint and is often overlooked until the condition becomes serious (Bruton, 1998).

Uncontrolled blood glucose resulting in hyperglycemic states contributes to the development of autonomic neuropathy that results in gastropathy. However, when a client develops gastropathy, further hyperglycemia can result due to poor gastric emptying. In a person with type 2 diabetes that does produce some insulin, the fed state triggers insulin secretion. But, if there is delayed emptying and absorption, a hypoglycemic state can result. When the glucose is finally absorbed, there is often late hyperglycemia. These patients often have very hard to control diabetes at this point as a result of gastropathy.

Those at risk for developing gastropathy are those who have had diabetes for more than 10 years and those who already have other types of neuropathy such as peripheral neuropathy. Gastropathy is diagnosed by history, which often includes early satiety, postprandial bloating, abdominal distention, and nausea and vomiting of undigested food. Also, patients whose glucose was under good control who now are out of control may have gastropathy. The test to diagnose gastropathy, radionuclide scintigraphy, uses a technetium Tc99m labeled meal, and scans are done at 15, 30, 60, and 120 minutes to measure gastric emptying (Bruton, 1998). It is estimated that about 50% of patients with long-standing type 1 or type 2 diabetes have gastric delays (Kong, Horowitz, Jones, Wishart & Harding, 1999).

Retinopathy

Retinopathy is the leading cause of new blindness in the 20-74 age group. During the first 20 years of the disease, nearly all patients with type 1 and more than 60% with type 2 diabetes develop retinopathy. It is estimated that 3.6% of patients with type 1 and 1.6% of those with type 2 were legally blind. "The natural history of the disease progresses

Table 12-4
Guidelines for Eye Examinations

Disease Process	Time Interval Recommendations
Type 1 Diabetes	Dilated and comprehensive eye examination by an ophthalmologist or optometrist 3-5 years after the onset of diabetes
Type 2 Diabetes	Initial examination shortly after diabetes diagnosis
Subsequently for both types	Annually by an ophthalmologist or optometrist who is knowledgeable and experienced in the diagnosis of retinopathy and is aware of its management
Less frequent exams	Every 2-3 years at the advice of the eye care professional with an initial normal eye exam
Macular edema, proliferative diabetic retinopathy, or non-proliferative diabetic retinopathy	Prompt care needed - referral to an ophthalmologist knowledgeable in treating and managing retinopathy

Note: From Fong et al. (2004).

from mild proliferative abnormalities characterized by increased vascular permeability, to moderate and severe nonproliferative retinopathy with vascular closure to proliferative diabetic retinopathy characterized by the growth of new blood vessels on the retina and posterior surface of the vitreous" (Fong et al., 2004, p. S84). Macular edema also occurs that includes retinal thickening from leaky blood vessels. Hypertension and cataract surgery can accelerate these changes. Macular edema impairs central vision. New vessels and fibrous tissues contribute to retinal detachment that produces severe and permanent vision loss.

The major predictor for the development of retinopathy is the duration of diabetes. The risk for development reaches 80% for patients with type 1 diabetes who have had the disease for more than 15 years. Up to 21% of patients with type 2 have retinopathy with initial diagnosis of diabetes (Fong et al., 2004).

The key to slowing or preventing the development of retinopathy is control of glucose with the avoidance of hyperglycemia. Intensive glucose control was shown to reduce the progression by 76% (Batchelder & Barricks, 1995). Blood pressure control is also important. In the U.K. Prospective Diabetes Study (1998), patients with type 2 diabetes who were hypertensive and had tight blood pressure control (BP < 150/80) and were on ACE inhibitors or beta blockers had a 34% reduction in retinopathy progression. This translates into a reduced risk of visual acuity deterioration in those patients that keep their blood pressure under control and are on ACE inhibitors or beta blockers as many renal patients are. Laser photocoagulation also significantly reduces severe visual loss in people who have some degree of retinopathy and are early in the disease. Unfortunately, retinopathy is often not detected until some loss of vision has occurred.

Patients with diabetes should be routinely evaluated to detect treatable retinopathy. This includes dilated indirect ophthalmoscopy with biomicroscopy. A guideline for frequency of examinations is based on the severity of the retinopathy. Recommendations are for annual eye exams for those affected, but for those not yet affected, yearly examinations may not be cost effective (Vijan, Hofer, & Hayward, 2000). Older people at risk for cataracts, glaucoma, age-related macular degeneration and other potentially blinding disorders need more frequent examinations. Often patients with renal failure have had diabetes for many years, or it has caused their nephropathy, so these patients would be candidates for yearly eye examinations. At the time of the eye exam, teaching needs to be done related to glycemic, blood pressure, and serum lipid control. All of these are factors in progressive retinal deterioration. The guidelines for eye examinations are listed in Table 12-4.

Neuropathy and Lower Extremity Ulceration

As diabetes progresses, patients are likely to develop peripheral vascular disease due to atherosclerotic plaques, and this is an important precursor to ulcer development. Neuropathy is nerve damage attributed to diabetes. Numbness and reduced thermal and pain sensation in the feet occur as peripheral neuropathy advances (Bild et al., 1989). Also, neuropathic foot deformities occur with the unopposed action of the extensor tendons, and this leads to clawing of the toes and prominence of the metatarsal heads. Because of maldistribution of pressure, ulcers are more prone to develop on the areas underlying the metatarsal heads. Infection of chronic ulcers is a major cause of gangrene and, in turn, amputation. When an insensate foot is subject to even minor trauma or increased pressure, as with ill-fitting shoes, an ulcer may develop.

Risks for foot ulcers are greater in those who have had diabetes for 10 years or more, have poor glucose control, or have cardiovascular or renal complications (Hill et al., 1996). People with diabetes who also have ESRD often are at even higher risk for foot ulcer development because of severe hypertension, prior exposure to steroids, altered calcium metabolism, and protein restriction (Hill et al., 1996). Foot lesions may be the single most mismanaged problem

Table 12-5
The Semmes Weinstein Monofilament Sensory Foot Examination

1. Provide a quiet atmosphere free of distractions

2. Place the filament on the client's hands and an explanation of the procedure given. The client should be able to feel the monofilament without looking.

3. Apply the monofilament perpendicular to the skin surface on the appropriate sites on the sole of the foot.

4. Apply enough pressure to cause the monofilament to bend for 2 seconds.

5. Do not apply the filament to wounds, calluses, scars, or necrotic tissue.

6. Ask the client if they feel the pressure.

7. Ask the client where they feel the pressure.

8. Apply the monofilament twice and once as a "sham" without touching to each site.

9. Protective sensation is present if the client answers 2 out of 3 correctly at each site.

10. If the client answers incorrectly 2 out of 3 times, protective sensation is absent and the client is at risk for ulceration.

Note: From Boulton, A.J.M, Connor, H., & Cavanagh, P.R. (2000).

facing patients with diabetes and chronic renal failure (Broersma, 2004). The rate of lower limb amputation among diabetic patients with ESRD is ten times greater than the diabetic population at large. Also, two thirds of patients with diabetes and ESRD die within 2 years following the first lower extremity amputation (Deery & Sangeorzan, 2001). Once an ESRD client with diabetes develops a foot ulcer, it is hard to treat because of impaired wound healing and increased susceptibility to infection in patients with poor glucose control. The amputation rate for patients with diabetes and ESRD is 10/100 versus 1.9/100 for patients with ESRD alone (Pugh, Gohdes, & Eggers, 1999). In patients with nephropathy, neuropathy is often present. Neil, Knuckey, and Tanenberg (2003) found that all of the participants in their study of foot care and shoe management in those with ESRD and diabetes had severe neuropathy as well as renal failure.

Patient Education: The Role of the Nephrology Nurse

Sloan (1999) found that the large majority of nephrology patients are amenable to assessment, advice, and education by nephrology nurses. Welch and Austin (1999) suggest that nurses have the capability to develop individual interventions for the stressors of HD patients, and they can alter patient outcomes by interventions. Nephrology nurses not only provide support but can also be instrumental in preventing some of the complications of diabetes and ESRD. The dialysis unit provides an excellent opportunity for frequent education and reinforcement as part of daily care and assessment. In patients with diabetes and renal disease, there should be a multidisciplinary effort involving specialists from nephrology and endocrinology. Nurses who provide the day-to-day clinical care will need to help patients sort through all the information related to their two inter-related diseases. The following areas are mainstays of

nephrology nursing and should be taught and reinforced at regular intervals.

Foot Care Practices

Since dialysis patients have consistent, interdependent interactions with dialysis nurses on a regular basis, this relationship between nurse and patient can serve as a basis for integrating preventive and self-care practices into a client's daily reality. An important result of diabetic neuropathy is the loss of the protective sensation in the feet and legs. Neuropathy involving the feet can be measured using a Semmes-Weinstein test (Semmes-Weinstein, 1987). The steps involved in this sensory examination are listed in Table 12-5. Loss of protective sensation using this test involves monofilaments, simple tools of graduated sizes, which provide a quick method of diagnosing neuropathy. The 10 g monofilament is used on multiple sites on the foot to assess sensory level (Cavanagh, Ulbrecht, & Caputo, 2001).

Those who have lost the protective sensation must be extra vigilant in their foot care and shoe management. Foot care and inspection should include the following:

Foot inspection. Patients with diabetes are instructed to examine their feet daily for reddened areas, blisters, corns, calluses, or open areas. Some patients have retinopathy or lack mobility or flexibility making foot inspection difficult.

Foot cleaning. The recommendation for foot cleaning includes once a day cleaning with warm water and thorough drying afterwards.

Nail cutting. Proper nail cutting requires cutting the nails straight across. It is suggested that for patients with diabetes, regular podiatric care should be sought so they were not cutting their own nails. Dangerous nail cutting practices can lead to ingrown toenails with a subsequent infection that leads to limb loss.

Going barefoot. Patients with diabetes are advised to

Table 12-6

Modified Siriraj Foot-Care Score Questionnaire (Total possible score – 20)

Question	Possible Scores
How often do you inspect your feet?	3= more than 5 times a week 2= 2-4 times a week 1= once a week or less 0= never
How often do you clean your feet?	2= twice a day 1= once a day 0= never
What do you use to clean your feet?	2= soap and water 1=water only 0= shower water hits them
Do you clean between your toes?	1= yes 0= no
Do you dry between your toes?	1= yes 0 = no
What do you do if your feet get dirty?	2= clean them right away 0= clean them next time I bathe
What do you use to cut your nails?	2= straight end nail clipper 1= blunt scissors 0= sharp scissors or knife
How do you cut your toenails?	2= straight across 0= cut the nail as much as possible
How often do you wear shoes when walking outside in the summer time?	2= always 1= most of the time 0= never
Do you ever go barefooted or sock footed in the house?	3= no 2= bedroom only 1= bathroom only 0= yes, everywhere

always wear foot protection and never to go barefoot. Cotton socks are also recommended at all times.

Patients who have ESRD and diabetes are at high risk for developing foot ulcers. On-going, nonjudgmental assessment of patients' foot care and shoe management knowledge is a mainstay of foot ulcer prevention. The Siriraj Foot Care Scale (Sruissadaporn et al., 1998) is a 10-item scale revised by Neil (2001) to reflect Western culture. It uses point values ranging from 0-3 to examine the self-care practices related to the foot. Items include foot inspection (1 question), foot cleaning (5 questions), nail care (2 questions), and going barefoot (2 questions). Items were based on standard foot care management techniques prescribed by the ADA and the Joslin Clinic Diabetes Teaching Guide (1983). This scale has a possible score of 20. A score below 15 indicates high risk for foot ulcer development. Table 12-6 displays this foot care questionnaire that is useful in assessing risk for foot ulcer formation.

Shoe Management

When an insensate foot is subject to even minor trauma or increased pressure, as with ill-fitting shoes, an ulcer may develop. Ensuring proper footwear is, thus, an important part of a treatment program for people with diabetes, even for those in the earliest stages of the disease. If there is evidence of neuropathy, wearing the right footwear is crucial. It is well known that footwear is a significant cause of ulceration. Shoes must accommodate dorsal deformities and cushion areas of high pressure. In particular, they should relieve excessive pressure on areas that are prominent, such as the metatarsal heads. Shoes must also reduce shock (the vertical pressure on the bottom of the foot due to the weight of the person) and shear (the horizontal movement of the foot within the shoe). Deformities of the foot resulting from loss of fatty tissue, hammertoes, and toe amputations must also be accommodated. Deformities need to be stabilized to relieve pressure and avoid further destruction (Lavery, Vela, Fleischli, Armstrong, & Lavery, 1997).

Shoe fit is critical in the prevention of foot ulcers. Despite its importance, this is usually left to the subjective

Table 12-7
Think FAST: Footwear Appropriateness Scoring Tool

SHOE CHARACTERISTIC

	Yes	No
1. Are the shoes the same shape as the feet?		
2. Is there at least 1/2 of an inch between the end of the toes and the end of the shoe when standing?		
3. Is the toe box deep enough to prevent deformity of the shoes by the toes AND the toes can move inside of the shoes?		
4. Are shoes wide enough to prevent stretching of the upper part of the shoe by the foot?		
5. Does the heel slide around in the heel cup?		
6. Is the heel cup firm and does not shift to the left or right when standing or walking?		
7. Is the heel of the shoe less than 1 inch in height?		
8. Is the sole of the shoe made of a material that would cushion the impact of walking?		
9. Is the shoe flexible at the base of the toe?		
10. Is the upper part of the shoe made from a material that facilitates ventilation?		
11. Is the shoe secured to the foot with laces, buckles or Velcro that allows for loosening or tightening while the shoe is being worn?		
12. Does the shoe provide protection by completely enclosing the foot?		
TOTAL		

How to use this tool
1. Use this tool as a guide to evaluate the appropriateness of commercial footwear worn by a person.
2. If the answer is yes to all of these questions, the shoe probably will not cause injury to the feet.
3. If the answer is no to any of the questions, the shoes may cause injury to the feet.
4. If the answer is no to more than one question, the shoes are likely to cause injury to your feet.

Note: Copyright - Dr. Craig L. Broussard, PhD, RN, CNS, CWS, CWCN, CHRNC, Clinical Consultants. Reprinted with permission.

opinion of the fitter and the wearer. When a person has insensate feet, they may not be able to feel the pressure of the shoe on their feet unless the shoe is tight. Therefore, it is important that shoes are professionally fit for the person who is insensate. Boussard (2001) developed the Footwear Appropriateness Scoring Tool (Table 12-7), a tool that is useful in assessing shoe fit. Items include the toe box being deep enough, the shoe box being wide enough, the heel not slipping in the shoe, the heel not being more that 1″ in height, and the materials the sole is made of cushioning the impact of walking. Also, good shoes must be secured with laces, buckles, or Velcro®. The neuropathic foot must be cushioned so that undo pressure does not occur on any part of the foot leading to a foot ulcer. Nephrology nurses can have an impact on shoe management by basic shoe assessment and recommendations to the client. Often, good athletic shoes with laces are adequate shoes if they fit properly. Patients should not wear open toe shoes and should always wear socks as an extra protection against foot ulcers.

Conclusion

Patients with diabetes and the comorbid condition of renal disease present a unique challenge to the health care community. A multidisciplinary approach to these two processes is essential for the proper management of both diseases. Diabetic nephropathy is preventable if patients are diagnosed early in the course of nephropathy, which requires early screening for the detection of microalbuminuria. Unfortunately, patients with type 2 diabetes may not know they have nephropathy until it has progressed to a point that is no longer reversible. Nephrology nurses can play an important role in the reinforcement of medical regimes and in early surveillance, especially in the area of blood glucose monitoring and foot and shoe management.

References

American Diabetes Association (ADA). (2004a). *What is pre-diabetes?* Retrieved December 4, 2004, from www.diabetes.org/diabetes prevention/pre-diabetes.jsp

American Diabetes Association (ADA). (2004b). Diabetes risk test. Retrieved September 12, 2005, from http://www.diabetes.org/risk-test.jsp

American Diabetes Association (ADA). (2004c). *Gestational diabetes.* Retrieved December 2, 2004 from www.diabetes.org/gestational-diabetes.jsp

American Diabetes Association (ADA). (2004d). *Diabetes symptoms.* Retrieved March 27, 2004, from www.diabetes.org/diabetes-symptoms.jsp

American Diabetes Association (ADA). (2004e). *Genetics of diabetes.* Retrieved December 2, 2004, from www.diabetes.org/genetics.jsp

Agarwal, R., & Levi, M. (1994). Selection of therapy for patients with end stage renal disease. In W.L. Henrich (Ed.), *Principles and practice of dialysis.* Baltimore: Williams and Wilkins.

Batchelder, T., & Barricks, M. (1995). The Wisconsin epidemiologic study of diabetic retinopathy. *Archives of Ophthalmology, 113,* 702-703.

Bloomgarden, Z.T. (2002). Diabetic ketoacidosis in patients with CHF and/or renal failure. *Medscape Diabetes & Endocrinology, 4*(1). Retrieved March 27, 2004, from www.medscape.com/viewarticle/430196_print

Bild, D.E., Selby, J.V., Sinnock, P., Browner, W.S., Braveman, P, & Showstack, J.A. (1989). Lower-extremity amputation in people with diabetes. *Diabetes Care, 12,* 24-31.

Bilous, R.W. (2003). Normal blood glucose in diabetes patients with chronic renal failure. *Medscape Diabetes & Endocrinology, 5*(2). Retrieved March 27, 2004, from www.medscape.com/viewarticle/461108_print

Boulton, A.J.M, Connor, H., & Cavanagh, P.R., (2000). The foot in diabetes. New York: John Wiley & Sons. Boussard, C. (2001). *Think FAST: Footwear appropriateness scoring tool.* Poster session presented at the 15th Anniversary Conference, Southern Nursing Research Society, Baltimore, MD.

Boussard, C.L. (2001). *The footwear appropriateness scale.* Poster presented at the Southern Nursing Research Society, Baltimore, MD.

Broersma, A. (2004). Preventing amputations in patients with diabetes and chronic kidney disease. *Nephrology Nursing Journal, 31,* 53-64.

Bruton, S.A. (1998). Diagnosing diabetic gastropathy: A primary care challenge. *Clinical Focus, 5,* 11-16.

Cavanagh, P.R., Ulbrecht, J.S., & Caputo, M.C. (2001). The biomechanics of the foot in diabetes mellitus. In J.H. Bowker & M.A. Pfeifer (Eds.), *Levin and O'Neal's the diabetic foot* (6th ed.). Philadelphia: Mosby. p 177-178.

Daugirdis, J.T., Blake, P.G., & Ing, T.I. (2001). *Handbook of dialysis.* New York: Lippincott, Williams & Wilkins.

Deery, H.G., & Sangeorzan, J.A. 2001. Saving the diabetic foot with special reference to the patient with chronic renal failure. *Infectious Disease Clinics of North America,* 15(3), 953-981.

DeMarchi, S., Cecchin, E., Camurri, C., Raimondi, A., Donadon, W., Lippi, U., & Tesio, F. (1983). Origin of glycosylated hemoglobin A1 in chronic renal failure. *International Journal of Artificial Organs,* 6(2), 77-82.

Diabetes and Kidney Disease. (2005). National Kidney Foundation. Retrieved September 12, 2005, from http://www.kidney.org/atoz/atozItem.cfm?id=37

Diagnosis and Classification of Diabetes Mellitus: American Diabetes Association (2005). *Diabetes Care, 28,* S37-42.

Fresenius Medical Care - Nutrition Education. (2003). *Diabetes and your renal diet.* (2003). Charlotte NC: Fresenius.

Fong, D.S., Aiello, L, Gardener, T.W., King, G.L., Blankenship, G., Cavallerano, et al. (2004). Retinopathy in diabetes. *Diabetes Care, 26*(1), 226-229.

Goldstein, D.E., Randie, R.L., Lorenz, R.A., Malone, J.I., Nathan, D.M., & Peterson, C.M. (2003). Tests of glycemia in diabetes. *Diabetes Care, 27,* S91-93.

Hill, M.N., Hilton, S.C., Ylitalo, M., Feldman, H.I., Holechek, M.J., & Benedict, G.W. (1996). Risk of foot complications in long-term diabetic patients with and without ESRD: A preliminary study. *ANNA Journal, 23,* 381-386.

Funnell, M.M., Hunt, C., & Kulkarni, K. (1998). *A core curriculum for diabetes education* (3rd edition). Chicago: American Association of Diabetic Educators.

Implications of the Diabetes Control and Complications Trial: American Diabetes Association. (2003). *Diabetes Care, 26,* S25-27. Retrieved September 12, 2005, from http://care.diabetes journals.org/cgi/content/full/26/suppl_1/s25

Joslin Clinic Diabetes Teaching Guide. (1983). In G.P. Kozak, C.S. Hoar, J.L. Towbotham, F.C. Wheelock, G.W. Gibbons, & D. Campbell (Eds.), *Management of diabetic foot problems.* Philadelphia: W.B. Saunders.

Kong, M., Horowitz, M., Jones, K.L., Wishart, J.M., & Harding, P.E. (1999). Natural history of diabetic gastroparesis. *Diabetes Care,* 22(3), 503-507.

K/DOQI Clinical Practice Guidelines for Cardiovascular Disease in Dialysis Patients. Retrieved September 12, 2005, from http://www.kidney.org/professionals/kdoqi/guidelines_cvd/guide 12.htm

Kumar, J., & Young, J.H. (1999). Diabetes mellitus and the kidney. *End Stage Renal Disease.* [Brochure] Denville, NJ: Psy-Ed Corporation.

Lavery, L.A., Vela, S.A., Fleischli, J.,G., Armstrong, D.G., & Lavery, D.C. (1997). Reducing plantar pressure in the neuropathic foot. A comparison of footwear. *Diabetes Care, 20*(11), 1706-10.

Lewis, E.J., Hunsicker, L.G., Bain, R.P., & Roche, R.D. (1993). The effect of angiotensin-converting-enzyme inhibition on diabetic nephropathy: The Collaborative Study Group. *New England Journal of Medicine, 329,* 1456-1462.

Montgomery, P.A. (1999). Gastrointestinal complications of diabetes mellitus. *Journal of Pharmaceutical Care in Pain and Symptom Management, 7*(2), 11-34.

Nakao, T., Matsumoto, H., Okada, T., Han, M., Hidaka, H., Yoshino, M., et al. (1998). Influence of erythropoietin treatment on hemoglobin A1c levels in patients with chronic renal failure on hemodialysis. *Internal Medicine, 37,* 826-830.

Neil, J.A. (2001). Assessment of foot care knowledge in rural persons with diabetes with and without foot ulcers. *Ostomy/Wound Management, 48,* 50-56.

Neil, J.A., Knuckey, C.J., & Tanenberg, R.J. (2003). Prevention of foot ulcers in patients with diabetes and end stage renal disease. *Nephrology Nursing Journal, 30,* 39-43.

Pfutzner, A., Kunt, T., Holberg, C., Mondok, A., Pahler, S., Konrad, T., et al. (2004). Fasting intact proinsulin is a highly specific predictor of insulin resistance in type 2 diabetes. *Diabetes Care, 27*(4), 682-687.

Pugh, J.A., Gohdes, D., Eggers P.W. (1999). *Lower extremity amputation rates are very high in diabetic ESRD patients* (Abstract 0770). Abstract presented at the 59th Annual Scientific Sessions of ADA, San Diego, CA.

Quillen, D.M. (2004). Medications for the treatment of type 2 diabetes. Retrieved November 26, 2004, from www.medscape.com/viewarticle/426540?src=search

Rabkin, R. (2003). Diabetic nephropathy. *Clinical Cornerstone, 5*(2), 1-11.

Sagarin, M, & McAfee, A. (2005). Hyperosmolar Hyperglycemic Nonketotic Coma. Retrieved September 12, 2005, from http://www.emedicine.com/emerg/topic264.htm

Semb, S. (2004). Nursing management: Diabetes mellitus. In S.M. Lewis, M.M. Heitkemper, & S.R. Dirksen (Eds.), *Medical-surgical nursing* (6th ed.), Baltimore: Mosby, Inc.

Semmes Weinstein Monofilaments. (1987). [brochure] Morgan Hill, CA: North Coast Medical.

Skyler, J.S. (2001). Diabetes mellitus: Old assumptions and new realities. In J.H. Bowker & M.A. Ppfeifer (Eds.) *Levin and O'Neil's the diabetic foot* (6th edition). Philadelphia: Mosby.

Sloan, R. (1999). Guarded alliance between hemodialysis patients and their health care providers. *ANNA Journal, 26,* 503-505.

Sruissadaporn, S., Ploybutr, S., Nittyanant, W., Vannasaeng, S., & Vichayanrat, A. (1998). Behavior in self-care of the foot and foot ulcers in Thai non-insulin dependent diabetes mellitus. *Journal of the Medical Association of Thailand, 31*(1), 29-36.

Taal, M.W., & Brenner, B.M. (2002). Combination ACEI and ARB therapy: Additional benefit is renoprotection? *Current Opinion in Nephrology Hypertension, 11,* 377-381.

Taylor, M.R. (1998). The diabetic patient. In J. Parker (Ed.), *Contemporary nephrology nursing* (pp. 465-478). Pitman, NJ: American Nephrology Nurses' Association.

UK Prospective Diabetes Study Group. (1998). Tight blood pressure control and risk of macrovascular and microvascular complications in type 2 diabetes. UKPDS, 38. *British Medical Journal, (317),* 708-713.

Vijan, S., Hofer, T.P., & Hayward, R.A. (2000). Cost-utility analysis of screening intervals for diabetic retinopathy in patients with type 2 diabetes mellitus. *Journal of the American Medical Association, 283,* 889-896.

Welch, J.L., & Austin, J.K. (1999). Factors associated with treatment-related stressors in hemodialysis patients. *ANNA Journal, 26,* 318-325.

Additional Readings

American Diabetes Association (ADA). (2004f). Frequently asked questions about diabetes. Retrieved November 26, 2004, from www.diabetes.org/pre-diabetes/faq.jsp

American Diabetes Association (ADA). (2004g). National diabetes fact sheet. Retrieved November 26, 2004, from www.diabetes.org/diabetes-statistics/national-diabetes-fact-sheet.jsp

Franz, M. (2003). *A core curriculum for diabetes education: Diabetes and complications* (5th ed.). Chicago: American Association of Diabetic Educators.

Waugh, N.R., & Robertson, A.M. (2003). Protein restriction for diabetic renal disease. *Cochrane Review of Abstracts: The Cochrane Library, 2.*

- Diabetes is defined as an alteration in the metabolism of carbohydrates, proteins, and fats. It is a multisystem disease related to a decrease in insulin production, insulin utilization, or both defects.

- Type 1 diabetes, formerly known as insulin dependent diabetes or juvenile diabetes, occurs most often in people under the age of 30. It results from a destruction of the pancreatic beta cells due to an autoimmune process. Type 2 diabetes is the most prevalent and usually occurs in people over age 40.

- Diabetes is responsible for 35% of renal failure. In fact, diabetes is the most common cause of renal failure. The clinical course leading to nephropathy differs in the two types of diabetes. The four stages leading to nephropathy are: microalbuminuria, macroproteinuria, chronic kidney disease, and ESRD.

- The chronic complications of diabetes are entities that lead to morbidity and mortality in patients with diabetes. Renal disease itself is often a complication of diabetes. In addition, the following are diabetic complications with emphasis on the client with renal failure.

- Management of the patients with diabetes and renal disease involves monitoring medications and blood pressure, checking blood glucose levels, and following dietary guidelines.

- The chronic complications of diabetes are entities that lead to morbidity and mortality in patients with diabetes. Renal disease itself is often a complication of diabetes.

- An important result of diabetic neuropathy is the loss of the protective sensation in the feet and legs. Neuropathy involving the feet can be measured using a Semmes-Weinstein test.

- Nephrology nurses not only provide support but can also be instrumental in preventing some of the complications of diabetes and ESRD. The dialysis unit provides an excellent opportunity for frequent education and reinforcement as part of daily care and assessment.

ANNP612

Diabetes and Kidney Disease: A Challenge in Chronic Disease Management

Janice A. Neil, PhD, RN

Contemporary Nephrology Nursing: Principles and Practice contains 39 chapters of educational content. Individual learners may apply for continuing nursing education credit by reading a chapter and completing the Continuing Education Evaluation Form for that chapter. Learners may apply for continuing education credit for any or all chapters.

Please photocopy this page and return to ANNA.
COMPLETE THE FOLLOWING:

Name: _____

Address:_____

City:_____ State: _____ Zip: _____

E-mail: _____

Preferred telephone: ☐ Home   ☐ Work: _____

State where licensed and license number (optional): _____

CE application fees are based upon the number of contact hours provided by the individual chapter. CE fees per contact hour for ANNA members are as follows: 1.0-1.9 - $15; 2.0-2.9 - $20; 3.0-3.9 - $25; 4.0 and higher - $30. Fees for nonmembers are $10 higher.

ANNA Member: ☐ Yes   ☐ No   Member # (if available) _____

☐ Checked Enclosed   ☐ American Express   ☐ Visa   ☐ MasterCard

Total Amount Submitted: _____

Credit Card Number: _____ Exp. Date: _____

Name as it appears on the card: _____

CE Evaluation Form
To receive continuing education credit for individual study after reading the chapter
1. Photocopy this form. (You may also download this form from ANNA's Web site, **www.annanurse.org**.)
2. Mail the completed form with payment (check) or credit card information to American Nephrology Nurses' Association, East Holly Avenue, Box 56, Pitman, NJ 08071-0056.
3. You will receive your CE certificate from ANNA in 4 to 6 weeks.

Test returns must be postmarked by **December 31, 2010.**

CE Application Fee
ANNA Member $15.00
Nonmember $25.00

EVALUATION FORM

1. I verify that I have read this chapter and completed this education activity. Date: _____

_____
Signature

2. What would be different in your practice if you applied what you learned from this activity? *(Please use additional sheet of paper if necessary.)*

_____
_____
_____
_____
_____
_____
_____
_____
_____
_____
_____

Evaluation	Strongly disagree				Strongly agree
3. The activity met the stated objectives.					
a. Describe the effect of diabetes mellitus on the renal system.	1	2	3	4	5
b. Discuss the management of the patient with both diabetes and renal disease.	1	2	3	4	5
c. Summarize the care needed for patients with complications of diabetes mellitus.	1	2	3	4	5
d. Outline an educational plan of care for a patient with diabetes mellitus and renal disease.	1	2	3	4	5
4. The content was current and relevant.	1	2	3	4	5
5. The content was presented clearly.	1	2	3	4	5
6. The content was covered adequately.	1	2	3	4	5
7. Rate your ability to apply the learning obtained from this activity to practice.	1	2	3	4	5

Comments _____

_____

8. Time required to read the chapter and complete this form: _____ minutes.

This educational activity has been provided by the American Nephrology Nurses' Association (ANNA) for 1.8 contact hours. ANNA is accredited as a provider of continuing nursing education (CNE) by the American Nurses Credentialing Center's Commission on Accreditation (ANCC-COA). ANNA is an approved provider of continuing education by the California Board of Registered Nursing, CEP 0910.

End Stage Renal Disease

Lori Candela, EdD, RN, APRN, BC, FNP
Kathy P. Parker, PhD, RN, FAAN

Chapter Contents

End Stage Renal Disease

Chapter 13

Lori Candela, EdD, RN, APRN, BC, FNP
Kathy P. Parker, PhD, RN, FAAN

E nd stage renal disease (ESRD) represents the end of the continuum of renal function, a point at which the progressive, irreversible loss of nephrons renders the kidneys unable to maintain metabolic homeostasis. As previously discussed, the degree of renal function is described in terms of glomerular filtration rate (GFR) (see Chapter 7). ESRD (renal failure in the chronic setting), by definition, is present when the GFR< 15 cc/minute (Stage V) (National Kidney Foundation [NKF], 2000b), a point at which renal replacement therapy becomes necessary.

ESRD continues to be a significant health problem in the United States population. By the end of 2002, there were over 300,000 patients with ESRD in the United States and the number of patients receiving treatment for kidney failure is increasing at a rate of approximately 2.5% per year (USRDS, 2004). The incidence of chronic renal failure is higher in the elderly. This finding may be related to the overall aging of the general population, the progressive loss of renal function with age, and the improved survival of patients with chronic diseases that have renal complications such as diabetes mellitus. However, although aging of the population may contribute to the growth of ESRD, it does not explain the overall six-fold increase in the problem over the last two decades, and increased research into other unique groups of ESRD patients is needed (USRDS, 2004). Although the reasons are unclear, the incidence of ESRD is higher in African Americans, Native Americans, and Hispanic Americans. Gender also seems to be a risk factor, as both the prevalence and incidence rates of ESRD have remained consistently 1.4 times higher in males than in females (USRDS, 2004), an observation possibly related to gender-related differences in the responsiveness of the renin-angiotensin system (Pechere-Bertschi & Burnier, 2004).

Whether treatment with dialysis or transplantation is indicated, ESRD remains a condition that extracts a serious toll from those with the illness and from society as a whole. As renal function diminishes, patients experience a myriad of physical and psychosocial problems that literally affect every aspect of their lives (Curtin, Bultman, Thomas-Hawkins, Walters, & Schatell, 2002; National Kidney Foundation [NKF], 2000c). In addition, the monetary cost of ESRD is substantial. Hospitalization is often required as part of treatment. Dialysis, if needed, must be provided on a regular basis. Drug regimens are expensive. The total estimated direct medical charges for ESRD alone, excluding the costs of care for patients with renal insufficiency, was over $17.0 billion during 2002 – 6.7% of the Medicare budget (USRDS, 2004).

Nurses are being called upon with increasing frequency to play key roles in the management of patients with ESRD. In addition, effective management of these patients requires continual collaboration, coordination, and communication among all members of the health care team in order to optimally manage the complex needs of these patients. This chapter focuses on the diverse clinical manifestations of ESRD. The pathophysiologic basis, clinical presentation, and selected medical treatments of these manifestations are described. Assessment parameters, nursing interventions, and expected outcomes are summarized in tables at the end of this textbook (see Appendices B, C, and D).

Fluid, Electrolyte, and Acid-Base Disturbances

ESRD is associated with a variety of disturbances in fluid, electrolytes, and acid-base balance and these are covered in detail in Chapter 5. Many of the features of uremia can be related to either accumulation or depletion of organic or inorganic ions that impair cell metabolism and stimulate abnormal hormonal responses (Bailey & Mitch, 2004). Once renal function falls below 25% of normal, the kidneys have a limited capacity to deal with excess fluid, electrolytes, and acid-base load, as well as stressors associated with volume and electrolyte loss. Table 13-1 shows the change in plasma concentration of the major solutes and the decreased ability of the kidney to concentrate urine in the face of progressive nephron loss (Koeppen & Stanton, 2001). The nursing care related to the management of fluid, electrolyte, and acid-base balance changes is summarized in Appendix B.

Metabolic and Endocrine Disturbances

In renal failure, the homeostasis of metabolic and endocrine systems depends on a variety of adaptive mechanisms, many of which are poorly understood. Unfortunately, these adaptations have numerous adverse systemic effects that result in the development of metabolic and regulatory disorders. The major abnormalities that occur include glucose intolerance, disturbances in protein and lipid metabolism, and alterations in endocrine function. In order to plan appropriate care, nurses should develop an understanding of the pathophysiologic basis and psychosocial responses associated with these changes (see Appendix B).

Glucose Intolerance

Glucose intolerance and insulin resistance develop in patients with ESRD (Bailey & Mitch, 2004; Mak, 2000; Massry & Smogorzewski, 2001b). Although baseline insulin levels are increased and the degradation of insulin is reduced when GFR falls to less than 20%, there is a decreased response or resistance to insulin (up to 60%) at the tissue level. Other factors that may also contribute to glucose intolerance include delayed insulin secretion after glucose ingestion, altered cellular metabolism secondary to acidosis, mode of dialysis, and gastrointestinal complications affecting intake and absorption (Mak, 2000). Although insulin and glucose metabolism are improved with regular dialysis, complete normalization does not always occur. However, the glucose intolerance is seldom severe enough

Table 13-1

Effects of Progressive Nephron Loss on the Plasma Concentration of Selected Solutes and Urine Concentrating Ability

	GFR (% of normal)				
	100	**65**	**33**	**20**	**10**
Plasma [Na^+] (mEq/L)	140	140	140	138	136
Plasma [K^+] mEq/L	4	4	4	4.5	5.5
Plasma [Ca^{++}] mg/dl	10	10	10	8.7	8.2
Plasma [Pi^-] mg/dl	4	4.2	4.3	5.2	5.8
Plasma [HCO_3^-] mg/dl	24	24	22	16	13
Plasma [creatinine] mg/dl	1	1.6	3.1	5.0	10.4
Plasma BUN mg/dl	14	18	29	46	82
Plasma pH	7.4	7.4	7.37	7.3	7.26
P_{osm} (mOsm/kg H_2O)	290	292	295	300	310
Max U_{osm} (mOsm/kg H_2O)	1200	1000	500	350	310
Min U_{osm} (mOsm/kg H_2O)	50	50	70	200	310

Note: From Koeppen & Stanton, (2003). Renal Physiology, St. Louis: Mosby, 3rd ed. p 182.

to result in extreme hyperglycemia and ketoacidosis. Nonetheless, the absence of glycosuria as a safety valve can result in the development of profound hyperglycemia in diabetic patients with ESRD.

Although glucose intolerance develops in many patients, the reduced metabolic clearance and degradation of insulin may actually decrease the insulin requirements of diabetics who develop renal failure, leading to hypoglycemia (Bailey & Mitch, 2004; Mak, 2000). This may be complicated by the fact that diabetic dialysis patients may also have a blunted response to the effects of low blood sugar. Thus, unless this problem is recognized and the insulin dosage is reduced, symptomatic hypoglycemia can develop. Appropriate nursing management of these patients includes a careful assessment of glucose levels and insulin requirements, maintenance of an adequate oral intake prior to dialysis, and use of a hemodialysate glucose level of 200 mg/dl to avoid hypoglycemia.

Glucose and insulin abnormalities in nondiabetic ESRD patients may play an important role in the pathogenesis of hyperlipidemia by impairing lipoprotein lipase activity and therefore may represent important risk factors for accelerated atherosclerosis (Massry & Smogorzewski, 2001b). Glycemic control also correlates with morbidity and mortality in diabetic ESRD patients and poor control is associated with vascular complications, malnutrition, and shortened survival (Tzamaloukas, Murata, Zager, Eisenberg, & Avasthi, 1993). Glycosated hemoglobin remains useful in assessing long-term control in diabetic ESRD patients.

Alterations of Protein Metabolism

There are a number of abnormalities in amino acid and protein metabolism in ESRD (Kopple, 2001). Protein synthesis is generally normal in early renal insufficiency but gradually decreases with progressive renal failure. Malnutrition, insulin resistance, metabolic acidosis, and

hyporesponsiveness to growth hormone are possible causes (Kopple, 2001). Clinical markers of poor protein metabolism include low serum levels of albumin, transferrin, and prealbumin, all of which are indicators of overall nutritional status. However, despite their clinical utility, these levels may still be insensitive to changes in nutritional status, do not necessarily correlate with changes in other nutritional parameters, and can be influenced by non-nutrition factors (infection, or inflammation, hydration, acidemia). Thus, the patient's clinical status (changes dialysis modality, acid-base status, and degree of protein losses) must be evaluated (NKF, 2000a).

Although protein restriction is often an important component of the treatment plan (Bailey & Mitch, 2004), it is important that patients with ESRD have adequate intake in order to avoid depleting their protein stores. Negative-nitrogen balance is associated with increased mortality (Carfray et al., 2000; Kaysen & Don, 2003; Steinman, 2000). Adequate energy intake in the form of calories is also important. In a restricted protein diet, as much of the protein as possible should be of high biological value (containing essential amino acids such as meat and fish). These essential amino acids are vital for protein synthesis. On the other hand, low biological value proteins (bread and cereals) provide few essential amino acids and their breakdown increases the BUN. Adequate dialysis is also important in the maintenance of appropriate protein metabolism.

Nursing care should begin with a careful assessment of eating habits, dietary preferences, and cultural influences on eating patterns. A dietary or nutritional support team consult is often crucial in conducting a thorough nutritional evaluation. Oral supplements or total parenteral nutrition are then prescribed after assessing the patient's unique needs. Multivitamin supplements are also frequently recommended. Nurses should continually monitor indicators of nutritional status, including weight, electrolytes, and albumin levels. Sources of protein depletion such as losses from wounds, drainage, or peritoneal dialysis should be identified and replaced. Patients and their families should also be educated regarding the importance of adequate nutritional intake (see Appendix B).

Alterations of Lipid Metabolism

Dyslipidemia is a common complication of patients with ESRD (Lacour, Massy, & Drueke, 2001). Although serum cholesterol is usually normal or only slightly elevated, serum triglyceride levels are frequently high (a condition referred to as Type IV hyperlipoproteinemia). The development of hypertriglyceridemia is believed to be related to decreased lipoprotein lipase activity and a reduced conversion of VLDL to LDL (Lacour et al., 2001). The use of high concentrations of glucose in peritoneal dialysate leads to an increase in the carbohydrate load and has been reported to aggravate hypertriglyceridemia in some patients. However, the glucose concentration of 100 to 200 mg/dl in hemodialysate does not appear to add to the carbohydrate load and has not been shown to make a significant contribution to lipid abnormalities. Other factors that may aggravate lipid abnormalities in some patients include the use of beta blockers and diuretics. Several endocrine disturbances in ESRD contribute to dyslipidemia, including increased glucagon levels, elevated parathyroid hormone, decreased testosterone, increased leptin levels, growth hormone resistance, and deficits in carnitine (Bailey & Mitch, 2004; Lacour et al., 2001).

The treatment of hypertriglyceridemia is important in the ESRD patient because of its relationship to the development of atherosclerosis and coronary artery disease, major causes of morbidity and mortality. Lowering the dietary intake of saturated fats and carbohydrates may be helpful. However, because of other dietary restrictions used in the treatment of renal failure patients, the usefulness of these additional dietary modifications may be limited. A carefully monitored program of exercise can help reduce triglyceride levels as can avoidance of drugs known to exacerbate hyperlipidemia such as beta adrenergic blocking agents. The use of antilipemic agents such as gemfibrozil or lovastatin has not been reported in large numbers of patients with chronic renal failure. Unfortunately, there are no randomized controlled intervention trials of chronic kidney disease patients showing that the treatment of dyslipidemia reduces the incidence of coronary vascular disease (NKF, 2000d).

Endocrine Disorders

A wide variety of endocrine abnormalities are known to develop in patients with ESRD as changes occur in the synthesis, secretion, and metabolism of various hormones, as well as alterations in their biologic activity (Daugirdas, Blake, & Ing, 2001; Bailey & Mitch, 2004) (see Table 13-2). Several of these abnormalities are covered in other appropriate sections of this chapter. For example, changes in insulin metabolism were previously discussed in the section entitled "Glucose Intolerance." Because alterations in erythropoietin and parathyroid hormone production cause numerous clinical symptoms contributing to the "uremic

Table 13-2

Summary of Endocrine Abnormalities in Dialysis Patients

Pancreas
  Insulin
    Postreceptor defect, insulin resistance
    Insulin binding, normal or reduced
    Impaired insulin secretion
    Decreased insulin catabolism
  Hyperglucagonemia
    Impaired glucagon degradation
    Augmented gluconeogenesis
Renin-angiotensin, aldosterone
  Angiotensin II, aldosterone levels usually normal or reduced
Catecholamines
  Controversial; resting levels high or low
  Reduced renal excretion and enzymatic degradation
  Decreased neuronal uptake
  Increased sympathetic nerve traffic (not found in nephrectomized patients)
Cortisol
  Increased total and free plasma levels
  Decreased degradation
  Decreased binding to cortisol-binding globulin
  IV dexamethasone required to suppress cortisol secretion
Thyroid
  Increased incidence of goiter and hypothyroidism
  Thyroxine and triiodothyronine levels tend to be low
  Thyroid-stimulating hormone usually normal; best test for hypothyroidism
Gonadal
  Serum total and free testosterone reduced (decreased production)
  Seminal fluid volume, sperm motility reduced
  Plasma luteinizing hormone and follicle-stimulating hormone levels normal
    Increase appropriately after clomiphene
    Fail to increase after estrogen stimulation
    Reduced gonadotropin pulsatility
  Serum prolactin levels 3-6 times normal
Growth hormone
  Immunoreactive growth hormone levels increased
  Insulin-like growth factor levels normal or increased, but bioactivitiy is reduced
  Recombinant human growth hormone therapy for children and malnourished adults
Parathyroid hormone, 1,25-dihydroxyvitamin D3
  Serum levels of parathyroid hormone increased
    Early cause is hypocalcemia
    Late cause is gland hypertrophy
  Serum levels of calcitriol reduced
    Reduced 1-hydroxylation by the kidney
      Structural damage
      Hyperphosphatemia

Note: From Daugirdas, J.T., & Ing, T.S. (1994). *Handbook of dialysis* (p. 492). Boston: Little, Brown and Company. Reprinted with permission.

syndrome," these abnormalities are covered in a subsequent section. Two additional endocrine-related problems commonly seen in the chronic renal failure population are hypothyroidism and sexual dysfunction, both of which are discussed below.

Although most dialysis patients are euthyroid, hypothyroidism occurs with increased frequency in this population (Bailey & Mitch, 2004). Symptoms include cold intolerance, lethargy, hoarseness, dry skin, and weight gain. However, the diagnosis is difficult to make on clinical features because dialysis patients often have cold intolerance and lethargy related to the uremic syndrome. T_3 and T_4 levels are of limited usefulness in making the diagnosis of hypothyroidism as baseline levels are commonly low in the dialysis patient. A TSH level over 20 microunits/ml is usually sufficient evidence that hypothyroidism is present and indicates the need for thyroxine therapy (Daugirdas et al., 2001).

Of the clinical complications that result from endocrine alterations, sexual dysfunction is one of the most upsetting to chronic renal failure patients (Fraser & Arieff, 2001; Massry, Bellinghieri, Savica, & Smogorzewski, 2001). Although not well-understood, the abnormalities are caused by dysfunction of the hypothalamic-pituitary-adrenal axis and are characterized by: a) elevated levels of luteinizing hormone (LH), follicle-stimulating hormone (FH), prolactin, and LH-releasing hormone; and b) decreased levels of testosterone in men and progesterone in women. Symptoms of sexual dysfunction include impotence, decreased libido, testicular atrophy, and reduced sperm count in men and amenorrhea, dysmenorrhea, frigidity, and decreased libido in women (Massry et al., 2001). Reproductive abnormalities also occur. Pregnancy is rare in uremic women who have a GFR less than 30 ml/min and spontaneous abortions, amenorrhea, and dysfunctional uterine bleeding are common. Men are frequently infertile from absent or decreased spermatogenesis.

A number of other abnormalities appear to be important in the development of impotence, including changes in the autonomic nervous system, impairment in arterial and venous systems of the penis, hypertension (and drugs associated with its treatment), and other endocrine abnormalities (Arieff, 2004). Elevated prolactin levels may cause galactorrhea in both sexes as well as amenorrhea in women and impotence in men (Massry et al., 2001). Agents such as bromocryptine decrease prolactin levels and may improve sexual functioning in men.

Treatment for sexual dysfunction should begin with a thorough history and physical examination. Laboratory tests that are frequently ordered include a complete blood count, a biochemical panel, a urinalysis and culture and sensitivity, and thyroid, testosterone, prolactin, FSH, and LH levels (Massry et al., 2001; Schmidt, Luger, & Horl, 2002). Correction of anemia with erythropoietin has also been shown to improve sexual function. Vacuum devices used to achieve erection and medications such as Viagra may be effective (Massry et al., 2001). Other treatments for impotence among men with ESRD include penile prostheses, direct injection of α-blocking agents, or other vasodilators into the penis (Arieff, 2004). Psychological counseling of the patient and partner is often helpful. It is also very important that nurses, themselves, obtain the education necessary to

Table 13-3
Potentially Toxic Compounds That Accumulate in Renal

Urea	Pyridine derivatives
Phenols	Guanidion compounds
Indoles	β-Microglobulin
Skatoles	Aliphatic amines
Hormones	Hippurate esters
Polyamines	Middle molecules
Trace elements	Aromatic amines
Serum proteinases	

Note: From Bailey & Mitch (2004), Table 48-3, p. 2143. Reprinted with permission.

ensure that they are comfortable and knowledgeable discussing issues of sex and sexuality.

Uremic Syndrome

The term *uremia* was first coined by P.A. Piorry to describe a condition caused by "contaminating the blood with urine" (Bailey & Mitch, 2004). Uremia results from the retention of substances that are normally excreted by the kidneys, including the end products of protein metabolism such as BUN. However, renal failure is also associated with the accumulation of several other potentially toxic substances such as guanido compounds, polyamines, phenols, indoles, and benzoates (Bailey & Mitch, 2004) (see Table 13-3). Additionally, much attention has been focused on the role of the middle nitrogenous molecules, compounds with a molecular mass of 500 to 3,000 daltons (Fraser & Arieff, 2001), in the development of uremic symptoms. Although it is known that these middle molecules are retained in patients with renal disease, their exact nature and pathophysiologic role remain to be defined. Several polypeptide hormone levels, including PTH (parathyroid hormone), insulin, glucagon, luteinizing hormone, and prolactin rise as renal failure progresses. In addition, as the kidneys continue to fail, production of erythropoietin (EPO) and 1,25 dihydroxycholecalciferol declines (Skorecki, Green, & Brenner, 2005).

The term uremic syndrome is used to describe the constellation of signs and symptoms associated with end stage renal failure. This condition affects multiple organ systems and thus reflects the complex role that the kidneys play in systemic regulation.

The clinical features of the uremic patient are generally more severe and develop more rapidly in acute renal failure patients as adaptive mechanisms have not had time to occur. In ESRD patients, the number and severity of symptoms may vary considerably depending on the rate of disease progression and compliance with medical therapy (Fraser & Arieff, 2001). The nurse must, therefore, carefully assess the patient's overall status and be very knowledgeable regarding the multisystemic manifestations of the uremic syndrome (see Appendix D).

Figure 13-1

Factors Potentially Contributing to Sleep Problems in Patients with End-Stage Renal Disease

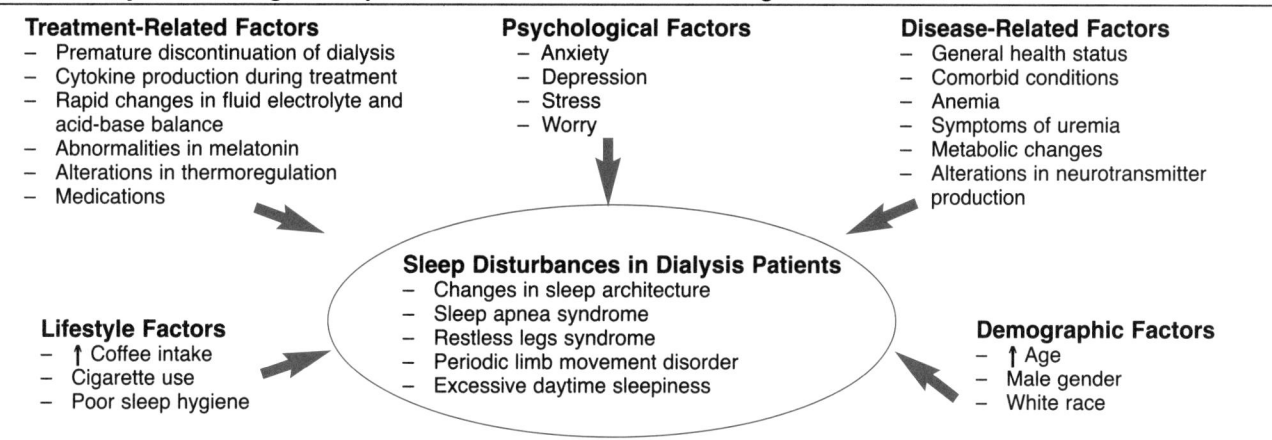

Treatment-Related Factors
- Premature discontinuation of dialysis
- Cytokine production during treatment
- Rapid changes in fluid electrolyte and acid-base balance
- Abnormalities in melatonin
- Alterations in thermoregulation
- Medications

Psychological Factors
- Anxiety
- Depression
- Stress
- Worry

Disease-Related Factors
- General health status
- Comorbid conditions
- Anemia
- Symptoms of uremia
- Metabolic changes
- Alterations in neurotransmitter production

Lifestyle Factors
- ↑ Coffee intake
- Cigarette use
- Poor sleep hygiene

Sleep Disturbances in Dialysis Patients
- Changes in sleep architecture
- Sleep apnea syndrome
- Restless legs syndrome
- Periodic limb movement disorder
- Excessive daytime sleepiness

Demographic Factors
- ↑ Age
- Male gender
- White race

Note: From Parker, K.P. (2003). Sleep disturbances in dialysis patients. *Sleep Medicine Reviews, 7*(2), 131-143. Used with permission.

Neurologic Manifestations

A variety of neurologic complications affecting the central, peripheral, and autonomic nervous systems are seen in patients with ESRD (Arieff, 2004). These abnormalities are believed to be related to the retention of uremic toxins, decreased cerebral blood flow, and reduced cerebral oxygen utilization (Arieff, 2004; Porth, 2004). Neurological changes vary directly with the rate at which renal dysfunction develops and often respond favorably to dialysis.

The term uremic encephalopathy has been used to describe the neurologic symptoms associated with advanced renal failure (Arieff, 2004; Fraser & Arieff, 2001). EEG abnormalities (slowed activity) increase with the degree of uremia and usually improve after about 6 months on dialysis (Arieff, 2004). However, even after the initiation and stabilization of renal replacement therapy, patients may continue to manifest subtle nervous system dysfunction, including impaired cognitive function, weakness, and peripheral neuropathy (dialysis dependent encephalopathy) (Arieff, 2004). Small intracerebral hemorrhages (strokes) and necrotic foci (risk factors for which include diabetes mellitus, uremia, hyperparathyroidism, smoking, hypertension, and elevated cholesterol and triglycerides) may contribute to the problem (Arieff, 2004). The earliest central nervous system (CNS) effects usually noted include reduced cerebral activity and alterations in mentation and cognition (Fraser & Arieff, 2001). Other CNS effects include headache, sluggishness, apathy, drowsiness, and insomnia accompanied by daytime drowsiness. As uremia worsens, somnolence, confusion, asterixis, seizures, and coma can develop. Behavioral alterations include personality changes, increased irritability, emotional lability, diminished sexual interest and performance, and depression (Arieff, 2004; Fraser & Arieff, 2001).

Although CNS effects are more apparent with increasing levels of uremia, a specific type of encephalopathy, including seizures, has been noted, particularly when dialysis therapy is first begun, and more often in young patients (Fraser & Arieff, 2001). This condition, referred to as dialysis disequilibrium syndrome (DDS), was initially thought to be related to a rapid fall in the osmolality of the blood during dialysis, resulting in cerebral edema. Later theories have focused on the role of the accumulation of organic acids during hemodialysis as cerebral spinal fluid (CSF) pH decreases, leading to brain swelling. Less-severe manifestations of this syndrome also occur in chronic dialysis patients causing symptoms such as headache, nausea, blurring of vision, muscular twitching and cramps (Arieff, 2004). Prevention of DDS includes adjustments in the length of time of dialysis and the addition of osmotically active solutes to dialysate (Arieff, 2004; Fraser & Arieff, 2001).

Dialysis dementia, a progressive, frequently fatal neurologic disease, was first described in 1972. The cause has been linked to contamination of dialysis water with aluminum and/or other trace elements such as tin, cobalt, manganese, iron, and magnesium (Arieff, 2004). It is sometimes associated with renal disease in children and may be related to the effects of uremia on a developing neurological system. Although it is seen less frequently today, isolated incidents still occur. Early manifestations of this problem include dysarthria and apraxia of speech with slurring, stuttering, and hesitancy. Later symptoms include personality changes, dementia, and seizures. Usually, the disease progresses to death within 6 months (Arieff, 2004; Fraser & Arieff, 2001).

Sleep complaints are common in ESRD, affecting up to 80% of patients. Chronic sleep disturbances negatively affect quality of life and functional health status (Parker, Kutner, Bliwise, Bailey, & Rye, 2003). The most common sleep disturbances reported are sleep apnea syndrome, restless leg syndrome, periodic limb movement disorder, and excessive daytime sleepiness (Parker, 2003; Parker, Bliwise, Bailey, & Rye, 2003). Figure 13-1 lists factors contributing to sleep disturbances in dialysis patients (Parker, 2003, p. 132).

Peripheral nervous system effects include paresthesias in the lower extremities that are symmetrical, slowly progressive, begin distally, and spread proximally. Typically, paresthesias affect the lower before the upper extremities (Arieff, 2004). Other complications include painful dysthesias (burning feet syndrome), decreases in deep tendon reflexes, gait

Table 13-4
Etiological Factors and Symptoms Related to Myocardial Calcification and Atherosclerosis

Etiological Factors leading to Myocardial Calcification and Atherosclerosis
Acidosis
Uremia
Anemia
Volume overload
Electrolyte disturbances: K^+, Ca^{++}, Mg^{++}
Hypertension
Nutritional deficiencies
Carbohydrate intolerance
Hyperlipidemia
Secondary hyperparathyroidism

Symptoms of Myocardial Calcification and Atherosclerosis
Congestive heart failure
Cardiomyopathy
Arrhythmias
Functional Murmurs

changes, and foot drop. Muscle twitching, myoclonic jerks, and restless legs are painful, annoying, and interfere with sleep. These abnormalities are related to demyelinization of the neural axon. Symptoms may be decreased through regular dialysis and reversed by restoration of renal function via transplant (Fraser & Arieff, 2001).

Patients with ESRD often experience a variety of disturbances related to autonomic nervous system (ANS) dysfunction. Among these include a decrease in the number of functioning eccrine sweat glands and a reduction in the volume of sweat. Others have reduced baroreceptor sensitivity, which may lead to paroxysmal hypertension, postural hypotention, persistent hypotension, and hypotensive episodes during hemodialysis. ANS dysfunction may also contribute to problems with gastrointestinal motility, impotence, and abnormal circadian variations of blood pressure (Campese, Tanasescu, & Massry, 2001). Depression of the cough reflex may also occur (Fraser & Arieff, 2001). The cranial nerves are also often affected, causing transient nystagmus, miosis, and facial asymmetry (Fraser & Arieff, 2001).

Nursing care should begin with a careful assessment of the patient's cognitive and neurologic function. It is important to identify those factors that would aggravate or cause deterioration of the neurologic status such as concomitant abnormalities in fluid, electrolyte, and acid-base disturbances. Changes in neurologic status are also associated with severe hypertension and cerebrovascular events. Deficiency of certain vitamins such as B12 and B6 can precipitate neurologic abnormalities. Adverse reactions to drugs such as antibiotics, antihypertensive agents, ritalin, and cimetidine can cause a variety of central and peripheral nervous system effects.

Cardiovascular Manifestations

The cardiovascular system is greatly affected by renal failure (see Table 13-4). By the time patients reach ESRD,

between 30%-45% have developed cardiovascular disorders. Anemia, hyperparathyroidism, hyperphosphotemia, and ongoing microinflammation associated with chronic renal disease are contributing factors as well as the more classic risk factors that include hypertension, dyslipidemia, sympathetic overactivity, and hyperchromocysteinemia.

Cardiovascular disease is the leading cause of morbidity and mortality and is responsible for 40%-45% of all deaths in the dialysis and renal transplant populations (McMahon & Parfrey, 2004; Skorecki et al., 2005).

Hypertension is very prevalent in all stages of renal failure (McMahon & Parfrey, 2004; Skorecki et al., 2005). As renal destruction progresses, salt and water continue to be retained, resulting in chronic state of extracellular fluid excess. Additionally, peripheral vascular resistance may be increased due to activation of the renin-angiotensin system, increased sympathetic activity, and dysfunction of endothelial cells (McMahon & Parfrey, 2004). Other mechanisms that may contribute to the high prevalence of hypertension in ESRD include stimulation of the sympathetic nervous system by the kidney, increased vascular sensitivity to vasopressors, enhanced endothelin release, high parathyroid hormone levels, and insulin resistance (Luke & Reif, 2001). Untreated hypertension leads to the development of coronary artery disease, congestive heart failure, peripheral artery disease, renal disease, and cerebrovascular disease (Porth, 2004). In the patient with chronic kidney disease (not yet on dialysis) with hypertension, acceleration is noted in both cardiovascular disease and loss of renal function. Blood pressure medications are, therefore, an important component of treatment. However, most antihypertensive agents may increase vascular instability and can cause profound hypotension during dialysis. Therefore, the administration of these drugs should be timed to minimize their action during the procedure.

Congestive heart failure is often present in ESRD. Causes include diastolic dysfunction (often due to left ventricular hypertrophy) and systolic failure (due to dilated cardiomyopathy) (McMahon & Parfrey, 2004; Parfrey & Foley, 2001). These conditions may be aggravated by other problems often associated with renal failure such as hypertension, anemia, and acidosis (Porth, 2004). A low pressure form of pulmonary congestion may be noted even without volume overload in the renal failure patient. The increased alveolar membrane permeability can by seen radiologically as a butterfly wing distribution and may respond well to dialysis (Skorecki, Green, & Brenner, 2005). The specific type of heart failure is diagnosed by electrocardiography, echocardiography, measuring biochemical markers such as ischemia (creatine phosphokinase and lactate dehydrogenase), nuclear scanning, and coronary angiography (McMahon & Parfrey, 2004). Treatment for systolic dysfunction primarily includes diuretics, beta-blockers, ACE inhibitors, and digoxin. For diastolic dysfunction, treatment of ischemia, b-blockers, long-acting nitrates, and calcium-channel blockers are often used (McMahon & Parfrey, 2004).

Cardiac arrhythmias, including both atrial and ventricular arrhythmias, may occur due to left ventricular hypertrophy, dilated cardiomyopathy, and coronary heart disease. Disturbances in sodium, potassium, calcium, magnesium, and hydrogen serum levels also contribute to the problem and may be worsened with rapid fluid shifts during dialysis (McMahon & Parfrey, 2004).

Cardiac valvular disease develops from valve calcification in the area of the annulus and leaflets. As many as 55% of dialysis patients have evidence of aortic valve calcification, which carries an increased risk of cardiovascular mortality. Mitral valve calcification may affect up to 39% of dialysis patients. Risk factors include abnormal calcium phosphate metabolism as well as left atrial dilation, duration of pre-dialysis systolic hypertension, duration of dialysis, and involvement of the posterior cusp (McMahon & Parfrey, 2004).

Uremic pericarditis is an inflammation of the pericardium, the serous membrane that surrounds the heart and the roots of the great blood vessels. In dialysis patients, it may result from bacterial, viral, or tubercular infections, diseases involving the serous membranes themselves (such as lupus), or to the uremia itself (Lundin, 2001). The condition may also be a sign of a failing kidney in transplant recipients. The pericardial inflammation can be widespread or localized. As the membranes of the pericardium thicken, vascularity to the area increases. Movement between the layers causes blood vessels to break and results in the development of a serosanguinous effusion. Life-threatening heart compression may result due to rapid fluid accumulation in the pericardium (tamponade) or from heart constriction secondary to chronic scarring and thickening of the pericardial membrane (Lundin, 2001). Clinical manifestations include chest pain in the precordial area (improved by sitting up and leaning forward), often with radiation to the neck, abdomen, back, or side. Changes in cardiac filling and venous return are responsible for a worsening of the pain with coughing, deep breathing, position changes, and swallowing. A pericardial friction rub is usually present. Auscultation reveals a harsh, scratchy sound best heard with the patient sitting forward. The absence of the rub does not preclude the presence of uremic pericarditis since patient position and/or the volume of the effusion may decrease or eliminate the sound altogether. Other symptoms may include tachycardia, hypotension, narrowing pulse pressure, and a paradoxical pulse. EKG changes reveal widespread ST elevation and new onset atrial arrhythmias, including atrial fibrillation, may be observed. An elevated white blood cell count and low grade fever may be present. Radiographs may reveal an enlarged cardiac silhouette and clear lung fields (Lundin, 2001). Regular dialysis and use of anti-inflammatory agents can be effective in relieving the pericardial inflammation (Porth, 2004). Severe constrictive pericarditis may necessitate drainage via pericardiocentesis or surgical placement of a pericardial window (Lundin, 2001; Porth, 2004).

Appropriate nursing management includes a careful assessment of the cardiovascular status of the patient and careful monitoring of fluid, electrolyte, and acid-base balance. Many cardiac medications require dosage adjustments in renal failure, and patients' responses to these agents may vary with electrolyte levels. Assessing the renal failure patient for other cardiovascular risk factors and providing education regarding risk factor reduction is also important.

Respiratory Manifestations

A variety of pulmonary complications are associated with the uremic syndrome. These complications include pulmonary edema, pleuritis with or without pleural effusion, and increased susceptibility to pulmonary infection. In addition, Kussmaul respirations secondary to metabolic acidosis are frequently encountered. Thus, a careful assessment of the pulmonary system is crucial in the management of these patients as prompt treatment is often required.

Pulmonary edema occurs frequently in patients with renal failure and is generally related to congestive heart failure and volume overload. Associated symptoms include shortness of breath, orthopnea, hypoxemia, dullness to percussion over the bases of the lungs, inspiratory crackles, and S_3 gallop on cardiac auscultation. Severe pulmonary edema is associated with pink-tinged frothy sputum and elevation of pCO_2 (Brashers, 2002).

Pleural inflammation and effusion are common in uremic patients. Congestive heart failure, infection, and salt and water retention all increase susceptibility (Gheuens, Daelemans, & De Broe, 2000). Additionally, the uremic patient is more susceptible to infection in the lungs and elsewhere due to peripheral blood lymphocytopenia, decreased cell-mediated immunity, and possibly reduced antibody production of the pleura (Morehead & Morris, 2001). Symptoms of uremic pleuritis include decreased breath sounds and dullness to percussion over the area (especially with effusion), pleuritic-type pain, low grade fever, and pleural and/or pericardial friction rub (Morehead & Morris, 2001). Thoracentesis may be done for diagnostic purposes or to relieve the pleural space of accumulating fluid. The use of antibiotics may be warranted if infection is present (Brashers, 2002). Proper dialysis will also help to decrease the incidence of uremic pleuritis.

Pulmonary calcification may be present in both dialyzed and nondialyzed renal failure patients. Causes are not fully understood but may include hyperparathyroidism. Often the calcifications do not appear on chest radiograph but may be noted with the use of tomography or radionuclide scanning. Symptoms are related to lung restriction and may include respiratory distress (Morehead & Morris, 2001).

Hematologic Manifestations

Anemia is a well-known complication of renal failure (Remuzzi, Schieppati, & Minetti, 2004). The problem generally worsens as renal function deteriorates, with the hemoglobin often dropping as low as 6-8 g/dL. Only 3% of patients exhibit a normal hematocrit by the time dialysis is begun. The anemia of renal failure is characterized by normocytic and nomochromic red blood cells (Remuzzi et al., 2004). Associated symptoms include tiredness, muscle fatigue, reduced exercise tolerance, poor concentration, impaired memory, decreased appetite, palpitations, angina, cold intolerance, and reduced libido (Macdougall, 2000; Van Wyck, 2001).

Although the major cause of the anemia is related to a decreased production of erythropoietin, other factors may play a role (Remuzzi et al., 2004). Hyperparathyroidism can promote anemia by directly suppressing erythroid progenitor cell growth and inducing marrow fibrosis, decreasing the pool of progenitor cells in the bone marrow. Iron and folate deficiency may also contribute to anemia. Iron loss is up to five times greater in uremic patients and is due to occult gastrointestinal bleeding, losses in the dialyzer, and ongoing phlebotomy. Folate and iron stores may be lowered due to dietary insufficiency, and removal with dialysis. In the uremic environment, the red blood cell lifespan is shortened as a result of low-grade hemolysis or hypersplenism. Anemia due to aluminum overload is uncommon today due to less use of aluminum containing phosphate binders and the use of water deionizers. Patients with microcytic anemia and normal iron stores should be evaluated for aluminum toxicity (Remuzzi et al., 2004).

Administration of recombinant human erythropoietin (r-HuEPO) has dramatically improved most patients by correcting anemia, increasing exercise tolerance, and improving subjective well-being, appetite, cognitive functioning, and overall quality of life (Remuzzi et al., 2004). When administered in doses of 50 to 150 U/kg IV or SQ from one to three times a week, it causes an increase in hematocrit, approaching normal limits within about 8 to 14 weeks. (Because of the length of time required for full effects, transfusions may be used instead of r-HuEPO to treat the anemia of ARF.) Adequate assessment of iron stores through measurements of ferritin, iron saturation, and transferrin are important, and iron adequate replacement (oral and IV) is essential (Fishbane & Paganini, 2000; Remuzzi et al., 2004). In addition, supplementation of folic acid, iron, and amino acids is often given to patients with renal failure to replace suspected dietary deficiencies or extra losses due to dialysis (Remuzzi et al., 2004). Androgens can increase the red cell mass in some anemic dialysis patients. However, because of the high incidence of side effects, r-HuEPO should be the primary therapy. Other interventions that may assist include improving dialysis clearance and increasing exercise (Fishbane & Paganini, 2000). Inadequate responses to r-HuEPO may result from infection, chronic blood loss, vitamin deficiencies, aluminum toxicity, hemoglobinopathies (thalassemia, sickle cell anemia), and malignancies (Remuzzi et al., 2004).

A bleeding tendency related to platelet dysfunction also develops in uremia manifested by easy bruising, GI bleeds, epistaxis, bleeding gums, and pericardial, retroperitoneal, and intracranial bleeding (Boccardo & Remizzi, 2001; Remuzzi et al., 2004). Uremic platelets display defective aggregation and adhesiveness related to a decreased availability of platelet factor 3 and an altered platelet response to clotting factor VIII (von Willebrand's factor) (Boccardo & Remizzi, 2001). The platelet count is usually in the normal range although dialysis may temporarily aggravate thrombocytopenia. The most reliable test to evaluate bleeding tendency is the bleeding time. Interventions that can improve the bleeding time include intensive dialysis, increasing the hematocrit, and treatment with cryoprecipitate, desmopressin, and estrogen (Remuzzi et al., 2004). Cryoprecipitate and desmopressin are believed to improve the bleeding time by supplying or inducing other forms of factor VIII. The mechanisms by which estrogen decreases bleeding time is poorly understood (Boccardo & Remizzi, 2001; Skorecki et al., 2005).

Uremia is also associated with immune system defects and include both humoral and cellular alterations. Neutrophils have impaired chemotaxis, adherence, and phagocytic action (Chatenoud & Latscha, 2001; Remuzzi et al., 2004). The result is that patients are more susceptible to infections, have increased severity of infection, and are predisposed to chronic infections such as hepatitis and tuberculosis (Chatenoud & Latscha, 2001; Horl, 2000). Finally, an association exists between the impaired immune system in uremic patients and increased risk for the development of cancer (Vamvakas & Heidland, 2001).

In summary, the hematologic manifestations of uremic syndrome have the potential to profoundly affect the health outcomes of patients with ESRD. Nursing management should begin with a careful assessment of hematologic parameters and evaluation of related signs and symptoms. Evaluation of the patient's status and response to treatment is an ongoing process.

Dermatologic Manifestations

ESRD patients may suffer from numerous types of skin disturbances. Skin color may be pale gray or yellow brown (depending on phototype), and changes are attributable to urochrome pigment depositions and anemia. Patients may also experience bullous lesions and bullous dermatosis (seen more commonly in males who have been on dialysis for a long period of time). Additionally, patients may develop pseudo-Kaposi's sarcoma in the area of arteriovenous shunts or fistulas or hands due to overflow of blood or insufficient blood drainage in the area (Babapour & Gurevitch, 2001; Naeyaert & Beele, 2000). Metastatic calcinosis can occur in uremia due to high levels of serum calcium phosphate and secondary hyperparathyroidism. The incidence is 58% in patients with hyperparathyroidism and 20% in those without hyperparathyroidism. Painful, erythematous nodules develop, usually on the buttocks, extremities, thighs, and abdomen. The condition carries a 50% mortality rate, usually from sepsis. Early treatment involves parathyroidectomy (Naeyaert & Beele, 2000).

Of all the skin disturbances, pruritus may be the most difficult for patients. Pruritus, an unpleasant, intense desire to scratch, affects between 37%-85% of patients on dialysis. Unlike non-renal failure patients who often present with generalized itching, uremic patients often can localize the area of itching. The exact cause is not known but may be related to excessive PTH, increased cutaneous mast cells, increased skin dryness, and dialysis components (Babapour & Gurevitch, 2001; Naeyaert & Beele, 2000).

Treatment for pruritus includes efforts to relieve dry skin with topical emollients that are best applied following a bath or shower when the skin is still wet. Exposure to ultraviolet light (UVB bands) has been reported to provide some relief after as little as 4-6 exposures. Medications that are useful in some patients include antihistamines, oral activated charcoal, and cholestyramine. Lidocaine, administered intravenously during dialysis may decrease symptoms for 24 hours (Naeyaert & Beele, 2000). Rarely, uremic crystals may be noted on the skin (uremic frost) (Skorecki et al., 2005). Dialysis may improve symptoms in some patients. Ironically, dialysis may worsen symptoms in others (Babapour & Gurevitch, 2001).

Nail changes can be seen in chronic dialysis patients

Figure 13-2
Causes of GI Bleeding in Renal Failure

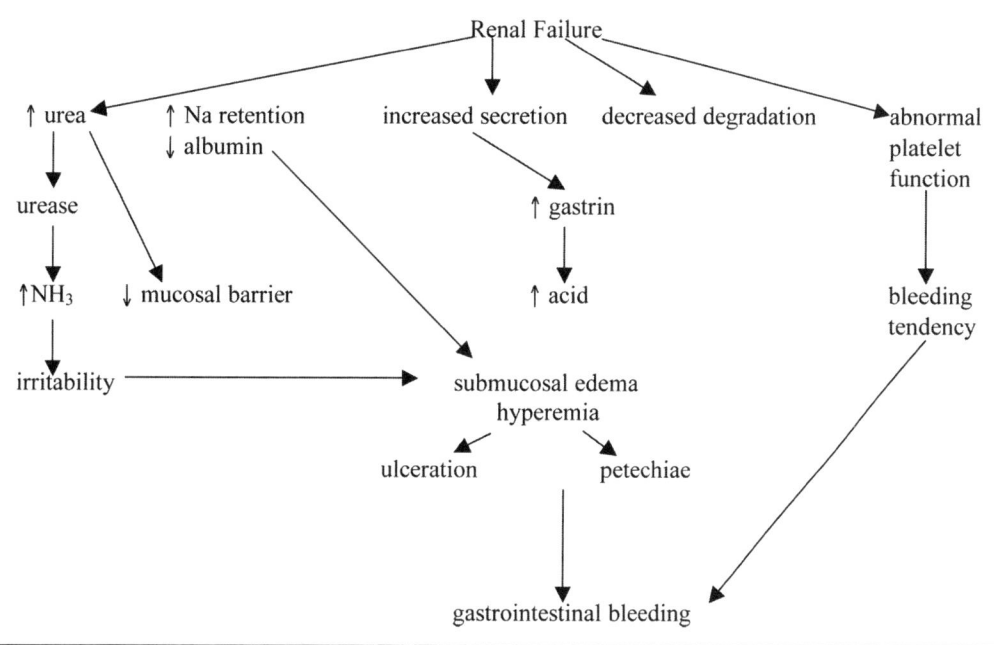

and renal failure patients not on dialysis. The nails, fingernails, and toenails become thin and brittle and are characterized by a white proximal nail bed and a red or brown discoloration of the distal nail bed (half-and-half nail). The cause of the nail changes is unknown but may be related to hypoalbuminemia (Babapour & Gurevitch, 2001; Naeyaert & Beele, 2000).

A thorough nursing assessment of the skin is critical in both acute and chronic renal failure patients. Prevention of skin breakdown from scratching is especially important as broken areas can provide a portal of entry for infection. Keeping the skin clean and moisturized and the finger nails short and well trimmed are important basic nursing interventions.

Gastrointestinal Manifestations

Despite advances with renal replacement therapies, ESRD patients may suffer from a host of gastrointestinal problems. A uriniferous breath odor, known as uremic fetor, may be present and is due to urea breakdown in saliva. Patients with uriniferous fetor may complain of a metallic, unpleasant taste in the mouth. Anorexia, nausea, hiccups, and vomiting may be present due to the central nervous effects in uremia (Skorecki et al., 2005). Heartburn and dyspepsia are commonly reported. Gastroesophageal reflux disease (GERD) is also common and may be due to alterations in the hormones that affect lower esophageal sphincter tone and a higher occurrence of hiatal hernia. Gastritis and peptic ulcer disease can develop and should be fully evaluated as to their causes, which may include *H. pylori,* use of ulcerogenic drugs, alcohol, and tobacco use. Elevated amylase levels are common in renal failure and are associated with decreasing GFR. Elevated lipase levels, also commonly observed, may be partially due to the stimulating effects of heparin on

lipoprotein lipase during dialysis (Nickl, 2001).

Gastrointestinal bleeding (upper or lower) is common and exacerbated by the bleeding tendency associated with uremia and/or the use of heparin during hemodialysis. The pathophysiological mechanisms in renal failure that may lead to gastrointestinal bleeding are depicted in Figure 13-2. Early institution of dialysis and prophylactic antacids and H_2 blockers may prevent problems.

Nursing care should begin with a thorough assessment of the oral cavity, abdomen, and bowel patterns. All vomitus and stool should be checked for occult blood, the presence of which can potentially increase the BUN. Good oral hygiene not only makes the patient more comfortable, but may also help enhance the appetite.

Skeletal-Muscular Manifestations

Bone disease occurs frequently in the renal failure patient and is referred to as renal osteodystrophy (Jani, Guest, & Lafayette, 2000; Martin, Gonzales, & Slatopolsky, 2004). The condition is both painful and debilitating but with proper medical and nursing care and compliance with medical therapy on the part of the patient, the devastating effects of renal bone disease can be prevented.

The two major types of renal osteodystrophy are high-bone turnover and low-bone turnover osteodystrophy (Martin et al., 2004; Porth, 2004). High-bone turnover osteodystrophy, also known as osteitis fibrosa cystica, is the most common form. As GFR falls, phosphate is retained and calcium levels fall, stimulating increased PTH levels (Jani et al., 2000). Lower active vitamin D levels, due to decreased kidney production of 1,25 dihydroxycholecalciferol further increases PTH. The high PTH and local cytokines, such as tumor necrosis factor-a, nitric acid, endothelin, and interleukin 1, 4, 6, and 11 result in increased osteoclast and osteoblast activity (Martin et al., 2004; Massry & Smogorzewski, 2001a). As bone resorption becomes more severe, bone density decreases and is replaced by coarser, porous bone (Porth, 2004). Fibrosis develops in the marrow space as bone marrow cells differentiate in fibroblast type cells (Jani et al., 2000).

Laboratory changes associated with high-turnover bone disease include marked elevations of alkaline phosphatase levels from bone destruction, elevated phosphorus levels, and increased PTH (Martin et al., 2004). Although hypocalcemia is typical, hypercalcemia can develop with progressive parathyroid disease. X-rays reveal subperiosteal bone reabsorption (bone thinning) most easily noted in the hands and clavicles. Bone biopsy is considered the gold standard for definitive diagnosis, although indications for the test are controversial. More frequently, empiric treatment designed to lower phosphate levels, normalize calcium levels, and suppress PTH (calcitriol) is begun (Jani et al., 2000; Massry & Smogorzewski, 2001a).

There are two major types of low-turnover bone disease. Osteomalacia is a condition characterized by decreased bone turnover with increased formation of unmineralized bone tissue. The second type is adynamic bone disease, which is characterized by decreased bone matrix formation, decreased numbers of osteoblasts and osteoclasts, and increased osteoid thickness (Jani et al., 2000; Martin et al., 2004; Massry & Smogorzewski, 2001a; Porth, 2004).

Common symptoms of both high and low bone turnover disease include bone tenderness, pruritus, muscle weakness (especially in the proximal muscles of the lower extremities), bone pain, spontaneous tendon rupture, fractures, skeletal deformity, and severe incapacity often involving the ribs, hips, pelvis, and vertebrae (Jani et al., 2000; Massry & Smogorzewski, 2001a; Porth, 2004). Metastatic and extraskeletal calcifications of the lung, shoulder joint, peripheral arteries, coronary arteries, skin, and eyes are also commonly observed (Martin et al., 2004).

A major focus of treatment for both high and low turnover renal osteodystrophy should be on prevention. Dietary phosphate reduction is crucial with a restriction of less than 800 mg/day in dialysis patients. Phosphate control with binders should be done to keep levels within normal limits. Calcium antacids have replaced the use of aluminum antacids to bind phosphate (Jani et al., 2000). Calcitrol therapy may be helpful in decreasing PTH levels but should not be used unless the phosphate level is < 6 mg/dL since high phosphate levels decrease the effectiveness of the calcitrol and may predispose the patient to metastatic calcification. Finally, parathyroidectomy may be necessary for severe hyperparathyroidism that is refractory to treatment (Jani et al., 2000; Martin et al., 2004).

Summary

Developments in the field of nephrology have presented the nursing profession with great challenges. Not only is the scientific and theoretical basis of the discipline exceedingly complicated, but the nursing management required by patients with end stage renal disease continues to grow in complexity with further scientific developments. A thorough understanding of the physiologic basis and human responses, both systemic and psychosocial, is essential in order to effectively plan appropriate nursing interventions and evaluate patient outcomes.

References

Arieff, A. I. (2004). Neurologic complications of renal insufficiency. In B.M. Brenner (Ed.), *Brenner & Rector's the kidney* (7th ed.) (Vol. 2, pp. 2227-2254). Philadelphia: W.B. Saunders.

Babapour, G. R., & Gurevitch, A. W. (2001). The skin in uremia. In S. G. Massry & R. J. Glassock (Eds.), *Massry and Glassock's textbook of nephrology* (4th ed.) (pp. 1377-1380). Philadelphia: Lippincott, Williams & Wilkins.

Bailey, J. L., & Mitch, W. E. (2004). Pathophysiology of uremia. In B. M. Brenner (Ed.), *Brenner & Rector's the kidney* (Vol. 2) (pp. 2139-2164). Philadelphia: W.B. Saunders.

Boccardo, P., & Remizzi, G. (2001). Hematopoietic system in uremia. Part 2. Bleeding and coagulation. In S. G. Massry & R. J. Glassock (Eds.), *Massry and Glassock's textbook of nephrology* (4th ed.) (pp. 1324-1329). Philadelphia: Lippincott, Williams & Wilkins.

Brashers, V.L. (2002). Alterations of pulmonary function. In K.L. McChance & S.E. Huether (Eds.), *Pathophysiology: The biological basis for disease in adults and children* (4th ed.) (pp. 1105-1144). St. Louis: Mosby.

Campese, V.M., Tanasescu, A., & Massry, S.G. (2001). Central and peripheral nervous system in uremia. Part 3. Autonomic nervous system. In S.G. Massry & R.J. Glassock (Eds.), *Massry and Glassock's textbook of nephrology* (4th ed.) (pp. 1287-1291). Philadelphia: Lippincott, Williams & Wilkins.

Carfray, A., Patel, K., Whitaker, P., Garrick, P., Griffiths, G.J., & Warwick, G.L. (2000). Albumin as an outcome measure in haemodialysis in patients: The effect of variation in assay method. *Nephrology Dialysis & Transplantation, 15*(11), 1819-1822.

Chatenoud, L., & Latscha, B.D. (2001). Immunological disturbances in uremia. In S.G. Massry & R.J. Glassock (Eds.), *Massry and Glassock's textbook of nephrology* (4th ed.) (pp. 1431-1438). Philadelphia: Lippincott, Williams & Wilkins.

Curtin, R.B., Bultman, D.C., Thomas-Hawkins, C., Walters, B.A., & Schatell, D. (2002). Hemodialysis patients' symptom experiences: Effects on physical and mental functioning. *Nephrology Nursing Journal, 29*(6), 562, 567-574; discussion 575, 598.

Daugirdas, J., Blake, P.G., & Ing, T. (2001). Handbook of dialysis. Philadelphia: Lippincott, Williams & Wilkins.

Fishbane, S., & Paganini, E. P. (2000). Hematologic abnormalities. In P. G. Daugirdas, T. S. Blake & T. S. Ing (Eds.), *Handbook of dialysis* (3rd ed.). Philadelphia: Lippincott, Williams & Wilkins.

Fraser, C.L., & Arieff, A.I. (2001). Nervous system manifestations of renal failure. In R.W. Schrier (Ed.), *Diseases of the kidneys and urinary tract* (7th ed.) (Vol. III) (pp. 2769-2794). Philadelphia: Lippincott, Williams & Wilkins.

Gheuens, E.O., Daelemans, R., & De Broe, M.E. (2000). Pulmonary problems in hemodialysis and peritoneal dialysis. In N.L. Lamiere & R.L. Mehta (Eds.), *Complications of dialysis.* New York: Marcel Dekker, Inc.

Horl, W.H. (2000). Immune dysfunction in hemodialysis and peritoneal dialysis patients. In N.L. Lamiere & R.L. Mehta (Eds.), *Complications of dialysis.* New York: Marcel Dekker, Inc.

Jani, A., Guest, S., & Lafayette, R.A. (2000). Arthopathies and bone disorders in hemodialysis and peritoneal dialysis patients. In N.L. Lamiere & R.L. Mehta (Eds.), *Complications of dialysis* (4th ed.). New York: Marcel Dekker, Inc.

Kaysen, G.A., & Don, B.R. (2003). Factors that affect albumin concentration in dialysis patients and their relationship to vascular disease. *Kidney International Supplement*(84), S94-97.

Koeppen, B.M., & Stanton, B.A. (2001). *Renal physiology* (3rd ed.). St. Louis: Mosby, Inc.

Kopple, J.D. (2001). Amino acid and protein metabolism in chronic renal failure. In S.G. Massry & R.J. Glassock (Eds.), *Massry and Glassock's textbook of nephrology* (4th ed.) (pp. 1356-1367). Philadelphia: Lippincott, Williams & Wilkins.

Lacour, B., Massy, Z., & Drueke, T.B. (2001). Metabolic and endocrine disturbances in uremia. Part 2. Lipid metabolism. In S.G. Massry & R.J. Glassock (Eds.), *Massry and Glassock's textbook of nephrol-*

ogy (pp. 1347-1356). Philadelphia: Lippincott, Williams & Wilkins.

Luke, R.G., & Reif, M.C. (2001). Cardiovascular system in uremia. Part 3. Hypertension. In S.G. Massry & R.J. Glassock (Eds.), *Massry and Glassock's textbook of nephrology* (4th ed.) (pp. 1305-1313). Philadelphia: Lippincott, Williams & Wilkins.

Lundin, P. (2001). Cardiovascular system in uremia. Part 1. Uremic pericarditis. In B.M. Brenner (Ed.), *Brenner & Rector's the kidney* (7th ed.) (Vol. 2, pp. 1292-1295). Philadelphia: Lippincott, Williams & Wilkins.

Macdougall, I.C. (2000). Hematological problems and their management in hemodialysis and peritoneal dialysis patients. In N.L. Lamiere & R.L. Mehta (Eds.), *Complications of dialysis.* New York: Marcel Dekker, Inc.

Mak, R.H. (2000). Impact of end-stage renal disease and dialysis on glycemic control. *Seminars in Dialysis, 13*(1), 4-8.

Martin, K.J., Gonzales, E.S., & Slatopolsky, E. (2004). Renal osteodystrophy. In B.M. Brenner (Ed.), *Brenner & Rector's the kidney* (7th ed.) (Vol. 2, pp. 2255-2305). Philadelphia: W.B. Saunders.

Massry, S.G., Bellinghieri, G., Savica, V., & Smogorzewski, M. (2001). Metabolic and endocrine disturbances in uremia. Part 6. Sexual dysfunction. In S.G. Massry & R.J. Glassock (Eds.), *Massry and glassock's textbook of nephrology* (4th ed.) (pp. 1371-1376). Philadelphia: Lippincott, Williams & Wilkins.

Massry, S.G., & Smogorzewski, M. (2001a). Calcium metabolism. Part 3. Dyscalcemias. In S.G. Massry & R.J. Glassock (Eds.), *Massry and Glassock's textbook of nephrology* (4th ed.) (pp. 326-340). Philadelphia: Lippincott, Williams & Wilkins.

Massry, S.G., & Smogorzewski, M. (2001b). Metabolic and endocrine disturbances in uremia. Part 1. Glucose and insulin metabolism. In S.G. Massry & R.J. Glassock (Eds.), *Massry & Glassock's textbook of nephrology* (4th ed.) (pp. 1342-1376). Philadelphia: Lippincott, Williams & Wilkins.

McMahon, L.P., & Parfrey, P.S. (2004). Cardiovascular aspects of chronic kidney disease. In B.M. Brenner (Ed.), *Brenner & Rector's the kidney* (7th ed.) (Vol. II, pp. 2189-2226). Philadelphia: W.B. Saunders.

Morehead, R.S., & Morris, P.E. (2001). Pulmonary complications of uremia. In S.G. Massry & R.J. Glassock (Eds.), *Massry and Glassock's textbook of nephrology* (4th ed.) (pp. 1314-1317). Philadelphia: Lippincott, Williams & Wilkins.

Naeyaert, J.M., & Beele, H. (2000). Dermatological problems in dialysis patients, including calciphylaxis. In N.L. Lamiere & R.L. Mehta (Eds.), *Complications of dialysis.* New York: Marcel Dekker, Inc.

National Kidney Foundation (NKF). (2000a). *Clinical practice guidelines for nutrition in chronic renal failure.* New York: Author.

National Kidney Foundation (NKF). (2000b). *K/DOQI clinical practice guidelines for chronic kidney disease evaluation. Part 4. Definition and classification of stages of chronic kidney disease. Guideline 1. Definition and stages of chronic kidney disease.* Retrieved from http://www.kidney.org/professionals/doqi/kdoqi/p4_classg2.htm

National Kidney Foundation (NKF). (2000c). *K/DOQI clinical practice guidelines for chronic kidney disease: Evaluation, classification, and stratification. Part 6. Association of gfr with complications in adults. Guidelines 12. Association of level of gfr with indices of functioning and well-being.* New York: Author.

National Kidney Foundation (NKF). (2000d). *K/DOQI clinical practice guidelines for managing dyslipidemias in chronic kidney disease.* New York: Author.

Nickl, N.J. (2001). Gastrointestinal tract in uremia. Part 1. Gastrointestinal abnormalities. In S.G. Massry & R.J. Glassock (Eds.), *Massry and Glassock's textbook of nephrology* (4th ed.) (pp. 1330-1333). Philadelphia: Lippincott, Williams & Wilkins.

Parfrey, P.S., & Foley, R.N. (2001). Cardiovascular system in uremia, part 2. Cardiomyopathy. In S.G. Massry & R.J. Glassock (Eds.), *Massry and Glassock's textbook of nephrology* (Vol. 4th) (pp. 1295-1304). Philadelphia: Lippincott, Williams & Wilkins.

Parker, K.P. (2003). Sleep disturbances in dialysis patients. *Sleep Medicine Reviews, 7*(2), 131-143.

Parker, K.P., Bliwise, D.L., Bailey, J.L., & Rye, D.B. (2003). Daytime sleepiness in stable hemodialysis patients. *American Journal of Kidney Disease, 41*(2), 394-402.

Parker, K.P., Kutner, N.G., Bliwise, D.L., Bailey, J.L., & Rye, D.B. (2003). Nocturnal sleep, daytime sleepiness, and quality of life in stable patients on hemodialysis. *Health and Quality of Life Outcomes, 1*(1), 68.

Pechere-Bertschi, A., & Burnier, M. (2004). Female sex hormones, salt, and blood pressure regulation. *American Journal of Hypertension, 17*(10), 994-1001.

Porth, C.M. (2004). *Essentials of pathophysiology: Concepts of altered health states.* Philadelphia: Lippincott, Williams & Wilkins.

Remuzzi, G., Schieppati, A., & Minetti, L. (2004). Hematologic consequences of renal failure. In B. M. Brenner (Ed.), *Brennor and Rector's the kidney* (7th ed.) (Vol. 2) (pp. 2165-2189). Philadelphia: W.B. Saunders.

Schmidt, A., Luger, A., & Horl, W.H. (2002). Sexual hormone abnormalities in male patients with renal failure. *Nephrology Dialysis & Transplantation, 17*(3), 368-371.

Skorecki, K., Green, J., & Brenner, B.M. (2005). Chronic renal failure. In D.L. Kasper, E., Braunwald, A.S. Fauci, S.L. Hauser, D.L. Longo & J.L. Jameson (Eds.), *Harrison's principles of internal medicine* (16th ed.). New York: McGraw-Hill.

Steinman, T.I. (2000). Serum albumin: Its significance in patients with ESRD. *Seminars in Dialysis, 13*(6), 404-408.

Tzamaloukas, A.H., Murata, G.H., Zager, P.G., Eisenberg, B., & Avasthi, P.S. (1993). The relationship between glycemic control and morbidity and mortality for diabetics on dialysis. *ASAIO Journal, 39*(4), 880-885.

United States Renal Data System (USRDS). (2004). *U.S. Renal data system, USRDS 2004 annual data report: Atlas of end-stage renal disease in the United States.* Bethesda, MD: National Institutes of Health, National Institute of Diabetes and Digestive and Kidney Diseases.

Vamvakas, S., & Heidland, A. (2001). Cancer in uremia. In S.G. Massry & R.J. Glassock (Eds.), *Massry and Glassock's textbook of nephrology* (4th ed.) (pp. 1439-1442). Philadelphia: Lippincott, Williams & Wilkins.

Van Wyck, D.B. (2001). Hematopoietic system in uremia. Part 1. Anemia. In S.G. Massry & R.J. Glassock (Eds.), *Massry and Glassock's textbook of nephrology* (4th ed.) (pp. 1318-1324). Philadelphia: Lippincott, Williams & Wilkins.

- ESRD continues to be a significant health problem in the United States population. By the end of 2002, there were over 300,000 patients with ESRD in the United States and the number of patients receiving treatment for kidney failure is increasing at a rate of approximately 2.5% per year (USRDS, 2004).

- Once renal function falls below 25% of normal, the kidneys have a limited capacity to deal with excess fluid, electrolytes, and acid-base load, as well as stressors associated with volume and electrolyte loss.

- Uremia results from the retention of substances that are normally excreted by the kidneys, including the end products of protein metabolism such as BUN. However, renal failure is also associated with the accumulation of several other potentially toxic substances.

- Sleep complaints are common in ESRD, affecting up to 80% of patients. Chronic sleep disturbances negatively affect quality of life and functional health status. The most common sleep disturbances reported are sleep apnea syndrome, restless leg syndrome, periodic limb movement disorder, and excessive daytime sleepiness.

- Congestive heart failure is often present in ESRD. Causes include diastolic dysfunction (often due to left ventricular hypertrophy) and systolic failure (due to dilated cardiomyopathy). These conditions may be aggravated by other problems often associated with renal failure such as hypertension, anemia, and acidosis.

- Administration of recombinant human erythropoietin (r-HuEPO) has dramatically improved most patients by correcting anemia, increasing exercise tolerance, and improving subjective well-being, appetite, cognitive functioning, and overall quality of life.

- A major focus of treatment for both high and low turnover renal osteodystrophy should be on prevention. Dietary phosphate reduction is crucial with a restriction of less than 800 mg/day in dialysis patients. Phosphate control with binders should be done to keep levels within normal limits.

ANNP613

End Stage Renal Disease

Lori Candela, EdD, RN, APRN, BC, FNP, and Kathy P. Parker, PhD, RN, FAAN

Contemporary Nephrology Nursing: Principles and Practice contains 39 chapters of educational content. Individual learners may apply for continuing nursing education credit by reading a chapter and completing the Continuing Education Evaluation Form for that chapter. Learners may apply for continuing education credit for any or all chapters.

Please photocopy this page and return to ANNA.
COMPLETE THE FOLLOWING:

Name: _____

Address:_____

City:_____State:_____Zip:_____

E-mail: _____

Preferred telephone: ☐ Home ☐ Work: _____

State where licensed and license number (optional): _____

CE application fees are based upon the number of contact hours provided by the individual chapter. CE fees per contact hour for ANNA members are as follows: 1.0-1.9 - $15; 2.0-2.9 - $20; 3.0-3.9 - $25; 4.0 and higher - $30. Fees for nonmembers are $10 higher.

ANNA Member: ☐ Yes   ☐ No   Member # (if available) _____

☐ Checked Enclosed   ☐ American Express   ☐ Visa   ☐ MasterCard

Total Amount Submitted: _____

Credit Card Number:_____ Exp. Date: _____

Name as it appears on the card: _____

CE Evaluation Form
To receive continuing education credit for individual study after reading the chapter
1. Photocopy this form. (You may also download this form from ANNA's Web site, **www.annanurse.org**.)
2. Mail the completed form with payment (check) or credit card information to American Nephrology Nurses' Association, East Holly Avenue, Box 56, Pitman, NJ 08071-0056.
3. You will receive your CE certificate from ANNA in 4 to 6 weeks.

Test returns must be postmarked by **December 31, 2010.**

CE Application Fee
ANNA Member $15.00
Nonmember $25.00

EVALUATION FORM

1. I verify that I have read this chapter and completed this education activity. Date: _____

_____
Signature

2. What would be different in your practice if you applied what you learned from this activity? *(Please use additional sheet of paper if necessary.)*

_____
_____
_____
_____
_____
_____
_____
_____
_____
_____
_____
_____
_____

Evaluation	Strongly disagree				Strongly agree
3. The activity met the stated objectives.					
a. Describe the pathophysiologic basis of two of the metabolic disturbances that occur with ESRD.	1	2	3	4	5
b. Discuss the psychosocial responses associated with two of the metabolic disturbances that occur with ESRD.	1	2	3	4	5
c. Relate the nursing implications of caring for patients with metabolic changes that occur with ESRD.	1	2	3	4	5
4. The content was current and relevant.	1	2	3	4	5
5. The content was presented clearly.	1	2	3	4	5
6. The content was covered adequately.	1	2	3	4	5
7. Rate your ability to apply the learning obtained from this activity to practice.	1	2	3	4	5

Comments _____

_____

8. Time required to read the chapter and complete this form: _____ minutes.

This educational activity has been provided by the American Nephrology Nurses' Association (ANNA) for 1.5 contact hours. ANNA is accredited as a provider of continuing nursing education (CNE) by the American Nurses Credentialing Center's Commission on Accreditation (ANCC-COA). ANNA is an approved provider of continuing education by the California Board of Registered Nursing, CEP 0910.

Client and Family Decision Making About Treatment Modalities for End Stage Renal Disease

Maryse Pelletier Hibbert, MN, RN
Isabelle Toupin, MN, RN
Cynthia Baker, PhD, MN, RN

Chapter Contents

Client and Family Decision Making about Treatment Modalities for End Stage Renal Disease

Chapter 14

Maryse Pelletier Hibbert, MN, RN
Isabelle Toupin, MN, RN
Cynthia Baker, PhD, MN, RN

This chapter will highlight the factors that influence the choice of renal replacement therapy, the decision making process regarding renal therapy as well as describe the impact of such decision on family members.

Factors Influencing Selection of Renal Replacement Therapy

There are three types of renal replacement therapies available to patients with end stage renal disease (ESRD): hemodialysis, peritoneal dialysis, and kidney transplant. There is no cure for ESRD and therefore, these treatment options are life prolonging. Studies have examined a wide number of medical and nonmedical factors influencing the selection of renal replacement therapy for ESRD. Medical factors have included survival rates, impact on the quality of life, and co-morbidity. The most common nonmedical influencing factors investigated have been comparative treatment costs, informational requirements of different dialysis modalities, patients' geographical proximity to treatment centers, and several psychosocial characteristics of patients and families.

Medical Factors

Earlier analyses of the comparative impact of peritoneal and hemodialysis on patients' survival have been controversial. Study findings were debated because of the confounding effects of co-morbid conditions, differences in treatment methods from one country to another, and differences in the statistical analyses used to estimate mortality rates (Prichard, 2000). More recent studies indicate that there is little difference between hemodialysis and peritoneal dialysis on patient survival (Diaz-Buxo, 1998; Prichard, 2000). Studies of the impact of treatment modalities on quality of life have been concerned with life style, personal preferences, aptitudes, and coping abilities (Diaz-Buxo, 1998). Quality of life offered by a given treatment modality has also been related to age, gender, race, income, and environment (Vecchi et al., 1994). Differences in quality of life of individuals on hemodialysis and peritoneal dialysis are not consistent. Prichard (2000) concludes that it is unclear whether modality per se has an important impact on the quality of life, but rather, modality should be chosen to match each patient's lifestyle and particular social set of circumstances.

The presence of significant comorbid conditions also influences the choice of treatment modality for certain individuals (Prichard, 1996). Co-morbid conditions such as hypertension, cardiovascular diseases, and diabetes are prevalent among people requiring dialysis for ESRD. In fact, diabetes is the leading cause of kidney failure in the United States (Holocheck, 2004). Alloati and co-investigators (2000) reported that hemodialysis is preferable in situations when glycemia is difficult to control or when there is severe

hypertension especially in the elderly. Maiorca, Cancarini, Zubani, Movilli, and Brunori (1996) argued that there is no evidence that survival rates among diabetics are higher on peritoneal dialysis than on hemodialysis. Although peritoneal dialysis is not suitable for all patients with ESRD, it is a viable therapy for those who can perform self-care and daily exchanges (4 to 5 times per day, 7 days per week) and who can fit therapy into their own routine. It allows the patient to be more mobile, causes less hemodynamic instability (i.e., hypotension, nausea, vomiting), and imposes fewer restrictions in food and fluid intake. There are illness factors that may preclude individuals from being able to choose peritoneal dialysis, including having a history of: severe pulmonary disease, multiple abdominal surgical procedures, chronic pancreatitis, back problems and/or diverticulitis, severe arthritis or poor hand strength, and recurrent abdominal wall or inguinal hernias (Holechek, 2004).

Nonmedical Factors

The cost of a given dialysis modality depends on the country where the therapy is dispensed and is also affected by the nature of the health care system (Prichard, 2000). For instance, the structure of the reimbursement plan in the United States explains in part the underutilization of peritoneal dialysis (Venkataramen & Nolph, 1999). In contrast, the health care policies in Canada and in the United Kingdom encourage the selection of peritoneal dialysis, which is less expensive for a national health care system than hemodialysis (Alloati et al., 2000). Hemodialysis is the most commonly used method of dialysis in the United States (Smeltzer & Bare, 2000).

In general, people with advanced chronic kidney disease are unfamiliar with dialysis and lack information about this therapy (King, 2000). Two studies investigated the patients' level of knowledge about dialysis during a predialysis program. Klang, Björvell, and Clyne (1999) found that individuals with ESRD had the least amount of knowledge about dialysis treatments. This study also found that none of these individuals had received information about other peoples' experiences with dialysis treatment. Gomez, Valido, Celadilla, Bernaldo deQuiros, and Mojon (1999) reported that among 304 individuals with ESRD, most had a better understanding of peritoneal dialysis than hemodialysis treatments. Individuals under the age of 65 were more knowledgeable about the various types of dialysis treatments than those over 65 years of age.

When faced with ESRD, most individuals require education about the advantages and the disadvantages of the various options available in order to choose a dialysis treatment modality (Venkataramen & Nolph, 1999). A study conducted by Devins, Mendelssohn, Barré, and Binik (2003) found that psycho-educational interventions in the predialysis phase extend the time period to initiating dialysis therapy. A survey conducted by the National Kidney Foundation in the United States of people with chronic renal failure found that the most common source of information about treatment options were nephrologists, followed by nurses, and then social workers (King, 2000). The manner in which information about dialysis is relayed to the patient and family may influence their choice of treatment modality.

A number of geographical factors have been examined in relation to dialysis treatment selection. For instance, living a long distance from the treatment center, having spent extensive time traveling to and from a center for hemodialysis, and lacking access to transportation have been associated with the selection of peritoneal dialysis (Little, Irwin, Marshall, Rayner, & Smith, 2001). Although most patients on hemodialysis undergo the procedure in a hospital or outpatient satellite settings, home hemodialysis is an option for some. Home hemodialysis requires a highly motivated patient who is willing to take responsibility for the procedure and is able to adjust each treatment to meet the body's changing needs (Holechek, 2004). It also requires the cooperation and commitment of a partner to assist the patient (Courts, 2000). Often the patient is not comfortable imposing on a family member's time and may not be comfortable with the presence of the dialysis machine in his or her home (Smeltzer & Bare, 2000). One of the main advantages of home hemodialysis is that it allows greater freedom in choosing dialysis times and requires no travel time when compared to hospital hemodialysis. Whether hemodialysis is performed at home or in a hospital, there are advantages to this mode of therapy, which may include less protein loss, rapid fluid removal, and rapid lowering of urea, creatinine, and potassium levels (Holechek, 2004). There are also potential complications associated with this treatment: (a) hypotension; (b) muscle cramps from rapid removal of sodium and water or from neuromuscular sensitivity; (c) loss of blood; (d) hepatitis B and C; (e) sepsis related to infections of vascular access; and (f) disequilibrium syndrome, which develops as a result of very rapid changes in the composition of the extracellular fluid (Holechek 2004; Smeltzer & Bare, 2000).

Kidney transplantation is another renal replacement therapy option for some individuals with ESRD. Kidneys for transplantation may be obtained from compatible blood type cadaver donors or from three categories of living donors such as: living-related donors who are genetically related individuals (e.g., close relatives), emotionally-related living donors but have no genetic link (e.g., spouses and friends), or altruistic living donors who are unknown to the recipient (Molzahn, Starzomski, & McCormick, 2003). An advantage of kidney transplantation compared to dialysis is that it reverses many of the pathophysiological changes associated with renal failure and eliminates the dependency on dialysis and accompanying dietary and lifestyle restrictions (Molzahn et al., 2003). Additionally, it has been well documented that transplantation in comparison to both CAPD and hemodialysis improves patients' and families' quality of life (Molzahn, 1991; Winsett & Hathaway, 1999). In one study using three measures of quality of life

(QoL), transplantation offered a higher QoL compared to CAPD, home or hospital hemodialysis (Molzahn, Northcott, & Dossetor, 1997). Using the 10-point Cantril Self-Anchoring Striving Scale, the average QoL score for renal transplant recipients was 7.4 compared to means in the range of $M = 5.3$ for patients receiving hemodialysis and $M = 5.7$ for patients on CAPD. The benefits of an organ transplant have been found to extend to family members because of the joy they experience from witnessing the recipient return to health and acquire a sense of normality in his or her daily life (Molzahn et al., 2003). Unfortunately, in the United States as in the rest of the world, there is a critical shortage of available kidneys for transplantation and as result, most individuals will need to initiate some form of dialysis treatment prior to receiving a transplant.

Decision making about renal replacement therapy is made by the patients, significant others, and/or physicians (Courts, 2000). While some patients have medical or psychological problems that preclude a particular dialysis modality or transplantation, the majority of the patients do have a choice. Psychosocial characteristics of patients influencing treatment modality selection include potential for treatment compliance, availability of social support, and life style factors. A survey of nephrologists in the United States, for instance, revealed that the patient's likelihood to comply with a treatment was the most important psychosocial consideration taken into account by nephrologists in recommending a dialysis modality (Thamer et al., 2000). In this study, nephrologists recommended peritoneal dialysis for 61% of the patients they considered to be likely to comply with the treatment. Patients' social support networks have also been taken into account. Nilsson and colleagues (1998) linked family, friends, and employers support with treatment choice. Hemodialysis and peritoneal dialysis have quite different effects on lifestyle. Two studies indicate the most important lifestyle advantage of hemodialysis for patients is more free time, whereas the most important lifestyle advantage of peritoneal dialysis is a greater control of one's treatment schedule and more flexibility (King 2000; Vecchi et al., 1994). This flexibility appears to be an influencing factor for people who continue working as several studies report that dialysis patients who are employed are more likely to be treated with peritoneal dialysis than with hemodialysis (Diaz-Buxo, 1998). Other factors that may influence treatment choice include: (a) the patient's need for autonomy, independence, and control; (b) the patient's fear of needles and blood, concerns about being tied to a machine, and threats to body image; (c) health care professionals' assessment that one type of treatment may be more or less effective or convenient for a particular individual; and (d) the patient's refusal or lack of motivation to assume self-care responsibilities for home dialysis and/or spouse or other family member's refusal to assist with dialysis care at home (Whittaker & Albee, 1996).

In summary, a multitude of factors has been taken into account in recommending or in selecting a dialysis treatment modality. The decision is exceedingly complex and it is the responsibility of the health care team to help the person find the treatment modality that most corresponds with his or her medical condition and lifestyle. The decision should be a shared one involving at the least, the nephrologist and the person with kidney failure (Moss, 2001).

Process of Making the Choice

The decision-making process is presented first from the perspective of the nephrologists and then from the perspective of patients with kidney failure and their families. A survey of American nephrologists and of members of the National Kidney Foundation Council on Dialysis identified patient preference as the most important factor in the decision-making process followed by quality of life, morbidity, and survival (Mendelssohn, Mullaney, Jung, Blake, & Mehta, 2001). Similarly, a study by Thamer and colleagues (2000) among nephrologists in the United States indicated that the patient's opinion was the most important consideration in determining dialysis treatment choice.

Several investigators have examined the decision-making process from the point of view of the person with kidney failure. A study conducted by Whittaker and Albee (1996) reported that the presence or absence of basic resources such as family support influenced the person's choice. A survey by King (2000) revealed that 29% of people with kidney failure believed that the best way to make the decision is in collaboration with one's family and with the nephrologist. Little and colleagues (2001) show that living with a supportive spouse influenced patients' selection of peritoneal dialysis as a treatment modality. A qualitative study described the selection of a treatment modality as an individual process in partnership involving three stages. In the first, patients keep comparing different treatment options in their mind over and over again until suddenly, in the second stage of the process, an external event occurs such as observing a person on dialysis carrying out the treatment or listening to a news program about dialysis that resonates with them. This produces a turning point moment of decision in which patients suddenly know which treatment modality they want. They stop comparing options and maintain their commitment to the particular modality chosen. Once this happens, however, a third phase begins in which patients open themselves to the possibility of other options in the future. In this last phase, although the treatment modality selected in the turning point moment appears to be the right choice for the patient and for the most part they will not waver from their decision, they do not necessarily see it as their final choice (Toupin, 2004). Ideally, adequate preparation for dialysis or transplantation requires at least 12 months of frequent contact with a renal team (Mendelssohn et al., 1999). Late referral to a nephrologist shortens the time for decision about treatment modality and placing a vascular access.

In summary, studies show that persons with chronic renal failure need informational support when selecting a dialysis treatment. Research has found that selecting a dialysis treatment modality is a process often involving several partners such as family members, other dialysis patients, and health care professionals. Surveys also indicate that the nephrology team believes that the preference of the person with renal failure should be the key factor in choosing a dialysis treatment.

Role of Nurses in Supporting Clients and Family

Nurses provide education and support when accompanying patients with renal failure and their families during the decision-making process. Churchill, Blake, Jindal, Toffelmire, and Goldstein (1999) underscore the importance for health care professionals to inform both the patient and family members about treatment options. In the present context of limited resources for the treatment of chronic renal failure, often a pre-dialysis team helps the patient and family prepare for ESRD. This multidisciplinary team, which includes physicians, nurses, social workers, and dietitians helps the patient and family understand the prognosis, treatment options, and symptom management, as well as the potential impact of the disease and its management on quality of life. Generally, pre-dialysis education programs are offered by nurses and are oriented towards helping patients understand and cope with the disease process. They also aim to facilitate treatment selection. One of their objectives is to increase understanding sufficiently to enable the person with kidney failure to make a judicious choice of a treatment modality (Coupe, 1998; Klang, Björvell, & Clyne, 1999).

The nurse provides support during the decision-making process and may accompany the person and family members through individual follow-up visits or phone calls. The support role may also involve showing the person the dialysis unit and introducing him or her to other persons who are already on dialysis. Recent studies have found that informal support from people who have lived similar experiences has a positive impact and is helpful in the decision-making process (Coupe, 1998; Klang et al., 1999; Toupin, 2004). The nurse should consider the possibility of matching the patient with people on dialysis of the same age, living arrangements, and employment status. It would also be helpful to ensure that the patient meets individuals on both hemodialysis and on peritoneal dialysis. Given their involvement in the decision-making process, the nurse should consider the possibility of including family members who will assist with dialysis in these meetings as well. Selecting a dialysis treatment modality is a difficult decision and stirs up feelings of uncertainty and anxiety. Patients and their families need to be able to count on the support of a well-qualified and experienced multidisciplinary team in which the nurse plays a significant role.

Once the decision is made about dialysis treatment, both the patient and family members need to integrate the demands of ESRD and its associated treatment regimens into their daily lives. A plethora of studies have been conducted about individuals on dialysis. However, information about their family members has been more limited even though they have been involved in providing emotional, physical, and technical support to individuals on various modes of renal replacement therapy for more than four decades. Collectively, the research and anecdotal reports published about these family members have focused on stressors, burden, quality of life, and adjustment of the marital dyad. Factors such as caregiver gender, age, and length of time assisting with dialysis care, as well as coping have been found to influence the family members' response and adjustment to ESRD, dialysis, and transplantation. The following section will describe the experiences of family members who live and/or assist an adult individual on various renal replacement therapies.

Impact of ESRD and Renal Replacement Therapy on Family Members

Involvement of the spouse or other family member is critical with dialysis; however, some family members may find this burdensome because the treatment necessitates modifications to lifestyles and daily routines. In some cases, spouses must assume new roles within the family such as sole income provider. In other cases, roles are reversed as the healthy spouse assumes responsibilities relinquished by the ill partner. Changes such as these can seriously compromise the spouse's psychological well-being, quality of life, and coping abilities (Friesen, 1997; Wagner, 1996).

Stressful Situations Associated with ESRD and Renal Replacement Therapy

The type of renal replacement therapy a person receives influences the kind of stressors family members experience. For example, stressors associated with assisting with home hemodialysis may include: dealing with the breakdown of the dialysis machine, inserting needles for dialysis (venipuncture), and being apprehensive about the fear that the individual could die while on the machine (Bryan & Evans 1980; Lowry & Atcherson 1984). Family members are often required to make rapid decisions that potentially could affect the life of the patient. Therefore, being at the front line of care when home alone and things are not going well with the ill person and/or dialysis treatment can be very stressful. Nephrology nurses have been identified to be a vital source of informational and emotional support during times of crisis. The family members are extremely grateful and thankful for having access to nephrology nurses when guidance is needed at home with dialysis treatment. Family members have described most nephrology nurses to be "kind," "concerned," and/or "fantastic," and many have expressed relief and comfort knowing that they are readily available (Pelletier-Hibbert & Sohi, 2000).

Stressors related to assisting with peritoneal dialysis center on assisting with pharmacologic interventions, doing diasylate exchanges, ordering all the dialysis supplies, as well as getting up many times during the night to trouble shoot (Pelletier-Hibbert & Sohi, 2000). Peritoneal dialysis requires self-care abilities on the part of the individual or assistance from a trained caregiver who is often a family member (Srivastava, 1988). However, the extent of a family member's level of involvement of assisting with dialysis is usually influenced by the individual's willingness and ability to participate in dialysis care. A few researchers have indicated that some individuals transfer total responsibility for peritoneal dialysis to a family member, usually a spouse, once they get home due to failing health or after losing interest in doing dialysis over an extended period of time (Friesen 1997; Pelletier-Hibbert & Sohi, 2000; Srivastava, 1988). Some family members may perceive themselves to be ill-prepared for the physical and emotional strains of assuming full responsibility for peritoneal dialysis treatment. In response, they may resent dialysis and feel anger and frustration towards the ill person. Campbell (1998) warns that health care professionals need to be aware that family members can experience burnout from the constant demands of the illness and its associated treatments, much the same as do individuals in the helping profession. Most family members assume caregiving responsibilities out of love, concern, marital vows, duty and/or lack of alternatives. For some family members, the notion of reciprocity motivates them to assist with dialysis care (Pelletier-Hibbert & Sohi, 2000).

Although the family members of individuals who receive center hemodialysis have no direct dialysis care responsibilities, they also experience a host of other challenges and struggles. For these family members, fitting commuting to and from the dialysis unit into a busy schedule, waiting at the center for dialysis treatment to be completed, and rearranging work schedules to drop off and pick up the patient after dialysis were found to have a significant impact on their time and energy (Bryan & Evans 1980; Lowry & Atcherson 1984; Pelletier-Hibbert & Sohi, 2000). As Campbell (1998) indicated, time is at a premium for these family members as they struggle to incorporate the many hours needed for dialysis treatment and transportation, time and energy that are taken away from other vital needs and tasks for survival, family maintenance, and/or fulfillment of responsibilities.

There are also stressors that are common to all family members regardless of the type of dialysis therapy. Planning and preparing meals to accommodate the dietary restrictions imposed by ESRD is stressful. Having to blend a variety of dietary regimens prescribed for other co-morbid illnesses such as diabetes and/or cardiovascular diseases may complicate meal preparation (Pelletier-Hibbert & Sohi, 2000). In addition, helping to support the individual with compliance issues related to dietary and fluid intake has also reported to be an enormous challenge for some family members (Campbell, 1998). Family members want to do their utmost to help the patient survive and improve their health and quality of life. In response, they may engage in the role of gatekeeper, which consists of making a plan of action to organize, to regulate, and to supervise patients' daily fluid and dietary intake, in order to ensure that they adhere to their prescribed regimen. Being involved in the role of gatekeeper entails more than just keeping an eye on, or making observations about, what and how much patients drink or eat. It is more like being on guard, night and day, to ensure that the patient does not drink too much or eat the wrong type of food. Despite their efforts, family members are aware that adhering to the prescribed fluid and dietary regimen can be a major challenge for patients. They often have firsthand experience with witnessing and managing the consequences of the patient's non-adherence to the prescribed regimen, such as shortness of breath, congestive heart failure, rapid weight gain, increased blood pressure, edema, and sometimes death. Being a gatekeeper is considered to be a stressful role; however, it is also perceived to be an important role that helps that person feel like he or she is doing something to shape the course of the illness.

Stressors experienced by kidney transplant recipients and their family members include the need to adjust to an intense and lengthy follow-up period, the regimens and side effects associated with immunosuppresant medications, worries about organ rejection, and uncertainty about how long the transplanted kidney will function (Sutton & Murphy, 1989; Starzomski & Hilton, 2000; Weems & Patterson, 1989; White, Ketefian, Starr, & Voepel-Lewis, 1990).

Whether kidney failure is sudden or insidious, family members report that the moment renal failure and dialysis treatment enters their lives, it is considered to be an intrusive stranger that creates a lot of uncertainty. Uncertainty is particularly stressful when it results from not knowing: (a) when the patient's health will take a turn for the worse, (b) whether dialysis treatment will effectively manage the illness symptoms and/or how the patient will feel after each dialysis treatment, (c) how long dialysis treatment will sustain life and whether the patient will die from kidney failure, and/or (d) when and if the patient will get a kidney transplant (Pelletier-Hibbert & Sohi, 2001). Brock (1987) studied uncertainty and information needs in family members of individuals on center hemodialysis. The author found that when family members had a good understanding of the illness and dialysis treatment, they experienced less stress associated with uncertainty. According to Brock, it is important for family members to have information at their disposal, because this will help them to give the illness a place in their lives. The caregiver's employment is often affected by the illness and its treatment. The unpredictable nature of the illness, the patient's deteriorating health, and/or the side effects of dialysis treatment may require that family members reduce their work hours from full-time to part-time, take unpaid leave, rearrange work hours, and/or decline job opportunities. This suggests that renal failure and its associated treatment affect employment more than employment affects the caregiving role.

The various sources of stressors imposed by ESRD and its associated regimens may increase the family members' burden, decrease their quality of life (QoL), and negatively affect their emotional and physical well-being. The following section will address these issues.

Burden and QoL

In general, the literature focusing on the burden and quality of life of caregivers of individuals on dialysis is scarce. Only five studies explicitly focused on investigating burden and/or quality of life in caregivers of individuals on CAPD (Dunn, Lewis, Bonner, & Meize-Grochowski, 1994), hospital hemodialysis (Belasco & Sesso, 2002; Lindqvist, Carlsson, & Sjodén, 2000), and/or waiting for a kidney transplant (Harris, Thomas, Wicks, Faulkner, & Hathaway, 2000; Wicks, Milstead, Hathaway, & Cetingok, 1997). No studies were found that focused specifically on burden in family members of patients on home hemodialysis.

Caregiver burden is a multidimensional phenomenon

reflecting the physical, psycho-emotional, social, and financial consequences of caring for an ill family member (George & Gwyther, 1986). Researchers studying caregiver burden differentiate between objective and subjective burden. Subjective burden focuses "on the perceived strain or stress associated with providing care, while objective burden refers to the disruptions in family life and the tasks and activities related to providing care" (Wicks et al., 1997, p. 528). Objective burden is tangible, while subjective burden is related to the caregiver's feelings about the tangible changes that occur as a result of assuming the caregiving roles. Caregiver burden is one of many factors that influences quality of life (QoL) in caregivers of individuals with ESRD. Spouses who experience poor QoL may not be in a position to support their ill partner (Dunn et al., 1994). Framing of caregiving as a burden puts forward a negative lens that until recently may have precluded the discovery of any rewards for the caregiver. Caring theorists suggest that caregiving may be rewarding, sustaining, and growth producing. Unfortunately, much of the literature on family members of individuals on dialysis has depicted a negative experience.

Dunn et al. (1994) investigated the QoL of spouses of CAPD patients, the relationship between QoL, severity of illness, socioeconomic status, marital adjustment, and coping ability, and the best predictors of QoL. The results showed that more than half (55%) of the family members experienced moderate to drastic changes in their quality of life since PD was initiated. Marital adjustment was the best predictor of QoL, followed by high income. Similarly, Belasco and Sesso (2002) found that, in general, caregivers of individuals on center hemodialysis experienced moderate amount of burden that resulted from drastic changes in both personal and social lives. Living with an individual who has both ESRD and diabetes can also create high levels of burden in caregivers. Wicks et al. (1997) explained that the high level of burden in these caregivers may be associated with significant deterioration in health of diabetics once dialysis begins which may further decrease the patients' ability to independently care for themselves. Consequently, they may need assistance from caregivers in various dimensions of life.

Lindqvist et al. (2000) explored health–related quality of life and coping of spouses of individuals on various renal replacement therapies. They studied 21 husbands and 34 wives of CAPD, center hemodialysis, and renal transplant individuals. The spouses of partners on hemodialysis rated themselves to experience more difficulty than the other two groups in being able to cope with the physical, social, and psychological aspects of their partners' illness and treatment. In contrast, the spouses of transplant recipients reported more satisfaction with their physical health, emotional well being, sleep patterns, and sexual functioning. Other studies about caregivers of those waiting for a kidney transplant have found that they experience little to no burden and report good to excellent QoL (Harris et al., 2000; Wicks et al., 1997). Differences between the findings of spouses of partners on dialysis and those of transplant recipients may be related to transplant recipients and candidates experiencing relatively stable health conditions when compared to individuals who are not eligible for transplantation (Wicks et al., 1997). Therefore, the spouses of transplant recipients and candidates may experience less interference occasioned by daily and long-term problems associated with ESRD and dialysis treatment and hence may experience less burden and more stable QoL (Molzahn, 1991; Starzomski & Hilton, 2000).

Psychological and Physical Responses to Stress

The psychological and physical outcomes of dealing with the stress of dialysis include fatigue, anxiety, and frustration. In a recent study (White & Grenyer, 1999), husbands and wives of partners on either hospital hemodialysis or CAPD reported feelings of sadness, resentment, guilt, and loss of partnership, sexual intimacy, and decreased quality of life. Along with dealing with the many changes in roles and responsibilities, family members may also experience stress from the significant changes in their relationship with the patient, as well as with extended families and long-time friends (Pelletier-Hibbert & Sohi, 2000). The many physiological, physical, and/or psychosocial limitations inherent in having kidney failure and being on dialysis may contribute to a loss of connectedness with the patient. Family members may experience a sense of emotional and physical detachment in their relationship with the patient. This loss of connectedness may be expressed in statements of missing the companionship, the sexual intimacy, expressions of affection (a valuable source of support), and missing the person as they had known them before the illness. For some family members, feelings of loneliness and aloneness are intricately linked with the loss of connectedness with the patient.

The Marital Context

The significance of marital and family context has long been recognized in ESRD. According to Devins, Hunsley, Mandin, Taub, and Paul (1997) "the condition may affect and be affected by, family life in many ways" (p. 326). However, controversy exists regarding the role of the marital dyad in the adjustment of each partner to the demands of ESRD and dialysis treatment. Some researchers have concluded that a spouse's adjustment is influenced by his or her ill partner's reaction to ESRD and dialysis treatment (Chowanec & Binik, 1989; Horsburg, Rice, & Matuk, 1998). Others, however, stipulated that a couple's adaptation to the demands of the illness and home hemodialysis rests heavily on the physical and psychological well-being and coping abilities of the spouse-caregiver (Brackney, 1979; Daneker, Kimmel, Ranich, & Peterson, 2001). Despite differences in perspectives, these researchers agree that spouses of partners with ESRD experience many of the same challenges and constraints encountered by the ill-partner and that ESRD and dialysis affects them as a couple.

Chowanec and Binik (1989) examined the relationship among chronic renal failure, marital functioning, and individual psychological well-being in 89 couples (n = 43 wives with ESRD and n = 46 husbands with ESRD), sampled from 5 groups of partners with varying stages of kidney disease and various renal replacement therapies. They

found increased marital role strain and decreased psychological well-being in couples with a spouse on dialysis, particularly those on home dialysis. This finding may be explained by the fact that people on either home hemodialysis or peritoneal dialysis and their caregivers bear a larger burden in terms of treatment responsibility and daily conduct of the therapeutic regimen in comparison to center hemodialysis and non-dialysis patients. Similarly, when spouses of partners on hospital hemodialysis or with a renal transplant were compared, spouses of dialysis partners experienced reduction in personal growth, especially loss of independence and changes in their social lives (Devins et al., 1997; Kaye, Bray, Gracely, & Levinson, 1989). In contrast, spouses of transplant recipients report significant enhancement in their personal growth. Being more directly affected by ESRD and dialysis treatment may account for the observed spousal differences in these studies.

Assisting with home hemodialysis has been found to adversely affect the lives and marital relationship of spouses. Friesen (1997) highlights three levels of spousal involvement with dialysis care: the *doers,* the *minimal assistant,* and *the joint doers.* The *doers* assume all the tasks of running the home hemodialysis while their partners play a passive role in their treatment. As a result, the *doers* experience moderate levels of resentment associated with being tied down and restricted in certain aspects of their lives. The *minimal assistants* work full-time, have young children, and even though they provide the least amount of assistance to their partner with dialysis, they express the strongest feelings of resentment toward their partner's disease and lifestyle changes imposed by dialysis. In contrast, the *joint partners* share the responsibilities of dialysis with their ill partner, and tend to be older and retired. Unlike the other two groups, the *joint partners* maintain activities outside the home, successfully accommodate home hemodialysis into their daily lives, and express little resentment toward dialysis in comparison to those spouses who are either under- or over-involved. They focus more on the normal aspects of their lives rather than how drastically their lives have been transformed by the demands of the illness and its associated treatments. The strong cooperative relationships between the partners influence their experience with dialysis, suggesting that a more cooperative approach to dialysis care is associated with better adjustment to the illness and its treatment with less anger and resentment. Additional observations by Friesen (1997) reveal that the *joint partners* tend to grow closer together as a couple, whereas the *doers* report a stable marital relationship. In contrast, the *minimal assistants* demonstrate marital relationships that are strained. Danaker et al. (2001) stipulated that "chronic illness may have a profound effect on a marriage, often creating new sources of marital tension or amplifying existing marital problems" (p. 840). Therefore, examination of predialysis marital relationship as a possible predictor of success with home dialysis could provide valuable information for screening home hemodialysis candidates or providing marital counselling prior to initiating dialysis. It is not known if nonmarried significant others would respond in the same manner to assisting with home hemodialysis because the few studies that included this group combined the analysis with spouse caregivers.

In other studies researchers found that a collaborative relationship between spouses during home dialysis influences each of the partner's adjustment to dialysis. Brackney's (1979) study of 12 male home hemodialysis patients and their wife-assistants found that the partner's physical health and adaptation to dialysis is enhanced when the spouse makes a positive emotional adjustment to home dialysis and collaborates on dialysis-related tasks. In turn, both partners' abilities to effectively assist with home dialysis care is dependent on each others' (a) ability to work cooperatively during dialysis, (b) emotional adjustment to home dialysis, and (c) physical health. Thus, it appears that the better the emotional adjustment to home dialysis and physical health of one spouse, the greater the efficacy of the other spouse to perform his or her dialysis-related duties. This suggests that emotional and health complaints from either partner may indicate that the couple needs additional support from health care professionals.

The patient's level of depression has been found to impact on the spouse's level of depression and marital satisfaction (Danaker et al., 2001). These researchers found that spouses who lived with highly depressed ill partners were more depressed, and spouses who received little to no support from the ill partner were also more depressed. Being depressed invariably depletes the spouses' coping resources, reduces their ability to provide support to the ill partner, and impairs their ability to carry out the caregiving role. Soskolne and Kaplan De-Nour (1989) have argued that health care professionals should not assume all spouses are reliable support systems for the patients because they too can be distressed.

It is clear from the review of the literature that living and assisting someone on dialysis can be challenging for most family members, especially those assisting with home dialysis. Spouses of individuals on home dialysis seem to encounter more changes in their marital, personal, and social lives than spouses of individuals on hospital hemodialysis or transplant recipients. However, the spousal adjustment to home dialysis can be enhanced by a collaborative relationship between the caregiver and care recipient. In addition, there is evidence to suggest that a caregiver's level of stress, burden, and quality of life as well as coping abilities varies according to the type of renal replacement treatment, the patient's ability to perform ADL, the patient's level of depression, and the presence of co-morbid illnesses such as diabetes in the patient. Other factors have been reported to influence the caregivers' abilities to integrate the demands and restrictions imposed by ESRD and dialysis treatment.

Factors Contributing to the Differential Impact of Caregiving

Factors found to influence the response of family members center on gender, age, length of time spent assisting with dialysis care, as well as the type of coping strategies used to manage the demands of ESRD, dialysis, and transplantation.

Gender Differences

In the few studies where gender differences in adjustment to ESRD and dialysis treatment of couples and spouse caregivers were examined, mixed results were found. Women's experiences as patients or partners were more negative (Blogg, O'Shaughnessy, & Cairns 1999; Chowanec & Binik, 1989; Devins et al., 1997; Lindqvist et al., 2000), and husbands as spouses experienced more difficulty adjusting (Soskolne & Kaplan De-Nour, 1989).

Gender differences in patients. Devins et al. (1997) found that couples in which the patient was a woman reported a decline in personal growth, whereas couples in which the patient was a man reported no change in this dimension. Similarly, Chowanec and Binik (1989) reported significant gender differences in psychological well-being, with female patients reporting more psychological distress and more marital role strain than male participants. However, no significant statistical differences were reported in either marital or psychological well-being of husbands and wives of individuals in either the dialysis and nondialysis groups.

Gender differences in spouse-caregivers. Only two studies compared gender differences in spouses. Blogg et al. (1999) found that when wife and husband caregivers were assessed about disruption to household routines, social life, and standard of living imposed by dialysis, husbands reported the least amount of distress. Blogg et al. explained that men living with women experiencing ESRD may encounter less disruption in their day-to-day lives "due to the continuance of the female patient's traditional social roles, such as maintaining the household routine and family life," while simultaneously assuming her responsibilities for sustaining home dialysis (p. 512). In contrast, Soskolne and Kaplan De-Nour (1989) compared the psychological distress and psychosocial adjustment of spouses and partners on center hemodialysis. They found that husbands in comparison to wife caregivers reported more psychological distress. Soskolne and Kaplan De-Nour explained that women have traditionally occupied a nurturing role, performed the essential household tasks and assumed major responsibility for the care of children, spouses and aged relatives. Therefore, when a woman is sick, her ability to perform these various roles is diminished, causing all family members to be affected, especially the spouses. Men may need to assist or take on additional and nontraditional responsibilities placed on them as partners, fathers, and/or caregivers, causing the healthy husband to feel distressed. The sample in most studies included mostly women, especially wife-caregivers. The focus is understandable given that women generally predominate in the caregiving role. However, in the few studies that included men and women caregivers, combined analysis or comparisons with very few men were conducted. Consequently, these studies were unable to discern the unique concerns, issues, and experiences of men. Several researchers over the past three decades have called for studies of male caregivers of individuals living with ESRD and assisting with home dialysis (Blogg et al., 1999; Brunier & McKeever, 1993; Danaker et al., 2001; Friesen, 1997).

Age of the Caregiver

The few studies that examined the caregiver's age as a predictor of distress and adjustment to ESRD and dialysis treatment showed mixed results. Harris et al. (2000) found no significant age differences in total burden or role strain between younger and older caregivers of individuals waiting for a kidney transplant. However, in four studies, younger spouses were found to experience more difficulties adjusting to changes imposed by ESRD and dialysis treatment (Blogg et al., 1999; Friesen, 1997; White, Richter, Koeckeritz, Lee, & Munch 2002). For example, Atcherson (1981) compared the adjustment of spouses under 45 years of age with those over 45 years of age during dialysis training sessions and 3 months after assisting their husbands with home hemodialysis. While both age groups reported being worried and nervous about dialysis during training, only the younger spouses reported ongoing difficulty with sleep and anxiety as well as more headaches, trouble with memory, nervousness, and tiredness after 3 months of assisting with dialysis. Similarly, in an Australian study by Blogg et al. (1999) it was found that spouses under the age of 45 experienced more personal distress (anxiety, depression, and fear associated with the caregiving role) and life upset (disruptions to household routine, social life and standard of living) than spouses between the age of 45 to 60 years or spouses greater than 60 years of age. Consistent with these studies, Friesen (1997) noted that younger spouses experienced the most resentment towards dialysis, participated the least in dialysis care, and had a particularly difficult time adjusting to the challenges and constraints imposed by ESRD and home dialysis. Similarly, White, Richter, et al. (2002) found that younger caregivers of individuals on home hemodialysis in comparison to older caregivers experienced more illness-induced stresses in their daily lives and more changes in lifestyle choices, financial status, and roles. These researchers explained that caregivers, especially younger persons, might feel more limited in career and social activities when they assume the caregiving role. Similarly, younger caregivers may experience more secondary role strains, such as work and child rearing and may have greater financial commitments; thus, caregiving may be more easily accepted at a later stage in life (Blogg et al., 1999; Friesen, 1997). Younger spouses have also expressed concerns about being insufficiently informed about their ill partner's diminished abilities to fulfill their needs and desires for intimacy. Others have experienced shattered hopes and dreams of being able to have children in the future (Pelletier-Hibbert & Sohi, 2001).

Length of Time Caregiving

Several longitudinal studies have explored the influence of the length of time living with someone with ESRD on the caregiver's distress. However, the results are inconsistent. Some studies report persistent caregiver distress, whereas others found that distress dissipates over time. For example, Lowry and Atcherson (1984) found that at 6 months after starting home hemodialysis, spouses continued to be easily angered with their ill-partner. According to the researchers, these persistent reactions may have been a reflection of feelings of deprivation associated with a variety of losses and changes imposed by the illness and dialysis. Lowry and Atcherson also found that depression, insomnia, and diminished ability to think were experienced by all spouses when they first began dialysis training sessions. However, with the exception of three spouses, all these symptoms disappeared at 6 months after initiating dialysis. In a more recent study about family members of individuals on hemodialysis, Belasco and Sesso (2002) found a small negative relationship between caregiver burden and length of time caregiving, suggesting that longer involvement in caregiving increases burden. Unlike previously discussed studies, Bryan and Evan's (1984) national survey of 198 home hemodialysis caregivers in the United States revealed that anxiety declined over time, with anxiety levels being higher during the first 2 years of caregiving than in later years. Caution must be applied in interpreting the results of this survey since measures to evaluate changes in anxiety levels were not reported. Similarly, Courts (2000) observed that the level of stress experienced by 14 spouses of home hemodialysis partners decreased over time. However it is not clear how stress was measured or how long they had assisted with dialysis. As might be anticipated, levels of concerns about ESRD and dialysis were generally highest during training for most caregivers. However, for some caregivers emotional and physical distress persisted for an extended period of time after initiating dialysis. Therefore, the impact of time on the caregiver's well-being may be an important deciding factor as to whether or not home hemodialysis may be an option for an individual. Since all studies focused on caregivers of patients on home hemodialysis, it is unknown how length of time spent assisting patients on peritoneal dialysis might be different or similar for the caregivers.

Coping Strategies

Only a few researchers have investigated coping as a predictor of the family member's adjustment to ESRD and dialysis. Only one study (Srivastava, 1988) was found that specifically investigated coping, while some investigators explored the relationship between coping and other variables (Dunn et al., 1994; Lindqvist et al., 2000) or identified themes of coping in qualitative studies (Flaherty & O'Brien, 1992; Pelletier-Hibbert & Sohi, 2001).

In three studies (Dunn et al., 1994; Lindqvist et al., 2000; Srivastava, 1988) coping strategies were explored using the *Jalowiec Coping Scale*. Spouses of partners on hemodialysis and peritoneal dialysis tend to use more emotion-focused coping strategies to manage their emotional responses to ESRD and dialysis treatment (Dunn et al., 1994; Lindqvuist et al., 2000). In comparison, Srivastava (1988) reported that spouses of individuals on CAPD used all of the following types of problem and emotion-focused coping strategies: accept the situation as it was, try to maintain control over the situation, and find out more about the situation. In addition, both men and women rated themselves to be coping well or very well, despite feelings that dialysis was very demanding and, in some cases was, the central focus of their lives. According to Lazarus and Folkman (1984), emotion-focussed strategies have been found to be helpful in situations that are distressing and appraised as unchangeable and beyond the individual's control.

Two qualitative studies demonstrated that the coping strategies used by family members of individuals with ESRD varied with the modality of renal replacement therapy. Findings from Flaherty and O'Brien (1992) showed that family members of individuals receiving center hemodialysis used a remote coping strategy, such as distancing themselves from the illness most often. In contrast, family members of individuals on CAPD used a distressed coping strategy, which included worrying. In comparison to the other two groups, family members of individuals on home hemodialysis only used the enfolded coping strategy, which entailed finding something positive in dialysis. Differences in the type of coping strategies used by family members may be due to the level of involvement required to assist with dialysis. In another study, Pelletier-Hibbert and Sohi (2001) identified that 41 family members of individuals on hospital and home hemodialysis or CAPD used the following four coping strategies: living each day as it comes, drawing on God's strength, finding positive meaning, and hoping for a transplant.

The results of these studies suggest that gender, age, length of time assisting with dialysis as well as coping strategies influence adjustment to ESRD, dialysis, and transplantation. However, the limited literature regarding these variables indicates that more inquiries into these areas are needed to help nurses better understand the challenges caregivers face. Such research could help nurses implement interventions to ease caregiver's distress, strengthen coping skills, and enable them to better meet their ill family member's needs without compromising their own health and quality of life.

Nursing Interventions

Family members have been involved with dialysis care for more than four decades. As can be seen from the literature review, the role of family members is crucial in the process and outcome of dialysis. In fact, Campbell (1998) has argued that good outcomes in all dimensions of dialysis care depend as much on the labors and support of family members as they do on technology and professional interventions. The escalation in the numbers of patients diagnosed with ESRD will continue as the 21st century unfolds. The fastest growing segment of the ESRD population is individuals 70 years of age and older and those with multiple comorbid conditions such as diabetes and cardiovascular disease. Caregivers are now expected to handle caregiving roles far more complex and often for a much longer duration than previous generations. If family caregivers are to continue to effectively assist with the technological demands and the physical and emotional components of caregiving, they must be adequately prepared to meet these challenges. Studies related to other caregiving situations have found that when caregivers perceive themselves to be well prepared to assume the caregiver role, less strain, burden, and depression are experienced (Archbold, Stewart, Greenlick, & Harvarth, 1990); self-efficacy and esteem are enhanced (Smith, 1994), and positive caregiving outcomes are experienced (Given, Given, Stommel, Collins, & King, 1992).

Caregivers need to be assessed for their physical and psychological well-being, coping abilities, as well as family and work-related responsibilities prior to the start of dialysis and followed up on every few months once dialysis has been initiated. This recommendation has been supported by other researchers (Brock, 1987; Campbell, 1998; Friesen, 1997). Educational, psychosocial, and economic issues surrounding ESRD and treatment options also need to be addressed. Meeting with caregivers prior to the start of dialysis would provide nurses with an opportunity to assess their understanding of the illness, the information they already possess, the kind of information they need or want, how they perceive the illness to impact their daily lives, and how they are coping. Such baseline information could be used to develop a framework to address their immediate and evolving needs or concerns.

For family members of center hemodialysis patients, follow-up strategies could be implemented while they wait for the patient's dialysis or follow-up visits to be completed, or while they participate in a training session for home dialysis care. For the caregivers whose presence is less visible around the dialysis unit, emotional support must extend beyond the boundaries of hospitals into the homes of caregivers. Researchers suggest that a phone call to and/or a separate interview with the caregiver every few months would be beneficial to determine the impact of the illness on their daily lives and to assess each of the caregiver's assumed responsibilities and levels of coping over the span of the family member's illness (Campbell, 1998; Dunn et al., 1984; Srivastava, 1988). The information gathered from the family members will provide a framework for consistent and individualized care and will guide the development of early and specific interventions to meet family members' unique needs during the course of the illness trajectory. Nurses could encourage information sharing between individuals in the decision-making process about treatment options and those already receiving dialysis. These exchanges could provide opportunities for individuals and family members to both receive and reciprocate support, while simultaneously preparing individuals and their family members to anticipate and prepare for the impact of ESRD and dialysis treatment on their daily lives.

In addition, Schneider (2004) suggests that renal nurses need to assess the level of physical fatigue in caregivers. This can be achieved by using a simple measure like the Fatigue Severity Scale (FSS), which can easily be administered. Interventions that focus on rest and respite may greatly benefit the caregivers.

The demands of the illness and dialysis treatment require that family members assume and adjust to new roles and responsibilities, learn new skills, and even give up aspects of their former lives. As familial roles change to accommodate the demands of ESRD and dialysis, both spouses may need assistance to learn how to effectively collaborate, communicate, and interact within the new context of their relationship. It is important to establish a mechanism for the evaluation of both the care recipient and caregiver's responses to ESRD and its associated treatment regimens. Renal care professionals need to capitalize on every opportunity to assess and respond to the tremendous emotional impact that an uncertain and stressful illness can have on renal family members in "an era where technological advances are sustaining life" (White & Grenyer, 1999, p. 1319). Renal care professionals' attention should be aimed specifically at those family members who lack social support, who are the "lone doers" in dialysis care, who travel great distances to the dialysis unit, and who juggle many roles and responsibilities.

Moreover, the caregivers' commitment to meeting challenges associated with dialysis may supersede addressing their own self-care needs. It is therefore vital for health care professionals to continue to focus on the family as the "unit of care" throughout the disease trajectory. Peterson (1985) stipulates that it is only by focusing on both the dual needs of the patient and his or her family that health care professionals will "be able to prevent a crisis from occurring rather than intervening only after the family has spent down their emotional and psychological resources" (p. 31). Support received from health care professionals can be a significant strategy that can contribute to reducing or avoiding crises in families. Nephrology nurses working in hemodialysis and home dialysis units have been singled out as being very helpful in providing informational and emotional support to family members (Campbell, 1998; Dunn et al., 1994; Friesen, 1997; Srivastava, 1988). Robinson (1998) asserts that families find nurses' invitations to engage in meaningful conversation about the effect of illness on their lives to be one of the most useful interventions in assisting families to move beyond and overcome problems. The capacity of nurses to be witnesses to the families' experiences with dialysis is central to providing care; it is the soul of clinical work with families. Nurses are in a position to be strong advocates for these family members when they are unable to be heard or understood.

References

Alloati, S., Manes, M., Paternoster, G., Gaiter, A., Molino, A., & Rosati, C. (2000). Peritoneal dialysis compared with hemodialysis in the treatment of end-stage renal disease. *Journal of Nephrology, 13*(5), 1-18.

Archbold, P., Stewart, B., Greenlick, M., & Harvarth, T. (1990). Mutuality and preparedness as predictors of caregiver role strain. *Research in Nursing & Health, 13,* 375-384.

Atcherson, E. (1981). Home hemodialysis and the spouse assistant. *AANNT Journal, 8,* 29-34.

Belasco, A., & Sesso, R. (2002). Burden and quality of life of caregivers of hemodialysis patients. *American Journal of Kidney Disease, 39*(4), 805-812.

Blogg, A., O'Shaughnessy, D., & Cairns, D. (1999). Levels and predictors of distress in home hemodialysis caregivers. *Dialysis & Transplantation, 28*(9), 507-517.

Brackney, B. (1979). The impact of home hemodialysis on the marital dyad. *Journal of Marital and Family Therapy, 5,* 55-60.

Brock, M.J. (1987). Uncertainty, information needs and coping effectiveness of renal families. *ANNA Journal, 14*(3), 242-246.

Brunier, G.M., & McKeever, P.T. (1993). The impact of home dialysis on the family: Literature review. *ANNA Journal, 20*(6), 653-659.

Bryan F.A., & Evans, R.W. (1980). Hemodialysis partners. *Kidney International, 17,* 350-356.

Campbell, A. (1998). Family caregivers: Caring for aging end-stage renal disease patients. *Advances in Renal Replacement Therapy, 5*(2), 98-108.

Chowanec, G.D., & Binik, Y.M. (1989). End stage renal disease and the marital dyad: An empirical investigation. *Social Science and Medicine, 28,* 971-983.

Churchill, D., Blake, P., Jindal, K., Toffelmire, B., & Goldstein, M. (1999). Clinical practice guidelines for initiation of dialysis: chapter 1, clinical guidelines for initiation of dialysis. *Journal of the American Society of Nephrology, Suppl. 13,* (10), S289-S291.

Coupe, D. (1998). Making decisions about dialysis options: an audit of patients' views. *EDTNA/ERCA Journal, 24*(1), 25-26.

Courts, N. (2000). Psychosocial adjustment of patients on home hemodialysis and their dialysis partner. *Clinical Nursing Research, 9*(2), 177-190.

Danaker, B., Kimmel, P., Ranich, T., & Peterson, R. (2001). Depression and marital dissatisfaction in patients with end-stage renal disease and in their spouses. *American Journal of Kidney Diseases, 38*(4), 839-846.

Devins, G., Hunsley, J., Mandin, H., Taub, K., & Paul, L. (1997). The marital context of end-stage renal disease: Illness intrusiveness and perceived changes in family environment. *Annals of Behavioral Medicine, 19*(4), 325-332.

Devins, G., Mendelssohn, D., Barré, P., & Binik, Y. (2003). Predialysis psychoeducational intervention and coping styles influences time to dialysis in chronic kidney disease. *American Journal of Kidney Diseases, 42*(4), 693-703.

Diaz-Buxo, J. A.(1998). Modality selection. *Journal of the American Society of Nephrology, 9,* S112-S117.

Dunn, S.A., Lewis, S.L., Bonner, P.N., & Meize-Grochowski, R. (1994). Quality of life for spouses of CAPD patients. *ANNA Journal, 21*(5), 237-257.

Flaherty, M., & O'Brien, M. (1992). Family styles of coping in end stage renal disease. *ANNA Journal, 19*(4), 345-366.

Friesen, D. (1997). A descriptive study of home hemodialysis spouse. *Dialysis and Transplantation, 26,* 310-325, 345.

George, L., & Gwyther, L (1986). Caregivers well-being: A multidimensional examination of family caregivers of demented adults. *The Gerontologist, 26*(3), 253-259.

Given, C., Given, B, Stommel, M., Collins, C., & King, S. (1992). The caregiver reaction assessment for caregivers of persons with chronic physical or mental impairments. *Research in Nursing Health, 15,* 271-281.

Gomez, C.G., Valido, P., Celadilla O., Bernaldo deQuiros A.G., & Mojon, M. (1999). Validity of a standard information protocol provided to end-stage renal disease patients and its effects on treatment selection. *Peritoneal Dialysis International, 19*(5), 471-477.

Harris, T., Thomas, C., Wicks, M., Faulkner, M., & Hathaway, D. (2000). Subjective burden in young and older African-American caregivers of patients with end-stage renal disease awaiting transplant. *Nephrology Nursing Journal, 27*(4), 383-391.

Holecheck, M.J. (2004). Nursing management: Acute renal failure and chronic kidney disease. In S.M. Lewis, M. McLean-Heitkemper, & S. Ruff-Dirksen (Eds.), *Medical- Surgical Nursing* (pp. 1210- 1246). St Louis: Mosby.

Horsburg, M., Rice, V., & Matuk, L. (1998). Sense of coherence and life satisfaction: Patient and spousal adaptation to home dialysis. *ANNA Journal, 25*(2), 219-230.

Kaye, J., Bray, S., Gracely, E., & Levinson, S. (1989). Psychosocial adjustment to illness and family environment in dialysis patients. *Family System Medicine, 7*(1), 77-89.

King, K. (2000). Patients' perspectives of factors affecting modality selection: A national kidney foundation patient survey. *Advances in Renal Replacement Therapy, 7*(3), 261-268.

Klang, B., Björvell, H., & Clyne, N. (1999). Predialysis education helps patients choose dialysis modality and increases disease-specific knowledge. *Journal of Advanced Nursing, 29*(4), 869-876.

Lazarus, R.S., & Folkman, S. (1984). *Stress, appraisal and coping.* New York: Springer Publishing Company.

Lindqvist, R., Carlsson, M., & Sjodén, P. (2000). Coping strategies and health related quality of life among spouses of continuous ambulatory peritoneal dialysis, haemodialysis, and transplant patients. *Journal of Advanced Nursing, 31*(6), 1398-1408.

Little, J., Irwin, A., Marshall, T., Rayner, H., & Smith, S. (2001). Predicting a patient's choice of dialysis modality: experience in a United Kingdom renal department. *American Journal of Kidney Diseases, 37*(5), 981-986.

Lowry, M., & Atcherson, E. (1984). Spouse-assistants adjustments to home hemodialysis. *Journal of Chronic Diseases, 37*(4), 293-300.

Maiorca, R., Cancarini, G.C., Zubani, R., Movilli, E., & Brunori, G. (1996). Differing dialysis treatment strategies and outcome. *Nephrol Dial Transplant, suppl 2,* 11, 134-139.

Mendelssohn, D., Barrett, J., Brownscombe, L., Ethier, J., Greenberg, D., Kanani, S., Levin, A., & Toffelmire, E. (1999). Créatinine élevée: Recommendations pour la prise en charge et la présentation à un néphrologue.*CMAJ-JAMC, 161*(4), 1-8.

Mendelssohn, D., Mullaney, S., Jung, B., Blake, P., & Mehta, R. (2001). What do American nephrologists think about dialysis modality selection? *American Journal of Kidney Diseases, 37*(1), 22-29.

Molzahn, A.E. (1991). Quality of life after organ transplantation. *Journal of Advanced Nursing, 16,* 1042-1047.

Molzahn, A., Northcott, H., & Dossetor, J. (1997). Perceptions of physicians, nurses, and patients regarding quality of life of patients with end-stage renal disease. *ANNA Journal, 24,* 247-253.

Molzahn, A., Starzomski, R., & McCormick, J. (2003). The supply of organs for transplantation: Issue and challenges. *Nephrology Nursing Journal, 30*(1), 17-26.

Moss, A.H., (2001). Shared decision- making in dialysis: The new RPA/ASN guidelines on appropriate initiation and withdrawal of treatment. *American Journal of Kidney Diseases, 37*(5), 1081-1091.

Nilsson, L., Anderberg, C., Ipson, R., Person, E., Anderson, G., & Lund, A. (1998). Quality decision making in dialysis. *EDTNA/ERCA Journal, 24,* 11-14.

Pelletier-Hibbert, M., & Sohi, P. (2000). The experiences of family members of individuals living with end-stage renal disease. Unpublished manuscript.

Pelletier-Hibbert, M., & Sohi, P. (2001). Sources of uncertainty and coping strategies used by family members of individuals living with end-stage renal disease. *Nephrology Nursing Journal, 28*(4), 411-417.

Peterson, K. (1985). Psychosocial adjustments of the family caregiver: Home hemodialysis as an example. *Social Work in Health Care, 10*(3), 15-32.

Prichard, S. (1996). Treatment modality selection in 150 consecutive patients starting ESRD therapy. *Peritoneal Dialysis International, 16,* 69-72.

Prichard, S. (2000). Decision process about options in renal therapy substitution: Selection versus election. *Nefrologia, 20*(3), 8-11.

Robinson, C. A. (1998). Women, families, chronic illness, and nursing interventions: From burden to balance. *Journal of Family Nursing, 4*(3), 271-290.

Smeltzer, S.C., & Bare, B.G. (2000). *Textbook of medical-surgical nursing.* Philadelphia: Lippincott.

Smith, C. (1994). A model of caregiving effectiveness for technologically dependent adults resident at home. *Advances in Nursing Science, 17*(2), 27-40.

Schneider, R. (2004). Chronic renal failure: Assessing the fatigue severity scale for use among caregivers. *Journal of Clinical Nursing, 13,* 219-225.

Soskolne, V., & Kaplan De-Nour, A. (1989). The psychosocial adjustments of patients and spouses to dialysis treatment. *Social Science & Medicine, 29* (4), 497-502.

Srivastava, R. (1988). Coping strategies used by spouses of CAPD patients. *ANNA Journal, 15*(3) 174-178.

Starzomski, R., & Hilton, A. (2000). Patient and family adjustment to kidney transplantation with and without an interim period of dialysis. *Nephrology Nursing Journal, 27*(1), 17-33, 52.

Sutton, T., & Murphy, S. (1989). Stressors and patterns of coping in renal transplant patients. *Nursing Research, 38*(1), 46-49.

Thamer, M., Hwang, W., Fink, N., Sadler, J., Wills, S., Levin, N., Bass, E., Levey, A., Brookmeyer, R., & Powe, N. (2000). US nephrologist's recommendation of dialysis modality: Result of a national survey. *American Journal of Kidney Disease, 36*(6), 1155-1165.

Toupin, I. (2004). Le processus de la prise décisionnelle face au premier choix d'une modalité de dialyse tel que vécu par la personne atteinte d'insuffisance rénale et un membre significatif de sa famille. Unpublished Master's thesis. University of Moncton, Canada.

Vecchi, A., Scalamogna, A., Columbini, M., Cesana, B., Cancarini, G.C., Catizone, L., Cocchi, R., Lupo, A., Viglino, G., Salomone, M., Segoloni, G.P., & Giangrande, A. (1994). Well being in patients on CAPD and hemodialysis. *The International Journal of Artificial Organs,* 17(9), 473-477.

Venkataramen, V., & Nolph, K. (1999). Socioeconomic aspects of peritoneal dialysis in north America: Role of non medical factors in the choice of dialysis. *Peritoneal Dialysis International, 19,* supplement 2, S419-S422.

Wagner, C. (1996). Family needs of chronic hemodialysis patients: A comparison of perceptions of nurses and families. *ANNA Journal, 23*(1), 19-28.

Weems, J., & Patterson, E. (1989). Coping with the uncertainty and ambivalence while awaiting a cadaveric renal transplant. *ANNA Journal, 16*(1), 27-31.

White Y., & Grenyer, B. (1999). The biopsychosocial impact of end-stage renal disease: The experience of dialysis patients and their partners. *Journal of Advanced Nursing, 30*(6), 1312-1320.

White, M., Ketefian, S., Starr, A., & Voepel-Lewis, T. (1990). Stress, coping, and quality of life in adult kidney transplant recipients. *ANNA Journal, 17*(6), 421-425.

White, N., Richter, J., Koeckeritz, J., Lee, Y., & Munch, K. (2002). A cross-cultural comparison of family resiliency in hemodialysis patients. *Journal of Transcultural Nursing, 13*(3), 218-227.

Whittaker, A. A., & Albee, B.J. (1996). Factors influencing patient selection of dialysis treatment modality. *ANNA Journal, 23*(4), 369-375.

Wicks, M., Milstead, E., Hathaway, D., & Cetingok, M. (1997) Subjective burden and quality of life in family caregivers of patients with end-stage renal disease. *ANNA Journal, 24*(5), 527-538.

Winsett, R., & Hathaway, D. (1999). Predictors of QoL in renal transplant recipients: Bridging the gap between research and clinical practice. *ANNA Journal, 26,* 235-240.

- Differences in quality of life of individuals on hemodialysis and peritoneal dialysis are not consistent. Prichard (2000) concludes that it is unclear whether modality per se has an important impact on the quality of life, but rather, modality should be chosen to match each patient's lifestyle and particular social set of circumstances.

- The cost of a given dialysis modality depends on the country and the nature of its health care system (Prichard, 2000). For instance, the structure of reimbursement in the United States explains in part the underutilization of peritoneal dialysis (Venkataramen & Nolph, 1999). In contrast, the health care policies in Canada and in the United Kingdom encourage the selection of peritoneal dialysis, which is less expensive for a national health care system than hemodialysis (Alloati et al., 2000).

- A number of geographical factors have been examined in relation to dialysis treatment selection. For instance, living a long distance from the treatment center, having spent extensive time traveling to and from a center for hemodialysis, and lacking access to transportation have been associated with the selection of peritoneal dialysis (Little, Irwin, Marshall, Rayner, & Smith, 2001).

- An advantage of kidney transplantation compared to dialysis is that it reverses many of the pathophysiological changes associated with renal failure and eliminates the dependency on dialysis and accompanying dietary and lifestyle restrictions (Molzahn et al., 2003). Additionally, it has been well documented that transplantation in comparison to both CAPD and hemodialysis improves patients' and families' quality of life (Molzahn, 1991; Winsett & Hathaway, 1999).

- A multitude of factors has been taken into account in recommending or in selecting a dialysis treatment modality. The decision is exceedingly complex, and it is the responsibility of the health care team to help the person find the treatment modality that most corresponds with his or her medical condition and lifestyle.

- Studies show that persons with chronic renal failure need informational support when selecting a dialysis treatment. Research has found that selecting a dialysis treatment modality is a process often involving several partners such as family members, other dialysis patients, and health care professionals.

- Nurses provide education and support when accompanying patients with renal failure and their families during the decision-making process. Churchill, Blake, Jindal, Toffelmire, and Goldstein (1999) underscore the importance for health care professionals to inform both the patient and family members about treatment options.

- Involvement of the spouse or other family member is critical with dialysis however; some family members may find this burdensome because the treatment necessitates modifications to lifestyles and daily routines. In some cases, spouses must assume new roles within the family such as sole income provider.

- Nephrology nurses have been identified to be a vital source of informational and emotional support during times of crisis. The family members are extremely grateful and thankful for having access to nephrology nurses when guidance is needed at home with dialysis treatment.

- The various sources of stressors imposed by ESRD and its associated regimens may increase the family members' burden, decrease their quality of life (QoL), and negatively affect their emotional and physical well-being.

- It is clear that living and assisting someone on dialysis can be challenging for most family members, especially those assisting with home dialysis. Spouses of individuals on home dialysis seem to encounter more changes in their marital, personal, and social lives, than spouses of individuals on hospital hemodialysis or transplant recipients.

- Factors found to influence the response of family members center on gender, age, length of time spent assisting with dialysis care, as well as the type of coping strategies used to manage the demands of ESRD, dialysis, and transplantation.

- The fastest growing segment of the ESRD population is individuals 70 years of age and older and those with multiple co-morbid conditions such as diabetes and cardiovascular disease. Caregivers are now expected to handle caregiving roles far more complex and often for a much longer duration than previous generations.

ANNP614

Client and Family Decision Making about Treatment Modalities for End Stage Renal Disease

Maryse Pelletier Hibbert MN, RN; Isabelle Toupin, MN, RN; and Cynthia Baker, PhD, MN, RN

Contemporary Nephrology Nursing: Principles and Practice contains 39 chapters of educational content. Individual learners may apply for continuing nursing education credit by reading a chapter and completing the Continuing Education Evaluation Form for that chapter. Learners may apply for continuing education credit for any or all chapters.

Please photocopy this page and return to ANNA.
COMPLETE THE FOLLOWING:

Name: _____

Address:_____

City:_____ State: _____ Zip: _____

E-mail: _____

Preferred telephone: ☐ Home   ☐ Work: _____

State where licensed and license number (optional): _____

CE application fees are based upon the number of contact hours provided by the individual chapter. CE fees per contact hour for ANNA members are as follows: 1.0-1.9 - $15; 2.0-2.9 - $20; 3.0-3.9 - $25; 4.0 and higher - $30. Fees for nonmembers are $10 higher.

ANNA Member: ☐ Yes   ☐ No   Member # (if available) _____

☐ Checked Enclosed   ☐ American Express   ☐ Visa   ☐ MasterCard

Total Amount Submitted: _____

Credit Card Number: _____ Exp. Date: _____

Name as it appears on the card: _____

CE Evaluation Form
To receive continuing education credit for individual study after reading the chapter
1. Photocopy this form. (You may also download this form from ANNA's Web site, **www.annanurse.org.**)
2. Mail the completed form with payment (check) or credit card information to American Nephrology Nurses' Association, East Holly Avenue, Box 56, Pitman, NJ 08071-0056.
3. You will receive your CE certificate from ANNA in 4 to 6 weeks.

Test returns must be postmarked by **December 31, 2010.**

CE Application Fee
ANNA Member $20.00
Nonmember $30.00

EVALUATION FORM

1. I verify that I have read this chapter and completed this education activity. Date: _____

_____
Signature

2. What would be different in your practice if you applied what you learned from this activity? *(Please use additional sheet of paper if necessary.)*

_____

_____

_____

_____

_____

_____

_____

_____

_____

_____

_____

Evaluation	Strongly disagree				Strongly agree
3. The activity met the stated objectives.					
a. Relate the impact of the diagnosis and treatment of renal disease on a patient and family to the nurse's ability to provide support and care.	1	2	3	4	5
b. Discuss the concerns that family members have about the patient's disease and choice of treatment.	1	2	3	4	5
c. Summarize the nursing interventions necessary to avoid a patient receiving differential treatment based on age, gender, coping strategies, and length of treatment.	1	2	3	4	5
4. The content was current and relevant.	1	2	3	4	5
5. The content was presented clearly.	1	2	3	4	5
6. The content was covered adequately.	1	2	3	4	5
7. Rate your ability to apply the learning obtained from this activity to practice.	1	2	3	4	5

Comments _____

_____

8. Time required to read the chapter and complete this form: _____ minutes.

This educational activity has been provided by the American Nephrology Nurses' Association (ANNA) for 2.1 contact hours. ANNA is accredited as a provider of continuing nursing education (CNE) by the American Nurses Credentialing Center's Commission on Accreditation (ANCC-COA). ANNA is an approved provider of continuing education by the California Board of Registered Nursing, CEP 0910.

Quality of Life and Chronic Kidney Disease: Living Long and Living Well

Anita E. Molzahn, PhD, RN

Chapter Contents

Quality of Life and Chronic Kidney Disease: Living Long and Living Well

Anita E. Molzahn, PhD, RN

One of our goals as nephrology nurses is to enhance the quality of life (QOL) of people with chronic kidney disease (CKD). While researchers struggle to develop a consistent definition of QOL, most of us understand that QOL reflects individuals' subjective assessment of how they perceive their lives, and that QOL can be rated from very good to very poor.

This chapter explores the concept of QOL as it relates to individuals with CKD. Methods to measure QOL, research findings regarding factors related and unrelated to QOL, and strategies for promoting QOL are presented. The chapter concludes with implications for nursing practice, education, and administration.

Overview of Quality of Life

The World Health Organization (WHO) defined QOL as "individuals' perceptions of their position in life in the context of the culture and value systems in which they live and in relation to their goals, expectations, standards and concerns" (WHOQOL Group, 1998, p. 551).

QOL is a broader concept than health status because it incorporates individuals' assessments of aspects of their lives that go beyond their well-being. For instance, a person's work, personal relationships, friendships, emotional state, and environment are integral to their QOL. Only the person him- or herself can assess his or her own QOL.

Why is QOL Important?

QOL is important, not only because is reflects life overall, but because it has a close relationship to health status, morbidity, and mortality (Lowrie, Curtin, LePain, & Schatell, 2003; Valderrabano, Jofre, & Lopez-Gomez, 2001). Survival is longer in people with a better QOL; similarly, better health status, and less morbidity are associated with higher QOL (Mapes, Bragg-Gresham, Bonner et al., 2004). As a result, QOL monitoring has been used in a wide range of outcome studies. It is no longer adequate to measure only morbidity and mortality associated with new therapies and treatments. QOL must be a paramount consideration as well.

Who Assesses QOL?

Although there is recognition that only the individual can assess his or her life, health care professionals often are asked to evaluate the QOL of the people for whom they provide care. Some of the original "QOL" measures, such as the Karnofsky scale (Karnofsky & Burchenal, 1949), involved physician ratings of the functional abilities of people. However, more recent research has shown that people on dialysis may have different assessments of their QOL than those assessments conducted by their health professionals. Molzahn, Northcott, and Dossetor (1997) found statistically significant differences and only moderately low correlations between the ratings of QOL of people with chronic renal disease and those of their health care professionals. In other words, the health care professionals' perceptions of their patients' QOL were not very accurate, if one assumes that

the individual knows his or her QOL best. Similarly, there are differences between ratings of people on dialysis about their QOL and ratings their family members provide about them (Perry, Nicholas, Molzahn, & Dossetor, 1995). In an analysis of research that involves proxies (someone to rate qualities or characteristics for another), it was found that proxies could only rate concrete observable symptoms and quality of services with any degree of accuracy (McPherson & Addington-Hall, 2003). Proxies cannot accurately rate subjective aspects of experience (including pain, depression, anxiety, and QOL).

If only the person him or herself can assess QOL, we, as nurses, need to discuss QOL with those in our care to determine what would make a difference to them. In other words, listening to the people that we care for is critical to enhancing their QOL. What will enhance the QOL of one person may not necessarily enhance the QOL of another. In fact, we may not even be aware of a change in a person's QOL, for the better or worse, unless he or she tells us and we are listening.

Living with Chronic Kidney Disease: The Experience

The experience of living with CKD involves many challenges. It is difficult for healthy individuals to truly understand the illness experience. The challenges of fluid and dietary restrictions, anemia, lack of energy, numerous symptoms, dependence on a machine or technology, countless medications, issues regarding body image, impairments in sexuality and fertility, and fear of death all contribute to the stress associated with the illness and treatment. Impairments in functioning and well-being begin long before kidneys fail (National Kidney Foundation [NKF]), 2002). Although transplantation offers hope, it, too, requires ongoing medical therapy.

A small but growing number of qualitative nursing studies address the experience of living with dialysis therapy. Qualitative research typically is used when little is known about a topic. However, as related to QOL, qualitative research provides a much richer description of life for people living with kidney disease. Although numerous studies compare QOL among treatment modalities, those studies do not usually help us to develop an understanding of the personal meaning of the experience for those receiving treatment, mostly because they are designed to answer more specific questions.

Rittman, Northsea, Hausauer, Green, and Swanson (1993), in a study of the lived experience of six people on dialysis, described a theme or pattern that they labeled *control: the meaning of technology*. They described how the participants in the study assumed a new understanding of being, maintained hope, "dwelled" in dialysis, and maintained control. Ritman and her colleagues also discussed how people on dialysis developed a "normal way of being," which involved "taking on a new understanding" (Rittman et al., 1993, p. 331). One man described moving from feeling like "being a pianist and having your hands cut off at the wrists" to moving to a state where "life is not much different [from what it was before]" (Rittman et al., 1993, p. 329). Another participant reported that coming for dialysis was like "brushing your teeth; it is just something you do and you don't think much about it" (p. 329); this participant had been on dialysis for 14 years, and he acknowledged that it took three years to reach that place. A number of authors (Nagle, 1998; O'Brien, 1983; Rittman et al., 1993) have discussed similar descriptions of the meaning of life for people on dialysis using technology.

Families also experience challenges in coming to terms with the illness. However, health care professionals do not always consider the impact of the treatment on the family. Hibbert discusses many of the issues for family members in Chapter 14 of this book. It is important to recognize that an individual's QOL is embedded within a network of relationships, including those of family members and care providers, and a person's QOL is greatly affected by the QOL of his or her spouse/partner (Dunn, Lewis, Bonner, & Meize-Grochowski, 1994). Although we commonly think about the support people on dialysis receive from family members, Cohen (1995) discussed the new set of supportive relationships that people receiving dialysis therapy developed with the staff. In the relationships nurses develop with the people that they care for, we can find many examples of meaningful encounters that have enhanced QOL. Some authors have described this relationship as similar to a psychotherapeutic patient/therapist relationship (Morehouse, Colvin, & Maykut, 2001).

Quality versus Quantity of Life

Early research on clinical outcomes associated with dialysis therapy focused on survival. Certainly, survival is important to people with CKD. However, it is not sufficient in and of itself. Mortality statistics associated with ESRD indicate that people treated with transplantation have better survival (and better QOL) than people treated with dialysis (United States Renal Data System [USRDS], 2003; Wolfe et al., 1999); in fact, on average, people with kidney transplants live twice as long as people on dialysis. Mortality risk factors for people with ESRD include age, number and type of co-morbid medical conditions, race, gender, nutritional status, and inflammation (USRDS, 2003). Approximately 50% of all deaths of persons on dialysis in all age groups are from cardiovascular complications (USRDS, 2003). Sepsis also is a frequent cause of death. However, despite these statistics, people with many risk factors have lived for many years with dialysis therapy, and indeed, seem to thrive.

Living Long and Living Well

What facilitates "living long and living well" on dialysis? While the average remaining life years of people on dialysis for a 50-year-old White male dialysis patient is 5.3 years (USRDS, 2003), many people live long and productive lives with renal replacement therapy. Variables such as co-morbidities, age, and complications are important factors from a statistical perspective. However, one cannot help but wonder whether social or personal characteristics are more amenable to change, and that such changes might make a difference in quality (and quantity) of life on dialysis. Curtin, Mapes, Petillo, and Oberley (2002) conducted a study of

people who survived on dialysis over 15 years and described an adaptation process that resulted in transformation. This transformation involved comprehensive active self-management on the part of the individual receiving therapy. According to all 18 long term survivors of dialysis that were interviewed, the process was arduous and involved a number of affirmations. The affirmations included acknowledging that "I want to live;" "I am still me;" "I am still valuable;" and "I am in control" (Curtin et al., 2002). It is important to note that effective self-management was a consistent manifestation of successful transformation in all of the participants. The researchers concluded by saying: "...comprehensive self-management included a positive and active endeavor to change what was changeable, control what was controllable, and to actively struggle to come to terms with the consequences of chronic illness" (p. 622). This is an area where nurses have a role. If we can assist those we care for to move along a path to the positive outcome of transformation and comprehensive active self-management, they will be well on the way to attaining an optimal QOL.

Measuring Quality of Life

It may be helpful for nurses to be familiar with some of the issues regarding measurement of QOL. One consideration in selecting an appropriate QOL measure is whether the measure is disease-specific or general (and appropriate for a general healthy population). Some researchers and clinicians prefer disease-specific measures of QOL because such measures include questions specific to the illness, and these items may be more sensitive in identifying changes in health status. However, disease-specific questionnaires also tap symptoms or aspects of the illness that are not necessarily reflective of the broad concept of QOL. In other words, the questions might measure something other than QOL. Some researchers suggest using both generic and disease-specific instruments, but that process may require more time and create greater burden for people completing the survey.

Another issue in choosing a QOL measure pertains to the subjective nature of QOL. Some researchers argue for an objective assessment. However, because QOL can only be rated by the individual, in light of his or her perceptions and experiences, objectivity is impossible.

There also are practical considerations in selecting a QOL measure, including length of the assessment, its reliability and validity, and its responsiveness to change. Whether QOL measures are used for research, quality improvement, or other purposes, it is important to examine the published literature pertaining to the questionnaire to ensure that it measures QOL (rather than some other concept such as depression, health status, functional status) and that it does so with accuracy (with reliability).

Popular Measures

Probably the best known measure of health-related QOL is the Medical Outcomes Survey Short Form (SF-36), which was developed for the Medical Outcomes Trust studies in the 1990s and has been extensively used and tested. Norms are available for various populations, and these provide useful comparative data. The SF-36 measures (a) physical function, (b) role limitation due to physical problems, (c) social func-

Table 15-1
Selected Quality of Life Measures

Measure	Domains	Access
Medical Outcomes Survey Short Form SF-36	• Physical function • Role Physical Social Function • Physical Pain • Mental Health • Role Emotional • Vitality • General Health	Documentation available at http://www.sf-36.org/tools/ Instruments available for use with a fee
KDQ	• Physical • Fatigue • Depression • Relationships with others • Frustration	Available free of charge from Dr. Laupacis at alaupacis@ices.on.ca
Kidney Disease Questionnaire KD-QOL	• SF-36 domains as above and • Symptoms/problems • Effects of kidney disease • Burden of kidney disease	Short form and scoring guide available at no charge with registration at http://gim.med.ucla.edu/kdqol
CHEQ (CHOICE Health Experiences Questionnaire)	• SF-36 • And 8 additional generic domains (cognitive functioning, sexual functioning, sleep, work, recreation, travel, finances, and general quality of life); and 6 ESRD-specific domains (diet, freedom, time, body image, dialysis access [catheters and/or vascular], and symptoms).	Available free of charge from Dr. Albert Wu at awu@jhsph.edu or Nancy Fink at nfink@jhsph.edu.
Flanagan's Quality of Life Scale QLS	• Physical and material well- being • Relationships with other people • Social, community, and civic activities • Personal development and fulfillment • Recreation • Independence.	Available free of charge from Dr. Carol Burkhardt at burckhac@ohsu.edu
Ferrans and Power's Quality of Life Index QLI	• Quality of life overall • Health and functioning • Psychological/spiritual • Social/economic • Family	Available free of charge from Dr. Ferrans at http://www.uic.edu/orgs/qli/
WHOQOL-100 WHOQOL-BREF (26 items)	• Physical • Psychological • Spiritual • Level of independence • Social • Environment	Available free of charge at http://www.who.int/evidence/assessment-instruments/qol/index.htm

tioning, (d) bodily pain, (e) general mental health, (f) role limitation due to emotional problems, (g) vitality, and (h) general health perceptions (Ware, Kosinski, & Keller, 1994). Used in a wide range of populations, it is applicable to physically healthy as well as to ill populations. However, it should be noted that although this measure is frequently referred to as a measure of health-related QOL, it is probably really a measure of health and functional status. Use of this measure requires a license and a fee in many cases.

Lapaucis, Muirhead, Keown, and Wong (1992) developed the Kidney Disease Questionnaire (KDQ), which consists of 26 questions in five dimensions: (a) physical symptoms, (b) fatigue, (c) depression, (d) relationships with others, and (e) frustration). A disease-specific measure, the KDQ was developed specifically for people receiving hemodialysis therapy. Hence, it would need revision before use with people on peritoneal dialysis or other therapies.

Another popular measure of QOL is the Kidney Disease Quality of Life Scale (KDQOL), which incorporates the SF-36 as well as a number of questions specific to symptoms of chronic renal disease (Hays, Kallich, Mapes, Coons, & Carter, 1994). A short form of this instrument and a scoring template are available free of charge online with registration (see http://www.gim.med.ucla.edu/kdqol/).

Similarly, the CHOICES Health Experiences Questionnaire (CHEQ) (Wu et al., 2001) is an instrument that augments the SF-36. The measure was designed to examine the differences between treatment modalities and dosages and can be used for people undergoing either hemodialysis or peritoneal dialysis. See Table 15-1 for a selection of additional QOL measures as well as additional details on the measures described above.

Resources for Selecting QOL Measures

A number of resources are available to nurses who participate in selecting an appropriate survey instrument to measure of QOL (e.g., Cagney et al., 2000; Edgell et al., 1996; Valderrabanno et al., 2001). It is important to remember that there is no perfect way to measure QOL, and that all measures have some limitations and margins of error. The purpose of measuring QOL should be considered, and it may be useful to critically reflect on whether the scores will provide the information or evidence that is being sought. In some cases, QOL measurement is used inappropriately or for the wrong reasons. For example, if the dosage of recombinant erythropoietin is increased, it is probably more appropriate to assess changes in hematocrit and functional status than to assess QOL. Similarly, if a corporation advertises high QOL of its patient population, it is worth considering that the case mix and selection of patients will have a significant impact on QOL scores. It is also worth remembering that any measurement has a margin of error, and that margin is still fairly large (50% or more with some instruments) for measurement of QOL. Hence, clinicians should not make life and death decisions on the basis of QOL scores alone.

Predictors of Quality of Life

Earlier in this chapter, there was discussion regarding what qualitative researchers have learned about QOL. Much other quantitative research addresses factors that contribute to QOL; some of the major factors found to be related to QOL include (a) transplantation, (b) erythropoietin therapy, (c) health and functional status, (d) ability to work, (e) social support, (f) co-morbidities, and (g) symptoms.

Transplantation

There is general agreement that transplantation offers a higher QOL than any of the available dialysis modalities (Molzahn et al., 1997; Terada & Hyde, 2002; USRDS, 2003; Waiser et al., 1998). This is the case, even when variables such as co-morbidities (e.g., diabetes, hypertension) and age are controlled.

However, transplantation is only a treatment modality. Although offering a better QOL than life on dialysis, transplantation has limitations when comparisons are made with the general population. Physical functioning after transplantation is not as good as in the general population, and long term kidney transplantation outcomes such as psychological status and general health perception are not as good as those of long term liver and heart transplant recipients (Karam et

al., 2003). Also, unfortunately, given the scarcity of organs at the present time, transplantation is not possible for many people with kidney failure.

Erythropoietin

The availability of recombinant erythropoietin was a major breakthrough for people with CKD. Clinical data show that after therapy with recombinant erythropoietin, peak oxygen consumption, an indicator of exercise ability, increases by about 50% as the hematocrit increases. Increases in exercise capacity, higher energy levels, and higher levels of activity are related to increased social and emotional well-being, improvements in sexual function, appetite, and sleep (Levin, 1992). Further, it has been found that QOL also increases with erythropoietin therapy (Evans, Rader, Manninen, & Cooperative Multicenter EPO Clinical Trial Group, 1990). Although some debate regarding the optimal hematocrit level may exist, there is little doubt that QOL increases as the hematocrit increases with this therapy (Mingardi, 1998).

Health and Functional Status

People who are healthier and who are able to function most effectively tend to have a higher QOL than those who are less healthy and have more difficulty managing activities of daily living. This is the case in people with renal disease as well as in individuals with other chronic illnesses (Molzahn et al., 1997; Painter, Carlson, Carey, Paul, & Myll, 2000). Although it may seem obvious, healthy and more independent people, on average, have a higher QOL.

Ability to Work

Of interest is the finding in some research that perceived *ability to work* was significant while actual employment status was not. People receiving dialysis therapy continue to have a low rate of employment, in the range of 20% to 40%, which has changed little from the rate reported in 1985 by Evans and colleagues. Molzahn, Northcott, and Hayduk (1996) observed that ability to work was an important predictor of QOL of people with end stage renal disease. Education and pre-dialysis employment are the best predictors of employment after start of dialysis (Curtin Oberley, Sacksteder, & Friedman, 1996). Better educated people who are working before they start dialysis are more likely to work after they have started with the therapy. Curtin et al. (1996) found that staff perceptions of patients' ability to work also was key. However, type of dialysis, length of time on dialysis, number of co-morbid conditions, and cause of renal failure were not found to be associated with employment status.

Despite a significantly better QOL after renal transplantation, the percentage of patients working remains unchanged (Waiser et al., 1998). The reasons for this finding have not been fully explored. However, possible explanations include patient concerns pertaining to health and disability insurance and fear of loss of benefits on return to work, even on a part-time basis. U.S. legislation, the Ticket to Work and Work Incentives Improvement Act of 1999 (Social Security Administration, 2004) has expanded work incentives and access to health insurance for people with disabilities who work in the United States (Center for Medicare and Medicaid Services, 2004), but this is not necessarily the case in other countries.

Co-morbidities

Diabetes mellitus and cardiovascular diseases are common co-morbid conditions associated with CKD. Because these diseases cause renal failure, separating the effects of these conditions on QOL from that of CKD is difficult. In a matched sample of people with co-morbid conditions, people with CKD reported a similar QOL to matched controls without CKD (Loos, Bincon, Frimat, Hanesse, & Kessler, 2003). These researchers found that the greatest deleterious effect on QOL is unplanned first dialysis. Nevertheless, patients with diabetes, regardless of reported QOL, have the lowest five year survival rates (USRDS, 2003), and hospital admission rates have increased for people with cardiovascular disease and end stage renal disease (ESRD).

Symptoms

People with ESRD experience a wide range of symptoms that cause them distress on a day-to-day basis (Thomas-Hawkins, 2000). In a study of symptom experiences relating to the general areas of fatigue/sleep, sexual concerns, and mobility, over 22 symptoms were identified as being of concern to the 307 people with kidney failure who agreed to participate. The most common symptoms reported included lack of energy, feeling tired, dry mouth/thirst, itchy skin, and difficulty falling asleep. The majority of these symptoms were found to be significantly related to either the mental or physical component scores of the SF-36 instrument (Curtin, Bultman, Thomas-Hawkins, & Schatell, 2002). In a recent study, Jablonski (2004) found that high levels of symptoms and low levels of symptom relief were linked to diminished QOL. Similarly, Killingworth and Van Den Akker (1996) found a relationship between symptom severity and QOL, and Merkus, Jager, Dekker, De Haan, and Boeschoten (1999) found that symptom burden predicted both physical and mental components of the SF-36.

From 50% to 80% of people on dialysis report sleep problems, such as delayed sleep onset, frequent awakening, restlessness, and daytime sleepiness (Parker, 1996). In a recent study (Iliescu et al., 2003), poor sleep was found to be directly related to lower QOL. Relatively little research has addressed interventions to improve the quality of sleep of those on dialysis. Daily nocturnal dialysis, nasal continuous positive airway pressure, or use of a nasal dilator have been suggested treatments for sleep snoring and obstructive sleep apnea, but these therapies are not easily accessible (Iliescu et al., 2003). Recently, Tsay, Rong, and Lin (2003) found that acupressure significantly decreased wake time, and participants (people with kidney failure) in their study experienced an improved quality of sleep at night and improved QOL over the control group. Further studies with larger sample sizes are warranted to explore whether other researchers make similar observations and to identify other strategies to improve sleep and affect QOL.

Fatigue also has been found to affect QOL. Srivastava (1986) found that higher levels of fatigue were linked to lower perceived QOL. The majority of patients in her study who reported a QOL of less than 90 (on a 100 point scale) indicated that their QOL would improve appreciably if their tiredness were relieved.

Restless leg symptoms among dialysis patients also have been found to be associated with lower QOL (Unruh et al., 2004). In a sample of 894 dialysis patients, 15% had severe symptoms of restless legs. This symptom was again associated with lower scores on the measure of QOL. As more research on symptoms and symptom management is conducted and published, we are likely to learn more about interventions that can minimize symptoms and enhance QOL.

Factors Thought to be Unrelated to Quality of Life

Research indicates that certain factors may be unrelated to QOL. These factors include age, gender, socioeconomic status, and race.

Age

A general but incorrect assumption persists that QOL decreases in older adults with kidney failure. This is not necessarily the case. There are conflicting findings pertaining to the relationship between age and QOL. A number of studies have shown that age is not a significant predictor of QOL scores in people with kidney failure when other important variables are controlled (Molzahn et al., 1997). Other researchers have found that age is positively related to satisfaction with life (Iacovides et al., 2002; Jablonski, 2004). That is, older adults on dialysis rated their QOL higher than did younger adults. Loos and colleagues (2003) noted, as might be expected, that older ESRD patients have lower QOL scores than do older controls without CKD. Thus, it is impossible to draw conclusions about the relationship between age and QOL of people with kidney failure at this time.

There has been considerable debate about how to study QOL of children. Many of the early studies of children with kidney failure report on such variables as school attendance, number of age-appropriate activities, and friendships. There has been concern about the QOL of children with kidney failure when they reach adulthood. In a recent Dutch study, adult dialysis patients whose kidney failure began in childhood (between 0 and 14 years of age) were found to have a normal QOL in the mental functioning domains as adults. However, in the physical domains of the SF-36, impairments were evident, as one might expect with the illness (Groothoff et al., 2003). It was speculated that a long period of renal replacement therapy facilitates adjustment but leaves patients with kidney failure at risk of impaired physical functioning. Again, further research pertaining to QOL of children on dialysis is warranted.

Gender

At this time, no evidence exists that QOL of women is significantly different than that of men with kidney failure. Neither Molzahn, Northcott, and Dossetor (1997) or Jablonski (2004) noted differences in QOL of men and women when other variables were controlled. Fewer women than men develop kidney failure. Approximately 47% of the ESRD population in the United States in 2001 was female (USRDS, 2003). Women on hemodialysis have better survival and QOL when compared with men when various demographic, medical, and treatment factors are controlled (Kimmel & Patel, 2003). However, there is some concern that women are less likely to be transplanted than men. Reasons for this are unknown but possible reasons may include the fact that men are less likely to be kidney donors and that there may be differences in antibodies between the genders (Wolfe et al., 2000). There also are differential living organ donation rates between men and women, with women being more likely to donate to a spouse or family member than men (Kayler et al., 2002). These barriers may have a negative overall impact on QOL of women with CKD because QOL is higher after transplantation than with dialysis therapy.

Socioeconomic Status

Although some people would assume that QOL is associated with socioeconomic status, there are no clear relationships between these two variables. For example, people in developing countries like India and China rate their QOL as high, or higher, than people in developed countries (WHOQOL Group, 1998). A Brazilian study reported that socioeconomic status was associated with QOL in people with kidney failure (Sesso, Rodrigues-Neto, & Ferraz, 2003). However, this finding is inconsistent and may reflect particular challenges associated with the economic disparities in Brazil. In the United States, socioeconomic status also may be related to race, and it is difficult to isolate the effects of either variable. Further research is warranted.

Race

In various cross-cultural studies of QOL in general populations, country of origin and race were not found to be important predictors of QOL. In one study from the UK (Bakewell, Higgins, & Edmunds, 2001), people of South Asian origin (from the Indian sub-continent) had a lower perceived QOL than White Europeans with kidney failure on peritoneal dialysis and after transplantation. No differences in QOL were found between Asian and White Europeans on hemodialysis (Bakewell et al., 2001). Although Jablonski (2004) found that non-Whites reported a higher QOL, reports of QOL in relation to race and ethnicity must be carefully examined, given potential differences in co-morbidities and socioeconomic status. At this time, it is impossible to draw conclusions.

Promoting Health and Quality of Life

Many nurses view their role as promoting health and QOL. Since QOL is subjective, and QOL is what the individual says it is, nurses must work collaboratively with the persons for whom they provide care to assess and optimize QOL. What we may perceive as improved QOL might not be what that individual would view as improved QOL. For instance, while nurses might emphasize the importance of fluid restriction to minimize weight gain, following this advice might not actually enhance that person's QOL (although it is likely to have other benefits). It is through listening to and understanding what is important to a person that we gain greater understanding about how to promote QOL and health for each individual.

No single strategy or plan will work for everyone. Nevertheless, some common interventions used to promote QOL and well-being are addressed in the following paragraphs. Support and encouragement, education, exercise, employment, and active self-management, other innovative

approaches to rehabilitation, and regular ongoing assessment of individuals and program evaluation are likely to be used at either the individual or facility level (Curtin, Klag, Bultman, & Schatell, 2002; Life Options Rehabilitation Program, 2003).

Support and Encouragement

People with kidney failure can and do benefit from social support. That support can come from many different people and places. Most often, family members and friends are identified as the sources of support, but nurses and other health care team members also provide support, as do members of church communities, community organizations, and peer support groups. Support has been linked to increased QOL and improved survival in a variety of chronic illnesses (Kimmel, Peterson, Wiebs, et al., 1998). Lack of social support has been found to be related to poorer QOL (Tell et al., 1995). The precise mechanisms of the effects of social support on health and QOL are the subject of active research for sociologists and many researchers have found that social support buffers or mediates the impact of negative life events. Nursing interventions or strategies that foster support of people with kidney disease and their families are likely to have a positive impact on QOL.

Education

Education is a commonly employed nursing strategy. Interventions to increase knowledge of people on dialysis have been found to be associated with positive outcomes, including better QOL, improved adherence to the treatment regime, increased sense of mastery, successful adaptation to stressors, and improved health and functional status (Devins & Binik, 1996; Korniewicz & O'Brien, 1994). However, increases in knowledge alone do not result in behavior changes. For example, we all know of people who continue to smoke despite knowledge of the deleterious effects of smoking on health status. Similarly, many people with kidney failure who know the need to follow specific dietary and fluid restrictions do not do so. They make choices of their own free will and nurses need to recognize their right to do so. An empowering relational approach to education may be more effective than the traditional behavioral approaches (Molzahn, 1996; Parse, 1998). Rather than reprimanding people who do not follow their diet, or developing contracts to facilitate adherence, approaches such as listening to the clients' perspectives about their unique struggles to manage and accommodate the limitations may result in a nurse-patient partnership to deal with the stressors clients face.

Exercise

In recent years, there has been increasing evidence of the benefits of exercise in maintaining the health and well being of people with CKD. Numerous studies have demonstrated that aerobic exercise training improves muscle strength, increases left ventricular systolic function, decreases depression, and reduces fatigue. With exercise, cardiovascular function, including resting heart rate, heart rate variability, and blood pressure (Deligiannis, Kouidi, & Tourkantonis, 1999) and improved lipid metabolism, glucose tolerance, and insulin sensitivity (Runyan & Atterbom, 1990)

Table 15-2
Sample Exercise Options

1. Some dialysis clinics have purchased stationary exercise bicycles that can be used during treatment.
2. A simple set of flexibility exercises (neck stretch, arm stretches, shoulder shrug and rotation, chest and upper back stretch, side stretch, and single knee pull, leg stretch, and calf stretch) are easy to complete and can be adapted for hemodialysis (see www.lifeoptions.org for useful diagrams and guidelines).
3. Other activities that maintain and improve flexibility include water exercises, T'ai chi, yoga, bowling, gardening and golf.
4. Strengthening exercises such as arm curls, arm extensions, lower leg extensions, straight leg extensions, seated marching, back leg swing, abdominal curl, chair push up, bench press, stair step, and chair squat can be conducted to increase strength, in sets of 10 repetitions. The number of repetitions can be increased for a total of three sets, and weights can be added to further increase strength.
5. Resistance machines can be used, for the same purpose as above.
6. Endurance can be developed with cardiovascular exercise. This can include walking, bicycling, stair stepping, swimming, aerobics, dancing, skating, basketball, or other sports. The three phases to a cardiovascular exercise session should consist of a warm up period, conditioning period and a cool down period.

are significantly improved. Improved QOL also has been observed with exercise in dialysis patients (Painter et al., 2000; Kouidi et al., 1997). Combined aerobic exercise and progressive strengthening exercises were found to improve physical functioning on a number of measures (DePaul, Moreland, Eager, & Clase, 2002). In general, higher levels of physical activity are associated with lower mortality rates of hemodialysis patients (Kutner, Brogan, & Fielding, 1997).

There are many options for exercise programs. These options range from educating patients about safe exercise, to referring patients to rehabilitation professionals, to establishing an on-site exercise program. Examples of exercise regimens are included in Table 15-2.

Goodman and Ballou (2004) studied perceived barriers and motivators to exercise in hemodialysis patients. They found that lack of motivation was the primary factor limiting dialysis patients' exercise. Other significant barriers to exercise level included lack of interest, fear of falling, and lack of access to exercise facilities. Motivators associated with exercise included belief in one's ability to be physically active, wanting to feel better, wanting to be less anxious, to have less pain, high expectations from family/friends, feeling healthy, knowing the value of increased exercise, and enjoying how exercise feels.

Often the most difficult aspect of exercise (for any of us) is maintaining the program or regimen. One strategy might be to encourage clients to put their goals and schedule in writing. Joining a class or exercising with someone else can facilitate regular participation. Exercise programs in health care facilities should start slowly and be fun. Variety in the program will keep people more motivated. At the facility level in Texas, one study showed that "exercise" is a rehabil-itation program and that there are fewer "exercise" programs than other kinds of rehabilitation programs in dialysis clinics (Curtin et al., 2002). This is an area where nurses can provide leadership.

The nurse's encouragement can help motivate the people to be physically active. In a study of 100 patient care staff, Painter et al. (2004) found that staff encouragement of physical activity was very important. The factors that predicted whether a staff member encouraged exercise activity were (a) professional training, (b) the perception that patients lacked motivation to exercise, (c) the perception that the staff member did not have the skills to motivate people to exercise, and (d) the perception that it was not a part of the job responsibility.

In other words, staff who believed in the benefits of exercise and were confident in their abilities and in the capability of the people that they cared for, were more likely to encourage exercise. There may be a need for more education of nephrology nursing staff about safe exercises, the benefits of exercise for their clients, and motivational techniques. Administrative support for exercise is key. Nurses are in an excellent position to encourage clients to think positively about the benefits of exercise, whether exercise is done in the clinic, in a rehabilitation program or fitness center, or at home.

Employment

Early in the history of maintenance hemodialysis therapy, employment and/or contribution to society was expected of all dialysis patients, and indeed, was one of the selection criteria for who was chosen to receive the new and scarce dialysis treatment. Although it is important for all of us to participate in meaningful activities, the goal of employment on dialysis may be unrealistic for everyone with kidney disease. For working age adults, meaningful activity can include paid employment. For others, attendance at an educational institution, work in the home (as a homemaker), or volunteer activity is personally important. Molzahn et al. (1996) found that the ability to work was more important than the actual employment status in predicting QOL. Similarly, Randolph (2001) noted that unemployment lowers QOL, and that there is a relationship in African American males between interpersonal trust, attachment style, religious conviction, and return to work.

In recent years in the United States, greater attempts have been made to support vocational rehabilitation of people with ESRD. The Life Options Rehabilitation Advisory Council offers an online booklet entitled *Employment: A Kidney Patients' Guide to Working and Paying for Treatment* (Life Options Rehabilitation Council, 2000) that advises people with CKD on employment and treatment matters. The issues pertaining to insurance, disability, and benefits are complex, and advice from a vocational rehabilitation counselor or nephrology social worker can be invaluable.

Active Self-Management

A number of studies have shown that people who engage in self-management of their disease and/or its treatment are more likely to enjoy a higher QOL (Horsburgh, 1999; Curtin & Mapes, 2001). People who live long and live well on dialysis are those that engage in comprehensive self-care management (Curtin et al., 2002).

Self-management is a process that people use to manage their conditions (e.g., take medications, follow diet); maintain, create, or change meaningful life roles; and deal with the emotional consequences of having a chronic illness (Lorig et al., 2000; Institute of Medicine [IOM], 2001). The term is used broadly, in many contexts, and sometimes to describe health education programs, health promotion programs, and patient behaviors. Lorig *et al.* (2000) identify the main skills associated with self-management as problem solving, decision-making, finding and using resources, forming partnerships with health care professionals, and taking action.

In a qualitative exploratory-descriptive study, Curtin and Mapes (2001) described six patient self-management strategies that people used who had lived for at least 15 years on dialysis. These strategies included (a) impression management, (b) selective symptom report and management, (c) vigilant oversight of care, (d) proposal of treatment by the individual, and (e) confrontation of the system (e.g., active self-advocacy and independent adoption of treatment use/use of alternative therapies). Each of these strategies is striking in that they are ways that patients have used to navigate the usual ways that care is delivered in dialysis facilities. For instance, impression management includes putting on a "happy face," not complaining unless it is really important, and trying to avoid having negative interactions with the staff. Curtin and Mapes (2001) quote one patient, "You know you have to be careful not to make them mad or get a reputation for being a troublemaker—then they might stick you or infiltrate your vessel on purpose. You know that's happened" (p. 389). In relation to selective symptom report or management, long term survivors commented, "I have to be really sick to say something" (p. 389). Although the participants in the study reported significant symptoms and major concerns, they prioritized their symptoms and kept many "minor" aches to themselves, sometimes to their detriment. With regard to vigilant oversight of care, all the respondents described considerable attentiveness to their care, and pointed out errors and poor technique to staff. They frequently found it necessary to suggest treatments, procedures, or interventions to their health care provider, but they did so "carefully." Respondents also reported active self-advocacy and confronting the system, pointing out errors and challenging professionals. Where possible, many of them independently changed medical treatment or adopted alternative therapies without seeking medical approval.

It is disturbing that people on dialysis feel that they need to go to these lengths to work around, rather than with health professionals. These reported self-management strategies suggest the need for change in nursing approaches. The character of the health care environment and the nature of the relationships among health care professionals and providers could be more honest and open, to promote and direct communication. The emphasis on compliance and adherence prevalent in dialysis centers today could be replaced with a caring philosophy or nursing theory that is more empowering and enables people receiving treatment to engage in active self-management. No simple recipe can be provided to change the prevailing culture in dialysis facilities. Health promotion approaches (Hartrick, Lindsey, & Hills, 1994), caring approaches (see Molzahn, 1996, for example), and theory-guided practice (see Parse, 1998, for example) all are approaches that could be used to facilitate self-management and promote collaborative partnerships with clients to achieve common goals and QOL, as defined by each individual.

Innovative Approaches to Rehabilitation

For a number of years, the Life Options Rehabilitation Program recognized dialysis facilities that offered innovative rehabilitation programs for people with kidney failure. Winning dialysis clinics reported a wide range of innovative programs and activities. Education and exercise programs were probably the most commonly reported. Curtin et al. (2002) conducted a survey of dialysis facilities in Texas to explore rehabilitation practices and their relationship to outcomes. They used the Life Options Unit Self-Assessment Tool (USAT) (Life Options Rehabilitation Council, 2000) to quantify facility rehabilitation efforts. The tool consists of a self-scored checklist of 100 possible rehabilitation activities organized around the '5 Es', namely encouragement, education, exercise, employment, and evaluation. Higher facility level scores on the USAT were associated with higher mean scores of dialysis patients in the facility on mental health functioning. No association was noted between rehabilitation interventions and physical functioning scores because too few Texas facilities offered exercise to show significance. Through creativity and new innovations, dialysis facilities can and should offer new programs, with the goal of increasing patient survival and improving QOL.

Evaluation

As new programs are started, evaluation of their effectiveness on outcomes is important. It is through ongoing research and evaluation that strategies to enhance the QOL can be carefully examined and programs modified to produce even better results. Rigorous study and evaluation builds nursing knowledge and contributes to evidence-based nursing practice.

QOL is a nursing-sensitive outcome, and while nurses do not and should not have control over many aspects of the lives of people with kidney failure, it is important to demonstrate whether the nursing and health promotion strategies that nurses use in provision of care are beneficial. QOL measurement can be a very useful strategy to examine the quality of care provided.

Program evaluation and quality improvement initiatives also are important. They will enhance the knowledge of nurses and other dialysis clinic personnel regarding the effectiveness of interventions. The extent to which the patients' QOL goals are being met can be monitored. By assessing which efforts are successful and which are not, techniques can be honed to further improve QOL, functioning, and well-being of those who entrust their lives to us.

Implications for Nursing

Promoting and maintaining health and QOL is an important nursing goal. People with kidney disease who have a higher QOL also will live longer and live better regardless of the treatment modality that they select. A number of strategies have been proposed to help promote QOL. These include offering support and encouragement, promoting self-management of the people we care for, working in partnership with them, promoting exercise programs, encouraging age-appropriate activities including work, offering educational programs, and evaluating care and programs. Because there is a high correlation between the QOL of a person with kidney disease and that of his or her spouse (Dunn et al., 1994), there will be benefits to the entire family unit if QOL is optimized for the person with kidney disease.

Education programs for nephrology nurses and other staff should emphasize the importance of QOL as the goal of care. They also should address the strategies that long term survivors of dialysis therapy use to manage their treatment (and manage their care providers!). An approach to QOL that acknowledges the individual's right to make choices would not only promote honesty, credibility, and integrity in the nurse-client relationship, but also would enable the health care professional to provide care without experiencing or communicating guilt and blame.

Although considerable research has been conducted on QOL of people with chronic kidney disease, there is still much to learn. Many possible future research questions have been identified in this chapter. In particular, we need more study on specific interventions and strategies that could enhance QOL.

In relation to implications for nursing administration, the role of leadership in promoting QOL is important. Many facilities and corporations are now monitoring QOL regularly. Some are advertising their clinics in terms of the QOL ratings. Although it may be difficult for any single clinic to make claims about QOL of their client population, recognizing that there are vast differences in case mix, sociodemographic characteristics, and other variables, it is in the best interest of facilities to promote the highest possible QOL of their clients. Supporting facility-wide programs to enhance QOL is a leadership responsibility that could have positive outcomes.

References

Bakewell, A.B., Higgins, R.M., & Edmunds, M.E. (2001). Does ethnicity influence perceived quality of life of patients on dialysis and following renal transplant? *Nephrology Dialysis Transplantation, 16,* 1395-1401.

Cagney, K.A., Wu, A.W., Fink, N.E., Jenckes, M.W., Meyer, K.B., Bass, E.B., et al. (2000). Formal literature review of quality-of-life instruments used in end-stage renal disease. *American Journal of Kidney Diseases, 36,* 327-336.

Center for Medicare and Medicaid Services. (2004). Ticket to work and work incentives improvement act. Retrieved November 8, 2004, from http://www.cms.hhs.gov/twwiia/

Cohen, J.D. (1995). *The experience of living on maintenance hemodialysis for 20 years and beyond: Impact on the patient and the family.* Unpublished doctoral dissertation. Union Graduate School, Health Psychology. UMI #pub9602208.

Curtin, R. B., & Mapes, D.L. (2001). Health care management strategies of long term dialysis survivors. *Nephrology Nursing Journal, 28,* 385-394.

Curtin, R.B., Bultman, D.V., Thomas-Hawkins, C., & Schatell, D. (2002). Hemodialysis patients' symptom experiences: Effects on physical and mental functioning. *Nephrology Nursing Journal, 29,* 562, 567-575, 598.

Curtin, R.B., Klag, M.J., Bultman, D.C., & Schatell, D. (2002). Renal rehabilitation and improved patients outcomes in Texas dialysis facilities. *American Journal of Kidney Diseases, 40,* 331-338.

Curtin, R.B., Mapes, D., Petillo, M., & Oberley, E. (2002). Long-term dialysis survivors: A transformational experience. *Qualitative Health Research, 12,* 609-624.

Curtin, R.B., Oberley, E.T., Sacksteder, P., & Friedman, A. (1996). Differences between employed and nonemployed dialysis patients. *American Journal of Kidney Diseases, 27,* 533-540.

Deligiannis, A., Kouidi, E., & Tourkantonis, A. (1999). Effects of physical training on heart rate variability in patients on hemodialysis. *American Journal of Cardiology, 84,* 197-202.

DePaul, V., Moreland, J., Eager, T., & Clase, C.M. (2002). The effectiveness of aerobic and muscle strength training in patients receiving hemodialysis and EPO: A randomized controlled trial. *American Journal of Kidney Diseases, 40,* 1219-1229.

Devins, G., & Binik, Y. (1996). Predialysis psychoeducational interventions: Establishing collaborative relationships between health services providers and recipients. *Seminars in Dialysis, 9,* 51-55.

Dunn, S.A., Lewis, S.L., Bonner, P.N., & Meize-Grochowski, R. (1994). Quality of life for spouses of CAPD patients. *ANNA Journal, 21,* 237-246, 257.

Edgell, E.T., Coons, S.J., Carter, W.B., Kallich, J.D., Mapes, D., Damush, T.M., et al. (1996). A review of health-related quality-of-life measures used in end-stage renal disease. *Clinical Therapeutics, 18,* 887-938.

Evans, R.W., Manninen, D.L., Garrison, L.P., Hart, L.G., Blagg, C.R., Gutman, R.A., et al. (1985). The quality of life of patients with end-stage renal disease. *New England Journal of Medicine, 312,* 553-559.

Evans, R.W., Rader, B., Manninen, D.L., & Cooperative Multicenter EPO Clinical Trial Group. (1990) The quality of life of hemodialysis recipients treated with recombinant human erythropoietin. *Journal of American Medical Association, 263,* 825-830.

Franke, G. H., Reimer, J., Philipp, T., & Heemann, U. (2003). Aspects of quality of life through end-stage renal disease. *Quality of Life Research, 12,* 103-115.

Goodman, E.D., & Ballou, MB (2004). Perceived barriers and motivators to exercise in hemodialysis patients. *Nephrology Nursing Journal, 31,* 23 - 29.

Gregory, D.M., Way, C.Y., Hutchinson, T.A., Barrett, B.J., & Parfrey, P.S. (1998). Patients' perceptions of their experiences with ESRD and hemodialysis treatment. *Qualitative Health Research, 8,* 764-783.

Groothoff, J.W., Grootenhuis, M.A., Offringa, M., Gruppen, M. P., Korevaar, J.C., & Heymans, H.S. (2003). Quality of life in adults with end-stage renal disease since childhood is only partially impaired. *Nephrology Dialysis Transplantation, 18,* 310-317.

Hartrick, G., Lindsey, E., & Hills, M. (1994). Family nursing assessment: Meeting the challenge of health promotion. *Journal of Advanced Nursing, 20,* 85-91

Hays, R.D., Kallich, J.D., Mapes, D.L., Coons, S.J., & Carter, W.B. (1994). Development of the Kidney Disease Quality of Life (KDQOL) instrument. *Quality of Life Research, 3,* 329-338.

Horsburgh, ME. (1999). Self-care of well adult Canadians and adult Canadians with end stage renal disease. *International Journal of Nursing Studies, 36,* 443-453.

Iacovides, A., Fountoulakis, K.N., Blaskas, E., Manika, A., Markopoulou, M., Kaprinis, G., et al. (2002). Relationship of age and psychosocial factors with biological rating in patients with end-stage renal disease undergoing dialysis. *Aging Clinical and Experimental Research, 14,* 354-360.

Iliescu, E.A., Coo, H., McMurray, M.H., Meers, C. L., Quinn, M.M., Singer, M.A., et al. (2003). Quality of sleep and health-related quality of life in haemodialysis patients. *Nephrology Dialysis Transplantation, 18,* 126-132.

Institute of Medicine (2001). Crossing the quality chasm: A new health system for the 21st century. Washington, DC: National Academies Press.

Jablonski, A.M. (2004). *The symptom experience of patients with end stage renal disease on hemodialysis.* Unpublished doctoral dissertation, Michigan State University.

Karam, V.H., Gasquet, I., Delvart, V., Hiesse, C., Dorent, R., Danet, C., et al. (2003). Quality of life in adult survivors beyond 10 years after liver, kidney, and heart transplantation. *Transplantation, 76,* 1699-1704.

Karnofsky, D.A., & Burchenal, J.H. (1949). The clinical evaluation of chemotherapeutic agents in cancer. In C.M. MacLeod (Ed.), *Evaluation of Chemotherapeutic Agents* (p. 196). Columbia: Columbia Univ. Press.

Kayler, L.K. Meier-Kriesche, H.U., Punch, J.D., Campbell, D.A., Leichtman, A.B., Magee, J.C., et al. (2002). Gender imbalance in living donor renal transplantation. *Transplantation, 73,* 248-252.

Killingworth, A., & Van Den Akker, O. (1996). The quality of life of renal dialysis patients. Trying to find the missing measurement. *International Journal of Nursing Studies, 33,* 107-120.

Kimmel, P.L., & Patel, S.S. (2003). Psychosocial issues in women with renal disease. *Advances in Renal Replacement Therapy, 10,* 61-70.

Kimmel, P.L., Peterson, R.A. Wiehs, K.L., Simmens, S.J., Alleyne, S., Cruz, I., & Veis, J.H. (1998). Psychosocial factors, behavioral compliance and survival in urban hemodialysis patients. *Kidney International, 54,* 245-254.

Korniewicz, D.M., & O'Brien, M.E. (1994). Evaluation of a patient hemodialysis education and support program. *American Nephrology Nurses Association Journal, 21,* 33-38.

Kouidi, E. Albani, M., Natsis, K., et al. (1998). The effects of exercise training on muscle atrophy in hemodialysis patients. *Nephrology Dialysis and Transplantation, 13,* 685-699.

Kouidi, E., Iacovides, A., Iordianidis, P. E., Vassiliou, S., Deligiannis, A., Lerodiakonou, C., et al. (1997). Exercise renal rehabilitation program: Psychosocial effects. *Nephron, 77,* 152-158.

Kutner, N.G., Brogan, D., & Fielding, B. (1997). Physical and psychosocial resource variables related to long term survival in older dialysis patients. *Geriatric Nephrology and Urology, 7,* 23-28.

Laupacis, A., Muirhead, N., Keown, P., & Wong, C. (1992), A disease specific questionnaire for assessing quality of life in patients on hemodialysis. *Nephron, 60,* 302-306

Levin, N.W. (1992). Quality of life and hematocrit level. *American Journal of Kidney Diseases, 20*(Suppl 1), 16-20.

Life Options Rehabilitation Program (1998). *Evaluation: Unit Self Assessment Manual for Renal Rehabilitation: A guide to the use and interpretation of the Life Options Unit Self Assessment Tool for renal rehabilitation.* Retrieved at http://www.lifeoptions.org/pdfs/usam.pdf on November 8, 2004.

Life Options Rehabilitation Program. (2003). Showcase of ideas. Retrieved November 8, 2004, at http://www.lifeoptions.org/profess/showcase/index.shtml

The Life Options Rehabilitation Advisory Council (2003). *Employment: A Kidney Patients' Guide to Working and Paying for Treatment.* Retrieved November 8, 2004, from http://www.lifeoptions.org/pdfs/empbk03.pdf

Loos, C., Briancon, S., Frimat, L., Hanesse, B., & Kessler, M. (2003). Effect of end-stage renal disease on the quality of life of older patients. *Journal of the American Geriatrics Society, 51,* 229-233.

Lorig, K., Holman, H., Sobel, D., Laurent, D., González, V., & Minor, M. (2000). *Living a healthy life with chronic conditions: Self-management of heart disease, arthritis, stroke, diabetes, asthma, bronchitis, emphysema and others* (2nd ed.). Boulder CO: Bull Publishing.

Lowrie, E.G., Curtin, R.B., LePain, N., & Schatell, D. (2003). Medical Outcomes Study Short Form 36: A consistent and powerful predictor of morbidity and mortality in dialysis patients. *American Journal of Kidney Diseases, 41,* 1286-1292.

Mapes. D.L. Bragg-Gresham, J.L., Bommer, J., Fukuhara, S., McKevitt, P., Wilkstrom, B., & Lopes, A.A. (2004) Health related quality of life in the Dialysis Outcomes and Practice Patterns Study (DOPPS). *American Journal of Kidney Disease, 44* (5 Suppl. 3), 54-60.

McPherson, C. J. & Addington-Hall, J. M. (2003). Judging the quality of care at the end of life: can proxies provide reliable information? *Social Science & Medicine, 56,* 95-109.

Meers, C., Singer, M.A., Toffelmire, E.B., et al. (1996). Self-delivery of hemodialysis care: A therapy in itself. *American Journal of Kidney Diseases, 27,* 844-847.

Merkus, M., Jager, K., Dekker, F., De Haan, R., & Boeschoten, E. (1999). Physical symptoms and quality of life of patients on chronic dialysis: Results of Netherlands Cooperative study on adequacy of dialysis (NECOSAD). *Nephrology Dialysis Transplantation, 14,* 1163-1170.

Mingardi, G. for the DIA-QOL Group. (1998). Quality of life and end stage renal disease therapeutic programs. *International Journal of Artificial Organs, 21,* 741-747.

Molzahn, A. E. (1996). Changing to a caring paradigm for teaching and learning. *American Nephrology Nurses Association Journal, 23,* 13-18.

Molzahn, A. E., Northcott, H. C., & Hayduk, L. (1996). Quality of life of patients with ESRD: A structural equation model. *Quality of Life Research, 5,* 426-432.

Molzahn, A.E., Northcott, H.C., & Dossetor, J.B. (1997). Quality of life of individuals with end stage renal disease: Perceptions of patients, nurses and physicians. *Nephrology Nursing Journal, 24*(3), 325-333.

Morehouse, R.E., Colvin, E., & Maykut, P. (2001). Nephrology nurse-patient relationships in the outpatient dialysis setting. *Nephrology Nursing Journal, 28,* 295-300.

Nagle, L. (1998). The meaning of technology for people with chronic renal failure. *Holistic Nursing Practice, 12* (4), 78-92.

National Kidney Foundation. (2002). KDOQI Clinical Practice Guidelines for chronic kidney disease: Evaluations, classifications and stratifications. *American Journal of Kidney Diseases, 39*(Suppl.1), S161-169.

O'Brien, M.E. (1983). *The courage to survive: The life career of the chronic dialysis patient.* New York: Grune & Stratton.

Painter, P., Carlson, L., Carey, S., Paul, S.M., & Myll, J. (2000). Physical functioning and health-related quality of life changes with exercise training in hemodialysis patients. *American Journal of Kidney Diseases, 35,* 482-492.

Parker, K. (1996). Dream content and subjective sleep quality in stable patients on chronic dialysis. *ANNA Journal, 23,* 201-213.

Parse, R.R. (1998). *The human becoming school of thought: A perspective for nurses and other health professionals.* Thousand Oaks, CA: Sage.

Perry, L. D., Nicholas, D., Molzahn, A.E., & Dossetor, J. B. (1995). Attitudes of dialysis patients and caregivers regarding advance directives. *American Nephrology Nurses' Association Journal, 22,* 457-463, 481.

Polaschek, N. (2003). The experience of living on dialysis: A literature review. *Nephrology Nursing Journal, 30,* 303-309, 313.

Randolph, C.Y. (2001). Correlates of psychological well-being and return to work decisions after the onset of end-stage renal disease. Unpublished Doctoral Dissertation, Catholic University of America.

Rittman, M., Northsea, C., Hausauer, N., Green, C., & Swanson, L. (1993). Living with renal failure. *ANNA Journal, 20,* 327-331.

Runyan, J.D., & Atterbom, H.A. (1990). Exercise and the hemodialysis patient. *Physician Assistant, 14*(4), 91-98.

Sesso, R., Rodrigues-Neto, J.F., & Ferraz, M.B. (2003). Impact of socioeconomic status on the quality of life of ESRD patients. *American Journal of Kidney Diseases, 11,* 186-195.

Social Security Administration (2004). The work site. Retrieved November 8, 2004, from http://www.socialsecurity.gov/work/Ticket/ticket_info.html

Srivastava, R.H. (1986). Fatigue in the renal patient. *American Nephrology Nurses Association Journal, 13,* 246-249.

Tell, G.S., Mittelmark, M.B., Hylander, B., Shumaker, S.A., Russell, G., & Burkart, J.M. (1995). Social support and health-related quality of life in black and white dialysis patients. *ANNA Journal, 22,* 301-308.

Terada, I., & Hyde, C. (2002). The SF-36: An instrument for measuring quality of life in ESRD patients. *EDTNA/ERCA Journal, 28*(2), 73-76, 83.

Thomas-Hawkins, C. (2000). Symptom distress and day-to-day changes in functional status in chronic hemodialysis patients. *Nephrology Nursing Journal, 27,* 369-379.

Tsay, S.L., Rong, J.R., & Lin, P.F. (2003). Acupoints massage in improving the quality of sleep and quality of life in patients with end-stage renal disease. *Journal of Advanced Nursing, 42,* 134-142.

United States Renal Data System (USRDS). (2003). USRDS 2003 Annual Data Report. Retrieved March 30, 2004, from http://www.usrds.org/2003/pdf/h_03.pdf. Bethesda MD: National Institute of Diabetes and Digestive and Kidney Diseases.

Unruh, M.L., Levey, A.S., D'Ambrosio, C., Fink, N.E., Powe, N.R., Meyer, K.B. (2004). Choices for health outcomes in caring for end-stage renal disease (CHOICE) study: Restless legs symptoms among incident dialysis patients: Association with lower quality of life and shorter survival. *American Journal of Kidney Diseases, 43,* 9000-9009.

Valderrabano, F., Jofre, R., & Lopez-Gomez, J.M. (2001). Quality of life in end-stage renal disease patients. *American Journal of Kidney Diseases, 38,* 443-464.

Waiser, J., Budde, K., Schreiber, M., Peibst, O., Koch, U., Bohler, T., et al. (1998). The quality of life in end stage renal disease care. *Transplant International, 11,* S42-S45.

Ware, J.E., Kosinski, M. & Keller, S.D. (1994). *Physical and mental health summary scales: A user's manual.* Boston: New England Medical Center.

White, Y., & Grenyer, B.F.S. (1999). The biopsychosocial impact of end-stage renal disease: The experience of dialysis patients and their partners. *Journal of Advanced Nursing, 30,* 1312-1320.

WHOQOL Group. (1998). The development of the World Health Organization WHQOOL-BREF Quality of Life Assessment. *Psychological Medicine, 28,* 551-558.

Wolfe, R.A., Ashby, V.B., Milford, E.L., Bloembergen, W.E., Agodoa, L.Y., Held, P.J., et al. (2000). Differences in access to cadaveric renal transplantation in the United States. *American Journal of Kidney Diseases, 36,* 1025-1033.

Wolfe, R.A., Ashby, V.B., Milford, E.L., Ojo, A.D., Ettenger, R.E., Agodoa, L.Y., et al. (1999). Comparison of mortality in all patients on dialysis, patients on dialysis awaiting transplantation, and recipients of a first cadaveric transplant. *New England Journal of Medicine, 341,* 1725-1730.

Wu, A. W., Fink, N.E., Cagney, K.A., Bass, E.B., Rubin, H.R., Meyer, K.B., et al. (2001). Developing a health-related quality-of-life measure for end-stage renal disease: The CHOICE Health Experience Questionnaire. *American Journal of Kidney Diseases, 37,* 11-21.

Quality of Life and Chronic Kidney Disease: Living Long and Living Well

Name of Resource	Brief Description	Where to Obtain Resource
American Association of Kidney Patients	The American Association of Kidney Patients has a number of educational materials for people on dialysis and their families.	http://www.aakp.org
Kidney School	Kidney School is an interactive web-based learning program in modules designed to help people learn more about living with kidney disease.	http://www.kidneyschool.org
Life Options Rehabilitation Program	This Web-site has information regarding rehabilitation for professionals and people with kidney disease and those receiving dialysis therapy. It includes valuable resource booklets for patients and professionals and a bibliography for professionals.	http://www.lifeoptions.org
MAPI Research Institute	The MAPI Research Institute in France is devoted to the study of health-related QOL. The Institute offers free newsletters on QOL and supports the QOLID database of instruments.	http://www.mapi-research-inst.com/
National Kidney Foundation	The National Kidney Foundation offers a number of publications for people on dialysis and transplant. There are publications such as *Fitness after Kidney Failure, Building Strength Through Exercise, Sexuality and Chronic Kidney Failure, Transplant Chronicle, Coping Effectively: A Guide for Patients and their Families*	http://www.kidney.org
QOLID Database	The QOLID database is a collaborative effort of several international organizations interested in patient reported outcomes. Over 400 QOL measures are described and sample instruments are available.	http://www.proqolid.org

- The World Health Organization (WHO) defined QOL as "individuals' perceptions of their position in life in the context of the culture and value systems in which they live and in relation to their goals, expectations, standards and concerns" (WHOQOL Group, 1998, p. 551).

- QOL is a broader concept than health status because it incorporates individuals' assessments of aspects of their lives that go beyond their well-being, such as a person's work, personal relationships, and friendships among other aspects. Only the individual person can assess his or her own QOL.

- Qualitative research typically is used when little is known about a topic. However, as related to QOL, qualitative research provides a much richer description of life for people living with kidney disease.

- Families also experience challenges in coming to terms with the illness. However, health care professionals do not always consider the impact of the treatment on the family.

- Mortality statistics associated with ESRD indicate that people treated with transplantation have better survival (and better QOL) than people treated with dialysis (United States Renal Data System [USRDS], 2003; Wolfe et al., 1999); in fact, on average, people with kidney transplants live twice as long as people on dialysis.

- What facilitates "living long and living well" on dialysis? Variables such as co-morbidities, age, and complications are important factors... however, are social or personal characteristics more amenable to change, and will such changes make a difference in quality (and quantity) of life on dialysis?

- It may be helpful for nurses to be familiar with some of the issues regarding measurement of QOL. One consideration in selecting an appropriate QOL measure is whether the measure is disease-specific or general (and appropriate for a general healthy population).

- Probably the best known measure of health-related QOL is the Medical Outcomes Survey Short Form (SF-36), which was developed for the Medical Outcomes Trust studies in the 1990s and has been extensively used and tested.

- Some of the major factors found to be related to QOL include (a) transplantation, (b) erythropoietin therapy, (c) health and functional status, (d) ability to work, (e) social support, (f) co-morbidities, and (g) symptoms.

- Research indicates that certain factors may be unrelated to QOL. These factors include age, gender, socioeconomic status, and race.

- Many nurses view their role as promoting health and QOL. Since QOL is subjective, and QOL is what the individual says it is, nurses must work collaboratively with the persons for whom they provide care to assess and optimize QOL.

- Promoting and maintaining health and QOL is an important nursing goal. People with kidney disease who have a higher QOL also will live longer and live better regardless of the treatment modality that they select.

ANNP615

Quality of Life and Chronic Kidney Disease: Living Long and Living Well

Anita E. Molzahn, PhD, RN

Contemporary Nephrology Nursing: Principles and Practice contains 39 chapters of educational content. Individual learners may apply for continuing nursing education credit by reading a chapter and completing the Continuing Education Evaluation Form for that chapter. Learners may apply for continuing education credit for any or all chapters.

Please photocopy this page and return to ANNA.
COMPLETE THE FOLLOWING:

Name: _____

Address:_____

City:_____ State: _____ Zip: _____

E-mail: _____

Preferred telephone: ☐ Home   ☐ Work: _____

State where licensed and license number (optional): _____

CE application fees are based upon the number of contact hours provided by the individual chapter. CE fees per contact hour for ANNA members are as follows: 1.0-1.9 - $15; 2.0-2.9 - $20; 3.0-3.9 - $25; 4.0 and higher - $30. Fees for nonmembers are $10 higher.

ANNA Member: ☐ Yes   ☐ No   Member # (if available) _____

☐ Checked Enclosed   ☐ American Express   ☐ Visa   ☐ MasterCard

Total Amount Submitted: _____

Credit Card Number: _____ Exp. Date: _____

Name as it appears on the card: _____

CE Evaluation Form
To receive continuing education credit for individual study after reading the chapter
1. Photocopy this form. (You may also download this form from ANNA's Web site, **www.annanurse.org.**)

2. Mail the completed form with payment (check) or credit card information to American Nephrology Nurses' Association, East Holly Avenue, Box 56, Pitman, NJ 08071-0056.

3. You will receive your CE certificate from ANNA in 4 to 6 weeks.

Test returns must be postmarked by **December 31, 2010.**

CE Application Fee
ANNA Member $15.00
Nonmember $25.00

EVALUATION FORM

1. I verify that I have read this chapter and completed this education activity. Date: _____

_____
Signature

2. What would be different in your practice if you applied what you learned from this activity? *(Please use additional sheet of paper if necessary.)*

_____

_____

_____

_____

_____

_____

_____

_____

_____

_____

_____

Evaluation	Strongly disagree				Strongly agree
3. The activity met the stated objectives.					
a. Discuss the quality of life issues that are concerns to people with renal disease.	1	2	3	4	5
b. Describe the predictors of quality of life that are pertinent to people with renal disease.	1	2	3	4	5
c. Relate those activities that promote health and quality of life that should be incorporated into a nursing plan of care.	1	2	3	4	5
4. The content was current and relevant.	1	2	3	4	5
5. The content was presented clearly.	1	2	3	4	5
6. The content was covered adequately.	1	2	3	4	5
7. Rate your ability to apply the learning obtained from this activity to practice.	1	2	3	4	5

Comments _____

_____

8. Time required to read the chapter and complete this form: _____ minutes.

This educational activity has been provided by the American Nephrology Nurses' Association (ANNA) for 1.8 contact hours. ANNA is accredited as a provider of continuing nursing education (CNE) by the American Nurses Credentialing Center's Commission on Accreditation (ANCC-COA). ANNA is an approved provider of continuing education by the California Board of Registered Nursing, CEP 0910.

End-of-Life Care in the Chronic Kidney Disease Population

Lesley C. Dinwiddie, MSN, RN, FNP, CNN
Elaine R. Colvin, BSN, RN, MEPD

Chapter Contents

End-of-Life Care in the Chronic Kidney Disease Population

Chapter 16

Lesley C. Dinwiddie, MSN, RN, FNP, CNN
Elaine R. Colvin, BSN, RN, MEPD

Controversies concerning exactly when human life begins and ends remain unresolved, but there is one irrefutable fact about human life – it will end. Paradoxically, dying is the one area of health care that receives comparatively little attention or preparatory planning. Perhaps this is because death is the one outcome that is ultimately not preventable.

Dying is a very important stage of life and usually is accompanied by alterations in physiological, psychological, and emotional health. Usually there are family dynamics compounding the complexity of care to be delivered in this stage. Even when death is anticipated, few patients and their families have participated in, or completed, advance care planning that could prevent or minimize much of the pain, distress, anxiety, and expense incurred by reactive medical interventions triggered by the dying process.

Certainly this phenomenon has not gone unrecognized or been bypassed by the health care professions or the nephrology community. (An expanded description of resources available on EOL and palliative care can be found in Price's 2003 article, Resources for Planning Palliative and End-of-Life Care For Patients with Kidney Disease, *Nephrology Nursing Journal*, 30[6], 649-56, 664).

Nephrology nursing, through the American Nephrology Nurses' Association (ANNA), has endorsed the American Nurses Association Code of Ethics, which includes interpretive statements related to nursing care at the end of life. ANNA participated in the formulation of the Guidelines for Shared Decision-Making in the Appropriate Initiation of and Withdrawal from Dialysis published by the Renal Physicians Association and the American Society of Nephrology (2002). In recognition of the decreased survival for end stage renal disease (ESRD) patients, further work was done by a multidisciplinary ESRD End of Life Task Force, under the sponsorship of the Robert Wood Johnson Foundation, to focus on how best to promote palliative care for ESRD patients as well as remove barriers to that care. After all, the purpose of renal replacement therapy is to allow patients to do what they want to do with the rest of their lives. This should include their deaths. *Author's Note: "Last Acts" is a movement begun in 1995 and sponsored by the Robert Wood Johnson Foundation to build a coalition between medical organizations, academic centers, the media, and the public. Last Acts functions primarily as an information resource on end-of-life issues, events, legislation and products; a connector with peer and complementary organizations; a community of people addressing the same issues; a catalyst to initiate or maintain end-of-life efforts; and a coalition that gets the word out to improve end-of-life care (www.lastacts.com).*

Overview of Nursing's Role

The purpose of this chapter then is to discuss the nephrology nurse's role in advance care planning, palliative care, and bereavement for the patient with chronic kidney disease (CKD). This will be accomplished by addressing the:

- *ethical basis* for end-of-life nursing care;
- *practice considerations,* which include a philosophical discussion of the need for all practicing nephrology nurses to be comfortable with their own mortality as well as that of their patients' and respect for decision-making that is contrary to their personal philosophy;
- *advance care planning;*
- *legal issues,* including advance directives, living wills, health care power of attorney, and do not resuscitate (DNR) orders;
- *administrative issues,* which include incorporation of advance care planning in the admission orders and long-term care plan plus policies and procedures for management of life-threatening events, DNR orders, and sudden death in the dialysis unit;
- *palliative care* for those patients who chose not to initiate dialysis, for those on dialysis who are failing to thrive, and for those who withdraw from dialysis;
- grief counseling for the bereaved family and staff.

Selected readings from the *Palliative Care Core Curriculum for Nephrology Fellowship Training Programs* (2003) have been suggested to supplement the text.

Ethical Basis for End-of-Life Care

The Ethical basis for end-of-life nursing care in nephrology is based on the American Nurses Association (ANA) *Code of Ethics for Nurses with Interpretive Statements* (2001), which asserts:

"Nursing care is directed toward meeting the comprehensive needs of patients and their families across the continuum of care. This is particularly vital in the care of the patients and their families at the end of life to prevent and relieve the cascade of symptoms and suffering that are commonly associated with dying.

Nurses are leaders and vigilant advocates for the delivery of dignified and humane care. Nurses actively participate in assessing and assuring the responsible and appropriate use of interventions in order to minimize unwarranted or unwanted treatment and patient suffering. The acceptability and importance of carefully considered decisions regarding resuscitation status, withholding and withdrawing life-sustaining therapies, forgoing medically provided nutrition and hydration, aggressive pain and symptom management and advance directives are increasingly evident. The nurse should provide interventions to relieve pain and other symptoms in the dying patient even when those interventions entail risks of hastening death. However, nurses may not act with the sole intent of ending a patient's life even though such action may be motivated by compassion, respect for patient autonomy, and quality of life considerations. Nurses have invaluable experience, knowledge, and

Table 16-1
Competencies Necessary for Nurses to Provide High-Quality Care to Patients and Families during the Transition at the End of Life

Recognize dynamic changes in population demographics, health care economics and service delivery that necessitate improved professional preparation for end-of-life care.

Promote the provision of comfort care to the dying as an active, desirable, and important skill, and an integral component of nursing care.

Communicate effectively and compassionately with the patient, family, and health care team members about end-of-life issues.

Recognize one's own attitudes, feelings, values, and expectations about death and the individual, cultural, and spiritual diversity existing in these beliefs and customs.

Demonstrate respect for the patient's views and wishes during end-of-life care.

Collaborate with interdisciplinary team members while implementing the nursing role in end-of-life care.

Use scientifically based standardized tools to assess symptoms — e.g., pain, dyspnea, constipation, anxiety, fatigue, nausea/vomiting and altered cognition. Not needed unless in a formerly published work experienced by patients at the end of life.

Use data from symptom assessment to plan and intervene in symptom management using state-of-the-art traditional and complementary approaches.

Evaluate the impact of traditional, complementary, and technological therapies on patient-centered outcomes.

Assess and treat multiple dimensions, including physical, psychological, social and spiritual needs, to improve quality at the end of life.

Assist the patient, family, colleagues, and one's self to cope with the suffering, grief, loss, and bereavement in end-of-life care.

Apply legal and ethical principles in the analysis of complex issues in end-of-life care, recognizing the influence of personal values, professional codes, and patient preferences.
Identify barriers and facilitators to patients' and caregivers' effective use of resources.

Demonstrate skill at implementing a plan for improved end-of-life care within a dynamic and complex health care delivery system.

Apply knowledge gained from palliative care research to end-of-life education and care.

Note: From American Association of Colleges of Nursing. (1999). *Reflections*, Fourth Quarter edition, p. 36.

insight into care at the end of life and should be actively involved in related research, education, practice, and policy development" (American Nurses Association, 2001).

No discussion of ethics related to nursing care at the end of life would be complete without a reiteration of the principles of beneficence, nonmalificence, and autonomy. Beneficence is literally interpreted from its Latin roots and means "do good," nonmalificence means "do no harm," and autonomy means self-governance. The interpretive statement cited above does give clear direction on legal and ethical issues, but nurses frequently must examine their practice and the collaborative practice of their team to assure that they are indeed doing "what is best for the patient" and not just following orders or policies. On the other hand, questioning a patient's decision to request a DNR order or withdraw from dialysis also may constitute "doing harm" if the nurse puts his/her own beliefs ahead of the patient's. The principle of autonomy to make such decisions is clearly protected in law

by the Patient Self-Determination Act (PSDA) of 1991, but such an emotionally charged issue can be undermined in practice when the nurse cannot sublimate his/her own beliefs when caring for the patient.

Practice Considerations

Practice considerations therefore must address the need for all practicing nephrology nurses to be comfortable with their own mortality as well as that of their patients. It has been said that one cannot truly live until one has confronted one's own mortality (anon). Avoiding the appropriate discussion of end-of-life care with patients is negligence. The other side of this problem becomes apparent when nurses feel that the dialysis they are performing is futile. Indeed, the frustration generated by this apparent futility has even been named "dialyzing the dead." A practice born of this sentiment is known as a "slow code," where a patient, deemed "as good as dead" who suffers cardiac arrest, is not given appropriate resuscitation. This is illegal and constitutes malpractice.

While nurses may feel that dialytic (Badzek, Cline, Moss, & Hines, 2000) or resuscitative therapy is inappropriate or futile, and that this is not the decision they would make for themselves or their loved ones, they cannot impose their beliefs on their patients and/or their patients' families.

Understanding patients' cultural norms and acknowledging their spiritual beliefs will help nurses fulfill their duty to respect any patient or family decision that is contrary to their personal philosophy. Of course this does not preclude the nurse's responsibility to provide all patients and their families with all the information about advance care planning. Unfortunately, many nurses avoid this responsibility in the dialysis unit (Perry, Swartz, Smith-Wheelock, Westbrook, & Buck, 1996). Perhaps this is because nursing education has not given sufficient weight to end-of-life care, neglecting to instill not only the knowledge but also the necessary competencies to assure high quality care for the dying patient (see Table 16-1 for a sample list of competencies by the American Association of Colleges of Nursing). Alternatively, appropriate education may have been received, but in this era of nursing shortage with high turnover and tight staffing, many aspects of quality care receive less than optimal attention due to time constraints.

Advance Care Planning

Advance care planning is that part of the long-term care plan in which we begin a process of understanding, reflecting, and developing a plan based on the patients' wishes for medical care in the future when they might not be able to make those decisions themselves. Not having an advance care plan is analogous to going into childbirth having made no arrangements or even discussing the process and then letting others decide the where, when, and how of the birth.

Through the advance care planning process of understanding, reflecting, and identifying the patients' values and beliefs, we can also help them choose the best person who would make health care decisions for them in the event they could not. These surrogates would also need to be taught how best to advocate for this patient (Pendergast, 2001). Discussing the potential scenarios while the patient is in reasonably good health and mentally competent assures the staff and family that the patient can make reliable decisions. Patients should also know that these wishes are not irrevocable and can be changed by them at any time.

These wishes may include:
- A preference of place such as home, hospital, or hospice.
- The extraordinary measures to prolong life such as cardiopulmonary resuscitation, an artificial airway, feeding tube, intravenous therapy, and continuation of dialysis though they are dying.
- The circumstances under which they would want all treatment abandoned such as a persistent vegetative state.

Legal Issues

To assure patients that their wishes will be known when they are dying, it is important to make an advance directive that may include an oral statement to a loved one or caregiver, a written document known as a living will, a health care power of attorney, and a DNR order if so desired.

- A *living will* is a legal document stating the patient's desires with regard to health care treatment during dying if the patient is unable to communicate those wishes.
- *A Health Care Power of Attorney (HCPA)* is a legal document that allows the patient to appoint another person or persons to make health care decisions in the event that the patient is unable to make them. This authority supersedes the authority of the next of kin in decisions concerning health but does not allow the person with the HCPA to make any financial or other business decisions for the patient.
- *Do Not Resuscitate (DNR) orders* vary across states but a DNR order is usually a distinctive one-page document that the patient carries to prevent institution of CPR in the event of cardiac arrest. It relieves emergency services, other health care personnel, and good Samaritans of the responsibility of not administering CPR that they would otherwise initiate. In a dialysis unit, those patients with DNR orders must be made known to the staff so that staff will abide by the patients' wishes.

Team approach. A team approach to advance care planning with discussions at the time of admission and in all long-term care planning is good care for the patient as it allows the patient to make more informed choices, achieve better palliation of symptoms, and work on life issues (Quill, 2000). The team approach also relieves the nurse of unilateral responsibility. There is evidence that advance care planning reduces the stress for the family both at the time of the patient's death and many months later (Tilden, Tolle, Nelson, & Fields, 2001). However, an identified barrier to the communication about advance directives is the unwillingness of the caregivers rather than the patient and family to discuss death and dying (Curtis, Patrick, Caldwell, & Collier, 2000; Perry et al., 1996). Having the primary physician or nurse practitioner involved is essential to assure clear communication and appropriate interventions in the event of a life-threatening episode or illness. In the scenario, where the patient does not have an advance care plan, the patient and/or his family may be approached using a "hope for the best" but "prepare for the worst" strategy to elicit wishes for treatment if dying (Norton, Tilden, Tolle, Nelson, & Eggman, 2003). These same authors stressed that communication with patients and families must be in terms that they clearly understand and that clinicians must be congruent in the information they give.

In reality in the dialysis unit, it is the social worker who initiates discussions about advance care planning (Perry et al., 1996), but it is the responsibility of the whole team to make sure that the planning is done and reviewed appropriately. Still, many patients are resistant to this discussion and say that they come to dialysis to live, not to discuss dying (Robert Wood Johnson Foundation, Moss et al., 2003). Making it clear that this is part of the admission process and the annual care plan for *all* patients may make it more acceptable. Recent work described by Briggs (2004) has been to shift the focus of advance care planning from a document driven, decision focused event to a relational, patient-centered process. This is achieved by using a technique Briggs calls the intervention interview, which builds and strengthens relationships with patients. In her summary of lessons learned from using this technique, Briggs says that advance care planning is hard work because intimacy among strangers is difficult to achieve and patients are often afraid to talk to their loved ones about this difficult subject. For nurses, listening is the intervention. Patients give us clues but we need to hear them. This learned technique may be a suitable skill for the advanced practice nurse or other appropriately educated and experienced caregivers.

Administrative Responsibilities

Administrative responsibilities in the care of the dying patient include incorporation of advance care planning in the admission orders and long-term care plan. Patient care conferences should always include a review of the status of advance care planning. If the patient has an advance directive, it should be reviewed with the patient and family to affirm or change the contents. Monthly continuous quality improvement (CQI) conferences should utilize the care plan and advance directive to assure that the staff are aware of any changes in the status of the patient and that appropriate planning and care is instituted as necessary.

All dialysis units should have policies and procedures for the management of cardiac arrest, with or without a DNR order. Ignoring a patient's DNR order so that the patient "does not die in the dialysis unit" is unethical and may constitute assault and battery (Kjervik & Badzek, 1998). Other policies and procedures should be in place to address the management of the patient who dies suddenly in the dialysis unit with instructions for the appropriate care of the body after death. All patients should have a funeral home arrangement made for this eventuality, and the dialysis unit must have a procedure for transporting the body to a suitable, designated private space in the dialysis unit to respectfully accommodate the body until it is transported to the funeral home (Castner, 2004).

Defining Palliative Care

Palliative care, according to *Dorland's Medical Dictionary (2003)*, affords relief but not cure (p. 1353). The World Health Organization definition states that, "Palliative care is an approach which improves the quality of life of patients and their families facing life-threatening illness, through the prevention, assessment, and treatment of pain and other physical, psychosocial and spiritual problems" (Von Gunten, Ferris, Portenoy, & Glajchen, 2001). A third definition, given to dialysis patients in focus groups exploring end-of-life care, notes that, "Palliative care focuses on easing pain and making life better for people who are dying and their loved ones. Palliative care means taking care of the whole person – not just their physical symptoms, but also their emotional and spiritual needs. It looks at death and dying as something natural and personal. The goal of palliative care is to keep dying people as pain-free and comfortable as possible, to help them maintain their dignity, and to provide them the best quality of life until the very end of life." The last definition is the one that perhaps best reflects the intent of the code of ethics for nurses.

Figure 16-1
Introducing Palliative Care in the Course of Illness

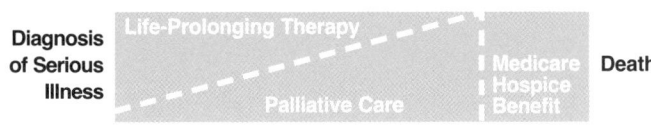

Knowing when to introduce palliative care can be challenging. In the majority of patients, it seems very difficult to identify that point in time when our kidney replacement therapy goes from being life-prolonging to death-denying. The answer becomes very clear, as you examine the graphic (see Figure 16-1) from the *Clinical Practice Guidelines for Quality Palliative Care* (2004). Palliative care begins at the diagnosis of serious illness and the institution of life-prolonging therapy and increases until it becomes the total mode of care prior to a patient's death.

Hospice

Synonymous with 100% palliative care is the term "hospice." Hospice has been associated with the terminal phase of cancer care because that was the patient population for whom it was created – but today any dying patient and family can benefit from this paradigm of palliative care where the treatment goal is comfort not cure. The dying CKD patient is very well suited to the services that hospice care offers regardless of the stage of disease. However, a recent Medicare Payment Advisory Commission Report (2004) states "beneficiaries with ESRD have low enrollment in the hospice benefit, despite their high mortality rate. For hospice patients with ESRD, ESRD may or may not be their terminal diagnosis. If ESRD is their terminal diagnosis, then dialysis needed on a palliative basis is considered a covered hospice service and would be paid through the per diem hospice rate. If, however, ESRD is not their terminal diagnosis, then Medicare would continue to cover their dialysis outside the hospice benefit, and their hospice coverage would not be liable."

Thus, the dying may be related to co-morbidities and/or general failure to thrive on dialysis. Patients or their families may choose not to begin dialysis in the former instance or withdraw from dialysis in the latter. All patients expressing a wish to withdraw from dialysis must carefully be screened for depression, pain, and treatable exacerbations of co-morbid illness. There are reported cases of seasonal affective disorder (SAD) that, until they are treated, lead patients to want to withdraw from dialysis. However, some patients choose to stay on dialysis even when they know they are dying. In such instances, the nephrology nurse partners with the hospice caregivers in giving palliative care. Regardless of dialysis status while in hospice, nurse practitioners (NPs) may now be the "attending physician" for patients who have enrolled in hospice (Buppert, 2004). It is extremely important that the patient who has withdrawn from dialysis continues to be followed by nephrology caregivers, both so that the patient will not feel abandoned but also because it is the nephrology team who knows the patient best and can thereby assure the highest level of care.

Treatment for the patient who has withdrawn from dialysis is directed at symptom relief without over-sedation, thus allowing the patient and family maximum opportunity to interact in comfort. In general, the dying from uremia is thought to be relatively pain-free with the patient progressing through periods of confusion to coma. However, if pain is present, it must be closely monitored and treated appropriately with medication, repositioning, massage, and guided imagery. Patients should be allowed to eat and drink at will, but appetite is usually suppressed and large fluid intake could induce pulmonary edema. Artificial means of feeding and hydration should not be started as the nutrients and fluid can exacerbate rather than relieve symptoms (DeVelasco & Dinwiddie, 1998; Pitorak, 2003). Pulmonary edema can be relieved, and the patient made more comfortable and less anxious, by hemofiltration treatments. Uremic frost, the accumulation of uric acid crystals on the skin from sweat, is not a symptom you would expect to see in this day and age of air conditioning. How long the patient will continue to live after withdrawal from dialysis is highly variable depending on the individual patient and his/her condition, but in the anuric patient it is rarely more than a matter of days.

Last but not least, the nurse's role with the dying CKD patient is to support and facilitate the quality of dying. Timely treatment of symptoms, reassuring family, facilitating communication between the patient and those he/she wants with them are very important acts of the nurse. Perhaps the hardest task for the nurse who knows this patient and the family well is to step back and let it be their time. It is not the nurse's place to give a patient "permission" to die – that is the prerogative of the family (Berns & Colvin, 1998).

Grief Counseling

CKD, like many chronic illnesses, leads to patients and their caregivers becoming well acquainted with each other over the years that they interact. Nowhere is this more apparent than in the dialysis unit. It is the only health care therapy where patients and staff interact at least three times a week through the foreseeable future. Indeed both nurses and patients have been known to remark that they see more of each other than they do their own families. Special bonds are also forged between patients over time because of their mutual experiences. So when a patient dies, both the patient's relatives and his/her dialysis family grieve. Often the death is unexpected, even when the patient is hospitalized, and so the remaining patients and staff must be told of the death in a kind and respectful manner. While there are many methods that dialysis facilities have used to do this, one that has been most acceptable is to reserve a small shelf in the reception area for a vase of flowers accompanied by an obituary or a card on which is written the patient's name and date of death (with permission from the family). Patients and staff then know of the death as soon as they enter the building and can both grieve and comfort each other. Requesting permission from the family to announce the death is not only respectful but complies with federal regulations regarding patients' privacy. Formal grief counseling for the bereaved family is not usually part of the nephrology nurses' practice being rather one of the many benefits of hospice care and a reason for encouraging patients and their families to seek hospice services for end-of-life care.

Conclusion

Even though survival rates for CKD patients are poor relative to other chronic diseases, we now use the term CKD5 interchangeably with ESRD because our incident patients should not view themselves as having a prognosis of terminal illness portending death. Therefore, in CKD patient care, we appropriately focus on quality of life for patients and their families. The prescribed therapy we give is designed to make them as physiologically well as possible so that they are able to have self-defined quality of life.

Quality of dying must be strived for as part of quality of life. Even though nephrology nurses are rarely involved with direct patient care in the final stages of dying, their responsibility is to promote quality of dying through a patient-centered, advance care planning process that benefits both the patient and the family. Certainly the manner in which a patient dies and the perceived quality of care that is given impacts our patients' loved ones. In the words of Dame Cicely Saunders, the founder of the first modern hospice, "How people die remains in the memories of those who live on." We, as nephrology nurses, have the responsibility and privilege to assure our patients and their families no less than excellent care at the end of life.

References

American Nurses Association, (2001). *Code of ethics for nurses with interpretive statements* (statement 1.3 pages 7-8).Washington, DC: American Nurses Association.

Badzek, L., Cline, H., Moss, A., & Hines, S. (2000). Inappropriate use of dialysis for some elderly patients: Nephrology nurses' perceptions and concerns. *Nephrology Nursing Journal, 27*(5), 462-470.

Berns, R., & Colvin, E. (1998). The final story: Events at the bedside of dying patients as told by survivors. *ANNA Journal, 25*(6), 583-587.

Briggs, L. (2004). Shifting the focus of advance care planning: Using an in-depth interview to build and strengthen relationships. *Journal of Palliative Medicine, 7*(2), 341-349.

Buppert, C. (2004). What is the current status of billing for NP hospice care. *Medscape, 6*(2).

Castner, D. (2004) Honoring DNR orders in the dialysis unit: Implementing a policy. *Nephrology Nursing Journal, 31*(1), 94-95.

Clinical Practice Guidelines for Quality Palliative Care. (2004). Executive Summary (p. 2). Retrieved from www.nationalconsensusproject.org

Curtis, J., Patrick, D., Caldwell, E., & Collier, A. (2000). Why don't patient and physicians talk about end-of–life care? *Archives of Internal Medicine, 160*, 1690-1696.

DeVelasco, R., & Dinwiddie, L. (1998). Management of the patient with end stage renal disease after withdrawal from dialysis. *ANNA Journal, 25*(6), 611-614.

Dorland's Illustrated Medical Dictionary. (2003). 30th edition, p. 1353. Philadelphia: W.B. Saunders Company.

Kjervik, D., & Badzek, L. (1998). Legal considerations at the end of life. *ANNA Journal, 25*(6), 593-597.

Medicare Payment Advisory Commission. (2004). *New approaches in Medicare.* Retrieved from http://www.medpac.gov/publications/congressional_reports/June04_Entire_Report.pdf

Moss, A. (2003). *Completing the continuum of nephrology care. End Stage Renal Disease Peer Workgroup, Recommendations to the Field. The Robert Wood Johnson Foundation.* Washington, DC: Renal Physicians Association.

Norton, S., Tilden, P., Tolle, S., Nelson, C., & Eggman, S. (2003). Life support withdrawal: Communication and conflict. *American Journal of Critical Care 12*(6), 548-555.

Pendergast, T. (2001). Advance care planning: Pitfalls, progress, promise. *Critical Care Medicine, 29*(2), N34-39 (suppl.).

Perry, E., Swartz, R., Smith-Wheelock, L., Westbrook, J., & Buck, C. (1996). Why is it difficult for staff to discuss advance directives with chronic dialysis patients. *Journal of the American Society of Nephrology, 7*(10), 2160-2168.

Pitorak, E.F., (2003). Care at the time of death. *American Journal of Nursing, 103*(7), 42-52.

Price, C.R. (2003). Resources for planning palliative and end-of life care for patients with kidney disease. *Nephrology Nursing Journal, 30*(6), 649-56, 664.

Quill, T. (2000). Initiating end-of-life discussions with seriously ill patients: Addressing the "elephant in the room." *Journal of the American Medical Association, 284*(19), 2502-2507.

Renal Physicians Association and American Society of Nephrology. (2002). *Shared decision-making in the appropriate initiation of and withdrawal from dialysis,* Clinical Practice Guideline. Washington, DC: Authors.

Robert Wood Johnson Foundation, Moss et al. (2003). ESRD Workgroup Final Report Summary on End-of-Life Care: Recommendations to the field. *Nephrology Nursing Journal, 30*(1), 58-63.

Additional Readings

Billings, J.A. (2000) Palliative Care. Recent Advances. *British Medical Journal, 321,* 555-558.

Braveman, C., & Cohen, L.M. (2002). Discontinuation of dialysis: The role of hospice and palliative care. *AAHPM Bulletin, 3*(1), 16-17.

Buckman, R. (1992). *How to break bad news: A guide for health care professionals.* Baltimore, MD: The Johns Hopkins University Press.

Cohen, L.M., Germain, M.J., Poppel., D.M., Woods, A.L., Pekow, P.S., & Kjellstrand, C.M. (2000). Dying well after discontinuing the life-support treatment of dialysis. *Archives of Internal Medicine, 160,* 2513-2518.

Cohen, L.M., & Germain, M.J. (2003). Palliative and supportive care. In H.R. Brady, & C.S. Wilcox (Eds.), *Therapy of nephrology and hypertension: A companion to Brenner's The Kidney* (2nd edition, pp. 753-756). Philadelphia: Elsevier Science.

Cohen, L.M., Dobscha, S.K., Hails, K.C., Morris, J.E., Pekow, P.S., & Chochinov, H.M. (2002). Depression and suicidal ideation in patients who discontinue the life-support treatment of dialysis. *Psychosomatic Medicine, 64,* 889-896.

Cohen, L.M., Reiter, G.S., Poppel, D.M., & Germain, M.J. (2001). Renal palliative care. In: J.M. Addington-Hall & I.J. Higginson (Eds.), *Palliative care for non-cancer patients.* New York: Oxford University Press.

Hijazi, F., & Holley, J.L. (2003). Cardiopulmonary resuscitation and dialysis: Outcome and patient's views. *Seminars in Dialysis, 16,* 51-53.

Hines, S.C., Glover, J.J., Holley, J.L., Babrow, A.S., Badzek, L.A., & Moss, A.H. (1999). Dialysis patients' preferences for family-based advance care planning. *Annals of Internal Medicine, 130,* 825-828.

Holley, J.L., Foulks, C.J., & Moss, A.H. (1991). Nephrologists' reported attitudes about factors influencing recommendations to initiate or withdraw dialysis. *Journal of the American Society of Nephrology, 1,* 1284-1299.

Jennings, B., Ryndes, T., D'Onofrio, C., & Baily, M.A. (2003, March-April). *Access to hospice care: Expanding boundaries, overcoming barriers.* Hastings Center Report – Special Supplement.

Kimmel, P.L., Emont, S.L., Newmann, J.M., Danko, H., & Moss, A.H. (2003). ESRD patient quality of life: Symptoms, spiritual beliefs, psychological factors, and ethnicity. *American Journal of Kidney Diseases, 42,* 713-721.

Leggat, J.E., Jr, Bloembergen, W.E., Levine, G., Hulbert-Shearon, T.E., & Port, F.K. (1997). An analysis of risk factors for withdrawal from dialysis before death. *Journal of the American Society of Nephrology, 8*(11), 1755-1763.

Moss, A.H., Holley, J.L., & Upton, M.B. (1993). Outcome of cardiopulmonary resuscitation in dialysis patients. *Journal of the American Society of Nephrology, 3,* 1238-1243.

Moss, A.H., Hozayen, O., King, K., Holley, J.L., & Schmidt, R.J. (2001). Attitudes of patients toward cardiopulmonary resuscitation in the dialysis unit. *American Journal of Kidney Diseases, 38,* 847-852.

Neu, S., & Kjellstrand, C.M. (1986). Stopping long-term dialysis: An empirical study of withdrawal of life-supporting treatment. *New England Journal of Medicine, 314*(1), 14-20.

Poppel, D., Cohen, L., & Germain, M. (2003). The Renal Palliative Care Initiative. *Journal of Palliative Medicine, 6,* 321-326.

Sekkarie, M.A., & Moss, A.H. (1995). Withholding and withdrawing dialysis: The role of physician specialty and education and patient functional status. *American Journal of Kidney Diseases, 31,* 464-472.

Singer, P.A. (1999). Advance care planning in dialysis. *American Journal of Kidney Diseases, 33,* 980-991.

Steinhauser, K., Christakis, N., Clipp, E., McNeilly, M., McIntyre, L. & Tulsky. (2000). Factors considered important at the end of life by patients, family, physicians and other providers. *Journal of the American Medical Association, 284*(19), 2476-2488.

Swartz, R.D., & Perry, E. (1999). Medical family: A new view of the relationship between chronic dialysis patients and staff arising from discussions about advance directives. *Journal of Women's Health Gender-Based Medicine, 8,* 1147-1153.

Swartz, R.D., & Perry, E. (1993). Advance directives are associated with "good deaths" in chronic dialysis patients. *Journal of the American Society of Nephrology, 3,* 1623-1630.

Tilden, V.P., Tolle, S.W., Nelson, C.A., & Fields, J. (2001). *Family decision making to withdraw life-sustaining treatments from hospitalized patients.* Nursing Research, 50(2), 105-115.

Von Gunten, C.F., Ferris, F.D., Portenoy, R.K., & Glajchen, M. (Eds.) (2001). *CAPD Manual: How to establish a palliative care program.* New York.

- Controversies concerning exactly when human life begins and ends remain unresolved, but there is one irrefutable fact about human life – it will end. Paradoxically, dying is the one area of health care that receives comparatively little attention or preparatory planning.

- Nephrology nursing, through the American Nephrology Nurses' Association (ANNA), has endorsed the American Nurses Association Code of Ethics, which includes interpretive statements related to nursing care at the end of life.

- No discussion of ethics related to nursing care at the end of life would be complete without a reiteration of the principles of beneficence, nonmalificence, and autonomy.

- Understanding patients' cultural norms and acknowledging their spiritual beliefs will help nurses fulfill their duty to respect any patient or family decision that is contrary to their personal philosophy.

- Advance care planning is that part of the long-term care plan in which we begin a process of understanding, reflecting, and developing a plan based on the patients' wishes for medical care in the future when they might not be able to make those decisions themselves.

- A team approach to advance care planning with discussions at the time of admission and in all long-term care planning is good care for the patient as it allows the patient to make more informed choices, achieve better palliation of symptoms, and work on life issues (Quill, 2000). The team approach also relieves the nurse of unilateral responsibility.

- Knowing when to introduce palliative care can be challenging. In the majority of patients, it seems very difficult to identify that point in time when our renal replacement therapy goes from being life-prolonging to death-denying... Palliative care begins at the diagnosis of serious illness and the institution of life-prolonging therapy and increases until it becomes the total mode of care prior to a patient's death.

- Synonymous with 100% palliative care is the term "hospice." Hospice has been associated with the terminal phase of cancer care because that was the patient population for whom it was created – but today any dying patient and family can benefit from this paradigm of palliative care where the treatment goal is comfort not cure.

Editor's Note: *Quality of dying must be strived for as part of quality of life. Even though nephrology nurses are rarely involved with direct patient care in the final stages of dying, their responsibility is to promote quality of dying through a patient-centered, advance care planning process that benefits both the patient and the family.*

ANNP616

End-of-Life Care in the Chronic Kidney Disease Population

Lesley C. Dinwiddie, MSN, RN, FNP, CNN; and Elaine R. Colvin, BSN, RN, MEPD

Contemporary Nephrology Nursing: Principles and Practice contains 39 chapters of educational content. Individual learners may apply for continuing nursing education credit by reading a chapter and completing the Continuing Education Evaluation Form for that chapter. Learners may apply for continuing education credit for any or all chapters.

Please photocopy this page and return to ANNA.
COMPLETE THE FOLLOWING:

Name: _____

Address:_____

City:_____ State:_____ Zip:_____

E-mail: _____

Preferred telephone: ☐ Home   ☐ Work: _____

State where licensed and license number (optional): _____

CE application fees are based upon the number of contact hours provided by the individual chapter. CE fees per contact hour for ANNA members are as follows: 1.0-1.9 - $15; 2.0-2.9 - $20; 3.0-3.9 - $25; 4.0 and higher - $30. Fees for nonmembers are $10 higher.

ANNA Member: ☐ Yes   ☐ No   Member # (if available) _____

☐ Checked Enclosed   ☐ American Express   ☐ Visa   ☐ MasterCard

Total Amount Submitted: _____

Credit Card Number: _____ Exp. Date: _____

Name as it appears on the card: _____

CE Evaluation Form
To receive continuing education credit for individual study after reading the chapter
1. Photocopy this form. (You may also download this form from ANNA's Web site, **www.annanurse.org**.)
2. Mail the completed form with payment (check) or credit card information to American Nephrology Nurses' Association, East Holly Avenue, Box 56, Pitman, NJ 08071-0056.
3. You will receive your CE certificate from ANNA in 4 to 6 weeks.

Test returns must be postmarked by **December 31, 2010.**

CE Application Fee
ANNA Member $15.00
Nonmember $25.00

EVALUATION FORM

1. I verify that I have read this chapter and completed this education activity. Date: _____

_____
Signature

2. What would be different in your practice if you applied what you learned from this activity? *(Please use additional sheet of paper if necessary.)*

_____
_____
_____
_____
_____
_____
_____
_____
_____
_____
_____
_____

Evaluation	Strongly disagree				Strongly agree
3. The activity met the stated objectives.					
a. Define palliative care	1	2	3	4	5
b. Discuss nursing's role in end-of-life care.	1	2	3	4	5
c. State the components of grief counseling that need to be included when planning care for patients and/or families dealing with end-of-life issues.	1	2	3	4	5
4. The content was current and relevant.	1	2	3	4	5
5. The content was presented clearly.	1	2	3	4	5
6. The content was covered adequately.	1	2	3	4	5
7. Rate your ability to apply the learning obtained from this activity to practice.	1	2	3	4	5

Comments _____

_____

8. Time required to read the chapter and complete this form: _____ minutes.

This educational activity has been provided by the American Nephrology Nurses' Association (ANNA) for 1.3 contact hours. ANNA is accredited as a provider of continuing nursing education (CNE) by the American Nurses Credentialing Center's Commission on Accreditation (ANCC-COA). ANNA is an approved provider of continuing education by the California Board of Registered Nursing, CEP 0910.

Clinical Management of the Renal Patient

UNIT 4

Unit 4 Contents

Nutrition and Chronic Kidney Disease

Jordi Goldstein-Fuchs, DSc, RD

Chapter Contents

Jordi Goldstein-Fuchs, DSc, RD

Chronic kidney failure is a disease syndrome where progressive, irreversible losses of the endocrine, excretory, and metabolic capacities of the kidney occur due to kidney damage. Once kidney damage has occurred, it cannot be reversed. Progression to end stage disease results in the need for kidney replacement therapy. Prediction as to whether an established chronic kidney disease will advance to end stage cannot always be accomplished. The pathophysiology of progressive kidney disease is an area of continued research (Goodman, London, Amann, Block, Giachelli, Hruska, et al., 2004; Redmond, McDevitt, & Barnes, 2004; Vattikuti & Toweler, 2004).

Nutritional management of chronic kidney disease (CKD) is an integral component of the medical care of both progressive and end-stage disease. Malnutrition, cardiovascular disease, bone disease, and anemia are the most common co-morbid conditions that accompany kidney disease, and they require both medical and nutritional intervention. Cardiovascular calcification and inflammation are now recognized to have a role in these co-morbid complications (Goodman et al., 2004, Kaysen, 2002).

Diet therapy has the potential to slow the progression of chronic kidney disease, compensates for impaired renal function and/or limitations of treatment modalities, has a major role in the management of the co-morbid conditions, and is a mainstay of therapy for malnutrition. The registered dietitian (RD) serves as an integral part of the renal health care team by assessing the patient's requirements and recommending the appropriate nutrition intervention. In addition, dietitians counsel patients and their families in the diet, follow patients for compliance, and help determine additional or changing nutritional needs (Wiggins, 2002). More recently, the RD plays a key role in bone disease management, assisting in the analysis of interventions that require intravenous vitamin D and phosphate-binding medications (Martin & Reams, 2003). The purpose of this chapter is to provide an overview of the components of nutrition care for the adult with established kidney disease, requiring peritoneal dialysis or hemodialysis replacement therapy, and post kidney transplantation.

NKF-Kidney Disease Outcomes Quality Initiatives (NKF-K/DOQI)

In an effort to provide evidence-based clinical practice guidelines for the care of patients with chronic kidney disease, the National Kidney Foundation (NKF) launched the Disease Outcomes Quality Initiatives (DOQI) in March 1995 (NKF-K/DOQI, 2000a). The guidelines have been completed for key components of care, including nutrition (NKF-K/DOQI, 2000a), anemia (NKF-K/DOQI, 2000b), chronic kidney disease (NKF-K/DOQI, 2002), dyslipidemia (NKF-K/DOQI, 2003a), bone disease (NKF-K/DOQI, 2003b), and hypertension (NKF-K/DOQI, 2004). Guidelines for the management of cardiovascular disease and diabetic kidney disease are in process. All of the guidelines are developed following a rigorous literature review procedure by an expert interdisciplinary panel selected in recognition of their expert-

Table 17-1
Stages of Chronic Kidney Disease (NKF-K/DOQI, 2002)

Stage	Description	GFR (ml/min/1.73m²)
1	Kidney damage with normal GFR	>90
2	Kidney damage with mild decrease in GFR	60 to 90
3	Moderate decrease GFR	30 to 60
4	Severe decrease GFR	15 to 30
5	Kidney failure	<15

ise in a given area. The results of the process, which often require review of more than 11,000 abstracts and articles, and a laborious data extraction process, are published in the *American Journal of Kidney Diseases*. Components of these clinical guidelines will be highlighted where relevant in this chapter because the K/DOQI guidelines provide the most current evidence-based clinical recommendations available. Additional information regarding the K/DOQI initiative can be found on the National Kidney Foundation Web site (www.kidney.org).

Definition of CKD

CKD is defined by the level of kidney function and whether there is evidence of kidney damage (NKF-K/DOQI, 2002). The CKD K/DOQI guidelines identify five stages of kidney disease, defined by the level of glomerular filtration rate (GFR) (see Table 17-1). While creatinine has traditionally been the standard of care to evaluate kidney function, the CKD K/DOQI guidelines determined that serum creatinine concentration alone should not be used to evaluate kidney function. The serum creatinine level is not an accurate index of kidney function by itself because the assumptions upon which the accuracy is based are not always valid. The reasons for this are:

- Creatinine is an ideal filtration marker whose clearance approximates GFR.
- Creatinine excretion rate is constant among individuals and over time.
- Measurement of serum creatinine is accurate and reproducible across clinical laboratories. As a result, clinical laboratories are being encouraged to report a GFR using available prediction equations along with the serum creatinine level.

Using this system, CKD is defined as kidney damage or a GFR <60 mL/min/1.73 m3 for ≥ 3 months (NKF-K/DOQI, 2002). Stages I-IV pertain to patients who do not require renal replacement therapy. Stage V is defined as kidney failure with a GFR < 15 (or dialysis dependent) (see Table 17-1).

Renal Physiology

The functional units of the kidneys are the more than 1 million nephrons within each kidney (Briggs & Schnermann, 1994). The glomerulus of the nephron selectively filters serum to remove waste products including solutes such as glucose, organic acids, and end products of metabolism, while preventing the loss of large protein molecules and red blood cells (Briggs & Schnermann, 1994). Glomerular diseases frequently result in urinary excretion of protein and subsequent hypoalbuminemia. A minimum urinary volume of approximately 600 ml (obligatory fluid) is required for the excretion of the average load of solids. About two-thirds of the solute load are nitrogenous wastes, consisting mostly of urea with smaller amounts of uric acid, creatinine, and ammonia. Accumulation of these protein metabolism end products to toxicity is the hallmark of renal insufficiency. The proximal tubules, the loop of Henle, the distal tubules, and the collecting duct of the nephron function primarily to maintain fluid and electrolyte balance, and acid-base homeostasis. With renal insufficiency, patients may easily dehydrate or become overloaded with fluid. In addition, the kidney often looses the ability to maintain normal serum phosphorus and potassium levels.

As an endocrine organ, the kidney is the chief source for renin, erythropoietin, and 1,25-dihydroxycholecalciferol $(1,25(OH)_2D_3)$ (Klahr,1998). The failure of the kidney to secrete these vital hormones results in the complications of hypertension, anemia, and renal osteodystrophy, respectively. Nutritional adjustments help prevent or decrease the severity of some of these complications.

Diet and Progression of Renal Failure

Studies completed in experimental models of renal disease have documented that high-protein diets lead to increased proteinuria, renal damage, and mortality, while dietary protein restriction results in improvements (Mitch, 1997). Application of the resulting hypothesis that dietary protein can delay, reverse, or halt CKD progression has not resulted in consistent beneficial effects. An example is the landmark multi-center clinical trial – the Modification of Diet in Renal Disease (MDRD) completed in the U.S. (Klahr et al., 1994). The MDRD study enrolled 840 CKD patients for intervention in diet and blood pressure. Two groups of patients were studied. Patients in Group A had GFRs in the range of 25-55 mL/min/1.73m2 and were randomized to a diet of ≥1g protein/kg/day or 0.6 g/kg/day. Mean blood pressures were maintained at 105 or 92 mmHg. Group B patients had GFRs in the range of 13-24 mL/min/1.73 m2 and were assigned diets that were 0.6 gm/kg/day or 0.3 g protein/kg/day plus a ketoacid supplement. Blood pressure goals were the same. Renal function was monitored for 2.2 years by measuring 125I-iothalamate renal clearance. Study results indicated that neither the low-protein diet nor blood pressure control decreased the loss of GFR. A low-protein diet was not found to be universally renal protective.

The *K/DOQI Clinical Practice Guidelines for Chronic Kidney Disease* (NKF-K/DOQI, 2002) include protein and calorie recommendations, which integrate the large body of data showing that protein energy malnutrition develops as a co-morbid condition of CKD and is associated with poor patient outcomes (Ikizler, Wingard, Harvell, Shyr, & Hakim, 1999; Kopple, 1994). While low protein may afford some protection from disease progression, inadequate protein and calorie intake is recognized to result in malnutrition in this patient population. The guidelines therefore try to balance these limitations.

These guidelines state that for individuals with a GFR < 25 ml/min who are not undergoing maintenance dialysis, the institution of a low-protein diet providing 0.60 g protein/kilogram body weight (kg) per day should be considered. However, if the individual cannot tolerate such a diet or as a result is unable to maintain an adequate intake of calories, then the individual should eat up to 0.75 grams of protein/kg/day.

- Regarding total energy intake: For individuals with a GFR < 25 ml/min who are not undergoing maintenance dialysis, 35 kilocalories (kcal)/kg/day is recommended for those younger than 60 years of age, and 30 to 35 kcal/kg for individuals 60 years of age and older.

Diet for Dialysis

The diet for dialysis compensates for lack of kidney function and dialysate losses, provides adequate nutrients for optimal health, and alleviates symptoms of uremia. The dietitian individualizes each patient's nutrition plan based on current nutritional status, pertinent serum laboratory values, and the treatment modality. Hemodialysis (HD) and peritoneal dialysis (PD) (either continuous ambulatory [CAPD] or continuous cyclic [CCPD]), affect nutritional status differently. The usual components of the diet that are modified are dietary sodium, potassium, phosphate, calcium, protein, calories, vitamins, and minerals. These values are integrated with nutritional status, dialysis adequacy information, and nutritional status assessment to provide individualized diet therapy.

Potassium

The kidney is the primary route for excretion of potassium. The average diet contains approximately 80 to 100 mEq (3,000 to 4,000 mg) potassium. Hyperkalemia occurs when serum levels exceed 6.0 mmol/L (6.0 mEq/L) (Beto & Bansal, 1992; Falkenhain, Hartman, & Hebert, 2004). The characteristic cardiac changes can be fatal. In CKD, dialysis treatments and decreased dietary potassium prevent hyperkalemia. HD removes approximately 100 to 200 mmol (100 to 200 mEq) per treatment, but serum levels rise rapidly between treatments if intake is not curtailed. The recommended dietary potassium depends on residual renal function; body size; the presence of anabolism, catabolism, or infection; and the potassium content of the dialysate. Patients achieve normal predialysis serum levels with a daily intake of approximately one mEq per kilogram ideal body weight or 38 to 80 mmol (38 to 80 mEq or 1,500 to 3,000 mg) daily (American Dietetic Association, 2002). Foods high in potassium include many fruits, vegetables, dairy products, and legumes. Table 17-2 categorizes fruits and vegetables by identifying them as being low, medium, or high in potassium content. To help patients limit their intake of these foods, dietitians must routinely reinforce the diet parameters.

Table 17-2

Potassium Content of Selected Fruits and Vegetables

All serving sizes are 1/2 cup unless otherwise noted.

Low-potassium (less than 150 mg)

Fruits

Apple (1)	Lime (1)
Apple juice	Lime juice
Applesauce	Papaya nectar
Apricot nectar	Peach (canned)
Blackberries	Peach nectar
Blueberries	Pear (canned)
Cranberries	Pear nectar
Cranberry juice cocktails	Pineapple
Fruit cocktail	Plums (1)
Gooseberries	Raspberries
Grape juice	Strawberries
Grapes	Tangerine (1)
Lemon (1)	Watermelon
Lemon juice	

Vegetables

Alfalfa sprouts	Eggplant
Bamboo shoots (canned)	Green beans
Bean sprouts	Lettuce (all types, 1 cup)
Beets (canned)	Mushrooms
Cabbage	Onions
Carrots	Radishes
Cauliflower	Summer squash
Corn	Water chestnuts (canned)
Cucumber	Watercress
Endive	

Medium-potassium (150-250 mg)

Fruits	*Vegetables*
Cherries	Asparagus
Cantaloupe	Broccoli
Figs (2 whole)	Celery
Grapefruit	Kale
Grapefruit juice	Mixed vegetables
Mango	Peas
Papaya	Peppers
Peach (fresh)	Summer squash
Pear (fresh)	Turnips
Rhubarb	Zucchini

High-potassium (more than 250 mg)

Fruits	*Vegetables*	
Apricots	Avocado	Pumpkin
Banana (1 small)	Bamboo shoots	Rutabagas
Dates (1/4 cup)	(fresh, raw)	Spinach
Honeydew melon	Beets (fresh)	Sweet potatoes
Kiwifruit	Brussels sprouts	Tomatoes
Nectarine	Chard	Tomato sauce,
Orange (1)	Greens (beet, col-	puree
Orange juice	lard, mustard, etc.)	Tomato juice
Prune juice	Kohlrabi	V-8 juice
Prunes (5)	Okra	Wax beans
Raisins	Parsnips	Winter squash
	Potatoes	Yams

Note: From American Dietetic Association (2002). A healthy food guide for people on dialysis. Chicago: American Dietetic Association.

Due to high weekly clearances, PD patients frequently do not require a dietary potassium restriction. The recommendation for dietary potassium will be dependent upon the individual's laboratory values (American Dietetic Association, 2002). The dietitian works within the renal team to individualize a patient's dietary potassium instructions. Some patients easily become hypokalemic, especially in response to poor dietary intake, diarrhea, or vomiting. If increased dietary intake is unsuccessful in raising the patient's serum potassium, potassium supplements may need to be used. Other patients may become hyperkalemic in response to excessive dietary intake, particularly those who are very active, and they need to restrict their dietary potassium.

While diet is thought of as the primary cause of hyperkalemia, there are a host of other conditions that may lead to high potassium levels, such as acidemia, some hormonal disturbances, and a variety of medications (Beto & Bansal, 1992).

Sodium and Fluid

Dialysis patients are unable to maintain sodium and water homeostasis and may be prone to edema, hypertension, and congestive heart failure (Falkenhain, Hartman, & Hebert, 2004). HD patients restrict their sodium and fluid intake to limit interdialytic weight gains to 2 kilograms or 0.3-0.5% of estimated dry weight. Recommendations are individualized according to the patient's urinary losses of sodium and 24-hour urinary volume. Anephric patients receive approximately 85-90 mEq (2,000 mg) sodium and 500 to 1,000 ml fluid daily.

Some HD patients frequently gain excessive amounts of fluid between treatments due to uncontrollable thirst. Causes of excess thirst include hyperglycemia, azotemia, inadequate dialysis, a high dietary intake of sucrose, and a high intake of salt. Salt is most frequently the cause. Only a 1% change in serum sodium will stimulate thirst. Many patients think of salt (sodium chloride) as the only source of sodium, but they may be unaware of the sodium in sources such as broth or bouillon, soy sauce, seasoning salts, convenience foods, deli foods, fast food restaurants, and preservatives for frozen, canned, or boxed food. The dietitian on the renal team works with patients to be aware of these hidden sources and to learn how to read labels where sodium content is listed. Methods to help patients achieve healthy lifestyle habits in regards to diet, fluid, and exercise have been reviewed in detail (Ford, Pope, Hunt, & Gerald, 2004; Burrowes & Cockram, 2004).

CAPD and CCPD result in greater sodium and fluid losses into the dialysate than hemodialysis due to the continual nature of peritoneal dialysis. Generally, restrictions of sodium and fluid are unnecessary. Patients learn how to monitor for both dehydration and overhydration and how to make the appropriate adjustments in their dialysis regimen. To treat fluid retention, patients infuse more concentrated dialysate solutions.

Phosphorus, Calcium, and Vitamin D

CKD creates a wide range of alterations in homeostasis of calcium and phosphorus, and in the metabolism of vitamin D. As glomerular filtration rate decreases and kidney

Table 17-3
NKF-K/DOQI Dietary Phosphate and Binder Recommendations (NKF-K/DOQI, 2003)

In CKD Patients (Stages 3 and 4):

5.1 If phosphorus or intact PTH levels cannot be controlled within the target range (see Guidelines 1, 3), despite dietary phosphorus restriction (see Guideline 4), phosphate binders should be prescribed (OPINION).

5.2 Calcium-based phosphate binders are effective in lowering serum phosphorus levels (EVIDENCE) and may be used as the initial binder therapy (OPINION).

In CKD Patients with Kidney Failure (Stage 5):

5.3 Both calcium-based phosphate binders and other noncalcium-, nonaluminum-, and nonmagnesium-containing phosphate-binding agents (such as sevelamer HCl) are effective in lowering serum phosphorus levels (EVIDENCE), and either may be used as the primary therapy (OPINION).

5.4 In dialysis patients who remain hyperphosphatemic (serum phosphorus > 5.5 mg/gL [1.78 mmol/L]) despite the use of either of calcium-based phosphate binders or other noncalcium-, nonaluminum-, nonmagnesium-containing phosphate-binding agents, a combination of both should be used (OPINION).

5.5 The total dose of elemental calcium provided by the calcium-based phosphate binders should not exceed 1,500 mg/day (OPINION), and the total intake of elemental calcium (including dietary calcium) should not exceed 2,000 mg/day (OPINION).

5.6 Calcium-based phosphate binders should not be used in dialysis patients who are hypercalcemic (corrected serum calcium of >10.2 mg/dL [2.54 mmol/L]), or whose plasma PTH levels are <150 pg/mL (16.5 pmol/L) on 2 consecutive measurements (EVIDENCE).

5.7 Noncalcium-containing phosphate binders are preferred in dialysis patients with severe vascular and/or other soft-tissue calcifications (OPINION).

5.8 In patients with serum phosphorus levels >7.0 mg/dL (2.26 mmol/L), aluminum-based phosphate binders may be used as a short-term therapy (4 weeks), and for one course only, to be replaced thereafter by other phosphate binders (OPINION). In such patients, more frequent dialysis should also be considered (EVIDENCE).

function becomes limited, decreased phosphorus excretion and increased dietary phosphorus retention lead to hyperphosphatemia (Malluche, Mawad, & Koszewski, 2002; Slatopolski, 2003). Generation of active vitamin D hormone (1,25-dihydroxycholecalciferol) is decreased along with a moderate decrease in ionized calcium, leading to over-stimulation of parathyroid hormone. Hyperparathyroidism can lead to bone disease, cardiovascular disease and/or mortality, and extraskeletal calcification of soft tissues such as blood vessels, lungs, joints, and kidneys (Slatopolsky 2003). Hyperphosphatemia can intensify hyperparathyroidism, leading to further secretion of parathyroid hormone (PTH) (Edwards 2002).

Hyperphosphatemia can be controlled via diet, phosphate binders, vitamin D therapy, and medical management of kidney function (Cupisti, Morelli, D'Alessandro, Lupetti, & Barsotti, 2003; Ford, Pope, Hunt, & Gerald, 2004). In CKD patients with elevated PTH levels and/or elevated serum phosphorus levels greater than 5.5, dietary phosphorus intake should be limited to 800 to 1,000 mg/day (NKF-K/DOQI 2003). Table 17-3 summarizes the K/DOQI dietary phosphorus restriction recommendations.

Several high-phosphorus foods are also high protein foods. As a result, patients must be followed closely by dietians to help insure adequate protein intake within recommended dietary guidelines. Patients are recommended to limit intake of dairy products, organ meats, nuts, and legumes to keep dietary phosphorus to a minimum. Table 17-4 identifies high-phosphorus food sources. Sargent and Lowrie (1982) have estimated that in a mixed diet, patients ingest 10.13 g phosphate for each 1 g protein. Patients with higher protein needs find it difficult to achieve adequate dietary protein while maintaining very low phosphate intakes.

Phosphorus-binding medications need to be taken with meals and snacks as dietary phosphate restriction is usually inadequate to manage serum levels of phosphorus or PTH within target range. Dietary restriction of phosphate is difficult as it is not a temporary intervention. Similar to dietary potassium, patients need to follow the dietary phosphate restriction long-term (Edwards, 2002). Nutrition education by the RD is critical for successful implementation of these recommendations (Ford, Pope, Hunt, & Gerald, 2004).

Several different types of phosphate binders are available to avoid hyperphosphatemia (see Table 17-5). There are three different types of calcium-based phosphate binders: calcium carbonate, calcium acetate, and calcium citrate. All three of them allow for at least 20% absorption of calcium. Calcium acetate is shown to have slightly higher phosphorus binding potential (Emmett, Sirmon, Kirkpatrick, Nolan, Schmitt, & Cleveland, 1991). Calcium phosphate binders can contribute to coronary artery calcification and should be monitored closely (Paret, 2003). In addition, the NKF-K/DOQI clinical guidelines for bone disease recommend non-calcium containing binders for dialysis patients with evidence of severe vascular and/or other soft-tissue calcification (see Table 17-3). In addition, the daily elemental calcium dose provided by calcium-based binders has been recommended to be limited to < 1,500 mg/day, and the total intake of elemental calcium, including dietary calcium, should not exceed 2,000 mg/day (NKF-K/DOQI, 2003a, b).

Magnesium carbonate is less frequently used as a phosphate binder. Magnesium carbonate can lead to hypermagnesemia and may a play a role in a dynamic bone disease. Aluminum hydroxide is a powerful phosphate-binding agent but can lead to osteomalacia, encephalopathy and aluminum toxicity (Cannata-Andia & Fernandez-Martin, 2002). If aluminum hydroxide is recommended as a binder in practice, it is generally recommended on a short-term basis. It should be noted that aluminum absorption is increased in the presence of citrate, including calcium citrate.

In response to concerns regarding elemental calcium intake, one non-calcium based binder is currently available – sevelamer hydrochloride. It is a non-mineral based phosphate binder that is a cationic polymer not absorbed but excreted in the feces. Sevelamer hydrochloride has been shown to be as effective at binding phosphorus as calcium carbonate and lowers cholesterol simultaneously (Chertow,

Table 17-4
Phosphate Content of Selected Foods

Food	Measure	Phosphorus (mg)	Protein (g)
Beans, black	1 cup	251	15
Soybeans, boiled	1 cup	421	29
Sunflower seeds	1 oz	322	6
Tofu, firm	100g	76	6
Cheese, cream	1 tbsp	15	1.09
Cheese, brie	1 oz	53	5.88
Milk, 2%	1 cup	232	8
Yogurt, low-fat	4 oz	162	6
Salmon	3 oz	282	21
Shrimp	3 oz	116	18
Peanuts, roasted	1 oz	147	8
Chocolate, semi-sweet	1 oz	37	1
Bread, wheat bran	1 slice	67	3.17
Caramel	1 package (2.5 oz)	81	3.27
Oat bran, raw	1 cup	690	16.26
Egg nog	1 cup	277	9.68

Table 17-5
Identification of Phosphate Binders and Calcium Content

Compound	Brand Name	Elemental Calcium (mg)
Calcium Carbonate	Tums EX	300
	Tums Ultra	400
	Oscal 500	500
	Calcichew	500
	Calci-Mix	500
	Caltrate 600	600
	Nephro-Calci	600
	Chooz Gum	200
Calcium Acetate	Phoslo	167
	Hil-Cal	113
Calcium Citrate	Citracal	76
Magnesium Carbonate	MagneBind 200	
	MagneBind	
Aluminum Hydroxide	AlternaGEL	
	Alu-Cap	
	Alu-Tab	
	Amphojel	
	Dialume	
Aluminum Carbonate	Basaljel	
Sevelamer HCL	Renagel	

2003; Logham-Adham, 1999). Advantages of sevelamer hydrochloride include that it can bind dietary phosphate without contributing to a positive calcium balance or resulting in hypercalcemia. It also binds to fatty acids and significantly lowers elevated low density lipoproteins (Chertow, 2003).

There is a constant search to find non-absorbable phosphate binders with maximum efficacy and no risk of mineral toxicity for chronic kidney disease patients. FDA approval has just been received for a lanthanum carbonate-based phosphate binder. Lanthanum cations are known to bind with phosphate anions and produce a product that is poorly absorbed by the gastrointestinal tract (Malluche, Mawad, & Koszewski, 2002). This product is planned for distribution in early 2005.

Hyperparathyroidism can be controlled in the CRF population by administration of active metabolites of vitamin D (Edwards 2002). Intravenous (IV) calcitriol and paricalcitol administered during dialysis suppresses PTH. However, both IV treatments increase intestinal calcium and phosphorus absorption and calcium mobilization from the bone, and should be limited with phosphorus and calcium levels above target range. Paricalcitol has been shown to mobilize less calcium and phosphorus from the bone than calcitriol (Malluche, Mawad, & Koszewski, 2002). Cinacalcet is a calcimimetic, recently approved by the FDA to suppress PTH. It works by binding to the calcium-sensing receptor, lowering PTH, serum calcium and phosphorus (Block, Martin, DeFrancisco, Turner, Avram, Suranyi et al., 2004). This pharmaceutical is recommended for the management of PTH and bone disease in patients who tend towards hypercalcemia and have demonstrated resistance to IV vitamin D therapy.

Table 17-6
Guidelines for Vitamin Supplements in Adults with Renal Disease

Vitamin	Nondialyzed Stage 3, 4, or 5 Chronic Kidney Disease	Chronic Hemodialysis	Chronic Peritoneal Dialysis
			Recommended Daily Intakes
Vitamin A	None	None	None
Vitamin E	400-800 IU	400-800 IU	400-800 IU
Vitamin K	None	None	None
Vitamin B1	1.1-1.2 mg	1.1-1.2 mg	1.1-1.2 mg
Riboflavin	1.1-1.3 mg	1.1-1.3 mg	1.1-1.3 mg
Vitamin B6	5 mg	10 mg	10 mg
Vitamin B12	2.4 µg	2.4 µg	2.4 µg
Vitamin C	75-90 mg	75-90 mg	75-90 mg
Folic acid	1 mg	1 mg	1 mg
Niacin	14-16 mg	14-16 mg	14-16 mg
Biotin	30 µg	30 µg	30 µg
Pantothenic acid	5 mg	5 mg	5 mg

Note: Modified from Chazot and Kopple (2005).

Other Vitamins and Minerals

Patients with renal disease are at increased risk for deficiencies of water-soluble vitamins, particularly vitamin C, folate, and pyridoxine (B6). Causes include altered intake of foods, drug-nutrient interactions, changes in retention and excretion patterns, interference in metabolism by uremic toxins, and losses to the dialysate (Chazot & Kopple, 2004). High doses of vitamin C may result in elevated plasma levels of oxalate. Supplementation should not exceed 75 to 90 mg/day, and supplementation with fat soluble vitamin A is not recommended. Studies have shown that patients develop hypervitaminosis A, which may result in bone resorption (Chazot & Kopple, 2004). Requirements for fat soluble vitamins E and K are thought to be similar to those of the general population. Patients need explanations as to why they take a special vitamin and instructions not to take multiple vitamins containing vitamin A or the standard form of vitamin D.

Vitamin formulations containing high dose folic acid have become available for the dialysis patient in response to the literature, suggesting that hyperhomocysteinemia is linked to cardiovascular disease and poor outcome in this patient population (Dennis & Robinson, 1996). The literature is controversial in this regard. Until the results of clinical trials currently in process are completed, it may be prudent to supplement in the range of 1 to 5 mg/day.

Vitamin supplements containing vitamin E, selenium, and zinc have also become available. Whether the higher cost of these supplements is warranted given results in a cardioprotective effects is not known. The potential for toxicity in each individual patient needs to be evaluated by the RD. A summation of suggested guidelines for vitamin supplements in adults with renal disease is shown in Table 17-6.

Iron metabolism plays an essential role in the anemia of CRF. Factors that contribute to anemia include failure of the kidney to secrete erythropoietin, blood loss of two to five liters per year from hemodialysis treatments, and possible binding of iron to the dialysis membrane (Frankenfield, Johnson, Wish, Rocco, Madore, & Owen, 2000). If left untreated, anemia can result in cardiac enlargement, ventricular hypertrophy, angina, heart failure, and malnutrition (Ma, Ebben, Hong, & Collins, 1999). Supplementation with recombinant human erythropoietin (rHuEPO) to replace the natural hormone dramatically decreases the incidence and severity of anemia seen prior to its availability. The K/DOQI recommended hematocrit and hemoglobin target levels are 33 to 36% and 11 to 12 g/dl, respectively (NKF-K/DOQI, 2000b). The general dose required for adult patients is 80 to 120 units rHuEPO/kg/week in two to three doses if administered subcutaneously. If the IV route is used, the general dosing is 120 to 180 units/kg body weight/week given over their dialysis sessions. The absolute dose depends on patient response (Albitar et al., 1995).

As a result of RHuEPO administration, most patients on dialysis replacement therapy will require iron replacement therapy (Nissenson & Strobos, 1999). This requirement is evaluated by monitoring serum ferritin and transferrin levels. Patients with iron deficiencies may not respond to erythropoietin. Patients may be prescribed oral iron supplements of 250 to 500 milligrams ferrous sulfate, or the equivalent ferrous fumerate or glutamate. However, IV iron administration has been observed to be more effective in treating iron deficiency anemia (Albitar et al., 1995).

Dietary requirements for other trace elements have not been well defined (Vanholder, Cornelis, Dhondt, & Lameire, 2004). Supplementation of the diet with zinc per day may improve dysgeusia (abnormal tastes), poor food intake, and impaired sexual function in some uremic patients. Increased body aluminum levels have been noted when patients are dialyzing without water purification systems or with high doses of aluminum-containing antacids. Therefore, use of aluminum-based antacids is discouraged (NKF-K/DOQI, 2003b). Elevated serum levels have been associated with anemia, osteomalacia, and dementia.

Protein and Energy

Protein intake must meet nutritional needs and compensate for any losses. Excessive intake enhances production of nitrogenous toxins while inadequate intake promotes protein malnutrition. Amino acid and protein losses occur with dialysis requiring a higher intake than needed for healthy adults. During HD, free amino acid losses average 4.5 to 7.7 grams and bound amino acid losses average 3.7 grams per treatment depending upon the type of dialyzer (Kalantar-Zadeh & Kopple, 2004). With CAPD and CCPD, both amino acids and albumin are lost across the peritoneal capillary membranes. Of the 4 to 15 grams lost daily, 50 to 80% is as albumin. Current protein recommendations for both patients on hemodialysis and peritoneal dialysis are 1.2 gms protein/kg body weight per day (NKF-K/DOQI, 2000a).

Quality of protein to meet essential amino acid (EAA) requirements is also important. Two-thirds of protein should be from HBV sources to assure that minimal EAA requirements are met. A strict vegan (plant products only) vegetarian diet can be difficult to plan using these guidelines. Dietitians generally work with combinations of legumes and soy products. The dietitian may recommend the use of calorically dense nondairy nutritional supplements added to a patient's usual intake to enhance vegan diets and to assure that all the EAA are provided.

Energy requirements for HD patients for weight maintenance, gain, and weight loss is an area of nutrition that is in need of further research. The number of studies that have actually measured energy expenditure in this patient population are limited in number and were completed in small numbers of patients (Ikizler, Wingard, Sun, Harvell, Parker, & Hakim, 1996; Ikizler, Pupim, Brouillette et al., 2002; Neyra, Chen, Un, Shyr, Hakim, & Ikizler, 2003; Monteon, Laidlaw, Shaib, & Kopple, 1986; Schneeweiss, Graninger, Stockenhuber, Druml, Ferenci, Eichinger et al., 1990). For example the study by Monteon et al. (1986) evaluated energy expenditure in 16 HD patients. Schneeweiss and colleagues (1990) measured energy expenditure in 25 HD patients. Both of these studies completed over 13 years ago, reported that resting energy expenditure in HD patients was not found to be different when compared to controls. In contrast, more recent studies by Ikizler et al. (1996, 1999, 2002) indicate that energy expenditure in this patient group is unique. Their results suggest that resting energy expenditure in HD patients is 1) greater than controls, 2) increased during dialysis when compared to pre- and post-HD, 3) higher during dialysis compared to non-dialysis day, and 4) increased during dialysis compared to controls. Their most recent study (2003) found that energy expenditure is greater in HD patients compared to patients with chronic kidney disease.

Therefore, there is conflicting data regarding energy expenditure in hemodialysis patients. The changes in dialysis treatment parameters such as type of dialyzer, blood flow rates, and dialysis treatment times could have an impact on energy expenditure and in part explain the difference in results reported in 1990 compared to the more recent data. However, even with consideration of these potential confounding factors, there is clearly a need for additional studies in this area.

Current energy recommendations for this patient population are based on an integration of data from studies that evaluated energy intake, energy measurements, and nitrogen balance. The *NKF-K/DOQI Clinical Practice Guidelines for Nutrition in Chronic Renal Failure* (2002) state the following: "The recommended daily energy intake for maintenance HD or patients with chronic PD is 35 kcal/kg body weight per day for those who are less than 60 years of age, and 30 to 35 kcal/kg body weight per day for individuals 60 years or older." This guideline statement is based on both evidence and opinion. The rationale for this energy guideline has been summarized as follows:

1. Studies evaluating calorie intake in hemodialysis patients have documented low energy intakes, averaging about 24 to 27 kcal/kg.
2. Resting energy expenditure (REE) studies have reported that hemodialysis patients have the same or slightly increased REE measurements compared to controls undergoing mild physical activity.
3. Nitrogen balance studies have indicated that at a calorie intake of 35 kcal/kg, neutral nitrogen balance is achieved with normalization of serum albumin and anthropometric measures.

For CAPD and CCPD patients, energy requirements are complicated by the use of dextrose as an osmotic agent in the PD fluids. Total energy intake recommended should include both the oral and the dialysate content. Grodstein, Blumenkrantz, Kopple, Moran, and Coburn (1981) proposed the following formula to calculate calories from absorbed dextrose:

$$Y = [(11.3\ X) - 10.9] \times L\ \text{dialysate} \times 3.7\ \text{kcal/g glucose}$$

The variable Y indicates the grams glucose absorbed per liter of dialysate, and X indicates the concentration of glucose (g/L). As much as 60 to 80% (100 to 250 g) of the dialysate dextrose can be absorbed and may account for more than one-third of the patient's daily caloric needs. It was initially thought that this extra energy source would aid the nutritionally compromised patient. However, there appears to be a spontaneous decrease in patients' intake in response to the dextrose load, precluding desired weight gains or reversals of malnutrition. Conversely, restriction of calories for weight reduction or weight maintenance in patients who are prone to obesity is complicated with high protein needs. In these patients, the dietitian often recommends the use of protein supplements to help replace protein losses, adding only minimal calories. The entire renal team can work together to encourage increased physical activity to prevent or help treat undesired weight gain.

Patients who have inadequate intake of protein and calories show a decrease in blood urea nitrogen (BUN), low serum proteins, particularly albumin, transferrin and prealbumin, and a low normalized protein catabolic rate (npcr). In stable patients, the npcr reflects dietary protein intake (Goldstein & Frederico, 1987). A summation of nutritional

Table 17-7
Nutrition Care Guidelines for Patients with CKD

Initial Nutrition Intervention

| Session: Initial | Length: 60-90 minutes | Time: Within 1 month of referral |

Factor	Interventions
Management Goals	1. Identify management goals of health care team. 2. Identify patient goals and expectations.
Nutrition Prescription	1. Calories – Individualized to maintain reasonable weight; use basal energy expenditure x activity factor (1.2-1.3) x stress factor; or use > 35 kcal/kg IBW or adjusted weight. 2. Protein – Based on creatinine clearance, GFR, urinary protein losses (0.6-1.0 g/kg IBW or adjusted weight), 50% from high biological value animal and/or plant sources. 3. Fats – For lipid abnormalities: fats, cholesterol, and carbohydrates adjusted per severity of risk factors (see Appendices G and H). 4. Sodium – Individualized, or 1-3 g/day. 5. Potassium – Individualized per lab values. 6. Phosphorus – Individualized, or 8-12 mg/kg IBW or adjusted weight; may require phosphate binder therapy. 7. Calcium – Individualized per calcium, phosphorus, and PTH lab values; use of vitamin D; and supplementation level. 8. Fluids – As desired to maintain appropriate hydration status. 9. Vitamin/mineral supplementation – As appropriate.
Self-Management Skills	1. Discuss simple definitions and examples of calories, protein, sodium, and other nutrients as appropriate (e.g., carbohydrates, fats, potassium, phosphorus, calcium, fluids). 2. Discuss basic dietary guidelines for renal insufficiency. 3. For diabetes, discuss basic dietary guidelines and timing of meals and snacks, if indicated. 4. Discuss laboratory tests and significance of results. 5. Discuss use and effect of phosphate binders, if prescribed. 6. Discuss food/drug interactions as indicated. 7. Discuss role and effect of diet and medications on renal function. 8. Discuss role of blood pressure control and blood glucose regulation in slowing the progression of renal failure. 9. Assess comprehension of education provided and projected compliance.
Functional Ability/Exercise	1. Provide necessary referrals for assistance with self-feeding and other activities of daily living (e.g., OT, PT, speech therapy). 2. Discuss exercise recommendations, if appropriate.
Behavioral Goals	1. Address eating and exercise behaviors. 2. Identify and summarize short-term behavioral goals that are specific and achievable. 3. Establish follow-up plan.
Communication	1. Document current nutritional status, plan of care, and goals of MNT. 2. Report recommendations/concerns to appropriate health care team member (e.g., MD, RN, pharmacist, social worker). 3. Provide information regarding nutrition prescription and dietary guidelines to referral source, extended care facility, home health care agencies, if appropriate.

Note: From Wiggins (2002).

care guidelines for CKD patients stages 1-5 are summarized in Tables 17-7 and 17-8.

Nutrition and Transplant

The overall goal of the post-transplant diet is to promote blood pressure control, prevent weight gain, normalize electrolyte imbalances, maximize bone density, control blood glucose levels, and promote overall good nutritional status

(Blue, 2002). While the renal transplant restores near normal kidney function, many metabolic challenges result (mainly as side effects of anti-rejection medication) that require special nutrition intervention. For example, 60% of renal transplant recipients develop hyperlipidemia. Approximately 40% of post-transplant mortality is due to cardiovascular death. Glucose intolerance is a common consequence and is associated with a higher risk for infection and decreased

Table 17-8

Nutrition Care Guidelines for Patients on Renal Replacement Therapy

Minimum Baseline Data Needed for Medical Nutrition Therapy

Factor	Data Needed
Laboratory Values with Dates (within 30 days of session)	1. BUN, creatinine 2. Albumin 3. Sodium, potassium, phosphorus, calcium 4. Serum glucose 5. Serum bicarbonate 6. PTH, if available 7. Hematocrit/hemoglobin 8. Ferritin, transferrin saturation 9. Dialysis adequacy and PET results 10. Urinalysis results (e.g., volume, urea, protein) 11. Others as appropriate (e.g., lipid profile, glycosylated hemoglobin, vitamin B12, folate)
Health Care Team's Goals for Patient	1. Patient prognosis 2. Expected outcome of nutrition therapy 3. Aggressive versus conservative measures
Medical History	1. Disease/condition causing *renal failure* 2. History of renal disease and treatment 3. Concurrent medical conditions (e.g., diabetes, cancer, HIV, cardiovascular disease, GI problems, hypertension, hyperlipidemia) 4. Any other medical or physical conditions with potential nutritional implications (e.g., surgery, infection, CVA, chemotherapy, blindness, neuropathies)
Medications/Therapies	1. Type of dialysis therapy and prescription 2. Diet order, tube-feeding order, parenteral nutrition order, and/or IDPN/IPN order 3. Any other treatments or therapies that may affect nutritional intake or status 4. Antihypertensives, diuretics 5. Anticoagulants 6. Phosphate binders 7. Vitamin/mineral supplements 8. Any other medications with food/drug interactions or nutritional impact (e.g., diabetes medications, GI medications, steroids)
Psychosocial Issues	1. Learning disabilities 2. Vision, hearing abilities 3. Cultural or language barriers 4. Mental status
Guidelines for Exercise	1. Medical clearance for exercise 2. Exercise limitations, if any

Note: From Wiggins (2002).

survival rates. Excessive weight gain exacerbates the hyperlipidemia and glucose intolerance, and may contribute to a metabolic syndrome increasing the risk of graft rejection. Table 17-9 summarizes long-term post-transplant complications.

During the post-transplant state, electrolyte imbalances may develop and include hypophosphatemia, which could contribute to a loss of bone density. Serum electrolytes should be closely monitored with appropriate intervention as indicated. Table 17-10 identifies the long-term post-transplant nutrition therapy recommended for adult kidney transplant recipients.

Nutritional Assessment

The renal dietitian assesses the patient's current nutritional status before recommending an appropriate diet. The assessment includes evaluation of clinical components, biochemical indices, body weight parameters, and body composition. Multiple measurements are required to evaluate all of these components (see Table 17-11). Parameters from each component are integrated together to evaluate and monitor each patient's nutritional status. These parameters have been discussed in detail elsewhere (Goldstein, 1998).

Another approach to nutrition assessment by integrating a larger number of different parameters is to use scoring systems.

Table 17-9
Long-Term Post-transplant Complications

Common Complications	Nutrition Therapy	Recommendations
Excessive weight	Appropriate calorie level for desired weight	1. Behavior modification 2. Exercise regimen of appropriate frequency, duration, and variety 3. Maintenance of adequate weight for height 4. Educate for side effects of medications
Hyperglycemia	Appropriate calorie level and carbohydrate distribution/restriction per American Diabetes Association guidelines	1. Appropriate weight status 2. Appropriate hypoglycemic medications 3. Adequate exercise 4. Diet education 5. Monitor glucose levels 6. Reduce corticosteroid doses as able
Hyperlipidemia	• American Heart Association guidelines with high fiber (-25 to 30 g/day) • < 30% of calories as fat • < 7 to 10% of calories as saturated fat • Weight loss, if indicated • Appropriate fat, cholesterol, and/or carbohydrate restrictions	1. Appropriate weight status 2. Adequate exercise 3. Behavior modification 4. Monitor lipid levels 5. Lipid-lowering drugs prn 6. Adjust immunosuppression drugs if able
Hypertension	Sodium-restricted diet	1. Appropriate weight status 2. Adequate exercise 3. Behavior modification 4. Monitor lipid levels
Osteoporosis	Adequate calcium, phosphorus, and vitamin D; supplement if needed; 1,000 to 1,500 mg calcium/day	1. Weight-bearing exercise 2. Maintenance of healthy lifestyle (no smoking) 3. Normal estrogen levels 4. Monitor vitamin and mineral levels prn

Note: From Blue (2002).

An example of such a system is the Subjective Global Assessment (SGA) (see Figure 17-1). The SGA process involves obtaining objective information by completing a medical history, physical examination, assessment of gastrointestinal symptoms, body weight patterns, and co-morbid conditions that affect nutritional requirements. Functional capacity is also evaluated. Subjective information is also reported, such as patient-reported food intake. Upon completion of the form, the patient is rated into one of three groups: well-nourished, mild-to-moderately malnourished, or severely malnourished. Nutrition intervention is then formulated. Whether the SGA is more useful as a screening and monitoring tool versus an assessment tool has yet to be determined. Determination for evidence of inflammation and cardiac calcification may need to be added for better sensitivity. Research is currently in process to validate the utility of the SGA in the hemodialysis patient population for nutrition assessment purposes. Results should be available in late 2005.

Malnutrition and Stage V CKD

Malnutrition is an important and modifiable risk factor for mortality in the patient receiving renal replacement ther-

apy. Multiple factors contributing to the development and persistence of malnutrition are summarized in Table 17-12. In addition to the serum albumin, serum cholesterol, creatinine, prealbumin, and phosphorus have all been identified to be important predictors of mortality (Block, Hulbert-Shearon, Levin, & Port, 1998; Chertow & Lazarus, 1997). Surveys report that 23 to 76% of patients on HD or PD show evidence of malnutrition (Chertow & Lazarus, 1997, Kalantar-Zadeh & Kopple, 2004). The importance of nutritional status on hemodialysis patient outcomes was first best demonstrated by the studies by Lowrie and Lew (1990). In a cross-sectional study of over 12,000 patients, this group showed that serum albumin was the most powerful predictor of death. While the normal range of serum albumin in most laboratories is 3.5 to 4.5 g/dl, values < 2.5 g/dl were associated with a risk of death 20 times that of the normal range, 4.0 to 4.5 g/dl. Additionally concerning was the finding that patients who had an albumin value in what was considered the normal range, 3.5 to 4.0 g/dl, had doubled the risk of death compared to those with an albumin in the range of 4.0-4.5 g/dl.

Over the subsequent 10 years, results from research has

Table 17-11
Components of Nutrition Assessment for Patients with CKD

1. Clinical	2. Food and Diet Intake	3. Biochemical	4. Body Weight	5. Body Composition
Physical examination	Diet history, food record or food frequency questionnaire	Visceral protein stores	History	Adipose stores
Nutrition assessment Scoring/screening Medical history	Appetite assessment	Static protein reserves	Actual	Lean body mass (skeletal muscle)
Psychosocial history	Quantitative food intake Qualitative food intake	Immune competence Vitamins, minerals and trace elements Fluid, electrolyte, and acid-base balance Anemia labs	Compared to standards Body mass index (BMI)	
Demographics Physical activity level Current medical/surgical issues	Food habits and patterns	Cardiovascular disease Lipid status, cardiac calcification Evidence of systemic inflammation	Weight change over time	
Prescribed medications Nutrient/drug interactions	Fluid intake/balance Lifestyle issues: physical activity	Bone disease labs	Goal weight	

Table 17-10
Long-term Post-transplant Nutrition Recommendations

Goals
1. Achieve or maintain desirable weight
2. Maintain acceptable blood glucose levels
3. Maintain cholesterol levels ≤200 mg/dL
4. Maintain normal blood pressure
5. Maintain optimal bone density
6. Minimize side effects of medications
7. Maintain healthy lifestyle

Nutrient Requirements	Recommendations
Calories	• 1.2-1.3 x BEE or adequate to maintain desirable weight
Protein	• 0.8-1.0 g/kg
Carbohydrate	• 45-50% total calories, 25-30 g dietary fiber per day
Fat	• ≤30% total kcal • ≤10% polyunsaturated • 10-15% monounsaturated • 7-10% saturated • <300 mg cholesterol/day
Fluid	• Ad lib
Vitamins	• RDA; supplement as needed
Minerals	• RDA; supplement or restrict as needed

Note: From Blue (2002).

Table 17-12
Factors Contributing to Malnutrition in CKD

1. Anorexia due to:
   a. nausea, emesis, medications
   b. uremia/uremic state of metabolism
   c. underdialysis
   d. accumulation of uremic toxins not completely removed by dialysis

2. Metabolic Acidosis
3. Endocrine disorders (insulin resistance, hyperparathyroidism, impaired response to IGF-1)

4. Comorbidity (infections, intercurrent illnesses)

5. Systemic inflammation

6. Reduced nutrient intake

7. Dialysis related:
   a. inadequate dose
   b. catabolism (bioincompatible membrane)
   c. loss of amino acids and protein into the dialysate
   d. reuse with bleach

8. Psychosocial:
   a. depression
   b. inability to purchase or prepare food adequately
   c. loss of/poor-fitting dentures

Figure 17-1
Subjective Global Assessment Scoring Sheet

Patient Name: _____ Patient ID: _____ Date: _____

Part 1: Medical History

	SGA Score		
	A	**B**	**C**

1. Weight Change

   A. Over change in past 6 months: kgs

   B. Percent change: _____ gain < 5% loss

                  _____% loss

                  _____>10% loss

   C. Change in past 2 weeks: _____ increase

                  _____ no change

                  _____ decrease

2. Dietary Intake

   A. Overall change: _____ no change

                  _____ change

   B. Duration: _____ weeks

   C. Type of change: _____ suboptimal solid diet _____ full-liquid diet

                  _____ hypocaloric liquids _____ starvation

3. Gastrointestinal Symptoms (persisting for >2 weeks)

   _____ none; _____ nausea; _____ vomiting; _____ diarrhea; _____ anorexia

4. Functional Impairment (nutritionally related)

   A. Overall impairment _____ none

                       _____ moderate

                       _____ severe

   B. Change in past 2 weeks _____ improved

                       _____ no change

                       _____ regressed

Part 2: Physical Examination

SGA Score			
Normal	**Mild**	**Moderate**	**Severe**

5. Evidence of: Loss of subcutaneous fat

                Muscle wasting

                Edema

                Ascites (hemo only)

Part 3: SGA Rating (check one)

   A. ☐ Well-Nourished   B. ☐ Mildly-Moderately Malnourished   C. ☐ Severely Malnourished

Note: From Baxter Healthcare Corporation (1993). Used with permission.

resulted in a new hypothesis that could potentially impact the evaluation of serum albumin as a nutrition assessment and monitoring tool. It has been determined that patients on dialysis replacement therapy have evidence of systemic inflammation. This is manifested through elevations in serum levels of pro-inflammatory cytokines such as tumor necrosis factor, interleukin-1, and interleukin-6 (Kaysen, 2002). These cytokines are associated with anorexia and muscle and fat wasting, generating an overall catabolic state of metabolism. In response to inflammation, hepatic synthesis of negative acute phase proteins increase, such as C Reactive Protein (CRP) (Kaysen, 2000). Serum levels of CRP have been used as a marker of systemic inflammation. Conversely, hepatic synthesis of acute phase proteins decreases, resulting in lowered serum levels. The serum albumin is one of several acute phase proteins. Therefore, hypoalbuminemia may be an effect of systemic inflammation rather than necessarily a change in protein and energy intake. In addition, if systemic inflammation induces a state of catabolism, intervention with aggressive diet and nutrition support may not be sufficient.

What factors trigger systemic inflammation is not currently clear. The hypothesis included the dialysis procedure itself, bioincompatible dialysis membranes, oxidative stress, or cardiovascular disease (CVD). CVD is the main cause of mortality in the hemodialysis patient population. It is hypothesized that a complex interplay between CVD and systemic inflammation are impacting nutritional status (Kaysen, 2000; O'Keefe & Daigle, 2002; Stenvinkel, Heimburger, Lindholm, Kaysen, & Bergstrom, 2000). The additive effects of systemic inflammation and potential catabolism resulting in weight loss, visceral muscle wasting, and poor outcome emphasizes the need to maintain strict and persistent nutritional assessment, monitoring, and interventions.

Nutritional Supplementation

To increase protein and energy in diets, dietitians increase the proportion of calorically dense foods in patients' diets (Karalis, 2002). The use of oral, enteral, and modular supplement products is common. For a program to be successful, it must be individualized, easy, and inexpensive for the patients. The dietitian can coordinate and facilitate this process. Some suggestions as to how this can be done are:
- Review nutritional parameters of all patients monthly and identify patients at risk.
- Educate patients on importance of nutrition in maintaining visceral stores in relation to patient outcomes.
- Give patients copies of their monthly serum chemistries, average interdialytic fluid gains, and weight changes.
- Work with usual food intake to increase protein and/or energy intake.
- Intervene early: within 1 month of indicators suggesting a deterioration in nutritional status.
- If supplements are needed, provide the patient with information regarding community resources for best product pricing.
- Follow patients closely to see that they are using the supplement.
- When necessary, involve the patient's family members to assure follow-through by the patients.

Intradialytic Parenteral Nutrition (IDPN)

When oral means are unsuccessful in correcting malnutrition, IDPN can be considered if the patient's insurance company will cover the cost. IDPN is potentially an anabolic therapy. The goal of IDPN is to restore nutritional status while the patient is unable to maintain an adequate intake to accomplish that goal. IDPN can serve as an effective alternative therapy for those HD patients who have not responded to, or who are not candidates for, oral or enteral nutritional therapy and cannot tolerate the fluid load of traditional parenteral nutrition (Cano, 2004; Goldstein & Strom, 1991).

IDPN therapy usually requires contract with an outpatient infusion pharmacy or company. The role of the company is to help determine if the patient qualifies for coverage and to provide the IDPN solutions. The IDPN solutions typically consist of amino acids, carbohydrate, and lipid. The nurses in the clinic infuse the formula directly into the venous drip chamber of the HD blood line. The infusion rate is determined by dividing the total IDPN solution volume by the patient's HD treatment time. Generally, it will not exceed 350 to 400 ml/hr. It is common to start with 500 ml amino acid and dextrose solution for the three treatments. On the first day that IDPN containing lipid is administered, nurses infuse the solution for 30 minutes and note any potential adverse reactions. If there are no side effects, lipids may be used in the solution thereafter. Lipids increase the calorie content of the solution dramatically. Nurses should take the solution out of the refrigerator in time for it to come to room temperature (about 30 minutes) and check the labels for dates and names to make sure the solution is current and is being given to the appropriate patient.

Most patients handle the formula without difficulty. There are some side effects, such as hyperglycemia, hypoglycemia, fluid overload, and a reaction to the lipids. Lipids should not be given to patients who report an egg allergy. If a reaction is going to occur, it is usually observed within the first 15 to 30 minutes after the test dose is administered. Symptoms observed include chest and back pain, dyspnea, dizziness, headache, nausea, and pressure over the eyes. Patients may experience wheezing, stridor, cyanosis, diaphoresis, fever, flushing, hypotension, or tachycardia. If a reaction is observed, stop the infusion immediately and alert the pharmacy.

Due to the high cost of IDPN and the CKD program, and with 93% of dialysis patients in the United States on the Medicare program, this therapy has been controversial. Foulks, Goldstein, Kelly, & Hunt (1991) suggest that IDPN (1) be reserved for malnourished patients who have not responded to intensive dietary counseling or oral supplementation, and (2) be administered for a minimum of 3 months. Current Medicare coverage dictates that patients meet the requirements for medical necessity. The policy, founded in the Medicare prosthetic device benefit, assumes that provision of parenteral nutrition administered only during dialysis would rarely be medically necessary. The nutrition assessment must show that the patient is severely malnourished, unable to absorb orally administered nutrients, and able to pass the test of permanence (require treatment for a minimum of 3 months) (Medicare/Medicaid, 1990).

Intraperitoneal Nutrition (IPN)

Nutritional dialysates, or IPN, have been shown to have positive effects in PD patients. These dialysates substitute amino acids for dextrose as the osmotic agent for one or two exchanges a day. Many studies have demonstrated that amino acid-based dialysates are safe and effective. Amino acids were first infused into the peritoneum in 1968 (Goldstein & Strom, 1991). In 1982, investigators reported an 80 to 90% absorption of amino acids after a 6-hour dwell of a 2-liter, 2% amino acid solution. This equaled 32 to 36 grams of amino acids. Bruno, Bagnis, Marangella, Rovera, Cantaluppi, and Linari (1989) documented an increased nitrogen balance after using a 1% amino acid solution once a day for 6 months (Wise, 1993). Compatibility of medications added to IPN depend on concentration of the mixture, length of storage, contact, and existence of other additives. Those medications that can be added safely to PD solutions are also compatible with the IPN solution.

Patient Education

The diet for CKD stages I-V is challenging for both the patient and the health care team. Nutrition education and continued reinforcement are essential aspects of medical management of the renal patient. Dietitians must balance the need to limit intake of nutrients with the need to provide adequate energy and protein to maintain or restore adequate nutritional status. The diet is a mainstay of therapy for the comorbid conditions that impact all stages of CKD: malnutrition, bone disease, anemia, and cardiovascular disease. Nutrition intervention should therefore start in the early phases of chronic kidney disease (Curtin, Becker, Kimmel, & Schatell, 2003). Nutrition care also plays a role in the prevention of kidney disease by addressing the common dietary risk factors associated with progressive CKD.

Uncontrolled diabetes mellitus and hypertension are the two largest causes of kidney failure. Forty percent of people with type-2 diabetes are predicted to develop kidney failure, and the majority with diabetic nephropathy will have a increased risk of cardiovascular disease (Lewis & Lewis, 2003). Death from cardiovascular morbidity is 9 to 10 times higher in the dialysis patient population when compared to that of the normal population (Wheeler, 1997). It is important for the dietitian and the patient to integrate the multifaceted nutritional recommendations to promote optimal health.

Adherence to a renal nutrition plan is not always achieved as a result of patient co-morbidities, social and familial conditions, and psychosocial limitations. Nutrition goals should encompass the least amount of change to one's preferred food choices and lifestyle. Reinforcement of the importance of an individual's nutrition plan by the health care team is a crucial part in making nutritional counseling successful (Cupisti et al., 2003). Educating CKD patients on the important nutritional adaptations that would most benefit health does not always influence self-management. Because CKD affects the physical, social, emotional, and cognitive aspects of a person, it is important that education also incorporates these same items. Motivation and empowerment of the patient is very important (Tsay & Hung, 2004).

Cultural Diversity

In the multicultural world of kidney disease, it is essential that health care practitioners understand and accept a vast range of cultural beliefs about health, food, and treatment (Nardi & Rooda, 2004). Diversity in culture can be seen throughout gender, religion, age, socioeconomic, occupation, and ritual differences. A dietitian can be more effective by working within patients' respective cultures to help them translate nutritional recommendations into daily life practices.

In 2003, the greatest percentage of ESRD patients were age 65 to 74. Since 1990, the rate of ESRD prevalence have nearly doubled in all races with Asians having the largest increase in incidence rate of the disease. CKD, stage 5, is most prevalent in Blacks and Native Americans. CKD, stage 5, occurs 4.4 times more often in Blacks and 3.5 times more often in Native Americans than in that of Caucasians. In addition, CKD, stage 5, is more common in males than in females (U.S. Renal Data Systems [USRDS], 2003).

With a rise in the number of culturally diverse dialysis clinics, health care practitioners have had to sensitize themselves to variations in the types of food important to their patients. Many resources are available to dietitians. Diet material for different cultures and ethnic groups is available through the American Dietetic Association's Web site (www.eatright.org).

Medical Nutrition Therapy

In January 2002, Medicare implemented the Medical Nutrition Therapy (MNT) program that provides reimbursement of nutrition care provided by Registered Dietitians to Medicare patients who have a diagnosis of chronic renal insufficiency or diabetes (Williams & Chianchiano, 2002). In response to this, the American Dietetic Association has published MNT protocols that detail the specific populations that can be served, the specifics regarding types of data to be collected within defined time frames, and types of interventions to be considered (Schiro-Harvey, 2002, Wiggins, 2002). A reproduction of a flow chart for the patient with a GFR in the range of 13 to 50 ml/min (which correlates to ranges within CKD stages 3 and 4) is shown as Figure 17-2.

Summary

The renal diet is an integral component of the patient's overall treatment. The diet is complex, and the challenge of caring for these patients continues to grow with advances in research and technology. Guidelines for dietary modifications continue to be made available and updated from the main organizations and resources dedicated to serving this patient population. These include the National Kidney Foundation, the Council on Renal Nutrition of the National Kidney Foundation, (www.jrnjournal.org), and the Renal Practice Group of the American Dietetic Association. The *Journal of Renal Nutrition* is the main professional research and clinical journal entirely committed to the specialty of nutrition and kidney disease. Results from research in the areas of nutrition assessment, metabolism, systemic inflammation, and cardiovascular disease will continue to challenge renal care practitioners as to how to best utilize nutrition intervention to improve patient outcomes. In the mean-

Figure 17-2
Flow Chart of Nutrition Care for Patients with CKD

Adult Pre-ESRD Flowchart

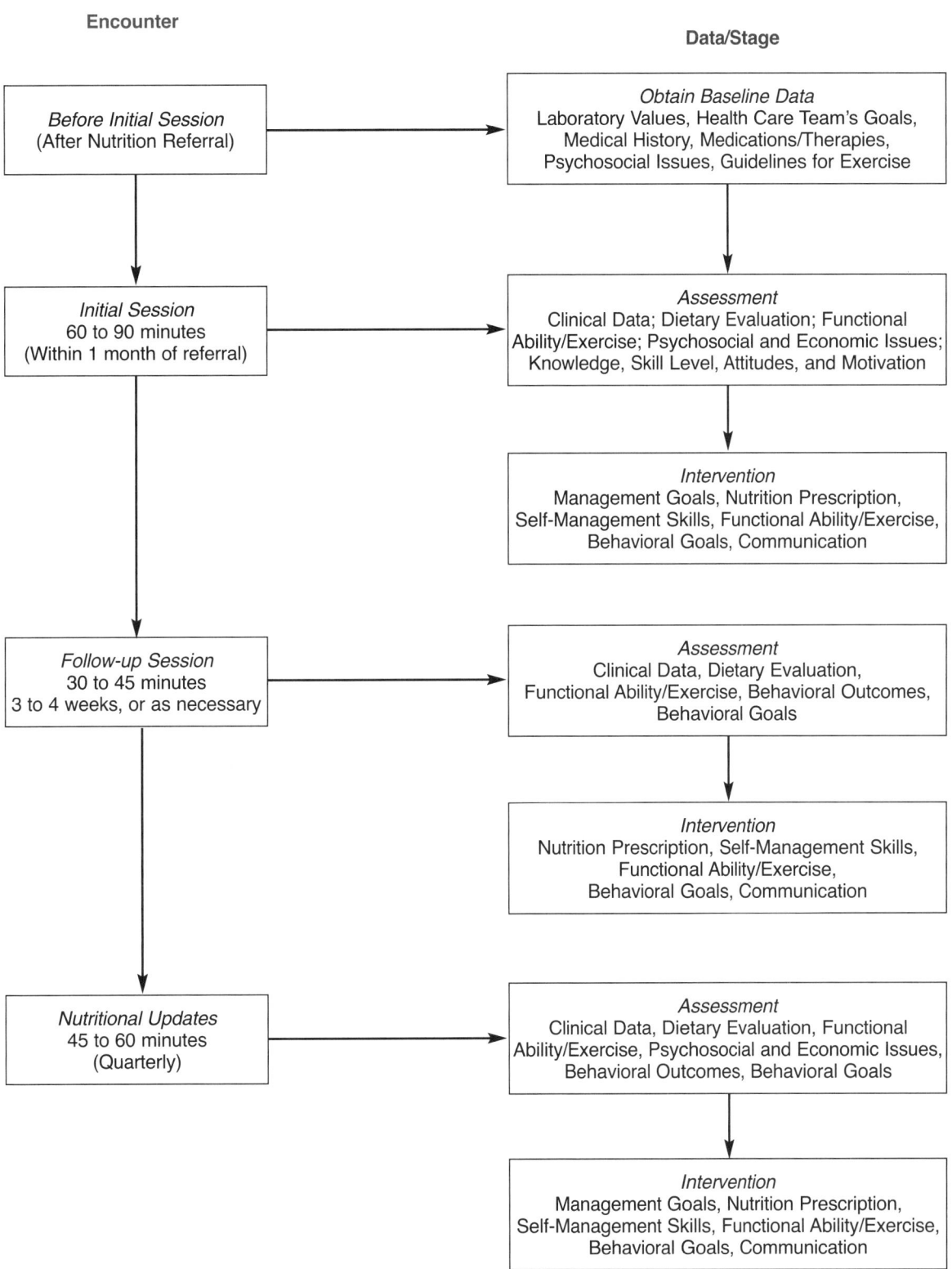

Encounter

Data/Stage

Before Initial Session
(After Nutrition Referral)

Obtain Baseline Data
Laboratory Values, Health Care Team's Goals,
Medical History, Medications/Therapies,
Psychosocial Issues, Guidelines for Exercise

Initial Session
60 to 90 minutes
(Within 1 month of referral)

Assessment
Clinical Data; Dietary Evaluation; Functional
Ability/Exercise; Psychosocial and Economic Issues;
Knowledge, Skill Level, Attitudes, and Motivation

Intervention
Management Goals, Nutrition Prescription,
Self-Management Skills, Functional Ability/Exercise,
Behavioral Goals, Communication

Follow-up Session
30 to 45 minutes
3 to 4 weeks, or as necessary

Assessment
Clinical Data, Dietary Evaluation,
Functional Ability/Exercise, Behavioral Outcomes,
Behavioral Goals

Intervention
Nutrition Prescription, Self-Management Skills,
Functional Ability/Exercise,
Behavioral Goals, Communication

Nutritional Updates
45 to 60 minutes
(Quarterly)

Assessment
Clinical Data, Dietary Evaluation, Functional
Ability/Exercise, Psychosocial and Economic Issues,
Behavioral Outcomes, Behavioral Goals

Intervention
Management Goals, Nutrition Prescription,
Self-Management Skills, Functional Ability/Exercise,
Behavioral Goals, Communication

Note: From Wiggins, K.L. (2002). *Guidelines for Nutrition Care of Renal Patients.* Renal Dieticians Dietetic Practice Group. Chicago: American Dietetic Association. Used with permission.

time, nutrition assessment, monitoring, patient education with continual reinforcement, and individualized diet application is among the best clinical outputs we can provide to all CKD patients.

References

Albitar, S., Meulders, Q., Hammond, H., Soutif, C., Bouvier, P., & Pollini, J. (1995). Intravenous versus subcutaneous dosing of epoetin alfa in hemodialysis patients. *American Journal of Kidney Disease, 26,* 331-340.

American Dietetic Association. (2002). *Medical nutrition therapy evidence based guides for practice. Chronic kidney disease (non-dialysis) medical nutrition therapy protocol.* Chicago: American Dietetic Association.

Beto, J., & Bansal, V.K. (1992). Hyperkalemia: Evaluating dietary and nondietary etiology. *Journal of Renal Nutrition, 2,* 28-29.

Block, G.A., Hulbert-Shearon, T.E., Levin, N.W., & Port, F.K. (1998). Association of serum phosphorus and calcium x phosphate product with mortality risk in chronic hemodialysis patient: A national study. *American Journal of Kidney Disease, 31,* 607-617.

Block, G.A., Martin, K.J., DeFrancisco, A.L.M, Turner, S.A., Avram, M.M., Suranyi, M.G., et al. (2004). Cinacalcet for secondary hyperparathyroidism in patients receiving hemodialysis. *The New England Journal of Medicine, 350,* 1516-1525.

Blue, L. (2002). Adult kidney transplantation. In J Hasse & L Blue (Eds), *Comprehensive guide to transplant nutrition* (pp. 44-57). Chicago: American Dietetic Association.

Briggs, J.P., & Schnermann, J.B. (1994). Overview of renal function. In A. Greenberg (Ed.), *Primer on kidney diseases* (pp. 1-16). Boston: Academic Press.

Bruno, M., Bagnis, C., Marangella, M., Rovera, L., Cantaluppi, A., & Linari, F. (1989). CAPD with an amino acid dialysis solution: A long-term, crossover study. *Kidney International, 35,* 1189-1194.

Burrowes J., & Cockram, D. (2004). Achieving patient adherence to diet therapy. In J. Kopple & S. Massry (Eds.), *Nutritional management of renal disease* (pp. 629-639). Philadelphia: Lippincott, Williams & Wilkins.

Cannata-Andia, J.B., & Fernandez-Martin, J.L. (2002). The clinical impact of aluminum overload in renal failure. *Nephrology Dialysis Transplant, 17*(2), 9-12.

Cano, N. (2004). Intradialytic parenteral nutrition: Where do we go from here? *Journal of Renal Nutrition, 14*(1), 3-5.

Chazot, C., & Kopple, J. (2004). Vitamin metabolism and requirements in renal disease and renal failure. In J. Kopple & S. Massry (Eds.), *Nutritional management of renal disease* (pp. 315-356). Philadelphia: Lippincott, Williams & Wilkins.

Chertow, G., & Lazarus, M. (1997). Malnutrition as a risk factor for morbidity and mortality in maintenance dialysis patients. In J. Kopple & S. Massry (Eds.), *Nutritional management of renal disease.* Philadelphia: Lippincott, Williams & Wilkins.

Chertow, G.M. (2003). Slowing the progression of vascular calcification in hemodialysis. *Journal of the American Society of Nephrology, 14,* S310-S314.

Cupisti, A., Morelli, F., D'Alessandro, C., Lupetti, S., & Barsotti, G. (2003) Phosphate control in chronic uremia: Don't forget diet. *Journal of Nephrology, 16*(1), 29-33.

Curtin, R.B., Becker, B., Kimmel, P.L., & Schatell, D. (2003). An integrated approach to care for patients with chronic kidney disease. *Seminars in Dialysis, Rehabilitation of Dialysis Patients, 16*(5), 399-402.

Dennis, V.W., & Robinson, K. (1996). Homocysteinemia and vascular disease in end stage renal disease. *Kidney International, 57,* S11-S17.

Edwards, R.M. (2002). Disorders of phosphate metabolism in chronic renal disease. *Current Opinion in Pharmacology, 2*(2), 171-176.

Emmett, M., Sirmon, M.D., Kirkpatrick, W.G., Nolan,C.R., Schmitt, G.W., & Cleveland, M.B. (1991). Calcium acetate control of serum phosphorus in hemodialysis patients. *American Journal of Kidney Disease, 17*(5), 544-550.

Falkenhain, M., Hartman, J., & Hebert, L. (2004). Nutritional management of water, sodium, potassium, chloride, and magnesium in

renal disease and renal failure. In J. Kopple & S. Massry (Eds.), *Nutritional management of renal disease* (pp.287-298). Philadelphia: Lippincott, Williams & Wilkins.

Ford, J.C., Pope, J.F., Hunt, A.E., & Gerald, B. (2004). The effect of diet education on the laboratory values and knowledge of hemodialysis patients with hyperphosphatemia. *Journal of Renal Nutrition, 14*(1), 36-44.

Foulks, C.J., Goldstein, D.J., Kelly, M.P., & Hunt, J.M. (1991). Indications for the use of intradialytic parenteral nutrition in the malnourished hemodialysis patient. *Journal of Renal Nutrition, 1,* 23-33.

Frankenfield, D., Johnson, C.A., Wish, J.B., Rocco, M.N., Madore, F., & Owen, W.F. (2000). Anemia management of adult hemodialysis patients in the U.S.: Results from the 1997 ESRD Core Indicators project. *Kidney International, 57,* 578-589.

Goldstein, D.J., & Frederico, C. (1987). The effect of urea kinetic modeling on the nutritional management of chronic hemodialysis patients. *Journal of the American Dietetic Association, 87*(4), 474-479.

Goldstein, D.J. (1998). Assessment of nutritional status. In W. Mitch & S. Klahr (Eds.), *Handbook of nutrition and the kidney* (pp. 45-86). Philadelphia: Lippincott-Raven.

Goldstein, J., & Strom, J.A. (1991). Intradialytic parenteral nutrition: Evolution and current concepts. *Journal of Renal Nutrition, 1,* 9-22.

Goodman, W.G., London, G., Amann, K., Block, G.A., Giachelli, C., Hruska, K.A., et al. (Vascular Calcification Work Group). (2004). Vascular calcification in CKD. *American Journal of Kidney Disease, 43*(3), 572-579.

Grodstein, G.P., Blumenkrantz, M.J., Kopple, J.D., Moran, J.K., & Coburn, J.W. (1981). Glucose absorption during continuous ambulatory peritoneal dialysis. *Kidney International, 19,* 564-567.

Ikizler, T.A., Wingard, R., Sun, M., Harvell, J., Parker, R., & Hakim, R. (1996). Increased energy expenditure in hemodialysis patients. *JASN, 7,* 2646-2653.

Ikizler, T., Wingard, R.L., Harvell, J., Shyr, Y., & Hakim, R. (1999). Association of morbidity with markers of nutrition and inflammation in chronic hemodialysis patients:A prospective study. *Kidney International, 55,* 1945-1951.

Ikizler, T.A., Pupim, L.B., Brouillette, J.R., et al. (2002). Hemodialysis stimulates muscle and whole body protein loss and alters substrate oxidation. *American Journal of Endocrinology and Metabolism, 282,* E107-E116.

Kalantar-Zadeh, K., & Kopple, J. (2004). Nutritional management of patients undergoing maintenance hemodialysis. In: J. Kopple & S. Massry (Eds.), *Nutritional management of renal disease* (pp. 433-466). Philadelphia: Lippincott, Williams & Wilkins.

Karalis, M. (2002). Ways to increase protein intake. *Journal of Renal Nutrition, 12*(2), 136-138.

Kaysen, G. (2002). Role of inflammation and its treatment in ESRD patients. *Blood Purification, 20*(1),70-80.

Kaysen, G. (2000). Malnutrition and the acute-phase reaction in dialysis patients-how to measure and how to distinguish. *Nephrology Dialysis Transplantation, 15*(10), 1521-1524.

Klahr, S. (1998). Effects of renal insufficiency on nutrient metabolism and endocrine function. In W. Mitch & S. Klahr (Eds.), *Handbook of nutrition and the kidney* (pp. 25-44). Philadelphia: Lippincott-Raven.

Klahr, S., Levey, A.S., Beck, G.J., Caggiula, A.W., Hunsicker, L., Kusek, J., et al. (1994). The effects of dietary protein restriction and blood pressure control on the progression of chronic renal failure: modification of diet in renal disease study group. *New England Journal of Medicine, 30*(13), 878-884.

Kopple, J.D. (1994). Effect of nutrition on morbidity and mortality in maintenance hemodialysis patients. *American Journal of Kidney Disease, 24,* 1002-1009.

Lewis, E.J., & Lewis J.B. (2003). Treatment of diabetic nephropathy with angiotensin II receptor antagonist. *Clinical and Experimental Nephrology, 7*(1), 1-8.

Loghman-Adham, M. (1999). Phosphate binders for control of phosphate retention in chronic renal failure. *Pediatric Nephrology, 13,* 701-708.

Lowrie, E.G., & Lew, N.L. (1990). Death risk in hemodialysis patients: the predictive value of commonly measured variables and an evaluation of death rate between facilities. *American Journal of Kidney Disease, 15*(5), 458-482.

Ma, J., Ebben, J., Hong, X., & Collins, A. (1999). Hematocrit level and associated mortality in hemodialysis patients. *Journal of the American Society of Nephrology, 10,* 610-619.

Malluche, H.M., Mawad, H., & Koszewski, N.J. (2002). Update on vitamin D and its newer analogues: Actions and rationale for treatment in chronic renal failure. *Kidney International, 62,* 367-374.

Martin, C., & Reams, R. (2003). The renal dietitian's role in managing hyperphosphatemia and secondary hyperparathyroidism in dialysis patients: A national survey. *Journal of Renal Nutrition, 13*(2), 133-136.

Mitch, W.E. (1997). Influences of diet on the progression of chronic renal insufficiency. In J. Kopple & S. Massry (Eds.), *Nutritional management of renal disease* (pp 317-340). Baltimore, MD: Williams & Wilkins.

Monteon, F.J., Laidlaw, S.T., Shaib, J.K., & Kopple, J.K. (1986). *Kidney International, 30,* 741-747.

Nardi, D.A., & Rooda, L.A. (2004). Diversity and patient care in a shrinking world. *Advances in Renal Replacement Therapy, 11*(1), 1-6.

Neyra, R., Chen, K.Y., Un, M., Shyr, Y., Hakim, R., & Ikizler, R. (2003). Increased resting energy expenditure in patients with end-stage renal disease. *Journal of Parenteral and Enteral Nutrition, 27*(1), 36-42.

Nissenson, A.R., & Strobos, J. (1999). Iron deficiency in patients with renal failure. *Kidney International, 55,* S18-S21.

NKF-K/DOQI. (2000a). Clinical practice guidelines for nutrition in chronic renal failure, *American Journal of Kidney Disease, 35*(Suppl. 2),:S1-S140.

NKF-K/DOQI. (2000b). Clinical practice guidelines for the treatment of anemia of chronic kidney disease. *American Journal of Kidney Disease, 37*(Suppl. 1), S182-S238.

NKF-K/DOQI. (2002). Clinical practice guidelines for chronic kidney disease: evaluation, classification, and stratification. *American Journal of Kidney Disease, 39*(Suppl. 1), S1-S000.

NKF-K/DOQI. (2003a). Clinical practice guidelines for managing dyslipidemias in chronic kidney disease. *American Journal of Kidney Disease, 41*(Suppl. 3), S1-S91.

NKF-K/DOQI. (2003b). Clinical practice guidelines for bone metabolism and disease in chronic kidney disease. *American Journal of Kidney Disease, 42*(Suppl. 3), S1-S202.

NKF-K/DOQI. (2004). Clinical practice guidelines on hypertension and antihypertensive agents in chronic kidney disease. *American Journal of Kidney Disease, 43*(Suppl. 1), S1-S290.

O'Keefe, A., & Daigle, N. (2002). A new approach to classifying malnutrition in the hemodialysis patient. *Journal of Renal Nutrition, 12*(4), 248-255.

Paret, C.L. (2003). Calcium containing phosphate binder use associated with accelerated atherosclerotic coronary calcification. *Journal of Renal Nutrition, 13*(4), 1-8.

Redmond, A,, McDevitt, M., & Barnes, S. (2004). Beta-1 integrins and glomerular injury. *Journal of Medical Investigation, 51*(1-2),1-13.

Sargent, J.A., & Lowrie, E.G. (1982). Which mathematical model to study uremic toxicity? National Cooperative Dialysis Study. *Clinical Nephrology, 17,* 303-314.

Schiro-Harvey, K. (Ed.). (2002). *National renal diet professional guide.* Chicago: American Dietetic Association.

Schneeweiss, B., Graninger, W., Stockenhuber, F., Druml, W., Ferenci, P., Eichinger, S., et al. (1990). Energy metabolism in acute and chronic renal failure. *American Journal of Clinical Nutrition, 52,* 596-601.

Slatopolsky, E. (2003). New developments in hyperphosphatemia management. *Journal of the American Society of Nephrology, 14,* S297-S299.

Stenvinkel, P., Heimburger, O., Lindholm, B., Kaysen, G.A., & Bergstrom, J. (2000). Are there two types of malnutrition in chronic renal failure? Evidence for relationships between malnutrition, inflammation and atherosclerosis (MIA syndrome). *Nephrology Dialysis Transplantation, 15*(7), 953.

Tsay, S., & Hung, L. (2004) Empowerment of patients with end-stage renal disease-a randomized controlled trial. *International Journal of Nursing Studies, 41*(1), 59-65.

U.S. Renal Data System (USRDS). (2003). *USRDS 2003 annual data report atlas.* Bethesda, MD: National Institutes of Health, National Institute of Diabetes and Digestive and Kidney Disease.

Vanholder, R., Cornelis, R., Dhondt, A., & Lameire, M. (2004). Trace element metabolism in renal disease. In J. Kopple & S. Massry (Eds), *Nutritional management of renal disease* (pp. 299-313). Philadelphia: Lippincott, Williams & Wilkins.

Vattikuti, R., & Toweler, D.A. (2004). Osteogenic regulation of vascular calcification: An early perspective. *American Journal of Physiology Endocrinology and Metabolism, 28*(5), 686-696.

Wheeler, D. (1997). Cardiovascular risk factors in patients with chronic renal failure. *Journal of Renal Nutrition, 7,* 182-186.

Wiggins, K.L. (2002). *Guidelines for nutrition care of renal patients. Renal Dietitians Dietetic Practice Group.* Chicago: American Dietetic Association.

Williams, M., & Chianchiano, J.D. (2002). Medicare medical nutrition therapy: Legislative process and product. *Journal of Renal Nutrition, 12*(1), 1-7.

- Nutritional management of chronic kidney disease (CKD) is an integral component of the medical care of both progressive and end-stage disease. Malnutrition, cardiovascular disease, bone disease, and anemia are the most common co-morbid conditions that accompany kidney disease, and they require both medical and nutritional intervention.

- In an effort to provide evidence-based clinical practice guidelines for the care of patients with chronic kidney disease, the National Kidney Foundation (NKF) launched the Disease Outcomes Quality Initiatives (DOQI) in March 1995 (NKF-K/DOQI, 2000a). The guidelines have been completed for key components of care, including nutrition (NKF-K/DOQI, 2000a), anemia (NKF-K/DOQI, 2000b), chronic kidney disease (NKF-K/DOQI, 2002), dyslipidemia (NKF-K/DOQI, 2003a), bone disease (NKF-K/DOQI, 2003b), and hypertension (NKF-K/DOQI, 2004).

- While creatinine has traditionally been the standard of care to evaluate kidney function, the CKD K/DOQI guidelines determined that serum creatinine concentration alone should not be used to evaluate kidney function. The serum creatinine level is not an accurate index of kidney function by itself because the assumptions upon which the accuracy is based are not always valid.

- Studies completed in experimental models of renal disease have documented that high-protein diets lead to increased proteinuria, renal damage, and mortality, while dietary protein restriction results in improvements (Mitch, 1997).

- The diet for dialysis compensates for lack of kidney function and dialysate losses, provides adequate nutrients for optimal health, and alleviates symptoms of uremia. The dietitian individualizes each patient's nutrition plan based on current nutritional status, pertinent serum laboratory values, and the treatment modality.

- The overall goal of the post-transplant diet is to promote blood pressure control, prevent weight gain, normalize electrolyte imbalances, maximize bone density, control blood glucose levels, and promote overall good nutritional status (Blue, 2002).

- Malnutrition is an important and modifiable risk factor for mortality in the patient receiving renal replacement therapy. Multiple factors contributing to the development and persistence of malnutrition are summarized in Table 17-11.

- To increase protein and energy in diets, dietitians increase the proportion of calorically dense foods in patients' diets (Karalis, 2002). The use of oral, enteral, and modular supplement products is common. For a program to be successful, it must be individualized, easy, and inexpensive for the patients. The dietitian can coordinate and facilitate this process.

- The diet for CKD stages I-V is challenging for both the patient and the health care team. Nutrition education and continued reinforcement are essential aspects of medical management of the renal patient. Dietitians must balance the need to limit intake of nutrients with the need to provide adequate energy and protein to maintain or restore adequate nutritional status.

- Guidelines for dietary modifications continue to be made available and updated from the main organizations and resources dedicated to serving this patient population. These include the National Kidney Foundation, the Council on Renal Nutrition of the National Kidney Foundation, (www.jrnjournal.org), and the Renal Practice Group of the American Dietetic Association.

Nutrition & Chronic Kidney Disease

Name of Resource	Brief Description	Where to Obtain Resource
Journal of Renal Nutrition Web site	The official Web site of the *Journal of Renal Nutrition* (JREN). The *JREN* is an interdisciplinary professional journal of the National Kidney Foundation Council on Renal Nutrition and the International Society on Nutrition & Metabolism in Renal Disease. Peer-reviewed and listed in Index Medicus, the *JREN* includes original research articles as well as material applicable for the clinical setting.	**www.jrnjournal.org**
National Kidney Foundation official Web site	The official site of the National Kidney Foundation (NKF) with links to the Council on Renal Nutrition (CRN), the largest organization of renal dietitians nationwide and around the world. Provides updates on the K/DOQI. A main source for information pertaining to kidney disease for both patients and professionals.	**www.kidney.org**
American Dietetic Association official Web site	The official site of the American Dietetic Association (ADA) that includes a link to the Dietitians Renal Practice Group (RPG). The ADA through the RPG and often in collaboration with CRN, is a source for new publications and information for use by the renal professional with patients.	**www.eatright.org**
iKidney.com - Worldwide Kidney Disease Community Web site	A Web site sponsored by Watson Pharma, Inc. that includes information regarding nutrition, pharmaceuticals and social issues. Often a source for recipes that are appropriate for patients as identified.	**www.ikidney.com**
Kidney School Web site	A Web site that provides education regarding all aspects of kidney disease. Excellent for patients.	**www.kidneyschool.org**
Centers for Medicare and Medicaid Services Web site	The Web site for reporting clinical performance measures (CPM) of the End-Stage Renal Disease (ESRD) program.	**http://cms.hhs.gov/esrd/1.asp**

ANNP617

Nutrition and Chronic Kidney Disease

Jordi Goldstein-Fuchs, DSc, RD

Contemporary Nephrology Nursing: Principles and Practice contains 39 chapters of educational content. Individual learners may apply for continuing nursing education credit by reading a chapter and completing the Continuing Education Evaluation Form for that chapter. Learners may apply for continuing education credit for any or all chapters.

Please photocopy this page and return to ANNA.
COMPLETE THE FOLLOWING:

Name: _____

Address: _____

City: _____ State: _____ Zip: _____

E-mail: _____

Preferred telephone: ☐ Home ☐ Work: _____

State where licensed and license number (optional): _____

CE application fees are based upon the number of contact hours provided by the individual chapter. CE fees per contact hour for ANNA members are as follows: 1.0-1.9 - $15; 2.0-2.9 - $20; 3.0-3.9 - $25; 4.0 and higher - $30. Fees for nonmembers are $10 higher.

ANNA Member: ☐ Yes ☐ No Member # (if available) _____

☐ Checked Enclosed ☐ American Express ☐ Visa ☐ MasterCard

Total Amount Submitted: _____

Credit Card Number: _____ Exp. Date: _____

Name as it appears on the card: _____

CE Evaluation Form
To receive continuing education credit for individual study after reading the chapter
1. Photocopy this form. (You may also download this form from ANNA's Web site, **www.annanurse.org.**)
2. Mail the completed form with payment (check) or credit card information to American Nephrology Nurses' Association, East Holly Avenue, Box 56, Pitman, NJ 08071-0056.
3. You will receive your CE certificate from ANNA in 4 to 6 weeks.

Test returns must be postmarked by **December 31, 2010.**

CE Application Fee
ANNA Member $15.00
Nonmember $25.00

EVALUATION FORM

1. I verify that I have read this chapter and completed this education activity. Date: _____

_____
Signature

2. What would be different in your practice if you applied what you learned from this activity? *(Please use additional sheet of paper if necessary.)*

_____
_____
_____
_____
_____
_____
_____
_____
_____
_____
_____

Evaluation	Strongly disagree				Strongly agree
3. The activity met the stated objectives.					
a. Compare and contrast the recommended diet for patients on dialysis with that recommended for patients having had a transplant.	1	2	3	4	5
b. Discuss nutritional supplementation that may be necessary in patients with renal failure.	1	2	3	4	5
c. Relate ways that cultural aspects of a patient's life may be included in a nutritional plan of care.	1	2	3	4	5
4. The content was current and relevant.	1	2	3	4	5
5. The content was presented clearly.	1	2	3	4	5
6. The content was covered adequately.	1	2	3	4	5
7. Rate your ability to apply the learning obtained from this activity to practice.	1	2	3	4	5

Comments _____

8. Time required to read the chapter and complete this form: _____ minutes.

This educational activity has been provided by the American Nephrology Nurses' Association (ANNA) for 1.8 contact hours. ANNA is accredited as a provider of continuing nursing education (CNE) by the American Nurses Credentialing Center's Commission on Accreditation (ANCC-COA). ANNA is an approved provider of continuing education by the California Board of Registered Nursing, CEP 0910.

Pharmacology of Renal Disease

Kristine Schonder, PharmD

Chapter Contents

Kristine Schonder, PharmD

Since the kidneys are responsible for the excretion of many medications, knowledge of pharmacology is essential for nurses working with patients with renal dysfunction. People with chronic kidney disease (CKD), especially those with renal failure, treated by either dialysis or transplantation, take numerous medications. The nurse is responsible for the safe administration of medications in hospitalized patients and for teaching dialysis patients about their therapeutic regimen. The purpose of this chapter is to describe the metabolism and elimination of pharmacologic agents and pharmacokinetics. Drug-induced renal disease is briefly addressed. The specific medications commonly used in CKD are also discussed.

Metabolism and Elimination of Pharmacologic Agents

Elaborate and complicated processes in the body have evolved to protect the body from the effects of external noxious influences. Medications are no different from any substance to which a person is exposed. To have an effect, the medication must reach the target tissue and attach to a receptor on the cell surface. Receptor stimulation will then set off a series of physiologic events that lead to the desired therapeutic effect. Unless a medication is directly infused into the bloodstream, it must be absorbed from the site of deposition. The medication must then be transported, or distributed to the target tissue, by means of cardiovascular circulation. A physiologic cleansing of foreign substances is initiated in the liver, resulting in degradation of drug to a less toxic or less fat-soluble form or elimination from the body in a water-soluble form via the kidneys or secretions.

Absorption

Medications administered intravenously reach the circulation immediately. However, with oral, dermal, or rectal

Table 18-1
Factors Affecting the Rate of Absorption

Factor	Comments
Solubility	Liquids are absorbed faster than solid dosage forms Aqueous solutions increase the rate of absorption, compared to oily solutions and suspensions.
Rate of dissolution	Applies to solid dosage forms Faster dissolution rates increase absorption
pH at the site of absorption	Acidic pH increases absorption of acidic compounds
Concentration of drug at the site of absorption	Higher drug concentration at the site increases absorption Lower drug concentration at the site decreases absorption
Circulation to the site of absorption	Increased blood flow increases rate of absorption Decreased blood flow decreases rate of absorption
Area of absorption surface	Large surface area (pulmonary alveoli, intestines, extensive skin surface) increases absorption Small surface area decreases absorption Edema decreases the rate of absorption
Physical characteristics of the drug	Nonionized form increases absorption Higher lipophilicity increases absorption Acidity of drug (acids better absorbed in acidic pH)
Route of administration	IV administration has most rapid effect Intramuscular administration is rapidly absorbed and bypasses first-pass liver metabolism Subcutaneous administration depends on nature of drug administered Aqueous solutions are rapidly absorbed Suspensions have slower absorption Pulmonary administration is rapidly absorbed Oral administration depends on nature of drug and dosage form (see solubility) Sublingual / buccal administration is rapidly absorbed and bypasses first-pass liver metabolism Rectal administration is variable and often incomplete. 50% of dose absorbed bypasses first-pass liver metabolism Topical administration depends on site of administration Mucous membranes associated with rapid absorption Skin absorption is proportional to the surface area applied. Oily vehicle can enhance skin absorption.

Table 18-2
Protein Binding of Drugs

Drugs that bind to: Albumin	Drugs that bind to: Alpha1-acid glycoprotein	Drugs that bind to: Albumin and Alpha1-acid glycoprotein
Benzodiazepines Ceftriaxone Clindamycin Clofibrate Dexamethasone Diazepam Dicloxacillin Ibuprofen Indomethacin Nafcillin Naproxen Phenytoin Probenecid Salicylic acid Sylfisoxazole Teniposide Thiopental Tolbutamide Valproic acid Warfarin	Bepridil Felodipine Flecainamide Perphenazine Phenobarbital Prazosin Rifampicin Risperidone Spironolactone Triazolam	Amitriptyline Bupivacaine Carbamazepine Diltiazem Disopyramide Erythromycin Imipramine Lidocaine Meperidine Methadone Nortriptyline Propranolol Quinidine Verapamil

routes of administration, absorption involves movement across cellular membranes (e.g., those lining both the absorptive surface and the blood vessel wall) and movement through intracellular spaces to reach the circulation. Local conditions can change the amount of medication that reaches the bloodstream; these conditions include pH, length of time the medication is in contact with absorptive surface, anatomic and physiologic condition of absorptive surface, and edema of the surrounding tissue. Although active and facilitated mechanisms can be present, movement of medication across surfaces is usually passive.

Oral absorption of medications can be reduced in the hospitalized patient due to physical removal by continuous or intermittent nasogastric suctioning, chemically neutralized gastrointestinal (GI) pH, altered peristalsis, intestinal villous atrophy, edematous bowel wall, and limited passage into the circulatory system because of poor perfusion of the intestines. In addition, physical medication interactions occur in the bowel lumen, hindering movement of medication through endothelial cell linings due to physical size.

Sublingual, intranasal, intramuscular, intravenous (IV), intraventricular, intracavitary, and epidural routes of administration have been developed to enhance absorption of medications, or to administer the agent directly to the site of action. Absorption of medications from intramuscular and subcutaneous injections may be affected by changes in tissue perfusion and movement through edematous tissue that may have physical distortions due to abnormal contents of fat and protein (see Table 18-1).

Distribution

Distribution of medication describes the transportation and deposition of a medication throughout the body. Very

Table 18-3
Factors Affecting Drug Distribution

Factor and Effect	Comments
Extent of Distribution	
Protein binding	High degree of protein binding decreases volume of distribution
Tissue binding affinity	High degree of tissue binding affinity decreases volume of distribution
Lipid solubility	Lipophilicity increases volume of distribution
Volume of body water	Increased body water increases volume of distribution
Rate of Distribution	
Membrane permeability	Increased permeability of the membrane increases volume of distribution
Blood perfusion	Increased blood perfusion increases volume of distribution

few medications can be directly administered to the site of need. Medication molecules that enter the bloodstream will be carried to their destination either in solution or attached to carrier molecules. Erythrocytes and serum proteins, such as albumin and alpha$_1$-acid glycoprotein, are common carriers of drugs (see Table 18-2). Medications that are bound to carrier molecules are inactive, but binding of medication is largely reversible. Detachment of medication occurs in areas of low concentration, such as the target tissue or tissue of elimination. Medications vary in their ability to bind to tissue based on chemical configuration and electrical charge. Chemicals may displace other chemicals if they are physically structured to attach better or have a stronger affinity for the binding site on the tissue or carrier molecules. Many different factors can affect both the rate and extent of drug distribution (see Table 18-3).

Various diseases can impair medication distribution. For example, poor perfusion of target tissue will limit the number of cells that are exposed to medication, while altered receptor binding will change the amount of medication attached to tissue. Receptors may be physically altered due to edema, malnutrition, or the competitive binding of other drugs or toxins. Since only free drug is active, potential for medication toxicity increases when decreased protein binding increases free serum concentrations of the drug, allowing tissues with functional receptors to bind more of the medication. Inflammation and loss of barrier integrity may allow medication to pass into otherwise drug-free areas, such as cerebral spinal fluid or the peritoneal cavity. Third spacing of fluid, in clinical situations such as ascites or massive edema, may result in additional volume into which medication can diffuse resulting in a need for higher dosage of medication to achieve therapeutic effects.

Metabolism

Medications are removed from the body through either of two major mechanisms. If the molecule is water soluble, the kidney will filter the chemical, or fluid lost through physiologic secretions will carry medication with it. If the medication is fat soluble, the medication must be altered to a water-soluble form that the kidney or secretions can remove. The liver is the most prolific organ that metabolizes or detoxifies medications, but all tissue can metabolize medications to a limited extent.

Enzymes are protein molecules that enhance the chemical transformation of various substances, both endogenous and exogenous. The numerous enzyme systems found in hepatocytes are adept at transforming chemicals whether they are medications or cellular waste products. Their effectiveness is limited by the physical environment of pH, temperature, and presence of synergistic substances called co-enzymes. Detoxification occurs by denaturing the fat-soluble chemical structure through reduction, demethylation, oxidation, or hydrolysis. Alternatively, the medication may be made more water-soluble by attaching a polar chemical molecule, such as glucuronide, sulfate, or glutathione. In renal failure, reduction and hydrolysis reactions are generally slowed, while glucuronidation, sulfated conjugation, and microsomal oxidation usually occur at a normal rate.

Rate of medication metabolism varies with the medication and the enzymes involved. Enzyme metabolism normally occurs at a defined rate. Enzymes are present in abundant concentration to allow metabolism of all molecules presented to the hepatocyte. Rarely, as in the case of alcohol or phenytoin, medication substrate will saturate the quantity of enzyme present, allowing drug accumulation to occur.

Certain enzymes are inducible, which means the synthesis of additional enzyme protein molecules. The best-

Table 18-4
Drugs that Affect Liver P450 Enzyme Function

Inducers of Drug Metabolism	Inhibitors of Drug Metabolism
Carbamazepine	Amiodarone
Ethanol	Azole antifungals (fluconazole, itraconazole, ketoconazole)
Phenobarbital	Cimetidine
Phenytoin	Clarithromycin
Rifampin	Diltiazem
Tobacco	Erythromycin
	Fluoroquinolone antibiotics (ciprofloxacin, levofloxacin, and others)
	Grapefruit juice
	Protease inhibitors (ritonavir, saquinavir, nelfinavir and others)
	Seratonin-reuptake inhibitors (SSRIs, fluoxetine, paraxetine, sertraline, and others)
	Verapamil

Note: This list is not all-inclusive. Other drugs can induce or inhibit drug metabolism by the cytochrome P450 enzyme system.

described example of inducible enzymes is the cytochrome P450 enzyme system, which can be induced by medications such as phenobarbital and rifampin. When an enzyme is induced, other medications that are metabolized by the same enzyme will be metabolized at a faster rate than normal, resulting in decreased levels than expected for the same dose in the absence of enzyme induction. Enzymes can also be inhibited by other medications that have a stronger affinity for the enzyme. The medication with the stronger affinity binds to the enzyme and does not allow the enzyme to metabolize other medications. As a result, other medications with weaker affinity for the enzyme will be metabolized at a slower rate than expected in the absence of enzyme inhibition, resulting in higher serum levels of the medication than expected for the same dose. Table 18-4 lists some of the more common drugs that affect the cytochrome P450 enzyme function.

The amount of medication metabolized may depend upon the ability of the body to deliver medication to the site of metabolism. Flow-dependent metabolism describes the ability of the liver to clear the blood of toxin so rapidly that the amount of medication metabolized can be determined principally by the rate of blood flow. Flow-dependent metabolism is synonymous with first pass effect, whereby oral medication entering the circulation in the GI tract immediately passes through the liver where the majority of medication is metabolized before reaching the systemic circulation. To thwart the first-pass effect, drugs that undergo rapid hepatic metabolism are often administered parenterally (Lehne, 2004).

Flow-independent metabolism is not influenced by blood flow. The amount of medication metabolized is limited by the inherent ability of hepatocyte detoxification. The amount of medication that can be cleared from blood will always be less than the amount of medication that is presented to the liver via blood flow (see Table 18-5).

Metabolic pathways that are influenced by blood flow are affected by diseases that reduce cardiac output or surgi-

Table 18-5
Relation of Drug Metabolism to Hepatic Blood Flow

Flow Dependent Metabolism	Flow Independent Metabolism
Fentanyl	Cyclosporine
Isoproterenol	Diazepam
Lidocaine	Digitoxin
Hydrocortisone	Erythromycin
Morphine	Phenytoin
Meperidine	Theophylline
Metoprolol	Warfarin
Nitroglycerin	
Propoxyphene	
Propranolol	
Verapamil	

cal revascularization that disrupts blood flow to the liver. Reduced protein binding increases the amount of free drug available for clearance and may increase the clearance of medication because the liver primarily extracts unbound medication. Hence, the patient may be at higher risk for toxicity due to elevated free concentration of drug, but the liver would also detoxify medications more rapidly. Diseases that affect hepatocyte function will also result in drug accumulation as the inherent ability to metabolize may change the relationship to one of flow-independent metabolism. Flow-independent pathways are primarily influenced by diseases that alter hepatocyte function.

Active metabolites may appear upon detoxification of parent compound. This may lead to prolonged therapeutic/toxic presence of medications such as meperidine or the benzodiazepines. In some cases, the drug administered is a pro-drug that must undergo first-pass metabolism to be converted to the active compound. An example is the angiotensin converting enzyme (ACE)-inhibitor, enalapril, which must be metabolized to enalaprilat to exert its activity in the body. In patients with diseases such as renal failure, where metabolism or elimination is impaired, adjustments to dosage may be required to prevent drug toxicity.

Elimination

Elimination is the final pathway by which a medication or its metabolite is removed from the body. The kidney is the main organ of elimination, while the liver can concentrate medication in bile. Minor routes of medication loss are through secretions, tears, and pulmonary gas exchange. Secretions of body fluids through wounds, burns, or drainage of compartmentalized collections (ascites) may result in enhanced clearance of medication from the body.

Medication elimination is influenced by three distinct activities of the kidney. Medications may be filtered at the glomerulus, reabsorbed from the lumen of the proximal and distal convoluted tubules, or actively secreted into the tubules. Filtration throughout the glomerulus is dependent on the protein binding of the drug, the molecular size and charge of the drug, glomerular integrity, and the number of functioning nephrons. Reabsorption is affected primarily by the number of functioning nephrons and urine pH, as is tubular secretion. For example, alkalinization of urine is use-

ful in phenobarbital and salicylate overdoses to enhance urinary excretion of medication. Certain medications, such as probenecid, can block the reabsorption of medications, such as penicillins and cephalosporins.

Renal disease will limit the amounts of water-soluble parent compound and metabolite that are removed from the blood. Diseases that affect glomerular filtration will limit the amount of excreted medication. Decreased perfusion of the kidney will reduce medication filtration, while inflammation of the glomerulus will allow large medication molecules to pass. Nephrotic syndrome is characterized by albumin loss that will carry bound medication into the urine. Changes in tubular integrity may alter secretion and reabsorption of molecules.

Bioavailability

The term bioavailability refers to the amount of drug that reaches the site of action. Bioavailability takes into consideration the other processes that the drug must undergo before reaching the site of action. Bioavailability will vary depending on the route of administration. For example, medications that are absorbed from the GI tract are first metabolized by enzymes in the mucosa. They are then presented to the liver for metabolization before it reaches the systemic circulation. In the case of drugs with flow-dependent metabolism, the bioavailability will be significantly reduced, whereas in drugs with flow-independent metabolism, bioavailability is increased. In some cases, the drug may be excreted into the bile, which diverts the drug away from the systemic circulation. On the other hand, medications that are absorbed transdermally reach systemic circulation immediately after crossing the skin barrier without first undergoing liver metabolism.

Pharmacokinetics

Medications behave in relatively reproducible manners once they enter the body. Mathematical models have been constructed to describe the behavior of molecules for the purpose of guiding dosage changes during periods of altered absorption, distribution, metabolism, and excretion. These models are referred to as pharmacokinetics.

Deterioration in the function of organs of metabolism and excretion will cause medication accumulation; while fluid shifts and altered tissue binding will change the concentration of free medication in the serum. The majority of medications are either relatively safe or minimally influenced by altered physiology. These agents can be prescribed with standard doses or adjusted based upon population nomograms. Selected agents are either extremely toxic or fluctuate dramatically in serum concentration with various pathologies in the body. Therapeutic drug monitoring has evolved to daily measurement of serum drug concentrations for some medications and adjustment of dosages based upon the patient status.

Receptor changes or competition for protein-binding sites can alter the active concentration of medications with significant protein binding. Medication interactions, such as aspirin and warfarin, or accumulation of uremic waste products will result in higher free concentrations of drug or additional binding to tissue receptors. Phenytoin is displaced from albumin in renal failure where free drug concentration can increase from 10% to 20% and may lead to toxicity.

Assay of free phenytoin levels has been recommended to better reflect dosage changes.

Medication elimination follows two basic forms. Linear elimination results when the body eliminates the same percentage of medication per unit time. The percent of medication removed is independent of the starting concentration. The amount of medication removed per unit of time will decrease as serum concentration decreases. If plotted on a log-linear graph, the serum concentration time curve will be a straight line throughout the dosing interval. Linear kinetics yield constant medication loss throughout the range of serum concentrations as well as the entire dosage interval. A percentage change in dose will yield an equivalent desired percentage change in serum concentration. Linear kinetics is also called first order kinetics.

Nonlinear elimination results when the body eliminates the same amount of medication per unit time while the percentage of medication removed changes. This pattern is due to a saturated elimination process, usually involving an enzyme that transforms the drug molecule. A saturated enzyme always functions at the maximum ability. Eventually, enough medication is eliminated to desaturate the enzymes, allowing a shift to linear kinetics. The serum concentration time relationship on a log-linear graph is a curve that initially reflects slow medication loss that increases until the linear portion of the curve is achieved. Dosage adjustments are not made on a ratio and proportion relationship as with linear kinetics. Because the majority of the dosage interval is spent in the nonlinear portion of the time curve, small amounts of medication will result in larger than expected changes in serum levels. Nonlinear kinetics is also called zero order kinetics.

Volume of Distribution and Clearance

Specific parameters to consider in adjustments of drug dosage are the volume of distribution and clearance. Volume of distribution and clearance are both affected by physiologic parameters and will change as the condition of the patient changes.

The volume of distribution is the apparent space in which a medication will disperse. This space is composed of fluid compartments and tissue binding sites. Volume of distribution is influenced by fluid shifts and accumulation. Volume of distribution of water-soluble medications is 0.25 mL/kg in euvolemia, but 0.15 mL/kg in dehydration, or as great as 0.35 mL/kg in fluid overload; that is, medication dosages should be reduced in dehydration, and dosage increases may be required in fluid overload. Gentamicin, for example, is sensitive to fluid shifts in the extracellular compartment. Intravascular blood volume has little impact on medications that are lipid soluble and do not distribute into fluid spaces.

Clearance is the amount of medication that can be removed from the blood in a defined period of time. Clearance is correlated to the function of the organ of elimination such as the liver or kidney, while volume of distribution is associated with fluid status and tissue binding efficiency.

Another pharmacokinetic parameter is the half-life or the time required for the serum concentration of a medica-

tion to fall by 50%. The half-life of a drug is dependent on the concentration of drug administered. Often, half-life is used to predict how frequently a drug should be dosed. Drugs with a shorter half-life are dosed more frequently than drugs with a longer half-life. Half-life is also used to determine when a drug reaches steady state, a term used to define the period when each subsequent dose of the drug will produce equivalent peak and trough serum concentrations. Steady state is generally achieved in five times the half-life. Disease processes will change parameters based upon physiologic alterations.

Pharmacodynamics

The relationship between drug concentration at the site of drug action and the physiologic response by the target tissue is called pharmacodynamics. A drug effect is produced when (a) there is a change in the physical environment of the bloodstream, such as pH or protein-binding changes, or (b) the drug attaches to a three-dimensional receptor found on the cell membrane or on an organelle within the cell. The interaction between drug and receptor causes a change in the structure of the cell surface that may open channels in the cell membrane through which electrolytes or other molecules can pass. Receptor stimulation also activates intracellular enzymes or releases intracellular chemicals that catalyze the desired physiologic response.

For most medications, the concentration at the receptor site determines the intensity of pharmacologic outcome. A dose response curve is generated for each medication during premarketing research to establish safe dosing ranges. Medication concentration and effect are proportional at low concentrations. Patient response to increasing doses is most evident with doses in the lower end of the dosing scale. As medication effect nears maximum, the receptors become saturated, and further increases in concentration have little to no benefit. Clinically, the chance of increasing toxicity is much greater with higher doses of a medication for the perceived benefit the patient may derive. The range in which the medication provides its effects is defined as the therapeutic index. The lower end of the therapeutic index is the minimal dose that is required for therapeutic effect; the higher end of the index is determined by the point at which the effect is seen at its maximum or the point at which toxicity occurs. Medications that have a narrow therapeutic index (i.e., a small range between minimal efficacy and toxicity) require close monitoring to optimize dose and clinical outcome.

Medications have a characteristic course of action. There is a delay that occurs after the administration of medication before the effect is seen. This delay is the time required to deliver medication to the site of action, bind medication to the receptor, and alter the cellular physiology to achieve desired outcome. A maximum or peak effect occurs when accumulation of medication at the receptor site is great enough to maximally bind to the receptor. The duration of medication effect reflects the elimination of medication from the central compartment and re-equilibration of medication molecules from receptor to the central compartment. Medication effect will diminish as receptor sites are evacuated until the concentration of drug becomes subtherapeutic. Although medication will remain in the body for at least five half-lives, medication effect will not be detectable once the concentration falls below the therapeutic level at the site of action.

Altered dynamic responsiveness is a poorly understood phenomenon. Not all patients react in the same way to equivalent doses or serum concentrations of the same drug. Differences in receptor structures, intracellular messengers, and feedback mechanisms have been proposed to account for individual differences.

Altered receptor binding is common with disease states. The three-dimensional proximity of structures of the cell membrane that define the receptor site can be altered in both design and chemical composition. Cell membranes can be physically distorted by malnourishment, edema, and inflammation. Antibodies may block the receptor or destroy the receptor site and cell. Antibodies can be produced by the body, such as insulin antibodies that block the site of insulin attachment, or can be administered exogenously as a medication, such as muromonab CD_3 that binds to the CD_3 receptor on T cells and causes cell lysis. Down regulation, a feedback mechanism that occurs after medication exposure, may decrease the number of receptors on the cell.

Altered responsiveness to receptor stimulation is common as disease may disrupt the intracellular chemical messenger system that is activated by the receptor. Stimulation of a cell surface receptor by a drug begins a cascade of chemical events that result in the anticipated outcome. Intracellular chemicals, such as electrolytes and cyclic AMP, may be depleted or functionally blocked by other molecules competing for binding sites. An example of this is the increased incidence of digoxin toxicity that occurs when intracellular potassium concentrations decrease.

Age can also affect the pharmacodynamic response to a medication. In advancing years, changes in dietary habits and tissue content of fat and proteins affect the chemical composition of the cell membrane. Failing physiologic reflexes may account for exaggerated or reduced pharmacologic effects, especially in the elderly. The inability of an organ system to detect or attenuate drug-induced changes could result in overwhelming drug effect and patient harm.

The metabolism and elimination of medications is clearly a complex process. Pathology in any number of areas can contribute to damage to the kidneys and drug-induced renal disease.

Drug Dosing Modifications in CKD

CKD poses many challenges in drug dosing. Because renal disease can affect other organ systems, each of the phases of drug distribution can be altered, including absorption, distribution, metabolism, and most notably, elimination.

Little is documented on the effects of renal insufficiency on absorption of drugs. Renal insufficiency can alter GI transit time and gastric pH or result in GI edema, vomiting and diarrhea, all of which can affect medication absorption. There are no definitive recommendations for drug dosing modifications as it relates to absorption of medications, but these factors should be taken into consideration when caring for the patient with CKD.

Drug distribution can also be altered in renal insuffi-

ciency due to changes in protein binding, tissue binding, and fluid balance. Accumulation of uremic organic acids can alter the protein binding of various medications. Protein binding of acidic compounds, such as phenytoin, salicylates, warfarin, and some antibiotics, is generally increased in end stage renal disease (ESRD). On the other hand, protein binding of basic drugs is less affected by uremia and may remain normal but can be increased, as with some benzodiazepines (e.g., clorazepate and diazepam) and serotonin-reuptake inhibitors (e.g., fluoxetine), or decreased, as with clonidine. The distribution of digoxin is reduced in renal failure because of alterations in tissue binding. Distribution of hydrophilic, or water-soluble, drugs may vary with changes in fluid balance.

Drug metabolism may be influenced by renal insufficiency, although the mechanism is not well understood. Alterations in the enzyme activity of the hepatocytes have been noted. However, definitive recommendations can only be made for those medications that are known to be affected by renal insufficiency-induced changes in metabolism.

Alterations in renal elimination are the best-recognized changes in pharmacodynamics that occur with renal insufficiency. The significance of these alterations and the subsequent actions that should be taken depend on a number of factors, such as the degree of renal insufficiency, the extent to which the medication is eliminated by the kidney, and the toxicities of the medication or the metabolite. As the degree of renal dysfunction increases, accumulation of the medication or metabolite increases and the need for dosage adjustment also increases. The exact point at which drug dosage adjustments are necessary varies with each medication. For many medications, those that are metabolized to inactive metabolites may require no dosage adjustment, even in the setting of complete renal failure. In general, most medications that have relatively minor toxicities or those that are metabolized to compounds with inactive metabolites or metabolites with minor toxicities do not require dosage adjustment until CKD progresses to the latter stages (e.g., Stages 4 and 5, glomerular filtration rate [GFR] < 30 mL/min/1.73 m²). However, those medications with severe toxicities, with toxicities that can occur at relatively low doses, or those that are metabolized to compounds with similar characteristics may need to be more aggressively adjusted based on renal dysfunction at a higher GFR.

Dosage adjustments in the setting of renal failure can involve decreasing the actual dose of the medication or increasing the interval at which it is administered, depending on the pharmacokinetics of the medication. As mentioned previously, renal insufficiency results in accumulation of the medication or its metabolites, which generally increases the elimination half-life of the medication from the body. Decreasing the dose or extending the dosing interval will allow for less total medication exposure in the setting of renal failure.

Dialyzability of Drugs

The dialyzability of drugs should be considered with any drug administered to patients receiving dialysis therapy. Dialysis therapy may or may not significantly affect the absorption and efficacy of a medication administered to a patient in renal failure. In general, if a medication is primarily excreted by the kidney, it is usually also removed by hemodialysis. However, peritoneal clearance of drugs varies because of the selectivity of the peritoneum. Therefore, the same cannot be said for peritoneal dialysis.

The effect of hemodialysis on the half-life of a medication is a function of the characteristics of the medication itself and the characteristics of the dialysis conditions. The molecular weight, particle size, volume of distribution, and protein binding affect the ability of the drug to pass through the dialysis membrane. Medications with a high molecular weight or large particle size cannot physically pass through the dialysis membrane, making them less likely to be removed by dialysis. Medications with a small volume of distribution will have a larger proportion contained in the vascular space compared to drugs with a large volume of distribution. This allows for a greater amount of medication with a small volume of distribution to be removed by dialysis compared to a large volume of distribution. Medications that are highly protein bound are less likely to be removed by dialysis, regardless of particle size, because the proteins themselves are not removed by dialysis. Only free drugs that are not protein

bound can be removed by dialysis. Medications with a high lipid affinity (fat-soluble drugs) are less likely to be removed by dialysis.

Dialysis conditions, such as the membrane permeability, pore size and surface area, perfusion, and dialysate flow rates will also affect the dialyzability of drugs. The extent of removal depends upon type of dialysis, length of dialysis, and type of filter used. The size of the medication molecule and extent of tissue binding establish the potential for drug removal, while the efficiency of dialysis will determine the extent of removal.

Dialysis techniques and filters have improved the removal of medication. Newer high efficiency filters will remove larger molecules, such as vancomycin. Chronic veno-venous or arterio-venous dialysis continuously remove medication over days rather than hours. Care must be used to interpret dosing charts that describe removal of medications by dialysis. The majority of information is dated and may not reflect current dialysis techniques. A search of the literature or contact with the pharmaceutical or dialyzer manufacturer may be helpful in guiding drug therapy when patients are using new dialysis devices.

Successful removal of drugs by dialysis is limited to medications and drugs in the blood, both in bound and free forms. However, because of the extensive distribution of many medications into fatty tissue, the drug will rapidly redistribute from tissue stores once dialysis is stopped. In cases of phenobarbital or theophylline overdose, this brief period of dialysis may be enough to stabilize the patient before serum drug levels again rise.

Artificial clearance of medication occurs with dialysis and presumably with plasmapheresis (see Table 18-6). As previously mentioned, dialysis devices will clear medication based upon type of dialysis and physical characteristics of the medication. Plasmapheresis of medication is a relatively unstudied phenomenon, but the treatment will remove some fraction of drug. In limited studies, the level of clearance has been low. The small volume of serum removed or "cleansed" contains only a small portion of total medication in the body. Medications that are heavily protein bound or lipophilic may be removed, but the majority of drug remains distributed throughout the body in other compartments. Clinically, medications that may be affected by dialysis or plasmapheresis should be held until the end of the procedure, or an additional dose should be given at the end of the treatment. Medications with a narrow therapeutic index may be best assessed by taking a serum concentration upon completion of the extracorporeal procedure.

Hemoperfusion with resins or activated charcoal has been successfully used to irreversibly bind water insoluble substances. It is the therapy of choice for removal of protein-bound medications.

Drug-Induced Renal Disease

One in every five cases of acute renal failure is associated with medication toxicity (Choudhury, 1997). With CKD, 1% to 20% of cases are associated with drug toxicity, depending on the region of the world reporting its experience. The kidneys are uniquely susceptible to medication toxicity due to a dependence on high blood flow for filtra-

Table 18-6
Drug Elimination through Artificial Clearance

Hemodialysis	Peritoneal Dialysis	Plasmapheresis
Acetaminophen	Aminoglycoside antibiotics	Digitoxin
Acyclovir	Ceftazidime	L-thyroxine
Allopurinol	Cefipime	Phenytoin
Aminoglycoside antibiotics	Enalapril	Propranolol
Azathioprine	Fluconazole	Salicylate
Aztreonam	Imipenem	Tobramycin
Chlorpheniramine	Lithium	
Fluconazole	Manitol	
Gabapentin	Phenobarbital	
Ganciclovir	Salicylate	
Imipenam	Sulfisoxazole	
Lithium		
Mannitol		
Meropenam		
Metformin		
Methylprednisolone		
Ofloxacin		
Pentazocine		
Phenobarbital		
Prednisone		
Procainamide		
Salicylate		
Sulfamethoxazole		
Sulfisoxazole		
Theophylline		
Trimethoprim		
Select ACE-inhibitors		
Select beta-blockers		
Select cephalosporins		
Select penicillins		

Note: This list is not all-inclusive. Other drugs can be removed by artificial clearance.

tion, a powerful ability to concentrate substrates, a large endothelial area that comes in contact with toxic substances, and a high metabolic activity that produces intracellular toxins.

The mechanisms of medication-mediated damage are multiple. As with other causes of renal disease, pathophysiology is divided into three categories: prerenal reasons for decreased perfusion, intrinsic renal disease (e.g., interstitial nephritis, glomerulonephritis, or acute tubular necrosis), and postrenal obstruction. In addition to direct toxic effects on renal tissue, altered physiologic effects are induced by medications that change fluid and electrolyte balance (e.g., diuretics) (Thatte, 1996).

Renal perfusion is affected by a number of mechanisms. Medications can reduce cardiac output by inducing hypovolemia (diuretics) and causing vasodilation (antihypertensives). Afferent arteriolar vasoconstriction will reduce the perfusion of the glomerulus, while efferent vasodilation will draw blood away from the glomerulus. Both actions decrease the glomerular filtration pressures and reduce the volume of glomerular filtrate. Nonsteroidal anti-inflammatory drugs (NSAIDs) reduce the synthesis of prostaglandins, which allows for afferent vasoconstriction thereby reducing glomerular filtration pressures in individuals with abnormal renal function. Angiotensin converting enzyme (ACE) inhibitors and angiotensin II receptor blockers (ARB) cause vasodilatation of the efferent arterioles, decreasing glomerular filtration pressure. This induces renal dysfunction despite increased renal blood flow by increasing cardiac output through afterload reduction. Cyclosporine can cause an intense generalized intrarenal vasoconstriction that can synergistically interact with NSAIDs and ACE inhibitors.

Drug-induced acute interstitial nephritis is a hypersensitivity reaction to a medication molecule that occurs in the renal interstitium. Common clinical signs and symptoms include hematuria (gross or microscopic), proteinuria, and pyuria. Occasionally, systemic manifestations of allergy, such as rash, fever, and arthralgia, are seen with interstitial nephritis. The most common diagnostic finding is the presence of eosinophils in the urine. Glomerular and vascular lesions are rarely seen in conjunction with interstitial nephritis.

Acute tubular necrosis (ATN) is a general term that covers many different conditions with similar manifestations. Damage may be confined to the proximal or distal convoluted tubule. Proximal tubular effects are seen most prevalently with aminoglycoside antibiotics, since the drugs can be concentrated in the renal cortex up to 20 times the serum concentration. Proximal lesions can be detected by urinary appearance of enzymes found in tubular cells (N-acetylglucosaminidase and alkaline phosphatase) or impaired proximal reabsorption of the filtered protein beta$_2$-microglobulin. Urinary magnesium and potassium losses are seen with proximal defects. Distal tubular damage is seen with platinum compounds (e.g., cisplatinum) used for cancer chemotherapy. Chronic administration disrupts the normal tubular functions and can lead to renal concentrating defects, potassium wasting, and distal renal tubular acidosis. Hydration, mannitol, and sodium loading have been used to lessen the toxic effects of drugs in the distal tubule. These treatments decrease the concentration of the medication

passing through the tubule, which decreases the toxic effects.

Medications may precipitate in the distal tubule but more frequently precipitate in the collecting ducts when water reabsorption concentrates the agent above its maximum solubility. When sulfonamides, methotrexate, and acyclovir precipitate, they can obstruct urine flow, leading to stasis and tubular cell death.

While all medications have some side effects, some medications can induce renal disease and failure. For many medications, there are multiple mechanisms through which renal damage can occur. For example, amphotericin B is an intense vasoconstrictor as well as a direct nephrotoxin to the proximal and distal tubules. Radiocontrast agents may cause systemic hypotension and direct nephrotoxicity, but they can also cause obstruction through precipitation of uric acid crystals. Clinical and laboratory findings may vary depending upon which mechanism is more prominent.

In rare instances, some medications, such as lithium, can cause chronic renal dysfunction (as well as acute renal failure) when taken over a long period of time. Patients may present with nonspecific symptoms such as nocturia, weakness, fatigue, nausea, or vomiting. Because the disease is largely asymptomatic, the damage occurs slowly and is not clinically detectable. Patients may not present with symptoms until 85% to 90% of renal function is lost. Long-term toxicity usually causes low-grade inflammation and deposition of scar tissue or occlusion of blood vessels. However, most drug-induced renal diseases involve all parenchymal elements. If the medication is stopped, deterioration of renal function is usually arrested.

Analgesic nephropathy refers to the chronic interstitial nephritis that occurs as a result of long-term use of acetaminophen, aspirin, and NSAIDs. Patients with analgesic nephropathy typically have consumed large amounts of analgesics in various combinations over a period of years. Reports of chronic disease with single agents are rare. The mechanism has been suggested to be a production of toxic metabolites. Acetaminophen metabolism in the liver produces a toxic metabolite that is rapidly neutralized by hepatocyte stores of glutathione. Depletion of glutathione in overdose situations has been fatal due to fulminant liver failure. Chronic analgesic use apparently causes similar renal cell damage that erodes viable tissue over a long period of time. The basic lesion is papillary necrosis seemingly due to damage and occlusion of the contiguous blood vessels leading to ischemic necrosis of the papillae. The renal tubules passing into the necrotic papillae are then blocked, leading to secondary atrophy of the overlying nephrons.

Commonly Used Drugs in Renal Insufficiency

Medication use in renal insufficiency can become quite complicated because of the many factors previously described. However, the complications associated with renal insufficiency necessitate the use of various medications for treatment and management.

Diuretics

Diuretics are often used to treat edema and hypertension that can cause or result from renal insufficiency. There are four primary categories of diuretics available: thiazide diuretics, loop (also referred to as "high ceiling") diuretics, potassium-sparing diuretics, and osmotic diuretics.

Thiazide diuretics include hydrochlorothiazide, chlorothiazide, chlorthalidone, indapamide, and metolazone. They work primarily by inhibiting reabsorption of sodium and chloride in the distal tubule, which promotes water loss. Thiazide diuretics can cause wasting of potassium, which may result in hypokalemia. They are used as the first-line agents to treat hypertension and can also be used to treat chronic heart failure (CHF) and edema of renal origin (e.g., nephrotic syndrome). The efficacy of thiazide diuretics is limited in patients with GFR < 30 mL/min/1.73 m²; therefore, their clinical utility in renal insufficiency is limited to those with early stages of CKD (e.g., Stages 1 – 3). However, thiazide diuretics, particularly indapamide and metolazone, can provide synergistic actions to enhance the activity of loop diuretics, further promoting water loss.

Loop or "high ceiling" diuretics include furosemide, bumetanide, and torsemide. These medications have greater clinical utility than thiazide diuretics in renal insufficiency, particularly in Stage 4; however, they are of little benefit in patients who have progressed to renal failure (Stage 5 CKD) with little or no urine output. Loop diuretics exert their activity by inhibiting reabsorption of sodium and chloride in the ascending loop of Henle, thus promoting water loss. The loop of Henle is one of the principal sites of sodium reabsorption in the nephron, making loop diuretics the most potent class of diuretics. Like thiazide diuretics, loop diuretics also cause wasting of potassium, often more significant than thiazide diuretics, which may also result in hypokalemia. Loop diuretics are often the primary diuretics used to control hypertension and edema in renal insufficiency. Oral doses are most often used for more gradual and sustained diuresis, while IV doses can be used to acutely promote rapid and significant water loss.

Potassium-sparing diuretics include spironolactone, amiloride, and triamterene. Spironolactone exerts its activity by competing with aldosterone in the distal tubules, thus increasing sodium, chloride, and water excretion while conserving potassium. Amiloride and triamterene work in a different manner by inhibiting the sodium/potassium active transport exchange pump in the distal tubule, resulting in retention of potassium and loss of sodium and water. These medications are weaker diuretics than thiazide and loop diuretics and are often used in combination with the others to prevent the development of hypokalemia. Use of these medications, however, should be limited to individuals with relatively normal renal function. Use potassium-sparing diuretics in renal failure often leads to the development of hyperkalemia because of the additive effect to the already decreased ability of the kidney to excrete potassium. Potassium-sparing diuretics should be used with caution in later stages of CKD (Stages 4 and 5).

Mannitol is an osmotic diuretic. Osmotic diuretics work by increasing the osmolarity of the plasma and renal tubular fluid, thereby preventing water reabsorption in the kidney. The increase in plasma osmolarity can extract water from the intracellular compartment, increasing arterial blood volume and renal blood flow. Osmotic diuretics are most often used in acute renal failure or to decrease intracranial pressure.

Water and electrolyte imbalances are the primary side effects of osmotic diuretics. Excessive water loss can disrupt sodium balance and lead to dehydration or hyponatremia. Osmotic diuretics should be used with caution in disease states prone to volume overload, such as CHF and ESKD.

Fluid and electrolyte imbalances are common complications associated with all classes of diuretics. Patients receiving diuretics should be closely monitored for response to the medication as they progress toward the achieved therapy goals. Monitoring parameters should include routine blood chemistries to identify electrolyte disorders, namely sodium, potassium, chloride, bicarbonate, calcium, and magnesium, as well as routine surveillance of fluid status to avoid dehydration.

Analgesics

Chronic pain is often difficult to manage in renal insufficiency because of the limitations of many of the pain medications in CKD. Analgesics can be discussed in terms of three distinct classes: non-narcotic drugs, narcotic drugs, and nonsteroidal anti-inflammatory drugs (NSAIDs).

Non-narcotic drugs include acetaminophen, aspirin (ASA), and tramadol. Acetaminophen should be considered the drug of choice of mild-to-moderate chronic pain in renal insufficiency, as it is metabolized by the liver and exerts little effect on the kidney. ASA, on the other hand, inhibits cyclooxygenase (COX), which in turn inhibits prostaglandin synthesis. Although use of aspirin has not been associated with renal damage, inhibition of prostaglandins can reduce renal blood flow and cause alterations in renal function. In addition, inhibition of the prostaglandin thromboxane A_2 reduces platelet aggregation, which can increase the tendency for bleeding. The inhibition of platelet aggregation is useful to prevent the development of clots in certain clinical situations, particularly in patients with myocardial infarction or in dialysis patients to prevent clotting of vascular access devices. Tramadol is a synthetic analgesic with weak opioid activity and non-opioid activity. It is used in patients with mild-to-moderate pain unrelieved by acetaminophen who cannot tolerate opioids. Tramadol is metabolized by the liver and exerts no effects on the kidney. It can be safely used in patients with renal insufficiency and requires no dosage adjustments.

NSAIDs include ibuprofen, ketoprofen, naproxen, and other medications and are widely used because of their availability over-the-counter. NSAIDs inhibit COX, which in turn inhibits prostaglandin synthesis, including the vasodilatory prostaglandins PGI_2, PGE_2, and PGF_2. Under normal circumstances in the kidney, these vasodilatory prostaglandins are produced in response to vasoconstriction caused by vasoactive hormones, such as angiotensin II, vasopressin, or endothelin, or in response to cytokines, ischemia, hypoxia, or other cellular disturbances to preserve renal blood flow and glomerular filtration. Additionally, these prostaglandins can increase renin release, diuresis, and natriuresis. With NSAID use, inhibition of these vasodilatory prostaglandins can potentiate nephrotoxicity in certain clinical situations, such as renal insufficiency, hepatic cirrhosis, CHF, hypertension, diabetes mellitus, sepsis, and hypovolemia. The most common side effects of NSAID use include sodium and

Table 18-7
Gabapentin Dosing Adjustment for CKD

GFR (mL/min/1.73 m2)	Total Daily Gabapentin Dose Range (mg)	Dose Frequency
> 60	900 – 3600	TID
30 – 59	400 – 1400	BID
15 – 29	200 – 700	QD
< 15	100 – 300	QD

Table 18-8
Gabapentin Supplemental Doses for Hemodialysis

Mainentance Range (mg/day)	Supplemental Dose (mg)
100 – 900	125
125 – 1200	150
150 – 1800	200
200 – 2400	250
300 – 3600	350

Note: Supplemental doses should be administered after each 4 hours of hemodialysis.

water retention and subsequent edema. Hyperkalemia and other electrolyte abnormalities can also result from NSAID use but are much less common. It is important that clinical assessment of any patient include the use of over-the-counter medications, particularly NSAID use. COX-2 inhibitors are a newer class of medications that work similarly to traditional NSAIDs and include celecoxib and valdecoxib. They differ from traditional NSAIDs by inhibiting only the COX-2 enzyme, which is more specific for pain and inflammation and has less effect on prostaglandin synthesis. The selectivity of the COX-2 inhibitors was thought to decrease the propensity toward renal dysfunction and GI mucosal injury. However, as clinical experience with these agents increases, it is becoming more evident COX-2 inhibition offers no greater protection against renal effects, with an incidence similar to the traditional NSAIDS. COX-2 inhibitors can also produce sodium and water retention and edema, similar to NSAIDs (Breyer, 2001).

Narcotic analgesics include a wide array of medications. The mechanisms of action vary by medication, but most often involve alterations in the pain threshold or the response to pain by the central nervous system (Ballantyne, 2003). Morphine sulfate is the drug of choice for patients with CKD who have acute pain. The dose should be reduced to 75% of the normal dose for patients with GFR 10–50 mL/min/1.73 m² and to 50% of the normal dose if the GFR is < 10 mL/min/1.73 m². The dosing intervals should remain the same. Codeine is also a drug of choice for pain management in CKD. Dosing adjustments in moderate-to-severe CKD are similar to morphine. Meperidine, however, should be avoided for long-term therapy because of the potential for the build-up of normeperidine, a metabolite that can accumulate in renal failure and cause seizures. Patients with CKD can receive a normal dose for the first dose, but should avoid repeated doses of meperidine. The dose of methadone does not need to be adjusted in renal failure because the elimination is thought to shift from renal elimination to fecal elimination in renal failure. However, the dosing interval may need to be extended. None of the narcotics are removed by dialysis to any extent. Therefore, supplemental doses are not required. However, narcotics can worsen constipation experienced by many patients with renal failure.

Other adjunctive agents are often used for neuropathic pain, particularly peripheral neuropathy caused by diabetes

(Holdcroft, 2003). Amitriptyline is a tricyclic antidepressant that is effective in controlling neuropathic pain. It is typically dosed at bedtime and does not need to be adjusted for renal dysfunction. Gabapentin is an anticonvulsant that can be used for neuropathic pain. Gabapentin is cleared renally and must be adjusted for renal insufficiency. Furthermore, patients receiving dialysis should receive supplemental doses with dialysis treatments. Dosing guidelines for gabapentin in CKD and dialysis are listed in Tables 18-7 and 18-8. Valproic acid is another anticonvulsant that may be used for neuropathic pain. The dose does not need to be adjusted for renal insufficiency. However, it should be noted that protein binding of valproic acid may be altered in renal failure.

Antihypertensives

Despite advances in the management of CKD, cardiovascular disease still remains the leading cause of mortality in CKD. Hypertension is present in approximately 50%–75% of patients with GFR < 60 ml/min/1.73 m² (National Kidney Foundation [NKF], 2002). An understanding of how hypertension occurs and what factors come into play is helpful in understanding management strategies. Factors associated with hypertension include retention of fluid and sodium, dysfunction of the renin-angiotensin system, increased activity of the sympathetic nervous system, changes in intracellular calcium, and reduced production of vasodilator substances by the kidneys. All antihypertensive medications have an equal ability to control blood pressure. The different mechanisms of action, however, result in different adverse effects and different effects on the kidney. The ideal antihypertensive agent in CKD is one that will also protect or improve renal function in addition to reducing blood pressure. It is important to remember the balance between blood pressure and kidney function. Increased blood pressure in the presence of renal impairment will continue to insult the already damaged kidney. However, overaggressive blood pressure reduction can impair renal function, particularly in those who have narrowed blood vessels and rely on higher than normal blood pressures to force blood through the circulatory system. The goal blood pressure for patients with CKD is < 130/80 mm Hg. Patients will often require two to three medications to reach this goal (NKF, 2004)

Angiotensin-converting enzyme inhibitors (ACEIs). ACEIs (e.g., captopril, enalapril, lisinopril, benazopril, ramipril, and others) interfere with the renin-angiotensin-aldosterone system (RAAS) and work by blocking angiotensin-converting enzyme (ACE), which is responsible for converting angiotensin I, a mild vasoconstrictor, to angiotensin II, a potent vasoconstrictor. Because of their effects on RAAS, ACEIs decrease sodium and water retention, peripheral resistance, and systemic vascular resistance and increase plasma volume, cardiac output, and renal blood flow. ACEIs should be considered the first drug of choice for hypertensive patients with CKD because of their effects in slowing the progression of kidney disease. They have been shown to slow the decline in GFR and decrease proteinuria in patients with both type 1 (Lewis, 1993) and type 2 diabetes mellitus (Ravid, 1993), as well as non-diabetic patients with CKD (Maschio, 1996; Gruppo Italiano di Studi Epidemiologici in Nefrologia [GISEN], 1997). ACEIs should be initiated early in the course of CKD and titrated to the maximum tolerable dose. In patients with renal failure or elderly patients, the initial starting dose should be reduced by 50% and then increased gradually.

ACEIs cause vasodilation in the efferent arterioles of the kidney, which can decrease glomerular pressure and cause a transient increase in serum creatinine. Generally, serum creatinine levels will return to baseline values within 1–2 weeks of therapy. For this reason, ACEIs should be used cautiously and monitored aggressively in patients with renal insufficiency. They should be avoided in patients with renal artery stenosis (RAS) because of the potential to precipitously drop glomerular pressure and induce renal failure. Orthostatic hypotension can occur when initiating or increasing the dose of ACEIs and patients should be monitored closely in these circumstances.

Because of their effects on aldosterone, ACEIs can result in hyperkalemia. Serum potassium levels should be closely monitored in patients receiving ACEIs, particularly those with CKD. The most common reason for discontinuation of ACEIs is the development of a non-productive cough. Alternative antihypertensive agents should be used if a cough develops, as this is a class phenomenon and switching to another ACEI agent will likely result in the same effect.

Angiotensin II receptor blockers (ARBs). ARB agents (e.g., losartan, valsartan, irbesartan, candesartan, and others) are the newest class of antihypertensive agents available. They exert their actions by blocking angiotensin II receptors, thereby inhibiting the vasoconstriction caused by angiotensin II. The resultant action is similar to ACEIs, but the ARBs differ mainly in their adverse effect profile. Like the ACEIs, ARBs have also been shown to decrease the progression of CKD (Brenner et al., 2001; Parving, 2001). For this reason, they are a suitable alternative and should be considered in patients with CKD who are unable to tolerate ACEIs. There is limited evidence that the addition of an ARB to an ACEI may result in a further decrease in kidney disease progression (Kincaid-Smith, 2002; Nakao, 2003); however, this has only been demonstrated in small studies and must be evaluated in larger clinical trials before the combination is used on a larger scale.

It is thought that the ACEI-induced cough is caused by the accumulation of bradykinin as a result of inhibition of the ACE enzyme. ARBs lack this effect on the ACE enzyme and

appear to have fewer tendencies to cause cough; however, cough has been reported in some patients receiving ARBs, though the incidence is much less than with ACEIs. Like ACEIs, ARBs can result in hyperkalemia, although the incidence appears to be less than the ACEIs, most likely due to the limited effect of ARBs on aldosterone.

Calcium channel blockers (CCBs). CCBs exert their activity by inhibiting the movement of calcium across vascular smooth cells, resulting in coronary and peripheral vasodilation and decreased systemic vascular resistance. CCBs can be divided into two categories: dihydropyridine CCBs and nondihydropyridine CCBs. The overall effect of the two categories on reducing blood pressure is similar, but they differ in their effects on the kidney.

Dihydropyridine CCBs (nifedipine, amlodipine, felodipine, nicardipine, and others) are more potent vasodilators than nondihydropyridine CCBs. In the kidney, dihydropyridine CCBs produce greater vasodilation in the afferent arteriole, resulting in a decrease in glomerular pressure, which has been shown to potentially worsen the progression of CKD (Lewis, 2001). For this reason, use of dihydropyridine CCBs should be used very cautiously in patients with CKD or avoided altogether. Side effects of dihydropyridine CCBs are usually more pronounced than the nondihydropyridine CCBs and include peripheral edema, dizziness, flushing, constipation, and headache. Of note, use of immediate release and sublingual nifedipine should be avoided in all patients, as this has been shown to increase mortality due to the rapid decrease and large fluctuations in blood pressure.

Nondihydropyridine CCBs (diltiazem and verapamil) have a greater ability to decrease cardiac contractility and slow cardiac conduction than the dihydropyridine CCBs. For this reason, they should be avoided in patients with left ventricular dysfunction, sick sinus syndrome, and second or third degree heart block. In the kidney, nondihydropyridine CCBs have beneficial effects on reducing proteinuria. Nondihydropyridine CCBs can also cause peripheral edema, dizziness, flushing, constipation, and headache, although these effects are generally seen less than with the dihydropyridine CCBs.

Beta-adrenergic blockers (β-blockers). Beta-adrenergic blockers (e.g., propranolol, atenolol, metoprolol, and others) block the sympathetic stimulation of $beta_1$-receptors in the heart and $beta_2$-receptors in the bronchi, peripheral blood vessels, and pancreas. β-blockers, in addition to diuretics, are considered to be first-line agents for the treatment of hypertension and myocardial infarction and are also indicated in patients with CHF. Some β-blockers are more selective for $beta_1$-receptors and are associated with fewer side effects. However, at higher doses all β-blockers lose specificity and will also block $beta_2$-receptors. In the kidney, β-blockers have the capability to reduce renal blood flow and GFR. Side effects of β-blockers include sedation, bradycardia, hypotension, and congestive heart failure, especially at high doses or if not monitored closely. Additionally, β-blockers can also mask hypoglycemic symptoms in diabetic patients. When discontinuing β-blockers, the dose should be gradually decreased to avoid rebound hypertension.

Centrally acting alpha₂-agonists. Centrally acting alpha₂-agonists (e.g., clonidine, methyldopa) decrease blood pressure by stimulating alpha$_2$-receptors in the brain, resulting in reduced sympathetic activity. The overall effect of these agents is to reduce systemic vascular resistance and heart rate. Because of its rapid onset of action, clonidine is useful in hypertensive urgencies to quickly reduce blood pressure. Side effects of central alpha$_2$-receptor agonists include somnolence and dry mouth. Rebound hypertension may occur with drug discontinuation or even decreased doses.

Direct vasodilators. Direct vasodilators (e.g., hydralazine, minoxidil) exert their effects by relaxing smooth muscle and reducing vascular resistance. The potent vasodilatory effect of these medications often produces a reflexive activation of the sympathetic nervous system, resulting in tachycardia and increased cardiac output. Generally, these medications are used in combination with other antihypertensive medications. Side effects include flushing, headache, dizziness, and palpitations. Hydralazine can also cause hypotension, an effect that is not generally seen with minoxidil. Minoxidil can cause excessive hair growth. This side effect may not be tolerable in some patients, particularly in women.

Alpha$_1$-receptor blockers. Alpha$_1$-receptor blockers (doxazosin, prazosin, and terazosin) decrease blood pressure by blocking the effects of norephinephrine in the arteries and arterioles, thereby inhibiting vasoconstriction and reducing systemic vascular resistance. However, alpha$_1$-receptor blockers should not be used as primary agents for the treatment of hypertension because of the increased risk of developing CHF (ALLHAT, 2000). Because of the results of this trial, alpha$_1$-receptor blockers should be reserved for treatment of benign prostatic hypertrophy to relax smooth muscle of the prostate and improve urine flow. Side effects of alpha$_1$-receptor blockers include orthostatic hypotension, syncope, and dizziness. Administering the dose at bedtime can minimize side effects.

Antihyperlipidemics

Hyperlipidemia plays a significant part in increasing the risk of cardiovascular disease in patients with CKD. Hyperlipidemia increases atherosclerotic cardiovascular disease in all individuals and contributes to the higher incidence of cardiovascular disease in CKD. Treatment of hyperlipidemia in CKD is important in reducing the overall risk of cardiovascular disease in patients with renal insufficiency. The NKF guidelines for the treatment of hyperlipidemia in CKD suggest that CKD should be considered a cardiovascular risk equivalent and that the target low-density lipoprotein (LDL) is < 100 mg/dL (NKF, 2003). There are several different types of medications that can be used to treat hyperlipidemia. Selection of an agent to use depends on a number of factors, most notably the lipid profile, as well as patient tolerability and preference.

HMG-CoA reductase inhibitors (statins). The statin medications (e.g., atorvastatin, lovastatin, pravastatin, simvastatin, and others) are now considered to be the mainstay of lipid lowering therapy. These drugs inhibit the final step in the synthesis of cholesterol by preventing the conversion of hydroxymethylglutaryl-coenzyme A (HMG-CoA), a precursor of cholesterol, to the final cholesterol product. The statins

are effective in lowering LDL cholesterol concentrations by altering the activity of the LDL-receptor and reducing LDL entry into circulation (Knopp, 1999). Additionally, the statins have favorable effects in lowering triglyceride concentrations and increasing beneficial high-density lipoprotein (HDL) concentrations.

Side effects of the statin medications include nausea, GI upset, muscle aches, and increased liver enzymes. Myopathy, which can manifest as rhabdomyolysis, and hepatotoxicity are rare but important side effects of statins. Patients should be monitored for signs of muscle aches and weakness. Liver function tests (LFTs) should also be regularly monitored. Statins should be used cautiously with drugs that inhibit the hepatic cytochrome P-450 enzyme system, as inhibition of these liver enzymes can increase statin levels and the risk for adverse effects, especially rhabdomyolysis.

Bile acid-binding resins. Bile acid-binding resins (cholestyramine, colestipol, and colesevelam) lower cholesterol by binding to bile acids in the intestine. This interrupts the enterohepatic circulation of bile acids, which increases the conversion of cholesterol to bile acids. The process also increases the production of cholesterol, which in turn increases triglyceride levels in the blood stream. The increase in triglyceride levels resulting from the use of bile acid-binding resins may limit their usefulness in patients who are prone to developing hypertriglyceridemia. Another limiting factor of bile acid-binding resins is the fact that they have less effect in lowering LDL levels compared to other agents. Currently, bile acid-binding resins are used clinically as adjunct therapy to statins to further lower LDL concentrations in patients who are receiving maximum doses of statin medications. Statins help to increase the effectiveness of bile acid-binding resins by inhibiting cholesterol production. Additionally, the combination of statins and bile acid-binding resins also further increases beneficial HDL levels.

Side effects of the bile acid-binding resins include bloating, gas, and constipation. Adusting the dose and increasing fiber intake can be helpful in managing constipation. In renal failure, cholestyramine causes chloride ions to be released in exchange for bile acids, which can lead to hyperchloremic acidosis. For this reason, cholestyramine should be used cautiously in patients with renal failure. It is also important to keep in mind that bile acid-binding resins can bind to other medications in the GI tract, particularly warfarin, digoxin, thyroxine, thiazide diuretics, folic acid, statins, cyclosporine, tacrolimus, mycophenolate mofetil, and others. Other medications should be separated by at least 2 hours before or 4 hours after the bile acid-binding resin is given to avoid the interaction.

Nicotinic acid (niacin). Nicotinic acid lowers cholesterol by inhibiting the mobilization of free fatty acids from peripheral tissues, which decreases hepatic synthesis of triglycerides. Niacin may also decrease the production of LDL. Furthermore, niacin increases beneficial HDL levels by up to 30%, which exceeds the ability of any other lipid-lowering agent. It appears that niacin is most effective at improving cholesterol profile when combined with other lipid lowering agents.

Side effects associated with niacin can be very problematic to patients. Flushing is the most common side effect, which is often intolerable to patients. Administering aspirin 325 mg 30 to 60 minutes prior to the dose of niacin decreases the severity of flushing, particularly with the first few doses. Most patients develop tachyphylaxis to the flushing, and aspirin pretreatment can be stopped after a few doses. Another significant side effect of niacin is hepatotoxicity, which occurs more frequently than with statins. LFTs should be aggressively monitored in patients receiving niacin. Sustained-release formulations of niacin can decrease the flushing side effects of niacin; however, the incidence of hepatotoxicity is increased with sustained-release preparations. Additionally, niacin may worsen glucose control in diabetic patients. Niacin should be used cautiously in patients with renal insufficiency, as there are few studies in CKD. Niacin is eliminated by the kidney to some extent; higher doses of niacin may accumulate in CKD leading to an increase in adverse effects.

Fibric acid derivatives (fibrates). Fibric acid derivatives (gemfibrozil and fenofibrate) increase fatty-acid oxidation in the liver and in muscle tissue. The result is decreased secretion of triglycerides. Fibric acid derivatives are the most effective drugs to lower triglycerides. Additionally, fibric acid derivatives also have a favorable effect on increasing beneficial HDL cholesterol and little effect on lowering LDL cholesterol.

Side effects associated with fibric acid derivatives include GI upset, abdominal pain, gallstones, and myositis. Fibric acid derivatives are excreted by the kidney and can accumulate in renal insufficiency, which can increase the risk of side effects, particularly myositis. Consequently, these drugs should be used cautiously in patients with CKD. Patients receiving warfarin should be monitored closely when initiating or increasing the dose of fibric acid derivatives, as the combination can increase warfarin levels and increase bleeding potential.

Vitamin Supplements

All patients with renal failure will need vitamin supplementation due to dietary restrictions and dialyzability of water-soluble vitamins. Specifically, vitamins that need to be replaced in dialysis patients include vitamins B_1, B_2, B_6, B_{12}, biotin, pantothenic acid, niacin, folic acid, and vitamin C. High doses of folic acid are sometimes used to treat hyperhomocysteinemia, which is a risk factor for cardiovascular disease. Specific vitamins that do not need to be replaced routinely in dialysis patients include the fat-soluble vitamins that are not removed by dialysis, such as vitamins A, E, and K. Vitamin preparations specifically designed for renal failure patients are available (e.g., Nephro-Vite®), but patients may also take less expensive over-the-counter products. Since most vitamins are water soluble, vitamin supplements should be taken after dialysis for the patient to receive the full therapeutic benefit.

Gastrointestinal (GI) Agents

Patients with CKD can have a variety of GI complaints as renal disease progresses. Complaints can range from varying degrees of nausea, caused by disease progression or often by other medications, to constipation, particularly in renal failure patients (Martin de Francisco, 2002).

Antacids

Antacids are frequently used to neutralize gastric acids. Calcium-containing antacids (Tums® and others) are more commonly used because of the added benefits of calcium supplementation. Magnesium and aluminum-based antacids can be used in patients with earlier stages of CKD (Stages 1 to 3) but are seldom used in renal failure (Stage 5) because of the risk of toxicity that can result from accumulation of magnesium and aluminum from these medications.

Histamine H_2 Receptor Antagonists (H_2-blockers)

Histamine H_2 receptor antagonists (H_2-blockers) inhibit the H_2 receptors found in the GI tract that are responsible for secreting acid in the stomach. H_2-blockers are often used to treat mild-to-moderate nausea or side effects from other medications. Cimetidine should be used with caution in renal failure due to the potential for mental confusion. Ranitidine has less propensity to cause mental confusion than cimetidine. The other H_2-blocking agents, famotidine and nizatidine, are not associated with mental status changes. The doses of all the H_2-blockers should initially be reduced in patients with GFR < 50 mL/min/1.73 m² and doses can be increased gradually based on the patient's response. Antacids can interfere with the absorption of H_2-blockers when taken simultaneously. With the availability of H_2-blockers over the counter, these agents are becoming more widely used. Nurses should be diligent in screening patients for use of any over-the-counter products because of the potential for drug interactions or adverse effects caused by these products.

Proton Pump Inhibitors (PPIs)

Proton pump inhibitors (PPIs) inhibit the proton pumps in the GI tract, which are responsible for secreting H⁺ ions (acid) into the stomach. Because they block the final pathway of acid secretion, PPIs are potent acid-blocking agents and are often used for moderate-to-severe nausea. These agents (omeprazole, lansoprazole, rabeprazole, pantoprazole and esomeprazole) are completely metabolized by the liver before they are excreted by the kidney. As such, no dosage adjustements are necessary in renal failure. Rare cases of interstitial nephritis have been reported with omeprazole. Omeprazole is also available over the counter.

Stool Softeners and Cathartics

Patients with CKD are often prone to constipation for a variety of reasons, such as decreased fluid intake, constipating effect of other medications, decreased mobility, etc.

Bulk forming agents. Bulk formers, such as methylcellulose and psyllium, stimulate peristalsis by increasing fecal mass. Because of fluid restrictions, patients with renal failure should limit the amount of water taken with these agents to half the recommended amount.

Hyperosmolar agents. Hyperosmolar agents, such as lactulose, sorbitol, and polyethylene glycol (PEG), are composed of sugar alcohols or other osmotic substances that draw water into the GI tract to increase frequency, weight, water content, and volume of stools. These agents are generally well tolerated by patients with CKD.

Stool softeners. Stool softeners, such as docusate and

senna, increase fluid penetration into the stool, softening the stool to ease GI transport. Docusate is generally well tolerated. Senna may cause cramping and diarrhea and should not be used long-term.

Saline cathartics. Saline cathartics, such as magnesium citrate and sodium phosphate, act as osmotic agents to draw water into the GI tract to stimulate peristalsis. Use of these agents in CKD is limited because of the high content of magnesium and phosphate contained in the products and the propensity for accumulation and toxicity.

Lubricants. Lubricating agents, such as mineral oil, soften and lubricate hard stools by preventing water absorption in the colon from the stool. Long-term use of mineral oil should be avoided as absorption of fat-soluble vitamins can be disrupted.

Enemas. A number of enema preparations can be used to evacuate the bowel. Use of enemas should be limited to the short-term because of potential mucosal damage and electrolyte depletion.

Sedatives and Hypnotics

Patients with CKD often have difficulty sleeping. Reasons for sleeplessness (e.g., depression) should be thoroughly explored before utilizing medications to induce drowsiness. Diphenhydramine, benzodiazepines (temazepam, lorazepam, oxazepam, diazepam and others), chloral hydrate, zolpidem, and zaleplon are often used as sedatives. In patients with CKD, these agents should be used at the lowest possible dose and increased gradually as the drugs may accumulate, leading to excessive sedation. It is important to note that all sedatives are approved for short-term management of insomnia and may not be suitable for long-term use, particularly in CKD because of the potential of drug accumulation. Zolpidem does not appear to require dosage adjustment in renal failure, but information is limited. Therefore, it should also be started at the lowest dose and increased gradually. There is no information on the use of zaleplon in renal failure and use should be avoided. Most of these medications are metabolized by the liver and are not removed by dialysis.

Antidepressants

Depression is a common, but often unrecognized, complication associated with CKD. Furthermore, depression is an important cause of mortality in patients with CKD (Lopes et al., 2002). Selective serotonin reuptake inhibitors (SSRIs), which include citalopram, escitalopram, fluoxetine, paroxetine, and sertraline, are the most commonly prescribed antidepressants today. All of the drugs in this class are extensively metabolized in the liver, making them safe for patients with CKD, requiring little or no dosage adjustments for declining renal function. The exceptions are citalopram, which is recommended to be used with caution in patients with severe renal failure, and paroxetine, which notes an increase in half-life with severe renal failure, although no dosage adjustment is recommended. All of the SSRIs are dosed once daily. Other antidepressants that are commonly used include venlafaxine and mirtazapine, both of which are eliminated via the kidneys to a higher degree. Doses of both venlafaxine and mirtazapine should be reduced as GFR falls

below 70 mL/min/1.73 m^2 and 40 mL/min/1.73 m^2, respectively. In severe renal failure with GFR < 10 mL/min/1.73 m^2, doses of both drugs should be reduced by 50%. Venlafaxine should be administered in two to three divided doses daily, although an extended release formulation is available that allows for once daily dosing. Mirtazapine should be taken once daily at bedtime because of the drowsiness associated with the drug.

Drug Therapy for the Management of Anemia

It is estimated that 800,000 adults have anemia (Hemoglobin [Hgb] < 11 g/dL) associated with CKD (Hsu, 2002). Hgb levels begin to decline when GFR < 79 mL/min/1.73 m^2 (Hsu, 2002). Anemia associated with CKD typically presents as a normochromic, normocytic anemia. The primary cause of anemia in CKD is a deficiency in erythropoietin (EPO) production. Several other factors can contribute to the development of anemia, including decreased red blood cell (RBC) survival, chronic blood loss (through blood sampling, dialysis, or GI losses), and iron and vitamin deficiencies (folate and B$_{12}$) (NKF, 2001). Workup for the treatment of anemia should begin when Hgb levels fall below 11 g/dL in pre-menopausal women and pre-pubertal patients, or below 12 g/dL in men and post-menopausal women to rule out other causes of anemia. It is essential that the workup for anemia in CKD patients include an analysis of iron stores to rule out iron deficiency as the cause for anemia. Some CKD patients with anemia may respond with an increase in Hgb and hematocrit (Hct) by repleting iron stores. Patients who do not respond to iron supplementation and do not have another obvious cause of anemia should be presumed to have anemia secondary to EPO depletion and begin EPO replacement therapy.

It is estimated that up to 90% of ESKD patients are receiving therapy for anemia (Hudson, 2002). In the past, blood transfusions were used to improve symptoms and to avoid severe tissue hypoxia that occurs in 25% to 50% of chronic renal failure patients. Unfortunately, patients who receive transfusions may develop iron overload; develop cytotoxic antibodies; experience transfusion reactions, such as flushing, urticaria, fever, and chills; or contract infections, such as HIV and hepatitis (although the risk is substantially decreased today). Recombinant human erythropoietin (rHuEPO) and its analogs and iron supplements are used to increase Hgb and Hct in CKD patients with anemia. The goal Hgb for patients with CKD is 11–12 g/dL.

Recombinant Human Erythropoietin (rHuEPO)

Recombinant human erythropoietin (rHuEPO) is indicated for the treatment of anemia associated with chronic renal failure, including patients on dialysis and not on dialysis. Prior to initiating therapy with rHuEPO, other potential causes of anemia should be ruled out, particularly vitamin B$_{12}$ or folate deficiencies and bleeding. In addition, the patient's iron status, including iron, iron binding capacity, percent transferrin saturation (TSat), and serum saturation, should be evaluated to ensure adequate iron stores. TSat should be at least 20% and ferritin at least 100 ng/mL before starting rHuEPO therapy. If iron levels are low, oral or IV iron treatment should be initiated.

rHuEPO doses should be individualized to the patient's response to therapy. Hgb and Hct values increase within 2 to 6 weeks after initiating rHuEPO. A more favorable pharmacodynamic response can be achieved with subcutaneous administration compared to IV administration. As a result, a subcutaneous dose of rHuEPO is generally two thirds the IV rHuEPO dose. Starting doses of rHuEPO are 80 to 120 units/kg/week subcutaneously or 120 to 180 units/kg/week intravenously. rHuEPO should be administered two to three times weekly. Patients receiving hemodialysis typically receive rHuEPO intravenously with each dialysis session for ease of administration. CKD patients not on dialysis or those receiving peritoneal dialysis should receive rHuEPO subcutaneously because of the more favorable response achieved. The dose of rHuEPO should be increased by 50% if the Hct has risen by < 2% over 2 to 4 weeks. Alternatively, the dose should be reduced by 25% if Hgb rises > 3 g/dL within 4 weeks of therapy or if Hgb exceeds the goal (11 - 12 g/dL in patients with CKD).

The most significant side effect of rHuEPO is hypertension. Patients with uncontrolled hypertension should not be treated with rHuEPO; blood pressure should be controlled before initiation of therapy. Blood pressure should be closely monitored in patients receiving rHuEPO therapy, and antihypertensive therapy should be initiated if appropriate to control hypertension caused by rHuEPO. Seizures have been reported as a potential side effect of rHuEPO; however, more recent information questions the causal relationship of rHuEPO and seizures (NKF, 2001). Therefore, rHuEPO therapy should not be withheld in patients with a seizure history. Thrombotic events have also been reported with rHuEPO therapy; however, the causal relationship has not been well established.

The most common cause of rHuEPO failure is iron deficiency. Several factors have been attributed to a delayed or diminished response to rHuEPO therapy, including infection, inflammation, chronic blood loss, osteitis fibrosa, aluminum toxicities, hemoglobinemias, folate or vitamin B_{12} deficiencies, multiple myeloma, malnutrition, or hemolysis. If an inadequate response is achieved in the absence of these factors, a hematology consult is warranted to determine the reason.

Darbepoetin Alfa

Darbepoetin alfa is a novel erythropoietin stimulating protein (NESP) that was approved in 2001 for the treatment of anemia associated with chronic renal failure, including patients on dialysis and not on dialysis. It is a hyperglycosylated analogue of rHuEPO that stimulates EPO production by the same mechanism. The presence of eight additional sialic acid side chains on the darbepoetin alfa molecule produces a longer half-life compared to rHuEPO. IV administration produces a half-life three times longer than rHuEPO; subcutaneous administration produces a half-life twice as long as rHuEPO. The longer half-life allows for less frequent dosing of darbepoetin alfa. Generally, once weekly or every other week administration is sufficient to achieve the same results as rHuEPO. As with rHuEPO, other causes of anemia should be ruled out, and the patient's iron status should be assessed prior to initiating darbepoetin alfa therapy.

Table 18-9
Erythropoietin – Darbepoetin Conversion Chart

Erythropoietin Dose (units per week)	Darbepoetin Dose (mcg)
Up to 10,999	25 mcg
11,000 to 17,999	40 mcg
18,000 to 33,999	60 mcg
34,000 to 59,999	100 mcg
60,000 – 89,999	150 mcg
> 90,000	200 mcg

Note: If erythropoietin is administered in doses divided twice weekly or three times weekly, darbepoetin should be administered as a once weekly dose. If erythropoietin is administered once weekly, darbepoetin should be administered every other week.

Darbepoetin alfa doses should be individualized to the patient's response to therapy. As with rHuEPO, a more favorable pharmacodynamic response can be achieved with subcutaneous administration compared to IV administration. However, initial dosing recommendations are the same for both routes of administration because of the long half-life of the drug. The recommended starting dose of darbepoetin alfa is 0.45 mcg/kg administered once weekly. The same principles generally apply for selection of patients for IV administration (hemodialysis patients) or subcutaneous administration (CKD patients not on dialysis or those receiving peritoneal dialysis). Doses should be individualized to achieve the same Hgb goal (11–12 g/dL in patients with CKD). If the Hct has risen by < 2% over 2 to 4 weeks, the dose of darbepoetin alfa should be increased by 25%. If the Hgb rises > 3 g/dL within 4 weeks of therapy or exceeds the goal, the dose can be decreased by 25% or the interval can be extended (i.e., once weekly dosing extended to every other week or every other week dosing extended to once monthly).

The side effects seen with darbepoetin therapy are the same as those seen with rHuEPO. Hypertension is the most significant side effect and should be treated with antihypertensive therapy as necessary. Factors that can contribute to a delayed or diminished response to darbepoetin therapy are the same as those listed previously for rHuEPO (see Table 18-9).

Iron Supplementation

Iron is necessary for the formation of Hgb. It is essential that iron stores be evaluated in patients who are initiating or receiving EPO replacement therapy. Ferritin levels should be maintained between 100 ng/mL and 800 ng/mL and TSat between 20% and 40% while receiving EPO therapy to ensure adequate response to therapy. As mentioned previously, the most common cause of failure to EPO therapy is iron deficiency. To maintain sufficient iron stores, iron supplementation is often needed in CKD patients receiving EPO replacement therapy.

Oral iron preparations. Oral iron preparations (ferrous sulfate, ferrous gluconate, ferrous fumarate, iron polysaccharide complex) are considered to be the first line of therapy for iron replacement. The dose of oral iron for replacement should provide 200 mg of elemental iron per day. The ferrous salts (sulfate, fumarate, and gluconate) are the least expensive form of oral iron replacement. The dose should be divided two to three times daily to minimize side effects. Most of the products that contain polysaccharide iron complex contain more elemental iron per dose, which can increase patient compliance by reducing the number of daily doses. However, these products are generally more expensive than the ferrous salts. Ascorbic acid (vitamin C) increases iron absorption. Some oral iron products include ascorbic acid in the formulation to capitalize on this interaction.

Side effects associated with oral iron preparations include constipation, diarrhea, nausea, vomiting, abdominal pain, and heartburn. Oral iron supplements are best taken on an empty stomach to increase absorption because iron absorption is dependent on an acidic pH in the GI tract. This, however, leads to an increase in GI-related side effects. In addition, any medications that can increase the pH of the GI tract will also alter oral iron absorption, such as antacids; phosphate binders, particularly calcium-containing binders; H_2-blockers; PPIs; and bile-acid binding resins. Oral iron supplementation can also decrease the absorption of other medications, particularly antibiotics, such as tetracyclines, sulfonamides, fluoroquinolones (e.g., ciprofloxacin, levofloxacin, ofloxacin, and others), and chloramphenicol. The dose of the antibiotics should be separated from oral iron doses by at least 2 hours to minimize the potential interaction.

Intravenous iron (IV) preparations. IV iron should be considered in patients who do not respond to oral iron supplementation. In general, oral iron supplementation is not adequate to maintain iron stores for erythrocyte production in patients receiving EPO therapy or dialysis, and most patients will require IV iron replacement.

Iron dextran. Iron dextran has long been the standard IV iron preparation. It is currently available in two formulations (INFeD® and DexFerrum®), which differ only in the molecular weight of the product. It was thought that the higher molecular weight of the iron product was associated with more adverse reactions compared to a lower molecular weight. Although more adverse effects have been reported with a higher molecular weight product that is no longer available, no clinical difference has been shown between the two products currently on the market. After injection, macrophages of the reticuloendothelial system remove iron dextran from the plasma. Ferric iron is then gradually released into the plasma, where it combines with transferrin. Transferrin transports the iron to the bone marrow to be incorporated into Hgb.

The dose of IV iron replacement needed to maintain adequate iron stores for EPO therapy is a total of 1 gram of elemental iron per course of therapy. Iron dextran provides 50 mg of elemental iron per mL. The typical dosage of iron dextran is approximately 100 mg weekly at the end of dialysis. Larger doses, up to 500 to 1000 mg iron dextran, can be administered at one time. This is particularly beneficial in CKD patients or those receiving peritoneal dialysis to decrease the number of infusions required to administer a full dose of iron replacment. A test dose is recommended because of the risk of anaphylaxis. Although anaphylactic reactions, known to occur following dextran injections, are usually evident within a few minutes, it is recommended that a period of an hour or longer lapse after the initial dose is given. Most facilities have a standard protocol for iron dextran administration that includes a test dose before each injection. Emergency equipment and medications (e.g., diphenhydramine and hydrocortisone) should always be within reach when the test dose is administered. The patient should be observed for other side effects such as pruritus, hypotension, and dyspnea. Iron dextran should be diluted and administered in a 0.9% sodium chloride solution, or it can be administered by a slow IV push no faster than 1 mL/min or diluted in an IV piggyback over 30 minutes.

The most significant side effect noted with iron dextran is anaphylactic reactions, which are life-threatening and manifest as hypotension, syncope, purpura, wheezing, dyspnea, and respiratory arrest. As described before, a test dose should be administered to determine the potential for anaphylaxis following iron dextran administration. However, anaphylactic reactions can occur in any patient despite no reaction to the test dose or even in patients who have received previous courses of iron dextran therapy. Therefore, it is important to closely monitor all patients who are receiving iron dextran therapy for any type of serious reaction during and following therapy. Other significant side effects of iron dextran therapy include delayed reactions, which manifest as arthralgias, myalgias, fever, headache, and lymphadenopathy. Other side effects include headache, dizziness, vomiting, and hypotension, which are often dose-related and can be decreased by prolonging the infusion time or decreasing the dose (Hudson, 2001).

Because of the significant side effects associated with iron dextran, newer IV iron products have been developed that are used more widely today than iron dextran.

Sodium ferric gluconate. Sodium ferric gluconate has been extensively used in Europe prior to its approval in the United States. Iron quickly dissociates from the complex and readily binds to transferrin for transport to the bone marrow to be incorporated into Hgb. Sodium ferric gluconate provides 12.5 mg elemental iron per mL. The dosage regimen approved to provide 1000 mg elemental iron per treatment course is 125 mg sodium ferric gluconate given during 8 consecutive dialysis sessions or clinic visits (usually weekly for 8 weeks). A test dose is not required before administration of sodium ferric gluconate infusions. The dose should be diluted in 100 mL of 0.9% sodium chloride administered over at least 15 minutes or can be administered as a slow IV push no faster than 12.5 mg/min (1 mL/min). Higher doses (up to 500 mg) have been administered over 3 to 5 hour infusions, although the incidence of side effects appears to be dose-related (Bastani, Jain, & Pandurangan, 2003).

Side effects associated with sodium ferric gluconate injections include anaphylactoid-type hypersensitivity reactions, manifesting with hypotension, pruritus, chest pain, and wheezing. The incidence of these reactions is very limited and none have been reported to be fatal. Other more common side effects include hypotension, flushing, nausea, vomiting, and diarrhea.

Iron sucrose. Like sodium ferric gluconate, iron sucrose was extensively used in Europe prior to its approval in the United States. Iron sucrose is dissociated by the reticuloendothelial system to sucrose and iron, which is taken up by transferrin and transported to the bone marrow. Iron sucrose provides 20 mg elemental iron per mL. The dosage regimen approved to provide 1000 mg elemental iron per treatment course is 100 mg iron sucrose given during 10 consecutive dialysis sessions or clinic visits (usually weekly for 10 weeks). A test dose is not required before administration of iron sucrose infusions. The dose can be administered as a slow IV push no faster than 20 mg/min (1 mL/min) or diluted in 100 mL of 0.9% sodium chloride administered over at least 15 minutes. Higher doses (up to 500 mg) have been administered over 3–4 hour infusions (Blaustein et al., 2003).

No anaphylactic or anaphylactoid-type reactions have been reported with the use of iron sucrose. Hypersensitivity reactions have been reported, manifesting as hypotension, wheezing, dyspnea, pruritus, or rash, but none of these reported incidences were life-threatening. Side effects that have been noted after administration of iron sucrose include hypotension, flushing, vomiting, and pruritus.

Drug Therapy for the Management of Electrolyte Disorders

Electrolyte disorders are common with the decline of renal function. Homeostasis of many of the electrolytes is dependent upon renal function. As CKD progresses, serum concentrations of various electrolytes become disrupted with deteriorating renal function. Renal elimination of phosphorus, potassium, sodium, and magnesium decreases, as does renal reabsorption of calcium. The resultant hyperphosphatemia, hyperkalemia, and hypocalcemia can lead to significant complications for the renal failure patient.

Hyperphosphatemia and Hyperparathyroidism

As renal disease progresses and phosphorus levels increase, hyperphosphatemia can lead to significant complications, namely cardiovascular disease, as well as secondary hyperparathyroidism and hypocalcemia, which can result in renal osteodystrophy. Phosphate binders become an essential addition to the medication regimen to reduce complications associated with renal disease. Phosphate binders should be taken within an hour after meals to decrease the amount of phosphate absorbed from the diet. The dose of the phosphate binder should be individualized to the patient to allow for variability in the diet and phosphate consumption, with smaller doses being administered with smaller meals and snacks and larger doses with larger meals. Routine monitoring of serum calcium and phosphorus levels is necessary to ensure adequacy of therapy and minimize toxicity to the patient. The goal phosphorus level in patients with ESKD is 2.7–4.6 mg/dL in patients with Stages 3 or 4 CKD and 4.5–5.5 mg/dL in patients with Stage 5 CKD. Serum calcium levels should be maintained at levels of 9–11.5 mg/dL in Stages 3 or 4 CKD and 8.4–9.5 mg/dL in Stage 5 CKD. The calcium-phosphorus product (Ca x Phos) should be maintained < 55 mg^2/dL^2 for any patient with CKD (NKF, 2003).

Aluminum and magnesium-based phosphate binders. Aluminum-based phosphate binders (aluminum hydroxide) have traditionally been used in the past to lower phosphate concentrations. Today, however, long-term use of these agents should be avoided to prevent aluminum toxicity. Aluminum toxicity usually manifests as organic brain disease, worsening renal osteodystrophy, and anemia. Magnesium-based phosphate binders should also be avoided in renal failure because of the potential for accumulation and toxicity (e.g., arrhythmias, hypotension, and diarrhea).

Calcium-based phosphate binders. Calcium-based phosphate binders are generally the first drugs of choice for lowering phosphorus concentrations in renal failure. They are particularly useful in patients with hypocalcemia as they will also increase calcium levels. The most commonly used agents are calcium carbonate and calcium acetate. Calcium carbonate is the least expensive of the two agents and is also the best absorbed of the two. However, phosphate binding is dependent on the amount of calcium in the GI tract not the amount absorbed. Therefore, calcium acetate binds a greater amount of phosphorus and is useful for patients who do not achieve adequate results with calcium carbonate. Calcium citrate has also been used but is not generally recommended as the citrate component of the product can increase aluminum absorption and contribute to toxicity. Side effects associated with the calcium-containing phosphate products are constipation and hypercalcemia.

Sevelamer. Sevelamer is a potent phosphate binder that does not contain calcium, aluminum, or magnesium. It is a cationic polymer compound that binds to phosphorus in the intestinal lumen. Sevelamer is not absorbed into the bloodstream but is eliminated via the GI tract with the bound phosphorus. Sevelamer is useful in patients with moderate-to-high calcium levels or who are not able to adequately decrease phosphate levels with calcium-containing products. Sevelamer provides added benefit to patients with CKD as it also lowers cholesterol levels by a mechanism similar to bile acid-binding resins. Side effects of sevelamer include constipation, nausea, dyspepsia, diarrhea, and flatulence. Sevelamer can also decrease the absorption of fat-soluble vitamins, such as vitamins A, D, E, and K and may bind to other medications when taken at the same time. Therefore, other medications should be administered 1 hour before or 4 hours after sevelamer.

Lanthanum. Lanthanum carbonate is a cationic element that is an effective phosphate binder. Lanthanum carbonate has a low solubility that readily dissociates in an acidic environment, such as the GI tract, making it available to bind to phosphate in the GI tract. The efficacy of lanthanum is similar to aluminum hydroxide with regard to phosphate binding ability. However, lanthanum is not absorbed from the GI tract and does not accumulate in patients with CKD. Likewise, lanthanum does not accumulate in bone like aluminum (Behets, Verberckmoes, D'Haese, & De Broe, 2004). Clinical trials demonstrate that lanthanum is well tolerated and have reported side effects that include nausea, vomiting, diarrhea, and abdominal cramps.

Vitamin D analogs. Vitamin D analogs are used to increase serum calcium levels in patients with hypocalcemia and to decrease parathyroid hormone levels and increase bone mineralization as treatment for renal osteodystrophy and secondary hyperparathyroidism. Targets for serum intact parathyroid levels are 30–70 pg/mL for Stage 3 CKD, 70–110 pg/mL for Stage 4 CKD and 150–300 pg/mL for Stage 5 CKD (NKF, 2003). When used for secondary hyperparathyroidism, vitamin D therapy should not be initiated in patients unless serum phosphorus levels are adequately controlled and corrected total serum calcium levels are normal. Because vitamin D is activated by the kidney, administration in patients with CKD must be provided in a form that does not require renal activation. Calcitriol is the activated form of vitamin D_3. It can be administered orally or intravenously. Paricalcitol is an activated form of vitamin D_2, typically found in plant sources, which differs slightly in structure from the vitamin D_3 normally found in the body from sunlight and meat sources. Currently, paricalcitol is only available in the IV form; however, an oral formulation is in Phase III trials. Doxercalciferol is a partially activated form of vitamin D_2, which requires final activation by the liver. It is available in capsule or IV forms.

Vitamin D analogs are well tolerated. The most significant side effect is hypercalcemia, caused by an increase in intestinal calcium absorption. Paricalcitol appears to have a lower risk of causing hypercalcemia compared to the other agents. Generally, IV vitamin D analog therapy is administered three times weekly with hemodialysis. Alternatively, oral vitamin D analogs may be administered daily or three times weekly. Vitamin D analog therapy must be monitored carefully and individualized to avoid hypercalcemia. The dose can be adjusted based on serum calcium levels and parathyroid hormone levels, depending on the indication for therapy.

Calcimimetics. Cinacalcet is a calcimimetic agent that is useful to decrease parathyroid levels with minimal effect on serum calcium concentrations. Cinacalcet increases the sensitivity of calcium receptors on parathyroid cells to inhibit excessive secretion of parathyroid hormone. Clinical studies to date demonstrate that cinacalcet produces a rapid decrease in parathyroid hormone levels, serum phosphorus, and the Ca x Phos product. The drug also decreases serum calcium levels (Cunningham, 2004). The role of cinacalcet in the treatment of secondary hyperparathyroidism is yet to be defined, although there is a definite role for patients who are not able to achieve goal levels of intact parathyroid hormone despite vitamin D therapy. It has been suggested that cinacalcet may also have a role as a first-line agent in patients who are naïve to vitamin D therapy (Cunningham, 2004). Few side effects have been reported for cinacalcet and include nausea, vomiting, and hypocalcemia.

Hyperkalemia

Hyperkalemia is a common complication in the latter stages of CKD (Stages 4 and 5). Decreased renal excretion of potassium is the primary cause of hyperkalemia in renal failure. However, other medications can also contribute to hyperkalemia, namely the ACE-inhibitors and ARBs, which are commonly used in CKD for their beneficial effects on the kidney. The development of ACE-inhibitor-induced hyperkalemia in the CKD patient may necessitate discontinuation of the ACE-inhibitor, thereby denying the patient of the reno-protective effects of the ACE-inhibitors to delay progression of renal disease. Prevention and management of hyperkalemia in the CKD patient is essential to providing optimal care to the patient.

Prevention of hyperkalemia can be achieved by avoiding those things that can cause an increase in total potassium body stores or decrease the elimination of potassium from the body. Patients are advised to avoid potassium-rich foods in their diet and potassium-containing salt substitutes to prevent hyperkalemia. Additionally, patients should avoid potassium supplements in the form of potassium replacement to prevent diuretic-induced hypokalemia or in the form of multivitamin supplements. The use of potassium-sparing diuretics can lead to hyperkalemia in CKD patients. If potassium-sparing diuretics are initiated in the earlier stages of CKD as treatment for other medical conditions, diligent follow-up must continue as CKD progresses and the patient moves to the later stages of kidney disease to avoid hyperkalemia. β-adrenergic blockers can interfere with potassium uptake into cells, which increases the risk of hyperkalemia.

Once renal failure occurs, the development of hyperkalemia is inevitable and must be treated to prevent cardiac complications. Dialysis is the primary modality used to decrease potassium levels in patients with renal failure. However, potassium levels can be significantly elevated before dialysis is initiated or between dialysis sessions. There are several strategies that can be used to decrease potassium levels in these situations. Loop diuretics can be used to promote renal potassium excretion in patients with residual renal function. It is important to note that colonic excretion of potassium plays a significant role in maintaining potassium homeostasis in patients with renal failure. Maintaining good bowel regimens and avoiding constipation are key steps in preventing the development of hyperkalemia in CKD patients. Use of stool softeners and cathartics, as described previously, plays an important role in the maintenance of potassium homeostasis.

Insulin and dextrose. Insulin and dextrose are often used to reverse life-threatening and symptomatic hyperkalemia. Insulin stimulates the sodium-potassium exchange pump found on cell membranes to increase intracellular potassium uptake. Dextrose aids in cellular uptake of potassium by providing the substrate on which insulin exerts its action and by directly stimulating insulin secretion from the pancreas. It also serves to decrease the risk of hypoglycemia that may be precipitated by insulin administration. Patients experiencing cardiac abnormalities should also be given calcium intravenously to stabilize the cardiac membrane. Generally, 10 units of regular insulin are given to acutely decrease serum potassium levels. Dextrose can be given as an infusion of 50% solution to prevent the development of hyperglycemia. Patients who are already hyperglycemic can receive smaller doses of dextrose, 5% to 10% infusions, to prevent the development of severe hyperglycemia or ketoacidosis.

Patients should be monitored for signs of hypoglycemia after receiving insulin injections and hyperglycemia after receiving dextrose infusions. Alterations in blood sugars should be appropriately managed. Patients should also be monitored for additional signs and recurrence of hyperkalemia. Repeat potassium levels within 2 to 4 hours can confirm the effectiveness of therapy or signal the need for additional therapy.

Beta$_2$ (β$_2$)-adrenergic agonists. β$_2$-adrenergic agonists (e.g., albuterol) can be used to acutely decrease serum potassium levels in symptomatic patients. Albuterol stimulates the sodium-potassium exchange pump found on cell membranes to increase intracellular potassium uptake. Additionally, it stimulates β_2-receptors in the pancreas to secrete insulin, which further promotes intracellular potassium uptake. The usual dose of albuterol administered is 20 mg via nebulizer or inhaler. The response to β_2-adrenergic agonist therapy is erratic because of underdosing often related to administration techniques. In addition, tachycardia can result from β_2-adrenergic stimulation, which can worsen cardiac abnormalities. For these reasons, β_2-adrenergic therapy is usually reserved as adjunctive therapy in patients already receiving insulin and dextrose therapy to provide synergistic effects on the sodium-potassium cellular pump.

Cationic exchange resins. Cationic exchange resins (e.g., sodium polystyrene sulfonate [SPS]) are used in the treatment of non-life-threatening hyperkalemia. SPS exchanges sodium ions for potassium ions in the GI tract. The amount of sodium and potassium exchanged varies by the route of administration. When administered orally, one gram of sodium is exchanged for 1 mEq of potassium. When administered rectally, one gram of sodium is exchanged for 0.5 mEq of potassium. SPS is available as a powder, which can be mixed with water or other liquid, or as a 70% sorbitol suspension. The sorbitol component of the suspension induces diarrhea, which further promotes potassium excretion. The usual dose of SPS is 15 to 60 grams orally or 60 to 100 grams rectally. Since the insoluble resin is not absorbed, there is no dosage adjustment required in renal failure, hepatic failure, or during dialysis. The effects of SPS can be expected within 6 hours after rectal administration and possibly longer after oral administration. Use of SPS is limited by the slow onset of action to patients with no cardiac abnormalities who are otherwise asymptomatic.

Side effects of SPS include loss of other electrolytes by direct exchange with SPS, as it is not selective exclusively for potassium, and by loss via diarrhea. Magnesium, calcium, and ammonium may also be lost with the administration of SPS. Other side effects include increased absorption of sodium, which can contribute to volume overload. The patient should be monitored for cardiac side effects associated with sodium reabsorption as well as weight gain, edema, hypertension, hypernatremia, pulmonary edema, and worsening left ventricular failure with CHF. Concomitant administration of magnesium-containing antacids can decrease the effectiveness of SPS by exchanging magnesium ions in place of potassium. It is important to monitor patients for hypokalemia, particularly in patients receiving digitalis because hypokalemia can increase the risk of digitalis toxicity.

Nursing implications center on the monitoring of maximum benefits of SPS with minimal side effects. A cleansing enema should be given after rectal administration of the SPS in sorbitol suspension because of the potential for colonic necrosis. Chilling the resin before oral administration increases the palatability of the suspension. The powder should be mixed with liquids to the patient's liking to increase compliance with therapy. Monitoring the patient's bowel patterns; assessing for hypoactive bowel sounds and/or ileus before administering SPS; and determining the effectiveness of stool softeners, laxatives, or cathartics will help prevent constipation, fecal impaction, and/or bowel necrosis.

Fludrocortisone. Fludrocortisone promotes aldosterone-mediated potassium elimination. Aldosterone stimulates the sodium-potassium exchange pump in the distal renal tubules, thereby increasing renal elimination of potassium. Aldosterone may also play a role in colonic elimination of potassium. Because of this, fludrocortisone may provide benefit to the management of intradialytic hyperkalemia (Imbriano, Durham, & Maesaka, 2003). The dose of fludrocortisone begins at 0.1 mg daily and can be titrated up to 0.3 mg daily to achieve the effect. Use of fludrocortisone is limited by its side effects, namely sodium and fluid retention, which can lead to hypertension, edema, and worsening of CHF. Patients should be slowly weaned from fludrocortisone if discontinuation is necessary to minimize the risk of adrenal insufficiency.

Summary

Because the kidney is responsible for elimination of many medications, pharmacokinetic and pharmacodynamic parameters can be significantly altered by CKD. As CKD progresses, the drug selection and monitoring become key in avoiding adverse reactions and slowing the progression of CKD. Understanding the pharmacology and pharmacodynamic principles associated with common medications used in CKD is essential for providing appropriate nursing care to the patient with CKD.

References

ALLHAT officers and coordinators. (2000). Major cardiovascular events in hypertensive patients randomized to doxazosin vs chlorthalidone: The antihypertensive and lipid-lowering treatment to prevent heart attack trial (ALLHAT). *Journal of the American Medical Association, 283*(15), 1967-1975.

Ballantyne, J.C. (2003). Opioid therapy for chronic pain. *New England Journal of Medicine, 349*(20), 1943-1953.

Bastani, B., Jain, A., & Pandurangan, G. (2003). Incidence of side-effects associated with high-dose ferric gluconate in patients with severe chronic renal failure. *Nephrology, 8*(1), 8-10.

Behets, G.J., Verberckmoes, S.C., D'Haese, P.C., & De Broe, M.E. (2004). Lanthanum carbonate: A new phosphate binder. *Current Opinion in Nephrology and Hypertension, 13*, 403-409.

Blaustein, D.A., Schwenk, M.H., Chattopadhyay, J., Singh, H., Daoui, R., Gadh, R., et al. (2003). The safety and efficacy of an accelerated iron sucrose dosing regimen in patients with chronic kidney disease. *Kidney International, 87*(Suppl.), S72-S77.

Brenner, B.M., Cooper, M.E., de Zeeuw, D., Keane, W.F., Mitch, W.E., Parving, H.H., et al. (2001). Effects of losartan on renal and cardiovascular outcomes in patients with type 2 diabetes and nephropathy. *New England Journal of Medicine, 345*(12), 861-869.

Breyer, M.D. (2001). Cyclooxygenase-2 selective inhibitors and the kidney. *Current Opinion in Critical Care, 7*, 393-400.

Choudhury, D. (1997). Drug-induced nephrotoxicity. *Medical Clinics of North America, 81*(3), 705-717.

Cunningham J. (2004). Achieving therapeutic targets in the treatment of secondary hyperparathyroidism. *Nephrology Dialysis and Transplantation, 19*(Suppl. 5), v9-v14.

Gruppo Italiano di Studi Epidemiologici in Nefrologia (GISEN). (1997). Randomized placebo-controlled trial of effect of ramipril on decline in glomerular filtration rate and risk of terminal renal failure in proteinuric, non-diabetic nephropathy. *Lancet, 349*(9069), 1857-1863.

Holdcroft, A. (2003). Management of pain. *British Medical Journal, 326*, 635-639.

Hsu, C.Y. (2002). Epidemiology of anemia associated with chronic renal insufficiency among adults in the United States: Results from the third National Health and Nutrition Examination Survey. *Journal of the American Society of Nephrology, 13*(2), 504-510.

Hudson, J.Q. (2001). Considerations for the optimal iron use for anemia due to chronic kidney disease. *Clinical Therapeutics, 23*(10), 1637-1671.

Hudson, J.Q. (2002). Advances in anemia management in chronic kidney disease. *Journal of Pharmacy Practice, 15*(6), 437-455.

Imbriano, L.J., Durham, J.H., & Maesaka, J.K. (2003). Treating interdialytic hyperkalemia with fludrocortisone. *Seminars in Dialysis, 16*(1), 5-7.

Kincaid-Smith, P. (2002). Randomized controlled crossover study of the effect on proteinuria and blood pressure of adding an angiotensin II receptor antagonist to an angiotensin converting enzyme inhibitor in normotensive patients with chronic renal disease and proteinuria. *Nephrology, Dialysis, and Transplantation 17*, 597-601.

Knopp, R.H. (1999). Drug treatment of lipid disorders. *New England Journal of Medicine, 341*(7), 498-511.

Lehne, R.A. (2004). *Pharmacology for nursing care* (6th ed., pp. 36-37). St. Louis: Saunders.

Lewis, E.J. (1993). The effect of angiotensin-converting enzyme inhibition on diabetic nephropathy. *New England Journal of Medicine, 329*(20), 1456-1462.

Lewis, E.J. (2001). Renoprotective effect of the angiotensin-receptor antagonist irbesartan in patients with nephropathy due to type 2 diabetes. *New England Journal of Medicine, 345*(12), 851-860.

Lopes, A.A., Bragg, J., Young, E., Goodkin, D., Mapes, D., Combe, C., et al. (2002). Depression as a predictor of mortality and hospitalization among hemodialysis patients in the United States and Europe. *Kidney International, 62*, 199-207.

Martin de Francisco, A.L. (2002). Gastrointestinal disease and the kidney. *European Journal of Gastroenterology & Hepatology, 14*(Suppl. 1), S11-S15.

Maschio, G. (1996). Effect of the angiotensin-converting enzyme inhibitor benazepril on the progression of chronic renal insufficiency. *New England Journal of Medicine, 334*(15), 939-955.

Nakao, N. (2003). Combination treatment of angiotensin-II receptor blocker and angiotensin-converting-enzyme inhibitor in non-diabetic renal disease (COOPERATE): A randomized controlled trial. *Lancet, 361*(9352), 117-124.

National Kidney Foundation (NKF). (2001). K/DOQI clinical practice guidelines for anemia of chronic kidney disease. *American Journal of Kidney Diseases, 37*(Suppl. 1), S1-S64.

National Kidney Foundation (NKF). (2002). K/DOQI clinical practice guidelines on chronic kidney disease: Evaluation, classification, and stratification. Kidney Disease Outcome Initiative. *American Journal of Kidney Diseases, 39*(Suppl. 1), S1-246.

National Kidney Foundation (NKF). (2003). K/DOQI clinical practice guidelines for bone metabolism and disease in chronic kidney disease. *American Journal of Kidney Diseases, 42*(Suppl. 3), S1-S202.

National Kidney Foundation (NKF). (2003). K/DOQI clinical practice guidelines for managing dyslipidemias in chronic kidney disease. *American Journal of Kidney Diseases, 41*(Suppl. 3), S1-S92.

National Kidney Foundation (NKF). (2004). K/DOQI clinical practice guidelines on hypertension and antihypertensive agents in chronic kidney disease. *American Journal of Kidney Diseases, 43*(Suppl. 1), S1-S290.

Parving, H.H. (2001). Irbesartan in patients with type 2 diabetes and microalbuminuria study group: The effect of irbesartan on the development of diabetic nephropathy in patients with type 2 diabetes. *New England Journal of Medicine, 345*(12), 870-878.

Ravid, M. (1993). Long-term stabilizing effect of angiotensin-converting enzyme inhibition on plasma creatinine and on proteinuria in normotensive type II diabetic patients. *Annals of Internal Medicine, 118*(8), 577-581.

Thatte, L. (1996). Drug-induced nephrotoxicity: The crucial role of risk factors. *Postgraduate Medicine, 100*(6), 83-106.

- CKD poses many challenges in drug dosing. Because renal disease can affect other organ systems, each of the phases of drug distribution can be altered, including absorption, distribution, metabolism, and most notably, elimination.

- The metabolism and elimination of medications is a complex process. Pathology in any number of areas can contribute to damage to the kidneys and drug-induced renal disease.

- Medications are removed from the body through either of two major mechanisms. If the molecule is water soluble, the kidney will filter the chemical, or fluid lost through physiologic secretions will carry medication with it. If the medication is fat soluble, the medication must be altered to a water-soluble form that the kidney or secretions can remove. The liver is the most prolific organ that metabolizes or detoxifies medications, but all tissue can metabolize medications to a limited extent.

- Volume of distribution and clearance are both affected by physiologic parameters and will change as the condition of the patient changes. The volume of distribution is the apparent space in which a medication will disperse. Clearance is the amount of medication that can be removed from the blood in a defined period of time.

- The complications associated with renal insufficiency necessitate the use of various medications for treatment and management including: diuretics, analgesics, antihypertensives, antihyperlipidemics, vitamin supplements, gastrointestinal agents, antacids, H2-blockers, proton pump inhibitors, stool softeners and cathartics, sedatives and hypnotics, and antidepressants.

- Anemia is a common problem associated with CKD. The primary cause of anemia in CKD is a deficiency in erythropoietin (EPO) production. Several other factors can contribute to the development of anemia, including decreased red blood cell (RBC) survival, chronic blood loss (through blood sampling, dialysis, or GI losses), and iron and vitamin deficiencies (folate and B_{12}).

- Electrolyte disorders are common with the decline of renal function. Homeostasis of many of the electrolytes is dependent upon renal function. As CKD progresses, serum concentrations of various electrolytes become disrupted with deteriorating renal function. Renal elimination of phosphorus, potassium, sodium, and magnesium decreases, as does renal reabsorption of calcium. The resultant hyperphosphatemia, hyperkalemia, and hypocalcemia can lead to significant complications for the renal failure patient.

- Because the kidney is responsible for elimination of many medications, pharmacokinetic and pharmacodynamic parameters can be significantly altered by CKD. As CKD progresses, the drug selection and monitoring become key in avoiding adverse reactions and slowing the progression of CKD.

Pharmacology of Renal Disease

Name of Resource	Brief Description	Where to Obtain Resource
Dialysis of Drugs	This booklet contains an extensive list of drugs indicating the dialyzability of each by hemodialysis, high-flux dialysis, and peritoneal dialysis and is available through Nephrology Pharmacy Associates.	Web link: http://www.nephrologypharmacy.com/pub_dialysis.html
K/DOQI Guidelines	The Kidney Disease Outcomes Quality Initiative (K/DOQI) has developed evidence-based practice guidelines for various aspects of kidney disease, including treatment of anemia, management of bone metabolism and disease, and management of hyperlipidemias in kidney disease.	Web link: http://www.nephrologypharmacy.com/pub_dialysis.html
The Drug Monitor – Renal Pharmacology	Renal therapeutics, diuretics, and information on renal dosing guidelines are discussed in this forum, along with clinical calculators and equations.	Web link: http://www.thedrugmonitor.com/renalpharmacology.html
iKidney.com	This is a useful website for patients and health care professionals that includes articles on many different aspects of living with kidney disease, medications, renal diet (including recipes) and other resources.	Web link: http://www.ikidney.com/iKidney/home.htm
Nephron.com	This website provides general renal information, calendars of events for renal associations, links to colleges and universities with nephrology departments, publications and other resources for health care professionals and patients.	Web link: http://nephron.com/

ANNP618

Pharmacology of Renal Disease

Kristine Schonder, PharmD

Contemporary Nephrology Nursing: Principles and Practice contains 39 chapters of educational content. Individual learners may apply for continuing nursing education credit by reading a chapter and completing the Continuing Education Evaluation Form for that chapter. Learners may apply for continuing education credit for any or all chapters.

Please photocopy this page and return to ANNA.
COMPLETE THE FOLLOWING:

Name: _____

Address:_____

City:_____State: _____Zip: _____

E-mail: _____

Preferred telephone: ☐ Home   ☐ Work: _____

State where licensed and license number (optional): _____

CE application fees are based upon the number of contact hours provided by the individual chapter. CE fees per contact hour for ANNA members are as follows: 1.0-1.9 - $15; 2.0-2.9 - $20; 3.0-3.9 - $25; 4.0 and higher - $30. Fees for nonmembers are $10 higher.

ANNA Member: ☐ Yes   ☐ No   Member # (if available) _____

☐ Checked Enclosed   ☐ American Express   ☐ Visa   ☐ MasterCard

Total Amount Submitted: _____

Credit Card Number: _____ Exp. Date: _____

Name as it appears on the card: _____

CE Evaluation Form
To receive continuing education credit for individual study after reading the chapter
1. Photocopy this form. (You may also download this form from ANNA's Web site, **www.annanurse.org**.)
2. Mail the completed form with payment (check) or credit card information to American Nephrology Nurses' Association, East Holly Avenue, Box 56, Pitman, NJ 08071-0056.
3. You will receive your CE certificate from ANNA in 4 to 6 weeks.

Test returns must be postmarked by **December 31, 2010.**

CE Application Fee
ANNA Member $25.00
Nonmember $35.00

EVALUATION FORM

1. I verify that I have read this chapter and completed this education activity. Date: _____

   _____
   Signature

2. What would be different in your practice if you applied what you learned from this activity? *(Please use additional sheet of paper if necessary.)*

   _____
   _____
   _____
   _____
   _____
   _____
   _____
   _____
   _____
   _____
   _____
   _____
   _____

Evaluation	Strongly disagree				Strongly agree
3. The activity met the stated objectives.					
a. Link the drug dosing modifications necessary in people with chronic kidney disease to their ability to metabolize and eliminate drugs.	1	2	3	4	5
b. Discuss reasons that commonly used drugs prescribed for people with renal insufficiency are required.	1	2	3	4	5
c. Summarize the drugs used for the treatment of anemia in patients with chronic kidney disease.	1	2	3	4	5
4. The content was current and relevant.	1	2	3	4	5
5. The content was presented clearly.	1	2	3	4	5
6. The content was covered adequately.	1	2	3	4	5
7. Rate your ability to apply the learning obtained from this activity to practice.	1	2	3	4	5

Comments _____
_____

8. Time required to read the chapter and complete this form: _____ minutes.

This educational activity has been provided by the American Nephrology Nurses' Association (ANNA) for 3.5 contact hours. ANNA is accredited as a provider of continuing nursing education (CNE) by the American Nurses Credentialing Center's Commission on Accreditation (ANCC-COA). ANNA is an approved provider of continuing education by the California Board of Registered Nursing, CEP 0910.

Contemporary Nephrology Nursing: Principles and Practice, Second Edition © — American Nephrology Nurses' Association 2006

Infections in the Hemodialysis Unit

Eileen Peacock, MSN, RN, CNN, CIC, CPHQ

Acknowledgments: *Portions of this chapter are reprinted from the following source: Alter, M.J., Tokars, J.L., Arduibo, M.J. & Favero, M.S. (2004). Nosocomial infections associated with hemodialysis. In C.G. Mayhall (Editor), Hospital epidemiology and infection control (3rd ed.) (pp. 1139-1160). Baltimore, MD: Williams & Wilkins.*

The Editors would also like to acknowledge the contributions to this chapter from the authors of Chapter 13, "Control of Infectious Diseases in the Renal Patient," which was published in the 1998 edition of this textbook. Those authors were: Janel Parker, MSN, RN, CNN; Linda Dickenson, BS, RN, CNN, CPHQ; Karen C. Wiseman, MSN, RN, CNN; Diane Alexander, MS, BSN, RN, CNN; and Eileen Peacock, MSN, RN, CNN, CIC, CPHQ.

Chapter Contents

Eileen Peacock, MSN, RN, CNN, CIC, CPHQ

Of the patients with end stage renal disease (ESRD) treated by maintenance hemodialysis in the United States, 91% are on hemodialysis (United States Renal Data System [USRDS], 2002). Chronic hemodialysis patients are at high risk for infection because the process of hemodialysis requires vascular access for prolonged periods. In an environment where multiple patients receive dialysis concurrently, repeated opportunities exist for person-to-person transmission of infectious agents, directly or indirectly via contaminated devices, equipment and supplies, environmental surfaces, or hands of personnel. Furthermore, hemodialysis patients are immunosuppressed, which increases their susceptibility to infection, and they require frequent hospitalizations and surgery, which increases their opportunities for exposure to nosocomial infections. This chapter provides a general overview of the major infectious diseases that can be acquired in the dialysis setting, describes epidemiologic and environmental considerations, as well as the most current infection control strategies recommended by the Centers for Disease Control and Prevention (CDC), Recommendations for Preventing Transmission of Infections Among Hemodialysis Patients, published in the April 27, 2001 issue of the Morbidity & Mortality Weekly Report (MMWR, Volume 50, No. RR-5). Important implications for the nephrology nurse are also discussed.

Bacterial Infections

The annual mortality rate among hemodialysis patients is 23%, and infections are the second most common cause, accounting for 14% of deaths (USRDS, 2002). Septicemia (11.1% of all deaths) is the most common infectious cause of mortality. In studies published during 1997-2000 that evaluated rates of bacterial infections in hemodialysis outpatients, bacteremia occurred in 0.63%–1.7% of patients per month and vascular access infections (with or without bacteremia) in 1.3%–7.2% of patients per month (Bonomo et al., 1997; Dobkin, Miller & Steibigel, 1978; Hoen, Paul-Dauphin, Hestin, & Kessler, 1998; Kaplowitz, Comstock, Landwehr, Dalton, & Mayhall, 1988;; Kessler, Hoen, Mayeux, Hestin, & Fontenaille, 1993; Bloembergen & Port, 1996; Stevenson et al., 2002; Tokars, Light, & Armistead, 2001). A review of four studies published during 2002 estimated that 1.8% of hemodialysis patients have vascular access associated bacteremia each month, amounting to 50,000 cases nationally per year (Tokars, 2002).

Because of the importance of bacterial infections in hemodialysis patients, the CDC initiated an ongoing surveillance project in 1999 (Tokars, Frank, Alter, & Arduino, 2002). All U.S. hemodialysis centers treating outpatients are eligible to enroll. Only bacterial infections associated with hospital admission or intravenous antimicrobial receipt are counted; since infections treated with outpatient oral antimicrobials are excluded, this system likely detects only the more severe infections. During 1999-2001, 109 centers reported data.

Rates of infection per 100 patient months were 3.2 for all vascular access infections (including access infections both with and without bacteremia), 1.8 for vascular-access associated bacteremia, 1.3 for wound infections not related to the vascular access, 0.8 for pneumonias, and 0.3 for urinary tract infections. Among patients with fistulas or grafts, wounds were the most common site of infection. Among patients with hemodialysis catheters, infections of the vascular access site were most common.

In a study of 27 French hemodialysis centers, 28% of 230 infections in hemodialysis patients involved the vascular access, whereas 25% involved the lung, 23% the urinary tract, 9% the skin and soft tissues, and 15% other or unknown sites (Kessler et al., 1993). Thirty-three percent of infections involved either the vascular access site or were bacteremias of unknown origin, many of which might have been caused by occult access infections. Thus, the vascular access site was the most common site for infection, but accounted for only one-third of infections.

Bacteria that cause infection can be either exogenous (i.e, acquired from contaminated dialysis equipment) or endogenous (i.e., caused by invasion of bacteria present in or on the patient). Endogenous pathogens first colonize the patient and later cause infection (CDC, 2001). Colonization means that the microorganisms have become resident in or on the body (e.g., *Staphylococcus aureus* [*S. aureus*] in the outer nasal passages; *Escherichia coli, Pseudomonas aeruginosa* in the stool); culture from the site is positive, but no signs or symptoms of infection exist. Colonization with potentially pathogenic bacteria is not uncommon in patients who are immunosupressed, have frequent exposure to antibiotics, or experience frequent or prolonged hospital admissions (CDC, 2001).

Transmission

Colonizing bacteria may persist for years without causing disease or harming their hosts, but can be spread to others by contact transmission. Transmission of bacteria may occur when microorganisms from an infected or colonized patient are transferred to the hands of a health care worker (HCW), who then touches another patient (CDC, 2001). Environmental surfaces such as countertops may also become contaminated. Transmission can then occur when a HCW touches a contaminated surface and then touches a patient (CDC, 2001). If a HCW's hands are not adequately cleaned and gloved before providing patient care, bacteria from the hands can transfer to the patient's vascular access site, blood line port, or catheter port. The bacteria are inadvertently introduced into the patient when the skin or access port is made patent by either a needle puncture or line connection (CDC, 2001). Infection then occurs as a result of the bacteria invading the body. Evidence exists that when the prevalence of colonization is less frequent, the prevalence of infection will also be less frequent (CDC, 2001). Asymptomatic carriers entering hospitals or other health care facilities may shed bacteria, even antibiotic resistant bacteria, for years but remain undetected, transmitting the colonized bacteria to others (Smith et al, 2004; Association for Professionals in Infection Control and Epidemiology [APIC], 2000).

Prevention of Transmission

The CDC *Recommendations for Preventing Transmission of Infections Among Hemodialysis Patients* (2001) are designed to prevent both colonization and the transmission of potential pathogens. Measures to prevent contact transmission of potential pathogens, whether from endogenous or exogenous sources, emphasize hand hygiene (i.e., hand washing or use of a waterless hand rub), glove use, and disinfection of environmental surfaces (CDC, 2001). Proper hand hygiene is a critical measure for preventing the transmission of potential pathogens. Good hand hygiene can result in a significant reduction in the carriage of potential pathogens on the hands, as well as a reduction in patient morbidity (CDC, 2002; APIC, 2000) and mortality related to nosocomial infection (APIC, 2000). Proper use of nonsterile disposable gloves also helps to reduce the potential for hand contamination of HCWs. The CDC (2002) has recommended that HCWs wear gloves to:

- reduce the risk of the HCW acquiring infections from patients
- prevent health care worker flora from being transmitted to patients
- reduce transient contamination of the HCW's hands by flora that can be transmitted from one patient to another

Even with glove use, hand washing is needed because pathogens deposited on the outer surface of gloves can be found on hands after the gloves are removed (Olsen et al., 1993; CDC 2001). Bacterial flora, known to colonize patients, have been cultured from the hands of more than 30% of HCWs who wore gloves during patient contact (CDC, 2002). Contamination may be possible due to defects in the gloves, leakage at the wrist, or contamination of the hands during glove removal (CDC, 2001). The gloves' integrity has known to vary on the basis of type and quality of glove material, intensity of use, and length of time used (APIC, 2000; CDC, 2002).

Exogenous pathogens also have caused numerous outbreaks, most of which resulted from inadequate dialyzer reprocessing procedures (e.g., contaminated water or inadequate disinfectant) or inadequate treatment of municipal water for use in dialysis. During 1995–1997, four outbreaks were traced to contamination of the waste drain port on one type of dialysis machine (CDC, 1998). Contaminated medication vials also are a potential exogenous source of bacterial infection for patients. In 1999, an outbreak of *Serratia liquefaciens* bloodstream infections and pyrogenic reactions among hemodialysis patients was traced to contamination of vials of erythropoietin. These vials, which were intended for single use, were contaminated by repeated puncture to obtain additional doses and by pooling of residual medication into a common vial (Grohskopf et al, 2001). Nephrology nurses need to be familiar with the infection prevention measures regarding medication preparation and distribution,

which include (CDC, 2001):

- Preparing medications in a room or area separated from the patient treatment area and designated for medication preparation.
- Not handling or storing used or contaminated supplies, equipment, or blood samples, in areas where medications are prepared.
- Intravenous medication vials labeled for single use should not be punctured more than once.
- Residual medication from two or more vials should not be pooled into a single vial.
- Common carts should not be used within the patient treatment area to prepare or distribute medications.
- When multiple dose medications vials are used (including vials containing diluents), prepare individual patient doses in a clean centralized area away from the treatment area and deliver separately to each patient.
- Do not carry medication vials, syringes, alcohol swabs in pockets.

Antimicrobial-Resistant Bacteria

Antibiotic resistance is widely acknowledged to be one of the most pressing medical problems facing the world today. In the United States alone, nearly 2 million patients acquire an infection in the hospital each year. Of those patients, about 90,000 die each year as a result of their infection. Alarmingly, more than 70% of the bacteria that cause hospital-acquired infections are resistant to at least one of the drugs most commonly used for treatment (NIAD, 2004). Treating resistant infections often requires the use of second and third choice drugs that may be less effective or more expensive (NIAD, 2004). Antimicrobial resistance may limit treatment choice presenting a challenge for the patient with drug allergies. The prognosis for a successful treatment outcome may be worse than with susceptible organisms, longer hospital stays may be required, along with special efforts to prevent transmission (APIC, 2000).

Drug resistance is the state of decreased or inhibited sensitivity to medications, such as antibiotics, that ordinarily cause death or inhibit growth of a cell. Resistance develops when bacteria find new ways to disarm the medications. Bacteria may be capable of changing their cell walls to keep drugs out (decreased drug permeability), altering the drug-receptor target site, and crossbreeding with related species transferring resistance factors from one bacterium to another. Resistance factors can spread between organisms, to different strains, and even to different species of bacteria (APIC, 2000). A key mechanism of antibiotic resistance is the ability of the bacteria to cause drug destruction. Resistant bacteria may be capable of producing enzymes to destroy or inactivate antibiotics (APIC, 2000). For example, one mechanism responsible for the resistance *of Staphylococcus aureus (S. aureus)* to β-lactamas antibiotics (penicillins) is the production of the bacterial enzymes, β–lactamases, by resistant bacteria. These enzymes are able to cause decomposition of the β-lactam ring; a vital part of the antibiotic structure. This ability of bacteria to produce β- lactamases is the most common resistant mechanism seen in penicillins and cephalosporins (USC, 2000).

Critical to the development of antimicrobial resistance is the bacteria's ability to adapt quickly to new environmental conditions, such as when an antibiotic is administered. A mutation that helps a bacterium to survive in the presence of an antibiotic quickly becomes predominant (NIAD a, 2004). For example, in the early 1940s when penicillin first became available for clinical use, it was not a challenge to effectively treat infection caused by *Staphylococcus aureus* (*S. aureus*). However, by the early 1950s, approximately 80% of these infections were resistant to penicillin, necessitating the development of new antibiotics. During the 1960s *S. aureus* infections were treated by administering the new antibiotics related to penicillin. These antibiotics were semi-synthetic penicillins (methicillin, oxacillin, and nafcillin) and first-generation cephalosoporins such as cephalothin. In less than 10 years, strains of *S. aureus* that were now resistant to methicillin and other semi synthetic penicillins were identified in England, Europe, and the United States (APIC, 2000). These resistant bacteria are commonly called methicillin-resistant *Staphylococcus aureus*, or MRSA. Due to exposure to several different antibiotics that have been used as treatment to fight infections, MRSA strains are also frequently resistant to many other classes of antibiotics such as tetracyclines and erythromycins, making vancomycin one of the limited few effective antibiotics available to treat such infections. The emergence of vancomycin-resistant *Staphylococcus* was not far behind. Resistance to all different kinds of antibiotics has been observed in organisms of all different species. Clinically important drug- resistant bacteria that cause infections include:

- **MRSA** - methicillin/oxacillin-resistant Staphylococcus *aureus*
- **MRSE** – methicillin/oxacillin-resistant Staphylococcus *epidermidis*, coagulase-negative staphylococcus (CNS)
- **VRE** - vanomycin-resistant enterococci
- **ESBLs** - extended-spectrum beta lactamases; resistant to cephalosporins and monobactams
- **PRSP** - penicillin-resistant Streptococcus *pneumoniae*
- **VISA** - vancomycin-intermediate Staphylococcus *aureus*
- **VSRA** - vancomycin-resistant Staphylococcus *aureus*

Hemodialysis patients have been in the forefront of the epidemic of antimicrobial resistance, especially vancomycin resistance. One of the earliest reports of vancomycin-resistant enterocci (VRE) was from a renal unit in London, England, in 1988 (Uttley et al., 1989). The prevalence of VRE stool colonization among dialysis patients has varied from 2.4% at three centers in Indianapolis, IN (Brady, Snyder, & Hasbargen, 1998) to 9.5% at a university hospital in Baltimore, MD (Roghmann et al., 1998). In one center with a prevalence of 9%, three patients developed VRE infections in 1 year (Fishbane et al., 1999). Among enterococci causing bloodstream infections in hemodialysis patients, 0-5% have been reported to be resistant to vancomycin (Tokars et al., 2002; Dopirak et al., 2002; Taylor et al., 2002).

Vancomycin resistance in staphylococci has also been reported in dialysis patients. Five of the first six U.S. patients with vancomycin intermediate-resistant *S. aureus* infections identified required dialysis (Fridkin, 2001). Additionally, the first patient found to be infected with a fully vancomycin resistant *S. aureus* strain was a chronic hemodialysis patient; vancomycin-resistant *S. aureus* was isolated from a foot wound and temporary catheter exit site (Chang et al., 2003).

Much has been done to curtail the development of antibiotic-resistant organisms. For example, the Centers for Disease Control and Prevention (CDC) recommend that vancomycin not be used when treating a *S. aureus* infection that is methicillin-sensitive. The CDC emphasizes the importance of appropriate antibiotic use and that vancomycin be used only when necessary. When appropriate, first-generation cephalosporins should be considered instead of vancomycin (CDC, 1995; Fogel et al., 1998).

Vancomycin is used commonly in dialysis patients, in part because vancomycin can be conveniently administered to patients when they come in for hemodialysis treatments. Prudent antimicrobial use is an important component of the CDC recommendations for preventing the spread of vancomycin resistance (CDC, 1995). This guideline states that vancomycin is *not* indicated for therapy (chosen for dosing convenience) of infections due to betalactamsensitive gram-positive microorganisms in patients with renal failure. Depending on the situation, alternative antimicrobials (e.g., cephalosporins) with dosing intervals greater than 48 hours, which would allow postdialytic dosing, could be used. Recent studies suggest that cefazolin given three times a week in the dialysis unit provides adequate blood levels and could be used to treat many infections in hemodialysis patients (Fogel et al., 1998; Marx, Frye, Matzke, & Golper, 1998).

Acceptable Use of Vancomycin

Situations in which the use of vancomycin is appropriate or acceptable:

- For treatment of serious infections due to beta-lactam resistant gram-positive microorganisms (e.g., MRSA). Clinicians should be aware that vancomycin may be less rapidly bactericidal than beta-lactam agents for beta-lactam susceptible staphylococci.
- For treatment of infections due to gram-positive microorganisms in patients with serious allergy to beta-lactam antimicrobials.
- When antibiotic-associated colitis (AAC) fails to respond to metronidazole (Flagyl) therapy or if AAC is severe and potentially life-threatening.
- Prophylaxis, as recommended by the American Heart Association, for endocarditis following certain procedures in patients at high risk for endocarditis.
- Prophylaxis for surgical procedures involving implantation of prosthetic materials or devices at institutions with a *high rate* of infections due to MRSA or methicillin-resistant *S. epidermidis* (CNS). A single dose administered immediately before surgery is sufficient unless the procedure lasts more than 6 hours, in which case the dose should be repeated. Prophylaxis should be discontinued after a maximum of 2 doses.

Discouraging Use of Vancomycin

Situations in which the use of vancomycin should be discouraged:

- Routine surgical prophylaxis.
- Empirical antimicrobial therapy for a febrile neu-

tropenic patient, unless there is strong evidence at the outset that the patient has an infection due to gram-positive microorganisms (e.g., inflamed exit of Hickman catheter), and the prevalence of infections due to beta-lactam resistant gram-positive microorganisms (e.g., MSRA) in the hospital is substantial.

- Treatment in response to a single blood culture positive for *coagulase-negative staphylococcus* (CNS), if other blood cultures drawn in the same time frame are negative, i.e., if contamination of the blood culture is likely. Because contamination of blood culture with skin flora, (i.e., *S. epidermidis; coagulase-negative staphylococcus* [CNS], may cause vancomycin to be inappropriately administered to patients). Phlebotomists and other HCWs who obtain blood cultures should be properly trained to minimize microbial contamination of specimens.
- Continued empirical use for presumed infections in patients whose cultures are negative for beta-lactam-resistant gram-positive microorganisms.
- Systemic or local prophylaxis for infection or colonization of indwelling central or peripheral intravascular catheters or vascular grafts.
- Selective decontamination of the digestive tract.
- Eradication of MRSA colonization.
- Primary treatment of AAC.
- Routine prophylaxis for patients on continuous ambulatory peritoneal dialysis (CAPD) (CDC, 1995).

Dialysis Precautions

For certain patients, including those infected or colonized with MRSA or VRE, contact precautions are used in the inpatient hospital setting. However, contact precautions are not recommended in hemodialysis units for patients infected or colonized with pathogenic bacteria for several reasons. First, although contact transmission of pathogenic bacteria is well-documented in hospitals, similar transmission has not been well-documented in hemodialysis centers. Transmission might not be apparent in dialysis centers, possibly because it occurs less frequently than in acute-care hospitals or results in undetected colonization rather than overt infection. Also, because dialysis patients are frequently hospitalized, determining whether transmission occurred in the inpatient or outpatient setting is difficult. Second, contamination of the patient's skin, bed clothes, and environmental surfaces with pathogenic bacteria is likely to be more common in hospital settings (where patients spend 24 hours a day) than in outpatient hemodialysis centers (where patients spend approximately 10 hours a week). Third, the routine use of infection control practices recommended for hemodialysis units (see Table 19-1), which are more stringent than the Standard Precautions routinely used in hospitals, should prevent transmission by the contact route (CDC, 2001).

Contact transmission can be prevented by hand hygiene (Boyce & Pittet, 2002), glove use, and disinfection of environmental surfaces. Infection control precautions recommended for all hemodialysis patients are adequate to prevent transmission for most patients infected or colonized with pathogenic bacteria, including antimicrobial-resistant strains (see Table 19-1). However, additional precautions should be

considered for treatment of patients who might be at increased risk for transmitting pathogenic bacteria. Such patients include those with either an infected skin wound with drainage that is *not* contained by dressings (the drainage does not have to be culture positive for MRSA or VRE or any specific pathogen) or fecal incontinence or diarrhea uncontrolled with personal hygiene measures. For these patients, consider using the following *additional* precautions:

- Staff members treating the patient should wear a separate gown over their usual clothing and remove the gown when finished caring for the patient.
- Dialyze the patient at a station with as few adjacent stations as possible (e.g., at the end or corner of the unit) (CDC, 2001).

Nephrology nurses are in a unique position to prevent the transmission and proliferation of drug resistant bacteria. There are several effective measures that can be easily implemented that will have a significant impact.

- Practice hand hygiene. Within health care facilities, drug-resistant bacteria are thought to be transmitted from patient to patient primarily through the contaminated hands of HCWs. Hand hygiene is the single most important infection control measure because it prevents transmission of pathogens via the hands of health care personnel (CDC, 2001).
- Partner with your patients. Per the CDC's *"Campaign to Prevent Antimicrobial Resistance in Dialysis Patients,"* a study of chronic hemodialysis patients has shown that a patient's hygiene practices have an important effect upon infection rates, especially access infections. Nephrology nurses must educate patients about hand washing, proper access care, and how to recognize signs and symptoms of infection. Patients should be encouraged to wash their hands upon entering and exiting the dialysis unit, to carefully wash their access arm prior to the treatment, and to use a glove if they hold their own vascular access site posttreatment to stop bleeding.
- Participate in your facility efforts to reduce the number of hemodialysis catheters. Catheters for hemodialysis are the most common factor contributing to bacteremia in dialysis patients (CDC, 2001). In fact, the relative risk for bacteremia in patients with dialysis catheters is sevenfold the risk for patients having AV fistulas.
- Perform follow-up to all cultures (see Table 19-2). Reviewing all cultures and the reported sensitivies (antibiotics that can be used to effectively treat the bacteria causing the infection) is vital to ensure appropriate and effective treatment, while preventing the bacteria from developing resistance to other antibiotics. Cultures should be obtained prior to starting the ordered antibiotics. Careful technique is required when obtaining a culture. Contamination of blood culture specimens and other patient specimens may lead to unnecessary antibiotic use. Antibiotics are usually ordered before the culture and sensitivity (C&S) results are available. The physician selects an antibiotic with an antimicrobial spectrum likely to target the bacteria causing the infection. This is called empiric

Table 19-1

Recommended Infection Control Practices for Hemodialysis Units

Infection Control Precautions for All Patients

- Wear disposable gloves when caring for the patient or touching the patient's equipment at the dialysis station; remove gloves and wash hands between each patient or station.

- Items taken into the dialysis station should either be disposed of, dedicated for use only on a single patient, or cleaned and disinfected before taken to a common clean area or used on another patient.
  - Nondisposable items that cannot be cleaned and disinfected (e.g., adhesive tape, cloth-covered blood pressure cuffs) should be dedicated for use only on a single patient.
  - Unused medications (including multiple dose vials containing diluents) or supplies (syringes, alcohol swabs, etc.) taken to the patient's station should be used only for that patient and should not be returned to a common clean area or used on other patients.

- When multiple dose medication vials are used (including vials containing diluents), prepare individual patient doses in a clean (centralized) area away from dialysis stations and deliver separately to each patient. Do not carry multiple dose medication vials from station to station.

- Do not use common medication carts to deliver medications to patients. Do not carry medication vials, syringes, alcohol swabs or supplies in pockets. If trays are used to deliver medications to individual patients, they must be cleaned between patients.

- Clean areas should be clearly designated for the preparation, handling and storage of medications and unused supplies and equipment. Clean areas should be clearly separated from contaminated areas where used supplies and equipment are handled. Do not handle and store medications or clean supplies in the same or an adjacent area to that where used equipment or blood samples are handled.

- Use external venous and arterial pressure transducer filters/protectors for each patient treatment to prevent blood contamination of the dialysis machines' pressure monitors. Change filters/protectors between each patient treatment, and do not reuse them. Internal transducer filters do not need to be changed routinely between patients.

- Clean and disinfect the dialysis station (chairs, beds, tables, machines, etc.) between patients.
  - Give special attention to cleaning control panels on the dialysis machines and other surfaces that are frequently touched and potentially contaminated with patients' blood.
  - Discard all fluid and clean and disinfect all surfaces and containers associated with the prime waste (including buckets attached to the machines).

- For dialyzers and blood tubing that will be reprocessed, cap dialyzer ports and clamp tubing. Place all used dialyzers and tubing in leak-proof containers for transport from station to reprocessing or disposal area.

Note: From CDC. (2001). Recommendations for preventing transmission of infections among chronic hemodialysis patients. *MMWR, 50*(No. RR-5), 1-43.

---

therapy. Gram stain results are often reported before the final culture results, and can aid the physician in determining if the empiric therapy will be effective. Inform the physician of the gram stain results as soon as possible. Culture and sensitivity results must also be reported to the physician as soon as possible. Based on the results, the physician may adjust the antibiotic to one that is more effective. Do not assume that the antibiotic ordered as empiric therapy will be effective as treatment. The physician will make that judgment based on the C&S findings. The CDC recommends vancomycin be used only when necessary; every effort should be made to avoid vancomycin use for the purpose of convenience dosing only. Stopping empiric therapy when cultures are negative can reduce antibiotic use and the chance of emergence of resistant organisms. If culture results are negative, notify the physician. A repeat culture and/or discontinuation of the antibiotic may be ordered. Because *S. epidermidis* (CNS) is a normal skin bacteria, often the physician will confirm the cultures have not been contaminated and that the results indeed reflect the patient's condition (see Table 19-3).

- Follow established policy and procedures for antibiot-

Table 19-2
Appropriate Culturing and Follow-up

- Cultures should be obtained prior to starting the ordered antibiotics. Careful technique is required when obtaining a culture. Contamination of blood culture specimens and other patient specimens may lead to unnecessary antibiotic use.

- Antibiotics are usually ordered before the culture and sensitivity (C&S) results are available. The physician selects an antibiotic likely to target the bacteria causing the infection. This is called empiric therapy.

- Gram stain results that are often reported before the final culture results can aid the physician in determining if the empiric therapy will be effective. Inform the physician of the gram stain results as soon as possible.

- Culture and sensitivity results must also be reported to the physician as soon as possible. Based on the results, the physician may adjust the antibiotic to one that is more effective. Do not assume that the antibiotic ordered as empiric therapy will be effective. The physician will make that judgment based on the C&S findings. The CDC recommends vancomycin is used only when necessary and not for convenience dosing.

- Stopping empiric therapy when cultures are negative can reduce antibiotic use and the chance of emergence of resistant organisms. If culture results are negative, notify the physician. A repeat culture and/or discontinuation of the antibiotic may be ordered.

ic storage, preparation and administration. Successful antimicrobial therapy does *not* solely depend on appropriate antibiotic selection. Nephrology nurses also play a critical role by ensuring prompt institution of the appropriate antibiotic(s), that antibiotics are given on time and as prescribed. The ability of an antibiotic to be effective is related to concentration, time, and synergy drug factors. Both the serum concentration of the drug and the organism exposure time to the drug must be optimal for the antibiotic to be effective. Antibiotics may also be prescribed in combination for their synergistic effect (i.e., an antibiotic that affects the bacteria at the cell wall and an antibiotic that affects protein synthesis) (APIC, 2000).

Vascular Access Infections

Access site infections are particularly important because they can cause disseminated bacteremia or loss of the vascular access. Local signs of vascular access infection include erythema, warmth, induration, swelling, tenderness, breakdown of skin, loculated fluid, or purulent exudate (Bonomo et al., 1997; Kaplowitz et al., 1998; Padberg, Lee & Curl, 1992; Tokars et al., 2002). In the CDC surveillance project, rates of access-associated bacteremia per 100 patient-months were 1.8 overall, and varied by access type: 0.25 for fistulas, 0.53 for grafts, 4.8 for permanent (tunneled, cuffed) catheters, and 8.7 for temporary (nontunneled, noncuffed) catheters (Tokars et al., 2001). Vascular access infections are caused (in descending order of frequency) by:
- *S. aureus* (32%-53% of cases)
- coagulase-negative staphylococci (CNS; 20%-32%)
- gram-negative bacilli (10%-18%), nonstaphylococcal
- gram-positive cocci (including enterococci; 10%-12%)
- fungi (<1%)

The proportion of infections caused by *S. aureus* is higher among patients with fistulas or grafts. The proportion caused by CNS is higher among patients dialyzed through catheters. Both bacteria are capable of biofilm formation (Donlan, 2001; Johannes et al., 2001). The bacteria can be spread through cross contamination and easily adheres to foreign bodies and biomaterials. The bacteria can gain access to the catheter by migration externally from the skin along the exterior catheter surface or internally from the catheter hub or port. Biofilm develop quickly and protect the bacterial inhabitants from antibiotics. Some biofilms have demonstrated strong resistance to conventional antibiotics, biocides, and hydrodynamic shear forces. Resistance to antimicrobial agents is an important feature of biofilm, making infections caused by bacterial biofilms difficult to eliminate and often requiring device (e.g., catheter) removal (Donlan, 2001; Johannes et al., 2001).

The primary risk factor for access infection is access type, with catheters having the highest risk for infection, grafts intermediate, and native arteriovenous (AV) fistulas the lowest (Hoen et al., 1998; Padberg et al., 1992; Tokars at al., 2002). Other potential risk factors for vascular access infections include:
- location of the access in the lower extremity
- recent access surgery
- trauma, hematoma, dermatitis, or scratching over the access site
- poor patient hygiene
- poor needle insertion technique
- older age
- diabetes
- immunosuppression
- iron overload

(Fan & Schwab, 1992; Bonomo et al., 1997; Besarab et al., 1998; Kaplowitz et al., 1998; Powe, Jaar, Furth, Herman, & Briggs, 1999).

Based on the relative risk of both infectious and noninfectious complications, it is recommended that native arteriovenous fistulas be used more commonly and hemodialysis catheters less commonly; a goal of no more than 10% of patients maintained with permanent catheter-based hemodialysis treatments is recommended (Bonomo et al., 1997; Kaplowitz et al., 1988; Besarab et al., 1998; NKF, 2001). To minimize infectious complications, patients should be referred early for creation of an implanted access, there-

Table 19-3
Identifying Cultures Contaminated from CNS

Clues to identify true coagulase-negative staph (CNS) bacteremia
- Occurrence of multiple positive blood culture sets
- Growth in both aerobic and anaerobic bottles
- Presence of foreign bodies in the patient, especially intravascular catheters & grafts
- Detection of positive blood cultures in less than 48 hours after cultures are obtained

Clues that blood cultures may be contaminated
- Only the aerobic bottle of a set is positive
- If two or more sets of blood cultures are done, but only one or a minority of bottles is positive
- The patient does not have a foreign body in place
- Delayed growth (longer than 48 hours) of a positive blood culture

Note: From APIC (2000).

by decreasing the time dialyzed through a temporary catheter. Additionally, permanent catheters should be used only in patients for whom implanted access is impossible. During 1995-2001, the percentage of patients dialyzed through fistulas increased from 22% to 30%, with most of the increase occurring since 1999 (Tokars et al., 2002; CDC, unpublished data). During the same period, use of grafts decreased from 65% to 44% of patients, and use of catheters increased from 13% to 25%; however, the rate of increase in catheter use appears to be slowing. Recommendations for preventing vascular access infections have been developed by the National Kidney Foundation (NKF, 2001) and the CDC (CDC, 2002) and recently summarized (Berns & Tokars, 2002). Selected recommendations for preventing hemodialysis-catheter associated infection include:
- not using antimicrobial prophylaxis before insertion or during the use of the catheter.
- not routinely replacing the catheter.
- using sterile technique (cap, mask, sterile gown, large sterile drapes, and gloves) during catheter insertion.
- limiting use of noncuffed catheters to 3-4 weeks.
- using the catheter solely for hemodialysis unless there is no alternative.
- restricting catheter manipulation and dressing changes to trained personnel.
- replacing catheter-site dressing at each dialysis treatment or if damp, loose, or soiled.
- disinfecting skin before catheter insertion and dressing changes (a 2% chlorhexidine-based preparation is preferred).
- ensuring that catheter-site care is compatible with the catheter material.

In hemodialysis patients, the Infectious Diseases Society of America has recommended treatment with nasal mupirocin in documented *S. aureus* carriers who have a catheter-related blood stream infection with S. aureus and continue to need the hemodialysis catheter (Mermel et al., 2001). Otherwise, the routine use of nasal mupirocin in patients with hemodialysis catheters is *not* recommended by either CDC or the National Kidney Foundation (NKF, 2001; CDC, 2002.)

Hepatitis B Virus (HBV)

HBV is the microbe that is most efficiently transmitted in the dialysis setting (CDC, 2001). Hepatitis B (HB) is the disease caused by the hepatitis B virus, a small DNA virus and member of the family Hepadnoviridae. The virus uses its own reverse transcriptase for replication (APIC, 2000). HBV has been classified into eight genotypes (A-H). Subtypes have now been identified within some genotypes. The predominate genotypes in the United States are A and C. Through ongoing research, more knowledge is being gained about HBV genotypes and their association to progression of the chronic carrier state, liver disease activity, and response to treatment (Fung & Lok, 2004).

The hepatitis B surface antigen (HBsAg) is a nonreplicating part of the virus that is produced in large quantities. In persons who recover from HBV infection, HBsAG is eliminated from the blood usually within 2-3 months (CDC, 2001). Antibody to the surface antigen is called surface antibody (anti-Hbs). The antibodies appear during convalescence. Generally, anti-Hbs and HBsAg are exclusive of each other, and the anti-HBs confers immunity and convalescence from infection with the HB virus (Parker, Dickenson, Wiseman, Alexander, & Peacock, 1998). The Dane particle of the HB virus has an interior core antigen (HBcAG), which can be detected in liver tissue only. Serological testing for HBcAG is not possible because HBcAg does not freely circulate in the blood (CDC, 2001). However, serological testing for the antibodies to the core antigen (anti-HBc) is available. Antibodies to the core antigen appear together in the IgM class (anti-HBc-IgM), during acute hepatitis B (usually about 4 to 6 months), and the IgG class (anti-HBc-IgG), during convalescence or chronic infection (Parker et al., 1998). After recovery from natural infection, most individuals will be positive for both anti-HBs and anti-HBc, whereas only anti-HBs develops in those successfully vaccinated against HBV (CDC, 2001).

The hepatitis E antigen (HBeAg) is part of the interior core antigen. It appears simultaneously with the HBsAg and denotes viral replication and high levels of circulating virus. The antibody to HBeAg indicates that viral replication is at a lower level, but it does not confer immunity (CDC, 2001; Parker et al., 1998).

Epidemiology

Hepatitis B virus (HBV) infection is a global health problem. Greater than 350 million people are infected worldwide (Edlich et al., 2003) and more than 250,000 chronic carriers die annually from HBV-related liver disease (Maynard, 1990). It is estimated 200,000 people acquire new HBV infections each year in the United States. Of those newly infected, 20,000–30,000 develop chronic hepatitis B. Approximately 1.25 million people in the United States now have chronic HBV infection, and 4,000 to 5,000 people die each year from hepatitis B-related chronic liver disease or liver cancer (CDC, 1991). Infection rates also differ among various racial and ethnic groups (CDC, 1991). For example, Asian Americans are infected at a higher rate than the general American population. Between 1 in 10 Asian Americans are thought to be chronically infected with HBV (Do, 2004).

During the early 1970s, HBV infection was endemic in dialysis units and outbreaks were common. Recommendations for the control of hepatitis B in hemodialysis centers were first published in 1977 (CDC, 1996), and by 1980, their widespread implementation was associated with a sharp reduction in incidence of HBV infection among both patients and staff members (Alter, Ahtone, & Maynard, 1983). The segregation of HBsAg-positive patients and their equipment from HBV-susceptible patients resulted in 70%-80% reductions in incidence of HBV infection among hemodialysis patients (Alter, Favero, & Maynard, 1986; Najem et al., 1981). The success of isolation practices in preventing transmission of HBV infection is linked to other infection control practices, including routine serological surveillance and routine cleaning and disinfection. Subsequently, the incidence and prevalence of HBV infection among chronic hemodialysis patients in the United States have dramatically declined, and by 2001, was 0.05% and 0.9%, respectively (CDC, unpublished data, 2001; Tokars, Miller, Alter, & Arduino, 2000). Only 2.9% of all centers reported patients with newly acquired infections, however, 26.5% of centers provided dialysis to one or more chronically infected patients (CDC, unpublished data, 2001). These chronically infected patients can serve as a reservoir for HBV transmission and outbreaks of HBV infections continue to occur among chronic hemodialysis patients.

Screening and Diagnostic Tests

Several well-defined antigen-antibody systems are associated with HBV infection, including HBsAg and antibody to HBsAg (anti-HBs); hepatitis B core antigen (HBcAg) and antibody to HBcAg (anti-HBc); and HBeAg and antibody to HBeAg (anti-HBe). Serologic assays are commercially available for all of these except HBcAg because no free HBcAg circulates in blood. One or more of these serologic markers are present during different phases of HBV infection (see Table 19-4) (Hoofnagle & Di Bisceglie, 1991). HBV infection also can be detected using qualitative or quantitative tests for HBV DNA. These tests are not FDA-approved and are most commonly used for patients being managed with antiviral therapy (Dienstag et al., 1999; Lai, Chien, & Leung, 1998; Najem et al., 1981).

The presence of HBsAg is indicative of ongoing HBV infection and potential infectiousness. In newly infected per-

sons, HBsAg is present in serum 30-60 days after exposure to HBV and persists for variable periods. Transient HBsAg positivity (lasting <18 days) can be detected in some patients during vaccination (CDC, 2001; Kloster, Kramer, Eastlund, Grossman, & Zarvan, 1995; Lunn, Hoggarth, & Cook, 2000). Anti-HBc develops in all HBV infections, appearing at onset of symptoms or liver test abnormalities in acute HBV infection, rising rapidly to high levels, and persisting for life. Acute or recently acquired infection can be distinguished by presence of the immunoglobulin M (IgM) class of anti-HBc, which persists for approximately 6 months. In persons who recover from HBV infection, HBsAg is eliminated from the blood, usually in 2 to 3 months, and anti-HBs develops during convalescence. The presence of anti-HBs indicates immunity from HBV infection. After recovery from natural infection, most persons will be positive for both anti-HBs and anti-HBc, whereas only anti-HBs develops in persons who are successfully vaccinated against hepatitis B. Persons who do not recover from HBV infection and become chronically infected remain positive for HBsAg (and anti-HBc), although a small proportion (0.3% per year) eventually clear HBsAg and might develop anti-HBs (CDC, 2001; McMahon et al., 1990).

Transmission

The chronically infected person is central to the epidemiology of HBV transmission. HBV is transmitted in the dialysis setting by percutaneous (i.e., puncture through the skin) or permucosal (i.e., direct contact with mucous membranes) exposure to infectious blood or to body fluids that contain blood. All HBsAg-positive persons are infectious, but those who are also positive for hepatitis B e antigen (HBeAg) circulate HBV at high titers in their blood (10^{8-9} virions/mL) (Alter et al., 1976; Shikata, Karasawa, & Abe, 1977). With virus titers in blood this high, body fluids containing serum or blood also can contain high levels of HBV and are potentially infectious. Furthermore, HBV at titers of 10^{2-3} virions/mL can be present on environmental surfaces in the absence of any visible blood and still cause transmission (Alter et al., 1976; Bond, Favero, & Petersen, 1981; CDC, 2001; Favero, Bond, Petersen, Berquist, & Maynard, 1974). HBV is relatively stable in the environment and remains viable for at least 7 days on environmental surfaces at room temperature (Alter et al., 1976; Bond et al., 1981; CDC, 2001; Favero et al., 1974).

HBsAg has been detected in dialysis centers on clamps, scissors, dialysis machine control knobs, and doorknobs (CDC, 2001; Favero et al., 1973). Thus, blood-contaminated surfaces that are not routinely cleaned and disinfected represent a reservoir for HBV transmission. Dialysis staff members can transfer virus to patients from contaminated surfaces by their hands or gloves or through use of contaminated equipment and supplies (CDC, 2001). Such examples of cross contamination can result in outbreaks. Most HBV infection outbreaks among hemodialysis patients have been related to cross-contamination to patients and include:

- environmental surfaces, supplies (e.g., hemostats, clamps), or equipment that were not routinely disinfected after each use.
- multiple dose medication vials and intravenous solu-

Table 19-4
Interpretation of Serologic Test Results for Hepatitis B Virus Infection

Serologic Markers				Interpretation
HBsAg*	Total Anti-HBc[†]	IgM[§] Anti-HBc	Anti-HBs[¶]	
–	–	–	–	Susceptible, never infected
+	–	–	–	Acute infection, early incubation**
+	+	+	–	Acute infection
–	+	+	–	Acute resolving infection
–	+	–	+	Past infection, recovered and immune
+	+	–	–	Chronic infection
--	+	–	–	False positive (i.e., susceptible), past infection, or "low-level" chronic infection
–	–	–	+	Immune if titer is ≥ 10 mIU/mL

*   Hepatitis B surface antigen·
[†]   Antibody to hepatitis B core antigen.
[§]   Immunoglobulin M.
[¶]   Antibody to hepatitis B surface antigen.
** Transient HBsAg positivity (lasting ≤ 18 days) might be detected in some patients during vaccination.

tions that were not used exclusively for one patient.
• medications for injection that were prepared in areas adjacent to areas where blood samples were handled.
• staff members who simultaneously cared for both HBV-infected and susceptible patients.
• failure to routinely screen patients for HBsAg or routinely review results of testing to identify infected patients.
• sharing of supplies, particularly multiple dose medication vials, among patients.
• Underutilization of the hepatitis B vaccine.
(Alter et al., 1983; Carl et al., 1983; CDC, 2001; Snydman et al., 1976; Kantor, Hadler, Schreeder, Berquist, & Favero, 1979; Niu et al., 1989).
HBV transmission among chronic hemodialysis patients also has been associated with hemodialysis provided in the

acute-care setting (CDC, 1996; CDC, 2001; Hutin et al., 1999). Transmission appeared to stem from chronically-infected HBV patients who shared staff members, multiple dose medication vials, and other supplies and equipment with susceptible patients. These episodes were recognized when patients returned to their chronic hemodialysis units, and routine HBsAg testing was resumed. Frequent serologic testing for HBsAg will detect patients recently infected with HBV quickly so isolation procedures can be implemented before cross-contamination can occur.

Transmission from HBV-infected chronic hemodialysis patients to patients undergoing hemodialysis for acute renal failure has not been documented, possibly because these patients are dialyzed for short durations and have limited exposure. However, such transmission could go unrecognized because acute renal failure patients are unlikely to be tested for HBV infection.

Other risk factors for acquiring HBV infection include injection drug use, sexual and household exposure to an HBV-infected contact, exposure to multiple sexual partners, male homosexual activity, and perinatal exposure. Dialysis patients should be educated about these other risks and, for those patients chronically infected with HBV, informed that their sexual partners and household contacts should be vaccinated against hepatitis B (CDC, 1991; CDC, 2001).

Chronic Carrier State

Persistence of HBsAg for more than 6 months indicates a chronic HBV carrier state (Juszczyk, 2000). In 5% of patients with acute hepatitis B, a chronic carrier state develops (Parker et al., 1998; CDC, 2001). Most adults with healthy immune systems recover completely from newly acquired HBV infection. These individuals have eliminated the virus from their blood and have produced antibodies providing protection from future infection (CDC, 2001). Patient age and immune system status at the time of infection influence the development of a chronic carrier state (Parker et al., 1998). HBV genotype may also play a role (Fung & Lok, 2004).

In infants and young children, most cases of newly acquired HBV infection result in chronic infection (CDC, 2001). Ninety percent of newborns and 29%-40% of children, who become infected, develop chronic HBV infection. Only 5%-10% of infected adults with a healthy immune system progress to a chronic carrier state (Parker et al., 1998; Juszczyk, 2000). Due to the immunosuppressive effects of ESRD, dialysis patients usually experience a mild illness but progress to a chronic carrier state at a rate of 40%-90% (Parker et al., 1998). The overall outcome of chronic HBV infection varies. In the absence of interferon alpha or lamivudine (Epivir; 3TC) therapy, an estimated 5-year survival of 86%-97% (chronic hepatitis) to 55% (chronic active hepatitis with cirrhosis), has been cited (Juszczyk, 2000). Causes of death related to chronic HBV infection include hepatocellular carcinoma, liver failure, and upper gastrointestinal bleeding (Parker et al., 1998).

Vaccine

The first official recommendations on the use of hepatitis B vaccine published in June 1982 by the Advisory Committee on Immunization Practices (ACIP) (CDC, 2002), recommended high-risk groups, including dialysis patients, receive the vaccine (CDC, 2001). Since that time, the prevalence of chronic HBV infection has decreased substantially among populations whose infection rates were high (see Table 19-5) (CDC, 2002). The first hepatitis B vaccine (Hepavax®) used in the United States was derived from plasma donors and produced anti-HBs in 95% of the vaccinated subjects (Parker et al., 1998). Vaccines are now produced by recombinant DNA technology. Plasma-derived HBV vaccine is no longer used in the United States. Two yeast recombinant vaccines are now available: Recombivax-HB® and Engerix® (Parker et al., 1998; CDC, 2001).

Hepatitis B vaccination is an essential component of prevention in the hemodialysis setting (Parker et al., 1998). Optimal use of the vaccine reduces the reservoir of infected persons, thereby decreasing opportunities for cross transmission and the infection of others. National surveillance data have demonstrated that independent risk factors among chronic hemodialysis patients for acquiring HBV infection include the presence of >I HBV-infected patient in the hemodialysis center who is not isolated, as well as a <50% hepatitis B vaccination rate among patients (CDC, 2001; Tokars, Miller, Moyer, & Favero, 1997). All susceptible patients and staff should receive the HBV vaccine (see Table 19-6). Protection against hepatitis B infection is complete for persons with a healthy immune system who develop protective antibody levels (anti-HBs 10 mIU/mL or greater) after receiving the complete series. Protection of these individuals persists even when antibody titers become undetectable (CDC, 2001). However, among dialysis patients who respond to the vaccine, protection is not maintained when antibodies fall below anti-HBs 10 mIU/mL. It is for this reason that dialysis patients who achieve protective antibody response levels should still be retested annually, and if levels fall below anti-HBs 10mIU/mL, a booster dose should be administered (see Table 19-7) (CDC, 2001).

Dialysis Precautions

HBsAg-positive patients should undergo dialysis in a separate room designated only for HBsAg-positive patients. They should use separate machines, equipment, and supplies, and most importantly staff members should not care for both HBsAg-positive and susceptible patients on the same shift or at the same time. Dialyzers should not be reused on HBsAg-positive patients. Because HBV is efficiently transmitted through occupational exposure to blood, reprocessing dialyzers from HBsAg-positive patients might place HBV-susceptible staff members at increased risk for infection.

HBV chronically-infected patients (i.e., those who are HBsAg positive, total anti-HBc positive, and IgM anti-HBc negative) are infectious to others and are at risk for chronic liver disease. They should be counseled regarding preventing transmission to others, their household and sexual partners should receive hepatitis B vaccine, and they should be evaluated (by consultation or referral, if appropriate) for the presence or development of chronic liver disease according to current medical practice guidelines. Persons with chronic liver disease should be vaccinated against hepatitis A, if susceptible.

HBV chronically-infected patients do not require any routine follow-up testing for purposes of infection control. However, annual testing for HBsAg is reasonable to detect the small percentage of HBV-infected patients who might lose their HBsAg.

Hepatitis C Virus (HCV)

Hepatitis C virus (HCV) infection is the most common chronic bloodborne infection in the United States. Infection with HCV is caused by a single-stranded RNA virus that is classified as a separate genus in the Flaviridae family (Hwang, 2001; Parker et al., 1998). There are at least six genotypes of the virus with each differing slightly in their DNA sequencing. Numerous subtypes of HCV also exist within each genotype. Multiple quasispecies may co-exist in a single infected individual. Different genotypes and subtypes have different geographical distributions. In the United States, 1a and 1b are the predominant genotypes in patients

Table 19-5
Achievements in Public Health: Hepatitis B Vaccination - United States, 1982-2002

- 1982 - The Advisory Committee on Immunization Practices (ACIP) publishes first official recommendations on use of hepatitis B vaccine for high risk groups.

- 1992 - ACIP recommends a comprehensive strategy to eliminate HBV transmission in the United States focusing efforts on universal childhood vaccination, prevention of perinatal transmission, vaccination of adolescents and adults in high-risk groups, and catch-up vaccinations for susceptible children in high-risk populations.

- 1994 - Congress enacts "Vaccines for Children", a national program to purchase vaccines for eligible children aged <19 years.

- 1995 - ACIP recommends routine vaccination of all adolescents aged 11-12 years who had not been previously vaccinated.

- 1995 - Rate of HBV infection in health-care workers declined by 95% since 1983.

- 1999 - ACIP recommends HBV vaccine for all unvaccinated children aged <19 years.

- 2000 - National coverage rate for hepatitis B vaccine among children aged 19-35 months increased from 16% in 1993 to 90%; rate for adolescents aged 13-15 years increased from near zero to 67%.

- 2002 - Approximately 44 states have by now, enacted laws mandating hepatitis B vaccination for children entering elementary schools and childcare centers. Thirty-four states enacted laws requiring vaccination for adolescents in middle school.

- 2002- Prevalence of chronic HBV infection substantially reduced since 1982 in populations whose infection rates previously were high.

Note: From CDC (2002).

Table 19-6
Doses and Schedules of Licensed Hepatitis B Vaccines for Hemodialysis Patients and Staff Members

Group	Recombivax HB™*			Engerix-B®†		
	Dose	Volume	Schedule	Dose	Volume	Schedule
Patients aged >20 years Predialysis§	10 µg	1.0 ml	0, 1, and 6 months	20 µg	1.0 ml	0, 1, and 6 months
Dialysis-dependent	40 µg	1.0 ml¶	0, 1, and 6 months	40 µg	2-1.0 ml doses at one site	0, 1, 2, and 6 months
Patients aged <20 years**	5 µg	0.5 ml	0, 1, and 6 months	10 µg	0.5 ml	0, 1, and 6 months
Staff members aged >20 years	10 µg	1.0 ml	0, 1, and 6 months	20 µg	1.0 ml	0, 1, and 6 months

* Merck & Company, Inc., West Point, Pennsylvania
† SmithKline Beecham Biologicals, Philadelphia, Pennsylvania
§ Immunogenicity might depend on degree of renal insufficiency
¶ Special formulation
** Doses for all persons aged <20 years approved by the U.S. Food and Drug Administration; for hemodialysis patients, higher doses might be more immunogenic

Note: All doses should be administered in the deltoid by the intramuscular route.

with chronic hepatitis C (Zein et al., 1996). The different genotypes and subtypes are also associated with different rates of disease progression, severity, and response to treatment. For example, certain studies have shown that patients with HCV genotype 1a or 1b had more severe liver disease and lower rates of response to interferon therapy than did patients with HCV genotype 2a or 2b (Alonso et al., 2003; Zein et al., 1996).

Epidemiology

Approximately 170 million people worldwide are infected with HCV (Afdhal, 2004). HCV infects nearly 3 million persons in the United States with the majority of infections acquired by intravenous drug use (Pearlman, 2004). Chronic infection is reaching 85% in some populations with the risk of progression to advanced liver disease as high as 20% to 30% within 10 to 20 years of infection (Hwang, 2001;

Table 19-7
Schedule for Routine Hepatitis B Testing

Schedule for Routine Testing for Hepatitis B Virus (HBV) and Hepatitis C Virus (HCV) Infections

Patient Status	On Admission	Monthly	Semi-Annual	Annual
All patients	HBsAg*, Anti-HBc (total)* Anti-HBs*, Anti-HCV, ALT[†]			
HBV susceptible, including non-responders to vaccine		HBsAg		
Anti-HBs positive ($\geq$10 mIU/mL), anti-HBc negative				Anti-HBs
Anti-HBs and anti-HBc positive	No additional HBV testing needed			
Anti-HCV negative		ALT	Anti-HCV	

*Results of HBV testing should be known before the patient begins dialysis
[†]HBsAg=hepatitis B surface antigen; Anti-HBc=antibody to hepatitis B core antigen; Anti-HBs=antibody to hepatitis B surface antigen; Anti-HCV=antibody to hepatitis C virus; ALT=alanine aminotransferase.

Hepatitis B Vaccination

- Vaccinate all susceptible patients against hepatitis B.

- Test for anti-HBs 1-2 months after last dose
  - If anti-HBs is <10 mIU/mL, consider patient susceptible, revaccinate with an additional three doses, and retest for anti-HBs.
  - If anti-HBs is >10 mIU/mL, consider immune, and retest annually.
    - Give booster dose of vaccine if anti-HBs declines to <10 mIU/mL and continue to retest annually

Management of HBsAg-Positive Patients

- Follow infection control practices for hemodialysis units for all patients.

- Dialyze HBsAg-positive patients in a separate room using separate machines, equipment, instruments, and supplies.

- Staff members caring for HBsAg-positive patients should not care for HBV susceptible patients at the same time (e.g., during the same shift or during patient change-over).

Pearlman, 2004). The prevalence of HCV infection is higher in African Americans and Hispanics than it is in white Americans (Afdhal, 2004).

Data are limited on current incidence and prevalence of HCV infection among chronic hemodialysis patients. In 2001, 62% of centers reported that they tested patients for antibody to HCV (anti-HCV) (CDC, unpublished data). In the centers that tested, the reported incidence was 0.29% and prevalence was 8.6% (range among ESRD networks, 5.7%-11.9%). Twelve percent of centers reported newly acquired

HCV infections among patients. Higher incidence rates have been reported from cohort studies of hemodialysis patients in the United States (<1-3%) and Europe (3-10%) (Fabrizi et al., 1994; Fabrizi et al., 1998; Forns et al., 1997; McLaughlin et al., 1997; Niu, Coleman, & Alter, 1993; Petrosilla et al., 2001; Pinto dos Santos, Loureiro, Cendorolgo, & Pereira, 1996). Higher prevalences (10%-36%) also have been reported from studies of patients in individual facilities (Niu et al., 1993; Sivapalasingam, Malak, Sullivan, Lorch, & Sepkowitz, 2002).

Table 19-8

Interpretation of Test Results for Hepatitis C Virus Infection

Anti-HCV-positive
- An anti-HCV-positive result is defined as anti-HCV screening-test-positive and recombinant immunoblot positive (RIBA®) or nucleic acid test (NAT) positive; or anti-HCV screening-test-positive, NAT negative, RIBA positive.
- An anti-HCV-positive result indicates past or current HCV infection.
- An HCV RNA-positive result indicates current (active) infection, but the significance of a single HCV RNA negative result is unknown; it does not differentiate intermittent viremia from resolved infection.
- All anti-HCV positive persons should receive counseling and undergo medical evaluation, including additional testing for the presence of virus and liver disease.
- Anti-HCV testing generally does not need to be repeated, once a positive anti-HCV result has been confirmed.

Anti-HCV-negative
- An anti-HCV negative result is defined as anti-HCV screening-test-negative*; or anti-HCV screening-test-positive, RIBA negative; or 3) anti-HCV screening-test-positive, NAT negative, RIBA negative.
- An anti-HCV negative person is considered uninfected.
- No further evaluation or follow-up for HCV is required, unless recent infection is suspected or other evidence exists to indicate HCV infection (e.g., abnormal liver enzyme levels in immunocompromised persons or persons with no other etiology for their liver disease).

Anti-HCV-indeterminate
- An indeterminate anti-HCV result is defined as anti-HCV screening-test-positive, RIBA indeterminate; or anti-HCV screening-test-positive, NAT negative, RIBA indeterminate.
- An indeterminate anti-HCV result indicates that the HCV antibody status cannot be determined.
- Can indicate a false positive anti-HCV screening test result, the most likely interpretation in those at low risk for HCV infection; such persons are HCV RNA negative.
- Can occur as a transient finding in recently infected persons who are in the process of seroconversion; such persons usually are HCV RNA positive.
- Can be a persistent finding in persons chronically infected with HCV; such persons usually are HCV RNA positive.
- If NAT is not performed, another sample should be collected for repeat anti-HCV testing (>1 month later).

*Interpretation of screening immunoassay test results based on criteria provided by the manufacturer.

Note: From CDC (2003).

Screening and Diagnostic Tests

FDA-licensed or approved anti-HCV screening test kits being used in the United States comprise three immunoassays; two enzyme immunoassays (EIA) and one enhanced chemiluminescence immunoassay (CIA) (CDC, 2003). FDA-licensed or approved supplemental tests include a serologic anti-HCV assay, the strip immunoblot assay (Chiron RIBA® HCV 3.0 SIA, Chiron Corp., Emeryville, California), and nucleic acid tests (NAT) for HCV RNA (including reverse transcriptase polymerase chain reaction [RT-PCR] amplification and transcription mediated amplification [TMA]).

Anti-HCV testing includes initial screening with an immunoassay. If the screening test is positive, an independent supplemental test with high specificity should be performed to verify the results. Among hemodialysis patients, the proportion of false-positive screening test results averages approximately 15% (CDC, 2003). For this reason, not relying exclusively on anti-HCV screening-test–positive results to determine whether a person has been infected with HCV is critical. Table 19-8 describes the interpretation of HCV testing results both for screening and diagnosis.

For routine HCV testing of hemodialysis patients, the anti-HCV screening immunoassay is recommended, and if positive, supplemental anti-HCV testing using RIBA. RIBA is recommended rather than a NAT because it is a serologic assay and can be performed on the same serum or plasma sample collected for the screening anti-HCV assay. In addi-

tion, certain situations exist in which the HCV RNA result can be negative in persons with active HCV infection. As the titer of anti-HCV increases during acute infection, the titer of HCV RNA declines (Busch et al., 2000). Thus, HCV RNA is not detectable in certain persons during the acute phase of their hepatitis C, but this finding can be transient and chronic infection can develop (Williams et al., 2002). In addition, intermittent HCV RNA positivity has been observed among persons with chronic HCV infection (Alter et al., 1992; Larghi et al., 2002; Thomas et al., 2000). Therefore, the significance of a single negative HCV RNA result is unknown, and the need for further investigation or follow-up is determined by verifying anti-HCV status. In addition, detection of HCV RNA requires that the serum or plasma sample be collected and handled in a manner suitable for NAT and that testing be performed in a laboratory with facilities established for this purpose. Although in rare instances, detection of HCV RNA might be the only evidence of HCV infection, a recent study conducted among almost 3,000 hemodialysis patients in the United States found that only 0.07% were HCV RNA positive but anti-HCV negative (CDC, unpublished data).

Transmission

HCV is most efficiently transmitted by direct percutaneous exposure to infectious blood, and like HBV, the chronically-infected person is central to the epidemiology of HCV transmission. Risk factors associated with HCV infection among hemodialysis patients include blood transfusions from unscreened donors and years on dialysis (Niu et al., 1993; Sivapalasingam et al., 2002). The number of years on dialysis is the major risk factor independently associated with higher rates of HCV infection. As the time patients spent on dialysis increased, their prevalence of HCV infection increased from an average of 12% for patients receiving dialysis <5 years to an average of 37% for patients receiving dialysis >5 years (Hardy, Sandroni, Danielson, & Wilson, 1992; Selgas et al., 1992; Niu et al., 1993; Sivapalasingam et al., 2002).

These studies, as well as investigations of dialysis-associated outbreaks of hepatitis C, indicate that HCV transmission most likely occurs because of inadequate infection control practices. During 1999-2000, CDC investigated three outbreaks of HCV infection among patients in chronic hemodialysis centers (CDC, unpublished data, 1999 and 2000). In two of the outbreaks, multiple transmissions of HCV occurred during periods of 16-24 months (attack rates: 6.6%-17.5%), and seroconversions were associated with receiving dialysis immediately after a chronically infected patient. Multiple opportunities for cross-contamination among patients were observed, including:

- equipment and supplies that were not disinfected between patient use.
- use of common medication carts to prepare and distribute medications at patients' stations.
- sharing of multiple dose medication vials, which were placed at patients' stations on top of hemodialysis machines.
- contaminated priming buckets that were not routinely changed or cleaned and disinfected between patients.
- machine surfaces that were not routinely cleaned and disinfected between patients.
- blood spills that were not cleaned up promptly (CDC, 1996).

In the third outbreak, multiple new infections clustered at one point in time (attack rate: 27%), suggesting a common exposure event. Multiple opportunities for cross-contamination from chronically-infected patients also were observed in this unit. In particular, supply carts were moved from one station to another and contained both clean supplies and blood-contaminated items, including small biohazard containers, sharps disposal boxes, and used vacutainers containing patients' blood.

Other risk factors for acquiring HCV infection include injection drug use, exposure to an HCV-infected sexual partner or household contact, multiple sexual partners, and perinatal exposure (Alter, 1997; Alter, 2002). The efficiency of transmission in settings involving sexual or household exposure to infected contacts is low, and the magnitude of risk and the circumstances under which these exposures result in transmission are not well defined.

Transplantation

Transplantation of the liver for ESRD caused by HCV is an appropriate treatment. Unfortunately, transplantation does not cure the infection. Approximately 93% of patients transplanted for liver disease due to HCV develop recurrent infection in the new liver. Eligibility for transplantation, therefore, depends on the severity of associated diseases rather than on the presence or absence of HCV (Parker et al., 1998).

Dialysis Precautions

HCV transmission within the dialysis environment can be prevented by strict adherence to infection control precautions recommended for all hemodialysis patients (see Table 19-1). Although isolation of HCV-positive patients is not recommended, routine testing for ALT and anti-HCV is important for monitoring the potential for transmission within centers and ensuring that appropriate precautions are being properly and consistently used. HCV-positive patients can participate in dialyzer reuse programs. Unlike HBV, HCV is not transmitted efficiently through occupational exposures. Thus, reprocessing dialyzers from HCV-positive patients should not place staff members at increased risk for infection. HCV-positive persons should be evaluated (by consultation or referral, if appropriate) for the presence or development of chronic liver disease according to current medical practice guidelines. They also should receive information concerning how they can prevent further harm to their liver and prevent transmitting HCV to others (CDC, 1998; NIH, 2000). Persons with chronic liver disease should be vaccinated against hepatitis A, if susceptible.

Human Immunodeficiency Virus (HIV) Infection

HIV causes immunosuppression of the host individual and the development of acquired immune deficiency syndrome (AIDS). The HIV virus infects cells of the human body by inserting RNA into blood cells. HIV primarily infects CD4+ T- lymphocytes, a white blood cell that regulates production of antibodies to fight invading viruses or bacteria. After the virus binds to the D4+ T-cell, HIV injects its RNA strands into the T-cell (Parker et al., 1998). HIV is a retro virus that uses an enzyme, reverse transcriptase, to reverse the flow of genetic information from the virus to the body cells. This allows the virus to reproduce a DNA copy of its RNA strand necessary for the virus to replicate (Parker et al., 1998). Viral replication continues throughout the course of HIV disease. Up to 10 billion virions are reproduced and cleared daily. The half-life of an HIV-infected CD4 cell is about 1.3 days. Although most CD4 cells turn over rapidly, some belong to a latent pool with a long half-life. Viral reproduction is associated with a decline in the number of CD4 cells over the years.

In the absence of effective antiretroviral treatment, viral replication exceeds the ability of the immune system to produce CD4 cells. A declining number of CD4 cells indicate that the HIV disease is advancing. As the CD4 cell count continues to fall to dangerously low levels, the individual is at increasing risk for opportunistic infections and neoplasms. Bacterial, fungal, and viral infections pose serious threats to individuals who are severely immunosuppressed, that is, have a CD4+ T-cell count less than 200 cells/uL (Parker et al., 1998). Pneumocystis carinii pneumonia (PCP), toxoplasmic encephalitis, mycobacterium avium complex, and fungal infections such as cryptosporidiosis and microsporidiosis are common among severely immunosupressed individuals

(Parker et al., 1998). Unfortunately the drugs used to treat opportunistic infections in HIV disease may also cause nephrotoxicity or electrolyte abnormalities.

Epidemiology

HIV was first reported in the United States in 1981 and has become a major worldwide epidemic. Since this time, more than 830,000 cases of AIDS have been reported in the United States. By 1987 it was the leading cause of death among U.S. men between the ages of 25 and 44. As many as 950,000 Americans may be infected with HIV. One-quarter of these individuals are unaware of their infection. The epidemic is growing most rapidly among minority populations and is a leading killer of African-American males ages 25 to 44 (Dean, Steele, Satcher, & Nakashima, 2005; Futterman, 2005). The number of women with HIV infection and AIDS has been increasing steadily worldwide. By the end of 2003, according to the World Health Organization (WHO), 19.2 million women were living with HIV/AIDS worldwide, accounting for approximately 50% of the 40 million adults living with HIV/AIDS (National Institute of Allergy and Infectious Diseases [NIAID], 2004). As of the end of 2002, an estimated 384,906 people in the United States were living with AIDS (CDC, 2002). During 1985–2001, the percentage of U.S. hemodialysis centers that reported providing chronic hemodialysis for patients with HIV infection increased from 11%–37%, and the proportion of hemodialysis patients with known HIV infection increased from 0.3%–1.5% (AAMI, 1993; CDC, unpublished data, 2001).

Testing

Specific antibody to HIV is produced shortly after infection. The exact time at which antibodies will be detectable depends on factors such as host and viral characteristics. Antibody may be present at low levels during early infection but not at the detection limit of some assays. Antibody can be detected in most individuals by 6 to 12 weeks after infection as shown by screening tests, usually the enzyme-linked immunosorbent assays/enzyme immunoassays (ELISA/EIA), and the confirmatory test called a Western blot. ELISA is the most commonly used test to screen for HIV infection. The Western blot is probably the most widely accepted confirmatory assay for the detection of antibodies to the retroviruses. The Western blot can distinguish the difference between the HIV antibody and other antibodies that react to the ELISA. Used in combination with the ELISA, repeatedly reactive results are considered 99% accurate (Parker et al., 1998).

During acute HIV infection and prior to the appearance of antibody, also known as the window period, HIV infection can be confirmed by the circulation of p24 antigen, or the presence of viral RNA or DNA. Although highly sensitive antibody assays exist to detect very low levels of HIV antibody in blood, the window period prior to appearance of antibody can rarely be shortened to less than 3 weeks. Since March 1985, all blood in the United States has been screened for HIV. This practice has almost eliminated the risk of contracting HIV through a blood transfusion in the United States (Parker et al., 1998). Routine testing of hemodialysis patients for HIV infection for infection control purposes is not necessary or recommended (CDC, 2001).

Transmission

HIV is transmitted by blood and other body fluids that contain blood. Sexual contact, needle sharing among IV drug abusers, and intrauterine transmission between mother and newborn infant are common routes of transmission. Compared to the HB virus, HIV is not transmitted efficiently through occupational exposure (CDC, 2001). In addition, no patient-to-patient transmission of HIV has been reported in U.S. hemodialysis centers. However, such transmissions have been reported in other countries; in one case, HIV transmission was attributed to mixing of reused access needles and inadequate disinfection of equipment (Velandia et al., 1995).

Vaccine Development

HIV is a retrovirus that is able to enter cells and hide from the immune system. The virus is always changing, confusing the immune system by changing some of its parts. To be effective a vaccine must recognize all the parts of the virus (Parker et al., 1998). However, there are lines of evidence to support the contention that a safe and effective vaccine against HIV infection is very possible (AIDS Vaccine Research Working Group [AVRWG], 2003). Several different approaches to vaccine design are being investigated. Many of the initial approaches focused on the HIV envelope protein, the primary target for neutralizing antibodies in HIV-infected individuals. More recent approaches to vaccine development include recombinant proteins, synthetic peptides, recombinant viral vectors, recombinant bacterial vectors, and recombinant particles. Only the whole-killed and live-attenuated HIV vaccine approaches have not progressed into clinical trials in uninfected individuals because the potential risk outweighs the potential benefits. A strong interest also remains regarding the development of a therapeutic vaccine that could offer benefit to individuals already infected with HIV (AVRWG, 2003).

Transplantation and HIV

HIV transmission following transplant of organs led to the development of guidelines for the procurement and transplantation of organs in 1994. These guidelines require blood from donors be tested for various strains of HIV. Several federal agencies' guidelines, state agencies' guidelines, and voluntary industry standards regarding organ donation and screening for HIV have significantly decreased the risk of infection with HIV following organ transplant (CDC, 1994; Parker et al., 1998).

Serious questions remain about the safety and efficacy of organ transplantation in people with HIV infection. Because immunosuppression after kidney transplantation could pose a serious risk for opportunistic infections, transplantation in patients with HIV is considered experimental. Study protocols for cadaveric renal transplantation are currently being used or considered by a few transplant centers with the goal of evaluating the impact of transplantation and immunosuppression, HIV disease progression, immune function and activity, as well as graft function and survival (Salifu et al., 2004).

HIV and Renal Failure

Renal disease is a relatively common but generally late complication of HIV disease (Abbott, Trespalacios, Agodoa, & Ahuja, 2003; Rao, 2001) and can result from direct kidney infection with HIV or from the adverse effects of the medications used to treat the disease. HIV-associated nephropathy (HIVAN) often includes proteinuria, rapidly progressive renal insufficiency and large kidneys. Patients with HIVAN receiving renal replacement therapy have a poor prognosis when compared to patients with all other causes of ESRD (Abbott et al., 2003; Kirchner, 2002; Rao, 2001). According to the U.S. Renal Data System (USRDS), HIVAN accounts for approximately 10% of new ESRD cases in the United States. HIVAN may also be the third leading cause of end-stage renal failure in Blacks between the ages of 20 and 64 (Winston, Burns, & Klotman, 2000). HIVAN among Blacks has been associated with intravenous drug use (IVDU), and it is estimated that 30%-60% of people with HIVAN have a history of IVDU. Although HIVAN has been associated with decreased patient survival after initiation of dialysis (Abbott et al., 2003), overall survival of patients with HIV who are receiving dialysis has shown an improvement over the years and is thought to be due to the introduction of potent and aggressive antiretroviral therapy (Ahuja, Grady, & Khan, 2002; Ifudu et al., 1997; Rao, 2001). Highly active antiretroviral combination therapy (HAART) dramatically suppresses viral replication and the appearance of drug resistance for relatively long periods of time (Locatelli et al., 2004; Winston, Klotman, & Klotman, 1999). HAART may also slow the progression of HIVAN to ESRD (Ross, & Klotman, 2002). The effectiveness of HAART is related to the combination of medications and their ability to disrupt HIV at different stages during viral replication. Public Health Service Guidelines (DHHS, 2004) recommend combinations of three or four antiretroviral drugs (reverse transcriptase inhibitors & a protease inhibitor) as first treatment for HIV. USRDS studies indicate only 58% to 61% of U.S. dialysis patients with HIVAN receive antiretroviral therapy and of those receiving therapy, only 59% were receiving more than one of the recommended antiretroviral drugs (Abbott et al., 2003). Study recommendations include future prospective studies to determine the efficacy and tolerability of HAART in patients with HIVAN and ESRD (Abbott et al., 2003).

Nephrology nurses caring for patients receiving HAART need to be aware that many antiretroviral medications are excreted primarily through the kidney. Dose adjustment may be prescribed for patients with renal insufficiency or those receiving renal replacement therapy. In addition, many of the drugs may cause renal-related side effects or may be contraindicated when other medications are prescribed. For example, the nucleoside reverse transcriptase inhibitors (NRTI's) have been known to cause life-threatening type B lactic acidosis (Justesen & Pedersen, 2000; Sheng et al., 2004; Tripuraneni et al., 2004; Walker, 2004). The nonnucleoside reverse transcriptase inhibitors (NNRTI's) as a class, are commonly associated with allergic/hypersensitivity reactions (Temesgen & Beri, 2004). The protease inhibitors interact dangerously with rifamycin derivatives (i.e., rifampin and rifabutin) used to treat tuberculosis. Rifamycins enhance the metabolism of protease inhibitors causing sub-therapeutic levels of the protease inhibitors. The protease inhibitors slow the metabolism of rifamycins, resulting in increased serum levels of rifamycins (Bergshoeff et al., 2003; CDC, 1996). Indinavir may cause crystalluria, nephrolithiasis, and indinavir-associated crystal-induced renal failure (Abbott, Swanson, Agodoa, & Kimmel, 2004; Dieleman et al., 2003). Certain protease inhibitors (i.e., ritonavir) are associated with hepatotoxicity, particularly in patients with underlying liver dysfunction or coinfected with hepatitis C or B virus (CDC, 2001; Sulkowski et al., 2000).

Dialysis Precautions

Infection control precautions recommended for all hemodialysis patients are sufficient to prevent HIV transmission between patients. HIV-infected patients do not have to be isolated from other patients or dialyzed separately on dedicated machines. HIV-infected patients can participate in dialyzer reuse programs. Because HIV is not transmitted efficiently through occupational exposures, reprocessing dialyzers from HIV-positive patients should not place staff members at increased risk for infection.

Hepatitis Delta Virus (HDV)

Hepatitis D virus (HDV) is an RNA virus that requires simultaneous infection with HBV. HDV replicates only in hepatocytes and has a complex interaction with HBV. HDV and HBV may concurrently infect an individual or superinfect a chronic HBsAg carrier (APIC, 2000; CDC, 2001). The clinical expression, incidence of fulminant hepatitis, and chronic carrier rate differ between coinfection and superinfection. Approximately 5% of coinfections result in chronic HBV and HDV infection; whereas the chronic carrier state HD results in more than 90% of those who survive the acute phase of HDV superinfection (Parker et al., 1998; APIC, 2000). Over 60% of patients with chronic HDV will develop cirrhosis. High mortality rates are associated with both types of infection (CDC, 2001).

Epidemiology, Transmission, and Diagnosis

Sources of infections for delta virus are intravenous drug use, homosexuality, blood transfusions, and heterosexual contact. Mode of transmission is identical to hepatitis B since HDV is dependent on HBV for survival. The prevalence of HDV infection is low in the United States, with rates of <1% among HBsAg-positive persons in the general population and >10% among HBsAg-positive persons with repeated percutaneous exposures (e.g., injecting-drug users, persons with hemophilia) (Hadler & Fields, 1991). Areas of the world with high endemic rates of HDV infection include southern Italy, parts of Africa, and the Amazon Basin (CDC, 2001).

Few data exist on the prevalence of HDV infection among chronic hemodialysis patients, and only one transmission of HDV between such patients has been reported in the United States (Lettau et al., 1986). In this episode, transmission occurred from a patient who was chronically infected with HBV and HDV to an HBsAg-positive patient after a massive bleeding incident; both patients received dialysis at the same station (CDC, 2001).

A serologic test that measures total antibody to HDV is commercially available and measures both IgG and IgM antibodies (CDC, 2001; Parker, 1998). Anti-HD levels will disappear in 1 to 2 years when the acute infection resolves. Chronic infection results in persistently high anti-HD levels (Parker et al., 1998).

Dialysis Precautions

Because HDV depends on an HBV-infected host for replication, prevention of HBV infection will prevent HDV infection in a person susceptible to HBV. Patients known to be infected with HDV should be isolated from all other dialysis patients, especially those who are HBsAg positive.

Preventing Transmission of Infections Among Chronic HD Patients

Preventing transmission among chronic hemodialysis patients of bloodborne viruses and pathogenic bacteria from both recognized and unrecognized sources of infection requires implementation of a comprehensive infection control program. The components of such a program include infection control practices specifically designed for the hemodialysis setting, including routine serologic testing and immunization, surveillance, and training and education. CDC has published recommendations describing these components in detail (CDC, 2001).

The infection control practices recommended for hemodialysis units (see Table 19-1) will reduce opportunities for patient-to-patient transmission of infectious agents, directly or indirectly via contaminated devices, equipment and supplies, environmental surfaces, or hands of personnel. These practices should be carried out routinely for all patients in the chronic hemodialysis setting because of the increased potential for blood contamination during hemodialysis and because many patients are colonized or infected with pathogenic bacteria.

Additional measures are required to prevent HBV transmission because of the high titer of HBV and its ability to survive on environmental surfaces (see Table 19-1). It is the potential for environmentally mediated transmission of HBV, rather than internal contamination of dialysis machines, that is the focus of infection control strategies for preventing HBV transmission in dialysis centers. For patients at increased risk for transmission of pathogenic bacteria, including antimicrobial-resistant strains, additional precautions also might be necessary in some circumstances. Nephrology nurses should consult the CDC recommendations for details on these practices (CDC, 2001). The following is a summary of selected issues not already discussed under the section (s), *Dialysis Precautions*:

Routine Testing

• All chronic hemodialysis patients should be routinely tested for HBV and HCV infection, and the results promptly reviewed so that potential episodes of transmission can be identified quickly and patients appropriately managed based on their testing results. Test results (positive and negative) must be communicated to other units or hospitals when patients are transferred for care. Routine testing for HDV or HIV infection for purposes of infection control is not recommended.

• Before admission to the hemodialysis unit, the HBV serologic status (i.e., HBsAg, total anti-HBc, and anti-HBs) of all patients should be known. For patients transferred from another unit, test results should be obtained before the patients' transfer. If a patient's HBV serologic status is not known at the time of admission, testing should be completed within 7 days. The hemodialysis unit should ensure that the laboratory performing the testing for anti-HBs can define a 10 mIU/mL concentration to determine protective levels of antibody.

• Routine HCV testing should include use of both a screening immunoassay to test for anti-HCV and supplemental or confirmatory testing with an additional, more specific assay. Use of NAT for HCV RNA as the primary test for routine screening is not recommended because few HCV infections will be identified in anti-HCV negative patients. However, if ALT levels are persistently abnormal in anti-HCV negative patients in the absence of another etiology, testing for HCV RNA should be considered. Blood samples collected for NAT should not contain heparin, which interferes with the accurate performance of this assay.

Disinfection, Sterilization, and Environmental Hygiene

Good cleaning, disinfection, and sterilization procedures are important components of infection control in the hemodialysis center. The procedures do not differ from those recommended for other health care settings (Favero & Bond; 1991; Favero & Boylard, 1995), but the high potential for blood contamination makes the hemodialysis setting unique. Additionally, the need for routine aseptic access of the patient's vascular system makes the hemodialysis unit more akin to a surgical suite than to a standard hospital room. Medical items are categorized as critical (e.g., needles and catheters), which are introduced directly into the bloodstream or normally sterile areas of the body; semicritical (e.g., fiberoptic endoscopes), which come in contact with intact mucous membranes; and noncritical (e.g., blood pressure cuffs), which touch only intact skin (Boyce & Pittet, 2002; Marx et al., 1998). Cleaning and housekeeping in the dialysis center has two goals:

• removal of soil and waste on a regular basis, thereby preventing the accumulation of potentially infectious material.

• maintenance of an environment that is conducive to good patient care.

Crowding of patients and overtaxing of staff members may increase the likelihood of microbial transmission. Adequate cleaning may be difficult if there are multiple wires, tubes, and hoses in a small area. There should be enough space to move completely around each patient's dialysis station without interfering with the neighboring stations. Where space is limited, elimination of unneeded items; orderly arrangement of required items; and removal of excess lengths of tubes, hoses, and wires from the floor can improve accessibility for cleaning. Because of the special requirements for cleaning in the dialysis center, staff should be specially trained in this task.

After each patient treatment, frequently touched environmental surfaces, including external surfaces of the dialysis machine, should be cleaned (with a good detergent) or disinfected (with a detergent germicide). It is the cleaning step that is important for interrupting the cross contamination transmission routes. Antiseptics, such as formulations with povidone iodine, hexachlorophene, or chlorhexidine, should not be used, because these are formulated for use on skin and are not designed for use on hard surfaces.

Wastes from a hemodialysis center that are actually or potentially contaminated with blood should be considered infectious and handled accordingly. Eventually, these items of solid waste should be disposed of properly in an incinerator or sanitary landfill, depending on state or local laws.

Standard protocols for sterilization and disinfection are adequate for processing any items or devices contaminated with blood. Historically there has been a tendency to use "overkill" strategies for instrument sterilization or disinfection and housekeeping protocols. This is not necessary. The floors in a dialysis center are routinely contaminated with blood, but the protocol for floor cleaning is the same as for floors in other health care settings. Usually, this involves the use of a good detergent germicide; the formulation can contain a low or intermediate level disinfectant.

Large blood spills should be cleaned to remove visible material, and then, the area should receive low to intermediate level disinfection following the directions of the germicide manufacturer. Blood and other specimens, such as peritoneal fluid, from all patients should be handled with care. Peritoneal fluid can contain high levels of HBV and should be handled in the same manner as the patient's blood. Consequently, if the center performs peritoneal dialysis, the same criteria for separating HBsAg positive patients who are undergoing hemodialysis apply to those undergoing peritoneal dialysis.

HBV has not been grown in tissue cultures, and without a viral assay system, studies on the precise resistance of this virus to various chemical germicides and heat have not been performed. However, the resistance of HBV to heat and chemical germicides may approach that of some other viruses and bacteria but certainly not that of the bacterial endospore or the tubercle bacillus. Further, studies have shown that HBV is not resistant to commonly used high level and intermediate level disinfectants (Bond et al., 1981; Sattar, Tetro, Springthorpe, & Giuliu, 2001).

Blood contamination of venous pressure monitors has been implicated in HBV transmission (CDC, 1993). Therefore, venous pressure transducer filters should be used; these filters should not be reused.

In single pass artificial kidney machines, the internal fluid pathways are not subject to contamination with blood. Although the fluid pathways that exhaust dialysis fluid from the dialyzer may become contaminated with blood in the event of a dialyzer leak, it is unlikely that this blood contamination will reach a subsequent patient. Therefore, disinfection and rinsing procedures should be designed to control contamination with bacterial rather than blood borne pathogens.

For dialysis machines that use a dialysate recirculating system (such as some ultrafiltration control machines and those that regenerate the dialysate), a blood leak in a dialyzer, especially a massive leak, can result in contamination of a number of surfaces that will contact the dialysis fluid of subsequent patients. However, the procedures that are normally practiced after each use — draining of the dialysis fluid, subsequent rinsing, and disinfection — will reduce the level of contamination to below infectious levels. In addition, an intact dialyzer membrane will not allow passage of bacteria or viruses. Consequently, if a blood leak does occur with either type of dialysis machine, the standard disinfection procedure used for machines in the dialysis center to control bacterial contamination will also prevent transmission of bloodborne pathogens.

Infectious disease prevention can be a challenge for the nephrology nurse caring for the immunosuppressed patient. Nephrology nurses involved in the quality improvement activities in their facility are vital to the ongoing study of ways to reduce the incidence of infection. Surveillance for infections and other adverse events is required to monitor the effectiveness of infection control practices, as well as training and education of both staff members and patients to ensure that appropriate infection control behaviors and techniques are carried out. Vaccine-preventable disease such as HBV also presents an opportunity for improvement. Nephrology nurses play a critical role in making sure patients understand the benefits of vaccination and are properly vaccinated against HBV, influenza, and pneumococcal disease. Surveillance data, such as HBV and HCV serologic testing results, vaccination status, episodes of bacterermia, loss of the vascular access caused by infection — including date of infection onset, site of infection, genus and species of the infecting organism — and antimicrobial susceptibility results of drug-resistant bacteria, should be maintained, trended, and discussed during quality improvement meetings (CDC, 2001). There should be an ongoing study of ways to improve prevention and control processes to reduce nosocomial infection rates to the lowest possible level (APIC, 2000). In each chronic hemodialysis unit, policies and practices should be reviewed and updated to ensure that infection control practices recommended for hemodialysis units are implemented and rigorously followed. Intensive efforts must be made to educate new staff members and reeducate existing staff members regarding these practices. Nephrology nurses must never underestimate the potential impact sound infection prevention and control measures can have on dialysis patient outcomes.

Tuberculosis: An Old Disease With a New Face

After decades of declining incidence, tuberculosis (TB) is again a major health concern in the United States. The presence of a large immunosuppressed population, due in part to the AIDS epidemic and the persistence and growth of TB globally have contributed to the increasing number of TB cases in the United States. Not only is TB back, but in many places it is back with a vengeance. Multi-drug resistant strains of TB are emerging that are resistant to many of the drugs commonly used to treat TB. Tuberculosis is of interest in the chronic dialysis setting. Chronic renal failure (CRF) and diabetes mellitus are identified as risk factors that increase the chance of developing clinical TB after infection with the tuberculosis bacillus.

Etiology

Tuberculosis is caused by the tubercle bacillus *Mycobacterium tuberculosis.* There are approximately 30 members of the genus *Mycobacterium,* only a few of which cause disease in humans.

TB is spread primarily by respiratory means. Although the disease can involve any organ, the lungs provide the primary route for infection. Whenever people with active pulmonary or laryngeal TB speak, sing, talk, cough or sneeze, thousands of tiny respiratory droplets are released into the air. The smallest of these droplets (known as droplet nuclei) dry and remain airborne for indefinite periods of time and may contain one to several mycobacteriums. Larger particles fall to the floor or other surfaces and are not sources of airborne transmission of the disease (Protic & Hardy, 1993; Riley & Nardell, 1993). Droplet nuclei are approximately 1 to 5 microns in size and are the most dangerous particles, because they are small enough to be readily inhaled by susceptible hosts and deposited into alveoli in the lungs. The upper respiratory tract is highly resistant to infection with TB, while infectious particles that enter the lower portions of the lungs will readily survive and multiply. Even a single droplet nuclei containing an infectious TB particle is enough to cause infection in a susceptible host (Lindberg, 1993; Riley & Nardell, 1993).

The number of bacilli exhaled by most infected patients is not large, although patients with cavitary disease, or laryngeal or endobronchial TB may be highly contagious. Infectiousness generally coincides with the numbers of infectious organisms in sputum, the extent of the pulmonary disease and the frequency of coughing. When presented to a host with a functional immune system, *M. tuberculosis* is a highly infectious but not highly virulent organism, so repeated, prolonged exposure is usually necessary for infection to occur. However, when the immune system is defective, it appears that infection can progress to active disease after short exposure times to small numbers of organisms (Protic & Hardy, 1993).

Pathophysiology

While similar in many ways to other bacteria, there are some characteristics peculiar to *M. tuberculosis* that is important to remember when caring for patients infected with TB. The first difference is the slow rate of reproduction of the bacilli when compared to other bacteria. *Escherichia coli,* a common pathogen, normally divide every 20-30 minutes and produce visible colonies after an overnight incubation period. *M. tuberculosis* has a mean doubling time of 12-24 hours and may require weeks of growth to produce a visible colony. This is significant because it can delay identification and diagnosis of the organism. In some cases (particularly when infection with drug-resistant strains is suspected) this slow growth can also delay drug-susceptibility tests, which may delay appropriate drug therapy.

Another unusual characteristic of *M. tuberculosis* is the structure of its cell wall. The cell wall contains an outer layer of fatty acids and waxes that are toxic to host cells and tissues and that make the bacilli hydrophobic (insoluble in water). This layer contributes to its slow growth rate and also serves to protect the organism from many antimicrobial

agents. In addition, the layer prevents the body's macrophages (cells that ingest foreign matter) from being able to completely destroy all of the invading bacilli. Since *M. tuberculosis* is able to remain viable within macrophages, it has an enhanced ability to remain inaccessible to several antitubercular drugs (Protic & Hardy, 1993). This is one reason why drug therapy for TB is prolonged.

Once an individual inhales tubercle bacilli into the alveoli, how the body reacts to the presence of the bacilli depends in part on the susceptibility of that person, how many particles were inhaled, and how virulent the organisms are. The lung tissue responds to the presence of the bacilli with inflammation, and the body's normal defense mechanisms attempt to eliminate the invader. Inflammation may lead to the development of nodules called primary tubercles. As cells gather around the tubercle, the outer portion becomes fibrosed, which leads to decreased blood flow and nutrition to the tubercle center. As the center becomes necrotic, the outer fibrosis acts to wall off the area of infection. This necrotic tissue becomes soft and cheesy in consistency, a process called caseation. Over time, this material may become either calcified or liquefied (liquefaction necrosis). At times the person infected with TB may cough up some of the liquefied material, leaving a hole or cavity in the lung tissue. On x-rays, these cavities are visible and are termed cavitary disease, which is suggestive of TB. Lymph nodes in the hilar region of the lung may be involved as they filter drainage from infected areas (Daniel, 1987; Phipps & Daly, 1983).

If the host has a competent immune system, further multiplication and spread of the organisms are halted, usually within 2-10 weeks of the initial infection. Alveolar macrophages, which ingest bacilli present in the alveoli of the lungs, spread throughout the host's body. However, viable bacilli remain in the host's macrophages in a dormant or resting state, and reactivation of the disease is possible at a later time. These people are considered to have TB infection or latent TB. Even though they have TB infection, they have no signs or symptoms of the disease and are not capable of transmitting TB to others at this point, although they will demonstrate a positive reaction to a purified protein derivative (PPD) skin test. People with latent TB have approximately a 10% risk during their lifetime of developing active (infectious and symptomatic) TB, with the greatest risk occurring within the first 2 years after infection.

When the host's defenses are inadequate and unable to check the spread of the bacilli, the person is said to have active TB disease. In this case, the individual would demonstrate clinical symptoms of TB and would be capable of spreading the infection to others. Many of the new cases of TB being seen now are in older people who were infected decades ago, and the disease emerges when the host's immune system is weakened and no longer able to contain the infection. Rates of TB are also increased in racial and ethnic minorities who have other risk factors for TB, such as birth in a country with high prevalence rates of TB, and in individuals with HIV infection, low socioeconomic status, and/or exposure in congregate settings (for example, prisons and shelters) (CDC, 1994a).

The HIV epidemic has played a key role in the resurgence of TB. HIV-positive patients with compromised immune systems have a much higher risk of developing active clinical disease after the initial infection, or of developing disease subsequent to earlier infection.

Multidrug-Resistant TB

Another cause for alarm is the increased incidence of TB that is resistant to at least two of the first-line drugs used to successfully treat TB. In the past, drug resistance was commonly the result of inappropriate or inadequate treatment of TB, but it appears now that multi-drug resistant TB (MDR-TB) is also being spread among patients by direct exposure, particularly in locations with large numbers of HIV-infected patients (Casey, 1993). Before the onset of the AIDS epidemic, drug resistance was most often seen in immigrants from countries in which TB is endemic. In these countries, antitubercular drugs may be available over the counter so patients may take only one drug, which they discontinue when symptoms subside. In situations like this where treatment is inadequate, only the most susceptible organisms are eliminated. When single drug therapy is employed for an insufficient length of time or when dosing schedules are erratic, the development of resistant strains will be encouraged. This type of resistance is known as secondary or acquired drug resistance.

Primary drug resistance occurs when only a few of the organisms present have an inherent resistance to one or more of the most commonly used antitubercular drugs. In this situation, drug resistance is a random event that occurs apart from any drug therapy.

To prevent the emergence of drug-resistant strains of TB, certain principles of drug therapy must be applied consistently to patients treated for TB. Appropriate drug regimens must contain several different drugs to which the organism is susceptible, and the dosing schedule must maintain sufficient drug concentrations at infection sites to inhibit or kill the organisms present. Drug regimens must also be continued long enough to ensure that all organisms are eliminated (CDC, 2003). Specific drug therapy for resistant strains of TB will depend on whether the organism is resistant to one or more of the drugs commonly used to treat TB. Some organisms are resistant to only one drug, while others show resistance to multiple drugs (American Thoracic Society/CDC, 2003).

Signs and Symptoms of TB

Pulmonary TB should be suspected in people who complain of fevers, chills, night sweats, fatigue, weight loss, decreased appetite, chest pain, prolonged and productive coughing (longer than 3 weeks duration), or hemoptysis. While these symptoms can be due to numerous factors, they are the classic symptoms of TB. Whenever patients present with any of these complaints, they should be viewed with suspicion for TB until that diagnosis is ruled out. If the disease presents at an extrapulmonary site, the symptoms will depend on the body sites/systems affected; risk factors for TB must always be considered when evaluating an ill person who may have been exposed to the disease (CDC, 1994a).

While extrapulmonary TB occurs more often in people with HIV, pulmonary TB is still the most common form of TB, including those with HIV. While HIV-negative patients have a 10% rate of extrapulmonary TB, patients with full-blown AIDS have a 70% rate of TB at sites other than the lung, and patients with HIV whose immune systems are not as impaired have a 24%-45% rate of extrapulmonary TB. Patients with HIV and extrapulmonary TB most often demonstrate lymphadenitis (inflammation of lymph nodes) and miliary disease (formation of tubercles throughout body organs due to dissemination of the bacilli through the bloodstream). These patients may complain of tender lymph nodes, fever, fatigue, and weight loss. People with extrapulmonary TB are not usually considered infectious unless they have an open abscess or draining lesion (Jo, 1993). Anyone who is suspected of having TB must be immediately placed in isolation and be referred for further evaluation, which should consist of a physical examination, a Mantoux tuberculin skin test, a chest x-ray, and sputum smears and cultures.

BCG Vaccine

In many countries where TB is endemic, bacillus Calmette-Guerin (BCG) vaccine is used in an effort to provide immunity to TB. It is not normally used in this country because of the low risk of infection and the lack of consistent evidence supporting its efficacy in preventing disease. BCG contains attenuated tubercle bacilli unable to produce disease. Eight major trials of the vaccine have demonstrated effective rates from 0-76%, with no explanations for the wide range of results (CDC, 1994a). One trial conducted in South India did not demonstrate a protective effect from the vaccine, even though two of what were believed to be the most potent strains available were used. There is evidence from a variety of other studies that BCG vaccine may provide some protection to infants and young children against the more serious forms of TB, although that protection does not appear to apply to adults (American Thoracic Society, 1994).

Even though there is no clear evidence supporting the effectiveness of the BCG vaccine, many countries where TB is endemic still use the vaccine, especially for infants. One disadvantage to using BCG is that it often leads to positive PPD skin test results in vaccinated individuals, which lessens the effectiveness of the skin test as a screening tool. There is currently no way to detect the difference between a positive reaction due to vaccination and a positive reaction due to TB infection. In those vaccinated with BCG, the probability that positive skin tests are due to TB infection increases:

1. as the size of the skin test reactions increase,
2. as the length of time between vaccinations and skin testing increases,
3. when patients were in contact with infectious TB disease,
4. when there are positive family histories of TB,
5. when chest x-rays show evidence of previous TB, or
6. when patients are from countries where TB is common.

In most situations, a history of BCG vaccination does not alter the guidelines for interpreting skin test results. Current CDC recommendations are that people vaccinated with BCG who demonstrate any of the previously listed risk factors for TB and who have positive skin tests be evaluated for TB. Once active TB has been ruled out, they may require preventive therapy. It cannot be overemphasized that BCG vac-

Table 19-9

Medical Conditions That Increase the Risk of Developing TB Disease Once Infection Has Occurred

- HIV infection

- Substance abuse (especially drug injection)

- Silicosis

- Recent infection with TB (within the past 2 years)

- Abnormal chest x-ray, which suggests previous TB (in a person who received inadequate or no treatment)

- Diabetes mellitus

- Prolonged corticosteroid therapy or other immunosuppressive therapy

- Hematologic and reticuloendothelial diseases (for example, leukemia, Hodgkin's disease)

- End stage renal disease

- Intestinal bypass or gastrectomy

- Chronic malabsorption syndromes

- Cancer of the head and neck

- Being > 10% below ideal body weight

Note: From Centers for Disease Control. (1994). Core curriculum on tuberculosis. Atlanta, GA: Author.

Table 19-10

Populations with a High Prevalence of TB Infection

- Close contacts of infectious tuberculosis cases

- Foreign-born persons from high-prevalence countries (Asia, Africa, Latin America)

- Medically underserved, low-income populations, including high-risk racial and ethnic groups

- The elderly

Note: From Centers for Disease Control. (1994). Core curriculum on tuberculosis. Atlanta, GA: Author.

Table 19-11

Groups to Screen with a Tuberculin Skin Test

- Persons with HIV infection

- Close contacts of infectious tuberculosis cases

- Persons with medical conditions that increase the risk of TB (see Table 19-8)

- Foreign-born persons from high prevalence countries

- Low-income populations, including high-risk minorities

- Alcoholics and intravenous drug users

- Residents of long-term care facilities (including prisons and nursing homes)

- Populations identified locally as being at increased risk for TB, such as health care workers in some areas/settings

Note: From Centers for Disease Control. (1994). Core curriculum on tuberculosis. Atlanta, GA: Author.

cination can never be assumed to be the cause of a positive skin test (CDC, 1994a).

Because of the lack of clear data demonstrating the efficacy of BCG, and the fact that use of BCG may interfere with future skin test results, the use of BCG is recommended in select situations.

Screening Methods for TB

Risk factors. Screening tests done in the U.S. are used to identify infected people who need preventive therapy to stop progression to active disease, and as a part of the work-up for those with signs or symptoms of active disease. It is recommended that screening be done in groups with disease and infection rates in excess of those found in the general population. Institutional screening is recommended for staff of all health care facilities and residents of long-term care institutions where TB cases are identified or where those populations have a high incidence of TB disease and infection. The Centers for Disease Control and Prevention (CDC, 1994a) guidelines currently recommend that all health care facilities establish a TB screening program for their health care workers. The Occupational Safety and Health Administration (OSHA) now mandate that employers develop and follow TB screening and control programs for all personnel. This should be done to determine whether the health care worker is infected with TB and to determine if TB is being transmitted within the facility.

To adequately assess the risk for exposure to TB within any facility or setting, it is important to be aware of the known risk factors associated with TB. Identified risk factors that increase the risk of a person developing clinically active TB after being infected are listed in Table 19-9. Although TB can occur within any population or group, certain subpopulations have been identified that have a higher-than-average risk for TB. These groups are listed in Table 19-10. Knowing exposure risks helps employers and caregivers design plans to minimize or prevent exposure to TB.

Groups and individuals who should be screened. Proper interpretation of test results and appropriate follow-up and care are necessary components of any screening program. Screening usually consists of the Mantoux purified protein derivative (PPD) skin test. OSHA now mandates that all health care facilities, nursing homes, drug rehabilitation centers, homeless shelters, and prisons develop and implement controls to protect workers and employees from TB. Current CDC (1994a) guidelines have listed groups that should be screened with tuberculin skin tests, and these are found in Table 19-11.

Included in these groups who should be screened are those who have medical conditions that increase their risk of

Table 19-12
Classification of TB Skin Test Results

An induration of 5 mm or more is considered a positive reaction in the following persons:	An induration of 10 mm or more is considered positive in the following persons:	An induration of 15 mm is considered positive for persons who do not have any risk factors for TB.
• HIV infected persons or persons suspected of having HIV • Close contacts of a person with infectious TB • Persons with abnormal chest x-rays • Persons who inject drugs and whose HIV status is unknown	• Foreign-born persons • HIV-negative persons who inject drugs • Medically underserved, low-income populations • Residents of long-term care facilities • Locally identified high-prevalence groups (for example, migrant farm workers or homeless persons) • Children 4 years old without any other risk factors	

Note: From Centers for Disease Control. (1994). Core curriculum on tuberculosis. Atlanta, GA: Author.

progression to clinical disease once TB infection has occurred. Nephrology nurses should note that CRF is a risk factor for the progression of TB infection to disease, and many CRF patients may have additional risk factors as well (such as diabetes, substance abuse, or corticosteroid therapy). CDC (1994a) recommends that tuberculin skin test screening be done in high-risk groups, which includes patients with CRF. Chronic renal failure is an immunocompromising condition with cutaneous anergy that can result in false negative tuberculin skin tests (MMWR, 2004). Anergy testing can help determine false positive TB skin tests.

TB outbreaks in dialysis facilities continue in the United States. In 2003 an outbreak of TB occurred in Nevada. A staff member became ill with pulmonary TB and exposed 400 patients and staff before it was diagnosed (MMWR, 2004). Other outbreaks have occurred in California and New Jersey. Studies in New Jersey and California have documented TB disease rates 6 to 11 times greater among hemodialysis patients than among the states' population.

TB skin testing. At the present time, tuberculin skin testing is the only means available to demonstrate whether or not a person has been infected with TB. It is important to remember that skin testing is valuable only as a screening test and is not appropriate for use as a diagnostic tool. The test is based on the body's immune responses; a person infected with TB will demonstrate a cell-mediated or delayed hypersensitivity reaction when given the PPD test because of antibodies they have formed in response to the TB infection. PPD testing uses a highly purified product that contains protein from actual tubercle bacilli. In North America, a standard intermediate-strength dose of 5 tuberculin units of PPD is used for skin-testing purposes. Multiple-puncture methods of skin testing are convenient but not appropriate because of decreased specificity.

The Mantoux test provides the most accurate results. Using a tuberculin syringe, 0.1 ml containing 5 units of PPD is injected intradermally with the needle bevel facing up, usually in the skin of the inner forearm. When properly performed, the injection should produce a pale, sharply raised wheal just underneath the skin surface that is 6 to 10 mm in diameter. If the injection is made too deeply into the tissues, results would be suspect because a reaction may be too deep to palpate and assess properly. If the injection is too shallow, not enough of the PPD may have been delivered to properly elicit a response. The reaction should be read and documented by designated, trained personnel 48 to 72 hours after the injection. Patient or health care worker self-reading and reporting of skin test results should not be accepted (CDC, 1994a).

When recording skin test results, the terms positive and negative are no longer considered appropriate. Instead, results should be recorded as the number of millimeters of induration (hardness) at the largest diameter of the induration. This should be measured perpendicularly to the long axis of the forearm at the injection site. All reactions, even those classified as nonreactive, should be recorded in millimeters (such as 0 mm of induration). The area of induration should be assessed by gently palpating the site. Redness or erythema are not diagnostic criteria and should not be used to interpret test results. Interpretation of skin tests results are based on risk factors of the person being tested. Table 19-12 provides current CDC (1994a) criteria for evaluating and classifying skin test reactions in different individuals.

It is possible that some people may demonstrate false-positive results to the tuberculin skin test. These false-positive reactions could be due to infections with mycobacterium other than *M. tuberculosis* or due to immunization with BCG. False-negative results are also a problem that can occur for several reasons. People recently infected with TB may not demonstrate a positive skin test because it takes approximately 2 to 10 weeks after the initial infection to mount an immune response. Anyone exposed to infectious TB should have an immediate skin test to determine their baseline status and then be retested 10 to 12 weeks later to determine if infection has occurred.

Another reason for false-negative readings is the time period that has elapsed since the initial infection. In some people, the ability to react to skin tests may wane over time. When given the skin test years after the initial infection, they may at first manifest a negative reaction. However, the skin test acts as a stimulant to the immune system and the person will demonstrate a positive reaction to subsequent skin tests. This type of reaction is termed the booster phenomenon, and it is useful when trying to distinguish between old and newly acquired infections. In some settings, people who have an initial negative test are given another test 1 to 3 weeks later. If the reaction to the second test is positive, it is probably a boosted reaction, meaning that the person is infected but the infection probably occurred a long time ago. If both skin tests are initially negative, then any subsequent positive skin tests would more likely be due to recent infection with TB, a process termed conversion. Two-step testing is especially useful in settings where testing will occur at periodic intervals, such as health care workers or nursing home residents.

An increasingly common cause for false-negative skin tests results is anergy, the inability of the body to react to skin tests because of immunosuppression. HIV is a common cause of anergy, although it can be caused by other medical conditions, such as viral or bacterial infections, chronic renal failure, corticosteroids, chemotherapy, stress or age. It is estimated that 1 in 10 people infected with TB is both anergic and asymptomatic (Lavin & Haidorfer, 1993). One way to test for anergy is to administer a delayed-type hypersensitivity antigen, such as Candida by the Mantoux technique when the PPD is administered. These antigens are used because most adults will have developed antibodies to them either through exposure, disease, or vaccination. If the person fails to respond to these antigens, including the PPD, then it is very likely that the person is anergic and the PPD results are suspect at best.

Diagnosis of TB

Anyone who demonstrates symptoms of TB must be referred immediately for further medical care and follow-up, which should include a thorough medical history, physical exam, Mantoux tuberculin skin test, chest x-ray, and sputum smear and culture (or smears and cultures from the affected site in extrapulmonary TB, if possible). The health department must be notified within 24 hours of any suspected or confirmed cases of TB. As was mentioned earlier, patients should be assessed for any risk factors that could increase the risk of acquiring TB or that may increase the risk of progression to active disease. Demographic factors, such as country of origin, age, ethnic or racial factors, occupation or living conditions, should be evaluated in this assessment. While physical examination does not definitively diagnose or confirm TB, it can provide valuable information regarding the patient's current health status and other factors that may determine the prescribed treatment regimen.

Chest x-rays are also important when evaluating TB symptoms, although radiologic findings are not diagnostic of TB. The usual x-ray view obtained is the posterior-anterior view, although other views (such as lateral or lordotic) may be necessary. In some instances, it may be necessary to obtain CT scans or other studies for evaluation. In pulmonary TB, the abnormalities seen usually occur in the apical and posterior segments of the upper lobe or in the upper segments of the lower lobe (CDC, 1994a). Parenchymal changes demonstrated by x-rays and commonly associated with TB include cavitation, parenchymal infiltration, and air-space consolidation (such as with endobronchial spread of TB), miliary nodules and pleural effusion (Schluger & Rom, 1994). However, lesions may be evident anywhere in the lung fields and may have markedly different appearances between patients, especially if they have HIV or are immunosuppressed due to other causes (CDC, 1994a). People with AIDS and TB tend to demonstrate more atypical chest x-ray features, such as predominantly lower lobe infiltrates, miliary patterns, mediastinal and/or hilar lymphadenopathy, and an absence of cavitary disease. On the other hand, some with AIDS and TB may present with normal chest x-rays in 10% of this population, even when sputum cultures are positive (Jo, 1993).

At the present time, sputum cultures are the only means available to definitively diagnose TB. Anyone suspected of having pulmonary or laryngeal TB should produce three sputum specimens on three different days, preferably early morning specimens. To ensure that patients are able to properly provide sputum samples (not saliva or mucous from the nose and throat), health care workers should coach and directly supervise them in obtaining at least the first specimens. For those unable to cough up an adequate sample, aerosol induction can be used to stimulate them to cough up sputum. Induced sputum samples are usually watery and resemble saliva, so it is crucial that this specimen be labeled "INDUCED" so lab personnel do not discard it due to its appearance. In other cases bronchoscopy may be required to obtain the necessary samples. Gastric aspiration is sometimes useful in obtaining swallowed sputum specimens, particularly in infants and young children unable to cough up sputum (CDC, 1994a).

Whenever patients are attempting to provide specimens, hazardous aerosols may be produced. All appropriate infection control measures must be taken to prevent anyone in close proximity from becoming infected. These infection control measures are beyond the scope of this article and are discussed in references listed at the end of the article. This would include procedures such as coughing to obtain specimens, sputum induction using aerosol treatments, bronchoscopy, or any other required diagnostic procedures (Domin, 1993).

Although TB is primarily a pulmonary disease, it must be remembered that TB can affect almost any site in the body. When the patient presents with extrapulmonary TB, specimens obtained will depend on the organs or tissues affected and can include urine, cerebrospinal fluid, and pleural fluid, pus, or tissue samples. Tissue samples should be placed in saline solution, not formalin, and must be delivered to the laboratory immediately (CDC, 1994a).

Smears can determine within 24 hours whether or not the infection is caused by acid-fast bacilli (AFB), but cannot distinguish between infections caused by *M. tuberculosis* or other mycobacterium. Complicating the diagnosis is the fact that many patients with TB have negative AFB smears. For this reason, cultures are necessary to provide a definitive diagnosis and determine drug susceptibility patterns of the infecting organism, and should be done on all specimens regardless of smear results. Since traditional methods of isolating the organism have taken anywhere from 6-12 weeks, many clinicians begin treatment for TB with only a presumptive diagnosis based on x-ray results, clinical signs and symptoms, and smear results.

A more rapid means of organism identification has been developed that uses a liquid, broth-based culture medium and automated radiometric techniques (the BACTEC system). Using this method, culture results may be available in as little as 2 weeks. Tests using nucleic acid probes in addition to BACTEC systems can provide even more rapid identification of organisms (Schluger & Rom, 1994).

A procedure known as restriction fragment length polymorphism (RFLP) has been developed that can fingerprint specific strains of *M. tuberculosis*. This test may be used to identify outbreaks and transmission patterns (CDC, 2002).

Follow-up bacteriologic testing should be done at least monthly to determine if patients are still contagious and to evaluate their clinical response to therapy. All initial isolates should be subjected to drug susceptibility testing, and these tests should be repeated on patients who do not respond clinically to therapy or who continue to have positive cultures after 2 months of therapy. To curtail the spread or further development of drug resistant strains, it is imperative to identify drug resistance early and implement appropriate and effective treatment. The CDC (2003) has identified groups of people who are at increased risk of drug resistance, and they include:

- those with a history of previous treatment with TB medications,
- close contact with known drug-resistant TB,
- foreign-born residents from areas where there is a high incidence of drug-resistant TB (such as Asia, Latin America, Africa),
- residents of geographic areas in the U.S. where the prevalence of isoniazid-resistant TB is documented to be 4% or greater,
- those whose smears or cultures remain positive after 2 months of therapy with TB drugs.

Drug Therapy for TB

Antituberculosis chemotherapy is designed to kill tubercle bacilli rapidly, minimize the potential for the organisms to develop drug resistance and sterilize the host's tissues (American Thoracic Society/CDC 2003). The achievement of these outcomes requires a combination of drugs that are administered for a period of time. Lack of adequate follow-through with the prescribed drug regimen is one of the main reasons for the current resurgence of TB and the increase of drug-resistant strains. Treatment for TB currently falls into three categories: preventive therapy, treatment of active disease, and treatment for drug-resistant strains.

Preventive therapy. Preventive therapy is prescribed for people infected with TB (but who do not have active, clinical disease) in order to prevent progression to active disease at some later date (latent TB). Certain groups, as outlined in Table 19-8, have a high risk of developing TB disease after

infection occurs. When prescribing preventive therapy, clinicians must consider the risk of developing TB and the potential risk of INH toxicity. Before preventive therapy is initiated, clinicians should (a) rule out the possibility of TB disease, (b) determine if the patient has a history of treatment for TB infection or disease, (c) assess for any contraindications to administering INH (such as previous INH-associated hepatic injury; reactions to INH, for example, drug fever, rash or arthritis; or acute or unstable liver disease of any cause), and (d) determine whether the patient is at high risk for adverse reactions to INH. INH is normally used alone for preventive therapy, and current CDC (2003) guidelines recommend a maximum daily dose of 5 mg/kg (300 mg) daily in adults or 15 mg/kg (900 mg) once, twice or three times weekly; in children, a maximum of 10-15 mg/kg not to exceed 300 mg daily or 20-30 mg/kg (900 mg) twice weekly for 6 to 12 months.. Anyone infected with HIV or who are immunosuppressed for other reasons should receive a full 12 months of therapy (American Thoracic Society, 2003). Some people with positive skin tests may not be candidates for preventive therapy; these groups would include: (a) those at high risk for adverse effects due to INH therapy, (b) those who cannot tolerate INH, (c) people likely to be infected with drug-resistant strains of TB, or (d) those who are highly unlikely to complete a full course of preventive therapy (such as the homeless or migrant farm workers).

Everyone should be thoroughly educated about TB infection and disease and instructed to seek medical care immediately if they develop any signs or symptoms of the disease. Although there are instances where alternative therapies may be necessary, there is no clinical data to document clinical efficacy of any drug other than INH as a preventive therapy.

Anyone receiving preventive therapy should be seen for follow-up on at least a monthly basis. Each patient should be evaluated for:

- Adherence to the prescribed treatment regimen (including pill counts and/or urine tests to determine if INH metabolites are present).
- Symptoms of hepatitis, such as nausea, loss of appetite, vomiting, persistently dark urine, yellowish skin, malaise, unexplained elevated temperature for more than 3 days, or abdominal tenderness, especially in the right upper quadrant.
- Symptoms of neurotoxicity, such as paresthesias of the hands or feet.

People with increased risk of hepatotoxicity due to INH should have a serum glutamic-oxaloacetic transaminase (SGOT or AST) drawn just prior to the start of therapy and monthly thereafter. Persons at increased risk of hepatotoxicity include those who: (a) are age 35 or older, (b) use other medications that may cause interactions, (c) use alcohol daily, (d) have chronic liver disease, (e) use intravenous drugs, (f) are pregnant, or (g) have discontinued use of INH in the past due to adverse effects. It should be noted that having a positive hepatitis B surface antigen is not necessarily a contraindication to preventive therapy with INH. There is evidence to suggest that women may be at increased risk for fatal hepatitis associated with use of INH. Some persons taking INH will demonstrate mild increases in liver enzymes, which tend to resolve even with continuance of INH therapy. Discontinuation of INH should be considered only if liver enzyme measurements exceed three to five times the upper limit of normal or if the patient reports symptoms of adverse reactions.

Peripheral neuropathy is associated with the use of INH; administration of pyridoxine has been shown to prevent INH-induced neuropathy, especially in persons predisposed to neuropathy due to other disease states (e.g., diabetes, renal failure, alcoholism, and infection) (American Thoracic Society/CDC, 2003).

Treatment of TB disease. There are four basic principles that underlie any treatment regimen prescribed for active TB disease. They are:

1. Provide the safest, most effective therapy in the shortest period of time possible.
2. Always use multiple drugs to which the organisms are susceptible.
3. Never add a single drug to a failing regimen.
4. Ensure that the patient adheres fully to the treatment regimen.

The American Thoracic Society/CDC (2003) currently recommends an initial drug regimen that includes at least four drugs: INH, rifampin, pyrazinamide, and either ethambutol or streptomycin. The rationale behind multi-drug therapy is to prevent emergence of resistant strains. Patients are usually most infectious before the diagnosis is made and before treatment is initiated, so it is imperative that drug therapy be started immediately, even before the diagnosis of TB is confirmed. Initial therapy will in part be determined by the patient's risk factors, clinical symptoms and medical history, and by the characteristics of TB found in that particular community (for example, number of cases overall, prevalence of drug-resistant strains, and predominance of high-risk populations). Once culture and drug sensitivity results are determined, the drug regimen can be tailored to the specific characteristics of the infective organisms.

Promoting patient adherence to the treatment regimen is the major determinant to the outcome of treatment. Since treatment for TB requires numerous drugs to be taken for prolonged periods, and since many people with TB are those whose socioeconomic status provides numerous barriers to treatment, compliance with the treatment regimen is the first and primary goal of all health care providers. No drug therapy will work if it does not enter the patient's body. Careful coordination of all available community health resources with patients is necessary to ensure compliance with therapy. Directly observed therapy (DOT) is the preferred initial strategy that should be used with any daily or intermittent treatment schedule. When DOT is used, a designated health care team member, family member, or other designated responsible person observes the patient actually ingesting the medication. For those individuals who self-administer their antitubercular drugs, there are some fixed-dose combinations of drugs that may enhance patient adherence and reduce the risk of inappropriate monotherapy. In the U.S., the Food and Drug Administration has licensed fixed-dose combinations of INH and rifampin (Rifamate®) and also combinations of INH, rifampin, and pyrazinamide (Rifater®) (American Thoracic Society/CDC, 2003).

Treatment of pulmonary TB. The duration of therapy depends on the drugs used, culture and drug susceptibility test results, and the patient's clinical response to therapy. There are treatment regimens that can be used for either 6 or 9 months. Most persons with untreated pulmonary TB can be adequately treated using either the 6 or 9-month regimen. INH and rifampin must be included in all drug regimens lasting 9 months or less, and all 6-month courses must contain INH, rifampin, and at least initially, pyrazinamide. The first-line drugs commonly used to treat TB are listed in Table 19-13.

Adults with positive smears or cultures should have a 6-month course that begins with INH, rifampin, and pyrazinamide for the first 2 months. Until drug susceptibility of the organism is known, the first 2 months of therapy should also include either ethambutol or streptomycin, unless it is certain that there is little chance of drug resistance. If the organism is susceptible to INH and rifampin, the remaining 4 months of treatment should consist of these two drugs. For patients unable to take pyrazinamide, it is acceptable to use a 9-month regimen of INH and rifampin; this regimen should include either ethambutol or streptomycin until drug sensitivities are known or there is known to be little chance of drug resistance. As mentioned previously, DOT is required with any daily or intermittent dosage schedule.

TB and HIV. Recommendations for the duration of TB treatment for persons also infected with HIV are with a few exceptions, the same as for non-HIV infected persons. However, HIV patients must be closely followed to assess clinical and bacteriological responses to treatment, since the prevalence of drug resistance in this population is higher. These patients also require close follow-up because they seem to have a higher incidence of adverse effects caused by antitubercular drug therapy (American Thoracic Society/CDC, 2003). Treatment periods should be lengthened if the clinical response is slow or suboptimal in any way. Adherence to the treatment regimen is especially critical in this population, and the CDC strongly recommends DOT for this group (CDC, 2003).

Extrapulmonary TB. The basic principles of pulmonary TB treatment apply to the treatment of TB at sites other than the lungs. A 6-month course of therapy is recommended for treatment except in tuberculous meningitis in which a 9-12 month course of drug therapy is recommended. The addition of corticosteriods is recommended for tuberculous pericarditis and tuberculosis meningitis. Surgery may at times be required to obtain specimens for diagnosis or to relieve cardiac compression (from constrictive pericarditis) or spinal cord compression (resulting from tubercular erosion of vertebrae). Cardiac constriction, resulting from tuberculous pericarditis, may be prevented by the use of corticosteroids, which may also decrease neurologic sequelae of TB meningitis, especially when administered early in the course of the disease. The type of follow-up to assessments to determine the response to therapy will depend on the site of the infection and its accessibility (American Thoracic Society/CDC, 2003).

Drug-resistant TB. Drug-resistance in newly diagnosed TB may be suspected by use of information regarding contact with known drug-resistant cases or living in a region in

Table 19-13
Information on First-Line TB Drugs

Drug and Route	Major Adverse Reactions	Recommended Monitoring	Considerations for Patients with CRF
Isoniazid (PO, IM)	Hepatic enzyme elevations; hepatitis; peripheral neuropathy; mild CNS effects; interactions with phenytoin	Baseline measurements of hepatic enzymes. Repeat studies if: - baseline results are abnormal - patient at high risk for adverse reactions - patient has symptoms of adverse reactions	Removed by both peritoneal and hemodialysis. Minor dosage adjustments may be required for patients with severe renal impairments. On hemodialysis days, give dose after dialysis treatment
Rifampin (PO, IV)	GI upset; rash; drug interactions; hepatitis; bleeding problems; flu-like symptoms	Baseline CBC, hepatic enzymes. Repeat studies if: - baseline results are abnormal - patient has symptoms of adverse reactions	Plasma concentrations not appreciably affected by peritoneal or hemodialysis.
Pyrazinamide (PO)	Hepatitis; rash; GI upset; joint aches; hyperuricemia; gout (rare)	Baseline uric acid, hepatic enzymes. Repeat studies if: - baseline results are abnormal - patient has symptoms of adverse reactions	Use with caution in patients with renal failure or diabetes.
Ethambutol (PO)	Optic neuritis	Baseline and monthly tests: - visual acuity - color vision	Removed by peritoneal dialysis. Removed to a lesser extent by hemodialysis; on hemodialysis days, give dose after treatment. Longer dosage intervals and lower drug doses with renal failure.
Streptomycin (IM)	Ototoxicity; renal toxicity	Baseline and repeat as needed: - hearing - renal function studies	Dosages for renal failure patients should be based on serum drug levels. Give half of normal dose after hemodialysis treatment. Removed by peritoneal and hemodialysis.

Note: Adapted from: Centers for Disease Control. (1994). Core curriculum on tuberculosis. Atlanta, GA: Author. Lentino, J., & Leehey, D. (1994). Infections. In J. Daugirdas & T. Ing (Eds.), Handbook of dialysis (2nd edition) (pp. 469-490). Boston: Little, Brown and Company.

which there are known cases of drug resistant TB. Drug resistance is proven only by drug-susceptibility testing. These patients require prolonged treatment regimens based on their medical history and drug-susceptibility studies. Many times these organisms are also resistant to other first-line drugs, such as ethambutol and streptomycin. Clinicians unfamiliar with the treatment of MDR-TB are strongly urged to consult experts in the care of these patients (American Thoracic Society, 2003). These patients frequently require treatment with several second-line drugs, which are less effective and can cause serious adverse effects, so close and continuous monitoring throughout the treatment period is mandatory when treating MDR-TB. There have been documented cases of MDR-TB being spread by direct contact, and since these strains are so difficult to treat, it is imperative that appropriate treatment be started as soon as possible and that adherence to treatment be ensured by whatever means are necessary. (American Thoracic Society/CDC, 2003)

Renal Insufficiency and ESRD

Renal disease complicates the management of TB. Antituberculosis medications may be cleared by the kidney and also by hemodialysis. Decreasing the dose of some anti-tuberculosis drugs is generally not the best way to treat TB because the peak serum concentrations needed for adequate therapy cannot be reached. The best alternative is to change the dosing interval. Drugs that are cleared by the kidneys in patients with creatinine clearance of less than 30 ml/minute and those receiving hemodialysis treatments are managed by increasing dosing intervals (see Table 19-14). Drugs affected by renal clearance include ethambutol (EMB) and pyrazinamide (PZA) and its metabolites. INH, EMB and PZA are cleared by hemodialysis, but only PZA and its metabolites have significant clearance requiring supplemental dosing after hemodialysis. If PZA is given after dialysis, supplemental dosing is not required. In general, antituberculosis drugs should be given after hemodialysis to avoid losses during hemodialysis treatment (American Thoracic Society/CDC, 2003).

Doses of streptomycin, kanamycin, amikaicin and capreomycin must be adjusted in patients with renal failure. Approximately 40% of the drug is removed with hemodialysis when the drugs are given just before hemodialysis. The dosing interval should be increased for these drugs. (American Thoracic Society/CDC, 2003).

Patients with ESRD may have additional clinical concerns, such as gastroparesis, that may affect the absorption of the TB drugs. In addition, patients may also be taking medications that interact with these drugs.

There is no data for patients on peritoneal dialysis. Drug removal mechanisms differ between hemodialysis and peritoneal dialysis, so it cannot be assumed that hemodialysis precautions apply to peritoneal dialysis.

The CDC recommends that after a known exposure to infectious TB disease, immunocompromised patients should receive treatment for presumptive latent TB (LTB1), regardless of skin testing result (MMWR, 2004).

Infectivity. Infectiousness of a patient with TB is directly related to the number of tubercle bacilli released into the air whenever that person coughs, talks, sings, or sneezes. Most patients are considered infectious if they are coughing, undergoing cough-inducing or aerosol-generating procedures or if they have sputum smears that demonstrate the presence of acid-fast bacilli and at the same time are not receiving therapy, have just started therapy, or have a poor clinical or bacteriologic response to therapy. Infectiousness may persist for weeks or even months in patients with drug-resistant TB. Once effective therapy is begun, patients are no longer considered infectious as long as they meet all of the following criteria: (a) they have been receiving adequate drug therapy for 2 to 3 weeks, (b) they demonstrate a favorable clinical response to therapy, and (c) consecutive sputum smears collected on three separate days are negative (American Thoracic Society/CDC, 2003).

Conclusion

In summary, people with end stage kidney disease have suppressed immune systems and are exposed to many infectious agents in hemodialysis units. A wide range of bacterial infections are common and Hepatitis B, C and D and HIV viruses pose significant challenges for both patients and nurses. There is also a resurgence of tuberculosis among people

Table 19-14

Drug Frequency Changes for Adult Patients with Reduced Renal Function and Adult Patients Receiving Hemodialysis

Drug	Change in Frequency?
Rifampin	No Change
Pyrazinamide	Yes
Ethambutol	Yes
Lavofkaxacin	Yes
Cycloserine	Yes
Ethionamide	No Change
p-Aminosalicylic acid	No Change
Streptomycin	Yes
Capreomycin	Yes
Kanamycin	Yes
Amikacin	Yes

with chronic kidney disease. Prevention of these infections and controlling transmission are key aspects of the role of the nephrology nurse. Addressing infection control in hemodialysis units not only protects patients and their families, but also nurses and other staff entering the facility. Further research to minimize the effects of these infections is needed.

References

Abbott, K.C., Trespalacios, F.C., Agodoa, L.Y., & Ahuja, T.S. (2003). HIVAN and medication use in chronic dialysis patients in the United States: Analysis of the USRDS DMMS Wave 2 Study. *BMC Nephrology, 1,* 4-5.

Abbott, K.C., Swanson, S.J., Agodoa, L.Y., & Kimmel, P.L. (2004). Human immunodeficiency virus infection and kidney transplantation in the era of highly active antiretroviral therapy and modern immunosupression. *Journal of the American Society of Nephrology, 15*(6), 1033-1039.

Afdhal, N.H. (2004). The natural history of hepatitis C. *Seminars in Liver Disease, 24*(Suppl 2), 3-8.

Ahuja, T, Grady, J., & Khan, S. (2002). Changing trends in the survival of dialysis patients with human immunodeficiency virus in the United States. *Journal of the American Society of Nephrology, 13*(7), 1889-1893.

AIDS Vaccine Research Working Group (AVRWG). (2003). National Institute of Allergy and Infectious Diseases. Washington, DC: National Institutes of Health.

Alonso, O., Loinaz, C. Abradelo, M., Perez, B., Manrique, A., Gomez, R.., Jimenez, C., Meneu, J.C., Garcia, I., & Moreno-Gonzalez, E. (2003). Changes in the incidence and severity of recurrent hepatitis C after liver transplantation over 1990-1999. *Transplant Proceedings, 35*(5), 1836-1837.

Alter, M.J. (1997). The epidemiology of acute and chronic hepatitis C. *Clinics in Liver Disease, 1,* 559-568.

Alter, M.J. (2002). Prevention of spread of hepatitis C. *Hepatology, 36*(5 Suppl. 1), S93-S98.

Alter, M.J., Ahtone, J., & Maynard, J.E. (1983). Hepatitis B virus transmission associated with a multiple-dose vial in a hemodialysis unit.

Annals of Internal Medicine, 99, 330-333.

Alter, M.J., Favero, M.S., & Maynard, J.E. (1986). Impact of infection control strategies on the incidence of dialysis-associated hepatitis in the United States. *Journal of Infectious Diseases, 153*, 1149-1151.

Alter, M.J., Margolis, H.S., Krawczynski, K., Judson, F.N., Mares, A., Alexander, W.J., et al. (1992). The natural history of community-acquired hepatitis C in the United States. *New England Journal of Medicine, 327*, 1899-1905.

Alter, H.J., Seeff, L.B., Kaplan, P.M., McAuliffe, V.J., Wright, E.C., Gerin, J.L., et al. (1976). Type B hepatitis: The infectivity of blood positive for e antigen and DNA polymerase after accidental needlestick exposure. *New England Journal of Medicine, 295*(17), 909-913.

American Thoracic Society. (1994). Treatment of tuberculosis and tuberculosis infection in adults and children. *American Journal of Respiratory and Critical Care Medicine, 149*, 1359-1374.

American Thoracic Society, Centers for Disease Control. (2003). Treatment for tuberculosis, American Thoracic Society, CDC, and Infectious Diseases Society. *MMWR Recommendations and Reports,* June 20, 2003/52 (RR11).

Association for Professionals in Infection Control and Epidemiology (APIC). (2000). *APIC text of infection control and epidemiology.* Washington, DC: Author.

Association for the Advancement of Medical Instrumentation (AAMI). (1993). American national standard. Reuse of hemodialyzers (ANSI/AAMI RD47-1993). Arlington, VA: AAMI.

Besarab, A., Bolton, W.K., Browne, J.K., Egrie, J.C., Nissenson, A.R., Okamoto, D.M., et al. (1998). The effects of normal as compared with low hematocrit values in patients with cardiac disease who are receiving hemodialysis and epoetin. *New England Journal of Medicine, 339*(9), 584-590.

Bloembergen, W.E., & Port, F.K. (1996). Epidemiological perspective on infections in chronic dialysis patients. *Advancements in Renal Replacement Therapy, 3*(3), 201-207.

Bond, W.W., Favero, M.S., & Petersen, N.J. (1981). Survival of hepatitis B virus after drying and storage for 1 week. *Lancet, 1*, 550-551.

Bonomo, R.A., Rice, D., Whalen, C., Linn, D., Eckstein, E., & Shlaes, D.M. (1997). Risk factors associated with permanent access-site infections in chronic hemodialysis patients. *Infection Control in Hospitals Epidemiology, 18*(11), 757-761.

Boyce, J.M., & Pittet, D. (2002). Guideline for hand hygiene in health care settings. Recommendations of the Healthcare Infection Control Practices Advisory Committee and the HIPAC/SHEA/APIC/IDSA Hand Hygiene Task Force. *American Journal of Infectious Control, 30*(8), S1-46.

Brady, J.P., Snyder, J.W., & Hasbargen, J.A. (1998). Vancomycin-resistant enterococcus in end stage renal disease. *American Journal of Kidney Diseases, 32*(3), 415-418.

Busch, M.P., Kleinman, S.H., Jackson, B., Stramer, S.L., Hewlett, I., & Preston, S. (2000). Nucleic acid amplification testing of blood donors for transfusion-transmitted infectious diseases: Report of the Interorganizational Task Force on Nucleic Acid Amplification Testing of Blood Donors. *Transfusion, 40*(2), 143-159.

Casey, K. (1993). Fighting MDR-TB. *RN, 56*, 26-30.

Centers for Disease Control and Prevention (CDC). (1977). *Hepatitis – control measures for hepatitis B in dialysis centers* (Viral Hepatitis Investigations and Control Series). [HEW Publication No. 78-8358]. Atlanta, GA: CDC.

Centers for Disease Control and Prevention (CDC). (1991). Hepatitis B virus: A comprehensive strategy for eliminating transmission in the United States through universal childhood vaccination. Recommendations of the Advisory Committee on Immunization Practices (ACIP) (No. RR-13). *Morbidity & Mortality Weekly Report, 40*, 1-25.

Centers for Disease Control and Prevention (CDC). (1993). *Outbreak of hepatitis B in a dialysis center.* Epidemic Investigation Report EPI 91-17. Atlanta, GA: CDC.

Centers for Disease Control and Prevention (CDC). (1994a). Guidelines for preventing transmission of human immunodeficiency virus through transplantation of human tissue and organs. *Morbidity and Mortality Weekly Report, 43*, (No. RR-8) 1-13.

Centers for Disease Control. (CDC) (1994b). *Core curriculum on tuberculosis - What the clinician should know* (3rd ed.). Atlanta, GA: Author.

Centers for Disease Control and Prevention (CDC). (1995). Recommendations for preventing the spread of vancomycin resistance (No. RR-12). *Morbidity & Mortality Weekly Report, 44*, 1-13.

Centers for Disease Control and Prevention (CDC). (1996). Outbreaks of hepatitis B virus infection among hemodialyis patients – California, Nebraska, and Texas, 1994. *Morbidity & Mortality Weekly Report, 45*, 285-289.

Centers for Disease Control and Prevention (CDC). (1998b). Outbreaks of gram-negative bacterial bloodstream infections traced to probable contamination of hemodialysis machines – Canada, 1995; United States, 1997; and Israel, 1997. *Morbidity and Mortality Weekly Report, 47*, 55-59.

Centers for Disease Control and Prevention (CDC). (2001). Recommendations for preventing transmission of infections among chronic hemodialysis patients (No. RR-5). *Morbidity & Mortality Weekly Report, 50*, 1-43.

Centers for Disease Control and Prevention (CDC). (2002). Guidelines for the prevention of intravascular catheter-related infections (No. RR-10). *Morbidity & Mortality Weekly Report, 51*, 11-29.

Centers for Disease Control and Prevention (CDC). (2003). Guidelines for laboratory testing and result reporting of antibody to hepatitis C virus (No. RR-3). *Morbidity & Mortality Weekly Report, 52*, 1-15.

Chang, S., Sievert, D.M., Hageman, J.C., Boulton, M.L., Tenover, F.C., Downes, F.P., et al. (2003). Infection with vancomycin-resistant Staphylococcus aureus containing the van A resistance gene. *New England Journal of Medicine, 348*(14), 1342-1347.

Dean, H.D., Steele, C.B., Satcher, A.J., & Nakashima, A.K. (2005). HIV/AIDS among minority races and ethnicities in the United States, 1999-2003. *Journal of the National Medical Association, 97*(7 suppl.), 5S-12S.

Dieleman, J.P., van Rossum, A.M., Stricker, B.C., Sturkenboom, M.C., de Groot, R., Telgt, D., et al. (2003). Persistent leukocyturia and loss of renal function in a prospectively monitored cohort of HIV-infected patients treated with indinavir. *Journal of Acquired Immune Deficiency Syndrome. 32*(2),135-142.

Dienstag, J.L., Schiff, E.R., Wright, T.L., Perrillo, R.P., Hann, H.W., Goodman, Z., et al. (1999). Lamivudine as initial treatment for chronic hepatitis B in the United States. *New England Journal of Medicine, 341*(17), 1256-1263.

Do, S. (2001, Summer-Fall). The natural history of hepatitis B in Asian Americans. Asian *American Pacific Island Journal of Health, 9*(2), 141-153.

Dobkin, J.F., Miller, M.H., & Steigbigel, N.H. (1978). Septicemia in patients on chronic hemodialysis. *Annals of Internal Medicine, 88*(1), 28-33.

Donlan, R.M. (2001). Biofilms and device-associated infections. *Emergency Infectious Diseases, 7*(2), 277-281.

Dopirak, M., Hill, C., Oleksiw, M., Dumigan, D., Arvai, J., English, E., et al. (2002). Surveillance of hemodialysis-associated primary bloodstream infections: The experience of 10 hospital-based centers. *Infection Control in Hospitals Epidemiology, 23*(12), 721-724.

Fabrizi, F., Lunghi, G., Guarnori, I., Raffaele, L., Crepaldi, M., Pagano, A., et al. (1994). Incidence of seroconversion for hepatitis C virus in chronic hemodialysis patients: A prospective study. *Nephrology Dialysis Transplantation, 9*(11), 1611-1615.

Fabrizi, F., Martin, P., Dixit, V., Brezina, M., Cole, M.J., Gerosa, S., et al. (1998). Acquisition of hepatitis C virus in hemodialysis patients: A prospective study by branched DNA signal amplification assay. *American Journal of Kidney Diseases, 31*(4), 647-654.

Fan, P.Y., & Schwab, S.J. (1992). Vascular access: Concepts for the 1990s. *Journal of the American Society of Nephrology, 3*(1), 1-11.

Favero, M.S., & Bolyard, E.A. (1995). Microbiologic considerations. Disinfection and sterilization strategies and the potential for airborne transmission of bloodborne pathogens. *Surgical Clinics of North America, 75*(6), 1071-1089.

Favero, M.S., & Bond, W.W. (1991). Chemical disinfection of medical and surgical materials. In S.S. Block (Ed.), *Disinfection, sterilization, and preservation* (4th ed.) (pp. 617-641). Philadelphia: Lea and Febiger.

Favero, M.S., Bond, W.W., Petersen, N.J., Berquist, K.R., & Maynard, J.E. (1974). Detection methods for study of the stability of hepatitis B antigen on surfaces. *Journal of Infectious Diseases, 129*(2), 210-212.

Favero, M.S., Maynard, J.E., Petersen, N.J., Boyer, K.M., Bond, W.W., Berquist, K.R., et al. (1973). Hepatitis-B antigen on environmental surfaces [Letter]. *Lancet, 2,* 1455.

Fishbane, S., Cunha, B.A., Mittal, S.K., Ruggian, J., Shea, K., Schoch, P.E. (1999). Vancomycin-resistant enterococci in hemodialysis patients is related to intravenous vancomycin use. *Infection Control in Hospitals Epidemiology, 20*(7), 461-462.

Fogel, M.A., Nussbaum, P.B., Feintzeig, I.D., Hunt, W.A., Gavin, J.P., & Kim, R.C. (1998). Use of cefazolin in chronic hemodialysis patients: A safe and effective alternative to vancomycin. *American Journal of Kidney Diseases, 32*(3), 401-409.

Forns, X., Fernandez-Llama, P., Pons, M., Costa, J., Ampurdanes, S., Lopez-Labrador, F.X., et al. (1997). Incidence and risk factors of hepatitis C virus infection in a hemodialysis unit. *Nephrology Dialysis Transplantation, 12*(4), 736-740.

Fridkin, S.K. (2001). Vancomycin-intermediate and resistant Staphylococcus aureus: What the infectious disease specialist needs to know. *Clinics in Infectious Diseases, 32*(1), 108-115.

Fridkin, S.K., Edwards, J.R, Courval, J.M., Hill, H., Tenover, F.C., Lawton, R., Gaynes, R.P., McGowan, J.E., Jr; Intensive Care Antimicrobial Resistance Epidemiology (ICARE) Project and the National Nosocomial Infections Surveillance (NNIS) System Hospitals. (2001). The effect of vancomycin and third-generation cephalosporins on prevalence of vancomycin-resistant enterococci in 126 U.S. adult intensive care units. *Annals of Internal Medicine, 135*(3), 175-183.

Fung, S.K., & Lok, A.S. (2004). Management of hepatitis B patients with antiviral resistance. *Antiviral Therapy, 9*(6), 1013-1026.

Futterman, D.C. (2005). HIV in adolescents and young adults: Half of all new infections in the United States. *Topics in HIV Medicine, 13*(3), 101-105.

Grohskopf, L.A., Roth, V.R., Feikin, D.R., Arduino, M.J., Carson, L.A., Tokars, J.I., et al. (2001). Serratia liquefaciens bloodstream infections from contamination of epoetin alfa at a hemodialysis center. *New England Journal of Medicine, 344*(20), 1491-1497.

Hardy, N.M., Sandroni, S., Danielson, S., & Wilson, W.J. (1992). Antibody to hepatitis C virus increases with time on hemodialysis. *Clinical Nephrology, 38*(1), 44-48.

Hoen, B., Paul-Dauphin, A., Hestin, D., & Kessler, M. (1998). EPIBAC-DIAL: A multicenter prospective study of risk factors for bacteremia in chronic hemodialysis patients. *Journal of the American Society of Nephrology, 9*(5), 869-876.

Hoofnagle, J.H., & Di Bisceglie, A.M. (1991). Serologic diagnosis of acute and chronic viral hepatitis. *Seminars in Liver Disease, 11*(2), 73-83.

Hutin, Y.J., Goldstein, S.T., Varma, J.K., O'Dair, J.B., Mast, E.E., Shapiro, C.N., et al. (1999). An outbreak of hospital-acquired hepatitis B virus infection among patients receiving chronic hemodialysis. *Infection Control in Hospitals Epidemiology, 20*(11), 731-735.

Hwang, S.J. (2001). Hepatitis C virus infection: An overview. *Journal of Microbial Immunologic Infections, 34*(4), 227-234.

Ifudu, O., Mayers, J.D., Matthew, J.J., Macey, L.J., Brezsnyak, W., Reydel, C., McClendon, E., Surgrue, T., Rao, T.K., & Friedman, E.A. (1997). Uremia therapy in patients with end-stage renal disease and human immunodeficiency virus infection: has the outcome changed in the 1990s? *American Journal of Kidney Diseases, 29*(4), 549-559.

Jo, H. (1993). Assessment and management of persons coinfected with tuberculosis and human immunodeficiency virus. *Nurse Practitioner, 18,* 42-49.

Justesen, U.S., & Pedersen, C. (2000). Lactic acidosis type B: A life-threatening adverse effect of antiretroviral therapy. *Ugeskr Laeger, 162*(35). 4664-4665.

Juszczyk, J. (2000). Clinical course and consequences of hepatitis B infection. *Vaccine, 18*(Suppl. 1), S23-S25.

Kantor, R.J., Hadler, S.C., Schreeder, M.T., Berquist, K.R., & Favero, M.S. (1979). Outbreak of hepatitis B in a dialysis unit, complicated by false positive HBsAg test results. *Dialysis and Transplantation, 8,* 232-235.

Kaplowitz, L.G., Comstock, J.A., Landwehr, D.M., Dalton, H.P., & Mayhall, C.G. (1988). A prospective study of infections in hemodialysis patients: Patient hygiene and other risk factors for infection. *Infection Control in Hospitals Epidemiology, 9*(12), 534-541.

Kessler, M., Hoen, B., Mayeux, D., Hestin, D., & Fontenaille, C. (1993). Bacteremia in patients on chronic hemodialysis. A multicenter prospective survey. *Nephron, 64*(1), 95-100.

Kloster, B., Kramer, R., Eastlund, T., Grossman, B., & Zarvan, B. (1995). Hepatitis B surface antigenemia in blood donors following vaccination. *Transfusion, 35*(6), 475-477.

Lai, C.-L., Chien, R.-N., Leung, N.W.Y., and the Asia Hepatitis Lamivudine Study Group. (1998). A 1-year trial of lamivudine for chronic hepatitis B. *New England Journal of Medicine, 339,* 61-68.

Larghi, A., Zuin, M., Crosignani, A., Ribero, M.L., Pipia, C., Battezzati, P.M., et al. (2002). Outcome of an outbreak of acute hepatitis C among healthy volunteers participating in pharmacokinetics studies. *Hepatology, 36*(4 Pt. 1), 993-1000.

Lettau, L.A., Alfred, H.J., Glew, R.H., Fields, H.A., Alter, M.J., Meyer, R., et al. (1986). Nosocomial transmission of delta hepatitis. *Annals of Internal Medicine, 104*(5), 631-635.

Lindberg, P. (1993). Improving hospital ventilation systems for tuberculosis infection control. In Plant Technology & Safety Management Series, *Controlling occupational exposure to tuberculosis.* Oakbrook Terrace, IL: Joint Commission on Accreditation of Healthcare Organizations.

Lunn, E.R., Hoggarth, B.J., & Cook, W.J. (2000). Prolonged hepatitis B surface antigenemia after vaccination. *Pediatrics, 105*(6), E81.

Marx, M.A., Frye, R.F., Matzke, G.R., & Golper, T.A. (1998). Cefazolin as empiric therapy in hemodialysis-related infections: Efficacy and blood concentrations. *American Journal of Kidney Diseases, 32*(3), 410-414.

Maynard, J.E. (1990). Hepatitis B: Global importance and need for control. *Vaccine,* Supplement, S 18-20.

McLaughlin, K.J., Cameron, S.O., Good, T., McCruden, E., Ferguson, J.C., Davidson, F., et al. (1997). Nosocomial transmission of hepatitis C virus within a British dialysis center. *Nephrology Dialysis Transplantation, 12*(2), 304-309.

McMahon, B.J., Alberts, S.R., Wainwright, R.B., Bulkow, L., & Lanier, A.P. (1990). Hepatitis B-related sequelae. Prospective study in 1400 hepatitis B surface antigen-positive Alaska native carriers. *Archives of Internal Medicine, 150*(5), 1051-1054.

Mermel, L.A., Farr, B.M., Sherertz, R.J., Raad, I.I., O'Grady, N., Harris, J.S., et al. (2001). Guidelines for the management of intravascular catheter-related infections. *Clinics in Infectious Diseases, 32*(9), 1249-1272.

Najem, G.R., Louria, D.B., Thind, I.S., Lavenhar, M.A., Gocke, D.J., Baskin, S.E., et al. (1981). Control of hepatitis B infection. The role of surveillance and an isolation hemodialysis center. *Journal of the American Medical Association, 245,* 153-157.

National Institute of Allergy and Infectious Diseases (NIAID). (2004). *The problem of antibiotic resistance.* NIAID Fact Sheet. Washington, DC: Author.

National Kidney Foundation (NKF). (2001). K/DOQI clinical practice guideline for vascular access, 2000. *American Journal of Kidney Diseases, 37*(Suppl. 1), S137-S181.

National Institutes of Health. (2000). *Chronic hepatitis C: Current disease management* (pp. 1-21). Bethesda, MD: National Institute of Diabetes and Digestive and Kidney Diseases.

Niu, M.T., Coleman, P.J., & Alter, M.J. (1993). Multicenter study of hepatitis C virus infection in chronic hemodialysis patients and hemodialysis center staff members. *American Journal of Kidney Diseases, 22*(4), 568-573.

Niu, M.T., Penberthy, L.T., Alter, M.J, Armstrong, C.W., Miller, G.B., & Hadler, S.C. (1989). Hemodialysis-associated hepatitis B: Report of an outbreak. *Dialysis and Transplantation, 18,* 542-555.

Padberg, F.T., Jr., Lee, B.C., & Curl, G.R. (1992). Hemo access site infection. *Surgery, Gynecology, and Obstetrics, 174,* 103-108.

Parker, J., Dickenson, L., Wiseman, K.C., Alexander, D., & Peacock, E. (1998). Control of infectious diseases in the renal patient. In J. Parker (Ed.), *Contemporary nephrology nursing* (pp. 347-402). Pitman, NJ: American Nephrology Nurses' Association.

Pearlman, B.L. (2004). Hepatitis C infection: A clinical review. *Southern Medical Journal, 97*(1). 364-373.

Petrosilla, N., Gilli, P., Serraino, D., et al. (2001). Prevalence of infected patients and understaffing have a role in hepatitis C virus transmission in dialysis. *American Journal of Kidney Diseases, 35*(5), 1004-1010.

Phipps, W., & Daly, B. (1983). Problems of the lower airway. In W. Phipps, B. Long, & N. Woods (Eds.), *Medical-surgical nursing: Concepts and clinical practice* (2nd. ed.) (pp. 1297-1307). St. Louis: C.V. Mosby Company.

Pinto dos Santos, J., Loureiro, A., Cendoroglo, N., & Pereira, B.J.G. (1996). Impact of dialysis room and reuse strategies on the incidence of hepatitis C virus infection in hemodialysis units. *Nephrology Dialysis Transplantation, 11*, 2017-2022.

Powe, N.R., Jaar, B., Furth, S.L., Hermann, J., & Briggs, W. (1999). Septicemia in dialysis patients: Incidence, risk factors, and prognosis. *Kidney International, 55*(3), 1081-1090.

Protic, J., & Hardy, D. (1993). Resurgence of tuberculosis and emergence of multidrug-resistant strains: Implications for health care personnel. In Plant Technology & Safety Management Series, *Controlling occupational exposure to tuberculosis.* Oakbrook Terrace, IL: Joint Commission on Accreditation of Healthcare Organizations.

Riley, R., & Nardell, E. (1993). Controlling transmission of tuberculosis in health care facilities: Ventilation, filtration, and ultraviolet air disinfection. In Plant Technology & Safety Management Series, *Controlling occupational exposure to tuberculosis.* Oakbrook Terrace, IL: Joint Commission on Accreditation of Healthcare Organizations.

Ross, M.J., Klotman, P.E., & Winston, J.A. (2000). HIV-associated nephropathy: Case study and review of the literature. *AIDS Patient Care STDS, 14*(12), 637-645.

Ross, M.J., & Klotman, P.E. (2002). Recent progress in HIV-associated nephropathy. *Journal of the American Society of Nephrology, 13*(12), 2997-3004.

Rao, T.K. (2001). Human immunodeficiency virus infection and renal failure. *Infectious Disease Clinics of North America, 15*(3), 833-950.

Sattar, S.A., Tetro, J., Springthorpe, V.S., & Giulivi, A. (2001). Preventing the spread of hepatitis B and C viruses: Where are germicides relevant? *American Journal of Infection Control, 29*(3), 187-197.

Schluger, N., & Rom, W. (1994). Current approaches to the diagnosis of active pulmonary tuberculosis. *American Journal of Respiratory and Critical Care Medicine, 149,* 264-267.

Selgas, R., Martinez-Zapico, R., Bajo, M,A,, et al. (1992). Prevalence of hepatitis C antibodies (HCV) in a dialysis population at one center. *Peritoneal Dialysis International, 12*, 28-30.

Shikata, T., Karasawa, T., & Abe, K. (1977). Hepatitis B antigen and infectivity of hepatitis B virus. *Journal of Infectious Diseases, 136,* 571-576.

Sivapalasingam, S., Malak, S.F., Sullivan, J.F., Lorch, J., & Sepkowitz, K.A. (2002). High prevalence of hepatitis C infection among patients receiving hemodialysis at an urban dialysis center. *Infection Control in Hospitals Epidemiology, 23*(6), 319-324.

Snydman, D.R., Bryan, J.A., London, W.T., Werner, B., Bregman, D., Blumberg, B.S., et al. (1976). Transmission of hepatitis B associated with hemodialysis: Role of malfunction (blood leaks) in dialysis machines. *Journal of Infectious Diseases, 134*(6), 562-570.

Sulkowski, M.S., Thomas, D.L., Chaisson, R.E., & Moore, R.D. (2000). Hepatotoxicity associated with antiretroviral therapy in adults infected with human immunodeficiency virus and the role of hepatitis C or B virus infection. *Journal of the American Medical Association, 283*(1), 74-80.

Taylor, G., Gravel, D., Johnston, L., Embil, J., Holton, D., & Paton, S. (2002). Prospective surveillance for primary bloodstream infections occurring in Canadian hemodialysis units. *Infection Control in Hospitals Epidemiology, 23*(12), 716-720.

Temesgen, Z., & Beri, G. (2004). *Immunoallergy Clinics of North America, 24*(3), 521-531.

Thomas, D.L., Astemborski, J., Rai, R.M., Anania, F.A., Schaeffer, M., Galai, N., et al. (2000). The natural history of hepatitis C virus infection: Host, viral, and environmental factors. *Journal of the American Medical Association, 284*(4), 450-456.

Tokars, J.I. (2002). Bloodstream infections in hemodialysis patients: Getting some deserved attention. *Infection Control in Hospitals Epidemiology, 23*(12), 713-715.

Tokars, J.I., Alter, M.J., Miller, E., Moyer, L.A., & Favero, M.S. (1997). National surveillance of dialysis associated diseases in the United States, 1994. *ASAIO Journal, 43*, 108-119.

Tokars, J.I., Frank, M., Alter, M.J., & Arduino, M.J. (2002). National sur-

veillance of dialysis-associated diseases in the United States, 2000. *Seminars in Dialysis, 15*(3), 162-171.

Tokars, J.I., Light, P., & Armistead, N. (2001). Vascular access infections among hemodialysis outpatients. *American Journal of Kidney Diseases, 37*, 1232-1240.

Tokars, J.I., Miller, E.R., Alter, M.J., & Arduino, M.J. (1998a). *National surveillance of dialysis-associated diseases in the United States, 1996* (pp. 1-59). Atlanta, GA: Centers for Disease Control and Prevention.

Tokars, J.I., Miller, E., Alter, M.J., & Arduino, M.J. (1998b). *National surveillance of dialysis-associated diseases in the United States, 1995.* Atlanta, GA: U.S. Department of Health and Human Services.

Tokars, J.I., Miller, E.R., Alter, M.J., & Arduino, M.J. (2000). National surveillance of dialysis-associated diseases in the United States, 1997. *Seminars in Dialysis, 13*(2), 75-85.

Tokars, J.I., Miller, E.R., & Stein, G. (2002). New national surveillance system for hemodialysis-associated infections: Initial results. *American Journal of Infectious Control, 30*(5), 288-295.

U.S. Department of Health and Human Services. (2004). *Guidelines for the use of antiretroviral agents in HIV-1 infected adults and adolescents.* Panel on Clinical Practice for Treatment of HIV infection. Washington, DC: Public Health Service.

U.S.Renal Data System (USRDS). (2002). *USRDS 2002 Annual data report: Atlas of end stage renal disease in the United States* (pp. 15-564). Bethesda, MD: National Institutes of Health, National Institute of Diabetes and Digestive and Kidney Diseases.

Uttley, A.H., George, R.C., Naidoo, J., Woodford, N., Johnson, A.P., Collins, C.H., et al. (1989). High-level vancomycin-resistant enterococci causing hospital infections. *Epidemiological Infections, 103*(1), 173-181.

Velandia, M., Fridkin, S.K., Cardenas, V., Boshell, J., Ramirez, G., Bland, L., et al. (1995). Transmission of HIV in dialysis center. *Lancet, 345*(8962), 1417-1422.

Williams, I.T., Gretch, D., Fleenor, M., et al. (2002). Hepatitis C virus RNA concentration and chronic hepatitis in a cohort of patients followed after developing acute hepatitis C. In H.S. Margolis, M.J. Alter, T.J. Liang, & J.L. Dienstag (Eds.), *Viral hepatitis and liver disease* (pp. 341-344). Atlanta, GA: International Medical Press.

Winston, J., Klotman, M.E., & Klotman, P.E. (1999). HIV-associated nephropathy is a late, not early, manifestation of HIV-1 infection. *Kidney International, 55*, 1036-1040.

Winston, J.A., Burns, G.C., & Klotman, P.E. (2000). Treatment of HIV-associated nephropathy. *Seminars in Nephrology, 20*, 293-298.

Additional Readings

Alter, M.J., Favero, M.S., Miller, J.K., Moyer, L.A., & Bland, L.A. (1990). National surveillance of dialysis-associated diseases in the United States, 1988. *ASAIO Journal, 36,* 107-118.

Alter, M.J., Favero, M.S., Petersen, N.J., Doto, I.L., Leger, R.T., & Maynard, J.E. (1983). National surveillance of dialysis-associated hepatitis and other diseases, 1976 and 1980. *Dialysis and Transplantation, 12,* 860-865.

Anderson, R.L., Holland, B.W., Carr, J.K., Bond, W.W., & Favero, M.S. (1990). Effect of disinfectants on pseudomonads colonized on the interior surface of PVC pipes. *American Journal of Public Health, 80,* 17-21.

Anonymous. (1974). Decrease in the incidence of hepatitis in dialysis units associated with prevention program: Public health laboratory survey. *British Medical Journal, 4,* 751-754.

Arduino, M.J. (1996). Microbiologic quality of water used for hemodialysis. *Contemporary Dialysis Nephrology, 17,* 17-19.

Arduino, M.J. (1997). What's new in water treatment standards for hemodialysis? *Contemporary Dialysis Nephrology, 18,* 21-24.

Arduino, M.J., Bland, L.A., Aguero, S.M., Carson, L., Ridgeway, M., Favero, M.S. (1991). Comparison of microbiologic assay methods for hemodialysis fluids. *Journal of Clinical Microbiology, 29,* 592-594.

Association for the Advancement of Medical Instrumentation (AAMI). (1992). *American national standard. Hemodialysis systems* (ANSI/AAMI RD5-1992). Arlington, VA: AAMI.

Association for the Advancement of Medical Instrumentation (AAMI). (2001). *American national standard. Water treatment equipment for hemodialysis applications* (ANSI/AAMI RD62-2001). Arlington, VA: AAMI.

Baz, M., Durand, C., Ragon, A., Jaber, K., Andrieu, D., Merzouk, T., et al. (1991). Using ultrapure water in hemodialysis delays carpal tunnel syndrome. *International Journal of Artificial Organs, 14*(11), 681-685.

Beck-Sague, C.M., Jarvis, W.R., Bland, L.A., Arduino, M.J., Aguero, S.M., & Verosic, G. (1990). Outbreak of gram-negative bacteremia and pyrogenic reactions in a hemodialysis center. *American Journal of Nephrology, 10,* 397-403.

Berns, J.S., & Tokars, J.I. (2002). Preventing bacterial infections and antimicrobial resistance in dialysis patients. *American Journal of Kidney Diseases, 40*(5), 886-898.

Bland, L., Alter, M., Favero, M., Carson, L., & Cusick, L. (1985). Hemodialyzer reuse: Practices in the United States and implication for infection control. *ASAIO Journal, 31,* 556-559.

Bland, L.A., & Favero, M.S. (1989). *Microbial contamination control strategies for hemodialysis systems* (No. 3, pp. 30-36). Oakbrook Terrace, IL: Joint Commission on Accreditation of Healthcare Organizations, Plant, Technology, and Safety Management Series.

Bland, L.A., & Favero, M.S. (1993). Microbiologic and endotoxin considerations in hemodialyzer reprocessing (Vol. 3, Dialysis 3) (pp. 293-300). Arlington, VA: AAMI Standards and Recommended Practices.

Bland, L.A., Ridgeway, M.R., Aguero, S.M., Carson, L.A., & Favero, M.S. (1987). Potential bacteriologic and endotoxin hazards associated with liquid bicarbonate concentrate. *ASAIO Journal, 33,* 542-545.

Bolan, G., Reingold, A.L., Carson, L.A., Silcox, V.A., Woodley, C.L., Hayes, P.S., et al. (1985). Infections with mycobacterium chelonei in patients receiving dialysis and using processed hemodialyzers. *Journal of Infectious Diseases, 152,* 1013-1019.

Bond, W.W., Favero, M.S., Petersen, N.J., & Ebert, J.W. (1983). Inactivation of hepatitis B virus by intermediate-to-high-level disinfectant chemicals. *Journal of Clinical Microbiology, 18,* 535-538.

Canaud, B., Bosc, J.Y., Leray, H., Morena, M., & Stec, F. (2000). Microbiologic purity of dialysate: Rationale and technical aspects. *Blood Purification, 18*(3), 200-213.

Carl, M., Francis, D.P., & Maynard, J.E. (1983). A common-source outbreak of hepatitis B in a hemodialysis unit. *Dialysis and Transplantation, 12,* 222-229.

Carson, L.A., Bland, L.A., Cusick, L.B., Collin, S., Favero, M.S., & Bolan, G. (1987). Factors affecting endotoxin levels in fluids associated with hemodialysis procedures. In S.W. Watson, J. Levin, & T.J. Novitsky (Eds.), *Detection of bacterial endotoxins with the limulus amebocyte lysate test* (pp. 223-234). New York: Alan R. Liss.

Carson, L.A., Bland, L.A., Cusick, L.B., Favero, M.S., Bolan, G.A., Reingold, A.L., et al. (1988). Prevalence of nontuberculous mycobacteria in water supplies of hemodialysis centers. *Applied Environmental Microbiology, 54,* 3122-3125.

Centers for Disease Control and Prevention (CDC). (1979). *Non-A, non-B hepatitis in a dialysis center – Nashville, Tennessee.* Epidemic Investigation Report EPI-78-96. Phoenix, AZ: CDC.

Centers for Disease Control (CDC). (1982). Recommendations of the Advisory Committee on Immunization Practices (ACIP): Inactivated hepatitis B virus vaccine. *Morbidity & Mortality Weekly Report, 31,* 317-322, 327-328.

Centers for Disease Control and Prevention (CDC). (1986a). Occupational exposures to formaldehyde in dialysis units. *Morbidity and Mortality Weekly Report, 35*(24), 399-401.

Centers for Disease Control (CDC). (1986b). Bacteremia associated with reuse of disposable hollow-fiber hemodialyzers. *Morbidity & Mortality Weekly Report, 35,* 417-418.

Centers for Disease Control and Prevention (CDC). (1987a). *Clusters of bacteremia and pyrogenic reactions in hemodialysis patients – Georgia.* Epidemic Investigation Report EPI 86-65. Atlanta, GA: CDC.

Centers for Disease Control and Prevention (CDC). (1987b). *Pyrogenic reactions in patients undergoing high-flux hemodialysis – California.* Epidemic Investigation Report EPI 86-80. Atlanta, GA: CDC.

Centers for Disease Control and Prevention (CDC). (1987c). *Pyrogenic reactions in hemodialysis patients on high-flux hemodialysis – California.* Epidemic Investigation Report EPI 87-12. Atlanta, GA: CDC.

Centers for Disease Control and Prevention (CDC). (1987d). Recommendations for prevention of HIV transmission in health-care settings. *Morbidity & Mortality Weekly Report, 36,* 1S-18S.

Centers for Disease Control and Prevention (CDC). (1991). *Pyrogenic reactions and gram-negative bacteremia in patients in a hemodialysis center.* Epidemic Investigation Report EPI 91-37. Atlanta, GA: CDC.

Centers for Disease Control and Prevention (CDC). (1992) Bacteremia in hemodialysis patients. Epidemic Investigation Report EPI 92-10. Atlanta, GA: CDC.

Centers for Disease Control and Prevention (CDC). (1998a). Recommendations for prevention and control of hepatitis C virus (HCV) infection and HCV-related chronic disease (RR-19). *MMWR Recommendations and Reports, 47,* 1-39.

Centers for Disease Control and Prevention (CDC). (1999). *Possible ongoing transmission of hepatitis C virus in a hemodialysis unit.* Epidemic Investigation Report EPI 99-38. Atlanta, GA: CDC.

Centers for Disease Control and Prevention (CDC). (2000a). *Transmission of hepatitis C virus in a hemodialysis unit.* Epidemic Investigation Report EPI 2000-64. Atlanta, GA: CDC.

Centers for Disease Control and Prevention (CDC). (2000b). *Transmission of hepatitis C virus among hemodialysis patients.* Epidemic Investigation Report EPI 2000. Atlanta, GA: CDC.

Domin, M. (1993). The new face of tuberculosis: Preventing nosocomial transmission in health care facilities. In Plant Technology & Safety Management Series: *Controlling occupational exposure to tuberculosis.* Oakbrook Terrace, IL: Joint Commission on Accreditation of Healthcare Organizations.

Favero, M.S. (1981). *Microbiological contaminants* (pp. 30-33). Proceedings of the Association for the Advancement of Medical Instrumentation Technology Assessment Conference: Issues in Hemodialysis. Arlington, VA: AAMI.

Favero, M.S. (1983). Distinguishing between high-level disinfection, reprocessing, and sterilization. In Association for the Advancement of Medical Instrumentation (AAMI), *Reuse of disposables: Implications for quality health care and cost containment. Technology assessment report* (No. 6) (pp. 19-23). Arlington, VA: AAMI.

Favero, M.S., & Bland, L.A. (1986). Microbiologic principles applied to reprocessing hemodialyzers. In N. Deane, R.J. Wineman, & J.A. Bemis (Eds.), *Guide to reprocessing of hemodialyzers* (pp. 63-73). Boston: Martinus Nijhoff.

Favero, M.S., Carson, L.A., Bond, W.W., & Petersen, N.J. (1971). Pseudomonas aeruginosa: Growth in distilled water from hospitals. *Science, 173*(999), 836-838.

Favero, M.S., Carson, L.A., Bond, W.W., & Petersen, N.J. (1974). Factors that influence microbial contamination of fluids associated with hemodialysis machines. *Applied Microbiology, 28,* 822-830.

Favero, M.S., & Petersen, N.J. (1977). Microbiologic guidelines for hemodialysis systems. *Dialysis and Transplantation, 6,* 34-36.

Favero, M.S., Petersen, N.J., Boyer, K.M., Carson, L.A., & Bond, W.W. (1974). Microbial contamination of renal dialysis systems and associated health risks. *Transactions of the American Society of Artificial Internal Organs, 20-A,* 175-183.

Favero, M.S., Petersen, N.J., Carson, L.A., Bond, W.W., & Hindman, S.H. (1975). Gram negative water bacteria in hemodialysis systems. *Health Laboratory Science, 12,* 321-334.

Gazenfeldt-Gazit, E., & Eliahou, H.E. (1969). Endotoxin antibodies in patients on maintenance hemodialysis. *Israel Journal of Medical Science, 5,* 1032-1036.

Gordon, S.M., Oettinger, C.W., Bland, L.A., Oliver, J.C., Arduino, M.J., Aguero, S.M., et al. (1992). Pyrogenic reactions in patients receiving conventional, high-efficiency, or high-flux hemodialysis treatments with bicarbonate dialysate containing high concentrations of bacteria and endotoxin. *Journal of the American Society of Nephrology, 2,* 1436-1444.

Gordon, S., Tipple, M., Bland, L., & Jarvis, W. (1988). Pyrogenic reactions associated with the reuse of processed hollow-fiber hemodialyzers. *Journal of the American Medical Association, 260,* 2077-2081.

Hadler, S.C., & Fields, H.A. (1991). Hepatitis delta virus. In R.B. Belshe

(Ed.), *Textbook of human virology* (pp. 749-765). St. Louis, MO: Mosby Year Book.

Hadler, S.C., Murphy, B.L., Schable, C.A., Heyward, W.L., Francis, D.P., & Kane, M.A. (1984). Epidemiological analysis of the significance of low-positive test results for antibody to hepatitis B surface and core antigens. *Journal of Clinical Microbiology, 19*(4), 521-525.

Henderson, L.W., Koch, K.M., Dinarello, C.A., & Shaldon, S. (1983). Hemodialysis hypotension: The interleukin hypothesis. *Blood Purification, 1*, 3-8.

Hindman, S.H., Favero, M.S., Carson, L.A., Petersen, N.J., Schonberger, L.B., & Solano, J.T. (1975). Pyrogenic reactions during hemodialysis caused by extramural endotoxin. *Lancet, 2*, 732-734.

Jackson, B.M., Beck-Sague, C.M., Bland, L.A., Arduino, M.J., Meyer, L., & Jarvis, W.R. (1994). Outbreak of pyrogenic reactions and gram-negative bacteremia in a hemodialysis center. *American Journal of Nephrology, 14*(2), 85-89.

Jochimsen, E.M., Frenette, C., Delorme, M., Arduino, M., Aguero, S., Carson, L., et al. (1998). A cluster of bloodstream infections and pyrogenic reactions among hemodialysis patients traced to dialysis machine waste-handling option units. *American Journal of Nephrology, 18*(6), 485-489.

Kantor, R.J., Carson, L.A., Graham, D.R., Petersen, N.J., & Favero, M.S. (1983). Outbreak of pyrogenic reactions at a dialysis center: Association with infusion of heparinized saline solution. *American Journal of Medicine, 74*, 449-456.

Keane, W.F., Shapirom F.L., & Raij, L. (1977). Incidence and type of infections occurring in 445 chronic hemodialysis patients. *Transactions of the American Society of Artificial Internal Organs, 23*, 41-47.

Klotman, M.E., & Klotman, P.E. (1998). AIDS and the kidney. *Seminars in Nephrology, 18*, 371-372.

Lai, C.-L., Lau, J.Y., Yeoh, E.-K., Chang, W.-K., & Lin, H.-S. (1992). Significance of isolated anti-HBc seropositivity by ELISA: Implications and the role of radioimmunioassay. *Journal of Medical Virology, 36*, 180-183.

Laude-Sharpe, M., Caroff, M., Simard, L., Pusineri, C., Kazatchkine, M.D., & Haeffner-Cavaillon, N. (1990). Induction of IL-1 during hemodialysis: Transmembrane passage of intact endotoxins (LPS). *Kidney International, 38*, 1089-1094.

Lavin, J., & Haidorfer, C. (1993). Anergy testing - A vital weapon. *RN, 56*, 31-32.

Levine, O.S., Vlahov, D., Koehler, J., Cohn, S., Spronk, A.M., & Nelson, K.E. (1995). Seroepidemiology of hepatitis B virus in a population of injecting drug users. Association with drug injection patterns. *American Journal of Epidemiology, 142*(3), 331-341.

Lonnemann, G. (2000). Chronic inflammation in hemodialysis: The role of contaminated dialysate. *Blood Purification, 18*(3), 214-223.

Lonnemann, G. (2001). Efficacy of ultra-pure dialysate in the therapy and prevention of hemodialysis-associated amyloidosis. *Nephrology Dialysis Transplantation, 16*(Suppl. 4), 17-22.

Lowry, P., Beck-Sague, C.M., Bland, L., Aguero, S.M., Arduino, M.J., Minuth, A.N. et al. (1990). Mycobacterium chelonae infections among patients receiving high-flux dialysis in a hemodialysis clinic, California. *Journal of Infectious Diseases, 161*, 85-90.

McMahon, B.J., Parkinson, A.J., Helminiak, C., Wainwright, R.B., Bulkow, L., Kellerman-Douglas, A., et al. (1992). Response to hepatitis B vaccine of persons positive for antibody to hepatitis B core antigen. *Gastroenterology, 103*(2), 590-594.

Murphy, J., Parker, T., Carson, L., Bland, L., & Solomon, S. (1987). Outbreaks of bacteremia in hemodialysis patients associated with alteration of dialyzer membranes following chemical disinfection (Abstract). *ASAIO Journal, 16*, 51.

Niu, M.T., Alter, M.J., Kristensen, C., & Margolis, H.S. (1992). Outbreak of hemodialysis-associated non-A, non-B hepatitis and correlation with antibody to hepatitis C virus. *American Journal of Kidney Diseases, 19*, 345-352.

Oliver, J.C., Bland, L.A., Oettinger, C.W., Arduino, M.J., Garrard, M., Pegues, D.A., et al. (1992). Bacteria and endotoxin removal from bicarbonate dialysis fluids for use in conventional, high-efficiency, and high-flux dialysis. *Artificial Organs, 16*, 141-145.

Pegues, D.A., Oettinger, C.W., Bland, L.A., Oliver, J.C., Arduino, M.J., Aguero, S.M., et al. (1992). A prospective study of pyrogenic reactions in hemodialysis patients using bicarbonate dialysis fluids fil-tered to remove bacteria and endotoxin. *Journal of the American Society of Nephrology, 3*, 1002-1007.

Petersen, N.J., Boyer, K.M., Carson, L.A., & Favero, M.S. (1978). Pyrogenic reactions from inadequate disinfection of a dialysis fluid distribution system. *Dialysis and Transplantation, 7*, 52, 57-60.

Petersen, N.J., Carson, L.A., Doto, I.L., Aguero, S.M., & Favero, M.S. (1982). Microbiologic evaluation of a new glutaraldehyde-based disinfectant for hemodialysis systems. *Transactions of the American Society of Artificial Internal Organs, 28*, 287-290.

Port, F.K., VanDeKerkhove, K.M., Kunkel, S.L., & Kluger, M.J. (1987). The role of dialysate in the stimulation of interleukin-1 production during clinical hemodialysis. *American Journal of Kidney Diseases, 10*, 118-122.

Roberts, C., & Antonoplos, P. (1998). Inactivation of human immunodeficiency virus type 1 (HIV-1), hepatitis A virus (HAV), respiratory syncytial virus (RSV), vaccinia virus, herpes simplex virus type 1 (HSV-1), and poliovirus type 2 by hydrogen peroxide gas sterilization. *American Journal of Infectious Control, 26*, 94-101.

Roghmann, M.C., Fink, J.C., Polish, L., Maker, T., Brewrink, J., Morris, J.G. Jr., et al. (1998). Colonization with vancomycin-resistant enterococci in chronic hemodialysis patients. *American Journal of Kidney Diseases, 32*(2), 254-257.

Rudnick, J.R., Arduino, M.J., Bland, L.A., Cusick, L., McAllister, S.K., Aguero, S.M., et al. (1995). An outbreak of pyrogenic reactions in chronic hemodialysis patients associated with hemodialyzer reuse. *Artificial Organs, 19*, 289-294.

Schiffl, H., Lang, S.M., & Bergner, A. (1999). Ultrapure dialysate reduces dose of recombinant human erythropoietin. *Nephron, 83*(3), 278-279.

Silva, A.E., McMahon, B.J., Parkinson, A.J., Sjogren, M.H., Hoofnagle, J.H., Di Bisceglie, A.M. (1998). Hepatitis B virus DNA in persons with isolated antibody to hepatitis B core antigen who subsequently received hepatitis B vaccine. *Clinics in Infectious Diseases, 26*(4), 895-897.

Snydman, D.R., Bryan, J.A., Macon, E.J., & Gregg, M.B. (1976). Hemodialysis-associated hepatitis: Report of an epidemic with further evidence on mechanisms of transmission. *American Journal of Epidemiology, 104*, 563-570.

Stamm, J.M., Engelhard, W.E., & Parsons, J.E. (1969). Microbiological study of water-softener resins. *Applied Microbiology, 18*, 376-386.

Stevenson, K.B., Adcox, M.J., Mallea, M.C., Narasimhan, N., & Wagnild, J,P. (2000). Standardized surveillance of hemodialysis vascular access infections: 18-month experience at an outpatient, multifacility hemodialysis center. *Infection Control in Hospitals Epidemiology, 21*(3), 200-203.

Stevenson, K.B., Hannah, E.L., Lowder, C.A., Adcox, M.J., Davidson, R.L., Mallea, M.C., et al. (2002). Epidemiology of hemodialysis vascular access infections from longitudinal infection surveillance data: Predicting the impact of NKF-DOQI clinical practice guidelines for vascular access. *American Journal of Kidney Diseases, 39*(3), 549-555.

Tokars, J.I., Alter, M.J., & Arduino, M.J. (1995). Nosocomial infections in hemodialysis units: Strategies for control. In H. Jacobsen, G. Striker, & S. Klahr (Eds.), *The principles and practice of nephrology* (pp. 337-357). St. Louis: Mosby.

Townsend, T.R., Wee, S.B., & Bartlett, J. (1985). Disinfection of hemodialysis machines. *Dialysis and Transplantation, 14*, 274-287.

Wang, S., Levine, R.B., Carson, L.A., Arduino, M.J., Killar, T., Grillow, F.G., et al. (1999). An outbreak of gram-negative bacteremia in hemodialysis patients traced to hemodialysis machine waste drain ports. *Infection Control Hospital Epidemiology, 20*, 746-751.

Welbel, S.F., Schoendorf, K., Bland, L.A., Arduino, M.J., Groves, C., Schable, B., et al. (1995). An outbreak of gram-negative bloodstream infections in chronic hemodialysis patients. *American Journal of Nephrology, 15*, 1-4.

- The annual mortality rate among hemodialysis patients is 23%, and infections are the second most common cause, accounting for 14% of deaths (USRDS, 2002). Septicemia (11.1% of all deaths) is the most common infectious cause of mortality.

- Proper hand hygiene is a critical measure for preventing the transmission of potential pathogens. Good hand hygiene can result in a significant reduction in the carriage of potential pathogens on the hands, as well as a reduction in patient morbidity (CDC, 2002) and mortality related to nosocomial infection.

- Antibiotic resistance is widely acknowledged to be one of the most pressing medical problems facing the world today. In the United States alone, nearly 2 million patients acquire an infection in the hospital each year. Of those patients, about 90,000 die each year as a result of their infection.

- Access site infections are particularly important because they can cause disseminated bacteremia or loss of the vascular access. Local signs of vascular access infection include erythema, warmth, induration, swelling, tenderness, breakdown of skin, loculated fluid, or purulent exudate .

- Hepatitis B virus (HBV) infection is a global health problem. Greater than 350 million people are infected world wide (Edlich et al., 2003) and more than 250,000 chronic carriers die annually from HBV-related liver disease (Maynard, 1990). It is estimated 200,000 people acquire new HBV infections each year in the United States.

- Hepatitis B vaccination is an essential component of prevention in the hemodialysis setting (Parker et al., 1998). Optimal use of the vaccine reduces the reservoir of infected persons, thereby decreasing opportunities for cross transmission and the infection of others.

- Hepatitis C virus (HCV) infection is the most common chronic bloodborne infection in the United States. Infection with HCV is caused by a single-stranded RNA virus that is classified as a separate genus in the Flaviridae family (Parker et al., 1998; Hwang, 2001).

- HIV was first reported in the United States in 1981 and has become a major worldwide epidemic. Since this time, more than 830,000 cases of AIDS have been reported in the United States. By 1987 it was the leading cause of death among U.S. men between the ages of 25 and 44. As many as 950,000 Americans may be infected with HIV.

- Infection control precautions recommended for all hemodialysis patients are sufficient to prevent HIV transmission between patients. HIV-infected patients do not have to be isolated from other patients or dialyzed separately on dedicated machines. HIV-infected patients can participate in dialyzer reuse programs.

- Few data exist on the prevalence of HDV infection among chronic hemodialysis patients, and only one transmission of HDV between such patients has been reported in the United States (Lettau et al., 1986) . . . A serologic test that measures total antibody to HDV is commercially available and measures both IgG and IgM antibodies (Parker, 1998; CDC, 2001). Anti-HD levels will disappear in 1 to 2 years when the acute infection resolves.

- After decades of declining incidence, tuberculosis (TB) is again a major health concern in the United States. The presence of a large immunosuppressed population, due in part to the AIDS epidemic and the persistence and growth of TB globally have contributed to the increasing number of TB cases in the United States.

- Anyone who demonstrates symptoms of TB must be referred immediately for further medical care and follow-up, which should include a thorough medical history, physical exam, Mantoux tuberculin skin test, chest x-ray, and sputum smear and culture (or smears and cultures from the affected site in extrapulmonary TB, if possible).

ANNP619

Infections in the Hemodialysis Unit

Eileen Peacock, MSN, RN, CNN, CIC, CPHQ

Contemporary Nephrology Nursing: Principles and Practice contains 39 chapters of educational content. Individual learners may apply for continuing nursing education credit by reading a chapter and completing the Continuing Education Evaluation Form for that chapter. Learners may apply for continuing education credit for any or all chapters.

Please photocopy this page and return to ANNA.
COMPLETE THE FOLLOWING:

Name: _____

Address:_____

City:_____State: _____Zip: _____

E-mail: _____

Preferred telephone: ☐ Home   ☐ Work: _____

State where licensed and license number (optional): _____

CE application fees are based upon the number of contact hours provided by the individual chapter. CE fees per contact hour for ANNA members are as follows: 1.0-1.9 - $15; 2.0-2.9 - $20; 3.0-3.9 - $25; 4.0 and higher - $30. Fees for nonmembers are $10 higher.

ANNA Member: ☐ Yes   ☐ No   Member # (if available) _____

☐ Checked Enclosed   ☐ American Express   ☐ Visa   ☐ MasterCard

Total Amount Submitted: _____

Credit Card Number: _____ Exp. Date: _____

Name as it appears on the card: _____

CE Evaluation Form
To receive continuing education credit for individual study after reading the chapter
1. Photocopy this form. (You may also download this form from ANNA's Web site, **www.annanurse.org.**)
2. Mail the completed form with payment (check) or credit card information to American Nephrology Nurses' Association, East Holly Avenue, Box 56, Pitman, NJ 08071-0056.
3. You will receive your CE certificate from ANNA in 4 to 6 weeks.

Test returns must be postmarked by **December 31, 2010.**

CE Application Fee
ANNA Member $30.00
Nonmember $40.00

EVALUATION FORM

1. I verify that I have read this chapter and completed this education activity. Date: _____

_____
Signature

2. What would be different in your practice if you applied what you learned from this activity? *(Please use additional sheet of paper if necessary.)*

_____
_____
_____
_____
_____
_____
_____
_____
_____
_____
_____
_____

Evaluation	Strongly disagree				Strongly agree
3. The activity met the stated objectives.					
a. Summarize implications of antimicrobial-resistant bacteria to nurses caring for dialysis patients.	1	2	3	4	5
b. Compare the dialysis precautions necessary because of concerns related to Hepatitis B to those related to Hepatitis C and HIV.	1	2	3	4	5
c. Describe the assessment findings and interventions that would be expected in a patient with ESRD who also has tuberculosis.	1	2	3	4	5
4. The content was current and relevant.	1	2	3	4	5
5. The content was presented clearly.	1	2	3	4	5
6. The content was covered adequately.	1	2	3	4	5
7. Rate your ability to apply the learning obtained from this activity to practice.	1	2	3	4	5

Comments _____

_____

8. Time required to read the chapter and complete this form: _____ minutes.

This educational activity has been provided by the American Nephrology Nurses' Association (ANNA) for 4.5 contact hours. ANNA is accredited as a provider of continuing nursing education (CNE) by the American Nurses Credentialing Center's Commission on Accreditation (ANCC-COA). ANNA is an approved provider of continuing education by the California Board of Registered Nursing, CEP 0910.

Renal Disease Across the Lifespan

Unit 5 Contents

The Child with Kidney Disease

Cyrena Gilman, MN, RN, CNN
Annette Frauman, PhD, RN, FAAN

Chapter Contents

The Pediatric Patient

Cyrena Gilman, MN, RN, CNN
Annette Frauman, PhD, RN, FAAN

This chapter will present an overview of care of the child with all stages of chronic kidney disease (CKD). No attempt will be made to repeat information that is identical to that for adult patients. The age range to be covered will include children from birth to 20 years. Although the American Academy of Pediatrics (AAP) defines the age range of pediatrics as birth to 21 years, much of the data, such as the United States Renal Data System (USRDS) related to children with end stage renal disease (ESRD), goes up to age 20. Pediatric nurses provide care to children and parents within the context of families. Therefore, additional emphasis will be given to families of children in this chapter.

Philosophy of Pediatric Renal Nursing

A philosophy about the care of children is an essential component of the pediatric nephrology nursing approach. The following philosophical assumptions guide this chapter.

Kidney disease, its symptoms, and the side effects of treatment present many impediments to attaining a normal lifestyle. Each of the treatment modalities commonly used for children with CKD imposes time constraints and limitations that detract from the ability to attend school and play as other healthy children do (Fielding & Brownbridge, 1999). Children with CKD and their families need as much normality in their lives as possible within these constraints and look to nurses for help with achieving as normal a lifestyle as possible.

Health care providers and family members should hold the same expectations for children with kidney disease as for healthy children of similar developmental levels. Providers should expect developmentally congruent behaviors from these children. Chronically ill children need to participate in their own treatment regimen, should not be indulged or treated specially based solely on having the illness, or be treated as a "poor thing" (Gilman & Frauman, 1979). Children who are frequently referred to as a "poor thing," verbally or in other ways, will soon come to believe it. They will not progress developmentally, will not become adequately socialized, and will not be prepared to become functional adults, whether sick or well at that stage of life. In order to avoid becoming a "poor thing," children must be encouraged to be as independent as possible for their developmental levels.

Brief History of Pediatric Nephrology Care

At one time, conservative management was the only modality available to children with CKD, and most children with CKD died. Occasionally children were kept alive with intermittent peritoneal dialysis (IPD), but the widely varying serum chemistries and frequent admissions to the ICU for painfully invasive procedures effectively prevented any semblance of normality in their lives. If renal function did not return, the treatment was discontinued, and again, most children died.

In the mid-to-late 1960s, a few centers began to attempt hemodialysis (HD) of children, usually adolescents, as a last resort to preventing death. In 1971, Dr. Kjellstrand and colleagues at the University of Minnesota determined that 10% of circulating blood volume could be spared in an extracorporeal circuit. Based on that discovery, medical equipment manufacturers began producing smaller hemodialyzers and bloodlines to accommodate pediatric patients with chronic renal failure. However, with chronic HD, diets were severely restricted, external arteriovenous shunts were frequently problematic, and intradialytic complications and anemia were widespread.

The peritoneum was not employed for renal therapy until 1948-1949. In 1960, Dr. Harold McDonald at the University of Michigan developed procedures for inserting peritoneal catheters with a trocar and automated delivery systems for peritoneal dialysate, which helped further the care of younger patients (McBride, 1984). However, Moncrief and Popovich's development of continuous ambulatory peritoneal dialysis (CAPD) in 1976 resulted in the widespread successful use of PD for treating pediatric patients. It was first used on a child in Toronto in 1978.

A working kidney transplant has been the goal for pediatric patients with CKD for many years (Alexander, 1990). Improved surgical techniques and better immunosuppressive medications have aided achieving that goal. However, none of the recent improvements in transplantation have been specific to pediatrics.

Epidemiological Data

The Medicare chronic renal failure program recorded the admission to services of 1,349 children between the ages of birth and 19 (incident patients) in 2001. Incident rates per million population were: 10 for ages 0-4, 8 for ages 5-9, 15 for ages 10-14, and 28 for ages 15-19. Males have higher incidence rates among children in all four age groups (USRDS, 2003). Prevalence rates per million population were 27 for ages 0-4, 43 for ages 5-9, 84 for ages 10-14, and 157 for children ages 15-19.

Treatment modalities for children differ sharply from those of adults, with far greater use of peritoneal dialysis (PD) and transplant as first modality, compared with adults (USRDS, 2003). After 2 years of treatment, 31% are receiving HD, 15.2% CAPD or continuous cycling peritoneal dialysis (CCPD), and 44.9% have a functioning transplant (USRDS, 2003). Comparisons of cohorts from 1987-1991 and 1992-1996 show that overall incident survival has not changed. However, mortality analyses show a 4% fall in annual mortality rates for children age 0-9 and a much larger decline of 21% for those children age 10-19 (USRDS, 2003).

Etiologies of CKD in Children

The etiologies of CKD are quite different in children than in adults. For example, diabetes and hypertension, two major causes of kidney disease in adults, are rarely causes of CKD in children. Prevalence rates for children with diabetes as a primary cause of kidney failure are 3 per 10 million popula-

Contemporary Nephrology Nursing: Principles and Practice, Second Edition © — American Nephrology Nurses' Association 2006   **459**

tion (USRDS, 2003). In contrast, for all kidney failure patients, the rate was 3,119. Diabetes does occur in children, but the degree of damage necessary to result in CKD usually takes more than 20 years to evolve, by which time the child has become an adult (Mogyorosi & Ziyadeh, 2001).

Serious kidney disease in children may result in hypertension, but essential hypertension is rarely seen in children. The most frequent causes of CKD in children can be broken down into two major categories: congenital and acquired (USRDS, 2003). Males predominate among pediatric patients, especially among those with obstructive conditions and other congenital/hereditary conditions (USRDS, 2003). Most frequently, CKD that has its onset between birth and age 5 is due to congenital disease. That which occurs between ages 6 and 10 is most often a result of urological defects, which are also congenital, and after age 12, glomerulonephritis is the most frequent cause of CKD in children.

Congenital

Malformations of the urinary tract are extremely common, probably related to the complex embryology of the kidney and urinary tract. The human kidney is first detectable in the fifth gestational week. It is initially composed of a small epithelial bud surrounded by undifferentiated mesenchymal stem cells. The ureteric bud is a branch from the mesonephric or Wolffian duct and forms the calyces, collecting tubules, and ureters. Each newly formed collecting tubule has a metanephric tissue cap at the distal end. Cells within this cap form small vesicles that give rise to s-shaped tubules. Capillaries grow into one end of the S and become glomeruli. The tubules with their glomeruli form nephrons (Sadler, 2000). Similarly, the embryonic cloaca differentiates into a male or female perineum, urinary bladder, and urethra, also through a complex process (Stephens, Smith, & Hutson, 2002). These complex processes can result in abnormalities at any stage. While many malformations are non-pathogenic, such as a solitary kidney, others result in a complete lack of renal function or obstructions of the urinary tract causing renal damage in fetal life.

Obstructive uropathy may be associated with dysgenesis, or damage may occur because of back pressure of urine and/or resulting infections of the urinary tract. Obstructions may occur at any point along the urinary tract, from the meatus to the renal pelvis. These may be formed of abnormal structures, misplaced vessels, or valves where there should be none. Abnormal innervation to the ureters, such as that seen in prune-belly syndrome and other obstructive uropathy, slows or causes cessation of the normal peristalsis of the ureter, resulting in an obstruction just as an ileus, or non-functioning bowel, causes gastrointestinal (GI) obstruction. Other congenital syndromes cause renal failure through abnormalities of the glomerulus, including Alport's syndrome, nail-patella syndrome, Fabry disease, and Charcot-Marie-Tooth syndrome (Stephens et al., 2002). Inherited errors of metabolism, such as cystinosis and oxalosis, also can cause renal failure in children and infants. Autosomal recessive polycystic kidney disease (ARPKD) is a congenital form of polycystic disease that only occurs in children.

Acquired

Many cases of acute glomerulonephritis in children follow infection with an organism, including group A beta hemolytic streptococci, and viruses such as varicella, Epstein-Barr, rubeola, and cytomegalovirus. Often, the precipitating organism is not identified. Pathology of the glomerulus results from infiltration of the tissues with antibodies, resulting in enlargement of the glomeruli and obliteration of capillary lumens. The degree of luminal obliteration correlates with decreased glomerular filtration rates. In some children, especially those with initially severe disease, progression to renal failure occurs, though often slowly. Hemolytic uremic syndrome also causes acute renal failure in children with resulting damage that may or may not be permanent.

Other types of glomerulonephritis cause damage to the glomerulus and the basement membrane with progression to end stage kidney disease in some cases. Collagen vascular diseases, malignancies, and hemoglobinopathies may cause CKD in children just as they do in adults. Increased understanding of the interaction between genetic factors and external insults, such as infection or toxins, is adding to our understanding of the causes, prognosis, and treatment of glomerular disorders (Dell, McDonald, Watkins, & Avner, 2004).

Effects of Renal Failure on Children

Many of the effects of renal failure on children and adults are identical; others are markedly different due in part to children's unique metabolic state that results from growth, their height-to-weight ratio, and their higher percentage of body water.

Cardiovascular

The cardiovascular effects of renal failure in children are similar to those seen in adults, including hypertension, which can result in retinopathy and encephalopathy if unchecked; circulatory overload; edema; congestive heart failure; pericarditis; and arrhythmias. Hypertension in children with CKD is usually caused by extracellular volume expansion and is controlled by ultrafiltration (UF) (Solhaug, Adelman, & Chan, 1992). Children also may have marked left ventricular hypertrophy with considerable lateral displacement of the point of maximum impulse (PMI) (Morris, Skinner, Wren, Hunter, & Coulthard, 1993). Recent evidence has indicated that, like adults, children with CKD are at greatly increased risk of cardiovascular disease (Chavers & Schnaper, 2001; Parekh, Carroll, Wolfe, & Port, 2002). In a study of deaths among pediatric patients, Parekh et al. (2002) report that 25% were cardiac-related. Children with CKD are at increased risk of cardiovascular disease due to vascular calcifications, hypertension, and hyperlipidemia (Chavers & Schnaper, 2001).

Cutaneous

The cutaneous effects of CKD on children are quite obvious upon even cursory observation. The overall appearance is relatively pale or sallow in spite of receiving erythropoietin. Accumulation of urinary pigments in the skin may occur, just as they do in the adult. The skin is somewhat less likely to be dry or scaly in younger children with CKD, and itching is less frequently observed than in adults.

As in adults, when dialysis is discontinued or is not possible, urea may be deposited on the skin as sweat evaporates. The resulting crystal formations resemble frost and are thus called uremic frost. Bruising is sometimes noted in children with CKD. This is due to the capillary fragility resulting from CKD and is a sequela of most of the treatment modalities requiring heparinization.

Gastrointestinal (GI)

Children with CKD are quite likely to suffer frequently from nausea and anorexia, sometimes progressing to vomiting. The anorexia may be due in part to changes in taste, particularly a constant metallic aftertaste, but is generally not well understood. The problem can be profound and interfere seriously with the child's nutritional needs. In addition, children with CKD, because of their compromised immune state, are susceptible to infections of the GI tract as well as to GI bleeds. Because children who have an infection of the urinary tract often experience nausea and vomiting, in contrast to the symptoms of frequency, urgency, and pain commonly seen in adults, these symptoms should be evaluated in children with that fact in mind.

Genitourinary

Children with CKD secondary to congenital causes are much more likely to have high-output renal failure than are adults. The ability of these children with CKD to concentrate their urine is greatly impaired, and they may have a fixed urinary specific gravity with a total inability to respond to fluctuations in fluid status. In these children, fluid is removed by the kidney(s), but the urine specific gravity is extremely low, and other substances are poorly excreted at best. Serum blood urea nitrogen (BUN), creatinine, and electrolyte levels may resemble those of oliguric or anuric patients. Children, especially those with nephrotic syndrome, can have extremely high urine proteins to the point that the urine will gel if refrigerated.

Female adolescents with CKD may experience amenorrhea and anovulation even after the onset of puberty, which is often greatly delayed. Some pediatric nephrologists may prescribe hormonal contraceptives to adolescent females to prevent menses in an attempt to minimize additional blood loss. They may not have a corresponding loss of libido, however, and may have difficulty with vaginal lubrication and painful intercourse, just as adults with renal failure do. Similarly, males have delayed puberty and may suffer from impotence and sterility. However, the adolescent sex drive is powerful, and loss of libido and sterility should not be depended on to inhibit either male or female adolescents. Despite decreased likelihood of pregnancy, sexually active adolescents with CKD need to use birth control measures. Choosing an appropriate method may not be easy because of the need to balance safety and efficacy. Barrier methods (diaphragm, condom) are safest, but may not be well accepted by adolescents and are likely to be ineffective due to sporadic use. Intrauterine devices are contraindicated, and hormonal contraceptive methods may not be well tolerated. Additionally, because of their suppressed immune system,

sexually transmitted diseases (STDs) are particularly hazardous for adolescents with CKD. They should be given information about preventive measures before they become sexually active. Hergenroeder and Brewer (2001) report that only 56% of pediatric nephrologists say they interview patients without parents present. The pediatric nephrologists also stated that they ask only 53% of male patients and only 55% of female patients about intercourse.

Hematologic

Like adults, anemia is a problem for children with CKD, though this problem has been considerably diminished with the advent of recombinant erythropoietin. Darbepoetin has not yet been approved for use in the pediatric patient population, but the decreased frequency of dosing schedule is as attractive to children and their families as it is to adults.

Children who are posttransplantation and receiving azathioprine should be carefully monitored for its effects on bone marrow function, including diminished thrombocytes, erythrocytes, and leukocytes. Many centers are discovering that oral iron supplements do not adequately maintain hemoglobin in the optimal range, especially for children receiving HD. In that event, intravenous (IV) iron supplements may be required. Administration of IV iron causes a significant increase in serum ferritin (Warady, Schaefer, Alexander, Firanek, & Mujais, 2004). In fact, a maintenance IV iron protocol of 2 mg/kg/wk for pediatric HD patients reduced the dose of erythropoietin needed to maintain optimal blood hemoglobin levels. It was also more economical; improved efficacy of erythropoietin doses resulted in a 26% reduction in cost (Morgan, Gautam, & Geary, 2001).

Metabolic

Children with CKD are more likely than adults to experience metabolic acidosis. However, the other metabolic effects of CKD, including azotemia, hyperkalemia, sodium retention or wasting, hypermagnesemia, hyperuricemia, and lipid abnormalities, are similar.

Neuromuscular

Neuromuscular effects of CKD on children are also similar to those seen in adults. However, problems with growth and development are particularly problematic. Fatigue, muscle wasting, and lethargy greatly interfere with the developmental drive of children and affect their ability to perform new skills and tasks. Other neuromuscular effects are discussed in the section on growth and development.

Pulmonary

The pulmonary effects of CKD in children are similar to those in adults. Because of the child's smaller size, a relatively small amount of excess fluid may result in pulmonary edema. Children with active glomerular disease may have pulmonary edema secondary to fluid shifts. Additionally, the hypercoagulable state of active nephrotic syndrome can contribute to pulmonary thrombus formation. The respiratory status of infants or children with pulmonary compromise may be worsened by retained peritoneal dialysate, retained fluid post HD, or excessive intradialytic weight gains.

Children with renal damage in utero may not produce

sufficient quantities of urine to produce adequate amnionic fluids (oligohydramnios), which results in pulmonary hypoplasia (Limwongse & Cassidy, 2004). These children may have compromised pulmonary function in addition to kidney disease after birth.

Skeletal

The effects of CKD on bone in children are devastating and include abnormalities of metabolism such as hypocalcemia, hyperphosphatemia, and hyperparathyroidism. Renal osteodystrophy is common along with pathologic fractures due to demineralized bone. Calcium salts may be deposited in soft tissue (around joints, in blood vessels, heart, lungs, and conjunctiva).

A particularly devastating effect of long-term renal failure and dialysis is the deposition of beta-2 microglobulin in the soft tissues and bones. As in adults, the longer one is on dialysis and exposed to elevated levels of beta-2 microglobulin, the more likely one is to have this type of amyloidosis. If a pediatric patient rejects several transplants at a young age and faces the remainder of life on some type of dialysis, development of beta-2 microglobulin bone disease is inevitable (McCarthy, Williams, & Johnson, 1994). McCarthy et al. (1994) found that CAPD patients are less likely to develop beta-2 microglobulin disease than are HD patients, and patients hemodialyzed against high-flux synthetic membranes have a lower incidence than those dialyzed against cellulose acetate membranes. The progression of amyloid deposition is delayed with synthetic membrane HD, but not prevented. The researchers found that most patients will begin to develop the syndrome after 4 or 5 years of therapy; when the number of "beta-2 microglobulin months" (the serum beta-2 microglobulin level times the number of months of dialysis) exceeds 1500, the disease will definitely be present. Only natural kidney function, whether from native kidneys or a transplant, can completely avoid this devastating problem.

Immune

Children with CKD, like adults, have long been noted to have decreased resistance with an increased incidence of bacterial, viral, and fungal infections. Uremic patients also have a much-higher incidence of malignancies than the normal population (Benfield & Michael, 1992). In a study of children receiving CAPD, significantly lower serum IgG levels were found than in the controls, but all levels were in the normal range. Additionally, these children had essentially normal responses to live virus vaccines for measles, mumps, and rubella (MMR) (Hisano et al., 1991).

Uremic patients have normal to slightly elevated granulocyte counts, but the migration and chemotaxic function of these cells is usually slightly abnormal. Phagocytosis, on the other hand, is typically normal (Benfield & Michael, 1992).

Numerous investigators have found widely varying results in studying the number and function of lymphocytes in uremic patients. Although normal levels of IgG, IgA, and IgM are found in uremic patients, seroconversion and antibody titer formation are usually impaired. Impaired T-cell function, increased suppressor cell activity, intrinsic monocyte/macrophage dysfunction, and abnormal production of

interleukin-2 have been demonstrated in uremic patients but are difficult to reproduce in animals with experimentally-induced uremia. Uremic patients also have been noted to have thymic atrophy at autopsy (Benfield & Michael, 1992).

The vitamin and mineral deficits associated with the malnutrition present in most uremic patients have serious effects on the immune system. Some kidney diseases are treated with long-term immunosuppressive medication before end stage kidney disease is reached. Thus, the impaired immune system function found in uremic patients is most likely influenced by many factors, not the uremic condition alone (Benfield & Michael, 1992).

Children with CKD require immunizations to prevent communicable disease just as other children do. However, live virus vaccines should not be given to immunosuppressed children, whether pre or posttransplant, necessitating that the MMR vaccine and varicella vaccine be given during treatment for early stage kidney disease or while undergoing dialysis. A need for repeat doses of varicella vaccine (Furth et al., 2003) and pneumococcal vaccines (Fuchshuber et al., 1996) in order to produce immunity has been reported. Laube et al. (2002) describe a suggested protocol for children with CKD that resulted in no infections with the diseases for which the children were immunized except for varicella.

It is critical that all live virus vaccines be given before transplantation, as the immune-suppressed child's response to these will be altered. As children with kidney failure often do not have, or do not see, a primary care provider, the responsibility for ensuring that this is done often devolves upon the pediatric nephrology nurse.

Growth and Development

Children with CKD have the same developmental needs as healthy children. They may need additional assistance from parents, health care providers, educators, and others to achieve their maximum potential at each of the developmental stages. Certainly prevention of developmental problems is preferred to intervention after they have occurred. The focus needs to be positive: Enhance what the child can do, encourage progress, and de-emphasize deficits or handicaps.

Children are usually approached based on the age they appear to be. For the child with short stature or delayed puberty due to CKD, this is inappropriate. In order to help the child with CKD achieve as normal a life as possible, the pediatric nephrology nurse must first determine exactly what developmental level the child has attained. In determining this, the whole child must be observed. The child's behavior; relationships with family, friends, and peers; fine and gross motor coordination; and coping mechanisms all help establish what his or her developmental levels in those domains are. In addition, the child's likes and dislikes, as well as abilities compared with other children of the same chronological age must be considered.

Children with CKD go through the same developmental stages that other children do. However, the rate at which they progress through the stages is often markedly delayed and not necessarily consistent across developmental domains. Generalized psychological assessment tools for younger children (birth to 6 years), such as the Denver Developmental Screening Test (DDST), the Goodenough Draw-A-Man test, and the Brazelton Scale for Infant Development, can help in establishing a developmental level. The Vineland Adaptive Behavior Scales can be used clinically to determine which social and adaptive skills the child possesses and, by implication, which ones need to be worked on next. It is an excellent idea to have testing conducted by a child psychologist using global measures such as the Bayley and the Weschler Intelligence Scale for Children (WISC). The evaluation should also include tests of neuropsychological function, such as Raven's Progressive Matrices; the Beery Developmental Test of Visuomotor Integration; and tests of vigilance, auditory memory, and reaction time, since these have been shown to be affected by CKD (Fennell et al., 1990). These tests will provide an in-depth examination of the child's developmental attainments, which can be used in patient education or in assisting the child and family to obtain appropriate school placement. If a clinical or developmental psychologist is not available on the team caring for the child, their services may sometimes be obtained through the school system, a nearby university's psychology department, or a child psychiatry facility. Children with CKD from birth are more likely to suffer from much more severe developmental disabilities than children who acquire the disease later (Crocker et al., 2002)

Physical growth and sexual maturation. Physical growth failure is perhaps the most pervasive developmental issue for children with CKD. Despite numerous studies, the mechanisms of growth failure are still not well understood (Watkins & Richards, 2004). Less than optimal nutrition; metabolic acidosis; fluid and electrolyte disturbances; disorders of calcium and phosphorus metabolism; medications used in treatment, especially corticosteroids; and decreased production and diminished ability to use hormones have all been implicated in growth failure (Mehls, Blum, Schaefer, Tonshoff, & Scharer, 1992). The anorexia common in children with renal insufficiency and failure undoubtedly contributes. Additionally, children with severe protein-wasting glomerular disease have a greater tendency toward malnutrition. Probably all of these factors and perhaps others are influential. How each or the combination results in growth failure is not well known.

In general, the earlier the onset of renal failure and the longer its duration, the more severe growth deficiencies will be. Therefore, children with congenital kidney disease will suffer greater growth retardation than those with acquired kidney disease. Height reductions are most profoundly affected in infancy and adolescence, the periods in which growth is most rapid. Once growth potential is lost in these time periods, it will probably never be regained (Mehls et al., 1992). Children with renal disease often have a relatively normal growth curve, but usually remain well below the 3rd percentile of normal parameters. Additionally, adult height is usually reduced by up to 2.5 standard deviations.

Puberty, with its rapid growth and maturation of secondary sex characteristics, is often delayed and its intensity diminished. In a 1990 study, Scharer noted that puberty was delayed in their subjects by an average of 2.5 years, and the growth attainment in the prepubertal growth spurt was significantly impaired.

Use of human growth hormone has become a standard treatment for children with CKD. Children with CKD have normal or elevated levels of the hormone but are apparently not able to use their natural supply. The administration of additional hormone does enhance growth as demonstrated by numerous studies (Benfield, Parker, Waldo, Overstreet, & Kohaut; 1993; Fine et al., 1994; Koch et al., 1989). The earlier growth failure is documented and treatment with growth hormone begun, the better the final height outcome (Fine, Sullivan, & Tejani, 2000).

In order for growth hormone to work most effectively, the pediatric patient's nutrition must be optimal. Anemia, metabolic acidosis, and renal osteodystrophy must be treated and corrected. The child must have remaining growth potential, which is shown by open epiphyses and a Tanner stage of less than 5. Ongoing monitoring of length or height, weight, growth velocity, bone age, and Tanner stage is essential during the administration of growth hormone therapy (Miller, Macdonald, Kolnacki, & Simek, 2004).

Cognitive development. The effects of CKD on cognitive development of infants have been the subject of a number of studies. These studies have primarily evaluated the efficacy of various treatment modalities in preventing detrimental effects of CKD on neurological development. Polinsky, Kaiser, and Stover (1987) concluded from a review of 15 of these studies that CKD most consistently affected gross motor and language development. Development of infants is improved after renal transplantation, with studies showing improvement on a variety of measures, including the DDST, the Bayley, and the Revised Yale Developmental Schedule. However, neonates with CKD continue to have developmental delays even after transplantation.

Studies of the effects of CKD on cognitive development in older children have used both global measures of intelligence (for example, Stanford-Binet, WISC-R) as well as specific neuropsychological measures such as tests of vigilance, auditory memory, and reaction time. Associations have been found between age at onset of CKD, length of time in renal failure, treatment method, and a variety of measures of cognitive development (Fennell et al., 1990). Based on their body of work, Fennell and colleagues (1990) have advanced the hypothesis that renal failure affects cognitive development in two ways: one that influences the acquisition of new skills and is less likely to improve after successful transplantation, and another that affects attention, speed of processing, and modulation of responses. This latter effect seems to be dependent on abnormal blood chemistries and is, thus, more susceptible to improvement after successful transplantation (Fennell et al., 1990). A 2000 study (Brouhard et al.) that compared 62 children with ESRD with sibling controls found that the average IQ percentile rank for the patients was significantly lower than their siblings. Patients also tended to score lower on achievement tests in spelling, arithmetic, and reading. A review article published in 1994 (Frauman & Myers, 1994) contains numerous references and further information.

School attendance in children with CKD has received some attention, mostly in children who have received successful transplantation. Studies of these children are optimistic. In 1991, Morel and colleagues reported that of 9 transplant recipients of school age, all were attending; of 48 older than high school age, 93% had graduated, and 60% had attended college or technical training. A German study reported a high school completion rate of 14% (Rosenkranz, Bonzel, & Bulla, 1992), while a European Dialysis and Transplant Association (EDTA) study reports that of 617 adult subjects receiving renal replacement therapy as children, 41% did not complete school and only 58% were employed (Ehrich et al., 1992).

Psychosocial development. The effects of CKD on psychosocial development are not as devastating as once feared. Children with CKD seem to be quite resilient psychologically, especially those with successful renal transplants. Children treated at home with either HD or PD fare better than those on incenter treatment. Psychosocial adjustment is better for those with transplants than for those on either mode of dialysis. Most studies of children with CKD as they approach adulthood have found few problems except in the areas of growth failure and the formation and maintenance of intimate relationships (Beck, Nethercut, Crittenden, & Hewins, 1986; Morel et al., 1991).

In a 1996 study, Frauman, Gilman, and Carlson found that scores on the Vineland Adaptive Behavior Scales, a measure of psychosocial development, were more than two thirds of a standard deviation below the age standard mean scores. Percentile ranks for subscales for communication, daily living skills, and socialization were 19, 21, and 23 respectively. There was no significant difference between the group of subjects with a functioning transplant and those who had returned to dialysis following a transplant failure.

Treatment Modalities

Hemodialysis (HD)

The number of pediatric patients on chronic HD has increased over the last decade due to loss of peritoneal membrane function in some children, loss of renal transplant function, or a home environment that is not suitable for either performing PD or maintaining a transplant (Goldstein, 2001). Children who are cared for at dialysis facilities that are primarily for adult patients are more likely to be on HD than PD. (Leonard, Donaldson, Ho, & Geary, 2003)

Techniques. The hallmark of pediatric HD is the requirement that only 10% or less of the child's circulating blood volume can be in the extracorporeal circuit. One calculates circulating blood volume based on the milliliters (ml) of blood per kilogram of body weight found in the patient's age group (see Table 20-1). Although there is a wide variation in volumes between the age groups, most pediatric dialysis centers multiply the child's weight in kilograms by 70-80 ml. The kidney and bloodlines whose combined volumes will not exceed 10% of that total are selected to make up the extracorporeal circuit. Generally speaking, the lower the factor selected, the lower the allowable extracorporeal volume and the safer the HD system.

Hemodialyzers are selected for pediatric patients based on extracorporeal blood volume, rate of solute removal or efficiency, and UF rate. Over the years, all types of dialyzer membranes (cuprophan, cellulose acetate, polyacrylonitrile, polymethylmethacrylate, and polysulfone) have been used

Table 20-1
Approximate Blood Volume by Age

Age	Total Blood Volume in ml/kg
Preterm infants	90-105
Term newborns	78-86
1-12 months	73-78
1-3 years	74-82
4-6 years	80-86
7-18 years	83-90
Adults	66-88

Note: From Gunn, V.L., & Nechyba, C. (2002).

with children. The newer generation of dialyzer membranes, such as polymethylmethacrylate and polysulfone, are currently favored because their improved biocompatibility is less likely to activate proinflammatory cytokines or leukocytes (Goldstein & Jabs, 2004). Each type of dialyzer has different permeability to larger solutes and different UF coefficients, which are important factors to be considered in making the choice (Gruskin, Baluarte, & Dabbagh, 1992).

Improved biocompatibility also reduces the occurrence of dialyzer first-use reactions, which had been reported to be more common in patients who are less than 30 years old (Gruskin et al., 1992). This has not generally been reported in pediatric dialysis literature. Reuse of dialyzers has been recommended to prevent this reaction, but most pediatric dialysis units do not have the facility arrangements, equipment, or staffing to successfully perform reuse. In addition, the small numbers of pediatric patients on HD tend to make reuse less of a cost benefit. Most importantly, the long-term effect of dialyzer reuse on pediatric patients is not known.

Smaller artificial kidneys provide lower clearances of BUN and creatinine and much lower UF rates. Modern volumetric HD machines make a lower UF rate less critical than it was when fluid removal was based solely on the staff-controlled transmembrane pressure and the kidney's in vitro UF rate. Due to their exacting fluid control, modern volumetric machines are the best to use for pediatric patients.

Central HD delivery systems, which mix and pipe the same dialysate to many different HD stations in a center, are almost never used for pediatric patients. Each child requires an individualized treatment plan. It is unlikely that a pediatric center will have many HD patients requiring the same dialysate formulations (Gruskin et al., 1992).

The blood flow rates in pediatric dialysis units are always individualized. Similar to extracorporeal volume, the flow rates are based on the pediatric dialysis patient's size. The maximum blood flow rate for a patient should be 400 ml/min/1.73 m^2 of body surface area (Goldstein & Jabs, 2004).

Pediatric dialysis centers should use a bicarbonate-based dialysate. This provides for a gentle, non-stressful treatment and is absolutely essential in the child with compromised liver function. The potassium level and calcium level of the acidified portion of the dialysate mixture can be individualized according to patient requirements.

All dialysate used on pediatric patients should contain dextrose. Children receive extra calories for energy from a high dextrose bath and also have fewer treatment side effects. The dextrose level should be in the 200-250 mg percentage range.

Children are best hemodialyzed with the use of non-invasive vascular monitoring (NIVM). By providing a visual readout of hemoglobin, hematocrit, percent blood volume change, and oxygen saturation, NIVM permits increased UF, allowing achievement of lower dry weight targets while reducing dialysis-associated morbidity (DAM) in pediatric patients. If blood volume is decreased less than 8% per hour in the first 90 minutes of UF and less than 4% per hour for the remainder of the treatment, there is no DAM in pediatric HD patients (Jain, Smith, Brewer, & Goldstein, 2001). In addition, NIVM also helps patient care staff differentiate symptoms caused by true UF problems from anxiety-related behaviors (Goldstein, 2001).

Continuous monitoring of the patient's weight with metabolic weight scales during a HD treatment was a hallmark of pediatric dialysis in the past. The advent of volumetric HD machines and NIVM would seem to obviate the need for concurrent metabolic weight monitoring during HD, but when dialyzing a very small child or infant, every available indicator of the patient's condition must be used. Weight monitoring is critical for HD of infants weighing less than 12 kg. Unfortunately, volumetric HD machines are accurate to only 50-100 ml. Placing digital scales under the infant's bed during HD may detect UF inaccuracies early on (Goldstein & Jabs, 2004). This allows the nursing staff to prevent potential problems rather than deal with the consequences.

Heparinization of the pediatric renal patient on HD is much different than for the adult. One unit's protocol calls for an initial bolus of heparin to be given based on the patient's weight, usually 5 units/kg for patients weighing less than 25 kg or 3 units/kg for patients weighing more than 25 kg. Then a continuous infusion of heparin, which can be full strength (1000 units/ml) or diluted (500 units /ml, 100 units /ml, or even 50 units /ml) depending on the child's weight as well, is administered over the entire treatment. The rate of the infusion starts out at 30 units/kg/hr for patients under 25 kg and up to 1000 units/hr for those over 25 kg. The rate is adjusted in order to keep the activated clotting times (ACTs) of blood taken from the venous blood tubing between 180 and 200 seconds. For "tight" heparinization, the clotting times should be kept at no more than 25% above the baseline or preheparinization value. The heparin infusion can be maintained throughout the treatment for children with catheters for blood vessel access. It is discontinued 30 to 120 minutes before completion of the treatment for children with arteriovenous fistulae (AVF) to allow ample time for the ACT to return to normal prior to needle removal.

ACTs are done frequently on the acute patient or the new chronic patient to ascertain the child's heparin needs. Although they remain basically the same, these needs tend to fluctuate much more during subsequent treatments than they do in adult patients. As a result, even long-term chronic HD patients need ACTs performed at least once or twice

per treatment. Infection or exposure to cigarette smoke, whether in the home environment or if the child takes up smoking, will markedly increase the child's heparin requirements. Children with acute renal failure may need higher doses of heparin at first since they have not had renal failure long enough for the normal clotting factors to be affected. Children being dialyzed or hemoperfused for drug overdoses or poisonings definitely will need more heparin than a child of similar size in renal failure. It is possible to do HD without using heparin. For patients with antibodies to heparin, one can do heparin-free dialysis by periodically flushing the circuit with saline. Anticoagulation with citrate is another alternative.

In an effort to decrease the amount of time required for each adult HD treatment, high-flux and high-efficiency HD modalities were developed in the late 1980s. More permeable hemodialyzer membranes, rapid blood flow rates, faster dialysate flow rates, and volumetric UF control were crucial to this progress. High-flux dialysis used a membrane that was permeable to solutes with a wide range of molecular weights, including the relatively heavy beta-2 microglobulin. High-efficiency dialyzers had membranes permeable to solutes in the low to middle molecular weight range; the upper limit is usually a molecular weight of 5000 (Keen & Gotch, 1991).

Although children have a smaller volume of distribution, they receive the same clearance of solutes as adults do, which leads to a much greater overall mass transfer of solutes. Furthermore, they achieve maximum clearance levels of solutes at relatively low blood flow speeds. It might be argued then, that children receive high-efficiency dialysis all the time (Harmon & Jabs, 1994).

Shortened HD treatment time is never appropriate for children. The very rapid blood flows required cannot be obtained from pediatric patients' access, and a short time on dialysis is not sufficient for meeting pediatric metabolic needs. Short-time dialysis does not provide adequate clearances to allow growth or sufficient time for complete middle molecule clearance.

The usual pediatric HD schedule is a 4-hour treatment three times a week unless severe fluid overload or metabolic problems, such as hyperkalemia or hyperphosphatemia, call for a longer treatment. Five or 6-hour treatments may be required occasionally. Many infants and toddlers may require HD 5-7 days a week to permit optimal nutrition and growth (Leonard et al., 2003; Shroff, Wright, Ledermann, Hutchinson, & Rees, 2003). For home HD patients, 3 hours every other day is an option that may be adequate; however, it results in only 21 hours on the machine every 2 weeks versus 24 hours every 2 weeks with the usual schedule.

Daily home HD would appear to be the future trend in HD therapy. Patients on daily dialysis feel and think better, have more energy and stamina, and have better control of blood pressure and serum phosphorus with few, if any, medications. They have a more liberal diet and fluid intake with few, if any, dialysis-related symptoms. There is more flexibility and freedom to the treatment schedule enhancing the patient's control of his or her own life. The improved quality of life has been documented in adults. It would likely be true in children as well. Unfortunately, the financial impact of daily dialysis is often prohibitive (Goldstein, 2001; Ouwendyk, Leitch, & Freitas, 2001).

A side benefit of the development of high-flux dialyzers was the discovery that they may help to control beta-2 microglobulin buildup in pediatric patients who are going to require long-term HD. Beta-2 microglobulin is removed by natural kidney function, removed partially by PD, and minimally removed by standard hemodialyzers. High-flux dialyzers will slow the rate of buildup but will not prevent amyloid deposition altogether. Neither will these synthetic membrane dialyzers remove beta-2 microglobulin already accumulated in the patient's body, so they will not cure bone disease or other side effects of that accumulation (McCarthy et al., 1994).

Access issues. Blood vessel access issues are, in some ways, the same for children as for adults. In the early days of pediatric HD, external shunts and AVFs were the most common accesses. Gradually, the use of single lumen subclavian catheters and single-needle dialysis became more common for acute HD. The development and rapid improvements in dual-lumen subclavian catheters caused their increased use in children because they allow more efficient HD. Now the trend is returning to AVFs as the primary access for children as well as for adults. However, a lack of experienced surgical support, a short time on HD before scheduled kidney transplant, and a wish to avoid frequent painful experiences, especially for smaller children, have caused many centers to continue using HD catheter access. In fact, the majority of children on chronic HD in the U.S. have a permanent catheter for access (Goldstein & Jabs, 2004). The catheters offer needleless therapy, which is a real plus for young children with tiny veins or for those with a needle phobia.

A recent study showed that young children on HD almost exclusively had percutaneous catheters as access. This is not in accord with the NKF-DOQI recommendations that only 10% of patients have catheters as HD access (Leonard et al., 2003). The recommended placement for HD access catheters is in the right internal jugular vein. This site has fewer thromboses and causes less stenotic changes in the superior vena cava than subclavian catheters do (Goldstein & Jabs, 2004). However, the subclavian vein is frequently used as an access site (Leonard et al., 2003).

Diligent sterile technique during attachment and detachment from HD and exacting exit site care both in the dialysis unit and at home can result in low catheter infection rates and long-term catheter function. Units need to insure that they are using the correct disinfectant for their permanent catheters. Silicone catheters degrade over time if povidone iodine is used on them. Teflon catheters react poorly to alcohol-based cleaners. Chlorhexidine is recommended by the Centers for Disease Control and Prevention (O'Grady et al., 2002) for exit site cleaning, and other disinfectants, such as electrolytic chloroxidizer, can be used on any type of catheter material.

Although a viable long-term access for pediatric patients, catheters can be problematic. Because of smaller veins, their function is much more likely to be positional in children than in adults. Pediatric patients with catheters may have to be coaxed into assuming and holding unusual positions throughout a treatment to ensure adequate blood flow

for the procedure. This is as difficult a task for a toddler whose coping mechanism is movement as it is for the adolescent who has lost autonomy and control during his developing independence.

After a HD treatment, catheter lumens are flushed with sterile normal saline, a sterile cap is applied, and 1,000-10,000 units/ml heparin is instilled in the lumen. Generally, 10,000 units/ml heparin is used for those patients weighing more than 30 kg (Moritz, Vats, & Ellis, 2003). It is important that the pediatric dialysis unit staff know the exact volume of each lumen of the catheter, as one should only instill that amount of heparin plus 0.1-0.2 ml more to ensure the entire lumen is heparinized. Unfortunately, the actual catheter lumen volume may vary within 0.2 ml of volume printed on catheter (Moritz et al., 2003).

Children who are admitted to the hospital may receive flushes with dilute heparin every 6 to 12 hours, depending on the frequency of using their catheter access for blood samples or medication administration. It is best if such use is avoided, as repeated catheter access by many different people increases the likelihood of infection. Sometimes there is just no way to avoid using the dialysis catheter for non-dialysis purposes. If flushes are needed in the hospital, the solution used should be only 50-500 units/ml depending on the patient's size. Bleeding can arise due to not aspirating heparin flush when accessing the catheter or not completely aspirating the flush. In addition, heparin can leach out of the catheter lumen into systemic circulation. Use of the appropriate size catheter for the child, using low concentration heparin solutions for smaller children, and having only experienced dialysis personnel access dialysis catheters can prevent such complications (Moritz et al., 2003).

Children who are outpatients should not have to use heparin flushes at home because of increased likelihood of bleeding due to excessive heparinization and of infection secondary to contamination. Some pediatric centers have found that instilling undiluted heparin at the end of a HD treatment will keep most catheters patent until the beginning of the next treatment. The heparin will be withdrawn from the catheter prior to the next HD treatment in order to prevent overheparinization. After each treatment, the catheter's exit site is cleaned and a sterile dressing is applied to the exit site. The dressing and the external catheter limbs are held in place with a transparent plastic dressing, such as Tegaderm® or Op-site®.

In spite of careful heparinization, catheters can clot. If a partial clot or fibrin collection forms, it can sometimes be cleared by using tissue plasminogen activator (TPA) in the catheter. The children call it "Drano® for catheters," and it can be that effective.

Children with HD catheters should not take showers, swim, or engage in activities likely to bump or pull on their catheters or exit sites. In addition, keeping cool enough to prevent perspiration from dislodging the sterile dressing is important, particularly in summer. Although they seem intricate, these precautions enhance long-term catheter function.

Acute and chronic dual-lumen HD catheters are the most prevalent pediatric accesses. However, some chronic HD patients are unable to tolerate the lifestyle changes necessary to keep a HD access catheter functioning well long term. Furthermore, the NKF-DOQI guidelines recommend AVFs as primary HD access on all patients. Children can have AVF created from natural veins or with polytetrafluoroethylene (PTFE) grafts if their own veins are too small. Leonard et al. (2003) found that 33% of children over 6 years of age had AVFs, and 24% had arteriovenous grafts (AVGs) after 6 months on HD. The 2000 ESRD Clinical Performance Measures (CPM) project found that 37% of teens had AVFs, 22% had AVGs, and 41% had a catheter for access (Frankenfield et al., 2002).

The best plan is to create a primary AVF for a child using microsurgical techniques. The surgeon needs to be sure the blood flow in the AVF is adequate for dialysis and for keeping the access patent. However, too high a flow volume through an AVF or AVG can cause decreased perfusion of the limb due to "steal syndrome." The incidence of dialysis access induced limb ischemia (DAILI) is 2%-4% in primary AVG or BGF in adults; the rate of occurrence is unknown in children (Shemesh, Olsha, Mabjeesh, & Abramowitz, 2001).

The discomfort associated with cannulating an AVF or AVG can be controlled with topical anesthetics or distraction techniques for most children. The best part of having an AVF or AVG is that once hemostasis is achieved at the end of a treatment and bandaids applied, the children are free to do most activities. Traumatizing or lacerating the fistula is to be avoided, but water sports and showers are permissible.

AVF can have the same malfunctions in children as in adults: clotting, insufficient flow, infection, aneurysm formation, and steal syndrome. A regular assessment of access flow by ultrasound dilution can detect early venous stenosis and allow early intervention to prevent loss of access function (Goldstein & Jabs, 2004). A complication of AV access unique to children is that the limb with the fistula may grow more slowly than the contralateral limb. Because of their small veins, it is also easier to compromise circulation in children and possibly cause the loss of the limb distal to the fistula.

Some children may experience repeated vascular access problems and may eventually lose all possible access sites. The long-term implications of this problem are greater in the pediatric patient who may have 50 or 60 years of HD therapy ahead of him than in the adult patient with only 10 or 20 years of additional life expectancy.

Staffing. One of the issues that makes pediatric dialysis much more expensive than adult dialysis is the high staff-to-patient ratio that is required to safely hemodialyze children. A child who weighs more than 25 kg and is physiologically and psychologically stable on HD probably needs no more attention than an adult. However, if physiological or psychological problems occur, that child may need a 1:2 or possibly even 1:1 staff-to-patient ratio. Children who weigh between 12 kg and 25 kg definitely require 1:1 staffing, especially if comorbidities, such as developmental delay, are present. Those weighing less than 12 kg may require 2:1 staffing. The increased need for IV medication administration during HD has also increased the need for nursing care (Goldstein & Jabs, 2004).

Young children should be desensitized to prepare for HD therapy whenever possible (Gilman & Frauman, 1982). Children who need HD acutely and who are very young or

Table 20-2
Pediatric Hemodialysis Complications

Patient Problems

Hyperkalemia
Hypocalcemia
Hypernatremia
Fluid overload
　　　Pulmonary edema
　　　Hypertension
　　　Edema
Muscle cramps
Fever

Minor Emergencies

Hypertension
Hypotension
Blood leaks from the dialyzer, tubing, or access
Machine malfunctions
Allergic reaction to initiation of dialysis

Major Emergencies

Air embolism
Cardiac arrest
Seizures
Spontaneous bleeding
Disequilibrium syndrome

have not been prepared for the treatment must be entertained and encouraged to remain in one place during the treatment. The very uncooperative child can be sedated, but children should never be restrained during an entire HD treatment.

HD of the acutely ill neonate is extremely labor intensive. Two registered nurses (RNs) skilled in neonatal HD, or one RN, one technician, and, possibly, the pediatric nephrologist, must be in the room throughout the HD session. A neonatologist, nurses from the neonatal intensive care unit (ICU), and a respiratory therapist may also need to care for the infant whether the dialysis is done in the neonatal ICU or in the pediatric dialysis unit. Constant observation and instantaneous response to correct physiological changes are vital to a successful treatment outcome. While not all of these professionals will be needed at any one time, instant accessibility to their expertise may be required at unpredictable moments.

Complications. The complications that arise in pediatric HD patients are essentially the same as for adult patients. The main difference with children is that their smaller size and metabolic sensitivity make such complications much more likely to occur. Additionally, a small child may not be able to communicate changes occurring during the treatment that may alert dialysis staff to potential problems. There are three categories of complications: patient problems, minor emergencies, and major emergencies (see Table 20-2).

As with adult patients, prevention is preferable to correction for any of these complications. The pediatric patient will require close observation and frequent assessment; blood pressures are usually taken once every 15 to 20 minutes. Children weighing less than 12 kg need a blood pressure taken every 5 minutes if receiving acute dialysis.

Neonates receiving HD may need one taken even more frequently.

Incenter versus home HD. Acute HD and chronic HD of the pediatric patient who weighs less than 25 kg should be done in a unit staffed and equipped to handle pediatric HD. However, for the child who will be on HD for the foreseeable future and who is larger than 25 kg, home HD is a reasonable option offered by some centers. Whether or not a family succeeds with home HD depends on their interest in accomplishing this treatment goal, their ability to learn the procedures, and the support they receive from their dialysis center. A complete training program that teaches sterile technique, machine function, trouble shooting, and minor machine maintenance, as well as basic HD operations and monitoring and adjustment skills is required. Many pediatric dialysis centers find that they have very few home HD candidates. In that instance, referring the pediatric patient to a well-established home HD program in an adult dialysis center is very appropriate instead of formulating a program for just one or two patients in the pediatric center. Physiologically, if the child is large enough to dialyze safely at home, he or she is large enough to dialyze safely in an adult unit.

Peritoneal Dialysis (PD)

There are many different techniques to use in performing PD. IPD, CAPD, and CCPD, which is sometimes called automated peritoneal dialysis (APD), are the ones routinely used with pediatric patients. The latter two modalities are sometimes called continuous peritoneal dialysis (CPD).

Techniques. *IPD.* IPD is commonly used for the acutely ill renal failure patient who requires frequent (every 1 to 2 hour) exchanges and, thus, uses large volumes of fluid each day. Most patients on IPD are dialyzed in the pediatric intensive care unit, are usually quite ill, and require constant nursing interventions in addition to their hourly PD exchanges. Fluctuations in their serum chemistries often require frequent adjustments to the composition of their peritoneal dialysate.

The main disadvantage to IPD is that it is usually done with an open system, one that has air vents and other openings that permit bacteria on dust motes and droplet nuclei to enter the system in spite of careful nursing techniques. This, combined with the numerous breaks in the system required by the recurring changes of fluid bags, increases the likelihood of developing peritonitis. Valeri, Radhakrishnan, Vernocchi, Carmichael, and Stern (1993) found a higher rate of peritonitis in the first 48 hours of IPD for patients on open systems. Many centers will try to convert the pediatric IPD patient to a closed CAPD system as quickly as possible after the patient's condition stabilizes to forestall the development of peritonitis.

CAPD. CAPD is a description of the method of performing this PD therapy, not a description of the patient who uses it. Just like the elderly diabetic with bilateral below-the-knee amputations, the infant who has not yet learned to walk can be very appropriately dialyzed with CAPD.

CAPD provides the opportunity for the most normal lifestyle for the pediatric dialysis patient who will not be transplanted in the foreseeable future. Being on CAPD requires few, if any, dietary restrictions and generally fewer medications than other renal replacement therapies. Children on CAPD who are doing well generally come to clinic only once a month, so they can remain in school almost full time.

The usual CAPD prescription is an exchange volume of 900-1100 ml of dialysate per meter squared of body surface area (BSA) given three to five times a day, depending on the child's residual renal function and catabolic rate (Warady, Morganstern, & Alexander, 2004). As is true with adult patients, the higher the percentage of dextrose in the PD solution, the more fluid removed. Children use the standard 1.5%, 2.5%, and 4.25% solutions, but their exact prescription varies with individual eating habits, residual renal function, blood pressure, and fluid status.

There are many different types of commercial systems available to deliver PD fluid to the patient. Most systems allow the patient to disconnect from the original dialysate container and fluid delivery tubing, keeping only a short transfer set attached until time for the next exchange. Several vendors offer mechanical devices to assist in performing the exchange quickly and accurately.

Each PD vendor offers several different types of systems, and each vendor attempts to make their systems user-friendly and resistant to user error. Almost any system can be adapted for the pediatric patient. The center must choose a vendor based on the quality of patient support services, reliability of supply sterility, supply availability, and cost-effectiveness.

The major disadvantage of CAPD is that it is unremitting. The exchanges must be done an average of four times a day every day for as long as the child is receiving that therapy. Unlike some adult patients who are only required to do exchanges on 6 days out of 7, children need all the exchanges they can get in order to optimize growth.

Some families adapt well to this requirement and treat CAPD as just another general body maintenance procedure, like taking a shower or brushing teeth. Other families find the relentless responsibility very tiring and look for different ways to lighten the burden. This might involve additional caretakers, such as extended family members or family friends being trained to do CAPD in order to relieve the parent. Usually the adult CAPD patient and one other helper are trained to do CAPD. A pediatric patient with divorced and remarried parents and a busy lifestyle may need up to six people trained to provide care. When training caregivers, it is best to require that they perform a minimum of one exchange a week so that their exchange technique will not degrade due to lack of use. One exchange a day is best for keeping skills sharp.

Children dialyzed on CAPD usually do very well. They grow, have the maximum possible time in school, have about the same energy level as their healthy peers, and enjoy diets with few restrictions. The children's serum chemistries remain in an acceptable range, and they generally feel good. As a result, many pediatric centers recommend CAPD as the dialysis treatment of choice for their pediatric patients.

APD. APD or CCPD operates on the same principles as CAPD. However, a machine is used to infuse the proper amount of dialysate, time the dwell period, and drain the dialysate from the body. The machines are designed to alarm if any of these procedures are not occurring properly or completely. The exchanges are done while the child is attached to the machine for 8 to 12 hours each night.

Many pediatric dialysis centers routinely start each child in CKD on CCPD because they feel the weight of parental responsibility in performing CAPD dialysis exchanges is excessive. Other centers use CCPD for temporary or permanent parental respite. It is more expensive than CAPD due to the use of more fluid but provides a viable alternative.

Children who develop recurrent hernias when walking around with CAPD fluid in their abdomen should be switched to CCPD. One 8-year-old with encopresis on CAPD was totally continent when changed to CCPD. In addition to fewer demands on family caregivers, CCPD requires fewer breaks in the closed PD system and, thus, decreases the likelihood of contamination. Children with frequent bouts of peritonitis on CAPD may have fewer episodes on CCPD.

The main disadvantage of CCPD is that clearances are decreased as dialysis takes place only during a 10- to 12-hour period instead of throughout the entire day. As a result, more fluid volume per day is required to get enough dialysis, which, in addition to the tubing sets and drain bags as well as machine rental or purchase price, results in a higher cost than CAPD. Often pediatric patients on CCPD run higher serum creatinines than children on CAPD or than they themselves did on CAPD. Sometimes an overday dwell or an additional exchange or two during the day may be needed to control the creatinine.

An important consideration in doing CCPD is that the child should not feel isolated from the family during the exchange time. Children whose cycler is kept in their bedroom and who are old enough not to be asleep during the entire procedure will hate the whole experience if the rest of the family spends the evening gathered in the family room (Hislop & Lansing, 1983).

Families who are able to switch back and forth between CAPD and CCPD are likely to be the most successful on CCPD. On a regular school night, doing CCPD at home is very appropriate. However, if the family wants to go to grandmother's for the weekend, it may be too much of a hassle to arrange to have a cycler moved for such a short time period. In that instance, the family can switch to CAPD for the weekend and feel free to travel without compromising the child's therapy (Hislop & Lansing, 1983). The development of smaller, more portable cyclers has permitted PD patients to travel more easily.

Choice of technique. Twardowski et al. developed the Peritoneal Equilibration Test (PET) as a means of determining an individual patient's peritoneal membrane solute transport rates. The Pediatric Peritoneal Dialysis Study Consortium (PPDSC) evaluated performing the test in children by using 1,100 ml of dialysate per m² body surface area (BSA) instead of the standard adult 2,000 ml of 2.5% dextrose peritoneal dialysate for the test exchange volume (Warady, Morganstern, et al., 2004). They found that characterizing children as high, high average, low average, or low transporters helps decide which type of PD will be most effective.

Generally speaking, high transporters do better with more frequent, shorter dialysis exchanges, such as found in APD. Low transporters need longer dwell times to get maximum benefit from an exchange. This happens more often in

CAPD. However, manipulating the number and frequency of exchanges or cycles as well as increasing the fill volume can be necessary to achieve optimal clearance and UF (Warady, Schaefer, et al., 2004).

Access issues. Chronic access for each type of PD is achieved with a Tenckhoff catheter. The choice of straight or curly, of one cuff or two, varies from center to center. Numerous studies have found that pediatric patients with double cuff swan-neck catheters placed with downward pointing exit sites have fewer episodes of peritonitis. However, the 2004 North American Pediatric Renal Transplant Cooperative Study's (NAPRTCS's) Annual Report states that the most common PD access at present is a curled catheter with a single cuff, and a straight tunnel with a lateral exit site (NAPRTCS, 2004). The exit site should be placed by a skilled operator in an area that the patient prefers, if he or she is old enough to make a choice, but away from previous surgical scars, ostomy sites, and the belt line (Harvey, 2001; Verrina, Honda, Warady, & Piraino, 2000).

A single preoperative dose of a first-generation cephalosporin before Tenckhoff placement helps prevent peritonitis. Omentectomy, or alternatively suturing the omentum to either the epigastrum or lateral abdominal wall, may improve catheter function. Suturing the Tenckhoff to the anterior abdominal wall can also prevent catheter malfunction. Delaying use of the catheter up to 10-15 days postplacement can help prevent leaks, but few pediatric centers delay first use routinely (Harvey, 2001).

Acute PD may be performed with a Tenckhoff catheter. However, if a child is too ill to withstand surgical placement of a Tenckhoff catheter, a nylon stylet-type catheter or a soft polyurethane or Teflon catheter is placed using Seldinger technique over a guide wire and a peel-away sheath. Both of these types of acute access are at higher risk for leaks or poor function (Chadha, Warady, Blowey, Simckes, & Alon, 2000; Warady, Morganstern, et al., 2004).

A nonfunctioning Tenckhoff catheter is extremely frustrating for patients, family, and caregivers. As with adults, poor positioning of the catheter, constipation, fibrin, omentum wrapping around the catheter, and adhesions from past abdominal surgeries have all been known to interfere with catheter function. Some children are hypersensitive to the catheter and get eosinophilia at the exit site or in the peritoneal cavity.

Children, particularly those not yet toilet trained, have a high risk of exit site and tunnel infections. For those still wearing diapers, a long subcutaneous tunnel with the exit site well away from the diaper area is strongly recommended (see Figure 20-1).

The exit site care procedure varies with each institution. Many require sterile dressings and sterile technique during weekly dressing changes until the catheter is well healed. Some are absolutely adamant about sterile technique and insist dressings be worn over the exit site at all times. Other units ask the patient to wash the well-healed exit site with an antibacterial soap during the daily shower and tape the transfer set to the abdominal skin to prevent pulling on the Tenckhoff at the exit site. Dressings may be optional in that event, though daily use of Mupirocin cream at the exit site, which is recommended to prevent exit site infections, would require a dressing to prevent rubbing it off on clothing (Verrina et al., 2000).

Originally it was thought that ostomy stomas, polycystic kidneys, prune belly syndrome, or recent abdominal surgery would be an absolute contraindication. Successful placement of Tenckhoff catheters in pediatric patients with these issues has occurred.

Complications. Children on PD run similar risks of complications as adults do. Infection and catheter malfunction are the most common. Poor dialysate flow in or out, pain on drain or fill, bleeding, and, rarely, perforation of the bladder or bowel can also occur.

Exit site infections are more prevalent in children still wearing diapers, but for the toilet-trained child they may be no more frequent than in the adult population. Tunnel infections are usually secondary to exit site infections. These infections can progress to peritonitis, or peritonitis can be the result of contaminations during the exchange procedure.

Breaks in the closed system rather than poor exchange technique are more often the cause of contamination. Children have been known to bite holes in the tubing or bag (teething babies are notorious chewers), stick needles through the solution transfer set, play tug-of-war with the dog using the solution transfer set, pull the tubing off the Tenckhoff when jumping out of a tree, or pull the spike out of a bag due to walking away while a parent is performing an exchange. Parents, too, can cause contaminations. One mother who was holding her baby while cooking dinner melted the solution transfer set when it rubbed on a stove burner. In short, if there is a way to cause a break in the system, someone will do it sooner or later.

Frequent episodes of peritonitis can cause the peritoneal membrane to thicken, thus reducing UF and solute movement efficiency. Membrane failure, which can be defined as insufficient UF with or without abdominal adhesions or decreased peritoneal surface area, may be severe enough to require a patient change from PD to HD (Andreoli et al., 1993). Some children with UF failure may need to be hemodialyzed intermittently (once or twice a week) for fluid removal while being maintained on PD.

Peritonitis caused by alpha streptococci or Pseudomonas aeruginosa leads to membrane failure more often than that caused by other bacteria. In addition, patients treated with PD for a long time will develop membrane failure, possibly due to damaging effects of prolonged exposure to hypertonic glucose. Decreased membrane function can begin as early as 24 months after initiation of PD. The exact duration of treatment before total membrane failure varies with individuals. It is further difficult to define as more children are transplanted than are peritoneally dialyzed for lengthy time periods (Andreoli et al., 1993).

A final complication of PD is family burnout. The continuous requirement for treatment interventions in the home, including daily PD exchanges, concomitant tube feedings, injections of erythropoietin and/or growth hormone, and medication administration put a great burden on home caregivers (Rigden, 1994). Treatment demands, along with the high stress level of modern society, such as two-income families, child care requirements, and the financial and social burdens of rearing a child with renal failure, can quickly lead

Figure 20-1
Infant's Tenckhoff Catheter Exit Site Located Well Away From the Diaper Area.

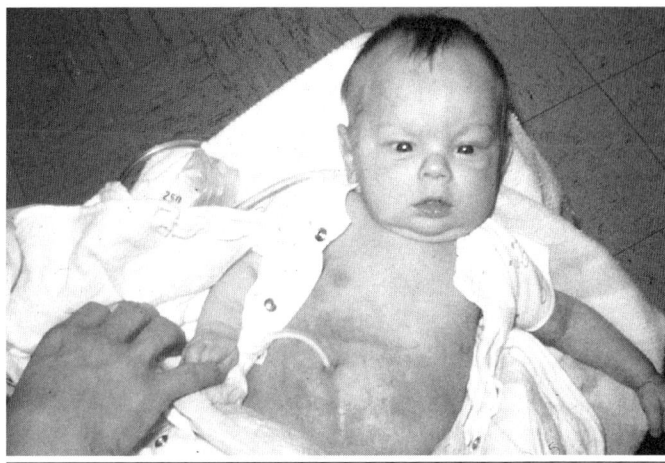

Photo courtesy of Riley Hospital for Children, Indianapolis, IN.

to mental, physical, and emotional exhaustion. If the caregiver is a single parent or perceives that few supportive resources are available, the progression to depletion will be much quicker. Pediatric renal nurses must be alert for signs of burnout and help families develop coping mechanisms or obtain respite to prevent serious side effects, such as poor exchange technique or cessation of dialysis altogether.

Incenter versus home PD. The benefit of CAPD or CCPD is that they are done in the home to maximize normality for the patient and family. Incenter PD done daily or nightly would require the child either to reside in the hospital or to sleep there each night, which would be a totally abnormal lifestyle.

Continuous Renal Replacement Therapies (CRRTs)

Techniques. CRRTs are the most recently developed treatment modalities being used on children. There are several forms of CRRT. Those used on children include continuous arteriovenous hemofiltration (CAVH), continuous venovenous hemofiltration (CVVH), continuous venovenous hemofiltration with dialysis (CVVHD), and continuous venovenous hemodiafiltration (CVVHDF). Slow continuous ultrafiltration (SCUF) and therapeutic plasma exchange (TPE) are also available but are infrequently used in the pediatric renal failure patient population. Consequently, they will not be discussed here.

While some centers have almost totally replaced acute HD in children with some form of CRRT, other centers use it only on the most critically ill patients — those who would be unlikely to survive the stress of intermittent HD treatments. Naturally, the center's choice in this matter is directly reflected in its survival statistics. Those using CRRT for almost all acute renal failure episodes have very good outcome statistics. Centers using CRRT only for ventilated patients in the pediatric intensive care unit with several major organ systems in failure in addition to the kidneys naturally have fewer successful outcomes.

The same volume considerations in pediatric HD apply

to the extracorporeal circuit in any of the CRRTs. No more than 10% of the child's circulating blood volume can be in the extracorporeal circuit at any one time. Blood prime may be required if the commercial set-up is not within the patient's 10% limit.

CAVH. CAVH provides the critically ill and hemodynamically unstable patient with safe, effective therapy through slow, continuous fluid and solute removal (Stapleton & Wright, 1992). The system has a built-in feedback loop:If the patient's blood pressure drops, the rate of UF will automatically decrease (Macias, Mueller, Scarim, Robinson, & Rudy, 1991). Along with improved fluid and electrolyte balance, CAVH also provides improved myocardial contractility in children with postoperative decreased cardiac output. Better pulmonary gas exchange, decreased central venous pressure (CVP), and reduced afterload with few changes in the mean arterial pressure (MAP) are additional benefits (Suddaby, Bell, & Murphy, 1990; Zobel et al., 1991).

CAVH for children is set up in the same manner as it is on adult patients. Just as in adults, a child must have an MAP of 60 mmHg and sufficient cardiac function to push the blood through the extracorporeal circuit in order for CAVH to be successful. Both an arterial and a venous access are required because it is the pressure differential that permits blood flow through the circuit and causes the filter to remove fluid from the circuit. Finding an arterial access with sufficient flow, particularly in the very small patient, is an extremely difficult task. In addition, the severely ill pediatric patient, especially the severely ill infant, is unlikely to be able to maintain an MAP sufficient to ensure adequate CAVH function.

In the early days of CAVH, some units compensated for lack of cardiac function by splicing a blood pump segment into the system and running the pump at a very low speed (2 to 5 ml per minute) to assist the flow through the circuit (Bell, 1988). Eventually this technique evolved into CVVH.

At about the same time, some adult units allowed filtrate to flow out by gravity, and replacement fluid inflow rate was increased or decreased to match the rate of outflow. Pediatric patients had to have the filtrate rate regulated by an IV pump or flow controller. This prevented too much fluid coming off too quickly, thus getting ahead of the replacement fluid rate and causing hypotension or shock.

Heparinization of the CAVH circuit attached to the pediatric patient is based, at least at the outset, on the patient's weight. An initial bolus of 20-40 u/kg is given, followed by a slow infusion of 10 u/kg/hr. The goal is to maintain the patient's ACT between 180-220 seconds in order to prevent clotting within the circuit. Because the flow rate within the circuit may be slow or may fluctuate, a higher level of heparinization may be required.

Studies have shown CAVH frequently provides inadequate solute clearance and causes serious complications with the vascular access. Therefore, it currently is rarely used (Benfield & Bunchman, 2004).

CVVH. CVVH offers the advantage of a blood pump to provide flow through the extracorporeal circuit and maintain system function. This means that an arterial access is not required, and the patient's MAP is not an issue. However, having a blood pump in the circuit makes it very easy to

entrain air in the system, thus requiring a venous drip chamber and foam detector to be added to the circuit.

In the past, units created their own adapted CVVH devices out of blood pumps, foam detectors, and IV pumps. These offered the flexibility of being able to use HD bloodlines of all sizes, thus creating very adaptable extracorporeal circuit volumes. However, these adapted systems lack a way to maintain blood temperature accurately within the circuit. Furthermore, using an IV pump as an ultrafiltrate monitor can cause an error rate as high as 30% (Benfield & Bunchman, 2004).

There are now five devices specifically for CRRT marketed in North America: B. Braun Diapact™CRRT; Baxter Accura and BM-25 systems; Gambro Prisma® System; and Edwards LifeScience Aquarius system. There are also two models of HD machines, the Fresenius 2008H and 2008K, that can be used for CRRT. While these commercial machines have variable blood flow rates, dialysate flow rates, and replacement fluid rates that can allow them to be flexible enough to use on many different patient sizes, only three of the CRRT systems have both adult volume and low-volume tubing available at present (Benfield & Bunchman, 2004). The HD machines can use any of the three sizes of blood tubing (adult, pediatric, and neonatal) available on the market. However, adult-sized tubing and the longer length of HD bloodlines increase the risk that the extracorporeal CRRT circuit volume will exceed the 10% limit on smaller children. Blood prime of the circuit will be necessary in that event.

There are three choices of anticoagulation for CVVH: none, heparin, and citrate. Many seriously ill patients will have clotting abnormalities, causing nephrologists to request no anticoagulation be administered. Unfortunately, this frequently results in clotting of the circuit after a relatively short use. Even patients with disseminated intravascular coagulation (DIC) or serious liver malfunction can manage to clot an extracorporeal circuit (Benfield & Bunchman, 2004). In addition, they are frequently receiving clotting factors and blood products that can readily clot off a filter or circuit.

Heparinization during CVVH can be a little tighter than that for CAVH, as the flow though the filter is easily maintained by the blood pump. A bolus of 20 units/kg is given when attaching the patient to a new system, which is followed by a continuous infusion of 20 units/kg/hr. The infusion is usually adjusted to keep the ACTs between 180-200 seconds, but they may be allowed to drop as low as 160 in children with bleeding tendencies. The infusion is generally diluted to 50 or 100 u/ml so that small amounts of heparin are infused via higher flow rates on the IV pumps. This results in greater dose accuracy and better mixing in the system than if very small amounts of fluid were used.

Citrate anticoagulation works by binding plasma calcium, thus interrupting the clotting cascade. Citrate is infused into the CVVH circuit before the filter at a rate that keeps the ionized calcium level of the circuit between 0.25 and 0.4 mmol/l. However, a second infusion of calcium into the patient at a site removed from the return of the CVVH circuit blood is needed to keep the patient's ionized calcium between 1.1-1.3 mmol/l. Besides bleeding, citrate anticoagulation can cause "citrate gap," a rise in total serum calcium

Figure 20-2
Continuous Venovenous Hemodiafiltration (CVVHD) in the Newborn Intensive Care Unit. Dialysate System Is on the IV Stand on the Right.

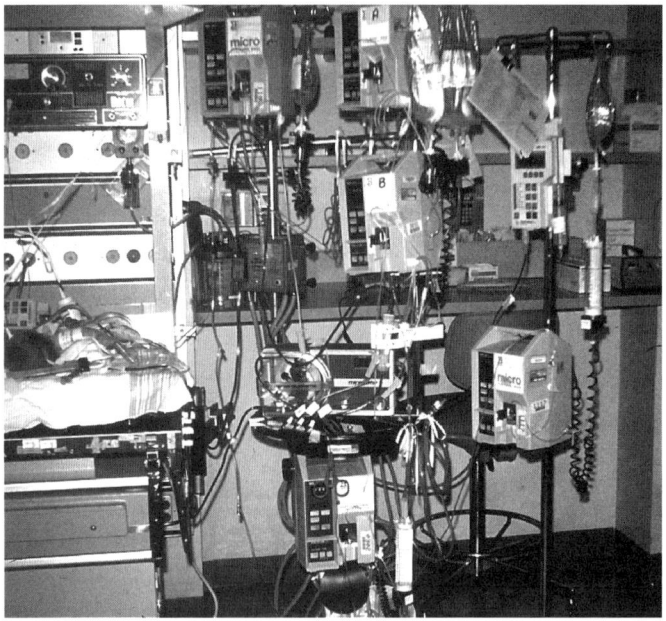

Photo courtesy of Riley Hospital for Children, Indianapolis, IN.

but a drop in ionized calcium, and metabolic alkalosis (Benfield & Bunchman, 2004).

CVVHD. If CVVH is not able to provide enough solute removal to control a patient's catabolic state, CVVHD can be begun. In this technique, dialysate, usually sterile 1.5% dextrose peritoneal dialysate, is pumped into the filter countercurrent to the blood flow (see Figure 20-2). The ultrafiltrate pump must be set high enough to withdraw the volume of dialysate plus the required volume of fluid to be removed. The dialysate works in the same manner as it does in HD to increase solute removal via diffusion (Benfield & Bunchman, 2004).

The dialysate used in CVVHD, as in PD, must be sterile because the large pores in the filter membranes would permit bacteria to travel across into the patient's blood. Septicemia would result if the dialysate used were only clean, as it is in HD. The rate of the dialysate flow is guided by the rates available on the pump used to remove both the filtrate and used dialysate from the filter, as well as the degree of solute clearance desired.

CVVHDF. CVVHDF provides solute removal by both convection and diffusion. It works in the same manner as CVVHD, but the rate at which dialysate is pumped through the UF compartment is at a much higher rate. It is both more complex and more costly to perform this technique (Benfield & Bunchman, 2004).

Access issues. As in all treatments involving extracorporeal circulation, blood vessel access is the biggest potential barrier to successful results.

The blood pump in CVVH permits the use of dual-lumen catheters in an internal jugular, subclavian, or femoral vein

in larger children. Either the acute or chronic type catheter may be used. In the past, Mauer and Lynch (1976) found that umbilical catheters worked well for neonatal HD, but more recent investigators have found that umbilical vessels do not permit sufficient blood flow for CVVH on neonates. They recommend, instead, the use of 6.5 or 7 French dual lumen catheters placed in the internal jugular, femoral, or subclavian veins (Bell, 1988; Thompson et al., 1991).

Complications. CVVH can present many complications. It presents the unique problem of continued UF even if the patient becomes hypotensive. Although the blood pump in the circuit increases the risk of drawing air into the system, the foam detector should prevent air embolism to the patient.

Patients receiving treatment run the risk of infection or bleeding due to either anticoagulation or coagulopathies. In addition, there can be clotting in the filter or circuit due to low flow or insufficient anticoagulation. Blood loss can occur from the circuit if system parts separate. Incorrect fluid replacements will lead to electrolyte imbalance, hypotension if too much fluid is removed, or hypertension if not enough fluid is removed. The increased fluid management accuracy of commercial systems over adapted systems should improve this problem.

Hemothorax or pneumothorax after a central venous catheter placement or impairment of circulation to a limb distal to access point may result in ischemic damage. Metabolic acidosis with citrate anticoagulation and lack of temperature control can also occur (Benfield & Bunchman, 2004).

Measuring Adequacy of Dialysis in Children

Adequate dialysis dose in children has not been identified due to the lack of research in this very small segment of the overall dialysis population and the lack of tools to measure quality of life in children (Goldstein, 2001). NKF-DOQI recommends a monthly Kt/V of 1.2 as a minimum delivered dialysis dose. However, it is hard to correlate pediatric clinical outcomes with a given Kt/V value.

Better, more appropriate outcome measures for children, such as urea reduction ratio (URR), serum PTH, nutrition, and development and growth as measured by median weight, height, and head circumference SDS are needed to assess dialysis adequacy especially in prepubertal patients (Shroff et al., 2003). Fatigue, exercise capacity, medication adherence, and school opportunities or barriers have been postulated as quality of life issues in children receiving chronic health care, but tools to measure these issues are not available (Goldstein, 2001). Nor do tools exist to measure pediatric patient function, well-being, or general health perception in the physical, psychological, and social domains of health-related quality of life (Warady, Morganstern, et al., 2004)

Normalized whole body clearance of urea is widely used in adult HD patients to assess adequacy of dialysis. If the patient's dietary protein intake is adequate, a Kt/V value of 1.2 or more is considered to indicate sufficient dialysis. Unfortunately, no studies have been done to determine that a Kt/V of 1.2 or greater will guarantee adequate dialysis and desired clinical outcomes in children.

Because of their higher nutritional needs and metabolic

Table 20-3
Pediatric Peritoneal Dialysis Adequacy Criteria

Parameters	Modalities		
	CAPD	CCPD APD with daytime dwell	NIPD APD with dry day
Total Kt/V in liters per week	> 2.0	> 2.1	> 2.2
Total Creatinine Clearance in liters per 1.73m2/week • For high/high average transporters • For low/low average transporters	> 60 > 50	> 63 > 52.5	> 66 > 55

Note: From Warady, B.A., et al., (2004).

requirements by weight, children require higher urea clearances than do adults. A greater postdialysis disequilibrium between intracellular fluid (ICF) and extracellular fluid (ECF) urea concentrations in children may skew the results if an immediate postdialysis blood sample were used as it is in adult patients. When Kt/V is calculated in pediatric HD, the postdialysis blood sample should be drawn 1 hour after the treatment is finished to allow full equilibration between ICF and ECF urea concentrations (Evans, Smye, & Brocklebank, 1992). However, waiting a full hour postdialysis can be very inconvenient for the patient, their family, and the dialysis unit. Fortunately, the equilibration is 69% complete at 15 minutes postdialysis so the equilibrated value can be estimated (Goldstein, 2001).

Sharma (2001) states that children getting intensive nutrition and higher dialysis clearances show normal or catch-up growth and normal puberty. However, a Network 1 study of clinical indicators showed exceeding dialysis adequacy recommendations did not improve patient morbidity. The adult standards of morbidity and mortality do not apply to children, so the group decided to look at hospitalization rates and need for antihypertensives. They found that patient age is the only variable that correlates with hospitalization rate; younger children are hospitalized more frequently. Dialysis adequacy also correlated inversely with age of the patient in kids treated with both PD and HD. The HD access type (catheter, AVF, or AVG) did not affect Kt/V in children receiving HD. All of the children were well-dialyzed, but greater than suggested Kt/V did not correlate with improvement in other clinical indicators (Brem, Lambert, Hill, Kitsen, & Shemin, 2001).

The ESRD CPM project in 2000 showed a mean Kt/V for adolescents on HD of 1.47; it was slightly higher in girls than boys. A similar pattern was noted for URR (Frankenfield et al., 2002).

A Kt/V of greater than 2.0/week is recommended for patients on CAPD; greater than 2.2/week, for those on APD. A total creatinine clearance is recommended based on the patient's peritoneal membrane characterization (Warady, Schaefer, et al., 2004) (see Table 20-3). Long-term multicenter studies of outcomes in well-dialyzed pediatric patients are needed to formulate recommendations for pediatric adequacy guidelines.

Transplantation

Transplantation is the treatment goal for all children with CKD. The optimal age for transplantation is somewhat controversial. Mortality is increased in recipients younger than age 2, but mortality is high in that age group receiving dialysis as well. Noncompliance with immune suppressive medications is an issue with adolescents, while growth is optimized in children receiving transplants prior to puberty (Smith & McDonald, 2000). Living related donor (LD) transplants are much more likely in children than adults, with 60% of children receiving kidneys from a parent (56% mothers, 44% fathers) (Benfield, 2003). Preemptive transplantation is more common in children than in adults because of the availability of living donors. In the U.S., approximately 20% of children receive preemptive transplants.

Obstructive uropathy and aplasia/dysplasia syndromes are the most common causes of renal failure requiring transplantation in children (Benfield, 2003). These conditions may require the child to undergo extensive urological intervention before transplantation is possible.

The pre-transplant workup should include evaluation for evidence of past infections with varicella, Epstein-Barr virus, cytomegalovirus, herpes simplex, toxoplasmosis, human immunodeficiency virus, and hepatitis A, B, and C. Many young children are naïve to these infections, and they may be transmitted through the use of an adult kidney in which these organisms are present (Benfield, 2003; Smith & McDonald, 2000). Immunizations, particularly the live virus vaccines including varicella, MMR, and in some countries, polio, should be given before transplantation and followed with serological studies to determine immunity.

The immune suppressive regimen in children is similar to that in adults. Drugs currently in use for immune suppression in children include corticosteroids, mycophenolate mofentil, cyclosporine, sirolimus, and tacrolimus. Corticosteroid use is tapered to every other day use to facilitate growth. Azothiaprine is less commonly used, decreasing from use in 85% of patients in 1993 to only 30% in 1996 (Benfield, 2003; Smith & McDonald, 2000).

Allograft survival has steadily improved with 94% of LD

grafts and 93% of cadaver donor (CD) grafts surviving to 1 year (Benfield, 2003). The most common cause for graft loss is chronic rejection, followed by acute rejection and vascular thrombosis. Recurrent disease is a problem in children, as in adults, but some of the underlying diseases are different. Diseases that can recur in children include focal segmental glomerulosclerosis (FSGS), hemolytic uremic syndrome, and primary oxalosis.

End-of-Life Care

Children may reach a point where treatment options have been exhausted, or particularly in the case of children with multiple handicaps or developmental delay, parents may decide that to proceed with further treatment is futile. Those providing care for the child and parents will need to continue, with a focus on palliation rather than treatment. A pediatric hospice can provide invaluable advice and skills through the dying process. Adult hospice agencies may have staff trained in the care of children and should be consulted if no pediatric hospice is available. Attention should be given to pain control if any is present, respiration, and skin care. Dietary restrictions should be removed, allowing the child to have foods and drinks that may have been long denied.

Specific Nursing Interventions

The purpose of nursing intervention for the child and family is to promote independence from health care providers; normality in lifestyle; and optimal emotional, physical, mental, and social development. Children and their parents must be an integral part of the care given. Prevention of problems is always to be preferred to intervening after the problem has occurred or worsened.

Nutrition

Nutritional needs of children with CKD are complex and require a great deal of attention from a multidisciplinary team of renal health care providers. Physicians are adept at determining the metabolic needs of children with CKD, dietitians are knowledgeable about determining the food and fluid intake that will meet those needs, but nurses and parents must implement a dietary plan that the child will actually consume. Most children need encouragement to eat enough nutrients and calories, but a few may need to be on restrictive diets. In that event, children must be prevented from eating the wrong things and encouraged to eat enough for energy and growth.

An additional consideration is the need to cope with school cafeterias, restaurants, birthday parties, and sleepovers while maintaining the child's dietary regimen. This needs to be done with sensitivity, perhaps allowing the child mild indiscretions and compensating either with dialysis or with greater restrictions during another part of the day. Often restaurants, theme parks, and other facilities will be happy to provide a nutritional analysis of the foods available; they need only to be asked. All parents and all children who are old enough to be making choices about food need to be aware of exactly what dietary restrictions or requirements are necessary and be taught to read food labels so that they can meet those needs. With the advent of mandatory food labels that specify the amounts of protein, sodium, potassium, and

other nutrients present, this task has become easier.

The major difference in renal dietary regimens for children is their need for sufficient nutrients, especially calories for growth; these must be superimposed on the requirements and restrictions inherent in a renal failure diet. Pure carbohydrates and pure fats are used for this purpose since these have little effect on renal function. Supplementing with polycose and other sugars, sometimes with the addition of concentrated medium-chain triglyceride (MCT) oils, is often necessary to provide adequate calories for growth. These substances may cause digestive problems such as poor absorption or diarrhea, and adjustments must be made accordingly. Additionally, in very small children or infants, nasogastric (NG), gastrostomy, or other tube feeding techniques may be needed to ensure adequate intake. Feeding by mouth is obviously preferable, but anorexia is common in chronically ill children. Severely anorexic teenagers may also have to be treated with tube feeding regimens.

Protein requirements for children with stage 1-4 CKD are identical to those for healthy children of the same height and age. These requirements rise slightly if HD is started (Johnson, 1993; McCann, 2002). Children treated with HD have dietary restrictions on intake similar to those of adults. However, what they eat, what they prefer to eat, and when and where they eat may differ widely. Just like other children of similar ages, children with CKD may develop strong attractions (fads) or aversions to certain foods. However, maintaining optimal nutrition is critical to enhancing growth and development. Helping parents and children come to agreement on how the dietary regimen will be handled will be most effective in resolving these issues.

Children receiving PD have fewer dietary restrictions than children on HD. They actually require higher than normal amounts of protein because of losses through the peritoneal membrane (McCann, 2002). Nutrition may be adversely affected, at least initially, by the feeling of fullness resulting from the dialysate in the abdominal cavity.

Nutrition after transplantation resembles that for healthy children. Again, the emphasis is on optimal nutrition. Steroid use may cause a great increase in appetite with resulting undesirable weight gain in some children. Additionally, sodium and fluid retention may be a problem for some children. As the steroid dosage is decreased to an alternate day regimen, these problems are likely to resolve.

Pharmacologic Concerns

Children with CKD receive most of the same medications as adults. However, medication dosages for children are always calculated on the basis of milligrams of medication per kilogram of body weight per day. Dosages are then divided as appropriate for the drug. When growth occurs, doses must be recalculated on a timely basis.

Tables indicating proper dosages are found in a variety of pediatric texts and must be used every time a new medication is given. As in adults, consideration must be given to the route of excretion of the drug and modified when the route is via the kidneys. Dialyzability of drugs is also a consideration, just as it is in adults. In addition, children may metabolize certain drugs differently than do adults, and a pediatric reference text should be consulted when giving drugs to children.

Children are often less able to articulate symptoms resulting from drug side effects; they must be observed carefully and questioned in terms they understand. Some adverse effects may be identified by laboratory testing.

One medication given much more frequently to children is Shohl's solution or bicitra. This is an acidic preparation that metabolizes to alkaline and buffers the metabolic acidosis so common in children. Both Shohl's solution and bicitra are preparations of sodium citrate and citric acid, with 1 mEq of acid per cc of solution. A pharmacist usually prepares these medications, and modifications can, thus, be made if necessary. This medication tastes vile; the colder it is when taken by mouth, the less offensive the taste to most people.

The actions, side effects, and risks of medications are the same in children as in adults. However, children come in many different sizes based on age, weight, and body surface area. In addition, there are individual differences in absorption, metabolism, and excretion of various medications (Betz & Sowden, 2004). Therefore, the first concern in medicating children is to ensure that the dosage is appropriate in mg/kg of body weight or in mg/m^2 of body surface area.

Second, it may be necessary to come up with different administration techniques for children. One may have to coax the uncooperative child to actually take oral medications. The medicines are often vomited, especially when the child is in renal failure. The nurse may need to find little tricks to prevent this outcome. For example, it may be necessary to numb the tongue by having the patient suck on flavored ice or a popsicle, or decrease taste sensation by holding the nose when taking oral medications (Hockenberry & Wong, 2004). Pills may be crushed between two spoons and mixed with ice cream, jelly, pudding, or honey. Some medications come in both pill and liquid forms. Be careful when mixing medications in food that the volume of food is not too great for the child to consume.

Parenteral medications require different injection sites than in adults, and needle lengths used should be based on the size of the child (Hockenberry & Wong, 2004). Pain control through use of topical anesthetic creams or application of ice to the injection site prior to injection administration is essential. Developmentally appropriate distraction techniques such as holding, blowing bubbles, singing, or solving riddles can also ease distress during injections.

Therapeutic Environment

Florence Nightingale, the fundamental nursing theorist, was the first to note how important a therapeutic milieu was to promote healing. She wrote that ventilation, food, light, cleanliness, noise level, and variety were important considerations in the care of the sick. She also noted that children "... are affected by the same things, but much more quickly and seriously...by want of fresh air, of proper warmth, want of cleanliness... by startling noises... by dullness and by want of light" (Nightingale, 1859, p. 72). Having access to natural air and light, such as a porch, patio, or play area is a real plus. It can be enormously reassuring for a child enduring a long hospitalization or even an extended clinic visit to be able to enjoy running, playing, or simply looking at an outdoor environment.

In addition to ensuring that a pediatric renal unit is clean, light, airy, and reasonably quiet, decorations must be planned keeping in mind the viewpoints of the children who will be the patients. The actual needs and preferences of the children should be considered, not just the adults' ideas of their areas of interest. Most pediatric renal units serve a wide range of ages, so providing age-appropriate decor can be a real challenge. The staff may need to decorate different parts of the unit with materials appropriate for each of the age groups coming to the unit.

One should keep in mind that younger children are very concrete, and pictures, posters, or murals of cartoons or other characters with missing or broken body parts will be very disturbing to them. Young children may assume that dialysis leads to the loss of body parts in that instance (Frauman & Gilman, 1989). Furthermore, some murals that look innocuous to an adult may be more frightening than entertaining for the very young child. Older children are at least bored or even insulted if the decor is focused on too young a theme. In addition, too young or too cheery a décor can demean children's very real concerns about their serious illness or imply denial that they experience pain or sadness about their disease (Hardgrove, 1980).

The ultimate goal in a pediatric renal unit is to "create a sense of caring, of gentleness, of beauty, of reassurance" (Hardgrove, 1980, p. 68). The use of color, carefully selected posters and murals, and, above all, the children's artwork can lead to a cheerful therapeutic environment. Hanging children's artwork makes them feel valued as well as in control of their environment. Holiday decorations made by the children and used repeatedly enhance their feelings of being valued and also give a sense of continuity in the unit. It also helps the staff remember the children who made the decorations and who may have been transplanted, recovered function, graduated to an adult dialysis unit, or died.

Patient safety must be a prime consideration when planning a pediatric renal unit. Space, lighting, electrical outlets' location and relationship to the emergency generator, location of electrical cords running to machines, handwashing facilities and hoppers for waste disposal, isolation capabilities for infectious patients, and washable walls and flooring must be carefully planned. The unit floor plan must be designed to maximize nursing care, prevent falls, and limit children's access to sharp instruments and hazardous chemicals.

Furniture in the pediatric renal unit must be appropriate for the various sizes of children served, yet allow staff to give care without intractable back pain. Tables and chairs, cribs, beds, and HD chairs must accommodate all sizes of children to be cared for. If small toilet facilities are not feasible, portable potty chairs or seat adapters for adult-size toilets must be available (Frauman & Gilman, 1989).

Play materials differentiate the pediatric renal unit from an adult unit. There must be appropriate materials for all ages of children served, but this does not mean that they must be complicated or expensive. Creative materials such as watercolors, scented markers, crayons and paper, or clay are particularly good choices. Books, puzzles, board games, card games, bubble makers, stacking toys, and other items for quiet play are also useful. Television, videotapes or DVDs, and computer games are good diversions that help time pass quickly, but they must not be allowed to take the place of interpersonal interactions with staff members or other children. Water play, finger painting, and tempera painting on easels are fun and creative, though messy. Cover-ups need to be handy to preserve clothing and contain messes.

Making appropriate decorations for each of the holidays, even made-up holidays like the dialysis unit's birthday, helps to relieve monotony and provides an opportunity for creativity and fun. The decorations made by patients and staff are almost always preferable. Flour and salt sculpting dough, paper for chains or cutouts, and paint are inexpensive materials to use for these projects. Bulletin boards, chalkboards, or the door into the unit can be decorated in holiday themes. Even the windows can be painted with washable paint to complete the decor.

The physical facilities, equipment, and supplies alone are not enough to ensure that the pediatric renal unit provides a therapeutic environment. Child and family-oriented care provided by a multidisciplinary staff with an attitude oriented to children is the most crucial element (Frauman & Gilman, 1989). Promoting normality in parent-child interactions, encouraging the child's participation in his or her care to the greatest possible extent, and incorporating siblings in the therapy are vital steps in that care.

Normal Life

Family Relationships

Children with complex physical problems often come from families with complex problems as well. Family relationships do not always conform to societal expectations, and they are not always what they seem on the surface. As there are many possible configurations for families, it is best to let the members define the scope of their particular family group (Frauman & Gilman, 1990). Careful assessment is necessary through both interviews and observations.

Children frequently live with a single parent, almost always the mother, putting a tremendous burden on one person to provide for all of the child's needs. If this parent is employed, she provides most or all of the family's income and health insurance coverage as well. Providing full-time care at home to the child with CKD is not an option. Clearly, help must come from somewhere. Enlisting the services of the social worker to obtain assistance with childcare; enhancing extended family support; and working with church and neighborhood groups, who then become in effect an extended family, may all be necessary. Often, older siblings become surrogate parents, which may lead to problems, especially during adolescence. Sometimes, the single parent may have to stop working and accept public assistance when available in order to provide the needed care for the child with CKD and siblings. Any single parent caring for a child with CKD will need exceptional assistance and support.

Stepparent families and families in which the mother has a live-in boyfriend are very common, especially in some cultural groups. The male figure's relationship with the child may range anywhere from virtually indistinguishable from that of a biological parent to nonexistent or even confronta-

tional. Often families are reluctant to share information about the relationship and feel inquiries are intrusive. Except in an urgent situation, it is probably best to assess the relationship over time and through observation as much as through direct questioning. Direct questions may cover a wide range of issues. For example, does the step-parent (or surrogate) bring the child to clinic or treatments? Does he or she participate in the care of the child or attempt to learn about the child's care? Does the person touch or hold the child? Is he or she patient with inevitable tears, or is the person angry and demanding of the child much of the time? The answers to these questions can provide valuable clues as to the nature of the relationship. Even if a stepparent or other companion is in the household, if the relationship with the child is strained or nonexistent, the parent will require support similar to that needed by a single parent.

Grandparents should neither be ignored nor expected to act as surrogate parents by the health care team. Ascertaining the relationships between grandparents, parents, and grandchildren is necessary, just as in assessing other family relationships. Grandparents who seem very involved in a crisis situation may not be able to maintain their support because of illnesses of their own or living some distance away. Routing information to grandparents through the parents is ideal, but this may not be possible when the parents are very young, poorly educated, or when the supply of bad news seems overwhelming. Grandparents' questions should be answered without betraying family confidences. Grandparents should also be involved in family teaching to the degree comfortable for them, the parents, and the child. A grandparent innocently handing a banana to a child on potassium restriction can be a dangerous situation. Other extended family members may also have very close ties to the child with CKD and, thus, must be considered by the nurse in planning care.

Siblings of the child with CKD are often not directly available to health team members for assessment or intervention. Helping parents to provide adequate care for the siblings without feeling constantly guilty can be difficult. Again, enlisting aid from all those available to provide support is necessary. It may be helpful to bring the sibling(s) to the clinic or the treatment facility to demystify what is happening to the child with CKD.

Psychosocial Care of Patient and Family

In caring for the child with CKD and the family, it is crucial to focus on keeping life as normal as possible for the entire family. The impact of CKD on the family unit can be devastating physically, psychologically, socially, and educationally (Soliday, Kool, & Lande, 2001; Watson, 1995). Upon receiving the diagnosis of CKD, the family will begin the grief process, which mourns the change in the child's health as well as the loss of a normal healthy child. Families come to realize that "...life...will never be the same again" (Dracopoulos & Weatherly, 1983, p. 141). The resulting anger, fear, and frustration can last a long time. In fact, pain often recurs as siblings and peers achieve normal developmental milestones. Family members are reminded that the child with CKD may not reach these milestones or may not reach them as easily; the child will always be different. When the child understands that chronic means forever, he or she may develop behavior problems. These problems along with the treatment demands, disruption of work, altered family life and relationships, and financial considerations leave all family members feeling overburdened and out of control (Dracopoulos & Weatherly, 1983).

In beginning to assist pediatric CKD patients and their families, nephrology nurses must ensure that they are presented with all possible treatment options and given assistance in making truly informed choices. Nephrology nurses must be sure that they have clear explanations of the goals and problems attached to each treatment modality (Rigden, 1994). Participation in formulating the treatment plan gives the family maximum control of the situation.

Children must also participate in planning and give their consent for treatment at a developmentally appropriate level (Gilman & Frauman, 1982). They should participate in their treatment or at least cooperate while someone else performs it. Parents will learn to care for the child initially but should gradually decrease their participation as the child matures and is able to take increasing responsibility for self-care. Remember, parents naturally have a hard time trusting anyone, even their own child, to do the required care as well as they have themselves over the years (Frauman & Gilman, 1985).

In coping with CKD, the family should avoid centering itself on the sick child. This is not a normal situation and will predictably lead to sibling resentment, fears, and guilt. Furthermore, family members should avoid personifying the child as the illness and parent(s) as the successful treatment. Thus, undesired outcomes will not be equated with parenting failure (Dracopoulos & Weatherly, 1983).

Family members should be encouraged to expect the child with CKD to make progress toward developmental milestones in the normal chronological order, if not at the usual ages. Making adaptations to assist the child's progress may be necessary. However, mastering self-care skills, going to school, participating in extracurricular activities as well as activities of daily living, finishing school, and progressing to employment are normal goals for all children. Working on these achievements helps family members to keep a perspective on the illness, to view the child as normal, and improves everyone's self-esteem (Frauman & Gilman, 1990). Expecting the child with CKD to assume the same kinds of household responsibilities that his or her healthy siblings do goes a long way toward decreasing anger and conflicts.

The nephrology nurse's goal should be to enhance the family's ability to care for the child without being intrusive or fostering dependence. Suggestions should be carefully phrased and interventions made in a nonjudgmental manner so that the family does not feel criticized, even by implication (Frauman & Gilman, 1990). One begins by identifying family strengths and weaknesses and the type and extent of support they are likely to require from the pediatric nephrology team (Rigden, 1994). It may be difficult to recognize the need for emotional support, as some families try to garner caregiver approval or to appear competent by hiding their stress from caregivers (Frauman & Gilman, 1990).

Anticipatory guidance should be offered at the critical events in the child's illness such as diagnosis, starting dialysis, or transplantation. At each of these events, the nurse will teach family members about how to care for the child. The nurse will explain everything that will be done, including how it works, how it feels, and why it is necessary in a manner appropriate to the child's and family's level of understanding.

Nurses should identify expected issues or problems at each of the critical events and help all family members deal with them. They can also help the family find effective coping mechanisms. Fostering and maintaining extended family relationships and friendships is helpful. Calling upon the family's past successes in dealing with problems is particularly effective. Facilitating networking with families of other children with CKD can enhance coping skills. Promoting open, honest, two-way communication between caregivers and family is crucial to success with these interventions (Frauman & Gilman, 1990; Rigden, 1994).

Play

Play is a very convenient intervention strategy when providing nursing care to children with CKD. Play can be used for assessment, patient teaching, and providing some much-needed pleasure to the child.

It is often difficult to gauge the emotional status of children receiving treatment for CKD. Small children, especially, have difficulty identifying and articulating their feelings of fear, anger, and frustration. Projective techniques using play, stories, and drawings can help nurses to understand what the child perceives and feels, making them thus able to intervene more appropriately (Gilman & Frauman, 1987).

Play activities can also be used to facilitate physical assessment. Drawing pictures on tongue blades and allowing children to explore equipment and examine parents or the nurse may make assessments less threatening, particularly when a child is first ill. Children will reciprocally play with the nurse during the assessment, such as during contests to determine who can open their mouth the widest. Having a focus for the child's eyes, such as a favorite toy or an adult doing something silly, will greatly facilitate eye examinations even in a very small child (Gilman & Frauman, 1987).

Teaching techniques based in play are probably the most effective methods used with children. Even a child who can read a brochure or booklet will learn better through demonstrations and games. Several computer games are now available to teach aspects of pediatric renal care.

Providing pleasure for the child is a goal of therapeutic play that should not get lost in the intense care necessary for these children. A play therapist or child life specialist can be invaluable in determining what games, toys, and play opportunities will be most useful for a given child.

School

School placement is a critical necessity for children with CKD. However, schools are often reluctant to have such children attend. Despite their misgivings, though, schools are required to provide education services for children with CKD and other chronic disorders. Federal legislation, including PL 94-142, PL 99-457, and the Individuals with Disabilities Education Act (IDEA), requires that all children receive an appropriate education in the least-restrictive environment.

Children with chronic conditions are considered to be at risk for developmental disabilities and may be eligible for services from birth to 5 years for that reason. Despite a variety of federal, state, and local case finding initiatives, parents may need to be quite assertive in securing these services for their child with CKD.

In addition, parents of children with CKD are often only offered services in handicapped classes or in homebound instruction. These may not be appropriate placements for an individual child. Appropriate placement should be determined on the basis of a thorough psychological evaluation and discussions with health care providers, parents, the child, and professional educators.

Decreased expectations of accomplishment for children with CKD may lead to diminished performance. Because the majority of children with renal failure survive to adulthood, they have the same need to develop independence as do other children; part of that independence is the ability to support oneself through meaningful employment. This is impossible without an adequate education. Such a concern may seem farfetched when thinking about a 3-year-old or an 8-year-old who doesn't have much energy, but all too soon the child becomes an adult without the needed knowledge and skills.

In addition, children with CKD need the social interaction preschool and school activities afford. Isolation from other children is not only lonely but may affect self-esteem and retard development of social and adaptive behaviors. Often parents and children discover a number of skills previously unidentified and sources of pleasurable activity not before tried. School placement is an absolute necessity for children with CKD, as necessary for future life as renal replacement therapy.

Special Occasions

Birthday parties, their own and those of other children, are a part of normal life for most children. Children with CKD need to have those same opportunities. For the child's own party, having refreshments, activities, and other aspects as much like their peers as possible is important. If serving hamburgers and French fries or pizza is the norm, then that must be done. If the child with CKD is on a restricted diet, smaller amounts or food cooked without salt can be provided unobtrusively. Going on an outing can be planned to follow a rest period if the child tires easily.

Travel is possible for children with CKD, but it requires considerable advance planning. For a child on dialysis, referral to another facility in the area to be visited is a necessity. The child on HD will need to be treated in the facility, and the child on PD will require services should there be a crisis with supplies or equipment or should peritonitis or other complications develop. The facility should preferably be a pediatric unit – most are accustomed to dealing with transient patients, especially those near frequent child tourist spots such as Disney, other theme parks, or national parks. Careful pre-arrangements need to be made with the receiving unit so that their requirements for staffing, equipment, and time are met. Plans must also be made regarding care of equipment and medications. Some equipment is very sensitive to movement, and many medications lose their efficacy in a hot car. If the child tires easily, flying or making short trips in the car may be needed. Sometimes sleeping while traveling prevents the child with CKD from arriving at a greatly desired destination in an extremely fatigued state.

Holidays may also require adaptation, and this may be hard for families with strong traditions for holiday food and activities. Working with the renal dietician to adapt family recipes will help as will planning activities for times when the child is feeling his or her best.

Camp is a normal activity for most children, and children with CKD are no exception. There are a number of special camps around the country designed exclusively for children with CKD. Camp facilities may include HD stations, PD exchange clean rooms, and medication dispensing areas. Alternatively, arrangements may be made with a nearby facility for dialysis treatments. Usually these camps accept children receiving all modalities of treatment, including conservative management. Ideally, the emphasis is usually on having fun and providing respite for parents rather than the pursuit of a therapeutic goal such as patient teaching. Children with CKD, especially those with a functioning transplant, may elect to attend a camp primarily for healthy children, such as scout camp or a religious camp. In that case, informing the camp staff and/or the camp nurse of the child's status and having locally available facilities for care is imperative.

Programs Assisting the Family

Financial

Medicare. Ever since Congress passed PL 92-603 in 1972, the CKD program of Medicare has covered anyone under age 65 if they have renal or kidney failure. Thus, children with CKD can indeed qualify for Medicare. Of course, it is highly unlikely that a child could meet the quarters-of-work requirement, so either one or both of the parents' work histories can be used.

Medicaid. If neither parent has sufficient work quarters to qualify for Medicare, a real likelihood with teenage parents of an infant with CKD, a family with a limited income may qualify for Medicaid. This program is administered differently in each state, but essentially it is designed to pay for medical expenses for persons unable to fund their own medical care. The extent of the coverage and the application process also vary from state to state; the pediatric dialysis unit social worker should be able to guide patients' families concerning local procedures. If a family exceeds the income levels to qualify for Medicaid, exceptions may be made if a high percentage of the family's income is spent on medical costs. The family should be encouraged to explore this possibility.

Supplemental Security Income (SSI). This federal program supports aged, disabled, or blind individuals with limited income and assets (including cash, land, personal property, and life insurance). The monthly payments can be a temporary measure until the patient qualifies for Social Security Disability, an unlikely event for the pediatric patient, or can be a permanent source of income. One applies for this program at the local Social Security Office. Information is also available at www.ssa.gov.

Handicapped Children's Assistance. This program will have different names, application procedures, and coverage in different states. Crippled Children's Assistance and Children with Special Health Care Needs are two examples. Many states offer assistance to families without access to health insurance with an affordable alternative administered by the state. Eligibility and availability vary from state to state. Generally, these programs help with the medical expenses arising from catastrophic diseases and may provide other services as well.

Private support. Local agencies, communities, and/or states may have private funds available to help specific beneficiaries, such as pediatric renal failure patients. These funds often arise in aid of a particular patient and then continue as a memorial to that patient. Churches or community groups may offer short- or long-term financial aid to a family (Dracopoulos & Weatherly, 1983). Some families even choose to start such a fund for themselves but should be warned that excessive fund-raising may affect their qualification for governmental assistance programs or programs funded by other sources.

Method I versus Method II payments. Families who will be performing any type of dialysis therapy at home are required to sign HCFA Form 382-U4 when a child has reached Stage V kidney disease and is certified by the physician on HCFA Form 2728. It is purely up to the family whether to select Method I or Method II for payments. However, most families are completely overwhelmed with the diagnosis of CKD and with their new responsibility to learn to care for the child at home. They frequently turn to the dialysis center staff for guidance in making this decision. One may reassure them that the net effect on the family by the choice of Method I or Method II is probably not very different. The backup support and care they receive from the dialysis center is the same. The kind of bills that will show up in their mailbox is the same. The major distinction is that they will be required to contact the vendor to arrange for supply delivery if they select Method II. For intelligent or medically sophisticated families, this is not a daunting concept. Those new to the medical system will probably find it much easier to select Method I and let the center do the supply procurement work.

Should the family become unhappy with their Method selection, it is always possible to change. However, the window opens for change only once each year on January 1. The treatment center should get the paperwork signed and submitted by mid-December so beginning the new Method at the first of the New Year is not problematic.

The undocumented family. Recent immigrants, especially those who are undocumented, face many challenges. For example, these families are not eligible for either Medicare or Medicaid coverage of ESRD care. Most facilities for children will try to find other sources of payment, such as private donations for dialysis. However, costs involved in transplantation can be prohibitive. It is not uncommon for transplant facilities to require prepayment of expenses for the transplant and the first year's postoperative care and medication in advance.

Often, services for the child are extremely limited or not available in their home country, so that returning to the homeland is not a welcome option.

Most often, English is not the family's first language. The child with CKD or a sibling may be called upon to be the family's translator, which is not an ideal arrangement. Most hospitals have translators available, but some smaller freestanding units may need to access translation services over the telephone.

Information Sources

When first presented with the diagnosis that their child has CKD, most families are overwhelmed. For many the next step is to gather as much information as they can find. The pediatric dialysis unit will have information about the specific treatment modality selected for the child, as well as how their unit functions in general. For information about kidney disease, all treatment modalities available, and sources of both financial and psychosocial assistance, parents may contact their local chapter of the National Kidney Foundation and the American Kidney Fund, or their local CKD Network office (The Renal Network, 2004).

The National Institute of Diabetes and Digestive and Kidney Disease (NIDDK), part of the National Institutes of Health (NIH), also has booklets, fact sheets, information packets, catalogs, and guides available at minimal prices. In addition, it offers comprehensive lists of professional-level articles available by treatment modality, as well as a newsletter, KU Notes, describing the latest developments and information available about kidney and urologic disease.

Most organizations, companies, professional societies, and special interest groups have informational Web sites. In addition, there are some chat rooms run by nephrology professionals and families of pediatric nephrology patients where pediatric patients and family members can exchange information with others in similar situations (See http://therenalnetwork.org/RenalLinks/OtherRenalLinks.html). As with most chronic illnesses, there is a real lack of instructional material available at a level appropriate for younger children. Several organizations, companies, and pediatric dialysis centers have identified this problem and are working on developing material at reading levels appropriate for preschool, school age, and teenage patients.

Summary

Care for children with CKD is a complex but rewarding nursing task. The pediatric nephrology patient is not just a tiny adult but a member of a special patient population with unique requirements. Children differ markedly from adults in their physiological responses to CKD, and treatment regimens differ considerably. Furthermore, the child with renal failure is not a discreet entity but part of a family unit.

In order to provide successful care, the pediatric nephrology nurse must recognize the total impact of renal failure on the child and all family members and plan to meet the needs of everyone in the family. Careful attention must be given to growth and development issues, nutrition, psychosocial support, and educational achievement, in addition to the special techniques required for performing successful renal replacement therapies on pediatric patients. Development of the child needs to be considered continually in every aspect of care, and adaptations must be made as the child matures. Because the child with CKD has a much longer total remaining life span than the adult CKD patient, the pediatric nephrology nurse's work has a far-reaching impact.

References

Alexander, S.R. (1990). Controversies in pediatric renal transplantation. *American Kidney Fund Letter, 7,* 5-21.

Andreoli, S.P., Langefeld, C.D., Stadler, S., Smith, P., Sears, A., & West, K. (1993). Risks of peritoneal membrane failure in children undergoing long-term peritoneal dialysis. *Pediatric Nephrology, 7,* 543-547.

Beck, A.L., Nethercut, G.E., Crittenden, M.R., & Hewins, J. (1986). Visibility of handicap, self-concept, and social maturity among young adult survivors of end stage renal disease. *Developmental and Behavioral Pediatrics, 7,* 93-96.

Bell, S.B. (1988). CAVH in pediatrics: Meeting the challenge. *ANNA Journal, 15,* 25-26.

Benfield, M.R. (2003). Current status of kidney transplant: Update 2003. *Pediatric Clinics of North America, 50,*1301-1343.

Benfield, M.R., & Bunchman, T.E. (2004). Management of acute renal failure. In E.D. Avner, W.E. Harmon, & P. Niaudet (Eds.), *Pediatric nephrology* (5th ed.) (pp. 1253-1266). Philadelphia: Lippincott Williams and Wilkins.

Benfield, M., & Michael, A.F. (1992). Immunology of uremia. In C.M. Edelmann (Ed.), *Pediatric kidney disease* (2nd ed.) (pp. 783-790). Boston: Little, Brown and Company.

Benfield, M., Parker, K.L., Waldo, F.B., Overstreet, S.L., & Kohaut, E.C. (1993). Treatment of growth failure in children after renal transplantation. *Transplantation, 55,* 305-308.

Betz, C.L., & Sowden, L.A. (2004). *Mosby's pediatric nursing reference* (5th ed.). St. Louis: Mosby.

Brem, A.S., Lambert, C., Hill, C., Kitsen, J., & Shemin, D.G. (2001). Clinical morbidity in pediatric dialysis patients: Data from the network 1 clinical indicators project. *Pediatric Nephrology, 16,* 854-857.

Chadha, V., Warady, B.A., Blowey, D.L., Simckes, A.M., & Alon, U.S. (2000). Tenckhoff catheters prove superior to cook catheters in pediatric acute peritoneal dialysis. *American Journal of Kidney Diseases, 35,* 1111-1116.

Chavers, B., & Schnaper, H.W. (2001). Risk factors for cardiovascular disease in children on maintenance dialysis. *Advances in Renal Replacement Therapy, 8,* 180-190.

Crocker, J.F.S., Acott, P.D., Carter, J.E.J., Lirenman, D.S., MacDonald, G.W., McAllister, M., Mc Donnell, M.C., Shea, S., & Bawden, H.N. (2002). Neuropsychological outcome in children with acquired or congenital renal disease. *Pediatric Nephrology, 17,* 908-912.

Dell, K.M., McDonald, R.A., Watkins, S.L., & Avner, E.D. (2004). Polycystic kidney disease. In E.D. Avner, W.E. Harmon, & P. Niaudet (Eds.), *Pediatric nephrology* (5th ed.) (pp. 675-699). Philadelphia: Lippincott Williams and Wilkins.

Dracopoulos, D.T., & Weatherly, J.B. (1983). Chronic renal failure: The effects on the entire family. *Issues in Comprehensive Pediatric Nursing, 6,* 141-146.

Ehrich, J.H., Rizzoni, G., Broyer, M., Brunner, F.P., Brynger, H., Fassbinder, W., Geerlings, W., Selwood, N.H., Tufveson, G., & Wing, A.J. (1992). *Nephrology Dialysis and Transplantation, 7,* 579-586.

Evans, J.H.C., Smye, S.W., & Brocklebank, J.T. (1992). Mathematical modeling of haemodialysis in children. *Pediatric Nephrology, 6,* 343-353.

Fennell, R.S., Fennell, E.B., Carter, R.L., Mings, E.L., Klausner, A.B., & Hurst, J.R. (1990). A longitudinal study of the cognitive function of children with renal failure. *Child Nephrology and Urology, 10,* 199-204.

Fielding, D., & Brownbridge, G. (1999). Factors related to psychosocial adjustment in children with end stage renal failure. *Pediatric Nephrology, 13,* 766-770.

Fine, R.N., Koch, V.H., Boechat, M.I., Lippe, B.H., Nelson, P.A., Fine, S.E., & Sherman, B.M. (1994). Growth after recombinant human growth hormone treatment in children with chronic renal failure: Report of a multicenter randomized double-blind placebo controlled study. *Journal of Pediatrics, 124,* 374-382.

Fine, R.N., Sullivan, E.K., & Tejani, A. (2000). The impact of recombinant human growth hormone treatment on final adult height. *Pediatric Nephrology, 14,* 679-681.

Frankenfield, D.L., Neu, A.M., Warady, B.A., Watkins, S.L., Friedman, A.L., & Fivush, B.A. (2002). Adolescent hemodialysis: Results of the 2000 ESRD clinical performance measures project. *Pediatric Nephrology, 17,*10-15.

Frauman, A.C., & Gilman, C.M. (1985). "Normal life" - A goal for the child with chronic renal failure. *ANNA Journal, 12,* 192-195.

Frauman, A.C., & Gilman, C.M. (1989). Creating a therapeutic environment in a pediatric renal unit. *ANNA Journal, 16,* 20-22, 26.

Frauman, A.C., & Gilman, C.M. (1990). Care of the family of the child with end stage renal disease. *ANNA Journal, 17,* 383-386, 401.

Frauman, A.C., Gilman, C.M., & Carlson, J.R. (1996). Rehabilitation and social and adaptive development of young renal transplant recipients. *ANNA Journal, 23,* 467-471,484.

Frauman, A.C., & Myers J.T. (1994). Cognitive, psychosocial, and physical development in infants and children with end stage renal disease. *Advances in Renal Replacement Therapy, 1,* 49-54.

Fuchshuber, A., Kuhnemund, O., Keuth, B., Lutticken, R., Michalk, D., & Auerfeld, U. (1996). Pneumococcal vaccine in children and young adults with chronic renal disease. *Nephrology Dialysis and Transplant, 11,* 468-473.

Furth, S.L., Hogg, R.J., Tarver, J., Moulton, L.H., Chan, C., & Fivush, B.A. (2003). Varicella vaccination in children with chronic renal failure. *Pediatric Nephrology, 18,* 33-38.

Gilman, C.M., & Frauman, A.C. (1979). Psychosocial care of the child in renal failure. *AANNT Journal, 6,* 143-148.

Gilman, C.M., & Frauman, A.C. (1982). Dialysis desensitization: Preparation of the very young child for chronic hemodialysis. *Dialysis and Transplantation, 11,* 660-661.

Gilman, C.M., & Frauman, A.C. (1987). Use of play with the child with chronic illness. *AANNT Journal, 14,* 259-261.

Goldstein, S.L. (2001). Hemodialysis in the pediatric patient: State of the art. *Advances in Renal Replacement Therapy, 8,* 173-179.

Goldstein, S.L., & Jabs, K. (2004). Hemodialysis. In E.D. Avner, W.E. Harmon, & P. Niaudet (Eds.), *Pediatric nephrology* (5th ed.) (pp. 1395-1410). Philadelphia: Lippincott Williams and Wilkins.

Gruskin, A.B., Baluarte, H.J., & Dabbagh, S. (1992). Hemodialysis and peritoneal dialysis. In C.M. Edelmann (Ed.), *Pediatric kidney disease* (2nd ed.) (pp. 827-916). Boston: Little, Brown and Company.

Gunn, V.L., & Nechyba, C. (2002). *The Harriet Lane handbook. A manual for pediatric house officers.* Philadelphia: Mosby.

Hardgrove, C. (1980). Children respond to therapeutic art. *Hospitals, 54,* 67-69.

Harmon, W.E., & Jabs, K. (1994). Hemodialysis. In M.A. Holliday, T.M. Barratt, & E.D. Avner (Eds.), *Pediatric nephrology* (3rd ed.) (pp. 1354-1372). Baltimore: Williams & Wilkins.

Harvey, E.A. (2001). Peritoneal access in children. *Peritoneal Dialysis International, 21,* S218-S222.

Hergenroeder, A.C., & Brewer, E.D. (2001). A survey of pediatric nephrologists on adolescent sexual health. *Pediatric Nephrology, 16,* 57-60.

Hisano, S., Miyazaki, C., Hatae, K., Kaku, Y., Yamane, I., Ueda, K., & Okamua, S. (1991). Immune status of children on continuous ambulatory peritoneal dialysis. *Pediatric Nephrology, 6,* 179-181.

Hislop, S., & Lansing, L. (1983). A comparison of pediatric home peritoneal dialysis modalities: The family point of view. *AANNT Journal, 11,* 22-23, 53.

Hockenberry, M.J, & Wong, D.L. (2004). *Wong's clinical manual of pediatric nursing.* St. Louis: Mosby.

Jain, S.R., Smith, L., Brewer, E.D., & Goldstein, S.L. (2001). Non-invasive intravascular monitoring in the pediatric hemodialysis population. *Pediatric Nephrology, 16,* 15-18.

Johnson, K.B. (Ed.). (1993). *The Harriet Lane handbook: A manual for pediatric house officers* (13th ed.). St. Louis: Mosby-Year Book, Inc.

Keen, M.L., & Gotch, F.A. (1991). Dialyzers and delivery systems. In M.G. Cogan & P. Schoenfeld (Eds.), *Introduction to dialysis* (2nd ed.) (pp. 1-44). New York: Churchill Livingstone.

Kjellstrand, C.M., Shideman, J.R., Santiago, E.A., Mauer, S.M., Simmons, R.L., & Buselmeier, T.J. (1971). Technical advances in hemodialysis of very small pediatric patients. *Proceedings of the Dialysis and Transplant Forum,* 124-132.

Koch, V.H., Lippe, B.M., Nelson, P.A., Boechat, M.I., Sherman, M.M., & Fine, R. (1989). Accelerated growth after recombinant human growth hormone treatment of children with chronic renal failure. *Journal of Pediatrics, 115,* 365-371.

Laube, G.F., Berger, C., Goetschel, P., Leumann, E., Neuhaus, T.J. (2002). Immunizations in children with chronic renal failure. *Pediatric Nephrology, 17,* 638-642.

Leonard, M.B., Donaldson, L.A., Ho, M., & Geary, D.F. (2003). A prospective cohort study of incident maintenance dialysis in children: An NAPRTC study. *Kidney International, 63,* 744-755.

Limwongse, C., & Cassidy, S.B. (2004). Syndromes and malformations of the urinary tract. In E.D. Avner, W.E. Harmon, & P. Niaudet (Eds.), *Pediatric nephrology* (5th ed.) (pp. 93-121). Philadelphia: Lippincott Williams & Wilkins.

Macias, W.L., Mueller, B.A., Scarim, S.K., Robinson, M., & Rudy, D.W. (1991). Continuous venovenous hemofiltration: An alternative to continuous arteriovenous hemofiltration and hemodiafiltration in acute renal failure. *American Journal of Kidney Diseases, 18,* 451-458.

McBride, P. (1984) The development of hemo- and peritoneal dialysis. In A.R. Nissenson, R.N. Fine, & D.E. Gentile (Eds.), *Clinical dialysis* (pp. 1-26). Norwalk, CT: Appleton-Century-Crofts.

McCann, L. (Ed.). (2002). *Pocket guide to nutrition assessment of the patient with chronic kidney disease* (3rd ed.). [Brochure]. New York: Council on Renal Nutrition of the National Kidney Foundation.

McCarthy, J.T., Williams, A.W., & Johnson, W.J. (1994). Serum beta-2 microglobulin concentration in dialysis patients: Importance of intrinsic renal function. *Journal of Laboratory and Clinical Medicine, 123,* 495-505.

Mehls, O., Blum, W.F., Schaefer, F., Tonshoff, B., & Scharer, K. (1992). Growth failure in renal disease. *Bailliere's Clinical Endocrinology and Metabolism, 6,* 665-685.

Miller, D., Macdonald, D., Kolnacki, K., & Simek, T. (2004). Challenges for nephrology nurses in the management of children with chronic kidney disease. *Nephrology Nursing Journal, 31,* 287-294.

Mogyorosi, A.M. & Ziyadeh, F.N. (2001). Diabetic nephropathy. In S.G. Massry & R.J. Glassock (Eds.), *Massry & Glassock's textbook of nephrology* (4th ed.) (pp. 874-895). Philadelphia: Lippincott Williams & Wilkins.

Morel, P., Almond, P.S., Matas, A.J., Gillingham, K.J., Chau, C., Brown, A., et al. (1991). Long-term quality of life after kidney transplantation in childhood. *Transplantation, 52,* 47-53.

Morgan, H.E.G., Gautam, M., & Geary, D.F. (2001). Maintenance intravenous iron therapy in pediatric hemodialysis patients. *Pediatric Nephrology, 16,* 779-783.

Moritz, M.L., Vats, A., & Ellis, D. (2003). Systemic anticoagulation and bleeding in children with hemodialysis catheters. *Pediatric Nephrology, 18,* 68-70.

Nightingale, F. (1859). *Notes on nursing: What it is and what it is not.* London: Harrison Publishing.

North American Pediatric Renal Transplant Cooperative Study (NAPRTCS). (2004). *2004 annual report.* Boston: Author.

O'Grady, N.P., Alexander, M., Dellinger, E.P., Gerberding, J.L., Heard, S.O., Maki, D.G., et al. (2002), Guidelines for the prevention of intravascular catheter-related infections. *Morbidity and Mortality Weekly Report, 51,* 1-26.

Ouwendyk, M., Leitch, R., & Freitas, T. (2001). Daily hemodialysis: A nursing perspective. *Advances in Renal Replacement Therapy, 8,* 257-267.

Parekh, R.S., Carroll, C.E., Wolfe, R.A., & Port, F.K. (2002). Cardiovascular mortality in children and young adults with end-stage kidney disease. *The Journal of Pediatrics, 141,* 191-197.

Polinsky, M.S., Kaiser, B.A., & Stover, J.B. (1987). Neurologic development of children with severe chronic renal failure from infancy. *Pediatric Nephrology, 1,* 157-165.

Rigden, S. (1994). Planning therapy. In M.A. Holliday, T.M. Barratt, & E.D. Avner (Eds.), *Pediatric nephrology* (3rd ed.) (pp. 1419-1422). Baltimore: Williams & Wilkins.

Rosenkranz, J., Bonzel, K.E., & Bulla, M. (1992). Psychosocial adaptation of children and adolescents with chronic renal failure. *Pediatric Nephrology, 6,* 459-463.

Sadler, T. W. (2000). *Langman's medical embryology* (8th ed.). Philadelphia: Lippincott Williams & Wilkins.

Sharma, A.K. (2001). Reassessing hemodialysis adequacy in children: The case for more. *Pediatric Nephrology, 16,* 383-390.

Shemesh, D., Olsha, O., Mabjeesh, N.J., & Abramowitz, H.B. (2001). Dialysis access induced limb ischemia corrected using quantitative duplex ultrasound. *Pediatric Nephrology, 16,* 409-411.

Shroff, R., Wright, E., Ledermann, S., Hutchinson, C., & Rees, L. (2003). Chronic hemodialysis in infants and children under 2 years of age. *Pediatric Nephrology, 18,* 378-383.

Solhaug, M.J., Adelman, R.D., & Chan, J.C.M. (1992). Hypertension in the child with chronic renal insufficiency or undergoing dialysis. *Child Nephrology and Urology, 12,* 133-138.

Soliday, E., Kool, E., & Lande, M.B. (2001). Family environment, child behavior, and medical indicators in children with kidney disease. *Child Psychiatry and Human Development, 31,* 279-295.

Smith, J.M. & McDonald, R.A. (2000). Progress in renal transplantation for children. *Advances in Renal Replacement Therapy, 7,* 158-171.

Stapleton, S., & Wright, J. (1992). Continuous arteriovenous hemofiltration: An alternative dialysis therapy in neonates. *Neonatal Network, 11,* 17-25.

Stephens, F.D., Smith, E.D., & Hutson, J.M. (2002). *Congenital anomalies of the kidney, urinary and genital tracts* (2nd ed.). London: Martin Dunitz.

Suddaby, E.C., Bell, S.B., & Murphy, K.J. (1990). Continuous hemofiltration in infants and children. *Pediatric Nursing, 16,* 79-82.

Thompson, G.N., Butt, W.W., Shann, F.A., Kirby, D.M., Henning, R.D., Howells, D.W., & Osborne, A. (1991). Continuous venovenous hemofiltration in the management of acute decompensation in inborn errors of metabolism. *The Journal of Pediatrics, 118,* 879-884.

The Renal Network. (2004). *Other renal links.* Retrieved from http://therenalnetwork.org/RenalLinks/OtherRenalLinks.html.

United States Renal Data System (USRDS). (2003). *United States Renal Data System 2003 annual data report* (NIH Publication No. 93-3176). Bethesda, MD: U.S. Government Printing Office.

Valeri, A., Radhakrishnan, J., Vernocchi, L, Carmichael, L.D., & Stern, L. (1993). The epidemiology of peritonitis in acute peritoneal dialysis: A comparison between open- and closed-drainage systems. *American Journal of Kidney Diseases, 21,* 300-309.

Verrina, E., Honda, M., Warady, B.A., & Piraino, B. (2000). Prevention of peritonitis in children on peritoneal dialysis. *Peritoneal Dialysis International, 20,* 625-630.

Warady, B.A., Morganstern, B.Z., & Alexander, S.R. (2004). Peritoneal dialysis. In E.D. Avner, W.E. Harmon, & P. Niaudet (Eds.), *Pediatric nephrology* (5th ed.) (pp. 1375-1394). Philadelphia: Lippincott Williams and Wilkins.

Warady, B.A., Schaefer, F., Alexander, S.R., Firanek, C., & Mujais, S. (2004). *Care of the pediatric patient on peritoneal dialysis – Clinical process for optimal outcomes.* [Brochure]. Deerfield, IL: Baxter Healthcare Corporation.

Watkins, S.L., & Richards, G.E. (2004). Evaluation of growth and development. In E.D. Avner, W.E. Harmon, & P. Niaudet (Eds.), *Pediatric nephrology* (5th ed.) (pp. 425-448). Philadelphia: Lippincott Williams and Wilkins.

Watson, A.R. (1995). Strategies to support families of children with end stage renal failure. *Pediatric Nephrology, 9,* 628-631.

Zobel, G., Stein, J.I., Kuttnig, M., Beitzke, A., Metzler, H., & Rigler, B. (1991). Continuous extracorporeal fluid removal in children with low cardiac output after cardiac operations. *The Journal of Thoracic and Cardiovascular Surgery, 101,* 593-597.

- Kidney disease, its symptoms, and the side effects of treatment present many impediments to attaining a normal lifestyle. Each of the treatment modalities commonly used for children with CKD imposes time constraints and limitations that detract from the ability to attend school and play as other healthy children do (Fielding & Brownbridge, 1999).

- Treatment modalities for children differ sharply from those of adults, with far greater use of peritoneal dialysis (PD) and transplant as first modality, compared with adults (USRDS, 2003).

- The most frequent causes of CKD in children can be broken down into two major categories: congenital and acquired (USRDS, 2003).

- Many of the effects of renal failure on children and adults are identical; others are markedly different due in part to children's unique metabolic state that results from growth, their height-to-weight ratio, and their higher percentage of body water.

- Renal failure in children will affect the following systems: cardiac, cutaneous, gastrointestinal, genitourinary, hematologic, metabolic, neuromuscular, pulmonary, skeletal, immune, and growth and development.

- The number of pediatric patients on chronic HD has increased over the last decade due to loss of peritoneal membrane function in some children, loss of renal transplant function, or a home environment that is not suitable for either performing PD or maintaining a transplant (Goldstein, 2001).

- There are many different techniques to use in performing PD. IPD, CAPD, and CCPD, which is sometimes called automated peritoneal dialysis (APD), are the ones routinely used with pediatric patients. The latter two modalities are sometimes called continuous peritoneal dialysis (CPD).

- CRRTs are the most recently developed treatment modalities being used on children. There are several forms of CRRT. Those used on children include continuous arteriovenous hemofiltration (CAVH), continuous venovenous hemofiltration (CVVH), continuous venovenous hemofiltration with dialysis (CVVHD), and continuous venovenous hemodiafiltration (CVVHDF). Slow continuous ultrafiltration (SCUF) and therapeutic plasma exchange (TPE) are also available but are infrequently used in the pediatric renal failure patient population.

- Living related donor (LD) transplants are much more likely in children than adults, with 60% of children receiving kidneys from a parent (56% mothers, 44% fathers) (Benfield, 2003). Preemptive transplantation is more common in children than in adults because of the availability of living donors. In the U.S., approximately 20% of children receive preemptive transplants.

- Children may reach a point where treatment options have been exhausted, or particularly in the case of children with multiple handicaps or developmental delay, parents may decide that to proceed with further treatment is futile. Those providing care for the child and parents will need to continue, with a focus on palliation rather than treatment.

- The purpose of nursing intervention for the child and family is to promote independence from health care providers; normality in lifestyle; and optimal emotional, physical, mental, and social development.

- Children with complex physical problems often come from families with complex problems as well. Family relationships do not always conform to societal expectations, and they are not always what they seem on the surface. As there are many possible configurations for families, it is best to let the members define the scope of their particular family group (Frauman & Gilman, 1990).

- Family members should be encouraged to expect the child with CKD to make progress toward developmental milestones in the normal chronological order, if not at the usual ages. Making adaptations to assist the child's progress may be necessary. However, mastering self-care skills, going to school, participating in extracurricular activities as well as activities of daily living, finishing school, and progressing to employment are normal goals for all children.

- Programs that are available to financially assist the family of a child with CKD include Medicare, Medicaid, Supplemental Security Insurance (SSI), and Handicapped Children's Assistance agencies. In addition, support services are available through the National Kidney Foundation (NKF) and the American Kidney Fund (AKF), or local CKD Network offices (The Renal Network, 2004). The National Institute of Diabetes and Digestive and Kidney Disease (NIDDK), which is part of the National Institutes of Health (NIH), also has booklets, fact sheets, information packets, catalogs, and guides.

ANNP620   **The Child with Kidney Disease**

Cyrena Gilman, MN, RN, CNN, and Annette Frauman, PhD, RN, FAAN

Contemporary Nephrology Nursing: Principles and Practice contains 39 chapters of educational content. Individual learners may apply for continuing nursing education credit by reading a chapter and completing the Continuing Education Evaluation Form for that chapter. Learners may apply for continuing education credit for any or all chapters.

Please photocopy this page and return to ANNA.
COMPLETE THE FOLLOWING:

Name: _____

Address:_____

City:_____State:_____Zip:_____

E-mail:_____

Preferred telephone: ☐ Home   ☐ Work: _____

State where licensed and license number (optional): _____

CE application fees are based upon the number of contact hours provided by the individual chapter. CE fees per contact hour for ANNA members are as follows: 1.0-1.9 - $15; 2.0-2.9 - $20; 3.0-3.9 - $25; 4.0 and higher - $30. Fees for nonmembers are $10 higher.

ANNA Member: ☐ Yes   ☐ No   Member # (if available) _____

☐ Checked Enclosed   ☐ American Express   ☐ Visa   ☐ MasterCard

Total Amount Submitted: _____

Credit Card Number: _____ Exp. Date: _____

Name as it appears on the card: _____

CE Evaluation Form
To receive continuing education credit for individual study after reading the chapter
1. Photocopy this form. (You may also download this form from ANNA's Web site, **www.annanurse.org**.)
2. Mail the completed form with payment (check) or credit card information to American Nephrology Nurses' Association, East Holly Avenue, Box 56, Pitman, NJ 08071-0056.
3. You will receive your CE certificate from ANNA in 4 to 6 weeks.

Test returns must be postmarked by **December 31, 2010.**

CE Application Fee
ANNA Member $25.00
Nonmember $35.00

EVALUATION FORM

1. I verify that I have read this chapter and completed this education activity. Date: _____

    _____
    Signature

2. What would be different in your practice if you applied what you learned from this activity? *(Please use additional sheet of paper if necessary.)*

    _____
    _____
    _____
    _____
    _____
    _____
    _____
    _____
    _____
    _____
    _____
    _____
    _____
    _____

Evaluation	Strongly disagree				Strongly agree
3. The activity met the stated objectives.					
a. Summarize the etiologies of CKD in children.	1	2	3	4	5
b. Describe the effects of renal failure in children.	1	2	3	4	5
c. Correlate the specific nursing interventions necessary to the treatment modality being used.	1	2	3	4	5
d. Generate a plan of care aimed at gaining a normallife for a child with CKD.	1	2	3	4	5
4. The content was current and relevant.	1	2	3	4	5
5. The content was presented clearly.	1	2	3	4	5
6. The content was covered adequately.	1	2	3	4	5
7. Rate your ability to apply the learning obtained from this activity to practice.	1	2	3	4	5

Comments _____
_____

8. Time required to read the chapter and complete this form: _____ minutes.

This educational activity has been provided by the American Nephrology Nurses' Association (ANNA) for 3.5 contact hours. ANNA is accredited as a provider of continuing nursing education (CNE) by the American Nurses Credentialing Center's Commission on Accreditation (ANCC-COA). ANNA is an approved provider of continuing education by the California Board of Registered Nursing, CEP 0910.

The Young and Middle Aged Adult with Chronic Kidney Disease

Leanne Dekker, MBA, MN, RN

Chapter Contents

The Young and Middle Aged Adult with Chronic Kidney Disease

Chapter 21

Leanne Dekker, MBA, MN, RN

Depending on the practice setting, nephrology nurses provide care to persons of all ages, as chronic kidney disease (CKD) and end stage renal disease (ESRD) can occur at any point in a person's life. Across the lifecycle, the prevalent cause of renal disease will differ as will the focus of care and the individualized nursing interventions required for quality care. The goal of nephrology nursing remains constant: to provide quality care supporting people with chronic kidney disease and their family to attain the highest possible quality of life.

In this chapter, the focus is on the care of the young and middle aged adult with chronic kidney disease. Young adults are those persons aged 20 to 44 years, while middle age is considered as the following 2 decades, the years between 45 and 64. The care requirement for these patients is important, as, collectively, patients aged 20 to 64 years represent 63.5% of the 406,000 people in the United States living with renal replacement therapy (hemodialysis, peritoneal dialysis, or a functional kidney transplant) in 2001 (United States Renal Data System [USRDS], 2003). Following an overview of the demographics of the patient population, the physiological and psychosocial implications of chronic renal failure and chronic disease in these two age groups are described. Nursing interventions directed towards supporting maximal health, well-being, and independence for this group of patients and their families are also presented.

Demographics

The USRDS reports that in 2001 the average age of persons undergoing treatment for ESRD in the United States was 58.7 years, an increase largely attributable to the growing number of persons beginning treatment at an older age. Small variations in the age of persons living with ESRD are found across ethnic groups with the average age being 58.9 years for Whites, 56.0 for Blacks, 57.0 for Native Americans, 58.2 for Asians, and 56.2 for Hispanics (USRDS, 2003). Despite the small increase in average age, in absolute numbers the largest segment of patients living with ESRD continues to be persons aged 45 to 65 years. In 2001, nearly 50% of patients beginning treatment were aged between 20 and 64 years, 12,753 (13.7%) in the 20 to 44 year range, and 33,332 (35.7%) in the 45 to 64 year age group (USRDS, 2003).

The growth in the ESRD population aged between 44 and 65 is projected to continue as the baby boomer generation reaches middle age. Some of this growth will be mitigated, as health promotion initiatives and targeted strategies to reduce the progression of chronic renal disease to ESRD continue. The USRDS (2003) reports that the incident rates for new patients commencing treatment appear to be leveling, with only a 1% increase in incidence noted between 2000 and 2001.

In terms of cause of renal disease, the incident rates for glomerulonephritis have declined 12% since peaking in 1995 (USRDS, 2003). However, diabetes and hypertension continue to drive growth in patient numbers. It is projected that by 2006 the number of patients with chronic renal failure from diabetes who are entering treatment will equal that of all other conditions. In a similar manner, the number of patients with renal failure resulting from hypertension grew 50% between 1990 and 2001 (USRDS, 2003). The USRDS projects continued growth in the number of young and middle aged adults receiving treatment, as patients are living longer with ESRD due to improvements in mortality and morbidity rates.

Mortality and Morbidity

Improvements in mortality and morbidity of young and middle aged adults with ESRD are impacting growth in patient numbers. Overall mortality decreased 10% since 1988 with the greatest gains found in the first 2 years following initiation of renal replacement treatment, where a reduction of 23% occurred since 1985 (USRDS, 2003). In contrast, mortality rates for vintage patients (those receiving treatment for 5 years or longer) decreased between 1988 and 1994, but has risen 12% since 1994. This shift in mortality suggests that the young and middle aged adult, while living longer with treatment, continues to experience a long-term survival less than that of the general population (USRDS, 2003). In the United States, life expectancy for the general population has risen by 0.2 years annually since 1971 (Arias, 2004). A person aged 45 years is projected to survive an additional 34.3 years (32 years if male; 36.3 years if female). In contrast, patients aged between 40 to 44 years undergoing dialysis treatment have a projected survival of 20% that of their healthy counterpart (7.4 years if male; 7.2 if female). Projected survival rates for transplant patients are higher: 20 years for males and 22.8 for females (USRDS, 2003). Similar reductions are found in projected survival for persons with ESRD aged 60-64 years, where the projected survival is 17.7 years (16.1 males; 19.5 females) for persons aged 65 years. The rate for patients on dialysis aged between 60 to 64 years is reduced to less than 4 years (3.9 males; 3.8 females), and transplant patients have a projected survival rate of less than 13 years (10.6 males; 12.8 years) (USRDS, 2003).

In terms of morbidity, hospitalization rates among ESRD patients have shown an overall reduction of 1% since 1993. This reduction is considered to be directly attributed to the 24% reduction in hospitalization for vascular access (USRDS, 2003). However, the reduction in hospitalization of ESRD patients for vascular access problems was countered by an increase of 13.5% in hospitalization for circulatory and 11.5% for respiratory reasons. The rate of hospitalization for ESRD patients aged 20 to 44 in 2001 was slightly less (1,874 per 1,000 patient years of treatment) than the hospitalization rate for those aged 45-64 years (1,973 per 1,000 patient years). Rates for transplant patients were markedly lower at 939 for the 20-44 year age group and 893 for those aged 45 to 64 (USRDS, 2003).

Health Belief Model and the Meaning of Chronic Illness

Research into the meaning of chronic illness has found that the term is not used consistently, primarily because of the diversity in what is termed a chronic illness. For example, some chronic illnesses are not severe enough to result in impairment or activity changes (Sidell, 1997). Three frameworks for understanding health behaviors and chronic illness within the context of chronic renal failure are particularly useful. These are the health belief model (Becker & Maiman, 1975), the illness trajectory framework (Strauss et al., 1984), and Dimond's (1984) work on the meaning of chronic illness.

Health Belief Model

The focus of the health belief model is on the individual's own perceptions of the threat to health and benefits and barriers to adopting a particular health behavior (Becker & Maiman, 1975). In this model, the person determines health actions based on the perceived likelihood of developing the health risk, complication, or illness. As well, the personal perspective of the severity of the illness is considered in terms of the impact on one's life. The model suggests that health behavior depends on how much an individual values a particular goal and on his or her judgment that a particular action will achieve that goal (Morgan, 2000; Ross, 2001). The concept of self-efficacy within the health belief model is also useful to understand behaviors supporting chronic illness care (Becker & Maiman, 1975).

Self-efficacy impacts behaviors related to chronic illness care, which include decisions on whether to adhere to the treatment regimen. In the same manner, adherence is seen as self-determined based on beliefs about the disease, its severity, and the perceived benefits of adhering to the prescribed treatment (Morgan, 2000). Kaveh and Kimmel (2001) agree indicating that the health care team must understand the patient's and family's expectations and attitudes regarding the illness when assisting the person in developing mutually agreed upon compliance goals.

Meaning of Chronic Illness

Strauss and colleagues (1984) assert that chronic illness is long-term, characterized by intrusiveness, complexity, and uncertainty; the focus may be on palliation rather than cure. This is the case with chronic renal failure, where people have lived for decades following initiation of dialysis or kidney transplant. Dimond (1984) describes a three-level schemata for understanding the meaning of chronic illness that is very applicable to people living with chronic renal failure. In Dimond's framework, chronic illness is understood within three contexts: clinical, social, and personal meaning. Clinical definitions are based on anatomical or physiological manifestations. Family, friends, co-workers, healthcare workers, and others who relate with the person form social definitions of the illness. The personal meaning of the illness is the meaning held by the individual living with the illness. All three meanings are influenced by age, gender, cultural expectations, and the degree of visibility of any impairment (Dimond, 1984).

In their work on chronic illness, Strauss and his colleagues (1984) describe how the concept of an illness trajec-tory can be used to encompass the physiological changes associated with the disease and to reflect the work associated with managing the disease and its manifestations. The illness trajectory is also useful when considering the impact the disease, its manifestations, and treatments will have on the individual and his or her family. Factors that will impact an individual's illness trajectory are uncertainty, the personal meaning given the illness, and the capacity to manage the work associated with the illness (Molzahn & Kikuchi, 1998).

The concepts of health belief model, the social and personal meanings of chronic illness, and the illness trajectory are useful to consider as nurses care for patients and families living with renal disease. Nephrology nurses encounter patients with renal disease or those at risk for renal disease across the course of the illness trajectory. Interventions are provided from prevention of renal disease and renal failure to end-of-life care for patients and their families. At each point, it is important to consider the individual's and family's meanings of chronic illness in developing, implementing, and evaluating nursing interventions.

Given the nature of chronic renal disease and the success of renal replacement therapy, people with ESRD will experience a number of life transitions within their individual illness trajectory. Living their lives with renal disease, children become adolescents, adolescents become young adults, adults enter middle age, and the middle aged become elderly. Thus, it is useful to consider the developmental framework developed by Erickson (1980) when determining nursing management of the young and middle aged adult with chronic renal failure.

Developmental Tasks of Adults

Erickson (1980) describes young adulthood as that time of life when the focus of growth and development is on establishing intimacy, developing intimate relationships and understanding with others. During this period of life, mutual enrichment exists in intimate interactions. Individual well-being is enhanced through affectionate or intellectually stimulating interactions with others (Erickson, 1980). Sidell (1997) suggests that chronic illness in the young adult may interrupt the process of establishing intimacy; however, the person's ability to adjust to the illness is influenced in turn by the degree to which intimacy has been established. In caring for adults with renal disease, consideration must be given to the effects of the illness on the partner. Decisions regarding children or additional children and career and job planning must be considered within the limitations or unpredictability of the illness (Sidell, 1997).

In contrast, the developmental task of an adult in middle age is to manage a crisis of generation versus stagnation (Erickson, 1980). During the years of 40 to 54, attention is placed on actions to aid the welfare of others and on establishing or guiding the next generation. Sidell (1997) suggests that chronic illness during middle age will re-awaken struggles or conflicts experienced in earlier adulthood and may add to the frustration of the midlife crisis. Chronic illness also brings fear of dying or early aging, all of which will impact how the person manages the illness (Sidell, 1997).

Transition of Care for Young Adults

Of particular importance to the discussion of the care of the young adult is the transition of an adolescent to the world of adult health care. Data from the USRDS (2003) suggest that children aged 10 to 14 years at initiation of renal replacement therapy have an 86.6% likelihood of living 10 years. Thus, attention should be placed on how to assist the older adolescent to move from receiving care in a pediatric to an adult setting.

There is limited information on the nursing management of the adolescent's transition to being an adult with a chronic disease. The goal of transitional health care for adolescents and young adults has been identified as optimizing health and facilitating the young person's capacity to attain his or her potential (Rosen, Blum, Britto, Sawyer, & Siegel, 2003). Successful transition requires the active involvement of the adolescent, his or her family, and the care team. The use of a step-driven protocol sensitive to the patient's developmental, cognitive, and social situation has been found to support successful transition (Myers, 2002; Rosen et al., 2003; Scal, Evans, Blozis, Okinow, & Blum, 1999). Therefore, a transition plan should support physical functioning and also include anticipatory guidance for social functioning (Scal et al., 1999).

Recommendations from the Society for Adolescent Medicine (Rosen et al., 2003) for transition care include identifying a health care provider to assume responsibility for the transition within the broader context of care coordination. In this role, provision is made to develop and maintain detailed and written transition plans that include a portable, assessable medical summary to facilitate the smooth collaboration and transfer of care among and between health professionals. It is also important to ensure that the same standards for primary and preventive health care are applied to young people with chronic conditions as to their peers. An important policy issue related to transition care is the need for comprehensive continuous health insurance made available to young people throughout adolescence and into adulthood (Rosen et al., 2003).

Healthy Lifestyles and Quality of Life

There is a growing awareness of the importance of controlling underlying disease processes and promoting exercise to support improved functional outcome and quality of life in adult patients with chronic renal failure (Kutner, Zhang, & McClellen, 2000; Rahman & Smith, 1998). Control of underlying diseases in certain patient subgroups, such as persons with diabetes mellitus and hypertension, is linked to reduced patient mortality and morbidity as well as slower progression of renal disease, delaying the need for renal replacement therapy (Rahman & Smith, 1998). Christensen and Ehlers (2002) note the growing body of evidence that patient education and ongoing health assessment will slow the progression of renal disease and reduce morbidity. This effect is believed to be related to the increased adherence to medication and treatment regimens resulting from increased knowledge. Perceived social and family supports are also thought to reduce patient mortality in persons with chronic renal failure (Christensen, Wiebe, Smith, & Turner, 1994; Kimmel et al., 1998).

Promotion of a Healthy Lifestyle

In 2000, the American government reaffirmed its Healthy People initiative by developing strategies to improve health and reduce disease in the population (Office of Health Promotion and Disease Prevention [OHPDP], not dated). This initiative, now entitled *Healthy People 2010*, identifies a series of health indicators that are important to consider within the context of the young and middle aged adult with chronic renal failure. These are physical activity, overweight and obesity, tobacco use, substance abuse, responsible sexual behavior, mental health, injury and violence, environmental quality, immunization, and access to health care. The *Healthy People 2010* initiative has a specific focus on CKD, outlining strategies to prevent kidney disease, delay kidney failure, and promote healthy lifestyles for persons with ESRD (OHPDP, n.d.).

It is important in persons with chronic diseases, such as renal failure, that general health status continues to be assessed and that age specific investigations are included in the health assessment. Australian researchers found that routine health assessments of patients undergoing dialysis are often ignored. Jang and colleagues (2001) surveyed 48 adult women undergoing hemodialysis and found that more than half had not had a regular gynecological examination in the previous 2 years and that more than a third of the women over 50 years of age had not had a mammogram in this period.

The American Academy of Family Physicians (AAFP) (2004) guidelines on recommended preventive services for adult women and for adult men provide a useful framework for regular health assessments of young and middle aged adults. It is important that routine screening for cancers be included in the health and physical assessment plan for patients with chronic renal failure. The AAFP recommends that adult women over the age of 40 receive periodic (annual or biannual) mammograms to screen for breast cancer. A Pap smear is recommended for all women who have ever had sex and have a cervix at least every 3 years to screen for cervical cancer. In terms of colorectal cancer, all adults over the age of 50 years should be screened annually using fecal occult blood testing, sigmoidoscopy, or colonoscopy. Adults with a family history of colorectal cancer should have a complete colonoscopy prior to age 50. The AAFP (2004) notes that insufficient evidence is available to recommend routine screening in men for prostate cancer using prostate specific antigen (PSA) testing or digital rectal examination.

Attention should also be placed on the continuation of regular immunizations and promotion of healthy lifestyles. The AAFP (2004) recommends routine screening for congenital rubella syndrome in women of childbearing potential, the provision of diphtheria boosters every 10 years after the age of 50, annual immunization for influenza, and the use of pneumococcal vaccination in adults with chronic disease.

Health assessment practices with this age group should also include counselling on birth control for women of childbearing years and their partners and screening for sexually transmitted diseases. While uncommon, research suggests that pregnancy can occur in 1-7% of women on chronic dialysis who are within childbearing years and that half of the infants born to women on chronic dialysis survive

(Holley & Reddy, 2003). As well, counseling on maintaining a healthy weight; engaging in regular exercise; and limiting tobacco, alcohol, and other substance use should be included in the periodic health assessment.

Functional Status

Research suggests functional status and quality of life are associated with the individual person's capacity to self-manage aspects of renal failure and its treatment (Curtin & Mapes, 2001; Curtin, Mapes, Petillo & Oberley, 2002; Curtin, Bultman, Thomas-Hawkins, Walters & Schatell, 2002; Lev & Owen, 1998). In addition, a focus on patient education and vocational counseling has been shown to increase levels of employment following initiation of dialysis (Rasgon et al., 1993).

The relationship between symptoms commonly experienced by dialysis patients and physical and mental functioning has been examined. Curtin, Bultman, and colleagues (2002) questioned 307 adult patients on the frequency of 47 symptoms commonly reported by people undergoing hemodialysis. Symptoms reported by the group that were suggested to impact physical and mental functioning clustered around fatigue, tiredness, sexuality, and mobility. More than 90% of participants reported lack of energy and feeling tired, while 70% experienced dry mouth and itchy skin. Based on these findings, the researchers suggest that the primary goals of patient care should focus on preservation of the highest possible functioning with strategies directed towards symptom management.

Day-to-day variation in functional status has been described. Thomas-Hawkins (2000) found that variations in functional status correspond to the person's hemodialysis schedule. In this research, adults on dialysis reported a lower score for participation in social and community activities on the second dialysis day of the week when compared to the preceding and subsequent non-dialysis days. However, no differences were found in the person's completion of activities of daily living across dialysis days and non-dialysis days.

Participation in Regular Exercise

Increased attention has been placed on the relationship between involvement in physical exercise, functional status, and quality of life for adults with ESRD. In addition to reducing mortality (Kutner, Brogan, & Fielding, 1997), regular exercise by patients on dialysis has been suggested to reduce depression, anxiety, and hostility. As well, regular exercise in this population is associated with improved social adjustment and increases the person's sense of independence and control, thus resulting in improved well being and quality of life (Kouidi et al., 1997; Painter, Carlson, Carey, Paul, & Myll, 2000). Dialysis patients who engage in a small amount of regular exercise, 1 hour twice a week for 5 months, report improved self-rated health and physical functioning and a reduction in bodily pain (Molsted, Eidemak, Sorensen, & Kristensen, 2004).

More research is required, however, as conflicting results on the impact of regular exercise on physiological measures are found. Kouidi and colleagues (1998) note that while muscle atrophy improved in hemodialysis patients undergoing regular exercise, no change was found in blood pressure, total cholesterol, high and low density lipoproteins, and triglycerides. In another study, it was found that regular exercise improved cardiovascular function of hemodialysis patients, serving to reduce heart rate variability and blood pressure (Deligiannis, Kouidi, & Tourkanonis, 1999).

Understanding what prevents and motivates an adult with chronic renal failure to engage in exercise is important. Goodman and Ballou (2004) used a convenience sample of adults receiving hemodialysis within one outpatient clinic to study the barriers and motivators to exercise. In this group of patients, participation in exercise was low. The majority (83%) of patients in this sample reported that they were less active now than prior to commencing hemodialysis, with nearly half reporting that that they engaged in mild exercise for less than 15 minutes in a typical week (Goodman & Ballou, 2004). Barriers to exercise included lack of motivation and interest in exercise, a fear of falling, and limited access to exercise facilities. Inactivity and disease specific changes in muscle mass also serve as reasons for not exercising (Goodman & Ballou, 2004; Kouidi et al., 1998).

In contrast, factors identified by adults with chronic renal failure that motivated them to exercise included a personal belief in one's ability to be physically active, the desire to feel healthy, and a belief that exercise will result in less pain and decreased anxiety (Goodman & Ballou, 2004). A sense of improvement in everyday life has also been found to motivate people to exercise (Molsted et al., 2004). Family expectations towards participation in exercise were also indicated as reasons for exercise by a group of hemodialysis patients (Goodman & Ballou, 2004).

Sexuality and Sexual Functioning

The psychological and physiological impact of renal disease and renal replacement therapy on sexuality and sexual functioning is important to young and middle aged adults. Adults with renal disease report reduced sexual functioning, especially immediately following commencement of renal replacement therapy (Binik & Mah, 1994; Milde, Hart, & Fearing, 1996; Zarifian, 1994). Patients described reduced frequency of intercourse, problems with erection and ejaculation, and a diminished sexual desire. Binik and Mah (1994) suggest that while increasing uremia will impact sexual functioning, other physiological and psychosocial factors are also in play regarding sexuality and sexual functioning in adults with renal disease. For example, the intrusiveness of chronic renal failure and renal replacement therapy were identified as factors in one's sexuality (Binik & Mah, 1994; Milde et al., 1996). In men, sexual dysfunction can be attributed to decreased testosterone levels and increased prolactin production. Women may experience a decreased libido, impaired fertility, and difficulty with achieving orgasm. In their work, Binik and Mah found that improved sexual functioning was reported following transplantation, but note that sexual functioning posttransplant did not reach the level held prior to renal disease.

Nephrology nurses working with young and middle aged adults must consider the impact that the renal disease and its treatment may be having on the person's sexual health. Milde and colleagues (1996) note that decreased sexual functioning can lead to fears about loss of love and approval, thus negatively impacting the family relationship. Molzahn (1998) recommends that assessment of sexual functioning be included as a standard component of the history and physical assessment of persons with renal disease. Questions on sexual functioning and satisfaction, when included in the assessment and presented in a non-judgmental manner, will support identification of sexual difficulties that are amendable to treatment. Early identification of sexual dysfunction will assist the person in accessing possible medical, surgical, social, psychological, educational, and behavioral interventions to support improved sexual functioning. A number of medications commonly used by patients in chronic renal failure are known to cause impotence, for example antihypertensives. Small changes in a person's medication regimen may improve sexual functioning (Zarifian, 1992).

Quality of Life

Since initiation of chronic dialysis therapy in the 1960s, attention has been placed on the quality of life of persons with chronic renal failure. Despite this, a clear understanding of the concept of quality of life for persons with chronic renal failure has not been attained. There are a number of reasons for this; however, the primary limitations to describing the concept relate to the diversity in defining and measuring the concept (Ferrans, 1996; Molzahn, 1998; Parsons & Harris, 2003). However, we use the term in health care and research as if we have a common definition and understanding. Molzahn (1998) notes that despite the multitude of articles published on quality of life in the past 30 years, it is difficult to draw conclusions or compare findings due to differences in definition, conceptualization and measurement of this concept.

There is increasing agreement that quality of life is a subjective concept, defined by the individual, and understood within the context of his or her personal life situation (Ferrans, 1996; Hagren, Pettersen, Severinsson, Lıtzén, & Clyne 2001; Molzahn, 1998). Ferrans (1996) notes that everyone perceives the impact of a specific health condition or treatment regimen differently. At an extreme, a treatment or chronic disease considered by one person as making his or her life not worth living may be viewed by another as simply a nuisance.

There also appears to be some agreement among researchers that differences in quality of life may be found across dialysis therapies and following transplantation. Research has suggested an improved quality of life following successful transplant when compared to undergoing dialysis therapy (for example, Baiardi et al., 2002; Evans et al., 1985; Gudex, 1995; Keogh & Feehally, 1999; Parsons & Harris, 1997). Other studies suggest that home therapies, such as home hemodialysis and continuous ambulatory peritoneal dialysis, result in a higher level of perceived quality of life than do dialysis therapy provided in a hospital or outpatient clinic setting (Churchill, Morgan, & Torrance, 1984). One group of researchers found that persons who returned to dialysis following a failed transplant reported the lowest quality of life (Johnson, McCauley, & Copley, 1982). However, more research is required to fully understand how treatment modality influences the quality of life experienced by the person with chronic renal failure.

Qualitative research examining the meaning of life on dialysis has provided some interesting insights into the life experience of the young and middle aged adult living with chronic renal failure. This is important, as the experience of being an adult with chronic renal failure and the complexity and ambiguity of this experience are shaped by both the disease and its treatment regimen (Polaschek, 2003). Polaschek (2003) found that men managing self-care hemodialysis at home face significant challenges. Managing the symptoms of the renal failure; living with the limitations associated with the treatment regimen; having increased dependence on family, caregivers, and health professionals; and facing an uncertainty in health status challenge these individuals.

Findings of research conducted on people using continuous ambulatory peritoneal dialysis (CAPD) are similar. In a study of 26 adult CAPD patients, Lindqvist, Carlsson, and Sjöjén (2000a) found that these adults were striving for normality and independence. This group of patients described how they strove to keep up appearances, worked to control their own life, attempted to manage losses and dependence on others, and dealt effectively as possible with concerns of physical health and self-esteem (Lindqvist et al., 2000a).

The metaphor of the dialysis machine as an actual and symbolic lifeline has been used by individuals undergoing hemodialysis to describe how they were holding on to life and avoiding death at a cost of reduced freedom (Hagren et al., 2001). Other adults with chronic renal disease described their life as dwelling in dialysis, living with and being at home in the dialysis unit (Rittman, Northsea, Hansauer, Green, & Swanson, 1993). For these people, maintaining hope was an important mechanism by which to find meaning in their life (Rittman et al., 1993). Access to a strong social support system has also been described as important to one's quality of life (Cormier-Daigle & Stewart, 1997).

Adjustment, Coping, and Adherence

In chronic renal failure, there is significant work associated with managing the illness. Dialysis treatments are intrusive, requiring significant time and impacting all aspects of the person's life. While medical factors are of primary importance in determining the dialysis modality to be used by the patient, the choice of therapy is also influenced by nonmedical factors. These include patient and provider preferences and judgments about which modality is likely to be associated with the most favorable patient adherence and quality of life (Christensen & Ehlers, 2002; Christensen & Moran, 1998).

When treatment modality decisions are made, the desired level of involvement and access to health care providers should be considered (Christensen & Ehlers, 2002). The person who receives hemodialysis in a hospital or outpatient clinic receives care in a relatively passive context. The equipment is set up and the treatment delivered by registered nurses, licensed vocational nurses, and dialysis technicians. In contrast, the home dialysis patient has an opportunity to be much more active in the treatment delivery and direction. However, home dialysis patients have substantively less contact with renal care providers. Peritoneal dialysis requires the patient to take an even more active role in the delivery of care, as the person performs the exchange procedure four or five times daily or throughout the night. A functional renal transplant allows a transition towards greater independence from health care providers (Christensen & Ehlers, 2002).

Adjustment and Adaptation to Chronic Renal Failure

Considerable attention has been placed on how individuals adjust and adapt to chronic renal failure and the required treatment regime. In an early study of 25 patients undergoing maintenance dialysis, Reichsman and Levy (1972) found that patients appear to move between three stages of adaptation. These stages are a honeymoon period following improvement of the clinical manifestations of the disease with dialysis, a period of disenchantment and discouragement as the person realizes that dependence on treatment is required for his or her life, and then adaptation and acceptance. The researchers suggest that people move through these stages at different times and may, in fact, regress from one stage to another depending on their health status (Reichsman & Levy, 1972). This early work on adaptation has led to more recent studies on the relationship between adaptation and adherence to the treatment regime and social support, vocational rehabilitation, morale, and social functioning among dialysis patients (Cormier-Daigle & Stewart, 1997; Pollin, 1994; Tell et al., 1995)

Pollin (1994) describes eight fears faced by a person with a chronic illness. These fears are loss of control, loss of self-image, loss of dependency, stigma, abandonment, expression of anger, isolation, and death. Adjustments to the chronic illness will occur at three points in the course of the illness. The three points of adjustment occur are at the time of diagnosis, during a flare up or exacerbation of the illness, and when the person must take action to manage his or her own care (Pollin, 1994). For adults with chronic renal failure, depending on the nature of the renal disease, these three levels may occur concurrently serving to impact the person's capacity for adjustment.

Research into adjustment and adaptation to renal disease has also considered the concepts of loss and grief for one's previous existence. These include loss and grief for one's health and one's former life in terms of control and independence. Factors found to influence loss and grief are age, gender, social support system, and health status prior to onset of the renal failure (Christensen et al., 1992; Sidell, 1997). Adults find entry into the medical world of nephrology care strange and frightening if the person has had little previous exposure. The language, schedules, and systems of interaction must be learned and accommodated (Sidell, 1997). Parsons and Harris (1997) note that vocational rehabilitation is an important aim of therapy for patients below retirement age. Pre-dialysis education and counseling were found to influence the person's ability to maintain employment while balancing their treatment regimen with their personal and employment roles.

Coping with Chronic Renal Failure

How people cope and adapt to a chronic illness, such as renal failure, is unique, individual, and difficult to define (Sidell, 1997). Adaptation is dynamic; there is no one exact point where it can be stated that the person has adapted. The person's capacity to cope and adjust to illness is influenced by multiple forces, may be achieved with individual creativity, and will occur at an uneven pace within the various spheres of life (Dimond, 1984). In general terms coping responses fall within two major categories, behavioral or cognitive (Dimond, 1984; Lazarus & Folkman, 1984; Pollin, 1994). Responses that can be categorized as behavioral or problem solving are those where the person seeks to change the situation by seeking information, learning to control symptoms, and planning for the short- and long-term future. In contrast, cognitive responses might include denial, minimalization, and partialization to control one's emotional response.

Pollin (1994) describes the work of coping with chronic illness as identifying the problem, assessing the situation, facing fears, finding a release for tension, and acknowledging and working within one's own coping style. The person and his or her family must then understand that adjustment ebbs and flows. Integration of the chronic illness into the life of the person and his or her family can take some time.

Welch and Austin (2001) examined the relationships between stressors, coping, and depression to test how coping behaviors impact depression experienced in adults with chronic renal failure. In their study, which involved adults who were receiving hemodialysis treatments in the Midwestern United States, they found that people who used avoidance coping behaviors were more likely to experience psychosocial stress and depression than patients identified as using problem-solving or social support coping behaviors. To further explain the variation in coping strategies used by this group of people, Welch and Austin (2001) suggest that the use of avoidance coping behaviors most likely reflects a long-standing habit in dealing with problems.

Adherence to the Treatment Regimen

It is suggested that 30 and 60% of dialysis patients do not adhere to diet, fluid intake, and medication regimens (Christensen & Ehlers, 2002; Gordon, Leon, & Sehgal, 2003; Kimmel et al., 1998; Rocco & Burkart, 1993). Non-adherence is most common in relation to fluid intake restrictions and somewhat less frequent for dietary or medication requirements. Conflicting results are found when examining the incidence of missed dialysis treatments. Kimmel and colleagues (1998) suggest that missing a dialysis treatment was relatively rare, occurring in less than 2% of scheduled treatments. However, others (e.g., Gordon et al., 2003; Rocco & Burkart, 1993) found a higher rate of skipped or shortened treatments.

To better understand the reasons for patients skipping or shortening hemodialysis treatments, Gordon and colleagues (2003) conducted follow-up interviews with patients identified as missing or shortening a treatment. In this sample of 168 patients from 29 different dialysis units, 10% of all hemodialysis treatments were skipped and 5.4% of the remaining treatments were shortened. The most commonly cited reason for shortening a treatment was for medical reasons, with 38% of loss time attributed to illness, cramping, or needing to use the bathroom. In contrast, life tasks such as conducting personal business or having a doctor's appointment were reasons given for 33% of the skipped treatments.

Transportation accounted for 10% of the shortened treatment time. As well, 19% of the shortened time related to patients choosing to end their treatment early because they disagreed with the dialysis prescription. Of interest, the study population was over represented with males and African Americans when compared to the total patient population of people receiving care at the 29 hemodialysis units sampled (Gordon et al., 2003).

Research into factors that support compliance and adherence to the treatment regimen for adults with chronic renal failure is limited and inconclusive (Hailey & Moss, 2000). The personality traits of self-efficacy and conscientiousness are suggested as having an association with an individual's capacity to successfully manage the medication and fluid restriction regimens of chronic renal failure and dialysis therapy (Christensen & Ehlers, 2002; Wiebe & Christensen, 1997). Individuals with an internal locus of control are also suggested to exhibit a more favorable regimen adherence (Christensen & Ehlers, 2002).

Another related concept is that of self-management, which is defined as an individual's effort to attain optimal health, prevent illness, recognize symptoms, and cope with or manage the chronic condition (Curtin & Mapes, 2001). In a study involving long-term hemodialysis adult patients (greater than 15 years on treatment), a number of self-management strategies were identified. These long-term patients described how they managed their interactions with staff and physicians to receive optimal care, reporting symptoms based on their intuitive feeling that something was not right and conducting a vigilant overview of care provided to ensure that treatments and interventions were performed correctly and safely. In addition to proposing or refusing treatments or interventions, the patients also disclosed that they independently adopted a new treatment or modified their medications (Curtin & Mapes, 2001).

Successful self-managed patients are described as persons with personal autonomy, who participate actively in their treatment and care regimen and value being listened to and seen as individuals (Hagren et al., 2001). Increased autonomy with self-care was also found in a qualitative analysis of the experience of six men undergoing self-care hemodialysis (Polaschek, 2003). These men stated a belief that engaging in self-care enhanced their independence and helped them maintain a more normal lifestyle. However, this was seen as a double-bind situation since self-care allowed them to be more autonomous but reinforced their dependence on dialysis.

Hailey and Moss (2000) assert that the influence of patient characteristics, which may be predictive of compliance or adherence to treatment, vary with the contextual circumstances in which the treatment occurs. They recommended that the focus on research into compliance and adherence be on development and evaluation of strategies to improve compliance rather than identification of factors seen to influence compliance.

These findings on self-management, adherence to treatment, medication, and fluid restriction regimens, while limited, provide insight into the challenges faced by adults with chronic renal failure. Nephrology nurses have an opportunity through the patient-nurse relationship to play a pivotal role in educating, counseling, and supporting patients to self-manage the chronic renal failure and its associated treatment regimens.

Family Support in Chronic Renal Failure

A reoccurring theme in literature on outcomes of patients with chronic renal failure is the importance of family support in relation to perceived quality of life and health status. Research about the role of family support is diverse, with studies examining stress and uncertainty associated with the diagnosis and treatment regimen, coping strategies of families, the impact of a parent's diagnosis on children, and the roles that family members may play in provision of treatment. Family support will help the adult with chronic renal failure manage the disease, its treatments, and the uncertainty of outcomes (Christensen et al., 1992; O'Brien, 1983).

Changes in family dynamics and relationships occur following the diagnosis of chronic renal failure. Using the family stress theory developed by McCubbin and Thompson (1987), Starzomski and Hilton (2000) examined family adjustment posttransplant. They suggest that following a diagnosis of a chronic, life-threatening disease, such as chronic renal failure, a family will try new coping methods, take in new information, and accommodate to the changes imposed by the illness. The family's capacity to adapt to the change imposed by the illness can be explained in some regard by the characteristics of the family, its resources, and its capabilities (Starzomski & Hilton, 2000).

Uncertainty and stress have been identified as factors that influence the family's ability to support the individual with chronic renal failure (Brock, 1987; Pelletier-Hibbert & Sohi, 2001; Srivastava. 1988). Forty-one family members of patients undergoing hemodialysis or peritoneal dialysis were asked to discuss their experience of living with a person with chronic renal failure (Pelletier-Hibbert & Sohi, 2001). Participants described how stress was created by the uncertainty caused from the unreliability of the person's health, complications of the dialysis treatment, the fear of the person dying, and the wait for a kidney. Coping strategies used by these family members included living each day as it comes, not planning for the future, hoping for a kidney transplant, and seeing small improvements in health status. For some participants the capacity to cope came from reliance in their faith and finding positive meanings in the illness (Pelletier-Hibbert & Sohi, 2001). In an earlier study, Brock (1987) found that knowledge and education about renal disease and its treatment did not reduce the level of uncertainty expressed by family members.

The relationship between family style and adaptation to renal disease has been considered. Flaherty and O'Brien (1992) found five distinct family styles (e.g., remote, altered, distressed, enfolded, and receptive) in a study of adaptation to chronic renal failure by the family. In the remote family style, family member responses suggested that their lives and family functioning had not been impacted or interfered with by the family member's chronic disease. In contrast, family members that fell into the altered family style group described major changes in roles and activities of family members following the diagnosis of chronic renal failure.

Sorrow and grief characterized the responses of participants considered within a distressed family style. Some participants suggested that the disease had strengthened the family bonds, and in this enfolded family style, the family members considered the disease a collective responsibility. The receptive family style included those participants whose responses included indicators of acceptance and adjustment to the diagnosis of chronic renal failure in their family member.

Impact on the Spouse and Marital Relationship

Limited research has been done on the impact to spouses and the marital relationship of the diagnosis and treatment of chronic renal failure. Most attention in this regard has been placed on the spousal role as caregiver and, in particular, providing hands-on assistance with the hemodialysis or peritoneal dialysis treatments (Brinker & Lichtenstein, 1981; Brunier & McKeever, 1993; Frank, 1988; Srivastava, 1988; Tell et al., 1995). Tell and colleagues (1995) note the importance of family and spousal support in providing tangible assistance to patients in terms of transportation, access to medical services, and assistance with personal care, for example. Brunier and McKeever (1993), in their review of the literature on home hemodialysis, found that female spouses frequently assumed the role of hemodialysis assistants, adding a new responsibility to the multiple roles in the family as spouse, homemaker, worker, and frequently primary care giver. As well, the spouse may be required to assume outside roles and responsibilities previously held by the sick partner (Brinker & Lichtenstein, 1981). The assumption of new roles and a requirement to shift between established roles may lead to conflict between spouses as levels of dependency and independence fluctuate and change (Frank, 1988).

Research into coping strategies and health-related quality of life found that spouses who perceived that they were handling their spouse's illness well reported improved physical and emotional health, a better family life, and slept better than did those spouses who reported difficulties in handling the spouse's diagnosis of chronic renal failure (Lindqvist, Carlsson, & Sjöjén, 2000b). In one study, the quality of life of spouses of transplant patients was seen as better when compared to that of spouses of hemodialysis or CAPD patients (Lindqvist et al., 2000b). However, the researchers suggest that the younger age of the transplant couples included in the sample may have influenced this finding. Other researchers (Chowanec & Binik, 1989) found no change in marital relations or psychological well being in couples following a spouse being diagnosed with chronic renal failure. More research is needed to fully understand the impact that chronic renal failure has on the marital relationship and the quality of life of spouses of young and middle aged adults with chronic renal failure.

Impact on Children of Parents with Chronic Renal Failure

Little is known about the adjustment of children to their parent's renal disease and its treatment. The findings of one study suggested that adolescents had difficulty adjusting to the parent's dialysis regimen (Schlebusch, Naidoo, & Kallmeyer, 1983). However, this finding is limited by a small sample. In this study, responses from eight adolescents with

a parent having chronic renal failure were compared to those of eight adolescents with healthy parents. Beanlands (1987) suggests that children may move through stages of adjustment following a parent's diagnosis. Children, she suggests, move from an information seeking stage to a stage of learning to live with the parent who is chronically ill. In Beanland's work, the children identified a stage of "getting sick" where a change in health status or a complication in the parent's treatment regimen would lead to concern and uncertainty by the child. Over time and with resolution of the complication (e.g., peritonitis), the child would move back into the "learning to live with it" stage. Molzahn and Kikuchi (1998) found in their study of the quality of life among children and adolescents with a parent undergoing dialysis that the participants experienced uncertainty and described fears associated with their parent's condition and the dialysis treatment.

Information needs, uncertainty, and fear about the future have also been found in research on children's reactions to a parent's terminal illness. In a study of adolescents' reaction to a parent's terminal cancer, the adolescent appeared to cope with the impending death using a variety of intellectual defenses, seeking information, and looking for meaning in the experience (Christ, Siegel, & Sperber, 1994). Monroe and Krause (1996) suggest that the capacity of children to understand information on a parent's illness may be greater than we assume and suggest that children be encouraged to express their understanding of the illness using pictures. They also suggest that care is taken to accommodate children into the hospital or caregiving environment recognizing that children will pick up on non-verbal cues. Reassurance, information on what is likely to occur, and involvement in nurturing an ill parent through simple tasks are suggested as strategies to assist a child in understanding the illness (Monroe & Kraus, 1996).

Developing Effective Nurse / Patient Relationships

Nephrology nurses have a unique opportunity through the nature of the practice setting to develop effective and meaningful therapeutic relationships with young and middle aged adults with chronic renal failure and their families. The following description of nurses in an outpatient hemodialysis unit illustrates the nature of the relationship. Nurses must have "the ability to listen, to teach, to not give up, but also to let go, to use humor to connect with patients, and to relieve tension" (Morehouse, Colvin & Maykut, 2001, p. 299). In the dialysis unit, patient care takes place in an open space, making interactions between nurses and patients, patients and patients, and nurses and nurses visible and public. This care environment is compared to that of a long-term support group with depth, reciprocity, and compassion characterizing the relationship (Morehouse et al., 2001). However, it is also important to view each person as an individual and to assist the person to feel comfortable and at ease in the setting. Trust occurs over time, and its development is facilitated by individualized care (Hagren et al., 2001).

Morgan (2000) concurs that individualized care is essential to the nurse-patient relationship in this practice setting. Use of individualized interventions may empower patients to assume responsibility for their health needs. Polaschek

(2003) believes that individualized care is essential in the nephrology practice setting that appears on first glance to be technology driven. However, the role of the nurse is to humanize the technology. The potential of nephrology nursing is in the nurse's capacity to respond to the patient as a person living with renal disease (Polaschek, 2003).

Nephrology nursing has also been depicted as a partnership of care between the nurse, the patient, and his or her family (Ziegert & Fridlund, 2001). Ziegert and Fridlund (2001) describe how the nurse may share in the patient's and family's movement between hope and despair as they master acute complications, uncertainty regarding transplant given the scarce supply of kidneys, and the final stage of life.

Education, shared decision-making, reinforcement, and follow-up are identified as interventions to help empower the young and middle aged adult with chronic renal failure (Quirk, 1998). Quirk (1998) suggests that continuity of care can help patients achieve positive outcomes. Effective communication with patients is an essential component of nephrology nursing practice, as communication is essential for teaching patients and families about the treatment regimen and to reinforce adherence (Courts, 1994; Holland, 1998; Morgan, 2000; Montemuro et al., 1994).

Bonner (2003) describes the expert nephrology nurse as being trusted, teaching others, and being seen as a role model. The expert nurse holds extensive clinical skills, has an inquiring mind, and constantly seeks knowledge and expertise to maintain his or her expert knowledge. As well, expert nephrology nurses are considered by their peers to be strong teachers, to deal with patients better than their colleagues, and to have the ability to take on more responsibility than others (Bonner, 2003). Bonner sees being trusted as both contributing to and depicting the expert nephrology nurse.

Little is known about the influence that the use of a particular model of nursing care may have on patient outcomes and care provided within the nephrology setting. Molzahn (1989) reported on a pilot project on primary nursing and compliance that found little change following implementation. However, she notes that in this pilot project nurses were responsible for directing the care (e.g., writing care plans) but were not always assigned to care for their primary patients. Morgan (2000) examined literature on adherence and found limited information on the model of care and patient adherence.

Nurses have a strong role to play in supporting patient choice regarding treatment modality. Nursing interventions include educating, counseling, and supporting adults and their families on potential treatment options. Nurses must focus on the advantages and disadvantages of each treatment modality specific to that individual patient, respecting factors related to the person's health status, medical condition, and social factors that might influence treatment selection. As the member of the interdisciplinary team that spends the most time with the patient and his or her family, nurses are pivotal to the success of the treatment plan (Compton, Provenzano, & Johnson, 2002).

Keeping and English (2001) describe the nurse's role as facilitating knowledge for patients and families through formal and informal learning strategies. Formal learning has a defined goal (e.g., learning to do a bag exchange for CAPD;

understanding and adhering to the medication regimen). In contrast, informal learning occurs on a continuum of intentionality and consciousness and is a byproduct of experience. The nephrology nurse acts to facilitate informal and incidental learning by creating a health care setting that provides for networking, modeling, and coaching of patients and families (Keeping & English 2001).

Pelletier-Hibbert and Sohi (2001) found that both patients and their families valued nurses providing information, spending time with them, and talking with patients and families about their experience. Quality care from the patients' and families' perspective included assessing the individual's and family's understanding of the illness, identifying sources of stress or uncertainty, examining the impact of illness and its treatment on their daily lives, and determining how they are coping. These factors serve to provide a framework for care over the span of the nurse-patient relationship (Pelletier-Hibbert & Sohi, 2001).

Summary

The care of the young and middle aged adult with chronic kidney disease offers interesting challenges to the nephrology nurse due to the diversity of this group of patients in terms of health status and life situation. This patient population, ranging in age from 20 to 65 years, has the potential to live a long, functional, and quality life with careful management of the renal failure, its treatment, and prevention of co-morbid conditions. The young and middle aged adult is challenged by the uncertainty, stress, and fear associated with this chronic disease. More information is needed on the manner that chronic renal failure and its treatment may influence health status, sexual functioning, family relationships, rehabilitation, social support, and perceived quality of life. Research into strategies to increase adherence and promote the use of effective coping behaviors is required to improve our understanding of the challenges faced by the young and middle aged adult with chronic renal failure.

Nephrology nurses are well positioned to support this patient group and their families to achieve a high quality of life through education, counseling, and skilled technical nursing interventions. The importance of considering each patient as an individual is emphasized since individualized care has been found to facilitate trust, learning, and quality clinical outcomes. Research about nursing care, nursing interventions, and nursing outcomes will increase understanding of the nursing care required by this complex patient group.

References

American Academy of Family Physicians (AAFP). (2004). *Periodic physical assessments. Recommendations of the American Academy of Family Physicians.* Available online at www.aafp.org/exam.xml

Arias, E. (2004). United States life tables 2001. *National Vital Statistics Reports, 52*(14), Hyattsville, MD: National Center for Health Statistics. Available online www.cdc.gov/nchs/data/nvsr/nvsr52/nvsr52_14.pdf.

Baiardi, F., Degli Espositi, E., Cocchi, F., Fabbri, A., Sturani, A., Valpiani, G., & Fusarol, M. (2002). Effects of clinical and individual variables on quality of life in chronic renal failure. *Journal of Nephrology, 15,* 61-67.

Beanlands, H. (1987). The experience of being a child in a family where one parent is on home dialysis. Unpublished masters thesis. University of Toronto, Toronto, ON.

Becker, H., & Maiman, L.A. (1975). Socio-behavioral determinants of compliance with health and medical care recommendations. *Medical Care, 13,* 10-24.

Binik, Y.M., & Mah, K. (1994). Sexuality and end stage renal disease: Research and clinical recommendations. *Advances in Renal Replacement Therapy, 1,* 198-209.

Bonner, A. (2003). Recognition of expertise: An important concept in the acquisition of nephrology nursing expertise. *Nursing & Health Sciences, 5,* 123-131,

Brinker, K.J., & Lichtenstein, V.R. (1981). Value of a self-help group in the psychological adjustment of end stage renal disease clients and their families. *AANNT Journal, 8,* 23-27.

Brock, M.J. (1987). Uncertainty, information needs, and coping effectiveness of renal families. *ANNA Journal, 17,* 242-245, 267.

Brunier, G.M., & McKeever, P.T. (1993). The impact of home dialysis on the family: Literature review. *ANNA Journal, 20,* 653-659.

Christ, G.H., Siegel, K., & Sperber, D. (1994). Impact of parental terminal cancer on adolescents. *American Journal of Orthopsychiatry, 64,* 604-613.

Christensen, A.J., & Ehlers, S.L. (2002). Psychological factors in end stage renal disease: An emerging context for behavioral medicine research. *Journal of Consulting and Clinical Psychology, 70,* 712-724.

Christensen, A.J., & Moran, P.J. (1998). The role of psychosomatic research in the management of end stage renal disease. *Journal of Psychosomatic Research, 44,* 523-528.

Christensen, A.J., Smith, T.W., Turner, C.W., Holman, J.M., Gregory, M.C., & Rich, M.A., (1992). Family support, physical impairment, and adherence in hemodialysis. An investigation of main and buffering effects. *Journal of Behavioral Medicine, 12,* 249-265.

Christensen, A.J., Wiebe, J.S., Smith, T.W., & Turner, C.W. (1994). Predictors of survival among hemodialysis patients. Effect of perceived family support. *Health Psychology, 13,* 521-526.

Chowanec, G., & Binik, Y. (1989). End stage renal disease and the marital dyad: An empirical investigation. *Social Science & Medicine, 28,* 971-983.

Churchill, D.N., Morgan, J., & Torrance, G.W. (1984). Quality of life in end stage renal disease. *Peritoneal Dialysis Bulletin, 4*(1), 20-23.

Compton, A., Provenzano, R., & Johnson, C.A. (2002). The nephrology nurse's role in improved care of patients with chronic kidney disease. *Nephrology Nursing Journal, 29,* 331-336.

Cormier-Daigle, M., & Stewart, M. (1997). Support and coping of male hemodialysis-dependent patients. *International Journal of Nursing Studies, 34,* 420-430.

Courts, N. (1994). Psychological interventions for patients receiving hemodialysis. *Urological Nursing 14*(2), 79-81.

Curtin, R.B., Bultman, D.C., Thomas-Hawkins, C., Walters, B.A.J., & Schatell, D. (2002). Hemodialysis patients' symptom experiences: Effects on physical and mental functioning. *Nephrology Nursing Journal, 29,* 562-574.

Curtin, R.B., & Mapes, D. L. (2001). Health care management strategies of long-term dialysis survivors. *Nephrology Nursing Journal, 28,* 385-394.

Curtin, R.B., & Mapes, D. L., Petillo, M., & Oberley, E. (2002). Long-term dialysis survivors: A transformational experience. *Qualitative Health Research, 12,* 609-624.

Deligiannis, A., Kouidi, E., & Tourkanonis, A. (1999). Effects of physical training on heart rate variability in patients on hemodialysis. *American Journal of Cardiology, 84,* 197-202.

Dimond, M. (1984). Identifying the needs of the chronically ill. In S.E. Milligan (Ed.), *Community health care for chronic physical Illness: Issues and models* (pp. 1-14). Cleveland: Case Western Reserve University.

Erickson, E. H. (1980). Themes in adulthood in the Freud-Jung correspondence. In N. J. Smelser & E. H. Erikson (Eds.), *Themes of work and love in adulthood* (pp. 43-74). Cambridge, MA: Harvard University Press.

Evans, R.W., Manninen, D.L., Garrison, L.P., Bragg, C.R., Gutman, R.A., Hull, A.R., & Lowrie, E.G. (1985). The quality of life of patients with end stage renal disease. *New England Journal of Medicine, 312,* 553-559.

Ferrans, C.E., (1996). Development of a conceptual model of quality of life. *Scholarly Inquiry for Nursing Practice: An International Journal, 10,* 293-304.

Flaherty, M., & O'Brien, M. (1992). Family styles of coping in end stage renal disease. *ANNA Journal, 19,* 345-349.

Frank, D.I. (1988). Psychosocial assessment of renal failure patients. *ANNA Journal, 15,* 207-210, 232.

Goodman, E.D., & Ballou, M.B. (2004). Perceived barriers and motivators to exercise in hemodialysis patients. *Nephrology Nursing Journal, 31,* 23-29.

Gordon, E.J., Leon, J.B., & Sehgal, A.R. (2003). Why are hemodialysis treatments shortened and skipped? Development of a taxonomy and relationship to patient subgroups. *Nephrology Nursing Journal, 20,* 209-217.

Gudex, C.M. (1995). Health-related quality of life in end stage renal failure. *Quality of Life Research, 4,* 359-366.

Hagren, B., Pettersen, I., Severinsson, E., Lützen, K., & Clyne, N. (2001). The haemodialysis machine as a lifeline: Experiences of suffering from end stage renal disease. *Journal of Advanced Nursing, 34*(2), 196-202.

Hailey, B.J., & Moss, S.B. (2000). Compliance behaviour in patients undergoing haemodialysis: A review of the literature. *Psychology, Health & Medicine, 5, 395-406.*

Holland, J. (1998). Integrating the role of the renal nurse case manager. *Nephrology News & Issues, 12*(1), 19-23.

Holley, J.L., & Reddy, S.S. (2003). Pregnancy in dialysis patients: A review of outcomes, complications, and management. *Seminars in Dialysis, 16,* 384-388,

Jang, C., Bell, R.J., White, V.S., Lee, P.S., Dwyer, K.M., Kerr, P.G., & Davis, S.R. (2001). Women's health issues in hemodialysis patients. *Medical Journal of Australia, 175,* 298-301.

Johnson, J.P., McCauley, C.R., & Copley, J.B. (1982). The quality of life of hemodialysis and transplant patients. *Kidney International, 3,* 286-291.

Kaveh, K., & Kimmel. P.L. (2001). Compliance in hemodialysis patients: Multidimensional measures in search of a gold standard. *American Journal of Kidney Diseases, 37,* 244-266.

Keeping, L.M., & English, L. M. (2001). Informal and incidental learning with patients who use continuous ambulatory peritoneal dialysis. *Nephrology Nursing Journal, 28,* 313-323.

Keogh, A.M., & Feehally, J. (1999). A quantitative study comparing adjustment and acceptance of illness in adults on renal replacement therapy. *ANNA Journal, 26,* 471-478, 500, 505.

Kimmel, P.L., Peterson, R.A., Weihs, K.L., Simmens, S.J., Alleyene, S., Cruz, I., et al. (1998). Psychosocial factors, behavioral compliance, and survival in urban hemodialysis patients. *Kidney International, 54,* 245-254.

Kouidi, E., Lacovides, A., Lordanidis, P., Vassilious, S., Deligiannis, A., Lerodiakonou, C., et al. (1997). Exercise renal rehabilitation program: Psychosocial effects. *Nephron, 77,* 152-158.

Kouidi, E., Albani, M., Natsis, K., Megalopoulos, A., Gigis, P., Guiba-Tziampiri, O., et al. (1998). The effects of exercise training on muscle atrophy in hemodialysis patients. *Nephrology Dialysis Transplant 13,* 685-699.

Kutner, N.G., Brogan, D., & Fielding, B. (1997). Physical and psychosocial resource variables related to long-term survival in older dialysis patients. *Geriatric Nephrology and Urology, 7*(1), 23-38.

Kutner, N.G., Zhang, R., McClellan, W.M. (2000). Patient-reported quality of life early in dialysis treatment: Effects associated with usual exercise activity. *Nephrology Nursing Journal, 27,* 357-367.

Lazarus, R.S., & Folkman, S. (1984). *Stress, appraisal, and coping.* New York: Springer.

Lev, E.L., & Owen, S.V. (1998). A prospective study of adjustment to hemodialysis. *ANNA Journal, 25,* 495-504.

Lindqvist, R., Carlsson, M., & Sjöjén, P. (2000a). Perceived consequences of being a renal failure patient. *Nephrology Nursing Journal, 27,* 291-297.

Lindqvist, R., Carlsson, M., & Sjöjén, P. (2000b). Coping strategies and health-related quality of life among spouses of continuous ambulatory peritoneal dialysis, haemodialysis, and transplant patients. *Journal of Advanced Nursing, 31,* 1398-1408.

McCubbin, H.I., & Thompson, A.I. (1987). *Family assessment inventories for research and practice.* Madison, WI: University of Wisconsin.

Milde, F.K., Hart, L.K., & Fearing, M.O. (1996). Sexuality and fertility concerns of dialysis patients. *ANNA Journal, 23,* 307-315.

Molsted, S., Eidemak, I., Sorensen, H.T., & Kristensen, J.H. (2004). Five months of physical exercise in hemodialysis patients: Effects on aerobic capacity, physical function, and self-rated health. *Nephron, 96,* 76-81.

Molzahn, A.E. (1998). Psychosocial impact of renal disease. In J. Parker (Ed.), *Contemporary nephrology nursing (pp. 271-281).* Pitman, NJ: American Nephrology Nurses' Association.

Molzahn, A.E. (1989). Primary nursing and patient compliance in a hemodialysis unit. *American ANNA Journal, 16,* 267-272.

Molzahn, A.E., & Kikuchi, J.F. (1998). Children and adolescents of parents undergoing dialysis therapy: Their reported quality of life. *ANNA Journal, 25,* 411-418.

Monroe, B., & Kraus, F. (1996). Children and loss. *British Journal of Hospital Medicine, 56,* 260-269.

Montemuro, M., Marin, L., Jakoson, S., Mohide, E., Beecroft, M., Porterfield, P., & Ollinger, D. (1994). Participatory control in chronic hospital-based hemodialysis patients. *ANNA Journal, 21,* 429-438.

Morehouse, R.E., Colvin, E., & Maykut, P. (2001). Nephrology nurse-patient relationships in the outpatient dialysis setting. *Nephrology Nursing Journal, 28,* 295-300.

Morgan, L. (2000). Methods to improve adherence to the treatment regimen among hemodialysis patients. *Nephrology Nursing Journal, 27,* 299-304.

Myers, P.S. (2002). Transitioning an adolescent dialysis patient to adult health care. *Nephrology Nursing Journal, 29,* 375-376.

Office of Health Promotion and Disease Prevention. (not dated). *Healthy People 2010.* Available at www.healthypeople.gov

O'Brien, M.E. (1983). *The courage to survive: The life career of the chronic dialysis patient.* New York: Grune & Stratton.

Painter, P., Carlson, L., Carey, S., Paul, S.M., & Myll, J. (2000). Physical functioning and health related quality of life changes with exercise training in hemodialysis patients. *American Journal of Kidney Disease, 35,* 482-492.

Parsons, D.S., & Harris, D.C. (2003). A review of quality of life in chronic renal failure. *Pharmacoeconomics, 12,* 140-160.

Pelletier-Hibbert, M., & Sohi, P. (2001). Sources of uncertainty and coping strategies used by family members of individuals living with end stage renal disease. *Nephrology Nursing Journal, 28,* 411-419.

Polaschek, N. (2003). Living on dialysis: Concerns of clients in a renal setting. *Journal of Advanced Nursing, 41,* 44-52.

Pollin, I. (1994). *Taking charge: Overcoming the challenge of long-term illness.* New York: Random House.

Quirk, B. (1998). Primary patient care in a chronic outpatient hemodialysis unit. *American ANNA Journal, 25,* 253-357.

Rahman, M., & Smith, M.C. (1998). Chronic renal insufficiency: A diagnostic and therapeutic approach. *Archives of Internal Medicine, 158,* 1743-1752.

Rasgon, S., Schwankowski, L., James-Rogers, A., Widrow, L., Glick, J., & Butts, E. (1993). An intervention for employment maintenance among blue collar workers with end stage renal disease. *American Journal of Kidney Diseases, 22,* 404-412.

Reichsman, F., & Levy, N. (1972). Problems in adaptation to maintenance hemodialysis. A four-year study of 25 patients. *Archives of Internal Medicine, 130,* 859-865.

Rittman, M., Northsea, C., Hansauer, N., Green, C. & Swanson, L. (1993). Living with renal failure. *ANNA Journal, 20,* 327-331.

Rocco, M.V., & Burkart, J.M. (1993). Prevalence of missed treatment and early sign-offs in hemodialysis patients. *Journal of the American Society of Nephrology, 4,* 1178-1183.

Rosen, D.S., Blum, R.W., Britto, M., Sawyer, S.M., & Siegel, D.M. (2003). Transition to adult health care for adolescents and young adults with chronic conditions. A position paper of the Society for Adolescent Medicine. *Journal of Adolescent Health, 33,* 309-311.

Ross, J.E. (2001). Developing a new model for cross-cultural research synthesizing the Health Belief Model and the theory of reasoned action. *Advances in Nursing Science, 23*(4), 1-15.

Scal, P., Evans, T., Blozis, S., Okinow, N., & Blum, R. (1999). Trends in transition from pediatric to adult health care services for young adults with chronic conditions. *Journal of Adolescent Health, 24,* 259-264.

Schlebusch, L., Naidoo, N.K., & Kallmeyer, J. (1983). Psychological effects of in-centre haemodialysis on the dialysand's adolescent children. *South African Medical Journal. 63*(10), 363-365.

Sidell, N.L. (1997). Adult adjustment to chronic illness: A review of the literature. *Health and Social Work, 33,* 5-12.

Srivastava, R. (1988). Coping strategies used by spouses of CAPD patients. *ANNA Journal, 15,* 174-178.

Starzomski, R., & Hilton, A. (2000). Patient and family adjustment to kidney transplantation with and without an interim period of dialysis. *Nephrology Nursing Journal, 27,* 17-32.

Strauss, A.L., Corbin, J., Fagerhaugh, S., Glaser, B.G., Maines, D., Suszek, B., & Wiener, C.L. (1984). *Chronic illness and the quality of life* (2nd Edition). Toronto, ON: C.V. Mosby Company.

Tell, G., Mittelmark, M., Hylander, B., Shumarker, S., Russell, G., & Burkart, M. (1995). Social support and health related quality of life in black and white dialysis patients. *ANNA Journal, 22,* 301-310.

Thomas-Hawkins, C. (2000). Symptom distress and day-to-day changes in functional status in chronic hemodialysis patients. *Nephrology Nursing Journal, 27,* 369-379.

United States Renal Data System (USRDS). (2003). *Annual data report. Atlas of end stage renal disease in the United States.* Available online www.usrds.org/research.htm

Welch, J.L., & Austin, J.K. (2001). Stressors, coping, and depression in haemodialysis patients. *Journal of Advanced Nursing, 33,* 200-207.

Wiebe, J.S., & Christensen, A.J., (1997). Conscientiousness, health beliefs, and patient adherence in renal dialysis. *Annals of Behavioral Medicine, 19,* 30-35.

Zarifian, A. (1994). Case study of the anemic patient: Epoetin alfa: Focus on sexual function. *ANNA Journal, 21,* 368-371.

Zarifian, A. (1992). Sexual dysfunction in the male end stage renal disease patient. Pathophysiology review. *American Nephrology Nurses Association Journal, 19,* 527-34.

Ziegert, K., & Fridlund, B. (2001). Conceptions of life situation among next-of-kin of haemodialysis patients. *Journal of Nursing Management, 9,* 231-239.

- The USRDS (2003) reports that in 2001 the average age of persons undergoing treatment for ESRD in the United States was 58.7 years, an increase largely attributable to the growing number of persons beginning treatment at an older age.

- Overall mortality in young and middle-aged adults decreased 10% since 1988 with the greatest gains found in the first 2 years following initiation of renal replacement treatment, where a reduction of 23% occurred since 1985 (USRDS, 2003). In contrast, mortality rates for vintage patients (those receiving treatment for 5 years or longer) decreased between 1988 and 1994, but has risen 12% since 1994.

- In terms of morbidity, hospitalization rates among ESRD patients have shown an overall reduction of 1% since 1993. This reduction is considered to be directly attributed to the 24% reduction in hospitalization for vascular access (USRDS, 2003).

- In the Health Belief Model (Becker & Maiman, 1975), the person determines health actions based on the perceived likelihood of developing the health risk, complication, or illness. As well, the personal perspective of the severity of the illness is considered in terms of the impact on one's life.

- Data from the USRDS (2003) suggest that children aged 10 to 14 years at initiation of renal replacement therapy have an 86.6% likelihood of living 10 years. Thus, attention should be placed on how to assist the older adolescent to move from receiving care in a pediatric to an adult setting.

- There is a growing awareness of the importance of controlling underlying disease processes and promoting exercise to support improved functional outcome and quality of life in adult patients with chronic renal failure (Kutner, Zhang, & McClellen, 2000; Rahman & Smith, 1998).

- Research suggests functional status and quality of life are associated with the individual person's capacity to self-manage aspects of renal failure and its treatment. In addition, a focus on patient education and vocational counseling has been shown to increase levels of employment following initiation of dialysis (Rasgon et al., 1993).

- The psychological and physiological impact of renal disease and renal replacement therapy on sexuality and sexual functioning is important to young and middle aged adults. Adults with renal disease report reduced sexual functioning, especially immediately following commencement of renal replacement therapy (Binik & Mah, 1994; Milde, Hart, & Fearing, 1996; Zarifian, 1994).

- Adaptation to a chronic illness is dynamic; there is no one exact point where it can be stated that the person has adapted. The person's capacity to cope and adjust to illness is influenced by multiple forces, may be achieved with individual creativity, and will occur at an uneven pace within the various spheres of life (Dimond, 1984).

- It is suggested that 30 and 60% of dialysis patients do not adhere to diet, fluid intake, and medication regimens (Christensen & Ehlers, 2002; Gordon, Leon, & Sehgal, 2003; Kimmel et al., 1998; Rocco & Burkart, 1993). Nonadherence is most common in relation to fluid intake restrictions and somewhat less frequent for dietary or medication requirements.

- Uncertainty and stress have been identified as factors that influence the family's ability to support the individual with chronic renal failure (Brock, 1987; Pelletier-Hibbert & Sohi, 2001; Srivastava. 1988).

- Limited research has been done on the impact to spouses and the marital relationship of the diagnosis and treatment of chronic renal failure. Most attention in this regard has been placed on the spousal role as caregiver and, in particular, providing hands-on assistance with the hemodialysis or peritoneal dialysis treatments.

- Nephrology nurses have a unique opportunity through the nature of the practice setting to develop effective and meaningful therapeutic relationships with young and middle aged adults with chronic renal failure and their families.

- Bonner (2003) describes the expert nephrology nurse as being trusted, teaching others, and being seen as a role model. The expert nurse holds extensive clinical skills, has an inquiring mind, and constantly seeks knowledge and expertise to maintain his or her expert knowledge.

- Nephrology nurses are well positioned to support this patient group and their families to achieve a high quality of life through education, counseling, and skilled technical nursing interventions. The importance of considering each patient as an individual is emphasized since individualized care has been found to facilitate trust, learning, and quality clinical outcomes.

ANNP621   ## The Young and Middle Aged Adult with Chronic Kidney Disease

Leanne Dekker, MBA, MN, RN

Contemporary Nephrology Nursing: Principles and Practice contains 39 chapters of educational content. Individual learners may apply for continuing nursing education credit by reading a chapter and completing the Continuing Education Evaluation Form for that chapter. Learners may apply for continuing education credit for any or all chapters.

Please photocopy this page and return to ANNA.
COMPLETE THE FOLLOWING:

Name: _____

Address:_____

City:_____ State: _____ Zip: _____

E-mail: _____

Preferred telephone: ☐ Home   ☐ Work: _____

State where licensed and license number (optional): _____

CE application fees are based upon the number of contact hours provided by the individual chapter. CE fees per contact hour for ANNA members are as follows: 1.0-1.9 - $15; 2.0-2.9 - $20; 3.0-3.9 - $25; 4.0 and higher - $30. Fees for nonmembers are $10 higher.

ANNA Member: ☐ Yes   ☐ No   Member # (if available) _____

☐ Checked Enclosed   ☐ American Express   ☐ Visa   ☐ MasterCard

Total Amount Submitted: _____

Credit Card Number: _____ Exp. Date: _____

Name as it appears on the card: _____

CE Evaluation Form
To receive continuing education credit for individual study after reading the chapter
1. Photocopy this form. (You may also download this form from ANNA's Web site, **www.annanurse.org**.)

2. Mail the completed form with payment (check) or credit card information to American Nephrology Nurses' Association, East Holly Avenue, Box 56, Pitman, NJ 08071-0056.

3. You will receive your CE certificate from ANNA in 4 to 6 weeks.

Test returns must be postmarked by **December 31, 2010.**

CE Application Fee
ANNA Member $20.00
Nonmember $30.00

EVALUATION FORM

1. I verify that I have read this chapter and completed this education activity. Date: _____

_____
Signature

2. What would be different in your practice if you applied what you learned from this activity? *(Please use additional sheet of paper if necessary.)*

_____
_____
_____
_____
_____
_____
_____
_____
_____
_____

Evaluation	Strongly disagree				Strongly agree
3. The activity met the stated objectives.					
a. State the mortality and morbidity rates for young and middle aged adults with chronic kidney disease.	1	2	3	4	5
b. Describe the implications of chronic kidney disease to young and middle adults as to their ability to adjust, cope and adhere to their regimen.	1	2	3	4	5
c. Relate the impact of chronic kidney disease on the families of people diagnosed with chronic kidney disease.	1	2	3	4	5
4. The content was current and relevant.	1	2	3	4	5
5. The content was presented clearly.	1	2	3	4	5
6. The content was covered adequately.	1	2	3	4	5
7. Rate your ability to apply the learning obtained from this activity to practice.	1	2	3	4	5

Comments _____

_____

8. Time required to read the chapter and complete this form: _____ minutes.

This educational activity has been provided by the American Nephrology Nurses' Association (ANNA) for 2.0 contact hours. ANNA is accredited as a provider of continuing nursing education (CNE) by the American Nurses Credentialing Center's Commission on Accreditation (ANCC-COA). ANNA is an approved provider of continuing education by the California Board of Registered Nursing, CEP 0910.

The Older Adult With Chronic Kidney Disease

Terran Mathers, DNS, RN

Chapter Contents

Terran Mathers, DNS, RN

Provision of care for the older individual is different from that of younger populations, because of the changes that occur as a result of the aging process itself, the numerous diseases that tend to occur within this cohort, and the problems encountered with the treatment received (Kane, Ouslander, & Abrass, 2004). These changes often coexist and are interrelated.

Due to demographic projections, more studies are being conducted on the older adult population than before. This group has been categorized in several ways, including as a homogenous group of those individuals over 65 years of age, and by chronologic subcategories (e.g., young-old of 50 to 70 years old, "elite-old" of 100 years and above [Ebersole, Hess, & Luggen, 2004, p. 13]). Today, however, neither of these subcategories provide an accurate description of the functional capabilities and unique needs of the older adult. Miller (2004) suggests that "the concept of functional age provides a more rational basis for care than the measurement of how many years have passed since the person was born" (p. 5).

The purpose of this chapter is to provide an overview of the older adult with chronic kidney disease (CKD) and to describe nursing care that will promote maximal functioning, health, comfort, and independence. It must be kept in mind that a holistic approach is needed to care for the nephrology patient, regardless of age. The care of the older adult encompasses not only the physical person, but the psychological, social, spiritual, and familial aspects.

Aging in Perspective

Demographics

From 1993 to 2003, the number of older Americans over the age of 65 has increased by 3.1 million, accounting for 9.5% of the population (American Association of Retired Persons [AARP], 2004). It is predicted that this trend will continue, and that this population will outnumber all others, between the years of 2010 and 2030, when the baby boomer generation reaches 65 years of age. Increases in longevity have been attributed to: attitude changes, healthier lifestyles, environmental changes, higher educational levels, greater use of assistive devices, avoidance of health-risk behaviors, improved diagnostic and therapeutic techniques, and decreased prevalence of chronic conditions (Fries, 2002; Lan, Melzer, Tom, & Guralnik, 2002). Other characteristics of interest for the older adult population are summarized in Table 22-1.

Chronic Illness and Aging

Chronic illness can be defined as the "irreversible presence, accumulation, or latency of disease states or impairments that involve the total human environment for supportive care and self-care, maintenance of function and prevention of further disability" (Lubkin, 1990, p. 6). Although great strides have been made to improve the overall health status of individuals, older adults have more chronic conditions than younger people (National Center for Health Statistics, 2004). Chronic conditions may also relate to the increased mortality rate of this population (see also Chapter 3).

Incidence and Prevalence of Renal Disease

The median age of a new patient initiating CKD therapy is 65, according to the 2002 data from United States Renal Data System (USRDS, 2004). The incident rate for this older population increased 8% in 2002 from the previous year. Since 1992, a 41% increase was noted in the 65-74 year old

Table 22-1
Characteristics Highlighting an Aging Population

	Males	Females
Life Expectancy	16.6 years over 65	19.5 years over 65
Marital Status		
Married	71%	41%
Widowed	14%	44%
Single (never married)	4%	4%
Divorced or separated/spouse absent	11%	10%
Living Arrangements		
Lives with spouse	71%	41%
Lives alone	19%	40%
Other	10%	19%
Median Income	$20,363	$11,845
Employed in labor force	18.3%	10.7%

Note: Adapted from The American Association of Retired Persons and USDHHS Administration on Aging, A Profile of Older American (2004), whose information is based on data from the U.S. Bureau of the Census.

group, while a 93% increase was evident in those patients 75 years of age and older. The highest prevalence rates since 1992 are for those patients ages 65-74, which is a 57% increase. Numbers have doubled for those of 75 years and older (USRDS, 2004).

Cardiovascular diseases are highest in the 65+ age group with ESRD who also have hypertension and diabetes, and have survived 1 year of dialytic therapy (USRDS, 2004). Studies in this area are ongoing as researchers try to determine appropriate diagnostic and therapeutic procedures for the prevention and treatment of these diseases. Practices are already being changed with the initiation of the K/DOQI Clinical Practice Guidelines for Cardiovascular Disease in Dialysis Patients, which include a recommended echocardiography soon after dialysis is initiated (USRDS, 2004).

Nursing Homes and Long-Term Care

Currently, only 4.5% of the elderly reside in nursing homes (AARP, 2004). As the general population gets progressively older, this percentage is expected to increase. Fifty percent of ESRD patients in nursing homes are 65 years of age and older, with a mean age of approximately 72 years (USRDS, 2004). Diabetics make up 50% of the population, and hypertension affects 1 out of 3 ESRD patients in these settings (USRDS, 2004). In an effort to assist clinicians working in alternative settings such as long-term care (LTC), the American Nephrology Nurses' Association (ANNA) released a learning module geared specifically toward the patient care providers taking care of CKD patients in settings outside of nephrology or dialysis (ANNA, 2004).

Goal of Medical Treatment

The general goal of treatment of an older adult with CKD is maintenance of health status at an optimal level of functioning. How this is accomplished depends on the individual's condition. Amount and types of medical treatment will fluctuate based on the decisions made by the multidisciplinary team in collaboration with the older adult and his/her family as active participants in the process.

Relevant Issues of Significance

Physiological Changes

The physiological and pathophysiological changes that occur with aging affect both internal and external structures in the human body (see Table 22-2). This may bring about adaptive responses to achieve even the smallest of activities of daily living, depending on the severity of the physiological change. The health care professional can assess whether the changes known to occur most often among older adults have occurred and can use this knowledge to develop an effective plan of care. For the older person with kidney disease, physiological changes can affect overall physical, psychological, and sociological functioning. For the purposes of this chapter, a brief overview of sensory, cardiovascular, respiratory, and renal changes associated with aging are presented, and the issue of frailty is highlighted.

Sensory. The five senses of hearing, vision, smell, taste, and touch are affected by the aging process, more in some individuals than others. Hearing and visual changes can alter

the way an individual perceives and comprehends information presented, while impaired smell and taste can affect nutritional status. Alterations in touch can interfere with manipulation and safety. Specific diseases such as diabetes and hypertension, which have effects on the functioning of the eyes, are addressed in detail in Chapters 6 and 12. These conditions are more prevalent in the older individual due to the physiological changes associated with aging.

Auditory deficiencies can occur from changes in air and/or bone conduction. Changes in air conduction result in difficulty with clarity of sounds, specifically with the discrimination of high-pitched sounds, while the changes in bone conduction cause diminished amplification of speech that is of normal volume (Ebersole, Hess & Luggen, 2004; Winchester, 2002). Causes for impairment may be attributed to genetics; nerve cell degeneration; intense noise exposure; trauma; ototoxic drugs (e.g., diuretics and chemotherapeutics); metabolic diseases in organs such as the kidney; vascular diseases; infections; and wax buildup in the ear canal (Weinstein, 2003). Consequences of hearing loss may include inhibition of verbal communication and contact with others, contributing to social isolation, depression, self-esteem disturbance, and misunderstanding by the patient of specific instructions (i.e., when and how to take medications) and educational information. These can ultimately decrease quality of life of the older adult and hinder patient care.

Normal physiological changes of the eyes that occur with aging can cause functional changes that bring difficulty in recognizing or seeing persons, places, and things. Some of the changes include: (a) changes in color perception (making it difficult to discriminate between greens and blues), (b) a decrease in peripheral vision and depth perception, (c) response to change in lighting, (d) refraction that affects the focusing on objects that are close (presbyopia), and (e) an increased sensitivity to glare (Miller, 2004). These problems, as in those of hearing, can have an effect on the care given elderly persons, including education and rehabilitation. *Healthy People 2010*, a national health promotion and disease prevention initiative, specifically identifies objectives to improve health related to hearing and vision (United States Department of Health and Human Services, 2000).

The sense of smell can serve several purposes for an older person: safety (to detect gas leaks or smoke), association with pleasant events of the past (cinnamon and Mom's pumpkin pie), and maintenance of nutritional status (stimulation of salivation and hunger) (Ebersole, Hess, & Luggen, 2004). Any deficiency in smell is a cause for concern, especially if the individual is living alone. Taste, which can also affect the nutritional status of the older adult, will be discussed later in this chapter, in the discussion of nutritional issues.

With aging, there is decreased tactile sensation. That is, the skin does not sense pressure changes or changes in the temperature as readily. This is a cause for concern for older adults since they may not be able to determine water temperature, sense when they have a firm grasp of something, or feel the pressure being exerted upon parts of the body. In the case of the dialysis patient, decreased sensation may contribute to skin breakdown when in a chair for long periods of time during a hemodialysis treatment. A peritoneal dialysis patient may not be able to connect the tubing to the bag of dialysate solution for treatment because of decreased touch sensitivity necessary for complete manual dexterity.

Cardiovascular system. Because of the increased number of chronic diseases as one grows older, it is difficult to determine if cardiovascular changes are disease-related or due to aging. Technological advancement is now allowing researchers to identify those older individuals who are free of cardiovascular disease, so that studies may be conducted to determine the affect that the aging process alone has on cardiovascular functioning. Controlling for other variables, including a person's lifestyle (i.e., smoking, nutrition, stress) and cultural influence can also affect research outcomes (Miller, 2004).

Cardiac complications are considered to be the leading cause of death in those patients with CKD (USRDS, 2004). According to Ismail, Hakim, Oreopoulos, and Patrikarea (1993), older age in a dialysis patient can be considered a risk factor for left ventricular hypertrophy, dilated cardiomyopathy, and ischemic heart disease. The impact of heart disease has been demonstrated in small studies conducted on patients ages 65 and older receiving dialytic therapy. Survival rates are shorter than those of the general dialysis population (Alpert, 1995). It is clear that nurses need to consider cardiovascular functioning in planning their care. Awareness of signs and symptoms, as well as the appropriate nursing interventions will assist nurses in caring for these individuals. Strategies may include the control of blood pressure, preventative measures accompanied with treatment for hyperparathyroidism, appropriate dialytic prescriptions, corrective action for anemia, and monitoring of pharmaceutical agents (see Chapter 18 for drug therapies). The K/DOQI Clinical Practice Guidelines for Cardiovascular Disease in Dialysis Patients (National Kidney Foundation, 2005), based on research evidence, provide direction for monitoring and control of cardiovascular complications.

Respiratory system. Several changes occur within the respiratory system that affect an older person, and can be of more concern if that person is on dialysis. The chest wall and musculoskeletal changes include the calcification of the costal cartilage, weakening of the respiratory muscles, and osteoporosis of the ribs and vertebrae. Because of these changes, there is a reduction in the efficiency of the respiratory system and the maximal inspiratory and expiratory force. This affects the supply of oxygen and removal of carbon dioxide, impacting vital organs, and tissue functioning (Miller, 2004).

The lungs become smaller with decreases in muscle tone, and the vasculature is affected. Gas exchange is compromised so that there is a decrease in arterial pO_2 (Miller, 2004). This age-related change, accompanied by complications of hemodialysis, can cause some difficulties for the older person. The individual with kidney disease is also usually anemic, resulting in decreased oxygen transfer within the body due to the smaller number of red blood cells.

The elastic recoil of the lungs is reduced somewhat with age, affecting expansion and retraction of the lungs. This results in an increase of the residual volume, while the forced expiratory volume is decreased. This change in recoil also affects airflow rates, with an overall decrease in the efficiency of the lungs (Miller, 2004).

Renal system. It is generally accepted that there is a progressive decline in overall renal functioning once a person reaches early adulthood, as a result of changes in renal structure and vasculature (Eaton & Pooler, 2004). Anatomical changes specific to the normal aging of one's kidneys include a decrease in the weight of the kidney and total renal mass, resulting primarily from the vascular changes in the cortex. There is a decrease in the cells within the glomeruli due in part to sclerosis, and a decrease in the tubules that experience some hypertrophy. The basement membranes of these two areas thicken, and the size of individual cells increase.

Accompanying the physiological changes noted above, are impairments in various areas of functioning. Some of these include: (a) decreases in the renal plasma flow (RPF) and glomerular filtration rate (GFR), which affects the filtration fraction ("calculated by dividing GFR by effective RPF") (Radke, 1994, p. 184); (b) decreased ability to concentrate urine; (c) decreased renin secretion (Seeley, Stephens, & Tate, 2006); (d) reduced sodium retention, thought to be related to changes in the renin-aldosterone system (Radke, 1994); (e) decrease in urinary excretion of calcium, thought to be partially related to the reduction in renal mass and serum calcium levels (Radke, 1994); (f) impaired potassium excretion due to a lowered aldosterone level (Eaton & Pooler, 2004); and (g) a reduction in vitamin D synthesis (Seeley, Stephens, & Tate, 2006). Normally, the kidneys adapt and function adequately as physiological changes occur within the human body. However, stress induced by acute and chronic illnesses may upset homeostasis, possibly resulting in renal failure for that individual.

Frailty. Older adults with chronic kidney disease also have a high prevalence of frailty (Shlipak et al., 2004). Frail older adults are individuals who lack functional reserve and are at risk for decline. Unintentional weight loss, self-reported exhaustion, measured weakness, slow walking speed, and low physical activity are all indicators of frailty. After adjusting for co-morbidity, chronic renal insufficiency was found to be significantly associated with frailty in a study of community dwelling older adults from 4 clinical centers in the United States (Shlipak et al., 2004). This suggests that frail elderly persons with kidney disease warrant special attention to preserve their independence and indeed survival.

Psychosocial Challenges and Realities

Theories of psychosocial development. Throughout one's life span, learning is accompanied by many behavior changes that occur due to adaptation to environmental factors. As with every stage of life, old age can be met and experienced with upheaval or serenity. Havighurst (1952) and Erikson (1963) are two theorists who are known for their work with psychosocial development associated with growing older. Havinghurst (1952) describes the developmental tasks of older adulthood as later maturity. He states that a developmental task is one that "arises at or about a certain period in the life of the individual, successful achievement of which leads to his happiness and to success with later tasks, while failure leads to unhappiness in the individual, disapproval by the society, and difficulty with later tasks" (p. 2). During this period of old age, the individual adjusts to phys-

Table 22-2
Expected Changes Related to the Aging Process

Understanding normal age-related changes is the foundation to understanding health and disease in older people. The following section highlights changes within each organ system that are known to decline with age.

Skin and connective tissue
- Loss of dermal thickness produces transparent, thin skin appearance.
- In the epidermis, melanocytes' (pigment-producing cells) number and activity decrease, making skin more sensitive to ultraviolet sunlight.
- Progressive loss of melanocytes in hair bulbs and decreased number of hair follicles result in greying and thinning of hair.
- Decrease in epidermis turnover contributes to slower wound healing.
- Sebaceous and sweat glands decrease in number, size, and function, therefore producing less oil and sweat.
- Decreased vascular bed and responsiveness (and sweating) predispose older people to hypothermia and hyperthermia.
- Decreased vitamin D_3 production and decreased exposure to sunlight may contribute to osteoporosis and osteomalacia.

Nervous System
- Moderate cortical atrophy.
- Loss of neurons in the neocortex, substantia nigra, and limbic system.
- Lipofuscin pigment accumulates primarily in glial tissues.
- Certain neurotransmitters decline.
- Binding sites for dopamine and serotonin decrease.
- Peripheral nerve fibers decrease in number and size.
  - Motor and sensory nerve conduction decreases.
  - A decrease in vibratory sensation in feet and ankles may occur.

Special senses
Vision
- Atrophy of periorbital tissue may cause upper and lower lids to droop.
- Visual activity may decrease due to changes in the retina or neural components.
- Loss of accommodation causes hyperopia.
- Nuclear sclerosis causes myopia.
- Decreased tear secretion may cause dryness of eyes.

Hearing
- Pure tone loss is greater at high frequencies than at low frequencies.
- Pitch discrimination declines primarily at very high and low frequencies.
- Speech discrimination declines and is worsened with background noise.

Smell
- Olfaction declines, causing poor detection and discrimination by the eighth decade.

Oral
- A reduction in the integrity of epithelial and connective tissue causes a thinning of the oral mucosa and affects bone pulpal tissues.
  - Blood supply is decreased.
  - Nerve innervation is compromised.
  - Tissue quality is modified.
  - Calcifitic tissue changes occur.
- A compositional change in the nature of saliva.
  - Altered sodium levels.
  - Increase in potassium.
  - Decrease in secretory proteins.
- A reduction in taste perception.
  - Increase in threshold potentials for salt and bitter tastes.
- Structural changes to the teeth.
  - Erosion.
  - Abrasion.
  - Attrition.
- Gingival recession.
  - Alveolar dehiscence.
  - Compromised spatial position of teeth.

Cardiovascular
- Conducting system loses cells and fibers and becomes infiltrated with fat.
- Heart rate at rest and achievable maximum declines [maximum HR = (220-age)].
- Increase in stroke volume (S.V.) compensates for lower heart rate (H.R.) and maintaining cardiac output (C.O.) [C.O. = H.R. x S.V.].
- Intrinsic contractile function declines.
- Vascular compliance decreases due to changes in the vessel walls with intima cellular proliferation and fibrosis and media elastin fragmentation and calcification.
- In Western and developed countries, systolic blood pressure increases with lower rate of increase in diastolic pressure.

Table 22-2 (continued)
Expected Changes Related to the Aging Process

Respiratory
- Lung elastic recoil decreases as a result of collagen and elastic changes.
- Chest wall compliance decreases due to stiffening of the chest wall.
- Respiratory muscle strength decreases.
- Lung volumes change as a consequence of the above changes.
  - Increase in residual volume and functional residual capacity.
  - Decrease in vital capacity and expiratory flow rates.
- Gas exchange.
  - Decrease in arterial pO_2, due to ventilation-perfusion mismatch.

Gastrointestinal
- Esophageal motility decreases due to lower amplitude contractions after swallowing (presbyesophages).
- Gastric mucosa thins, acid-producing parietal cells atrophy, and gastric acid secretion decreases.
- Small and large intestinal mucosa atrophies, reducing absorptive surface area and decreasing the ability to absorb sugars, calcium, vitamin B_{12}, and iron.
- Liver decreases in size but maintains function; however, the microsomal enzyme function declines.

Renal
- Renal mass decreases with primarily cortical losses of nephrons, glomeruli, and capillaries.
- Renal plasma flow decreases.
- Glomerular filtration rate (GFR) falls.
- Creatinine clearance progressively declines 1% per year after age 40 with no change in serum creatinine levels, because creatinine generation also decreases.
- Ability to retain sodium (Na) declines.
- Ability to concentrate urine declines.

Musculoskeletal
- Decrease in muscle weight compared to total body weight.
- Decreased muscular strength and endurance associated with decrease in number of muscle fibers.
- Hyaline cartilage water content declines.
- Bone loss is universal, but rate is highly variable; loss is more rapid in women after menopause than in men.

Hematopoietic
- Overall red cells, hemoglobin, hematocrit, white cells, and platelets maintain normal values and functions.
- Active bone marrow decreases and marrow fat increases but remains adequate for hematopoiesis.

Immune System
- Thymic involution begins about age of puberty.
- Number of T- and B-lymphocytes does not change.
- T-lymphocyte function declines.
  - Decreased response to skin tests.
  - Production of interleukin-2 is reduced.
- B-lymphocyte function is not as clear.
  - Immunoglobulins IgM and perhaps IgG levels decline.
  - Immunoglobulin production to a challenge (vaccine or antigen) is lowered response and shortened duration.

Endocrine
- Progressive decline in carbohydrate tolerance.
  - Primary defect in insulin resistance as post-receptor defect.
- Metabolic clearance rate of thyroid hormone decreases but thyroxine (T4) levels are normal.

Genital/Sexual Function
Women
- With menopause, rapid decline of estrogen and progesterone.
- Hormonal changes cause atrophic changes of uterus, vagina, external genitalia, and breasts.
- Sexual activity decreases, but exact role of biologic changes and sociocultural factors are unknown.

Men
- Testosterone levels remain level.
- Prostate gland increases in size due to hyperplasia.
- Erectile and ejaculatory function declines; postejaculatory refractory period increases.
- Sexual response is delayed due to reduced penile sensitivity and increased threshold for tactile stimulation.

Note: From Stanford, E.P., & Schmidt, M.G. (1991). Guidelines for education: Geriatric health care professionals (pp. 18-20). Used with permission. Diane L. Schneider, MD, UCSD School of Medicine, prepared this for the San Diego Geriatric Education Center publication.

ical changes, retirement, living with the spouse who has retired, changes in income, establishment of living arrangements that are physically satisfactory, and affiliation with one's peers while also assimilating social roles and obligations.

Erikson (1963) looks at life as a continuum with four major phases subdivided into eight stages. A review of the last phase of old age pertains to individuals 60 or more years of age. This phase is further categorized into ego integrity versus despair. Ego integrity refers to individuals' sense of peace, as well as their view of satisfaction with past life and self. They are able to let go and look toward the future with contentment. Despair, on the other hand, is experienced by individuals who wish they could go back to earlier days and change the past.

Stressors of aging. As an individual grows older, changes and transitions take place that are considered stressors. These can be viewed as positive or negative, depending on the effect they have on the individual. Specific stressors for older individuals include those that affect them psychologically, but these are often overlooked because old age is often portrayed as a time of tranquility and contentment. Common emotional reactions for this age group include grief, guilt, loneliness, rage, depression, helplessness, and anxiety (Butler, Lewis, & Sunderland, 1998). Situational crises, such as widowhood, marital problems, sexual problems, financial difficulties, physical changes and discomfort, disability, hospitalization, death and dying (of loved ones and concern for self) (Butler et al., 1998), ageist attitudes, retirement, and relocation (Miller, 2004), can add stress to the lives of older adults.

The impact of life events are important to consider because they can have an effect on the overall well-being of individuals. Miller (2004) has differentiated the meaning of life events as they occur within older individuals' lives from those of younger adults. She believes that:

1. Events for an older person are frequently associated with loss;
2. Several events are more likely to occur within a short time span;
3. They last for a longer period of time; and,
4. Powerlessness is often felt by the individual (p. 140).

Sexuality. Sexuality is often overlooked as an important aspect of life of the older person. Whether it is by offering a hug, holding of hands, flirting, a sexual fantasy, or sexual intercourse, older individuals have as much a right to express their sexual feelings as any other human being. Dysfunction in this area of behavioral responses can be attributed not only to the aging process and physiological changes, but also societal attitudes and myths regarding sexual expression, chronic illnesses, lack of a partner, lack of knowledge/education regarding methods of sexual expression, and medications/drugs and alcohol (Ferrini & Ferrini, 2000).

Aging physiology and sexual responses. As with other body systems, the reproductive system changes as one grows older, causing a need for adaptations in sexual activity. For females, sexual response changes include: slower vaginal lubrication with a decreased amount produced, a thinning of the vaginal lining, less flexibility of the vagina, and a decrease in the intensity of orgasms. Males experience: a decrease in the urgency of the sex drive; a longer time to have an erection, with the penis also not as firm as in previous years; loss of erection prior to orgasm; more stimulation needed for ejaculation, which is then less forceful (if one does ejaculate) with a smaller amount of semen; and a longer refractory period (Byer & Shainberg, 1991).

Societal attitudes and myths. There are an array of societal myths and stereotypes pertaining to sexuality of the older adult population. Two common misconceptions are:

1. Sex is not practiced by older adults. Contrary to popular beliefs, sexual activity occurs well into the ninth decades by some individuals. People who were most active sexually in their younger years tend to be the most active in later years.
2. Older individuals do not enjoy sex. Unless severely compromised by physical difficulty and inhibitions, older adults can enjoy sex as much as younger adults. Sexual drive can differ for individuals from one time to another (as in younger life), and each person has individual sexual desires and needs (Ebersole, Hess & Luggen, 2004).

Chronic illnesses. Individuals are more susceptible to chronic illnesses as they grow older. The older nephrology patient may be dealing with not only renal failure, but also other illnesses that may be causing sexual dysfunction. The diseases may be neurologic, vascular, endocrine, musculoskeletal or psychological in nature (Nusbaum, Hamilton, & Lehahan, 2003) and may include such diseases as diabetes, arthritis, cardiovascular conditions, and mental illness.

Lack of partner or spouse. Lack of a sexual partner tends to be more of a problem for women than men. Women outlive men, so there are fewer males from which to choose (Ferrini & Ferrini, 2000).

Education. It is important that information regarding physiological changes in the normal aging process and any usual occurring changes brought about by a disease be shared with the patient and his/her partner. Knowing what is normal will help relieve some of the guilt often experienced by older individuals when sexual activity and relationships are hindered. Education also involves dispelling myths, and introducing alternative methods for expressing sexuality such as changes in coital positions and alternate ways to express intimacy. Information on the availability of medical and surgical interventions, if necessary, should also be provided.

Medications/drugs and alcohol. Many pharmacological agents and alcohol can have an effect on sexual activity, both physically and psychologically. Some of the medications that can have an adverse effect are included in the following classifications: antihypertensives, lipid-lowering agents, antihistamines, psychotropics, anxiolytics, anticholinergics, and diuretics (just to name a few) (Nusbaum, Hamilton, & Lenahan, 2003). Blood levels indicative of large amounts of alcohol intake also correlate with diminished sexual performance, including temporary impotence for men with a potential for loss of erections if the intake is chronic (Ferrini & Ferrini, 2000), and reduced libido and orgasms by women (Ferrini & Ferrini, 2000; Miller, 2004).

Sexual counseling. Sexual counseling is best addressed by professionals who have received specific training and are skilled in this area. This may be any member of the multidisciplinary team, including nurses, social workers, and

Table 22-3

Sexual Counseling of the Geriatric Nephrology Patient - The PLISSIT Model

Levels of Counseling	Purpose	Patient Outcomes
Permission	Allows patients to discuss sexual concerns openly and without hesitation, with reassurance from health care professionals.	Understanding that the sexual problems encountered are normal and that sexual activity is still permitted.
Limited **I**nformation	Provides patients with reading materials in layman's terms concerning sexual changes related to renal disease and the aging process. These are then discussed with health care professionals.	Patients are reassured through written information and have a more thorough understanding of the effects of renal disease accompanied by aging as it relates to sexual activity.
Specific **S**uggestions	Suggestions are presented by health care professionals for improving the sexual problems of patients.	The strategies provided allow patients alternatives from which to choose for expressing sexuality.
Intensive **T**herapy	Assistance is provided by certified sex therapists.	Patients benefit from therapists educated in the field of sex therapy when the previous three levels are unsuccessful.

Note: Adapted from the Hartford Institute for Geriatric Nursing "Try This" series by Wallace (2000).

nephrologists. Because talk about sexual activity was usually taboo for older persons during their earlier years, it is often the health care provider who needs to first mention sexual activity and potential problems. Physical assessment and a sexual history may reveal problems that could be reversed through some minor interventions, or even through surgery, if it is of a more serious nature. An approach suggested by Wallace (2000) that is often used in sexual counseling is PLISSIT. This four-step method could be used with older nephrology patients as well, and is summarized in Table 22-3.

Depression. Although depression is less frequent among older adults than those who are younger, it has been identified as the most common functional psychiatric disorder for the older individual (Ebersole, Hess & Luggen, 2004). Some possible causes of depression include: poor health, loss, medication, drug and substance abuse, failure to thrive, loneliness, isolation, increasing dependence, and inability to perform activities of daily living.

In a recent study, it was found that the level of depressive affect of older adults was lower than for younger individuals (Kimmel et al., 2000). This does not negate the fact that assessment for depression is an important aspect of nursing care. Assessing the older adult with CKD for depression can be difficult, because the cause is not always readily recognized and the measures of depression are often confounded with physical changes experienced by all people with renal disease (e.g., sleep problems, lack of energy) (Kimmel, 2002).

Coping with life. Growing old can be a challenge for any individual. How one accepts these challenges will help to determine the state of mind and body, which in turn can cause a fluctuation in the individual's self-esteem. A self-

esteem disturbance may be identified in such life circumstances as retirement, loss of spouse, physical disability, impact of ageism associated with negative stereotypes, decreased social interaction, and loss of control over environmental issues.

The psychological well-being of individuals will depend on the effectiveness of coping strategies. Individuals will experience life events from different perspectives, thereby adding, maintaining and discarding defense mechanisms as the situations dictate, depending on the personal perceptions that they have of each event. Denial, projection, fixation, regression, displacement, counterphobia, and idealization have been identified as the main ones used by older people (Butler et al., 1998).

Problems that may surface if a crisis situation ensues and usual coping mechanisms are not effective include depression, loneliness, isolation, and a lowered self-esteem. Researchers have shown that psychiatric morbidity is not higher in people on hemodialysis compared to continuous ambulatory peritoneal dialysis (CAPD) (Lordanidis et al., 1993). Little research, however, has been conducted pertaining to specific coping strategies of older adults with kidney disease because they are often grouped together with middle-aged individuals.

Spirituality. When considering the spirituality of an older person, background assessment should include not only the physical, psychological, and social aspects of life, but also the individual's cultural, religious, and ethnic background. Spirituality is a broader concept than religion. Reed (1991) describes healthy spirituality as that which "fosters a concern for others and self, a sense of meaning and enjoyment in life, commitment to purposes greater than the self, a sense of relatedness, and a means for moving through a debilitating sense of guilt, anger, and anxiety" (p. 17). Spirituality often gives meaning to life's experiences, and assists people in coping with difficult life circumstances. Spirituality of older adults with CKD has not been specifically studied, but Walton (2002), in a grounded theory study of hemodialysis patients aged 36 to 78 years found that categories of spirituality were faith, presence, and receiving and giving back. Participants described spirituality as a life-giving force, full of awe, wonder, and solitude that inspired one to strive for balance in life. In a quantitative study, Kimmel, Emont, Newmann, Danko and Moss (2003) found that scores on the Spiritual Beliefs Scale were correlated with quality of life scores of people with ESRD. Clinical practice also suggests that spirituality is important to many older adults with CKD, and may help them deal with the challenges associated with the illness and treatment.

Comprehensive Nursing Assessment and Interventions

A detailed patient-specific, accurate, and comprehensive assessment of the older person provides information necessary to analyze individual strengths and weaknesses. Alterations of functioning may be pinpointed through an integration of physical, psychological, and social data. The assessment should encompass genetics, culture, and nutrition as well as adaptation to changes in health and functioning, outside support, spiritual beliefs, living arrangements, economic status, recent life situations, and disease/illness (Campbell, 1995). The assessment may be conducted by means of observations, interviews, and physical assessment and include both subjective and objective data. Knowing the expected changes that occur with normal aging, as noted in Table 22-2, can help to identify what is abnormal. The aging process has a multitude of diverse presentations.

Nursing Strategies/Adaptations

Assessment of the older person is conducted in much the same manner as with other age groups. There are, however, several adaptations that should be taken into account. These include time, environmental conditions, and communication techniques. Other factors that need to be included within these are sensory deficits and cognitive changes.

Time. Time of day is a consideration that may mean the difference between obtaining accurate and specific information from that which is given too quickly. Older people may not do well at certain times of day, and it is important to establish times suitable for them. Sleep patterns are different in older adults, with some taking a nap during the afternoon. For those older individuals already receiving dialysis therapy, the best assessment time may be just before the treatment. Because older individuals tend to tire easily, have slower functioning, a longer history to share, and more problems to discuss, multiple interviews for shorter periods of time may also assist in eliciting the needed data (Eliopoulos, 2001).

Environmental conditions. It is important to consider the environmental setting during an interview. The room should be well lit, but without the brightness of direct sunlight and florescent lights which can cause an irritating glare for elderly individuals (Eliopoulos, 2001). Chairs should be padded slightly and have a straight back for comfort. Have available pillows and blankets, especially when patients are lying on an examination table or are having a dialysis treatment, and minimize the length of time they need to be in this position, if at all possible. Room temperature should be at a comfortable level, keeping in mind that these individuals chill easily due to the decrease in the amount of body fat. Extraneous noises should be kept to a minimum, especially if there is a hearing problem. And, finally, allowing for as much privacy as feasible will produce an atmosphere conducive for an effective exchange of information and assessment (Campbell, 1995; Eliopoulos, 2001).

Communication techniques. The basic skill of listening is necessary for assessment. The nurse should be positioned so as to allow the elderly individual to lip read to accommodate for hearing loss if this should be the case. Give the older individual enough time to express herself/himself. Use open-ended questions to extract the individual's perceptions and viewpoints (Eliopoulos, 2001). Many older adults like to reminisce, and although the nurse can gain insight into the background of the individual's problems (Campbell, 1995), it may also be necessary to also redirect the questioning. Use understandable lay terms, refraining from medical jargon and terms that may not be understood. At times, it will be necessary to use family members to assist with signs and symptoms, because the elderly tend to underreport some information, such as problems with mental clarity, for fear that they may be seen as senile. However, initial interviews of individuals should be conducted when they are alone so as to obtain information directly from them and to prevent interference from family members who often try to provide the answers. If the individual requests that another family member be present, this should be accommodated. If not, the family can still be approached separately for their input. Where language is a barrier, interpreters may be needed to facilitate the interaction. The nurse must also be aware of and respect ethnic and cultural differences in perceptions relating to health (Campbell, 1995).

Observing nonverbal communication and outward physical appearance of the individual by the nurse cannot be overemphasized. This in itself may answer many questions or lead to effective assessment that otherwise may be overlooked. Even simple observations of physical mobility, such as moving from one position to another, may indicate some problems not identified by the patient (Eliopoulos, 2001).

Assessment Tools and Interventions

An array of assessment tools specific to the older population is available (Ebersole, Hess & Luggen, 2004). Key points that need to be addressed in the assessment of the older person include: chief concerns, health history, medication history, recent life changes, daily activities, cognitive patterns, and support systems. It is up to the nurse to decide what assessment tools would be useful and which would best facilitate the care planning of the patient within the nephrology facility. To obtain a holistic overview of the patient, the nephrology nurse must not only review the information obtained by the nephrologist, but also use this information to obtain further data. Collaborative assessment facilitates the care of these patients for optimal outcomes and includes specifics concerning the physical, psychological, and social functioning of the individual.

Figure 22-1
Strategies to Enhance Self-Esteem

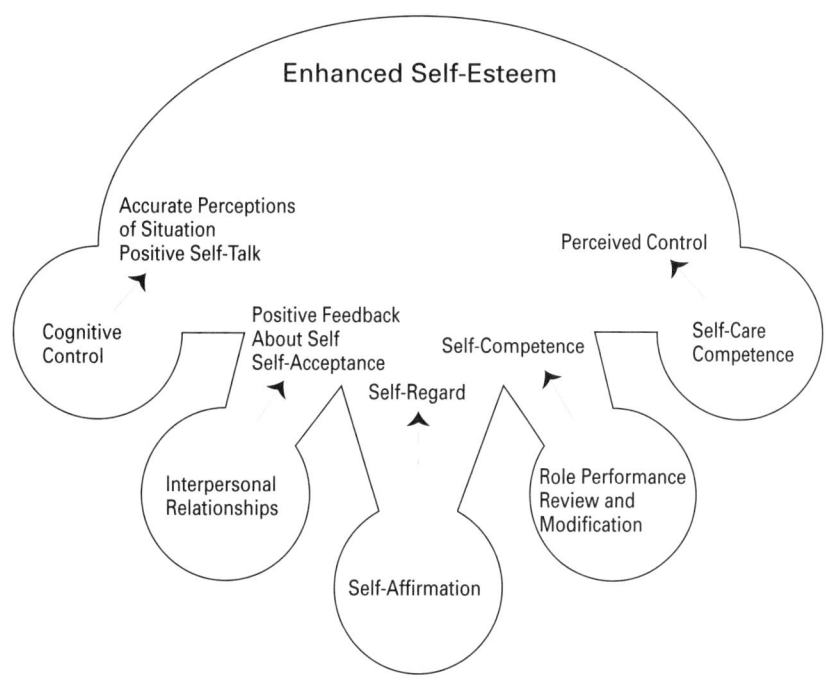

Note: From Miller, J. (2000). Enhancing self-esteem. In J. Miller (Ed.), *Coping with chronic illness: Overcoming powerlessness* (3rd ed.) (pp. 505-521). Philadelphia: F.A. Davis Company. Reprinted with permission.

Physical data. A health history, physical assessment, and laboratory data are components of the assessment of the physical aspect of an individual. In addition to objective data, it is also necessary to obtain subjective input from the patient and from the other health team members. Developing medical and nursing diagnoses can be a challenging process. The older person often presents with signs and symptoms that can be attributed to multiple factors, making it difficult to pinpoint a specific problem. Assessment of physical data is ongoing and is often interrelated with both psychological and social behavioral manifestations. Campbell (1995) has suggested points to consider when identifying physiological and psychological problems:

- there is a proven decline in the biological makeup of an older individual of tissues and organ systems;
- depression has an impact on psychological functioning; and
- psychological changes can be the result of changing pathophysiology (Foreman & Gradowski, 1992).

As noted by Campbell (1995), the cognitive functioning of an individual can be affected physiologically by "cardiovascular problems, metabolic disorders, hematological disorders, neurological disorders and deficits, and iatrogenic disorders" (p. 91). Physical data, such as bruising, can also be useful to identify problems such as falls, which are more frequent in the elderly (Tideiksaar, 2002).

Interventions are dependent on the diagnoses and the specific problems identified. Education and then follow-up assessment may encompass such things as need for medication changes, potential side effects, significance of laboratory values, support groups and counseling, the disease process, and self-care.

Psychological/emotional data. The nephrology nurse must keep in mind that older adults with CKD may have experienced major changes as a result of the renal disease. Nephrology nurses should explore individuals' problems and their perceptions of these problems. Through the use of therapeutic communication with an emphasis on open-ended questions and utilization of listening skills, the nurse can facilitate verbalization of the person's thoughts and feelings. In collaboration with the individual, attempts can be made to explore alternatives, problem-solve, and find solutions. As an advocate, the nurse should also collaborate with the interdisciplinary team and elicit appropriate assistance, thereby helping these individuals to acquire and use the various resources available to solve or gain control of their problems.

Several interventions are suggested to promote psychological well-being of the older individual. These include:
1. Education – Evaluating first the emotional readiness, or motivation to learn as well as the experiential readiness, or the background knowledge, values and attitudes of an individual will assist in developing the instructional content and methods specific to the needs of a particular indi-

vidual. Also, the needs and goals of the older person should be elicited and taken into consideration.

2. Enabling and empowerment - Through this process, assistance is provided to individuals to help gain control over specific aspects of their lives. Nephrology nurses can facilitate this process through encouragement of independence and self-care for the older nephrology adult. Positive and constructive feedback is important in this process to encourage continuing personal growth and development, as well as an optimal level of functioning.

3. Enhancement of self-esteem – Miller (2000) suggested five strategies that an individual can use to increase personal self esteem: cognitive control, interpersonal relationships, self-affirmation, role performance review and modifications, and self-care competence (p. 514). These are noted in Figure 22-1 with accompanying outcomes that can be used for evaluation purposes. Although not specific to the older individual, these ideas could be used to assist the older adult to move toward a more positive view of self. The nurse needs to identify the strengths and abilities of each individual person with emphasis on these qualities.

4. Support groups – Participation in support groups may help older adults with CKD to express their feelings and anxieties, eliciting feedback and problem-solving solutions from others who have experienced similar situations. They may be in the form of groups specific to certain conditions and circumstances such as CKD, widowhood, or depression. Educational groups about a certain interest of the patient, or groups formed based on age of the participants, such as senior citizen activity groups, may also be useful. Other ideas for groups may include reminiscing, remotivation, music and dance, guided autobiography, and travel clubs. Groups are often not used by the older adult due to financial concerns, transportation, time restraints of the dialysis treatments, and even lack of knowledge about the availability of resources. Interventions could be directed toward removing barriers so participation is possible.

5. Social support networks – Social support systems can provide older adults with a sense of well-being and give meaning to their lives. Family, group, peer, or individual counseling can provide a means of support during troubled times of anger, confusion, depression, and anxiety. All of these support systems, of course, depend on availability at the time of need. Family support may be marginal, especially if members are not living within the same geographic area. There are also family members who hinder the individual's progress and independence. Utilization of this kind of support needs to be facilitated to that person's best advantage.

Many nursing interventions depend on the cognitive functioning of the individual. When the nurse assesses cognitive functioning, she does so to determine whether there is a progressive change in the mental status of the individual, and to help determine what interventions may be useful to the individual. Tools such as the Short Portable Mental Status Questionnaire (SPMSQ) by Pfeiffer (1974), the Mini-Mental Status Exam (Folstein, Folstein, & McHugh, 1975), and the Confusion Assessment Method Instrument (CAM) (Waszynski, 2001) are valuable assessment instruments for cognitive status.

Social/functional data. Indicators of social functioning of an individual include degree of competence, independence, and autonomy. Health problems can reduce socialization, leading to isolation, loneliness, and depression (Eliopoulos, 2001). During the social assessment, consideration should be given to the social support network, family support, financial status, independence with regard to activities of daily living and functional ability, image, cognitive functioning, and environmental adequacy (Kaiser, 1990).

A social assessment consists of basic identifying data about the person such as full name, address, telephone number, next of kin, insurance information, and use of other outside agencies. The nurse should identify the environmental adequacy of living conditions, compatibility of the physical condition of the residence with the needs of the patient, security of the home and neighborhood, and the availability of a support network (i.e., neighbors, family and friends) and means of transportation for activities other than dialysis treatments. Financial status is also of great importance, because without monetary support, many social activities, whether recreational in nature or of necessity such as doctors' appointments, cannot be accomplished. Often, this information is obtained by the social worker in a dialysis facility, but is of great importance for the nurse to be aware of in the plan of care.

Functional status can have a great impact on the socialization of the individual. According to Nelson and Mayfield (1994), "functional assessment is a systematic attempt to objectively measure performance in the areas of daily living, activities of daily living (ADL), instrumental activities of daily living (IADL), mental status, social status, and economic resources" (p. 120). Functional deficits may not always be something that older individuals are aware of because they tend to deteriorate slowly and make adaptations accordingly. Requesting a description of a typical day from the individual may assist the nurse in identifying situations that can be addressed through simple interventions. It is useful to identify the routine of ADLs such as eating, grooming and dressing, transferring self from one area to another, and toileting. It is also important to know what they can do with regard to IADLs such as shopping, housekeeping chores, and transportation. In addition to verbal and written accounts, the nurse must observe how well the patient is accomplishing tasks. Observations of transfer from a wheelchair to the dialysis chair, walking with or without mechanical assistance, and even noting the method of transportation and timeliness with appointments are important assessments. Several tools may be utilized to assess the overall functional status: The Katz Index of Independence in Activities of Daily Living (ADL) (Shelkey & Wallace, 1998), the Fall Assessment Tool (Farmer, 2000), and the Instrumental Activities of Daily Living (IADL) (Lawton & Brody, 1969).

Interventions are dependent upon the specific areas of need as identified by the assessments above. Several suggestions include:

1. Identification of resources – To facilitate socialization, nurses can provide the older adult with a list of community resources, based on the interests of the patient, to facilitate socialization. Participation can be encouraged by helping the individual understand why particular

groups and activities have been suggested, and providing informational literature about them. The activities may involve developing new skills or hobbies, or personal sharing with others about a skill already mastered. Budget restraints may be somewhat relieved if information is provided about a community class on financial management, by talking with appropriate financial advisors, or through referral for financial assistance. Maintaining or increasing functional status and independence could be facilitated through established physical therapy programs with a goal of maximizing optimal level of functioning.

2. Provision of necessary assistance – Everyday living can be eased in a number of ways, from hiring a home aide who can assist with the shopping or housecleaning, or mechanical assistance in the form of a wheelchair or walker.

Renal Replacement Therapies

Since the initiation of Medicare funding in 1972 and the Federal Age Discrimination Act of 1975, the number of older adults treated for CKD has increased in the United States. There is still much concern about ethical, economic, and social considerations when placing an individual on some form of renal replacement therapy (RRT). As with younger patients, the quality of an older individual's life is of utmost importance. These viewpoints are incorporated within the following discussion of each of the three modalities of hemodialysis (incenter and home), peritoneal dialysis, and transplantation. Withholding dialysis can also be considered an option and more information about this can be found in Chapter 16.

Hemodialysis

In-center hemodialysis remains the primary form of RRT chosen for the older adult (USRDS, 2004). Both internal and external physical changes due to the aging process, other chronic conditions, and mental impairments can make it difficult for the individual to function without assistance, and this setting and mode of treatment provides the necessary support. With home hemodialysis, which is the least used of all the dialytic therapies, the physical and emotional support of another individual is essential during the time of treatment. Often that other person is the spouse, who may also be of an older age and may not be capable or willing to assume the responsibilities of caring for a sick partner. Hemodialysis offers more control of the physical conditions of anorexia and malnutrition, and less stress on pulmonary function when compared to peritoneal dialysis.

Hemodialysis necessitates the creation of a vascular access and attainment of good vascular access can be particularly challenging in the older adult. Arteriovenous fistulae (AVF) are the access of choice. In April of 2004, a national initiative by the Centers for Medicare and Medicaid Services (CMS) was launched to increase the use of AVF in all hemodialysis patients (Compton, 2005). However, given the poor vasculature of some older adults, other forms of vascular access may be required.

When dialyzing the older person, a lower cardiac reserve and autonomic dysfunction may make ultrafiltration more difficult. The body does not always respond effec-

tively to the volume shifts, resulting in hypotension whose "sequelae may include seizures, cerebral infarction, myocardial ischemia, aspiration pneumonia, and vascular access thromboses" (Ismail et al., 1993, p. 762). Careful monitoring of the dry weight and ultrafiltration of no more than 1 L/hr has been recommended for the older nephrology adult (Ismail et al., 1993). Hemodynamic monitoring systems may also be useful in monitoring older adults with cardiovascular instability. Older adults with CRF who have a decreased cardiac or pulmonary reserve may also be at risk for hypoxemia, which occurs for most individuals at the beginning of the hemodialysis treatment; oxygen therapy may be useful in such a situation.

Older adults are at risk for gastritis induced by the uremia and specific drugs. Subdural hematomas due to falls can be complicated by systemic heparinization used in the hemodialysis treatment. They are also more prone to infections due to a compromised immune system (Ismail et al., 1993).

Peritoneal Dialysis

Peritoneal dialysis is the second most common dialytic therapy used by older adults (USRDS, 2004). Reasons for selecting this modality are based on physical as well as psychosocial considerations, which all have a bearing on the individual's functional capacity as well as the quality of life.

Because continuous ambulatory peritoneal dialysis offers less fluctuation in levels of fluid and toxins, it is particularly useful for those that have a diminished cardiovascular reserve (Wizemann, Timio, Martin, & Kramer, 1993). There is also a homeostasis exhibited with the blood chemistries, including the maintenance of a higher hematocrit.

Maintenance of independence and self-care can be viewed as an advantage of this dialytic therapy. Peritoneal dialysis can also be selected for the dependent person who has some form of support with the treatment. In addition to family members, assistance may be available from paid helpers in the home, in nursing homes, and in adult day care centers that offer care specific to peritoneal dialysis (Nissenson, Diaz-Buxo, Adcock, & Nelms, 1990).

Sensory losses of eyesight and touch, and difficulty with manual dexterity could create difficulties for older adults using peritoneal dialysis, but technological advances may help them compensate. However, there is also a potential for respiratory distress with the pressure of the fluid in the peritoneal cavity.

Transplantation

The 2004 Annual Data Report indicated that approximately 18% of individuals needing some form of RRT over 65 years of age had been transplanted (USRDS, 2004). According to the statistical data of the USRDS (2004), the probability of a patient on dialysis over the age of 65 getting a transplant is .08. It is unlikely for a dialysis patient over 75 to be considered for a transplant. Some nephrologists still believe that transplantation is a high risk for older patients. For instance, intestinal ischemia has been found to be a more common complication of transplantation in older adults, both early and later posttransplantation, leading to an increase in morbidity and mortality (Dee, Butt, &

Ramaswamy, 2002). Conclusions were that individuals over 40 years of age who had received a cadaver kidney and had abdominal symptoms posttransplant are at greater risk for this complication. Further, given the shortage of cadaveric donor organs, there seems to be some reluctance to transplant older adults. Although the United Network of Organ Sharing (UNOS) has a policy of nondiscrimination, which has facilitated the transplant of individuals over 65, there are still considerable ethical concerns among nephrology professionals as to the appropriateness of this procedure for someone late in life. This is especially evident when it concerns young living related donor kidneys to older persons.

Nevertheless, the success rate of transplantation in older adults is increasing. One of the factors contributing to this success is the preoperative selection and evaluation of the patient. Although the criteria are basically the same as that for any other CKD patient, special evaluation procedures may be employed to assess the older adult for complications that may preclude transplantation. For example, there may be a need for additional invasive cardiac testing, gall bladder evaluation, lower GI exams/studies, and mammograms (females).

Because of changes in pharmacokinetics in older adults, lower dosages of immunosuppressants are usually indicated. With this change, the graft survival rates have increased.

Conservative Treatment

Not all people choose RRT; some choose conservative or palliative care. Some people start dialysis and then choose to withdraw (see Chapter 16 for end of life care). Quality of life concerns and fear of being a burden on others (Maddocks, 1995) are factors that contribute to this situation. ANNA was involved in developing guidelines with the Renal Physicians' Association (RPA) and American Society of Nephrology (ASN) regarding this issue (RPA/ASN, 2002) (see also Chapter 16).

Discontinuation of any medical regime usually occurs when the physician and/or patient see continuation of treatment as a burden rather than a benefit. A decrease in neurological and functional status is often the main reason that the decision is made to withhold or withdraw from dialysis (Holley, Faulks, & Moss, 1991). Other issues that come into the decision-making process include factors affecting quality of life, such as major events in life (other than a diagnosis of renal disease), having an effect on one's coping abilities (McCormick, 1993). Regardless of the reasons, the nephrology nurse has the responsibility to respect an individual's right to self-determination, and to provide information, support, and comfort to the person who decides to discontinue dialysis treatment. Consideration should be given to the competency of the patient, the fact that the patient is voluntarily making the decision without coercion, and that the patient is well informed of the consequences accompanying the discontinuation of treatment (McCormick, 1993).

Informed consent and advance directives play a significant role in the demonstration of autonomy and decision making by the patient. According to McCullough, Rhymes, Teasdale, and Wilson (1995), "a meaningful informed consent process creates a common ground between beneficence-based and autonomy-based clinical ethical judgment"

(p. 577). To achieve this, a nine-step process has been proposed by these same authors from a physician perspective, and is one that can be easily adapted for use with the older person with CKD. These steps (as adapted) include the following:

1. Patient understanding of renal disease, the alternative treatments available, and prognosis of each;
2. Enhancement of patient knowledge through correction of statements made concerning renal disease and the alternative treatments;
3. Explanation regarding the patient's condition and the treatments according to the nephrologist's best clinical judgment;
4. Enhancement of cognitive understanding by the physician and supportive efforts of the nurse to the patient;
5. Identification of the patient's values and beliefs;
6. Evaluation of alternatives by the patient, with clarification by the nephrologist and nurse;
7. Preferences identified by the patient, based on personal values and beliefs;
8. Recommendation made by the nephrologist, keeping patient preferences and own clinical judgment in mind; and,
9. Plan is mutually agreed upon.

In the informed consent and communication process, three components are critical: all information is provided, the patient makes the decision freely and without coercion, and the patient making the decision is competent (Cassel, 1990, p. 41). The informed consent process would be conducted by the nephrologist and reinforced by the nephrology nurse, fostering choice and control by the patient. Should patients be unable to make their own decisions and participate in the process above, another may speak on the patient's behalf. This is often the next of kin or someone who has been designated in writing as the Durable Power of Attorney for Health Care (known as advance directive) by the patient. This representative indicates how they feel the patient would respond if s/he was able to do so, makes any wishes of the patient known, and participates in the decision-making process. Another form of advance directive is that of the Living Will, written by the patient prior to a state of incompetence, of his wishes regarding any form of aggressive treatment. Many older patients prefer that family members be the surrogate decision makers (Shawler, High, Moore, & Velotta, 1992). It is important, however, that nurses provide guidance in these matters, encouraging the older adult person to discuss personal concerns and wishes with family members so that the preferred method of treatment will be carried out. Staff members need to also be aware of the wishes of the patient, so that appropriate patient care is provided (Miller, 2004).

Who Makes the Choice?

The older patient should be well informed of the advantages and disadvantages of the options available for renal failure treatment. If capable of making decisions, the patient, along with the family and health care professionals, should choose the method that will maximize quality of life and optimize functioning. Consideration should be given to physical, sociological, and psychological issues and needs when making the choice.

Nutritional Considerations

Like other people with CKD, older individuals also face dietary restrictions. A nutritional issue for this population includes attaining adequate caloric intake with the dietary restrictions in potassium, phosphorus, sodium, fluid, and sometimes protein. Dietary restrictions and listings of foods recommended/contraindicated in each of these areas have already been addressed in Chapter 17.

The dietary management and nutritional status specific to that of an older adult with CKD can be a complex issue. People develop patterns of eating habits, based on tradition, ethnic background, religious preferences, and personal food habits (Ebersole, Hess & Luggen, 2004). No matter what has influenced their current dietary intake, malnutrition is cited as a common problem among the older population due to a deficiency of essential nutrients and calories with deviations in dietary patterns (Ebersole, Hess, & Luggen, 2004). Specific factors having an effect on nutritional status include physiological status, psychosocial and economic issues, environmental and functional considerations, and pathological conditions associated with digestion and nutrition (Miller, 2004). Proper assessment, education, and individual monitoring are necessary in each of these areas for the prevention of malnutrition and assurance of proper nutritional intake.

Physiological Status

Sensory changes occur with aging. Two of these, specifically taste and smell, can affect the appetite. There is a decrease in the number of taste buds (which are located on the tongue, plate, and tonsils) affecting sensitivity to sour, salty, and bitter tastes. The ability to detect sweet tastes is usually maintained (Miller, 2004). Olfactory changes that occur include a decrease in the sensory cells of the mucosa and those at the olfactory bulb located at the brain (Ebersole, Hess, & Luggen 2004). In addition to the problems associated with renal disease, these losses can make it difficult for an individual to obtain proper nutritional intake if the food is not palatable, or does not smell good.

Other factors that affect nutritional intake include smoking and medications. Saliva production, diminished by medications and disease, can have an effect on the digestion process occurring in the mouth, which in turn can have an effect on the amounts and kinds of food ingested. Constipation (possibly due to medications and a lowered activity level) and dental changes (periodontal gum disease and infections, missing dentures, or ill-fitting dentures) can make it difficult to chew food. Dentures cover the secondary taste areas of the palate, making it difficult to taste the food. Lactose intolerance, impaired vitamin D metabolism, vitamin B_{12} deficiency, dementia, hypothyroidism, diabetes, atrophic gastritis, and upper respiratory diseases are all conditions that can interfere with nutritional intake (Bromley, 2000; Finkel et al., 2001; Morley, 2002).

Psychosocial and Economic Issues

Psychosocial considerations can contribute to malnutrition. Isolation and loneliness, depression, and bereavement, although not exclusive to the older adult, can have serious consequences within this population if not identified. Also, those individuals who are confused, forgetful, and/or disoriented tend to receive improper nutrition.

As an individual grows older, changes in financial status frequently occur. This can cause a strain on the individual when the lower income needs to cover medications, medical bills, housing repairs, and other necessities of life, as well as food. This can lead to a decrease in food purchases, as well as an increase in consumption of inappropriate foods and drinks that are bought at a lower cost. The consumption of alcohol also makes it difficult to maintain adequate nutrition necessary with a renal diet.

Environmental and Functional Considerations

Transportation may be a physical impediment to the purchase of food because the older individual is unable to get to the grocery store or, if able to walk, fears going out alone. Preparation of the food once it is purchased can also be a difficult task, depending on the physical abilities of the older adult. A person with strict financial constraints may live in substandard housing without a refrigerator to store certain items or may not own a stove on which to prepare a meal (Ebersole, Hess, & Luggen, 2004).

Pathological Conditions

Often older persons have more than one chronic condition, and this in itself may present difficulties with eating. Stiles (1993) lists the following complications and their sequelae, which all can have an effect on nutritional status: Parkinson's disease (shaking), alcoholism (depressant), swallowing disorders (inability to swallow foods necessitating other means of feeding), cancer (nausea and vomiting), cardiopulmonary disease (restricted diet), diabetes (restricted diet), drug-nutrient interactions (medications cause anorexia, or the drug interferes with nutrient absorption), malabsorption syndromes (inability to absorb adequate calories and nutrients), surgery or trauma (difficulty eating depending on cause and/or increased need for caloric intake to potentiate healing process), recurrent infections (increases need for caloric intake for healing, which is already a difficult process to maintain), and renal disease (restricted diet and uremia, which can have a negative effect on appetite).

Addressing Nutritional Issues

While dietitians are essential members of the interdisciplinary renal team, the nephrology nurse must also be aware of the issues pertaining to the nutritional status of the older CKD patient. Accurate assessment of those areas identified in the previous sections is necessary to facilitate adequate nutritional intake. Educating the older person and family members is important. Family and friends may be providing meals and therefore need specific education.

Guidelines proposed by Henrich (1990) to assess the nutritional status of the elderly dialysis patient include: monitoring of weight loss, indicated as the "best predictor of insidious malnutrition" (p. 340); and attention to a low serum albumin level, the protein catabolic rate, protein intake, and energy stores measured by triceps skin fold. Since prevention of malnutrition is the primary goal for older adults undergoing dialysis, it is important to liberalize the diet when possible to assure adequate intake of protein and energy

(Burrowes, 2003). Consistency in monitoring laboratory values, as well as physiological status, psychosocial and economic issues, environmental and functional abilities, and pathological conditions is a step toward stabilizing nutritional status and increasing quality of life.

Drug Therapy

There are several considerations that must be taken into account when medicating the older person. One of these is polypharmacy, which often accompanies chronic illnesses, and is a common occurrence especially among this population. LeSage (1991) describes polypharmacy as the "concurrent use of several different drugs" which may be of the same therapeutic class, to treat "coexisting disease or a single illness" (p. 274). Other definitions describe polypharmacy as the use of five or more drugs or the use of at least one unnecessary drug (Carlson, 1996; Hanlon, Weinberger, & Samsa, 1996). Thirty-four percent of prescription drugs are consumed by older persons, with those aged 65 to 69 averaging 13.6 prescription medications per year (American Society of Consultant Pharmacists, 2000). This often leads to confusion regarding an already complex drug regimen, which can result in devastating consequences for the older individual. LeSage (1991) has identified other causes for potential complications with drug use:

1. Misdiagnosis of an ailment;
2. More than one prescriber who does not know what others have already given the patient, leading to duplicate medications and drug interactions;
3. Self-medication with over-the-counter drugs and drugs of other individuals without consultation with health care professionals;
4. Hoarding of medications that have been discontinued, for "later use if necessary"; and,
5. Failure to accurately assess the individual for underlying causes of a problem sometimes leading to the treatment of one drug's side effects with another drug. As the body ages, changes occur in pharmacodynamics (drug effects at site of action) and pharmacokinetics (absorption, distribution, metabolism, and excretion of a drug) that can lead to morbid adverse effects (Roberts, Snyder, & Friedman, 1996). Because of these changes, along with the practices of drug usage of the older patient, there is always the danger of health risks and complications.

Pharmacodynamics

Two types of pharmacodynamic alterations have been identified in the older adult population. The first of these are changes at the cellular level (Roberts, Snyder & Friedman, 1996). There may be an increased or decreased sensitivity to a drug due to the number of receptors as well as the attraction of the drug to the receptors (Kane et al., 2004). The second pharmacodynamic alteration is that of "homeostatic vitality" (Schwertz & Buschmann, 1989, p. 31). That is, the response of the body with adverse drug reactions may interfere with the primary intention of the drug. Serious adverse reactions have been demonstrated with cardiovascular and psychotropic drugs (Bates, Miller, & Cullen, 1999; Kane et al., 2004). Reactions from these and other drugs have also been noted in the respiratory, thermo-regulatory, and renal

systems (Roberts, Snyder, & Friedman, 1996).

As new drugs are released and prescribed, research must continue in the area of pharmacodynamic alterations in the older adult population. While this information is available for some drugs and dosages have been adjusted accordingly, research is still needed for dosage requirements of specific drugs (Kane et al., 2004).

Pharmacokinetics

As an individual ages, physiological and anatomical changes occur in the gastrointestinal tract, the site of most *absorption* of oral drugs. Changes associated with aging include decreased gastrointestinal motility and decreased secretion of gastric acid as well as a decline in blood flow and decreased surface area of the intestine (Ebersole, Hess & Luggen, 2004; Gerber & Brass, 1990). Despite these changes, research has shown that absorption of oral drugs is not significantly affected as one ages (Roberts, Snyder, & Friedman, 1996). Absorption of drugs administered by intramuscular injection or topical administration may be affected by decreases in tissue perfusion and skin hydration of older adults (Roberts, Snyder & Friedman, 1996).

Plasma protein binding and body composition determine drug *distribution* within the body. Throughout the aging process, serum albumin, total body water, and lean body mass tend to decline. On the other hand, body fat increases, with a greater amount in men than women. These changes cause alterations in both the half-life of a drug as well as volume of distribution (Kane et al., 2004).

The *metabolism* of drugs in the liver and enzyme activity based on environmental factors has made it difficult to predict changes specific to the older adult in this area. Studies are needed that take into account specific factors such as gender, smoking, combinations with other drugs, and even atmospheric pollutants and their effect on the metabolism of specific drugs consumed by the older person. Assumptions cannot be made that an older individual metabolizes drugs at the same rate as a younger one (Kane et al., 2004).

Older adults are at high risk for toxic effects and enhanced actions of a drug when *excretion* is affected, specifically drugs that are dependent on the kidney for this process. These drugs have been found to have a longer half-life, be eliminated from the body more slowly, and reach a higher concentration (Kane et al., 2004). As the glomerular filtration rate (GFR) declines, the clearance of a drug is decreased. The loading dose of a drug usually remains the same, but the drug regimen will be altered in one of three ways: reduced dosages at the same intervals; same dosages but administered less frequently; or, alterations in both the dosages and intervals (Roberts, Snyder, & Freidman, 1996).

Adherence

Studies of older individuals have shown that non-adherence to medications correlates with the number of medications or doses prescribed. That is, the greater the number or doses prescribed, the less likely it is that an individual will follow the regimen (Barat, Andreasen, & Damsgaard, 2001; Gray, Mahoney, Blough, 2001; Donnan, MacDonald, & Morris, 2002). Lack of adherence to medication regimens (with overuse, under use, or misuse) may occur for any one or several of the following reasons: uncomfortable side effects experienced by the drugs, inability to read the labels correctly or open the bottles with ease, belief that more than the prescribed dosage may have a better effect, financial constraints to purchase the prescribed medications, memory lapses regarding whether a particular medication has been taken, transportation problems obtaining the medications, inability to open the drug bottle, and misunderstanding of the use of a particular medication, appropriate times and dosages prescribed. Knowledge deficits regarding the foods that can alter a drug's reactions or drugs that can alter absorption of nutrients leading to malnutrition are also important considerations. All of these factors can have a significant influence on the therapeutic medication levels of the individual.

Nursing Interventions

The older adult with CKD is particularly vulnerable to problems with medications not only because of the aging process, but the fact that excretion of drugs is affected by the nonfunctioning kidneys. Dialytic therapy may be the only means by which to eliminate the drugs. Knowledge of the specifics of each drug taken by these patients, including dosages, therapeutic levels and actions, potential side effects, and adverse reactions, as well as a general understanding of the effects of renal failure on drug excretion and pharmacogeriatrics, is necessary for effective patient care. A change in the individual should not be attributed to old age, but should automatically alert the nurse to careful evaluation of the medications taken by the individual. The following assessments should be considered:

1. A complete medical history and list of personal physicians.
2. A drug history, including a listing of the medications, dosages, and times of administration for each medication, versus what they are supposed to be taking. Identify all prescription and nonprescription drugs, those they take belonging to other individuals, and those prescribed by each of their other physicians.
3. Appropriate serum levels of specific medications to assure that the therapeutic levels are maintained, as well as those serum values affected by medications.
4. Mental status examination.
5. Effects and reactions to each medication with documentation of findings to provide for effective follow-up.
6. The patient's overall understanding of the individualized drug regimen, and educating them (repeatedly if necessary) on the important aspects of each drug including his/her responsibility to help monitor the effects and report any unusual problems.
7. Compliance with regard to under use, misuse, and nonuse of drugs, taking into account any changes with physical, psychological, social, and economic status.
8. Use of one pharmacy to assist in the control of the drug regimen.
9. Use of alternative methods (such as stress reduction methods, diet therapy, and psychotherapy) to reduce the need for the number of drugs.
10. Assurance that the older adult understands the reasoning for change of dosage and discontinuation of medications, discouraging hoarding while encouraging compliance.
11. Simplifying the drug regimen as much as possible, using daily dosage where possible rather than multiple doses per day.

It is the responsibility of all members of the health team to promote effective pharmacotherapy. Communication and thorough individualized care planning and understanding are necessary to ensure one's safety and enhance quality of life.

Education - Adaptation for Life's Changes

Providing education to an older population can be a challenging, yet rewarding experience. The educator must individualize teaching based on the needs of each older adult. When planning an educational session, three areas are important to consider: the person to be instructed, the teaching environment, and the instructional design of the presentation. Elements of these three areas are highlighted in Table 22-4.

Gerogogy is the term applied to the teaching of older persons. As the individual grows older, the following factors must be kept in mind by the educator: multiple and significant individual roles, lifestyle based on values, beliefs and attitudes of past experiences, developmental level, recent and remote educational experiences, financial commitment, and definitive educational goals (Polson, 1993). Factors that may influence learning include the individual's reading ability, knowledge about the topic to be presented including personal perceptions and misconceptions, ethnic and cultural backgrounds, religious practices, meaningfulness of the material to be presented, a need for concrete ideas and tasks, and timing of the instruction. The cognitive, affective, and psychomotor domains of learning need to be considered. When examining cognition, orientation to time, place and person are assessed. Affectively, one's attitude and feelings with regard to physical health and status, the medical regime and/or proposed topic of discussion are assessed by observation and direct questioning. Observing psychomotor skills gives a nurse feedback regarding functional status of the neurological and musculoskeletal systems combined.

Physical and pathophysiological changes associated with aging can have a significant impact on the teaching methods utilized and the individual's readiness for learning. The physiological changes can affect comprehension as well as the ability to participate in the learning process. The effects of aging on the central nervous system, however, can slow down the processing, requiring a little more time for comprehension and resulting in an increase in response time (Dellasega, Clark, McCreary et al., 1994).

Environmental Conditions

It is important that the teaching environment is conducive to learning. The ideal location for receiving instruction is one which is familiar to the patient such as the home (Dellasega, 1990). In the case of the patient on dialysis, the facility is familiar to the patient, and can be considered a good location for instruction, with some accommodations.

Table 22-4
Considerations for teaching elderly patients with CRF.

Patients
- Assess their immediate concerns and priorities.
- Assess their personal values and lifestyle.
- Determine their reading level.
- Determine their mental status.
- Assess any physical disabilities (i.e., visual, auditory, or musculoskeletal impairments).
- Determine the appropriate time for reviewing information.
- Assess for medications that influence alertness and comprehension.

Environment
- Provide an area with adequate lighting.
- Provide an area that is comfortable.
- Provide an area conducive to concentration.

Instructional Design
- Use multimedia methods such as pamphlets, audiotapes, and videotapes.
- Use written materials with large type and bold print.
- Use posters.
- Allow patients to control the pace of the presentation.
- Keep educational sessions short (30 minutes or less).
- Reinforce information using different approaches.

Note: From Mathers, T. (1995). Epoetin alfa - Focus on the geriatric patient (Educational supplement sponsored by Amgen, Inc.). *ANNA Journal, 22*(5), 494-497. Adapted from Stewart & Walton (1992) and Matheson (1994). Reprinted with permission.

These may include appropriate lighting without glare, few distractions and minimal background noise, padded straight back chairs and adjustable table heights, a comfortable and relaxing temperature, adequate ventilation, privacy if possible, and an organized and neat work area (Dellasega, Clark, McCreary, Helmuth, & Schan, 1994; Matheson, 1994).

Instructional Systems Design

Variables relevant to the enhancement of learning and improved performance make up an instructional systems design (ISD) model. According to Rossett (1995), the ISD is consists of the following steps: analysis, design, development, use, and evaluation. Analysis or needs assessment is a part of every phase of the process. This is comparable to that of the nursing process. Table 22-5 reflects this comparison.

Analysis. The first step in designing a program is the conduct of a needs assessment of the older adult. Identification of any mental, physical, or psychological conditions, and the patient's attitudes, values, or beliefs about the disease process or topic of presentation may alert the instructor to factors that will facilitate or even impede the learning process. Once accomplished, the educator can then proceed to design an individualized program with teaching methods and techniques to communicate pertinent information that is needed to attain mutual and realistic goals.

Design and development. Information from the needs assessment will help the educator design the program and develop appropriate and meaningful material. Utilization of multimedia methods such as pamphlets, audiotapes, and videotapes (for some patients), written materials with large

Table 22-5
Comparison of the Nursing Process (NP) and Instructional Systems Design (ISD)

NP	Common Descriptors	ISD
Assess	Determination of patient's needs	Analyze
Plan	Development of appropriate interventions	Design and Develop
Intervene	Implementation of meaningful measures	Use
Evaluate	Analysis of outcomes	Evaluate

type and bold print, and poster presentations, all well organized, relevant, simple, and concrete, can facilitate learning (Matheson, 1994; Stewart & Walton, 1992). It has been suggested that building on previous knowledge will facilitate learning for the older person (Theis, 1991).

Use. Throughout the implementation of the plan, educational sessions should be well organized and kept to a maximum of 30 minutes in length for the older patient (Matheson, 1994). Material should be presented at a comfortable pace controlled by the patient so that s/he may absorb the information without feeling rushed, and then reinforced (Matheson, 1994).

Evaluation. Although identified as the last step in the instructional design model, evaluation should also be continuous throughout the implementation process. The patient can be evaluated for understanding of the information being presented and for any previously unidentified problems. Evaluation at the end of a session can then provide feedback of knowledge gained and that yet to be achieved. Further plans for other sessions are based on this evaluation.

Educational Outcomes

Assessing and making accommodations in the three areas of concern, namely the patient, environment, and instructional design, will facilitate nursing care for the older adult. If also accompanied by support and respect, rapport can be established between the older adult and the educator, and a working relationship fostered leading toward optimal achievement of both the individual's goals and the overall educational goals for that person.

Rehabilitation and the Older Adult

Rehabilitation has the goal of improving the physical capabilities of the individual and improving quality of life (Blagg & Fitts, 1994). Rehabilitation of the older adult patient can be a challenge to both the health care professional as well as the individual. According to Stineman and Granger (1994), rehabilitation programs are comprised of some key elements to facilitate the care of this population. These include:

1. A reduction in disabling effects if rehabilitation is initiated early;
2. Identification of needs of the older adult population;
3. Physical and verbal exchange between patients and staff;
4. Establishment of rapport, to include the patient, family and team members;
5. A balance of the various treatment modalities;
6. Environmental and equipment adaptations with personal prescriptions and appropriate patient training;
7. Educational programs;
8. An interdisciplinary team approach with communication between and among the rehabilitation team and with others in all phases of the process, including the referral phase and postrehabilitation follow-up; and,
9. A program based on realistic individual goals and expectations, reemphasized in each stage of the rehabilitation process.

As a first step toward rehabilitation, assessment of this population must include their sense of control and health outlook (Kutner, Cardenas, & Bower, 1992). Personal strengths and weaknesses need to be identified. The patient's physical ability, social functioning, sense of well-being, and perspective on what constitutes a quality life must also be taken into account (James-Rogers, 1994). All of this can be accomplished if age-appropriate tools are used. Then, keeping in mind the five core objectives of encouragement, education, exercise, employment, and evaluation established by the Life Options Advisory Council (Medical Education Institute, 1995), and the fact that individuals become less homogenous as they grow older, the rehabilitation program can be individualized according to identified needs and goals.

Active participation is required for any rehabilitation program to be successful. Many times this involves encouragement from the physician, staff, family, and peers, and even other patients who form a support for the individual. Psychological status of the older adult patient can also be improved by encouraging the individual to engage in activities that promote a healthy outlook on life.

Education is very important to include in this aspect of care. Helping these individuals to understand their disease, its treatment and what is happening with regard to care facilitates an improvement in overall well-being.

Physical exercise is an important component of all rehabilitation programs, including those of older adults. The capacity for exercise is reduced as chronic kidney failure progresses, so it is suggested that rehabilitation be started as early as possible in the course of this disease process (Blagg & Fitts, 1994). Decrease in exercise and activity specific to the dialysis patient have been attributed to fatigue, time restraints, and hospitalizations, to include access surgeries (Blagg & Fitts, 1994). As exercise programs with the older adult are initiated, physiological changes, endurance, and functional capacity need to be monitored. Suggested exercises to slow the rate of physical degeneration include walking, swimming, and bicycling.

Employment is broadly defined. Although the number of older workers is increasing (Shrey & Hursh, 1994), there are still those who view themselves as retired. These are the ones that need to consider vocational and recreational activities. Work may include the responsibilities of being a homemaker, a volunteer worker, a gardener, or activities such as painting, swimming, or golfing. Recognition and praise for one's achievements will enhance self-worth and well-being.

Evaluation is continuous throughout the rehabilitation process and needs to be accompanied by outcome analysis. This will assist the team in determining whether the program established for a particular patient or a facility is appropriate.

Caregivers

The family is the most common source of emotional and material support. Although we often view older individuals as recipients of care, they are frequently giving to the rest of the family. In this sense, they may provide support in the form of being good listeners, giving advice, providing financial support and child care, providing a home for divorced children, serving as family historians, and providing religious stability and cultural identification (Ebersole, Hess & Luggen, 2004).

Reversal of roles within the family may be due to the increased dependency of older persons, where children provide the care for parents. The stress of caring for individuals with a chronic illness such as renal disease cannot be underestimated. Older individuals may be dependent on others to accomplish such tasks as remembering medication, needing transportation to treatment centers and physicians' appointments, and needing assistance in activities of daily living. The experience can be overwhelming and even devastating for anyone.

Beach (1993) pointed out various themes that emerged in the literature with respect to caregivers. These were related to balancing the older person's needs with other daily activities, hindering the social activities of caregivers, limited assistance by other family members (i.e., siblings and children) to assist in the provision of care, and use of institutions when exhausted physically and/or emotionally. Subjective experiences were categorized into three specific areas that the health care providers need to be mindful of when considering the caregivers: role strain, sense of self, and problem solving/coping (Beach, 1993).

It is important for the nurse to aid the patient in identifying those who can be of assistance and then to mobilize these resources. As one grows older, some key members in the family may be lost and others are less accessible. Children may live in other areas of the country. Spousal support may be available, but more often than not, spouses are also older individuals who may have their own health problems that interfere with giving care to the partner. In addition, personal health may be neglected when emphasis is placed on the care of the spouse. It is also important to keep in mind the physical and emotional status of the caregivers. Caregivers need information on sources of support for themselves, including counseling and knowledge about respite care, so that quality time and care can be given to the dependent older adult.

Gerontological Research

Nurses need to be aware of current research findings and be ready to adjust assessments, plans, interventions, and evaluations to facilitate quality patient care with effective outcomes. A review of the literature reveals that, until recently, nephrology nursing research has often integrated the older adult subjects (ages 65 and older) as part of the overall adult population, instead of viewing them as a separate group. Research is not without problems when older adults are considered. Adaptations in tools are sometimes required, and ethical issues that pertain to older adult participants need to be considered.

Nevertheless, research in the field of gerontological nephrology nursing is growing. As long as appropriate measurements are utilized and the research is conducted in a rigorous manner, it will continue to provide guidelines for the future. Nephrology nursing research that contributes to innovative approaches to optimize quality of life and provide better care to the older adult population is sorely needed.

Summary

It is the responsibility of every nephrology nurse caring for older adults to know about their special needs. This includes being knowledgeable about the changes that occur with aging as well as the changes that occur with renal disease. As the number of older patients increase, a holistic perspective must be integrated into the framework and maintained for the enhancement of quality care. If specific services needed by an individual cannot be provided by the dialysis facility and nephrology health care providers, then resources in the form of outside community services must be considered.

References

Alpert, M. (1995). Cardiovascular risks for hemodialysis and peritoneal dialysis patients. *Nephrology News & Issues, 9*(5), 12,14,16,18.

American Association of Retired Persons [AARP]. (2004). *A profile of older Americans: 2003.* Washington, DC: Program Resources Department, American Association of Retired Persons (AARP) and Administration on Aging (AoA), U.S. Department of Health and Human Services.

American Nephrology Nurses' Association [ANNA]. (2004). Chronic kidney disease: What every nurse should know. Module 1: Stage 5 chronic kidney disease – Hemodialysis in the long-term care setting. Pitman, NJ: American Nephrology Nurses' Association.

American Society of Consultant Pharmacists. (2000). Senior care Pharmacy: The statistics. *Consultant Pharmacist, 15,* 310.

Barat, L., Andreasen, E., & Damsgaard, E. (2001). Drug therapy in the elderly: What doctors believe and patients actually do. *British Journal of Clinical Pharmacology, 51,* 615-622.

Bates, D., Miller, E.B., & Cullen, D. (1999). Patient risk factors for adverse drug events in hospitalized patients. *Archives of Internal Medicine, 159,* 2553-2560.

Beach, D. (1993). Gerontological caregiving: Analysis of family experience. *Journal of Gerontological Nursing, 19*(12), 35-41.

Blagg, C., & Fitts, S. (1994). Dialysis, old age, and rehabilitation. *Journal of the American Medical Association, 271*(1), 67-68.

Bromley, S. (2000). Smell and taste disorders: A primary care approach. *American Family Physician 61*(2), 427-436.

Burrowes, J. (2003). Nutrition assessment and management of elderly dialysis patients. *Topics in Clinical Nutrition, 18*(4), 280-287.

Butler, R., Lewis, M., & Sunderland, T. (1998). *Aging and mental health: Positive psychosocial and biomedical approaches* (5th ed.). (L. Sharp & C. Geldis, Eds.). New York: Macmillan Publishers.

Byer, C., & Shainberg, L. (1991). *Dimensions of human sexuality* (3rd ed.). Dubuque, IA: William C. Brown.

Campbell, J. (1995). Assessment. In M. Hogstel (Ed.). *Geropsychiatric nursing* (2nd ed.) (pp. 73-95). St. Louis: Mosby Year Book.

Carlson, J. (1996). Perils of polypharmacy: 10 steps to prudent prescribing. *Geriatrics, 51,* 26-35.

Cassel, C. (1990). Ethical problems in geriatric medicine. In C. Cassel, D. Riesenberg, L. Sorensen, & J. Walsh (Eds.), *Geriatric medicine* (2nd ed., pp. 38-47). New York: Springer- Verlag.

Compton, A. (2005). National vascular access improvement initiative: Fistula first. *Nephrology Nursing Journal, 32*(2), 221-222.

Dee, S., Butt, K., & Ramaswamy, G. (2002). Intestinal ischemia: A significant early postoperative complication after renal transplantation. *Archive of Pathology & Laboratory Medicine, 126*(10), 1201-1204.

Dellasega, C. (1990). Self-care for the elderly diabetic. *Journal of Gerontological Nursing, 16*(1), 16-20.

Dellasega, C., Clark, D., McCreary, D., Helmuth, A., & Schan, P. (1994). Nursing process: Teaching elderly clients. *Journal of Gerontological Nursing, 20*(1), 31-38.

Donnan, P., MacDonald, T., & Morris, A. (2002). Adherence to prescribed oral hypoglycemic medication in a population of patients with type 2 diabetes: A retrospective cohort study. *Diabetic Medicine, 19,* 279-284.

Eaton, D.C., & Pooler, J. (2004). *Vander's renal physiology* (6th ed.). New York: McGraw Hill.

Ebersole, P., Hess, P., & Luggen, A. (2004). *Toward healthy aging: Human needs and nursing response* (6th ed.). St. Louis: Mosby.

Eliopoulos, C. (2001). *Gerontologic Nursing* (5th ed.). Philadelphia: Lippincott William and Wilkins.

Erikson, E. (1963). *Childhood and society.* New York: W. W. Norton.

Farmer, B. (2000). *Try This Series: Best Practices in Nursing Care to Older Adults – Fall Risk Assessment.* Hartford: The Hartford Institute for Geriatric Nursing. Retrieved October 18, 2005, from www.hartfordign.org

Ferrini, A., & Ferrini, R. (2000). Sexuality. In A. Ferrini, & R. Ferrini (Eds.), *Health in later years* (3rd ed.). Madison, WI: Brown & Benchmark.

Finkel, D., Pedersen, N., & Larsson, M. (2001). Olfactory functioning and cognitive abilities: A twin study. *Journal of Gerontology: Psychological Sciences, 56B,* 226-233.

Folstein, M., Folstein, S., & McHugh, P. (1975). Mini-mental state: A practical method for grading the cognitive state of patients for the clinician. *Journal of Psychiatric Research, 12,* 189-198.

Foreman, M., & Gradowski, R. (1992). Diagnostic dilemma: Cognitive impairment in the elderly. *Journal of Gerontological Nursing,*

18(9), 5-12.

Fries, J. (2002). Successful aging: An emerging paradigm of gerontology. *Clinics in Geriatric Medicine, 18*, 371-382.

Gerber, J., & Brass, E. (1990). Drug use. In R. Schrier (Ed.), *Geriatric medicine* (pp. 91-103). Philadelphia: W.B. Saunders Company.

Gray, S., Mahoney, J., & Blough, O. (2001). Medication adherence in elderly patients receiving home health services following hospital discharge. *Annals of Pharmacotherapy, 35*, 539-545.

Hanlon, J., Weinberger, M., Samsa, G. (1996). A randomized, controlled trial of a clinical pharmacist intervention to improve inappropriate prescribing in elderly outpatients with polypharmacy. *American Journal of Medicine, 100*, 428-437.

Havinghurst, R.J. (1952). Developmental tasks and education. New York: David McKay.

Henrich, W. (1990). Dialysis considerations in the elderly patient. *American Journal of Kidney Diseases,* 16(4), 339-341.

Holley, J., Faulks, C., & Moss, A. (1991). Nephrologists' reported attitudes about factors influencing recommendations to initiate or withdraw dialysis. *Journal of the American Society of Nephrology, 1*, 1284-1288.

Lordanidis, P., Alivanis, P., Iakovidis, A., Dombros, N., Tsagalidis, I., Balaskas, E., Derveniotis, V., Ierodiakonous, C., & Tourkantonis, A. (1993). Psychiatric and psychosocial status of elderly patients undergoing dialysis. *Peritoneal Dialysis International, 13* (Suppl. 2), S192-S195.

Ismail, N., Hakim, R., Oreopoulos, D., & Patrikarea, A. (1993). Renal replacement therapies in the elderly: Part 1, hemodialysis and chronic peritoneal dialysis. *American Journal of Kidney Diseases, 22*(6), 759-782.

Ismail, N., Hakim, R., & Helderman, H. (1994). Renal replacement therapies in the elderly: Part II. Renal transplantation. *American Journal of Kidney Diseases, 23*(1), 1-15.

James-Rogers, A. (1994). Rehabilitation and the elderly dialysis patient. *Dialysis & Transplantation, 23*(9), 517-518.

Kaiser, F. (1990). Principles of geriatric care. *American Journal of Kidney Diseases, 16*(4), 354-359.

Kane, R., Ouslander, J., Abrass, I., & Itmar, B. (2004). *Essentials of clinical geriatrics* (5th ed.) New York: McGraw-Hill.

Kimmel, P.L. (2002). Depression in patients with chronic renal disease: What we know and what we need to know. *Journal of Psychosomatic Research, 53*, 951-956.

Kimmel, P.L., Emont, S.L., Newmann, J.M., Danko, H., & Moss. A.H. (2003). ESRD patient quality of life: Symptoms, spiritual beliefs, psychosocial factors, and ethnicity: *American Journal of Kidney Diseases, 42*, 713-721.

Kimmel, P., Peterson, R., Weihs, K., Simmens, S., Alleyne, S., Cruz, I., & Veis, J. (2000). Multiple measurements of depression predict mortality in a longitudinal study of chronic hemodialysis patients. *Kidney International, 57*, 2093-2098.

Kutner, N., Cardenas, D., & Bower, J. (1992). Rehabilitation, aging and chronic renal disease. *American Journal of Physical Medicine and Rehabilitation, 71*(2), 97-101.

Lan, T-Y., Melzer, D., Tom, B., & Guralnik, J. (2002). Performance tests and disability: Developing an objective index of mobility-related limitation in older populations. *Journal of Gerontology: Medical Sciences, 57*, M294-M301.

Lawton, M., & Brody, E. (1969). Assessment of older people: Self-maintaining and Instrumental Activities of Daily Living. *Gerontologist, 9*, 179-186.

LeSage, J. (1991). Polypharmacy in geriatric patients. *Nursing Clinics of North America, 26*(2), 273-289.

Lubkin, I.M. (1990). *Chronic illness: Impact and interventions.* Boston: Jones and Bartlett.

Maddocks, I. (1995). Management of the dying patient. In W. Reichel (Ed.), *Care of the elderly: Clinical aspects of aging* (4th ed.) (pp. 561-569). Baltimore: Williams & Wilkins.

Matheson, L. (1994). Improving patient outcomes: Educating the elderly. *Dialysis & Transplantation, 23*(9), 514-516.

McCormick, T. (1993). Ethical issues in caring for patients with renal failure. *ANNA Journal, 20*(5), 549-555.

McCullough, L., Rhymes, J., Teasdale, T., & Wilson, N. (1995). Preventive ethics in geriatric practice. In W. Reichel (Ed.), *Care of the elderly: Clinical aspects of aging* (4th ed.) (pp. 573- 586).

Baltimore: Williams & Wilkins.

Medical Education Institute. (1995, September/October). Bridges to renal rehabilitation: Focus on the 5 E's. *Renal Rehabilitation Report, 3*(5), 5-10.

Miller, J. (2000). Enhancing self-esteem. In J. Miller (Ed.), *Coping with Chronic Illness: Overcoming Powerlessness* (3rd ed.) (pp. 505-521). Philadelphia: F.A. Davis.

Miller, C. (2004). *Nursing for wellness in older adults: Theory and practice* (4th ed.). Philadelphia: Lippincott Williams and Wilkins.

Morley, J. (2002). Pathophysiology of anorexia. *Clinics in Geriatric Medicine, 18*, 661-674.

National Center for Health Statistics. (2004). *Health, United States, 2004* (DHHS Publication No. 2004-1232). Hyattsville, MD: U.S. Department of Health and Human Resources.

National Kidney Foundation. (2005). K/DOQI clinical practice guidelines for cardiovascular disease in dialysis patients. Retrieved October 18, 2005, from http://www.kidney.org/professionals/kdoqi/guidelines_cvd/methods.htm

Nelson, M., & Mayfield, P. (1994). Health assessment. In M. Hogstel (Ed.), *Nursing care of the older adult* (3rd ed.). Fort Worth, TX: Delmar Publishers.

Nissenson, A., Diaz-Buxo, J., Adcock, A., & Nelms, M. (1990). Peritoneal dialysis in the geriatric patient. *American Journal of Kidney Diseases, 16*(4), 335-338.

Nusbaum, M. Hamilton, C., & Lenahan, P. (2003). Chronic illness and sexual functioning. *American Family Physician, 67*(2), 347-354.

Pfeiffer, E. (1974). A short portable mental status questionnaire for assessment of organic brain deficit in elderly patients. *Journal of the American Geriatrics Society, 23*(10), 422-441.

Polson, C. (1993, September). *Teaching adult students.* Idea Paper No. 29, Center for Faculty Evaluation and Development, Division of Continuing Education, Kansas State University.

Radke, K. (1994). The aging kidney: Structure, function, and nursing practice implications. *ANNA Journal, 21*(4), 181-190.

Reed, P. (1991). Spirituality and mental health in older adults: Extant knowledge for nursing. *Family and Community Health, 14*(2), 14-25.

Roberts, J., Snyder, D., & Friedman, E. (1996). *Handbook of pharmacology of aging.* Boca Raton, FL: CRC Press.

Rossett, A. (1995). Needs assessment. In G. Anglin (Ed.), *Instructional technology: Past, present, and future.* Englewood, CO: Libraries Unlimited.

Renal Physicians Association and American Society of Nephrology (2002). *Shared decision making in the appropriate initiation and withdrawal from dialysis: Clinical practice guideline.* Washington DC: Authors.

Schwertz, D., & Buschmann, M. (1989). Pharmacogeriatrics. *Critical Care Nursing Quarterly, 12*(1), 26-37.

Seeley, R., Stephens, T., & Tate, P. (2006). *Anatomy and Physiology* (7th ed.). Boston: McGraw-Hill.

Shawler, C., High, D., Moore, K., & Velotta, C. (1992). Clinical considerations: Surrogate decision making for hospitalized elders. *Journal of Gerontological Nursing, 18*(6), 5-11.

Shelkey, M., & Wallace, M. (1998). *Try This Series: Best Practices in Nursing Care to Older Adults – Katz Index of Independence in Activities of Daily Living (ADL).* Hartford: The Hartford Institute for Geriatric Nursing. Retrieved October 18, 2005, from www.hartfordign.org

Shrey, D., & Hursh, N. (1994). Protecting the employability of the working elderly. In G. Felsenthan, S. Garrison, & F. Steinberg (Eds.). *Rehabilitation of the aging and elderly patient* (pp. 487-496). Baltimore: Williams & Wilkins.

Shlipak, M.G., Stehman-Breen, F., Fried, L.F., Song, X., Siscovick, D., Fried, L., Psaty, B.M., & Newman, A.B. (2004). The presence of frailty in elderly persons with chronic renal insufficiency. *American Journal of Kidney Diseases, 45*, 861-867.

Stewart, K. & Walton, R. (1992). Teaching the elderly. *Nursing 92, 22*(10), 66, 68.

Stiles, N. (1993, July 13). Sanders Brown Summer Series Workshop: Geriatric nutrition, Lexington, KY.

Stineman, M., & Granger, C. (1994). Outcome studies and analysis: Principles of rehabilitation that influence outcome analysis. In G. Felsenthan, S. Garrison, & F. Steinberg (Eds.). *Rehabilitation of the aging and elderly patient* (pp. 511-522). Baltimore: Williams & Wilkins.

Theis, S. (1991). Using previous knowledge to teach elderly clients. *Journal of Gerontological Nursing, 17*(8), 34-38.

Tideiksaar, R. (2002). *Falls in older people: Prevention and management* (3rd ed.). Baltimore: Health Professions Press.

United States Department of Health and Human Services. (2000). *Healthy People 2010: National Health Promotion and Disease Prevention Objectives.* Retrieved October 18, 2005, from http://www.healthypeople.gov

United States Renal Data System [USRDS]. (2004). USRDS 2004 Annual Data Report. Bethesda, MD: National Institutes of Health.

Wallace, M. (2000). *Try This Series: Best Practices in Nursing Care to Older Adults – Sexuality.* Hartford: The Hartford Institute for Geriatric Nursing. Retrieved October 18, 2005, from www.hartfordign.org

Walton, J. (2002) Finding a balance: A grounded theory study of spirituality in hemodialysis patients. *Nephrology Nursing Journal, 29,* 447–457.

Waszynski, C. (2001). *Try This Series: Best Practices in Nursing Care to Older Adults – Confusion Assessment Method (CAM).* Hartford: The Hartford Institute for Geriatric Nursing. Retrieved October 18, 2005, from www.hartfordign.org

Weinstein, B. (2003). A primer on hearing loss in the elderly. *Generations, 27*(1), 15-18.

Winchester, J.F. (2002). Special clinical problems in geriatric patients. *Seminars in Dialysis,* 15(2), 116 – 120.

Wizemann, V., Timio, M., Martin, A., & Kramer, W. (1993). Options in dialysis therapy: Significance of cardiovascular findings. *Kidney International, 43*(Suppl.), S85-S91.

Young, G., Kopple, J., Lindholm, B., Vonesh, E., De-Vecchi, A., Scalamagna, A., Castelnova, C., Oreopoulos, D., Anderson, G., & Bersgtrom, J. (1991). Nutritional assessment of CAPD patients: An international study. *American Journal of Kidney Diseases, 17,* 462-471.

- Care for the older individual differs from that of the younger population due to changes which occur as a result of the aging process. The number of these individuals is increasing when compared to the total population, and will continue to do so.

- The increase in longevity can be attributed to: attitude changes, healthier lifestyles, environmental changes, higher educational levels, greater use of assistive devices, avoidance of health-risk behaviors, improved diagnostic and therapeutic techniques, and decreased prevalence of chronic conditions.

- The median age of a new patient initiating CKD therapy is 65 (USRDS, 2004), with cardiovascular diseases greatest in the 65+ age group of patients with ESRD.

- As the general population gets progressively older, the percentage of elderly residing in nursing homes is expected to increase; this will increase the number of elderly CKD patients residing in nursing homes.

- Issues of concern for the elderly include those related to physiology and psychosocial perspectives. Points addressed that are of a physiological nature include changes in the five senses, cardiovascular system, respiratory system, and the renal system. Psychologically, grief, guilt, loneliness, rage, depression, helplessness, and anxiety are expressed by the elderly (Butler, Lewis, & Sunderland, 1998).

- A comprehensive nursing assessment of the older adult should include adaptations in time, environmental conditions, and communication techniques. The tools used to obtain the assessment depends on which would best facilitate the care planning of the patient.

- The primary form of RRT chosen for the elderly patient is in-center hemodialysis, with the second most common dialytic therapy being peritoneal dialysis.

- Malnutrition is a common nutritional problem among the elderly. Proper assessment of nutrition involves consideration of physiological status, psychosocial and economic issues, environmental and functional considerations, and pathological conditions.

- It is important to consider three specific areas when preparing to educate the geriatric nephrology person: the patient, the environmental conditions, and the instructional design. Comparable to the nursing process, the Instructional Systems Design model, according to Rossett (1995), consists of an analysis, design and development, use, and evaluation.

- Rehabilitation can play a role in the quality of life of an older adult. Incorporating the core objectives of encouragement, education, exercise, employment, and evaluation, as identified by the Life Options Advisory Council, will promote this perspective of nephrology care for the older person.

- Emotional and material support is given through a family system, and it is important to identify those who can be of assistance to the dependent older adult, and then mobilize theses resources. Concern for the caregiver's welfare and its effect on the care of the older person is also important.

The Older Adult with Renal Disease

Name of Resource	Brief Description	Where to Obtain Resource
American Journal of Nursing (AJN) Series: Nursing Care of Older Adults: A New Look at the Old Issues: Volume 104 Number 8, August 2004 Through Volume 106 Number 12, December 2006	The American Journal of Nursing (AJN), in collaboration with the Gerontological Society of America (GSA) has developed this series on the nursing care of older adults. It is available in print as well as webcast on the Web site provided. CE credits can be applied for that meet recertification requirements for specific nursing associations and RN relicensure.	Medical Library (Print Version) http://www.nursingcenter.com (PDF version; webcast)
American Journal of Nursing (AJN) AJN's Older Adult Forum	This online forum allows individuals to talk with authors of the "Nursing Care of Older Adult's: A New Look at the Old" series, colleagues, or other experts regarding gerontological patient care.	http://www.nursingcenter.com
American Nephrology Nurses' Association Online Modules	The geriatric web resource is designed to assist nephrology nurses to become more adept at recognizing the unique aspects of caring for the aged. It is a continuation of ANNA's work with the Nurse Competence in Aging (NCA) initiative.	http://www.annanurse.org/aging
Hartford Institute for Geriatric Nursing	This institute is a nurse-led institute whose purpose is to provide knowledge about and improvement of health care for older Americans. Not only is the systems in which nurses learn and work influenced by the work of this institute, but also the competence of the nurse caring for older adults.	http://www.hartfordign.org
Healthy People 2010	Healthy people 2010 is a national governmental and organizational (public, private, non-profit) collaborative effort whose overall goals are to increase the quality and years of healthy life and to eliminate health problems. Contains 467 science-based objectives and 10 Leading Health Indicators which can all be applied to the elderly: physical activity, overweight and obesity, tobacco use, substance abuse, responsible sexual behavior, mental health, injury and violence, environmental quality and immunization, and access to health care.	Medical Library http://www.healthypeople.gov (PDF version)
Merck Institute on Aging and Health Online Resource: Nurse's Notes for Healthy Aging	The purpose of this Web site is to educate health care professionals as well as the general public about research findings and utilization of these findings to improve the aging process.	http://www,miahonline.org/resources/nursesnotes/index.html

The Older Adult with Renal Disease

Name of Resource	Brief Description	Where to Obtain Resource
Nurse Competence in Aging Online informational center	This Web site, customized by individual nurses, provides practice information on care of older adults. Specifics may be obtained on geriatric topics, patient signs and symptoms, and specialty practice areas. A "Try This Series" provides assessment tools for this cohort.	http://www.GeroNurseOnline.org
The Gerontological Society of America Online informational center	This gerontological society is a professional organization that provides individuals (practitioners, researchers, educators, and policy makers) opportunities to use basic and applied research for the purpose of improvement of the quality of life as one ages. "Explore the Issues" and webcasts available.	http://www.geron.org
The Merck Manual of Geriatrics Editors: M.H.Beers, M.D. and Robert Berkow, M.D. Copyright: 2000-2005	This manual (available in print and online) provides information regarding diseases, including treatments, drugs and dosages for older adults. The internet format provides the flexibility for the authors to update information as needed.	Medical Library http://www.merck.com/mrkshared/mm_geriatrics/contents.jsp

ANNP622

The Older Adult with Chronic Kidney Disease

Terran Mathers, DNS, RN

Contemporary Nephrology Nursing: Principles and Practice contains 39 chapters of educational content. Individual learners may apply for continuing nursing education credit by reading a chapter and completing the Continuing Education Evaluation Form for that chapter. Learners may apply for continuing education credit for any or all chapters.

Please photocopy this page and return to ANNA.
COMPLETE THE FOLLOWING:

Name: _____

Address:_____

City:_____ State: _____ Zip: _____

E-mail: _____

Preferred telephone: ☐ Home ☐ Work: _____

State where licensed and license number (optional): _____

CE application fees are based upon the number of contact hours provided by the individual chapter. CE fees per contact hour for ANNA members are as follows: 1.0-1.9 - $15; 2.0-2.9 - $20; 3.0-3.9 - $25; 4.0 and higher - $30. Fees for nonmembers are $10 higher.

ANNA Member: ☐ Yes ☐ No Member # (if available) _____

☐ Checked Enclosed ☐ American Express ☐ Visa ☐ MasterCard

Total Amount Submitted: _____

Credit Card Number: _____ Exp. Date: _____

Name as it appears on the card: _____

CE Evaluation Form

To receive continuing education credit for individual study after reading the chapter

1. Photocopy this form. (You may also download this form from ANNA's Web site, **www.annanurse.org**.)

2. Mail the completed form with payment (check) or credit card information to American Nephrology Nurses' Association, East Holly Avenue, Box 56, Pitman, NJ 08071-0056.

3. You will receive your CE certificate from ANNA in 4 to 6 weeks.

Test returns must be postmarked by **December 31, 2010.**

CE Application Fee

ANNA Member $25.00

Nonmember $35.00

EVALUATION FORM

1. I verify that I have read this chapter and completed this education activity. Date: _____

   _____
   Signature

2. What would be different in your practice if you applied what you learned from this activity? *(Please use additional sheet of paper if necessary.)*

   _____

   _____

   _____

   _____

   _____

   _____

   _____

   _____

   _____

   _____

   _____

   _____

Evaluation	Strongly disagree				Strongly agree
3. The activity met the stated objectives.					
a. Relate the physiologic and psychosocial changes that occur with aging to the assessment findings in patients receiving RRT.	1	2	3	4	5
b. Discuss the nutritional considerations of caring for elderly patients with CKD.	1	2	3	4	5
c. Summarize the information that the nurse must be aware of when giving medications to the elderly with CKD.	1	2	3	4	5
d. Generate a plan of education for an elderly patient diagnosed with CKD.	1	2	3	4	5
4. The content was current and relevant.	1	2	3	4	5
5. The content was presented clearly.	1	2	3	4	5
6. The content was covered adequately.	1	2	3	4	5
7. Rate your ability to apply the learning obtained from this activity to practice.	1	2	3	4	5

Comments _____

_____

8. Time required to read the chapter and complete this form: _____ minutes.

This educational activity has been provided by the American Nephrology Nurses' Association (ANNA) for 3.0 contact hours. ANNA is accredited as a provider of continuing nursing education (CNE) by the American Nurses Credentialing Center's Commission on Accreditation (ANCC-COA). ANNA is an approved provider of continuing education by the California Board of Registered Nursing, CEP 0910.

Hemodialysis

Unit 6 Contents

Hemodialysis Technology

Carolyn E. Latham, MSN, MBA, RN, CNN
Based on previous edition by Patricia Baltz Salai, MSN, RN, CNN, CRNP

Chapter Contents

emodialysis (HD) is used extensively throughout the world to treat patients with acute and chronic renal failure. In the U.S., HD is the most commonly used treatment modality for patients requiring renal replacement therapy. According to the United States Renal Data System (USRDS), 92% of dialysis patients receive HD compared to 8% receiving peritoneal dialysis (PD) (USRDS, 2003).

Introduction to HD

The widespread use of this modality has been made possible by extraordinary scientific contributions of many talented individuals and the worldwide exchange of ideas, knowledge, and expertise. It is hard to imagine a time without the common availability of this life saving treatment. However, the following passage, from a very reputable medical textbook of its time, reveals that HD has not always been available or accessible:

"The use of the artificial kidney and other techniques of extrarenal dialysis have little place in the management of chronic renal failure...on rare occasions, it may be helpful in tiding him over an acute exacerbation," (Relman, 1959, p. 1060).

There have been remarkable advances in the field since the above medical textbook was published. These developments have continued over the years and have led to more effective HD supplies, equipment, and techniques.

This chapter will describe the fundamental HD principles and prevalent components of HD systems. It will discuss the use of HD technology from preparation to post-treatment maintenance. The nursing care of a patient receiving HD therapy will be reviewed including pre- and post-treatment assessment, monitoring response to therapy, and communication among the multidisciplinary team.

HD Defined

HD is one type of therapy that uses dialysis, a process in which substances move across a semipermeable membrane to remove unwanted solutes and fluid and restore acid base and electrolyte balance. The semipermeable membrane separates two opposing solutions and allows certain substances to pass while restricting the passage of others. In HD, an artificial kidney contains the semipermeable membrane, a solution path for blood and a fluid compartment for the dialyzing fluid or dialysate. Electrolytes and fluid are able to pass through the membrane pores while the passage of larger substances such as red blood cells and albumin is restricted provided the membrane is intact. This artificial kidney, along with other essential components of the HD system, is able to replace most but not all of the functions of the natural kidney.

The natural kidney maintains acid base and electrolyte balance, controls fluid volume, removes waste products, contributes to blood pressure control, maintains red blood cells, and promotes bone maintenance through specialized cells in the kidney. The innate human kidneys work continuously maintaining homeostasis 24 hours per day.

The terms artificial kidney, dialyzer, hemodialyzer, and dialyzer filter are used synonymously to indicate the medical device that is key in attempting to substitute for normal renal

Table 23-1
Replacement Therapy for Normal Kidney Functions

Normal Kidney Functions	Replacement Therapy
Electrolyte restoration	Hemodialysis
Acid-base correction	Hemodialysis
Waste removal	Hemodialysis
Fluid balance	Hemodialysis and diet
Renin-angiotensin/BP control	Medication
Erythropoeitin/RBC production	Medication
Vitamin D activation/bone maintenance	Medication

functions. The replacement functions occur intermittently, however, only during the dialysis sessions for a total of about 12 to 48 hours per week. In contrast to the human kidney, the HD process is unable to achieve the functions involving hormone secretion, such as blood pressure control, erythropoietin production, or bone maintenance. These functions must be supported with pharmacologic agents as illustrated in Table 23-1.

HD Principles, Concepts, and Terms

HD relies on key principles to allow the removal of substances and fluid as well as correcting acid base and electrolyte balance. These key principles include ultrafiltration (UF), osmosis, diffusion, and convection. There are also concepts and terms that are applied to the HD process such as clearance, permeability, molecular weight, dialyzer efficiency, and flux. These will be discussed in more detail, as they are critical in understanding the technological aspects of the therapy.

Fluid Removal

Ultrafiltration (UF). UF is the process through which body water removal is accomplished during dialysis. It is the movement of a solvent, a liquid capable of dissolving another substance or solute, from one area to another because of a pressure or concentration difference. In HD, UF, the transfer of fluid from the blood to the dialysate through the dialyzer membrane, is due primarily to a pressure gradient (transmembrane pressure) existing between the blood and dialysate compartments (Association for the Advancement of Medical Instrumentation [AAMI], 2003).

Osmosis. Osmosis, although not as significant for fluid removal during HD, is important in understanding fluid shifts that can occur as a result of HD. Osmosis is the passage of a solvent (fluid) through a semipermeable membrane to establish equilibrium in the amount of liquid on either side of the membrane. This fluid shift is created by a concentration difference for water across the membrane. Water will move from an area of greater water concentration to lesser water concentration. When there is a concentration difference, osmosis occurs until a pressure difference develops that is great enough to oppose this; the osmotic pressure is the required pressure great enough to oppose the osmotic effect (Guyton, 1986).

In dialysis, osmotic gradients may be established by adding substances such as glucose to the dialysate to draw water from the blood to the dialysate. Although useful in PD, this has limited clinical usefulness in HD for fluid removal because it is difficult to estimate and unpredictable (Lancaster, 1979).

However, as a result of the HD process, osmotic gradients can create movement of body fluid from the interstitial or intracellular compartments. For example, when fluid is removed from the blood, fluid in turn moves from the interstitial space to the blood resulting in refilling of the interstitial space from fluid moving out of the intracellular spaces (Kaufman, Polaschegg, & Levin, 1993).

UF via hydrostatic pressures. The hydrostatic or hydraulic pressure has the most significant influence on UF during HD. Hydrostatic pressure is the pressure that a liquid exerts against the wall of its container. From an UF perspective, the blood circuit is generally considered exerting positive pressure against the membrane while negative pressure is exerted from the dialysate side.

The positive hydrostatic pressure on the blood side acts to push water from the blood across the semipermeable membrane to the dialysate compartment. Although the blood side is commonly regarded as exerting a positive pressure, there are areas of the extracorporeal blood circuit and within the blood compartment of the dialyzer where negative pressures are generated. These pressures will be explained in more detail in later sections.

On the dialysate side, negative pressure can be created by the dialysis machine. This negative pressure on the dialysate side acts as a vacuum and pulls water from the blood compartment through the membrane and into the dialysis compartment for removal. Current HD equipment technology with controlled and more reliable methods of fluid removal has the added capability of generating positive pressure on the dialysate side to prevent excessive UF when needed. With conventional or low-flux dialyzers, the generation of negative pressure on the dialysate side is sufficient. However, when using high-flux dialyzers, the controlled UF technology allowing either positive or negative pressure is critical and required.

The ability of the hemodialyzer to remove body water varies widely among devices and is determined primarily by the UF capability of the membrane being used. This capability is expressed as the UF coefficient (K_{UF}), which is a measurement of the water flux or the permeability of the dialyzer membrane to water. The K_{UF} is one of the defining characteristics of high-flux versus low-flux dialyzers, which will be discussed in more detail later. The UF coefficient describes the amount of water a dialyzer membrane will permit to pass during a given period of time at a specified pressure. For hemodialyzers, it is expressed as ml/hr/mm Hg TMP. This measures the volume of water in milliliters (ml) that will pass through the membrane during 1 hour (hr) per each millimeter of mercury (mmHg) transmembrane pressure (TMP) (Salem & Mujais, 1993).

The TMP exerted on the dialysis membrane can be determined by subtracting the dialysis solution pressure exerted from the machine from the blood compartment pressure (Ismail & Hakim, 1991). Both the blood compartment pressure and the

dialysis solution pressure are measured in mmHg. According to AAMI (2003), the TMP which can be expressed by the following equation:

$$TMP = (P_{Bi} + P_{Bo})/2 - (P_{Di} + P_{Do})/2 - P_{oncotic}$$

$P_{oncotic}$ = oncotic pressure created by plasma proteins
P_{Bi} = pressure at the arterial (inlet) port of a hemodialyzer blood compartment
P_{Bo} = pressure at the venous (outlet) port of a hemodialyzer blood compartment
P_{Di} = pressure at the inlet port of a hemodialyzer dialysate compartment
P_{Do} = pressure at the outlet port of a hemodialyzer dialysate compartment

The actual amount of fluid removed during HD is a function of both the ability of the dialyzer to remove the fluid and the TMP influenced by the settings of the HD machine to exert a certain amount of pressure. The amount of UF removed during the HD treatment is referred to as the UF rate.

Backfiltration. UF involves the movement of fluid from the blood compartment to the dialysate compartment. With conventional dialyzers with low UF coefficients, normal TMP, and fluid removal requirements, fluid moves from the blood side to the dialysate side. However, when dialysis is performed using a dialyzer with a high UF coefficient (i.e., high-flux dialyzer) and the patient requires minimal fluid removal, and the TMP is low, the pressure on the blood side near the outlet (venous end) may be lower than the dialysate pressure at its inlet and backfiltration occurs (Klinkman, Ebbighausen, Uhlenbusch, & Vienken, 1993). Backfiltration refers to the movement of fluid from the dialysis fluid compartment into the blood and commonly occurs when using high-flux dialyzers (see Figure 23-1).

A clinical concern related to backfiltration is the potential transport of contaminants present in the dialysate across the membrane into the blood (Hoenich, Ghezzi, & Ronco, 2004; Soltys, Zydney, Leypoldt, Henderson, & Ofsthun, 2000). Although pyrogen exposure and endotoxemia is a danger for all HD methods, the use of high-permeability membranes has been associated with theoretically higher risk (Canaud & Krieter, 2005).

Endotoxins, the major component of the outer cell wall of gram-negative bacteria, are lipopolysaccharides and are the most common pyrogenic organisms (AAMI, 2004). Endotoxins can acutely activate both humoral and cellular host defenses, leading to an acute syndrome characterized by fever, shaking chills, hypotension, multiple organ failure, and even death if allowed to enter the circulation in a sufficient dose (AAMI, 2004). Long-term exposure to low levels of endotoxin has been implicated in a chronic inflammatory response, which may contribute to some of the long-term complications seen in HD patients (AAMI, 2003).

Solute Removal

In HD, in addition to UF, clearance or removal of solutes from the blood through the semipermeable membrane can occur simultaneously (Lazarus, Denker, & Owen, 1996). The clearance or solute transport out of the blood during HD can result from diffusion, convection, or adsorption.

Clearance. The term "clearance" is used by nephrologists when assessing the ability of the natural kidneys to

Figure 23-1
Backfiltration Occurs When the Blood Pressure Near the Outlet Is Lower Than the Dialysate Pressure at its Inlet.

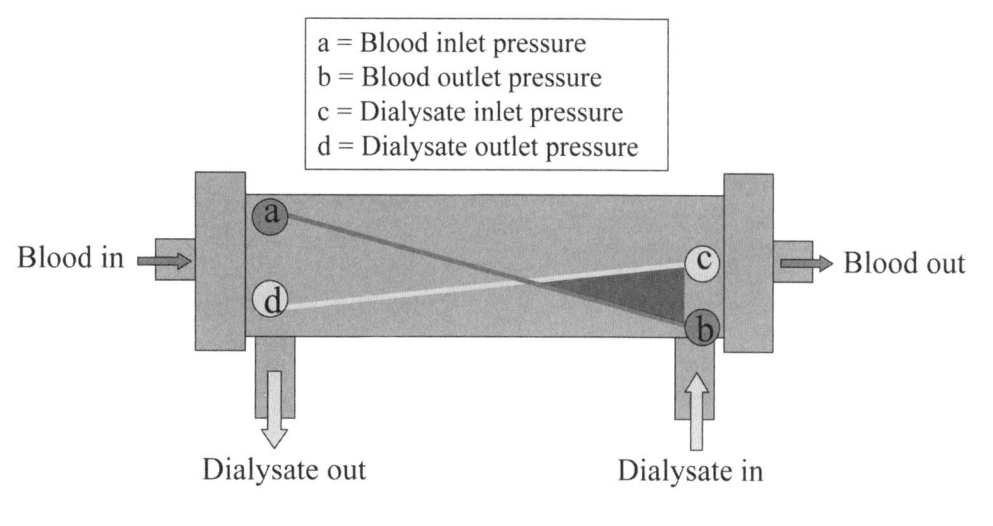

a = Blood inlet pressure
b = Blood outlet pressure
c = Dialysate inlet pressure
d = Dialysate outlet pressure

Blood in →

Blood out

Dialysate out   Dialysate in

remove metabolic waste products from the blood stream. It is also used in HD to describe the ability of a dialyzer to remove a specific solute. It is a measure of net flux of a given solute across the hemodialyzer membrane that is expressed as the number of milliliters of blood completely cleared of a solute per unit of time (AAMI, 2003).

Clearance is stated as a volume flow measurement in ml/minute and is expressed in relationship to a specific blood flow rate. For example, a urea clearance of 320 at a blood flow rate of 400 ml/min reflects the dialyzer's capability of removing all urea from 320 ml of blood every time 400 ml of blood passes through the dialyzer in a minute. The dialyzer's ability to clear various solutes is one measure used to compare the performance capabilities of dialyzer devices.

Dialyzer clearance can be measured in vitro or in vivo. The published clearance values stated on product literature are often reported as in vitro values. In vitro device testing in a non-clinical or laboratory setting involves non-animal testing and is used to evaluate specific chemical, physical, and immunological properties of devices including performance characteristics (McCarthy, 2004). In vitro measurements, because they are performed without blood cells or plasma protein, are not affected by protein absorption. In vitro measurements, when performed using aqueous solutions without red blood cells or plasma proteins, are not affected by changes in the membrane permeability due to factors such as protein absorption, clotting, or channeling of blood.

In vivo values are obtained in a clinical setting while patients are dialyzing and are often less than the in vitro values; this difference may be minimal to as much as 20% less than the clearance achieved in vitro at the same pump speeds and dialysate flow rates (Renal Physicians Association [RPA], 1993; Saha & Van Stone, 1992). The difference is dependent on membrane changes in the clinical situation such as protein adsorption and patient's hematocrit when blood comes in contact with the membrane.

Table 23-2
Molecular Weights of Common Substances

Substance	Molecular Weight (MW) *in daltons*
NaCl	58
Urea	60
Calcium	111
Creatinine	113
Glucose	180
Inulin	5200
Vitamin B12	1355
B2M	11,800
Cytochrome C	12,400
Retinol binding protein	21,000
Factor D	25,000
Albumin	69,000
Endotoxins	Wide range up to 30,000

During HD, there are many factors that influence clearance including: the size and properties of the solute; dialyzer membrane characteristics such as polymer, thickness, consistency, pore size; and surface area (SA) and shape or configuration of hollow fibers (Leypoldt et al., 2003). Dialyzer design and flow dynamics can also impact clearance as well as clinical parameters such as dialysis treatment frequency, length, blood and dialysate flows, and vascular access function. Strategies to maximize the clearance of solutes during treatment will be discussed in later sections of this chapter.

Dialyzer membranes vary in their ability to remove or clear solutes. The size or weight of the solute is very important in relation to the dialyzability, the ability of the solute to

Figure 23-2
Diffusion

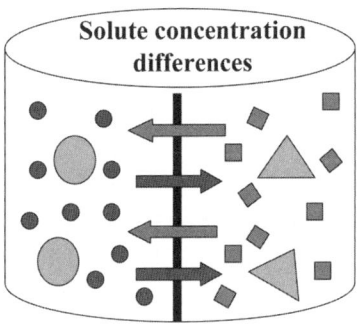
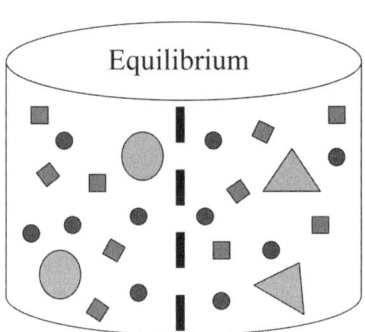

be cleared during dialysis. The molecular weight or the sum of the atomic weights of all the atoms in a molecule solute is measured in daltons, representing the atomic mass unit (Weast, 1983). Table 23-2 lists the molecular weights of substances commonly measured to define a dialyzer's ability to clear a substance in relation to dialysis.

As long as the dialyzer membrane is intact, the goal is to allow certain sized solutes through the membrane to be removed while preventing larger sized particles such as albumin and red cells from passing through. The size of the particle can also help predict the medications that may or may not be dialyzable. Generally, solutes less than 5,000 daltons can freely pass through the pores of most dialyzer membrane types (Soltys et al., 2000). However, solutes that are 10,000 to 20,000 daltons are usually too large to pass through low-flux membranes but can pass through high flux (Soltys et al., 2000). Solutes greater than 40,000 daltons are usually too large to pass through any intact dialysis membrane (Soltys et al., 2000).

The sieving coefficient (SC) is the permeability of dialysis membranes to a particular solute and is defined as the ratio of solute concentration in the ultrafiltrate to that of the plasma (Ismail, Brouillette, & Mujais, 1999). A SC of one for a given substance represents free transport through the membrane while a value of zero indicates the membrane is impermeable for this substance.

Diffusion. All substances including water molecules and dissolved particles are in constant motion. The continued movement of molecules among each other, whether in liquid or gas, is called diffusion (Guyton, 1986).

A concentration difference occurs when the number of solutes on one side of the membrane is greater than the number of solutes on the other side. The concentration difference between the two sides of the membrane establishes a solute concentration gradient across the membrane. This driving force causes solutes to move across the membrane from the more concentrated side to the less concen-

trated side (Keshaviah, 1991). The movement occurs until the concentrations are equal (see Figure 23-2).

During HD, solutes move between the blood and the dialysis solution compartments. The primary mechanism for toxin removal by HD is diffusion across the dialyzer's semipermeable membrane (Keshaviah, 1991). Solutes highly concentrated in the blood of a uremic patient, such as urea, creatinine, and potassium, move into the dialysis solution as these substances are absent or present in low concentrations in the dialysate (Ismail & Hakim, 1991). At the same time, solutes that are present in a higher concentration in the dialysis solution than in the patient's blood move through the membrane from the dialysis solution into the blood (see Figure 23-3). This is often referred to as back-diffusion (Klinkmann, Ebbighausen, Uhlenbusch, & Vienken, 1993).

Several factors affect diffusion, particularly the rate at which it occurs during HD. These factors include membrane SA and thickness; the number of pores in the membrane; the concentration gradient between the blood and the dialysis solution; blood and dialysate flow rates; solution temperatures; membrane resistance; and the molecular size, weight, and charge of the solutes (Ismail & Hakim, 1991). Blood flow and dialysate flow are typically arranged in a counter current configuration to allow for maximal concentration gradients between blood and dialysate at any point along the length of the fibers (Ismail et al., 1999) (see Figure 23-4). During the HD procedure, the dialysate is warmed to maintain warmth of the blood circuit and enhance the diffusion of solutes. Both blood and dialysate form an unstirred thin layer on each side of the semipermeable membrane that molecules must cross (Ismail et al., 1999). These unstirred layers act to decrease the effective concentration gradient and thus decrease the rate of diffusion.

Convection (Solute drag). In addition to diffusive clearance, solutes can move with the water as water moves

Figure 23-3
Movement of Solutes Across Hemodialyzer Membrane

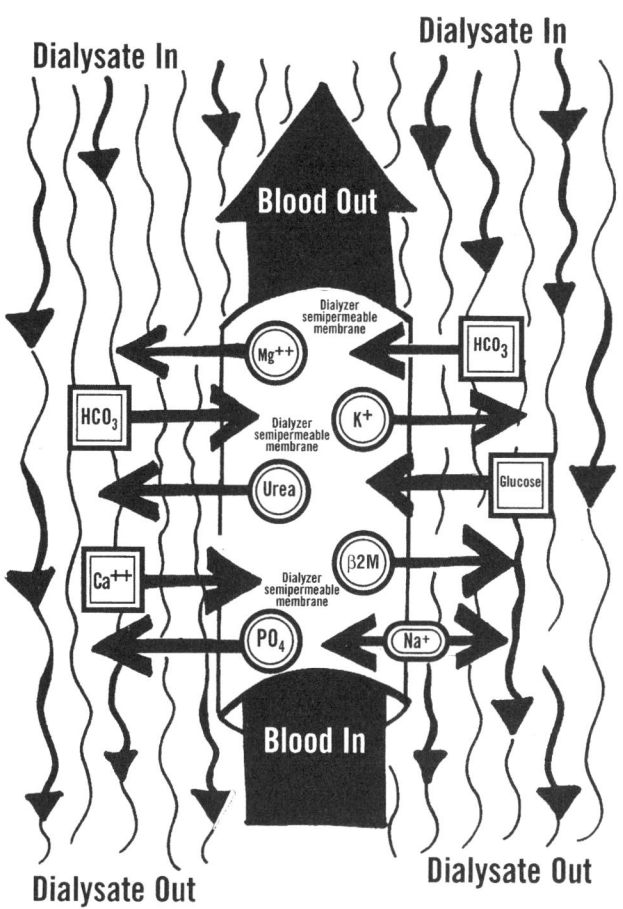

Solutes in greater concentration in the blood such as K+ and urea move to the dialysate while solutes in greater concentration in the dialysate move from the dialysate compartment to the blood.

Figure 23-4
Counter Current Configuration of Blood and Dialysate

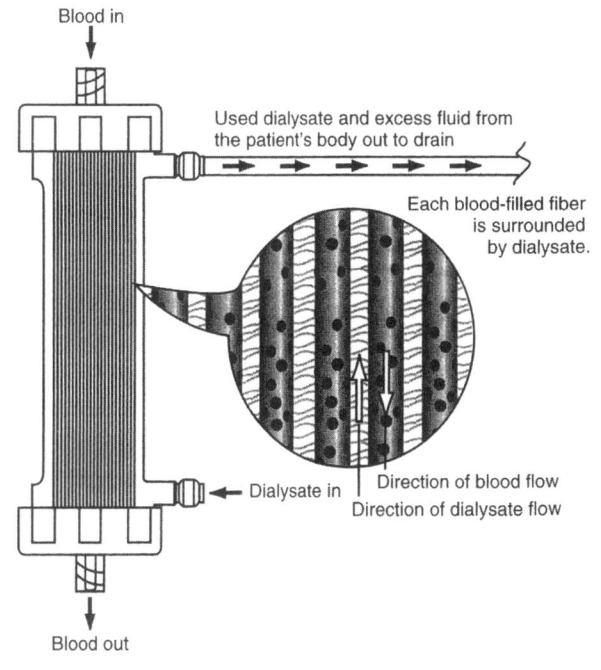

Note: Used with permission from the Amgen copyrighted *Core Curriculum for Dialysis Technicians*, 2nd edition, Blood and dialysate flow: Countercurrent directions.

across the semipermeable membrane of the dialyzer. This convective movement is also referred to as solute drag, as the solutes are being "dragged" across the membrane with the water as it moves across the membrane. The driving force for convective transport is the pressure difference across the membrane (TMP). UF affects the clearance of larger solutes more than small solutes.

Components of the HD System

The HD system includes the dialyzer to filter the blood and the dialysis machine used to proportion and monitor the dialysate fluid as well as pump and monitor the blood flowing through the extracorporeal circuit. The extracorporeal blood circuit includes blood tubing to deliver blood from the patient's access to the dialyzer and return the blood from the dialyzer back to the patient's access. Needles or catheters are used to provide blood from the patient's vascular access to the blood tubing. The dialysate circuit includes the mixing and delivery system used to cre-

ate the dialysate, which is made from water and electrolyte/buffer solution. The water used for HD must be purified prior to use necessitating special water treatment systems that are also vital components of the HD treatment.

The Dialyzer

Structure. Today, there are two types of dialyzer construction: hollow fiber or parallel plate. Both the parallel plate and hollow fiber dialyzers are designed with two internal compartments, one to contain blood and the other for dialysis solution. The two compartments are separated by a semipermeable membrane.

There are four ports on the dialyzer, two for blood and two for dialysate. Blood enters the dialyzer through the inlet port (arterial blood port), flows through the blood compartment, and leaves the dialyzer via the outlet (venous) port on the opposite end. Dialysis solution enters through the inlet dialysate port on the dialyzer, flows through the dialysate compartment, and exits the dialyzer through the outlet dialysate port. To create the counter current flow of blood and dialysate, the blood inlet and dialysate outlet are on the same end of the dialyzer so the blood exits on the same end of the dialyzer where the dialysate enters. As previously mentioned, this creates the maximum concentration gradient to enhance diffusion.

Parallel plate dialyzer. Although parallel plate dialyzers were used extensively in the past, currently, they are not commonly used in the U.S. The parallel plate dialyzer utilizes multiple parallel sheets of membrane and support structures resembling a series of flat, hard plastic plates

Figure 23-5
Parallel Plate Hemodialyzer

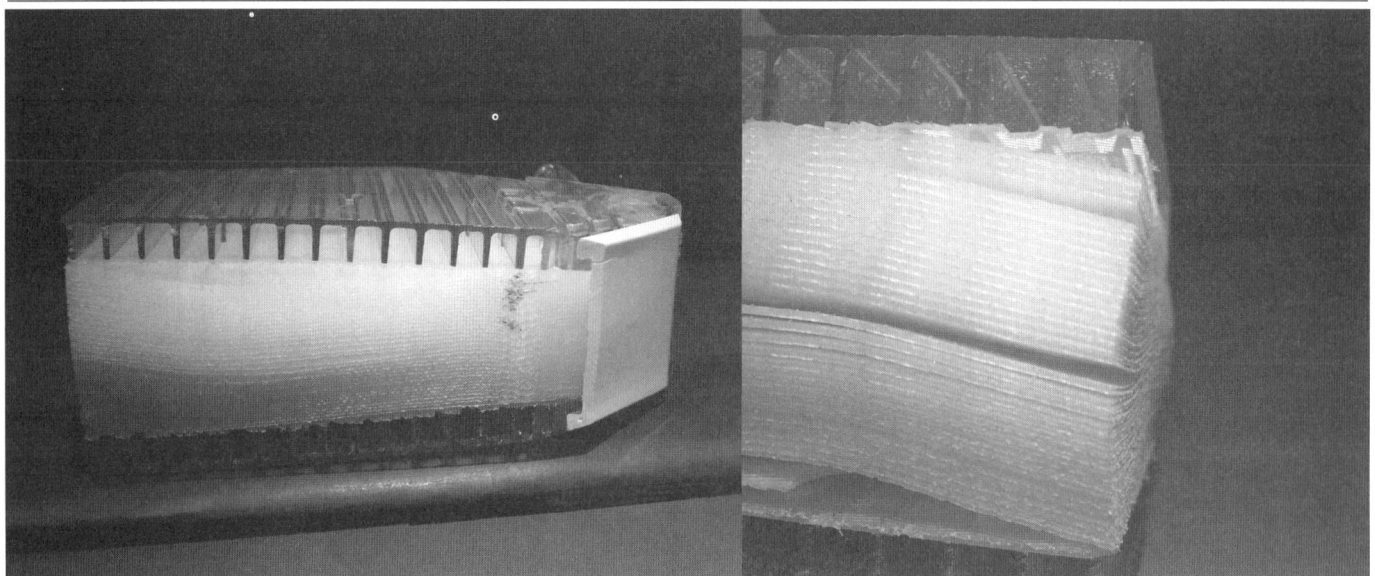

Note: Photograph courtesy of Carolyn Latham, Russell Dimmitt, and Kim Tecca.

Figure 23-6
Hollow Fiber Hemodialyzer: Bundle of Fibers and Plastic Cylinder

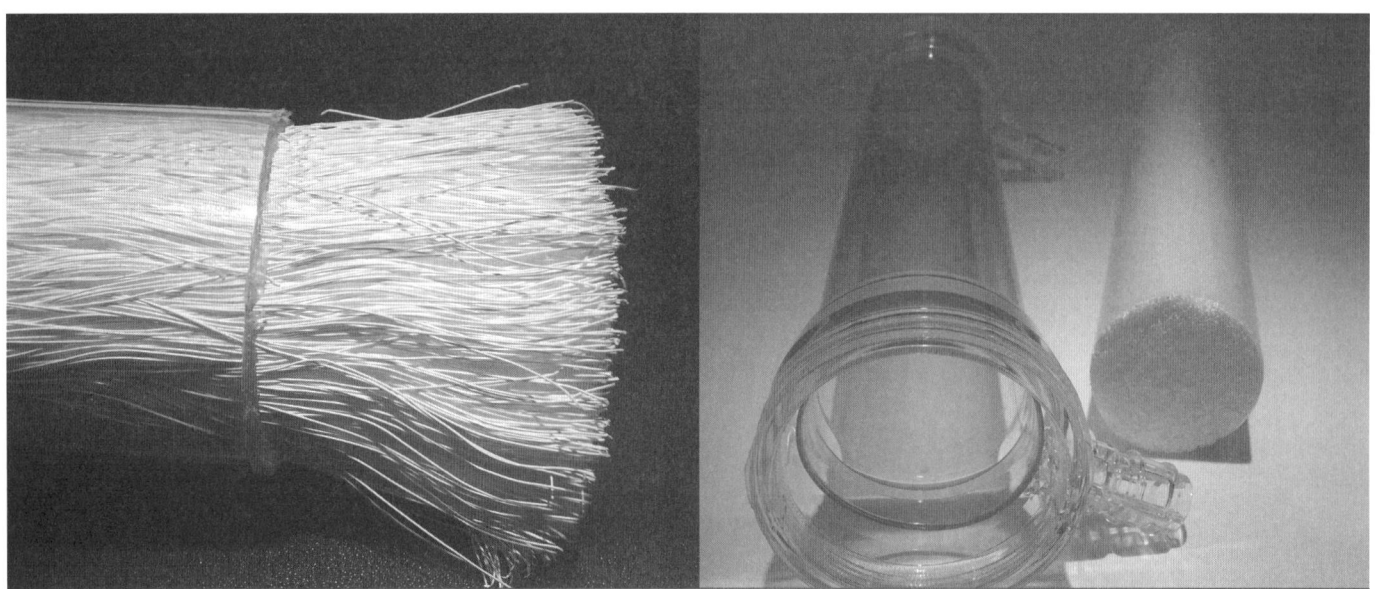

Note: Photograph courtesy of Carolyn Latham, Russell Dimmitt, and Kim Tecca.

sandwiched with sheets of thin plastic membranes on top of one another (see Figure 23-5). The dialyzer is designed so blood and dialysis solution pass through alternate spaces between the membrane sheets (Daugirdas, Van Stone, & Boag, 2001).

Hollow fiber dialyzer. The hollow-fiber or capillary dialyzer is the most common construction and utilizes thousands of capillary tubules with the semi-permeable membrane forming the wall of each tubule and resembles a bundle of hair or thin straws housed inside a rigid, clear plastic cylinder (see Figure 23-6).

In the hollow-fiber dialyzer, the blood flows through the inside of the fibers while the dialysate flows around the outside of the fibers. The bundle of thin hair-like fibers is held in place at each end of the dialyzer by polyurethane potting material. The function of the potting material is to form a tight seal between the blood and the dialysate compartments while holding the fibers in place (Ismail et al., 1999). During the manufacturing process, the end of the potting material is cut sharply to open up the end of the fibers so blood can flow through. A sharp and smooth cut is desired to promote smooth flow of blood and decrease residual blood. Rigid caps made of polystyrene, polycarbonate, or other materials are on each end of the dialyzer

Table 23-3
Dialyzer Membrane Polymers

Membrane Type	Material
Cellulosic	
	• Cuprammonium cellulose (Cuprophan®) • Cuprammonium rayon • Modified cellulose acetate • Saponified cellulose ester • Regenerated cellulose
Modified	
Substituted with acetate	• Cellulose diacetate (CA, CDA) • Cellulose triacetate (CTA)
Cellulosynthetic	• DEAE-substituted cellulose and cellulose (Hemophan®)
Coated	• Cuprammonium rayon coated with polyethylene glycol (PEG) • Regenerated cellulose coated with vitamin E
Synthetic	
	• Polyacrylonitrile and methacrylate (PAN) • Polyacrylonitrile and methallyl sulfonate (AN-69®) • Polyamide, polyarylethersulfone, and polyvinylpyrrolidone (Polyflux) • Polycarbonate • Polyethylene polyvinyl alcohol (EVAL) • Polymethylmethacrylate (PMMA) • Polysulfone (PS)

and contain inlet (arterial) and outlet (venous) blood ports onto which the inlet and outlet blood tubing is connected. The header end caps may be removable or non-removable, depending on the manufacturer, and may or may not be constructed with removable o-rings (see Figure 23-7).

Membrane. The performance of the dialyzer is dependent to a large degree on the membrane material (polymer) and manufacturing (fabrication) process that controls the membrane microstructure. The performance is measured in terms of the removal of unwanted solutes and excess fluid from the patient and interactions between the membrane device and the cellular and soluble components of the blood (Radovich, 1995).

Polymer. The polymer is the chemical composition of the semipermeable membrane. The membrane polymer properties influence the biocompatibility, the hydrophobic or hydrophilic nature, water content, and protein absorption capabilities of the membrane. The adsorbed proteins can affect the underlying permeability of the membrane and thus can influence solute and fluid removal.

There are numerous membranes on the market today but three primary categories, including cellulosic, modified cellulosic, and synthetic. The modified cellulosic category can be further subdivided into substituted and coated. The substituted subcategory has also been further classified into those substituted with acetate and those with a synthetic material; the latter also being referred to as cellulosynthetic (Ajuria & Kimmel, 2004). These coated, substituted, and cellulosynthetic dialyzer membranes, are also referred to as semi-synthetic (see Table 23-3).

Membranes used in the U.S. have changed dramatical-

Figure 23-7
Dialyzer Header Cross-Section

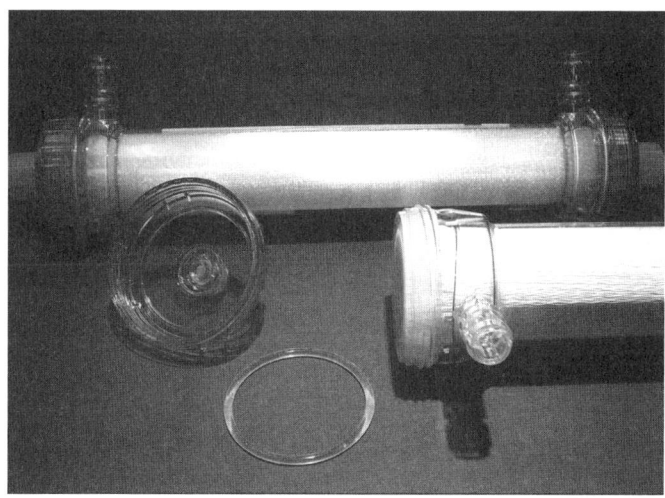

Note: Copyright, 2005, Fresenius Medical Care. Reprinted with permission.

ly in the last 10 years with synthetic high-flux dialyzers being used more commonly (Collins, Liu, & Ebben, 2004). According to the USRDS (1997), the use of synthetic membranes had increased from 9% in 1990 to 55% in 1996, while the use of cellulosic membranes had decreased from 70% in 1990 to 22% in 1996 with the use of modified cellulosic membranes remaining fairly unchanged. According to Centers for Medicare and Medicaid Services (CMS) (2003), the usage of high-flux dialyzers increased from about 30% in 1993 to 85% in 2002.

Cellulosic. Cellulose-based membranes, derived from cotton or wood, contain hydroxyl groups, providing surface for complement activation and associated intradialytic leukopenia, indices of bioincompatibility (Ajuria & Kimmel, 2004; Boure & Vanholder, 2004; Ismail et al., 1999). These cellulosic membranes are also referred to as natural, from their cotton derivative (Boure & Vanholder, 2004), or unmodified or unsubstituted. They include cuprammonium cellulose (Cuprophan®), cuprammonium rayon, saponified cellulose ester, and modified cellulose acetate.

Modified cellulosic (semi-synthetic). Substituted cellulosic membranes were created to reduce complement activation and improve their biocompatibility. The modification also increased the hydrophobic nature in some with resulting increased permeability to water and larger weight substances. Substituted cellulosic membranes contain polymers in which the hydroxyl groups are replaced with acetyl groups, such as diacetate or triacetate, or with synthetic tertiary amino groups, diethylamino ethyl (DEAE), referred to as cellulosynthetic (Ajuria & Kimmel, 2004; Ismail et al., 1999; Radovich, 1995). Cellulosic membranes can also be altered by coating the membrane with substances such as cuprammonium rayon coated with polyethylene glycol (PEG) or cellulose coated with vitamin E.

Synthetic. Synthetic membranes are glassy engineering plastics or vinyls that have been associated with less dialysis-related leukopenia as well as a low degree of complement activation (Gutch & Stoner, 1993; Hoenick, 1988). Examples include polyacrylonitrile (PAN), copolymer of polyacrylonitrile, and sodium methallyl sulfonate (AN 69®); polysulfone (PS); polyamide (PA); blend of polyarylethersulfone, polyamide, and polyvinylpyrrolidone (Polyflux); and polymethylmethacrylate (PMMA).

Microstructure. The membrane microstructure or morphology is controlled during the manufacturing process to obtain the desired permeability and mechanical strength (Radovich, 1995). The microstructure defines the pore density and the pore size distribution in the membrane (Radovich, 1995). This determines removal of low and high molecular weight substances by diffusion and convection as well as fluid removal. The pore size represents the size of microscopic openings between polymer chains. The pore size distribution signifies the number of small pores compared to larger pores. The porosity characterizes the total fraction of membrane that is open and reflects the size, number, and distribution of pores.

Symmetric or homogenous membrane structures have the same porosity and pore size distribution throughout the wall from the fiber lumen surface to the fiber's outer surface (Radovich, 1995). Examples include cellulose, cellulose diacetate, and triacetate (Radovich, 1995). Asymmetric or heterosporous membranes, such as AN69, polyflux, PMMA, or polysulfone, can have a thin, dense lumen surface with much higher porosity and larger pore sizes in the remaining membrane (Radovich, 1995).

Hydrophilic membranes absorb and hold water in contrast to hydrophobic membranes that do not absorb water but increase water permeability. The amount of protein adsorbed varies with membrane type and can contribute to the removal of substances (Boure & Vanholder, 2004). The protein adsorption can influence cellular interactions and activation processes and transport capabilities (Radovich, 1995).

Surface area (SA). The SA of the dialyzer is stated in square meters and reflects the total membrane area. As the SA of the dialyzer increases, the space available for contact between the blood and the dialysis solution increases. As the amount of contact increases, diffusion increases. The numerous dialyzers available for HD vary in SA, allowing for selection of dialyzer according to patient need. Most are in the .8 to 2.0 m² range.

Water and Large Solute Permeability (Flux)

Water permeability is affected by the manufacturing process and the polymer. The UF capability is affected by porosity, SA, and hydrophilic versus hydrophobic properties.

Hemodialyzers are classified into high and low-flux dialyzers based on water and large solute permeability. High-flux dialyzers have been defined as having a mean clearance of β2 microglobulin of > 20 mL/min and an UF coefficient K_{UF} > 14 mL/h/mmHg during the first use or over the lifetime of the dialyzer with a given reprocessing method (AAMI, 2003; Cheung et al., 2003). Low-flux dialyzers are also referred to as conventional dialyzers and have been defined as having a mean clearance of β2 microglobulin < 10 mL/min (Cheung et al., 2003). The Food and Drug Administration (FDA) uses water permeability to differentiate between high-flux and low-flux dialyzers, with a K_{UF} of > 8 mL/h/mmHg defining high flux (AAMI, 2003).

The manufacturer reported UF coefficients of dialyzers are commonly reported as in vitro or ex vivo measurements. As with differences between in vitro and in vivo clearance data, true in vivo UF coefficients have been found to range 5%-30% lower than in vitro measurements reported by manufacturers (Daugirdas, Van Stone, et al., 2001). This difference is thought to be due to blood protein and hematocrit variances among patients as well as to such factors as excessive protein layering and partial dialyzer fiber clotting (Ismail et al., 1999).

Studies have shown mixed benefits of high-flux therapy. Studies showing various benefits of high-flux therapy include but are not limited to improved lipoprotein profiles (Josephson, 1992; Seres, Strain, Hashim, Goldberg, & Levin, 1993), improved cardiac function (Churchill et al., 1993), improved patient survival (Hornberger, Chernew, Petersen, & Garber, 1992), reduced dialysis associated amyloidosis (Winchester, Salsberg, & Levin, 2003), and improved patient symptoms (Churchill et al., 1992). However, there have also been studies showing no significant difference between high and low flux in various areas (Cheung et al., 2003, Ottosson, Attman, & Knight-Gibson, 2001). The HEMO study, a large multicenter clinical trial, demonstrated that randomization to high-flux dialysis did not significantly alter the primary outcome of an all-cause mortality (Cheung et al., 2003). The HEMO study did show, however, a statistically significant decrease in cardiac deaths associated with high-flux dialysis (Cheung et al., 2003).

Small Solute Permeability (Efficiency)

Dialyzers can also be classified by their ability to remove small solutes, referred to as low molecular weight solutes such as urea and creatinine. The term low molecular weight **solute** can be confused with low molecular weight **proteins** that are 500 to 60,000 daltons and are often referred to as middle molecules or larger sized substances (Clark & Winchester, 2003).

The term high efficiency is used to define dialyzers that can remove high amounts of small solutes and is commonly measured by urea clearance. Both high-flux and low-flux dialyzers can also be high-efficiency dialyzers. The flux refers to the large molecular weight substances and water while efficiency refers to the ability to remove low molecular weight (small) substances. Efficiency of a dialyzer can also be defined by its urea KoA, the mass transfer coefficient representing the maximum urea removal capacity of a dialyzer (Leypoldt & Cheung, 2001). The efficiency of a dialyzer can be impacted by the SA, porosity, and blood and dialysate flows. The same factors that influence clearance and diffusion described earlier can impact efficiency as this defines the ability to clear small solutes primarily by diffusion.

Flow Dynamics

Optimal dialyzer design characteristics allow smooth blood flow with lower propensity to cause clotting, minimal channeling of dialysate, and low resistance at the level of the membrane. The efficiency of the membrane and dialysate contact depends on dialysate and blood flow dynamics and can be impacted by dialyzer design.

Channeling of dialysate can occur as a result of nonuniform dialysate flow distribution. Spacer yarns have been added to optimize the packing density of fibers and to allow more uniform distribution of dialysate flow (Ismail et al., 1999). Crimping of fibers has also been introduced to maximize the blood and dialysate contact time.

Unstirred fluid layers on either the blood or dialysate side of the membrane can decrease the effective concentration gradients at the membrane surface (Ajuria & Kimmel, 2004). The thickness of the unstirred layers can be affected by dialysis solutions, blood flow rates, and dialyzer design. Transport depends on efficiency of contact between the blood and membrane interface and the membrane and dialysate interface.

Sterilization methods. The most common sterilization methods for hemodialyzers include: (a) steam/heat, (b) gamma irradiation, (c) ethylene oxide, and (d) electron beam. The sterilization methods used are dependent on the dialyzer membrane as dialyzer membrane materials react differently to the various sterilization methods.

Biocompatibility. Biocompatibility in HD can be defined as the sum of specific interactions between blood and the artificial materials of the HD circuit (Hakim, 1993). The biocompatibility can be influenced by all components of the HD system such as dialysis membranes, sterilants, blood tubing, dialysate, as well as the patient's susceptibility (Hakim, 1993).

Biocompatibility of the dialyzer is influenced by the polymer blend, manufacturing process, dialyzer design, materials used for fabrication, as well as sterilization, the membrane area, and reuse status of the dialyzer. A biocompatible dialyzer membrane is one with minimization of negative interactions between the membrane device and the cellular and soluble components of the blood. Studies have shown large and statistically significant dialyzer membrane differences (Hakim et al., 1996; Levin & Zasuwa, 1993). When blood encounters the HD membrane, reactions such as complement activation; triggering of the coagulation cascade; as well as activation of cellular components such as neutrophil granulocytes, monocytes, lymphocytes, and platelets are initiated (Ismail et al., 1999). Studies have supported improved survival and recovery from acute renal failure, lower morbidity and mortality, decreased incidence of infection, and decreased amyloid bone disease with use of more biocompatible dialyzers (Ismail & Hakim, 1991).

Reuse Versus Single Use

Dialyzers can be designed for single use or reuse, also called reprocessing. Any dialyzer intended for reuse must be labeled for reuse in accordance with the FDA. In accordance with the FDA requirements, manufacturers must provide instructions for safe and effective reuse and in vitro and in vivo performance data as dialyzer characteristics such as clearance may be affected by reuse (AAMI, 2003).

Dialyzer reuse. The reuse of hemodialyzers has been practiced in the U.S. for greater than 20 years and in 2000 practiced in approximately 78% of the dialysis units (Collins et al., 2004). The prescription to reuse remains the sole responsibility of the patient's physicians (AAMI, 2003). Reuse can be done using either a manual or automated process. Reuse programs must meet regulatory requirements including training and education and quality measures. The AAMI (2003) has developed recommended practice standards for reprocessing including considerations for record keeping, personnel health, qualifications and training, patients, equipment, physical plant, environmental safety, materials and supplies, procedural steps, patient monitoring, quality control, and assurance.

There are various germicides and/or heat used for reuse including: formaldehyde, heat and citric acid, peracetic acid, and glutaraldehyde. Collins et al. (2004) studied mortality and hospitalization risks according to various reuse practices using data on reuse practices from the annual survey of HD units conducted by the Centers for Disease Control and Prevention (CDC). They found for the 1998-1999 period, reuse practices were not associated with a survival advantage or disadvantage. They looked at formaldehyde with bleach and without bleach, glutaraldehyde with bleach and without bleach, peracetic acid with and without bleach, and no reuse.

Preprocessing. AAMI (2003) recommends preprocessing, subjecting the dialyzer to the reuse process before first use, to establish the original total cell volume (TCV) to be used as the reference TCV for subsequent reprocessing whenever possible. TCV, the solution volume needed to fully prime the blood compartment, is the sum of the fiber bundle volume (FBV) and the header volume (AAMI, 2003). When this is not possible, AAMI recommends a

Figure 23-8
Typical Hemodialysis System

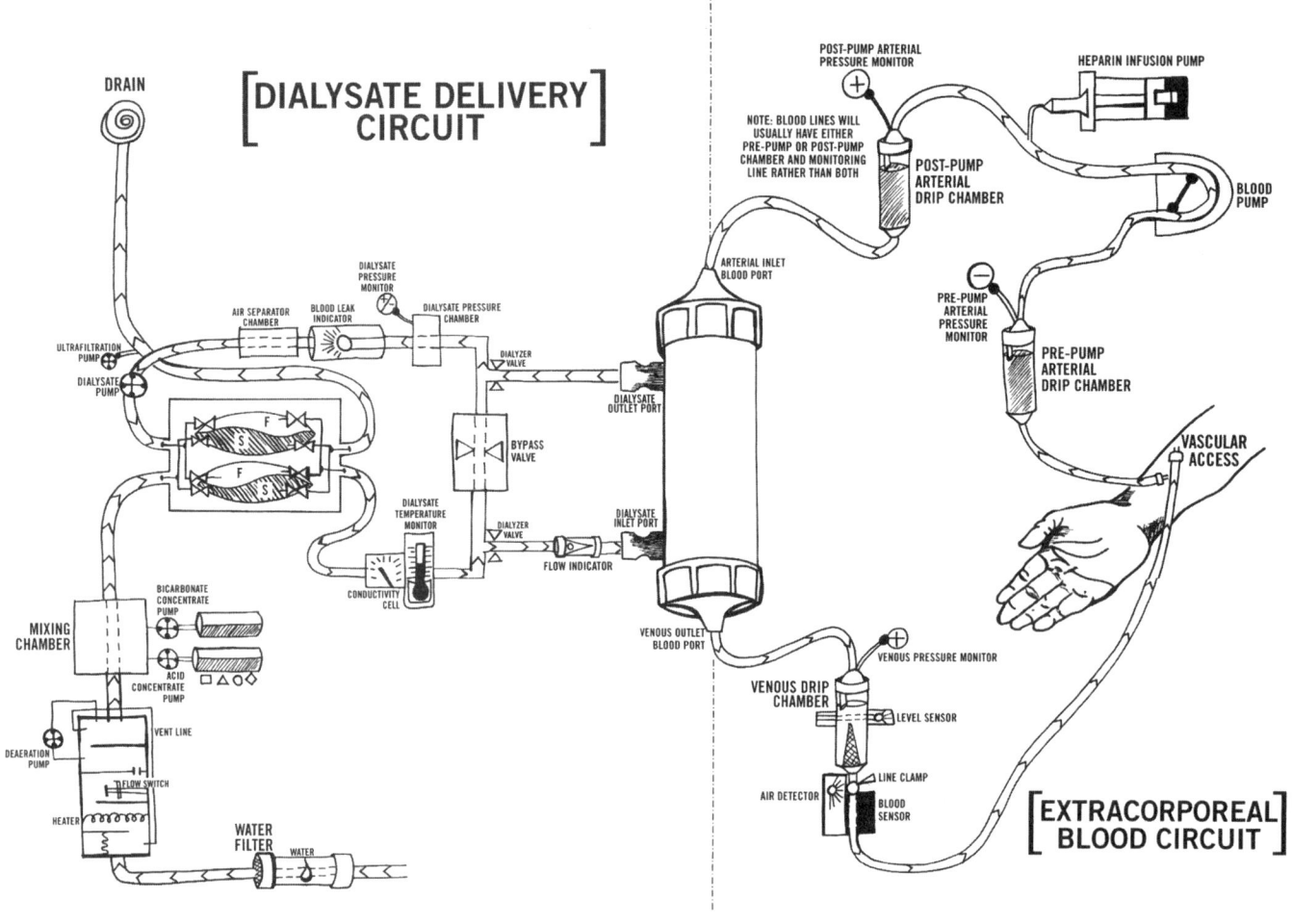

Note: Diagram courtesy of Carolyn Latham and Mark Rolston.

method referred to as volume averaging of the lot. The TCV of dialyzers can vary from values used to develop the original manufacturer's literature, from lot to lot, and from dialyzer to dialyzer within a lot (AAMI, 2003).

Reuse process. The reuse process involves rinsing, cleaning, testing for dialyzer performance, disinfection, and germicide removal (Kaufman & Levin, 2001). After the dialyzer is first used during treatment, the dialyzer is then reprocessed. Dialyzers should be reprocessed within 2 hours post HD treatment to inhibit bacterial growth or refrigerated and not allowed to freeze (AAMI, 2003).

Precleaning is commonly practiced and includes removal of gross deposits of blood products before rinsing and cleaning with a reprocessing machine. Cleaning agents, including hydrogen peroxide, sodium hypochlorite, peracetic acid, or other chemicals, must not have any significant adverse effects on the structural integrity and performance of the dialyzer (AAMI, 2003). Chemical germicides or other procedures used for disinfecting dialyzers must have been shown to accomplish at least high-level disinfection (AAMI, 2003). The water used to prepare the germicide solution must be purified in accordance with

regulatory and AAMI requirements.

Tests of dialyzer performance are done to check the integrity of the membrane, its clearance, and UF capabilities. Inspection is done after reuse and again prior to use. The dialyzer should not be used if it has an abnormal or unaesthetic appearance such as overall brownish or black discoloration, if there are clots visible in the header, or if bands of clotted fibers are present (Kaufman & Levin, 2001). The dialyzer is checked, preferably with the patient, to make certain that it is the proper dialyzer belonging to the patient. The dialyzer is tested for the presence and proper disinfectant concentration. After priming, it is tested for disinfectant residual to make sure the disinfectant has been properly removed from the dialyzer prior to being used for treatment. Inadequate rinsing of the disinfectant prior to use may result in fatal patient adverse reactions.

Monitoring of the patient includes observation for symptoms such as fever and chills, which may indicate contamination of the dialyzer. The nurse should also observe for dialyzer failures such as leaks, deviation in UF rates, progressive increase in the patient's serum creatinine, or deterioration in the patient condition such as development of uremic symptoms (Kaufman & Levin, 2001). Dialyzer failures are recorded in the facility's complaint investigation log and should be included in the quality management program.

Extracorporeal Blood Circuit

The extracorporeal circuit includes the needle or catheter placed in the patient's vascular access, blood lines that transport the patient's blood to and from the dialyzer, the dialyzer, and components of the HD equipment that monitor and pump the blood through the system. The saline, saline administration tubing, heparin pump, and heparin line attached to the heparin syringe inserted into the heparin pump are also components of the extracorporeal blood circuit. The volume of blood contained within the dialyzer and blood tubing varies on type of dialyzer and blood tubing set and usually ranges from approximately 150-280 ml.

Bloodlines. Bloodlines are pliable tubing that allow for a constant flow of blood through the extracorporeal blood circuit, transporting the blood from the patient's vascular access site to the dialyzer (arterial blood tubing) and from the dialyzer back to the patient's access (venous blood tubing). The arterial blood tubing is color coded with red while the venous blood tubing is color-coded with blue. Along the main bloodlines, there are various ports and smaller line segments for infusing and administering medications, drawing of blood, and monitoring for pressures and air. The bloodlines are shown in Figure 23-8, which diagrams the components of a typical HD system. The volume of blood usually contained in bloodlines can vary according to the type but usually ranges from 100-150 ml, representing a little over half of the overall blood volume. The remaining blood volume in the extracorporeal circuit is contained in the dialyzer and is usually between 60-120 ml.

Blood pump and blood pump segment. A roller-style blood pump moves blood from the patient's vascular access, through the dialyzer, and back to the patient. This device is necessary to overcome the resistance in the dialyzer and the vascular access and does so by creating positive pressure within the extracorporeal system. The pump is an integral part of the HD equipment and propels the blood through the pliable tubing by means of sequential action of rollers compressing the tubing (AAMI, 1994). It is important that periodic pump calibration is performed to assume stable and accurate blood flow rates.

The blood pump segment is part of the arterial blood tubing and is supplied with a specific internal diameter. Blood pump segments are supplied in different internal diameters so it is critical that the blood pump internal diameter setting on the machine match the internal diameter specification of the blood tubing segment. Dimensions of blood tubing sets, including pump segment diameter that may be used with the machine, are described by the manufacturers (AAMI, 2003).

The volume of blood flowing through the extracorporeal circuit per minute is dependent on the number of revolutions per minute of the blood pump, the diameter of the pump segment, the negative pressure within the circuit, and the adequacy of the patient's vascular access (Curtis &

Varughese, 2000). Blood flows used during HD usually range from 300-500 ml/min but can be lower or higher depending on the functional status of the vascular access, prescription, and pump capabilities. The displayed blood flow rate may overstate the actual blood flow rate depending on bloodline tubing fatigue and the prepump arterial pressure representing the adequacy of the vascular access blood flow. This difference can be 10% from set values (Fan & Schwab, 1993).

Pressure monitoring. In the extracorporeal blood circuit positive pressure is generated from the blood pump segment through to the end of the venous patient connector. Negative pressure is generated from the arterial limb of the vascular access to the blood pump. Monitoring of the various pressures throughout the extracorporeal circuit is important in guarding against or detecting clotting, disconnections, kinking or obstruction of blood tubing, or dysfunction of the vascular access. Pressures should be monitored continuously throughout the treatment. All alarms should be responded to promptly and action taken to correct the problem. Alarms should be checked pre-dialysis to ensure they are in working condition; alarms should be set and maintained per manufacturer's instruction and/or facility policy and procedure.

The monitoring devices measure the pressures in mmHg and alarms ensure that pressures remain within specific acceptable limits. The monitoring lines are bloodline segments that are connected to an internal transducer (pressure monitor) located on the inside of the dialysis machine via a transducer protector (TP). The TPs are fluid barriers, preventing saline and blood from entering the machine. They are used to prevent cross contamination from one patient's blood to another's. It is important that they remain dry as they may not function properly if wet. Any wet TP should be replaced immediately and inspected; if fluid is visible on the side of the TP that faces the machine, it should be reported to a qualified person who can open the machine and check for contamination after the treatment is completed (FDA, 1999). If contamination has occurred, the machine should be taken out of service and disinfected before further use (FDA, 1999).

The venous pressure monitor measures the positive pressure in the extracorporeal circuit distal to the hemodialyzer caused by the resistance of blood flowing back to the patient through the venous bloodline segment, drip chamber, and the patient's access. Although a low venous pressure alarm can signal that something has caused a lower pressure, such as a bloodline disconnect, the monitors are not capable of completely preventing blood loss or even exsanguinations (AAMI, 2003). The venous pressure monitor may not be sufficiently sensitive to detect the change in pressure that occurs when a venous needle accidentally pulls out because the magnitude of the pressure drop across the needle is much greater than that of the pressure in the blood access (AAMI, 2003). Therefore, the patients' vascular access needs to be visible at all times during the dialysis treatment to facilitate observation that the needles or catheters are in place and bloodline and access device connections are secure and intact.

High venous pressure alarms may indicate bloodline

Table 23-4

Typical Hemodialysis Dialysate Composition
(Dialysate Formed From Acid Concentrate, Bicarbonate Concentrate and Purified Water)

Component	Typical Range	Derived From
Acetic acid (acetate)	2-4 mEq/L	Acid (A) concentrate *(Note: The acetic acid in this dialysate is not to be confused with acetate concentrate or dialysate)*
Bicarbonate	35 mEq/L	Bicarbonate (B) concentrate
Calcium	2.5-3.5 mEq/L	Acid (A) concentrate
Chloride	98-124 mEq/L	Acid (A) concentrate
Dextrose	200 mg/dl	Acid (A) concentrate
Magnesium	0.5-1.0 mEq/L	Acid (A) concentrate
Potassium	2.0-3.0 mEq/L	Acid (A) concentrate
Sodium	135-145 mEq/L	Acid (A) concentrate Bicarbonate (B) concentrate

obstructions such as kinks, closed clamps, clots in the drip chambers, or access malfunction. Pressures outside of the high and low alarm limits activate audible and visual alarms, a mechanism that minimizes UF to avoid hemoconcentration, shuts off the blood pump, and clamps the venous return line (AAMI, 2003).

Arterial pressure monitors measure the pressure within the arterial bloodline either pre-pump or post-pump. Pre-pump monitors measure the pressures in the arterial bloodline segment between the vascular access and the blood pump. This segment, under negative pressure, is a source of passive entry of air into the blood circuit and is a high-risk segment (Corea, Pittard, Gardner, & Shinaberger, 1993).

The pre-pump pressures are an indication of the adequacy of the vascular access in delivering blood. Low alarms are triggered for increasing (high) negative pressure and can signify decreasing blood pressures, insufficient flow of blood from access, or a kink in the blood tubing between the patient and monitoring site. This pressure is helpful in ensuring the blood pump is set at a rate the access can supply. High negative (lower pressures) pre-pump arterial pressures may lead to the generation of micro bubbles, and contribute to the lower than expected blood flow, and hemolysis (Francos et al., 1983; Graves, 2001; Sands, Glidden, Jacavage, & Jones, 1996; Sweet, McCarthy, Steingart, & Callahan, 1996).

High alarms (less negative pressure) can be triggered by leaks between the patient and monitoring site, as pressure is generally negative in this segment and the air being pulled into the circuit causes the pressures to move upward, less negative. A high alarm can also be triggered because of decreasing blood pump speeds or the saline line clamp being opened, which can also move the pressures to being less negative.

Post-pump arterial monitors measure the pressures between the blood pump and the blood compartment of the dialyzer and can detect clotting in the dialyzer. The pressures are positive as the blood is being pushed through the system against the resistance of the blood tubing, the dialyzer, and the vascular access. Low alarms (less positive)

can indicate line separation, decrease in blood pump speed, or occlusion in the bloodline between the blood pump and the monitoring site. High alarm conditions can be triggered by increased blood viscosity from UF, infiltrations of the venous needle, increases in the blood pump speed, kinks or clotting in the bloodline between the monitoring site and the patient, and clotting in the dialyzer.

Air detector. The air detector on the HD machine is a sensor device and alarm system that detects air or foam in the extracorporeal circuit before the blood is returned to the patient (AAMI, 2003). The purpose of the detector is to prevent air that may have inadvertently entered the blood circuit from being returned to the patient, as air may be lethal. The air detector relies on the correct placement of the venous blood tubing set to function correctly. The venous bloodline drip chamber is placed in a drip chamber level-sensing device while the venous blood tubing is mounted in the line-sensing device distal to the drip chamber where a clamping device is also located. It is imperative that the venous line connected to the patient be securely fitted inside this clamping device during a dialysis treatment. If the line is removed briefly for troubleshooting purposes, the clinician should never leave the patient's side without re-engaging the venous line and drip chamber into the correct position of the air detector and reactivating the alarm. The air detector alarm system, if properly engaged, will activate audible and visual alarms, stop the blood pump and occlude the venous line, and reduce UF if air is detected.

During equipment maintenance procedures a device resembling a segment of venous blood tubing with drip chamber can be used and is referred to as a "dummy chamber or device." It is important that this device is never substituted for the venous blood tubing attached to the patient as it will prevent the air detector and line-clamping device from preventing air to reach patient. It is dangerous to use this device in the clinical setting and is better if restricted to use during maintenance procedures rather than set up or other procedures in the clinical setting.

Heparin pump. The heparin pump allows for the continuous infusion of heparin into the blood circuit gradually over the course of the treatment or can be used to administer bolus doses. Most heparin pumps can accommodate various syringe types determined by the manufacturer. For the heparin pump to work properly, it is important to ensure it is appropriately mounted and connected to the heparin line. To ensure accurate dosage, the heparin tubing must be primed with heparin before use.

Dialysate Circuit

Dialysis solution (dialysate). Dialysate is the aqueous fluid containing the electrolytes and often dextrose that is intended to exchange solutes with blood during HD (AAMI, 2004). Dialysate is also referred to as dialysis solution or dialyzing fluid and is made from treated water and concentrate that is delivered to the dialyzer by the dialysate proportioning and delivery system of the dialysis machine. The concentrations of electrolytes and dextrose (if used) in the final dialysate solution are prescribed by the nephrologist and will be addressed in a later section. Table 23-4 lists the common components of dialysis solutions.

It is important to understand the difference between the dialysis solution and the dialysis concentrate. The dialysis concentrate is fluid containing high concentrations of electrolytes that must be diluted with purified water to form dialysate. It is available in various formulations and concentration dilution ratios. It can come in liquid or powder form and can be placed at the point of use (at the dialysis station) or prepared in a separate area and centrally delivered to the dialysis station and proportioning machine depending on the concentrate type.

The most commonly used concentrate solutions are a combination of bicarbonate (base or part B), used as a buffer, and acidified (acid or part A) concentrates of electrolytes such as sodium, potassium, magnesium, calcium chloride, and often dextrose. The bicarbonate solutions are prone to bacterial growth. Concentrates are supplied for different mixing ratios: 35X, 36.83X, 45X, and 36.1X and are indicated on each concentrate container. This determines how the acid, bicarbonate, and treated water components will be mixed or proportioned by the dialysate delivery systems in the dialysis machine. It is imperative that the correct formulas are used so the final dialysate is correct. Caution must be taken when receiving or retrieving concentrate containers to visibly ensure the correct solution is selected by carefully reading the label on the container. Failure to use the correct concentrates can result in serious adverse events including patient death.

Dialysate Delivery Systems

The proportioning system is a critical component of the HD machine and is used to proportion water and concentrate(s) to prepare, de-aerate, warm, monitor, and deliver dialysate to the dialyzer (AAMI, 2003). It also performs a critical role in UF.

Various types of dialysate delivery systems have been used over the years. These systems have included the batch system, central and individual proportioning systems, and regenerative (sorbent) dialysate systems. The most common system used today is the individual proportioning system

and will be described in more detail below. Other systems have become either obsolete or are used less frequently.

Dialysate errors have been reported as hazards in HD. Therefore, in-line conductivity monitors are required for proportioning dialysate supply systems. Conductivity is a measure of the conduction of the electrolytes in the dialysate. Monitoring includes in-line conductivity cells to control and monitor each proportioning system plus a conductivity monitor to monitor the final dialysate delivered to the hemodialyzer (AAMI, 2003). Because the electrical conductivity is determined by the ionic content of the dialysate, it is, therefore, an indirect measure of the function of the proportioning system (Lazarus et al., 1996).

Conductivity alarms will trigger interruption of the dialysate flow by diverting dialysate to the drain until the alarm condition is corrected. It will also activate visible and audible alarms that can be muted. Unfortunately, clinicians may rely on conductivity alarms to signal when the concentrate solution container has emptied. When this happens, there is an interruption in dialysate flow to the dialyzer and a potential loss in dialyzer efficiency. It is better to replace the concentrate solution before the container is empty and triggers the dialysate alarm.

The proportioning systems are also equipped with water de-aeration systems to minimize any air in the dialysate as dissolved air in the dialysate circuit may adversely affect the dialysis system monitors and sensors, dialyzer efficiency, UF control, and patient safety (AAMI, 2003). It may also cross the membrane and enter the blood causing foaming and possible air embolism in the patient (AAMI, 2003).

The temperature of the dialysate maintains a physiologic range through the use of heat exchangers and/or immersed heater elements to warm the water before it is mixed with concentrate (Lazarus et al., 1996). Heating the dialysate water helps to de-aerate, facilitates mixing with concentrate, and prevents patients from becoming hypothermic during treatment (Lazarus et al., 1996). Failure to maintain dialysate temperature within the physiological range has caused patient complications such as hemolysis, chills, hypothermia, and clotting of the hemodialyzer. Temperature limits are usually set for 35°–37° C. The high temperature limit of 42° C is common in dialysis machines because protein denaturation and hemolysis can take place above a temperature of 45° C. Temperature alarms have both visual and audible alarms for immediate recognition of the alarm condition. If a temperature alarm is triggered, it will interrupt delivery of the dialysate to the dialyzer and divert it to the drain until the situation is resolved.

HD systems have a blood leak detector and alarm device to detect blood in the dialysate, which initiates audible and visual alarms, diverts the flow of dialysate to the drain, and stops the blood pump automatically (AAMI, 2003). Blood in the dialysate is an indication that there may be a leak in the dialyzer allowing for the passage of potentially dangerous substances in the dialysate, such as bacteria, to pass into the patient's blood and allow blood loss into the dialysate.

Today, most machines incorporate UF controllers that allow the machines to be used with high-flux dialyzers

(AAMI, 2003). Current HD systems incorporate a variety of UF control systems. Two UF control systems in widespread practice for single pass dialysate systems include flow sensor systems, which simultaneously measure the dialysate inflow and outflow rates, and volumetric balancing systems, which use matched diaphragm pumps (Lazarus et al., 1996). Volumetric balancing systems equally proportion dialysate to and from the dialyzer. Fluid removal is obtained by the use of an UF pump to generate negative pressure. UF control systems display the UF rate, the UF time, current volume removed, and target UF volume.

TMP monitors are also incorporated into dialysis machines. In systems without UF, the operator calculates and sets the TMP, observes the blood compartment and dialysate pressures periodically during the treatment, and adjusts the TMP as necessary.

Because high volumes of highly conductive fluids are used in conjunction with an electrical device, such as the HD machine, safety features have been built into equipment design to prevent electrical accidents to users and to protect the machine from damage. It is important to prevent damage or correct damage to any of the protective structures. These include components that shield electrical grounds, machine accessory outlets, and panel seams from liquid spills. It is important that the protective covering or panels, also referred to as a chassis, are maintained in proper condition without rust or other damage.

Ancillary Devices

Single needle devices. These devices, uncommonly used, allow dialysis with only a single blood pathway. A solitary line from the vascular access attaches to a Y tube connector, which, in turn, attaches to the bloodlines. Intermittently, blood is withdrawn from and returned to the patient. Two single needle systems used today are the pump/clamp and double pump systems. Time, pressure, and volume can be used for controlling the single needle cycles (Polaschegg & Levin, 2004).

Other ancillary devices. Other devices may also be used such as automatic blood pressure monitoring devices, blood volume monitoring devices, continuous dialysate biochemical monitors, dialysis quantification monitors, access flow, pressure or recirculation monitoring capability, patient data cards, continuous blood volume monitoring, and blood temperature control modules (Polaschegg & Levin, 2004).

Water Treatment for Dialysis

During each HD treatment, patients are exposed to more than 120 l of water. This is about 20 to 30 times the average person's exposure to water. Because HD patients are exposed to an enormous amount of water, the contact involves direct access to their bloodstream via the dialyzer membrane, and there is an inability to excrete water-related toxins in urine, it is critical that the purity of the water used for HD be known and controlled (AAMI, 2001; Daugirdas, Van Stone, et al., 2001). This requires specially treated water beyond the normal municipal treatment of tap water. In fact, the various chemicals used to make tap water safe for drinking and general use can be harmful and

even lethal if the same tap water was used for HD. Table 23-5 summarizes potentially toxic substances and contaminants in water, possible causative factors, and related adverse effects (AAMI, 2001; Selenic et al., 2004; Ward, 1993, 2002).

Water treatment-related adverse effects are extremely serious, and they can affect multiple patients at one time with devastating and fatal results. The importance of appropriate water treatment systems, components, and associated monitoring and maintenance activities cannot be overstated. With advances in technology such as the increased utilization of high permeability (flux) devices, prevalence of dialyzer reuse, and the common use of bicarbonate dialysis, the importance of higher levels of water quality is apparent (Ismail et al., 1999).

The AAMI has established minimum standards for water used for HD and reprocessing (AAMI, 2001, 2003). The CMS have also incorporated AAMI standards into the Federal Conditions for Coverage of Suppliers of End Stage Renal Disease Services (CMS, 1998). The AAMI standards outline maximum allowable limits for substances and microbiological contaminants in water used for dialysate, HD, and reuse and are updated periodically.

The physician in charge of dialysis has the ultimate responsibility for selecting the water treatment system and for the ongoing maintenance of the system. Clinical and technical associates responsible for monitoring and maintaining the system need to be knowledgeable and competent in water treatment and related standards.

The following strategies have been successfully employed to provide safe water that meets or exceeds current water standards and avoid water-related problems and disasters: (a) strict adherence to appropriate water system designs; (b) re-evaluation of all components in the water treatment system when water consumption is increased or changes; (c) training and competency assessment programs for medical, clinical, and technical associates incorporating acceptable ranges and action thresholds, appropriate action, and follow-up required for unacceptable results and the importance of reporting unusual findings, (d) strict adherence to monitoring water system components and performance including chloramine removal; (e) comprehensive quality management programs incorporating quality control, assurance, and improvement including trend analysis; (f) good communication between the dialysis facility and municipal water company, particularly regarding any changes to condition of public water; (g) security for water treatment rooms; (h) restriction of replacement of components of water system while patients are dialyzing; and (i) emergency planning and training (Ward, 2002).

Water treatment systems should be designed to minimize bacterial growth. Strategies include using a distribution loop, avoiding stagnant flows by appropriately sizing pipes and not using dead ends, pressurizing tanks, or multiple branches; including bacterial control devices such as ultrafilters; and regularly and adequately disinfecting and surveying processes of the water treatment and distribution systems (Ward, 1993, 2002).

Because of the importance of monitoring for bacterial growth, the collection timing and methods are critical to

Table 23-5
Potentially Toxic Substances and Contaminants in Water

Toxic Substances, Contaminants	Potential Cause(s), Contributing Factors	Adverse Effect
Aluminum (Added to municipal water supply when colloidal matter is high making the water turbid)	Inadequate water treatment due to fouling of RO membranes and cartridge filters; increase in aluminum in municipal water; lack of communication between municipal water supplier and dialysis facility; RO failure; Al containing acid concentrate pump; cement lined pipes	*Patient:* Dialysis encephalopathy, bone disease, anemia, death
Calcium (Added to municipal water supply to increase pH to reduce corrosion and limit leaching of lead and copper into water supply)	Water softener failures. Hard water contains high concentrations of calcium and magnesium.	*RO Equipment:* The hard water causes scaling on membranes leading to premature failing of RO membrane *Patient:* Hypercalcemia; hard water syndrome.
Chloramines (Chlorine and chloramines are added to municipal water supply for disinfection)	Increase in municipal water levels; RO capacity increases without increasing sizing of carbon; infrequent or improper monitoring of chloramines; insufficient action when thresholds exceeded; lack of knowledge of action required; lack of policies and procedures; backwashing carbon beds rather than replacing; inadequate empty-bed contact time	*Equipment:* Damaging to thin film RO membranes *Patient:* Hemolysis, anemia, headaches, hypotension, chest pain, cardiac arrest, methemoglobinemia
Copper (Can leach from copper and brass piping)	Use of copper or brass piping and/or parts in the water distribution system	*Patient:* Flushing, chills, headache, vomiting, methemoglobinemia, hemolysis
Disulfides (Sulfate-reducing bacteria converting sulfate to disulfides)	Improperly maintained reverse osmosis unit membranes creating anaerobic environment promoting bacterial growth	*Patient:* Gastrointestinal, cardiovascular, respiratory and central nervous system effects, death
Endotoxin (Released from cell wall of bacteria)	Use of water not meeting AAMI standards; storage tank with post-tank deionizer; inadequate microbial surveillance; inadequate disinfection; tap water used in reuse process	*Patient:* Pyrogenic reactions. S/S: reactions 1-2 hr into treatment, shaking & chills, fever, nausea, vomiting, mayalgia, hypotension
Fluoride (Added to municipal water supply to prevent dental caries)	Deionizer exhaustion; improper sizing of deionizers for water demand and deionizer exchange cycle; on-line resistivity monitors fitted with visual alarm only with no audible alarm; staff unfamiliar with type of visual alarm; accidental increase in municipal water supply levels	*Patient:* Severe pruritis, nausea, burning sensation, headache, syncope, fatal cardiac arrhythmias
Sodium Azide (Used as chemical preservative in non-medical use ultrafilters)	Leaching of chemical preservatives from inadequately rinsed ultrafilters; lack of knowledge of ultrafilters containing sodium azide	*Patient:* Blurred vision, abdominal pain, headache, life-threatening hypotension
Nitrates (Found in some well water; due to bacterial contamination, agricultural fertilizers)	Have been found in home dialysis environments when well water was used and was contaminated with urine from domestic animals	*Patient:* Hemolysis, hypotension, methemoglobinemia, nausea
Zinc (Can leach from galvanized iron pipes)	Can leach from galvanized iron and brass pipes.	*Patient:* Nausea, fever hemolysis and anemia

the success of a surveillance program. According to the CDC (Arduino, 2001), microbial monitoring should be performed: (a) after a suspected pyrogenic reaction or bacteremia, (b) after modification to the water treatment system, (c) at least weekly for new water treatment systems, and (d) at least monthly for established water treatment systems. Sample collection techniques for water used to prepare dialysate should include collecting the sample close to where dialysate is mixed, through a sampling spigot, allowing water to run through the spigot for 30-60 seconds before collecting the sample using a sterile container (Arduino, 2001). Sample collection techniques for water used to reprocess dialyzers should include collecting water from the water supply line used to rinse dialyzers, prepare dialyzer disinfectant, and operate the dialyzer reprocessing system (Arduino, 2001). The water should flow for 30 to 60

Figure 23-9
Schematic of Reverse Osmosis Membrane

ENLARGED SCHEMATIC OF REVERSE OSMOSIS MEMBRANE

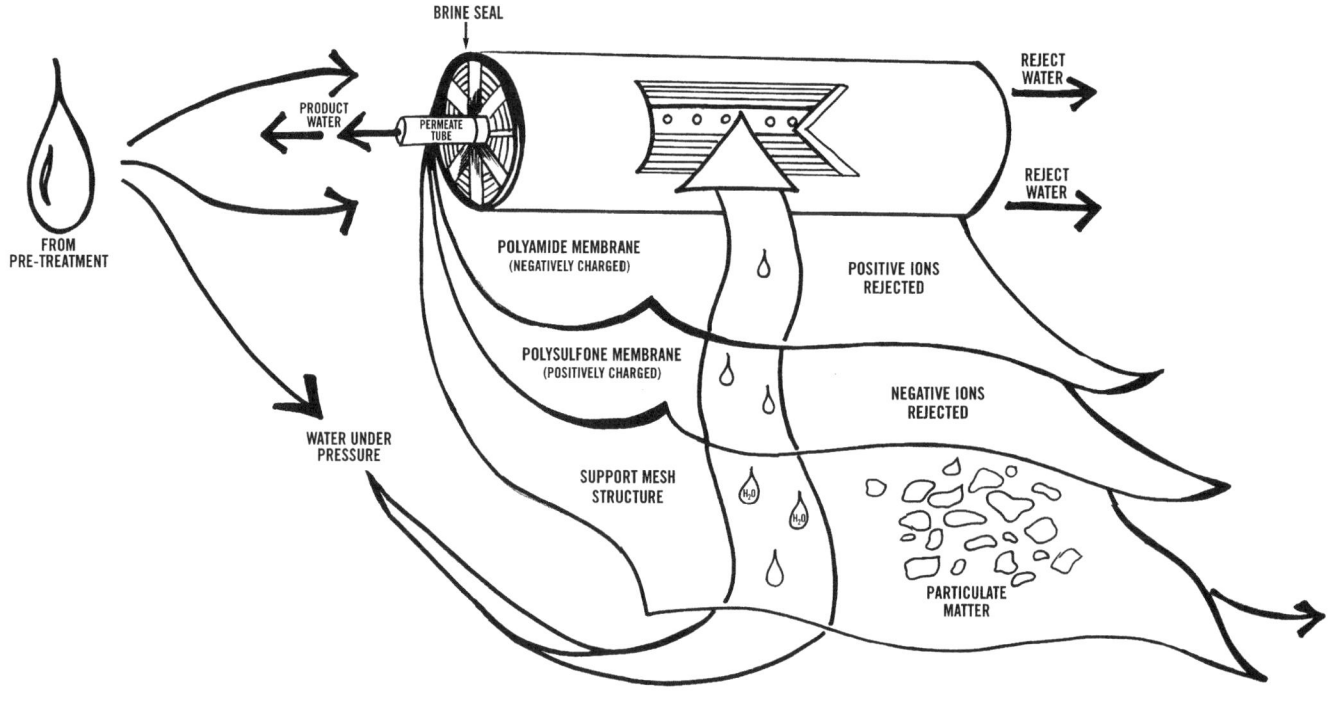

Note: Illustration courtesy of Mark Rolston.

seconds, avoiding collecting samples from tubing connected to spigots and quick connect devices and using a sterile endotoxin-free container (Arduino, 2001).

If cultures are positive, they should be repeated to confirm the result. Appropriate action including disinfection is warranted if the repeat assay confirms original results (Arduino, 2001). Bacterial surveillance should be recorded and trended and incorporated into quality improvement activities. Disinfection strategies include: chemical germicides, aqueous formaldehyde, sodium hypochlorite, hydrogen peroxide, peracetic acid, ozone, chlorine dioxide, and hot water pasteurization > 80° C.

Methods of water purification. There are several methods for purifying or treating the water to be used for HD, dialysate preparation, or reprocessing. Whatever system is employed, the product water must be below regulated limits at the correct temperature, pressure, and flow rate for operation of the facility's equipment, including equipment for dialyzer reprocessing and dialysate concentrate preparation (Ward, 1993). The most common method is reverse osmosis (RO) where water is pressured across a tight membrane that removes greater than 90% of the impurities (Ahmad, 1999). An alternative treatment method is the use of deionization (DI). RO and DI systems will be described as well as additional components.

RO. This method uses a semipermeable membrane to

Figure 23-10
Deionization

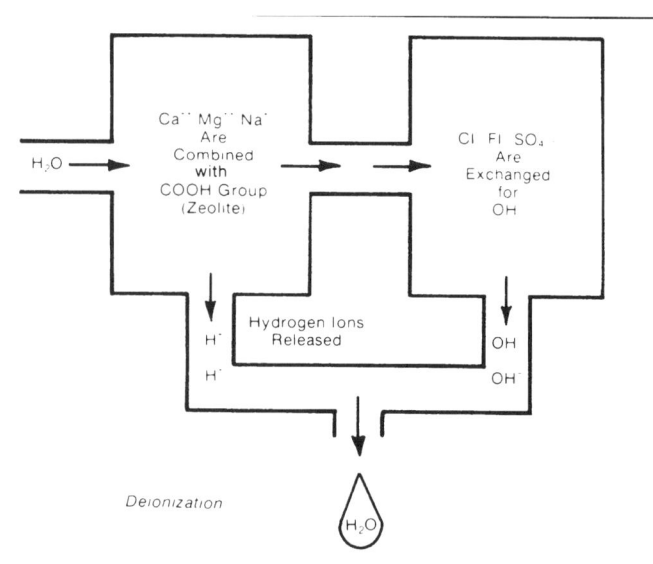

Deionization

Note: From Wick, G.S. , & Parker, J. (1998). Hemodialysis. In J. Parker (Ed.), *Contemporary Nephrology Nursing* (p. 537). Pitman, NJ: American Nephrology Nurses' Association. Reprinted with permission.

remove both organic matter and electrolytes from the water (see Figure 23-9). As water is pushed through the membrane, the passage of smaller molecular weight substances such as sodium and chloride is restricted due to the extremely small size of the membrane's pores. In this manner, more than 90% of impurities are removed. Bacteria and viruses are also rejected by the membrane, so the product water approaches distilled quality (Gutch & Stoner, 1993; Van Stone, 1994).

Water softening. Hardness of water is produced primarily by calcium and magnesium. The water softening process replaces calcium and magnesium ions with sodium ions while the water passes through an exchange resin bed. This exchange occurs on a milliequivalent per milliequivalent basis. Thus, for example, for each calcium ion (++) removed, two sodium ions (+) are exchanged. This process results in a higher quality water that extends the life of the RO membrane (Gutch & Stoner, 1993).

DI. The DI process uses an ion-exchange resin similar to that in a water softener (see Figure 23-10). The resin used for DI results in the substitution of ions and cations with H+ and OH-. The deionizer is either a "mixed bed" or "dual bed" depending on whether the two types of resins are together in one tank or in separate tanks. In the anion bed, chloride, fluoride, sulfates, nitrates, bicarbonate, and other negatively charged ions are exchanged for hydroxide ions (OH-). In the cation bed, positively charged ions such as calcium, magnesium, and sodium are exchanged for hydrogen ions (H+). The hydrogen and hydroxide ions combine to form water molecules (Cappelli & Inguaggiato, 2004; Gutch & Stoner, 1993). The ion exchange beds tend to exhaust suddenly. Therefore, standby beds are necessary so a conversion can be made. The life of the beds depends upon water composition and/or the volume of water moving through the system.

Carbon tanks. Carbon tanks contain activated charcoal that adsorbs chlorine and chloramines onto the carbon particles. Monitoring should be performed prior to each patient shift for chlorine/chloramines breakthrough to protect patients from potential exposure. Since the carbon has a high affinity for organic material, it can be contaminated with bacteria if not serviced or exchanged frequently (Ismail et al., 1999). Two carbon tanks in series are recommended, with each tank having an empty bed contact time of at least 5 minutes at the maximum product water flow rate for a total EBCT of at least 10 minutes (AAMI, 2001).

Pressure gauges. Pressure gauges are used to monitor the flow of water through various components of the water treatment system. These monitors need to be monitored for changes in the pressures. The expected pressures and actionable changes or delta pressures should be defined and clearly communicated to the staff.

Storage tank. If a storage tank is used, it should be of minimum size with a tight-fitting lid with filtered air vent and conical bottom with drain at lowest point.

The HD Prescription

The HD prescription is a set of physician orders that include but are not limited to the dialysis dose, dialyzer, dialysate, fluid removal, profiling such as sodium or UF,

anticoagulation, medications, standing orders for complications, and laboratory testing.

Amount of Dialysis (Dialysis Dose)

Medical orders related to the dialysis dose include the length and frequency of treatment, the dialyzer type and size, blood flow and dialysate rates, and the frequency and type of laboratory testing to monitor the dose delivered. The nephrologist determines the amount of dialysis based on the individual patient needs. Patient specific factors that determine the dialysis dose include the patient's size (body water volume), residual urea clearance, fluid gains between dialysis, and pregnancy (Kumar & Depner, 2004).

A stable chronic HD patient's dosing needs will be different than a new patient first dialyzing with severe azotemia or hyponatremia, for whom disequilibrium syndrome is a risk. For these patients, a shortened treatment length, a slower blood flow rate, concurrent dialysate flow, and a lower efficiency dialyzer may be prescribed.

The urea kinetic model of Kt/V has become the preferred method for determining the prescribed dialysis dose and for measuring the delivered dose; it more accurately reflects urea removal compared to URR and can be used to assess a patient's nutritional status and modify the dialysis prescription for a patient who has residual renal function (O'Connor & Wish, 2004).

Formal urea kinetic modeling (UKM), currently the most accurate method for measuring Kt/V, is preferred by the National Kidney Foundation (NKF) *K/DOQI Clinical Practice Guidelines*, but has not received universal application because of the availability of simpler Kt/V formulas (O'Connor & Wish, 2004).

Dialysis Solution

Dialysate sodium. Dialysate sodium is typically 135-145 mEq/L. If the patient has marked predialysis hypernatremia or hyponatremia, dialysate sodium may be prescribed accordingly. Solutions with a sodium level of 3-4 mEq/L lower than serum sodium may cause the blood returning to the patient to be hyponatremic compared to the interstitial fluid. This will result in water leaving the hypernatremic blood and moving into the interstitial and intracellular spaces, causing a rapid decrease in circulating blood volume even with low UF rates. This could lead to hypotension or cramps and could contribute to or exacerbate disequilibrium. Thus, the dialysate sodium is typically kept at or slightly above plasma level (Bregman, Daugirdas, & Ing, 2001; Daugirdas & Kjellstrand, 2001; Ismail & Hakim, 1991).

Dialysate sodium levels greater than 140 mEq/L have, at times, been associated with increased thirst, increased interdialytic weight gains, and hypertension. Studies have shown that high and variable sodium dialysate can be used successfully in preventing and treating dialysis disequilibrium (Jenson, Dobbe, Squillace, & McCarthy, 1994). In a typical HD treatment using variable sodium, the patient initially dialyzes with a dialysate sodium concentration of 145 mEq/L. Throughout the treatment, the dialysate sodium is decreased in steps to 138-140 mEq/L for the final hour. This feature allows the patient to have the benefits of a high sodium dialysate, such as fewer intradialytic symptoms and hypotension. It also has been shown to decrease the need for nursing interventions throughout the treatment because the patient is more stable. Decreasing the dialysate sodium to 138-140 mEq/L for the final hour reduces the risk of high interdialytic weight gains and blood pressure that have often been associated with high dialysate sodium levels of 145 mEq/L or higher (Jenson et al., 1994).

Bicarbonate. In bicarbonate and acid solution, the usual level of bicarbonate is 35 mEq/l (Daugirdas & Kjellstrand, 2001) with lower levels possibly indicated for quotidian nocturnal HD (Hollon & Ward, 2005).

Potassium. The most commonly prescribed potassium is 2 mEq, but the nephrologist may prescribe different levels of dialysate potassium based on the individual patient's needs (Daugirdas & Kjellstrand, 2001). For example, for patients on digitalis, higher potassium levels may be prescribed. Zero potassium dialysate is rarely prescribed due to the risk of lowering serum potassium too rapidly, resulting in arrhythmias. Also, correction of severe acidosis during HD may cause a shift of potassium, into the cells, further lowering the serum potassium and possibly leading to arrhythmias as well.

Calcium. The calcium in the dialysate commonly prescribed is 2.5 to 3.5 mEq/L. If the patient has predialysis hypocalcemia, a higher dialysate calcium may be prescribed to avoid the ionized calcium from being lowered further (Daugirdas & Kjellstrand, 2001; Ismail & Hakim, 1991).

Dextrose. Dextrose is routinely prescribed for all patients to reduce the incidence of hypoglycemia during dialysis. A typically prescribed amount is 200 mg/dL (Daugirdas & Kjellstrand, 2001).

Fluid Removal

The patient's target weight is also a part of the prescription. Normally, fluid removal needs will vary with each dialysis session and is based on the target or dry weight of the patient. Fluid removal calculations should always take prime and rinse volumes into account.

Isolated UF can be a safe method of fluid removal in dialysis if large amounts of water need to be removed although fatal complications have occurred. Isolated UF is also referred to as sequential UF and involves bypassing the dialysate solution to drain, only allowing UF to take place. A typical sequential UF prescription is for an hour in the beginning of the treatment. This technique should be prescribed by the physician if used. Hyperkalemia can be an adverse effect of this isolated or sequential UF.

Delivering the Prescription

Ongoing evaluation of treatment parameters and successful delivery of the prescribed treatment are very important in making sure the patient meets clinical targets and receives satisfactory therapy. Nephrology nurses play a critical role in ensuring that HD patients receive the treatment that has been prescribed and that medical information is communicated back to the nephrologist when the prescription is not attained or patient goals cannot be met.

Levin and colleagues (1991) described the requirements for ensuring adequate therapy: (a) an appropriate prescription, (b) a high level of nursing expertise, (c) an efficiently operating HD machine, (d) satisfactory access to the circulation, (e) an informed patient, and (f) ongoing data collection and review. Assuming the dosing prescription is adequate, there are strategies that can be used to overcome obstacles in achieving the prescribed dialysis dose and targeted Kt/V (see Table 23-6).

Currently, the nephrology health care team looks at several indicators in addition to Kt/V to determine adequacy of and patient response to therapy. Measurements such as hematocrit and albumin, as well as assessment of patient symptoms, fluid volume status, bone disease, and functional status and well-being are examined in conjunction with Kt/V to determine the patient's response to therapy and to individualize the HD prescription. The multidisciplinary health care team should routinely monitor to see that the patient attains the targeted Kt/V and other quality indicators. This should also be reviewed during the multidisciplinary care planning process.

Anticoagulation During HD

During a HD treatment, the patient's blood comes into contact with access needles, extracorporeal blood tubing including drip chambers, and the dialyzer membrane. Any of these interactions may initiate clotting of the blood, especially in conjunction with exposure of blood to air in drip chambers (Hertel, Keep, & Caruana, 2001). This may lead to blood clots within the blood tubing, drip chambers, dialyzer fibers, or header. Clot formation in the extracorporeal circuit begins with a coating of the surfaces by plasma proteins followed by platelet adherence and aggregation, thromboxane A$_2$ generation, and activation of the intrinsic coagulation cascade, which leads to thrombin formation and fibrin deposition (Hertel et al., 2001). In addition, the propensity of intradialytic clotting is influenced by the blood flow through the dialyzer; the extent of recirculation in the extracorporeal circuit; the amount of UF; and the length, diameter, and composition of the bloodlines (Lazarus et al., 1996). Anticoagulation agents and methods are part of the medical prescription for HD.

Patient specific variables that influence thrombogenicity and determine the requirements for anticoagulants include the presence of congestive heart failure, malnutrition, neoplasia, blood transfusions, and comorbid coagulopathies, such as disseminated intravascular coagulation or warfarin therapy (Lazarus et al., 1996).

Heparin anticoagulation. Anticoagulation with heparin is the usual method of preventing clotting in the extracorporeal system because of its low cost, ease of administration, simplicity of monitoring, and relatively short biologic half-life. The anionic mucopolysaccharide heparin is the most widely used anticoagulant for dialysis (Lazarus et al., 1996). Heparin was one of the key developments that made HD possible (Hertel et al., 2001). A German investigator, George Haas, is the physician credited with first using heparin in dialysis in 1928 (McBride, 1979).

The half-life of heparin is 30 to 120 minutes (Hertel et al., 2001). Porcine heparin works by bonding to circulating antithrombin III, resulting in a rapid inactivation of clotting

Table 23-6
Strategies for Achieving Prescribed Dialysis Dose

Obstacle (Potential causes of ↓Kt/V)	Strategy	Rationale
Dialysate flow in countercurrent direction due to error in connecting dialysate tubing	Ensure countercurrent dialysate flow; verify during treatment; correct discrepancies	Countercurrent flow of blood and dialysate promotes diffusion by increasing concentration gradients
Inadequate blood flow rates due to improper setting of blood pump	Verify correct blood flow rate during treatment; correct discrepancies	Solute clearance increases as blood flow rates increase and are reduced with reduction in blood flow rate
Inadequate blood flow rates due to insufficient vascular access	Monitor pre-pump arterial pressures to detect excessive negative pressures. Monitor and report access malfunction; refer for correction of access problem.	Negative arterial pressures (>250) may signal access malfunction or inability of access to deliver set blood flow; also indicates a difference between setting and actual blood flow
Inadequate dialysate flow rates due to improper settings or lack of concentrate solution	Verify dialysate flows are correct and in accordance with prescription. Ensure adequate amount of dialysate solution for treatment length	Solute clearance increases as dialysate flow increases; lack of concentrate solution causes and interruption of dialysate flow through dialyzer and decreases clearance.
Shortened treatments due to patients failing to comply because of lack of knowledge or other factors such as transportation or personal commitments	Teach patients and staff importance of receiving length of treatment prescribed. Explore causes; seek assistance as necessary; intervene	Patients and staff may not understand the impact on mortality and hospitalization. Staff may inadvertently encourage nonadherence.
Interruptions in dialysis due to complications and alarms conditions	Measure liters process Record on and off times accurately. Document disruptions in therapy.	Alarm conditions can result in stopping of blood pump or interruption in dialysate flow; both will decrease clearance
Incorrect laboratory specimens (wrong day or time, timing of draws, diluted or clotted specimens)	Supervise laboratory collection timing and techniques.	Incorrect laboratory specimen collection methods can lead to inaccurate results.
Clotting of dialyzer fibers	Give appropriate anticoagulant dose. Monitor for proper levels of blood in drip chambers. Monitor for clotting.	Clotting of fibers reduces effective surface area for blood and dialysate contact and reduces clearance. Unnecessary air/blood interface in drip chambers can promote clotting.
Improper priming of dialyzers	Prime (rinse) dialyzers per policy and procedure and manufacturers' IFU.	Air in hollow fibers can lead to inadequate filling of hollow fibers decreasing effective surface area for urea clearance

factors I, IX, XI, and XII (Hertel et al., 2001).

When monitoring an appropriate heparin prescription, the nurse should also be aware that concomitant use of some other medications may alter the effects of heparin. The use of oral anticoagulants, salicylates, cephalosporins, and nonsteroidal anti-inflammatory drugs may enhance the effects of heparin and place the patient at risk for bleeding if the heparin dose is not adjusted. The reverse is true of digitalis, tetracyclines, nicotine, and antihistamines, which counteract the heparin effect. Patients using those medications may need more heparin during dialysis. The nurse should also be aware that the patient's heparin requirements may increase with the use of recombinant erythro-

poietin and the resultant increase in hematocrit (Breiterman-White, 1995).

Undesired effects include pruritus, allergy, osteoporosis, hyperlipidemia, thrombocytopenia, and excessive bleeding (Hertel et al., 2001). For patients who are allergic, develop unwanted effects, or have bleeding tendencies, alternative anticoagulation methods including anticoagulation-free methods have been developed (Hertel et al., 2001).

Heparin can be prescribed in various amounts depending on patient needs and techniques dependent on physician preference. There are three methods of heparin anticoagulation. These include: (a) systemic routine; (b) fractional, tight, or minimal heparinization; and (c) regional heparinization in which only the extracorporeal dialytic circuit is anticoagulated by the administration of heparin into the arterial line and protamine into the venous line and is rarely used today (Hertel et al., 2001; Lazarus et al., 1996).

Techniques for tight or minimal heparinization, regional heparin anticoagulation, and regular systemic heparinization may use blood tests for clotting times to determine dosage and effects of anticoagulation. There are several methods for testing clotting times. Whole blood partial thromboplastin time (WBPTT) is a test that accelerates the blood clotting time by adding a reagent called thrombofax to the blood. The mixture is then heated and tilted every 5 seconds until a clot forms. The prolongation of the WBPTT is linearly related to the heparin dose given during dialysis (Caruana & Keep, 1994).

The time constraints of HD are such that the partial thromboplastin time cannot be used to monitor the effectiveness of anticoagulation in the outpatient setting (Lazarus et al., 1996). Either no direct measure of the intensity of anticoagulation is performed or an activated clotting time (ACT) is used (Lazarus et al., 1996). In this assay, whole blood is mixed with an activator of the extrinsic clotting cascade such as kaolin, diatomaceous earth, or ground glass, and the time necessary for the blood to first congeal is monitored (Lazarus et al., 1996). The normal range is 90-140 seconds. As for partial thromboplastin time, the dialysis facility that performs this routine assay must be federally certified for its performance (Lazarus et al., 1996).

Routine heparin prescriptions are for patients who are at a normal risk for bleeding and are not considered at an unusually higher risk for bleeding. Systemic heparinization is commonly based on 50-100 units/kg of heparin initiation bolus with the continuous dose at about 1,000 units per hour (Lazarus et al., 1996). The target ACT is approximately 50% above baseline values (Lazarus et al., 1996). Techniques for routine heparin prescriptions include administering a heparin bolus followed by a constant infusion or giving a heparin bolus followed by repeated bolus doses as necessary or giving a single bolus (Hertel et al., 2001; Lazarus et al., 1996). The heparin bolus should be given using a systemic technique, waiting 3-5 minutes after injecting the heparin to allow heparin to disperse before initiating dialysis, and starting the blood pump. It is also important that heparin be administered after both needles are satisfactorily placed in the access for dual needle venipuncture.

Tight, minimal, or fractional heparinization is prescribed for patients who are at slight risk for bleeding. The best method for administration of a tight heparin prescription is the initial bolus followed by a constant infusion (Hertel et al., 2001). The constant infusion technique avoids the rise and fall in clotting times that occurs with the repeated bolus method (Hertel et al., 2001). A commonly prescribed dose for fractional heparinization is 10-50 units/kg of heparin administered initially followed by 500-1,000 units per hour (Lazarus et al., 1996). The target ACT is 25% (fractional) or 15% (tight fractional) above baseline (Lazarus et al., 1996).

Today, regional heparinization is rarely prescribed for patients at risk for bleeding. A typical prescription includes: 500 units of heparin initially, 500-750 units infused into the arterial line, 3.75 mg/h of protamine infused into the venous line, ACT maintained for the patient at baseline level and for the dialytic circuit at 10 seconds or longer. Because of heparin's longer half-life in comparison to protamine, an additional 50 mg of protamine should be given at the end of dialysis (Lazarus et al., 1996).

Heparin-free dialysis. Heparin-free dialysis is the method of choice for patients who are actively bleeding, are at high risk for bleeding, or in whom the use of heparin is contraindicated (e.g., patients with heparin-induced thrombocytopenia) (Hertel et al., 2001). This technique involves periodically rinsing the dialyzer with 50-250 ml of saline while occluding the blood inlet line, usually every 15-30 minutes (Hertel et al., 2001; Lazarus et al., 1996). The periodic rinsing is necessary to allow inspection of the dialyzer for evidence of clotting and may reduce the propensity for dialyzer clotting (Hertel et al., 2001). Usually, the blood flow is prescribed as high as possible to reduce potential clotting.

Regional citrate anticoagulation. Regional citrate anticoagulation is an alternative to heparin-free dialysis. Since calcium is required in the coagulation process, lowering of the ionized calcium level of the blood in the extracorporeal circuit anticoagulates the blood. The extracorporeal ionized calcium level is lowered by infusion of trisodium citrate into the arterial bloodline (Hertel, 2001). The process is reversed by a simultaneous infusion of calcium chloride into the venous blood to avoid returning blood with a very low calcium level to the patient, which would be very dangerous (Hertel et al., 2001). A dialysate solution containing no calcium is prescribed (Hertel et al., 2001). Advantages over heparin-free dialysis include: clotting almost never occurs, the blood flow rate does not need to be high, the patient is not at risk for bleeding due to heparin, and saline flushes are not required (Hertel et al., 2001). Disadvantages include: serum calcium level must be monitored throughout the treatment and two intravenous infusions are required, one of citrate and one of calcium carbonate (Hertel et al., 2001). Citrate metabolism generates bicarbonate, so use of this technique will result in a greater than usual increase in serum bicarbonate during the treatment. Therefore, it should be used with extreme caution in patients at risk for alkalemia. The patient should be monitored for signs and symptoms of hypocalcemia (Hertel et al., 2001).

Assessing anticoagulation therapy. Prior to the administration of heparin, the patient should be assessed regarding any events or changes in condition that have occurred since the last dialysis treatment. Any signs of bleeding or potential for risk of bleeding should be noted before administration and a physician notified. Examples of these events include any open or closed injuries; falls; bruising and contusions; hemorrhaging including the eye; surgical, dental, or biopsy procedures that have been performed or will be performed; and pericarditis. This information should be documented and communicated to other clinicians involved in the patient's care.

During a HD treatment, visual inspection of the dialyzer is important in assessing the effects of anticoagulation. Visual signs of clotting in the system include extremely dark blood, shadows, or black streaks in the dialyzer and clot formation in the drip chambers and the headers of the dialyzer. Other signs of clotting are the rapid filling of the transducer filters with blood, indicating increased pressure within the system, and a venous chamber that fills repeatedly with blood or foam (Breiterman-White, 1995). Changes can also be seen in the arterial and venous pressures, depending upon where the clotting is occurring in the extracorporeal circuit. If a post-pump arterial pressure monitor is used, an increasing pressure reading can signify clotting. If post-pump arterial pressure monitors are not used, clotting in the dialyzer and venous line can be reflected in an increased venous pressure. A clotted venous needle can also cause both the post-pump arterial and venous pressures to be elevated (Breiterman-White, 1995; Caruana & Keep, 1994). It is useful to note the amount of clotting in the dialyzer after dialysis. A few clotted fibers or some clots in the header are not unusual; however, large amounts of clotting are indicative of a need for increased anticoagulation. In programs doing reuse, total cell volume testing can provide information related to dialyzer clotting during dialysis (Caruana & Keep, 1994).

The Use of HD Technology

Predialysis Treatment

Equipment preparation. Dialysis systems should be prepared according to policies and procedures Manufacturer recommendations or instructions for use (IFU) are part of the labeling of medical devices and provide valuable information on the proper use of the equipment. Each medical device also contains an important lot number that permits tracing of manufacturing history and is valuable if a medical device error or malfunction occurs.

All machine safety checks should be performed as well as checking the conductivity and pH with an independent meter. In line conductivity monitors that are internal components of the delivery system can fail, typically as a result of the corrosion of critical components of electrodes; therefore, it is mandatory that the conductivity be checked manually before the machine is used for treatment to ensure the internal conductivity monitor is working correctly (Lazarus et al., 1996).

Thorough rinsing of the HD equipment and dialyzer is critical during setup. The machine should be rinsed of disinfectants using treated water and tested for residual disinfectant in the machine. Priming or rinsing of the dialyzer with normal saline aids in removing air and manufacturing residuals and sterilants such as ethylene oxide for single use dialyzers and disinfectants used during reprocessing for reused dialyzers. Failure to remove manufacturing residuals or ethylene oxide can cause dialyzer reactions. Failure to remove reuse disinfectants or air can lead to death. There are two common priming techniques. One involves a one pass rinsing of the dialyzer and the other involves recirculation of the priming fluid. The manufacturer of the dialyzer will provide instructions on the methods that can be used with their product. The facility policy and procedure will further define the methods and steps to be taken for priming. During the priming procedure, it is important to maintain aseptic technique preserving sterility of the ends of the bloodlines that will be connected to the patient's access.

After priming, the dialysis should be initiated within 5 to 10 minutes. If the system sits longer, it may leach ethylene oxide into the rinsing fluid. If more than 10 minutes elapse, the dialyzer should be rinsed briefly a second time just prior to use (Daugirdas, 1994). If a reprocessed dialyzer has been primed and recirculated and the residual disinfectant test performed, if recirculation is stopped for any length other than immediately prior to initiation, the system will require additional recirculation and retesting.

Patient assessment and preparation. Vital signs and weight are important components of the predialysis assessment. The predialysis weight should be compared with the postweight from the previous treatment and with the patient's estimated dry weight (EDW). Other parameters such as blood pressure, pulse, respirations, temperature, the presence or absence of edema, signs of bleeding, complaints of pain, unusual weakness, or other symptoms as well as an interdialytic history should be evaluated. Any large weight gain accompanied by dyspnea and orthopnea should prompt a complete cardiorespiratory examination including auscultation of the lungs, assessment of the patient for edema, and auscultation of the heart. Cardiac or respiratory signs of volume overload without an accompanying large weight gain should prompt a reassessment of the patient's EDW. Unusual signs and symptoms should be reported to the patient's nephrologist for potential changes in the prescription or plan of care. The nephrologists may want to hold antihypertensive medications prior to HD for patients with hypertension who are prone to hypotension during the treatment.

The interdialytic history is a very important part of the nursing assessment. It can provide valuable information that is helpful in interpretation of physical findings. For example, a brief interdialytic dietary history can be helpful in interpreting the interdialytic weight gain in the reassessment of the patient's EDW. The patient should be asked: if he or she has experienced any unusual symptoms including pain in any areas, bleeding, swelling, redness, or drainage from access site(s); has sustained any injuries such as contusion; has had any accidents such as falls; or has noticed any signs of bleeding such as hemorrhaging of the eyes or unusual bruising. As patient care technicians and licensed practical/vocational nursing personnel often participate in data collection, they need to be taught what to report to the registered nurse.

Vascular access assessment and preparation. The patient's access site should be examined for patency and signs of infection prior to each dialysis. Blood sampling is done via the access needle for arteriovenous fistula (AVF) and AV grafts (AVG) prior to heparinization as heparin interferes with some tests. Blood sampling through the catheter should be done only after removal of heparin from and adequate flushing of the catheter lumen. It is important that the correct laboratory specimen tubes and collection methods are done in accordance with the lab tests ordered.

Beginning the Treatment

Once the vascular access has been prepared, heparin administered as ordered, and the recirculated saline in the extracorporeal circuit has been replaced with fresh saline, the treatment is ready for initiation. The refreshed priming solution in the system can be either given to the patient or removed as explained below.

If the patient is to receive the prime, both the arterial and venous bloodlines should be connected to the access prior to starting the blood pump. The blood flow rate is started slowly, allowing the circuit and dialyzer to fill gradually while examining to ensure extracorporeal pressures and the vascular access are satisfactory. If no problems are detected, the blood flow rate is set at the prescribed rate.

If the patient is not to receive the saline in the system because of volume overload or other medical reasons, the procedure is different and requires great caution because of the potential for exsanguination. Because of this potential lethal complication, this practice has either been eliminated in facilities or has been restricted to special circumstances. The arterial bloodline is connected to the access, and the priming fluid is allowed to drain from the circuit while it is being displaced by blood until the blood reaches the venous air trap (chamber). At that time, the venous line is connected to the access. The clinician must always be attentive at the patient's side while the blood is replacing the prime solution. It is critical the clinician is not distracted or does not leave until the venous bloodline is attached because of the potential for severe blood loss and exsanguinations leading to death. Once both bloodlines are attached to the access, the blood flow rate is initially increased slowly to evaluate the blood flow to and from the access and through the system. If satisfactory and there are no unusually high pressures or problems with the access, such as infiltration of the needles, the blood flow rate is increased to the prescribed level.

Bloodlines are examined for appropriate clamping of any administration lines that could allow air to enter the system, clamps on monitoring lines are in open position, arterial and venous pressures are noted, all limits are set, and drip chambers are examined for appropriate levels. The air detector setting is verified to ensure it is set, and the venous bloodline is in the correct position prior to leaving the patient's side. This is a critical step to prevent the possibility of air entering the patient leading to potentially fatal air embolus. Also, verify that all settings are correct and that the heparin infusion pump is set and on if applicable.

It is also very important prior to leaving the patient's side to ensure the access is secure and visible to prevent severe blood loss and lethal exsanguinations in the event of line disconnect or needle displacement.

Intradialytic Monitoring

Blood circuit. Nursing management related to arterial pressure monitoring or alarm situations includes assessment of the problem to determine the cause of pressure changes or alarms as well as troubleshooting the problem.

If a pre-pump arterial pressure alarm occurs, the nurse should reduce the blood flow rate to the point that inflow suction decreases enough to allow the alarm to stay off.

This will allow the nurse time to ascertain the problem and correct it. The nurse should first ensure that the patient's blood pressure is not unusually low. If it is, it should be corrected by fluid replacement and/or reduction in the UF rate. If the problem is not hypotension, needle position should be suspected. The arterial needle should be repositioned by moving it up or down slightly or by rotating it to change the position of the bevel. An attempt to restore the blood flow to the previous rate is appropriate after adjustment of the needle. Needle adjustment can be attempted again if the low arterial pressure is still present (Van Stone, 1994).

The nurse may consider placement of another arterial needle and dialyze through it in an attempt to achieve a greater blood flow rate. The original needle can be left in place with a syringe attached and clamped to the end until the treatment is completed, unless infiltration has occurred. If the suction cannot be corrected, dialysis can be continued at a slower blood flow rate with an increase in treatment time to compensate for this as ordered. The observations and interventions should be documented in the patient's medical record.

Venous pressure or outflow pressure is also monitored on the blood circuit. High blood flow rates when using a smaller gauge needle can result in higher venous pressures as can clotting in the venous blood line, in the filter of the venous air trap, in the venous needle, or in the venous limb of the vascular access. Stenosis or spasm in the venous limb of the access or at the graft vein anastomosis of an AVG can cause an increased pressure. An improperly positioned venous needle and kinked venous bloodline should always be ruled out (Van Stone, 1994).

If clotting of the venous line or filter is the reason for the increased pressure, it can be confirmed by rinsing of the line with saline. If necessary, a new venous line can be primed and substituted for the clotted one. The presence of obstruction, such as clotting in the venous needle or venous limb of the access, can be confirmed by irrigating the venous needle or port with a syringe of normal saline and noting the resistance. To evaluate for stenosis the same type of test can be performed as with arterial pressure, occluding the access between the arterial and venous needles. In this case, if the venous pressure rises when the access is occluded, it suggests that stenosis downstream is causing the outflow obstruction (Van Stone, 1994).

As previously mentioned, the extracorporeal blood circuit is armed with an air detector that constantly monitors the blood returning to the patient for the presence of air. The danger of air accidentally entering the blood circuit is greatest between the arterial access site and the blood pump where the pressure within the system is negative. Common sites of air entry include around the arterial needle, if it is slightly loose or leaky; a broken pump segment on the tubing; and the infusion set connected to a normal saline infusion. The administration of albumin or medications in vented bottles can lead to air entering the system and; therefore, vented bottles should be prohibited in the dialysis setting. Rather, the solutions can be transferred to plastic solution bags without venting. Any administration ports or lines on saline administration lines must be capped with either injection ports, syringes, or other closed caps and clamped and secured to reduce the possibility of air accidentally entering the system. The patient is also at extreme risk of an air embolus if an air rinse is used to return the patient's blood at the end of a treatment. For this reason, rinsing the blood back using saline is the most common practice.

Dialysate circuit. Conductivity and temperature are continuously monitored on the dialysate circuit. A properly functioning bypass valve, which diverts dialysate away from the dialyzer, will protect the patient from dialysate with an abnormal conductivity or temperature. The dialysate is also monitored for the presence of hemoglobin, which would indicate a blood leak inside the dialyzer. Small blood leaks cannot always be discerned by observing the dialysate line. False alarms do occur and may be due to air bubbles within the dialysate lines. A blood leak should always be confirmed with a test of the effluent using a test strip such as those used to test for hemoglobin in the urine. If a blood leak is confirmed, the dialysate compartment pressure should be set to -50 mmHg or lower to minimize the entry of bacteria or endotoxin from the dialysate into the bloodstream. Small leaks in hollow fiber dialyzers may seal themselves off. However, if they do not seal off, the blood can usually be returned and dialysis discontinued or restarted with a new circuit (Daugirdas, Ross, & Nissenson, 2001). The dialysate compartment of the dialyzer should be periodically inspected to ensure adequate filling. If concentrate jugs are used at the station, they should be periodically monitored to ensure an adequate supply. A continuous flow of concentrate to the proportioning machine is more desirable to avoid interruptions in the flow of dialysate through the hemodialyzer.

Patient monitoring. The patient's vital signs, including blood pressure and pulse, should be monitored periodically during the treatment along with machine parameters discussed above. The frequency is based on the patient's condition and can be as often as every 10 to 15 minutes during acute HD and at 30 to 45 minute increments for most stable, chronic in-center patients. The patient should also be monitored for HD complications. The patient's access should also be monitored to ensure it is visible during the treatment.

Termination of the HD Treatment

The blood in the extracorporeal circuit is returned to the patient by displacing it in the circuit with normal saline. The patient usually receives 100-300 ml of normal saline during the rinseback procedure. When the venous bloodline is light pink, the normal saline infusion is stopped. If the patient's blood pressure is low at the end of the treatment, more normal saline can be infused as necessary per MD order and/or facility policies and procedures to raise the blood pressure. Use of air to return blood to the patient is not recommended because of the high incidence of air embolism with this procedure, as described above. Once the blood is returned to the patient, the needles are removed from the AVF or graft, and venous stasis is achieved with the application of pressure to the venipuncture sites. If a catheter was used for dialysis, the catheter

lumens are rinsed with normal saline and heparinized before the caps are replaced and the limbs clamped.

Postdialysis Patient Assessment

The patient's vital signs and blood pressure should be reassessed. The postdialysis weight should be compared with the preweight and the target weight. If weight loss is greater or less than anticipated, nursing measures should be taken. The calculations related to UF requirements should be reviewed for errors, such as failure to include the priming solution or rinse solution. The dialyzer should be observed for signs of clotting that could reduce dialyzer permeability. The patient should be assessed for any dizziness, orthostatic hypotension, or other complaints. Any unusual postdialysis bleeding from the vascular access should be evaluated. The postdialysis findings should be documented in the health record and communicated to other clinicians involved in the care of the patient.

Postdialysis Processes

Blood work. Serum samples obtained immediately postdialysis can give information regarding urea removal, correction of acidosis, and normalization of electrolytes. However, movement of these substances between body fluid compartments will continue after dialysis is completed.

Postdialysis Equipment Care

After the treatment, the dialysis machine is stripped of the disposable blood circuit equipment such as bloodlines, intravenous bags, and syringes. If the center performs dialyzer reuse, the dialyzer is prepared for this procedure. If reuse is not employed, the dialyzer is discarded with the other disposable equipment. After use, the machine is rinsed with treated water to remove all dialysate from the circuit.

After the rinse is completed, disinfection of the machine is performed. If chemical disinfectants are used, they should be selected based on the compatibility with the materials used in the device and in accordance with the manufacturers' IFU. Each manufacturer is required to provide information about the chemicals that are known to be compatible with the device (AAMI, 2003).

Summary

The patient receiving HD presents many challenges for the nephrology nurse. The foundation of practice for nephrology nurses caring for the HD patient is a strong knowledge base in the principles of HD, the technological components of the therapy, strategies for safe and effective treatments, as well as optimizing therapy and the ongoing assessment of patient response to therapy. As our knowledge and treatment technologies advance, extra effort must be made to maintain a high level of clinical and technical expertise. Nephrology nursing is a unique and wonderful specialty that requires an understanding of the intricate relationships among patient assessment, equipment intervention, and patient outcomes. Moving toward the goals for optimal dialysis therapy allows nephrology nurses the opportunity to utilize the highest level of nursing commitment and expertise in the delivery of HD.

References

Ahmad, S. (1999). *Manual of clinical dialysis.* London, UK: Science Press Ltd.

Ajuria, J., & Kimmel, P. (2004). Choice of the hemodialysis membrane. In W. Henrich (Ed.), *Principles & practice of dialysis* (pp. 1-15). Philadelphia, PA: Lippincott, Williams & Wilkins.

Arduino, M. (2001, May). Biological principles of water treatment for hemodialysis. In R. Hakim (Chair), *Preparing for the future: Learning from the past.* Presented at the 4th Annual Medical Conference of Renal Care Group, New Orleans, LA.

Association for the Advancement of Medical Instrumentation (AAMI), American National Standards Institute, Inc. (1994). *Hemodialyzer blood tubing* (ANSI/AAMI RD17). Arlington, VA: Author.

Association for the Advancement of Medical Instrumentation (AAMI). (2001). *AAMI Standards and recommended practices: Dialysis.* Arlington, VA: Author.

Association for the Advancement of Medical Instrumentation (AAMI), American National Standards Institute, Inc. (2003). *Hemodialysis systems* (ANSI/AAMI RD5). Arlington, VA: Author.

Association for the Advancement of Medical Instrumentation (AAMI), American National Standards Institute, Inc. (2004). *Dialysate for hemodialysis* (ANSI/AAMI RD52). Arlington, VA: Author.

Boure, T., & Vanholder, R. (2004). Which dialyzer membrane to choose. *Nephrology Dialysis Transplantation, 19*(2), 293-296.

Bregman, H., Daugirdas, J., & Ing, T. (2001). Complications during hemodialysis. In J. Daugirdas, P. Blake, & T. Ing (Eds.), *Handbook of dialysis* (3rd ed., pp. 148-168). Philadelphia: Lippincott, Williams & Wilkins,

Breiterman-White, R. (1995). A review of heparin use in hemodialysis and peritoneal dialysis. *ANNA Journal, 22*(5), 491-493.

Cappelli, G., & Inguaggiato, P. (2004). Water treatment for contemporary hemodialysis. In W. Horl, K. Koch, R. Lindsay, C. Ronco, & J. Winchester, (Eds.), *Replacement of renal function by dialysis* (5th ed., pp. 491-503)., AA Dordrecht, The Netherlands: Kluwer Academic Publishers.

Caruana, R.J., & Keep, D.M. (1994). *Anticoagulation.* In J.T. Daugirdas & T.S. Ing (Eds.), *Handbook of dialysis* (2nd ed.) (pp.13-29). Boston: Little, Brown.

Centers for Medicare & Medicaid Services (CMS). (1998). *Subparts S-T (reserved). Subpart U: Conditions for coverage suppliers of end-stage renal disease (ESRD) services,* (42 CFR Chapter IV) (10/1/98 ed.). Retrieved November 17, 2005, from http://www.gpoaccess.gov/nara

Centers for Medicare & Medicaid Services (CMS). (2003). 2003 Annual Report, End Stage Renal Disease Clinical Performance Measures Project. Department of Health and Human Services, Centers for Medicare & Medicaid Services, Center for Beneficiary Choices, Baltimore, Maryland, December 2003.

Cheung, A.K., Levin, N.W., Greene, T., Agodoa, L., Bailey, J., Beck, G., et al. (2003). Effects of high flux hemodialysis on clinical outcomes: Results of the hemo study. *Journal of the American Society of Nephrology, 14,* 3251–3263.

Churchill, D., Bird, D., Taylor, D., Beecroft, M., Gorman, J., & Wallace, J. (1992). Effect of high-flux hemodialysis on quality of life and neuropsychological function in chronic hemodialysis patients. *American Journal of Nephrology, 12,* 412-418.

Churchill, D., Taylor, D., Tomlinson, C., Beecroft, M., Gorman, J., & Stanton, E. (1993). Effect of high-flux hemodialysis on cardiac structure and function among patients with end-stage renal failure. *Nephron, 65,* 573-577.

Clark, R., & Winchester, J. (2003). Middle molecules and small-molecular weight proteins in ESRD: Properties and strategies for their removal. *Advances in Renal Replacement Therapy, 10*(4), 270-278.

Collins, A.J., Liu, J., & Ebben, J.P. (2004). Dialyzer reuse-associated mortality and hospitalization risk in incident Medicare hemodialysis patients, 1998-1999. *Nephrology Dialysis Transplantation, 19*(5), 1245-1251.

Corea, A., Pittard, J., Gardner, P., & Shinaberger, J. (1993). Management of safety monitors on hemodialysis machines. In A. Nissenson & R. Fine (Eds.), *Dialysis therapy* (2nd ed.) (43-49). Philadelphia: Hanley & Belfus.

Curtis, J., & Varughese, P. (Eds.). (2000). *Dialysis technology: A manual for dialysis technicians* (2nd ed.). Dayton, OH: National Association of Dialysis Technicians/Technologists.

Daugirdas, J.T. (1994). Chronic hemodialysis prescription: A urea kinetic approach. In J.T. Daugirdas & T. S. Ing (Eds.), *Handbook of dialysis* (2nd ed., pp. 192-220). Boston: Little, Brown.

Daugirdas, J., & Kjellstrand, C. (2001). Chronic hemodialysis prescription: A urea kinetic approach. In J. Daugirdas, P. Blake, & T. Ing (Eds.), *Handbook of dialysis* (3rd ed.) (pp. 121-147). Philadelphia, PA: Lippincott, Williams & Wilkins.

Daugirdas, J., Ross, E., & Nissenson, A. (2001). Acute hemodialysis prescription. In J. Daugirdas, P. Blake, & T. Ing (Eds.). *Handbook of dialysis* (3rd ed.) (pp. 102-120). Philadelphia: Lippincott, Williams & Wilkins.

Daugirdas, J., Van Stone, J., & Boag, J. (2001). Hemodialysis apparatus. In J. Daugirdas, P. Blake, & T. Ing (Eds.), *Handbook of dialysis* (3rd ed.) (pp. 46-66). Philadelphia: Lippincott, Williams & Wilkins.

Fan, P., & Schwab, S. (1993). Single-patient hemodialysis machines. In A. Nissenson & R. Fine (Eds.), *Dialysis therapy* (2nd ed.) (pp. 35-38), Philadelphia: Hanley & Belfus, Inc.

Francos, G., Burke, J., Besarab, A., Martinez, J., Kirkwood, R., & Humme, L. (1983). An unsuspected cause of acute hemolysis during hemodialysis. *American Society of Artificial Internal Organs, 29,* 140-145.

Graves, G., (2001). Arterial and venous pressure monitoring during hemodialysis. *American Nephrology Nursing Journal, 28*(1), 23-28.

Gutch, C., & Stoner, M. (1993). *Review of hemodialysis for nurses and dialysis personnel* (5th ed.). St. Louis, MO: C.V. Mosby Company.

Guyton, A. (Ed.). (1986). *Textbook of medical physiology* (7th ed.). Philadelphia: W.B. Saunders Company,

Hakim, R. (1993). Clinical implications of hemodialysis membrane biocompatibility. *Kidney International, 44,* 484-494.

Hakim, R., Held, P., Stannard, D., Wolfe, R., Port, F., Daugirdas, J., et al. (1996). Effect of the dialysis membrane on mortality of chronic hemodialysis patients. *Kidney International, 50,* 566-570.

Hertel, J., Keep, D., & Caruana, R. (2001). Anticoagulation. In J. Daugirdas, P. Blake, & T. Ing (Eds.), *Handbook of dialysis* (3rd ed.) (pp. 182-198). Philadelphia: Lippincott, Williams & Wilkins.

Hoenick, N. (1988). Comparison of membranes used in treatment of end stage renal failure. *Kidney International, 33*(24), S44-S48.

Hollon, J. & Ward, R. (2005). Acid-base homeostasis in dialysis patients. In A. Nissenson & R. Fine (Eds.), *Clinical dialysis* (4th ed.) (pp. 553-575). New York: The McGraw-Hill Companies, Inc.

Hornberger, J., Chernew, M., Petersen, J., & Garber, A. (1992). A multivariate analysis of mortality and hospital admissions with high-flux dialysis. *Journal of the American Society of Nephrology, 3,* 1227-1237.

Ismail, N., Brouillette, J., & Mujais, S. (1999). Hemodialysis technology. In H. Malluche, B. Sawaya, R. Hakim, M. Sayegh, & N. Ismail (Eds.), *Clinical nephrology & transplantation* (pp. 1-38). Landshut, Germany: Bosch-Druck.

Ismail, N., & Hakim, R. (1991). Hemodialysis. In D.Z. Levine (Ed.), *Care of the renal patient* (2nd ed.) (pp 220-246). Philadelphia: Saunders.

Jacobson, E.D. (1999). *CDRH safety alerts, public health advisories, and notices. FDA safety alert: Potential cross-contamination linked to hemodialysis treatment.* Rockville, MD: U.S. Food and Drug Administration (FDA), Center for Devices and Radiological Health.

Jenson, B.M., Dobbe, S.A., Squillace, D.P., & McCarthy, J.T. (1994). Clinical benefits of high and variable sodium concentration dialysate in hemodialysis patients. *ANNA Journal, 21*(2), 115-120.

Josephson, M. (1992). Improvement of plasma lipoprotein during high flux dialysis. *American Journal of Kidney Disease, 20,* 361-366.

Kaufman, A.M., & Levin, N.W. (2001). Dialyzer reuse. In J. Daugirdas, P. Blake, & T. Ing (Eds.), *Handbook of dialysis* (3rd ed., pp. 169-181). Philadelphia: Lippincott, Williams & Wilkins.

Kaufman, A., Polaschegg, H., & Levin, N. (1993). Common clinical problems during hemodialysis. In A. Nissenson & R. Fine (Eds.).

Dialysis therapy (2nd ed.) (pp. 109-113). Philadelphia: Hanley and Belfus, Inc.

Keshaviah, P. (1991). Technology and clinical application of hemodialysis. In H. Jacobson, G. Striker, & E. Klahr (Eds.), *The principles & practice of nephrology* (pp. 740-749). Philadelphia: B.C. Decker.

Klinkmann, H., Ebbighausen, H., Uhlenbusch, I., & Vienken, J. (1993). High-flux dialysis, dialysate quality, and backtransport. In V. Bonomini (Ed.), *Contributions to nephrology: Vol. 10. Evolution in dialysis adequacy* (pp. 89-97). Basel: Karger.

Kumar, V., & Depner, T. (2004). Approach to hemodialysis kinetic modeling. In W. Henrich (Ed.), *Principles and practice of dialysis* (pp. 82-102). Philadelphia: Lippincott, Williams & Wilkins

Lancaster, L. (Ed.). (1979). *The patient with end stage renal disease.* New York: John Wiley & Sons.

Lazarus, J.M., Denker, B., & Owen, W. (1996). Hemodialysis. In B. Brenner (Ed.), *The kidney* (5th ed.) (pp. 2424-2506). Philadelphia: W.B. Saunders Co.

Levin, N., Gotch, F., Bednar, B., Gallagher, N., & Peterson, G. (1991). Kinetics and quality assurance: Prescription therapy through kinetic modeling. *ANNA Journal, 18*(3), 269-290.

Levin, N., & Zasuwa, P. (1993). Relationship between dialyzer type and signs and symptoms. *Nephrology Dialysis Transplantation, 8*(Suppl. 2), 30-39.

Leypoldt, J., & Cheung, A. (2001). Increases in mass transfer-area coefficients and urea Kt/V with increasing dialysate flow rate are greater for high-flux dialyzers. *American Journal of Kidney Diseases, 38*(3), 575-579.

Leypoldt, J., Cheung, A., Chiranthavat, T., Gilson, J., Kamerath, C., & Deeter, R. (2003). Hollow fiber shape alters solute clearances in high flux hemodialyzers. *ASAIO Journal,* pp. 81-87.

McBride, P. (1979), *Genesis of the artificial kidney.* Deerfield, IL: Travenol Laboratories, Inc.

McCarthy, T. (2004). *Animal models in medical device development and qualification.* (Reference paper Vol. 10-2). Charles River Laboratories. Retrieved December 1, 2004, from www.criver.com/techdocs/meddev.html

O'Connor, A., & Wish, J. (2004). Hemodialysis adequacy and the timing of dialysis initiation. In W. Henrich (Ed.), *Principles and practice of dialysis* (3rd ed.) (pp. 111-127). Philadelphia: Lippincott Williams & Willkins.

Ottosson, P., Attman, P., & Knight-Gibson, C. (2001). Do high-flux dialysis membranes affect renal dyslipidemia? *American Society of Artificial Internal Organs, 47,* 229-234.

Polaschegg, H., & Levin, N. (2004). Hemodialysis machines and monitors. In W. Horl, K. Koch, R. Lindsay, C. Ronco, & J. Winchester, (Eds.), *Replacement of renal function by dialysis* (5th ed.) (pp. 325-449)., AA Dordrecht, The Netherlands: Kluwer Academic Publishers.

Radovich, J. (1995). Composition of polymer membranes for therapies of end stage renal disease. In V. Bonomini & Y. Berland (Eds.), *Contributions to nephrology: Vol. 113. Dialysis membranes: Structure & predictions.* (pp. 11-24). Basel: Karger.

Relman, A.S. (1959). The nephrotic syndrome: Uremia. In R.L. Cecil & R.F. Loeb Eds.), *A textbook of medicine* (10th ed.). Philadelphia: W.B. Saunders Company.

Renal Physicians Association (RPA) Working Committee on Clinical Practice Guidelines. (1993, December). *Clinical practice guideline on adequacy of hemodialysis. Clinical practice guideline, number 1.* Washington, DC: Author.

Saha, L.K., & Van Stone, J.C. (1992). Differences between KT/V measured during dialysis and KT/V predicted from manufacturer clearance data. *The International Journal of Artificial Organs, 15*(8), 223-230.

Salem, M., & Mujais, S. (1993). Technical and functional considerations in choosing hollow-fiber dialyzers. In *Dialysis therapy* (2nd ed.). Philadelphia: Hanley & Belfus, Inc.

Sands, J., Glidden, D., Jacavage, W., & Jones, B. (1996). Differences between delivered and prescribed blood flow in hemodialysis. *American Society of Artificial Internal Organs, 42*(5), M717-M719.

Selenic, D., Alvarado-Ramy, F., Arduino, M., Holt, S., Cardinali, F., Blount, B., et al. (2004). Epidemic parenteral exposure to volatile sulfur-containing compunds at a hemodialysis center. *Infection Control and Hospital Epidemiology, 25*(3), 256-261.

Seres, D., Strain, G., Hashim, S., Goldberg, I., & Levin, N. (1993). Improvement of plasma lipoprotein profiles during high-flux dialysis. *Journal of the American Society of Nephrology, 3,* 1409-1415.

Soltys, P.J., Zydney, A., Leypoldt, J.K., Henderson, L.W., & Ofsthun, N.J. (2000). Potential of dual-skinned, high-flux membranes to reduce backtransport in hemodialysis. *Kidney International, 58,* 818-828.

Sweet, J., McCarthy, S., Steingart, R., & Callahan, T. (1996). Hemolytic reactions mechanically induced by kinked hemodialysis lines. *American Journal of Kidney Disease, 27*(2), 262-266.

United States Renal Data System (USRDS). (1997). *1997 Annual Data Report.* Bethesda, MD: United National Institutes of Health, National Institute of Diabetes and Digestive and Kidney Diseases.

United States Renal Data System (USRDS). (2003). *2003 Annual Data Report: Atlas of end stage renal disease in the United States.* Bethesda, MD: United National Institutes of Health, National Institute of Diabetes and Digestive and Kidney Diseases.

Van Stone, J.C. (1994). Hemodialysis apparatus. In J. Daugirdas & T. Ing (Eds.), *Handbook of dialysis* (2nd ed.) (pp. 30-52). Boston: Little, Brown.

Ward, R. (1993). Water treatment for in-center hemodialysis, including verification of water quality and disinfection. In A. Nissenson & R. Fine (Eds.), *Dialysis therapy* (2nd ed.) (31-38). Philadelphia: Hanley & Belfus.

Ward, R., (2002, May). Water disasters, pitfalls, and water precautions. In R. Hakim (Chair), *The right start in continuum of care.* Presented at the 5th Annual Medical Conference of Renal Care Group, Dallas, TX.

Weast, R.C. (Ed.). (1983). *Handbook of chemistry and physics* (64th ed.). New York: CRC Press.

Winchester, J., Salsberg, J., & Levin, N. (2003). Beta-2 microglobulin in ESRD: An in-depth review. *Advances in Renal Replacement Therapy, 10*(4), 279-309.

Additional Readings

Association for the Advancement of Medical Instrumentation (AAMI), American National Standards Institute, Inc. (1996). *Hemodialyzers* (ANSI/AAMI RD16). Arlington, VA: Author.

Association for the Advancement of Medical Instrumentation (AAMI), American National Standards Institute, Inc. (2003). *Reuse of hemodialyzers* (ANSI/AAMI RD47 & RD47/A1). Arlington, VA: Author.

Henrich, W. (Ed.). (2004). *Principles and practice of dialysis* (3rd ed.). Philadelphia: Lippincott, Williams & Wilkins.

- Hemodialysis (HD) is used extensively throughout the world to treat patients with acute and chronic renal failure. In the U.S., HD is the most commonly used treatment modality for patients requiring renal replacement therapy.

- HD is one type of therapy that uses dialysis, a process in which substances move across a semipermeable membrane to remove unwanted solutes and fluid and restore acid base and electrolyte balance.

- The key principles of HD are UF, osmosis, diffusion, and convection. They enable the removal of substances and fluid as well as correcting acid-base and electrolyte imbalance.

- Ultrafiltration is the process through which body water removal is accomplished during dialysis. It is the movement of a solvent, a liquid capable of dissolving another substance or solute, from one area to another because of a pressure or concentration difference. In HD, it is accomplished primarily through hydrostatic pressure.

- Diffusion is the movement of solutes, through a semipermeable membrane, from an area of greater concentration to an area of lesser concentration. The primary mechanism for toxin removal by HD is diffusion.

- Clearance refers to removal of a substance from the bloodstream during a specific unit of time. It is an empirical measurement of the volume of blood that is totally cleared of a particular substance per unit of time (1 minute). Clearance or solute transport out of the blood during HD can result from diffusion, convection, or adsorption.

- The HD system is composed of two circuits: the extracorporeal circuit and the dialysate circuit. The HD system includes the dialyzer to filter the blood and the dialysis machine used to proportion and monitor the dialysate fluid as well as pump and monitor the blood flowing through the extracorporeal circuit.

- The dialysate circuit includes the mixing and delivery system used to create the dialysate; the dialysate is made from purified or treated water and an electrolyte/buffer solution. The dialysate is part of the dialysis prescription and includes electrolytes such as sodium, chloride, potassium, and magnesium.

- The extracorporeal circuit includes the needle or catheter placed in the patient's vascular access, blood lines that transport the patient's blood to and from the dialyzer, the dialyzer, and components of the HD equipment that monitor and pump the blood through the system.

- Today, there are two types of dialyzer construction: the parallel plate and the most commonly used hollow fiber dialyzer. The hemodialyzer is designed with two internal components, one to contain blood and the other for dialysis solution. The two compartments are separated by a semipermeable membrane.

- There are three primary types of dialyzer membranes: cellu-losic, modified, and synthetic. The modified group can be further subdivided into substituted with acetate, cellulosynthetic, and coated.

- Water and large solute permeability defines the "flux" of the dialyzer. Dialyzers are classified as high or low flux. Dialyzer efficiency is defined by small solute permeability and is frequently measured by urea clearance.

- Biocompatibility is influenced by all components of the hemodialysis system such as dialysis membranes, sterilants, blood tubing, dialysate and the patient's susceptibility. It is influenced by the polymer blend of the membrane, manufacturing process, dialyzer design, materials used for fabrication as well as sterilization and reuse status.

- During hemodialysis, the patient's blood is exposed to more than 120 liters of water. This is greater than 20 times the amount the average person would normally take in orally in a 24-hour period. Thus, substances that are not harmful in drinking water may be harmful in dialysis water. Substances in the water have direct access to the patient's bloodstream, so it is very important that the purity of water used for hemodialysis be known and controlled.

- Monitoring of the various pressures throughout the extracorporeal circuit is important in guarding against or detecting clotting, disconnections, kinking or obstruction of blood tubing or dysfunction of the vascular access.

- The HD prescription is a set of physician orders that include but are not limited to the dialysis dose, dialyzer, dialysate, fluid removal, profiling such as sodium or UF, anticoagulation, medications, standing orders for complications, and laboratory testing.

- An adequate hemodialysis prescription is only the beginning of an adequate treatment. Ongoing evaluation of treatment parameters as well as successful delivery of the prescribed treatment is very important. Nephrology nurses have a most crucial role in ensuring that hemodialysis patients receive the treatment that has been prescribed.

- Levin described the requirements for ensuring adequate therapy: an appropriate prescription, a high level of nursing expertise, an efficiently operating hemodialysis machine, satisfactory access to the circulation, an informed patient, and ongoing data collection and review.

- The foundation of practice for nephrology nurses caring for the HD patient is a strong knowledge base in the principles of HD, the technological components of the therapy, strategies for safe and effective treatments, as well as optimizing therapy and the ongoing assessment of patient response to therapy.

Hemodialysis Technology

Name of Resource	Brief Description	Where to Obtain Resource
Name of Resource **NKF-K/DOQI Clinical Practice Guidelines for Hemodialysis Adequacy: Update 2000** *Author: National Kidney Foundation K/DOQI Work Group on Hemodialysis Adequacy* **American Journal of Kidney Diseases (AJKD)**, Vol. 37, No. 1, Suppl. 1, January 2001)	**Brief Description** This document includes the revised and updated versions of the DOQI guidelines originally published in 1997 on **hemodialysis adequacy**. Guidelines are included in the following areas: • Measurement of hemodialysis adequacy • Hemodialysis dose • Blood urea nitrogen (BUN) sampling • Hemodialyzer reprocessing and reuse • Hemodialysis dose troubleshooting • Maximizing patient adherence to the hemodialysis prescription	**Where to Obtain Resource** AJKD article - Medical library Information regarding these guidelines and other guidelines are available through the National Kidney Foundation's Kidney Disease Outcome Quality Initiative NKF-K/DOQI website: http://www.kidney.org/professionals/kdoqi/guidelines or www.kdoqi.org
U.S. Food and Drug Administration (FDA) MedWatch Program	MedWatch is the FDA's safety information and adverse reporting program. Information can be obtained regarding medical device safety alerts as well as medical device reporting requirements and instructions	Department of Health and Human Services Food and Drug Administration MedWatch; HFD-410 5600 Fishers Lane Rockville, MD 20857 Phone: 888-INFO-FDA (1-888-463-6332) Fax: 301-827-7241 http://www.fda.gov/medwatch
Handbook of Dialysis (3rd Edition – 2001) (Paperback) *Editors: J. Daugirdas, P. Blake, & T. Ing.*	This is a pocket-sized handbook including information on numerous aspects of dialysis including several chapters specific to hemodialysis.	Medical bookstore or Lippincott Williams & Wilkins 530 Walnut Street Philadelphia, PA 19106 USA http://www.lww.com
Association for the Advancement of Medical Instrumentation (AAMI) Standards Publications ANSI/AAMI RD5:2003 ANSI/AAMI RD16:1996; RD16/A1:2002 ANSI/AAMI RD17:1994 ANSI/AAMI RD 47:2002; RD47/A1:2003 ANSI/AAMI RD52:2004 ANSI/AAMI RD61:2000 ANSI/AAMI RD62:2001	Guidelines pertaining to hemodialysis developed by AAMI are available as follows: RD5: Hemodialysis systems, 3rd edition RD16: Hemodialyzers, 2nd edition and amendment RD17: Hemodialyzer blood tubing, 2nd edition and amendment RD47: Reuse of hemodialyzers, 3rd edition and amendment RD52: Dialysate for hemodialysis RD61: Concentrate for hemodialysis RD 62: Water treatment equipment for hemodialysis applications	Association for the Advancement of Medical Instrumentation 1110 N. Glebe Road, Suite 220, Arlington, VA 22201-4795 Phone: 703-525-4890 Fax: 703-525-1067 http://www.aami.org

ANNP623

Hemodialysis Technology

Carolyn E. Latham, MSN, MBA, RN, CNN

Contemporary Nephrology Nursing: Principles and Practice contains 39 chapters of educational content. Individual learners may apply for continuing nursing education credit by reading a chapter and completing the Continuing Education Evaluation Form for that chapter. Learners may apply for continuing education credit for any or all chapters.

Please photocopy this page and return to ANNA.
COMPLETE THE FOLLOWING:

Name: _____

Address: _____

City: _____ State: _____ Zip: _____

E-mail: _____

Preferred telephone: ☐ Home   ☐ Work: _____

State where licensed and license number (optional): _____

CE application fees are based upon the number of contact hours provided by the individual chapter. CE fees per contact hour for ANNA members are as follows: 1.0-1.9 - $15; 2.0-2.9 - $20; 3.0-3.9 - $25; 4.0 and higher - $30. Fees for nonmembers are $10 higher.

ANNA Member: ☐ Yes   ☐ No   Member # (if available) _____

☐ Checked Enclosed   ☐ American Express   ☐ Visa   ☐ MasterCard

Total Amount Submitted: _____

Credit Card Number: _____ Exp. Date: _____

Name as it appears on the card: _____

CE Evaluation Form
To receive continuing education credit for individual study after reading the chapter
1. Photocopy this form. (You may also download this form from ANNA's Web site, **www.annanurse.org**.)
2. Mail the completed form with payment (check) or credit card information to American Nephrology Nurses' Association, East Holly Avenue, Box 56, Pitman, NJ 08071-0056.
3. You will receive your CE certificate from ANNA in 4 to 6 weeks.

Test returns must be postmarked by **December 31, 2010.**

CE Application Fee
ANNA Member $25.00
Nonmember $35.00

EVALUATION FORM

1. I verify that I have read this chapter and completed this education activity. Date: _____

_____
Signature

2. What would be different in your practice if you applied what you learned from this activity? *(Please use additional sheet of paper if necessary.)*

_____

_____

_____

_____

_____

_____

_____

_____

_____

_____

_____

_____

_____

Evaluation	Strongly disagree				Strongly agree
3. The activity met the stated objectives.					
a. Explain the principles of hemodialysis.	1	2	3	4	5
b. Diagram the components of a hemodialysis system.	1	2	3	4	5
c. Describe the interventions necessary by the nurse to assure adequacy and safety of hemodialysis treatments.	1	2	3	4	5
4. The content was current and relevant.	1	2	3	4	5
5. The content was presented clearly.	1	2	3	4	5
6. The content was covered adequately.	1	2	3	4	5
7. Rate your ability to apply the learning obtained from this activity to practice.	1	2	3	4	5

Comments _____

_____

8. Time required to read the chapter and complete this form: _____ minutes.

This educational activity has been provided by the American Nephrology Nurses' Association (ANNA) for 3.8 contact hours. ANNA is accredited as a provider of continuing nursing education (CNE) by the American Nurses Credentialing Center's Commission on Accreditation (ANCC-COA). ANNA is an approved provider of continuing education by the California Board of Registered Nursing, CEP 0910.

Vascular Access for Hemodialysis

Randee Breiterman White, MS, RN, CNN

Chapter Contents

Randee Breiterman White, MS, RN, CNN

Access to the blood stream is the weak link in hemodialysis (HD) adequacy. Without a well functioning vascular access, optimal HD can never be provided. The results of a poor vascular access can be devastating for the patient, as the outcome of inadequate dialysis over time can be the development of irreversible co-morbidities and/or death (Sehgal, Dor, & Tsai, 2001; Sehgal et al., 1998). A well-functioning vascular access requires dedication to assessment, monitoring, tracking, and timely intervention when needed. The following chapter will describe the types of vascular access available today along with their advantages and shortcomings and review the various methods for assessment, monitoring, and interventions commonly provided.

History of Dialysis Access

To briefly review, the first dialysis access was developed by Scribner and Quinton in 1960 and has been the basis for all vascular access since (Quinton, Dillard, & Scribner, 1960). It consisted of Teflon® tubes, one placed in an artery and one in a vein, exiting through the skin and joined together by a Teflon loop. Femoral vein cannulation was first described the following year by Shaldon. It wasn't until 1966 that Brescia and colleagues first described the internal arteriovenous fistula (AVF) as we know it today (Brescia, Cimino, Appel, & Hurwich, 1966). Since then, many variations on the original Scribner and equally as many variations on the AVF have been tried. For those lacking in adequate native vessels, materials used to construct bridge grafts have included bovine carotid artery (Richie, Johnson, Walker, & Ginn, 1972), umbilical cords (Mindich, Silverman, Elguezabal, & Levowitz, 1975), preserved saphenous vein (Piccone et al., 1975), expanded polytetraflouroethylene (ePTFE) (Tellis, Kohlberg, Bhat, Driscoll, & Veith, 1979), and polyurethane (Matsuda et al., 2003). The use of catheters became easier when Uldall, in 1979, developed a catheter that allowed for repeated puncture of the subclavian vein (Uldall, Woods, Bird, & Dyck, 1979). In the 1980s, interventional radiology began to assist in the management of the non-surgical maintenance and surveillance of vascular access (O'Reilly, Hansen, & Rosental, 1978; Reilly, Pearson, Watkin, & Wood, 1982; Turmel-Rodriguez, Pengloan, & Bourquelot, 2002). In 1983 the long-term tunneled catheter for HD was introduced, and patients who had no options for traditional vascular access could now be dialyzed regularly (Schanzer, Kaplan, Bosch, Glabman, & Burrows, 1986). Ultimately, the *National Kidney Foundation/Dialysis Outcome Quality Initiative (NKF-DOQI) Clinical Practice Guidelines for Vascular Access* were published in 1997 leading to quality improvement and maintenance programs for vascular access nation wide (National Kidney Foundation [NKF], 1997).

K/DOQI Guidelines

The NKF-DOQI guidelines were established in an effort to standardize practice for the creation, maintenance, surveillance, and quality improvement of dialysis vascular access. HD and vascular access experts reviewed thou-

Table 24-1
Pertinent Issues when Evaluating for Vascular Access Type and Location

- Previous central venous catheters: associated with central vein stenosis
- Dominant arm: use of non-dominant arm has less impact on self-care
- Pacemaker use: associated with central vein stenosis
- Severe congestive heart failure: access affects cardiac output and vascular flow dynamics
- Arterial or venous peripheral catheters: previous damage to vasculature
- Diabetes mellitus: previous damage to vasculature
- Anticoagulant therapy or coagulopathies: increased thrombotic events or decreased hemostasis
- Previous circulatory access: site availability
- Heart valve disease or prosthesis: increased co-morbidity with infection
- Previous arm, neck, or chest surgery: previous damage to vasculature
- Anticipated renal transplant from living donor: impacts type of access chosen
- Co-morbid conditions: affects choice of access type

sands of pieces of literature from studies to anecdotal notes. Scientifically proven facts were separated from opinion, and guidelines were developed that addressed all aspects of dialysis vascular access from site selection to revision of existing access. These guidelines have been updated continuously and have now become the standard upon which access care across the world is based. Throughout this chapter, the K/DOQI guidelines will provide the underlying principles (Eknoyan et al., 2001).

Access Selection

Patient History

In order to optimize the choice for type and placement of dialysis vascular access, a careful history and physical should be done (see Table 24-1). Patient history should elicit whether the patient has had any previous instrumentation that might have caused scarring or obliteration of the veins usually used for vascular access. Previous instrumentation (e.g., central vein catheter use or pacemaker wires) can scar the central vein enough to cause stenosis or obliteration of flow (see Figure 24-1). This can cause swelling of the access arm to the extent that the access is unusable. The use of peripherally inserted central catheters (PICC) or arterial lines can also scar veins that would ordinarily be used to create vascular access (Teruya, Abou-Zamzam, Limm, Wong, & Wong, 2003). Any time the patient has had previous chest, neck, or arm surgery, including previous vascular access, one should be cautious in assuming that the vasculature of that area is intact (Huber & Seeger, 2003; NKF, 1997).

History of disease is important in the assessment, as vas-

Figure 24-1
Collateralization of the Subclavian Vein Due to Occlusion (arrow)

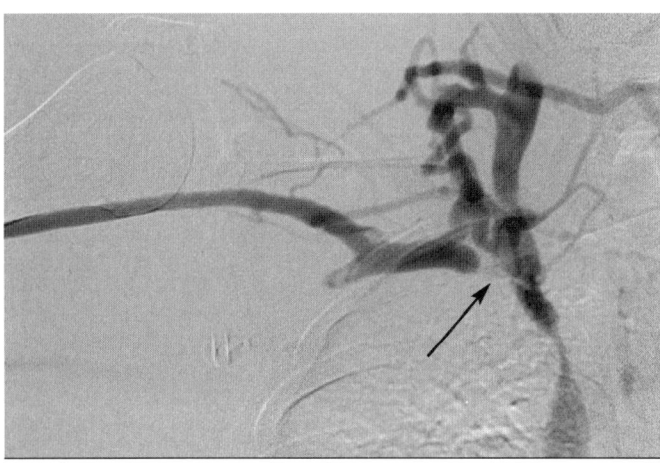

Table 24-2
The Allen Test

1. Have patient clench fist of one hand to produce pallor.
2. Compress both radial and ulnar arteries to occlude arterial flow to the hand.
3. Have patient open fist.
4. Release pressure on the ulnar artery and count the number of seconds it takes for color to return to the hand and all the fingers. More than 3 seconds indicates decreased ulnar artery flow.
5. Repeat the procedure, this time releasing pressure on the radial artery to evaluate radial arterial flow.
6. Repeat the procedure on the opposite hand.

cular disease and coagulopathies will impact the likelihood that a vascular access will remain functional. For instance, diabetes mellitus causes peripheral vascular disease, and lupus and multiple myeloma are two disease states that have renal and coagulopathic sequalae.

Special consideration should be used when assessing for type of vascular access in certain patients. In a patient with severe congestive heart failure, the placement of a vascular access may increase vascular return to the right side of the heart and cause exacerbation of the disease (MacRae, Pandeya, Humen, Krivitski, & Lindsay, 2004). The existence of any type of prosthetic device, especially heart valves, can be of concern as the risk of infection varies with type of access. Placement of central catheters is especially risky in the patient with prosthetic heart valves for this reason. In the patient expecting a living related transplant, the use of leg vasculature may be contraindicated, as stenosis occurring in those veins may make them unavailable at a later date for the transplant to be successful.

Finally, it is always wise to try to use the non-dominant arm for vascular access. When the patient is being dialyzed, the access arm will be unavailable for use, and if any access complications occur, it is always better to have the non-dominant arm affected.

Physical Exam

A thorough physical exam to evaluate arterial and venous blood supply in both extremities should be done. Evaluation of arterial flow includes assessment of peripheral pulses by palpation, bilateral upper arm blood pressures, and the performance of an Allen test (see Table 24-2). Evaluation of venous blood supply includes an assessment for edema, comparison of extremity circumference, inspection for collateral vein development, and examination for any evidence of previous trauma or instrumentation for central or peripheral catheters that may have damaged targeted vasculature. If there is evidence of any of the aforementioned, diagnostic studies should be performed to determine the underlying cause prior to any decision about placement of vascular access (Malovrh, 2003a; Malovrh, 2003b).

Diagnostic Studies

There are multiple diagnostic studies available ranging from the simple non-invasive to the more difficult and costly. The literature is replete with overwhelming evidence that vein mapping greatly increases the likelihood of successful vascular access placement even in young, otherwise healthy individuals with normal appearing veins and arteries (Allon et al., 2001; Ascher et al., 2000). The preferred method of vein mapping is with non-invasive venous Doppler. Vein size can be determined and the evidence of stenosis and/or thrombosis ruled out. The drawback to Doppler ultrasound is that the central veins cannot be visualized and stenosis and/or thrombosis can only be inferred based upon waveforms. If there is any indication that there may be a problem with the central veins, more definitive diagnostics such as magnetic resonance imaging (MRI) or magnetic resonance venography (MRV) may be done. Radiological venogram can be performed in patients for whom renal function is no longer an issue. Although less expensive than either MRI or MRV, the use of intravenous (IV) contrast should be avoided in patients not yet on dialysis due to nephrotoxicity (Andrew & Berg, 2004). If venography is unavoidable in these patients, gadolinium or carbon dioxide is available for contrast, but neither provide the clear pictures that conventional IV contrast can provide (Sam et al., 2003). Should arterial flow in the targeted extremity be of concern, Doppler ultrasound should be employed to evaluate the underlying cause. If more detail is required, an arteriogram and magnetic resonance arteriography (MRA) with the attendant risks for contrast-induced nephrotoxicity are the other choices. If the use of contrast cannot be avoided, there are some mixed data that show that the use of acetylcysteine solution prior to the procedure may be useful in minimizing renal damage (Bagshaw & Ghali, 2004).

Types of Vascular Access

External AV Shunts

Although external AV shunts are used infrequently, there still may be times when they are useful (Coronel et al., 2001). The external AV shunt was the first of the shunts developed and today is only used in cases of emergent need for continuous renal replacement therapy (CRRT) and inability to place either central or femoral lines. The original shunt itself consisted of two rigid Teflon® tips, one placed in an artery and one in a nearby vein, to which silastic tubing is attached and brought to the skin surface through separate puncture wounds. The silastic tubes were then connected with an additional piece of silastic to form a continuous circuit. More recently these have been used as two silastic tubes anchored to the walls of the vessel with a Dacron® patch (Coronel et al., 2001).

There are several advantages to using an external AV shunt. Only local anesthesia is required for placement, it can be used immediately, no venipuncture is required, and high blood flow rates are easily obtainable. Unfortunately, placing an external AV shunt renders the utilized artery and vein unusable for further access due to damage to the vasculature. In addition, there is a high rate of complications, so these are typically used for only short periods of time and/or as a final attempt at vascular access. As opposed to other forms of vascular access, placement depends upon availability of undamaged vessels and is usually in the upper extremity if needed for CRRT and/or the need for therapy is limited and the lower extremity if there is any possibility of chronic renal failure in order to preserve vasculature for more permanent vascular access (Hartigan & White, 2001).

The most frequent complication associated with the external AV shunt is thrombosis. This can be due to misalignment of the cannula tips within the vessel, bending of the vessel wall, arterial narrowing close to the cannula tip, recent thrombi, fibrosis at the cannula tip, inadequate anticoagulation, pressure on the area caused by a tight bandage or garment, hypotension, or bending of the shunt connector. Aspiration of the clot or embolectomy may be attempted (Coronel et al., 2001).

Other complications that can occur with an external AV shunt are infection, skin erosion, and dislodgement of the cannula tips. Infection usually begins as local cellulitis at the cannula insertion sites and is almost inevitable. If not treated early, local infection can progress to sepsis. In malnourished individuals, infection at the insertion site can lead to skin erosion and possible hemorrhage. Dislodgment of the cannula tips is life threatening due to the risk of hemorrhage (Coronel et al., 2001).

Daily shunt care with meticulous attention to aseptic technique is required. Any signs or symptoms of infection including an elevated white blood cell count should prompt suspicion of shunt infection. Blood pressure measurements and blood draws should be avoided in the shunt extremity. A dressing should cover the shunt at all times with the loop of the shunt exposed in order to confirm patency without removing the dressing. Bull dog clamps should always be attached to the dressing for immediate availability should the shunt disconnect accidentally. In order to prevent accidental disconnection, any connections should always be taped, and tension on the cannula should be avoided during the HD treatment.

The conscious patient with an external shunt should be taught how to perform daily dressing care and to keep the area clean and dry. As with any vascular access, the patient should be able to assess patency, know the signs and symptoms of infection, and know who to call to report problems to. Finally, the patient should be able to demonstrate emer-

gency care for the dislodgement or separation of shunt cannulas.

Native AVF

The most desirable vascular access is the native AVF. According to the K/DOQI guidelines, 50% of all patients new to dialysis should have an AVF placed and, ultimately, 40% of all patients in any given HD unit should have a functioning AVF. Each time a patient needs a new access created, an AVF should be considered. An AVF is the surgical creation of an anastomosis between an artery and a vein that allows the arterial blood to flow through the vein. Over time, this causes venous enlargement and thickening of the vein wall, a process known as arterialization. The increase in vein size enables the insertion of large bore needles into the venous portion of the fistula to remove and return blood for HD. The arterial anastomosis of the AVF is never cannulated. The sites for creation of an AVF are only limited by the patient's available vasculature and skills of the clinician creating the anastomosis (Berman & Gentile, 2001; Bonforte, Zerbi, & Surian, 2004; Burkhart & Cikrit, 1997; Dixon, Novak, & Fangman, 2002; Goldstein & Gupta, 2003; Hazinedaroglu et al., 2004; Weyde, Krajewska, Letachowicz, & Klinger, 2002).

The AVF is usually placed in anticipation of the need to start HD within the following several months. K/DOQI guidelines recommend timing for the placement of an AVF either be when the patient's glomerular filtration rate (GFR) as measured by creatinine clearance is 25 ml/min or less or when the serum creatinine reaches 4 mg/dl. Optimally, it is best to place an AVF 6-12 months before the start of HD therapy or as far in advance as possible to allow time for maximum maturation of the vein before use. Unlike synthetic vascular access, there is no evidence that early placement of an AVF leads to the development of earlier vascular access complications (NKF, 2001).

Advantages. Compared to other types of vascular access, there are several major advantages of the AVF. Primarily, the incidence of clotting and infection are much less than with synthetic bridge grafts and external devices. There is no concern for allergic response as with synthetic bridge grafts. Because the AVF is native vasculature, the cannulation points will heal rather than seal with a fibrin plug as in the synthetic bridge graft. Lastly, a well-developed and maintained AVF has the greatest longevity and lowest incidence of complications than any other type of vascular access for HD (Gibson et al., 2001; Huber, Carter, Carter, & Seeger, 2003).

Disadvantages. Disadvantages of an AVF are few. The major disadvantage is the length of time required for maturation before the fistula can be safely cannulated and used. Length of time to maturation depends upon the quality of the vessels, the anastomosis, and how well the patient exercises the fistula extremity. The skills required to create and cannulate the AVF differ from those required to implant and cannulate a synthetic bridge graft. Special training is required, and skill in cannulating one type of access does not equate with skill in cannulating the other.

Placement. Placement site for an AVF is clearly outlined in the K/DOQI guidelines in order of priority. See Table 24-3

Table 24-3
Placement of Access in Order of Preference by Type

		Advantages	Disadvantages
1	Wrist: radial cephalic	Easy to create Longer patency rate Fewer complications Lower morbidity	Failure to mature Long maturation time Lower blood flow Negative cosmetic impact
2	Elbow: brachial cephalic	Higher blood flow Easily cannulated Longer patency rate Cosmetically easier to hide under clothing	More difficult to create Increased arm swelling Increased incidence of steal
3	Forearm AVG	Large surface area Preserves upper arm vasculature for future access Easy to cannulate Less time to mature than AVF Shorter patency rate	Smaller outflow vessels may increase rate of thrombosis Increased pain and swelling More interventions required Negative cosmetic impact Increased pain and swelling
4	Transposed brachial basilic	Patency better than AVG	Two operations required
5	Upper arm AVG	Less time to mature than AVF Large surface area Easy to cannulate Larger outflow veins improve flow Cosmetically easier to hide under clothing Shorter patency rate	Increased pain and swelling More interventions required Impacts future use of upper arm vasculature

Note: Adapted from NKF (2001). *K/DOQI clinical practice for vascular access guidelines 3 & 4.*

for most frequently used sites and placement priority. There are several configurations that can be used in the creation of an AVF (Bruns & Jennings, 2003; Cull et al., 2002; Gormus, Ozergin, Durgut, Yuksek, & Solak, 2003; Hossny, 2003; Konner, 2003). The non-dominant arm is the preferred extremity in order to allow the patient freedom of dominant arm movement while on HD. Pre-AVF patient education regarding the avoidance of venipunctures and blood pressure measurements in the targeted arm will help to preserve the vasculature so that the best possible site can be chosen for AVF placement (Malovr, 2003a).

Complications. Complications of AVF can be divided into early and late failure. Early failure is usually caused by non-development of the vein or disturbances in blood flow dynamics within the vein. Early failure rates tend to be higher in women, older patients, and patients with diabetes, although there is evidence that careful preoperative evaluation and the use of diagnostic evaluation for suitable veins can enable even these patient populations to benefit from AVF placement (Allon et al., 2000; Feldman et al., 2003; Lok & Oliver, 2003; Malovrh, 2002). Non-development can be the result of insufficient vasculature, such as poor arterial flow, small vein size, or because the vessels are so deep they cannot be cannulated. In this case, there is a weak or absent thrill or bruit and surgical revision is required. A disruption in normal blood flow dynamics can be the result of a stenosis or stricture in the vein or multiple collateral veins in the vein chosen for arterialization. The presence of multiple collateral veins in the vessel chosen for arterialization allows so much runoff into these veins that the vein engorgement required to develop arterialization never occurs. Doppler

ultrasound or venography can be done to visualize collateral blood flow and determine which veins should be surgically ligated to allow development of the primary outflow vein (Faiyaz et al., 2002).

Failure due to venous stricture in the primary vein can cause venous hypertension, which can result in sore thumb syndrome or subclavian vein syndrome. In sore thumb syndrome, the vein stricture proximal to the anastomosis causes blood to flow down the thumb and the thumb veins become engorged as outflow is impeded. The result can be throbbing or pulsing of the distal veins accompanied by edema that can extend to the entire hand. Eventually the nail bed can become cyanotic with serous drainage. Ligation of the distal venous limb with a side-to-side anastomosis or performing an end-to-end or side-to-end anastomosis has virtually eliminated this complication (Konner, 2003). Subclavian vein syndrome results from venous engorgement when there is a subclavian vein stricture. Engorgement of the arm veins can result in swelling of the arm, neck, and face on the affected side. Diagnosis of venous hypertension is made by clinical assessment followed by either Doppler ultrasound or fistulography. Usually the latter is chosen as balloon angioplasty or stenting may be performed to attempt a reduction in the degree of stenosis (Neville, Abularrage, White, & Sidawy, 2004).

Late failure of an AVF can be caused by thrombosis, infection, or high output cardiac failure. K/DOQI recommends that AVF failure rate due to thrombosis should be less than 0.25 episodes per patient year. Thrombosis can be caused by stenosis of the outflow vein without collateral circulation, hypotension, volume depletion, hypercoagulability,

Table 24-4
Signs and Symptoms of Impending Thrombosis

- Change in quality of the bruit
- Difficulty cannulating
- Difficulty maintaining intradialytic blood flow
- Increase in venous pressure
- Decrease in arterial pressure
- Prolonged bleeding after needles are removed
- Unexplained increase in BUN and/or serum creatinine
- Unexplained decrease in Kt/V
- Black blood syndrome: blood becomes increasingly darker as recirculation causes the same blood to pass through the dialyzer and hemoconcentration occurs
- Absence of pulse on palpation
- Absence of bruit on auscultation

or occlusive compression of the access. Thrombosis can be anticipated with several clinical signs and symptoms (see Figure 24-4). Percutaneous transluminal angioplasty (PTA) can be used to treat stenoses, and prevention is the best treatment for either hypotension or volume depletion. If a hypercoagulable state is suspected, low dose anticoagulation may be utilized. There are mixed reports of success with the use of antithrombotics (Kaufman, 2000; O'Shea, Lawson, Reddan, Murphy, & Ortel, 2003). Unfortunately these have been shown to increase the risk of bleeding in the HD population, making this an alternative for only a select group of patients. Thrombosis of the AVF has, until recently, meant the demise of that access and the surgical creation of another. In the last few years, the use of lytic agents and PTA to restore patency in the thrombosed AVF has become more common, with a primary patency rate of over 90% and long-term patency over 80% (Liang et al., 2002; Schon & Mishler, 2000; Schon & Mishler, 2003).

Infection of the AVF is rare and per K/DOQI guidelines should not exceed 1%. Infection is usually caused by inattention to aseptic technique during cannulation or poor patient hygiene. Signs and symptoms include pain, inflammation, or drainage anywhere along the course of the AVF. Any fever of unknown origin should trigger a thorough inspection of the AVF, and usually, antibiotics are quite effective in the treatment of an infected AVF. Venous cannulation distal to the inflammation should be avoided. If septic emboli are suspected, the AVF should be surgically explored and a takedown may be indicated.

High output cardiac failure results from the AVF creating a decrease in peripheral resistance, which results in increased cardiac output (MacRae et al., 2004). This usually occurs in the setting of the development of a large AVF in combination with severe anemia or pre-existing cardiovascular disease. Signs and symptoms occur with the patient at or near their dry weight and include pulmonary crackles, tachycardia, shortness of breath, and jugular vein distention. Peripheral edema may or may not be present along with confusion and hypoxemia. Treatment of high output cardiac failure is surgical. Flow through the AVF must be decreased either by an attempt at banding or by ligating and eliminating the AVF altogether. When high output cardiac failure is

suspected, the cardiopulmonary status of the patient should be carefully assessed at each HD treatment. Hemoglobin and hematocrit should be monitored carefully to prevent exacerbation due to anemia. If the patient becomes symptomatic, when the patient is not receiving HD, the AVF extremity may be wrapped with an ace bandage to increase peripheral resistance taking care not to completely occlude the flow. The patient will need to know how to: remove and reapply the ace bandage; modify daily activities until the problem is corrected; minimize interdialytic weight gains, as this will exacerbate the problem; and report any change in symptoms immediately.

Assessment. Assessment of the AVF should include inspection for approximation of the suture line in the first postoperative week and from the immediate postoperative period on, any signs or symptoms of infection, the presence of edema, any areas of induration, and the presence of collateral veins. A thrill should be palpable at the anastomosis and a bruit audible along the length of the primary vein. As the AVF matures, the thrill should become more palpable along the length of the vein. With the application of a tourniquet, dilated veins should be easily appreciated. Poorly defined veins, hardened areas within the vein that might signify previous hematoma, or aneurysmal dilatations, should be avoided for cannulation. In order to identify problems early, documentation should begin with the first inspection of a new AVF and should be standardized to include the condition of the anastomosis and the ease of cannulation, the size and condition of the veins, the distance from the anastomosis that the bruit is audible, the degree of maturation and presence of collateral veins, where needles were placed for the HD treatment, and how long it took for bleeding to cease after the treatment ended (Hartigan & White, 2001).

Cannulation technique. Cannulation of an AVF takes a certain amount of skill. The most commonly approved method of skin preparation precannulation is to have the patient wash the area with an antibacterial soap before applying 10% povidone iodine, 2% clorhexidine, or 70% alcohol to the cannulation site. A tourniquet should be used to cannulate the AVF regardless of vessel size. This prevents trauma to the vessel intima. The angle of needle insertion should be 25-30 degrees or less. A steeper angle should be used in people with a deeper access. A steeper angle of insertion increases the risk of nicking the back wall of the vessel and infiltration. The angle of the needle should be flattened as soon as flashback is obtained again to prevent nicking of the back of the vein. Needle sites should be changed with each HD session in order to promote the use of the largest fistula surface area available. This increases the longevity of the fistula and prevents the development of aneurysmal dilatation of the AVF. Cannulation toward the anastomosis for the arterial flow and away from the anastomosis for the venous return with the needles placed at least 1.5-2 inches apart minimizes the amount of recirculation that will occur.

Another technique for cannulation of an AVF is "buttonhole" or "constant site" cannulation. Originally described by Twardowski and Kubara (1979), the repeated cannulation into the same site creates a tunnel of scar tissue over a period of 2-3 weeks. After the buttonhole has been created, a dull needle is used for future cannulation (Buttonhole Needle Sets, Medisystems Corporation). The buttonhole technique was originally used in AVF with limited sites for cannulation. Additional advantages of this technique include less painful cannulation, decreased chance of infiltration, and ease of cannulation for home HD patients. It is recommended that the area chosen for each buttonhole be relatively straight and easily accessible to the patient that might wish to self-cannulate (Twardowski, 1995; Twardowski & Kubara, 1979). There are no data available regarding the use of the buttonhole technique with synthetic vascular access. Regardless of cannulation technique, needles should be securely taped to the patient's arm and bloodlines secured to the patient's arm or clothing to prevent accidental dislodgement (Brouwer, 1995; NKF, 1997). The access should remain visible at all times during dialysis to facilitate frequent assessment by the nursing staff.

Patient education. Patients who are candidates for AVFs should hear early in their pre-HD education that venipuncture and blood pressure measurements in the targeted arm should be avoided. After placement of the AVF, this should continue. About 10-14 days postoperatively, after the suture line is well approximated and provided there is no drainage and minimal swelling, exercises to help maturation of the AVF can be started. A light tourniquet can be applied above the level of the AVF and a rubber ball, rolled up sock, or commercially available handgrip is squeezed for 5-10 minutes four to five times a day. If the patient watches television, the exercises should be done each time the commercials come on for the duration of the commercials. A full day's exercises can be accomplished during a 2-hour program, and this is a good way for the patient to remember to complete them. The patient should be taught how to palpate the AVF for a thrill, to avoid sleeping on or wearing anything tight on the access extremity, how to recognize and report signs and symptoms of infection, and how to stop any bleeding that may occur. It is important the patient understand that this is his or her lifeline and that ultimate control belongs to him or her. The patient is responsible for ensuring the HD staff cleanse the area properly and rotate sites when cannulating. If possible, the patient should learn how to self-cannulate (Hartigan & White, 2001; Malvohr, 2003a).

AV Bridge Grafts

An AV bridge graft is a biologic, semibiologic, or synthetic conduit implanted subcutaneously and interposed between an artery and a vein. Biologic grafts are created from a saphenous vein or other transplanted native vessel. Semibiologic grafts are bovine heterografts – bovine carotid artery or mesenteric vein that has been treated to remove proteins (Johnson & Kenoyer, 1974; Richie, Withers, Petracek, & Conkle, 1978) or modified human umbilical vein graft – a human umbilical vein that has been treated to destroy collagen cells and then covered with a Dacron mesh. Synthetic grafts are created from polytetraflouroethylene (PTFE) (Butler, Baker, & Johnson, 1977; Raju, 1987) or expanded polytetraflouroethylene (ePTFE) (Baker, Johnson, & Goldfarb, 1976). PTFE is the most frequently used synthetic material for HD access. These are most commonly referred to as grafts or synthetic AV grafts (AVG). Needles are insert-

ed into the graft material in a way that is similar to the cannulation of an AVF in order to remove and return blood during the HD procedure. AVGs are generally used when the patient's vasculature is unable to support the creation and/or maturation of an AVF or after the failure of an AVF.

K/DOQI guidelines recommend AVGs be placed 3-6 weeks prior to the start of HD, usually in anticipation of the need to start HD within the following several weeks.

Advantages. There are several advantages of a graft over an AVF. A graft can usually be used as soon as the operative swelling decreases and the subcutaneous tunnel tissue adheres to the graft material (NKF, 2001). Therefore, a graft can be functional in 2-3 weeks as opposed to the months required in the use of an AVF. In the elderly, diabetic, or malnourished patient, healing may take somewhat longer. The length of the graft can be used for cannulation so there may be more total surface area available for cannulation than with an AVF. The size of the graft and its blood flow are not dependent upon maturation but instead upon the size of the graft used for implantation (Paulson, Ram, & Zibari, 2002). Lastly, cannulation of a large bore graft can sometimes be easier than cannulation of even a mature small peripheral vein, even after it has matured.

Disadvantages. Unfortunately, there are as many disadvantages as advantages to the use of synthetic grafts. There is a high incidence of infection as compared to AVFs. Because the graft is synthetic, it will act as a site for colonization should bacteria enter the bloodstream for any reason (Raju, 1987). There is always the potential for an allergic response to the synthetic graft material. There is an increased rate of thrombosis (Back & White, 2002; Beathard, 2002), and puncture sites don't heal, they merely seal. In-growth of collagen into the graft material helps to stabilize the graft and allows this sealing action. Early use of the AVG before the adherence of subcutaneous tunnel tissue into the wall of the graft increases the potential for bleeding and hematoma formation along the tunnel, which can potentially ruin the access (Back & White, 2002; NKF, 2001). The slightly roughened areas along the walls of the graft that develop over time from multiple punctures result in platelet aggregation that ultimately can lead to thrombosis (Back & White, 2002; Mickley, 2004) (see Figure 24-2). Neo-intimal hyperplasia occurs at the graft vein anastomosis and is the most frequent cause of graft stenosis and subsequent thrombosis (Mickley, 2004; Roy-Choudhury et al., 2001). Reports of primary patency rates range from 23% to 38% at 1 year (Gibson et al., 2001; Miller, Carlton, Deierhoi, Redden, & Allon, 2000) with most grafts requiring balloon angioplasty or surgical revision about every 12-18 months. The average lifespan for the use of the same surgical site is from 3-5 years, a much shorter survival span than with an AVF (Lilly et al., 2001; Palder et al., 1985).

Placement. A graft can be placed between any suitable artery and vein as long as it can be placed in a subcutaneous location superficially enough to be seen and cannulated easily (Paulson et al., 2002). The K/DOQI recommendations are to begin with the forearms and work proximally as necessary (see Table 24-3). Usually one begins with a forearm loop, the arterial and venous anastomoses being at the antecubital space. When the forearm loop must be abandoned, an upper

Figure 24-2
Note the Roughened Areas of the Synthetic Graft Where Platelet Aggregation Can Occur

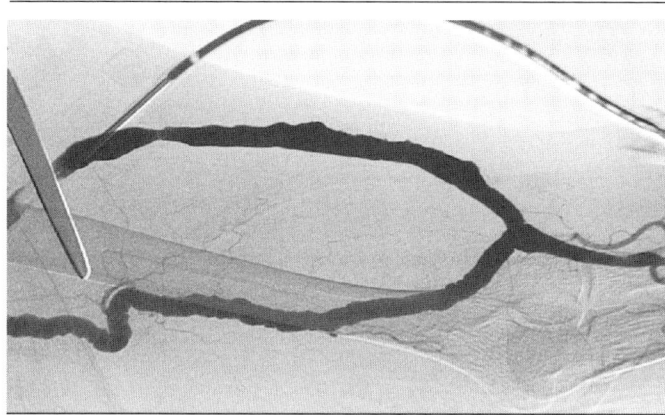

Figure 24-3
Long Area of Stenosis at the Venous Anastomosis

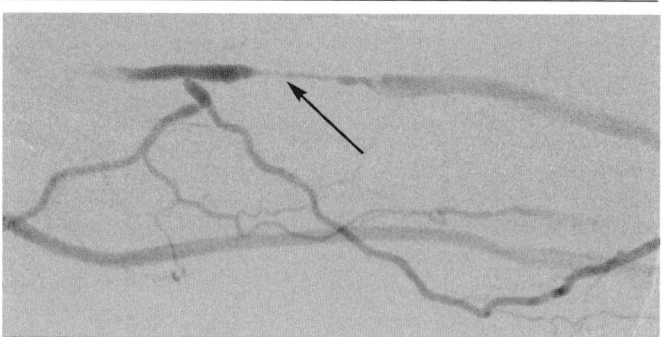

arm curved can be placed. Grafts can be placed in the thigh but pose a greater risk for ischemia and infection due to increased arterial size and proximity to the groin (Miller, Robbin, Barker, & Allon 2003; Tashjian et al., 2002).

Complications. Thrombosis is the most frequent graft complication and can occur from anatomic or non-anatomic causes. K/DOQI recommends that AVG failure due to thrombosis should not exceed 0.5 episodes per patient year. Anatomically, stenosis, or narrowing of a vein due to intimal hyperplasia, can occur in the outflow vein or proximal veins that drain the graft and accounts for more than 80% of all graft thromboses (Kanterman et al., 1995; Roy-Choudhury et al., 2001). Venous anastomosis stenosis is the most commonly found stenosis (see Figure 24-3). Because of the change in flow dynamics within the stenosed graft, the quality of the bruit will change, there may be difficulty in cannulation, it may be difficult to maintain the prescribed blood flow during the HD treatment, venous pressure may increase or arterial pressure decrease, and there may be prolonged bleeding after needles are removed (Paulson et al., 2002). The occurrence of any of these should prompt investigation of the cause. The diagnosis can be made by percent recirculation > 10% (see Table 24-5), seeing a downward trend in Kt/V measurements or access flow measurements, Doppler ultrasound, or fistulogram. The fistulogram has become the gold standard for determining the presence and location of vascular access stenosis (O'Reilly et al., 1978; Schwab, 1999). The increased use of prospective surveillance of all vascular access has led to a decrease in the use of recirculation studies, and in many cases, either Doppler ultrasound or fistulogram is performed when downward trends in Kt/V or access flow begin to occur (Paulson et al., 2002). Treatment is by PTA or surgical revision depending upon the stenosis location, severity, and response to PTA (Aburahma, Hopkins, Wulu, & Cook, 2002; Clark & Rajan, 2004). Although patient situation and needs must be taken into account, K/DOQI recommendations are for surgical revision if angioplasty is required more than twice within 3 months. Stents may be useful for recurring stenoses in selected patients.

Thrombosis can also occur from nonanatomic causes such as hypotension, volume depletion, hypercoagulable states, or occlusive compression of the access. Diagnosis of a nonanatomic cause for thrombosis is made in the absence of an anatomic finding on Doppler ultrasound or fistulogram. Treatment of the nonanatomic thrombosis addresses the causative factor and centers on prevention of reoccurrence. Prevention of hypotension/volume depletion during the HD treatment can be accomplished by frequently reassessing dry weight, avoidance of excessive ultrafiltration, the use of ultrafiltration or sodium modeling, and assessment of the patient's antihypertensive regimen. Referral for a hypercoagulopathic workup may be made if no other contributing factors can be identified. However, there are many physiological causes for enhanced thrombosis in the HD patient and, in particular, with the use of AVGs (Back & White, 2002; Casserly & Dember, 2003). Antithrombotic therapy may be indicated in select circumstances (Kaufman, 2000; O'Shea et al., 2003).

AVG infection is second only to the rate of infection in HD catheters. K/DOQI recommends that the rate of infection in AVG not exceed 10%. Infection usually occurs due to a break in aseptic technique during cannulation or poor hygiene and care of the access extremity and also can occur from bacterial seeding from another infected site in the body (Raju, 1987, Ready, 2002). Signs and symptoms of graft infection include redness, pain, swelling, or drainage from any area of the graft. Usually, but not always, graft infection is accompanied by fever and chills or rigor. Any unexplained temperature in a patient with a graft in place should be investigated, as there is evidence that even without any clinical signs, abandoned grafts can be a source of infection (Nasar & Ayus, 2000; Sheikh-Hamad & Ayus, 1998). Suspicion of infection in an abandoned or asymptomatic AVG can be investigated with the use of an Indium scan (Ayus & Sheikh-Hamad, 1998; Sheikh-Hamad & Ayus, 1998). Complications that can occur as a result of graft infection are thrombosis, septic emboli, endocarditis, sepsis, and possible erosion of the skin over the area of infection with resultant hemorrhage (Minga, Flanagan, & Allon, 2001; Ready, 2002). Diagnosis is usually made by clinical exam and blood and/or site cultures. Treatment of graft infection starts with antibiotics. In the presence of bacteremia or if the infection involves the graft itself, surgical excision is the treatment of choice. After completion of antibiotic therapy and negative blood cultures, a new vascular access can be placed.

A pseudoaneurysm can occur anywhere along the

course of a graft as a result of unsealed needle puncture sites and/or poor hemostasis (Back & White, 2002). This is an unusual dilatation of the graft that can be prevented by rotating needle sites and applying even pressure to the puncture site and underlying graft when needles are removed post HD treatment (Brouwer, 1995). Diagnosis of pseudoaneurysm is made by clinical assessment, Doppler ultrasound, or fistulogram. Treatment is by surgical revision only if the pseudoaneurysm is rapidly expanding, exceeds two times the diameter of the graft, threatens the viability of the overlying skin, or is infected (NKF, 2001).

Steal syndrome is a graft complication that requires immediate attention. It is so called because the graft diverts blood flow or steals blood from the distal portion of the limb causing ischemia. This occurs more commonly in the diabetic, the elderly, those with preexisting peripheral vascular disease, and in those with multiple previous vascular accesses in the same extremity. Signs and symptoms include pain distal to the anastomosis, numbness, tingling, pallor, and poor capillary refill in the affected fingers and hand. These problems usually become worse during the dialysis treatment as even more blood is shunted away from the affected area (Wilson, 2002). Any or all of the aforementioned may be present with increasing severity over time and possible progression to ischemic fingertips. Diagnosis is usually made on the basis of symptoms, although arterial Dopplers may be used to provide conclusive evidence in mild cases. Treatment may be to ligate the vascular access in order to restore circulation the hand. If possible, a distal revascularization and interval ligation can be done (Knox, Berman, Hughes, Gentile, & Mills, 2002). For mild steal, comfort measures include keeping the hand warm, placing the hand in a dependent position during the dialysis treatment to facilitate arterial flow, and encouraging the patient to perform hand exercises to maintain blood supply.

Lastly, when a needle passes through the graft during cannulation, it can create a fistula between the graft and an underlying vein. Blood is then shunted from the AVG to the underlying vein thus disturbing the blood flow pattern. Signs and symptoms include a strong pulsation in the area of the graft that was previously not present. Diagnosis is made through clinical assessment, Doppler flow studies, and/or fistulogram. Referral should be made to a vascular surgeon, and treatment can range from observation to surgical revision.

Assessment. Assessment of the AVG should include inspection for approximation of the suture lines in the first postoperative week and from the immediate postoperative period on, any signs or symptoms of infection. Edema and ecchymosis should be expected as a result of the tunneling required during operative placement of the graft material. The swelling may persist for 1-3 weeks, gradually decreasing as the subcutaneous trauma subsides. A thrill should be palpable at the arterial anastomosis and along the length of the AVG. As the swelling decreases, the bruit should become more palpable along the length of the graft. Hardened areas along the graft length that might signify remaining postoperative hematoma should be avoided during cannulation. In order to identify problems early, documentation should begin with the first inspection of a new AVG and should be

standardized to include the condition of the anastomosis and the ease of cannulation, the size and condition of the graft, the distance from the anastomosis that the bruit is audible, where needles were placed for the HD treatment, and how long it took for bleeding to cease after the treatment ended.

Cannulation technique. Different from an AVF where direction of blood flow is easily determined, the direction of blood flow in a forearm loop AVG will depend on how the surgeon configured the graft. Although the most common forearm loop configuration results in the venous end of the graft being on the thumb side, this is not always the case. It is, therefore, important to determine direction of flow prior to the first use of the AVG. There are several ways to accomplish this. Auscultation will usually reveal a stronger bruit close to the anastomosis on the arterial side of the graft. Momentarily occluding the AVG at the midportion should reveal a diminished bruit and thrill on the venous side. After cannulation, if mid graft pressure is applied, the flashback should remain on the arterial side and greatly diminish or disappear on the venous side. The arterial side of the AVG will maintain a pulse (Brouwer, 1995). The most commonly approved method of skin preparation pre-cannulation is to have the patient wash the area with an antibacterial soap before applying 10% povidone iodine, 2% clorhexidine, or 70% alcohol to the cannulation site. An AVG should never be cannulated if there is no evidence of a thrill or bruit as lytic therapy is contraindicated in recently cannulated access.

Early cannulation of an AVG carries the risk of dissection of graft material and hemorrhage into the tunnel. Until granulation tissue has had time to incorporate into the wall of the graft, cannulation should be performed carefully to prevent damage to either the AVG or the peripheral circulation. If significant swelling still exists, the skin on both sides of the graft material should be gently depressed in order to displace the edema and enable palpation of the graft itself. The needles should be taped carefully to the skin as they can easily be displaced as the edema resettles into the surrounding tissue. Early cannulation of an AVG should only be performed by the most experienced clinicians. Cannulation of an AVG is similar to that of an AVF with the notable exception of needle angle. The angle of needle insertion should be approximately 45 degrees. A lesser angle of insertion increases the risk of dragging the cutting edge of the needle along the course of the graft, and a steeper angle increases the risk of perforating the back wall of the graft. If the AVG is not easily cannulated, probing is not recommended as the bottom or side of the graft material can be punctured and hemorrhage into the tunnel can ensue. The needle should be removed and pressure should be applied until hemostasis occurs prior to trying to cannulate again. The angle of the needle should be flattened as soon as flashback is obtained again to prevent nicking of the back of the AVG (Hartigan & White, 2001). Needle sites should be rotated with each HD session with 50% of the surface area of the AVG being used for arterial cannulation and 50% for venous cannulation. This will increase the longevity of the AVG and help to prevent the development of pseudoaneurysms. Most nurses use retrograde cannulation (toward the arterial anastomosis for the arterial flow and toward the venous anastomosis for the venous return) with the needles placed at least 1.5-2 inches apart. This minimizes the amount of recirculation that will occur. Antegrade cannulation with needle tips at least 1-1.5 inches apart is also acceptable. Needles should be securely taped to the patient's arm and bloodlines secured to the patient's arm or clothing to prevent accidental dislodgement (Brower, 1995; NKF, 2001). The access should remain visible at all times during dialysis to facilitate frequent assessment by the nursing staff.

Patient education. Postoperatively, the patient should be instructed to elevate and abduct the affected extremity and to use the extremity as much as possible to facilitate venous return and minimize swelling. Patients should hear that venipuncture and blood pressure measurements in the affected arm should be avoided. The patient should be taught how to palpate the AVG for a thrill, to avoid sleeping on or wearing anything tight on the access extremity, how to recognize and report signs and symptoms of infection, and how to stop any bleeding that may occur. The patient should be taught the importance of prophylactic antibiotics before any invasive procedure, including dental work, and counseled to keep the dialysis staff informed should such a procedure be scheduled. It is important the patient understand that this is his or her lifeline and that ultimate control belongs to him or her. The patient is responsible for ensuring the HD staff cleanse the area properly and rotate sites when cannulating. If possible, the patient should learn how to self-cannulate (Hartigan & White, 2001).

Central Venous Catheters

Central venous catheters for HD are large bore double lumen catheters constructed of rigid or semi rigid material that are placed percutaneously. The ports are designated as arterial (red) or venous (blue) with the arterial lumen ending proximal to the venous in order to minimize recirculation of the blood (Schwab & Beathard, 1999).

There are many HD catheters on the market and all are similar (Wentling, 2004). In single catheters with double lumens, multiple side holes and large bore lumens allow a large volume of blood flow. Twin catheters that are placed side by side have the advantage of minimizing recirculation even more as the catheter tips can be placed where desired and side holes are circumferential (Perini et al., 2000). In addition, in the case of thrombus, infection, or malfunction, each catheter can be removed independently (Wivell et al., 2001). Catheters for short-term and long-term use have a slightly different design and have different indications (Ash, 2001; Depner, 2001).

Short-term catheters are placed when use is for 1-3 weeks or less, usually when immediate access to the bloodstream is needed. They can be used temporarily for HD, plasmapheresis, when a peritoneal dialysis (PD) patient is recovering from peritonitis that required removal of the PD catheter, temporarily after renal transplantation, or for other renal replacement therapies for acute renal failure. They are commonly used after removal of a permanent access because of infection or while waiting for a thrombectomy or revision of an existing vascular access (Oliver, 2001; Schwab & Beathard, 1999).

Long-term catheters, or chronic tunneled cuffed catheters, are usually used if temporary access is required for

Table 24-5
Procedure for Drawing Noninvasive Two Needle Stop Flow Percent Recirculation

1. Measure within the first 30 minutes after prescribed blood flow is established
2. Turn off ultrafiltration
3. Blood samples are drawn simultaneously from arterial (A) and venous (V) lines and labeled as such
4. Stop blood pump and clamp arterial line
5. Separate the arterial needle and bloodline
6. Withdraw 10 ml blood from arterial line, keep sterile, set aside
7. Within 30 sec draw 5 ml from arterial needle line and label systemic sample (S)
8. Return the 10 ml of sterile blood that was set aside
9. Reconnect arterial bloodline and needle
10. Unclamp the line and resume dialysis
11. Measure blood urea nitrogen levels in the three samples
12. Compute recirculation: % recirc = 100(S-A)/(S-V)
13. If % recirc > 10% refer for angiography or ultrasound

longer than 3 weeks, such as when there is a prolonged course of acute renal failure; if a prolonged course of antibiotics is required prior to replacement of an AVG or PD catheter; or while waiting for an AVF to mature. In addition, these catheters can be used when there are no longer any options for traditional vascular access because of lack of available sites remaining for placement or because of peripheral vascular disease (Weijmer & ter Wee, 2004; Work, 2002). K/DOQI defines a chronic catheter as one being in place for more than 3 months and recommends that they be used on less than 10% of the patients in a given HD unit (NKF, 2001). Unfortunately, as HD has improved, patients are living longer and running out of sites for permanent access, and catheter use has increased. Whereas catheters began as a temporary solution for access need, they are increasingly used as the patient's primary access (Butterly & Schwab, 2001).

Advantages. The advantages of short-term catheters are that they can be easily placed at the bedside in the internal jugular, femoral, or subclavian vein and can be used immediately after placement is confirmed by chest X-ray (Weijmer, Vervolet, & ter Wee, 2004).

Long-term catheters are usually made of a softer material than temporary catheters in order to minimize damage to tissues as they stay in place so much longer. The long-term catheter is tunneled subcutaneously and enters the circulation at the vein rather than at the skin insertion site to minimize migration of microorganisms. A Dacron cuff encircling the catheter at the level of the subcutaneous tissue anchors the catheter and also acts to prevent microbial migration along the tunnel created by the catheter (Deutsch & White, 2002).

Disadvantages. Unfortunately, short-term catheters are easily infected, uncomfortable for the patient, and are associated with a high incidence of vein stenosis. Disadvantages that accompany tunneled cuffed catheter use are the same as for short-term catheters. In addition, these catheters must be placed either in the operating room or under ultrasound guidance in radiology. The risk of central vein stenosis or occlusion is greater as the catheter usually stays in place so much longer. Despite the cuff placement, infection remains a significant risk and removal of a cuffed catheter is a little more invasive as the cuff has to be dissected away from ingrown tissue.

Placement. Short-term catheters are usually placed at the bedside using sterile technique. Preferred placement is into the internal jugular vein, followed by the femoral, and lastly the subclavian vein. A catheter placed into the internal jugular vein may be left in place up to 3 weeks. There is less risk of pnuemothorax during insertion and the bleeding site is easily compressible after removal. Although there is a lower rate of central vein stenosis with the internal jugular placement, the dressing is difficult to secure and the infection and thrombosis rates are similar to that of other placement sites (Weijmer & ter Wee, 2004).

Short-term femoral vein catheters are generally removed within 3 to 5 days as they are easily infected if left in longer. The femoral vein is easily cannulated and the risk of insertion complications is low. In addition, the femoral vein catheter may be used immediately after placement. Unfortunately, the short-term femoral catheter is very uncomfortable for the patient as a straight leg, supine position must be maintained (Weijmer & ter Wee, 2004). Femoral vein catheters are contraindicated with iliofemoral thrombosis, deep vein thrombosis, or iliofemoral bypass.

The subclavian vein placement is the least preferred although the dressing is easily secured and the catheter may be left in place for several weeks. There is a higher risk of pneumothorax, it must be placed with the patient in a recumbent position, and thus is difficult to place in a patient with shortness of breath. In addition, the artery is not compressible if punctured during placement and there is a high rate of thrombosis and stenosis. Because of the high rate of subclavian vein stenosis, this site should be avoided if the patient will need permanent access in the future (Schwab et al., 1988; Weijmer et al., 2004).

Typically, tunneled cuffed catheters enter the skin below the level of the clavicle and are tunneled subcutaneously up to the level of the vein. As with temporary catheters, internal jugular placement is the site of choice, with subclavian vein placement resulting in increased incidence of subclavian vein stenosis. Unless fluoroscopy is used during placement of the catheter, placement must be confirmed with chest x-ray prior to use (Work, 2002). Use of the femoral vein is possible, but the incidence of infection is much higher with this site and should only be used as a last resort. There are other placement options such as the translumbar or transthoracic placement into the vena cava, but these are used infrequently and usually only if all other options for vascular access have been exhausted (Deutsch & White, 2002; Smith, Ryan, & Reddan, 2004).

Complications. Complications of catheter use can be categorized into early and late. Early complications are those associated with the placement procedure itself. Central vein catheter complications include pneumothorax, hemothorax, arterial puncture, tissue perforation of the brachial plexus, trachea, superior vena cava or myocardium, sheared catheter

with embolization, and dysrhythmias (Teichgraber, Gebauer, Benter, & Wagner, 2003). Inadvertent femoral artery puncture can cause a retroperitoneal bleed evidenced by a drop in blood pressure or decreased pulses in the affected extremity. Per K/DOQI guidelines, catheter insertion complications such as pneumothorax, air embolism, hemothorax, or hematoma requiring evacuation should not exceed 2%.

Late complications are those associated with catheter use and are more varied. Air embolism can occur as a complication of the HD treatment (see the chapter on Hemodialysis) or from the patient shearing the catheter above the level of the catheter clamps at a location other than the dialysis unit. Patient teaching regarding catheter care should always include emergency management of a cut catheter.

Infection is a common complication seen with the use of catheters and can be as simple as an exit site infection or as complicated as line sepsis. Exit site infections occur in 8% - 20% of catheters and are characterized by pus or cellulitis at the site. The patient will often complain of pain at the site. Topical antibiotics are required and drainage from the tunnel should always be cultured so that the appropriate parenteral antibiotics can be administered. For persistent exit site or tunnel infection, the catheter may need to be removed (Saad, 2001). Although K/DOQI recommends that systemic infection should be less than 10% at 3 months in those patients with catheters and less than 50% at 1 year, catheter-related septicemia occurs in 2%-20% of all catheters. Colonization occurs primarily from the exit site, although the source may also be a distant focus that seeds the catheter. There may be pus or cellulitis at the exit site, fever and shaking chills are common, and the patient will have clinical signs of sepsis. Unless another source of infection can be identified, prompt removal of the catheter is required along with administration of broad spectrum parenteral antibiotics until the organism can be identified. The catheter can be replaced after 24-48 hours in a new site unless the patient remains clinically septic, in which case in and out femoral catheterization may be required until blood cultures are negative (Granata, D'Intini, Bellomo, & Ronco, 2004; Saad, 2001). Bacterial endocarditis is increasingly being seen as a complication of catheter sepsis (Marr et al., 1998). There has been some recent success with the instillation of an antibiotic lock solution into the lumen of the catheter at the termination of HD. This seems to eliminate the bacterial biofilm that develops on the catheter within days of placement and coats the inner lumen of the catheter (Krishnasami et al., 2002; Weijmer et al., 2004).

Thrombus is another common complication of dialysis catheters. A mural thrombus occurs along the vein wall, usually at the catheter insertion site, and is commonly due to epithelial injury. A thrombus in the catheter itself can occur along the inner lumen of the catheter. A fibrin sheath can develop along the external surface of the catheter forming a sleeve from the point of venous blood entry into the catheter and extending around the tip of the catheter (Xiang, Verbeken, Van Lommel, Stas, & De Wever, 2001) (see Figure 24-4). Diagnosis of thrombus is usually considered when there is difficulty maintaining blood flow during the HD treatment or when there is difficulty aspirating or flushing the catheter. A Doppler ultrasound or angiogram can be used to confirm the presence and location of the thrombus. Thrombolytic agents can be instilled into the catheter to lyse the intracatheter thrombus (Clase, Crowther, Ingram, & Cina, 2001; Little & Walshe, 2002). If unsuccessful, the catheter may need to be exchanged. If a fibrin sheath is present, removing and exchanging the catheter using the same entry site without disrupting the sheath will not remedy the problem. The new catheter will simply slide into the old fibrin sheath like putting a hand in a glove. Usually a wire with a balloon attached is placed through the old catheter, the catheter is removed, the balloon is inflated to break up the sheath, and then a new catheter is placed over the wire. Alternatively, fibrin stripping can be attempted. This is a procedure most commonly performed in radiology by threading a snare up through the aorta, encircling the catheter, and stripping the sheath off (Teichgraber et al., 2003). Persistent mural thrombus or catheter tip thrombus may require systemic thrombolytic therapy, especially if a tip thrombus is large enough to cause serious consequence if it breaks off during removal of the catheter (Beathard, 2001; Clase et al., 2001).

Stenosis of the catheterized vessel occurs as the catheter comes in contact with the vessel wall and causes trauma and scarring. Scarring begins to occur very quickly and, thus, the recommendation is that catheters be used only when absolutely necessary and other type of access created as quickly as possible. Stenosis of the vessel remains asymptomatic until the lumen of the vessel becomes narrow enough to cause venous hypertension. At this point the arm on the affected side becomes swollen and chest wall collaterals begin to develop (Schwab et al., 1988). Stenosis is diagnosed by Doppler ultrasound or angiogram and can be remedied by either balloon angioplasty or stenting. Unfortunately, stenotic lesions are prone to reoccur and frequently require intermittent angioplasty or stenting to maintain vein patency (Gray et al., 1995). Development of a central vein stenosis can limit the use of the involved extremity for future access.

Catheter malposition can affect the quality of HD received. This can be seen if the catheter abuts the vein wall, becomes kinked, has an improperly placed constricting suture, or if the catheter has moved from the proper position after placement. Diagnosis is usually made by chest x-ray or angiogram, and catheter replacement or suture removal usually remedies the problem (Deutsch & White, 2002, Teichgraber et al., 2003).

Assessment. Catheter dressing changes should be done only by trained dialysis staff per specific HD unit protocol. There are many studies comparing dressing types and cleansing techniques for HD catheters (Gillies et al., 2003; Little & Palmer, 1998; Mann, Otlikowski, Gurrin, & Keil, 2001). The NKF-DOQI recommendations (NKF, 2001) state that skin disinfection should be done with chlorhexidine or povidone iodine and povidone iodine or mupirocin ointment should be applied to the catheter exit site. Catheter manufacturers have recommendations for the application of exit site ointments as interactions may occur depending upon the catheter material. A sterile occlusive dressing should cover the catheter insertion site and should be changed each dialysis treatment by dialysis staff. Not only does this help to

Figure 24-4
Thrombus and Fibrin Sheath on Twin Catheters

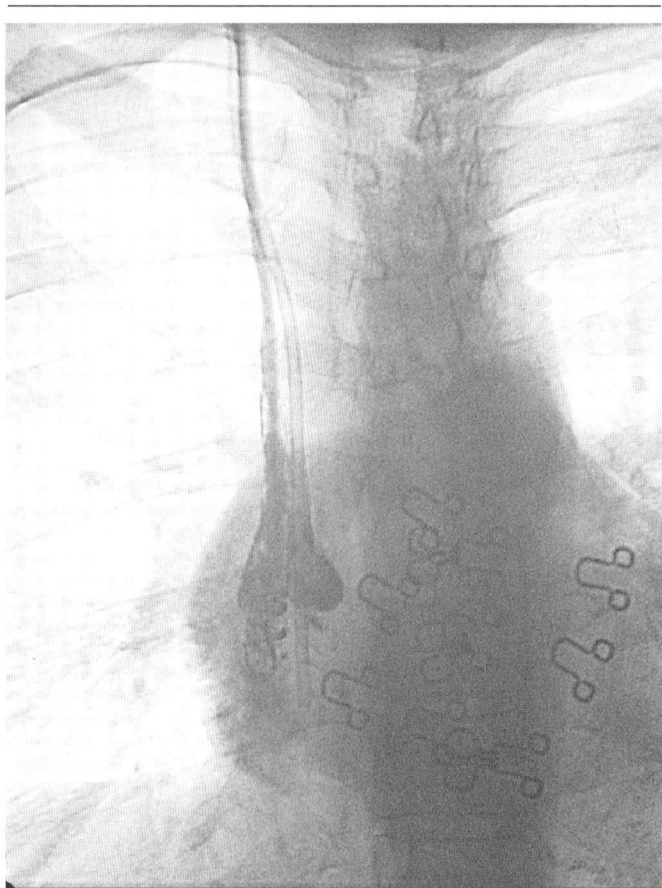

minimize the incidence of infection, but it also affords the opportunity to assess the insertion site. The insertion site should be assessed for redness or drainage and any drainage should be cultured. The tunnel should be assessed for redness and tenderness. Debris should be cleaned from the exit site with hydrogen peroxide, and povidone iodine should be applied and allowed to dry before re-applying the dressing. The dressing should be applied so that it does not pull on the catheter, and it should be labeled with the date, the words "do not flush," the amount of heparin and saline instilled per lumen, and the nurse's initials. The dialysis catheter should not be used for interdialytic infusions except in extreme circumstances with a specific doctor's order. Documentation should include the type and location of the catheter, any assessment findings, and interventions performed (NKF, 2001).

Using a catheter. Aseptic technique should be used when initiating or terminating HD using a catheter. Sterile 4x4s saturated in povidone iodine should be applied to both ports for 5 minutes prior to opening the catheter at both initiation and termination of the treatment. Because of the high incidence of nasal carriage of *staphylococcus aureus* (SA) and methicillin resistant *staphylococcus aureus* (MRSA) in HD patients and staff, both nurse and patient should wear a mask to minimize droplet contamination whenever opening the catheter ends. Before using the catheter, the indwelling solution should be aspirated, and after catheter use it should be flushed with normal saline prior to instilling whatever solution is being used. The most common instillation is a heparin saline mix with the dose dependent upon physician preference, unit protocol, and patient condition. It is important that the volume be equal to or slightly more than the volume of the internal lumen of the catheter (NKF, 2001). Information on lumen volumes is available from the manufacturer or distributor or may be found imprinted on the lumens of some catheters.

During use, there are several interventions that can be attempted to remedy low blood flows. Examining the catheter shaft for kinking, lowering the patient's head to increase central venous pressure, asking the patient to cough during aspiration of the catheter, changing the patient's position, and applying pressure to the exit site with a dressing in place are all interventions that may be attempted. If a temporary catheter is not sutured in place, one can attempt to rotate the catheter shaft. Reversing the bloodlines so that the arterial line is attached to the venous port and vice versa may be used as a last resort to improve blood flow (Hartigan & White, 2001). Ultimately, the use of fibrinolytic agents or a catheter change by the physician or interventional radiologist may be required.

Cuffed catheter removal should be done with the patient in a supine position by surgery or radiology, usually by whoever placed it. The supine position increases the pressure in the vein and inhibits the entrance of air into the vessel when the catheter is removed. Manual pressure should be applied to the site for 20 minutes then the exit site covered with povidone iodine ointment to air seal the site. After a sterile dressing is applied, the patient can resume a sitting position but should be observed for at least another 30 minutes.

Patient education. The patient must be given careful instructions about catheter care in order to optimize use and decrease the incidence of infection or catheter loss. The dressing must be kept clean and dry, and the catheter should remain taped to the skin or under the dressing. End ports and clamps should be bridge taped to prevent accidental disconnection. The patient should hear that they have the responsibility for ensuring that only dialysis personnel use the catheter and that they should insist that masks are worn when catheter care is being provided. Education regarding signs and symptoms of infection and how and to whom these should be reported should be given verbally and in writing for the patient to post at home in a place it can be easily seen. The patient should be able to demonstrate clamping the catheter in case of accidental cutting and the application of direct pressure for accidental removal of the catheter (Hartigan & White, 2001).

Subcutaneous Port Devices

Over the last several years subcutaneously placed metal ports attached to double lumen tunneled catheters have been introduced to the market (Beathard & Posen, 2000; Canaud et al., 1999; Levin et al., 1998; Schwab et al., 2002). These were modeled after the ports originally used for chemotherapy in the oncology population. There are several types available, all of which are accessed by some type of large bore needle. In the HD population subcutaneous ports are most often used in patients for whom there are no alter-

natives to long-term more permanent vascular access. Unfortunately, these have not been used in large populations and little data is available regarding long-term use.

The LifeSite is the port most consistently in use at this time. The LifeSite is made of a stainless steel/titanium alloy. It is a dome shaped valve that contains a pinch clamp that opens and closes when a standard 14-gauge dialysis needle is inserted or removed. The device is attached to a single lumen catheter and both port and catheter are internalized. The pinch clamp prevents access to the bloodstream unless the dialysis needle is in place. When the needle is removed, the pinch clamp closes, preventing blood leakage. Because each port has a single valve and catheter, two must be implanted. Each is cannulated using the buttonhole technique. The valve and buttonhole are irrigated with an antimicrobial solution before and after each use using a 25 gauge needle. The smaller needle cannot open the LifeSite valve, preventing inadvertent instillation of the antimicrobial solution into the bloodstream.

The LifeSite system has been evaluated in several clinical studies looking at blood flow rates, infection, device survival, complications, and ease of use from both a nursing and patient perspective. In all respects, data obtained showed similar outcomes to those of other dialysis catheters on the market. Dialysis staff and patients gave positive feedback related to ease of use and pain free cannulation. Unfortunately, infection rates have also proven similar to that of other dialysis catheters (Beathard & Posen, 2000; Moran, 2000; Rayan, Terramani, Weiss, & Chaikof, 2003; Ross, Narayan, Bergeron, Worthington, & Strom, 2002; Schwab et al., 2002). In addition, Rayan et al. (2003) report that traditional markers of line infection, such as pain and redness at the site, occurred in only 5 out of 17 patients. Infection in the remaining patients initially presented as sepsis.

Advantages. There are several advantages to the use of a subcutaneous device. As the entire device is internalized, the skin remains a barrier to infection. The ports themselves are made of metal and are durable so that replacement is minimal. There are no external limbs, decreasing the risk of contamination or damage by the patient. Additionally, patients concerned with cosmetic issues may prefer this type of access. In the small studies available, dialysis staff felt that there were few difficulties in using port devices and patient satisfaction was high (Beathard & Posen, 2000; Canaud et al., 1999).

Disadvantages. The disadvantages of long-term use of subcutaneous ports are similar to those of the central venous catheter. The catheter portion of the device is inserted into a central vein, and thus, although access to the catheter by dialysis personnel is different, catheter access to the circulation is the same. Port insertion must be done by someone well versed in the placement technique. An improperly placed port is difficult to access and can result in unnecessary pain for the patient and the possibility of hematoma formation (Moran & Prosl, 2004). There are specific needles required for use of some ports (Canaud et al., 1999). Unfortunately, the fact that subcutaneous ports are entirely internalized means that surgical or radiological intervention is required should problems arise. Increasingly, the interventional radiologist is becoming involved in the placement, intervention, and removal of some ports (Schwab et al., 2002).

Placement. The preferred site for port placement is in the upper chest with the cannulas placed in the internal jugular vein. Placement priority is similar to that of conventional tunneled HD catheters.

Complications. Complications of subcutaneously placed port devices are similar to those of central venous catheters with the addition of the immediate post placement issues related to wound healing. During insertion, an incision is made and the port is placed into a pocket created in the subcutaneous tissue. For placement of dual ports, two separate pockets are required to ensure stabilization of each device. Bleeding into the pocket, or the collection of fluid around the port device postoperatively, makes cannulation difficult, and the resulting fluid collection becomes an excellent medium for infection. A port placed too close to the surface of the skin can result in skin erosion over the surface of the port, but a port placed too deeply may be difficult to access (Moran & Prosl, 2004).

Use of improper needles can cause bleeding as can the use of the port by inexperienced personnel. Pocket hematomas are easily infected and can result in the loss of the access. The irrigation of the pocket with an antibiotic solution, alcohol, or a combination of both has been used with mixed results in treating port infections. Repeated positive cultures are cause for removal of the port device.

Assessment. The skin on and around the port should be inspected at each dialysis treatment for any signs of redness or swelling. Any signs of infection should be followed up with prophylactic antibiotics.

Use. Strict aseptic technique is required when accessing or de-accessing a port. Skin disinfection per unit protocol is essential in reducing the risk of infection. Only staff members knowledgeable about the proper accessing/de-accessing technique should be allowed to use the port.

Patient education. As with the use of catheters, meticulous attention to aseptic technique is imperative. Thorough knowledge of the device and recommended cannulation technique will help decrease complications. Any suspicion of infection should immediately be treated with intravenous antibiotics as infected ports must be surgically removed.

Patient teaching should be similar to that with centrally placed catheters. Interdialytic infusions should not be allowed, and only personnel familiar with the device should use it. The use of masks and aseptic technique will help to decrease the chance of infection. The patient should be taught how to inspect the site daily for signs of redness or infection. In addition, the patient should be taught the signs and symptoms of infection and to whom and how to report should they experience any problems.

Access Surveillance

Because of the dynamic state of vascular access in any given patient, every dialysis facility should establish some organized approach for the assessment of vascular access, diagnosis of complications, and the tracking of interventions performed (NKF, 2001). Goals are to increase the lifespan of each vascular access, improve the detection of significant stenosis before they occur, improve the early referral of patients for angioplasty or operative revision, and decrease the use of central lines.

Assessment

Surveillance begins with a clinical assessment performed and documented at least weekly. Persistent swelling, prolonged bleeding after needles are pulled, thrombosis or clots pulled from the needle during cannulation, any signs or symptoms of infection, change in appearance, increase in venous pressure or decrease in arterial pressure, or any temperature in the AVG patient should raise suspicion. Any alteration in the characteristics of the bruit or thrill should be evaluated. A thrill should be palpable at the arterial, mid, and venous portions of the access and a bruit should be audible. A palpable pulse without thrill indicates a low flow state. Intensification of the bruit is an indication of stricture or stenosis. Changes in temperature of the affected limb, especially of the hand or fingers, and of course any numbness, tingling, or pain should be evaluated.

Access Monitoring

There are several ways that access monitoring can be performed. Monitoring that can be done in the dialysis unit while the patient is dialyzing includes ultrasound dilution, dynamic venous pressure, static venous pressure, and recirculation studies.

Ultrasound dilution measures time transit as a bolus of saline is injected into the bloodlines and passes through an ultrasound detector clamped to the bloodlines. This method of measuring access flow has become the gold standard. Small ultrasound sensors are clipped onto both the arterial and venous bloodlines and normal saline is injected into the bloodline either from the patient's saline bag or by direct injection. A laptop computer is used to perform calculations based upon the amount of time it takes for the saline dilute blood to pass through the sensors. Measurements can be obtained for delivered blood flow, access recirculation, access flow, and cardiac output. Routine monitoring of vascular access with ultrasound dilution has been shown to decrease hospital days, thrombosis rate, missed treatments due to thrombosis, and the number of catheters used (McCarley et al., 2001). Advantages of ultrasound dilution include the accuracy and standardization of measurements, the ease of testing, and the ability to perform the testing while the patient is dialyzing. Disadvantages include the special equipment required (Transonic Systems, Inc., 2001).

Dynamic venous pressures can be measured at the beginning of every dialysis treatment by recording the venous pressure at QB 200 ml/min during the first 2-5 minutes of the treatment. Measurements should be obtained with the same size needle each time. Once a baseline is established, three successive measurements must exceed this in order for the change to be to be considered significant. Factors that can easily confound dynamic venous pressure measurements are needle placement or labile blood pressure of the patient (Segal & Weitzel, 2004). Static venous pressure is the venous pressure measurement at 0 QB expressed as a ratio with the mean arterial pressure. Static venous pressure is calculated using the venous drip chamber pressure added to the difference in height in cm between the venous drip

Table 24-6
K/DOQI Recommendations for Access Patency

	AVF	AVG	Tunneled Catheter
Thrombosis	Excluding failures in first 2 months of use: < 0.25 episodes/pt year	< 0.5 episodes/pt year	
Infection	< 1% over use life	< 10% over use life	< 10% at 3 months < 50% at 1 year
Primary access failure	No recommendations	30 day primary failure: Forearm straight < 15% Forearm loop < 10% Upper arm < 10%	< 5 % unable to deliver blood flow > 300 ml/min
Cumulative patency*	No recommendations	70% at 1 year 60% at 2 years 50% at 3 years	No recommendations due to variety of catheters in use

Note: * Cumulative patency – the number of AVF/AVGs that remain patent over a given time period.

chamber transducer and the venous needle in the access and normalized to systolic blood pressure (Dember, Holmberg, & Kaufman, 2002). Once again, the drawbacks to using static venous pressure monitoring are the effects of needle placement and blood pressure and, in this case, the accuracy of measurements and computations. The advantages to using static or dynamic venous pressures are that either is fairly reliable, readily available, and inexpensive to obtain. Both are less predictive of stenoses in native venous fistulae as opposed to bridge grafts due to collateral vessel development that can allow runoff and, thus, prevent higher venous pressures from developing (Segal & Weitzel, 2004). When using static or dynamic venous pressures to monitor vascular access, measurements should be done every 1 to 2 weeks and documented so that trends can be identified and investigated.

Recirculation studies are more predictive of stenosis in native fistulae. Any recirculation in a fistula or synthetic vascular access over 10% should be investigated by angiogram. Other monitoring methods that can be used include Doppler flow and magnetic resonance (MR). Both are too expensive to be done frequently and neither can be performed with the patient on dialysis. Doppler is a good predictor of stenosis, but results can be operator dependent, while MR is very accurate. Both are used more often in assessing access dysfunction rather than in routine access screening.

Data Tracking

In any setting, it is important to track access monitoring results and interventions or revisions performed for each access on each patient. Urea reduction ratio, Kt/V, angiograms or other diagnostics, clinical assessment, incidence of thrombosis, and incidence of infection are examples of the kinds of access monitoring that should be tracked for trend analysis. Each dialysis center should have a method for tracking access creation, complications, and interventions performed. The tracking of interventions performed should include the procedure performed, thrombectomy, angioplasty, or surgical revision, and the outcomes achieved. K/DOQI recommendations for patency can be seen in Table 24-6.

Figure 24-5
Graft AV fistulae

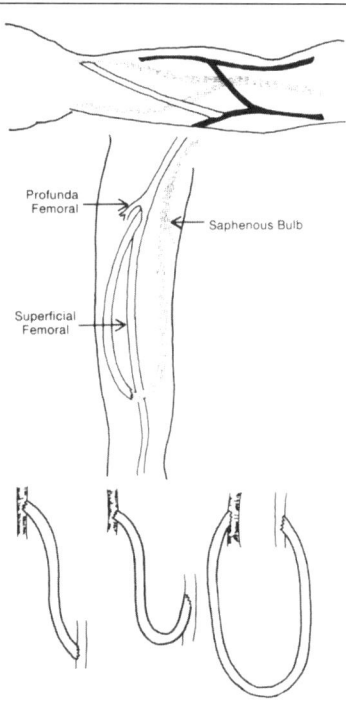

Top: graft interposed between radial artery and basilic vein. Middle: graft interposed between superficial femoral artery and saphenous vein. Bottom: various arrangements for AV grafts (straight, curved, loop).

Note: From Hartigan, M.F., & Thomas-Hawkins, C. (1995). Circulatory access for hemodialysis. In L.E. Lancaster (Ed.). (1995). *ANNA Core Curriculum for Nephrology Nursing* (3rd ed., p. 271). Pitman, NJ: American Nephrology Nurses' Association. Reprinted with permission.

Each HD unit should have its own policies regarding the kind of routine monitoring that should be performed. A monitoring program for AVFs and grafts will permit early detection and treatment of stenoses and prevention of thromboses. Tracking primary failure rates and complications of vascular access can be an important tool to determine the presence of center specific variables such as patient demographics, comorbidities, premature cannulation, or surgical inexperience. Primary access failure is defined as failure of patency within the first 30 days of creation of the vascular access. There is no proposed standard for failure rate of AVFs. The primary failure rate for AVGs is dependent upon location of the graft with forearm straight grafts being less than 15%, forearm loop grafts less than 10%, and upper arm grafts less than 5%. Primary failure of a catheter is defined as inability to deliver a blood flow of > 300 ml/min during the first use of the catheter. The primary failure rate recommended by K/DOQI for catheters is no more than 5%. Tracking cumulative patency rates of vascular access refers to the number of accesses that remain patent during a given time period. There are no recommended guidelines for AVF patency. It is recommended that the cumulative patency rate for AVGs be 70% at 1 year, 60% at 2 years, and 50% at 3 years. Catheters have a patency rate that is extremely variable depending upon the type of catheter used, and thus, there are no recommendations for catheter patency.

Conclusion

Circulatory access to the bloodstream has always been a challenge for the dialysis population. Although many advances have been made over the years, many variables remain obstacles to obtaining and maintaining optimal vascular access. As the dialysis population continues to grow and older patients with increasingly complex comorbidities progress to dialysis, access will become even more difficult. Consistent dedication to assessment, monitoring, tracking, and timely intervention when needed will help prolong useful access life.

References

Aburahma, A.F., Hopkins, E.S., Wulu, J.T., & Cook, C.C. (2002). Lysis/balloon angioplasty versus thrombectomy/open patch angioplasty of failed femoropopliteal polytetraflouroethylene bypass grafts. *Journal of Vascular Surgery, 35*(2), 307-315.

Allon, M., Lockhart, M.E., Lilly, R.Z., Gallicho, M.H., Young, C.J., Barker, J., et al. (2001). Effect of preoperative sonographic mapping on vascular access outcomes in hemodialysis patients. *Kidney International, 60*, 2013-2020.

Allon, M., Ornt, D.B., Schwab, S.J., Rasmussen, C., Delmez, J.A., Greene, T., et al. (2000). Factors associated with the prevalence of arteriovenous fistulas in hemodialysis patients in the HEMO study. *Kidney International, 58*, 2178-2185.

Andrew, E., & Berg, K.J. (2004). Nephrotoxic effects of X-ray contrast media. *Journal of Toxicology: Clinical Toxicology, 42*(3), 325-332.

Ascher, E., Gade, P., Hingorani, A., Mazzariol, F., Gunduz, Y., Fodera, M., et al. (2000). Changes in the practice of angioaccess surgery: Impact of dialysis outcome and quality initiative recommendations. *Journal of Vascular Surgery, 31*, 84-92.

Ash, S.R. (2001). The evolution and function of central venous catheters for dialysis. *Seminars in Dialysis, 14*(6), 416-424.

Ayus, J.C., & Sheikh-Hamad, D. (1998). Silent infection in clotted hemodialysis access grafts. *Journal of the American Society of Nephrology, 9*, 1314-1317.

Back, M.R., & White, R.A. (2002). Biologic response to prosthetic dialysis grafts. In S.E. Wilson (Ed.), *Vascular access principles and practice* (pp. 61-73). Philadelphia: Mosby.

Bagshaw, S.M., & Ghali, W.A. (2004). Acetylcysteine for prevention of contrast induced nephropathy after intravascular angiography: A systematic review and meta analysis. *BMC Medicine, 2*(1), 38.

Baker, L.D., Johnson, J.M., & Goldfarb, D. (1976). Expanded polytetraflouroethylene (PTFE) subcutaneous arteriovenous conduit: An improved vascular access for chronic hemodialysis. *Transcriptions of the American Society of Artificial Internal Organs,* (Vol. XXII), 382-387.

Beathard, G.A. (2001). Catheter thrombosis. *Seminars in Dialysis, 14*(6), 441-445.

Beathard, G.A. (2002). Angioplasty for arteriovenous grafts and fistulae. *Seminars in Nephrology, 22*(3), 202-210.

Beathard, G.A., & Posen, G.A. (2000). Initial clinical results with the LifeSite hemodialysis access system. *Kidney International, 58*(5), 2221-2227.

Berman, S.S., & Gentile, A.T. (2001). Impact of secondary procedures in autogenous arteriovenous fistula maturation and maintenance. *Journal of Vascular Surgery, 34*(5), 866-871.

Bonforte, G., Zerbi, S., & Surian, M. (2004). The middle arm fistula: A new native arteriovenous vascular access for hemodialysis patients. *Annals of Vascular Surgery, 18*(4), 448-452.

Brescia, M.J., Cimino, J.E., Appel, K., & Hurwich, B.J. (1966). Chronic hemodialysis using venipuncture and a surgically created arteriovenous fistula. *New England Journal of Medicine, 275*(20), 1089-1092.

Brouwer, D.J. (1995). Cannulation camp: Basic needle cannulation training for dialysis staff. *Dialysis and Transplantation, 24*(11), 606-612.

Bruns, S.D., & Jennings, W.C. (2003). Proximal radial artery as inflow site for native arteriovenous fistula. *Journal of the American College of Surgeons, 197*(1), 58-63.

Burkhart, H.M., & Cikrit, D.F. (1997). Arteriovenous fistulae for hemodialysis. *Seminars in Vascular Surgery, 10*(3), 162-165.

Butler, H.G., Baker, L.D., & Johnson, J.M. (1977). Vascular access for chronic hemodialysis: Polytetrafluoroethylene (PTFE) versus bovine heterograft. *The American Journal of Surgery, 134*, 791-793.

Butterly, D.W., & Schwab, S.J. (2001). Catheter access for hemodialysis: An overview. *Seminars in Dialysis, 14*(6), 411-415.

Canaud, B., My, H., Morena, M., Lamy-Lacavalerie, B., Leray-Moragues, H., Bosc, J., et al. (1999). Dialock: A new vascular access device for extracorporeal renal replacement therapy. Preliminary clinical results. *Nephrology Dialysis Transplantation, 14*(3), 692-698.

Casserly, L.F., & Dember, L.M. (2003). Thrombosis in end stage renal disease. *Seminars in Dialysis, 16*(3), 245-256.

Clark, T.W.I., & Rajan, D.K. (2004). Treating intractable venous stenosis: Present and future therapy. *Seminars in Dialysis, 17*(1), 4-8.

Clase, C.M., Crowther, M.A., Ingram, A.J., & Cina, C.S. (2001). Thrombolysis for restoration of patency to haemodialysis central venous catheters: A systematic review. *Journal of Thrombosis and Thrombolysis, 11*, 127-136.

Coronel, F., Herrero, J.A., Mateos, P., Illescas, M.L., Torrente, J., & del Valle, M.J. (2001). Long-term experience with the Thomas shunt, the forgotten permanent vascular access for hemodialysis. *Nephrology Dialysis and Transplantation, 16*, 1845-1849.

Cull, D.L., Spence, M.T., Carsten, C.G., Youkey, J.R., Snyder, B.A., Sullivan, T.M., et al. (2002). The fistula elevation procedure: A valuable technique for maximizing arteriovenous fistula utilization. *Annals in Vascular Surgery, 16*, 84-88.

Dember, L.M., Holmberg, E.F., & Kaufman, J.S. (2002). Value of static venous pressure for predicting arteriovenous graft thrombosis. *Kidney International, 61*, 1899-1904.

Depner, T.A. (2001). Catheter performance. *Seminars in Dialysis, 14*(6), 425-431.

Deutsch, L., & White, G.H. (2002). Central venous cannulation for hemodialysis access. In S.E. Wilson (Ed.), *Vascular access principles and practice* (pp. 114-131). Philadelphia: Mosby.

Dixon, B.S., Novak, L., & Fangman, J. (2002). Hemodialysis vascular access survival: Upper arm native arteriovenous fistula. *American Journal of Kidney Diseases, 39*(1), 92-101.

Eknoyan, G., Levin, N.W., Eschbach, J.W., Golper, T.A., Owen, W.F., Schwab, S., et al. (2001). Continuous quality improvement: DOQI becomes K/DOQI and is updated. *American Journal of Kidney Diseases, 37*(1), 179-194.

Faiyaz, R., Abreo, K., Zaman, F., Pervez, A., Zibari, G., & Work, J. (2002). Salvage of poorly developed arteriovenous fistulae with percutaneous ligation of accessory vein. *American Journal of Kidney Diseases, 39*(4), 824-827.

Feldman, H.I., Joffe, M., Rosas, S.E., Burns, J.E., Knauss, J., & Brayman, K. (2003). Predictors of successful arteriovenous fistula maturation. *American Journal of Kidney Diseases, 42*(5), 1000-1012.

Gibson, K.D., Gillen, D.L., Caps, M.T., Kohler, T.R., Sherrard, D.J., & Stehmen-Breen, C.O. (2001). Vascular access survival and incidence of revisions: A comparison of prosthetic grafts, simple atogenous fistulas, and venous transposition fistulas from the United States Renal Data System Dialysis Morbidity and Mortality Study. *Journal of Vascular Surgery, 34*(4), 694-700.

Gillies, D., O'Riordan, E., Carr, D., O'Brien, I., Frost, J., & Gunning, R. (2003). Central venous catheter dressings: A systematic review. *Journal of Advanced Nursing, 44*(6), 623-632.

Goldstein, L.J., & Gupta, S. (2003). Use of the radial artery for hemodialysis access. *Archives of Surgery, 138*, 1130-1134.

Gormus, N., Ozergin, U., Durgut, K., Yuksek, T., & Solak, H. (2003). Comparison of autologous basilica vein transpositions between forearm and upper arm regions. *Annals of Vascular Surgery, 17*, 522-525.

Granata, A., D'Intini, V.D., Bellomo, R., & Ronco, C. (2004). Vascular access for acute extracorporeal renal replacement therapies. In C. Ronco & N.W. Levin (Eds.), *Hemodialysis vascular access and peritoneal dialysis access* (pp. 159-177). New York: Karger.

Gray, R.J., Horton, K.M., Dolmatch, B.L., Rundback, J.H., Anaise, D., Aquino, A., et al. (1995). Use of wallstents for hemodialysis access-related venous stenosis and occlusions untreatable with balloon angioplasty. *Radiology, 195*(2), 479-484.

Hartigan, M.F., & White, R.B. (2001). Circulatory access for hemodialysis. In L.E. Lancaster (Ed.), *Core curriculum for nephrology nursing* (4th ed.) (pp. 305-329). Pitman, NJ: American Nephrology Nurses Association.

Hazinedaroglu, S., Karakayali, F., Tuzuner, A., Ayli, D., Demirer, S., Duman, N., et al. (2004). Exotic arteriovenous fistulas for hemodialysis. *Transplantation Proceedings, 36*, 59-64.

Hossny, A. (2003). Brachiobasilic arteriovenous fistula: Different surgical techniques and their effects on fistula patency and dialysis related complications. *Journal of Vascular Surgery, 37*(4), 821-826.

Huber, T.S., Carter, J.W., Carter, R.L., & Seeger, J.M. (2003). Patency of autogenous and polytetraflouroethylene upper extremity arteriovenous hemodialysis accesses: A systematic review. *Journal of Vascular Surgery, 38*(5), 1005-1011.

Huber, T.S., & Seeger, J.M. (2003). Approach to patients with "complex" hemodialysis access problems. *Seminars in Dialysis, 16*(1), 22-29.

Johnson, J.M., & Kenoyer, M.R. (1974). Bovine graft arteriovenous fistula for hemodialysis. *The American Journal of Surgery, 128*, 728-731.

Kanterman, R.Y., Vesely, T.M., Pilgrim, T.K., Guy, B.W., Windus, D.W., & Picus, D. (1995). Dialysis access grafts: Anatomic location of venous stenosis and results of angioplasty. *Radiology, 195*(1), 135-139.

Kaufman, J.S. (2000). Antithrombotic agents and the prevention of access thrombosis. *Seminars in Dialysis, 13*(1), 40-46.

Knox, R.C., Berman, S.S., Hughes, J.D., Gentile, A.T., & Mills, J.L. (2002). Distal revascularization-interval ligation: A durable and effective treatment for ischemic steal syndrome after hemodialysis access. *Journal of Vascular Surgery, 36*(2), 250-256.

Konner, K. (2003). The initial creation of native arteriovenous fistulas: Surgical aspects and their impact on the practice of nephrology. *Seminars in Dialysis, 16*(4), 291-298.

Krishnasami, Z., Carlton, D., Bimbo, L., Taylor, M.E., Balkovetz, D.F., Barker, J., et al. (2002). Management of hemodialysis catheter-related bacteremia with an adjunctive antibiotic-lock solution. *Kidney International, 61*, 1136-1142.

Levin, N.W., Yang, P.M., Hatch, D.A., Dubrow, A.J., Caraiani, N.S., Ing, T.S., et al. (1998). New access device for hemodialysis. *ASAIO Journal, 44*(5), M529-M531.

Liang, H., Pan, H., Chung, H., Ger, L., Fang, H., Wu, T., et al. (2002). Restoration of thrombosed Brescia-Cimino dialysis fistulas by using percutaneous transluminal angioplasty. *Radiology, 223*(2), 339-344.

Lilly, R.Z., Carlton, D., Barker, J., Saddekni, S., Hamrick, K., Oser, R., et al. (2001). Predictors of arteriovenous graft patency after radiologic intervention in hemodialysis patients. *American Journal of Kidney Diseases, 37*(5), 945-953.

Little, K., & Palmer, D. (1998). Central line exit sites: Which dressing? *Nursing Standard, 12*(48), 42-44.

Little, M.A., & Walshe, J.J. (2002). A longitudinal study of the repeated use of alteplase as therapy for tunneled hemodialysis catheter dysfunction. *American Journal of Kidney Diseases, 39*(1), 86-91.

Lok, C.E., & Oliver, M.J. (2003). Overcoming barriers to arteriovenous fistula creation and use. *Seminars in Dialysis, 16*(3), 189-196.

MacRae, J.M., Pandeya, S., Humen, D.P., Krivitski, N., & Lindsay, R.M. (2004). Arteriovenous fistula - associated high-output cardiac failure: A review of mechanisms. *American Journal of Kidney Diseases, 43*(5), e17-e22.

Malovrh, M. (2003a). Approach to patients with end stage renal disease who need an arteriovenous fistula. *Nephrology Dialysis and Transplantation, 18*, v50-v52.

Malovrh, M. (2003b). The role of sonography in the planning of arteriovenous fistulas for hemodialysis. *Seminars in Dialysis, 16*(4), 299-303.

Malovrh, M. (2002). Native arteriovenous fistula: Preoperative evaluation. *American Journal of Kidney Diseases, 39*(6), 1218-1225.

Mann, T.J., Otlikowski, C.E., Gurrin, L.C., & Keil, A.D. (2001). The effect of the biopatch, a chlorhexidine impregnated dressing on bacterial colonization of epidural catheter exit sites. *Anesthesia Intensive Care, 29*(6), 600-603.

Marr, K.A., Kong, L., Fowler, V.G., Gopal, A., Sexton, D.J., Conlon, P.J., et al. (1998). Incidence and outcome of staphylococcus aureus bacteremia in hemodialysis patients. *Kidney International. 54*(5), 1684-1689.

Matsuda, H., Miyazaki, M., Oka, Y., Nakao, A., Choda, Y., Kokumai, K., et al. (2003). A polyurethane vascular access graft and a hybrid polytetrafluoroethylene graft as an arteriovenous fistula for hemodialysis; comparison with an expanded polytetrafluoroethylene graft. *Artificial Organs, 27*(8), 722-727.

McCarley, P., Wingard, R.L., Shyr, Y., Pettus, W., Hakim, R.M., & Ikizler, T.A. (2001). Vascular access blood flow monitoring reduces access morbidity and costs. *Kidney International, 60*, 1164-1172.

Mickley, V. (2004). Stenosis and thrombosis in haemodialysis fistulae and grafts: The surgeon's point of view. *Nephrology Dialysis and Transplantation, 19*, 309-311.

Miller, P.E., Carlton, D., Deierhoi, M.H., Redden, D.T., & Allon, M. (2000). Natural history of arteriovenous grafts in hemodialysis patients. *American Journal of Kidney Diseases, 36*(1), 68-74.

Miller, C.D., Robbin, M.L., Barker, J., & Allon, M. (2003). Comparison of arteriovenous grafts in the thigh and upper extremities in hemodialysis patients. *Journal of the American Society of Nephrology, 14*, 2942-2947.

Mindich, B.P., Silverman, M.J., Elguezabal, A., & Levowitz, B.S. (1975). Umbilical cord vein fistula for vascular access in hemodialysis. *Transactions of the American Society of Artificial Internal Organs, 21*, 273-280.

Minga, T.E., Flanagan, K.H., & Allon, M. (2001). Clinical consequences of infected arteriovenous grafts in hemodialysis patients. *American Journal of Kidney Diseases, 38*(5), 975-978.

Moran, J.E. (2001). Subcutaneous vascular access devices. *Seminars in Dialysis, 14*(6), 452-457.

Moran, J.E., & Prosl, F. (2004). Totally implantable subcutaneous devices for hemodialysis access. In C. Ronco & N.W. Levin (Eds.), *Hemodialysis vascular access and peritoneal dialysis access* (pp. 178-192). New York: Karger.

Nasar, G.M., & Ayus, J.C. (2000). Clotted arteriovenous grafts: A silent source of infection. *Seminars in Dialysis, 13*(1), 1-3.

Neville, R.F., Abularrage, C.J., White, P.W., & Sidaway, A.N. (2004). Venous hypertension associated with arteriovenous hemodialysis access. *Seminars in Vascular Surgery, 17*(1), 50-56.

National Kidney Foundation (NKF). (1997). *NKF-DOQI clinical practice guidelines for vascular access* (pp. 17-78). New York: NKF.

National Kidney Foundation (NKF). (2001). K/DOQI clinical practice guidelines for vascular access: Update 2000. *American Journal of Kidney Diseases, 37*(Suppl.1), S137-S181.

O'Reilly, R.J., Hansen, C.C., & Rosental, J.J. (1978). Angiography of chronic hemodialysis arteriovenous grafts. *American Journal of Roentgenology, 130*(6), 1105-1113.

O'Shea, S.I., Lawson, J.H., Reddan, D., Murphy, M., & Ortel, T.L. (2003). Hypercoagulable states and antithrombotic strategies in recurrent vascular access site thrombosis. *Journal of Vascular Surgery, 38*, 541-

548.

Oliver, M.J. (2001). Acute dialysis catheters. *Seminars in Dialysis, 14*(6), 432-435.

Palder, S.B., Kirkman, R.L., Whittemore, A.D., Hakim, R.M., Lazarus, M., & Tilney, N.L. (1985, August). Vascular access for hemodialysis patency rates and results of revision. *Annals of Surgery,* 235-239.

Paulson, W.D., Ram, S.J., & Zibari, G.B. (2002). Vascular access: Anatomy, examination, management. *Seminars in Nephrology, 22*(3), 183-194.

Perini, S., LaBerge, J.M., Pearl, J.M., Santiestiban, H.L., Ives, H.E., Omachi, R.S., et al. (2000). Tesio catheter: Radiologically guided placement, mechanical performance, and adequacy of delivered dialysis. *Radiology, 215,* 129-137.

Piccone, V.A., Jr., Lee, H., Ramos, S., Ahmed, N., DiScala, V., Hammanci, M., et al. (1975). Preserved allografts of dilated saphenous vein for vascular access in hemodialysis: An initial experience. *Annals of Surgery, 182*(6), 727-732.

Quinton, W., Dillard, D., & Scribner, B.H. (1960). Cannulation of blood vessels for prolonged hemodialysis. *Transcription of the American Society of Artificial Internal Organs, 6,* 104-113.

Rayan, S.R., Terramani, T.T., Weiss, V.J., & Chaikof, E.L. (2003). The LifeSite hemodialysis access system in patients with limited access. *Journal of Vascular Surgery, 38*(4), 714-718.

Raju, S. (1987). PTFE grafts for hemodialysis access techniques for insertion and management of complications. *Annals of Surgery, 206*(5), 666-673.

Reilly, D.T., Pearson, H.J., Watkin, E.M., & Wood, R.F. (1982). Phlebography in the salvage of dialysis fistulae. *Clinical Radiology, 33*(5), 569-575.

Richie, R.E., Johnson, H.K., Walker, P., & Ginn, E. (1972). Creation of an arteriovenous fistula utilizing a modified bovine artery graft: Clinical experience in fourteen patients. *Proceedings of the Clinical Dialysis and Transplant Forum, 2,* 86-88.

Richie, R.E., Withers, E.H., Petracek, M.R., & Conkle, D.M. (1978). Vascular access for chronic hemodialysis: Use of bovine xenografts to create arteriovenous fistulas. *Southern Medical Journal, 71*(4), 386-388.

Ross, J.J., Narayan, G., Bergeron, E.K., Worthington, M.G., & Strom, J.A. (2002, July). Infections associated with use of the LifeSite hemodialysis access system. *Clinical Infectious Diseases, 35,* 93-95.

Roy-Choudhury, P., Kelly, B.S., Miller, M.A., Reaves, A., Armstrong, J., Nanayakkara, N., et al. (2001). Venous neointimal hyperplasia in polytetrafluoroethylene dialysis grafts. *Kidney International, 59*(6), 2325.

Saad, T.F. (2001). Central venous catheters: Catheter-associated infection. *Seminars in Dialysis, 14*(6), 446-451.

Sam, A.D., Morasch, M.D., Collins, J., Song, G., Chen, R., & Pereles, F.S. (2003). Safety of gadolinium contrast angiography in patients with chronic renal insufficiency. *Journal of Vascular Surgery, 38*(2), 313-318.

Schanzer, H., Kaplan, S., Bosch, J., Glabman, S., & Burrows, L. (1986). Double lumen, silicone rubber, indwelling venous catheters. A new modality for angioaccess. *Archives in Surgery, 121*(2), 229-232.

Schon, D., & Mishler, R. (2000). Salvage of occluded autologous arteriovenous fistulae. *American Journal of Kidney Diseases, 36*(4), 804-810.

Schon, D., & Mishler, R. (2003). Pharmacomechanical thrombolysis of natural vein fistulas; reduced dose of TPA and long-term follow up. *Seminars in Dialysis, 16*(3), 272-275.

Schwab, S.J. (1999). Vascular access for hemodialysis. *Kidney International, 55*(5), 2078.

Schwab, S.J., & Beathard, G. (1999). The hemodialysis catheter conundrum: Hate living with them, but can't live without them. *Kidney International, 56,* 1-17.

Schwab, S.J., Quarles, L.D., Middleton, J.P., Cohan, R.H., Saeed, M., & Dennis, V.W. (1988). Hemodialysis-associated subclavian vein stenosis. *Kidney International, 33,* 1156-1159.

Schwab, S.J., Weiss, M.A., Rushton, F., Ross, J.P., Jackson, J., Kapoian, T., et al. (2002). Multicenter clinical trial results with the LifeSite hemodialysis access system. *Kidney International, 62*(3), 1026-1033.

Segal, J.H., & Weitzel, W.F. (2004). Monitoring techniques of vascular access. In C. Ronco & N.W. Levin (Eds.), *Hemodialysis vascular access and peritoneal dialysis access* (pp. 216-227). New York: Karger.

Sehgal, A.R., Dor, A., & Tsai, A.C. (2001). Morbidity and cost implications of inadequate dialysis. *American Journal of Diseases, 37*(6), 1223-1231.

Sehgal, A.R., Snow, R.J., Singer, M.E., Amini, S.B., DeOreo, P.B., & Cebul, R.D. (1998). Barriers to adequate delivery of hemodialysis. *American Journal of Kidney Diseases, 31*(4), 593-601.

Sheikh-Hamad, D., & Ayus, J.C. (1998). The patient with a clotted PTFE graft developing fever. *Nephrology Dialysis Transplantation, 13,* 2392-2393.

Smith, T.P., Ryan, J.M., & Reddan, D.N. (2004). Transhepatic catheter access for hemodialysis. *Radiology, 232*(1), 246-251.

Tashjian, D.B., Lipkowitz, G.S., Madden, R.L., Kaufman, J.L, Rhee, S.W., Berman, J., et al. (2002). Safety and efficacy of femoral-based hemodialysis access grafts. *Journal of Vascular Surgery, 35,* 691-693.

Teichgraber, U.K., Gebauer, B., Benter, T., & Wagner, H.J. (2003). Central venous access catheters: Radiological management of complications. *Cardiovascular and Interventional Radiology, 26,* 321-333.

Tellis, V.A., Kohlberg, W.I., Bhat, D.J., Driscoll, B., & Vieth, F.J. (1979). Expanded polytetraflouroethylene graft fistula for chronic hemodialysis. *Annals of Surgery, 189*(1), 101-105.

Teruya, T.H., Abou-Zamzam, A.M. Jr., Limm, W., Wong, L., & Wong, L. (2003). Symptomatic subclavian vein stenosis and occlusion in hemodialysis patients with transvenous pacemakers. *Annals of Vascular Surgery, 17*(5), 526-529.

Transonic Systems Inc. (2001). *Equipment instructions.* Ithica, NY: Transonic Systems Inc.

Turmel-Rodrigues, L., Pengloan, J., & Bourquelot, P. (2002). Interventional radiology in hemodialysis fistulae and grafts: A multidisciplinary approach. *Cardiovascular and Interventional Radiology, 25*(1), 3-16.

Twardowski, Z.J. (1995). Constant site (buttonhole) method of needle insertion for hemodialysis. *Dialysis & Transplantation, 24*(10), 559-560, 576.

Twardowski, Z.J., & Kubara, H. (1979). Different sites versus constant sites of needle insertion into arteriovenous fistulas for treatment by repeated dialysis. *Dialysis & Transplantation, 8*(10), 978-980.

Uldall, P.R., Woods, F., Bird, M., & Dyck, R. (1979). Subclavian cannula for temporary hemodialysis. *Proceedings of the Clinical Dialysis and Transplant Forum, 9,* 268-272.

Weijmer, M., Vervolet, M.G., & ter Wee, P.M. (2004). Compared to tunneled cuffed hemodialysis catheters, temporary untunnelled catheters are associated with more complications already within 2 weeks of use. *Nephrology Dialysis Transplantation, 19*(3), 670-677.

Weijmer, M., & ter Wee, P.M. (2004). Temporary vascular access for hemodialysis treatment current guidelines and future directions. In C. Ronco & N.W. Levin (Eds.), *Hemodialysis vascular access and peritoneal dialysis access* (pp. 94-111). New York: Karger.

Wentling, A.G. (2004). Hemodialysis catheters: Materials, design, and manufacturing. In C. Ronco & N.W. Levin (Eds.), *Hemodialysis vascular access and peritoneal dialysis access* (pp. 114-127). New York: Karger.

Weyde, W., Krajewska, M., Letachowicz, W., & Klinger, M. (2002). Superficialization of the wrist native arteriovenous fistula for effective hemodialysis vascular access construction. *Kidney International, 61,* 1170-1173.

Wilson, S.E. (2002). Autologous arteriovenous fistulas direct anastomosis for hemodialysis access. In S.E. Wilson (Ed.), *Vascular access principles and practice* (pp. 82-90). Philadelphia: Mosby.

Wivell, W., Bettmann, M.A., Baxter, B., Langdon, D.R., Remilliard, B., & Chobanian, M. (2001). Outcomes and performance of the Tesio twin catheter system placed for hemodialysis access. *Radiology, 221,* 697-703.

Work, J. (2002). Hemodialysis catheters and ports. *Seminars in Nephrology, 22*(3), 211-219.

Xiang, D.Z., Verbeken, E.K., Van Lommel, A.T.L., Stas, M., & De Wever. I. (2001). Sleeve related thrombosis a new form of catheter related thrombosis. *Thrombosis Research, 104,* 7-14.

- A well-functioning vascular access requires dedication to assessment, monitoring, tracking, and timely intervention when needed.

- The National Kidney Foundation/Dialysis Outcome Quality Initiative (NKF-DOQI) *Clinical Practice Guidelines for Vascular Access* were established in an effort to standardize practice for the creation, maintenance, surveillance, and quality improvement of dialysis vascular access.

- In order to optimize the choice for type and placement of dialysis vascular access, a careful history and physical should be done.

- The external arteriovenous (AV) shunt was the first of the shunts developed and today is only used in cases of emergent need for continuous renal replacement therapy (CRRT) and inability to place either central or femoral lines.

- An arteriovenous fistula (AVF) is the surgical creation of an anastomosis between an artery and a vein that allows the arterial blood to flow through the vein.

- An AV bridge graft is a biologic, semibiologic, or synthetic conduit implanted subcutaneously and interposed between an artery and a vein.

- Central venous catheters for HD are large bore double lumen catheters constructed of rigid or semi rigid material that are placed percutaneously.

- In the HD population subcutaneous ports are most often used in patients for whom there are no alternatives to long-term more permanent vascular access.

- Because of the dynamic state of vascular access in any given patient, every dialysis facility should establish some organized approach for the assessment of vascular access, diagnosis of complications, and the tracking of interventions performed. Goals are to increase the lifespan of each vascular access, improve the detection of significant stenosis before they occur, improve the early referral of patients for angioplasty or operative revision, and decrease the use of central lines.

- Access surveillance begins with a clinical assessment performed and documented. Persistent swelling, prolonged bleeding after needles are pulled, thrombosis or clots pulled from the needle during cannulation, any signs or symptoms of infection, change in appearance, increase in venous pressure or decrease in arterial pressure, or any temperature in the AVG patient should raise suspicion.

- Consistent dedication to assessment, monitoring, tracking, and timely intervention when needed will help prolong useful access life.

ANNP624

Vascular Access for Hemodialysis

Randee Breiterman White, MS, RN, CNN

Contemporary Nephrology Nursing: Principles and Practice contains 39 chapters of educational content. Individual learners may apply for continuing nursing education credit by reading a chapter and completing the Continuing Education Evaluation Form for that chapter. Learners may apply for continuing education credit for any or all chapters.

Please photocopy this page and return to ANNA.
COMPLETE THE FOLLOWING:

Name: _____

Address:_____

City:_____ State: _____ Zip: _____

E-mail: _____

Preferred telephone: ☐ Home   ☐ Work: _____

State where licensed and license number (optional): _____

CE application fees are based upon the number of contact hours provided by the individual chapter. CE fees per contact hour for ANNA members are as follows: 1.0-1.9 - $15; 2.0-2.9 - $20; 3.0-3.9 - $25; 4.0 and higher - $30. Fees for nonmembers are $10 higher.

ANNA Member: ☐ Yes   ☐ No   Member # (if available) _____

☐ Checked Enclosed   ☐ American Express   ☐ Visa   ☐ MasterCard

Total Amount Submitted: _____

Credit Card Number:_____ Exp. Date: _____

Name as it appears on the card: _____

CE Evaluation Form
To receive continuing education credit for individual study after reading the chapter
1. Photocopy this form. (You may also download this form from ANNA's Web site, **www.annanurse.org.**)

2. Mail the completed form with payment (check) or credit card information to American Nephrology Nurses' Association, East Holly Avenue, Box 56, Pitman, NJ 08071-0056.

3. You will receive your CE certificate from ANNA in 4 to 6 weeks.

Test returns must be postmarked by **December 31, 2010.**

CE Application Fee
ANNA Member $20.00
Nonmember $30.00

EVALUATION FORM

1. I verify that I have read this chapter and completed this education activity. Date: _____

   _____
   Signature

2. What would be different in your practice if you applied what you learned from this activity? *(Please use additional sheet of paper if necessary.)*

   _____
   _____
   _____
   _____
   _____
   _____
   _____
   _____
   _____
   _____
   _____
   _____
   _____
   _____
   _____

Evaluation	Strongly disagree				Strongly agree
3. The activity met the stated objectives.					
a. Describe the process used to select the appropriate access type and site for a given patient.	1	2	3	4	5
b. Compare and contrast the various types of vascular access devices available as to advantages and disadvantages, complications, and patient education needed.	1	2	3	4	5
c. Discuss the nursing assessments and interventions needed to increase the lifespan of each type of vascular access.	1	2	3	4	5
4. The content was current and relevant.	1	2	3	4	5
5. The content was presented clearly.	1	2	3	4	5
6. The content was covered adequately.	1	2	3	4	5
7. Rate your ability to apply the learning obtained from this activity to practice.	1	2	3	4	5

Comments _____

8. Time required to read the chapter and complete this form: _____ minutes.

This educational activity has been provided by the American Nephrology Nurses' Association (ANNA) for 2.8 contact hours. ANNA is accredited as a provider of continuing nursing education (CNE) by the American Nurses Credentialing Center's Commission on Accreditation (ANCC-COA). ANNA is an approved provider of continuing education by the California Board of Registered Nursing, CEP 0910.

Hemodialysis: Prevention and Management of Treatment Complications

Karen C. Robbins, MS, RN, CNN
Based on previous edition by Patricia Baltz Salai, MSN, RN, CNN, CRNP

Chapter Contents

Complications of hemodialysis (HD) therapy are omnipresent challenges for nurses to prevent and manage. Adverse events requiring intervention are estimated to occur in 20%-30% of dialysis treatments and have an unfavorable effect on quality of life for hemodialysis patients (Stefandis, Stiller, Ikonomov, & Mann, 2002). Long-term cardiovascular problems are also correlated with recurrent adverse events during HD (Stefandis et al., 2002). Complications experienced by dialysis patients consist of those occurring during therapy and those that evolve over time – months to years – of chronic therapy (Levin & Ronco, 2002). The former will be the focus of this chapter.

The most common complications of hemodialysis treatments are, in descending order of frequency: hypotension (20%-30%), muscle cramps (5%-20%), nausea and vomiting (5%-15%), headache (5%), itching (5%), chest pain (2%-5%), back pain (2%-5%), and fever and chills (< 1%) (Bregman, Daugirdas, & Ing, 2001). These and other complications of this therapy are discussed in detail in this chapter and are listed in Table 25-1.

Estimated Dry Weight

Many of the intradialytic complications are related to efforts to achieve the estimated dry weight (EDW). There is, unfortunately, no standard measure of dry weight. It is typically achieved through trial and error and is an ongoing process. It is described as the lowest weight a patient can tolerate without the development of symptoms or hypotension, a definition that still stands (Henderson, 1980). It is the weight, postdialysis, where all or most excess body fluid has been mobilized and removed without untoward effects of therapy (Daugirdas & Kjellstrand, 2001) or orthostatic hypotension (Negrea, 2003). The development of intradialytic symptoms at weight below EDW or chronic volume overload with poor blood pressure (BP) control at weight above EDW reflect the imprecision of this measure (Jaeger & Mehta, 1999).

The use of volumetric or ultrafiltration (UF) controlled dialysis equipment provides more precise management of fluid removal. Ensuring accurate weights before and after hemodialysis (HD) is critical to the ongoing assessment of the EDW, especially when the patient weighs himself or herself. Compare the pretreatment weight with the previous posttreatment weight and the EDW. A predialysis weight near or below the previous postdialysis weight or EDW may suggest that the patient has lost weight, has experienced difficulty eating, had gastrointestinal losses, or that EDW has not yet been reached in a new patient. Consider the BPs and pulse before, during, and after treatments as another indicator of the accuracy of the EDW. Low BPs or a rapid pulse may indicate a low volume state. The EDW should be re-visited. The nursing assessment includes evidence of edema, focusing on the entire patient. If, for example, a patient is confined to bed or a recumbent position, assessment for edema should include the sacral area, as edema is present in dependent areas. Someone who is upright or sitting much of the time would likely present with edema in the extremities.

Bioimpedence spectroscopy is a noninvasive and sensitive indicator of total body water, measuring the distribution of that water in the intracellular fluid (ICF) and extracellular fluid (ECF) compartments (Shulman, Heidenheim, Kianfar, Shulman, & Lindsay, 2001). The height and weight of each subject must be extremely accurate as well as the circumference of each body part on which bioimpedence is measured. For this measurement, electrodes are placed over areas where circumference has been measured and measurements are taken before HD and after varying periods of UF. This measurement has been used during dialysis to determine the distribution of water and how it shifts during a dialysis treatment. Resistance of body fluid compartments is measured reflecting the state of hydration. The hydration state is a measurement of total body water in proportion to lean (non-lipid) body volume mass and can yield a ratio of resistance that reflects the ICF and ECF relative blood volume. Because patients on HD accumulate excess ECF, this can be used as a more objective measure of EDW. By using bioimpedence, many dialysis patients were found to have high ratios of ICF to ECF after dialysis, suggesting that dry weight had not been achieved (Shulman et al., 2001).

An incorrectly high EDW may contribute to hypertension. As much as 80% of hypertension may be secondary to hypervolemia (Jaeger & Mehta, 1999). If patients are in a chronic state of fluid overload due to failure to reach the actual EDW, they are at risk for hypertension and cardiovascular disease (Shulman et al., 2001). Cardiovascular disease and cerebrovascular accidents are the leading causes of mortality in dialysis patients, and hypertension is linked to the disease progression (Jaeger & Mehta, 1999). Congestive heart failure, pulmonary edema, and left ventricular hypertrophy/left ventricular dilatation are all linked with increased mortality and hypertension (Jaeger & Mehta, 1999). Inaccurate overestimation of dry weight, then, has significant consequences.

An EDW that is set too low can lead to repeated episodes of intradialytic complications as when patients have gained real body weight. The estimated weight loss is no longer achievable, and repeated attempts to reach it may cause dialysis treatments to become so unpleasant it could jeopardize the patient's ability or willingness to adhere to the dialysis prescription (Jaeger & Mehta, 1999).

Accurate estimation of dry weight is, thus, paramount in performing HD with patient focused outcomes. Recognizing that bioimpedence measurement is not widely available, a stepwise reduction of targeted weight is a model for determining EDW (Levin & Ronco, 2002). The steps in this approach include a "challenge" to the EDW in small increments (e.g., 0.2-0.3 kilograms) until symptoms become evident. The use of blood volume monitors provides additional data that can be used to evaluate the fluid shifts from the ECF to the intravascular space (Daugirdas, Van Stone, & Boag, 2001).

Table 25-1
Hemodialysis Complications

Complication	Etiology	Signs/Symptoms	Prevention	Treatment
Hypotension	Reduction in cardiac output Decrease in systemic vascular resistance Splanchnic vasodilatation due to food ingestion Anemia Low dialysate sodium Antihypertensive medications Hypoalbuminemia Aggressive UF Acetate dialysate Unstable cardiovascular status	Low BP (may be associated with nausea, vomiting, diaphoresis, or cold clammy skin) Warm feeling (early sign) Dizziness Tachycardia Loss of consciousness and seizures	Ensure accurate pre-dialysis weights Frequent assessment of EDW Withhold antihypertensive medications prior to dialysis Monitor hematocrit Teach patient to restrict interdialytic fluid intake Teach patient early signs and symptoms of hypotension α adrenergic blockers Cool dialysate Sodium profiling UF profiling	Place patient in head back position Trendelenburg position only in extreme circumstances Reduce UF rate If necessary to reverse low BP, administer normal saline and/or osmotic agents
Muscle Cramps	Excess fluid removal Hypo-osmolality Hypotension ↑ extra cellular shifts in extremities to preserve central blood volume	Pain Tightness in muscle group	Frequent assessment of EDW Use of dialysate with appropriate sodium and potassium concentrations Sodium modeling, UF profiling Use of osmotic agents	Stretching of affected muscles Application of heat to muscle group Volume expansion, if indicated
Chest Pain Arrhythmias (e.g. atrial fibrillation)	Anemia Coronary artery spasm Arteriosclerotic heart disease Severe volume depletion	Pain or tightness in chest Pain may be accompanied by diaphoresis, nausea, dyspnea	Monitor hematocrit Utilize appropriate UF target Assess and treat volume depletion Frequent assessment of EDW	Administer nitroglycerin and related drugs as ordered Administer oxygen as indicated Temporarily decrease UF rate Discontinue dialysis, if severe ↓ blood flow rate
Fever/Chills	Infection Pyrogens/Endotoxins	Temperature elevation during or shortly after dialysis (infection) Temperature elevation within first 45-75 minutes of dialysis (pyrogen/endotoxin exposure) Cold feeling Involuntary shaking Rarely, hypotension	Proper water treatment, disinfection of equipment, reuse procedures, and preparation of dialysate Clean technique in preparation of dialysate and system Preparation of extracorporeal circuit limited to 2 hours prior to initiation of dialysis treatment	Assess for signs and sources of infection Obtain blood cultures, inlet and outlet dialysate and water cultures Administer antipyretics and antibiotics as ordered

Table 25-1
Hemodialysis Complications (continued)

Complication	Etiology	Signs/Symptoms	Prevention	Treatment
Dialysis Disequilibrium	Rapid decrease in BUN Rapid pH changes Electrolyte shifts Possible shift of fluid into CSF→7 cerebral edema	Occur during or soon after dialysis Headache Nausea, vomiting Hypertension Restlessness Increased pulse pressure Decreased sensorium Convulsions Coma Death	Slower urea removal during dialysis (short treatments, less efficient dialyzer, slow BFR, lower dialysate flow) High sodium dialysate/sodium modeling Administration of an osmotic agent Assessment for signs and symptoms	Early recognition of signs and symptoms Termination of the dialysis treatment, if necessary Treat symptoms supportively
Acute Hemolysis	Hypotonic or hypertonic dialysate solutions High dialysate temperature Blood exposure to toxins such as copper, chloramines, nitrates, formaldehyde, or bleach Rarely, RBC trauma from roller pump or high negative pressure in circuit	Chest and/or back pain Dyspnea Clear or translucent blood in venous blood line Localized burning and pain in access return site Dysrhythmias Hyperkalemia Acute decrease in hematocrit Pink plasma in centrifuged blood	Alarms in working order Appropriate check of dialysate temperature and conductivity prior to dialysis Regular preventive maintenance of monitors and alarms Monitor pre-pump arterial pressure Proper water preparation for dialysis If appropriate, test for bleach and formaldehyde in system	Discontinue dialysis without reinfusing blood Monitor vital signs Assess for dysrhythmias, dyspnea, hypotension Administer oxygen, as indicated Check hematocrit, electrolytes If appropriate, replace volume or transfuse
Air Embolism	Defective or disarmed air detector Loose connection or leak in the extracorporeal circuit prior to blood pump Empty air-vented IV containers attached to circuit prior to blood pump	Dependent on position of patient when air infused Feeling and sight of air rushing into circulation Chest pain Dyspnea Coughing Cyanosis Visual problems Confusion Hemiparesis Death	Correct use of air detector Secure all connections Return patient's blood with saline rinse, and not air rinse During dialysis, administer normal saline as a bolus rather than a continuous infusion Observe infusion sites carefully	Stop infusion of air immediately Place patient in Trendelenburg position on left side Assess vital signs Administer oxygen Notify physician
Dialyzer Reaction	Type A: Hypersensitivity to dialyzer sterilant Uncertain	Type A: Acute bronchoconstriction Initially, feeling of uneasiness, agitation, chest tightness, dyspnea, nausea Coughing, wheezing Urticaria, facial edema Respiratory stridor	Type A: Use of a dialyzer with a different sterilant	Type A: Symptom management If severe, terminate dialysis without reinfusing blood
	Type B: Complement activation by dialyzer membrane Reduced with reuse	Type B: Back pain Chest pain Hypotension	Type B: Use of biocompatible membrane Reuse of cellulosic membranes	Type B: Supportive care/symptom management (e.g., administer oxygen via nasal cannula) Termination of dialysis rarely required

Table 25-1
Hemodialysis Complications (continued)

Complication	Etiology	Signs/Symptoms	Prevention	Treatment
Dysrhythmias	Electrolyte and pH changes Removal of antiarrhythmic medications with dialysis	Irregular pulse Possible hypotension	Dialysate potassium at least 2 mEq/liters for patients on digitalis Monitor heart rate and rhythm Monitor EKG in high risk patients	Administer antiarrhythmic agents as ordered Discontinue dialysis for severe symptomatic dysrhythmias Treat symptoms supportively
Cardiac Arrest	Electrolyte imbalance Dysrhythmias Myocardial infarction Cardiac tamponade Large air embolism Hemolysis Exsanguination Hyperthermia	Absence of pulse Lack of spontaneous respiratory effort Unresponsiveness	Prevent conditions that can lead to cardiac arrest Careful assessment of patient during dialysis EKG monitoring for high risk patients	Begin CPR as appropriate Discontinue dialysis and return blood to patient, if appropriate
Seizures	Dialysis disequilibrium Electrolyte imbalances Hypotension Dialysate composition errors	Convulsions May be unresponsive	Avoid/counteract large drop in BUN Frequent monitoring of BP Support BP throughout treatment	Support airway, as necessary Replace volume, if indicated Administer anticonvulsant medications as ordered
Exsanguination	Accidental or traumatic separation of blood lines, needles dislodged from access site, or caps loosened from dialysis catheter Dialysis membrane rupture with failure of blood leak detector Rupture of AVF anastomosis or aneurysm	Obvious source of bleeding Shock Seizures Cardiac arrest	Secure all bloodline and access connections/caps Carefully secure needles with tape Ensure conditions that allow visualization of extracorporeal circuit at all times Ensure properly functioning blood detector and pressure alarms Place blood lines in pump properly	Stop bleeding at any site Return all appropriate blood to patient If blood loss significant, administer volume expander, oxygen, and possibly transfuse Notify physician
Dialysis Encephalopathy	Accumulation of aluminum in body from water used to prepare dialysate or large quantities/long-term use of aluminum-based phosphate binders	Speech disturbances Myoclonus Seizures Gait changes Intellectual deterioration EEG changes Osteodystrophy Anemia	Use appropriately treated water for dialysis Use non-aluminum phosphate binders Assess for early signs and symptoms	Early recognition of signs and symptoms Serum aluminum chelation to decrease body aluminum stores

Table 25-1
Hemodialysis Complications (continued)

Complication	Etiology	Signs/Symptoms	Prevention	Treatment
Neutropenia	Use of cellulosic dialyzer membranes Activation of complement cascade and neutrophil accumulation in pulmonary vasculature	Hypotension Nausea/vomiting Chest pain	Use of biocompatible dialyzer	Draw all CBCs prior to dialysis
Hypoxemia	Hypoventilation secondary to acetate dialysate Intrapulmonary diffusion block due to neutrophil aggregation in lungs	Possible dyspnea, cyanosis in already compromised patients	Use of biocompatible dialyzer Use of bicarbonate dialysate	Administer oxygen
Amyloidosis	Repeated immune stimulation with long-term dialysis on cellulosic membranes β_2M synthesis exceeds that removed by dialysis	Carpal synovial amyloid deposits Cystic bone deposits Carpal Tunnel Syndrome	Use of biocompatible membrane dialyzers	Treat symptomatically
Interleukin-1 Stimulation	Interaction between dialyzer membrane and monocytes during dialysis	Long-term catabolic changes over the years of muscle, fat, connective tissue, and the liver resulting, in part, in wasting and negative nitrogen balance Transient elevation of body temperature during dialysis Headache	Possibly reduced with biocompatible membranes Possibly reduced with reuse	Treat symptomatically

Hypotension

Intradialytic hypotension (IDH) is the most common complication of HD, occurring in 20% to 30% of dialyses by some reports (Bregman et al., 2001) and as high as 25%-50% of all treatments in other reports (Schreiber, 2001). IDH is characterized by an abrupt drop in BP equal to or greater than 30 mm Hg in normal or hypertensive patients, predialysis. A predialysis systolic blood pressure (SBP) less than 100 mm Hg with a decrease of less than 30 mm Hg also constitutes IDH. Its etiology is multifactorial and cannot be explained by a single, underlying mechanism (Schreiber, 2001).

IDH sequelae can range from subtle complaints to life-threatening events. The manifestations can range from mild, "not feeling well" to more moderate visual complaints, nausea and vomiting, decreased mental status, posttreatment malaise, and fatigue. Serious vascular complications from IDH can include cerebral infarction, cardiac ischemia, vascular access thrombosis, nonocclusive mesenteric ischemia, and arrhythmias (Schreiber, 2001). Even though data link hypertension to cardiovascular and cerebrovascular events,

the impact of hypotension on cerebrovascular insults is not as clear. A variety of strategies may be employed to prevent or treat hypotension, with varying degrees of effectiveness. Prophylaxis is clearly preferable to responding to IDH episodes, as it can affect morbidity and mortality (Schreiber, 2001).

One study linked increased mortality with HD-associated hypotension (Shoji, Tsubakihara, Fujii & Imai, 2004). Specifically, significant and independent risk factors for 2-year mortality were linked with the lowest SBP during dialysis and the fall of the SBP when standing from the supine position postdialysis. The fall in BP was appreciably greater in patients with diabetes, although this was not correlated with mortality rates as it was in those without diabetes. The authors speculate that the mortality is likely related to hypotension, leading to damage to vital organs including the brain and heart (Shoji et al., 2004).

Hypotension can develop from intrinsic factors such as changes in body chemistry from the treatment itself. Intrinsic causes of hypotension include: hypovolemia from a slower rate of capillary refilling than the UF rate; vasoconstriction resulting from heat retention secondary to the fluid shifts from UF (although vasodilatation may follow); autonomic dysfunction that limits vasoconstriction; and diastolic dysfunction that limits cardiac output as hypovolemia decreases ventricular filling. Extrinsic factors inducing hypotension include medications and the physical components of dialysis such as dialyzer membranes and acetate or low calcium dialysate (Levin & Ronco, 2002). Uncommon causes of IDH include pericardial tamponade, myocardial infarction, occult hemorrhage, septicemia, arrhythmias, dialyzer reaction, hemolysis, and air embolism (Bregman et al., 2001).

Intrinsic Causes of IDH

Excess fluid that accumulates in the various body compartments in patients with compromised kidney function must be removed during HD with UF. As the blood circulates through the extracorporeal circuit, fluid is removed from the blood or the intravascular compartment. The rate of fluid removal and refilling of nonprotein bound water from the interstitial space to the intravascular compartment will determine the change in blood volume. As the blood volume contracts, the plasma protein concentration increases, increasing the oncotic pressure. This, in combination with a decreased capillary hydrostatic pressure, enables fluid to move from the interstitium to the intravascular space (Leunissen, Kooman, & van der Sande, 2000; Levin & Ronco, 2002).

Hypotension becomes a clinical problem when it occurs too frequently. It may interfere with the patient's ability to tolerate dialysis and the goals of keeping the patient free of uremic symptoms and excess fluid.

The most common cause for IDH is a rapid decrease in blood volume and a decrease in cardiac output (Bregman et al., 2001). The mean arterial pressure (MAP) is determined by the peripheral vascular resistance (PVR) and the cardiac output (CO). The CO is a function of stroke volume and heart rate. Stroke volume depends upon the plasma volume and myocardial contractility (Diroll & Hlebovy, 2003). During HD, a decrease in plasma volume will lead to decreased BP if compensatory changes in heart rate, PVR, or myocardial contractility do not occur. When the UF rate is high because of a large weight gain, fluid may be removed from the vascular space at a rate faster than plasma refilling (fluid moves in from intracellular and interstitial fluid compartments). Maintenance of blood volume during HD depends upon rapid refilling of the blood compartment from surrounding compartments. If the plasma refilling rate is low and the patient is unable to maintain adequate or increased PVR, hypotension will result (Bregman et al., 2001).

Decreased BP during dialysis is chiefly a reflection of the large amount of fluid relative to plasma volume that is removed during an average HD treatment. These rapid decreases in blood volume can be due to large interdialytic weight gains of greater than 3% of the body weight, resulting in the need for a high UF rate to accomplish a large fluid removal during a short dialysis treatment. As the patient approaches his or her EDW, the rate at which the blood compartment refills from surrounding spaces is diminished. A decrease in blood volume will result in a decrease in cardiac filling, leading to a decrease in cardiac output, and ultimately a decrease in BP.

Studies by Shulman et al. (2001) suggest that fluid compartment shifts are not the same throughout the body. Central blood volume (CBV) (cardiopulmonary circulation and great vessels) is preserved, while extracellular shifts and reductions are greatest in the legs followed by the arms. CBV is thought to have a direct effect on the maintenance of BP (Prakash, Reddan, Heidenheim, Kianfar, & Lindsay, 2002). Factors that affect fluid shifts also include reduced plasma osmolality, as it impedes plasma refilling. The patient's nutritional status and serum albumin level are significant in determining this plasma osmolality.

Blood volume depletion causes a state in which CO is limited by cardiac filling. Any minor decrease in PVR can precipitate a drop in BP because the CO cannot increase enough to compensate. Use of acetate-containing dialysate solution can lead to vasodilatation (Bregman et al., 2001).

Lack of vasoconstriction can also cause hypotension during HD. Hypotension during HD is a common problem in diabetic patients due to autonomic neuropathy and coexisting vessel disease. Arteriolar constriction in response to volume depletion is impaired (Tzamaloukas & Friedman, 2001). Thus, patients with diabetes have a decreased ability to maintain their BP during HD.

Core body heating is a powerful stimulus for vasodilatation, resulting in both arterial and venous vasodilatation. In the Gotch hypothesis, it is stated that an increase in body temperature during HD is a result of UF (Maggiore, 2002). The UF causes peripheral vasoconstriction and heat accumulation in the body. Heat accumulation alters thermal homeostatic mechanisms and jeopardizes cardiovascular tolerance to UF (Maggiore, 2002; Schneditz, Ronco, & Levin, 2003). The core temperature continues to increase if the heat does not dissipate, eventually leading to vasodilatation. Thermodynamic stability can be enhanced with controlled maintenance of the core temperature. This appears to be more effective in those patients who have a lower initial temperature (Levin & Ronco, 2002; Maggiore, 2002). Even though the changes experienced may be less than 1 degree C, modest deviations from the normal temperature can provoke large changes in the circulation (Maggiore, 2002). The dialyzer membrane type – cellulosic or non-cellulosic, low or high flux – has no bearing on this hemodynamic response resulting from fluid removal (Maggiore, 2002). Patients who experience hypotensive episodes may benefit from altered dialysate temperature (see "Cool Dialysate" under "Strategies to Prevent IDH," in this chapter).

Splanchnic vasodilation results from the ingestion of food immediately prior to or during HD. Dilation causes an increase in capacity of those blood vessels, resulting in a decrease in systemic BP. This food effect lasts at least 2 hours (Bregman et al., 2001). Patients prone to hypotension during HD should be discouraged from eating immediately prior to or during HD to avoid hypotension (Bregman et al., 2001, Levin & Ronco, 2002).

Tissue ischemia that occurs during hypotension causes the release of adenosine. Adenosine blocks the release of norepinephrine from sympathetic nerve terminals and also has intrinsic vasodilator properties. Thus, hypotension can perpetuate itself through this release of adenosine and its effects. This tissue ischemia effect may also be the reason that anemic patients are prone to hypotension (Bregman et al., 2001).

Cardiac factors are common causes of decreased BP during HD. The heart's ability to maintain or increase CO in response to volume depletion plays a major role in prevention of hypotension. Hypertrophy and dilatation of the left ventricle, increased age, atherosclerosis, and coronary artery disease can all limit this response. Diastolic dysfunction secondary to a stiff hypertrophied heart results in the inability to maintain CO in response to a minor decrease in filling pressures. Decreased cardiac reserve can also be due to the chronic high output state secondary to the anemia of chronic renal failure and the presence of an arteriovenous fistula (AVF) or arteriovenous graft (AVG) (Leunissen et al., 2000). The venous system contains more than 80% of the total blood volume. As a result of UF and changes in the venous capacity, cardiac filling may decrease, leading to decreased cardiac output and IDH. Uremic autonomic neuropathy or the use of beta blockers can also inhibit responses necessary to increase the BP, such as an increase in the pulse rate (Bregman et al., 2001).

Diroll and Hlebovy (2003) describe a different scenario involving two principles: the Frank Starling mechanism and Laplace's Theorem. Cardiac output can be decreased when the muscle itself becomes overstretched as occurs with hypervolemia. The greater the heart muscle is stretched during filling, the greater the force of the contraction, increasing the volume of blood entering the aorta: the Frank Starling mechanism. When muscle fibers are stretched beyond a point that contraction is no longer enhanced, stroke volume decreases and heart failure is the result. The premise of Laplace's Theorem is that tension in the wall of a chamber (e.g., the left ventricle) increases as the radius of the chamber increases. The myocardium demand for oxygen is a reflection of the tension in the chamber. When the radius is dilated to such an extent that the demand for oxygen can no longer be met, CO declines and the efficacy of the heart as a pump begins to fail. Thus, increased intravascular volume may increase the tension in the myocardium to such a degree that it cannot pump effectively. The tendency to decrease UF may be just the opposite of what is most needed namely contraction of the volume and decreasing left ventricular dilation, so the CO can be increased.

Dialysis-related carnitine disorder (DCD) can contribute to hypotension. Carnitine, an essential cofactor in normal fatty acid metabolism, must bind with fatty acids to enter the mitochondrial matrix for energy production. Carnitine also binds with the byproducts of fatty acid metabolism to enhance their removal from the mitochondria. Hence, carnitine is necessary for cardiac and skeletal muscle function. A blunted response to erythropoietin therapy, cardiomyopathy, skeletal muscle dysfunction evident by generalized fatigability, and hypotension are manifestations of this disorder (Eknoyan, Latos, & Lindberg, 2003). Clearly, these manifestations are inter-related and play a role in hypotension. Ninety percent of the carnitine is in muscle and 10% in the blood. Seventy percent of that 10% is removed with HD and the effect is cumulative, rendering the patient more and more deficient in carnitine over time (Eknoyan et al., 2003).

Extrinsic Causes of IDH

Acetate leads to peripheral vasodilatation. Patients who are cardiac compromised due to a decrease in left ventricular function are especially prone to hypotension. Acetate should not be used as a buffer in this population because of the vasodilatation resulting from the acetate (Leunissen, et al., 2000).

Excessive UF rates bringing the patient below his or her EDW or to a target weight set too low can lead to hypotension both during and after the HD treatment. Inaccurate weights result in inappropriate UF calculations, thus removal of inappropriate amounts of fluid. Failure to use UF controllers can put the patient at risk for errors in fluid removal and postdialysis weights below the EDW. Without a UF controller, fluid removal can fluctuate considerably, causing transient rapid UF rates and resultant hypotension (Bregman et al., 2001). If a UF controller is not available, less permeable dialyzers must be used so that changes in transmembrane pressure (TMP) will cause smaller changes in actual fluid removal.

Dialysate sodium levels can also affect the patient's intradialytic BP. When dialysate sodium is less than plasma sodium, the blood returning to the patient from the dialyzer will be hypotonic in relation to fluid in surrounding spaces. To maintain equilibrium, water will leave the blood compartment, causing an acute decrease in blood volume. This effect is most pronounced early in the treatment. Excessive sodium removal secondary to inappropriately low dialysate sodium levels, such as less than 136 mEq/liter, reduces plasma sodium level and further exacerbates plasma volume reduction during UF (Bregman et al., 2001).

Many antihypertensive medications, such as hydralazine, impair vasoconstriction. Beta blockers decrease cardiac contractility and limit the increase in heart rate that should occur. Patients may be told to hold medications until completion of the HD treatment. Vasoactive medications (e.g., antihypertensives, narcotics, and angiolytics) should be withheld before HD, particularly in patients susceptible to hypotension, as this can influence the vascular response to hypovolemia (Leunissen et al., 2000).

Peripheral vascular resistance (PVR) may be acutely decreased during HD because of many vasoactive substances that can be administered during dialysis or released by the cells. Aggregation of neutrophils in the extracorporeal system and sequestration of neutrophils in the lungs may produce pulmonary hypertension and a fall in CO and BP (Leunissen et al., 2000). Release of cationic proteins and release of chemical inflammatory mediators from cells may induce acute allergic and potent vasodilatory effects. Interleukin-1 is released in response to exposure of whole blood to cellulose membranes (Leunissen et al., 2000). This release of interleukin-1 and its effects will be discussed in greater detail later in the chapter.

Nursing Management of IDH

Nursing management of IDH should focus on early detection, measures to support or restore BP, and prevention. Early detection is the key to prevention of serious consequences resulting from hypotension. Making patients aware of the signs and symptoms of hypotension that they should report to the patient care staff will help in early detection of the problem. Other important measures are close observation of the patient and monitoring vital signs more frequently in patients prone to hypotension.

Trendelenberg Position

When IDH is discovered, the patient may be placed in the Trendelenberg position if respiratory status allows. Initiated by Friedrich Trendelenberg in the 1870s to improve surgical accessibility to the pelvic organs, it was embraced as a strategy to treat shock from a variety of causes as well as hypotension (Fink, 1999). The "autotransfusion" of this maneuver appears to stabilize the BP for perhaps 10 minutes as the body restabilizes itself in this position. However, the Trendelenberg position has been shown to increase intracranial and intraocular pressures, cause cardiac overload and pulmonary compromise, increase myocardial oxygen consumption, and increase the risk of gastric aspiration. The risk of airway occlusion is especially high in obese patients. It has the additional disadvantage of blocking the body's attempt at autoregulation. Elevating the legs 30 to 45 degrees, flexing at the hip with the trunk remaining horizontal, with the head level with the trunk or elevated slightly on a pillow is suggested as an alternative to Trendelenberg. This position does not displace the abdominal organs that compromises ventilation, overload of the heart, or risk cerebral edema (Fink, 1999). The use of this strategy for IDH should be revisited for its appropriateness as a routine maneuver to effectively manage hypotension.

UF Rate

Other strategies to immediately deal with IDH include decreasing the UF rate to as near zero as possible. It can be resumed at a later time, possibly at a slower rate, once vital signs have stabilized. Slowing of the blood flow rate may help in limited instances (e.g., when cardiac output is poor) (Bregman et al., 2001). A decrease in blood flow rate as well as a decrease in dialysate negative pressure results in a decrease in pressure in the blood compartment of the dialyzer with parallel plate dialyzers. If acetate dialysate is being used, then a decrease in blood flow rate will reduce transfer of acetate to the patient. When a UF controller is not available, slowing of the blood flow rate makes it easier to limit the amount of UF. If a hollow fiber dialyzer, bicarbonate dialysate, and a UF controller are being used, then a decrease in the blood flow rate should not be done initially unless the hypotension is severe or unresponsive to other measures (Bregman et al., 2001).

Volume Replacement

Reversal of hypotension can often be accomplished with a bolus of normal saline solution, 100 ml or more, as necessary, rapidly administered via the extracorporeal circuit. As an alternative, hypertonic sodium chloride, hypertonic glucose, mannitol, hydroxyethyl starch (HES), or albumin solutions can be used to treat the low BP (Bregman et al., 2001). Some studies have suggested that hypertonic sodium chloride is less effective than hyperoncotic preparations of albumin or HES (van der Sande, Luik, Kooman, Verstappen, & Leunissen, 2000). The use of hypertonic sodium chloride has

the risk of increased thirst contributing to increased interdialytic weight gains. There is some concern about the use of mannitol or HES because of the problem of accumulation due to their longer half-lives and the continued hyperoncotic effects of fluid shifts between dialysis treatments (Bregman et al., 2001; Leunissen et al., 2000; Levin & Ronco, 2002). This could pose the risk of the development of increased intravascular volume, exacerbating hypertension with the possibility of congestive heart failure or pulmonary edema, particularly in the longer interim between HD treatments. Unless muscle cramps are present, hypertonic sodium chloride seems to be no more effective than normal saline solution and avoids the increased thirst associated with hypertonic saline. Nasal oxygen administration may be of benefit by helping to prevent tissue ischemia and improve myocardial function (Bregman et al., 2001).

Dialysate Sodium Levels

A dialysis machine with an UF controller should be used whenever possible, especially in patients with a propensity for hypotension. Dialysate sodium level should be at or above the patient's plasma sodium level, and bicarbonate dialysate should be used anytime the patient dialyzes with a high blood flow rate or with a high-efficiency or high flux dialyzer. In selected patients prone to hypotension, the dialysate solution temperature may be decreased to 34-36 degrees centigrade during HD. This may need to be done only when the patient has had a large interdialytic weight gain (Bregman et al., 2001).

Strategies to Prevent IDH

Dialysate Buffer

Acetate has been shown to have a cardiopressant action in patients with impaired cardiac function. It is a direct vasodilator and decreases precapillary arteriolar vasoconstriction. Acetate interferes with capillary refilling by increasing the capillary hydrostatic pressure thus lowering BP and altering refilling. The use of bicarbonate dialysate is recommended as the buffer of choice, especially in those patients with known cardiovascular instability (Levin & Ronco, 2002).

Cool Dialysate

While the core temperature of the individual patient may influence the efficacy of this strategy, a cool dialysate temperature may improve hemodynamic stability (Bregman et al., 2001; Hoeben, Abu-Alfa, Mahnensmith, & Perazella, 2002, Levin & Ronco, 2002). Patients with lower "normal" temperatures may tolerate the cooler dialysate better than those whose temperatures are higher. Dialysate temperatures of 37°C are warmer than almost all HD patients, thus, the dialysate temperature adds to the warming of the patient. The cooler dialysate appears to dissipate some of the heat generated from UF. An increase in venous tone, vascular resistance, and cardiac contractility all help to support BP. Perhaps most important is the preservation of central blood volume and cardiac output in maintaining BP. Temperature recommendations vary from 34°-36° C. An automated means of controlling the dialysate temperature integrated into the dialysis equipment is an option on some machines. It entails a module to monitor the temperature in the arterial and venous bloodlines and adjust the dialysate temperature as programmed into the equipment. Complaints of being cool/cold and, possibly, shivering are the only side effects associated with cool dialysate. If shivering develops, it may offset or minimize the benefits of this approach (Bregman et al., 2001; Hoeben et al., 2002; Leunissen et al., 2000; Levin & Ronco, 2002; Maggiore, 2002; Schneiditz, et al., 2003).

Adrenergic Agonist

Patients with diabetes often have autonomic neuropathy leading to impaired arteriolar vasoconstriction in response to UF and volume depletion (Tzamaloukas & Friedman, 2001). Patients with a tendency for hypotension, whether diabetic or not, may respond to an alpha-adrenergic agonist, such as midodrine. This drug, an oral agent, is given 15 to 30 minutes before HD and may help avert IDH episodes. It may be repeated midway during therapy, as its results are time limited. Some studies suggest the combination of cool dialysate and midodrine have an additive effect, while other studies have not found such an effect (Bregman et al., 2001; Hoeben et al., 2002).

Sodium Profiling

Hypotensive episodes may be diminished by sodium profiling (Leunissen et al., 2002). Shifting fluid from the ICF to ECF to improve efficiency of UF is enhanced by an increase in the dialysate sodium. The osmolarity between ICF and ECF compartments are steady under stable state conditions. A high dialysate sodium during UF causes a decline in the ICF and expansion of the ECF. This is induced by an increase in the ECF osmolarity from the higher dialysate sodium concentration. Thus, hypovolemic symptoms may be averted as there is rapid refilling of the vascular space, albeit at the expense of a sodium load (Stefandis et al., 2002). Various profiles exist in dialysis equipment and offer different changes in the delivered dialysate sodium. As with hypertonic sodium chloride, sodium profiling has been shown to increase inter-dialytic weight gains secondary to increased thirst (Laut, D'Avella, Reynaud, & Li, 2002).

Hypertonic saline may be used in the absence of sodium modeling with the intent to achieve the same outcome – avert hypotension secondary to hypovolemia. A large portion of hypertonic sodium chloride is retained, even when given 2 hours before the end of HD, with 78% being retained when given even 1 hour prior to the end of therapy. This leads to the vicious cycle of increased thirst, increased inter-dialytic weight gain, and the need for excessive UF with the risk for hypotension or muscle cramps (Stefandis et al., 2002).

These strategies are controversial and must be evaluated on a patient per patient basis, as they are not appropriate for all patients.

UF Profiling

While sodium profiling is useful in moving fluid between compartments (i.e., from the ICF eventually to the intravascular space), UF profiling facilitates movement of fluid from the intravascular compartment into the dialysate,

with UF as the outcome (Wilson, 2004). UF profiling varies the rate of fluid removal, permitting the vascular space to refill. This can be done manually by varying the UF goal to increase or decrease the UF rate. Some dialysis equipment contains UF profiles programmed in the software, while others may allow for creation of individualized UF rates according to the patient's individual response to HD. Rapid UF, especially in patients with a compromised cardiovascular system, may not be well tolerated (Leunissen et al., 2000). The risk of symptomatic IDH near the end of treatment may be reduced if the UF rate is lower. The rate of blood volume change is dependent upon the rate of refilling of the intravascular space from the ICF. While the total volume of fluid to be removed is usually determined prior to treatment initiation, the UF rate need not be constant. Whether done manually or by an electronic UF profiling program, varying the UF rate may be employed to avert IDH (Stefandis et al., 2002).

Blood Volume Monitoring

Monitoring of blood volume and the changes that occur over the course of the dialysis treatment can be observed using an optical technique that measures the changes in the quality of light passing through the blood line (Daugirdas et al., 2001). This provides a measure of blood volume changes. As fluid is removed from the intravascular compartment at a greater rate than capillary refilling, the red blood cells become more concentrated resulting in an increasing hematocrit. If fluid is shifting at roughly the same rate as UF, a steady profile will be displayed. This profile may present an opportunity to increase the rate of UF until a change in the blood volume is reflected by an increased hematocrit or decreased blood volume. This may, in some patients whose blood volume changes rapidly, allow for the anticipation of hypotensive events with intervening actions to prevent or abort such occurrences before reaching a true hypotensive state. Blood volume monitoring must not be used at the exclusion of other objective assessment tools. A "typical patient profile" may seem to emerge with individual patients, but caution must be used as this may vary from one treatment to the next. Factors influencing this profile include serum albumin, tissue hydration, and the presence of diabetes (blood glucose levels and its effect upon osmosis and fluid shifts). As the sophistication of these monitors evolves, feedback to vary UF rate or sodium concentration may become available in an effort to avert untoward intradialytic events (Leunissen et al., 2000).

Isolated Ultrafiltration

IDH resulting from UF and decreased intravascular volume during HD is also associated with losses from diffusion. Isolated ultrafiltration (IU) removes iso-osmolar fluid from the systemic circulation via convection across the semi-permeable membrane with either high flux or conventional membranes. Clearance via diffusion does not take place. The purpose of IU is to remove excess fluid from the vasculature without significantly changing the blood solute concentrations while maintaining the patient's BP. Primarily water, low-molecular weight solutes, and electrolytes are removed at concentrations about the same as plasma levels (Mulloy,

Caruana, Kozeny, & Ing, 2002).

IU is performed with the same HD machine and extracorporeal circuit, including the dialyzer, as the HD treatment. Application of positive pressure to the blood side or negative pressure to the dialysate side of the dialyzer membrane creates a transmembrane pressure that generates the formation of ultrafiltrate (Mulloy et al., 2002). Although different equipment accomplishes this in different ways, the principle of removing fluid without circulating dialysate through the dialyzer is consistent (Sigler, Teehan, Daugirdas, & Ing, 2001). The efficacy of IU or sequential UF (i.e. IU carried out either immediately before or after HD) was demonstrated as early as 1975, with the principle of IU having been used to treat edematous patients as early as 1952 (Mulloy et al., 2002).

The membrane sieving coefficient of a solute determines the degree to which solutes are removed. Unlike UF with dialysis and its attendant diffusion, the solute composition of the blood is essentially unchanged with IU. There may be a slight hemoconcentration effect with an increase in the hematocrit, plasma proteins, and plasma oncotic pressure, but little change occurs in electrolytes. There may be a minor change in the blood pH with a slight decrease in the plasma bicarbonate concentration after the removal of 1-3 liters of ultrafiltrate over 1 to 2 hours (Mulloy et al., 2002).

Circulatory stability is better with IU than with UF during HD (Mulloy et al., 2002). The effects of osmolality, total peripheral resistance, and blood temperature may account for the differences in the outcomes of various modes of UF. The decrease in plasma osmolality during HD but not in IU probably contributes to the drop in BP. An increased heart rate, a small increase in total peripheral resistance, and a lower BP reveal circulatory instability during HD. The BP and heart rate are stable during IU from an increase in total peripheral resistance, even with continued fluid losses. A lower core body temperature may promote peripheral vasoconstriction, as the temperature of blood returning to the patient is slightly lower with IU than with conventional HD. This is another reminder that lowering the dialysate temperature may be a successful strategy to use during HD to avoid IDH (Mulloy et al., 2002).

Large amounts of fluid can be removed during IU; the rate of fluid removal is dependent upon several factors. The amount of overhydration, the degree of cardiovascular stability, and the rate of refilling from the interstitium into the vascular space all influence the rate of fluid removal. It may be possible to remove 2-4 liters of fluid in 1.5 to 3 hours with IU in extremely edematous patients. Because the solute removal in IU is essentially isotonic, conventional dialysis should be carried out if there is the need to correct the solute concentration. It is important to add the IU time to the regularly prescribed dialysis time. Failure to do so may lead to poor dialysis adequacy (Mulloy et al., 2002).

Muscle Cramps

Muscle cramps occur in about 5% to 20% of HD treatments, especially near the end of the dialysis session (Bregman et al., 2000). They are most common after a large fluid gain when a patient requires rapid UF during HD. The cramps commonly accompany a hypotensive episode although they can occur alone. The pathophysiology of dialysis-associated muscle cramps is not well understood, but extracellular volume contraction associated with a rapidly changing osmolality may cause the cramping as well as tissue ischemia and carnitine deficiency (Leunissen et al., 2000; Levin & Ronco, 2002). Hypokalemia has been implicated as well (Leunissen et al., 2000).

It is also possible that fluid shifts do not occur consistently in all body compartments. Central blood volume (cardiopulmonary circulation and great vessels) is preserved while fluid shifts are greater from the periphery, especially the lower limbs and somewhat less in the upper limbs. Hence, more ECF is removed from the peripheral compartments than from the trunk. This suggests that muscle cramps, during and immediately after dialysis, may occur as the central blood volume is preserved at the expense of the peripheral blood volume (Shulman et al., 2001).

Severe and prolonged cramps, beginning during the latter part of dialysis and persisting after the treatment ends, can occur when the patient is dehydrated or below his or her EDW. Use of a low sodium dialysate that acutely lowers the plasma sodium concentration can result in constriction of blood vessels in an isolated muscle group (Bregman et al., 2001). When hypotension and muscle cramps occur at the same time, the hypotension may respond to volume expansion, but cramps may persist. The UF rate can be temporarily decreased, and muscle bed blood vessels can be dilated by the administration of normal saline, hypertonic sodium chloride, or hypertonic glucose solutions. The disadvantage of using normal saline is that weight reduction during HD will be less. A disadvantage of hypertonic sodium chloride (10 ml of 23%) is hyperosmolality, resulting in postdialysis thirst (Bregman et al., 2001). The use of hypertonic glucose (50 ml of 50%) is better in non-diabetics (Bregman et al., 2001). Stretching of the muscles through dorsiflexion of the foot, either manually or by standing, may help relieve the cramps. While a patient's innate response to cramps in the feet or legs is to stand, caution should be exercised. If the muscle cramps are accompanied by hypotension, standing may evoke profound orthostatic hypotension and should be avoided until the patient's BP is known. Application of heat to the muscle group can also help, if available, although it does not provide immediate relief. Prevention of hypotensive episodes will eliminate the majority of cramping episodes. Frequent assessment of EDW to ensure accuracy is of utmost importance.

Chest Pain

HD may aggravate existing heart disease (Murphy & Parfrey, 2002). Chest pain occurring in 1%-4% of dialysis treatments results from coronary artery disease, anemia, and severe decrease in intravascular volume (Bregman et al., 2001). Mild chest pain during HD, sometimes associated with mild back pain, cannot always be explained and must be differentiated from dialysis associated complications (e.g., hemolysis or Type B dialyzer reaction) (Bregman et al., 2001; Negrea, 2003). Nursing management includes administration of oxygen, reduction of the blood flow, reduction of UF rate to zero until the BP increases, and discontinuation of dialysis if chest pain is severe (Nicholls, 2001). If present, volume depletion is treated with normal saline or other volume expanders. Nitroglycerine should be given only if the patient's BP is acceptable. Place the patient in a reclining position and anticipate that BP will decrease following the administration of nitroglycerine (Nicholls, 2001).

Assessment of the patient to determine the appropriate EDW and UF goal are proactive measures to prevent chest pain. Measures to maintain adequate hematocrit, such as recombinant human erythropoietin or darbapoietin alfa, maintenance of iron stores, and transfusions as necessary, will help prevent chest pain secondary to anemia. Nitroglycerine and related maintenance drugs should be prescribed as needed for the patient with coronary artery disease.

Fever and Chills

Fever and chills during HD can occur for a number of reasons. Fever can be related to infection, pyrogens, endotoxin, or endotoxin fragments (Levin & Ronco, 2002; Negrea, 2003). Endotoxins are lipopolysaccharides derived from the outer membrane of Gram-negative bacteria. Because of their high molecular weight, it is possible that only fragments of the endotoxins can pass the dialytic membrane. Dialysate components, namely water and bicarbonate, are the most common source of this contamination. Lipopolysaccharides cause the release of pyrogenic cytokines from monocytes and endothelial cells that generate a cascade of clinical sequelae (Levin & Ronco, 2002).

Fever that occurs during HD should be aggressively explored with infection as the primary consideration. Bacteremia is a result of vascular access infection 50% to 80% of the time, with catheters responsible for them most often and arteriovenous fistulae least often (Negrea, 2003). The febrile reaction occurs during dialysis, with or without interdialytic fever, as bacterial diffusion is more disseminated from the release of the catheter with the HD procedure (Levin & Ronco, 2002).

Chills are defined as a cold feeling with involuntary shaking, sometimes accompanied by fever, hemodynamic instability, myalgias, and headache (Levin & Ronco, 2002). Fever and chills occurring during the course of dialysis are most likely secondary to a pyrogenic reaction when the patient is afebrile prior to HD. Nursing management of this problem includes assessment of the patient for signs and sources of infection, such as access, respiratory, urinary tract, and so forth. Obtaining cultures of blood, dialysate, and water is important. Limulus amoebocyte lysate (LAL) assay should also be performed to determine the presence of endotoxin in water and/or dialysate that can cross the membrane leading to a pyrogen reaction. A positive LAL assay indicates that endotoxin has crossed the dialysis membrane and blood cultures will likely be negative as intact organisms are not the cause of the febriel reaction (Amato, 2005). Antipyretics should be administered for patient comfort. In an undiagnosed febrile reaction, empiric treatment with antibiotics may be considered until culture results are known.

Careful disinfection of equipment, especially in high flux dialysis, can help prevent febrile reactions. The bicarbonate powder used to generate the sodium bicarbonate dialysate

concentrate can be contaminated with bacteria, molds, and/or pyrogens, creating the need for proper disinfection of all areas contacted by the solution (Pittard, 2002). Other equipment preparation, such as proper reuse procedures, is also important. Proper disinfection of the water system, dialysis equipment, and concentrate containers is essential (Bregman et al., 2001). The focus of the disinfection program is to prevent the proliferation of bacteria rather than reacting in response to their excessive proliferation to an unacceptable level (i.e., above an action level) (Association for the Advancement of Medical Instrumentation [AAMI], 2004). The action levels for water and various types of dialysate are defined by current AAMI Standards (AAMI, 2004; Amato, 2005).

Dialysis Disequilibrium Syndrome

Dialysis disequilibrium syndrome (DDS) is a set of systemic and neurologic symptoms, often associated with characteristic EEG findings, occurring during or soon after a HD treatment. It often occurs when a severely uremic patient is dialyzed aggressively (Bregman et al., 2001). It is also common in elderly and pediatric populations, patients with severe metabolic acidosis, and pre-existing brain damage (Levin & Ronco, 2002).

The etiology of DDS is controversial. Perhaps the most common theory is that edema in the brain develops due to a gap in the rate of removal of urea from the blood and that of cerebrospinal fluid. This disequilibrium between these areas leads to a transfer of water into brain cells. The cerebrospinal fluid becomes acidotic from intracerebral accumulation of osmolytes (Levin & Ronco, 2002). Some attribute this acute change in pH of the cerebral spinal fluid during HD as the cause of the syndrome (Bregman et al., 2001). Increased levels of cerebral edema, especially in the posterior parietooccipital areas, have been demonstrated by magnetic resonance imaging even in HD patients demonstrating no manifestations of DDS (Sheth, Wu, Messé, Wolf, & Kasner, 2003).

DDS was more problematic when patients with a high blood urea nitrogen (BUN) were commonly subjected to prolonged dialysis. Milder forms may still be seen in acute and chronic dialysis patients.

Signs and symptoms of mild disequilibrium syndrome include headache, hypertension, restlessness, nausea, and vomiting. Headache is a common symptom associated with HD (5%), and nausea and vomiting also occur in 5% to 15% of routine HD treatments (Bregman et al., 2001). Therefore, some episodes of disequilibrium go unrecognized. Although most nausea and vomiting in stable patients are associated with hypotension, they can also be an early manifestation of DDS. As the syndrome progresses or becomes more severe, seizures, decreased sensorium, and coma can occur. Death may even result (Bregman et al., 2001). Since the diagnosis is one of exclusion, other sources of the presenting symptoms such as uremia, hyponatremia, hypoglycemia, cerebral vascular accident, or subdural hematoma must be ruled out (Sheth et al., 2003).

Nursing management of mild disequilibrium syndrome includes recognition of early signs and symptoms. While the simplest approach is to prevent DDS by reducing the efficiency of HD (by decreasing the blood and dialysate flows) and the treatment time, early recognition remains important (Levin & Ronco, 2002). Since nausea, vomiting, restlessness, blurry vision, and headache are nonspecific symptoms, it is difficult to be certain that they are secondary to disequilibrium. If these mild symptoms occur in an extremely uremic patient, measures should be taken to decrease the efficiency of the dialysis treatment as described above. Plasma urea reduction should be limited to 30% (Bregman et al., 2001). This action also decreases the pH change. Hyperosmolar agents such as hypertonic sodium chloride or glucose solutions or mannitol can be administered to decrease movement of water out of the plasma. A dialysate sodium concentration less than 140 mEq/L may exacerbate any cerebral edema (Bregman et al., 2001). Dialysate sodium greater than 140 mEq/L has been found to be useful in maintaining a higher serum osmolality during HD, thus preventing or alleviating some of the symptoms and discomforts associated with disequilibrium (Bregman et al., 2001). However, adverse effects secondary to a high dialysate sodium, such as high interdialytic weight gains and elevated BP, have limited its use for this complication. Both high and variable sodium dialysate levels have been successful in reducing dialysis disequilibrium symptoms without significant adverse effects. If none of these measures is effective, the treatment may need to be terminated earlier than planned if symptoms persist (Bregman et al., 2001).

The occurrence of signs and symptoms of severe disequilibrium such as seizures, obtundation, or coma necessitates the immediate termination of the dialysis treatment. Seizures are treated with maintenance of the airway and ventilation. Mannitol administered intravenously may be of benefit. Coma is treated supportively and usually subsides within 24 hours if due to disequilibrium (Bregman et al., 2001; Levin & Ronco, 2002).

Acute Hemolysis

Acute hemolysis during HD is a medical emergency and is almost always due to a problem with the dialysis solution. Overheated dialysate from malfunctioning equipment can lead to this emergent problem. Hypotonic or hypertonic dialysis solution from insufficient or excessive concentrate to water ratio can also lead to hemolysis. Water/dialysis solution contamination with metals, organic substances, and inorganic substances in the water used to prepare the dialysate can cause hemolysis. These contaminants include zinc, copper from pipes, nitrates, chlorine, and chloramines from the water supply, as well as bleach and formaldehyde used to disinfect the water system and HD machines (Amato, 2001). Kinking of the bloodline immediately before the blood pump is a source of mechanically induced hemolysis (Levin & Ronco, 2002). In rare instances, hemolysis can be caused by erythrocyte trauma in an improperly occluded roller blood pump or excessive negative pressure in the extracorporeal circuit (Behrens, 2001; Bregman et al., 2001).

Signs and symptoms of hemolysis include chest pain or tightness, back pain, and dyspnea. The patient may also complain of burning in the access return site and experience hypotension. A port wine or cherry pop appearance of the blood in the venous line postdialyzer indicates excessive hemolysis. Centrifuged samples of hemolyzed blood will show a pink discoloration of the plasma. If massive hemolysis is not detected early, hyperkalemia may occur due to the release of potassium from ruptured red blood cells. This can lead to electrocardiographic abnormalities reflecting altered myocardial function, muscle weakness, and the possibility of cardiac arrest. Laboratory results may also reveal a marked decrease in hematocrit and hyponatremia (Bregman et al., 2001).

Nursing management of gross hemolysis includes immediate halting of the blood pump and clamping the arterial and venous blood lines. HD should be terminated without returning hemolyzed blood to the patient. The patient's vital signs should be monitored, and the nurse should be alert for signs of arrhythmias; which would indicate administration of oxygen is indicated. Volume replacement should also be given if necessary. Blood samples for hemoglobin, hematocrit, and electrolytes should be obtained, and the nurse should anticipate possible treatment for hyperkalemia or low hematocrit. Once stabilized, the patient should be assessed for the need for continued HD. He or she also should be evaluated for the need for continued observation for delayed hemolysis, which may occur for some time after the treatment ends. Dialysate samples should be collected for analysis to determine its role in the complication (Bregman et al., 2001). If the hemolysis develops in an isolated patient, HD may be resumed when the source of hemolysis has been corrected. If, however, it occurs in more than one machine simultaneously, the entire shift of patients must be removed from dialysis until the source can be identified. In this case, the water treatment or dialysate central delivery system is suspect as the cause (Behrens, 2001; Levin & Ronco, 2002).

Occult hemolysis is more difficult to diagnose in the absence of a visible change in the appearance of the blood. Haptoglobin, an acute phase protein, binds hemoglobin and is freed during intravascular hemolysis. Its absence or a decrease below the normal level may suggest hemolysis. However, the interpretation of haptoglobin results must occur in the context of the patient's comorbid conditions that can alter the level (e.g., folate deficiency, hypersplenism, sickle cell anemia, estrogen therapy, and liver disease). Plasma free hemoglobin measures hemoglobin that is not attached to red blood cells and is characteristically elevated with hemolysis. Other laboratory findings suggesting hemolysis include elevated lactate dehydrogenase (LDH) resulting from the freeing of the enzyme from ruptured red blood cells. As with haptoglobin, recognize that many other factors can lead to an elevated LDH level (Behrens, 2001).

Prevention of hemolysis is accomplished with appropriate dialyzer bypass mechanisms on the HD machine to protect the patient from temperature or conductivity deviation in the dialysis solution. The conductivity and temperature monitors must be working properly to alert the nurse and trigger the bypass mechanism. Proper preventive maintenance will ensure that these devices are functioning adequately to safeguard the patient. Proper water preparation and monitoring of pre-pump arterial pressures are also measures that may prevent hemolysis. Checking the bloodlines to ensure there are no kinks will protect patients from this possible complication (Behrens, 2001).

Air Embolism

Air embolism is a potentially fatal complication of HD that must be detected and treated immediately to avert disastrous outcomes (Bregman et al., 2001). Dialysis equipment includes air detectors on the venous line postdialyzer to prevent this complication (Levin & Ronco, 2002).

The amount of air injected, the rate of injection, the size of the bubbles, and the point of entry determine the clinical severity of an air embolism. An air embolism can be caused during HD if air enters the extracorporeal circuit via a faulty connection at the arterial needle, the pre-pump arterial tubing segment, or the inadvertent open end of a central venous catheter. The air detector on the blood circuit should protect the patient; current equipment should not allow the disabling of the air detector during HD. If the alarm is disarmed or malfunctioning, air may move through the venous bloodline, past the air detector, and into the patient (Levin & Ronco, 2002).

Signs and symptoms of an air embolus depend somewhat upon the position of the patient at the time the air enters the blood stream. In patients who are seated or in bed with head elevated, air will tend to pass up the jugular vein into the cerebral venous system without entering the heart. This causes obstruction of cerebral venous return with loss of consciousness, seizures, and possibly death. If the patient is recumbent, air tends to enter the heart and form foam in the right ventricle, which then passes on into the lungs. At this point the patient will exhibit dyspnea, cough, and chest pain. In a patient lying on the right side, the air may go to the pulmonary arteries, resulting in acute pulmonary hypertension. Some air may also pass into the left ventricle with resulting arterial embolism to the brain and the heart. This can cause arrhythmias and acute neurologic dysfunction. The patient may exhibit sudden dyspnea, cyanosis, respiratory arrest, and loss of consciousness. If the patient is in Trendelenberg position at the time the air enters, air will pass to the lower extremities, causing patchy cyanosis (Bregman et al., 2001; Levin & Ronco, 2002).

Regardless of patient position, foam or air pockets can be found in the venous blood line, and the patient may call out in alarm at the feeling of air rushing into the venous system. If air has entered the heart, a churning sound may be heard on auscultation of the heart (Levin & Ronco, 2002).

Nursing management of an air embolus includes immediate clamping of venous bloodline and halting of the blood pump to discontinue infusion of air into the patient. The patient should immediately be placed into Trendelenberg position on his or her left side with chest and head tilted downward. This traps air in the right ventricle, away from the pulmonary valve. Cardiorespiratory support by administration of 100% oxygen by mask or via endotracheal tube, if patient is unconscious, may be indicated. In severe cases, aspiration of air from the ventricle with a percutaneously inserted needle may be attempted by the physician. Monitoring of vital signs is crucial (Bregman et al., 2001). While normobaric oxygen can be beneficial, hyperbaric oxygen therapy is an additional aid (Levin & Ronco, 2002).

The nephrology nurse has a vital role in prevention of air embolism during HD. Preventive measures include use of the air detector at all times, securely locking luer connections, and administration of normal saline in bolus form rather than a continuous infusion unless it is via an infusion pump with infusion volume limits. Vented intravenous bottles, rarely used, should not be used in the extracorporeal circuit if at all possible. The heparin infusion should always be administered into the blood line at a point after the blood pump (Bregman et al., 2001).

Dysrhythmias

Arrhythmias are common in HD, originating from both patient and treatment-related factors. Patient-related factors include age, left ventricular hypertrophy, coronary artery disease, heart and/or lung failure, decrease in the extracellular fluid volume, electrolyte and acid-base abnormalities, digoxin use, sympathetic dysfunction, and possibly, phosphate and parathyroid hormone levels (Leunissen et al., 2000; Levin & Ronco, 2002;). Factors related to treatment are shifts of potassium, calcium, and acid base balance. Hypovolemia and resulting sympathetic stimulation contribute to arrhythmias (Leunissen et al., 2000; Levin & Ronco, 2002). Some studies have shown complex ventricular arrhythmias occurring in more than 50% of patients on dialysis. The clinical significance of these arrhythmias is unclear. The development of more severe atrial and ventricular tachycardias can occur (Leunissen et al., 2000).

Hypokalemia places the heart at increased risk for arrhythmias due to an increased ratio between intracellular and extracellular potassium. This causes a negative membrane potential that can lead to arrhythmias, especially in those patients on digoxin. Digoxin increases the heart's sensitivity to rapid changes in potassium and is a known risk factor in potentially dangerous arrhythmias (Leunissen et al., 2000; Levin & Ronco, 2002).

Nursing management includes the use of appropriate dialysate potassium levels. In a patient on digoxin, dialysate potassium should never be less than 2 mEq/L. It has been suggested that a modulated potassium concentration can maintain a more constant gradient by varying the dialysate concentration throughout the treatment (Levin & Ronco, 2002). The patient's pulse and BP should be monitored for changes and cardiac monitoring for EKG changes as necessary. Antiarrhythmic drugs should be administered as ordered.

Cardiac Arrest

The major cause of death among HD patients is cardiac disease, accounting for 45% of all mortality. Sudden cardiac death may be implicated in 60% of that mortality. The obstructive nature of coronary artery disease coupled with electrolyte shifts during HD, left ventricular hypertrophy, and abnormal cardiac ultrastructure may contribute to the risk of sudden death. Acute myocardial infarction is responsible for approximately 20% of that mortality (Herzog, 2003). Karnik et al. (2001) found an incidence of 7 cardiac arrests per 100,000 HD treatments. Forty percent survived the initial cardiac arrest, while 60% expired within 48 hours of the event. Cardiac arrest during HD can occur for a number of reasons, and it must be decided quickly if the cardiorespiratory arrest is due to intrinsic disease or technical errors. Technical errors include air embolism, unsafe dialysate composition, overheated dialysate, line separation and severe hypotension, or exposure to the sterilant in the dialyzer. If it is a result of air in the lines (air embolus), grossly hemolyzed blood, or hemorrhage from line separation, this should be quickly apparent (Levin & Ronco, 2002). Other causes of cardiac arrest include electrolyte imbalances, dysrhythmias, myocardial infarction, cardiac tamponade, and profound shock. Signs and symptoms include absence of apical or carotid pulse, respiration, and asystole or ventricular fibrillation as demonstrated on a cardiac monitor (Keen, Lancaster, & Binkley, 2001; Levin & Ronco, 2002).

If there is no reason to suspect dialysate abnormalities or other technical problems, nursing management is supportive, with initiation of cardiopulmonary resuscitation (CPR), discontinuation of HD, and prompt return of the blood to the patient. The access lines should be left in place to be available for fluid and medication administration. If, however, the arrest occurs at the initiation of treatment, the blood should not be returned to the patient, as a technical problem is suspect. CPR and other supportive measures are carried out. A sample of dialysate as well as a sample of the patient's blood should be sent for electrolyte analysis. The dialyzer and bloodlines should be saved for the possible need for further analysis. The dialysis machine should be removed from patient care so it can be checked to rule out any equipment malfunction (Keen et al., 2001; Levin & Ronco, 2002). Prevention of causes, as well as careful patient assessment before and during dialysis, are important nursing measures. Cardiac monitoring should be considered for high-risk patients on HD (Keen et al., 2001).

Seizures

Seizures occur in less than 10% of chronic HD patients, while they occur more frequently in acute HD patients (Khosla & Swartz, 2002). The incidence is greater in children than adults. Seizure activity typically occurs during, immediately after, or within 12-24 hours after HD (Khosla & Swartz, 2002).

Some seizure activity is the result of predictable characteristics of HD. There are patients who have a greater risk for developing seizure activity during HD, and there are interventions prior to or during HD that may decrease that risk. Neuromuscular irritability from uremia and destabilizing factors of HD are factors in the development of seizure activity. HD-related characteristics that may provoke seizures include: uremic toxicity, dialysis disequilibrium and accompanying acid-base changes, hypoxemia, hemodynamic instability including rapid changes in BP, intracranial bleeding hastened by the use of heparin, too rapid transfusion in children, and removal of anticonvulsants by HD (Khosla & Swartz, 2002).

Patient characteristics that predispose patients to seizures can be identified, and clearly patients with a known seizure history are at risk. Microvascular disease, such as hemolytic uremic syndrome, atheroembolism, and severe hypertension, increases the risk. Myocardial infarction or severe cardiomyopathy may elevate the risk due to the decreased cardiac output and resulting hypoperfusion. Encephalopathy from uremia or liver dysfunction also places the patient at risk of seizures (Khosla & Swartz, 2002).

Interventions before dialysis include assessment for evidence of intracranial bleeding, cardiac function including arrhythmias, identification of hypocalcemia, and possible preventive use of anticonvulsants. If any of these conditions is present, forms of less aggressive therapy such as peritoneal dialysis or continuous veno-venous hemofiltration, may be more appropriate (Khosla & Swartz, 2002).

If HD is the therapy to be initiated, nursing management includes measures to minimize osmotic changes during HD as described in the discussion of DDS. The use of a higher dialysate sodium level (levels > 140 mEq/L), sufficient glucose (approximately 200 mg/dL), and an osmotic agent can be effective, especially if the BUN is greater than 130. Seizures can also be prevented with avoidance of a rapid decrease in BUN or blood glucose. Measures to prevent this rapid reduction in BUN are presented in the DDS discussion. These include use of a smaller dialyzer, reduction of dialysate flow, and even co-current rather than counter-current dialysate flow to slow the rate of solute clearance. If the patient is hypocalcemic, the use of a higher calcium dialysate may help reverse this or, at the very least, reduce the risk of seizure activity. The use of oxygen may be indicated for patients with underlying cardiac or respiratory disease. Bicarbonate dialysis rather than acetate containing buffers improves hemodynamic and neuromuscular stability. Synthetic membranes that are more biocompatible that do not activate inflammatory mediators will further reduce the potential for seizures (Khosla & Swartz, 2002; Nicholls, 2001).

Seizures should be treated by the immediate cessation of HD and support for a patent airway. Blood samples should be drawn for glucose, calcium, and other electrolytes thought to be relevant. If hypoglycemia is suspected, intravenous dextrose should be administered (Khosla & Swartz, 2002; Nicholls, 2001).

If a patient is at high risk for seizures, administration of an anticonvulsant medication should be considered. If the patient's routine anticonvulsant medication is dialyzable, then an additional dose during HD may be necessary. Patients vulnerable to seizures, despite prophylactic measures, may be better served by alternate replacement therapies (Khosla & Swartz, 2002).

Exsanguination

Exsanguination during HD can occur due to breaks in the extracorporeal system or due to access problems. Separation of the bloodlines, needle dislodgement, and dialyzer rupture are potential causes. Arterial and venous pressure alarms on the HD blood circuit should alert the nurse to these problems because of the resultant rapid decline in system pressures when a break occurs in the system (Daguirdas et al., 2001). Access problems can include rupture of the AVF or AVG, aneurysm, pseudoaneurysm, anastamosis, or separation of a catheter from the catheter cap (Besarab & Raja, 2001; Keen et al., 2001). Failure to connect the venous bloodline to the patient when dumping the normal saline prime at treatment initiation can also lead to exsanguination.

Signs and symptoms include obvious bleeding, leading to shock and seizures. Nursing management involves minimizing the blood loss by clamping both sides of the separated bloodline, catheter, or ruptured dialyzer and stopping the blood pump. Pressure should be applied to any bleeding site. Symptoms should be treated with oxygen, volume expanders, and blood replacement in a timely manner as indicated. Prevention includes securing all connections and luer locks, catheter caps, and needles with tape. Facilities may consider implementing a taping protocol that is designed to ensure that to the extent possible, needles are safely secured. Visualization of the entire extracorporeal circuit is important throughout the dialysis treatment. Use of appropriate pressure monitors and blood leak detectors can cause early detection of problems and prevent exsanguination (Keen et al., 2001).

Dialysis Encephalopathy

Dialysis encephalopathy is a neurologic disorder that occurs primarily in patients who have been receiving chronic HD for many years. Aluminum toxicity from the use of aluminum-containing phosphorous binders is generally accepted as the cause of this progressive disorder. Currently, the availability of alternate and effective phosphorous binders coupled with water treatment that effectively removes aluminum from the water supply makes frank aluminum overload rare. Another factor contributing to aluminum overload is iron depletion. Binding sites on transferrin become available in the presence of iron depletion leading to increased binding of aluminum to the receptor sites. More effective use of iron therapy has made these sites less available for aluminum (D'Haese & DeBroe, 2001; Keen et al., 2001).

Early neurologic signs and symptoms include speech disturbances, such as dysarthria, aphasia, stuttering or stammering, and can progress to personality changes, gait changes, myoclonus, seizures, and progressive dementia (Keen et al., 2001). Other evidence of aluminum toxicity may be found, such as microcytic hypochromic anemia, in the absence of iron deficiency as the aluminum occupies the binding sites for iron on transferrin. Aluminum-associated bone disease (osteomalacia) may be present. Plasma aluminum levels of greater than 200 µg/mL is strongly suspicious, and toxicity cannot be ruled out at a level as low as or less than 100 µg/mL. Rises in plasma aluminum of more than 200 µg/mL after a desferoxamine (Desferal®, "DFO") stimulation test is very suggestive of an increased tissue burden of aluminum. A rise of more than 400 µg/mL is highly predictive. A bone biopsy from the iliac crest with stain for aluminum is diagnostic. Aluminum toxicity does not necessarily need to be debilitating or fatal if there is early diagnosis and treatment (D'Haese & DeBroe, 2001).

Management includes chelation of aluminum with DFO. Concurrent administration of intravenous iron during DFO therapy should be avoided as chelation of iron will occur; this would negate any benefits of the iron therapy and failure to achieve chelation of aluminum. DFO is continued until basal levels of aluminum are only slightly increased and there is only a small rise of 20-30 µg/mL after DFO administration. One gram of DFO is given intravenously two times per week during the last 30 minutes of the HD treatment. The best management, however, is prevention. Use of appropriately-treated water for HD is an important factor in prevention. Substitution of aluminum-based gels with other phosphorous binders is recommended (D'Haese & DeBroe, 2001; Keen et al., 2001).

Hypoxemia

The PO_2 drops anywhere from 5 to 30 mm Hg during HD. This fall is not clinically significant unless the patient has pre-existing pulmonary or cardiac disease for whom this may be dangerous. There are several possible reasons for this drop in PO_2. Hypoventilation is almost always implicated. Acetate dialysate can result in loss of CO_2 from the blood passing through the dialyzer. This leads to hypocapnia, which causes the patient to hypoventilate slightly. Contributing to this is CO_2 consumption during acetate metabolism. Conversely, bicarbonate dialysate has elevated CO_2 levels so it does not cause hypocapnia. Bicarbonate, however, can cause alkalosis, particularly if the dialysate bicarbonate level is greater than 35 mEq/L. Transfer of bicarbonate from the dialysate to the blood can result in metabolic alkalosis, which is a well-known cause of hypoventilation and hypoxemia (Bregman et al., 2001).

Intrapulmonary diffusion block secondary to leukocyte (neutrophil) aggregation in the pulmonary vasculature can also result in hypoxemia. Some studies have suggested that the alveolar to arterial oxygen gradient is increased very early during HD as a result of neutrophils in the capillaries. Supplemental oxygen should be administered during dialysis to acutely-ill patients or those whose clinical course might be compromised by even mild hypoxemia. Nasal oxygen is usually sufficient to prevent hypoxemia (Bregman et al., 2001).

In high-risk patients, a dialyzer made of substituted cellulose or synthetic materials can reduce complement activation and neutrophil aggregation in the pulmonary vasculature. Bicarbonate dialysate should be used with a bicarbonate level low enough to not result in alkalemia (Bregman et al., 2001).

Hemodialysis-Related Amyloidosis

Dialysis-related amyloidosis (DRA) is a complication in patients undergoing long-term HD. Amyloid consists primarily of β_2 microglobulin (β_2M). β_2M is the subunit protein in DRA. It is found in most biological fluids, including serum, urine, and synovial fluid, and has a molecular weight of 11,800 daltons. The glomeruli normally filter β_2M and it is catabolized after proximal tubular reabsorption. The rate of β_2M synthesis exceeds that removed by different dialysis modalities so that levels are elevated up to 60-fold in HD patients. When there is more residual renal function, these levels may be less elevated, but they increase when the glomerular filtration rate is less than 2.1 mL/minute. β_2M is 20% to 40% lower in patients on PD or patients on HD using high flux, polysulfone dialyzers rather than low-flux, cellulose-based dialyzers (Acchiardo, 2002; Kay & Hano, 2001).

Duration on dialysis and the occurrence of DRA are closely correlated. Acchiardo (2002) reports that 21% of patients exhibited amyloid deposits within the first 2 years on HD and more than 90% of patients had deposits after 7 years. Over 95% of HD patients have shoulder pain and carpal tunnel syndrome when on HD 19 years or longer (Kay & Hano, 2001). A study of post mortem examinations of HD patients revealed β_2M deposition in large joints even in the absence of clinical symptoms (Acchiardo, 2002).

Carpal tunnel syndrome due to amyloid infiltration of the β_2M protein is a frequent complication of long-term therapy. The median nerve is compressed at the wrist as it passes through the carpal tunnel where β_2M deposits are found (Kay & Hano, 2001). The incidence of carpal tunnel syndrome is 20% to 25% after 5 years on dialysis, and after 10 years, the incidence is approximately 50%. It is usually bilateral, progressive, and requires surgery for relief of symptoms that include numbness, hypoesthesia, paresthesias, and amyotrophy (Acchiardo, 2002). Pain in the fingers tends to worsen at night, during HD, and with repeated flexion and extension of the wrist (Acchiardo, 2002; Kay & Hano, 2001). Worsening of pain during HD may result from a vascular access-induced steal phenomenon causing median nerve ischemia. The increase in extracellular fluid in the interdialytic period may also compress the median nerve (Kay & Hano, 2001). Other symptoms include shoulder pain, joint stiffness, soft tissue swelling, and effusion. Knees, ankles, elbows, and hips are targets for DRA (Acchiardo, 2002).

The most successful therapy is kidney transplantation, as the functioning organ vigorously excretes large amounts of β_2M. Retreat of symptoms may also be attributed to the anti-inflammatory effects of steroid therapy (Acchiardo, 2002). In the absence of a transplant, splinting the affected wrist in a neutral position, especially during HD and at night, may provide some relief of symptoms. Steroid injection into the carpal tunnel provides permanent relief for about 30% of patients. If symptoms cannot be alleviated with these strategies, surgical decompression may be required and yields improvement in 90% of the patients. Unfortunately, carpal tunnel syndrome will recur in most patients within 2 years, as the underlying etiology remains (Kay & Hano, 2001).

Biocompatible membranes known to clear more β_2M should be used whenever possible to retard the progression of DRA (Acchiardo, 2002; Kay & Hano, 2001).

Membrane Biocompatibility

Dialyzer Reactions

Biocompatibility has been defined as the absence of inflammatory process when one is in contact with "non-self components" (Hakim, 2002). Blood comes in contact with a variety of materials as it travels through the extracorporeal system – bloodlines, dialyzing membrane, and remnants from its sterilization – many "non-self" components (Leunissen et al., 2000).

Dialyzer reactions include anaphylactic reactions as well as many less severe reactions of uncertain origin. These events, sometimes called "first use syndrome," occur in patients dialyzed with a new dialyzer as opposed to a reprocessed dialyzer. However, similar reactions occur with reused dialyzers. Dialyzer reactions are described in two categories – Type A and Type B – type B reactions are much less frequent than in years past (Bregmen et al., 2001).

Type A reactions. A Type A dialyzer reaction is more severe than a Type B reaction. Although milder symptoms such as dyspnea, feeling of warmth at the fistula site or throughout the body, and a sense of impending doom are common initial symptoms, anaphylaxis, cardiac arrest, and death may ensue. Somewhat milder cases may present with itching, urticaria, cough, sneezing, watery eyes, or gastrointestinal symptoms such as abdominal cramping or diarrhea (Bregman et al., 2001). Angioedema may also develop as a component of this reaction. Type A reactions occur during the first 5 to 10 minutes (maximum 20) of the HD session (Keen et al., 2001; Leunissen et al., 2000). Severe reactions are infrequent but represent a major cause for concern. The most severe cases have some features in common. The symptoms, starting within a few minutes of the initiation of HD, rapidly progress to complaints of feeling hot and flushed and the patient may become anxious and agitated. Dyspnea, itching, wheezing, chest pain, back pain, abdominal pain, nausea and diarrhea, and, in some cases, the feeling of impending death are common signs and symptoms. The patient's BP may be low or high. Cardiorespiratory arrest is rare. These severe reactions have occurred in patients with every type of dialyzer membrane. The reaction may be immunologic or toxic in nature (Bregman et al., 2001).

The etiology of Type A reactions varies. Ethylene oxide (ETO), a gas sterilant, was implicated initially in about two thirds of patients because they were found to have elevated serum titers of immunoglobulin E (IgE) antibodies to ETO-altered proteins (Bregman et al., 2001). ETO was used by manufacturers to sterilize almost all hollow fiber dialyzers in the 1980s, and it tended to accumulate in the potting compound inside the dialyzer. ETO reactions are less common because manufacturers are taking care to remove it, while some have changed potting compound materials to reduce absorption of ethylene oxide (Bregman et al., 2001). Adequate rinsing and priming in preparing the dialyzer for therapy is critical to avoid Type A reactions.

Reactions mediated by the bradykinin system were initially reported in patients both dialyzed with the AN69 membrane and treated with angiotensin-converting enzyme (ACE) inhibitors. The negatively charged AN69 membrane activates the bradykinin system, and effects are magnified because of the ACE inhibitors since the angiotensin-converting enzyme inactivates bradykinin. It is unclear to what extent ACE inhibitors and other PAN-based membranes or non-PAN membranes cause the same type of reaction. ACE inhibitors may be just amplifying a dialyzer reaction occurring by some other mechanism (Bregman et al., 2001).

Type A reactions have occurred with high-flux dialyzers used with bicarbonate dialysate, which may implicate contamination of the dialysate. Bacterial or endotoxin contamination of the water used to reprocess dialyzers or mix the bicarbonate have been implicated in anaphylactic-type dialyzer reactions. The cause, however, is often unknown (Bregman et al., 2001).

Occasionally, allergic reactions have been associated with heparin. These reactions have usually been mild, but some reactions to heparin have reportedly led to anaphylaxis. When a patient seems to be allergic to all dialyzers, and dialysate contamination has been ruled out, a heparin allergy should be considered and a trial of heparin-free dialysis or citrate anticoagulation initiated (Bregman et al., 2001).

Complement has been associated with acute increase in pulmonary artery pressure during dialysis with unsubstituted cellulose membrane. Complement activation may be a cause of anaphylactic Type A reactions, but this is not firmly established (Bregman et al., 2001).

Nursing management of a Type A reaction is based on symptom management. HD should be stopped immediately and bloodlines clamped. The blood in the lines and dialyzer should not be returned to the patient and the system discarded. Immediate cardiorespiratory support may be required in an anaphylactic reaction. Intravenous antihistamines, steroids, or epinephrine may be given according to the severity of the reaction. Patient education regarding signs and symptoms is important in early recognition and intervention (Bregman et al., 2001; Keen et al, 2001).

Prevention of Type A reactions can be accomplished by proper rinsing of the dialyzers prior to use to rid them of residual ETO and other allergens. Gamma-radiated or steam sterilized dialyzers may present a viable option to ETO sterilized dialyzers. Administration of antihistamines before dialysis may help in patients demonstrating possible sensitivity. Placing the patient on a reuse program and reprocessing new dialyzers prior to the first use may enhance removal of noxious substances prior to HD. Avoidance of the use of AN69 dialyzers in patients taking ACE inhibitors may be beneficial (Bregman et al., 2001; Leunissen et al., 2000).

Type B reactions. Type B reactions are nonspecific and less severe than Type A. They occur later in dialysis, usually 20 to 40 minutes, and are associated with back or chest pain. The etiology is unknown. Complement activation has been implicated, but its role has never been proven. If reuse is beneficial in preventing this reaction, it is not known if this effect is due to the protein coating of the membrane from previous uses resulting in increased biocompatibility, or due to washout of potentially toxic substances from the dialyzer during previous uses and reprocessing (Bregman et al., 2001; Leunissen et al., 2000).

Nursing management of a Type B dialyzer reaction is supportive in nature. Oxygen per nasal cannula should be administered. Myocardial ischemia is common, so any angina should be treated promptly. Dialysis can usually be continued because symptoms typically abate after the first hour (Bregman et al., 2001). In more severe cases, it may be necessary to stop dialysis (Leunissen et al., 2000).

Prevention of Type B reactions can be accomplished by placing the patient on a reuse program, although benefits of reuse are controversial. Changing to a different dialyzer membrane that will cause less complement activation, such as substituted cellulose (cellulose acetate) or a synthetic membrane, may help (Bregman et al., 2001). However, one study found no difference between a biocompatible versus bioincompatible membrane (Leunissen et al., 2000).

Neutropenia/Complement Activation

Dialyzer membranes made of unsubstituted cellulose will have many exposed hydroxyl groups on their surfaces that can activate the complement cascade in the blood flowing through the dialyzer. The complement fragments will then cause circulating neutrophils to migrate to the lungs where they will localize next to the blood vessel walls, resulting in neutropenia. After 30-60 minutes of HD, the circulating neutrophil count will again rise to normal levels or even above normal. Substituted cellulose membranes have

the hydroxyl groups chemically covered, so they cause much less activation of complement resulting in less neutropenia. This neutrophil accumulation in the pulmonary vasculature is a recognized phenomenon during HD and has been implicated in the hypoxemia that occurs in some patients early in HD. Most synthetic membranes cause little neutropenia or complement activation (polysulfone, polycarbonate, polymethylmethacrylate) (Bregman et al., 2001).

Signs and symptoms such as nausea and vomiting, hypotension, chest pain, and back pain may be due to neutropenia and complement activation, but this is controversial. The majority of patients on cellulose acetate membranes do not experience these symptoms (Bregman et al., 2001).

Complement activation may delay recovery of renal function in acute renal failure because it causes sequestration of neutrophils in the glomeruli. The white blood cell count may also be transiently reduced by 50%-80% during dialysis with a cellulose membrane. Thus, all complete blood counts (CBCs) should be drawn before treatment (Bregman et al., 2001).

Hemodialysis-Related Interleukin-1 Stimulation

HD causes an interaction between the dialyzer membrane and monocytes in the patient's blood that may result in a local inflammatory response. This response leads to increased monocyte production and induction of interleukin-1 (IL-1) that is likely enhanced by complement activation from blood-membrane interaction. Complement activation increases the transcription of IL-1 and tissue necrosing factor (TNF). Cellulosic or cellulose-base membranes activation of complement enhances activation of monocytes and increases production of IL-1. Microbial content of the dialysis solution may also contribute to this IL-1 production. An increased level of IL-1 can cause long-term systemic effects as well as acute changes during and shortly after the HD procedure. Acetate dialysate may play a role in the formation of IL-1 as well (Hakim, 2002).

Cytokine production may be implicated in the acute and chronic metabolic and inflammatory changes seen in HD patients. Healthy subjects given IL-1 developed fever, sleepiness, anorexia, myalgia, arthralgia, headache, and gastrointestinal disturbances. When given larger doses, they also experienced hypotension. TNF administered in low dosages to healthy subjects is associated with hypotension, leukopenia, and metabolic dysfunction. In vitro studies have demonstrated a high synergism between IL-1 and TNF. Thus, the "interleukin hypothesis" was based upon the similarity of signs and symptoms resulting from HD and those associated with IL-1 administration (Pereira & Cheung, 2000). All of these manifestations of IL-1 and TNF are familiar as symptoms patients undergoing HD experience.

Cytokines may have a role in accelerated atherosclerosis and cardiovascular morbidity in HD patients as they are thought to lead to proliferation of vascular smooth muscle cells, stimulation of platelet-derived growth factor, and atherosclerotic plaques. IL-1 increases the production of amyloid that may add to the amyloidosis associated with $\beta_2 M$ so cytokines may contribute to bone, articular, and periarticular diseases (Pereira & Cheung, 2000).

Acute phase proteins generated by the liver are stimulated, albumin synthesis suppressed, proteolysis of muscle, and a negative nitrogen balance all result from the actions of IL-1, TNF, and interleukin-6. IL-1 and TNF appetite suppressant effects are likely due to their effect on hepatic metabolism. This combination may account, in part, for some of the wasting seen in long-term HD patients. Hence, IL-1 is implicated in mortality and morbidity of HD patients (Pereira & Cheung, 2000). The use of biocompatible membranes and the avoidance of cellulose-based membranes appears to be desirable in order to minimize the severity of these problems.

Summary

Complications arising from HD are frequent. It is critical to understand the underlying etiology of complications as well as the proactive strategies to prevent or minimize these complications. This sound knowledge base in managing complex interactions is necessary to respond to challenging situations and to anticipate patients' responses to interventions. This prepares nephrology nurses to promote their ultimate goal of achieving positive patient outcomes.

References

Acchiardo, S.R. (2002). Dialysis amyloidosis. In A.R Nissenson & R.N. Fine (Eds.), *Dialysis therapy* (pp. 417-419). Philadelphia: Hanley & Belfus, Inc.

Amato, R.L. (2005). Water treatment for hemodialysis – updated to include the latest AAMI standards for dialysate (RD52:2004). *Nephrology Nursing Journal, 32*(3), 151-167.

Amato, R.L. (2001). Water treatment for hemodialysis, including the latest AAMI standards. *Nephrology Nursing Journal, 28*(6), 619-629.

Association for the Advancement of Medical Instrumentation (AAMI). (2004). AAMI standards on CD – Dialysis edition, Version 4.0. Arlington, VA: AAMI.

Behrens, J. (2001). Assessing anemia secondary to hemolysis in hemodialysis patients. *Nephrology Nursing Journal, 28*(2) Suppl., 253-256.

Besarab, A., & Raja, R.M. (2001). Vascular access for hemodialysis. In J.T Daugirdas., P.G. Blake, & T.S. Ing (Eds.), *Handbook of dialysis* (3rd ed., pp. 67-101). Philadelphia: Lippincott Williams & Wilkins.

Bregman, H., Daugirdas, J.T., & Ing, T.S. (2001). Complications during hemodialysis. In J.T. Daugirdas, P.G. Blake, & T.S. Ing (Eds.), Handbook of dialysis (3rd ed.) (pp. 148-168). Philadelphia: Lippincott Williams & Wilkins.

Daugirdas, J.T., & Kjellstrand C.M. (2001). Chronic hemodialysis prescription: A urea kinetic approach. In J.T. Daugirdas, P.G. Blake, & T.S. Ing (Eds.), *Handbook of dialysis* (3rd ed.) (pp. 121-147). Philadelphia: Lippincott Williams & Wilkins.

Daugirdas, J.T., Van Stone, J.C., & Boag J.T. (2001). Hemodialysis apparatus. In J.T. Daugirdas, P.G. Blake, & T.S. Ing (Eds.), *Handbook of dialysis* (3rd ed.) (pp. 46-66). Philadelphia: Lippincott Williams & Wilkins.

D'Haese, P.C., & DeBroe, M.E. (2001). Aluminum toxicity. In J.T. Daugirdas, P.G Blake, & T.S. Ing (Eds.), *Handbook of dialysis* (3rd ed.) (pp. 548-561). Philadelphia: Lippincott Williams & Wilkins.

Diroll, A., & Hlebovy, D. (2003). Inverse relationship between blood volume and blood pressure. *Nephrology Nursing Journal, 30*(4), 460-461.

Eknoyan, G., Latos D.L., & Lindberg, J. (2003). Practice recommendations for the use of L-carnitine in dialysis-related carnitine disorder: Carnitine Consensus Conference. *American Journal of Kidney Diseases, 41*(4), 868-876.

Fink K.C. (1999). Is Trendelenberg a wise choice? *Journal of Emergency Nursing, 25*(1), 60-62.

Hakim, R.M. (2002). Biocompatibility of dialysis membranes. In A.R. Nissenson & R.N. Fine (Eds.), *Dialysis therapy* (pp. 110-115). Philadelphia: Hanley & Belfus, Inc.

Henderson, L.W. (1980). Symptomatic hypotension during hemodialysis. *Kidney International, 17*, 571-576.

Herzog, C.A. (2003). Cardiac arrest in dialysis patients: Approaches to alter an abysmal outcome. *Kidney International, 63*(Suppl. 84), S197-S200.

Hoeben, H., Abu-Alfa, A.K., Mahnensmith, R., & Perazella M.A. (2002). Hemodynamics in patients with intradialytic hypotension treated with cool dialysate or midodrine. *American Journal of Kidney Diseases, 39*(1), 102-107.

Jaeger, J.O., & Mehta, R.L. (1999). Assessment of dry weight in hemodialysis: An overview. *Journal of the American Society of Nephrology, 10*(2), 392-403.

Karnik, J.A., Young, B.S., Lew, N.L., Herget, M., Dubinsky, C., Lazarus, M., & Chertow G.M. (2001). Cardiac arrest and sudden death in dialysis units. *Kidney International, 60*, 350-357.

Kay J., & Hano J.E. (2001). Musculoskeletal and rheumatic diseases. In J.T. Daugirdas, P.G. Blake, & T.S. Ing (Eds.), *Handbook of dialysis* (3rd ed.) (pp. 637-651). Philadelphia: Lippincott Williams & Wilkins.

Keen, M.L., Lancaster, L.E., & Binkley, L.S. (2001). Hemodialysis. In L.E.Lancaster (Ed.), *Core curriculum for nephrology nursing,* (4th ed.) (pp. 255-303). Pitman, NJ: American Nephrology Nurses' Association.

Khosla, N., & Swartz R.D. (2002). Hemodialysis-associated seizure activity. In A.R. Nissenson & R.N. Fine (Eds.), *Dialysis therapy* (pp. 180-182). Philadelphia: Hanley & Belfus, Inc.

Laut, J., D'Avella, J., Post, J., Reynaud A., & Li, L. (2002). Sodium modeling increases interdialytic weight gain in hemodialysis patients. *American Society of Nephrology,* Abstract presentation.

Leunissen, K.M.L., Kooman, J.P., & van der Sande, F.M. (2000). Acute dialysis complications. In N. Lameire & R.L. Mehta (Eds.), *Complications of dialysis* (pp. 69-88). New York: Marcel Dekker, Inc.

Levin, N.W., & Ronco, C. (2002). Complications during hemodialysis: Common clinical problems during hemodialysis. In A.R. Nissenson & R.N. Fine (Eds.), *Dialysis therapy* (pp. 171-179). Philadelphia: Hanley & Belfus, Inc.

Maggiore Q. (2002). Isothermic dialysis for hypotension-prone patients. *Seminars in Dialysis, 15*(3), 187-190.

Mulloy, L.L, Caruana, R.J., Kozeny, G.A., & Ing, T.S. (2002). Isolated ultrafiltration. In A.R. Nissenson & R.N. Fine (Eds.), *Dialysis therapy* (pp. 166-169). Philadelphia: Hanley & Belfus, Inc.

Murphy, S.W., & Parfrey, P.S. (2002). Management of ischemic heart disease, heart failure, and pericarditis in hemodialysis patients. In A.R. Nissenson & R.N. Fine (Eds.), *Dialysis therapy* (pp. 353-358). Philadelphia: Hanley & Belfus, Inc.

Negrea, L.A. (2003). Complications of hemodialysis. In D.E. Hricik, R.T. Miller, & J.R. Sedor (Eds.), *Nephrology secrets* (2nd ed.) (pp. 183-185). Philadelphia: Hanley & Belfus, Inc.

Nicholls, A.J. (2001a). Heart and circulation. In J.T. Daugirdas, P.G. Blake, & T.S. Ing (Eds.), *Handbook of dialysis* (3rd ed.) (pp. 583-600). Philadelphia: Lippincott Williams & Wilkins.

Nicholls, A.J. (2001b). Nervous system. In J.T. Daugirdas, P.G. Blake, & T.S. Ing (Eds.), *Handbook of dialysis* (3rd ed.) (pp. 656-666). Philadelphia: Lippincott Williams & Wilkins.

Pereira, B.J.G., & Cheung, A.K. (2000). Complications of bioincompatibility of hemodialysis membranes. In N. Lemeire & R.L. Mehta (Eds.), *Complications of dialysis* (pp. 41-68). New York: Marcel Dekker, Inc.

Pittard, J. (2002). Safety monitors in hemodialysis. In A.R. Nissenson & R.N. Fine (Eds.), *Dialysis therapy* (pp. 171-179). Philadelphia: Hanley & Belfus, Inc.

Prakash S., Reddan D., Heidenheim A.P., Kianfar C., & Lindsay R.M. (2002). Central, peripheral, and other blood volume changes during hemodialysis. *ASAIO Journal, 48*(4), 379-382.

Schneditz, D., Ronco, C., & Levin N. (2003). Temperature control by the blood temperature monitor. *Seminars in Dialysis, 16*(6), 477-482.

Schreiber, M.J. (2001). Clinical dilemmas in dialysis: Managing the hypotensive patient, setting the stage. *American Journal of Kidney Diseases, 38*(4), Suppl. 4, S1-S10.

Sheth, K.N., Wu., G.F., Messé, S.R., Wolf, R.L., & Kasner, S.E. (2003). Dialysis disequilibrium: Another reversible posterior leukoencephalopathy syndrome? *Clinical Neurology and Neurosurgery, 105*, 249-252.

Shoji, T., Tsubakihara, Y., M. Fujii, M., & Imai, E. (2004). Hemodialysis-associated hypotension as an independent risk factor for two-year mortality in hemodialysis patients. *Kidney International, 66*(3), 1212-1220.

Shulman, T, Heidenheim, A.P, Kianfar, C., Shulman, S.M., & Lindsay, R.M. (2001). Preserving central blood volume: Changes in body fluid compartments during hemodialysis. *ASAIO Journal, 47*(6), 615-618.

Sigler, M.H., Teehan, B.P., Daugirdas, J.T., & Ing, T.S. (2001). Slow continuous therapies. In J.T. Daugirdas, P.G. Blake, & T.S. Ing (Eds.), *Handbook of dialysis* (3rd ed.) (pp. 199-230), Philadelphia: Lippincott Williams & Wilkins.

Stefandis, I., Stiller, S., Ikonomov, V., & Mann, H. (2002). Sodium and body fluid homeostasis in profiling hemodialysis treatment. *The International Journal of Artificial Organs, 25*(5), 421-428.

Tzamaloukas, A.H., & Friedman, E.A. (2001). Diabetes. In J.T.Daugirdas, P.G.Blake, & T.S. Ing (Eds.), *Handbook of dialysis* (3rd ed.) (pp. 453-465), Philadelphia: Lippincott Williams & Wilkins.

van der Sande, F.M., Luik, A.J., Kooman, J.P., Verstappen, V., & Leunissen, K.M.L. (2000). Effect of intravenous fluids on blood pressure course during hemodialysis in hypotensive-prone patients. *Journal of the American Society of Nephrology, 11,* 550-555.

Wilson, S. (2004). UF profiles and sodium modeling. iKidney.com. Retrieved May 21, 2004, from www.ikidney.com/iKidney/Community/Pro2Pro/Nurses/UFProfilesandSodiumModeling.htm

Suggested Readings

Emili, S., Black, N.A., Paul, R.V., Rexing, C.J., & Ullian, M.E. (1999). A protocol-based treatment for intradialytic hypotension in hospitalized hemodialysis patients. *American Journal of Kidney Diseases, 33*(6), 1107-1114.

van der Sande, F.M., Kooman, J.P., Konings, C.J., & Leunissen, K.M.L. (2001). Thermal effects and blood pressure response during post dilution hemodialfiltration and hemodialysis: The effect of replacement fluid and dialysate temperature. *Journal of the American Society of Nephrology, 12*(9), 1916-1920.

- Adverse events requiring intervention are estimated to occur in 20%-50% of hemodialysis treatments.

- The accuracy of the estimated dry weight is critical in preventing complications of hemodialysis.

- Hypotension is the most commonly occurring intradialytic complication at a rate of 20%-50% of all hemodialysis treatments. Strategies to prevent hypotension include use of bicarbonate dialysate, sodium profiling, ultrafiltration profiling, cool dialysate, alpha adrenergic agonists, isolated ultrafiltration, biocompatible membranes, and administration of L-carnitine in those patients demonstrating a carnitine deficiency.

- Fluid shifts may not occur consistently in all body compartments. Central blood volume appears to be preserved at the expense of maximum shifting of fluid in the lower extremities first, followed by upper extremities. This may explain the occurrence of muscle cramps in the lower extremities.

- Blood volume monitoring may allow for early identification of fluid volume shifts so that hypotension or other complications related to decreased intravascular volume can be avoided.

- Trendelenberg position for intradialytic complication management may be detrimental as a routine strategy to treat intradialytic hypotension. Its use should be limited to extreme emergencies.

- Chest pain occurring during hemodialysis should be differentiated from dialysis associated complications.

- Fever and chills developing during hemodialysis may be related to vascular access infection, most commonly from a central venous catheter. Technical problems should also be considered.

- Urea clearance should be minimized to 30% in dialysis disequilibrium syndrome to avoid development of untoward sequelae from too rapid clearances.

- Acute, gross hemolysis is a medical emergency. Occult hemolysis is a challenge to identify.

- Cardiac arrest on hemodialysis has an abysmal prognosis: 60% of patients experiencing cardiac arrest while on hemodialysis will expire within 48 hours.

- Exsanguination on hemodialysis can almost always be prevented with fastidious attention to technical aspects of hemodialysis.

- Using bicarbonate dialysate in lieu of acetate dialysate can aid in prevention of intradialytic complications.

- Hemodialysis-related amyloidosis progresses more slowly in patients with even slight residual renal function. Duration on dialysis and the occurrence of dialysis-related amyloidosis are closely related. Patients benefit from the use of polysulfone dialyzers or other biocompatible membrane rather than cellulose-based membranes.

- Nursing assessment before, during, and after hemodialysis is a major deterrent to intradialytic complications.

ANNP625

Hemodialysis: Prevention and Management of Treatment Complications

Karen C. Robbins, MS, RN, CNN

Contemporary Nephrology Nursing: Principles and Practice contains 39 chapters of educational content. Individual learners may apply for continuing nursing education credit by reading a chapter and completing the Continuing Education Evaluation Form for that chapter. Learners may apply for continuing education credit for any or all chapters.

Please photocopy this page and return to ANNA.
COMPLETE THE FOLLOWING:

Name: _____

Address:_____

City:_____ State: _____ Zip: _____

E-mail: _____

Preferred telephone: ☐ Home   ☐ Work: _____

State where licensed and license number (optional): _____

CE application fees are based upon the number of contact hours provided by the individual chapter. CE fees per contact hour for ANNA members are as follows: 1.0-1.9 - $15; 2.0-2.9 - $20; 3.0-3.9 - $25; 4.0 and higher - $30. Fees for nonmembers are $10 higher.

ANNA Member: ☐ Yes   ☐ No   Member # (if available) _____

☐ Checked Enclosed   ☐ American Express   ☐ Visa   ☐ MasterCard

Total Amount Submitted: _____

Credit Card Number:_____ Exp. Date: _____

Name as it appears on the card: _____

CE Evaluation Form
To receive continuing education credit for individual study after reading the chapter
1. Photocopy this form. (You may also download this form from ANNA's Web site, **www.annanurse.org.**)
2. Mail the completed form with payment (check) or credit card information to American Nephrology Nurses' Association, East Holly Avenue, Box 56, Pitman, NJ 08071-0056.
3. You will receive your CE certificate from ANNA in 4 to 6 weeks.

Test returns must be postmarked by **December 31, 2010.**

CE Application Fee
ANNA Member $25.00
Nonmember $35.00

EVALUATION FORM

1. I verify that I have read this chapter and completed this education activity. Date: _____

_____
Signature

2. What would be different in your practice if you applied what you learned from this activity? *(Please use additional sheet of paper if necessary.)*

_____
_____
_____
_____
_____
_____
_____
_____
_____
_____
_____
_____
_____

Evaluation	Strongly disagree				Strongly agree
3. The activity met the stated objectives.					
a. List complications that challenge nurses involved in providing hemodialysis therapy.	1	2	3	4	5
b. Relate the basis of complications of hemodialysis therapy to the management and patient care necessary.	1	2	3	4	5
c. Devise strategies to help prevent complications of hemodialysis therapy.	1	2	3	4	5
4. The content was current and relevant.	1	2	3	4	5
5. The content was presented clearly.	1	2	3	4	5
6. The content was covered adequately.	1	2	3	4	5
7. Rate your ability to apply the learning obtained from this activity to practice.	1	2	3	4	5

Comments _____

_____

8. Time required to read the chapter and complete this form: _____ minutes.

This educational activity has been provided by the American Nephrology Nurses' Association (ANNA) for 3.1 contact hours. ANNA is accredited as a provider of continuing nursing education (CNE) by the American Nurses Credentialing Center's Commission on Accreditation (ANCC-COA). ANNA is an approved provider of continuing education by the California Board of Registered Nursing, CEP 0910.

Home Dialysis Therapies

Lori Harwood, MSc, RN, CNeph(C)
Rosemary Leitch, RN, CNeph(C)

Chapter Contents

Home Dialysis Therapies

Chapter 26

Lori Harwood, MSc, RN, CNeph(C)
Rosemary Leitch, RN, CNeph(C)

ome dialysis is an optimal option for patients requiring renal replacement therapy. These therapies are more cost effective than in-center therapies, and the benefits to patients are well documented. Despite this evidence for these therapies, home hemodialysis (HHD) is often only available as a secondary treatment choice and with little support in traditional hemodialysis (HD) centers (Branson & Moran, 2004). It is timely to include a chapter on home therapies in this textbook, as there is a renewed interest in longer HD times, more frequent HD, and home modalities. Peritoneal dialysis (PD) is an extremely important home dialysis modality and is discussed in this chapter but it is detailed elsewhere in this textbook. The focus of this chapter is mainly on HHD.

Utilization of Home Dialysis Therapy

More than a quarter of a million individuals in the United States (U.S.) are on dialysis (United States Renal Data System [USRDS], 2003). Of those, 92% are treated with HD and 8% with PD (USRDS, 2003). Superior patient and economic outcomes are documented with home therapies, yet in recent years, only a few patients were on home dialysis. The prevalence of individuals on HHD is 0.4% - 0.6%, and PD is slightly higher at 8.4% - 10.4% (USRDS, 2003). Internationally, New Zealand and Australia lead in numbers of patients on home therapies with the majority of patients on home dialysis (USRDS, 2003).

History of Home Dialysis

In 1960 several technologies combined to secure long-term HD as an option for end stage renal disease (ESRD) therapy. Dr. Belding Scribner developed the Teflon arteriovenous shunt that resulted in an access that could be used for repetitive dialysis (Scribner, Buri, Caner, Hegstrom, & Burnell, 1960). Equipment modifications such as the Kiil dialyzer (Penreas, Cole, Tu, & Scribner, 1961) and the change in practice for nurses to perform HD without the constant presence of a physician (Murray, Tu, Albers, Burnell, & Scribner, 1962) made HD possible. The number of patients requiring HD continued to grow, as did the cost.

HHD was first used in the early 1960s (Blagg, 1997) as a means to provide a more cost-effective form of HD. The first documented case of a HHD patient was in Japan in 1961, under the care of Dr. Yuke Nose (Nose, 1965). The first person to receive HHD in the United States was a 15-year-old teenage girl, assisted by her mother, in 1964 (Curtis, Cole, Fellows, Tyler, & Scribner, 1965). The decision to dialyze at home was made because a committee, mandated to ration the resources of HD based on established criteria, refused to dialyze her due to her age. The advantages of HHD were soon realized, and the number of patients on this form of dialysis steadily began to increase. In 1973, when the Medicare End Stage Renal Disease Program came into effect, 40% of all U.S. HD patients were on HHD (Blagg, 1997). With the Medicare program more individuals became eligible for HD and it became their right to choose whether or not to receive HD.

The growth of HHD continued until the early 1980s and then started to decline. Several factors have been associated with this decline in HHD including: the increased age and co-morbidities of patients requiring dialysis and the decreased numbers of low risk patients who would be more suitable for HHD (Blagg, 2000; Mackenzie & Mactier, 1998); better re-imbursement for the physician and the HD facility in settings other than the home (Lindsay & Leitch, 2004), thus the creation of greater numbers of regional in-center HD units (Mackenzie & Mactier, 1998) and for profit free-standing units; and the sociodemographic changes in the family and in the workplace, which have decreased the amount of assistance available to help with HHD (Mackenzie & Mactier, 1998). Many of the helpers themselves were elderly and unable to assist in the home (Blagg, 2000). Due to the decline in prevalence of home therapies many younger nephrologists have very little experience with HHD (Blagg, 2000) and, thus, are unlikely to create new home dialysis programs.

Patients are often fearful of the HD technology (Blagg, 2000) compared to simpler PD methods. The ease and short training time of continuous ambulatory peritoneal dialysis (CAPD) and continuous cyclic peritoneal dialysis (CCPD) have also decreased the number of those who perhaps would have chosen HHD. PD became a mainstream treatment for ESRD in 1976 (Blagg, 1997). For those wanting a home therapy PD continues to be an alternative.

Benefits of Home Dialysis

Patient Outcomes

The benefits to patients dialyzing in the home are many. They include more flexibility in dialysis schedules, thus more opportunity for adequate dialysis; convenience; no transportation issues; more time with the family; less time in the hospital setting; increased knowledge regarding dialysis and personal health; independence; and control over personal treatment. Studies have revealed that HHD has better patient survival (Grant, Rodger, Howie, et al., 1992; Jacobs & Selwood, 1996; Mailloux et al., 1996; Woods, Port, Stannard, Blagg, & Held, 1996), provides better quality of life (Bremer, McCauley, Wrona, & Johnson, 1989; Evans et al., 1985; Kutner, Brogan, & Kutner, 1986; McFarlane, Bayoumi, Pierratos, & Redelmeier, 2003; Ting, Kjellstrand, Freitas, Carrie, & Zarghamee, 2003), offers greater independence and opportunity for rehabilitation (Oberley & Schatell, 1996) and decreased hospitalization (Ting et al., 2003) than other forms of dialysis.

Financial Implications of Home Dialysis

Home dialysis therapies are more cost effective than in-center treatment largely due to the cost savings of personnel performing the dialysis. A Canadian study compared the cost of hospital HD, HHD, self-care HD, and CAPD (Goeree, Manalich, Grootendorst, Beecroft & Churchill, 1995). It was found that average costs per patient year were highest for hospital HD and lowest for CAPD and HHD. Two other Canadian studies concluded that nocturnal HD (McFarlane et al., 2003) and short daily HD (Kroeker, Clark, Heidenheim, Kuenzig, Leitch, & Meyette, 2003) performed in the home were less costly than conventional in-center HD. Mackenzie and Mactier (1998), in an analysis of the cost of their dialysis program in the United Kingdom (UK) over a 2-year period in the 1990s, also concluded that HHD was more cost effective than treating the same number of patients in an in-center therapy.

Paying for the health care professional to perform the HD in the home has also been shown to be cost effective. An evaluation of four in-center HD patients who were changed to staff-assisted home hemodialysis (SAHHD) was conducted. Despite paying for the personnel performing the dialysis, SAHHD was determined to be cost effective (Agraharkar, Du, Ahuja, & Barclay, 2002). These patients also showed improvements in the dialysis core indicators and experienced fewer hospitalizations. This modality may be of particular benefit for those with a terminal illness who are severely debilitated and require ambulance transportation to and from in-center dialysis.

HHD is the least costly compared to other dialysis modalities. Another important factor to consider when assessing for patient suitability is also the high "upfront" costs associated with the equipment and water installation. The concept of "pay back" with HHD is the period in which the higher initial costs of training and start up are exceeded by the greater long-term costs savings of HD (Mackenzie & Mactier, 1998). This has been estimated to be 14.4 months in the U.S. (Delano, Feinroth, Feinroth, & Friedman, 1981) and 14.2 months in the UK (Mackenzie & Mactier, 1998).

HHD Modalities

Conventional, Short Daily, and Nocturnal HD

Conventional refers to HD performed three times a week, each treatment for 2.5 to 5 hours. Conventional HD (CHD) can be done in-center or in the home. Short daily HD refers to HD, performed five to seven times a week, each treatment for 1.5 to 3 hours with a high efficiency dialyzer. Short daily HD can be done in-center or in the home. Nocturnal dialysis refers to HD performed 5 to 7 nights per week, each treatment for 6 to 10 hours while the patient sleeps. Nocturnal HD is generally considered a home therapy but some programs do this in-center thrice weekly.

Short daily HD (SDHD) therapy was first introduced in Los Angeles, CA, in 1967 (DePalma, Pecker, & Maxwell, 1969) and Brooklyn, NY, in 1975 (Manhor, Louis, Gorfien, & Lipner, 1981). These two programs performed SDHD in-center. The first to perform SDHD in the home was in Bologna, Italy, in 1972 (Bonomini, Mioli, Albertazzi, & Scolari, 1972). These three programs are considered the trailblazers of SDHD. The U.S. programs encountered problems with financial support, as Medicare reimbursed only three treatments a week, as well as problems with logistics and technology. Other parts of the world, especially Italy, were able to continue to have current SDHD programs. Some of these problems were improved in the 1980s and, thus, programs were developed throughout the world (Kjellstrand, 1998).

Nocturnal home HD (NHHD) therapy, also referred to as quotidian or "more frequent dialysis" was pioneered in 1994, in Toronto, Canada, where patients received long, nightly HD in the home (Uldall et al., 1994). In 1997, Lynchburg Nephrology Dialysis, Inc. started a Nightly Home Hemodialysis program in the United States modeled after the Toronto program (Lockridge et al, 2004). As of this writing, there are several other centers who have also started programs, and a new level of interest in home dialysis has been generated.

Solute Removal with More Frequent Dialysis

The NKF-KDOQI guidelines recommend the minimal delivery dose of HD should be a Kt/V of 1.2 or a urea reduction ratio of 65% per treatment (National Kidney Foundation [NKF], 2000). Recent evidence in the HEMO study (Eknoyan et al., 2002) suggests the futility of increasing the dialysis dose beyond the NKF-KDOQI guidelines. In this study there was no association between increased Kt/V and patient survival. These findings raise the question – why have such benefits been observed with short daily dialysis and nocturnal dialysis?

The answer lies in the achievement of optimal dialysis using a modality that is the most efficient at removal of all uremic toxins by the most physiological method with the least impact on the patient's daily life (Buoncristiani, Cairo, Giombini, & Bonforte, 1989). The best dialysis treatment is one that is efficient and continuous. Intermittent HD is efficient but not continuous. PD is continuous but not efficient (Lindsay et al., 2001).

As a measure of the physiological impact of the dialysis treatment Valek and Lopot (1989) introduced the concept of time-averaged deviation (TAD) of urea blood concentrations and time-averaged concentration (TAC) (Buoncristiani, Fagugli, Quintaliani, & Kulurianu, 1997). In a person with normal renal function the TAD of urea blood concentration remains steadily at zero. A dialysis modality would be considered physiological if the TAD is as low as possible. This can only be achieved through continuous dialysis treatments such as CAPD and CCPD. Therefore, unphysiological treatments have high TAD, which increases with the duration between sessions and the efficiency of sessions. TADs have remained high the last 20 years of HD due to the traditional acceptance of thrice weekly dialysis and the introduction of high efficiency dialyzers (Buoncristiani et al., 1997).

SDHD performed six times a week for only 2 hours has a higher weekly removal of urea than longer treatments of 4 hours, three times a week. Most (60-65%) of the removal with conventional HD of urea occurs in the first half of the session with a low efficiency dialyzer (Buoncristiani et al., 1997). Therefore, if the session is decreased to 2 hours the removal of urea will be reduced by 35% and 40% (Buoncristiani et al., 1997). However, by doubling the number of dialysis treatments per week the theoretical gain is in the order of 20% to 30% (Buoncristiani et al., 1997). This gain may be more with the use of a high efficiency dialyzer, where up to 75% of urea reduction can take place in the first half of a treatment (Buonicristiani et al., 1997). The removal of urea per treatment and per week, therefore, decreases and blunts somewhat but not completely the above-mentioned gain, which is beneficial. Thus, increasing the frequency of dialysis is more physiological for the patient than increasing the length of dialysis treatments. The result is that in the first 2-3 weeks on a daily therapy the predialytic serum urea levels decrease until a near steady state is achieved (Buonicristiani et al., 1997).

Clinical Advantages of More Frequent Home Hemodialysis

Buoncristiani, Cairo, Giombini, Quintaliani, and Bonforte (1989) noted dramatic patient improvement in 536 patients treated with 90-minute short daily home hemodialysis (SDHHD). A double lumen single needle was used in 80% of the treatments with a blood pump speed of 275 mls/min. Outcomes included a significant rise of hemoglobin and hematocrit, perfect control of acid-base equilibrium with normal serum bicarbonate levels, excellent intradialytic cardiovascular stability, the disappearance of intradialytic symptoms with ultrafiltration as high as 1.5 Kg/h, and the ability to achieve dry weight. Patients reported experiencing significant improvement in all aspects studied: general well being, painful symptoms, post-dialytic asthenia, work ability, family and social life, degree of rehabilitation, and sexual potency.

Kjellstrand and Ting (1998) described similar results in their experience with SDHHD reporting highly significant early improvement in quality of life (QOL) indicators, well being, as well as greater strength and endurance. Medications to treat anemia and hypertension were reduced as were hospitalizations. Treatments were more stable and patients experienced less cramping and had fewer hypotensive episodes. Patients also reported increased energy levels, more time with family, and less time associated with dialysis.

In 1998, Pierratos and colleagues published their 3-year experience with NHHD. At the time of publication, 12 patients had been on the therapy for up to 34 months. NHHD was performed 6-7 nights a week for 8-10 hours, with a low surface area polysulfone dialyzer, a central venous catheter (CVC), a blood pump speed of 300 ml/min, and a dialysate flow of 100 to 300 mls/min. Anticoagulation was achieved with heparin at an average hourly rate of 1100 ± 300 u/h with no initial bolus. All patients used a dialysate with potassium at 2 mEq/L and bicarbonate 28 to 32 mEq/L. Dialysate calcium levels were individualized according to serum calcium levels. Patients reported initial sleep problems that improved in less than a week. The ultrafiltration was very well tolerated with a maximum ultrafiltration rate of 400 ml/hour. Patients who previously had intradialytic symptoms became asymptomatic, and antihypertensive medications were reduced. Patients also reported improvements in pruritus, nausea, postdialytic symptoms, and energy levels. Appetites improved and diets were liberalized. Protein intake and protein catabolic rate increased. Predialysis serum urea and creatinine progressively decreased. Phosphate levels returned to normal serum levels, and the need for phosphate binding medications was eliminated. In fact, some patients required phosphate supplementation in the dialysate. Hemoglobin levels and erythropoietin (EPO) use did not change significantly. There was also greater removal of Beta2-microglobulin, which is associated with secondary amyloidosis, carpal tunnel syndrome, and arthropathy. In the

3 years of nocturnal dialysis no episode of hemodynamic instability was experienced that would require the presence of a helper, thus making it safe therapy for patients without assistants. Similarly, data collected on 28 patients over 5.5 years of experience revealed similar findings to those reported by Perratos et al. (Lockridge et al., 2004). A more recent study reported that enhancing the uremic clearance by NHHD resulted in a rise in hemoglobin and reductions in EPO requirements (Schwartz, Pierratos, Richardson, Fenton, & Chan, 2005).

In London, Ontario, Canada, the first study comparing patient outcomes of SDHHD and NHHD with matched conventional HD controls was conducted by Lindsay (2003). The results showed that some outcomes were better with SDHHD and others with NHHD. More importantly, both more frequent dialysis modalities were superior to conventional in-center HD in the following areas: fluid management, interdialytic symptoms (Heidenheim, Muirhead, Moist, & Lindsay, 2003), blood pressure management (Nesrallah, Suri, Moist, Kortas, & Lindsay, 2003) nutritional status (Spanner, Suri, Heidenheim, & Lindsay, 2003), phosphate levels (Lindsay et al., 2003), and urea clearance (Suri, Depner, Blake, Heidenheim & Lindsay, 2003).

Home Hemodialysis Program Requirements

Policies and Procedures

A home dialysis unit must first determine policies and procedures to follow when offering various home modalities. Ting, Leitch, and Ouwendyk (2004) pose many of the questions that need to be addressed. What is the maximum capacity of each type of modality? Is monitoring necessary for nocturnal dialysis? Is the type of vascular access a limiting factor? How will non-compliance be handled? Can the patient dialyze alone? Will a dependent patient relying solely on an assistant be allowed to be at home? Will staff-assisted HHD be an option? It is essential that multidisciplinary team members be convinced that HHD is a valuable treatment option and is involved in the development of policies and procedures. Answers to these questions must be consistent with the in-center and chronic kidney disease (CKD) program but tailored to suit the home environment. Having a consistent approach can help in patient selection and assist a patient to make the decision regarding modality. The commitment by management to provide appropriate equipment, training, support staff, and space is essential to the establishment of a successful program.

HHD programs require the following:

- Professional, knowledgeable, trustworthy training staff designated for home dialysis
- Hemodialysis equipment suitable for home patient use
- Defined patient responsibilities and program expectations
- Biomedical/technical support for equipment and water installation and maintenance
- On-call nursing and medical support
- Multidisciplinary team– includes physician, nursing, dietary, social work, and pharmacists
- Follow-up clinics
- Peer support (e.g., Kidney Foundation)

- Supply delivery service
- Suitable teaching environment – quiet, comfortable, minimum of interruptions
- Appropriate nurse-patient ratio for teaching
- Outline of training schedule including expected time commitment
- Appropriate teaching material

Patients and Home Hemodialysis

Patient Suitability for Home Hemodialysis

Prior to patient acceptance for home hemodialysis, an assessment or interview with a home dialysis nurse is imperative. This interview provides an opportunity for the patient to communicate expectations and for the nurse to determine if the patient would be able to function in the home. The determination of patient and family suitability involves many factors.

Introduction of treatment options. It is prudent to determine who may be suitable for HHD as early as possible in an attempt to promote self-care prior to the patient "settling in" and becoming accustomed to the full-care environment. Once they have become dependent on others for care and have developed social interactions in the unit, it can be difficult to convince patients of the benefits of self-care. Explaining all therapy options in the CKD clinic can serve as the initial step to get the patient to consider HHD (Lindsay & Leitch, 2004). Choosing a home dialysis modalities has been significantly correlated to longer durations of follow-up in a CKD clinic (Piccoli et al., 2005). Ideally, patients should begin dialysis in the home training unit. Patients involved in their own care experienced increased control of their disease and time for daily activities. Outlining practical benefits such as decreased travel time and expenses, scheduling flexibility, increased time with their family, and employment often captures interest in home dialysis. Explanations of physical benefits of frequent dialysis therapy, increased survival of the HHD patient and the potential to enjoy a better QOL must be included in discussions (Agraharkar et al., 2002; Woods et al., 1996). Essential to the discussion are the potential disadvantages of HHD that include time required for set-up and cleaning, responsibilities, supply management, medication administration, and stress. Some patients do not want to see the HD equipment in their home and find it a constant reminder of their chronic illness. Also, patients starting frequent dialysis at home have nothing with which to compare it. They don't understand the symptoms associated with conventional dialysis. But more importantly, some of them have difficulty accepting their disease and have no transition time to do that. Providing the opportunity for interaction with those already on home HD may help to alleviate some of these fears.

HHD is not an option suited to everyone. The responsibilities can be overwhelming and the physical requirements demanding. An assistant for the more debilitated patient may not be available or the home may be unsuitable. Patients require a high motivational level and may find that they are quite dependent upon the social support enjoyed in the dialysis center and would find the isolation at home unacceptable. They may prefer to leave their medical management to the dialysis staff instead of taking on this responsibility (Ting et al., 2004).

Assessment interview. If the patient and family have agreed to pursue HHD, pre-training assessment is necessary. The purpose is to identify any existing and potential health-related concerns prior to undertaking an expensive, time-consuming training period and to prevent patients failing on this modality (Lindsay & Leitch, 2004). Selecting appropriate candidates with a thorough assessment will contribute to success in the training period (Chow & Bennett, 2001).

Chow and Bennett (2001) developed a tool to assist in the assessment of patients for home dialysis. This tool measures six domains: (a) physical stability; (b) nutritional stability, (c) communication, (d) ability to maintain self care, (e) psychological suitability, and (f) social support. The tool has been proven to be reliable for assessment of patients for home dialysis.

The person and the assistant (if applicable) must meet with the home dialysis nurse and social worker to discuss the many aspects of home dialysis. Benefits, responsibilities, and the expectations of the program as well as the stressors of home dialysis are reviewed. Discussion includes such practicalities as training time commitments, accommodation requirements, and childcare and employment schedules. Meeting with the patient provides the home dialysis nurse the opportunity to determine the person's physical strength to handle the equipment and supplies, dexterity, vision, and communication skills. Addressing such issues as ability to read, color blindness, and hearing difficulties assists the nurse in making adjustments to training material and teaching tools in preparation for training (Lindsay & Leitch, 2004). The person's emotional and psychological suitability will be assessed prior to training with the assistance of the social worker and the nephrologist. Depression is common in patients with ESRD and can interfere with learning (Lindsay & Leitch, 2004). Training may need to be delayed until after treatment for depression.

Information regarding patient responses to previous dialysis treatments can be obtained from the referring unit. Although dialysis-related problems are important, they should not necessarily prevent the patient from entering the training program especially if daily dialysis is an option. More frequent dialysis is tolerated much better with fewer interdialytic symptoms experienced than with conventional therapy. The individual must be stable during their training period treatments to limit undesirable situations in the home setting (Lindsay & Leitch, 2004). If an assistant is used, the patient and assistant must be able to work as a team. Both the patient and assistant will need to be given the opportunity to discuss fears and concerns separately (Courts, 2000). When it is determined from all perspectives that the patient is suitable, a home visit is organized to assess the installation requirements. After the technical and clinical teams have ascertained feasibility, the training process can begin.

Psychosocial concerns and patient and family adjustment. It is well established that QOL is improved with home dialysis. Compared to in-center patients, HHD patients report higher life satisfaction (Stark, 1985) and psychosocial adjustment, lower levels of anxiety and HD stressors (Courts & Boyette, 1998), and more opportunity for employment

(Oberley & Schatell, 1996) particularly for young adult males (Burton, Canzona, Lindsay, & Palmer, 1985).

While it is important to acknowledge the benefits of home dialysis, it is of equal importance to explore those reasons that some patients do not do well on a home therapy. The application of this information will assist in the assessment of suitability and will help identify indicators for those at risk for failure so that the team can provide for earlier supportive interventions.

Anxiety, as it relates to the home dialysis treatment therapy, was shown to be a significant cause for HHD failure (Richmond, Lindsay, Burton, Conley & Wai, 1982). Depression, regardless of the home therapy, was noted to be an independent risk factor for living or dying. As well, stress scores were reported to be a predictor of failure to return to in-center therapy (Wai, Richmond, Burton, & Lindsay, 1981). This study highlights the importance of multi-disciplinary support required for the success of the patient receiving dialysis in the home.

A few publications are authored by home dialysis patients, sharing their positive experiences with home dialysis (Cagle et al., 1999; Harper, 1997; Piccoli et al., 2000). Common themes in their accounts include improvements in physical status, increased control of his or her life, and more time spent with family. Two poignant examples follow:

"The main reason I chose home hemodialysis was that it would allow me to continue to work, since my dialysis facility did not have an evening shift. I worked for the first 15 years on dialysis. This allowed me to remain a contributing member of society and gave meaning to my life. It also helped to make dialysis a necessary chore rather than the focus of my life" (Harper, 1997, p. 10).

"I used to think of myself as being sick with a not-too-promising future. Now I feel well, have confidence, energy and a feeling of well being that is hard to convey to others. I feel that NHHD [nocturnal home hemodialysis] *has given me my life back"* (Cagle et al., 1999, p. 75).

Patients deciding to change to or start with a home therapy do so with careful consideration of both the possible clinical advantage and personal preferences of home dialysis (Piccoli et al., 2000). Personal motivations of patients are focused on three areas: (a) the search for the best dialysis treatment, (b) confidence in their caregivers' opinion, and (c) the logistics of coordinating the dialysis treatments around work and other life commitments (Piccoli et al., 2000). The distance to a dialysis center, observation of other dialysis patients, suggestions by spouse, and physician recommendations are also determinants of choosing a home dialysis therapy (Courts, 2000). Younger adult females who are looking after young children in the home tend to prefer CAPD to HHD (Burton et al., 1985).

Patients and families often experience uncertainty and fear of the unknown when considering a home dialysis modality. Common fears described by patients in this situation include being a burden to the family, self-cannulation, and access survival. Since home dialysis takes place in the "home," it is advisable to include the family in the decision for this modality. Children may experience fear of the HD machine, the sounds it makes, and may resent the time required for the parent to dialyze. Providing an opportunity

to see the machine before equipment enters the home and allowing them to do minor chores to assist with the therapy will serve as a method of including them in the home dialysis process.

HHD is stressful for both the patient and caregiver and requires a strong relationship as it impacts on the entire family (Courts, 2002). A review of literature published in 1993 reviewed 48 research and anecdotal accounts of HHD since 1967 (Brunier & McKeever, 1993). This review reported that partners of HHD patients share many of the chronic disease-related problems and find home dialysis as stressful and complex as the patients. They often continue with all the responsibilities they previously handled in addition to home dialysis. Partners may also experience the same reactions that the patient exhibits such as anger, denial, anxiety, and depression. Caregivers have also reported fatigue and ill effects to their own health status due to the burden of caregiving (Luk, 2002) as well as feeling isolated and not supported by health care providers (Luk, 2002; Wellard & Street, 1999). Courts (2000) reported that regardless of these negative findings, partners preferred dialysis at home to transplant or in-center HD.

Patient and Family Education

HHD education programs. Historically, in the early years of HHD, it was customary for the teaching facility to develop all of the patient education materials. Today, most HD equipment suppliers have a variety of teaching tools already established and available for use. Established HHD programs also are generally willing to share instruction material. Web sites are available for patient education as well as information provided by organizations such as the Kidney Foundation. It is, therefore, beneficial to investigate and incorporate or adapt existing material (Leitch & Ouwendyk, 2004).

Home dialysis nurses are patient educators and need to apply adult learning principles and education theory for effective teaching programs. It is beyond the scope of this chapter to include comprehensive detail on this topic; however, Wick and Robbins (1998) have published a chapter on education theories and principles for effective patient education.

The training period. The training period serves as the final opportunity to determine if home dialysis is feasible: Can the person perform the treatment safely and competently with minimal problems, maintain the equipment, and know when to call for advice? It also provides an ideal situation for the home dialysis nurse and ESRD patient to develop a rapport that fosters independence as well as establishes a support network. This is essential once the person is managing their own treatment in the home setting, as the home dialysis nurse must trust the person to inform the unit of concerns. Failure to do so could put the individual's health in jeopardy.

The time required for training completion will vary considerably with each person. Influencing factors include the cognitive, emotional, and physical state of the patient; age; motivation; previous experience; nurse/patient ratio; and modality. If SDHHD is chosen, this therapy allows for more practice with the actual dialysis treatment (Leitch &

Table 26-1
Practical Tips for Patient Education Sessions

Training sessions:
- are well organized so as not to waste time.
- are flexible to accommodate a variety of ages and education levels.
- occur during dialysis and on non-dialysis days if able.
- build on previously learned material to allow for repetition.
- identify individual learning styles and alter presentation of material accordingly.
- recognize saturation point to indicate time to stop.
- allows for testing of material and provides opportunity for return.
- provide demonstration, ongoing feedback.
- may or may not involve an assistant depending upon unit policies.
- allow for simple documentation of sessions.

Table 26-2
Ideas for Successful Patient Education

- The ESRD patient has decreased concentration (10-15 minutes at a time).
- Individuals can generally learn seven new pieces of information at a time.
- Adults learn better when information is in meaningful context.
- More learning occurs when readers must interact, such as fill in blanks, circle choices.
- Demonstration and discussion are the methods of choice.
- Patients are most comfortable in an informal setting that allows the nurse and learner the opportunity to relate one to one.
- Have fun – provide cartoons, relate past experiences.
- If at first you don't succeed, re-evaluate. Maybe someone else should try. The goal is to get the patient home.
- Keep open communication. Discuss concerns with the patient. They may be too stressed or too unwell to learn, and if so, involve social work, nephrologist.
- Keep alternate options in mind. Temporary trial in a limited care setting to gain self-confidence.
- Assess the working relationship of the patient and spouse (Is it conducive to learning?).

Figure 26-1
Longitudinal View of a Dialyzer

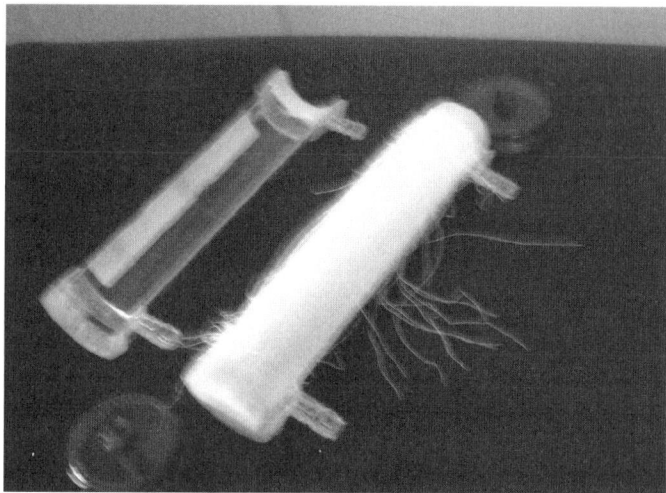

Ouwendyk, 2004) and, possibly, the elimination of the need for an assistant. Training time can be shortened considerably if the patient has learned to cannulate their access prior to commencing training or if they are already on a self-care program. In the London Daily Dialysis Study, training time varied from as little as a mean of 13.63 training days for those already performing self-care dialysis, to a mean of 21 training days for patients who were previously on an in-center therapy and had more physical limitations (Leitch et al., 2003). Regardless, it is important to adjust the training period to suit the individual patient's needs (Leitch & Ouwendyk, 2004). Investing the required time during training pays in the long run as patients will become more confident. Practical tips for patient education sessions are summarized in Table 26-1 and ideas for successful patient teaching in Table 26-2.

Often a family member may participate as an assistant and should therefore undergo training with the patient and accept a level of responsibility depending upon the ability of the patient. Preferably, the patient should manage the bulk of the treatment, but in some circumstances the helper may actually do everything. The training period provides an opportunity to observe how they work together and if the relationship might support home dialysis. Couples who have a troubled relationship prior to the introduction of home dialysis should be closely monitored to decide if home dialysis is advisable; bad relationships are not improved by HHD. For those who have a compatible relationship, it provides an opportunity to strengthen it.

Patient education material. Principles of patient education need to be taken into consideration when selecting and using educational material. Educational material given to patients needs to be well organized and concise, written in short units with adequate amounts of white space to ensure that the learner is not overwhelmed. Subheadings need to be highly visible and appropriate, the font size should be large enough for easy reading, and lines should be double or triple spaced. The communication of the technical and medical terminology associated with HD must be presented in a format easy for patients to understand. A glossary should be included in the patient material. Patient education material is considered appropriate for patients when it is written at a grade 6 level. If developing your own education material, various instruments are available in the literature and through computer programs to the assess readability level. Wherever possible, illustrations should be included, which will enhance the written text. Patient education material should be culturally sensitive.

A teaching plan is necessary to provide organization, feedback, and documentation for the chart, tailored to the individual. Adopting the principles of adult learning is desirable. Adults do not like to waste time; want to be treated as co-learners; prefer immediate, positive feedback; and like accomplishments recognized and rewards provided. It is important to "emphasize the do's and minimize the don'ts" to provide encouragement and foster a positive learning atmosphere.

When teaching about the complications of dialysis and problem-solving skills, various teaching tools can be used to

Figure 26-2
Set-up Guide. Flip Chart Format

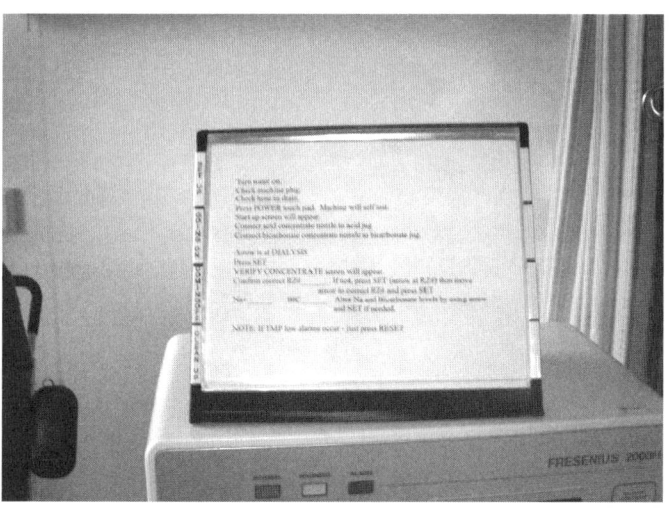

simulate actual situations encountered. The following is a list of teaching tools that can assist in simulation of dialysis related problems:

- dialyzer cut in half to demonstrate blood and dialysate pathways (see Figure 26-1)
- red food dye to simulate blood for practice situations
- rubber arm for cannulation practice
- milk in the dialysate to simulate a blood leak (check with technical department)
- soap in the extracorporeal circuit to simulate air and foam in blood pathway.
- visual aids such as posters, videos, set-up guide – flip chart format, computers (see Figure 26-2)
- Glo Germ® to demonstrate the importance of hand-washing
- role playing

Content of home hemodialysis education programs. A well-established program at Sacred Heart Kidney Centre, Spokane, WA, uses a program consisting of eight learning modules, referred to as blocks, which cover all aspects of

Figure 26-3
Content of Patient Education

Module	Content
Block 1	• Training orientation including signing consent forms, completing admission forms, updating care plans, reviewing medications, compiling list of supplies, issuing of the training manual • Demonstration of hand washing, blood pressure and weight monitoring, dialyzer preparation, coming off dialysis and machine sterilization and documentation
Block 2	• Use of the blood access device and hemodialysis equipment • Set-up of a reused dialyzer, preparation of a needle or catheter, venipuncture, and initiation of dialysis • Recognition of infection and daily access care
Block 3	• Review of dialysis equipment and water treatment • Equipment alarms that stops the blood pump, cause by-pass and alert to power failure • Manual operation of the blood pump and heparin pump • Establishing patient dry weight, calculation of ultrafiltration • Demonstration of water and machine testing and documentation
Block 4	• Explanation of medical problems of the dialysis patient • Review of significant lab values • Reuse troubleshooting, recirculation for short term interruption • Reverse osmosis procedures • Blood sampling
Block 5	• Management of dialysis problems such as hematomas, pyrogen reaction, power failure, cramps, hypotension, clotting, inadequate blood flow and vessel spasm. • Medication administration • Demonstration of medication administration and documentation, reuse dialyzer set-up, venipuncture, recirculation and starting and completing a dialysis treatment as well as demonstrate setting and resetting of alarms.
Block 6	• Review of all home dialysis obligations including home schedule, inventory and ordering of supplies, partner vacation, illness, travel, follow-up care and back up. • Must be competent with all procedures and successfully complete a final examination
Block 7 and 8	• Experience dialyzing in a mock home setting for 2 weeks or at least 6 treatments without staff intervention. • Meet with the team and receive approval for a final plan for home dialysis • Monthly machine maintenance (equipment technicians) instruction • Home visit by technician and nurse for 1st treatment at home

Note: Adapted from Stevens (1996).

Figure 26-4
**First Short Hour Daily HHD Patient
and Spouse London, Canada Daily
Dialysis Study**

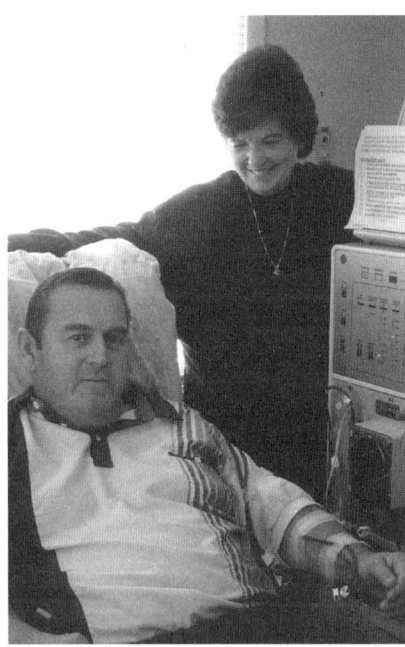

Note: Photo courtesy of Lori Harwood. Used
with permission.

home dialysis. Each block consists of theory, practical application, and uses the instruction manual and other teaching
aids to enable the patient and/or assistant to reach the goal
of successful completion of each section. Return demonstration and testing of procedures learned is included in each
block. Dialyzing independently for several hours during the
last week of training provides patients with the opportunity
to "be on their own" in a controlled environment and bol-
sters their self-confidence. It also gives the nurse a chance to
be sure that the patient is ready to dialyze at home independently. Once the patient and/or assistant has completed
all eight blocks, the first HHD treatment occurs with the
training nurse and technician visiting to ensure that all safety systems are in place. The training program also includes
weekly team meetings to identify any problems encountered.
Figure 26-3 is an outline of the learning units as described by
Stevens (1996).

Management of the Patient in the Home

Once the patient concludes training, an initial home
visit organized around the first treatment is recommended.
This visit is easily managed when the patient is on either conventional or SDHHD but is slightly more difficult for the
NHHD patient. An evening visit to ensure supplies and safety equipment is in place combined with phone calls can
serve as a modified home visit for these patients or a shorter
treatment during the daytime hours (Ouwendyk, Leitch, &
Freitas, 2001). Ongoing home visits are essential to validate
how the patient and assistant and other family members are
coping with HHD on a long-term basis (see Figure 26-4).
Visits should take place at least twice a year.

Telephone communication is a way of providing support
from a distance between home visits. The frequency can
decrease as comfort and self-confidence increases. On call
nursing support (24 hours) has been found to be particularly
important for the patient on nocturnal dialysis who may need
assistance during the night.

Clinic appointments enable the care provider to see firsthand how the patient is managing and provide an opportunity for the multidisciplinary team to assess the patient. There
is considerable variability in the frequency of clinic visits.
Those patients with a higher acuity should be seen more
often.

Laboratory testing should take place on a regular basis
depending on unit protocols or as individual needs dictate.
Patients usually learn to use a centrifuge to ensure proper
testing pre- and post-dialysis. Training needs to include the
proper handling of the centrifuge and blood samples
(Ouwendyk et al., 2001).

Patients are required to perform minor regular maintenance and disinfection of the HD machine and water system,
which is monitored by the technical department. They may
also be instructed in water sampling if this becomes their
responsibility. The biomedical technician repairs the
machine and water system in the home, when necessary,
and provides regular biomedical preventative maintenance.

Patients can be successfully instructed to administer a
variety of medications at home depending upon unit policies, safety considerations, and reimbursement issues. This
instruction would include reason for use, side effects,
method of administration, and precautions. In the U.S., only
erythropoietin is given in the home, and in Canada, vitamin
D, intravenous iron, and some antibiotics can be administered intradialyticly in the home.

Testing of the patient's knowledge for handling problem
situations should be done annually. This can be done on a
formal or informal basis depending upon unit policies and
patient needs. Testing ensures that knowledge attained during training is maintained at a level so as to ensure proper
handling of problem situations. Role-playing and demonstration serve as an effective method to accomplish this.

The physician provides an important link between the
home dialysis center and the home patient. Correspondence
is essential to inform the physician of concerns and ongoing
treatment plans. It is neither necessary nor appropriate for
the home dialysis unit to provide primary care such as yearly physicals, health screening, or immunization, although
patients tend to prefer this.

Home dialysis supplies may be delivered to the patient's
home by an outside service. Monitoring the success of the
delivery service is important to ensure that the patient is
maintaining an adequate and correct supply in the home.

Support groups, either local, regional, or national, provide an opportunity for sharing of information and patient
and family support. Information and referrals can be provided by the social worker or home dialysis nurse. The goal of
the home dialysis unit is to provide a network of support for
the person with ESRD and their family. Careful planning and
monitoring can enable home dialysis to continue for many
years.

Safety concerns with HHD. Safety is essential for the
patient dialyzing in the home setting, and all possible pre-

Figure 26-5
Moisture Sensors

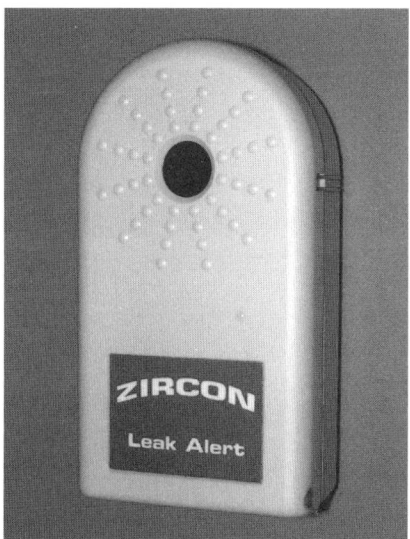

Figure 26-6a
IV 3000® Dressing

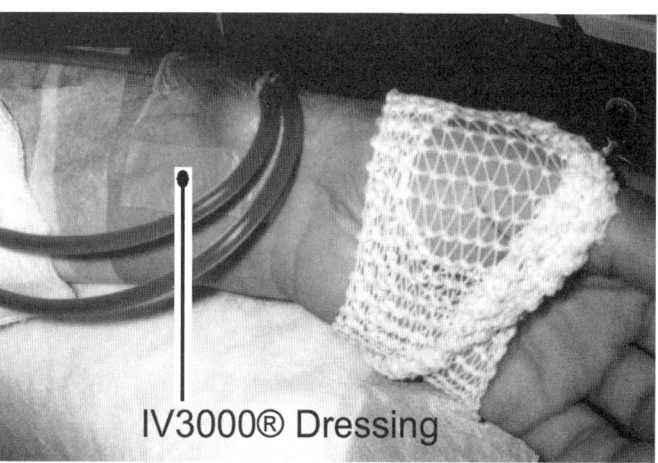

Figure 26-6b
Immobile NT® Dressing

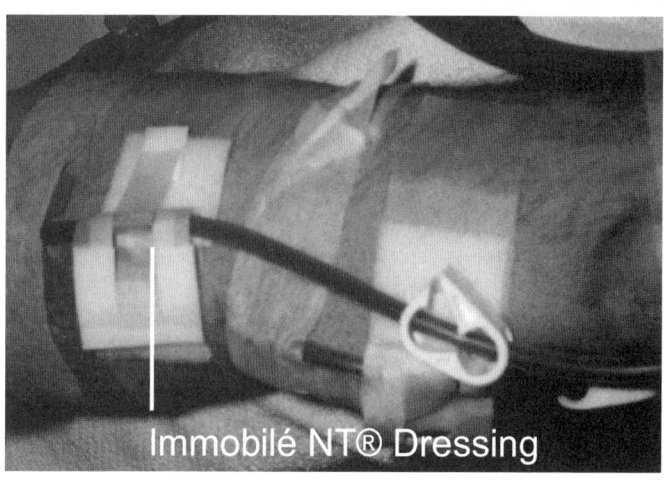

Figure 26-6c
Immobile FST® Dressing

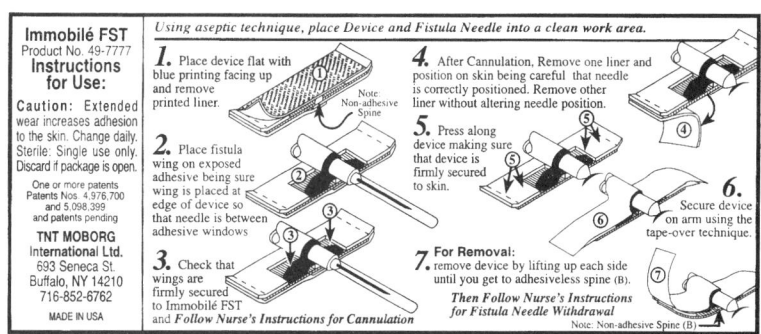

ventative measures must be taken to ensure the treatment is performed correctly and with a minimum of problems (Leitch & Ouwendyk, 2004). If problems do occur, the patient and assistant (if applicable) must be able to handle the situation to prevent any serious and potentially fatal situations.

During the training period, emphasis is placed on the importance of eliminating as many risks as possible and handling emergencies such as sudden hypotension and cramping, blood leaks, air embolism, large blood loss, infections, and power failure. Patients must be able to demonstrate and discuss appropriate actions to be taken should any of these emergencies occur. Careful observation during machine preparation can often detect defects in lines and dialyzers and allow correction prior to the patient actually commencing dialysis.

Information needs to be easily accessible in the event of an emergency. Posters or flip chart instructions for the most critical emergencies should be visible to allow for immediate direction in case of panic. Instructions should be concise with a minimum of steps. If patients believe they cannot cope with the situation, they are advised to shut the machine off, infuse saline in the event of hypotension, clamp both access limbs and blood lines, and call the on-call nurse/system established for advice. A well-indexed training manual will allow quick access for step-by-step instructions. It is essential for the patient dialyzing alone to have phone numbers for emergency assistance visible and the phone within reach. Emergency disconnection supplies and pictorial instructions must be handy and visible for emergency personnel if required (fire or unconscious patient) (Ouwendyk et al., 2001). In case of a

power failure a flashlight with spare batteries must also be within reach to illuminate the extracorporeal circuit during manual retransfusion. Moisture sensors placed strategically under the dialyzer and at the back of the machine will detect blood and dialysate leaks (see Figure 26-5). Enuresis monitors can also be attached to the bloodlines to assist in detecting any accidental blood loss or needle dislodgement. To prevent needle dislodgement, dressings such as IV 3000® (see Figure 26-6a),

Figure 26-6d
Burnet®

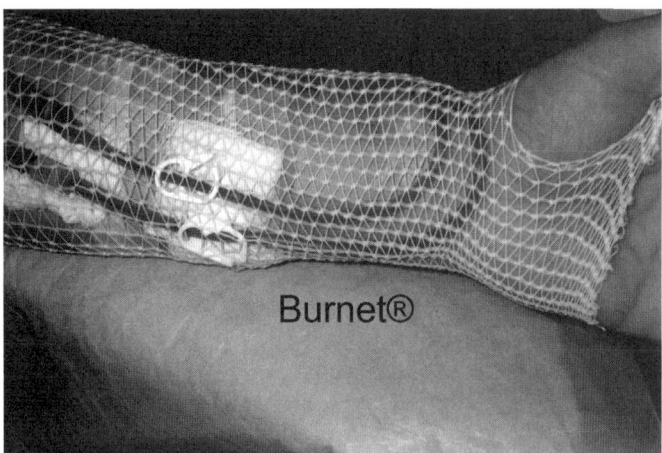

Figure 26-7
SecureCath™

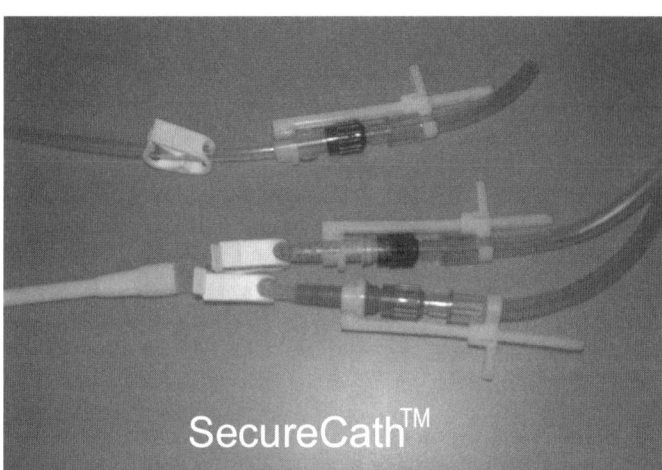

Immobile NT® (see Figure 26-6b), and Immobile FST® (see Figure 26-6c) can be used. Needles may also be secured using tape. The tape is placed over the wing of the fistula needle, under and across the wing in a "V" and then around the entire arm. A tube-like sock (see Figure 26-6d) is then placed over the needles to help contain the lines and prevent tapes from being removed by bedclothes. Adequately securing of the needles is essential for nocturnal dialysis (Ouwendyk et al., 2001). Specific locking devices are also used to prevent disconnection of the CVC from the bloodlines. Examples of these are Lock Box® and SecureCath® (see Figure 26-7) (for use with Fresenius® bloodlines only), which are used primarily with nocturnal dialysis. The Lock Box® is used in conjunction with the Interlink® (see Figure 26-8). This system prevents air entry through the CVC during connection and disconnection if the patient omits clamping the CVC. Air embolism will not occur as the cap remains on the CVC the entire time, thereby eliminating this complication (Ouwendyk et al., 2001). Discussion regarding the containment of pets during dialysis, particularly for the nocturnal patient, is required to avoid the risk of puncturing blood lines with their teeth, thereby creating large blood loss.

Home visits provide an opportunity to ensure that patients are prepared to handle emergencies and have the appropriate safety measures in place. Frequent dialysis treatment modalities have increased safety at home by decreasing and even eliminating episodes of cramping and hypotension, and many patients have been able to successfully demonstrate their capability to perform dialysis independently. These safety interventions have enabled patients who live alone to enjoy the benefits of home dialysis in a safe environment. In our experience, patients have been able to manage safely at home for years without the occurrence of catastrophic events.

Remote monitoring. When NHHD was initiated by Uldall et al. (1994), patient safety was yet to be determined with this new modality. Remote monitoring of the patient dialyzing while they slept was initiated to enhance patient safety and ensure patient compliance. The HD machine was connected either via phone modem or Internet connection to a

Figure 26-8
Lock Box® and Interlink System®

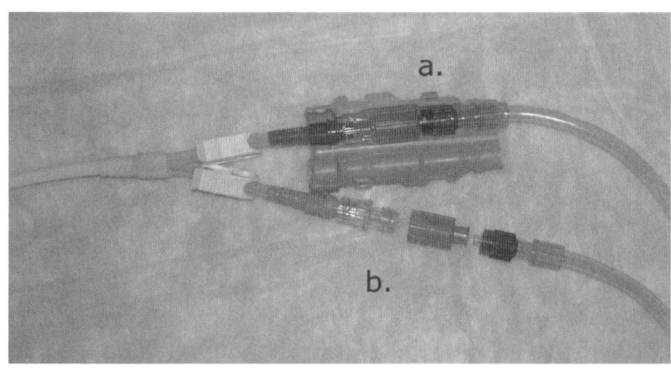

central station located within the hospital. Trained observers monitored machine parameters and alarm conditions while the patient slept and alerted the patient by phone if alarm conditions were not corrected in a timely manner or if machine parameters (such as venous, arterial pressures) were not within pre-determined limits. If the patient did not respond to the phone call then emergency services were notified to check on the patient. Since that time, in view of the absence of major problems, many patients are no longer monitored or are only monitored for an initial 3-month period. If no problems occur, then monitoring can be discontinued. Patients must be able to demonstrate that they are stable during the dialysis treatment and are awakened by alarms. Individual programs will need to decide whether monitoring is required, as it remains a controversial issue. Patients can be lured into a false sense of security when monitoring is in place. In actuality the monitor has limitations, as the individuals viewing the monitors can only phone the patient and alert emergency personnel who may take several minutes to reach the patient depending upon where the person lives. However, it does offer an opportunity for quality improvement monitoring to validate how many times a patient is dialyzing (Ouwendyk et al., 2001). Patients also have mixed views on monitoring. Some patients believe that monitoring is an intrusion, as they must communicate to the staff if they change nights off or alter treatment time. Others feel more comfortable knowing someone is monitoring the treatment. Some states, like New York, require home monitoring. Monitoring also increases the cost of NHHD, but this may be alleviated by the use of central monitoring where many machines in a wide geographical area can be observed by minimal staff. The case for nocturnal remote monitoring is yet to be decided and remains the decision of the home dialysis program.

Respite care. Building respite into a home dialysis program is essential. For the dialysis patient and the caregiver, the everyday tasks of home dialysis can become mundane, overwhelming, and lead to burnout. As the dialysis patient's age increases, so does the age of caregivers who often have their own health problems. Caregivers need to know that it is common to require a "vacation" from home dialysis or that they may become ill and should not feel guilty if they cannot perform the duty of assistant. This could be managed by having a home-helper periodically go into the home or have the patient come to the in-center unit. Home dialysis nurses can increase the frequency of home visits and offer telephone counseling to support the patient and caregiver during this difficult time and ensure proper resources are in place. Access flow monitoring using the ultrasound dilution method could be organized at the same time for patients with an arterio-venous fistula (AVF) or arterio-venous graft (AVG) to have the patient receive dialysis at the home dialysis center. It should be explained to the patient that it is in their best interest to encourage the assistant to take a break thereby avoiding "burn-out."

HHD patients can return to the in-center unit or to home dialysis center for temporary dialysis to provide some respite to the caregivers. Reassure patients and their caregivers that this is common, is important, and that their commitment as a caregiver is not being judged. The assistance from the multi-disciplinary team, particularly the social worker, is instrumental to support the patient and caregiver.

Equipment Requirements for HHD

The following equipment considerations need to be addressed for HHD: (a) dialysis machine, (b) water purification system, (c) home installation requirements, (d) technical staffing and equipment, (e) nightly monitoring and staffing (Francoeur & Digiambatista, 2001). HD machines are designed primarily for in-center use and, therefore, tend to be large and technical with many additional functions, which are unnecessary in the home. Unlike CCPD, these machines are generally not made specifically for home dialysis. HHD programs require technical support staff with experience in modifications required for home dialysis. Ideally, home machines must have easy- to-read screens, controls accessible from a seated or lying position, and must be safe and simple to operate (Lindsay & Leitch, 2004). Variable dialysate flows, volumetric control, and the ability to adapt to single needle dialysis are required. If there is a need for patient monitoring, the equipment also requires external communication capacity for remote monitoring or downloading. Undoubtedly, as the number of people receiving home dialysis increases, the number and types of machines available for home therapy will increase.

Home Installation

Installation of equipment for HHD requires a logical, structured approach and must include the patient in the planning. Patient awareness of their responsibilities and cost implications must be very clear, as adaptations to the home for home dialysis may be required. Who will do the actual work within the home? Who will provide insurance for the equipment and any damages that may be incurred in the home from equipment malfunction? Who will be responsible if the home requires significant upgrading to meet standards for installation? Are there special funds available for assistance if required? If a home is not suitable, will the patient consider relocating to allow this therapy to be instituted? These are only a few of the questions that need to be addressed by each HD program as policies and guidelines for HHD are established (Lindsay & Leitch, 2004).

Once the patient has been assessed and deemed suitable for HHD a site visit should follow to determine the suitability of the home. It is advisable not to begin any home modifications until the training period has progressed to a point where the team is reasonably certain that home dialysis will proceed. Modality selection also needs to be established prior to installation to determine where the machine will actually be located in the home. NHHD requires the equipment to be installed in a sleeping area, while CHD and SDHHD allow for a more flexible location. Individual equipment requirements will vary depending upon the design of the equipment (i.e., equipment has been developed specifically for home dialysis therapy that does not require continuous water infusion or drainage).

Home Assessment

The following criteria require assessment by a qualified individual during the site visit as suggested by Mehrabian, Morgan, Schlaeper, Kortas, and Lindsay (2003). Home ownership must be established to determine whether permission is necessary from a landlord, and if so, this should be obtained in writing. Adherence to municipal bylaws and renovation permits must be followed. Criteria for home assessment (Mehrabian et al., 2003) includes:

*   Access to the area of installation requires measurement of doors, safety of stairways, proximity of driveway to entrance for delivery of equipment and supplies. If possible, equipment should be installed on the ground level. If the installation is to be on a second level, can the equipment be easily managed?
*   Supply storage space must be adequate for the frequency of supply delivery and adhere to necessary environmental requirements.
*   Telephone service must be in place and accessible in the dialysis room if the patient dialyzes alone. If external monitoring is required, a second line is necessary for modem or internet connection.
*   Electrical supply must be adequate for the equipment requirements and must meet code standards.
*   Plumbing in the home must meet municipal codes and allow access to drains and vent pipes.
*   Water supply must be potable and have adequate pressure for the equipment requirements.

- Samples must be taken for chemical and bacteriological levels, which will vary depending upon source. This information will assist in determining water treatment requirements.
- Floor covering should be discussed, as it is advisable to have a water resistant surface due to the possibility of spills.
- Waste disposal requirements of municipalities may vary. If a septic system is utilized, can it handle the extra water volume and disinfectant used to sterilize the equipment? Is there a limit to the amount of garbage allowed per household? What are the requirements for disposal of biohazardous wastes?
- Cleanliness needs to be assessed to determine if there is an increased risk of infection in the home environment and to determine what needs to be done to remedy the situation if a problem is apparent.

In spite of this seemingly long list of requirements, home dialysis installation generally proceeds with minimal problems. Identifying problems and communication of concerns up-front can alleviate many problems and subsequent stressful situations for the patient who is already preoccupied with the training program. Once the installation plan is established, technical co- ordination with the home dialysis nurse guarantees that the home will be ready once training is complete.

Water Treatment

Proper water treatment is necessary to guarantee the safety of the HHD patient, and this is accentuated with more frequent dialysis. In CHD, patients are exposed to approximately 360 L/wk, or more than 25 times the average drinking water exposure (Mehrabian et al., 2003). NHHD patients are exposed to approximately 864 L/wk of water. Therefore, the water treatment equipment installed for HHD in the patient's home is a critical component to prevent the occurrence of disastrous situations.

The home dialysis program is ultimately responsible for the quality of water delivered for HHD and its continued monitoring. Standards established by The Association for the Advancement of Medical Instrumentation (AAMI), and the Canadian Standards Association must be followed when policies are established by the program. Although water treatment is seldom the responsibility of the nephrology nurse, it is advisable to have a basic understanding of the water treatment system to assist in troubleshooting should problems occur in the home setting. Generally, patient instruction for the system in the home and the maintenance required is the responsibility of the technical department. Cost of water required for the treatment needs to be

addressed with the patient, and if a problem arises, some utilities have actually given discounts for the home dialysis patient.

Water Management in the Home

Components of water management in the home have been summarized in Table 26-3. The first step in water management is to establish the requirements for water testing. This testing includes water hardness, chemical analysis, bacteria and endotoxin levels, and chlorine/chloramine content (Sterling, 2002). Qualified personnel must perform testing correctly, as incorrect results can lead to very expensive treatment requirements as well as increased patient risk (Sterling, 2002).

The water treatment method is then decided based on the test results, national standards, and costs. Some systems require major capital costs, while others require ongoing operational costs. The patient must manage the system chosen easily with workload kept to a minimum. The dialysis modality also needs to be taken into consideration, as various flow rates may dictate a preference for the method utilized (Mehrabian et al., 2003). It is essential that the home dialysis program ensure proper management of the water system if they are hiring outside agencies. The water service provider must provide ongoing testing results to the facility once the patient is at home at a frequency determined by the dialysis provider. Patient education material should include a numbered diagram of the system for troubleshooting and future reference should alterations be required.

The HHD unit should inform the local water distribution centers of the presence of a HHD system and requirements in their region so that any interruptions of service as well as potential water problems can be relayed in a timely fashion to the appropriate persons. This could be vital in the event of water contamination. A back-up plan for dialysis should be in place if the patient is unable to dialyze at home. An ongoing disinfection and maintenance program of the water system must be established. Patients are instructed to perform duties as determined by the program. This may also include obtaining water samples for routine testing and transporting them to a local laboratory.

The water treatment components used in HHD are similar to those used at in-center HD units but on a smaller scale and may include some or all of the following: pre treatment filters, water softener, carbon filtration, reverse osmosis, deionization systems (Roshto, 2000), ultra violet irradiation, and indwelling dialysate filters (Levin, 2001). Regardless of the system used, the production of the highest quality water that meets national guidelines must be guaranteed. The water treatment components should be a reasonable cost with a minimum of work required by the patient. Methods to attain "ultrapure" water are currently being investigated.

Clinical problems associated with poor water quality include pyrogenic reactions with high levels of endotoxin. Elevated serum C-reactive protein (CRP) levels are a marker of generalized inflammation and can be an indicator of poor water quality, therefore regular CRP monitoring in the HHD patient should be considered (Lindley, Lopot, Harrington, & Elseviers, 2001).

Table 26-3
Components of Water Management

- Water testing
- The water treatment method
- Water service providers
- Patient education
- Awareness of local water distribution centers
- Disinfection and maintenance program

Vascular Access and Home Hemodialysis

Adequate vascular access is one of the most important components of HD therapy. Dialysis adequacy can be easily monitored in a dialysis unit using routine urea kinetic monitoring, access flow monitoring, and dynamic pressure monitoring. Monitoring dialysis adequacy is not as simple for the person dialyzing at home. Newer HD equipment may have online monitoring of dialysis adequacy and access flow monitoring. If the equipment is not too complicated, assessment may be performed in the home. The patient must be trained in the proper care and management of the access that is being used (Leitch & Lindsay, 2004), as this is literally the patient's lifeline. Access care and management is a vital component of home dialysis training and support.

A properly functioning access must be in place prior to the initiation of the training period to prevent unnecessary stress and costly training delay. The achieved blood flows must be adequate for the selected modality. Long, slow nocturnal dialysis can be successful with flows as low as 150 mls/min, whereas short daily dialysis and conventional dialysis require much higher flows (400-500 mls/min) to obtain sufficient urea reduction rates (50% and 65%) (Ouwendyk et al., 2001). Vascular access may actually dictate which modality is practiced in the patient with limited access options.

Types of Vascular Access

Experience has shown that the person practicing HHD can successfully manage a range of vascular access. In the earlier years of home dialysis, the Scribner shunt and saphenous vein graft as well as the much-preferred AVF were used. This list now includes AVG and the tunneled CVC. Perhaps the greatest advantage for the home patient is the fact they are always the constant; present for every treatment, remembering the idiosyncrasies of their own access as opposed to the numerous individual nurses encountered in a dialysis unit. Patients are able to monitor venous and arterial pressures and are aware of variations or trends in values. Education focuses on the importance of reporting any deviations to the dialysis unit to enable further assessment with access flow devices or radiological intervention.

Tunneled CVCs were initially the only access used for nocturnal dialysis in the Toronto, Canada study (Uldall et al., 1994) due to the fear of needle dislodgment. Since then, access options have been expanded to include the AVF and AVG. Ideally, the CKD patient has a permanent access in place prior to initiating HD, but if this is not the case, education must include the risks and the importance of avoiding an indwelling catheter as a long-term access and stressing the value of a permanent vascular access. Once a person is comfortable utilizing a CVC for access, it is difficult to change to the needle access as they are naturally resistant to inflicting any discomfort and also appreciate the time saved without waiting for hemostasis to occur at the termination of treatment.

Cannulation instruction need not be the sole responsibility of the home dialysis training nurse. This instruction can begin in the in-center unit as long as proper instruction is given. Nurses who are willing to begin the instruction and follow home unit cannulation guidelines can initiate instruction weeks prior to the training period. Earlier instruction will

Table 26-4
Guidelines for Access Management in the Home

- Insist on meticulous technique (proper hand washing and cleansing of the access, as well as the basic principles of infection prevention as outlined in K/DOQI). The patient, prior to termination of the treatment, must use handwipes, as they are unable to obtain access to a sink while receiving treatment. Pets may be living in the home and their presence during initiation and termination of treatment must be discouraged.
- Instruct the patient to recognize the signs and symptoms of infection and promptly report to enable timely treatment. Patients have been able to successfully administer antibiotics at home once the treatment has begun, and they have received detailed instruction in the administration and side effects.
- Training includes basic troubleshooting for all accesses – flushing catheters, repositioning, needles.
- Advise the person to call the unit if they are having problems with needle access at home. Occasionally problems occur and the patient loses confidence. Determine a limit for the number of cannulation attempts for an individual treatment to avoid damage to the access. A visit to the unit or home visit will help instill confidence and provide an opportunity for assessment and if further intervention is warranted
- Safety is stressed for all types of access (prevention of air embolism and accidental disconnection).

allow for extended practice. Decreasing the stress associated with cannulation will contribute to patients' learning once the home training begins. There are many devices on the market that can be used to assist in this instruction, and manufacturers of vascular access devices often provide excellent educational material including videos. Patients who are already comfortable with the procedure are often willing to provide peer support and should be enlisted. Guidelines for access management in the home are listed in Table 26-4.

The Impact of More Frequent HD on Vascular Access

One of the greatest concerns expressed with the introduction of frequent dialysis is the potential harm that may be incurred by the vascular access due to more frequent punctures and accessing of the circulatory system increasing the potential for infection. Current research does not support this hypothesis. In fact, studies have reported fewer complications such as infection. Access longevity with more frequent dialysis compares favorably to CHD (Kjellstrand & Ting, 1998; Lindsay et al., 2001; Quintaliani et al., 2000; Twardowski, 1996). The reason for these findings is unclear but Kenley (1996) speculates it may be due to better blood pressure control, less hemoconcentration, or improvement of uremic thrombopathy. Twardowski (2004) explains that in the case of hypotensive episodes, the sudden reduction of fistula blood flow causes suction and damage of the tunica intima, the innermost coat of a blood vessel, by the inflow needle. Suction leads to intimal damage and contributes to

Figure 26-9
Button-Hole Cannulation Sites (AVF)

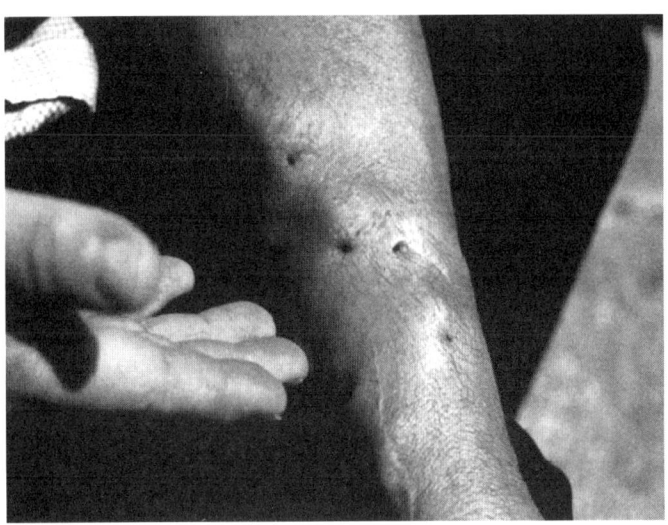

Table 26-5
Button-Hole Method of Cannulation

1. Scrub access limb at the sink using antibacterial soap and friction.
2. Select two sites at least 2 inches apart for initial cannulation (a straight section the length of the needle with easy accessibility for the patient), then use for subsequent cannulation.
3. Clean area with an appropriate antiseptic.
4. Remove button "plug" or scab using a sterile needle or sterile forceps. (This occurs after the initial cannulation and from then on.)
5. Clean area again with antiseptic.
6. Perform cannulation using the same angle as previous cannulation.
7. Once blood flashback has occurred, advance the needle leveling out as you go. If resistance is met, gently rotate the needle back and forth as you proceed.
8. Secure needle.

stenosis and thrombosis. The daily use of the access with less hypotension and more heparin administration may also be an important reason for this improvement.

Ting (2000) studied 30 patients who were converted from CHD to short daily six times per week dialysis. Problems were tracked by access type for the 12 months prior to short daily dialysis and for 388 patient-months on short hour daily dialysis. Access problems that were reported included aneurysms, pseudoaneurysms, or stenoses in AVF and AVG in areas that were punctured; infections in puncture sites or taped areas requiring antibiotic therapy; mechanical failure of a catheter; and catheter-related infections requiring antibiotic treatment, including sepsis, serious tunnel or exit-site infections. Problems not related to use were excluded. Ting (2000) concluded that frequent dialysis does not appear to have an adverse effect on access (AVF, AVG, and catheters) outcomes.

Single needle dialysis, which previously has been used for acute HD or desperate situations when dialysis is imperative and only one site for access is possible, is now being used routinely for NHHD and is resulting in adequate dialysis. Thus, concerns for risk to the access are probably unfounded as the number of punctures using single needle is the same as for conventional hemodialysis (Leitch & Lindsay, 2004). Future studies with larger sample sizes are required to provide more evidence on this subject.

Constant-Site (Button-Hole) Method

The button-hole technique has been used for many years in Europe and was initiated for patients who had limited access cannulation sites. Patients report less pain, easier cannulation, and fewer complications including infection (Ouwendyk et al., 2001, Scribner 1984, Twardowski, 1995). The use of the constant-site method for accessing the AVG has not been reported in the literature. With the button-hole cannulation method, needles are inserted into exactly the same site and angle thereby creating a scarred tunnel. Consecutive needle access then follows this tract and the needle literally

"slips" into the AVF. Teaching this method also seems to be simpler, as two sets of "buttons" (see Figure 26-9) are developed and the person need not be concerned with rotating sites to less familiar areas. The same sites can be used for many months and even years and are only abandoned if bleeding occurs around the site during dialysis (Scribner, 1982).

Both steel needles and Teflon catheters have been used for the constant-site method. After the initial breaking-in period (2–3 weeks), steels can be switched to a duller edged needle so as not to tear the adjacent tissues and cause bleeding (Twardowski, 1995). This method is ideally suited for the home patient, as the same person is performing the cannulation and able to use the required angle of insertion, whereas multiple staff in the unit setting may not be as successful. To establish and develop a button site, select one site for the arterial and one for the venous return. Once these sites are established, proceed to a second set, which serve as back up (Peterson, 2002). Sites may also be alternated every other treatment so the patient maintains a comfort level cannulating all four buttonholes. See Table 26-5 for the button hole cannulation method for HHD.

The AVFs vary in development, some are short and tortuous, others long and straight. The constant-site method seems to be the preferred method for the very short fistula where cannulation sites are minimal. Long straight fistulas are also suited to this option as well as the rope-ladder method where there is equal distribution of punctures along the length of the fistula vein (Kronung, 1984). The most important parameter is the number of punctures per unit area to prevent aneurysm formation and stenosis, which does not occur if these methods are correctly performed (Kronung, 1984).

The Role of the HHD Nurse

Implications for Practice, Education, and Research

An essential component of nursing practice includes patient education and support. A large portion of the home dialysis nurses' role is allotted to these two activities. Patients and families walk in the door frightened, apprehensive, and often overwhelmed by the diagnosis of ESRD. Managing their own treatments outside the hospital setting may seem an unattainable goal. HHD provides the patient with the opportunity to "be the best they can be." Our responsibility as professional health care providers is to assist the patient in meeting this need and to serve as a role model. Patient relationships provide a very rewarding experience for the home dialysis nurse where many skills are combined to reach the ultimate goal of successful HHD for the ESRD patient.

Once training is complete and the patient is at home, the training nurse then takes on the role of supporter and evaluator. It is essential that the patient and assistant (if applicable) have developed a rapport with the home dialysis nurse so they will feel comfortable reporting any changes and concerns to the nurse.

Home dialysis nursing provides autonomy and flexibility and challenges the nurse to explore new and nontraditional methods. Some nursing research has been conducted about home dialysis. However, many opportunities exist for future nursing research, particularly with the trend toward more frequent dialysis.

Two studies (Courts, 2000; Courts & Boyette, 1998) explored total HD stressors for HHD patients in comparison to other forms of home therapies using Baldree, Murphy and Power's (1982) stressors scale. The results of both studies indicate that patients on HHD report fewer HD stressors. However, the authors do not report the specific stressors that home dialysis patients experience. This tool was designed for use with in-center HD patients. The need exists for adaptation of this tool to reflect the home dialysis experience with reliability and validity. Knowledge of patient stressors would be very useful information to apply to education and support patients on home therapies.

In Brunier and McKeever's (1993) comprehensive review, it was concluded that the psychological aspects of the stressors and coping have been well studied; however, the societal, gender, and economic factors have not been addressed. In those studies, the majority of caregivers helping with home dialysis were women who did this in addition to maintaining the household. Recent studies confirm that the majority of caregivers for home hemodialysis continue to be women (MacKenzie & MacTier, 1998), who are over 55 years of age (Courts, 2000; Luk, 2002; White & Greyners, 1999; Quinan, 2005). The societal, gender, and economic factors remain issues which are understudied in home hemodialysis.

As previously stated, patients take their health care professional's opinion into consideration when deciding on a home modality. It is interesting to note that even renal programs with home dialysis often are not mentioning this option to patients. Data from the 1997 USRDS morbidity and mortality (Wave 2) study revealed that 75% of in-center HD patients said they were not offered home HD or PD. Of those, 50% reported if given the choice they would have chosen a home therapy. A later study conducted by Mehrotra, Marsh, Vonesh, Peters, and Nissenson (2005) surveyed individuals who had recently started hemodialysis and 66% reported not being presented with the option of PD and 88% were not presented with HHD. When nephrologists

were surveyed, they reported that home dialysis therapies were underused compared to full-care and in-center HD (Mendelssohn, Mullaney, Jung, Blake, & Mehta, 2001). Nurses with their knowledge of the patient and families are in a position to raise the possibility of home dialysis to the team and educate patients about the various options.

Patients' fears and concerns when deciding on a dialysis modality are well known. Further exploration of why patients do not choose a home therapy may have clinical application that would optimize future numbers on home therapies.

Home dialysis nursing is focused on patient education and preparation for home dialysis therapies. For such a large component of the role, only one reliable and valid tool (Chow & Bennett, 2001) has been published to assist nurses in their assessment of suitability of patients for home therapies. The use of this tool or others similar to it will guide practice and increase efficiencies in this process.

HHD programs are generally small and specialized often with only one or two nurses. Thus, published quantitative nursing studies often have small sample sizes. To achieve adequate sampling nurses will need to explore other options such as multi-centered studies. The small number of patients in the various home programs may be more suited to qualitative methodologies where the sample size tends to be smaller. There is also an absence of longitudinal nursing studies with this population.

The Future of Home Dialysis

The trend toward more frequent dialysis has nephrologists predicting a revival in HHD with a growth of 20% of the current dialysis population changing to more frequent HHD if there was appropriate reimbursement (Lindsay & Leitch, 2004; Twardowski, 1995). The future of HHD most certainly lies in the funding of this modality and technology to simplify the process in the home while PD continues to be a popular home therapy.

Summary

Home dialysis is an important option to provide to the ESRD patient. Many positive patient outcomes have been demonstrated as well as cost efficiencies. Home dialysis provides patients with more control over their dialysis schedule. Patients on the daily forms of dialysis have significant physical improvements that allow them to continue in their previous roles. A National Institute of Health study involving multiple centers performing home dialysis is scheduled to begin in the fall of 2005. Hopefully, with the data obtained from this study, the U.S. government will provide reimbursement for centers at a level that will allow many more dialysis units to start home training programs. It is essential to perform an assessment of the patient's needs as well as those of the caregiver to determine if home HD is an appropriate therapy. Careful assessment during the training period assists the multidisciplinary team to identify those patients who are suitable candidates and make a decision based on what modality is best for the patient and family. Home dialysis nurses are essential members of a health care team to provide care for the home dialysis patient.

References

Agraharkar, M., Du, Y., Ahuja, T., & Barclay, C. (2002). Comparison of staff-assisted hemodialysis with in-center hemodialysis and in-hospital hemodialysis. *Hemodialysis International, 6,* 58-62.

Baldree, K.S., Murphy, S.P., & Powers, M.J. (1982). Stress identification and coping patterns in patients on hemodialysis. *Nursing Research, 32,* 107-112.

Blagg, C.R. (1997). The history of home hemodialysis: A view from Seattle. *Home Hemodialysis International, 1*(1), 1-7.

Blagg, C.R. (2000). What went wrong with home hemodialysis in the United States and what can be done now? *Hemodialysis International, 4,* 55-58.

Bonomini, V., Mioli, V., Albertazzi, A., & Scolari, P. (1972). Daily-dialysis programme: Indications and results. *Proceedings of European Dialysis Transplant Association, 9,* 44-52.

Branson, M., & Moran, J. (2004). Supporting home dialysis therapies. The well bound model. *Nephrology News and Issues, 18*(3), 24-29.

Bremer, B.S., McCauley, C.R., Wrona, R.M. & Johnson, J.P. (1989). Quality of life in end stage renal disease: A reexamination. *American Journal of Kidney Diseases, 12,* 200-209.

Brunier, G., & McKeever, P.T. (1993). The impact of home dialysis on the family: Literature review. *ANNA Journal, 20*(6), 653-659.

Buoncristiani, U., Cairo, G., Giombini, L., Quintaliani, G., & Bonforte, G. (1989). Dramatic improvement of clinical-metabolic parameters and quality of life with daily dialysis. *International Journal of Artificial Organs, 12*(1 Suppl. 24), 133-136.

Buoncristiani, U., Fagugli, R., Quintaliani, G., Kulurianu, H. (1997). Rationale for daily dialysis. *Home Hemodialysis International, 1,* 12-18.

Burton, H.J., Canzona, L., Lindsay, R.M., & Palmer, S. (1985). Adaptation to home dialysis - The Ontario experience: Final report. Ontario, Canada: University of Western Ontario Press.

Cagle, J., Horsley, M., Scott, H., Scott, C., Lattimer, C., & Smith, S.W. (1999). Nocturnal home hemodialysis: Patients' personal experiences. *Home Hemodialysis International, 3,* 75-79.

Chow, J., & Bennett, L. (2001). Pre-training assessment tool (JPAT) - A pilot study. *EDTNA/ERCA Journal, XXVII*(1), 37-41.

Courts, N.F. (2000). Psychosocial adjustment of patients on home hemodialysis and their dialysis partners. *Clinical Nursing Research, 9*(2), 177-190.

Courts, N.F., & Boyette, B.G. (1998). Psychosocial adjustment of males on three types of dialysis. *Clinical Nursing Research, 7*(1), 47-63.

Curtis, F.K., Cole, J.J., Fellows, B.J., Tyler, L.L., & Scribner, B.H. (1965). Hemodialysis in the home. *American Society of Artificial Internal Organs, 11,* 7-10.

Delano, B.G., Feinroth, M.V., Feinroth, M., & Friedman, E.A. (1981). Home and medical centre haemodialysis. Dollar comparison and pay-back period. *Journal of the American Medical Association, 246,* 230-232.

DePalma, J.R., Pecker, E.A., & Maxwell, M.H. (1969). A new automatic coil dialyzer system for daily dialysis. *Proceedings of the European Dialysis Transplant Association, 6,* 26-34.

Eknoyan, G., Beck, G.J., Cheung, A.K., Daugirdas, J.T., Greene, T., Kusek, J.W., et al. (2002). Effect of dialysis dose and membrane flux in maintenance hemodialysis. *New England Journal of Medicine, 347*(25), 2010-1019.

Evans, R.W., Manninen, D.L., Garrison, Lo.P., Hart, L.G., Blagg, C.R., Gutman, R.A., et al. (1985). The quality of life of patients with end stage renal disease. *New England Journal of Medicine, 312,* 553-559.

Francoeur, R., & Digiambatista, A. (2001). Technical considerations for short daily home hemodialysis and nocturnal home hemodialysis. *Advances in Renal Replacement Therapy, 8*(4), 268-272.

Grant, A.C., Rodger, S.C, Howie, C.A. et al. (1992). Dialysis at home in the west of Scotland: A comparison of hemodialysis and continuous ambulatory peritoneal dialysis in age- and sex-matched controls. *Peritoneal Dialysis, 12,* 365-368.

Goeree, R., Manalich, J., Grootendorst, P., Beecroft, M.L., & Churchill, D. (1995). Cost analysis of dialysis treatments for end stage renal disease (ESRD). *Clinical Investigative Medicine, 18*(6), 455-464.

Harper, G. (1997). Home hemodialysis: A patient's perspective. *Home Hemodialysis International, 1*(1), 8-11.

Heidenheim, P., Muirhead, N., Moist, L., & Lindsay, R.M. (2003). Patient quality of life on quotidian hemodialysis. *American Journal of Kidney Diseases, 42*(1 Suppl. 1), S36-S41.

Jacobs, C., & Selwood, N.H. (1996). Renal replacement therapy for end stage renal failure in France. Current status and evolutive trends over the last decade. *American Journal of Kidney Disease, 25,* 188-195.

Kenley, R. (1996). Tearing down the barriers to daily home hemodialysis and achieving the highest value renal therapy through holistic product design. *Advances in Renal Replacement Therapy, 3*(2), 137-146.

Kjellstrand, C. (1998). A brief history of daily hemodialysis. *Home Hemodialysis International, 2,* 8-11.

Kjellstrand, C., & Ting, G. (1998). Daily dialysis: Dialysis for the next century. *Advances in Renal Therapy, 5*(4), 267-274.

Kroeker, A., Clark, W.F., Heidenheim, P., Kuenzig, L., Leitch, R., & Meyette, M. (2003). An operating cost comparison between conventional and home quotidian hemodialysis. *American Journal of Kidney Diseases, 42*(1 Suppl. 1), 49-55.

Kronung, G .C. (1984). Plastic deformation of cimino fistula by repeated puncture. *Dialysis and Transplantation, 13*(10), 635-638.

Kutner, N.G., Brogan, D., & Kutner, M.H. (1986). End stage renal disease treatment modality and patients' quality of life. *American Journal of Nephrology, 6,* 396-402.

Leitch, R., & Lindsay, R.M. (2004). Vascular access. In R.M. Lindsay (Ed.) *Daily and Nocturnal Hemodialysis* (pp. 48-54). Basel, Switzerland: Kargel.

Leitch, R., & Ouwendyk, M. (2004). Patient training and education. In R.M. Lindsay (Ed.) *Daily and Nocturnal Hemodialysis* (pp. 39-47). Basel, Switzerland: Kargel.

Leitch, R., Ouwendyk, M., Ferguson, E., Clement, L., Peters, K., Heideneheim, P., & Lindsay, R.M. (2003). Nursing issues related to patient selection, vascular access, and education in quotidian hemodialysis. *American Journal of Kidney Diseases, 42*(1 Suppl. 1), S56-S60.

Levin, R., (2001) The role of water in dialysis: Why does it need to be more than "clean?" *Nephrology News and Issues, 15*(2), 21-23.

Lindley, E.J., Lopot, F., Harrington, M., & Elseviers, M.M. (2001). Treating and monitoring water for dialysis in Europe. *Nephrology News and Issue, 15*(2), 27-35.

Lindsay, R.M. (2003). Introduction. *American Journal of Kidney Diseases, 42,* (1 Suppl. 1), S3-S4.

Lindsay, R.M., Alhejaili, F, Nesrallah, G., Leitch, R., Clement, L., Heidenheim, A.P., & Kortas, C. (2003). Calcium and phosphate balance with quotidian hemodialysis. *American Journal of Kidney Diseases, 42*(1 Suppl. 1), S24-S29.

Lindsay, R.M., Kortas, C., and the Daily/Nocturnal Dialysis Study Group (2001). Hemeral (daily) dialysis. *Advances in Renal Replacement Therapy, 8*(4) 236-249.

Lindsay, R.M., & Leitch, R. (2004). Home hemodialysis. In W.L. Horl, K.M. Koch, R.M. Lindsay, C. Ronco, & J.R. Winchester (Eds.), *Replacement of Renal Function by Dialysis* (5th ed., pp. 1553-1566). London, England: Kluwer Academic Publishers.

Lockridge, R., Spencer, M., Craft, V., Pipkin, M., Campbell, D., McPhatter, L., et al. (2004). Nightly home hemdialysis: Five and one-half years of experience in Lynchburg, Virginia. *Hemodialysis International, 8,* 61-69.

Luk, W. (2002). The home care experience as perceived by the caregivers of Chinese dialysis patients. *International Journal of Nursing Studies, 39*(3), 269-277.

Mackenzie, P., & Mactier, R.A. (1998). Home haemodialysis in the 1990s. *Nephrology, Dialysis and Transplantation, 13,* 1944-1948.

Mailloux, L.U., Kapikian, N., Napolitano, B., Mossey, R.T., Bellucci, S.G., Wilkes, B.M., et al. (1996). Home hemodialysis: Patient outcomes during a 24-year period of time from 1970 through 1993. *Advances in Renal Replacement Therapy, 3*(2), 112-119.

Manhor, N.L., Louis, B.M., Gorfien, P., & Lipner, H.I. (1981). Success of frequent short hemodialysis. *Transactions of the American Society of Artificial Internal Organs, 27,* 604-609.

McFarlane, P.A., Bayoumi, A.M., Pierratos, A., & Redelmeier, D.A. (2003). The quality of life and cost utility of home nocturnal and conventional in-center hemodialysis. *Kidney International, 46,* 1004-1011.

Mehrabian, S., Morgan, D., Schlaeper, C., Kortas, C., & Lindsay, R.M. (2003). Equipment and water considerations for the provision of quotidian home hemodialysis. *American Journal of Kidney Diseases, 42*(1 Suppl. 1), S66-S70.

Mehrotra, R., Marsh, D., Vonesh, E., Peters, V., & Nissenson, A. (2005). Patient education and access of ESRD patients to renal replacement therapies beyond in-center hemodialysis. *Kidney International, 68*(1), 378-390.

Mendelssohn, D.C., Mullaney, S.R., Jung, B., Blake, P.G., & Mehta, R.L (2001). What do American nephrologists think about dialysis modality selection? *American Journal of Kidney Disease, 37*(1), 22-29.

Murray, J.S., Tu, W.H., Albers, J.B., Burnell, & Scriber, B.H. (1962). A community hemodialysis center for the treatment of chronic uremia. *Transactions of the American Society of Artificial Internal Organs, 8*, 315-319.

Nesrallah, G., Suri, R., Moist, L., Kortas, C., & Lindsay, R.M. (2003). Volume control and blood pressure management in patients undergoing quotidian hemodialysis. *American Journal of Kidney Diseases, 42*(1 Suppl. 1), S13-S17.

NKF-KDOQI Hemodialysis Adequacy Work Group. (2000). *Practice guidelines for hemodialysis adequacy.* National Kidney Foundation.

Nose, Y. (1965). Discussion. *American Society of Artificial Internal Organs, 11*, 15.

Oberley, E., & Schatell, D.R. (1996). Home hemodialysis: Survival quality of life and rehabilitation. *Advances in Renal Replacement Therapy, 3*, 147-153.

Ouwendyk, M., Leitch, R., & Freitas, T. (2001). Daily hemodialysis: A nursing perspective. *Advances in Renal Replacement Therapy, 8*(4), 257-267.

Peterson, P., (2002). Fistula cannulation: The buttonhole technique. *Nephrology Nursing Journal, 29*(2), 195.

Piccoli, G.B., Bechis, F., Iacuzzo, C., Amania, P., Iadarola, A.M., Mezza, E., et al. (2000). Why our patients like daily dialysis. *Hemodialysis International, 4*, 47-50.

Piccoli, G.B., Mezza, E., Burdese, M., Consiglio, V., Vaggione, S., Mastella, C., et al. (2005). Dialysis choice in the contest of an early referral policy: There is room for self care. *Journal of Nephrology, 18*(3), 267-275.

Pierratos, A., Ouwendyk, M., Francoeur, R., Vas, S., Dominic, S., Raj, C., et al. (1998). Nocturnal hemodialysis: Three-year experience. *Journal of the American Society of Nephrology, 9*, 859-868.

Prenreas, J.P., Cole, J.J., Tu, W.H., & Scribner, B.H. (1961). Improved technique of continuous flow hemodialysis. *American Society of Artificial Internal Organs, 7*, 27-36.

Quinan, P. (2005). Home hemodialysis and the caregivers' experience: A critical analysis. *CANNT Journal, 15*(1), 25-32.

Quintaliani, G., Buoncristiani, U., Fagugli, R., Kulurianu, H., Ciao, G., Rondini, L., et al. (2000) Survival of vascular access during daily and 3 times a week hemodialysis. *Clinical Nephrology, 53*(5), 372-377.

Richmond, J.M., Lindsay, R.M., Burton, H.J., Conley, J., & Wai, L. (1982). Psychological and physiological factors predicting the outcomes on home haemodialysis. *Clinical Nephrology, 17*(3), 109-113.

Roshto, B. (2000). Dialysis water treatment 101: The fundamentals of planning a system for maximum safety and efficiency. *Contemporary Dialysis and Nephrology, 21*(12), 26-27.

Schwartz, D.I., Pierratos, A., Richardson, R.M., Fenton, S.S., & Chan, C.T. (2005). Impact of nocturnal home hemodialysis on anemia management in patients with end-stage renal disease. *Clinical Nephrology, 63*(3), 202-208.

Scribner, B.H. (1982). Circulatory access – Still a major concern. *Proceedings of the EDTA, 19*, 95-98.

Scribner, B.H. (1984) The overriding importance of vascular survival.

Dialysis and Transplantation, 13(10), 625.

Scribner, B.H., Buri, R., Caner, J.E.Z., Hegstrom, R., & Burnell, J.M. (1960). The treatment of chronic uremia by means of intermittent hemodialysis: A preliminary report. *American Society of Artificial Internal Organs, 6*, 114-122.

Spanner, E., Suri, R., Heidenheim, P., & Lindsay R.M. (2003). The impact of quotidian hemodialysis on nutrition. *American Journal of Kidney Diseases, 42*(1 Suppl. 1), S30-S35.

Stark, C.R. (1985, March/April). Home and in-center hemodialysis patients – A descriptive study. *Journal of Nephrology Nursing, 77-79.*

Sterling, M. (2002). The end result: Tips for ensuring safe and accurate water testing for dialysis patients. *Contemporary Dialysis and Nephrology, 23*(12) 30-32.

Stevens, J.E. (1996). Home hemodialysis – Yes, it can be learned. *Advances in Renal Replacement Therapy, 3*(2), 120-123.

Suri, R., Depner, T.A., Blake, P., Heidenheim, P., & Lindsay, R.M. (2003). Adequacy of quotidian hemodialysis. *American Journal of Kidney Diseases, 42*(1 Suppl. 1), S42-S48.

Ting, G.O. (2000). Blood access outcomes associated with short daily hemodialysis. *Hemodialysis International, 4*, 42-46.

Ting, G.O., Kjellstrand, C., Freitas, T., Carrie, B.J., & Zarghamee, S. (2003). Longer-term study of high comorbidity ESRD patients converted from conventional to short daily hemodialysis. *American Journal of Kidney Diseases, 42*(5), 1020-1035.

Ting, G.O., Leitch, R., & Ouwendyk, M. (2004). Patient recruitment and selection. In R.M. Lindsay (Ed.), *Daily and Nocturnal Hemodialysis* (pp. 29-38). Basel, Switzerland: Kargel.

Twardowski, Z.J. (2004) Blood access in daily hemodialysis. *Hemodialysis International, 8*(1) 70-76.

Twardowski, Z.J. (1996). Daily home hemodialyis: A hybrid of hemodialysis and peritoneal dialysis. *Advances in Renal Replacement Therapy, 3*(2) 124-132.

Twardowski, Z.J. (1995). The future of daily dialysis. *Seminars in Dialysis, 8*(5), 263-265.

Uldall, R., Francoeur, R., Ouwendyk, M., Wallace, L., Langos, V., Ecclestone, A., & Vas, S. (1994). Simplified nocturnal hemodialysis: A new approach to renal replacement therapy. *Journal of American Society of Nephrology, 5*, 80.

United States Renal Data System (USRDS). (1997). Annual data report. Bethesda, MD: The National Institute of Health, National Institute of Diabetes and Digestive and Kidney Diseases.

United States Renal Data System (USRDS). (2003). Annual data report. Bethesda, MD: The National Institute of Health, National Institute of Diabetes and Digestive and Kidney Diseases.

Valek, A., & Lopot, F. (1989). Uraemic toxins and blood purification strategies. *Contribution to Nephrology, 70*, 178-187.

Wai, L., Richmond, J., Burton, H., & Lindsay, R.M. (1981). The influence of psychosocial factors on survival of home dialysis patients. *Lancet, 2*, 1155-1156.

Wellard, S., & Street, A. (1999). Family issues in home-based care. *International Journal of Nursing Practice, 5*(3), 359-364.

White, Y., & Greyner, B. (1999). The biopsychosocial impact of end stage renal disease: The experience of dialysis patients and their partners. *Journal of Advanced Nursing, 30*(6), 1312-1322.

Wick, G.S., & Robbins, K.C. (1998). Patient education. In J. Parker (Ed.), *Contemporary nephrology nursing* (pp. 837-852). Pitman, NJ: Anthony J. Jannetti Inc.

Woods, J.D., Port, F.K., Stannard, D., Blagg, C.R., & Held, P.J. (1996). Comparison of mortality with home hemodialysis and center hemodialysis: A national study. *Kidney International, 49*, 1464-1470.

- Home dialysis is the most cost-effective form of dialysis.

- Patient outcomes and quality of life are better on home dialysis compared to in-center therapies.

- More frequent dialysis virtually eliminates interdialytic symptoms and has superior patient outcomes.

- Patient benefits to home dialysis include opportunity for adequate dialysis, convenience, no transportation issues, more time with family, less time in hospital setting, independence, control, and more knowledge regarding dialysis.

- More frequent HD and CAPD are more physiological than conventional HD.

- HHD machines must have easy-to-read screens; accessible controls from a seated or lying position; be safe and simple to operate; and have variable dialysate flows, volumetric controls, and the ability to adapt to single needle dialysis.

- Home suitability must be assessed by a qualified individual.

- Components of water management for HHD includes water testing, water treatment, a water service provider, patient education, and a disinfection and maintenance program.

- Home therapies should be discussed as early as possible in the CKD stages.

- The time required for patient education will vary for each patient depending on the cognitive, emotional, and physical state of the patient; age; motivation; previous experience; and modality chosen.

- Systems for safely dialyzing in the home need to be implemented and monitored with a well-indexed training manual, phone numbers, and a flashlight that is visible and within reach. Emergency disconnection supplies and pictorial instructions must be handy and visible for emergency personnel if required.

- Specific dressings can be applied to prevent accidental dislodgement of the needles during nocturnal dialysis.

- There is no evidence to suggest that frequent cannulation with daily dialysis contributes to access complications.

- The constant-site method of cannulation has been shown to be advantageous for patients on HHD.

- Respite care is important in supporting individuals during periods of stress, illness, or coping difficulties to prevent burnout and ensure success with home dialysis.

Home Dialysis Therapies

Name of Resource	Brief Description	Where to Obtain Resource
Print Resources Christopher, B. & Anderson, C. Home preparation and installation for home hemodialysis. In A.R. Nissenson & R. Fine (Eds.) *Dialysis Therapy* (3rd ed., pp. 87-89).	This chapter is based on experience at the North West Kidney Centre, Seattle, where they have the most home hemodialysis experience in the US and highlights home installation.	Medical Library Publisher, Hanley & Belfus, Inc. Philadelphia, PA ISBN 1-56053-426-5
Lindsay, R.M., & Leitch, R. (2004). Home hemodialysis. In W.L. Horl, K.M. Koch, R.M. Lindsay, C. Ronco, & J.R. Winchester (Eds). *Replacement of Renal Function by Dialysis* (5th ed., pp. 1553-1566). London, England: Kleuver Academic Publishers.	The authors describe this chapter as a "how to for home hemodialysis."	Medical Library This article has contact information of the author.
Schatell, D. (2005). Home dialysis: Home dialysis central and what you can do today. *Nephrology Nursing Journal, 32*(2), 235-237.	This article discusses the resources available for various home dialysis modalities on the web site.	Nephrology Nursing Journal
Chow, J., & Bennett, J. (2001). Pre-training assessment tool (JPAT) - A pilot study. *EDTNA/ERCA Journal, XXVII*(1), 37-41.	This is a tool that has been proven to be reliable for assessing suitability of potential home dialysis patients.	Medical Library This article has contact information of the author.
Web sites Patient Education	Content includes information regarding patient education, adult education and learning styles.	http://www.hsph.harvard.edu/healthliteracy/materials.html http://www.engr.ncsu.edu/learningstyles/ilsweb.html http://www.vark-learn.com/english/index.asp
Home Dialysis Central	This web site provides patient and professional information and support for home dialysis modalities.	http://www.homedialysis.org
Equipment Moisture Detector Zircon Electronic Water Detector Zircon Corporation 1580 Dell Avenue Campbell, CA 95008 USA E-mail: customer.service@zircon.com	Used to detect dialysate leaks.	Company

Home Dialysis Therapies

Name of Resource	Brief Description	Where to Obtain Resource
HemoSafe Patient Connector Clip for Hemodialysis Fresenius 95 Lexington Ave Lexington, MA 02420 (800) 662-1237	Used to prevent disconnection from blood lines to CVC.	Company
Lock Box Humber River Regional Hospital, 200 Church Street Weston, Ontario Canada M9N 1N8	Used to prevent disconnection from blood lines to CVC.	Company
Interlink System Baxter Health Care Deerfield, IL Becton Dickinson, Franklin Lakes, NJ	Used to prevent disconnection from blood lines to CVC and air entry.	Company
Immobile NT & Immobile FST Dressings T.N.T. Moborg International Limited 693 Seneca St. Buffalo, NY 142 10 www.moborg.com	Dressings used to prevent needle dislodgement.	Company
BurnNet Glenwood Laboratories Oakville, Ontario Canada	Covering of dressing used to keep dressing adhered during sleep.	Company
IV 3000 Dressing Smith and Nephew Medical Limited, Hull HU3 2BN England.	Dressings used to prevent needle dislodgement.	Company
Glo-Germ Co. P.O. Box 537 MOAB, UT 84532 (801) 259-6034	Used to demonstrate the need for handwashing during patient teaching.	Company

ANNP626

Home Dialysis Therapies

Lori Harwood, MSc, RN, CNeph(C); and Rosemary Leitch, RN, CNeph(C)

Contemporary Nephrology Nursing: Principles and Practice contains 39 chapters of educational content. Individual learners may apply for continuing nursing education credit by reading a chapter and completing the Continuing Education Evaluation Form for that chapter. Learners may apply for continuing education credit for any or all chapters.

Please photocopy this page and return to ANNA.
COMPLETE THE FOLLOWING:

Name: _____

Address:_____

City:_____ State: _____ Zip: _____

E-mail: _____

Preferred telephone: ☐ Home   ☐ Work: _____

State where licensed and license number (optional): _____

CE application fees are based upon the number of contact hours provided by the individual chapter. CE fees per contact hour for ANNA members are as follows: 1.0-1.9 - $15; 2.0-2.9 - $20; 3.0-3.9 - $25; 4.0 and higher - $30. Fees for nonmembers are $10 higher.

ANNA Member: ☐ Yes   ☐ No   Member # (if available) _____

☐ Checked Enclosed   ☐ American Express   ☐ Visa   ☐ MasterCard

Total Amount Submitted: _____

Credit Card Number: _____ Exp. Date: _____

Name as it appears on the card: _____

CE Evaluation Form
To receive continuing education credit for individual study after reading the chapter
1. Photocopy this form. (You may also download this form from ANNA's Web site, **www.annanurse.org.**)
2. Mail the completed form with payment (check) or credit card information to American Nephrology Nurses' Association, East Holly Avenue, Box 56, Pitman, NJ 08071-0056.
3. You will receive your CE certificate from ANNA in 4 to 6 weeks.

Test returns must be postmarked by **December 31, 2010.**

CE Application Fee
ANNA Member $15.00
Nonmember $25.00

EVALUATION FORM

1. I verify that I have read this chapter and completed this education activity. Date: _____

_____
Signature

2. What would be different in your practice if you applied what you learned from this activity? *(Please use additional sheet of paper if necessary.)*

_____
_____
_____
_____
_____
_____
_____
_____
_____
_____
_____
_____

Evaluation	Strongly disagree				Strongly agree
3. The activity met the stated objectives.					
a. State the benefits of home hemodialysis.	1	2	3	4	5
b. Describe the home hemodialysis modalities, vascular access, and equipment needed.	1	2	3	4	5
c. Analyze the role of the home hemodialysis nurse.	1	2	3	4	5
4. The content was current and relevant.	1	2	3	4	5
5. The content was presented clearly.	1	2	3	4	5
6. The content was covered adequately.	1	2	3	4	5
7. Rate your ability to apply the learning obtained from this activity to practice.	1	2	3	4	5

Comments _____

_____

8. Time required to read the chapter and complete this form: _____ minutes.

This educational activity has been provided by the American Nephrology Nurses' Association (ANNA) for 1.0 contact hour. ANNA is accredited as a provider of continuing nursing education (CNE) by the American Nurses Credentialing Center's Commission on Accreditation (ANCC-COA). ANNA is an approved provider of continuing education by the California Board of Registered Nursing, CEP 0910.

UNIT 7

Peritoneal Dialysis

Unit 7 Contents

Technical Aspects of Peritoneal Dialysis

Elizabeth Kelman, MEd, RN, CNeph(C)
Diane Watson, MSc, RN, CNeph(C)

Chapter Contents

Chapter 27

Technical Aspects of Peritoneal Dialysis

Elizabeth Kelman, MEd, RN, CNeph(C)
Diane Watson, MSc, RN, CNeph(C)

Peritoneal dialysis (PD) is a treatment that uses a natural membrane for fluid and solute exchange. The goals of therapy include removal of waste products, management of fluid, and regulation of acid-base and electrolyte imbalances. To achieve these goals, a dialyzing solution or dialysate is instilled into the peritoneal cavity for a period of time known as the dwell period. Following this dwell, the fluid or effluent (containing substances such as urea, creatinine, electrolytes, and amino acids) is drained and replaced with fresh dialysate. This fill, dwell, and drain process is referred to as an "exchange." Peritoneal dialysis developed into a home therapy, although "home" may be a nursing home or complex care facility depending on each individual's co-morbidities, choices, abilities, and support structures. The success of PD can be attributed to the combined efforts of researchers, individuals on peritoneal dialysis, and health care professionals who, in collaboration with the industrial community, have realized the potential benefits of the treatment. Despite a slow start in comparison with hemodialysis, PD has evolved into a modality that equals hemodialysis in long-term outcomes.

In this chapter, historical highlights of PD will be reviewed as a foundation for understanding the current treatment. The anatomy and physiology of the peritoneum will be discussed with reference to its capacity as a dialysis membrane. Basic requirements for the treatment will be presented, including prescriptive approaches, dialysis solutions, delivery systems, and intraperitoneal medication administration. Strategies for measuring adequacy of dialysis will be summarized with inclusion of the controversy in establishing targets for assessment. The intent is to provide nurses with a basis for assessing individuals for PD as well as appreciating the technical requirements for optimal dialysis outcomes. It is beyond the scope of this chapter to provide protocols for PD. The practice of peritoneal dialysis incorporates principles of asepsis that nurses utilize in developing procedures for treatment delivery. This area requires further nursing collaboration to promote evidence-based practice through research and dialogue within nephrology nursing organizations both nationally and internationally.

Choosing the Treatment Option for Dialysis

Peritoneal dialysis has been the treatment used for a wide range of people with ESRD, from the very young to the very old. It is thought that the daily removal of wastes and fluids provides a gentle, well-tolerated and efficient approach to dialysis. Oreopoulos, Lobbedez, and Gupta (2004) detailed the advantages of PD compared to hemodialysis as "decreased mortality rate with the exception of older female diabetics, preservation of residual renal function, reduced health care costs, life enhancement of independent living, better hemoglobin levels with reduced EPO and transfusions, and reduced incidence of bacteremia" (p. 88). People generally prefer the more liberal diet offered with PD, although it is not without restrictions.

There are specific populations for whom PD has been advocated. For example, individuals with cardiac instability may have significant benefits from daily gentle fluid removal. Those with diabetes may be able to utilize intraperitoneal rather than subcutaneous insulin to achieve glycemic control. The resultant reduction in needle punctures may contribute to improved quality of life. It has also been hypothesized that people with multiple myeloma benefit from the removal of light chains in the effluent (Prichard & Bargman, 2000). An interesting finding by Katz, Sofianou, Butler, and Hopleu (2001) was the recovery of renal function in individuals with malignant hypertension on PD. These authors described an advantage for recovery in people treated with continuous ambulatory peritoneal dialysis (CAPD) compared to those treated with hemodialysis, and they attributed this finding to the improved blood pressure control associated with CAPD.

While generally used with chronic kidney disease, PD plays a role as an acute intervention. Hajarizadeh, Rohrer, Herrmann, and Cutler (1995) studied PD in individuals with acute renal failure in association with ruptured aortic aneurysms. The authors reported advantages of using a dialysis treatment that did not require central venous cannulation and anticoagulation. Additional benefits included reduced cardiac instability and early identification of bleeding complications via the peritoneal cavity. These benefits also contributed to improved renal recovery and survival in individuals with acute renal failure secondary to cholesterol embolization treated with PD (Gillerot, Sempoux, Pirson,& Devuyst, 2002; Rao, Passadakis & Oreopoulos, 2003; Siemons, van den Heuvel, Parizel, Buyssens, De Broe & Cuykens, 1987).

Body habitus has been a controversial issue regarding selection of PD for individuals considered to be above average weight. There are theoretical concerns about infectious risks of catheters in skin folds and the effect on healing in obese individuals. The adequacy of dialysis and the impact of the glucose load have also been cited as concerns. There are no easy guidelines for determining the suitability of the candidate for the treatment. In a study of prevalent individuals on PD, Johnson, Herzig, Purdie, et al. (2000) noted that obesity was associated with a reduced risk of death. In their review, the authors felt that the higher body mass index created a protective effect from the energy reserves. In other studies, risks associated with peritonitis in overweight individuals were examined. Piraino, Bernardini, Centa, Johnston, and Sorkin (1991) reported on trends of increasing peritonitis rates but did not find statistically significant differences in this population. In a retrospective review of 242 incident individuals on CAPD, Afthentopoulos and Oreopoulos (2000) found that people who weighed more than 80 kilograms actually had fewer hospitalization days than those between the weights of 60 to 80 kilograms. Peritonitis rates, technique survival, and morbidity were comparable between the two groups; however, McDonald, Collins, Rumpsfield, and Johnson (2004) found an increased rate of peritonitis in individuals classified as overweight and obese. This finding was from an analysis of data collected by the Australia and New Zealand Dialysis and Transplant (ANZDATA) registry from 1991 to March 2003. McDonald, Collins, and Johnson (2003) believed that careful monitoring with recognition of infectious risks and weight reduction programs might prove beneficial to this group although they did not find evidence in the current literature to support these strategies. Thus, although opinion varies as to the suitability of PD for individuals with high body mass indices, there remains no definitive answer, and more studies are required to determine the feasibility of PD in overweight individuals.

While PD is suitable for a diverse population, there are relative contraindications to the therapy, which include previous multiple abdominal surgeries, diverticular disease, and cognitive or physical impairment affecting psychomotor skills. The presence of adhesions from previous abdominal surgeries or inflammatory processes may impair the membrane as a dialyzing surface; however, peritoneal catheter and membrane function can only be analyzed after initiation of treatment and may be difficult to predict. The adage, "You don't know until you try," is applicable here, as ultrafiltration capability and solute clearance can only be determined after catheter placement. Polycystic kidney size may affect the ability to cope with PD exchange volumes, but many individuals with polycystic kidney disease (PKD) have been successfully managed with PD. Diverticular disease, which has been associated with PKD as well as other etiologies, can theoretically pose a risk for bowel perforation or microperforation and peritonitis. In a review of 535 patients from 1994 to 1999, Pandya, Friede, and Williams (2004) concurred with Hadimeri, Johansson, Haraldsson, and Nyberg's previous findings (1998) that the risk of peritonitis did not increase for people with PKD.

A number of reports have indicated that individuals with physical and cognitive challenges can perform PD either independently or with assistance (Bentley, 2001; Carey, Chorney, Pherson, Finkelstein, & Kliger, 2001; Shokar, 2001; Smith, Sica, & Stacy, 1986; Wang, Izatt, Dalglish, Jassal, Bargman, Vas et al., 2002). Modifications in the training program and equipment design can be undertaken to facilitate the learning process for individuals faced with challenges such as visual impairment, paralysis, and amputations. Despite successes, there are also documented accounts of dilemmas that can occur. In a letter to the editor, Chow, Szeto, and Li (2003) shared a photograph of a peritoneal catheter cut by an individual with dementia who found the tube obstructive and did not appreciate the purpose of the treatment. In response, Moss reiterated the belief that careful consideration must be given in assessing the best treatment options for individuals with advanced cognitive impairment (Chow, Szeto, Li, & Moss, 2003).

History of Peritoneal Dialysis

Historically, dialysis was proposed as a temporary process until recovery of renal function. With the realization that kidney damage could be irreversible, dialysis developed into a life-support treatment. Use of the peritoneal cavity has been described as early as 1743 by Stephen Hales. He reported on Warrick's approach to treating a woman with ascites by infusing a solution of Bristol water and claret into the peritoneal cavity in an attempt to "close the mouths of the lymphatic system" (Drukker, 1983). Other clinical experiences included the delivery of fluid via the peritoneal space to dehydrated children by Blackfan and Maxcy in 1918, and the first documented use of dialysis in renal failure in 1923 by Ganter (Drukker, 1983; Gokal, 2000). Ganter based his efforts on experiences with animal studies in which he used a peritoneal lavage method. Ganter's work had been preceded by other scientists in their studies of transport characteristics for fluid and solute across membranes.

In 1877, Wegener noted that cold solution instilled into animals' peritoneal cavities decreased animals' body temperatures (McBride, 1984). Additionally, he described the use of increasing return volumes through the infusion of concentrated sugar solutions. This work was furthered by Starling, who in 1884, showed that return volumes could be varied based on the infusion of isotonic and hypotonic solutions (Gokal, 2000). In 1895, Orlow demonstrated changes in fluid volumes, effluent returns, and serum chloride levels, fueling the notion that not only fluid could be varied, but that the peritoneum could be used to affect blood constituents (McBride, 1984). Putnam's publications in 1927-1928 detailed poor survival outcomes when sodium chloride concentrations of greater than 1% were instilled into animals. Prior to Putnam's studies, Clark demonstrated that dextrose solutions were a useful means of removing fluid; this contrasted with sodium chloride based on the slower diffusion of dextrose into the blood (Drukker, 1983). From these results and other investigative work, the basic principles governing peritoneal dialysis emerged with an emphasis on volume, dialysis solutions' compositions, temperature, and dwell time of fluid in the cavity.

In the ensuing decades, progressive developments included utilization of PD in humans, implantable peritoneal catheters, commercially prepared dialysis solutions, improved delivery systems, and dialysis prescriptions. Modifications in delivery systems simplified the treatment and contributed to reductions in infections. Prescriptions for dialysis became more scientifically based as research continued into the form and function of the peritoneum. In Table 27-1, a few of the achievements in advancing the field of PD are detailed.

Anatomy and Physiology of the Peritoneal Membrane

Waniewski, Heimbürger, Werynski, and Lindholm (1996) described the peritoneal membrane as "a complex and complicated system of membranes and pores, which may be described as a distributed, multilayer, heteroporous, and topographically non-uniform structure with intramembrane compartments and possible specific biological transport characteristics" (p. S63). The complexity of this statement clearly highlights the intricacies of this marvelous living structure with intended biological functions other than the provision of a membrane for purposes of dialysis. The word *peritoneum* originates from the Greek meaning "to stretch around." this term aptly describes the structure of the peritoneum, which enfolds the abdominal organs and lines the abdominal wall. The lining facing the abdominal wall is the parietal surface while that which encompasses the organs is called the visceral surface. The area between these two

Table 27-1

Historical Highlights in Evolution of Peritoneal Dialysis

Date	Highlights	Investigators/Nurses	Significance
1923	First peritoneal dialysis with variable volume and dwell times; done x 1 treatment; stopped and patient death ensued	Ganter	Despite initial improvement, realization that more than one treatment is required
1936	First continuous peritoneal dialysis	Wear, Sisk, and Trinkle	Patient survival with dialysis; recovered from ARF
1940s	Use of gravity for delivery and removal of solutions	Kop	10/21 treated successfully
	2 catheters used for inflow/outflow	Seligman, Fine, and Frank	Improved treatment with enhanced flow
1950s	Development of IPD	Grollman	Flexible catheter
	Development of plastic delivery set and catheter	Maxwell	Treatment more accessible
	First chronic peritoneal dialysis (1956)	Ruben	Use of implanted catheter; 24-hour treatment once per week
1960s	Home dialysis with removable catheter	Boen	Use of a machine for dialysis solution delivery
	Still to supply water developed; later, water purification system (1969)	Tenckhoff	Simplifying system for home management
	Production of "Lasker" cycler, simplified machine allowed for hanging and warming solutions	Lasker	Further simplified and allowed for further expansion
1970s	Development of "long dwell equilibrated peritoneal dialysis"	Moncrief, Popovich, Sorrels	Improved solute and fluid removal, used glass bottles for dialysis solutions
	Developed and evaluated CAPD clinically	Nolph, Prowant	Proved efficacy of treatment but noted risk of peritonitis
	Introduction of portable plastic bag & tubing set	Oreopoulos, Izatt, Clayton	Decreased peritonitis rates; treatment more accessible
1980s	Intraperitoneal insulin	Khanna, Diaz-Buxo	Improved diabetic management
	Y-set with flush before fill	Buoncristiani	Decreased peritonitis related to touch contamination
	Adaptation of cycler for daily dialysis	Diaz-Buxo	Alternate approach to management with CCPD
	Introduction of assist devices/systems for improving management including disconnect systems	Collaborative work with industry	System more portable and accessible
	Membrane physiology and transport characteristics/adequacy of dialysis	Twardowski, Dobbie, Topley, Bargman	Scientific basis for clinical practice
1990s	Adequacy studies, including first randomized study	Maiorca; Churchill, Khanna,Lo, Szeto, Twardowski	Continued debate on adequacy of dialysis

Note: Adapted from: Drukker (1983); Gokal (2000); Maiorca & Cancarini (1999); McBride (1984); Moncrief & Popvich (1981); Oreopoulos, Khanna, Williams, & Vas (1982); Venkataraman & Nolph (2002); http://www.ISPD.org.

Figure 27-1
The Peritoneal Membrane

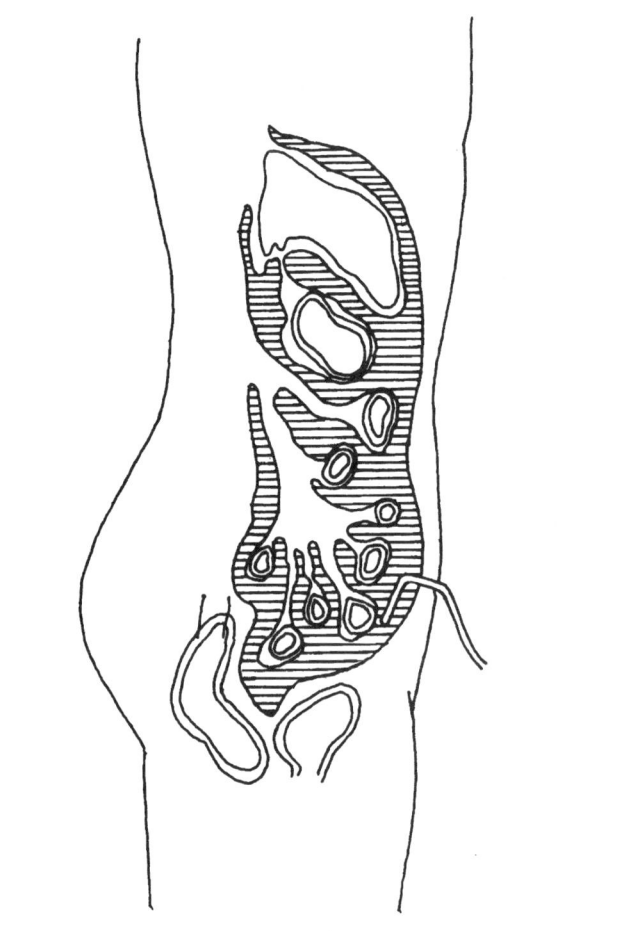

surfaces is the peritoneal cavity, which contains about 50 to 100 mL of fluid. This fluid acts as a lubricant to reduce friction between the organs. Potentially, the cavity can accommodate more volume as is seen in people with liver failure who can amass large amounts of ascites in this space.

Although primarily pictured as a two-walled continuous structure, there are points where the visceral lining folds over itself as many as four times, whereas the parietal lining exists as a single layer. Most of the small intestine is attached to the posterior abdominal wall by a double fold of the membrane. The fold away from the posterior abdominal wall resembles a fan and supports the blood vessels, lymphatics, and nerves supplying the small intestine; this section is called the mesentery. The lesser and greater omentum are also peritoneal structures, with the former extending from the liver to the stomach, and the latter hanging like an apron over the intestines (Burkart, Daeihagh, & Rocco, 2003). The peritoneal membrane is illustrated in Figure 27-1.

The size of the membrane has been estimated to be 1.72 to 2.08 m^2 in adults (Gotloib, Shostak, & Wajsbrot, 2000). In simpler terms, this has been described as roughly the same as the body surface area. In infants, the membrane is "twice that of an adult when scaled to body weight" (Warady, Alexander, Balfe, & Harvey, 2000). In adults, the visceral

membrane represents 80% of the peritoneal surface and the parietal accounts for 20%. Despite the size of the membrane, the effective surface area for dialysis is considered to be less and is related to the "dialysate to membrane" contact and blood perfusion (Krediet, 2000). Anatomically, the membrane differs between men and women. In men, the membrane is an enclosed structure but in women, the mucosal linings of the fallopian tubes are continuous with the peritoneum; thus, the fallopian tubes open into the peritoneal cavity (Wikipedia, 2005).

Structurally, the peritoneum consists of three layers. The monolayer facing the peritoneal cavity is the mesothelium, with microvilli covering its surface. These microvilli increase the effective surface area to allow exchange between the fluid in the peritoneal cavity and the cells. According to Di Paolo and Sacchi (2000), the greatest numbers of microvilli are present in the areas of greatest friction between the abdominal organs. Fang, Qian, Yu, and Chen (2004) emphasized the importance of the mesothelium in terms of its secretory functions in both maintaining structural and defensive properties of the peritoneum. Below the mesothelium are the basement membrane (which has a negative charge) and the interstitium (composed of collagen, fibers, lymphatic vessels, and capillaries). These two layers form support structures. The negative charge may constitute a barrier to some large molecules, including protein (Di Paolo & Sacchi, 2000). The membrane can be adapted for dialysis purposes because of the blood compartment in the interstitium, the presence of a semi-permeable membrane, and the potential for a dialysate compartment in the peritoneal cavity.

Blood flow to the capillaries differs between the visceral and parietal surfaces. Celiac and mesenteric vessels supply the visceral membrane with blood returned via the portal system. The intercostal, epigastric, and lumbar arteries supply the parietal membrane with return via the caval system. The blood vessels can be utilized for administration of intraperitoneal medications, which will be absorbed through the portal system and metabolized by the liver. Normally, only a small portion of the blood vessels are perfused with a blood flow of 50 to 100 ml/min. Also of importance to the dialysis procedure is the physiologic reabsorption of fluid from the cavity via the lymphatic system. The lymphatics remove fluid and cellular debris, including organisms, thereby protecting the cavity from infection. This uptake from the lymphatics influences the amount of fluid for actual removal from the body during dialysis, reducing the net fluid removed by 40% to 50% (Khanna, 2002). The primary site for lymphatic absorption is in the subdiaphragmatic space, and it is estimated to be "greater than 1.0 ml/min" or approximately 1.2 liters per day (Khanna, 2002, p. 232). Lymphatic uptake of fluid from the peritoneal cavity is governed by the effect of inspiration and expiration on the mesothelial cells and lymphatic vessels. Thus, there is continuous lymphatic uptake of the fluid with replenishment of the lubricant in the cavity by lamellar bodies located in the mesothelial cells (Dobbie, 1996).

In addition to the lymphatic system, the peritoneal cavity also has a defense system against infection in the form of cells, such as macrophages, leukocytes, mesothelial cells, and fibroblasts. These cells are involved in the activation of an inflammatory response to foreign matter and microorganisms (Brunkhorst, 2002). Macrophages in the peritoneal cavity are responsible for ingesting or phagocytosing foreign material (including bacteria) and are assisted in the identification by the presence of opsonins such as IgG and C_3. Small numbers of neutrophils are normally present, but they can be increased in the event of infection to aid in killing microorganisms. Mesothelial cells also participate in regulation of the inflammatory response through the production of mediators such as interleukins, Tumor Necrosis Factor-α and prostaglandins (Faull, 2000). Fibroblasts found in the interstitial layer also participate in the reactive process and play a role in structural changes in the peritoneum (Coles, Williams, & Topley, 2000). The proliferation of cells in the inflammatory response not only assists in killing the microorganisms, but also can be clinically helpful in diagnosing an inflammatory state. While the cells and mediators influence the inflammatory response, the peritoneum's protective role is also evident in its ability to wall off areas of infection. This occurs, for example, in appendicitis when peritoneum encases the infected area in an attempt to control spread of microorganisms throughout the abdominal cavity. Unfortunately, this can result in abscess formation.

There is an old adage in design that "form follows function." In the case of the peritoneal membrane, the original functions of the membrane can be summarized as friction reduction, nutrient transport and defense against infection; the peritoneum form is uniquely designed to accomplish these functions. Nephrology has reversed the adage and utilized the specialized form to expand the functions to act as a dialyzing membrane; thus, "function follows form." Given that the membrane is living tissue, function can alter the structure with its transformation into a dialysis membrane. Before discussing changes in peritoneal anatomy associated with dialysis in the individual with renal failure, the fundamentals of membrane transport applied to dialysis will be delineated.

Basic Transport Processes Applied to the Peritoneal Membrane

The PD process is mainly dependent on three main principles of transport: diffusion, osmosis, and convection. These transport processes produce ultrafiltration and solute movement leading to the removal of wastes and excess substances normally excreted by the kidneys in their homeostatic role. Among the wastes are small water soluble compounds such as urea and creatinine with molecular weights less than 500 daltons, protein-bound solutes less than 500 daltons, and middle molecules that are greater than 500 daltons (Kjellstrand, 1981; Vanholder & Glorieux, 2003 ; Vanholder, Gloreieux, De Smet, 2003;). β_2 microglobulin is an example of a middle molecule that is thought to contribute to the uremic state. The peritoneum is then capable of transporting a range of molecular weight substances, including urea (60 daltons), creatinine (113 daltons), glucose (180 daltons), β_2 microglobulin (11,800 daltons), and albumin (68,000 daltons). It is noteworthy that flow across the membrane is bidirectional, with solutes and water able to move back and forth between blood and dialysate.

Diffusion is defined as the movement of solutes from an area of high concentration to an area of low concentration across a semi-permeable membrane with the goal of equilibrating solute concentration. Factors affecting diffusion include molecular size of the solute, surface area, and permeability characteristics of the membrane, as well as length of time in contact with the membrane. Examples of solutes removed by diffusion with PD include urea, creatinine, and potassium. Urea represents a relatively small solute and is readily diffusible across the peritoneum. When dialysis solution is infused with a dwell time of 4 hours, there will be close to complete equilibration with the blood. In individuals with renal failure, goals of dialysis include regulation of electrolytes. The majority of these individuals have normal-to-high serum potassium levels. Since commercially manufactured dialysate does not contain potassium, the expectation is that potassium will follow its concentration gradient from blood to dialysate with eventual equilibration of the dialysate potassium concentration to the plasma concentration. As the dialysate is discarded, a net loss of potassium occurs. In individuals with hypokalemia, addition of potassium to the dialysate prevents further loss.

Osmosis refers to the movement of a solvent such as water through a semi-permeable membrane from a low solute concentration to a high solute concentration. Eventually, this process results in an equilibration of the solute concentrations on both sides of the membrane. The number of osmoles of solute per liter of a solution is defined as the *osmolarity* (Willatts, 1987). The capacity of the solutes to effectively exert an osmotic effect is defined as the *tonicity of the solution* (Preston, 2002). If two solutions are separated by a semi-permeable membrane, the solution with the higher osmolarity will promote movement of water (solvent) from the other compartment in an effort to equilibrate the solute concentration in both compartments. Figure 27-2 illustrates the effect of a semipermeable membrane on water movement.

In PD, glucose, a crystalloid, is utilized as the primary osmotic agent through varying the concentration available in dialysate. Thus, a high glucose concentration has the capacity to move more fluid across the membrane towards the glucose side than a lower glucose concentration. *Isotonic solutions* approximate the osmolarity of blood (285 to 295 mOsm/L), while *hypotonic solutions* are less concentrated and *hypertonic solutions* are more concentrated than blood. In PD, this osmotic principle is applied through the use of four strengths of glucose, representing hypotonic, isotonic, and hypertonic solutions as detailed in Table 27-2. The fluid removed over and above the instilled volume is called the *ultrafiltrate*. By combining the physical properties of diffusion and osmosis, PD can accomplish some of the fundamental functions previously accomplished by the kidneys, those of waste and fluid removal.

In addition to diffusion and osmosis, *convective transport* also occurs. In convection, more solutes are removed with greater volumes of fluid removal; this is known as *the solvent drag effect*. Unlike diffusion, convection does not rely on a concentration gradient. Sodium transport is influenced by convective transport, diffusion, and osmosis.

After initial instillation of dialysate, particularly hypertonic solutions, movement of water without solutes occurs

Figure 27-2
Two solutions separated by a semi-permeable membrane.

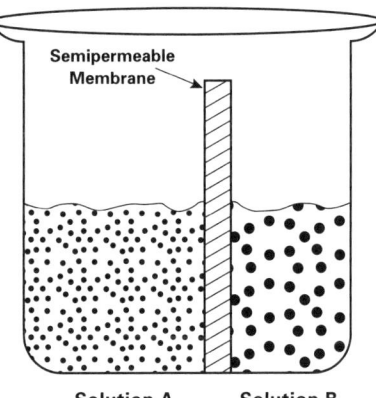

Solution A   Solution B

Solution A contains small particles which readily diffuse through the membrane. Glucose molecules in Solution B will exert an osmotic effect.

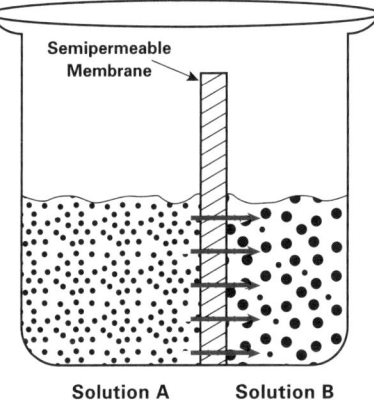

Solution A   Solution B

This shows diffusion with movement of particles from high to low concentration.

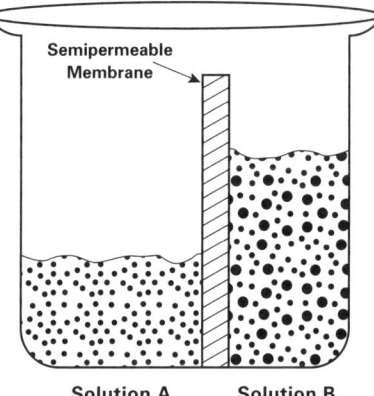

Solution A   Solution B

This shows the osmotic effect with the shift of water from A to B in response to the increased glucose content in B. Remember that over time, the glucose molecules can move from B to A, and this will reduce the osmotic effect for continued water movement from A to B.

Table 27-2
Osmotic Effect of Standard Solutions for PD

Strength of Solution*	Osmolarity	Effect of 2 L infused volume with 60 minute dwell time**
0.5%	296 mOsm/L	Hypotonic, fluid movement from dialysate to blood with less effluent returns expected from inflow volume
1.5 %	346 mOsm/L	Slightly hypertonic but clinically used as an isotonic solution to maintain fluid status or remove approximately 50-150 mL
2.5%	396 mOsm/L	Hypertonic, remove approximately 100-300 mL
4.25%	485 mOsm/L	Hypertonic, remove approximately 300-400 mL

*dextrose monohydrate concentrations
**Approximate effluent returns expected for volume infused; actual drain volumes will reflect individual variations in the peritoneum's structure and transport capabilities

Note: Adapted from Korbet & Kronfol, 2001, p. 337. 0.5% may not be available in the United States.

through channels specific to water transport, known as aquaporins. This effect is referred to as *sodium sieving*. With short dwells of 2 to 4 hours, this sieving effect has the potential to cause hypernatremia with greater water removal than sodium. With longer dwell periods, sodium removal occurs because the dialysate's sodium concentration has been diluted by water. This enhances the concentration gradient and promotes the shift of sodium from the blood to the dialysate. Movement of sodium with water can also occur by convection resulting in removal of sodium with the drained fluid. Since clearance for sodium is time-dependent, dwell time has an impact in the amount removed.

Models of Peritoneal Transport

In 1923, Putnam described the peritoneum as a living structure with holes punched into it, which allow the passage of large solutes. He also noted one of the limitations of this living structure in terms of inflammation permitting passage of proteins. Later, in a now classic model, Nolph described potential barriers to transport, while the membrane's capacity for water and solute transport were defined further by the three-pore model (Rippe, Simonsen, & Stelin, 1991; Rippe, 1993; Waniewski et al., 1996; White & Granger, 2000). Although Putnam's model may be easier to comprehend, these later models reflect the complexities of the peritoneum.

Nolph's model of 6 barriers to movement permitted a

graphic representation of transport across the capillaries to the peritoneal cavity. In considering movement of solutes and water across the capillary, the first barrier was thought to be a stagnant fluid layer against its wall after which the endothelium and basement membrane were encountered as potential resistances to flow. The next two barriers were postulated to be the interstitium and mesothelium, with the final resistance described as a stagnant fluid layer against the mesothelial surface. Nolph's classic model served to define the complexities of peritoneal transport and offers possible explanations for the time required for solute and water transport across a living structure (Twardowski, 2005).

The three-pore model described transport through varying pore sizes (Rippe, Venturoli, Simonsen, & de Arteaga, 2004). In this model, there are a large number of small pores responsible for the transport of low molecular weight solutes with radii in the range of 40 to 50Å. Urea and creatinine with radii of 2 to 3Å are easily transported through the small pores, as is glucose. A small number of larger pores with radii greater than 150Å permit transport of larger molecules such as protein. Researchers have also postulated the existence of ultra small pores responsible for the movement of water, and this concept has been further developed with evidence of water channels known as Aquaporin-1 in the peritoneal blood vessels (Blake & Daugirdas, 2001; Gotloib, Shostak, & Wajsbrot, 2000; Venturoli & Rippe, 2001; White & Granger, 2000). Krediet, Lindholm, and Rippe (2000) noted that these channels are likely the equivalent of the ultra-small pores first described in the three-pore model of transport and are responsible for water transport. Krediet emphasized that of the described resistances to flow, the primary barriers were the endothelial cells of the vascular wall (Krediet, 1997; Krediet, 1999; Krediet, Lindhome, & Rippe, 2000). Models of transport formulate the principles for performing PD based on structural findings and their influence on the targeted products for removal in the individual with renal failure. The living nature of the membrane also has an impact on transport because changes in structure and function occur over time.

Studying the peritoneum is difficult, but through biopsies attained at autopsy or surgical interventions, researchers have been able to describe anatomical changes in the peritoneum in PD and have collated their findings in the International Peritoneal Biopsy Registry. Structural changes within the peritoneum after initiation of dialysis have been described as loss of microvilli on the mesothelial surface, thickening of the basement membrane and interstitium, and a "tanned" appearance (Coles et al., 2000; Dobbie, Lloyd,& Gall, 1990; Fang, Qian, Yu & Chen, 2004; Schreiber, 1996). This tanned appearance may be related to the effect of oxidation products of dextrose. Yung and Davies (1998) commented that damage of the peritoneal mesothelium occurs after "persistent infection or the prolonged exposure to dialysis fluids," with "resultant denudation of cells on the mesothelial surface" (p. 2166). These structural changes can alter transport characteristics of the membrane such as ultrafiltration. Mortier, De Vriese, and Lameire (2003) described increased vasculature as the basis for increased solute movement and attributed this to the peritoneum's response to infection and inflammation.

Despite changes in the peritoneum over time, there are reports of long-term survival over 10 years (Islam, Briat, Soutif, Barnouin, & Pollini, 1997; Maitra et al., 2000) and even more than 20 years (Oreopoulos, 1999a). Thus, the peritoneum's unique ability to be adapted as a dialyzing membrane through the application of transport principles has permitted treatment alternatives for individuals with renal failure. Understanding the peritoneum's structure and function remains challenging as new research is undertaken to define and describe the peritoneum's capacity for dialysis.

Assessing Peritoneal Membrane Characteristics

A recent focus in PD has been toward developing clinical tools for measuring clearance across the membrane. This effort has led to a classification system that uses an evidence-based approach for determining appropriate prescriptions for delivering PD. Solute and water transport are assessed through measurement of the individual membrane's capacity to equilibrate a standard load of solute in a given amount of water. This is known as the peritoneal equilibration test (PET). It is important to recognize that the PET is not a measure of adequacy of solute removal during dialysis but an indication of the pattern of solute and water transport. Thus, PET results provide the clinician with individual membrane characteristics. This facilitates selection of prescriptions that provide the most efficient dwell time for removal of fluids and wastes based on the known solute transport over time.

The PET is a measurement of the transport characteristics of the peritoneum and defines membrane function in a continuum from slow transport to rapid transport of solutes. It should be noted that previously, transport was defined as low to high; however, trends are to redefine these terms, thus the terms "slow and rapid" transporters will be used here. While a rapid transporter does move solutes at rapid rate, large amounts of solute removal are not always associated with the measured amounts found in the effluent. This may be related to the fact that less volume is returned as a result of the rapid reabsorption of glucose and concomitant reduction in water movement. In contrast, a slow transporter may take longer to move substances across the membrane but have large ultrafiltrate volumes.

Determining the status of the membrane as a slow or rapid transporter is then done by measuring the differences between dialysate and plasma concentrations after a 4-hour dwell. To obtain the required blood and dialysate samples, a volume of fluid is instilled into the peritoneal cavity and left for a period of 4 hours. During this time, blood samples are taken at the midpoint (2 hours) and fluid samples taken at 0, 2, and 4 hours. Equilibration between the plasma and fluid is then determined by dividing the amount of a solute within the dialysate returns by the plasma level for a given solute. This is referred to as the D/P ratio and can be expressed as a percentage of clearance. Table 27-3 details the instructions for performing the PET. Twardowski (2002) developed a protocol that has become a recognized standard for carrying out the PET (Prowant & Schmidt, 1991). In an effort to standardize reporting of results among populations, strict adherence to the guidelines is recommended. If variations are used, then the reporting method should detail the alterations in order to interpret and compare results.

Table 27-3
Performing PET

Timing of step	Steps

CAPD – evening pre test If on APD – two options	Instill 2 liters of 2.5% dextrose solution for 8 to 12 hours
	  a. Omit the cycler night pretest and instill volume as per CAPD
	  b. Start the cycler earlier and/or shorten it to allow an 8 to 12-hour dwell

Morning of test	Drain overnight dwell, preferably in a standing position and measure returns Instill 2 liters of 2.5% dextrose over 10 minutes Roll from side to side after every 400 ml infused for good mixing
0 Hour	Record time when fill is completed Drain 200 ml into drain bag, mix, draw 10 ml sample Reinfuse remaining solution
2 hours	Repeat steps used at 0 hour to take effluent sample Take blood sample for urea, creatinine, and glucose
4 hours	Have individual stand and drain; mix sample Take 10 ml sample of effluent Send all 3 samples of effluent for urea, creatinine & glucose measurement (*Correction factor for interference by glucose needs to be done by lab to get true dialysate creatinine value)
Results of effluent and blood reported	Calculate D/P for urea and creatinine for 0, 2, and 4 hours and plot on graph Calculate D/Do G for glucose and plot on graph

Note: Adapted from Schmidt & Prowant (1991).

The D/P ratios have been established for urea and creatinine. Higher ratios reflect more rapid transport across the membrane. For example, a dialysate urea level at 4 hours of 80 mg/dl (28.56 mmol/L) and a plasma urea level of 90 mg/dl (32.13 mmol/L) would yield a D/P of 0.89 or 89% (see Table 27-4). Urea as a small solute tends to equilibrate up to 100% in an average transporter (Satko & Burkart, 2002), whereas creatinine as a larger molecule requires more time for equilibration; at 4 hours, one might expect a clearance of approximately 65%. Table 27-5 summarizes the transport characteristics based on PET results, while Figure 27-3 illustrates the curves for glucose and creatinine transport. The D/P of glucose is not measured due to the absorption of glucose from the dialysate. Instead, glucose in the dialysate is meas-

Table 27-4
Calculation of D/P for Urea

Dialysate Urea = 80 mg/dl Serum Urea = 90 mg/dl
D/P= 80 mg/dl/90 mg/dl = 0.89 (or 89%)

ured at the beginning and end of dwell. The glucose curve then represents the glucose reabsorption rate with the expectation that less glucose is present in the dialysate at the end of 4 hours due to its movement from the peritoneal cavity to blood. This is defined as the D/D_0. D refers to the dialysate glucose at the end of the dwell period. D_0 is the initial dialysis glucose concentration immediately after infusion, at time "0." Therefore, rapid transporters would absorb glucose faster than slow transporters.

As discussed earlier, structural changes of the membrane over time have been demonstrated. These alterations are likely related to the dialysis process and/or inflammatory changes associated with infection. Because of the increased use of hypertonic solutions in the event of these changes, the standard bag strength of 2.5% currently used for the PET may underestimate ultrafiltration failure (Krediet, 1999). For patients in whom this is suspected, a PET using a higher glucose concentration (i.e., 3.86% in Europe or 4.25% in North America) may be used to assess loss of ultrafiltration (Cara et al., 2005; Pride et al., 2002). Returns of less than 400 ml with a 4.25% after 4 hours are considered indicative of loss of ultrafiltration capacity (Khanna, 2002; Krediet, 1999).

Of significance is the finding that rapid transporters dissipate the osmotic agent in the dialysate, quickly resulting in decreased ultrafiltration or fluid removal. To compensate for this, shorter dwell times may be recommended to offset the effect and allow for maximal ultrafiltration before the osmotic effect is diminished. Despite the fact that slow transporters remove solutes slowly, studies have shown that this group has less morbidity and mortality than rapid transporters (Agarwal et al, 2000; Chung et al., 2000; Heaf, 2000; Szeto, Law, Wong, Leung, & Li, 2001;Voinescu, Khanna, & Nolph, 2002). Initially, if guidelines were strictly followed, many individuals who were slow transporters would have been converted to hemodialysis. In reality, these individuals have good clinical outcomes. These results led to the realization that there are compensations, likely in the form of middle molecule clearance and water removal, which have positive effects on outcome. It is postulated that although rapid transporters have excellent permeability for solute clearance, they experience loss of ultrafiltration capacity due to reabsorption of the osmotic agent, glucose. This inability to remove water efficiently predisposes rapid transporters to fluid overload, hypertension, and heart failure, and the extra glucose reabsorption may contribute to anorexia (Heaf, 2000). Additionally, although rapid transporters may move solute more quickly, the volume of ultrafiltrate produced is less than that of slow transporters. Despite the slower diffusive process, the volume produced in low transporters is greater with the maintenance of the osmotic gradient. More volume contains more solute, so the actual difference in amount of solute removed between rapid and slow transporters may not be significant in the long term.

Figure 27-3
Peritoneal Equilibration Curves

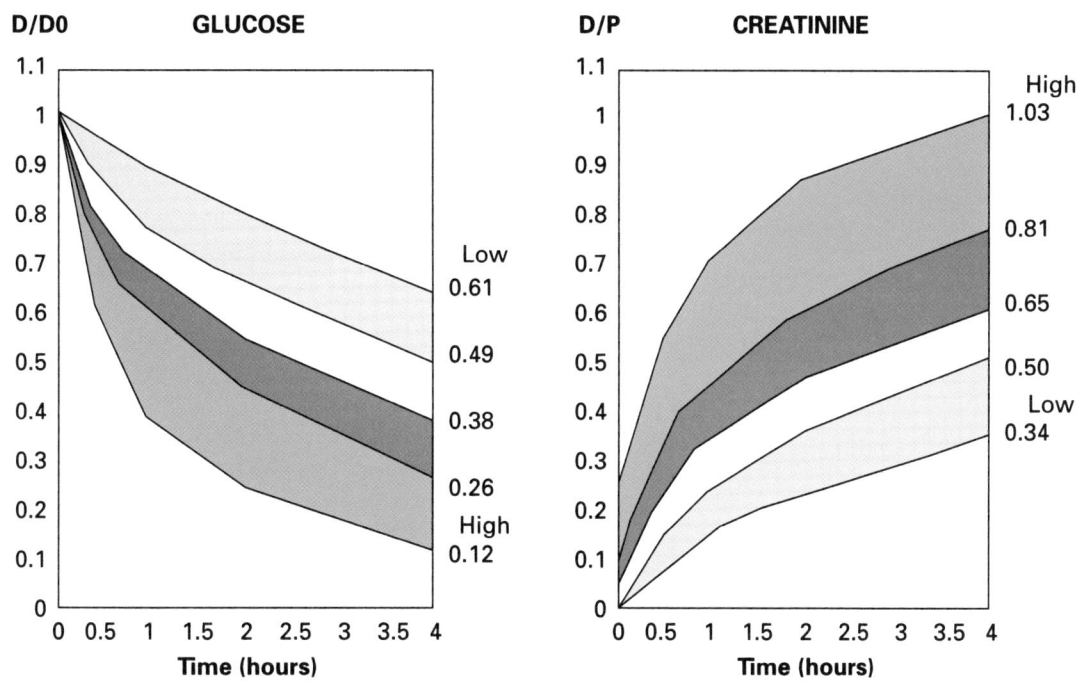

Peritoneal equilibration test curves for corrected creatinine dialysate to plasma (D/P) ratios (right figure) and dialysate glucose to dialysis solution glucose ratios at time 0 (D/DO) (left figure); determined from 103 equilibration studies in 86 patients.

Note: From Prowant, B.F., & Schmidt, L.M. (1991). The peritoneal equilibration test: A nursing discussion. *ANNA Journal, 18*, 361-366. Used with permission.

Table 27-5
Membrane Classification from PET results

Membrane Classification	4 hour D/P Cr	4 hour D/P Urea	4 hour D/Do Gl	Ultrafiltrate Net volume
Slow transporter	< 0.49	Low	High	High
Slow average transporter	0.50 – 0.64	Low average	High average	High average
Rapid average transporter	0.65 – 0.81	High average	Low average	Low average
Rapid transporter	>0.82	High	Low	Low

Note: Adapted from Basics of Peritoneal Dialysis Course, ISPD.

Results of PET can also assist in clinical problem solving. In cases of peritoneal fluid leak, PET results can assist in determining the cause of decreased fluid returns. If the clearance is unchanged from previous measurements, then the possible explanation for sustained clearance with decreased volume is that the peritoneal fluid is leaking out of the peritoneal space into other tissues and/or that increased lymphatic reabsorption has occurred. Thus, further investigations can be conducted to rule in or out other etiologies of a change in ultrafiltration volume. The PET requires a careful and purposeful protocol. Errors in collection techniques can adversely affect the results; a short summary of common errors is listed in Table 27-6.

According to current guidelines, PET should be done as a baseline to determine membrane characteristics and then performed serially. The National Kidney Foundation Dialysis Outcomes Quality Initiative (NKF/DOQI) guidelines recommend the timing and frequency of performing PET. The current recommendation is that the initial PET should be done 1 month post-initiation of PD because it is known that membrane characteristics tend to fluctuate in the first month of dialysis (Johnson et al., 2004; Satko & Burkart, 2002). Additionally, a period of 1 month should elapse after treatment of peritonitis before reassessing membrane characteristics. Because of the inflammatory response, the membrane

Table 27-6
Possible Errors in PET

Procedural Errors	Incomplete drainage of overnight exchange Timing not adhered in collection of samples Intraabdominal mixing not completed
Collection Errors	Inadequate sampling Mixing of fresh dialysate with effluent
Post-procedure	Labeling errors (for example, 0 hour sample labeled as 2 hour sample) Calculations not performed correctly Incorrect volume of returns measured

Note: Adapted from Uttley and Prowant (2000).

becomes more permeable and increases solute reabsorption transiently during an active infection, so the PET should never be carried out during a peritonitis episode. While PET is a measure of the permeability of the peritoneum, adequacy studies are used to assess the effectiveness of the dialysis. The approach to determining adequacy and current clinical tools will be described in the next section on equipment and prescriptive approaches to the PD treatment.

Applying the Principles to the Dialysis Prescription

The basic components of a PD prescription include the following: volume of exchange, number of exchanges, dwell time, dialysate solution composition, target weight reflecting euvolemia, and if required, intraperitoneal medications. The method by which the prescription may be delivered is categorized broadly as *continuous ambulatory peritoneal dialysis* (CAPD) or *automated peritoneal dialysis* (APD). CAPD indicates that a portable bag delivery system is used to perform the exchanges on a daily basis. APD refers to the use of a machine for delivering the exchanges either on a daily or intermittent basis. Daily dialysis is preferred for long-term treatment or chronic dialysis due to superior effectiveness. However, for short intervals, intermittent therapy may be provided in specific circumstances requiring peritoneal membrane rest, or dry periods with no dialysis for healing purposes. In presenting the therapeutic options, a review of an automated intermittent form of IPD will be discussed, followed by the development of daily dialysis options such as CAPD, continuous cyclic peritoneal dialysis (CCPD), and variations on CCPD.

Intermittent Peritoneal Dialysis (IPD)

As described in the "History of Peritoneal Dialysis" section of this chapter, Maxwell's introduction of a peritoneal catheter and the availability of commercial PD solutions made it feasible to perform *intermittent peritoneal dialysis* (IPD) for individuals with renal failure. Rapid exchanges were used initially with dialysate infusion and removal approximately every $1/2$ to 2 hours. The fluid was exchanged manually and was labor-intensive for nursing personnel. The treatments were delivered 2 to 3 times per week, with a total weekly treatment time of approximately 40 hours. IPD is still used in critical care settings and as an alternative for provid-

ing dialysis to patients who have had recent abdominal surgery (such as peritoneal catheter implantation, hernia repair, and transplant nephrectomy) or who have developed a peritoneal leak of fluid. The supine position used for this treatment has benefits related to incision healing and low intraabdominal pressure. Following catheter implantation, patients can be maintained on IPD with dialysis scheduled for 12 hours three times per week, or 20 hours twice per week (hence, the term *intermittent*).

With the development of cycling machines based on Lasker's design, an automated system facilitated the growth of PD in both the hospital and home settings. The machines were programmed to deliver a prescribed number of exchanges with dwell times of 5 minutes for 1-liter volumes and 10 minutes for 2-liter volumes. Up to 8 bags could be hung in a set, allowing the machine to deliver and drain fluid in a cyclic fashion over long periods of time. Additionally, the *cycler*, as it became known, had the advantage of automatically warming dialysis solutions. This was considered advantageous for improving blood flow, and hence, clearance as well as individuals' comfort levels. Prior to this, warm water baths were used to prepare the fluid but have since fallen out of favor because of infectious risks associated with water contamination. The treatment of IPD predated studies in membrane clearance that later demonstrated the inefficiency of short dwell periods in removing middle molecules in comparison with longer dwell periods. While it is now accepted that IPD is not a good choice for long-term management, it had its place in dialysis history as a means of sustaining numerous people with renal failure in the pre-CAPD/CCPD era. Now, IPD is used selectively in the acute care setting, rather than with chronic patients, according to the requirements of the individual with renal failure. The clinical knowledge gained from IPD was useful in establishing PD as a home and self-care option.

Continuous Ambulatory Peritoneal Dialysis (CAPD)

In 1975, Moncrief and Popovich were challenged to provide PD for an individual with renal failure who was unable to perform the then-standard treatment options of hemodialysis or IPD (Cameron, 2002). They developed a formula that provided an adequate clearance of wastes and fluid with five 2-liter exchanges daily with dwell times of at least 3 hours (Venkataraman & Nolph 2002). The target was stabilization of the urea level to 70 mg/dl (24.99 mmol/L). At that time, the original system in the United States relied on glass bottles of dialysis solution. While feasible, the system was cumbersome and associated with a high rate of peritonitis in the range of 1 every 10 weeks (Oreopoulos, Khanna, Williams, & Vas, 1982). Nolph studied the clinical application of this prescription and obtained results indicating effectiveness; however, the glass bottles provided an obstacle to making it practical for home use. In 1977, Oreopoulos further developed the process that became known as CAPD with the adaptation of existing plastic dialysis bags and dialysis tubing sets available in Canada. Early rates of peritonitis were high, but advantages of this approach to daily dialysis were clear and led to further clinical work popularizing the new technology. Oreopoulos and co-researchers (1982) cited the benefits of CAPD as "excellent biochemical control with steady state, improvement of anemia, minimal dietary and fluid restrictions, improvement in the well-being of the patients, and freedom from machine and electrical outlets, which allows patients to travel long distances for long periods" (p. 293). Disadvantages included infection and complications associated with intraabdominal pressure.

The original CAPD prescriptions reflected Popovich and Moncrief's proposal of 2 liters five times a day; however, adaptations have been made based on the findings of individual membrane characteristics. Volumes and number of exchanges may be adjusted. In the early prescriptions, exchanges consisted of two 4-hour dwells, one 6-hour dwell and one 10-hour dwell overnight. Currently, prescriptions take into account individual lifestyles and are comprised of 3 to 4 exchanges during the day and one overnight dwell. Although the long dwell could result in fluid reabsorption, it is accepted that middle molecules require additional time for removal. Thus, the combination of shorter and longer dwell times optimizes solute clearances as well as ultrafiltration. Another option to add exchanges is to use a device that performs an exchange at night while the individual is sleeping.

The first CAPD system used tubing with a spike on one end for attaching the solution bag, and the other end connected to the peritoneal catheter. The tubing with the bag attached remained connected to the individual performing dialysis. The inflow bag, once emptied, was folded up, still attached, and at the end of the dwell period was then unfolded and used as a drain bag with the next exchange. The bag was then discarded, and a full bag spiked for the next inflow. Table 27-7 details some of the designs used in attempts to reduce touch contamination during connection procedures. Some of these variations included disinfectants, in-line filters, and assist devices for bag connection using either heated copper wafers or ultraviolet light. One of the developments by Buoncristiani was the Y-set, which was a disconnect system. From this work came the *flush before fill* concept, which dramatically decreased the existing peritonitis rates; this philosophy has been advocated as a fundamental recommendation for dialysis practice (Bazzato et al., 1993; Burkart, Hylander, Durnell-Figel, & Roberts, 1990; Holley, Bernardini & Piraino, 1994; Maiorca & Cancarini, 1990; Shetty & Oreopoulos, 1994; Smith, 1997).

Continuous Cyclic Peritoneal Dialysis (CCPD)

Continuous cyclic peritoneal dialysis (CCPD) was developed as an alternative to CAPD. Diaz-Buxo, Walker, and Farner (1981) and Nakayawa, Price, Sinebraugh, and Suki (1981) proposed the use of a cycler for delivering dialysis overnight and freeing the person from exchanges during the day. They applied the CAPD prescription in reverse, with the bulk of exchanges done overnight, and the final exchange held for a long-day dwell. This free-day period has proven particularly advantageous to both pediatric and geriatric populations who may rely on assistance for management. The shorter nocturnal dwell times are also recommended for rapid transporters to enhance fluid removal prior to reabsorption of the glucose with the longer dwells associated with CAPD. Additionally, the exchange volumes may be adjusted to enhance clearances (Enoch, Aslam, & Piraino,

2002). For example, an individual who tolerates a 2-liter volume at night while supine and a 1-liter volume during the day may also be able to increase the night exchanges to 2.5 liters with a day dwell of 1.5 liters. Any additional volume in PD can add substantially to the clearances.

CCPD can be further adapted to include day exchanges that will increase clearance or decrease the effect of fluid absorption with long dwells. This approach is useful in rapid transporters who tend to absorb fluid with the long-day dwell.

Nocturnal Intermittent Peritoneal Dialysis (NIPD)

Despite the acknowledgment that continuous exchanges either at night or through the day are preferred for enhanced clearance, there are some individuals who do not tolerate a long dwell when ambulatory, such as patients with severe back pain or large hernias. *Nocturnal Intermittent Peritoneal Dialysis* (NIPD) is an option in which fluid is delivered at night and the patient is left dry during the day. In combination with residual renal function, this approach may be effective; however, declines in renal function may make it more difficult to control uremic symptoms necessitating a change in therapies. A disadvantage of this system is that clearance is decreased with the loss of the continuous 24-hour process.

Tidal Volume Peritoneal Dialysis (TVPD)

Twardowski (2002) described *tidal volume peritoneal dialysis (TVPD)* as an approach designed to ensure a constant presence of dialysate contact with the membrane. Previously described methods for CAPD, CCPD, and IPD are based on an intermittent flow of fluid. Thus, during fill and drain, there are periods when the membrane to dialysate contact is minimal. The purpose of TVPD is to maintain a more continuous exchange effect by leaving a constant reservoir or *reserve* of fluid in the cavity by only removing a portion with each drain. A volume of solution is exchanged and a proportion called the *tidal drain volume* is drained. After this, another volume known as the *tidal fill volume* is instilled to bring the reserve volume up to the desired exchange volume. Generally, the tidal volume is up to 50% of the total volume. For example when using a 2-liter exchange, the reservoir could be 1 liter with another liter exchanged as the tidal volume. Similar to other PD prescriptions, Twardowski (2002) found that the efficiency of TVPD is related to the dose delivered; thus, improved clearances were observed with larger volumes such as 3-liter exchanges in comparison with 1-liter exchanges. A prediction of the anticipated ultrafiltration volume is calculated into the prescription based on the observed drain amounts with varying strengths of solution. Ultrafiltrate can then be removed during the drain period. If not calculated correctly, an individual could deplete the fluid reserve if too much dialysate is drained or alternatively, begin to accumulate large volumes in the cavity. This accumulation can contribute to a sense of fullness and discomfort. The accuracy of the predicted ultrafiltrate per exchange is important in minimizing fluctuations in the reserve volume. Overall advantages of TVPD are noted as fewer machine alarms because of better fluid flow and reduced infusion pain for those individuals who experience dry pain with methods that empty the

Table 27-7
Development of CAPD Delivery Systems

Timeline	System	Advantages	Disadvantages
1970s	Spike set – first variation on previous manual set for exchanges	Portable system	Required spiking into bag; increased risk of touch contamination. Same flow line for fill and drain. Constantly connected to delivery system.
1980s	O-Z set	Recessed spike with disinfectant, first variation to address touch contamination. Used for teaching blind individuals self-care CAPD.	No longer required to wear bag and tubing but still connected to device, same flow line for fill and drain.
1980s	Y-set	First disconnect system, patients not required to remain connected to bag system. Introduction of flush before fill concept which reduced peritonitis rates.	First system used a bleach disinfectant to cleanse the tubing between exchanges; risk of accidental infusion of sodium hypochlorite into peritoneal cavity.
1980s to present	Alternate disconnect sets (company specific)	Variety of systems on the market including a transfer set attached to the peritoneal catheter, a disposable bag and tubing delivery set with option of bag pre-attachment to decrease risks of infection. Addition of disinfectant into capping method for transfer set.	Increased cost initially.
1980s to present	Assist devices	Variety of aids on market.	Designed to decrease touch contamination. Facilitate self-care for individuals. Address specialized needs of individuals (for example, co-existing morbidities such as stroke, visual impairment, arthritis, neuropathy)

cavity prior to refilling. *Dry pain* refers to the sensation of discomfort expressed by some individuals when the cavity is empty of dialysate. This sensation is most noticeable at the end of drain and beginning of fill; thus, the application of tidal volume with the reserve of fluid ensures that the cavity is never completely empty of fluid (Agrawal & Nolph 2000).

Continuous Flow Peritoneal Dialysis (CFPD)

Earlier researchers had identified constant flow as a means of delivering dialysate based on the placement of two catheters: one for inflow and one for outflow. Diaz-Buxo (2001) has modified this concept through the use of a dual lumen catheter with one lumen for inflow and the other for outflow. This approach allows for continuous flow of dialysate either through a system of fresh dialysate or single pass method (Frieda & Issad, 2003). Alternatively, the dialysate can be recirculated through a hemodialysis system

and the regenerated fluid used to achieve continuous flow (Amerling, Glezerman, Savransky, & Dubrow, 2003). According to Diaz-Buxo (2001), the potential advantages of this method include improved solute clearance and ultrafiltration with shorter cycling times. Potential disadvantages are related to the lack of clinical experience in determining the effect of high dialysate flow rates on the peritoneum, as well as risks of "over-distension or dehydration" (Diaz-Buxo, 2001, p. 376). As with TVPD, evaluation of the ultrafiltration patterns is imperative in determining the appropriate prescription.

In preparing people for decision-making regarding treatment options, lifestyle issues may affect choice of APD versus CAPD. For example, a shift-worker performing self-care PD may opt for CCPD in order to accommodate the work patterns. Inability to cope with automated devices may favor the choice of CAPD for individuals in matching treatments to their specific capabilities. Although the initial treatment can be based on individual assessment, changes in therapy may need to occur with loss of residual renal function when a greater emphasis on membrane characteristics may direct choices in treatment. For example, an individual with slow transport characteristics who initiated CCPD and then experienced a loss of renal function may require a change to CAPD in order to enhance solute clearance. Changes in therapy are influenced by the clinical assessment of individuals and control of uremic symptoms. The selection of the PD method is a composite of individual peritoneal membrane characteristics, lifestyle issues, cost factors, availability of equipment and experienced support required for the treatment.

Composition of Peritoneal Dialysis Solutions

Basic to the PD prescription is the type of dialysis solution recommended for use in both CAPD and APD. The desirable solution for PD should achieve the goals of dialysis without adverse effects, while preserving and maintaining peritoneal function. Cost-effectiveness and environmental disposal are equally important to availability and storage issues for individuals performing dialysis. To be effective for dialysis, the solution must be a balanced composition of an osmotic agent, electrolytes (including sodium, chloride, calcium and magnesium), and a buffer in a balance that facilitates fluid removal, electrolyte regulation, and correction of metabolic acidosis in renal failure.

The most widely used solutions for dialysis are glucose-based with lactate as a buffer. A wide variety of alternate products have been studied to perform the functions of fluid and solute removal, however, glucose and lactate-based solutions currently remain the basics of PD. Although these solutions have been used for decades with decreasing adverse effects related to quality control in industry, realization that glucose may be detrimental to the long-term survival of the peritoneum has become an issue of concern for practitioners. As a result, research on biocompatibility of solutions has been a major focus in the attempt to enhance outcomes through preservation of peritoneal integrity as a dialyzing surface (Miyata, Devuyst, Kurokawa & Van Ypersele de Strihou, 2002; Vardhan, Zweers, Gokal, & Krediet, 2003).

Although electrolyte composition is variable according to manufacturer, a standard formula for eletrolytes in the dialysate is:

      Sodium 132 mEq/L,
      Magnesium 1.5 mEq/L
      Chloride 102 mEq/L
      Calcium, either 2.5 mEq/L or 3.5 mEq/L

Additionally, the dialysate contains osmotic agents and buffers, which will be described below.

Osmotic Agents: Glucose, Icodextrin, and Amino Acids

Glucose. Glucose has been the mainstay of osmotic agents in use largely because of its availability and low cost; however, studies have shown that glucose can have deleterious effects on membrane function (Crawford-Bonadio & Diaz-Buxo, 2004; Jorres, 2003; Mortier, De Vriese & Lameire, 2003; Tauer et al.,, 2005; Wieslander, Linden &

Kjellstrand, 2001; Zheng, Ye, Yu, Bergstrom & Lindholm, 2001). This effect is related to the production of glucose degradation products (GDPs) during the sterilization process and the breakdown of glucose over time to advanced glycosylation end-products (AGEs), which are felt to deposit in the peritoneal tissues and blood vessel walls (Stigant & Bargman, 2002). Ha and Lee (2000) studied the effect of glucose and suggested that it was a pathogenic factor contributing to peritoneal membrane fibrosis in long-term dialysis. Glucose also has an impact on blood vessel walls with changes that appear similar to the vascular changes of diabetic microangiopathy; these may be important in the ultrafiltration failure described in individuals with long-term exposure to glucose (Krediet, Zweers, van de Wal, & Stujik, 2000). High glucose concentrations have also been shown to impair the host defenses of the peritoneal cavity; in particular, the phagocytic response is reduced while the GDPs also may suppress cell function (Holmes, 2002). Gokal and Mallick (1999) described weight gain, hyperinsulinemia, and hyperlipidemia as metabolic effects associated with glucose absorption that is in the range of 100 to 300 grams per day (Gokal & Mallick, 1999; Mistry & Gokal, 1994).

Icodextrin. In the Multi-Centre Investigation of Icodextrin in Ambulatory Peritoneal Dialysis Study (MIDAS) in the United Kingdom, the use of icodextrin, an alternative to glucose, was studied (Johnson et al., 2003; Mistry, Gokal, & Peers, 1994). Icodextrin is a starch-derived glucose polymer that metabolizes to maltose and has a molecular weight of 13,000 to 19,000 Daltons (Cooker, Holmes, & Hoff, 2002). With an osmolality of 282 – 286 mOsm/L, icodextrin is isoosmotic to uremic blood. The advantage, however, over glucose is that ultrafiltration is maintained by a colloid osmotic effect since the icodextrin is not readily reabsorbed across the peritoneum (Cooker et al, 2002, Frampton & Ploskar, 2003; Ho-dac-Pannekett et al., 1996). Icodextrin is most effective with long dwell periods of 8 to 12 hours because of the sustained effect on water removal (Gokal, 1999; Johnson et al., 2001; Johnson et al, 2003). This solution can be used for the overnight dwell with CAPD or the long-day dwell in CCPD. For shorter dwells, conventional dialysate will ultrafilter faster so icodextrin must be instilled with an appropriate dwell time. Maltose and other oligosaccharides are metabolic products of icodextrin, which accumulate in the blood. Although the clinical significance of these byproducts is not known, the recommendation is to limit the number of icodextrin exchanges to one per day, both to avoid excess levels and to promote the best utilization of the icodextrin with long dwells (Diaz-Buxo, 2005).

In individuals with diabetes, there is a risk of reading a falsely elevated blood glucose if the blood glucose is measured using a device that does not differentiate maltose from glucose. These devices may indicate that the blood glucose is higher than it actually is because both maltose and glucose are measured. If this "artificially high" glucose reading is treated, there is a potential for hypoglycemia (Riley, Chess, Donovan, & Williams, 2003). Glucose-specific methods avoid the interference by maltose but glucose dehydrogenase pyroloquinolinequinone-based methods measure the maltose as glucose and can overestimate the blood glucose level (Johnson et al., 2003; Riley et al., 2003). Nurses should check with the supplying company of meters to ensure the method of glucose interpretation will avoid this misinterpretation. This potential risk must also be communicated to institutions where individuals may be hospitalized, and measures should be taken to either rely on venous blood glucose levels or capillary levels tested with the appropriate device.

Complications of icodextrin therapy have also included occurrences of allergic skin reactions including psoriasiform rashes; blisters on sun-exposed areas and acute, dermal exfoliation (Johnson et al., 2003; Kannyet al., 2004, Goldsmith, Jayawardene, Sabharwal, & Cooney, 2000). Resolution of these responses occurs after cessation of icodextrin, in a range from 48 hours to 6 weeks. The product monograph recommends that people who are allergic to cornstarch and/or dextran should not use icodextrin.

There have been reports of sterile or culture negative bacterial peritonitis with the use of icodextrin. Sterile peritonitis refers to an inflammatory process without an identifiable organism on effluent cultures. Cloudy fluid returns and abdominal pain are associated with an inflammatory response. Borras, Martin, and Fernandez (2004) reported on sterile peritonitis in a cluster of 6 patients receiving icodextrin and attributed this to contamination in the solution manufacturing process. This has also been previously reported by other clinicians (Heering, Brause, Plum, & Grabensee, 2001; Pinerolo, Porri, & D'Amico, 1999; Reichel, Schultze, Dietze, Mende, 2001). Seow, Iles-Smith, Hirst, and Gokal (2003) and Basile, De Padova, Montanaro, and Giordano (2003) attributed the observed episodes to higher than normal peptidoglycan levels. Peptidoglycan is a substance found in cell walls of gram-positive organisms, which is capable of activating macrophages (Seow et al., 2003). Peptidoglycan was believed to produce an inflammatory response with the risk of relapse in individuals sensitized by the presence of this substance. Martis et al. (2005) reported on peptidoglycan contamination with *Alicyclobacillus* in a batch of solution. Product recall, evaluation and introduction of new screening protocols were undertaken to address the manufacturing issues.

Poulopoulos, Lam, and Cugelman (2004) also reported the presentation of 5 patients with sterile peritonitis; however, in this group, the etiology was attributed to a chemical reaction rather than manufacturing process.

Robertson, Huxtable, Blakemore, Williams, and Donovan (2001) described that individuals using an icodextrin dialysate system with povidone-iodine noted a blue-black line instead of the usual yellowish-brown stain associated with the disinfectant in the tubing. As the effluent is drained out, this color disappeared. The cause of the color change may be a reaction between the iodine in the disinfectant and the icodextrin, which has similarities to starch as a similar color change is reported with combining iodine and starch.

Amino acids. Protein and amino acid loss occurs into the peritoneal fluid, with the average daily protein loss estimated at 8 to 10 gms and amino acid loss at 3 to 4 gms (Hung et al., 2004; Jones et al., 1998; Pollock, Cooper, Ibels & De Kantzow, 2000). Amino acids can be used as a replacement for glucose as an osmotic agent with the intent to pro-

vide a source of protein rather than carbohydrate while achieving ultrafiltration. In some countries, this solution is available as a 1.1% amino acid solution (not currently available in U.S.). Adverse effects noted with the amino acid solution can include pain on inflow related to the acidity of the solution and metabolic acidosis (Alsop, 1994). To decrease this effect, the content of the standard amino acid solution was changed from a lactate of 35 to one of 40 mmol in solution (Pollock et al., 2000).

Kopple et al. (1995) described findings from an in-hospital balance study in which 19 individuals were dialyzed with 1 or 2 exchanges of amino acids. These authors believed that the dialysis solution had the potential to improve protein malnutrition in individuals with low oral intake. It was found, however, that if the individual did not ingest enough calories, a risk existed for converting the amino acids to waste products rather than actually using them for tissue repair and growth. Bruno, Gabella, and Ramello (2000) reviewed 15 clinical studies reported between the years 1983 to 1999 and concluded that amino acids could offer benefits if specific conditions, such as adequate caloric intake and correction of acidosis, were met. They advocated the use of amino acid solutions in individuals in whom malnutrition was an outcome of inadequate protein intake. In a 3-year randomized trial, Li et al. (2003) found that amino acids presented "a means to improve the nutritional status in high-risk patients" (p. 173), however they were not able to demonstrate a significant difference in patient survival.

In delivering amino acids, the solution ideally should be administered during the daytime, as studies have shown better results when given in conjunction with caloric intake (Faller et al., 1995; Hung et al., 2004). Dombros, Prutis, Tong et al. (1990) demonstrated that amino acids given at night did not have an effect in treating malnutrition. Although two exchanges of amino acids may be used daily (Rocco & Blumenkrantz, 2001), the general approach is to prescribe one. The 1.1% amino acid solution is felt to be comparable to a 1.5% dextrose solution in terms of ultrafiltration (Pollock et al., 2000). Plasma urea and bicarbonate levels should be followed as well as nutritional markers in assessing the clinical response to amino acid solutions.

Buffers: Lactate, Acetate, and Bicarbonate

To treat metabolic acidosis, buffers have been added to dialysate solutions. Acetate and lactate were the original buffers that are converted in the liver to bicarbonate after absorption across the peritoneum. However, despite controversial evidence, acetate was discontinued as an additive due to concerns about sclerosing of the peritoneum. Lactate concentrations are either 35 or 40 mEq/L with a pH of approximately 5.5. Schröder (2004) noted that the low pH of these lactate solutions has been associated with inflow pain as well as damaging effects on the mesothelium and macrophages. As with the hypertonic glucose, the acidic nature of these solutions can interfere with the peritoneal cavity's host defenses.

In developing a more biocompatible solution, the introduction of bicarbonate into the dialysate is a focus of industry (Heimburger & Mujais, 2003). The challenge is that bicarbonate cannot be pre-mixed because there is potential for the bicarbonate to cause precipitation of calcium. Through creation of bags with compartments, bicarbonate can be separated from the remaining solutes until immediately before instillation when mixing can occur.

The emphasis on developing more physiological dialysate solutions is to improve viability of the peritoneal membrane and to enhance PD as a long-term dialysis modality (Hjelle, Miller-Hjelle, & Dobbie, 1995; Holmes & Faict, 2003, Passlick-Deetjen, Schaub, & Schilling, 2002).

Intraperitoneal Medications

Having set the prescription, another aspect of peritoneal management is the administration of intraperitoneal (IP) medications. The peritoneum has been shown to be an effective route for drug administration for insulin and antibiotics.

Potassium

Although not routinely added to dialysate, intraperitoneal KCl has been used for individuals with hypokalemia. Two to four mEq of KCl/liter can be added intraperitoneally to inhibit further potassium losses into the dialysate (Diaz-Buxo, 2005). Spital and Sterns (1985) reported on findings from a study of five individuals on CAPD who were given an exchange containing 20 mEq/L of potassium. They found that the dose was well tolerated and resulted in a gradual increase in the plasma potassium level. Bargman (2000) noted that in a controlled hospital setting, up to 20 mEqKCl/L can be added IP for treatment of severe hypokalemia. Bargman adds a cautionary note that since the effect of this increased concentration of potassium on the peritoneal membrane is unknown, the use of this dose should only be in "urgent settings" (Bargman, 2000, p. 617).

Heparin

Heparin is utilized for prevention of fibrin formation, which could potentially block the catheter. IP heparin is not absorbed to the point of having a systemic anticoagulation effect (Bailie, Johnson, Mason, & St. Peter, 2004), thus is safe to use in moderate doses, such as 500-1000 u/L. For management of peritonitis, an inflammation of the peritoneal cavity which promotes fibrin formation, increased doses of heparin (such as 1000u/L), are recommended both to prevent fibrin formation and minimize the opportunity for bacteria to colonize on available fibrin.

Insulin

Short-acting insulin administered IP has proven effective in achieving glycemic control; however, there are both advantages and disadvantages associated with this route of administration. For individuals with diabetes, the opportunity to reduce or eliminate subcutaneous injections is an attractive one, and IP insulin has been found to decrease fluctuations of blood glucose levels compared to subcutaneous insulin (Quellhorst 2002). Another advantage is that IP insulin is more physiologic in its absorption via the portal system (Khanna & Oreopoulos, 1989; Diaz-Buxo, 2005). This results in more rapid and even absorption when compared to the subcutaneous route of administration (Quellhorst, 2002).

Disadvantages have been related to increased requirements of insulin given its adsorption to plastic tubing, dilution by the dialysate, and varying absorption rates dependent on dwell times (Farina, 2004; Quellhorst, 2002). There is also a potential increased risk of infection with additional manipulations of the system to add the insulin. However, early studies suggested that there is no statistically significant difference in the rate of peritonitis between people with diabetes and those without diabetes (Khanna & Oreopoulos, 1989; Madden, Zimmerman, & Simpson, 1982).

To ensure total injection of insulin into the dialysate, the needle must be of adequate length (greater than or equal to 1.5 inches or 3.8 cm) to penetrate the injection cap and barrier (Tzamaloukas & Friedman, 2001). Generally, the amount of insulin administered is greater than the previous subcutaneous dose given the adherence to plastic. Wideröe, Smeby, Berg, Jörstad, and Svartas (1983) demonstrated an absorption rate of 35%, compared to the larger percentage of 65% adsorbed to the plastic, whereas Fine, Parry, Araino, and Dent (2000) described 17% to 66% absorption rate of insulin, and the adsorption was 14% +/-5%. Methods have been described for administration in CAPD and APD. The practice with CAPD has been to double the 24-hour subcutaneous requirements to account for adsorption to tubing and then divide this amount among the exchanges to determine a basal dose. By using a sliding scale to increase or decrease the insulin requirements based on blood sugar results, the insulin dose can be further adjusted until an adequate basal dose is determined. Some individuals continue to use a sliding scale for self-adjustment of insulin in addition to the basal dose. Generally, the intraperitoneal requirement is two to three times the previous subcutaneous dose (Diaz-Buxo, 1999; Tzamloukas & Friedman, 2001). Quellhorst, (2002) reduced the amount of required insulin by instilling the medication into an empty peritoneal cavity with normal saline prior to infusing the dialysis exchange but found that this method required more steps and equipment than instilling insulin with the dialysate. Diaz-Buxo (1999) recommended dividing the calculated dose into 85% for day exchanges and 15% for night exchange for CAPD. For APD, Diaz-Buxo recommends giving 50% of the insulin for night exchanges and 50% of the insulin for daytime exchanges. If the prescription for CCPD includes a mid-day exchange, then the recommendation is to modify the administration by dividing it equally among all exchanges.

While the IP route for insulin is feasible, many practitioners and people on PD continue to use the option of subcutaneous insulin. The dose needs to be adjusted for the increased caloric load associated with glucose solutions for dialysis. In the initial stages of adjusting the insulin, close monitoring with capillary blood glucose levels is required. Sliding scales for insulin can be utilized to determine the dose requirements.

Antibiotics

Antibiotics may be given IP for both peritonitis and other infections as therapeutic blood levels can be achieved through this route (Bailie, Johnson, Mason & St. Peter, 2004). The ISPD has developed IP antibiotic dosing recommenda-

Figure 27-4
Double Bag System

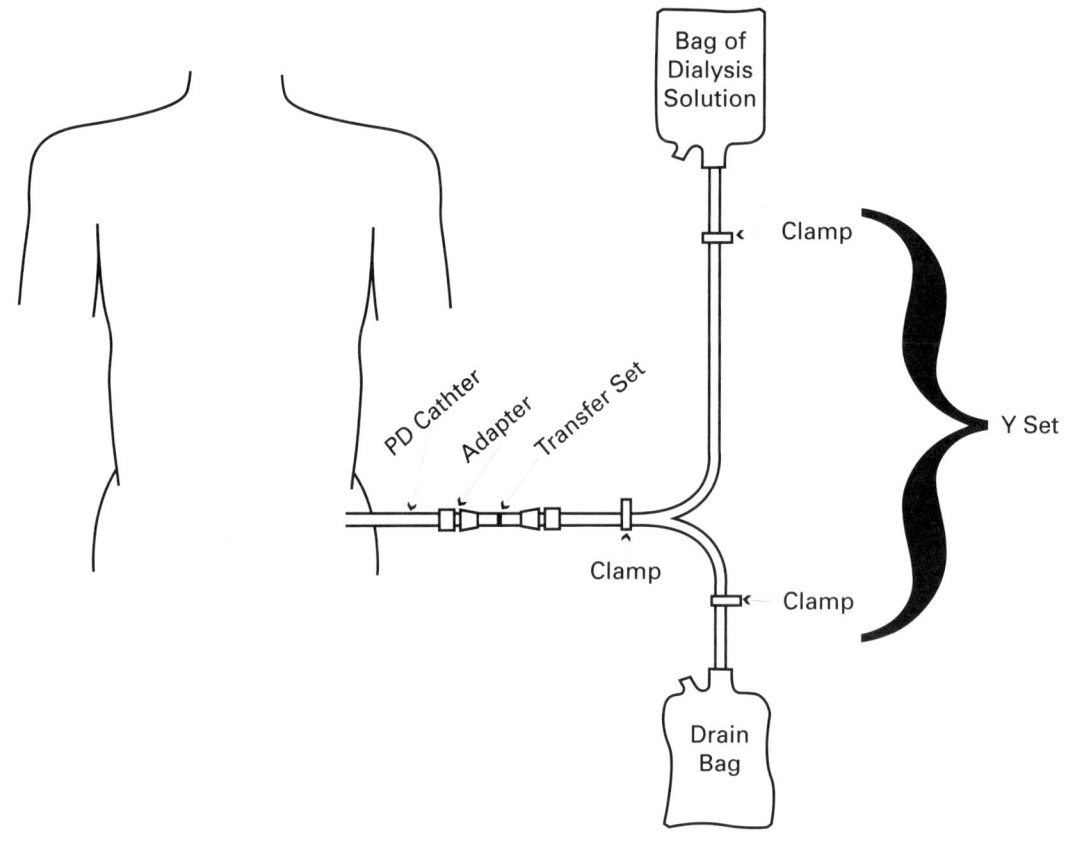

tions for IPD and APD and continuous dosing for CAPD (Piraino, 2005). Bailie et al. (2004) have suggested that further study in the area of APD and intraperitoneal antibiotics are required because APD may result in greater clearances of the medications.

Other Medications

Sodium bicarbonate IP has been used to raise the pH of dialysate for individuals who experience abdominal cramping relative to the acidity. IP xylocaine can be used for managing abdominal discomfort related to the dialysate. Diaz-Buxo (2005) suggests the use of 5 mL/L of 1% or 2% xylocaine for infusion pain. Prior to using medications to alleviate pain, it is important to determine treatable causes for the discomfort. For the treatment of gastroparesis, metoclopromide and erythromycin have been used IP (J. M. Bargman, personal communication, December 1, 2004). In early studies, the use of IP erythropoietin, either undiluted or diluted in dialysate, was investigated. Since diluted IP erythropoietin required higher doses of the medication, the undiluted route was found to be more cost-effective (Bailie et al, 2004; Bargman, Jones, & Petro, 1992; Lui, Chung, Leung, Chan, & Lai, 1990).

Practical Aspects of Peritoneal Dialysis

Regardless of the prescription for PD, protocols form the basis for directing the steps in performing the actual treatment. Aseptic principles are the foundation for reducing infectious risks and should be incorporated when developing protocols. It is recognized that unit-specific protocols are in place, and introducing change may be difficult particularly if peritonitis rates are satisfactory with the given practice. Thus, a wide range of practices may be found internationally, reflecting the experience of practitioners. While it is recognized that hygienic practices (such as handwashing) are instrumental in reducing infection rates, controversy exists over other practices (such as use of gloves and masks for exchanges).

Figueiredo, Poli de Figueiredo, and d'Avila (2000) reported peritonitis rates in two groups of individuals performing CAPD, one group using masks (N=24) and one without masks (N= 40). Peritonitis rates were 1.0 episode per year for the group using masks and 0.94 episodes per year for the group without masks. This difference did not reach statistical significance; however, the researchers believed that larger studies were needed to review the cost benefit of non-masking with the outcomes for infection. De Vecchi and Scalamogna (2001) were not convinced by the findings, and they conducted interviews with individuals with peritonitis in their unit. Of 324 episodes of peritonitis,

22 individuals who missed masking presented with gram-positive peritonitis. The researchers believe that masking should remain in the procedure, as the predicted cost benefit in reducing mask use would not be compensated for by the cost of peritonitis. This is supported by Piraino's (1998) review of peritonitis in which she considers masking to be an acceptable step in the procedure for decreasing risks of infection. On the other hand, Figueiredo, Poli de Figueiredo, and d'Avila (2001) further reported on their 5-year experience with 94 patients for whom the bag exchange procedure did not include masking; their results were consistent with other centers' peritonitis rates. In this publication, they stressed the value of hand washing, education with respect to risk factors for infection, and consistent teaching methods. Masking remains a unit-specific policy; all ramifications, including appropriately fitting masks and effectiveness of protection for the time involved for the exchanges, should be considered.

While it is generally recognized that a consistent approach with adherence to aseptic techniques is essential in promoting safe practice, the paucity of literature in nephrology nursing makes it difficult to make a statement regarding this issue. Protocols for connecting and disconnecting procedures, delivery set changes, warming of dialysate solutions, and medication injection must also be developed using research and experience-based best practice.

Equipment for performing dialysis is based on the prescription. For all forms of dialysis, the individual requires an implantable catheter that is connected via a locking device to a transfer set. The transfer set is tubing that remains attached to the catheter and is used for connecting the delivery set to the dialysis solution. This tubing should be changed per manufacturer's recommendations at regular intervals or as necessary if contaminated. Aseptic technique should be followed for any procedures involving exposure of the catheter end. A variety of delivery sets exist for instilling and draining. One example for CAPD is a double bag system that has a pre-attached bag of dialysis solution and a drainage bag (see Figure 27-4). Daly et al. (2002) reviewed literature on CAPD administration sets and concluded that the preferred system for bag exchanges should be the double bag system, which has been proven to reduce peritonitis rates. For CCPD, a cycling machine and tubing sets for fluid delivery are required, as well as a means for effluent disposal either through a bag, tank or drain system. Some tubing sets require clamps for the exchange process, but care must be taken that these clamps do not have "teeth," which can damage the tubing or catheters (Burrows & Prowant, 1998).

For the injection of medication into ports of bags, cleansing of the ports with a disinfectant is completed prior to injection, and adequate time should be allowed for the specific disinfectant to be effective. This time will vary according to the disinfectant's properties.

Cyclers for APD have built-in warming devices, but for CAPD, options for warming fluid are required as part of the equipment. Most individuals prefer to warm the solution prior to instillation. Room temperature or cold fluid can cause pain and discomfort on inflow, causing chills and

Table 27-8
Sample Guideline for Bag Selection

If > 0.5 kg below TW	use 0.5%
If TW ± 0.5 kg	use 1.5%
If >0.6 to 1.0 kg above TW	use 2.5%
If >1.0 kg above TW	use 4.25%

Note: Must be adjusted according to individual weight loss patterns.

abdominal cramping. It is recommended that only dry heat methods be used because water baths for solution have been associated with peritonitis from water contamination. Dry heat can include warming blankets, heating pads, commercial warming devices, and microwave ovens. Controversy remains regarding the use of microwaves because PD solution manufacturers do not recommend them; burns have been associated with overheating of bags. Despite this, researchers in this area have made suggestions for the proper use of microwaves. Armstrong and Zalatan (1992) suggested that heating bags by microwave was possible if times were established for heating with minimum and maximum external temperatures. They also recommended mixing the heated solution prior to infusing. Deutschendorf, Wenk, Lustagarten, and Mason (1994) conducted *in vitro* studies to assess if microwave warming affected the components of the solution. They did not find statistically different degradation products, and precipitate was not observed microscopically. They did comment, however, that with a non-rotating plate, "hot spots" were detected particularly at ports. Manufacturers' recommendations are also available and should be consulted, especially with the development of new dialysis solutions. For example, icodextrin and amino acid-based solutions should not be heated in a microwave oven.

A scale is also required for weight assessment to determine the target goal for fluid removal. A consistent approach to weighing a person should be established, either after each CAPD exchange or alternatively, on a daily basis. The target weight should specify if the individual is weighed with fluid indwelling or drained. Thus, an individual on CAPD with 2-liter exchanges could have a target set of 65 kg (full) indicating that the weight is done with a 2-liter volume of fluid in the peritoneal cavity. It may be helpful to provide the novice with guidelines for selecting bag strengths. A sample of a teaching tool is found in Table 27-8.

A blood pressure apparatus is needed for the assessment of blood pressure both in relation to fluid balance and treatment of hypo or hypertension. The blood pressure apparatus should be assessed in the training unit to validate the measurements obtained.

For people with diabetes, capillary blood sugar monitoring devices will be required. For individuals using icodextrin solution, the device should meet the requirements described under the section on peritoneal dialysis solutions.

Practical Aspects of Volume of Exchange and Bag Strength Selection

Volume of exchange is an important determinant of dialysate flow rates, which in turn, affect clearance. Dialysate-to-membrane contact is a reflection of the effective surface area used for dialysis. Volumes are adjusted to achieve the maximal volume effective for dialysis clearance and comfort level. For an individual initiating dialysis, a smaller exchange volume may be used and compensated for with an increased number of exchanges. One-liter exchanges may be advisable as a starting volume for IPD for catheter break-in, with a gradual increase up to the desired volume. In a blinded study, Sarkar, Bernardini, Fried, Johnston, and Piraino (1999) assessed individuals with volumes of exchange of 2, 2.5, and 3 liters, and found that most subjects were not able to note the difference in exchange volume. Ventura, Amato, Correa-Rotter, and Paniagua (2000) also described that many people can tolerate the 2.5 to 3.0 L volume for dialysis. In APD, the increase of volume can generally be done in increments of 100 mL, whereas in CAPD, the tendency is to base the increase on the available options of 1, 1.5, 2, 2.5, and 3-liter bags. The volume also affects intra-abdominal pressure, which is highest in the sitting position and lowest in the supine pressure (Enoch et al., 2002). Thus, adjustments to exchange volume may reflect the application of this knowledge. For example, an individual with a hernia receiving CCPD may tolerate an inflow volume of 2 liters at night and 1.5 liters during the day to reduce pressure in the upright position.

When selecting bag strengths for fluid removal, nurses, using guidelines, can adjust the osmotic concentration based on fluid assessment including weight, blood pressure, lung auscultation, presence of edema, and symptoms such as shortness of breath. The sample guideline in Table 27-8 is not intended as a standard but may be useful in determining an initial approach to bag selection. The guidelines may require adjustment in the presence of membrane thickening or reduced ultrafiltration capacity; that is, the 1.5% may remove less fluid, and the individual may require a combination of 2.5% and 4.25% solutions. A weight may be done before each CAPD exchange to determine bag selection, or alternatively, a daily weight may be used to select the bag strengths for the day. With APD, sets of bags are hung, with one set for CCPD/NIPD, and more than one set for IPD. Again, weight is used to determine the required combination of bags.

One of the perceived benefits of PD is often viewed as a more liberal oral fluid intake with the daily dialysis regimen. In light of the research on advanced glycosylation end products, health care practitioners may elect to reintroduce fluid restrictions in an attempt to control the use of hypertonic solutions. Alternate solutions such as icodextrin and amino acids may be used to reduce the number of glucose solutions required. It is important that these solutions have an extended dwell period for maximal effectiveness.

Following selection, the bags should be inspected for strength, composition, volume, clarity, and integrity. Defective bags should be reported to the manufacturer in the interest of quality control. If the defect occurs during the warming process, the method of heating used should be re-examined. In assessing individuals during training, literacy and numeracy skills should be incorporated into the initial assessment. Some systems are color-coded for the identification of differing composition of solutions, and the individual's ability to discern color differences should be noted. If there are reading or identification challenges, then alternate methods of coding the bags should be considered for safe selection and use. For example, if someone is not able to read the labels, bag strengths could be identified with different colored labels (i.e., red for 4.25%). This would require assistance from someone with literacy skills.

PD exchanges have been done in the home, in the car, at work, on vacation and at school. People have maintained active lifestyles and reported experiences of dialyzing while camping and hiking. Regardless of the location, efforts should be made to keep the environment clean, dust free, well-ventilated, and disruption-free to ensure consistent safe practice for optimal outcomes. Household pets should be restricted from the room designated for PD.

Measuring Adequacy of Dialysis

The term *adequacy* has been coined to represent effective control of uremic symptoms in an individual with renal failure. People are considered to be well dialyzed when they describe a sense of wellness, good appetite, energy, and mental acuity if there is no underlying dementia. People who are not well dialyzed may develop uremic symptoms, including nausea, anorexia, pruritus, fatigue, and decreased mental acuity. It should be remembered that no type of dialysis can completely replace the functions of the kidney, and likely can only approximate a GFR of 20 or so, thus emphasis must be placed on accomplishing the best possible dialysis for each individual.

While PET is a measurement of transport characteristics of the peritoneal membrane, adequacy studies are a measurement of the effectiveness of the dialysis process. As with PET, it is recommended that a standard approach be taken to adequacy studies for comparison of results. In measuring adequacy in people on PD, both peritoneal and residual renal clearances are determined in a 24-hour period. It has been found that residual renal clearance is better preserved on PD when compared with hemodialysis; this is largely related to the steady state achieved with less fluctuation in blood pressure and renal perfusion (Lameire, 1997; Oreopoulos, 1999b). Nonetheless, residual renal clearance decreases over time, necessitating re-evaluation of the PD prescription. Effluent and urine are collected and sent for analysis with the data obtained used to tabulate the weekly clearances of both urea and creatinine. Kt/V is the clearance over time divided by volume, and in PD, is calculated using urea. Adequacy studies produce a numerical interpretation of the effectiveness of dialysis and are tempting to use as a measurement of successful dialysis through the attainment of pre-determined targets. The National Kidney Foundation Dialysis Outcomes Quality Initiative (NKF-DOQI) established evidence and opinion-based clearance goals in 1997; however, because of further analysis of clinical practice, the original targets have been redefined. Recently, emphasis on the clinical assessment of the individual on PD has taken

Table 27-9
Adequacy Test for CAPD

Timing of Steps	Steps
Morning of collection	Fully drain and discard overnight dwell
24-hour period	Collect all bag exchanges.
Day post collection	Pool and mix effluent. * (*Alternately, weigh each bag and take aliquot from each bag – for 2 liter return, take 2 ml; for 2.3 liter return, take 2.3 ml to ensure representative sample.) Measure volume. Take sample. Send sample for creatinine, urea, glucose and protein Send blood sample (drawn pre, during or post collection) for urea and creatinine.
Results available	Calculate clearances

Note: Adapted from ISPD guidelines*

Table 27-10
Adequacy Test for CCPD

Day of study	Collect all effluent from overnight cycler. If additional day, exchanges may be collected on the day before or after the collection. Sample representative of 24-hour period. Weigh volume or alternatively, may record volume from machine. Day exchanges not drained by machine should be weighed separately. Send samples for urea, creatinine, glucose, and protein Blood sample close proximity to collection for urea, creatinine.
Results available	Calculate clearances

Note: Adapted from ISPD guidelines.

Table 27-11
Errors in Adequacy Testing

Pre procedure	Individual has not been following prescribed dialysis schedule pre collection Dialysis during time of test is not representing actual dialysis done
Collection errors	Missing volume of solution (for example, not collected, clamps not placed properly with loss of fluid) Aliquots not taken properly Incomplete urine collection Timing not recorded properly Collection of samples is done either greater than or less than 24 hours
Lab errors	Creatinine not corrected for glucose in lab
Calculation errors	Incorrect entry for computer programs

Note: Adapted from Uttley & Prowant (2000).

Table 27-12
Calculations for PD Adequacy Kt/V

24 hour dialysate urea/serum urea + 24 hour urine urea/serum urea

Volume *

*Volume based on Watson Formula, accounts for age, weight, and gender

CrCl Peritoneal Clearance + Renal Clearance**

Peritoneal clearance = 24 hour dialysate creatinine/serum creatinine x 24 hour dialysate volume in L x 7 days

**Calculated residual renal clearance – may be based on average of urea and creatinine clearance.

precedence in the literature on adequacy. This in part, is due to the controversy over the appropriate solute to measure adequacy in PD.

Guidelines for conducting adequacy studies for both individuals on CAPD and CCPD are shown in Tables 27-9 and 27-10. Frequency recommendations for performing these studies are found in DOQI guidelines; however, other resources (such as the Canadian Society of Nephrology [CSN] and Caring for Australians in Renal Impairment [CARI]) differ somewhat in recommendations. Since results depend on accurate collection methods, it is imperative to follow the standardized approach to minimize errors in the collection process, serum measurements, and calculations.

Common errors to avoid are detailed in Table 27-11. The formulas for determining Kt/V and creatinine clearance are found in Table 27-12, and there are computer programs for the analysis of findings from the adequacy studies.

Burkart (2000) emphasized that each 1 ml/min of residual renal clearance is equivalent to a CrCl of 10 L/week and a Kt/V of about 0.25 based on body surface area. This translates into the equivalent of approximately one additional exchange of 1.5 liters daily. In measuring the residual renal clearance, the average of urea and creatinine clearance is calculated because in advanced renal failure, urea clearance underestimates and creatinine clearance overestimates the glomerular filtration rate (Blake & Diaz-Buxo, 2001; Chandna & Farrington, 2004). With decline in renal function, creatinine is both filtered and then secreted, with the concentration in the urine representing more than what was originally filtered. The opposite is true for urea, which is both filtered and reabsorbed, leading to less urea in the urine than filtered through the remaining functional glomeruli. Since the clearance represents glomerular filtration, it is important to take this alteration into account when calculating the clearance.

Current Targets for Kt/V and CrCl

The original NKF-DOQI guidelines for Kt/V were 2.0, 2.1, and 2.2 respectively for CAPD, CCPD, and NIPD. The targets for creatinine clearance, based on L/week/body surface of 1.73 m², were 60, 63, and 66 respectively for CAPD, CCPD, and NIPD (NKF-DOQI, 1997). Since publication of these guidelines, further research has yielded differing opinions on the targets because they were difficult to attain, particularly in those with declining residual renal function. Research findings suggest that slow transporters had better outcomes than rapid transporters despite lower Kt/V and CrCl results. As a result, the Canadian Society of Nephrology established targets of Kt/V of 2.0 for CAPD/CCPD and NIPD (Blake et al, 1999). Furthermore, a CrCl of 60 L/wk was adopted for rapid transporters and a clearance of 50 L/wk for slow transporters (Blake & Diaz-Buxo, 2001). In 2000, the NKF-DOQI guidelines elected to follow a similar pattern for CAPD while maintaining the previously recommended standards for CCPD and NIPD.

The Canada-USA (CANUSA) Peritoneal Dialysis Study Group (1996) found that the relative risk (RR) of death was decreased with increases in Kt/V and creatinine clearance in a study of 680 individuals in 14 centers. Churchill (1998) reported that "the relative risk of death was decreased by 6% for a 0.1 greater weekly Kt/V and by 7% for a 5l/1.73 m² greater weekly CCr" (p. 159). Additional findings included increased RR of death in individuals who were rapid transporters and increased hospitalization and technique failure for individuals with decreased serum albumin levels (Canada-USA (CANUSA) Peritoneal Study Group, 1996; Churchill, 1998). The CANUSA study used total clearances, including both peritoneal and renal clearances to calculate the relative risk of death; however, further research determined that peritoneal clearances could not be considered equivalent to renal clearances (Diaz-Buxo, 2005). Bargman, Thorpe, and Churchill (2001), in their reanalysis of the data from CANUSA, determined that residual renal function was more important in "the survival advantage of peritoneal dialysis over hemodialysis" (p. 2161) and further that, peritoneal and renal clearances could not be considered equivalent. These investigators also noted that the advantage of renal clearance would be lost as renal function declined. They predicted that the eventual loss of "critical glomerular filtration rate" would occur within 2 to 3 years of peritoneal dialysis (Bargman, Thorpe, & Churchill, 2001).

ADEMEX, a prospective, randomized trial in which the effect of increased peritoneal small-solute clearances on clinical outcomes were studied, challenged treatment guidelines for people on CAPD. Using a control group with 4 exchanges of 2-liter volume daily, the study group had prescriptions modified to achieve a peritoneal clearance of greater than 60 L/wk/1.73 m² (Paniagua et al., 2002). In this study, no survival benefit was found with increasing targets. Although there were limitations to this study, Churchill, in Churchill, Diaz-Buxo, Gokal, Piraino, Shrikanth, & Teitelbaum (2003), congratulated the researchers "on moving from observational studies to hypothesis testing studies" (p. 369) but believed

that exclusion of people with cardiac disease led to a younger, healthier population in this study. He agreed, however, with Gokal in Churchill et al. (2003) that it was not necessary to work towards a pre-determined target applicable universally as suggested by the guidelines. Lo et al. (2003), also looking at adequacy, detailed a randomized study of three groups with Kt/V of 1.5 to 1.7, 1.7 to 2.0, and greater than 2, and found that there was no survival difference among the groups. The lowest study group, however, did exhibit more problems clinically such as inadequate ultrafiltration and inadequate dialysis leading to withdrawal from the study. Additionally, this group required more anemia intervention with the use of erythropoeitin (Lo et al., 2003). From this study, a minimal target of 1.7 was suggested, but the upper expected target was not addressed. Lo et al. (2003) also caution about extrapolating the results to other populations given that their population was "a relatively homogeneous racial population with low comorbidity and mortality and was limited to patients with low residual renal function" (p. 655).

Szeto, Wong et al. (2001) showed that in 140 individuals with anuria, an increase in dialysis was associated with better clinical outcomes. In this study, the average exchanges were 2 liters three times daily, with an average Kt/V of 1.73. This study showed a 6% increase in the relative risk of death with a 0.1 unit decrease in Kt/V. The conclusion was that the optimal dose of PD is yet to be determined, although the association made was that higher Kt/V results lead to better survival. In the study, three exchanges of 2-liter volumes were used. Researchers have noted that survival with this dialysis dose may be better in Asians than other races such as Caucasians because of smaller body size (Li & Szeto, 2001; Wang et al., 2003).

The issues of adequacy and targets for optimal dialysis will continue to be debated, and careful follow-up of programs for management are required. Underlying this is the consensus by world experts that clinical assessment must remain forefront in the review of individuals receiving PD. Churchill et al. (2003) detailed the debate on adequacy through summarizing the literature and providing opinions on the expected targets. By reviewing DOQI, CANUSA, ADEMEX, and the Hong Kong studies by Szeto, Wong et al. (2001) and Lo et al. (2001), recommendations were made to emphasize clinical assessment given that optimal targets are not well defined. In Churchill et al. (2003), Piraino suggested simplifying the goals by aiming for a minimum Kt/V of 1.8 for all prescriptions. In their discourse, Gokal and Shrikanth believed that "some patients do well with a Kt/V less than 2.0; if they are doing well, there is no need for either transfer to HD or a higher dialysis dose" (p. 372). Diaz-Buxo (2003) emphasized the need to determine other indicators in association with clearance, such as fluid-volume status, nutrition, and medical treatment. There is general agreement that for individuals achieving higher targets, lowering the dialysis prescription should not be undertaken. In summary, adequacy provides insights into clearance of urea and creatinine, but the results should be taken into consideration with clinical assessment of indicators of uremic control. From a nursing perspective, Prowant (2001) also promoted the close assessment of individuals for "signs of underdialysis and malnutrition" (p. 446) in monitoring the effectiveness of PD. It is further urged "that we should never get so caught up in the adequacy numbers that we forget to look at and listen to the patient" (Prowant, 2001, p. 446).

The results obtained from adequacy studies can be used as a guide to assess the efficacy of dialysis, but the overall assessment of the individual must be a major consideration in adjusting prescriptions. For individuals who are not meeting the established targets, changes in therapy can be recommended. Changes in the peritoneal membrane that impair transport characteristics can lead to reduced clearances, thus it behooves practitioners to assess adequacy at regular intervals.

Since a component of adequacy is the residual renal function, declines in urine output can affect Kt/V and CrCl to the extent that people who were once meeting targets are no longer able to do so. It is important to be cognizant of factors that can negatively affect renal function. Thus, aminoglycosides, non-steroidal analgesics, and radio-contrast dyes should be avoided in individuals with residual renal function in an attempt to preserve function (Bargman & Golper, 2005; Chandna & Farrington, 2004).

To improve adequacy, people on CAPD have the option of increasing the volume and frequency of exchanges. Thus, a change from 2 liters four times per day to 2.5 liters four times per day can enhance clearance, as can an increase to five exchanges per day. In recommending changes, the effect on lifestyle and adaptability to increased volumes needs to be considered.

For individuals on APD, including a day exchange, increasing the volume of exchange, or increasing the total hours on the cycler overnight can be used as modifications to enhance clearance. These measures are better options than simply increasing the number of exchanges at night since increasing the number will reduce dwell time and affect clearance of larger molecules.

The adequacy results should also be examined in light of the individual's membrane characteristics. For someone starting on PD, membrane characteristics are not known since the PET is done after a stabilization period on treatment. If the individual has residual renal function, either treatment choice may be effective, but as the kidneys deteriorate further, a review of the selected prescription can be undertaken. A transfer from one prescription to another (for example, CAPD to CCPD or CCPD to CAPD) can lead to improved achievement of targets. Again, these changes should only be made with concurrent assessment of how the individual is feeling in terms of uremic symptom control.

Global Utilization of PD

Although highly effective, relatively simple, and potentially inexpensive, PD has not been embraced worldwide. In some countries, such as India, transplantation is the predominant treatment for ESRD because ordinary individuals and families cannot afford dialysis. Unfortunately, in a great number of countries worldwide, the costs and resources required for maintenance dialysis, such as clean water and electricity, are prohibitive; thus, those with ESRD are not provided with dialytic therapy. It is estimated that 114 of the world's 230 countries offer access to dialysis treatment (PDServe, 2004).

At the end of 2000, there were over 1 million individuals on dialysis worldwide, with only approximately 15% on PD. There is a wide variation in distribution of dialysis modality from country to country. Mexico has the highest utilization of PD, with approximately 81% of ESRD patients on PD (Cueto-Manzano, 2003), while other countries, such as Japan, report less than 5% on PD (Kurokawa, Nangaku, Igani, & Miyata, 2002). These variations stem from a number of reasons, largely fiscal, and include differences in remuneration, costs of transportation of supplies, and support of governmental or private health insurance plans.

PD offers an extremely effective form of renal replacement therapy without the need for highly sophisticated, costly and exceedingly high technology equipment, and therefore should be the obvious choice for dialytic therapy, particularly if focusing on patient-centered care, with increased patient autonomy. Nevertheless, paradoxically, PD is identified as being more expensive in some countries, such as India, Pakistan, Romania, and Sri Lanka, and is offered to only 2% of those with ESRD in India (Jha, 2004; Li & Chow, 2001; Sakhuja & Sud, 2004; Ursea, Mircescu, Constantinovici, & Verzan, 1997). However, Hong Kong reports that PD is 55% less costly than HD (Li & Chow, 2001). Some countries, such as Mexico and Hong Kong, have a policy of "PD first" due to decreased costs and philosophy (Cueto-Manzano, 2003; Lo et al., 2001). In Hong Kong, PD is the treatment for 82% of dialysis patients in the public health system, with HD reserved for those for whom PD is contraindicated (Lo et al., 2001). These authors also looked at reasons for patients declining PD in their population, and interestingly, cultural attitudes played a large part. The primary reason for not accepting dialysis was, "Lived long enough, accept death," noting that "death at an advanced age is regarded as honorable" (Lo et al., 2001).

Other important issues come into play as well, such as physician and nurse willingness to promote PD. For example, in Japan, it is noted that reimbursement is the same for HD and PD. The fees for HD support the machines, supplies, hospitals, clinics, and health care professionals, whereas a majority of the reimbursement for PD goes straight to the providers of the PD fluids and supplies. This leaves little incentive for health care providers to promote PD (Kurokawa, Nangaku, Igani & Miyata, 2002). In the U.S., there is already an infrastructure of a large number of HD facilities that must be filled in order to remain solvent, thereby creating an incentive to keep patients on HD in such facilities (Nissenson, 2002). Nissenson (2002) also noted that as PD use has declined in the U.S., there are fewer adequately trained physicians and nurses supporting PD, resulting in further decline of PD. In a study of factors affecting the use of PD in a center in India, Mahajan, Tiwari, Kalra, Bhowmik, and Agarwal (2004) identified that only 3.3% of their patients chose PD because of the independent lifestyle, and none of the nephrologists or nephrology fellows routinely presented PD as a treatment option to their predialysis patients.

The cost of dialysis treatment is difficult to quantify and compare because there are a variety of variables, such as costs of labor, supplies, drugs, and shipping costs. Li and Chow (2001) attempted such a comparison in Asian countries. Not only were raw costs analyzed, but they were compared to the country's wealth, reflected by the Gross National Income (GNI) of individual countries. It was sobering to see the extreme disparity between the cost of PD and the average annual income of individuals, with Sri Lanka being worst off, having dialysis costs 4,683% higher than the GNI. These authors also identified that in some countries, such as India, Pakistan, and Sri Lanka, there is no governmental support for PD at all (Li et al., 2001). It also must be remembered that in some countries, health care requirements may be much more fundamental than provision of dialysis, and the health care needed for the whole population may be as basic as clean drinking water and control of disease (Correa-Rotter, 2001).

Korea now has an on-line registry program that is invaluable in collecting data in that country. It is a secure site to which only nephrology professionals have access. They report 17.7% of individuals with ESRD are on PD, with PD experiencing the largest increase rate (17.5%) (Kim, Jin, & Bang, 2003).

Peeters, Rublee, Just, and Joseph (2000) reviewed literature regarding dialysis in Western European countries and found that although less costly, PD was also generally used less than HD. This varied from country to country, with 8% to 11% PD usage in France, Italy, Germany, and Spain, and 45% in the United Kingdom. Again, discrepancies in reimbursement existed between HD and PD, as well as reimbursement to physicians, decreasing the incentive to prescribe PD (Peeters et al., 2000). Additionally, they found that there was no universal set of "rules" to estimate the costs to compare from country to country.

Locatelli et al. (2001) report an analysis of ESRD and renal replacement therapy in three Baltic countries, Lithuania, Estonia, and Latvia (2001). They found a wide variation in PD use, with Estonia utilizing PD for 20.4% of those with ESRD, and Latvia and Lithuania with significantly less, 9% and 4% respectively. They note that the need outweighs the supply, and suggest that a solution to develop the RRT program might be in providing PD (Locatelli et al., 2001).

Lack of comparable data regarding PD from countries around the world highlights the importance of national registries for ESRD, as well as guidelines for reporting costs. Nephrology nurses and professionals must make an effort to address the need for education regarding the simplicity and effectiveness of PD to meet the growing demand for dialysis worldwide.

References

Afthentopoulos, I.E., & Oreopoulos, D.G. (2000). Is CAPD an effective treatment for ESRD patients with a weight over 80 kg? *Clinical Nephrology, 47*(6), 389-393.

Agarwal, D.K., Sharma, A.P., Gupta, A., Sharma, R.K., Pandey, C.M., Kumar, R., et al. (2000). Peritoneal equilibration test in Indian patients on continuous ambulatory peritoneal dialysis: Does it affect patient outcome? *Advances in Peritoneal Dialysis, 16,* 148-151.

Agrawal, A., & Nolph, K.D. (2000). Advantages of tidal peritoneal dialysis. *Peritoneal Dialysis International, 20*(S2), S98-S100.

Alsop, R.M. (1994) History, chemical and pharmaceutical development of icodextrin. *Peritoneal Dialysis International*, 14 (Suppl 2), S5-S12.

Amerling, R., Glezerman, I., Savransky, E., & Dubrow, A. (2003). Continuous flow peritoneal dialysis: Principles and applications. *Seminars in Dialysis, 16*(4), 335-340.

Armstrong, S., & Zalatan S.J. (1992). Microwave warming of peritoneal dialysis fluid. *ANNA Journal, 19*(6), 535-540.

Bailie, G.R., Johnson, C.A., Mason, N.A., & St. Peter W.L. (2004). Peritoneal dialysis: A guide to medication use 2004. Retrieved November 30, 2004, from www.nephrologypharmacy.com/downloads/peritoneal

Bargman, J.M. (personal communication, December 1, 2004).

Bargman, J.M., Golper, T.A. (2005). The importance of residual renal function for patients on dialysis. *Nephrology, Dialysis, Transplantation, 20,* 671-673.

Bargman, J.M., Thorpe, K.E., & Churchill, D.N. (2001). Relative contribution of residual renal function and peritoneal clearance to adequacy of dialysis: A reanalysis of the CANUSA study. *Journal of American Society of Nephrology, 12*(10), 2158-2162.

Bargman, J.M., Jones, J.E., & Petro, J.M. (1992). The pharmacokinetics of intraperitoneal erythropoietin administered undiluted or diluted in dialysate. *Peritoneal Dialysis International, 12*(4), 369-372.

Basile, C., De Padova, F., Montanaro, A., & Giordano, R. (2003). The impact of relapsing sterile icodextrin-associated peritonitis on peritoneal dialysis outcome. *Journal of Nephrology, 16,* 384-386.

Bazzato, G., Landini, S., Fracasso, A., Morachiello, P., Righetto, F., & Scanferla, F., et al. (1993). Why the double-bag system still remains the best technique for peritoneal fluid exchange in continuous ambulatory peritoneal dialysis. *Peritoneal Dialysis International, 13*(S2), S152-S155.

Bentley, M.L. (2001). A touch technique peritoneal dialysis procedure for the blind and visually impaired. *CANNT Journal, 11*(2), 32-34.

Blake, P.G., Bargman, J.M., Bick, J., Cartier, P., Dasgupta, M.K., Fine, A., Lavoie, S.,D., Spanner, E. & Taylor, P.A. (1999). Guidelines for adequacy and nutrition in peritoneal dialysis in peritoneal dialysis. *Journal of American Society of Nephrology, 10,* S287-S321.

Blake, P.G., & Daugirdas, J. (2001). Physiology of peritoneal dialysis. In J.T. Daugirdas, P.G. Blake, & T.S. Ing (Eds.), *Handbook of dialysis* (3rd ed.) (pp. 281-296). Philadelphia: Lippincott Williams & Wilkins.

Blake, P.G., & Diaz-Buxo, J. (2001) Adequacy of peritoneal dialysis and chronic peritoneal dialysis prescription. In J.T. Daugirdas, P.G. Blake, & T.S. Ing (Eds.), *Handbook of dialysis* (3rd ed.) (pp. 343-360). Philadelphia: Lippincott Williams & Wilkins.

Borras, M., Martin, M., & Fernandez, E. (2004). Letter to the editor. *Peritoneal Dialysis International, 24*(1), 87-88.

Brunkhorst, R.R. (2002). Host defenses in APD. *Seminars in Dialysis, 15*(6), 414-417.

Bruno, M., Gabella, P., & Ramello, A. (2000). Use of amino acids in peritoneal dialysis solutions. *Peritoneal Dialysis International, 20*(S2), S166-171.

Burkart, J.M. (2000). Adequacy of dialysis. In R. Gokal, R. Khanna, R. Krediet & K. Nolph (Eds.) *Textbook of peritoneal dialysis* (pp. 465-499). Dordrecht: Kluwer Academic Publishers.

Burkart, J.M., Daeihagh, P., & Rocco, M.V. (2003). Peritoneal dialysis. In B.M. Brenner (Ed.). *The kidney* (7th ed.) (pp. 2625-2674). Philadelphia: W. B. Saunders Company.

Burkart, J.M., Hylander, B., Durnell-Figel, T., & Roberts D. (1990) Comparison of peritonitis rates during long-term use of a standard spike versus ultraset in continuous ambulatory peritoneal dialysis. *Peritoneal Dialysis International, 10*(1), 41-43.

Burrows, L., Prowant, B.F. (1998) Peritoneal dialysis. In J. Parker (Ed.) *Contemporary nephrology nursing* (pp. 605-659). Pitman, NJ: American Nephrology Nurses' Association.

Cameron, J.S. (2002). *Peritoneal dialysis transformed: CAPD* . In J.S. Cameron. A History of the Treatment of Renal Failure by Dialysis. Oxford University Press (p. 273-275).

Canada-USA (CANUSA) Peritoneal Dialysis Study Group (1996). Adequacy of dialysis and nutrition in continuous peritoneal dialysis: association with clinical outcomes. *Journal of the American Society of Nephrology, 7*(2), 198- 207.

Cara, M., Virga, G., Mastrosimone, S., Girotto, A., Rossi, V., D'Angelo, A., Bonfante, L. (2005). Comparison of peritoneal equilibration test with 2.27% an 3.86% glucose dialysis solution. *Journal of Nephrology*, 18(1), 67-71.

Carey, H.B., Chorney, W., Pherson, K., Finkelstein, F.O., & Kliger, A.S. (2001). Continuous peritoneal dialysis and the extended care facility. *American Journal of Kidney Diseases, 37*(3), 580-587.

Chandna, S.M., & Farrington, K. (2004). Residual renal function: Considerations on its importance and preservation in dialysis patients. *Seminars in Dialysis, 17*(3), 196-201.

Chow, K.M., Szeto, C.C., Li, P.K., & Moss, A.H. (2003). Peritoneal dialysis in patients with dementia. *American Journal of Kidney Disease, 42*(1), 212.

Chung, S.H., Chu, W.S., Lee, H.A., Kim, Y.H., Less, I.S., Lindholm, B., et al. (2000). Peritoneal transport characteristics, comorbid disease and survival in CAPD. *Peritoneal Dialysis International, 20*(5), 541-547.

Churchill, D.N. (1998). Implications of the Canada-USA (CANUSA) study of the adequacy of dialysis on peritoneal dialysis schedule *Nephrology Dialysis Transplantation, 13*(S6), 158-163.

Churchill, D.N., Diaz-Buxo, J.A., Gokal, R., Piraino, B., Shrikanth, S., & Teitelbaum, I. (2003). How much peritoneal dialysis is needed for optimal outcomes? *Seminars in Dialysis, 16*(5), 367-375.

Coles, G.A., Williams, J.D., & Topley, N. (2000). Peritoneal inflammation and long-term changes in peritoneal structure and function. In R. Gokal, R. Khanna, R. Krediet, & K. Nolph (Eds.), *Textbook of peritoneal dialysis* (pp. 565-583). Dordrecht: Kluwer Academic Publishers.

Cooker, L.A., Holmes, C.J., & Hoff, C.M. (2002). Biocompatability of icodextrin. *Kidney International, 62*(S81), S34-S45.

Correa-Rotter, R. (2001). The cost barrier to renal replacement therapy and peritoneal dialysis in the developing world. *Peritoneal Dialysis International, 21*(Supl. 3), S314-317.

Crawford-Baonadio, T.L., Diaz-Buxo, J. A. (2004). Comparison of peritoneal dialysis solutions. *Nephrology Nursing Journal, 31*(5), 500-507, 520.

Cueto-Manzano, A. (2003). Peritoneal dialysis in Mexico. *Kidney International, 63*(Suppl. 83), S90-S92.

Daly, C., Campbell, M., Cody, J., Grant, A., Donaldson, C., Vale, L., et al. (2002). Double bag or Y-set versus standard transfer systems for continuous ambulatory peritoneal dialysis in end-stage renal disease. *Evidence Based Nursing, 5*(1), 14.

Deutschendorf, A.F., Wenk, R.E., Lustgarten, J., & Mason P. (1994) Control of microwave heating of peritoneal dialysis solutions. *Peritoneal Dialysis International, 14*(2), 163-167.

De Vecchi, A.F., & Scalamogna, A. (2001). Does a face mask prevent peritonitis? *Peritoneal Dialysis International, 21*(1), 95-96.

Diaz-Buxo, J.A. (1999). Peritoneal dialysis prescriptions for diabetic patients. *Advances in Peritoneal Dialysis, 15*, 91-95.

Diaz-Buxo, J.A. (2001). Evolution of continuous flow peritoneal dialysis and the current state of the art. *Seminars in Dialysis, 14*(5), 373-377.

Diaz-Buxo, J.A.(2003). How much peritoneal dialysis is needed for optimal outcomes? *Seminars in Dialysis, 16*(5), 367-375.

Diaz-Buxo, J.A. (2005). Clinical use of peritoneal dialysis. In A.R. Nissenson & R.N. Fine (Ed.), *Clinical Dialysis* (4th ed.) (pp. 421-489) New York: McGraw-Hill Companies, Inc.

Diaz-Buxo, J.A., Walker, P.J., & Farner, C.D. (1981). Continuous cyclic peritoneal dialysis – A preliminary report. *Artificial Organs, 5*, 157-162.

Di Paolo, N., & Sacchi, G. (2000). Atlas of histology. *Peritoneal Dialysis International, 20*(S3), 9-86.

Dobbie, J.W. (1996). Surfactant protein A and lamellar bodies: A homologous secretory function of peritoneum, synovium, and lung. *Peritoneal Dialysis International, 10*(6), 574-581.

Dobbie, J.W., Lloyd, J.K., & Gall, C.A. (1990). Categorization of ultrastructural changes in peritoneal mesothelium, stroma and blood vessels in uremia and CAPD patients. *Advances in Peritoneal Dialysis, 6*, 3-12.

Dombros, N.V., Prutis, K., Tong, M., Anderson, G.H., Harrison, J., Sombolos, K., et al. (1990). *Peritoneal Dialysis International, 10*, 79-84.

Drukker, W. (1983). Peritoneal Dialysis: A historical review. In W. Drukker, F.M. Parsons, & J.F. Maher (Eds.) *Replacement of renal function* (pp 410-439). Boston: Martinus Nijhoff Publishers.

Enoch, C., Aslam, N., & Piraino, B. (2002). Intra-abdominal pressure, peritoneal dialysis exchange volume and tolerance in APD.

Seminars in Dialysis, 15(6), 403-406.

Faller, B., Aparicio, M., Faict, D., De Vos, C., de Précigout, V., Larroumet, N., et al. (1995). Clinical evaluation of an optimized 1.1% amino-acid solution for peritoneal dialysis. *Nephrology, Dialysis Transplantation, 10*(8), 1432-1437.

Fang, W., Qian, J., Yu, Z., & Chen, S. (2004). Morphological changes of the peritoneum in peritoneal dialysis patients. *Chinese Medical Journal, 117*(6), 862-866.

Farina, J. (2004). Peritoneal dialysis and intraperitoneal insulin: How much? *Nephrology Nursing Journal, 31*(2), 225-226.

Faull, R.J. (2000). Peritoneal defenses against infection: Winning the battle but losing the war?" *Seminars in Dialysis, 13*(1), 47-53.

Figueiredo, A.E., Poli de Figueiredo, C.E., & d'Avila, D.O. (2000). Peritonitis prevention in CAPD: To mask or not? *Peritoneal Dialysis International, 20*(3), 354-358.

Figueiredo, A.E, Poli de Figueiredo, C.E., & d'Avila, D.O. (2001). Bag exchange in continuous ambulatory peritoneal dialysis without use of a face mask: Experience of five years. *Advances in Peritoneal Dialysis, 17*, 98-100.

Fine, A., Parry, D., Ariano, R., & Dent, W. (2000). Marked variation in peritoneal absorption in peritoneal dialysis. *Peritoneal Dialysis International, 20*(6), 652-655.

Frieda, P., & Issad, B. (2003). Continuous flow peritoneal dialysis: Assessment of fluid and solute removal in a high-flow model of "fresh dialysate single pass." *Peritoneal Dialysis International, 23*(4), 348-355.

Frampton, J.E., & Plosker, G.L. (2003). Icodextrin: a review of its use in peritoneal dialysis. *Drugs, 63* (19), 2079-2105.

Gillerot, G., Sempoux, C., Pirson, Y., & Devuyst, O. (2002). Which type of dialysis in patients with cholesterol crystal embolism? *Nephrology Dialysis Transplant 17*, 156 -158.

Gokal, R. (1999). Fluid management and cardiovascular outcome in peritoneal dialysis patients. *Seminars in Dialysis, 12*(2), 126-132.

Gokal, R. (2000). History of peritoneal dialysis. In R. Gokal, R.Khanna, R. Krediet, & K. Nolph (Eds.), *Textbook of peritoneal dialysis* (pp.1-17). Dordrecht: Kluwer Academic Publishers.

Gokal, R., & Mallick, N.P. (1999). Peritoneal dialysis. *The Lancet 353*, 823-828.

Gokal, R. & Shrikanth, S.(2003). How much peritoneal dialysis is needed for optimal outcomes? *Seminars in Dialysis, 16*(5), 367-375.

Goldsmith, D., Jayawardene, S., Sabharwal, N., & Cooney, K. (2000). Allergic reactions to the polymeric glucose-based peritoneal dialysis fluid icodextrin in patients with renal failure. *The Lancet, 355*(9207), 897.

Gotloib, L., Shostak, A., & Wajsbrot, V. (2000). Functional structure of the peritoneum as a dialyzing membrane. In R. Gokal, R.Khanna, R. Krediet, & K. Nolph (Ed.), *Textbook of peritoneal dialysis* (pp. 37-106). Dordrecht: Kluwer Academic Publishers.

Ha, H., & Lee, H.B. (2000). Effect of high glucose on peritoneal mesothelial cell biology. *Peritoneal Dialysis International, 20*(S2), S15-S18.

Hadimeri, H., Johansson, A.C., Haraldsson, B., & Nyberg, G. (1998). CAPD in patients with autosomal dominant polycystic kidney disease. *Peritoneal Dialysis International, 18*(4) 429-432.

Hajarizadeh, H., Rohrer, M.J., Herrmann, J.B., & Cutler, B.S. (1995). Acute peritoneal dialysis following ruptured abdominal aortic aneurysms. *The American Journal of Surgery, 170*, 223-226.

Heaf, J. (2000). Pathogenic effects of a high peritoneal transport rate. *Seminars in Dialysis, 13*(3), 188-193.

Heimburger, O., & Mujais, S. (2003). Buffer transport in peritoneal dialysis. (2003) *Kidney International, 64*(S88), S37-S42.

Heering, P., Brause, M., Plum, J., & Grabensee, B. (2001). Peritoneal reaction to icodextrin in a female patient on CAPD. *Peritoneal Dialysis International, 21*, 321-322.

Hjelle, J.T., Miller-Hjelle, M.A., & Dobbie, J.W. (1995). The biology of the mesothelium during peritoneal dialysis. *Peritoneal Dialysis International, 15*(S7), S22-S23.

Ho-dac-Pannekeet, M.M., Schouten, N., Langendijk, M.J., Hiralall, J.K., de Waart, D.R., Struijk, D.G., Krediet, R.T. (1996). Peritoneal transport characteristics with glucose polymer based dialysate. *Kidney International, 50* (3), 979-986.

Holley J.L., Bernardini, J., & Piraino, B. (1994). Infecting organisms in continuous ambulatory peritoneal dialysis patients on the Y set.

American Journal of Kidney Disease, 23(4), 569-573.

Holmes, C.J. (2002). Abnormalities of host defense mechanisms during peritoneal dialysis. In A.R. Nissenson & R.N. Fine (Ed.), *Dialysis therapy* (3rd ed.) (pp. 235-239). Philadelphia: Hanley & Belfus, Inc.

Holmes, C.J., & Faict, D. (2003). Peritoneal dialysis solution biocompatibility: Definitions and evaluation strategies. *Kidney International, 64*(S88), S50-S56.

Hung, G.C., Hung, S.Y., Chou, K.J., Fang, H.C., Hung, Y.M., Lee, P.T., et al. (2004). Amino acid-containing peritoneal dialysis solution administration in malnourished patients: Comparison between daytime and overnight use. *Dialysis & Transplantation, 33*(2), 74-79.

Islam, M.S., Briat, C., Soutif C., Barnouin, F., & Pollini J. (1997). More than 17 years of peritoneal dialysis: A case report. *Advances in Peritoneal Dialysis, 13,* 98-103.

ISPD. (2001). ISPD Basics of Peritoneal Dialysis Course, ISPD Symposium June 26 2001, Montreal (Now available on www.e-dialysis.org).

Jha, V. (2004). End-stage renal care in developing countries: The India experience. *Renal Failure, 26*(3), 201-208.

Johnson, D.W., Agar, J., Collins, J., Disney, A., Harris, D.C.H., Ibels, L., et al. (2003). Recommendations for the use of icodextrin in peritoneal dialysis patients. *Nephrology, 8,* 1-7.

Johnson, D.W., Arndt, M., O'Shea, A., Watt, R., Hamilton, J., & Vincent, K. (2001). Icodextrin as salvage therapy in peritoneal dialysis therapy with refractory fluid overload. *BMC Nephrology, 2*(1), 2.

Johnson, D.W., Herzig, K.A., Purdie, D.M., Chang, W., Brown, A.M., Rigby, R.J., et al. (2000). Is obesity a favorable factor in peritoneal dialysis patients? *Peritoneal Dialysis Bulletin, 20*(6), 715-721.

Johnson, D.W., Mudge, D.W., Blizzard, S., Arndt, M., O'Shea , A., Watt, R., et al. (2004). A comparison of peritoneal equilibration tests performed 1 and 4 weeks after PD commencement. *Peritoneal Dialysis International, 24*(5), 460-465.

Jones, M.R., Gehr, T.W., Burkart, J.M., Hamburger, R.J., Kraus, Jr., A.P., Piraino, B.M., et al. (1998). Replacement of amino acid and protein losses with 1.1% amino acid peritoneal dialysis solution. *Peritoneal Dialysis International, 18*(2), 210-216.

Jorres, A. (2003). Glucose degradation products in peritoneal dialysis: from bench to bedside. *Kidney & Blood Pressure Research, 26,* 113-117.

Kanny, G., Durand, P.Y., Morisset, M., Chanliau, J., Moneret-Vautrin, D.A., & Kessler, M. (2004). Immunochemical analysis of peritoneal dialysate in a patient with hypersensitivity to icodextrin. *Peritoneal Dialysis International, 23*(4), 405-406.

Katz, I.J., Sofianou, L., Butler, O., & Hopley, M. (2001). Recovery of renal function in black South African patients with malignant hypertension: Superiority of continuous ambulatory peritoneal dialysis over hemodialysis. *Peritoneal Dialysis International, 21*(6), 581-586.

Khanna, R. (2002). Lymphatics and peritoneal dialysis. In A.R. Nissenson, & R.N. Fine (Eds.), *Dialysis therapy* (pp. 231-233). Philadelphia: Hanley & Belfus, Inc.

Khanna, R., & Oreopoulos, D.G. (1989). Peritoneal dialysis in diabetic end-stage renal disease. *Journal of Diabetes Complications, 3*(1), 12-17.

Kim, S.Y., Jin, D.C., & Bang, B.K. (2003). Current status of dialytic therapy in Korea. *Nephrology, 8,* S2-S9.

Kjellstrand, C.M. (1981). Do middle molecules cause uremic intoxication? *American Journal of Kidney Disease, 1*(1), 51-56.

Kopple, J.D., Bernard, D., Messana, J., Swartz, R., Bergstrom, J., Lindholm, B., et al. (1995). Treatment of malnourished CAPD patients with an amino acid-based dialysate. *Kidney International, 47*(4), 1148-1157.

Korbet, S.M., Kronfol, N.O. (2001). Acute peritoneal dialysis prescription. In J.T. Daugirdas, P.G. Blake, & T.S. Ing (Eds.), *Handbook of dialysis* (3rd ed.) (pp. 333-342). Philadelphia: Lippincott Williams & Wilkins.

Krediet, R.T. (1997). Evaluation of peritoneal membrane integrity. *Journal of Nephrology, 10*(5), 238-244.

Krediet, R.T. (1999). The peritoneal membrane in chronic peritoneal dialysis. *Kidney International, 55*(1), 341-356.

Krediet, R.T. (2000). The physiology of peritoneal solute transport and ultrafiltration. In R. Gokal, R.Khanna, R. Krediet, & K. Nolph (Eds.), *Textbook of peritoneal dialysis* (pp. 135-172). Dordrecht: Kluwer Academic Publishers.

Krediet, R.T., Zweers, M.M., van der Wal, A.C., & Struijk, D.G. (2000). Neoangiogenesis in the peritoneal membrane. *Peritoneal Dialysis International, 20*(S2), S19.

Kurokawa, K., Nangaku, M., Igani, R., & Miyata, T. (2002). Perspectives of chronic renal failure. *Nephrology, 7,* S145-S150.

Lameire, N.H. (1997). The impact of residual renal function on the adequacy of dialysis. *Nephron, 77,* 13-28.

Li, F.K., Chan, L.Y., Woo, J.C., Ho, S.K., Lo, W.K., & Chan, T.M. (2003). A 3-year, prospective, randomized, controlled study on amino acid dialysate in patients on CAPD. *American Journal of Kidney Disease, 42*(1), 173-183.

Li, P., Chow, M. (2001). The cost barrier to peritoneal dialysis in the developing world – An Asian perspective. *Peritoneal Dialysis International, 21*(Suppl 3), S307-S313.

Li, P.K., Szeto, C.C. (2001). Adequacy targets of peritoneal dialysis in the Asian population. *Peritoneal Dialysis International, 21*(S3), S378-S383.

Lo, W.K., Ho, Y.W., Li, C.S., Wong, K.S., Chan, T.M., Yu, A.W., et al. (2003) Effect of Kt/V on survival and clinical outcome in CAPD patients in a randomized prospective study. *Kidney International, 64,* 649-656.

Lo, W.K., Li, F.K., Choy, C.B.Y., Cheng, S.K., Chu, W.L., Ng, S.Y., et al. (2001). A retrospective survey of attitudes toward acceptance of peritoneal dialysis in Chinese end stage renal failure patients in Hong Kong – From a cultural point of view. *Peritoneal Dialysis International, 21*(Suppl 3), S318-S321.

Locatelli, F., D'Amico, M., H., Dainys, B., Miglinas, M., Luman, M., et al. (2001). The epidemiology of end-stage renal disease in the Baltic countries: An evolving picture. *Nephrology Dialysis Transplant, 16,* 1338-1342.

Lui, S.F., Chung, W.W., Leung, C.B., Chan, K., & Lai, K.N. (1990). Pharmacokinetics and pharmacodynamics of subcutaneous and intraperitoneal administration of recombinant human erythropoietin in patients on continuous ambulatory peritoneal dialysis. *Clinical Nephrology, 33*(1), 47-51.

Madden, M.A., Zimmerman, S.W., & Simpson, D.P. (1982). Continuous ambulatory peritoneal dialysis in diabetes mellitus: The risks and benefits of intraperitoneal insulin. *American Journal of Nephrology, 2*(3), 133-139.

Mahajan, S., Tiwari, S.C., Kalra, V., Bhowmik, D.M., & Agarwal, S.K. (2004). Factors affecting the use of peritoneal dialysis among the ESRD population in India: A single-center study. *Peritoneal Dialysis International, 24*(6), 538-541.

Maiorca, R., & Cancarini, G.C. (1990). Experiences with the Y-system. In Z.J. Twardowski, K.D. Nolph, & R. Khanna (Eds.), *Peritoneal dialysis: New concepts and applications* (pp. 167-190). New York: Churchill Livingstone Inc.

Maiorca, R., & Cancarini, G. (1999). Thirty years of progress in peritoneal dialysis. *Journal of Nephrology, 12*(S2), S92-S99.

Maitra, S., Burkart, J., Fine A., Prichard, S., Bernardini, J., Jindal, K.K., et al. (2000). Patients on chronic peritoneal dialysis for ten years or more in North America. *Peritoneal Dialysis International, 20*(S2), S127-S133.

Martis, L., Patel, M., Giertych, J., Mongoven, J., Taminne, M., Perrier, M.A., Mendozo, O., Goud,N., Costigan, A., Denjoy, N., Verger, C., & Owen. W.F. (2005). Aseptic peritonitis due to peptidoglycan contamination of pharmacopoeia standard dialysis solution. *Kidney International* 67(4), 1609-1615.

McBride, P. (1984). The development of hemo- and peritoneal dialysis. In A.R. Nissenson, R. N. Fine, & D.E. Gentile (Eds.), *Clinical dialysis* (pp. 1-28). Norwalk, Connecticut: Appleton-Century-Crofts.

McDonald, S.P., Collins, J.F., & Johnson, D.W. (2003). Obesity is associated with worse peritoneal dialysis outcomes in the Australia and New Zealand patient populations. *Journal of American Society of Nephrology, 14*(11), 2894-2901.

McDonald, S.P., Collins, J.F., Rumpsfield, M., & Johnson, D.W. (2004). Obesity is a risk factor for peritonitis in the Australian and New Zealand peritoneal dialysis patient populations. *Peritoneal Dialysis International, 24*(4), 340-346.

Mistry, C.D., & Gokal, R. (1994). The use of glucose polymer (icodextrin) in peritoneal dialysis: An overview. *Peritoneal Dialysis International, 14*(S3), S158-161.

Mistry, C.D., Gokal, R., & Peers, E. (1994). A randomized multicenter clinical trial comparing isosmolar icodextrin with hyperosmolar glucose solutions in CAPD. MIDAS study group. Multicenter investigation of icodextrin in ambulatory peritoneal dialysis. *Kidney International, 46*(2), 496-503.

Miyata, T., Devuyst, O., Kurokawa, K., & Van Ypersele de Strihou, C. (2002). Toward better dialysis compatibility: Advances in the biochemistry and pathophysiology of the peritoneal membrane. *Kidney International, 61*, 375-386.

Moncrief, J.W., & Popvich, R.P. (1981). *CAPD Update* (pp. 135-137). New York: Masson Publishing USA, Inc.

Mortier, S., De Vriese, A.S., & Lameire, N. (2003). Recent concepts in the molecular biology of the peritoneal membrane – Implications for more biocompatible dialysis solutions. *Blood Purification, 21*(1), 14-23.

Nakayawa, D., Price, C., Sinebraugh, B., & Suki,W. (1981). Continuous cyclic peritoneal dialysis: A viable option in the treatment of chronic renal failure. *Transactions of the American Society of Artificial Internal Organs, 27*, 55-57.

Nissenson, A.R. (2002). Why are fewer patients using peritoneal dialysis? *aapkRENALIFE, 18*(3). Retrieved November 15, 2004, from http://www.aakp.org/AAKP/RenalifeArt/2002/fewerperitoneal.htm

Oreopoulos, D.G. (1999a). Long-term CAPD for twenty years: Mrs. K.M. shows the way. *Peritoneal Dialysis International, 19*(3), 195-196.

Oreopoulos, D.G. (1999b). The optimization of continuous ambulatory peritoneal dialysis. *Kidney International, 55*, 1131-1149.

Oreopoulos, D.G., Khanna, R., Williams, P., & Vas, S.I. (1982). Continuous ambulatory peritoneal dialysis. *Nephron, 30*, 293-303.

Oreopoulos, D.G., Lobbedez, T., & Gupta, S. (2004). Peritoneal dialysis: Where is it now and where is it going? *The International Society of Artificial Organs, 27*(2), 88-94.

Pandya, B.K., Friede, T., & Williams, J.D. (2004). A comparison of peritonitis in polycystic and non-polycystic patients on peritoneal dialysis. *Peritoneal Dialysis International, 24*(1), 79-81.

Paniagua, R., Amato, D., Vonesh, E., Correa-Rotter, R., Ramos, A., Moran, J., & Mujais, S. (2002). Effects of increased peritoneal clearances in peritoneal dialysis: ADEMEX, a prospective, randomized, controlled trial. *Journal of the American Society of Nephrology, 13*, 1307-1320.

Passlick-Deetjen, J., Schaub, T.P., & Schilling. (2002). Solutions for APD: Special considerations. *Seminars in Dialysis, 15*(6), 407-413.

Peeter, P., Rublee, D., Just, P.M., & Joseph, A. (2000). Analysis and interpretation of cost data in dialysis: review of Western European literature. *Health Policy, 54*, 209-227.

PDServe. (2004) A global view of peritoneal dialysis. Retrieved November 10, 2004, from http://www.pdserve.com/pdserve/pdserve.nsf/Content/Global+View+of+PD

Pinerolo, M.C., Porri, M.T., & D'Amico, G. (1999). Recurrent sterile peritonitis at onset of treatment with icodextrin solution. *Peritoneal Dialysis International, 19*(5), 491-492.

Piraino, B. (1998). Peritonitis as a complication of peritoneal dialysis. *Journal of the American Society of Nephrology, 9*(10), 1956-1964.

Piraino, B., Bernardini, J., Centa, P.K., Johnston, J.R., & Sorkin, M.I. (1991). The effect of body weight on CAPD related infections and catheter loss. *Peritoneal Dialysis International, 11*(1), 64 -68.

Pollock, C.A., Cooper, B.A., Ibels, L.S., & De Kantzow, E. (2000). In R. Gokal, R. Khanna, R. Krediet, & K. Nolph (Eds.), *Textbook of peritoneal dialysis.* (pp. 515-543). Dordrecht: Kluwer Academic Publishers.

Poulopoulos, V., Lam, L., & Cugelman, A. (2004). Sterile peritonitis due to icodextrin: Experience from a Canadian center. *Peritoneal Dialysis International, 24*(1), 88-89.

Preston, R.A. (2002). *Acid-Base, fluids and electrolytes made ridiculously simple.* Miami: MedMaster, Inc.

Prichard, S.S., Bargman, J.M. (2000). The use of peritoneal dialysis in special situations. In R. Gokal, R. Khanna, R. Krediet & K. Nolph (Eds)., *Textbook of peritoneal dialysis.* (pp. 748-749). Dordrecht Kluwer Academic Publishers.

Pride, E.T., Gustafson, J., Graham, A., Spainhour, L. Mauck, V., Brown, FP., & Burkart, J.M. (2002). Comparison of a 2.5% and a 4.25% dextrose peritoneal equilibration test. *Peritoneal Dialysis International, 22*(3), 365-370.

Prowant, B.E., & Schmidt, L.M. (1991). The peritoneal equilibration test: A nursing discussion. *ANNA Journal, 18*(4), 361-366.

Prowant, B.F. (2001). Clarifying K/DOQI's guideline targets for peritoneal dialysis adequacy. *Nephrology Nursing Journal, 28*(4), 445-447.

Quellhorst, E. (2002). Insulin therapy during peritoneal dialysis: Pros and cons of various forms of administration. *Journal of the American Society of Nephrology, 13*(1), S92-S96.

Rao, P., Passadikis, P.,& Oreopoulos, D.G. (2003). Peritoneal dialysis in acute renal failure. *Peritoneal Dialysis International, 23*(4), 320-322.

Reichel, W., Schulze, B., Dietze, J., & Mende W. (2001). A case of sterile peritonitis associated with icodextrin solution. *Peritoneal Dialysis International, 21*, 414-415.

Riley, S.G., Chess, J., Donovan, K.L., & Williams, J.D. (2003). Spurious hyperglycaemia and icodextrin in peritoneal dialysis fluid. [Clinical review: Lesson of the week]. *British Medical Journal, 327*, 608-609.

Rippe, B. (1993). A three-pore model of peritoneal transport. *Peritoneal Dialysis International, 13*(S2), S35-S38.

Rippe, B., Simonsen, O., & Stelin, G. (1991). Clinical implications of a three-pore model of peritoneal transport. *Advances in Peritoneal Dialysis, 7*, 3-9.

Rippe, B., Venturoli, D., Simonsen, O., & de Arteaga, J. (2004). Fluid and electrolyte transport across the peritoneal membrane during CAPD according to the three-pore model. *Peritoneal Dialysis International, 24*(1), 10- 27.

Robertson, S., Huxtable, H., Blakemore, C., Williams, G., & Donovan, K.L. (2001). The icodextrin blackline sign. *Peritoneal Dialysis International, 21*(6), 621-623.

Rocco, M.V., & Blumenkrantz, M.J. (2001). Nutrition. In J.T. Daugirdas, P.G. Blake, & T.S. Ing (Eds.) *Handbook of dialysis* (3rd ed.) (pp. 420-445). Philadelphia: Lippincott, Williams & Wilkins.

Rostand, S.G. (1983). Profound hypokalemia in continuous ambulatory peritoneal dialysis. *Archives of Internal Medicine, 143*(2), 377-378.

Sakhuja, V., & Sud K (2003). End-stage renal disease in India and Pakistan: Burden of disease and management issues. *Kidney International, 83*(Suppl), S115-S118.

Sarkar, S., Bernardini, J., Fried, L., Johnston, J.R., & Piraino, B. (1999). Tolerance of large exchanges by peritoneal dialysis patients. *American Journal of Kidney Disease, 35*(6), 1136-1141.

Satko, S.G., & Burkart, J.M. (2002). Determination of CAPD and CCPD prescriptions. In A.R. Nissenson & R.N. Fine (Eds.) *Dialysis therapy* (3rd ed.) (pp. 221-233). Philadelphia: Hanley & Belfus, Inc.

Schmidt, L.M., & Prowant, B. (1991). How to do a peritoneal equilibration test. *ANNA Journal, 18*(4), 368-370.

Schreiber, M.J. (1996). Membrane viability in the long-term peritoneal dialysis patient. *Peritoneal Dialysis International, 17*(S3), S19-S24.

Schröder, C.H. (2004). Optimal peritoneal dialysis: Choice of volume and solution. *Nephrology Dialysis Transplantation, 19*(4), 782-784.

Seow, Y.Y.T., Iles-Smith, H., Hirst, H., & Gokal, R. (2003). Icodextrin-associated peritonitis among CAPD patients. *Nephrology Dialysis Transplantation, 18*, 1951-1952.

Shetty A., & Oreopoulos D.G. (1994). Connecting devices in CAPD and their impact on peritonitis. *Journal of Post Graduate Medicine, 40*, 179-184.

Shokar, S. (2001). Keep it simple: Teaching totally blind patients using Baxter's Twin Bag peritoneal dialysis system. *CANNT Journal, 11*(4), 8.

Siemons, L., van den Heuval, P., Parizel, G., Buyseens, N., De Broe M.E., Cuykens, J.J. (1987). Peritoneal dialysis in acute renal failure due to cholesterol embolization: two cases of recovery of renal function and extended survival. *Clinical Nephrology, 28*, 205 - 208.

Smith, B., Sica, D.A., & Stacy, W. (1986). Peritoneal dialysis in spinal cord injury. *Nephron, 44*(3), 245-248.

Smith, C.A. (1997). Does flush before fill decrease the incidence of peritonitis in our cycler population? *CANNT Journal, 7*(2), 20-22.

Spital, A., & Sterns, R.H. (1985). Potassium supplementation via the dialysate in continuous ambulatory peritoneal dialysis. *American Journal of Kidney Diseases* 6(3), 173-176.

Stigant C.E., & Bargman J.M. (2002). What's new in peritoneal dialysis: Biocompatibility and continuous flow peritoneal dialysis. *Current Opinion in Nephrology and Hypertension, 11*(6), 597-602.

Szeto, C.C., Law, M.C., Wong, T.Y., Leung, C.B., & Li, P.K. (2001). Peritoneal transport status correlates with morbidity but not longitudinal change of nutritional status of continuous ambulatory peritoneal dialysis patients: A 2-year prospective study. *American Journal of Kidney Disease, 37*(2), 329-336.

Szeto, C.C, Wong, T.Y.H., Chow, K.M., Leung, C.B., Law, M.C., Wang, A.Y.M., et al. (2001). Impact of dialysis adequacy on the mortality and morbidity of anuric Chinese patients receiving continuous ambulatory peritoneal dialysis. *Journal of the American Society of Nephrology, 12*(2), 355-360.

Tauer, A., Bender, T.O., Fleischman, E.H., Niwa, T., Jorres, A., Pischetsrieder, M. (2005). Fate of the glucose degradation products 3-deoxyglucosone and glyoxyal during peritoneal dialysis. Retrieved on June 27, 2005 from *Molecular Nutrition & Food Research* 49, DOI 10.1002/mnfr.200400111.

Twardowski, Z.J. (2002). Tidal peritoneal dialysis. In A.R. Nissenson & R.N. Fine (Eds.). *Dialysis therapy* (pp. 225-228). Philadelphia: Hanley & Belfus, Inc.

Twardowski, Z.J. ((2005). Physiology of peritoneal dialysis. In A.R. Nissenson & R.N. Fine (Ed.), *Clinical Dialysis* (4th ed.) (pp. 421-489). New York: McGraw-Hill Companies,Inc.

Tzamaloukas, A.H., & Friedman, E. (2001). In J.T. Daugirdas, P.G. Blake, & T.S. Ing (Eds.) *Handbook of dialysis* (3rd ed.) (pp. 453-465). Philadelphia: Lippincott, Williams & Wilkins.

Ursea, N., Mircescu, G., Constantinovici, N., & Verzan, C. (1997). Nephrology and renal replacement therapy in Romania. *Nephrology Dialysis Transplant, 12*, 684-690.

Uttley, L., & Prowant, B. (2000). Organization of a peritoneal dialysis programme – the nurses' role. In R. Gokal, R.Khanna, R. Krediet, & K. Nolph (Eds.), *Textbook of peritoneal dialysis* (pp. 363-386). Dordrecht: Kluwer Academic Publishers.

Vanholder. R.C. & Glorieux, G.L. (2003). An overview of uremic toxicity. *Hemodialysis International, 7*(2), 156-161.

Vanholder, R.C., Glorieux, G.L., De Smet, R.V. (2003). Back to the future: middle molecules, high flux membranes, and optimal dialysis. *Hemodialysis International, 7*(1), 52-57.

Vardhan, A., Zweers, M.M., Gokal, R., & Krediet, R. (2003). A solutions portfolio approach in peritoneal dialysis. *Kidney International, 64*(S88), S114-S123.

Venkataraman, V., & Nolph, K.D. (2002). Utilization of PD modalities: Evolution. *Seminars in Dialysis, 15*(6), 380-384.

Ventura, M.J., Amato, D., Correa-Rotter, & Paniagua, R. (2000). Relationship between fill volume, intraperitoneal pressure, body size and subjective discomfort perception in CAPD patients. *Peritoneal Dialysis International, 20*(2), 188-193.

Venturoli, D., & Rippe, B. (2001). Transport asymmetry in peritoneal dialysis: Application of a serial heteroporous peritoneal membrane model. *American Journal of Renal Physiology, 280*, F599-F606.

Voinescu, C.G., Khanna, R., & Nolph, K.D. (2002). High peritoneal transport: A blessing or curse? *Advances in Peritoneal Dialysis, 18*, 106-111.

Wang, T., Izatt, S., Dalglish, C., Jassal, S.V., Bargman, J., Vas, S., et al. (2002). Peritoneal dialysis in the nursing home. *International Urology Nephrology, 34*(3), 405-408.

Wang, T., Tziviskou, E., Chu, M., Bargman, J., Jassal, V., Vas, S., Oreopoulos, D.G. (2003). Differences in survival on peritoneal dialysis between oriental Asians and Caucasians: one center's experience. *International Urology and Nephrology, 35*(2), 267-274.

Waniewski, J., Heimbürger, O., Werynski, A., & Lindholm, B. (1996). Paradoxes in peritoneal transport of small solutes. *Peritoneal Dialysis International, 16*(S1), S63-S69.

Warady, B.A., Alexander, S.R., Balfe, J.W., & Harvey, E. (2000). Peritoneal dialysis in children. In R. Gokal, R.Khanna, R. Krediet, & K. Nolph (Ed.), *Textbook of peritoneal dialysis* (pp. 667-708). Dordrecht: Kluwer Academic Publishers.

White, R., & Granger, N. (2000). The peritoneal microcirculation in peritoneal dialysis. In R. Gokal, R.Khanna, R. Krediet, & K. Nolph (Ed.), *Textbook of peritoneal dialysis* (pp. 107-133). Dordrecht: Kluwer Academic Publishers.

Wideröe, T., Smeby, E.G., Berg, K.J., Jörstad, S., & Svartas, T.M. (1983). Intraperitoneal (125 I) insulin absorption during intermittent and continuous peritoneal dialysis. *Kidney International, 23*, 22-28.

Wieslander, A., Linden, T., Kjellstrand, P. (2001). Glucose degradation products in peritoneal dialysis fluids: how they can be avoided. *Peritoneal Dialysis International* 21 (S3), S119-S124.

Wikipedia (2005). Peritoneum. Retrieved June 19, 2005, from http://wikipedia.org/wiki/Peritoneum

Willatts, S.M. (1987). *Lecture notes on fluid and electrolyte balance.* Oxford: Blackwell Scientific Publications.

Yung, S., & Davies, M. (1998). Response of the human peritoneal mesothelial cell to injury: An *in vitro* model of peritoneal wound healing. *Kidney International, 54*, 2160-2169.

Zheng, Z., Ye, R., Yu, X., Bergstrom, J., Lindholm, B. (2001). Peritoneal dialysis solutions disturb the balance of apoptosis and proliferation of peritoneal cells in chronic dialysis model. *Advances in Peritoneal Dialysis, 17*, 53-57.

Additional Readings

Canadian Society of Nephrology. (2004). Clinical Practice Guidelines Retrieved October 17, 2004, from http://csnscn.ca/local/files/guidelines/CSN-Guidelines-1999.pdf

Caring for Australians with Renal Impairment (CARI) (2004) Dialysis adequacy: monitoring patients on peritoneal dialysis. Retrieved November 30, 2004, from http://www.kidney.org.au/cari/dialysis_adequacy_008_pub.php

International Society of Peritoneal Dialysis. http://www.ISPD.org

- Peritoneal dialysis (PD) is a treatment that uses a natural membrane for fluid and solute exchange. The goals of therapy include removal of waste products, management of fluid, and regulation of acid-base and electrolyte imbalances.

- Peritoneal dialysis has been the treatment used for a wide range of people with ESRD, from the very young to the very old. It is thought that the daily removal of wastes and fluids provides a gentle and efficient approach to dialysis, which is well tolerated.

- Historically, dialysis was proposed as a temporary process until recovery of renal function. With the realization that kidney damage could be irreversible, dialysis developed into a life-support treatment.

- The peritoneal membrane is described as "a complex and complicated system of membranes and pores, which may be described as a distributed, multilayer, heteroporous, and topographically non-uniform structure with intramembrane compartments and possible specific biological transport characteristics."

- The peritoneal dialysis process is mainly dependent on three main principles of transport: diffusion, osmosis, and convection.

- Diffusion is defined as the movement of solutes from an area of high concentration to an area of low concentration across a semi-permeable membrane with the goal of equilibrating solute concentration.

- Osmosis refers to the movement of a solvent such as water through a semi-permeable membrane from a low solute concentration to a high solute concentration.

- Studying the peritoneum is difficult, but through biopsies attained at autopsy or surgical interventions, researchers have been able to describe anatomical changes in the peritoneum in PD.

- A recent focus in peritoneal dialysis has been toward developing clinical tools for measuring clearance across the membrane. This effort has led to a classification system that uses an evidence-based approach for determining appropriate prescriptions for delivering peritoneal dialysis.

- The PET is a measurement of the transport characteristics of the peritoneum and defines membrane function in a continuum from slow transport to rapid transport of solutes.

- The basic components of a PD prescription include the following: volume of exchange, number of exchanges, dwell time, dialysate solution composition, target weight reflecting euvolemic weight, and if required, intraperitoneal medications. The method by which the prescription may be delivered is defined as continuous ambulatory peritoneal dialysis (CAPD) or automated peritoneal dialysis (APD).

- Continuous cyclic peritoneal dialysis (CCPD) was developed as an alternative to CAPD.

- Nocturnal intermittent peritoneal dialysis (NIPD) is an option in which fluid is delivered at night and the patient is left dry during the day.

- Tidal volume peritoneal dialysis (TVPD) is defined as an approach designed to ensure a constant presence of dialysate contact with the membrane.

- Continuous flow peritoneal dialysis (TVPD) allows for continuous flow of dialysate either through a system of fresh dialysate or single pass method.

- Basic to the PD prescription is the type of dialysis solution recommended for use in both CAPD and APD. The desirable solution for PD should achieve the goals of dialysis without adverse effects, while preserving and maintaining peritoneal function.

- Regardless of the prescription for PD, protocols form the basis for directing the steps in performing the actual treatment. Aseptic principles are the foundation for reducing infectious risks and should be incorporated when writing or revising protocols.

- Volume of exchange is an important determinant of dialysate flow rates, which in turn, affect clearance. Dialysate-to-membrane contact is a reflection of the effective surface area used for dialysis.

- One of the perceived benefits of PD is often viewed as a more liberal oral fluid intake with the daily dialysis regimen.

- The term adequacy has been coined to represent effective control of uremic symptoms in an individual with renal failure. Adequacy studies are a measurement of the effectiveness of the dialysis process.

- Although highly effective, relatively simple, and potentially inexpensive, PD has not been embraced worldwide. In some countries, transplantation is the predominant treatment for ESRD because ordinary individuals and families cannot afford dialysis.

ANNP627   **Technical Aspects of Peritoneal Dialysis**

Elizabeth Kelman, MEd, RN, CNeph(C), and Diane Watson, MSc, RN, CNeph(C)

Contemporary Nephrology Nursing: Principles and Practice contains 39 chapters of educational content. Individual learners may apply for continuing nursing education credit by reading a chapter and completing the Continuing Education Evaluation Form for that chapter. Learners may apply for continuing education credit for any or all chapters.

Please photocopy this page and return to ANNA.
COMPLETE THE FOLLOWING:

Name: _____

Address:_____

City:_____State: _____Zip: _____

E-mail: _____

Preferred telephone: ☐ Home   ☐ Work: _____

State where licensed and license number (optional): _____

CE application fees are based upon the number of contact hours provided by the individual chapter. CE fees per contact hour for ANNA members are as follows: 1.0-1.9 - $15; 2.0-2.9 - $20; 3.0-3.9 - $25; 4.0 and higher - $30. Fees for nonmembers are $10 higher.

ANNA Member: ☐ Yes   ☐ No   Member # (if available) _____

☐ Checked Enclosed   ☐ American Express   ☐ Visa   ☐ MasterCard

Total Amount Submitted: _____

Credit Card Number: _____ Exp. Date: _____

Name as it appears on the card: _____

CE Evaluation Form
To receive continuing education credit for individual study after reading the chapter
1. Photocopy this form. (You may also download this form from ANNA's Web site, **www.annanurse.org**.)
2. Mail the completed form with payment (check) or credit card information to American Nephrology Nurses' Association, East Holly Avenue, Box 56, Pitman, NJ 08071-0056.
3. You will receive your CE certificate from ANNA in 4 to 6 weeks.

Test returns must be postmarked by **December 31, 2010.**

CE Application Fee
ANNA Member $25.00
Nonmember $35.00

EVALUATION FORM

1. I verify that I have read this chapter and completed this education activity. Date: _____

_____
Signature

2. What would be different in your practice if you applied what you learned from this activity? *(Please use additional sheet of paper if necessary.)*

_____
_____
_____
_____
_____
_____
_____
_____
_____
_____
_____
_____
_____

Evaluation	Strongly disagree				Strongly agree
3. The activity met the stated objectives.					
a. Describe the basis for using the peritoneal membrane for dialysis.	1	2	3	4	5
b. Compare the different types of peritoneal dialysis.	1	2	3	4	5
c. Relate the composition of peritoneal dialysis solutions to aspects of volume exchange.	1	2	3	4	5
4. The content was current and relevant.	1	2	3	4	5
5. The content was presented clearly.	1	2	3	4	5
6. The content was covered adequately.	1	2	3	4	5
7. Rate your ability to apply the learning obtained from this activity to practice.	1	2	3	4	5

Comments _____
_____

8. Time required to read the chapter and complete this form: _____ minutes.

This educational activity has been provided by the American Nephrology Nurses' Association (ANNA) for 3.5 contact hours. ANNA is accredited as a provider of continuing nursing education (CNE) by the American Nurses Credentialing Center's Commission on Accreditation (ANCC-COA). ANNA is an approved provider of continuing education by the California Board of Registered Nursing, CEP 0910.

Peritoneal Dialysis Access

Barbara F. Prowant, MS, RN, CNN

Chapter Contents

Barbara F. Prowant, MS, RN, CNN

The success of chronic peritoneal dialysis (PD) depends upon a permanent, safe access to the peritoneal cavity (Gokal et al., 1998). Ash (2003) asserts that chronic PD catheters are the most successful of all transcutaneous access devices, as they survive for years rather than weeks or months; however, the incidence of catheter-related problems and infections is still too high, and these complications are the primary reasons for catheter removal in both pediatric and adult populations (Twardowski & Nichols, 2000; Verrina et al., 1993). Twardowski points out that prevention of infections (and good catheter function) have three prerequisites: optimal catheter design, appropriate implantation technique, and good care post implantation (Twardowski, Nichols, Nolph, & Khanna, 1992). This chapter will address these prerequisites as well as common infectious and noninfectious catheter complications.

History of PD Access

During the early experimentation with PD, access to the peritoneal cavity was achieved with devices designed for other medical purposes. These early access devices included metal needles, metal and glass cannulas, and even Foley catheters (Twardowski, 2004). There were frequent problems with access including leaks, infection, and catheter occlusions. Table 28-1 outlines the history of the development of catheters designed specifically for PD. Major advances were the use of flexible materials for the catheter tubing, the addition of small side holes along the distal catheter, and the use of catheter cuffs. Improvements in implantation techniques, such as the creation of a subcutaneous tunnel, the use of a stylet for catheter insertion, and use of a lateral or paramedical insertion site (rather than midline), also contributed to improved outcomes.

During the 1960s, two groups used "buttons" implanted in the abdominal wall so that a catheter could be inserted through the button for each chronic dialysis treatment (Boen, Mulinari, Dillard, & Scribner, 1962; Malette, McPhaul, Bledsoe, McIntosh, & Koegel, 1964), but the incidence of peritonitis was high. Boen also developed a method of repeated puncture, but this was associated with frequent pericatheter leaks (Boen, Mion, Curtis, & Shilipetar, 1964). Jacob and Deane (1967) inserted a Teflon rod, the "Deane's prosthesis," into the catheter track between dialyses so that repeated punctures were not required. In the 1970s, subcutaneous catheters punctured for each dialysis were developed in efforts to avoid exit-site infections (Gotloib et al., 1975; Stephen, Atkin-Thor, & Kolff, 1976).

More recently, innovations in catheter design have included silver-coated (Dasgupta, 1994; Crabtree et al., 2003) and antibiotic-bonded catheters (Trooskin, Donetz, Baxter, Harvey, & Greco, 1987; Trooskin, Harvey, Lennard, & Greco, 1990) in attempts to reduce bacterial colonization and subsequent infections; a catheter with a short intraperitoneal segment implanted 3-4 cm over the pubic bone so that the catheter will drain regardless of tip posi-

Table 28-1
History of the Development of Chronic Peritoneal Dialysis Catheters

1946 – Frank, Seligman, and Fine first used a subcutaneous tunnel.

1948 – Rosenak and Oppenheimer developed an access specifically for PD, a flexible stainless steel coil attached to a rubber drain.

1949 – Dérot and colleagues reported the use of polyvinyl tubing for a PD catheter.

1952 – Grollman et al. used a polyethylene catheter with side holes in the distal end.

1953 – Legrain and Merrill used polyvinyl tubing for their PD catheter.

1959 – Maxwell and colleagues introduced a nylon catheter with tiny distal perforations;
 – Doolan and colleagues designed a polyvinyl catheter with ridges to prevent obstruction of drain holes
 – The catheters from Maxwell et al. and Doolan, et al. were both inserted with trocars.

1964 – Gutch noted less irritation with silicon rubber catheters;
 – Palmer, Quinton, and Gray developed a silicone rubber catheter with a coiled intraperitoneal segment.

1965 – Weston and Roberts invented a stylet catheter, inserted without a trocar, which required a smaller incision and track and, thus, reduced the risk of leaks. This is still used for acute renal failure.

1968 – The first catheter cuffs of Dacron® polyester were used by McDonald and colleagues (a single cuff and Teflon® skirt);
 – Tenckhoff and Schechter introduced a double-cuffed catheter. The "Tenckhoff" catheter is still widely used and is the prototype for almost all modern catheters.

Note: From Twardowski, Z.J. (2004). History and development of the access for peritoneal dialysis. *Contributions to Nephrology, 142,* 387-401.

tion (Chiaramonte et al., 1992); and a "self-locating" catheter with a tungsten weight at the distal end (Di Paolo et al., 1996); however, these are not commercially available or widely used. The recent renewed interest in continuous flow PD has stimulated the development of an experimental double-lumen PD catheter (Diaz-Buxo, 2002; Ronco, Wentling, Amerling, Cruz, & Levin, 2004).

Catheters for Acute PD

Acute PD catheters are made of nylon or polyethylene and are straight and relatively stiff with numerous side holes in the distal portion. They do not have cuffs, but have wings that can be sutured to the skin to secure the catheter. Acute catheters are not recommended for patients who are

Figure 28-1
Straight and Coiled Double-Cuff Tenckhoff Catheters

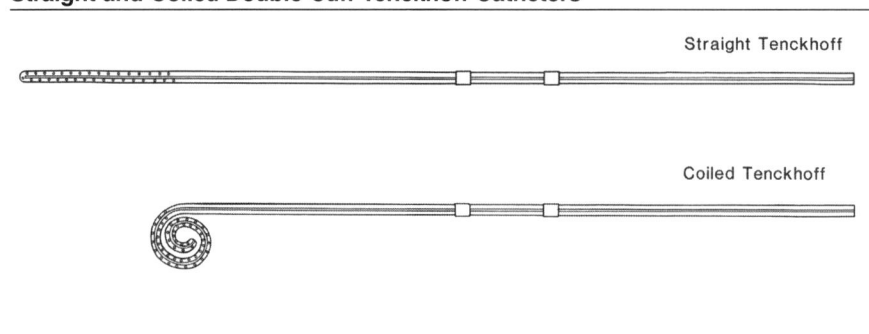

extremely obese or those who have had previous abdominal surgery because adhesions increase the risk of organ perforation.

Acute Catheter Insertion

Acute catheters typically come in a kit with all of the supplies required for insertion. These catheters can be placed at the bedside or in a treatment room, used immediately, and removed at the bedside. Frequently, a nurse assists with the procedure, acting as the circulating nurse. Acute catheters are inserted through a small midline skin incision just below the umbilicus. A large bore needle or the catheter and internal stylet are pushed through the abdominal wall while the patient holds a deep breath and tenses the abdomen. When the peritoneum is entered there is a decrease in resistance and often an audible "pop." The abdomen is pre-filled with saline or dialysis solution, and then the catheter is advanced into the peritoneum, toward the pelvis. If resistance is felt or the patient complains of pain, the catheter is pulled back and redirected. The catheter is fixed in place by suturing the wings or a disc to the skin surface. Absorbent sterile dressings are applied and are not changed unless they become saturated (Twardowski & Nichols, 2000).

Semi-rigid acute catheters have a number of potential complications. One is pre-peritoneal placement, where the catheter is not in the peritoneal space. This results in slow dialysis solution inflow, pain on inflow, localized swelling, and poor, if any, drain flow. Pre-peritoneal placement is treated by removing the catheter and reinserting a new catheter at another site (Zappacosta, 2002). The risk of organ perforation is greater with the semi-rigid catheters both during insertion and during dialysis therapy (see Surgical Complications, below).

Acute catheters have more drainage problems than chronic catheters. There is also a risk of the sutures becoming dislodged and losing the catheter in the peritoneal cavity, and the risk of a kinked internal segment breaking off.

Since acute catheters have no barriers to prevent bacteria from migrating into the peritoneal cavity, the risk of infection is great. Fluid may leak along the catheter track, further increasing the infection risk, as the dextrose-rich dialysis solution provides an excellent growth medium for bacteria. Limiting the time the catheter is left in place reduces the risk of infection, so rigid acute catheters are only used for up to 3 days (Ash, 2002). When acute dialysis is required for more than 3 days, a chronic catheter, typically a single-cuff Tenckhoff catheter, is used.

Chronic Dialysis Catheters

The most commonly used chronic catheters are made of silicone rubber tubing with a radiopaque stripe. They have a 4.9 mm or 5.0 mm external diameter, a 2.6 mm internal diameter, and one or two Dacron® polyester cuffs. Functionally, the catheter has 3 segments: the external segment; the tunnel segment, which passes through the subcutaneous fat and muscle; and the intraperitoneal segment. These catheters have an open end and multiple 0.5 mm to 1 mm side holes in the intraperitoneal segment starting 8-10 cm from the tip in straight catheters and 16 cm from the tip in coiled catheters (Ash, 2003; Twardowski, 2004).

A well-functioning catheter should not take more than 10 minutes to fill and 15 minutes to drain two liters (Verger, 2004). The longer and more curved the catheter is, the longer it will take to infuse and drain (Graff, Joffe, & Ladefoged, 1992), so coiled catheters will take a bit more time to drain and fill for each exchange compared to straight catheters, and a presternal catheter will take a little more time than an abdominal catheter; however, these differences are not clinically significant (Prowant & Ponferrada, 1998).

The Flex-Neck™ catheter (Medigroup, Inc., Naperville, IL) is made of a more flexible silicone and has a larger inner diameter (3.5 mm) and, therefore, faster flow rates, and can be bent to facilitate placement of the exit site. PD catheters are also made of polyurethane (see Cruz® catheter, Figure 28-9); these catheters also have larger lumens and faster flow rates.

Double-cuff catheters have longer survival and lower infection rates compared to single-cuff catheters in both adult and pediatric patients (Lindblad, Hamilton, Nolph, & Novak, 1988; U.S. Renal Data System [USRDS], 1992; Warady, Sullivan, & Alexander, 1996), so they are almost universally used for chronic dialysis.

The Tenckhoff catheter (Tenckhoff & Schechter, 1968) is the most widely used catheter throughout the world. It may have either a straight or coiled intraperitoneal segment (see Figure 28-1). Tenckhoff recommended implantation of the catheter with an arcuate (curved) subcutaneous tunnel so that both the external and the intraperitoneal segments are

Figure 28-2
**Schematic of the Subcutaneous Catheter Tract with a
Single-Cuff Tenckhoff Catheter**

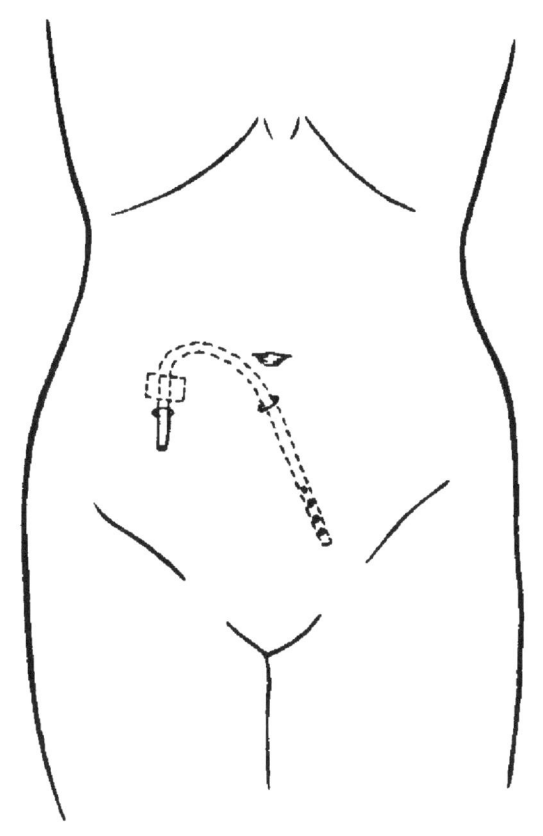

Note: From Tenckhoff (1974). Used with permission from the University of Washington.

Figure 28-3
Straight and Coiled Swan-Neck Catheters

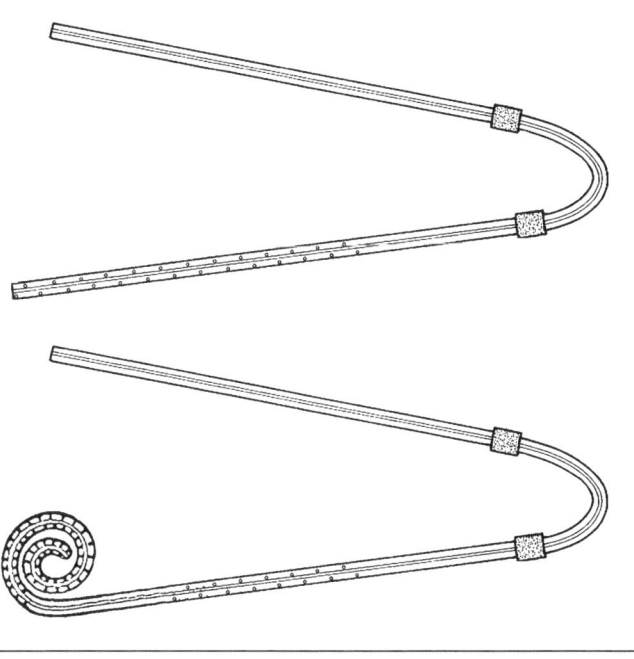

Figure 28-4
**The Stencils Markings for Right and Left Swan-Neck
Catheters Are Mirror Images of One Another**

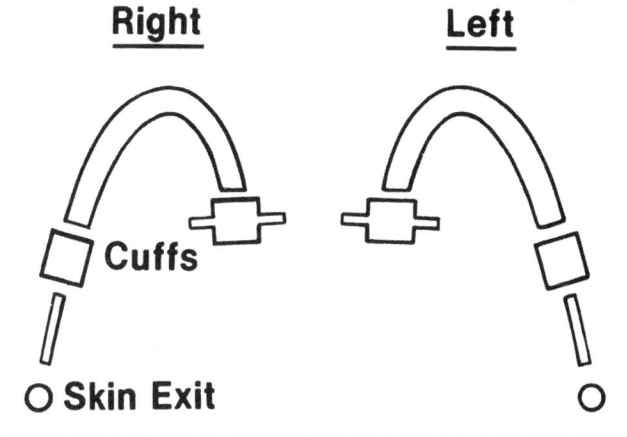

directed caudally (see Figure 28-2) (Tenckhoff, 1974). The Tenckhoff catheters are prototypes for almost all of the recently developed catheters.

Coiled catheters are sometimes referred to as "curled" or "spiral" catheters. The coiled intraperitoneal segment offers several advantages (Twardowski, 2004). Infusion pain is less frequent because with the coiled design more of the solution flows through the side holes, and the flow through the main lumen is within the coil and not aimed directly toward the peritoneum. Also, there is not the poking effect sometimes experienced from the tip of a straight catheter. Coiled catheters have a lower incidence of outflow failure than straight catheters (Ash, 2002), as they are not as likely to migrate, and in one study had significantly higher survival than straight Tenckhoff catheters (Nielsen, Hemmingsen, Friis, Ladefoged, & Olgaard, 1995). A study of 18 centers by the Pediatric Peritoneal Dialysis Study Consortium found that the majority of pediatric centers (88%) used coiled catheters (Neu, Kohaut, & Warady, 1995).

"Swan-neck" peritoneal catheters have a molded arc between the subcutaneous and deep cuffs (see Figure 28-3) to enable both the external and the intra-abdominal segments to be directed downward with minimal tension on

the catheter (Twardowski, Prowant, Khanna, Nichols, & Nolph, 1990). A stencil (see Figure 28-4) may be used to mark the position of the cuffs and tunnel on the skin prior to surgery. Swan-neck catheters may have either straight or coiled intra-abdominal segments, which are identical to those of Tenckhoff catheters. Clinical experience with swan-neck catheters documents a decreased incidence of cuff extrusion (Eklund, Honkanen, Kala, & Kyllönen, 1995) and catheter tip migration (Gadallah, Mignone, Torres, Ramdeen, & Pervez, 2000; Nebel, Marczewski, & Finke, 1991), complications that occur when a straight silastic catheter with "shape memory" is inserted with a curved tunnel. It has been found that catheters with a permanent

Figure 28-5
The Moncrief-Popovich Catheter

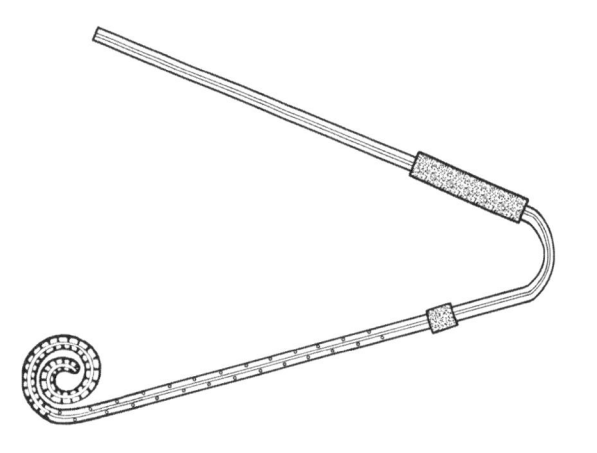

Figure 28-6
The Toronto Western Hospital Type 2 Catheter
(Note the flange and bead at the deep cuff)

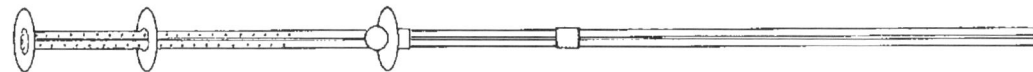

Figure 28-7
Swan-Neck Missouri Straight and Coiled Catheters
(Note the angled flange and bead at the deep cuff)

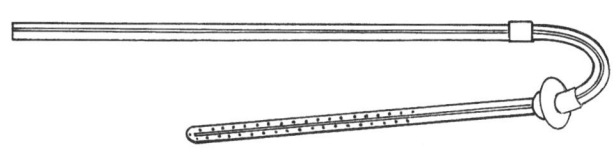

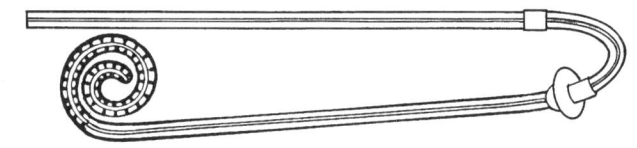

bend had a significantly lower rate of peritonitis than other catheters (Eklund et al., 1995; USRDS, 1992). Eklund et al. (1995) and Twardowski et al. (1990) found a lower incidence of exit-site infection compared to catheters with straight subcutaneous segments. The swan-neck catheters also have improved survival compared to Tenckhoff and Toronto Western catheters (Twardowski & Nichols, 2000) and are probably second to the Tenckhoff as the most widely used.

The Moncrief-Popovich catheter is a double-cuffed, swan-neck, coiled catheter with a longer (2.5 cm) subcutaneous cuff (see Figure 28-5) (Moncrief et al., 1993). This catheter is used with the Moncrief-Popovich implantation technique in which the external segment is buried under the skin for several weeks until there is strong tissue ingrowth into the subcutaneous cuff. Then, in a second surgical procedure, the external cuff is "exteriorized," and the

catheter can be used for dialysis (Moncrief et al., 1993). An article reviewing 10 years of clinical experience with the Moncrief-Popovich catheter found that in all but one series the rates of exit-site infection and peritonitis were similar or lower than those of other catheters. It concluded that use of the catheter and technique reduce infectious complications in PD (Dasgupta, 2002); however, a recent randomized, controlled study found that "subcutaneous burying of the distal catheter segment...does not reduce the risk of contracting peritonitis or exit-site infection" (Danielsson, Blohmé, Tranæus, & Hylander, 2002, p. 211). It is interesting to note that the Moncrief implantation technique has been used successfully with presternal catheters (Kubota et al., 2001).

Toronto Western Hospital Type 2 (TWH-2) catheters (see Figure 28-6) or simply "Toronto catheters" have two silicone rubber discs on the intraperitoneal segment to curtail migration and a polyester flange at the base of the deep cuff with a silicone "bead" close to the flange to provide a groove for a purse string suture (Ponce et al., 1982). The parietal peritoneum is tightly sutured between the bead (or "ball") inside the peritoneum and the flange outside the peritoneum.

The swan-neck Missouri catheter (see Figure 28-7) incorporates both the arced swan-neck subcutaneous segment of the swan-neck catheters and the flange and bead design at the deep cuff of the TWH-2 catheters (Twardowski et al., 1990). The flange and bead are slanted at a 45° angle,

Figure 28-8
The Swan-Neck Presternal Peritoneal Dialysis Catheter

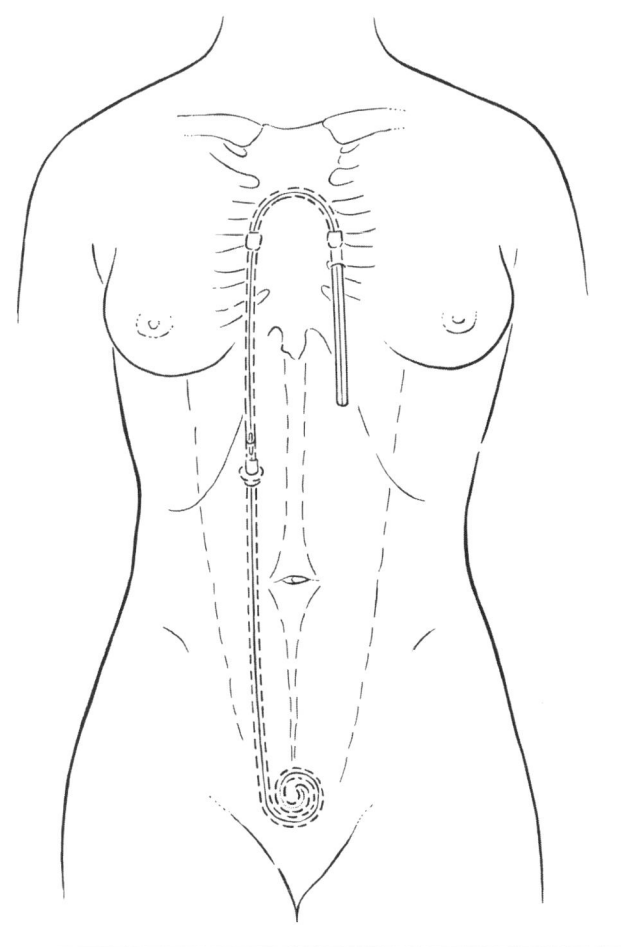

Note: Reprinted with permission from *American Journal of Kidney Diseases*, 27, 99-105, 1996. Twardowski, Z.J., Prowant, B.F., Pickett, B., Nichols, W.K., Nolph, K.D., & Khanna, R. Four-year experience with swan neck presternal peritoneal dialysis catheter.

requiring the catheters for the right and the left sides to be mirror images of one another.

The presternal catheter (see Figure 28-8) is a further variation of the swan-neck Missouri catheter (Twardowski et al., 1992). This catheter, designed to exit on the chest, has two sections connected by a titanium connector at the time of implantation. The distal part of the catheter is composed of a coiled intra-abdominal segment, the deep cuff and part of the tunnel segment. The proximal part of the catheter is composed of the remaining tunnel segment, an arcuate subcutaneous segment with two cuffs, and the external segment. The rationale for the presternal catheter is that the chest wall has far less motion than the abdomen, and this will decrease piston-like movement of the catheter within the sinus track. Furthermore, there is less subcutaneous fat on the chest, so location of the catheter exit in the presternal area should both facilitate healing and reduce the migration of organisms into the sinus tract. The prester-

Figure 28-9
The Cruz® or "Pail Handle" Catheter

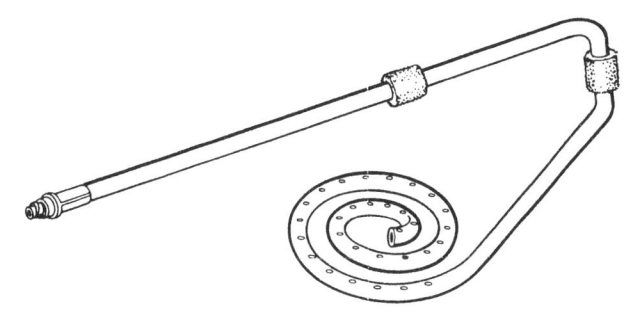

nal exit site is also further away from the groin, ostomies, and diapers; thus, there should be less cross-contamination. Although initial indications for use of the presternal catheter were obesity, abdominal stomas, and previous problems with other catheters, adult patients are also choosing this catheter electively (for reasons of body image and patients who prefer tub baths), and presternal catheters have been used successfully in pediatric patients (Chadha, Jones, Ramirez, & Warady, 2000; Warchol, Roszkowska-Blaim, Latoszynska, Jarmolinski, & Zachwieja, 2003).

Presternal catheters had excellent survival in the initial series, 86% at 3 years (Twardowski, Prowant, Nichols, Nolph, & Khanna, 1998). Other outcomes are similar to those observed with abdominal swan-neck catheters. Although exit-site infection rates tended to be lower for presternal than for swan-neck abdominal catheters, the difference was not statistically significant (Twardowski, 2002a).

The Cruz® or "pail handle" catheter (see Figure 28-9) (Cruz, 1992) is made of polyurethane and has two 90° bends (one just outside the exit site and one behind the subcutaneous cuff), instead of an arc, so that both external segment and intraperitoneal catheter segments are pointed downward. The catheter wall is thinner, making the inner diameter larger (3.1 mm), resulting in faster flow rates (Cruz, 1997). Because of the larger inner diameter, a special adapter must be used. The catheter is available with or without a permanently bonded pre-attached adapter. Insertion of a catheter with the adapter already in place requires a larger exit-site wound and tunnel track and was associated with more infectious complications in a series of 63 catheters (Crabtree, Siddiq, Chung, & Greenwald, 1998).

The T-fluted catheter (Ash & Janle, 1993) has a unique design. The fluted intraperitoneal segment forms a "T" with the tubing that passes through the abdominal wall and forms the external segment (see Figure 28-10). The intraperitoneal segment of this silicone catheter lies against the parietal peritoneum and has four flutes or grooves along the entire intraperitoneal length to channel the dialysis fluid as it infuses and drains. Early data indicate that these catheters have a somewhat shorter drain time and lower intraperitoneal residual volume compared to Tenckhoff catheters (Ash et al., 2002).

Figure 28-10
The T-fluted Catheter

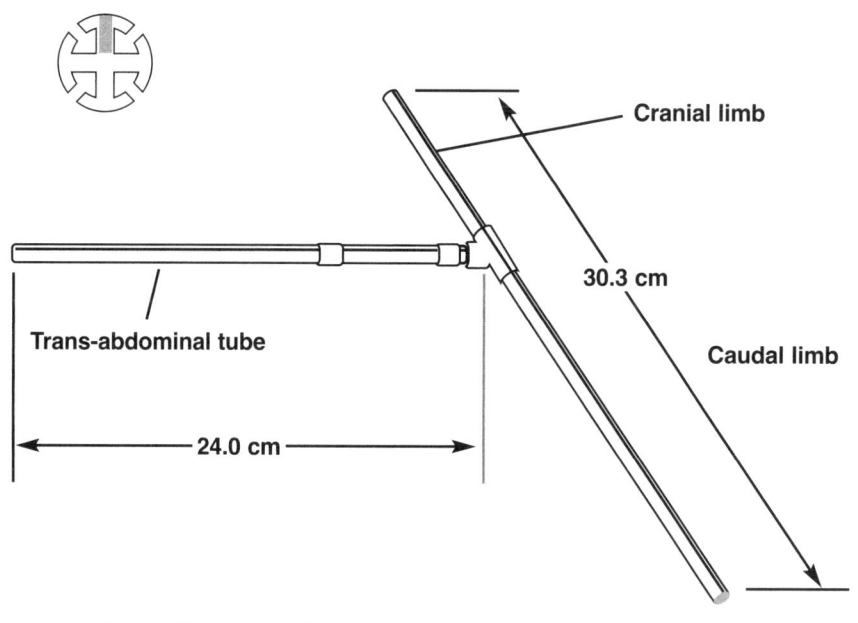

Note: Drawing provided by and used with permission of Medigroup, Inc.

Chronic Catheter Insertion

Preoperative Care

Preoperative patient education should include a review of why the patient requires dialysis, the type of PD catheter that will be implanted, where the catheter will be placed, a brief explanation of what to expect postoperatively, and an overview of catheter procedures and care.

Culturing the patient for *Staphylococcus aureus* (*S. aureus*) nasal carriage, defined as one positive culture, may also be a part of the preoperative protocol. *S. aureus* carrier status is a major risk factor for *S. aureus* catheter-related infections. Studies have shown that treating the nasal carriage with cyclical rifampin or nasal mupirocin reduced *S. aureus* exit-site infections to one third of the previous rate (Mupirocin Study Group, 1996; Perez-Fontan, 1993; Ritzau, Hoffman, & Tzamaloukas, 2001). Use of topical mupirocin at the catheter exit site resulted in a similar reduction in infections (Bernardini, Piraino, Holley, Johnston, & Lutes, 1996; Zimmerman et al., 1991). A meta-analysis of 10 randomized, controlled or cohort studies of mupirocin use in dialysis patients found a 62% reduction of *S. aureus* exit-site infections and a 66% reduction in *S. aureus* peritonitis (Tacconelli et al., 2003). The International Society for Peritoneal Dialysis (ISPD) catheter guidelines recommend that patients who are *S. aureus* nasal carriers *may* receive prophylaxis for nasal carriage but then go on to recommend application of mupirocin to the exit site as part of daily care (Gokal et al., 1998).

Catheter guidelines (Gokal et al., 1998) recommend that the catheter exit site be determined preoperatively. The patient should be assessed in both supine and upright positions, and the exit site should not be located under the belt-line, on a scar, or in abdominal fat folds (Purcell, 1993). Ideally, the exit site should be positioned where the patient can see it and reach it for exit-site care. The exit site is marked on the skin with a permanent marker. A stencil to guide the marking of the exit site and the catheter cuffs is available for swan-neck catheters.

Recommended preoperative skin preparation is a shower with chlorhexidine soap on the morning of the surgery (Gokal et al., 1998). Excessive hair should be removed with electric clippers.

Infection remains the major cause of impaired surgical wound healing. Although there have been conflicting reports of the efficacy of prophylactic preoperative antibiotics in preventing catheter-related infections, the use of prophylactic antibiotics is recommended in the consensus guidelines (Gokal et al., 1998). Prophylactic antibiotics pre catheter insertion significantly reduced the risk for postoperative peritonitis in adults (Gadallah et al., 2000), and pediatric patients who received perioperative antibiotics (from 12 hours preoperatively to 3 hours postoperatively) had significantly less early peritonitis than patients who did not receive antibiotics (Sardegna, Beck, & Strife, 1998). A prospective Network 9 study found that the use of prophylactic antibiotics was associated with a significantly lower risk of long-term peritonitis and of peritonitis with concomitant exit-site infection (Golper et al., 1996). Guidelines recommend that an antibiotic with staphylococcal coverage (e.g. a first generation cephalosporin) be given 1 hour preoperatively and 6-12 hours postoperatively (Gokal et al., 1998). It is important that the antibiotic be present in the blood and tissues before the catheter is implanted. Vancomycin should not be used for prophylaxis because of the emergence of vancomycin-resistant organisms (Gokal et al., 1998).

To reduce the risk of organ perforation, it is critical that the bowel and bladder are not distended at the time of surgery. Bowel preparation protocols vary but include the use of laxatives and/or enemas. If the patient is unable to empty the bladder prior to the procedure, catheterization is recommended.

Implantation Techniques

Detailed descriptions of catheter implantation techniques have been published elsewhere (Ahmad, 1999; Ash, 2002, 2003; Burkart, 1998; Cruz, 1996; Rodrigues, Cabrita, & Nogueira, 2004; Twardowski & Nichols, 2000). This discussion will simply describe and differentiate the three most common placement methods: "blind insertion" using a trocar, implantation by surgical dissection, or peritoneoscopy.

Wet cuffs provide better tissue ingrowth compared to dry cuffs that contain air (Poirier, Daly, Dasse, Haudenschild, & Fine, 1986). So, immediately before implantation the catheter should be immersed in sterile saline and the cuffs gently squeezed to remove air and then thoroughly soaked. Ahmed (1999) also recommends that the catheter be flushed with 30-50 ml of saline to remove any particulate matter.

Blind insertion is similar to the technique used for acute catheters and is usually performed by the nephrologist. An incision is made through the skin and subcutaneous tissue and the rectus muscle fibers are separated. Then, while the patient holds a deep breath and tenses the abdomen, the parietal peritoneum is punctured with a trocar or needle. The peritoneum is filled with saline or dialysis solution, and the catheter is passed into the peritoneal cavity using a stiffening stylet or guide wire. This is the least used method because of the greater risks of vessel or organ perforation. The technique should not be used in patients who have had multiple abdominal surgeries or intra-abdominal adhesions. Blind insertion also has a greater risk of early leaks, so is not recommended for patients who require immediate PD. Surgical backup is necessary in case of complications.

Implantation by surgical dissection (a mini-laparotomy) is most common. It is required for the Toronto Western, swan-neck Missouri, and presternal catheters as these have flanged cuffs at the peritoneum. After a skin incision is made, the tissues are dissected under direct vision and bleeding is controlled with electrocautery. A small incision is made in the deep fascia and the peritoneum, and the parietal peritoneum is lifted to create an air space between it and the visceral peritoneum. The catheter is introduced on a stiffening stylet or with forceps and directed by feel toward the deep pelvis. If the catheter tip is in a good position, the patient may feel pressure on the rectum. A purse-string suture is placed through the peritoneum, deep fascia and the posterior rectus sheath, and catheter cuff to close

the peritoneal incision snugly and hold the catheter in place. The purse-string suture is placed between the flange and bead in Missouri swan-neck and Toronto Western catheters.

Peritoneoscopic implantation uses a "peritoneoscope" to insert the catheter under direct visualization of the peritoneal cavity. This technique is useful if the patient has had previous abdominal surgeries or abdominal adhesions. The scope is placed and a trocar is introduced into the peritoneum. Six hundred to 1000 mL of air is injected to create a pneumoperitoneum, then a catheter guide is advanced and positioned under continuous observation, and the catheter is inserted through the guide. The cuff is placed in the muscle using hemostats. This procedure enables the operator to identify anatomical landmarks and to avoid the omentum and adhesions. Peritoneoscopic placement may reduce the risk of organ perforation. A meta-analysis found that complications with peritoneoscopy are similar to those with surgical dissection, but infection rates were lower (Ash, 2003). Two randomized, controlled studies found longer catheter survival with peritoneoscopic placement compared to surgical dissection (Gadallah et al., 1999; Pastan et al., 1991).

Catheter patency (inflow and outflow) should be tested before closing the insertion incision to ensure that there is adequate inflow and outflow without leakage (Verger, 2004). This allows for repositioning the catheter, if necessary, to correct drain problems.

Creation of the subcutaneous tunnel is similar for all methods of insertion. An incision is made at the desired skin exit, and a trocar or "tunneler" device the same size as the catheter is passed through the subcutaneous fat to the primary incision. Achieving the correct tunnel size is important for good clinical outcomes. If the tunnel is too tight, it does not allow drainage of necrotic tissue and may cause tissue edema, which decreases local tissue perfusion and delays healing. If the incision is too large, healing is prolonged because there is a larger wound to repair. When sutures are used to close the skin around the catheter, there is increased risk of infection. The tip of the catheter is pulled through the tunnel and through the exit site. Then the incision is closed and the operative sites covered with several layers of absorbent gauze dressings and secured with a semipermeable dressing, which also immobilizes the catheter (Twardowski & Nichols, 2000).

Guidelines for Catheter Implantation

Peritoneal catheter insertion should be done by a competent experienced operator and take place in the operating room under sterile conditions. Although either local anesthesia with sedation or general anesthesia can be used, general anesthesia should be avoided when possible because it predisposes to vomiting and constipation, and requires voluntary coughing postoperatively (Twardowski & Nichols, 2000). Coughing, vomiting, and straining all increase intra-abdominal pressure and, thus, increase the risk of early leaks and delayed healing. When local anesthesia is used, the patient receives sedation prior to and during the procedure (Twardowski & Nichols, 2000). With local anesthesia, the patient can confirm the position of the catheter tip by telling the surgeon where pressure is felt as the catheter tip is advanced.

There are several points of general agreement on the proper location of catheters (Ash, 2002, 2003; Gokal et al., 1998): (a) the peritoneal incision should be lateral or para-median, (b) the deep cuff should be in the musculature of the abdominal wall (i.e. within the medial or lateral border of the rectus sheath), (c) the intraperitoneal segment should be between the parietal and visceral peritoneum with the tip directed toward the right or left pelvic gutter, (d) the catheter tip location in the left pelvic gutter is preferred, as migration is more likely on the right side due to the upward peristalsis of the ascending segment of the large bowel, (e) the subcutaneous cuff should be located approximately 2 cm from the skin exit site, and (f) the exit site should be directed downwards. Downward directed exit sites were associated with significantly lower risk of peritonitis with concomitant exit and tunnel infection in the Network 9 study (Golper et al., 1996) and in a national pediatric study (Warady et al., 1996).

Dialysis nurses sometimes accompany patients to surgery and participate by ensuring that the patient receives the correct catheter, encouraging use of the preferred exit site, preparing the heparinized solution for checking catheter patency, and making sure that the catheter is capped and secured and that appropriate dressings are applied.

Surgical Complications

Perforation of abdominal organs is the most serious complication associated with PD catheter insertion. Blind insertion methods and constipation increase the risk of bowel perforation. Signs and symptoms of bowel perforation include a foul smelling, turbid dialysate with particulate matter, and profuse watery diarrhea. Treatment includes discontinuing dialysis, removing the catheter, and use of antibiotics to clear infection. The actual bowel puncture is usually managed nonsurgically (Zappacosta, 2002). Another PD catheter can be placed after the infection has cleared and the bowel has healed.

Bladder perforation can usually be avoided by emptying the bladder preoperatively. When bladder perforation occurs, it manifests as an increase in the volume of voidings with correspondingly lower PD drain volumes and the "urine" tests positive for glucose. Bladder perforation requires insertion of a urinary catheter and removal of the PD catheter. Zappacosta (2002) reports success in replacing the PD catheter and resuming dialysis immediately, while leaving the urinary catheter in place for at least 1 week.

Bleeding into the peritoneal cavity with resulting pink-tinged dialysate occurs post catheter insertion and is usually benign. Intraperitoneal heparin is given to prevent the formation of clots that could obstruct the catheter. The amount of bleeding and the color saturation of the dialysate should gradually diminish over subsequent dialysis drains or irrigations.

Small amounts of blood may make the effluent hazy; therefore, bleeding can be confused with peritonitis. Cell counts are useful for the differential diagnosis because the

white blood cell (WBC) count will not be elevated if the turbidity is due to bleeding.

More severe bleeding with clots and red effluent is rare and requires further evaluation. Hematocrits of $\geq 2\%$ or red blood cell counts of 60,000 cells per cubic centimeter indicate significant bleeding (Ash et al., 1995). Perforation of a major abdominal vessel results in grossly bloody dialysate effluent, a fall in hematocrit, and signs of shock. Zappacosta (2002) recommends managing hemorrhage with rapid exchange PD without heparin, supportive care, and transfusions if necessary, and states that most bleeds resolve within 24 hours. However, emergency exploratory surgery may be required to ligate the bleeding vessels (Ash et al., 1995).

Dialysate leaks are most likely to occur during the first month after catheter implantation. Exit-site leaks occur before there is tissue ingrowth into the catheter cuffs and predispose the patient to infections. Pericatheter leaks are more likely in both adults and children (Patel, Mottes, & Flynn, 2001) if the catheter is used immediately after placement. Leaks present as moisture or fluid at the exit site, which can be differentiated from serous drainage from the newly created catheter tunnel and exit site by measuring the dextrose content of the drainage with a dextrose stick. Early leaks are treated by discontinuing PD for a period of at least 14 days and restarting PD with lower exchange volumes (Schwenk, Charytan, & Spinowitz, 2002).

Most patients experience some degree of pain during the postoperative period. It is important to differentiate incisional pain from discomfort from catheter poking and pain related to dialysis exchanges. Typically, mild analgesics and comfort measures are effective in managing pain post catheter implantation.

Catheter Break-In

The longer the period before catheter use, the better the healing and the lower the risk of complications (Gokal et al., 1998). When possible, it is recommended that any PD be delayed for 1-3 days. In this case, the peritoneal cavity is flushed with heparinized (500-1000 u/L) saline or dialysate with in-and-out or hourly exchanges until clear. Then the catheter is "locked" with heparinized solution and capped. Verger (2004) suggests that normal saline may be less irritating than dialysis solution for catheter irrigations.

If immediate dialysis is required, supine dialysis with small infusion volumes (500-1500 mL) is necessary to minimize the intra-abdominal pressure in order to reduce the risk of dialysate leaks. The dialysate volume is gradually increased over 2-3 days. Continuous ambulatory peritoneal dialysis (CAPD) is not recommended for 10 to14 days after catheter implantation.

If dialysis is not initiated immediately, it has been traditionally been recommended that the catheter be flushed or irrigated with heparinized saline or dialysis solution regularly (typically weekly) to maintain patency and check function. Intermittent irrigation is not absolutely necessary to maintain catheter patency, as evidenced by the experience with the buried Moncrief-Popovich catheters. It does, however, provide an opportunity to evaluate catheter function and drain flows, and allows for early intervention for poorly functioning catheters.

Healing Post Catheter Implantation

At 1-week post implantation, well-healing PD catheter exit sites typically have a scab and a small amount of serous or bloody drainage. The surrounding skin is pale pink or pink. The visible sinus is lined with white tissue and has drainage similar in characteristics to the external drainage. In well-healing exits, epidermis starts to enter the sinus within 2-3 weeks and progresses steadily to cover at least half the sinus by 4-6 weeks (Twardowski & Prowant, 1996a). The new epithelium appears fragile and is pale pink or white in Caucasians. By the third week, there is no drainage or just minimal moisture deep in the sinus. As the sinus heals and granulation tissue develops, vessels become visible and/or the surface appears mottled – partly white and partly pink. The color of this granulation tissue gradually changes to pink.

The granulation tissue of a healthy sinus produces an exudate of WBCs and serum with opsonins. This prevents bacteria that normally colonize the sinus from invading the tissue and causing infection.

Although in the past it was commonly believed that the epidermis reached the subcutaneous cuff, observations of catheter tunnels removed from patients showed that in almost all human PD catheter tunnels, the epithelium stops a few millimeters from the exit site (Twardowski et al., 1991).

Exit sites that become infected very early do not show the normal progression of healing, or the progression of epidermis into the sinus stops or even regresses. Drainage becomes purulent and the granulation tissue becomes slightly or frankly exuberant. In the absence of healing, the exit is considered infected even if the purulent drainage and/or exuberant granulation tissue are present only in the sinus tract (Twardowski & Prowant, 1996a).

Exit Site Care

The single most important goal of exit-site care is to prevent exit-site infections. Exit-site care also provides an opportunity to assess the exit site and tunnel for signs of infection. Since there have been few controlled research studies evaluating elements of exit-site care procedures, there is no consensus regarding the best cleansing agents or optimal procedure; therefore, the recommendations for exit-site care are based on broad principles, related research (e.g., post surgical wound healing), clinical experience, and expert opinion.

Exit-Site Care Post Catheter Implantation

For post implantation care, the overall goal is to protect the exit site and promote healing, as the open wound is at greater risk for infection than a healed, healthy exit site. Specific goals of post implantation care are to minimize bacterial colonization during the first few weeks, and to avoid exit-site trauma and traction on the cuffs by immobilizing the catheter (Prowant & Twardowski, 1996).

Elements of exit-site care post catheter implantation are outlined in Table 28-2. The guidelines recommend that postoperative exit care procedures using aseptic technique (masks and gloves) be continued until the exit site is healed (Gokal et al., 1998). Typically, the exit site is healed and

Table 28-2
Principles of Exit-Site Care Post Catheter Implantation

- Restrict postoperative dressing changes to trained staff

- Frequent dressing changes during the first 2-3 weeks are not necessary unless dressings are wet; weekly dressing changes are recommended

- Aseptic technique using masks, gloves, and sterile supplies is required

- A mild, non-irritating agent should be used to clean the exit and surrounding skin

- Strong disinfectants should be kept out of the actual wound and away from the catheter

- Sterile water or normal saline should be used to rinse the exit

- The exit site should be dried

- Mupirocin calcium or another antibiotic may be applied for prophylaxis (avoid with polyurethane catheters)

- An absorbent, sterile dressing (e.g., several layers of gauze) should be placed over the exit site

- Semipermeable dressings should not be used alone as they trap moisture at the exit site and have been associated with increased incidence of infections

- The catheter must be immobilized

- The progression of healing should be evaluated and documented at each dressing change by staff

Note: Adapted from Prowant, B.F. & Twardowski, Z.J. (1996). Recommendations for exit care. *Peritoneal Dialysis International, 16*(Suppl. 3), S94-S99.

healthy within 4-6 weeks post catheter insertion (Twardowski & Prowant, 1996a); however, several groups of patients are at risk for slow healing. Systemic risk factors for poor wound healing include malnutrition, obesity, diabetes mellitus, corticosteroids, and uremia (Lewis, 2000). Surgical complications such as a catheter track that is wider than necessary, a hematoma in the tunnel, contamination of the wound, and infection also put patients at risk for delayed healing (Newman et al., 1993; Twardowski & Prowant, 1997).

In the absence of significant drainage, weekly dressing changes are recommended for the first 2 to 3 weeks in order to minimize manipulation of the catheter and to reduce the risk of contaminating the exit site, resulting in exit-site colonization (Gokal et al., 1998; Prowant & Twardowski, 1996). In a study of exit-site healing post catheter implantation, Twardowski and Prowant (1996a) found that early colonization of the exit was the most important risk factor for early infection; 75% of exit sites with early infections were colonized by week 1; 100% by week 2. In contrast, 60% of catheters that were not infected early were not yet colonized at week 2, and 40% were still not colonized at week 3. Catheters with early colonization also had higher rates of peritonitis and increased risk of catheter removal for exit or tunnel infection.

Although there is no consensus regarding the optimal cleansing agent for post implantation exit-site care, there is evidence that strong oxidants such as povidone iodine and hydrogen peroxide are cytotoxic and delay wound healing (Lineaweaver et al., 1985). If these agents are used for cleansing the exit site, care should be taken to use them only on intact skin surrounding the exit site and not in the exit-site wound. Alternative cleansing agents include normal saline and dermal wound cleansers, which are not harmful to the granulation tissue. An added advantage is that these agents do not require rinsing.

The use of prophylactic antibiotics at the exit site, particularly mupirocin calcium ointment, to promote healing has been widely practiced in recent years and shown to prevent early infections post catheter insertion (Prakashan et al., 2001). The ISPD Guidelines state, "As a maneuver to prevent exit-site infections, application of mupirocin to the exit site as part of the daily routine is advocated" (Gokal et al., 1998, p. 24).

In a recent prospective, double-blind randomized study of both incident and prevalent patients, Bernardini et al. (2005) found that gentamicin cream applied to the exit site during routine care was significantly more effective than mupirocin ointment in preventing both exit-site infections and peritonitis.

Exit-site dressings during the healing period should be absorbent, as most patients have some drainage for the first few weeks. Semipermeable dressings should not be used alone because they allow moisture to accumulate at the exit site (Twardowski & Prowant, 1996a).

Although immobilization is mandatory to minimize catheter movement during healing and to prevent tension on the catheter and accidental trauma, no method has been shown to be more effective than any other in securing the catheter. Tape, semipermeable dressings, and immobilizing devices can been used. No one technique works for all patients, so the immobilization technique must be individualized.

It has been recommended that patients do not bathe or shower in the early weeks post catheter implantation to avoid colonization with water-borne organisms (Gokal et al., 1998; Prowant & Twardowski, 1996).

Finally, the guidelines recommend that "in tropical or subtropical areas, sweating may affect the frequency of early dressing changes, which should be done when the exit site is wet, when the patient feels itchy under the taped skin, or when the stickiness of the tape is lost" (Gokal et al., 1998, p. 19).

Chronic Exit-Site Care

The primary goal of chronic exit-site care is to prevent infections. A secondary goal is to identify exit-site problems early so that interventions can be initiated promptly. Elements of catheter care procedures for a healed exit site are outlined in Table 28-3. Exit-site care procedures for infants and children are similar to those for adult PD patients (Neu et al., 1995; Prowant, Warady, & Nolph, 1993).

Table 28-3
Principles of Chronic Exit-Site Care

* Routine care should be done frequently, daily or every other day

* Care should be done whenever the exit site becomes wet or dirty

* Good handwashing is the first step of good exit-site care

* Assess the exit site and tunnel before cleaning the exit site

* Antibacterial soap is appropriate for cleaning the exit; mild medical-grade disinfectants may be used, if preferred
  ◦ the cleansing agent may need to be individualized due to sensitivities and allergies
  ◦ liquid soap is recommended because it reduces the risk of cross-contamination
    ▪ containers should not be refilled
    ▪ some units recommend that the soap dispenser be reserved exclusively for exit-site care

* Crusts, scabs, and cuticle should not be forcibly removed

* Chlorinated tap water may be used to rinse the exit
  ◦ untreated well water should be avoided
  ◦ remove aerators from faucets as these typically harbor gram-negative organisms

* Pat the exit site dry with a clean washcloth or towel; sterile supplies are not necessary

* Apply topical antibiotic (Gokal et al., 1998).

* Dressings have not been shown to benefit healthy exits; however, they may help keep the exit clean and protect it from trauma

* Secure or immobilize the catheter to prevent accidental trauma

Note: Adapted from Prowant, B.F., & Twardowski, Z.J. (1996). Recommendations for exit care. *Peritoneal Dialysis International*, *16*(Suppl. 3), S94-S99.

The optimal frequency of exit-site care has not been established. Although it is generally recommended that exit care be performed daily, we once surveyed our patients with healthy, mature exit sites and found that care was performed daily, every other day, or even once or twice weekly. Healthy exit sites probably do not require the same frequency of care as healing or equivocal exits; however, care must be done routinely to reduce resident bacteria, and daily care is generally recommended (Gokal et al., 1998).

A large multicenter study found lower exit-site infection rates when exit sites were cleaned with a povidone iodine solution rather than pure soap without an antibacterial agent (Luzar et al., 1990). Similarly, Wong et al. (2002) found lower rates with a chlorhexidine soap compared to pure liquid soap. Two other studies found lower rates of exit-site infection with over-the-counter antibacterial soap than with povidone iodine (Hasbargen, Rodgers, Hasbargen, Quinn, & James, 1993; Prowant et al., 1988). The data from these studies indicate that the use of an antibacterial agent for routine exit-site care reduces the risk of exit-site infections.

There have been documented cases of peritonitis with Pseudomonas species in PD patients from contaminated poloxamer-iodine solutions (Goetz & Muder, 1989; Parrott et al., 1982) and hexachlorophene, so it is important that soaps or solutions designated for exit-site care not be transferred from one container to another.

Vinegar rinses (acetic acid 2%) following showering have been used successfully to prevent infections when well water was contaminated with Pseudomonas organisms (Bishop, Harris, & Hays, 1996).

Topical mupirocin at the catheter exit site has been advocated as a strategy to prevent exit-site infections (Gokal et al., 1998) and is widely used. Local application of mupirocin has been shown to significantly reduce the rate of both exit-site infections and peritonitis (Bernardini et al., 1996; Casey et al., 2000). There are problems, however, with chronic use of mupirocin ointment. Resistant organisms have developed (Annigeri et al., 2001; Connolly, Noble, & Phillips, 1993; Rosales, Pérez-Fontán, Rodríguez-Carmona, & García-Falcón, 2001); however, they have not been frequent and a recent review concludes "that we can continue its [mupirocin] use with annual surveillance" (Thodis et al., 2003, p. 698). Structural changes in the silicon catheters of patients using mupirocin daily or 2-3 times weekly have been reported (Khandelwal et al., 2003; Weaver & Dunbeck, 1994), so it is important to keep the ointment from direct contact with the catheter. There are reports of discoloration and cracks and loose cuffs in polyurethane catheters, as well as catheter deformity related to use of mupriocin ointment at the exit site (Crabtree, 2003).

As noted above, Bernardini et al. (2005) found that gentamicin cream applied to the exit site during routine care was significantly more effective than mupirocin ointment in preventing both exit-site infections and peritonitis. An additional advantage of gentamicin cream is that it is much less expensive than mupirocin ointment.

A nursing survey of PD patients in Spain found that "none of the patients followed all of the recommendations [for exit-site care] given during the educational programme" (Gruart, Andreu, & Gil, 1999, p. 20). The authors surmised that this "noncompliance" could be due to either a misunderstanding or difficulty adapting the recommendations to their lifestyles. They go on to recommend that the exit-site care procedure should, within reasonable limits, be adjusted to suit the patient's daily habits. This study has several other implications for nursing care. When teaching patients to perform exit-site care, we need to address the motivation for following exit-site care procedures, that is, to prevent infections and ultimately to prolong catheter life. Patients may need periodic review and reinforcement of the procedure for exit-site care. Also, nurses need to query patients regarding the elements of the procedures they use for routine exit-site care, rather than assume that they are following the recommended procedure.

Exit-Site Assessment and Classification

It is recommended that patients or their dialysis partners assess the exit site and tunnel prior to routine exit-site care, and that a nurse or physician assesses the exit site and tunnel at routine clinic visits (Prowant & Twardowski, 1996). All patients and dialysis caregivers should know the signs and symptoms of exit-site infection and understand that these should be reported promptly to the PD team.

Good lighting and magnification are essential for effective exit-site assessment. A lighted, hand-held magnifying lens works well. External attributes included in the assessment include induration; skin color at the exit site; the presence of crusts, scabs, and exuberant granulation tissue ("proud flesh"); and the amount and characteristics of any drainage. The visible sinus track should be assessed for the extent of epithelium, the presence of exuberant granulation tissue, and the amount and characteristics of drainage. A checklist type form outlining exit-site characteristics aids in standardizing the assessment and documentation.

From the features noted in the exit-site assessment, the exit-site status can be classified. The classification scheme developed by Twardowski and Prowant (1996b) is outlined in Table 28-4. Other scoring systems assign a numerical code to each attribute, and the total score indicates whether or not the exit is infected (Holley & Moss, 1988; Schröder, 2001; Teixidó & Arias, 1998). A mature, healthy exit site that would be classified as perfect is shown in Figure 28-11. An infected exit site is shown in Figure 28-12.

Features of a traumatized exit depend on the intensity of the trauma and the time until the examination. Common features of trauma include: pain or tenderness, bleeding, and scab formation. It is important to encourage patients to report trauma, as prophylactic antibiotic therapy can prevent subsequent infection (Twardowski & Prowant, 1996c).

Since there are resident bacteria on the skin at the exit site, positive cultures alone are not evidence of an infection. Therefore, it is important to make a clinical determination that an exit site is infected. Chronic infections (> 4 weeks duration) are more likely than acute infections to have exuberant granulation tissue and may not have the erythema, pain, and induration seen in acute infections (Twardowski & Prowant, 1996c).

The subcutaneous catheter tunnel should also be assessed for signs of infection - tenderness, induration, and inflammation. The subcutaneous cuff should be palpated and gently squeezed in an effort to express exudate externally (Holley & Moss, 1988; Twardowski & Prowant, 1996c).

Risk Factors for Exit-Site Infection

As mentioned above, *S. aureus* nasal carriage is a major risk factor for catheter-related infections; however, prophylactic antibiotic therapy significantly reduces the incidence of infections.

In well-healed, healthy exit sites, trauma is probably the greatest risk factor for exit-site infection and cuff infection (Twardowski & Prowant, 1996c). Sources of exit-site trauma are outlined in Table 28-5. Trauma has been defined as "anything that breaks the integrity of the skin at the exit site or the epithelium or granulation tissue in the sinus" (Prowant & Twardowski, 1996, p. 596). Pulls on the catheter are particularly likely to cause physical trauma to the exit site, as they may disrupt tissue ingrowth at the sub-

Table 28-4
PD Catheter Exit-Site Classification Scheme

Perfect Exit Site

The following features are present in various combinations:
- exit color is natural, pale pink, or somewhat darker than natural skin tone
- no external drainage
- crust is absent, small, or there may be specks of crust on dressing
- strong, mature epithelium (epidermis) covers the entire visible sinus
- sinus is dry or exudate is barely visible
- drainage is clear or thick

The following features must be absent:
- granulation tissue
- fragile (mucosal) epidermis
- red, bright pink or purplish color
- crust which is large and/or difficult to remove

Equivocal Exit Site

The following features are present in various combinations:
- exit color may be bright pink, or red < 13 mm in diameter
- crust or scab may be large, difficult to detach
- dried exudate on the dressing
- plain or slightly exuberant granulation tissue around exit
- epithelium absent in sinus, or covers only part of the sinus
- slightly exuberant granulation tissue in the sinus
- purulent or bloody drainage only in the sinus (cannot be expressed outside)

The following features must be absent:
- pain or swelling
- erythema >13 mm
- purulent or bloody drainage externally
- distinctly exuberant granulation tissue ("proud flesh")

Good Exit Site

The following features are present in various combinations:
- exit color natural, dark, pale pink or purplish; pink discoloration <13 mm in diameter (border to border including catheter)
- no external drainage
- crust is absent, small, or there may be specks of crust on dressing
- strong mature epithelium (epidermis) at sinus rim
- epithelium deeper in sinus may be fragile, mucosal
- plain granulation tissue beyond the epithelium
- sinus is dry or exudate is barely visible
- drainage is clear or thick

The following features must be absent:
- pain or swelling
- any red color
- external drainage (even after pressure on the sinus or manipulation of the catheter)
- exuberant granulation tissue (even slightly exuberant)
- purulent or bloody drainage in the sinus

Infected Exit Site

The following features are present in various combinations:
- tenderness, soreness, pain
- swelling, induration
- erythema (bright pink or red) >13 mm diameter
- purulent or bloody external drainage, spontaneously or after pressure on sinus and/or wet exudate on dressing
- exuberant granulation tissue ("proud flesh") at the exit (Figure 28-14)
- crust or scab at the exit
- epithelium absent in sinus, or covers only part of the sinus
- exuberant granulation tissue in the sinus
- purulent or bloody drainage in the sinus
- crust or scab in the sinus

External Cuff Infection (Without Exit-Site Infection)

The following features are typically present:
- the tissue over or around the cuff may be indurated, tender or inflamed
- intermittent or chronic external drainage (sometimes seen only after pressure on the cuff)
- drainage purulent, bloody or "gluey"
- epithelium covers most or all of the visible sinus
- epithelium may be intermittently or chronically macerated
- there may be exuberant granulation tissue ("proud flesh") barely visible deep in the sinus

On external examination the exit may appear completely normal

Note: Adapted from Twardowski, Z.J., & Prowant, B.F. (1996b). Classification of normal and diseased exit sites. *Peritoneal Dialysis International, 16*(Suppl. 3), S32-S50.

cutaneous cuff. Trauma severe enough to cause tenderness, pain, or bleeding typically results in deterioration of the exit site and increases the incidence of exit-site infection. Catheters or extension tubings have been caught in car and shower doors, drawers, and recliners. There have been reports of infants pulling on catheters and kicking the exit site and of pets chewing and pulling on tubings. Since it is impossible to imagine or list every possible source of trauma, it is important that patients understand that they must protect the catheter at all times.

Local care post trauma includes cleansing blood from the exit site, since extravasated blood is a good medium for bacterial growth. Prophylactic antibiotic treatment for traumatized exits can markedly reduce the incidence of subsequent infection. In a study of 13 cases of exit-site trauma, only 2 of 9 patients who received a short course of oral antibiotic therapy developed exit-site infection compared to 3 of 4 patients who did not receive prophylactic antibiotic therapy (Twardowski & Prowant, 1996c). Twardowski (2002b) recommends a cephalosporin or a quinolone and

Figure 28-11
A Healthy PD Catheter Exit Site

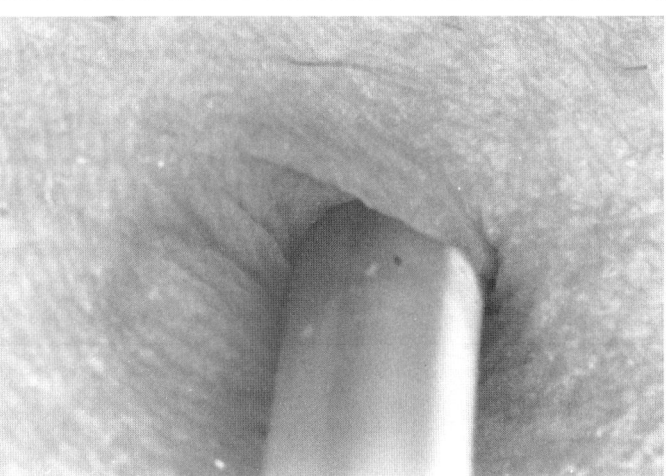

Figure 28-12
An Infected PD Catheter Exit Site

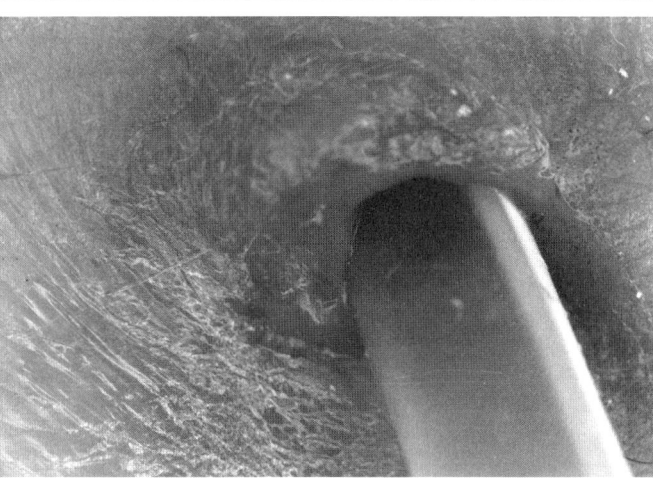

Table 28-5
Sources of Exit-Site Trauma

- Tension or pulling on the catheter
  - anchoring the catheter too tautly
  - anchoring the catheter in an unnatural position
  - accidental pulls on catheter or tubing
  - excessive movement or tension during procedures

- Pressure against the exit site
  - belts, seatbelts
  - tight clothing
  - prolonged leaning against the exit site
  - sleeping on the exit site
  - accidental blunt trauma

- Allergy to cleansing agent

- Irritation from tape or adhesive

- Overly vigorous exit-site care; forcibly removing a crust or scab

- Scratching or picking at the exit

Note: Adapted from Prowant, B.F., & Twardowski, Z.J. (1996). Recommendations for exit care. *Peritoneal Dialysis International, 16*(Suppl. 3), S94-S99.

Table 28-6
Guidelines for Preserving Peritoneal Catheter Integrity

- Use only the recommended size adapter

- Keep cleansing agents, disinfectants, antibiotics, or ointments away from the catheter

- Coil or fix the external catheter segment loosely to avoid kinking or bending

- Do not use scissors to remove exit-site dressings

- Use only nontraumatic, untoothed clamps on the catheter and/or use a gauze compress between the clamp and the catheter to protect it

- Do not use a syringe and needle to sample dialysate through the catheter wall

- Avoid using the abdomen for subcutaneous injections

- If patient is scheduled for abdominal surgery, notify the surgeon of catheter location and/or mark the location of the tunnel and deep cuff

- Never pin the catheter to clothing

- Do not use the catheter for other purposes – delivery of parenteral nutrition, medications, etc.

Note: Adapted and expanded from Verger, C. (2004). Maintenance of functioning PD access and management of complications. *Contributions to Nephrology, 142,* 410-421.

suggests that antibiotics be continued for 7 days after the exit site achieves a healthy appearance.

An extruding catheter cuff is a source of chronic irritation and a risk factor for exit-site infection (Twardowski & Nichols, 2000). Patients with cuff extrusions should be encouraged to protect the exit site from contamination, do meticulous exit-site care, and to report signs or symptoms of exit-site infection promptly.

Gross contamination of the exit site is also a risk factor for exit infection. Tenckhoff (1974) stressed that the exit site should be kept clean and dry to reduce the number of microorganisms. There are several strategies to prevent gross contamination of the exit site. These include wearing a dressing when exit is likely to become dirty or wet, avoiding submersion in water – especially in hot tubs and whirlpools (and particularly during exit-site healing and infection), using a waterproof dressing or barrier when swimming, swimming only in well-chlorinated pools, and performing exit-site care whenever the exit site is wet and immediately after swimming or submersion (Prowant, 1996).

In a single center review, 40% of pediatric patients with gastrostomy tube-related skin infections developed PD catheter exit-site infections with the same organism within the first few days after the gastrostomy tube infection. In contrast, the same study found that the use of diapers did not increase the incidence of exit-site infection (Levy, Balfe, Geary, Fryer-Keene, & Bannatyne, 1990). It is critical that the PD catheter exit site is out of the diaper area and away from other ostomy sites and gastrostomy tubes to prevent cross-contamination (Harvey, Braj, & Balfe, 1998).

Chronic Care of the PD Catheter

Table 28-6 summarizes guidelines for preserving peritoneal catheter integrity. A major goal of care for the catheter is to protect it from caustic agents and accidental trauma. Iatrogenic damage occurs when catheters are occluded with toothed clamps, accidentally cut with scissors or scalpels, and pinned to gowns, etc.

Catheter-Related Complications

Discomfort Related to the PD Catheter

The most common catheter-related complaint shortly after postoperative healing is that the patient can feel the catheter poking, particularly when the peritoneal cavity is empty. This typically resolves within a few weeks and can usually be managed by leaving 200 to 300 ml of dialysis solution in the peritoneal cavity when the patient is not dialyzing. When the discomfort does not resolve within a few weeks, treatment options include catheter repositioning or use of tidal PD (Twardowski, 2002c)

Some patients also complain of infusion pain. This is related to the "jet effect" of the rapid infusion of dialysis solution in catheters with a straight intra-peritoneal segment. Slowing the infusion rate can alleviate infusion pain.

Catheter Malfunction

There are two types of catheter obstructions – one-way, where the catheter can be used for infusion, but does not drain well, and two-way, where the catheter will neither infuse nor drain adequately, if at all. The nursing management is aimed at determining the cause of the problems and correcting the underlying cause(s).

A two-way malfunction is most commonly caused by kinks or clamps on the tubing or catheter and by clots. The nurse should inspect the entire length of the catheter, extension set, and tubing for closed clamps, kinks, or visible fibrin or clots. Kinks must be straightened and clamps opened appropriately to allow flow. It is also possible for the catheter to have an internal kink. Both lateral and posterior-anterior x-rays of the abdomen are required to confirm or rule out an internal kink.

PD catheters can become occluded with blood or fibrin clots. Blood clots are most common shortly after catheter placement (see Surgical Complications, above), but fibrin clots can occur at any time during the course of PD therapy. To prevent catheter obstruction, intraperitoneal heparin (250-500 u/L) is added to the dialysis solution when there are signs of bleeding, during peritonitis, and when there is visible fibrin (Daugirdas, Blake, & Ing, 2001). Occasionally, there is a patient with fibrin formation in every drain bag. Daily addition of heparin to the overnight or longest dwell exchange may prevent catheter obstruction (Zappacosta & Perras, 1984).

Treatment for clotted catheters includes catheter irriga-

tion, mechanical removal of the clot, and the use of thrombolytic agents (Daugirdas et al., 2001). Some clots can be dislodged by squeezing the bag of dialysis solution to increase the pressure. The goal is to dislodge the fibrin clot and detach fibrin from the tip and side holes of the catheter. Another approach is to irrigate the catheter using dialysis or saline solution in a large syringe. First, solution is flushed vigorously through the catheter, and then if the catheter does not drain spontaneously, attempts can be made to gently aspirate the catheter. The aspiration should be stopped if pressure is felt, so that adjacent tissue will not be pulled into the catheter (Verger, 2004).

Historically, streptokinase and urokinase were the thrombolytics used for peritoneal catheter obstruction by thrombi (Benevent, Peyronnet, Brignon, & Leroux-Robert, 1985; Wiegmann et al., 1985). Streptokinase was less expensive but had a higher risk of anaphylactic reactions (Daugirdas et al., 2001), so urokinase was more widely used. When urokinase was taken off the market in the U.S. for a period of time, this prompted the use of tissue plasminogen activator (tPA) for peritoneal catheter obstruction (Sahani et al., 2000). Before tPA is administered, the system is checked for kinks or clamps and an attempt is made to irrigate the catheter. Additionally, catheter position may be checked by abdominal x-ray. Then, 1 mg/ml of tPA is infused in an amount sufficient to fill the catheter and allowed to dwell for 1-2 hours (Zorzanello, Fleming, & Prowant, 2004). The solution is then aspirated and an attempt is made to drain by gravity. If the occlusion is resolved, the catheter is flushed with heparinized solution before resuming routine dialysis.

A one-way catheter malfunction can be caused by catheter kinks, malposition or migration, omental wrapping of the catheter, or entrapment of the catheter between loops of bowel. First, the assessment should evaluate bowel function and determine if the patient is constipated. If constipation is not present or is corrected and the problem remains, catheter malposition is likely. The catheter can be moved upward, out of the pelvis by peristalsis; this is more likely when the catheter tip is located on the right side (de la Cruz, Dimkovic, Bargman, Vas, & Oreopoulos, 2001), or the catheter can be caught up and trapped by the omentum. Simple catheter tip migration generally presents as adequate inflow and poor outflow when the patient is upright, but good outflow when the patient assumes a supine or side-lying position. An abdominal x-ray will document the catheter position. If the catheter has migrated upwards on the left side, the peristalsis of the descending colon may bring it back down; however, catheters translocated to the right upper abdomen usually do not return, because peristalsis of the ascending colon continues to push the tip upwards.

Laxatives or enemas may be given to correct constipation. Laxatives may also be used to stimulate peristalsis in an effort to bring catheters displaced to the left upper quadrant back down into the pelvis. Catheter repositioning may be attempted using a flexible metal device inserted through the catheter or by peritoneoscopy or surgery (Daugirdas et al., 2001).

Use of radiopaque contrast infused through the

Figure 28-13
A Nylon Tie in Place Over the Catheter/Adapter Junction to Prevent Accidental Loss of the Adapter

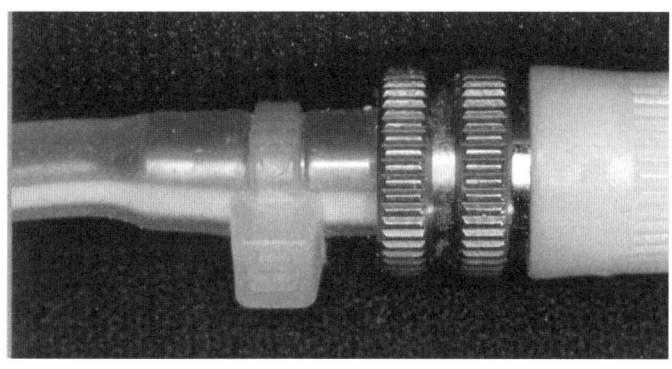

catheter (using sterile technique) may demonstrate omental wrapping, characterized by occlusion of some or all of the catheter openings. Contrast media infused through the catheter remains near the catheter, trapped by the omentum, and does not disperse through the peritoneal cavity. If the impedance to flow is significant, partial omentectomy may be indicated, either surgically or laparoscopically.

It is possible for a newly implanted catheter to have a pinpoint hole or linear defect resulting in a subcutaneous or external leak; however, catheter defects are more typically the result of long-term wear.

Cuff Extrusion

The primary cause of cuff extrusion is placement of the subcutaneous cuff too close to the exit site. Anchoring of the catheter too tautly or in any formation other than its natural shape also increases the risk of cuff extrusion. Catheter resilience or "shape memory" causes the catheter to slowly assume its original shape, which may push the cuff out of the sinus. This is a problem when a straight catheter is implanted with an arcuate tunnel.

Cuff extrusion frequently causes an exit-site infection, which is difficult to completely resolve until the cuff has completely extruded. The converse is also true. Cuff infection can cause cuff extrusion via tissue retraction around the cuff. Once the cuff is completely extruded, it can be shaved from the catheter, if necessary, to avoid skin irritation.

Damage to the Catheter

As catheters age, the material may deteriorate and become brittle. The catheters may crumble or crack, or break into two pieces. These problems are most likely to occur near the exit site where the catheter material is exposed to cleansing agents, antibiotics, and ointments or creams. Cracks may also develop at or near the adapter where the weight of the adapter causes the catheter to bend. The edge of the adapter may wear against the catheter, eventually damaging it. Cracks can also occur along the radiopaque stripe.

The single-piece, barbed catheter adapters, used before the introduction of the two-piece locking adapters, could become dislodged or fall out completely. This is due to the use of an inappropriate size adapter, stretching of the silastic tubing, or the adapter being accidentally pulled out of the catheter. An innovation to prevent accidental separation was placement of a nylon band over the catheter/adapter junction (see Figure 28-13). These bands were used successfully for many years (Schmidt, Craig, Prowant, & Twardowski, 1990).

In order to avoid contamination of the peritoneal cavity and subsequent peritonitis, patients should understand that a broken or leaking catheter should be covered with a sterile dressing and clamped immediately. The damaged catheter should not be used for dialysis exchanges. When damage to the catheter is at the distal end of the external segment, it can be easily repaired by cutting off the damaged segment and inserting a new adapter. When damage is close to the exit site, the catheter must be removed or have an extension added. Catheters with 2-3 cm of remaining external length can be lengthened with a 15 cm extension commercially available in a repair kit (Peri-Patch® Repair Kit, Tyco Healthcare, Mansfield, MA). A procedure for repairing the catheter is outlined in Table 28-7. The procedure can be modified to cut off the damaged segment of the catheter and/or to replace an adapter. A short course of prophylactic antibiotics is recommended (Usha et al., 1998).

Exit-Site and Tunnel Infections

Exit-site infection is a serious complication that can lead to tunnel infection, peritonitis, and catheter loss. The likelihood of sequelae increases with the intensity of symptoms. For instance, catheters with only erythema at the exit site rarely require removal; however, if there is purulent drainage from the exit site the risk of catheter removal is over 20% (Piraino, 1996a). Infectious complications account for > 75% of PD catheter removals (Gokal et al., 1998).

Distribution of Organisms

S. aureus has consistently been identified as the leading cause of exit site and tunnel infections (about 60% of infections) (Burkart, 1996; Piraino, 1996a). Cultures of catheter infections often grow multiple organisms, typically the second most frequent etiology of catheter infections. *Staphylococcus epidermidis,* enteric gram-negative organisms, and *Pseudomonas aeruginosa* (*P. aeruginosa*) are less common, each responsible for about 10% of catheter infections (Burkart, 1996; Piraino, 1996a). A few infections do not grow organisms on culture, and 1-3% of infections are fungal. *S. aureus* and *P. aeruginosa* exit-site infections are difficult to cure and can result in tunnel infections, peritonitis, and catheter loss. For treatment of these infections, Piraino (1996a) recommends extended courses of antibiotic therapy, the addition of oral rifampin for *S. aureus*, and removal of the subcutaneous catheter cuff, if indicated.

Nursing Care of Inflamed and Infected Exits Sites

Nursing care of an infected exit site has four major components – assessment, cauterization of exuberant granulation tissue, appropriate modifications in the exit-site care regimen, and patient education. Principles of

Table 28-7
Procedure for Extension or Repair of a Silastic PD Catheter

Supplies
- Peri-Patch Repair Kit®
- Drapes
- Scalpel blade
- Scalpel handle
- Sterile gloves
- PD transfer set
- Scissors
- Povidone iodine solution
- Mask
- Surgical cap (optional)

Key Steps
- When damage is reported, instruct patient to cover the area with sterile gauze and clamp catheter

At the outpatient clinic or emergency room:
- Mask, scrub hands, and don sterile gloves
- Prepare the damaged area of catheter:
  - disinfect area with two 1-minute scrubs using povidone iodine scrub
  - soak area in povidone iodine solution for 5 minutes
  - place disinfected catheter on sterile drape
- Prepare catheter repair kit
- Place a Beta-Cap® clamp on catheter extension tubing (do not close)
- Cut the old catheter proximal to the damaged area
- Allow approximately 10 ml of dialysate to flow out
- While draining, insert the barbed Teflon connector into the original peritoneal catheter
- Close the clamp on the catheter extension
- Dry connection site (the distal catheter and Teflon connector) with sterile gauze
- Wrap the mold around the barbed connector, fill with silicone glue and secure with the locking ring
- Place appropriate adapter in the extended catheter
- Connect to a new transfer set (PD may be resumed)
- Remove the mold after 72 hours

Note: Adapted from Usha, K., Ponferrada, L., Prowant, B.F., & Twardowski, Z.J. (1998). Repair of chronic peritoneal dialysis catheter. *Peritoneal Dialysis International, 18*(4), 419-423.

nursing care for an infected catheter exit site are outlined in Table 28-8.

Assessment of the inflamed exit site includes visual inspection, palpation of the deep cuff, obtaining pertinent history from the patient, and obtaining exit-site cultures. Pertinent history includes a description of any recent trauma, bleeding, irritation, or pain at the exit site; a determination of when the first symptoms of infection occurred; and a description of current exit-site care procedure as well as the frequency of care. The exit site should be assessed, classified, and cultures obtained prior to cleaning the exit site. When exudate is present, the drainage should be cultured rather than the skin at the exit site. This will increase the likelihood that the organisms grown on culture are

Table 28-8
Principles of Nursing Care for the Infected Exit Site

- Culture exudate (not skin); if exudate is not visible, gently squeeze the subcutaneous cuff and pull gently on the catheter in an attempt to express exudate
- Cauterize all exuberant granulation tissue and slightly exuberant granulation tissue in the sinus
- Increase frequency of exit care to daily or BID
- Topical soaks may be used as an adjunct to antibiotic therapy
- Do not use cytotoxic agents on external granulation tissue or in the sinus
- Do not forcibly remove crusts or scabs
- Use sterile dressings
- Immobilize the catheter
- Reassess exit at least every other week
- Do not submerge the exit

Note: Adapted from Prowant, B.F., & Twardowski, Z.J. (1996). Recommendations for exit care. *Peritoneal Dialysis International, 16*(Suppl. 3), S94-S99.

those responsible for the infection and not simply resident bacteria. Holley and Moss (1988) found that by tugging gently downward on the catheter while squeezing the subcutaneous cuff, they could express drainage from the sinus that was not seen otherwise.

Cauterization of exuberant granulation tissue ("proud flesh") facilitates healing. This is done by gently touching the granulation tissue with the tip of a silver nitrate stick. Care should be taken not to touch healthy tissue. The cauterized granulation tissue turns a grayish-white. One application may be sufficient for an equivocal or acute infection, but several cauterizations, once or twice weekly, may be required for a chronic infection. As the exit site heals, there is often a grayish discoloration of the skin around the exit site.

Changes in care for the infected exit site include increased frequency of care. Daily or twice daily care is generally recommended. Changing the cleansing agent is also common. It may be necessary to change the cleansing agent if it is irritating or if it is a medical antiseptic that is cytotoxic. Topical soaks have been used as an adjunct to antibiotic therapy. Strauss, Holmes, Nortman, and Friedman (1993) described the use of warm hypertonic saline compresses applied for 5-10 minutes three times daily along with antibiotic therapy to resolve "complicated" infections. Leung, Mok, Yu, and Au (2001) used a 1:1 solution of vinegar and sterile water as an adjunct to oral antibiotic therapy for *P. aeruginosa* infections. Sodium hypochlorite, normal saline, dilute hydrogen peroxide, and even povidone iodine and 70% alcohol solutions have also been used for exit-site soaks (Prowant et al., 1993); however, the efficacy of these has not been established, and as mentioned above, some of these solutions may actually damage tissue and delay healing. Soaks may be helpful;

however, in softening, large irritating crusts and scabs can develop over "proud flesh." Finally, some have recommended treating the infected exit site as an open wound and returning to a more conservative exit-site care procedure similar to that used for care post catheter implantation. This would include the use of sterile dressings.

Medical Treatment of Exit-Site Infections

Except where noted otherwise, the following recommendations for antibiotic therapy for infected exit sites are based on the ISPD 1998 update of practices for optimum access (Gokal et al., 1998).

Treatment of Equivocal Exit Sites

Equivocal exit sites may improve with silver nitrate cauterization alone or with topical antibiotic therapy combined with cauterization of any exuberant granulation tissue. Mupirocin, Neosporin®, and gentamicin ointment or gentamicin ophthalmic solution have been used and recommended, depending on the causative organism(s); however, Piraino (1996b) cautions against the use of Neosporin because of a high rate of contact hypersensitivity. Povidone-iodine ointment has also been used successfully (Hirsch & Jindal, 2003; Waite, Webster, Laurel, Johnson, & Fong, 1997). Since there is minimal drainage, a topically applied antibiotic stays at the exit site rather than being washed away by exudate, as occurs in acute infections. However, if there is not improvement within 2 weeks, a change to systemic antibiotics is indicated. For equivocal infections, it is recommended that therapy be continued for an additional week after the exit site achieves a healthy appearance.

Treatment of Acute infection

Recommended treatment of acute exit-site infections is immediate, systemic antibiotic therapy to cover gram-positive organisms with adjustment of the antibiotic when culture results are obtained. Specifically, a first generation cephalosporin is recommended for gram-positive organisms and a quinolone for gram-negative organisms, reserving vancomycin use for methacillin-resistant *S. aureus*. Exuberant and slightly exuberant granulation tissue should be cauterized. It is important to reevaluate the exit site periodically to determine the response to treatment. If the infection does not improve, the antibiotic can be changed or a second, synergistic antibiotic added. Rifampin is frequently added for staphylococcal infections. Most acute infections respond to treatment. Therapy should be continued for an additional week after the exit site achieves a healthy appearance (Gokal et al., 1998; Twardowski & Prowant, 1997).

Treatment of Chronic Infections

Exuberant granulation tissue is frequently present in chronic infections (see Figure 28-14) and may require repeated cauterization. A combination of synergistic antibiotics is recommended for chronic infections rather than a single agent in order to avoid the emergence of resistant organisms. Response to treatment is slow, and follow up every 2 weeks is recommended. Both bacterial flora and sensitivities may change during prolonged treatment, so the exit site should be recultured at each visit if there has been no improvement on appropriate therapy. Antibiotic treatment and local care should be continued until the exit site achieves a healthy appearance and can be classified as a "good" exit. If the exit site becomes equivocal and remains so, a topical antibiotic can replace systemic antibiotics.

Diagnosis and Treatment of Tunnel and Cuff Infections

Tunnel infections typically involve the subcutaneous catheter cuff and are also referred to as cuff infections. Symptoms of tunnel infection include erythema, tenderness, and/or edema over the cuff or along the subcutaneous tunnel with or without exudate. Positive findings on ultrasound examination of the tunnel are helpful in diagnosing tunnel and cuff infections. Ultrasonography can be used to determine the presence and severity of infection as well as to evaluate the response to treatment (Vychtil, Lilaj, Lorenz, Hörl, Haag-Weber, 1999). Negative ultrasound findings, however, do not rule out an infection.

Tunnel infections respond to antibiotic therapy slowly, and a complete cure without recurrence is not likely. Cuff shaving and tunnel revision procedures prolong catheter life for several weeks or months, but eventually up to half of the catheters are removed for cuff infection, often with concurrent peritonitis (Scalamogna, De Vecchi, Maccario, Castelnovo, & Ponticelli, 1995; Twardowski & Prowant, 1996c; Twardowski, 2002b). In a series of 41 cuff-shaving procedures, Scalamogna et al. (1995) noted that cuff shaving was effective for all *S. epidermidis* infections and half of *S. aureus* infections but was ineffective in gram-negative infections. There are several different "cuff shaving" procedures. In the simplest procedure, the subcutaneous cuff can be removed without revising either the exit site or tunnel. More aggressive procedures include opening the tunnel and debriding surrounding tissue and/or moving the tunnel and creating a new exit site.

Catheter Outcomes

Infectious complications remain the primary reason for catheter removal followed by catheter malfunction (Verrina et al., 1993); however, catheter survival rates have slowly improved due to improvements in catheter design, surgical technique, and catheter care. Burkart (1998) suggests that the lowest acceptable catheter survival rate is 80% at 1 year. Survival rates as high as 90% and 95% (Eklund et al., 1995; Lye, Kour, van der Straaten, Leong, & Lee, 1996) have been reported.

Removal of PD Catheters

Removal of an acute, uncuffed catheter is a simple procedure. The anchoring sutures are cut and the catheter is pulled out, an antibiotic ointment is applied, and the skin opening is covered with a sterile dressing.

Indications for removal of chronic PD catheters are listed in Table 28-9. Because there is tissue ingrowth into the subcutaneous and intramuscular catheter cuffs, catheters must be removed by careful surgical dissection. Ash (2003) provides a detailed step-by-step description of the surgical technique for removal of a double-cuff catheter. General

Table 28-9
Indications for Removal of a Chronic PD Catheter

- Peritonitis
  - fungal peritonitis
  - fecal peritonitis
  - peritonitis with concurrent chronic exit/site tunnel infection
  - peritonitis that does not resolve

- Chronic tunnel infection

- Catheter-related sepsis

- Encapsulating peritoneal sclerosis

- Malfunctioning catheter

- Broken catheter

- Unresolved catheter leak
  - external
  - subcutaneous

- Unresolved pleuro-peritoneal communication

Note: Adapted from Prowant, B.F., & Twardowski, Z.J. (1996). Recommendations for exit care. *Peritoneal Dialysis International, 16*(Suppl. 3), S94-S99.

Figure 28-14
Exuberant Granulation Tissue at the Exit Site During a Chronic Infection

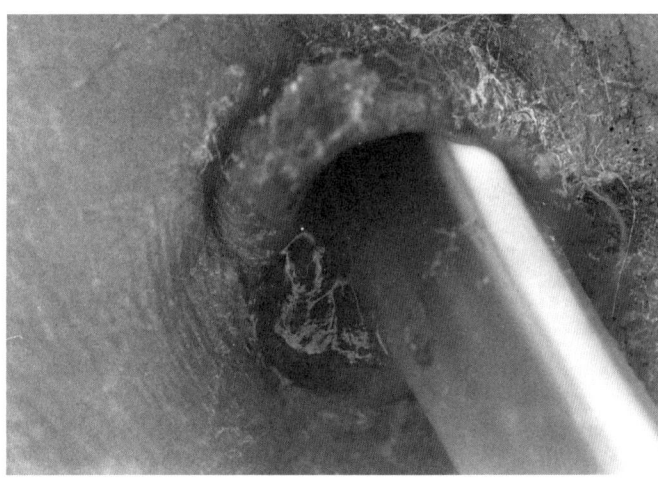

anesthesia is recommended for patients with catheters implanted in the belly of the rectus muscle and patients with swan-neck Missouri and Toronto Western catheters (Twardowski & Nichols, 2000). It is critical that all portions of the cuffs be removed, as residual Dacron® material may serve as a nidus for chronic infection. The opening at the deep cuff and peritoneum is closed with sutures. The skin incision may be closed or may be packed and left open to heal by secondary intention in the case of exit or tunnel infection. Twardowski and Nichols (2000) report good results with calcium-sodium alginate fiber dressings (Kaltostat® Wound Dressing, ConvaTec, Woerden, The Netherlands), as the fibers absorb exudate, control minor bleeding, and protect the wound from contamination.

In many cases, catheter removal and replacement can be done at the same time. This is ideal for malfunctioning or malpositioned catheters and has also been used successfully during infectious complications (Swartz, Messana, Reynolds, & Ranjit, 1991). Placement of the new catheter precedes removal of the infected catheter. The consensus peritonitis treatment guidelines (Keane et al., 2000) recommend the simultaneous procedure for relapsing peritonitis believed due to biofilm formation on the intra-abdominal catheter segment (primarily coagulase negative Staphylococcus) or to tunnel infections (primarily *S. aureus*). The guidelines also recommended that this approach be used only after effective antibiotic therapy when the effluent WBC is < 100/μL. Simultaneous replacement is not recommended for peritonitis episodes due to Pseudomonas species, fungi, or mycobacterium, or when an intra-abdominal abscess or intra-abdominal source of peritonitis is suspected (Keane et al., 2000).

Summary

Since the resurgence of PD in the 1970s, there has been ongoing research focused on improving PD access. New catheters, improved implantation techniques, antibiotic prophylaxis, and attention to catheter and exit-site care have decreased the incidence of catheter-related infections and increased catheter survival. Yet, there is still a paucity of prospective randomized studies comparing outcomes of new catheter designs, techniques for exit-site care, and treatment strategies for catheter-related infections. Research addressing these and other clinical aspects of PD catheters will provide a body of evidence to further enhance practice and improve outcomes.

References

Ahmad, S. (1999). *Manual of clinical dialysis.* London: Science Press.

Annigeri, R., Conly, J., Vas, S.I., Dedier, H., Prakashan, K.P., Bargman, J.M., Jassal, V., & Oreopoulos, D. (2001). Emergence of mupirocin-resistant *Staphylococcus aureus* in chronic peritoneal dialysis patients using mupirocin prophylaxis to prevent exit-site infection. *Peritoneal Dialysis International, 21*(6), 554-559.

Ash, S.R. (2002). Peritoneal access devices and placement techniques. In A.R. Nissenson & R.N. Fine (Eds.), *Dialysis therapy* (3rd ed., pp. 45-50). Philadelphia: Hanley & Belfus.

Ash, S.R. (2003). Chronic peritoneal dialysis catheters: Overview of design, placement, and removal procedures. *Seminars in Dialysis, 16*(4), 323-334.

Ash, S.R., Carr, D.J., & Diaz-Buxo, J.A. (1995). Peritoneal access devices: Hydraulic function and biocompatibility. In A.R. Nissenson, R.N. Fine, & D.E. Gentile (Eds.), *Clinical Dialysis,* (3rd ed.) (pp. 295-321). Norwalk, CT: Appleton & Lange.

Ash, S.R., & Janle, E.M. (1993). T-fluted peritoneal dialysis catheter. *Advances in Peritoneal Dialysis, 9,* 223-226.

Ash, S.R., Sutton, J.M., Mankus, R.A., Rossman, J., de Ridder, V., Nassvi, M.S., & Ross, J. (2002). Clinical trials of the T-fluted (Ash Advantage) peritoneal dialysis catheter. *Advances in Renal Replacement Therapy, 9*(2), 133-143.

Benevent, D., Peyronnet, P., Brignon, P., & Leroux-Robert, C. (1985). Urokinase infusion for obstructed catheters and peritonitis (Letter). *Peritoneal Dialysis Bulletin, 5,* 77.

Bernardini, J., Piraino, B., Holley, J., Johnston, J.R., & Lutes, R. (1996). Randomized trial of *Staphylococcus aureus* prophylaxis in peritoneal dialysis patients: Mupirocin calcium ointment 2% applied to the exit site versus cyclic oral rifampin. *American Journal of*

Kidney Diseases, 27(5), 695-700.

Bernardini, J., Bender, F., Florio, T., Sloand, J., Palmmontalbano, L., Fried, L., & Piraino, B. (2005). Randomized, double-blind trial of antibiotic exit site cream for prevention of exit site infection in peritoneal dialysis patients. *Journal American Society of Nephrology, 16*(2), 539-545.

Bishop, D., Harris, D., & Hays, F. (1996). Effective, inexpensive exit-site care (Abstract). *Peritoneal Dialysis International, 16*(Suppl. 2), S49.

Boen, S.T., Mion, C.M., Curtis, F.K., & Shilipetar, G. (1964). Periodic peritoneal dialysis using the repeated puncture technique and an automatic cycling machine. *Transactions American Society Artificial Internal Organs, 10,* 409-414.

Boen, S.T., Mulinari, A.S., Dillard, D.H., & Scribner, B.H. (1962). Periodic peritoneal dialysis in the management of chronic uremia. *Transactions American Society Artificial Internal Organs, 8,* 256-265.

Burkart, J.M. (1996). Significance, epidemiology, and prevention of peritoneal dialysis catheter infections. *Peritoneal Dialysis International, 16*(Suppl. 1), S340-S346.

Burkart, J.M. (1998). Strategies for optimizing peritoneal dialysis catheter outcomes: Catheter implantation issues. *Journal of the American Society of Nephrology, 9,* S130-S136.

Casey, M., Taylor, J., Clinard, P., Graham, A., Mauck, V., Spainhour, L., Brown, P., & Burkart, J. (2000). Application of mupirocin cream at the catheter exit site reduces exit-site infections and peritonitis in peritoneal dialysis patients. *Peritoneal Dialysis International, 20,* 566-574.

Chadha, V., Jones, L.L., Ramirez, Z.D., & Warady, B.A. (2000). Chest wall peritoneal dialysis catheter placement in infants with a colostomy. *Advances in Peritoneal Dialysis, 16,* 318-320.

Chiaramonte, S., Bragantini, L., Brendolan, A., Conz, P., Crepaldi, C., Dell'Aquila, R., Feriani, M., Milan, M., Ronco, C., & La Greca, G. (1992). Long-term experience with the Vicenza catheter. In K. Ota, J.F. Maher, J.F. Winchester, & P. Hirszel (Eds.), *Current concepts in peritoneal dialysis* (pp. 160-163). Amsterdam: Excerpta Medica, Elsevier Science Publishers.

Connolly, S., Noble, W.C., & Phillips, I. (1993). Mupirocin resistance in coagulase-negative staphylococci. *Journal of Medical Microbiology, 39,* 450-453.

Crabtree, J.H. (2003). Clinical biodurability of aliphatic polyether based polyurethanes as peritoneal dialysis catheters. *ASAIO Journal, 49*(3), 290-294.

Crabtree, J.H., Burchette, R.J., Siddiqi, R.A., Huen, I.T., Hadnott, L.L., & Fishman, A. (2003). The efficacy of silver-ion implanted catheters in reducing peritoneal dialysis-related infections. *Peritoneal Dialysis International, 23*(4), 368-374.

Crabtree, J. H., Siddiqi, R.A., Chung, J.J., & Greenwald, L.T. (1998). Long-term experience with polyurethane, pail handle, coiled tip peritoneal dialysis catheters. *ASAIO Journal, 44*(4), 309-313.

Cruz, C. (1992). Clinical experience with a new peritoneal dialysis access device (the Cruz™ catheter). In K. Ota, J.F. Maher, J.F. Winchester, & P. Hirszel (Eds.), *Current concepts in peritoneal dialysis* (pp. 164-169). Amsterdam: Excerpta Medica, Elsevier Science Publishers.

Cruz, C. (1996). Implantation techniques for peritoneal dialysis catheters. *Peritoneal Dialysis International, 16*(Suppl. 1), S319-S321.

Cruz, C. (1997). The Cruz catheter and its functional characteristics. *Peritoneal Dialysis International, 17*(Suppl. 2), S146-S148.

Danielsson, A., Blohmé, L., Tranæus, A., & Hylander, B. (2002). A prospective randomized study of the effect of a subcutaneously "buried" peritoneal dialysis catheter technique versus standard technique on the incidence of peritonitis and exit-site infection. *Peritoneal Dialysis International, 22*(2), 211-219.

Dasgupta, M. K. (1994). Silver peritoneal catheters reduce bacterial colonization. *Advances in Peritoneal Dialysis, 10,* 195-198.

Dasgupta, M. K. (2002). Moncrief-Popovich catheter and implantation technique: The AV fistula of peritoneal dialysis. *Advances in Renal Replacement Therapy, 9*(2), 116-124.

de la Cruz, M.C., Dimkovic, N., Bargman, J.M., Vas, S.I., & Oreopoulos, D.G. (2001). Is catheter function influenced by the side of the body in which the peritoneal dialysis catheter is placed? (Letter). *Peritoneal Dialysis International, 21*(5), 526.

Daugirdas, J.T., Blake, P.G., & Ing, T.S. (Eds.). (2001). *Handbook of dialysis* (3rd ed.). Philadelphia: Lippincott Williams & Wilkins.

Dérot, M., Tanret, P. Roussillon, J., & Bernier, J.J. (1949). La dialyse péritonéale dans le traitement de l'urémie aiguë. *Journal of Urology, 55,* 113-121.

Diaz-Buxo, J.A. (2002). Streaming, mixing, and recirculation: Role of the peritoneal access in continuous flow peritoneal dialysis (clinical considerations). *Advances in Peritoneal Dialysis, 18,* 87-90.

Di Paolo, N., Petrini, G., Garosi, G., Buoncristiani, U., Brardi, S., & Monaci, G. (1996). A new self-locating peritoneal catheter. *Peritoneal Dialysis International, 16*(6), 623-627.

Doolan, P. D., Murphy, W. P. Jr., Wiggins, R. A., Carter, N. W., Cooper W. C., Watten, R. H., & Alpen, E. L. (1959). An evaluation of intermittent peritoneal lavage. *American Journal of Medicine, 26,* 831-844.

Eklund, B.H., Honkanen, E.O., Kala, A.-R., & Kyllönen, L.E. (1995). Peritoneal dialysis access: Prospective randomized comparison of the swan neck and Tenckhoff catheters. *Peritoneal Dialysis International, 15*(8), 353-356.

Frank, H.A., Seligman, A.M., & Fine, J. (1946). Treatment of uremia after acute renal failure by peritoneal irrigation. *Journal of the American Medical Association, 130*(11), 703-705.

Gadallah, M.F., Mignone, J., Torres, C., Ramdeen, G., & Pervez, A. (2000). The role of peritoneal dialysis catheter configuration in preventing catheter tip migration. *Advances in Peritoneal Dialysis, 16,* 47-50.

Gadallah, M.F., Pervez, A., El-Shahawy, M.A., Sorrells, D., Zibari, G., McDonald, J., & Work, J. (1999). Peritoneoscopic versus surgical placement of peritoneal dialysis catheters: A prospective randomized study on outcome. *American Journal of Kidney Diseases, 33*(1), 118-122.

Gadallah, M.F., Ramdeen, G., Mignone, J., Patel, D., Mitchell, L., & Tatro, S. (2000). Role of preoperative antibiotic prophylaxis in preventing postoperative peritonitis in newly placed peritoneal dialysis catheters. *American Journal of Kidney Diseases, 36*(5), 1014-1019.

Goetz, A., & Muder, R.R. (1989). *Pseudomonas aeruginosa* infections associated with use of povidone-iodine in patients receiving continuous ambulatory peritoneal dialysis. *Infection Control and Hospital Epidemiology, 10*(10), 447-450.

Gokal, R., Alexander, S., Ash, S., Chen, T.W., Danielson, A., Holmes, C., Joffe, P., Moncrief, J., Nichols, K., Piraino, B., Prowant, B., Slingeneyer, A., Stegmayr, B., Twardowski, Z., & Vas, S. (1998). Peritoneal catheters and exit-site practices toward optimum peritoneal access: 1998 update. *Peritoneal Dialysis International, 18*(1), 11-33.

Golper, T.A., Brier, M.E., Bunke, M., Schreiber, M.J., Bartlett, D.K., Hamilton, R.W., Strife, F., & Hamburger, R.J. for the Academic Subcommittee of the Steering Committee of the Network 9 Peritonitis and Catheter Survival Studies. (1996). Risk factors for peritonitis in long-term peritoneal dialysis: The Network 9 peritonitis and catheter survival studies. *American Journal of Kidney Diseases, 28*(3), 428-436.

Gotloib, L., Nisencorn, I., Garmizo, A.L., Galili, N., Servadio, C., & Sudarski, M. (1975). Subcutaneous intraperitoneal prosthesis for maintenance peritoneal dialysis. *Lancet, 1*(7920), 1318-1320.

Graff, J., Joffe, P., & Ladefoged, S.D. (1992). An assessment of the flow rate within peritoneal dialysis catheters, using a standardized in vitro technique. *Advances in Peritoneal Dialysis,* 294-297.

Grollman, A., Turner, L. B., & McLean, J. A. (1951). Intermittent peritoneal lavage in nephrectomized dogs and its application to the human being. *Archives of Internal Medicine, 87*(3), 379-390.

Gruart, P., Andreu, L., & Gil, A. (1999). The influence of hygienic practices to the exit site/tunnel on peritoneal catheter infections. *EDTNA/ERCA Journal, 25*(2), 19-21.

Gutch, C.F. (1964). Peritoneal dialysis. *Transactions ASAIO, 10,* 406-407.

Hasbargen, B.J., Rodgers, D.J., Hasbargen, J.A., Quinn, M.J., & James, M.K. (1993). Exit-site care – Is it time for a change? *Peritoneal Dialysis International, 13*(Suppl. 2), S313-S315.

Harvey, E., Braj, B., & Balfe, J.W. (1998). Prevention, diagnosis, and treatment of PD catheter exit-site and tunnel infections in children. In R.N. Fine, S.R. Alexander, & B.A. Warady (Eds.), *CAPD/CCPD in children* (2ⁿᵈ ed.) (pp. 349-367). Boston: Kluwer Academic Publishers.

Hirsch, D.J., & Jindal, K.K. (2003). Local care of *Staphylococcus aureus* exit-site infection precludes antibiotic use. *Peritoneal Dialysis International, 23*(3), 301-302.

Holley, J.L., & Moss, A.H. (1988). Improved diagnosis of CAPD exit-site infections with catheter manipulation and the use of a grading system. *Advances in Continuous Ambulatory Peritoneal Dialysis, 4,* 177-180.

Jacob, G.B., & Deane, N. (1967). Repeated peritoneal dialysis by the catheter replacement method: Description of technique and a replaceable prosthesis for chronic access to the peritoneal cavity. *Proceedings European Dialysis Transplant Association, 4,*136-140.

Keane, W.F., Bailie, G.R., Boeschoten, E., Gokal, R., Golper, T.A., Holmes, C.J., Kawaguchi, Y., Piraino, B., Riella, M., & Vas, S. (2000). Adult peritoneal dialysis-related peritonitis treatment recommendations: 2000 update. *Peritoneal Dialysis International, 20*(4), 396-411. Erratum in (2000). *Peritoneal Dialysis International, 20*(6), 828-829.

Khandelwal, M., Bailey, S., Izatt, S., Chu, M., Vas, S., Bargman, J., & Oreopoulos, D. (2003). Structural changes in silicon rubber peritoneal dialysis catheters in patients using mupirocin at the exit site. *International Journal of Artificial Organs, 26*(10), 913-917.

Kubota, M., Kanazawa, M., Takahashi, Y., Io, H., Ishiguro, N., & Tomino, Y. (2001). Implantation of presternal catheter using Moncrief technique: Aiming for fewer catheter-related complications. *Peritoneal Dialysis International, 21*(Suppl. 3), S205-S208.

Legrain, M., & Merrill, J.P. (1953). Short-term continuous transperitoneal dialysis: A simplified technique. *New England Journal of Medicine, 248*(4), 125-129.

Leung, D.K.-C., Mok, W.F.-M., Yu, D.M.-W., & Au, T.-C. (2001). Use of distilled white vinegar dressing supplemental to oral antibiotics in the management of *Pseudomonas aeruginosa* exit-site infection in continuous ambulatory peritoneal dialysis. *Hong Kong Journal of Nephrology, 3*(1), 38-40.

Levy, M., Balfe, J.W., Geary, D., Fryer-Keene, S., & Bannatyne, R. (1990). Exit-site infection during continuous and cycling peritoneal dialysis in children. *Peritoneal Dialysis International, 10*(1), 31-35.

Lewis, S.M. (2000). Inflammation and infection. In S.M. Lewis, M.M. Heitkemper, & S.R. Dirksen, *Medical-surgical nursing* (5th ed.) (pp. 189-211). St. Louis: Mosby.

Lindblad, A. S., Hamilton, R. W., Nolph, K. D., & Novak, J. W. (1988). A retrospective analysis of catheter configuration and cuff type: A National CAPD Registry report. *Peritoneal Dialysis International, 8*(2), 129-133.

Lineaweaver, W., Howard, R., Soucy, D., McMorris, S., Freeman, J., Crain, C., Robertson, J., & Rumley, T. (1985). Topical antimicrobial toxicity. *Archives of Surgery, 120,* 267-270.

Luzar, M.A., Brown, C.B., Balf, D., Hill, L., Issad, B., Monnier, B., Moulart, J., Sabatier, J.-C., Wauquier, J.-P., & Peluso, F. (1990). Exit-site care and exit-site infection in continuous ambulatory peritoneal dialysis (CAPD): Results of a randomized multicenter trial. *Peritoneal Dialysis International, 10*(1), 25-29.

Lye, W.-C., Kour, N.-W., van der Straaten, J.C., Leong, S.-O., & Lee, E.J.C. (1996). A prospective randomized comparison of the swan neck, coiled, and straight Tenckhoff catheters in patients on CAPD. *Peritoneal Dialysis International, 16*(Suppl. 1), S333-S335.

Malette, W.G., McPhaul, J.J., Bledsoe, F., McIntosh, D.A., & Koegel, E. (1964). A clinically successful subcutaneous peritoneal access button for repeated peritoneal dialysis. *Transactions American Society of Artificial Internal Organs, 10,* 396-399.

Maxwell, M.H., Rockney, R.E., Kleeman, C.R., & Twiss, M.R. (1959). Peritoneal dialysis. I. Technique and applications. *Journal of the American Medical Association, 170*(8), 917-924.

McDonald, H.P. Jr., Gerber, N., Mishra, D., Wolin, L., Peng, B., & Waterhouse, K. (1968). Subcutaneous Dacron and Teflon cloth adjuncts for silastic arteriovenous shunts and peritoneal dialysis catheters. *Transactions American Society of Artificial Internal Organs, 14,*176-180.

Moncrief, J.W., Popovich, R.P., Broadrick, L.J., He, Z.Z., Simmons, E.E., & Tate, R.A. (1993). The Moncrief-Popovich catheter: A new peritoneal access technique for patients on peritoneal dialysis. *ASAIO Journal, 39,* 62-65.

Mupirocin Study Group. (1996). Nasal mupirocin prevents *Staphylococcus aureus* exit-site infection during peritoneal dialysis. *Journal of the American Society of Nephrology, 7*(11), 2403-2408.

Nebel, M., Marczewski, K., & Finke, K. (1991). Three years of experience with the swan-neck Tenckhoff catheter. *Advances in Peritoneal Dialysis, 7,* 208-213.

Neu, A.M., Kohaut, E.C., & Warady, B.A. (1995). Current approach to peritoneal access in North American children: A report of the Pediatric Peritoneal Dialysis Study Consortium. *Advances in Peritoneal Dialysis, 11,* 289-292.

Newman, L.N., Tessman, M., Hanslik, T., Schulak, J., Mayes, J., & Friedlander, M. (1993). A retrospective view of factors that affect catheter healing: Four years of experience. *Advances in Peritoneal Dialysis, 9,* 217-222.

Nielsen, P.K., Hemmingsen, C., Friis, S.U., Ladefoged, J., & Olgaard, K. (1995). Comparison of straight and curled Tenckhoff peritoneal dialysis catheters implanted by percutaneous technique: A prospective randomized study. *Peritoneal Dialysis International, 15*(1), 18-21.

Palmer, R. A., Quinton, W. E., & Gray, J. E. (1964, March 28). Prolonged peritoneal dialysis for chronic renal failure. *Lancet, 15,* 700-702.

Parrott, P.L., Terry, P.M., Whitworth, E.N., Frawley, L.W., Coble, R.S., Wachsmuth, I. K., & McGowan, J.E., Jr. (1982, September 25). Pseudomonas aeruginosa peritonitis associated with contaminated poloxamer-iodine solution. *Lancet, 2*(8300), 683-685.

Pastan, S., Gassensmith, C., Manatunga, A.K., Copley, J.B., Smith, E.J., & Hamburger, R.J. (1991). Prospective comparison of peritoneoscopic and surgical implantation of CAPD catheters. *Transactions American Society of Artificial Internal Organs, 37,* M154-M156.

Patel, U.D., Mottes, T.A., & Flynn, J.T. (2001). Delayed compared with immediate use of peritoneal catheter in pediatric peritoneal dialysis. *Advances in Peritoneal Dialysis, 17,* 253-259.

Pérez-Fontán, M., Garcia-Falcón, T., Rosales, M., Rodríguez-Carmona, A., Adeva, M., Rodríguez-Lozana, I., et al. (1993). Treatment of staphylococcus aureus nasal carriers in continuous ambulatory peritoneal dialysis with mupirocin: Long term results. *American Journal of Kidney Diseases, 22*(5), 708-712.

Piraino, B. (1996a). Peritoneal catheter exit-site and tunnel infections. *Advances in Renal Replacement Therapy, 3*(3), 222-227.

Piraino, B. (1996b). Exit-site care. *Peritoneal Dialysis International, 16*(Suppl. 1), S336-S339.

Poirier, V.L., Daly, B.D.T., Dasse, K.A., Haudenschild, C.C., & Fine, R.E. (1986). Elimination of tunnel infection. In J.F. Maher & J.F. Winchesters (Eds.), *Frontiers in Peritoneal Dialysis,* (pp.210-217). New York: Field, Rich and Associates.

Ponce, S.P., Pierratos, A., Izatt, S., Mathews, R., Khanna, R., Zellerman, G., & Oreopoulos, D.G. (1982). Comparison of the survival and complications of three permanent peritoneal dialysis catheters. *Peritoneal Dialysis Bulletin, 2*(2), 82-86.

Prakashan, K.P., Annigeri, R.A., Chu, M., Bargman, J.M., Vas, S.I., & Oreopoulos, D.G. (2001). Local application of mupirocin at the peritoneal catheter exit site prevents early postoperative infections and should become standard practice. *Peritoneal Dialysis International, 21*(5), 526-527.

Prowant, B.F. (1996). Nursing interventions related to peritoneal catheter exit-site infections. *Advances in Renal Replacement Therapy, 3*(3), 228-231.

Prowant, B.F., & Ponferrada, L.P. (1998). Clinical drain flow rates of Tenckhoff and swan-neck catheters (Abstract). *Peritoneal Dialysis International, 18*(Suppl. 1), S39.

Prowant, B.F., Schmidt, L.M., Twardowski, Z.J., Griebel, C.K., Burrows, L.K., Ryan, L.P., & Satalowich, R.J. (1988). Peritoneal dialysis catheter exit-site care. *ANNA Journal, 15*(4), 219-222.

Prowant, B.F., & Twardowski, Z.J. (1996). Recommendations for exit care. *Peritoneal Dialysis International, 16*(Suppl. 3), S94-S99.

Prowant, B.F., Warady, B.A., & Nolph, K.D. (1993). Peritoneal dialysis catheter exit-site care: Results of an international survey. *Peritoneal Dialysis International, 13*(2) 149-154.

Purcell, M.E. (1993). Preoperative peritoneal catheter abdominal marking. *ANNA Journal, 20*(1), 83.

Ritzau, J., Hoffman, R.M., & Tzamaloukas, A.H. (2001). Effect of preventing *Staphylococcus aureus* carriage on rates of peritoneal catheter-related staphylococcal infections. Literature synthesis. *Peritoneal Dialysis International, 21*(5), 471-479.

Rodrigues, A., Cabrita, A., & Nogueira, C. (2004). Techniques of peritoneal catheter insertion. In C. Ronco & N.W. Levin (Eds.), *Hemodialysis vascular access and peritoneal dialysis access. Contributions to nephrology, 142*, 402-409.

Ronco, C., Wentling, A.G., Amerling, R., Cruz, C., & Levin, N.W. (2004). New catheter design for continuous flow peritoneal dialysis. *Contributions to Nephrology, 142*, 447-461.

Rosales, M., Pérez-Fontán, M., Rodríguez-Carmona, A., & García-Falcón, T. (2001). Increasing resistance to mupirocin of *Staphylococcus aureus* (SAu) strains isolated from peritoneal dialysis (PD) patients and their partners. Long-term study (Abstract). *Peritoneal Dialysis International, 21*(Suppl. 2), S128.

Rosenak, S.S., & Oppenheimer, G.D. (1948). An improved drain for peritoneal lavage. *Surgery, 23*, 832-833.

Sahani, M.M., Mukhtar, K.N., Boorgu, R., Leehey, D.J., Popli, S., & Ing, T.S. (2000). Tissue plasminogen activator can effectively declot peritoneal dialysis catheters (Letter). *American Journal of Kidney Diseases, 36*(3), 675.

Sardegna, K.M., Beck, A.M., & Strife, C.F. (1998). Evaluation of perioperative antibiotics at the time of dialysis catheter placement. *Pediatric Nephrology, 12*, 149-152.

Scalamogna, A., DeVecchi, A., Maccario, M., Castelnovo, C., & Ponticelli, C. (1995). Cuff-shaving procedure. A rescue treatment for exit-site infection unresponsive to medical therapy. *Nephrology Dialysis Transplantation, 10*(12), 2325-2327.

Schmidt, L.M., Craig, P.S., Prowant, B.F., & Twardowski, Z.J. (1990). A simple method of preventing accidental disconnection at the peritoneal catheter adapter junction (Letter). *Peritoneal Dialysis International, 10*, 309-310.

Schröder, C. H. (2001). Validation of a scoring system for exit-site evaluation. *Peritoneal Dialysis International, 21*(6), 623-624. Erratum in (2003). *Peritoneal Dialysis International, 23*(1), 99.

Schwenk, M.H., Charytan, C., & Spinowitz, B.S. (2002). Dialysate leaks. In A.R. Nissenson & R.N. Fine (Eds.), *Dialysis therapy* (3rd ed.) (p. 271). Philadelphia: Hanley & Belfus.

Stephen, R.L., Atkin-Thor, E., & Kolff, W.J. (1976). Recirculating peritoneal dialysis with subcutaneous catheter. *Transactions American Society of Artificial Internal Organs, 22*, 575-585.

Strauss, F.G., Holmes, D.L., Nortman, D.F., & Friedman, S. (1993). Hypertonic saline compresses: Therapy for complicated exit-site infections. *Advances in Peritoneal Dialysis, 9*, 248-250.

Swartz, R., Messana, J., Reynolds, J., & Ranjit, U. (1991). Simultaneous catheter replacement and removal in refractory peritoneal dialysis infections. *Kidney International, 40*, 1160-1165.

Tacconelli, E., Carmeli, Y., Aizer, A., Ferreira, G., Foreman, M.G., & D'Agata, E.M.C. (2003). Mupirocin prophylaxis to prevent *Staphylococcus aureus* infection in patients undergoing dialysis: A meta-analysis. *Clinical Infectious Diseases, 37*(12), 1629-1638.

Teixidó, J., & Arias, N. (1998). Catheter exit site: Photographic diagnostic table based on graded attributes (criteria) (Abstract). *Peritoneal Dialysis International, 18*(Suppl. 1), S40.

Tenckhoff, H. (1974). *Chronic peritoneal dialysis: A manual for patients, dialysis personnel and physicians.* Seattle, WA: University of Washington School of Medicine.

Tenckhoff, H., & Schechter, H. (1968). A bacteriologically safe peritoneal access device. *Transactions American Society of Artificial Internal Organs, 14*, 181-187.

Thodis, E., Passadakis, P., Ossareh, S., Panagoutsos, S., Vargemezis, V., & Oreopoulos, D.G. (2003). Peritoneal catheter exit-site infections: Predisposing factors, prevention, and treatment. *International Journal of Artificial Organs, 26*(8), 698-714.

Trooskin, S.Z., Donetz, A.P., Baxter, J., Harvey, R.A., & Greco, R.S. (1987). Infection-resistant continuous peritoneal dialysis catheters. *Nephron, 46*(3), 263-267.

Trooskin, S.Z., Harvey, R.A., Lennard, T.W.J., & Greco, R.S. (1990). Failure of demonstrated clinical efficacy of antibiotic-bonded continuous ambulatory peritoneal dialysis (CAPD) catheters. *Peritoneal Dialysis International, 10*(1), 57-59.

Twardowski, Z.J. (2002a). Presternal peritoneal catheter. *Advances in Renal Replacement Therapy, 9*(2), 125-132.

Twardowski, Z.J. (2002b). Peritoneal catheter exit-site and tunnel infections. In A.R. Nissenson & R.N. Fine (Eds.), *Dialysis therapy* (3rd ed.) (pp. 239-244). Philadelphia: Hanley & Belfus.

Twardowski, Z.J. (2002c). Tidal peritoneal dialysis. In A.R. Nissenson & R.N. Fine (Eds.), *Dialysis therapy* (3rd ed.) (pp. 225-228). Philadelphia: Hanley & Belfus.

Twardowski, Z.J. (2004). History and development of the access for peritoneal dialysis. *Contributions to Nephrology, 142*, 387-401.

Twardowski, Z.J., Dobbie, J.W., Moore, H.L., Nichols, W.K., DeSpain, J.D., Anderson, P.C., Khanna, R., Nolph, K.D., & Loy, T.S. (1991). Morphology of peritoneal dialysis catheter tunnel. Macroscopy and light microscopy. *Peritoneal Dialysis International, 11*(3), 237-251.

Twardowski, Z.J., & Nichols, W.K. (2000). Peritoneal dialysis access and exit-site care including surgical aspects. In R. Gokal, R. Khanna, R.T. Krediet, & K.D. Nolph (Eds.), *Textbook of peritoneal dialysis* (2nd ed.) (pp. 307-361). Dordrecht: Kluwer Academic Publishers.

Twardowski, Z.J., Nichols, W.K., Nolph, K.D., & Khanna, R. (1992). Swan neck presternal ("bath tub") catheter for peritoneal dialysis. *Advances in Peritoneal Dialysis, 8*, 316-324.

Twardowski, Z.J., & Prowant, B.F. (1996a). Exit-site healing post catheter implantation. *Peritoneal Dialysis International, 16*(Suppl. 3), S51-S70.

Twardowski, Z.J., & Prowant, B.F. (1996b). Classification of normal and diseased exit sites. *Peritoneal Dialysis International, 16*(Suppl. 3), S32-S50.

Twardowski, Z.J., & Prowant, B.F. (1996c). Exit-site study methods and results. *Peritoneal Dialysis International, 16*(Suppl. 3), S6-S31.

Twardowski, Z.J., & Prowant, B.F. (1997). Current approach to exit-site infections in patients on peritoneal dialysis. *Nephrology Dialysis Transplantation, 12*, 1284-1295.

Twardowski, Z.J., Prowant, B.F., Khanna, R., Nichols, W.K., & Nolph, K.D. (1990). Long-term experience with Swan Neck Missouri catheters. *ASAIO Transactions, 36*(3), M491-M494.

Twardowski, Z.J., Prowant, B.F., Nichols, W.K., Nolph, K.D., & Khanna, R. (1998). Six-year experience with swan neck presternal peritoneal dialysis catheter. *Peritoneal Dialysis International, 18*(6), 598-602.

Usha, K., Ponferrada, L., Prowant, B.F., & Twardowski, Z.J. (1998). Repair of chronic peritoneal dialysis catheter. *Peritoneal Dialysis International, 18*(4), 419-423.

U.S. Renal Data System (USRDS). (1992). Excerpts from the 1992 USRDS Annual Report. VI. Catheter-related factors and peritonitis risk in CAPD patients. *American Journal of Kidney Diseases, 20*(5 Suppl. 2), 48-54.

Verger, C. (2004). Maintenance of functioning PD access and management of complications. *Contributions to Nephrology, 142*, 410-421.

Verrina, E., Perfumo, F., Zacchello, G., Edefonti, A., Bassi, S., Capasso, G., Caringella, D.A., Castellani, A., Longo, L., Rinaldi, S., Viglino, G., & Cantaluppi, A. (1993). Chronic peritoneal dialysis catheters in pediatric patients: Experience of the Italian registry of pediatric chronic peritoneal dialysis. *Peritoneal Dialysis International, 13*(Suppl. 2), S254-S256.

Vychtil, A., Lilaj, T., Lorenz, M., Hörl, W.H., & Haag-Weber, M. (1999). Ultrasonography of the catheter tunnel in peritoneal dialysis patients: What are the indications? *American Journal of Kidney Diseases, 33*(4), 722-727.

Waite, N.M., Webster, N., Laurel, M., Johnson, M., & Fong, I.W. (1997). The efficacy of exit-site povidone-iodine ointment in the prevention of early peritoneal dialysis-related infections. *American Journal of Kidney Diseases, 29*(5), 763-768.

Warady, B.A., Sullivan, E.K., & Alexander S.R. (1996). Lessons from the peritoneal dialysis patient database: A report of the North American Pediatric Renal Transplant Cooperative Study. *Kidney International, 49*(Suppl. 53), S68-S71.

Warchol, S., Roszkowska-Blaim, M., Latoszynska, J., Jarmolinski, T., & Zachwieja, J. (2003). Experience using presternal catheter for peritoneal dialysis in Poland: A multicenter pediatric survey. *Peritoneal Dialysis International, 23*(3), 242-248.

Weaver, M.E., & Dunbeck, D.C. (1994). Mupirocin (Bactroban®) causes permanent structural changes in peritoneal dialysis (PD) catheters (Abstract). *Peritoneal Dialysis International, 14*(Suppl. 1), S20.

Weston, R.E., & Roberts, M. (1965, May 15). Stylet-catheter for peritoneal dialysis. (Letter). *Lancet, 14,* 1049.

Wiegmann, T.B., Stuewe, B., Duncan, K.A., Chonko, A., Diederich, D.A., Grantham, J.J., Savin, V.J., & MacDougall, M.L. (1985). Effective use of streptokinase for peritoneal catheter failure. *American Journal of Kidney Diseases, 6*(2), 119-123.

Wong, F.S.-Y., Chan, W.-K., Chow, N.-Y., Tsui, Y.-T., Yung, J.C.-U., & Cheng, Y.-L. (2002). Comparison of exit-site infection with the use of pure liquid soap and chlorhexidine soap in daily exit-site care. *Hong Kong Journal of Nephrology, 4*(1), 54-59.

Zappacosta, A.R. (2002). Complications of acute peritoneal catheter insertion. In A.R. Nissenson & R.N. Fine (Eds.), *Dialysis therapy* (3rd ed.) (pp. 51-53). Philadelphia: Hanley & Belfus.

Zappacosta, A.R., & Perras, S.T. (1984). *CAPD: Continuous ambulatory peritoneal dialysis.* Philadelphia: J.B. Lippincott.

Zimmerman, S.W., Ahrens, E., Johnson, C.A., Craig, W., Leggett, J., O'Brien, M., Oxton, L., Roecker, E.B., & Engeseth, S. (1991). Randomized controlled trial of prophylactic rifampin for peritoneal dialysis-related infections. *American Journal of Kidney Diseases, 18*(2), 225-231.

Zorzanello, M.M., Fleming, W.J., & Prowant, B.F. (2004). Use of tPA in peritoneal dialysis catheters: A literature review and one center's experience. *Nephrology Nursing Journal, 31*(5), 534-537.

Readings

Gokal, R., Khanna, R., Krediet, R.T., & Nolph, K.D. (Eds.). (2000). *Textbook of Peritoneal Dialysis* (2nd ed.). Dordrecht: Kluwer Academic Publishers.

Nissenson, A.R., & Fine, R.N. (Eds.). (2005). *Clinical Dialysis* (4th ed., Chapters 13-19). New York: McGraw-Hill.

Ronco, C., & Levin, N.W. (Eds.). (2004). *Hemodialysis Vascular Access and Peritoneal Dialysis Access. Contributions to Nephrology, 142.* Basel: Karger.

- The success of chronic peritoneal dialysis (PD) depends upon a permanent, safe access to the peritoneal cavity (Gokal et al., 1998). Ash (2003) asserts that chronic PD catheters are the most successful of all transcutaneous access devices, as they survive for years rather than weeks or months.

- Acute PD catheters are made of nylon or polyethylene and are straight and relatively stiff with numerous side holes in the distal portion. They do not have cuffs, but have wings that can be sutured to the skin to secure the catheter. Acute catheters are not recommended for patients who are extremely obese or those who have had previous abdominal surgery because adhesions increase the risk of organ perforation.

- Double-cuff catheters have longer survival and lower infection rates compared to single-cuff catheters in both adult and pediatric patients (Lindblad, Hamilton, Nolph, & Novak, 1988; U.S. Renal Data System [USRDS], 1992; Warady, Sullivan, & Alexander, 1996), so they are almost universally used for chronic dialysis.

- The Tenckhoff catheter (Tenckhoff & Schechter, 1968) is the most widely used catheter throughout the world. It may have either a straight or coiled intraperitoneal segment (see Figure 28-1). The Tenckhoff catheters are prototypes for almost all of the recently developed catheters.

- Preoperative patient education should include a review of why the patient requires dialysis, the type of PD catheter that will be implanted, where the catheter will be placed, a brief explanation of what to expect postoperatively, and an overview of catheter procedures and care.

- Dialysis nurses sometimes accompany patients to surgery and participate by ensuring that the patient receives the correct catheter, encouraging use of the preferred exit site, preparing the heparinized solution for checking catheter patency, and making sure that the catheter is capped and secured and that appropriate dressings are applied.

- Perforation of abdominal organs is the most serious complication associated with PD catheter insertion. Blind insertion methods and constipation increase the risk of bowel perforation. Signs and symptoms of bowel perforation include a foul smelling, turbid dialysate with particulate matter and profuse watery diarrhea.

- The longer the period before catheter use, the better the healing and the lower the risk of complications (Gokal et al., 1998). When possible, it is recommended that any PD be delayed for 1-3 days. Continuous ambulatory peritoneal dialysis (CAPD) is not recommended for 10-14 days after catheter implantation.

- The single most important goal of exit-site care is to prevent exit-site infections. Exit-site care also provides an opportunity to assess the exit site and tunnel for signs of infection. Since there have been few controlled research studies evaluating elements of exit-site care procedures, there is no consensus regarding the best cleansing agents or optimal procedure.

- The primary goal of chronic exit-site care is to prevent infections. A secondary goal is to identify exit-site problems early so that interventions can be initiated promptly. Elements of catheter care procedures for a healed exit site are outlined in Table 28-3. Exit-site care procedures for infants and children are similar to those for adult PD patients (Neu et al., 1995; Prowant, Warady, & Nolph, 1993).

- It is recommended that patients or their dialysis partners assess the exit site and tunnel prior to routine exit-site care, and that a nurse or physician assesses the exit site and tunnel at routine clinic visits (Prowant & Twardowski, 1996). All patients and dialysis caregivers should know the signs and symptoms of exit-site infection and understand that these should be reported promptly to the PD team.

- There are two types of catheter obstructions – one-way, where the catheter can be used for infusion, but does not drain well, and two-way, where the catheter will neither infuse nor drain adequately, if at all. The nursing management is aimed at determining the cause of the problems and to correct the underlying cause(s).

- As catheters age, the material may deteriorate and become brittle. The catheters may crumble or crack, or break into two pieces. These problems are most likely to occur near the exit site where the catheter material is exposed to cleansing agents, antibiotics, and ointments or creams.

- Catheter survival should be >80% at one year. Infections are the primary reason for catheter removal. Cuffed catheters require surgical removal. Simultaneous replacement and removal is ideal for malfunctioning catheters and can be used for some episodes of relapsing peritonitis after effective antibiotic therapy.

ANNP628

Peritoneal Dialysis Access

Barbara F. Prowant, MS, RN, CNN

Contemporary Nephrology Nursing: Principles and Practice contains 39 chapters of educational content. Individual learners may apply for continuing nursing education credit by reading a chapter and completing the Continuing Education Evaluation Form for that chapter. Learners may apply for continuing education credit for any or all chapters.

Please photocopy this page and return to ANNA.
COMPLETE THE FOLLOWING:

Name: _____

Address:_____

City:_____State: _____Zip: _____

E-mail: _____

Preferred telephone: ☐ Home   ☐ Work: _____

State where licensed and license number (optional): _____

CE application fees are based upon the number of contact hours provided by the individual chapter. CE fees per contact hour for ANNA members are as follows: 1.0-1.9 - $15; 2.0-2.9 - $20; 3.0-3.9 - $25; 4.0 and higher - $30. Fees for nonmembers are $10 higher.

ANNA Member: ☐ Yes   ☐ No   Member # (if available) _____

☐ Checked Enclosed   ☐ American Express   ☐ Visa   ☐ MasterCard

Total Amount Submitted: _____

Credit Card Number: _____ Exp. Date: _____

Name as it appears on the card: _____

CE Evaluation Form
To receive continuing education credit for individual study after reading the chapter
1. Photocopy this form. (You may also download this form from ANNA's Web site, **www.annanurse.org**.)
2. Mail the completed form with payment (check) or credit card information to American Nephrology Nurses' Association, East Holly Avenue, Box 56, Pitman, NJ 08071-0056.
3. You will receive your CE certificate from ANNA in 4 to 6 weeks.

Test returns must be postmarked by **December 31, 2010.**

CE Application Fee
ANNA Member $20.00
Nonmember $30.00

EVALUATION FORM

1. I verify that I have read this chapter and completed this education activity. Date: _____

_____
Signature

2. What would be different in your practice if you applied what you learned from this activity? *(Please use additional sheet of paper if necessary.)*

_____
_____
_____
_____
_____
_____
_____
_____
_____
_____
_____
_____
_____

Evaluation	Strongly disagree				Strongly agree
3. The activity met the stated objectives.					
a. Describe a plan of care through all phases of chronic PD catheter insertion.	1	2	3	4	5
b. Relate peritoneal dialysis catheter-related complications to the symptoms that will be noted by the nurse.	1	2	3	4	5
c. Summarize the interventions to be used in the treatment of site infections seen with peritoneal dialysis catheters.	1	2	3	4	5
4. The content was current and relevant.	1	2	3	4	5
5. The content was presented clearly.	1	2	3	4	5
6. The content was covered adequately.	1	2	3	4	5
7. Rate your ability to apply the learning obtained from this activity to practice.	1	2	3	4	5

Comments _____
_____

8. Time required to read the chapter and complete this form: _____ minutes.

This educational activity has been provided by the American Nephrology Nurses' Association (ANNA) for 2.6 contact hours. ANNA is accredited as a provider of continuing nursing education (CNE) by the American Nurses Credentialing Center's Commission on Accreditation (ANCC-COA). ANNA is an approved provider of continuing education by the California Board of Registered Nursing, CEP 0910.

Preventing and Managing Complications of Peritoneal Dialysis

Elizabeth Kelman, MEd, RN, CNeph(C)
Diane Watson, MSc, RN, CNeph(C)

Chapter Contents

Preventing and Managing Complications of Peritoneal Dialysis

Chapter 29

Elizabeth Kelman, MEd, RN, CNeph(C)
Diane Watson, MSc, RN, CNeph(C)

In determining the choice of dialysis modality, individuals are faced with life-altering decisions. Through information and counseling, health care professionals can assist people with renal disease in making informed choices. Direct involvement in the decision making to choose a treatment option will facilitate the commitment to the selected therapy; however, as with any medical treatment, there are risks as well as benefits. Even while maintaining a sense of hope, the disclosure of complications may prove overwhelming. For those who select peritoneal dialysis (PD), the risk of peritonitis will be a reality; for a minority, rare complications associated with hydrothorax or encapsulating peritoneal sclerosis (EPS) may be encountered. The key to the management of complications is in prevention, identification, and early intervention; moreover, maintaining confidence in the therapy will be integral to the outcome for individuals engaged in self-care practices.

Complications to the therapy including those related to metabolism, increased abdominal pressure, and infection are outlined. Definition, assessment, intervention, and preventive measures are discussed in relation to the described complications. Through increased awareness of both the risks and benefits of PD, nurses can support individual choices regarding selection of the most appropriate treatment modality in either the home or institutional setting.

Assessment and Prevention of Complications

In considering an individual for PD, age, co-morbidities, medications, and learning capabilities should be taken into account in preparing for the treatment and minimizing risks associated with the catheter implantation and dialysis procedure. Diabetes, malnutrition, and friable tissues can affect post-operative wound healing, resulting in post-catheter implantation incisional leaks with initiation of dialysis. Similarly, medications such as steroids may slow healing of the incision, while anticoagulation may result in hematomas and bruising post-operatively. Thus, measures to enhance healing should include early catheter insertion, before dialysis is required, or adaptation of the technique to smaller, more frequent exchanges in situations when PD is required before the healing process is complete. Adjustment of anticoagulants in the pre-operative period is required to decrease post-operative bleeding complications that can contribute to hematomas with an associated risk of infection and delayed wound healing. The dietitian should be consulted for nutritional assessment and management of those who are malnourished to enhance oral intake to maintain nutrition required for wound healing.

In assessing individuals for PD, it is also important to determine their daily bowel patterns. Limitations in dietary intake of fiber, fluid restrictions, gastroparesis, and medications, such as antacids, narcotics, phosphate binders, and calcium channel blockers, can all contribute to the development of constipation. Risks associated with constipation include discomfort, anorexia, peritoneal catheter outflow problems, and migration across the bowel wall of organisms linked to enteric peritonitis (Piraino, 1998). Nakamura et al. (2004) reported the occurrence of a perforated colon in an individual with chronic constipation on PD. Thus, nephrology nurses must be vigilant in monitoring bowel patterns. Measures to establish a bowel regimen for the prevention of complications related to constipation should be incorporated into teaching plans. Additionally, diarrhea can pose a risk for peritonitis and requires assessment and treatment.

Non-Infectious Complications

Non-infectious complications encompass those conditions related to increased abdominal pressure, effluent appearance, metabolism, including fluid and electrolyte imbalances, and malnutrition. To determine the root causes through investigation of symptoms and patterns is part of the "detective work" of PD.

Some important symptoms individuals describe include pain and shortness of breath. Some signs reported by individuals are wet dressings, weight changes, bulging (hernias), and changes in the effluent, either in volume or appearance. It is vital to assess each symptom and sign to determine the appropriate interventions for maintaining PD.

Non-Infectious Causes of Pain

Abdominal pain related to PD may result from a variety of causes, such as catheter position, presence or lack of fluid in the peritoneal cavity, or dialysis technique. Pain can occur with inflow, dwell, or outflow, and like any pain experienced, it is important for nurses to identify the location, character, contributing and relieving factors, frequency, and duration in order to assist with diagnosis and management.

Pain associated with catheter position. As the PD catheter is positioned freely in a space surrounded by motile bowel and fluid, it is possible for movement of the catheter to occur. The internal location of the catheter, particularly if it is pressing on visceral structures such as the liver or rectum, can contribute to abdominal pain. This may occur immediately after catheter implantation or with position shifts at any time.

Mobilizing a catheter back into the pelvic gutter may relieve pain associated with its location. Potentially, inducing peristaltic activity of the bowel with the administration of laxatives and enemas can accomplish this position shift. This strategy may be effective whether or not the individual is constipated. Occasionally, manipulation of the catheter by interventional radiology may be required if other interventions are not successful. Displacement of the catheter can also occur with omental wrapping and is associated with obstruction and poor fluid outflow. In this instance, options including surgical laparotomy with omentectomy (Nicholson, Burton, Donnelly, Veitch, & Walls, 1991;

Reissman, Lyass, Shiloni, Rivkind, & Berlatzky, 1998; Rinaldi et al., 2004) and laparoscopic interventions with omentectomy or omentopexy, defined as suturing of the omentum to the abdominal wall, have been used (Crabtree & Fishman, 2005; Flanigan & Gokal, 2005; Lee & Donovan, 2002; Ogunc, 2001; Ogunc, Tuncer, Ogunc, Yardimsever, & Ersoy, 2003).

Pain occurring towards the end of the drain cycle is referred to as outflow pain. This describes pain associated with a relatively empty peritoneal cavity when the majority of the dialysate has been drained. The discomfort occurs due to the catheter's position or irritation of the peritoneal wall by the catheter without the fluid "cushion." Outflow pain may be more prevalent during periods of acute inflammation such as peritonitis; thus, it is important to note if the pain is new or if the individual normally experiences such discomfort with draining. To minimize the effect, a residual volume of 200 to 300 mL of fluid may be left indwelling. Generally, once the fill cycle is started, the pain resolves although the sensation can persist for a short time after refilling has commenced.

Occasionally, males experience a sensation of pain radiating to the penis after peritoneal catheter insertion. People on PD may also complain of rectal pain, particularly if they have a small frame and the catheter is quite deep in the pelvis. The catheter tip may irritate the nerve plexus thereby causing discomfort in that area. As dialysis progresses or with bowel movements, the catheter may migrate away from the point of pain sensation; however, if there is no improvement, dialysis with a residual volume may be utilized to "float" the catheter away from the point, or the catheter may require repositioning. Pain due to catheter position should always be attended to, as it is reversible and generally easily remedied. Repositioning or replacing the catheter may alleviate the problem if other measures fail.

Pain associated with dialysis technique. While abdominal pain is the most commonly associated pain, some individuals may describe back pain caused by increased abdominal pressure. People with prior back injuries or diseases affecting the spine may be at greater risk for developing discomfort. It may be helpful in this case to minimize the volume of the day dwell to reduce intra-abdominal pressure and pull on the lumbar area when the individual is upright. Continuous cyclical peritoneal dialysis (CCPD) may be an alternative for individuals as well as back supports and strengthening exercises. Overnight exchanges with dry day may be used; however, this approach negates the benefits of dialyzing for 24 hours.

Shoulder pain can occur as a referred pain via the phrenic nerve and may range from a mild presentation to severe pain. The cause of shoulder pain can be related to air entry into the peritoneal cavity, infusion pain with malposition of the catheter (Maaz, 2004), or dialysate composition. Air may be introduced into the peritoneal cavity with catheter insertion techniques using air infusion for visualization or can occur in small increments during bag changes if the tubing set is not flushed prior to infusion of dialysate. Treatment options include the application of heat locally as well as analgesics. Additionally, some people

may describe shoulder pain on changing from a supine position to sitting or standing and find that resuming the supine position relieves the discomfort. If the pain is related to intraperitoneal air accumulation, the air can be removed during the drain phase by placing the individual in a knee-chest position with hips elevated or in a Trendelenberg position (Maaz, 2004). The temperature of the dialysate fluid can also create abdominal discomfort or cramps.

As described in the previous chapter, peritoneal dialysate solutions can be warmed to normal body temperature (refer to Chapter 27 for discussion on heating methods). Overheated dialysate can cause pain and damage to the peritoneal membrane. Room temperature or cool solutions may be associated with chills and cramps. Using the back of the hand to assess the temperature of the bag can be done prior to inflow remembering that the internal fluid temperature will be warmer than that experienced through touching the bag's surface.

Pain associated with dialysate composition. The acidity of the standard dialysate can also contribute to discomfort. With PD solutions, the pH can be raised with the addition of bicarbonate. Dorval, Legault, Lessard, and Roy (2000) studied the effect of altering the pH in an *in vitro* study. They found that "a final concentration of $NaHCO_3$ of 11 mmol/L (i.e., 25 mL of 7.5% $NaHCO_3$ in a 2-L bag of solution) is probably adequate, since the pH approaches a more physiological level of 7.0 while the sodium concentration remains around 137 mmol/L" (p. 793). The development of commercially prepared bicarbonate dialysate with normal pH has provided an alternative to the lactate solutions. The production of bags with separate compartments allows mixing of the bicarbonate with the dextrose-electrolyte components immediately prior to infusion. Before this innovation, lactate was the preferred buffer since precipitation of solutes occurs with pre-mixed bicarbonate-electrolyte formulas. Mactier et al. (1998) reported reduced infusion pain with the use of bicarbonate and bicarbonate/lactate solutions although the combined buffer dialysate was more effective than the single buffer solution. Tranaeus (2000) reported similar findings in a study group of 70 people trialing a bicarbonate/lactate dialysate compared to 30 people using a lactate-based solution. Forty-one percent of the people using bicarbonate/lactate had less infusion pain than those using a lactate based solution.

Effects of Increased intra-Abdominal Pressure

The presence of fluid in the intraperitoneal space leads to increased intra-abdominal pressure. The highest pressure is noted in the sitting position and the least in the supine position. Additionally, coughing and straining can add to the abdominal wall pressure (Bargman, 2000). This increased pressure can be associated with leaks of peritoneal fluid. Potentially, fluid can leak through anatomical areas of weakness, which may occur between the pleural and peritoneal spaces or patent processus vaginalis. Additionally, fluid can leak into the soft tissue if there are pre-existing defects or alterations related to prior surgeries (Bargman, 2000; Schwenk, Charytan, & Spinowitz, 2002).

Gastric effects of PD. Decreased appetite related to the presence of the fluid, reflux, and delays in gastric emptying have also been postulated as complications with PD; however, the relationship of gastric symptoms to the presence of dialysate remains a controversial issue (Shay, Schreiber, & Richter, 1999). It should be noted that delayed gastric emptying has been reported in individuals with uremia as well as those on hemodialysis (De Schoenmakere, Vanholder, Rottey, Duym, & Lameire, 2001; Strid, Simren, Sotzer, Abrahamsson & Bjornsson, 2004).

In individuals not on PD, gastroesophageal reflux disease (GERD) as a result of increased pressure can occur in pregnancy and chronic constipation (Ray, Secrest, Ch'ien, & Corey, 2002); therefore, the presence of the intra-abdominal fluid may contribute to symptoms related to GERD. A survey of 92 people on PD and 91 on hemodialysis (HD) demonstrated a significant association between cough and self-reported heartburn in people on PD, leading the authors to conclude that the increased intra-abdominal pressure could be a contributing factor to these symptoms (Min et al., 2000).

Delayed gastric emptying has also been identified as a concern in PD although, it is not clear if the effect is due to the volume of solution, the dialysate composition, or increased serum glucose levels (Schoonjans et al., 2002; Van Vlem et al., 2002). Hubalewska et al. (2004) felt that dialysate volume was not the cause of slower gastric transit, although other studies have suggested that delays in the movement of indigestible solids can be attributed to the presence of dialysate in the abdomen (Brown-Cartwright, Smith, & Feldman, 1988; Schiff, Mücke, Sorodoc, & Brendel, 2000). Kim et al. (1999) found delayed gastric emptying during dwell particularly among individuals with body surface areas less than 1.5 m^2 and recommended adjustment of the dialysis prescription to smaller exchange volumes or the use of nightly intermittent peritoneal dialysis (NIPD).

Bargman (2000) in reviewing the literature on gastric effects of PD concluded that risk factors exist for individuals who have "lower esophageal sphincter pressure and delayed gastric emptying" (p.621), and thus, interventions should be taken to reduce symptoms. For individuals experiencing increased heartburn, regurgitation, or disturbed sleep patterns, a trial of smaller exchange volumes may be used to determine if these symptoms are volume-related. Other measures include dietary review to avoid caffeine, alcohol, spicy foods, and acidic juices; intake of smaller, more frequent meals; maintenance of an upright position after food intake; and regular bowel movements (Ray et al., 2002). The treatment of delayed gastric emptying in diabetes can include dietary adjustments and pharmacological agents such as prokinetic drugs including erythromycin and metoclopramide. Use of medications may be related to side effects, including bacterial resistance with erythromycin and central nervous system (CNS) effects of metoclopramide (Akheel, Rattansingh, & Furtado, 2005; Nephrology Pharmacy Associates, 2003).

Extraperitoneal leaks. Dialysate leakages may occur and can be related to delays in wound healing in the immediate post-catheter implantation period or later, with weight loss and associated poor skin turgor. Dialysate fluid can also track into weakened areas of the abdomen and adjacent tissues leading to subcutaneous and genital leaks. Although not always associated with hernias, the individual should be examined for hernias. Leakages into the subcutaneous tissues may be more difficult to see overtly but are associated with "bulges" or loss of symmetry, which are more noticeable in a standing position (Bargman, 2000). Another clue to leaks is that there may be decreased ultrafiltration (UF) volumes. Scrotal or labial swelling can be uncomfortable and embarrassing, and nursing staff should be sensitive during assessment and counseling.

After ruling out allergies to radio-contrast dye, the addition of dye to the peritoneal fluid is useful for computed tomography (CT) imaging to diagnose suspected fluid leaks (Bargman, 2000; Hawkins, Homer, Murray, Voss, & van der Merwe, 2000; Schwenk, Charytan, et al., 2002). After infusing the dialysate mixed with dye via the PD catheter, the individual should be ambulatory for about 30 minutes with a combination of walking and sitting in order to increase the intra-abdominal pressure for better imaging results (Bargman, 2004). Ogunc and associates (2003) recommended the addition of 100 mL of contrast to 2 liters of peritoneal dialysate. A PD nurse should inject the dye using standard sterile technique for adding medications.

In a study of symptomatic and non-symptomatic individuals on PD, Karahan and colleagues (2002) demonstrated the effectiveness of instilling contrast dye into the dialysate fluid and having individuals ambulate for 30 minutes prior to the imaging. Of 64 patients, the authors were able to detect a complication in 68% of the symptomatic group as well as 22% in the non-symptomatic group. Treatment modifications were made based on the findings of leaks and/or hernias.

Lam et al. (2004) described three case reports involving retroperitoneal leaks, a rarely reported phenomenon. The acute loss of UF led the authors to a diagnosis of leakage that is impossible to detect on physical examination. The leaks appeared to occur slowly. People may report diminished drained volumes following long dwells, but good UF with short dwells. This is related to the rate at which the leak is occurring. This finding also occurs with membrane failure, so a PET should be done to rule out a rapid transport state. Lam et al. (2004) further reported successful outcomes by utilizing intermittent peritoneal dialysis (IPD) for an 8-week period. With the dry intervals, the three people resumed continuous ambulatory peritoneal dialysis (CAPD) without any re-occurrence of this unusual complication.

Hernias. Hernias may also develop primarily from increased pressure without accompanying fluid leaks. Hernias, including incisional, inguinal, umbilical, epigastric, and ventral wall hernias, have been documented with an estimated occurrence of 20%-30% (Bargman, 2000; Bargman, 2001). Factors predisposing individuals to hernia formation are related to multiparity; anatomically weak areas including umbilical regions, inguinal canals, and linea albea; and previous surgical sites (Enoch, Aslam, & Piraino, 2002; Lupo et al., 1988). Tokgöz and colleagues (2003) demonstrated a correlation of small body size and increased risk of hernia formation. In addressing the formation of hernias at the peritoneal catheter insertion site, Spence, Mathews, Khanna, and Oreopoulos (1985) demonstrated improved healing and reduced incidence of hernia formation by changing from a midline to paramedian incision for PD catheter insertion. Of interest, some studies have shown that hernia formation is not related to the exchange volume in PD (Afthentopoulos, Rao, Bhaskaran, & Oreopoulos, 1997; Patterson, Whelan, & Schwab, 1988).

Two types of inguinal hernias can occur: indirect and direct. In order to understand the difference in these hernias, it is important to understand the specific anatomy of the area. The testes are originally in the abdomen and are encased in peritoneum. The peritoneum enters or invaginates into the inguinal canal allowing the testes to begin the descent into the scrotal sac. This channel of peritoneum or "processus vaginalis peritonei" usually closes at birth; however, it can remain open in a percentage of men. Additionally, women have a similar structure for the round ligament of the uterus. The existence of a patent processus vaginalis can predispose people to fluid leaks and bowel herniation with the addition of fluid into the peritoneal cavity (Health Guide for the Perplexed, 2005). Unilateral or bilateral swelling can then be seen in the groin or scrotal sac. Rarely, indirect hernias through a patent processus vaginalis can also occur in women. The hernia will manifest as swelling in the labia. On the other hand, a direct hernia is the result of direct pressure of the hernia on an area of weakness leading to protrusion through the inguinal canal.

Decreasing the volume of exchanges and adjusting the frequency may be used as temporary interventions prior to surgical repair or may become permanent adaptations for people who are poor surgical risks. Thus, a change to CCPD with a lower fill volume during the day or NIPD with a dry day period may be treatment options. For surgery, individuals should be well dialyzed pre-operatively to allow for a longer rest period post-operatively prior to reinitiating PD. When re-started, dialysis should be either via IPD or small exchange volumes with CAPD/CCPD. Decreasing the volume without compensating with additional exchanges can result in increased uremic symptoms; thus, clinical assessment of the response to a change in prescription must be monitored and the dialysis adjusted. In most cases, it is unnecessary to transfer the patient to HD for hernia repair.

In planning care of the individual, the nurse should also consider the use of devices such as scrotal or abdominal supports. Education regarding the risks of hernia strangulation should be given. The highest risk of strangulation is associated with small hernias, especially umbilical (Bargman, 2000). Indicators of potential strangulation include the inability to reduce the hernia or increased tenderness and should be reported immediately to avert serious consequences.

Hydrothorax. A rare complication is leakage of peritoneal fluid into the pleural space (Singh, Vaidya, Dale, & Morgan, 1983). This is referred to as a hydrothorax or pleuroperitoneal leak.

Shortness of breath and diminishing volumes of dialysate effluent are associated with the loss of fluid into the lung (Rudnick, Coyle, Beck, & McCurdy, 1979). The incidence rate is 2% in people on PD (Hughes, Ketchersid, Lenzen, & Lowe, 1999; Mak et al., 2002; Szeto & Chow, 2004). This complication can occur within hours to years of initiating PD and is more likely to occur in the right lung (Szeto & Chow, 2004).

In dialyzing individuals, nurses should be suspicious of hydrothorax in the event of sudden shortness of breath immediately after initiating dialysis accompanied by diminished fluid returns. Assessment findings include dullness on lung percussion and absent breath sounds over the area of fluid accumulation (Bargman, 2000; Hughes et al., 1999). The physical onset of this complication may be dramatic and frightening, thus reassurance and support will be needed to assist the individual while working to relieve the accompanying respiratory distress. Changing from a supine to an upright position and draining the peritoneal fluid can be helpful. Since hydrothorax can also occur as a later complication of PD, nurses should consider this possibility for people reporting shortness of breath not relieved by the use of hypertonic solutions. Weight gains, decreasing returns of dialysate, and increasing shortness of breath associated with hydrothorax may initially be mistaken for fluid overload, thus a complete assessment is critical in anyone with these symptoms. A chest x-ray is useful in differentiating fluid overload from hydrothorax since the fluid accumulation generally occurs in one lung as opposed to both.

Chow, Szeto, and Li (2003) described etiologies for this complication including congenital diaphragmatic defects, lymphatic drainage disorders, acquired anatomic defects, and pleuroperitoneal pressure gradients. These authors suggest that the heart and pericardium protect the left lung from this complication. Thus, areas of weakness or "blebs" can succumb to the addition of peritoneal fluid by allowing this area to open with subsequent movement of peritoneal fluid into the pleural space. Bargman (2000) further elaborated that this communication between peritoneal and pleural spaces may be open at the initiation of PD, which accounts for the immediate presentation, whereas later development occurs with either ongoing pressure or an event that removes the pre-existing barrier between the surfaces. Additionally, there may be a "one-way passage … with a valve-like defect" (Bargman, 2000, p. 612), which explains the persistence of hydrothorax after draining the effluent from the peritoneal cavity. Gagnon and Daniels (2004) proposed that hydrothorax may occur as a result of an embryonic remnant known as the pneumatoenteric recess and infracardiac bursa. If this persists after embryonic development, a potential channel for fluid movement could occur between the peritoneal cavity and right pleural space.

To confirm the diagnosis, a pleural tap may be done to compare the fluid content with serum. The expectation is a higher fluid glucose level and lower protein content compared to serum. Lactate can also be found if lactate-based solutions were instilled (Hughes et al., 1999). In a comprehensive review of published reports on hydrothorax from 2001 to 2003, Szeto and Chow (2004) noted that there are reports of "borderline chemical values" (p. 316) and further added that a "glucose gradient of more than 50 mg/dL (2.7 mmol/L) had 100% sensitivity and specificity in confirming a diagnosis of pleuro-peritoneal communication" (p. 316). To more effectively detect the actual point of fluid entry, CT or nuclear scans have been used (Spadaro, Thakur, & Nolph, 1982); however, radionuclide scanning has been suggested as the preferred investigative test for delineating the fluid pathway (Bargman, 2001; Chow et al., 2003). For this approach, Bargman (2001) has suggested the addition of technetium-labeled albumin colloid (5 mCi) with views taken at intervals of 10 minutes over half an hour followed by views in 2-3 hours if the leak was not identified in the earlier views. Also, the individual should be ambulatory to increase pressure and movement of the tracer (p. 403).

Immediate treatment consists of alleviating the symptoms by draining the peritoneal fluid to reduce further accumulation in the pleural space. Thoracentesis may be performed for relief of symptoms, particularly if the hydrothorax is massive, or may be used as an adjunct to diagnosis (Nassberger, 1982; Schwenk, Spinowitz, & Charytan, 2002). Treatments of hydrothorax have included resting the space with resultant spontaneous closure, decreasing volume of instillation for exchanges, sealing the leak with pleurodesis, and surgical closure (Bargman, 2000; Chow et al., 2003; Leblanc, Ouimet, & Pichette, 2001; Mak et al., 2002; Nomoto et al., 1989; Schwenk, Spinowitz, et al., 2002; Singh et al., 1983). While small volume PD such as IPD has been used with some success, other individuals require temporary transfer to HD.

Pleurodesis requires placement of a chest tube and instillation of an irritant, which results in inflammation and ultimately scarring, thus sealing of the leak with scar tissue. PD may be resumed in approximately 3 weeks post pleurodesis (Bargman, personal communication, 2004). Substances used for this purpose include talc, autologous blood, tetracycline, fibrin glue, hemolytic streptococcal preparation, or OK-432 (Chow et al., 2003; Schwenk et al., 2002). Surgical procedures with direct visualization of the leak can also be used to allow suturing or closure with chemical agents. Video-assisted approaches during surgery have been described which improve the localization of the area for pleurodesis (Szeto & Chow, 2004; Halstead, Lim, & Ritchie, 2002; Tsunezuka, Hatakeyama, Iwase, & Watanabe, 2001).

The re-initiation of PD will require inflow of small volumes under observation with increasing volume if no signs and symptoms of hydrothorax are seen. Individuals may be understandably hesitant to resume treatment and require support during the reintroduction of PD.

Hemoperitoneum

Hemoperitoneum refers to the presence of blood in the PD effluent. While the appearance can be alarming, the presence of bloody effluent can be related to a range of factors from benign to serious ones. Of importance in assessing an individual with hemoperitoneum is the determination of active bleeding versus the presence of transient red cells in the fluid. Decreasing serum hemoglobin in the presence of hemoperitoneum will assist in diagnosing active bleeding or substantial blood loss. Hemoperitoneum is visible when even a small amount of blood is present in the effluent; thus, the equivalent of 2 ml of blood in 1 liter of peritoneal fluid is enough to produce bloody effluent (Bargman, 2000; Nace, George, & Stone, 1985). Post-operatively, hemoperitoneum is observed with the initial exchanges and clears with flushing. Since this is an expectation after surgery, this hemoperitoneum is considered a minor event; however, Mital, Fried and Piraino (2004) in a review of 292 peritoneal catheter placements in 263 people found a major bleeding complication rate of two per cent. These major bleeding episodes were primarily associated with anticoagulation. Hemoperitoneum can also be noted after abdominal surgical procedures such as hernia repairs. Generally, with flushing, the effluent returns become increasingly lighter in appearance from red to light pink to clear. If the returns remain dark red, investigation may be required particularly if the individual's condition is changing and associated with hypotension, abdominal discomfort, and decreasing hemoglobin levels.

Bloody effluent also occurs commonly with menstruation or ovulation in women. Women of childbearing age should be counseled ahead of time as to this potential finding. Menstrual hemoperitoneum can occur if there is endometrial tissue in the peritoneal cavity at the time of menstruation or a few days before vaginal blood flow. This is due to retrograde reflux through the Fallopian tubes, which traverses the peritoneal cavity. Hemoperitoneum may also be associated with ovulation and occur mid menstrual cycle (Bargman, 2000; Greenberg, Bernardini, Piraino, Johnston, & Perlmutter, 1992).

Other conditions reported with hemoperitoneum have included anticoagulation, ovarian or renal cyst rupture, trauma or accidental injury to the abdominal contents, splenic rupture, malignancies, pancreatitis, encapsulating peritoneal sclerosis (EPS), dialysis-related amyloidosis with colon perforation, spontaneous abortion, and cytomegalovirus infection (Dozio et al., 2001; Fraley, Johnston, Bruns, Adler, & Segel, 1988; Harnett, Gill, Corbett, Parfrey, & Gault, 1987; Hou, 2001; Kanagasundaram, Macdougall, & Turney, 1998; Min et al., 1997; Ohtani, Imai, Komatsuda, Wakui, & Miura, 2000; Pollock, 2003).

Potential risks associated with hemoperitoneum include worsening anemia, catheter obstruction, and peritonitis. Thus, in managing individuals with hemoperitoneum, monitoring of symptoms and hemoglobin levels will assist in determining the severity of the finding. In managing an initial event of hemoperitoneum, flushes may be used to determine if the blood can be cleared. Since heparin does not cross the peritoneal membrane to exert an anticoagulant effect, the administration of intraperitoneal heparin can be used to prevent the catheter from becoming obstructed (Gokal et al., 1998). If the hemoperitoneum does not clear or if the individual develops hemodynamic instability, further investigation and referral to either gynecology or surgery is warranted.

Hemoperitoneum is a disturbing finding for individuals performing their own PD, and reassurance must be given as to the cause and interventions for the episode. Including this potential complication in teaching sessions will prepare people for the occurrence, but nurses should be sensitive to the fear an individual may feel on seeing bloody effluent for the first time.

Cloudy Effluent in Non-Infectious State

Cloudy effluent returns are generally considered to be infectious; however, it is important for nurses and patients to be aware of the exceptions. By having cloudy fluid analyzed for both cell constituents and infectious organisms, the reason for the alteration in clarity can be determined. If the effluent white cell count is below 100/mm^3, the cloudiness may be attributed to something other than infection.

When cloudy effluent occurs shortly after catheter implantation without clinical signs of peritonitis and a positive culture report, allergic eosinophilic peritonitis may be responsible (Ashgar, Woodrow, & Turney, 2000; Oh et al., 2004). Normally, this cloudiness will resolve spontaneously over 4-6 weeks (Leehey, Gandhi, & Daugirdas, 2001). In this setting, the cell counts show a high percentage of eosinophils without high total white cell counts. This can also be elicited as allergic responses to medications given intraperitoneally (IP), such as vancomycin, gentamicin, cefazolin, and thrombolytic agents (Rocklin & Teitelbaum, 2001; Steiner, 2002). Allergic responses have also been linked to plastics or plasticizers in the bags and/or tubing or even a component of the dialysate, such as occurs with contamination of commercially produced solutions (Rocklin & Teitelbaum, 2001; Williams & Foggensteiner, 2002). In Chapter 27, the appearance of cloudy effluent with the use of icodextrin solutions has been discussed. Both dialysis solutions and medications given IP, such as amphotericin and vancomycin, have been studied with the resultant finding of impurities in batches of preparations. Early recognition of this problem as well as documentation of lot numbers used can assist in the control of such occurrences. Daugirdas and colleagues (1987) also described the presentation of eosinophilic fluid with the entry of air into the peritoneal cavity. Leehey et al. (2001) further described case reports of high eosinophilic counts in infectious peritonitis caused by fungi and parasites.

Chyloperitoneum is effluent that has the appearance of a milky white fluid. It is caused by the accumulation of "lymph with emulsified fat from intestinal absorption following digestion" (Currier, 1995, p. 157). Bargman (2001) describes this phenomenon as intermittent, particularly since it is associated with high dietary fat intake. The presence of chyle in the peritoneum is most frequently associated with impairment of the lymphatic drainage system secondary to neoplasm (Bargman, 2000). Other causes of chyloperitoneum include trauma such as peritoneal catheter insertion, cardiopulmonary resuscitation, pancreatitis, superior vena cava syndrome, congenital "leaky lymphatics," tuberculosis, and the calcium-channel blocker manidipine (Bargman, 2000; Currier, 1995; Huang, Chen, Chen, & Tsai, 1996; Perez Fontan, Pombo, Soto, Perez Fontan, & Rodriguez-Carmona, 1993; Rocklin, Quinn, & Teitelbaum, 2000; Rocklin & Teitelbaum, 2001). On analysis, the fluid has a high triglyceride level (Bargman, 2001; Rocklin et al., 2000). Since high fat intake is associated

with chyloperitoneum, a diet with reduced long chain fatty acids may be effective (Bargman, 2001; Cárdenas & Chopra, 2002, Levy & Wenk, 2001; McCray & Parrish, 2004).

Cloudy fluid has also been observed in individuals with metastases. In the absence of infection and with findings of lymphocytes, further investigations may reveal a malignancy such as lymphoma and adenocarcinoma (Bargman, Zent, Ellis, Auger, & Wilson, 1994; Jobson & Adams, 1983; Vlahakos, Rudders, Simon & Canzanello, 1990). The peritoneal effluent can be sent for cytologic examination to investigate for presence of malignant cells.

Changes in color but not clarity can occur with the degree of uremia, as higher urea concentrations may tend to create a deeper amber color in the effluent. If given fluorescine for eye studies, people may notice that the effluent has a greenish-yellow, almost neon appearance, which will dissipate with subsequent exchanges. Additionally, drugs such as rifampin may cause an orange discoloration of the fluid. Carter, Garris, and Ullian (1996) described the phenomenon of rusty discoloration of peritoneal fluid in an individual who was receiving rifampin and then given intravenous (IV) iron dextran.

Fibrin in the effluent can contribute to haziness leading to the observation of fibrin strands or clumps in drainage bags left sitting out for a period of time and could be alarming to the individual on PD. The nurse might then recommend the use of heparin to prevent fibrin formation and clumping.

It is important to understand the nature and reasons for cloudy effluent and take a logical systematic approach to rule out infection, then to establish the likely cause of cloudy effluent. Cloudy effluent should be presumed to be peritonitis and treated accordingly. Treatment can be altered once cell counts are known.

Complications Associated with Metabolism and Nutrition

Fluid volume imbalances. Recent literature suggests that people on PD may exhibit effects of overhydration including left ventricular hypertrophy and hypertension, while some patients may have fluid overload, which is not easily detected (Enia et al., 2001; Khandelwal et al., 2003a; Konings, Kooman, van der Sande, & Leunissen, 2003); however, both fluid volume excess and fluid volume deficit can occur at varying times with changes in health status.

Fluid control is an outcome of both intake and output. Thus, fluid volume excess may be related to increased intake of fluid and/or salt (Wright et al., 2004), loss of residual renal function, inappropriate bag strength selection, non-performance of exchanges, and loss of UF capability either transiently or permanently (Tzamaloukas et al., 1995). Bargman (2004) cautions that peritoneal membrane failure may not always be responsible for UF loss and recommends that mechanical causes resulting in low effluent returns, such as pleural or abdominal wall leaks should be investigated and treated. If, however, true fluid volume excess either as a sole complication or accompanying a dialysate leak is present, reassessment of target weight, intake, and bag strengths utilized should be undertaken. For removal of excess fluid, hypertonic dextrose solutions or icodextrin may be utilized. For people with diabetes, increased use of hypertonic solutions may lead to greater thirst if blood sugars are not adequately controlled and, thus, perpetuate the problem of increased fluid intake. Adjustment of hypoglycemic agents is required to maintain glycemic control. Other factors contributing to hyperglycemia, such as infection and dietary patterns, should be included in the assessment.

Fluid volume deficit may occur through decreased oral intake or increased losses. These losses may be incorrect bag selection leading to excess UF or loss from other sources such as vomiting and/or diarrhea. In assessing the fluid status, decreased blood pressure with a postural drop can be an indicator of fluid deficit; however, orthostatic hypotension can occur both as a consequence of autonomic neuropathy and as the side effect of some antihypertensive medications. Hypotension can also occur in states of decreased effective circulatory volume when large amounts of fluid are shifted into the interstitial spaces due to hypoalbuminemia or congestive heart failure. Thus, the blood pressure should be interpreted with other indicators of fluid volume deficit such as decreased skin turgor, dry mucous membranes, and weight changes.

The concept of target weight is difficult, and some individuals have tried using hypertonic solutions in an attempt to decrease overall body weight leading to severe fluid dehydration. As well, in the first few months of dialysis, people may actually feel better, have increased oral intake, and begin to gain flesh weight. If, however, they continue to dialyze to the originally prescribed target weight, they could be at risk of developing signs and symptoms of fluid deficit. Careful analysis of the problem and re-education is required to avoid this misunderstanding of the concept of body weight. The selection of bag strengths must also be adjusted with concurrent illness such as gastroenteritis when less UF is required to maintain fluid balance. If hypotonic solutions are available, they can be used, or if the individual is able to maintain oral intake, salt solutions such as bouillon cubes or soup may help to restore balance.

Sodium imbalances. Both imbalances of sodium excess and depletion have been documented with hyponatremia related to fluid volume excess and malnutrition. Hypernatremia has been noted particularly with rapid exchanges such as those used with IPD or rapid cycles on automated peritoneal dialysis (APD). As discussed in Chapter 27, this is related to aquaporin I channels, which lead to water removal. Without long dwells, the diffusive removal of sodium is reduced and this can result in a hypernatremic state in people using APD prescriptions compared to those on CAPD (Khandelwal et al., 2003a). The use of longer dwell periods overnight and the addition of a day dwell can be used to increase sodium removal (Khandelwal et al., 2003b).

Gokal (1999) and Khandelwal et al. (2003b) described the use of salt restrictions although the authors agree that consensus as to the degree of salt restriction has not been reached. A range of daily intake from 100 to 200 mEq of sodium per day was suggested with the greatest restriction for those with hypertension (Gokal, 1999; Khandelwal et al., 2003b).

Hyponatremia can occur due to the dilutional effect of excess water intake on serum sodium concentration. In states of hyperglycemia, the shift of water from the cell to the extracellular space can also dilute the serum sodium (Prichard, 2001). Additionally, loss of potassium from cells can have a similar effect due to the replacement of the lost intracellular potassium with sodium (Bargman, 2000).

Potassium imbalances. Due to continuous loss of potassium with PD, approximately 10% to 30% of individuals develop hypokalemia (Prichard, 2001). This can be compounded at times of decreased oral intake or increased losses with vomiting or diarrhea. While increased dietary potassium intake is recommended, other measures include the administration of potassium supplements orally and IP potassium chloride. The addition of 3-4 mEq/L of potassium chloride IP will prevent further losses via the effluent but will not compensate for continuing losses (see Chapter 27 for additional recommendations). In determining the route of administration, the balance between the risks of increased breaks in the system through the addition of medication versus the ability to manage oral medications must be considered. Again, increasing intake with food sources is preferred, and Burrowes (2004), in a review of ethnic and cultural foods, includes the potassium content of foods associated with cultural preference that can be incorporated into the treatment of hypokalemia.

Hyperkalemia can also occur in a percentage of individuals and is most likely related to dietary intake, although increased catabolic activity can also raise serum potassium. Dietary restrictions and cation exchange resins can be used to resolve this imbalance; however, the use of increased numbers of exchanges may also be indicated as a treatment for faster removal of the excess potassium. Another potential cause of hyperkalemia is insulin deficiency with resultant hyperglycemia. Due to redistribution of the potassium, serum levels may be high until the hyperglycemia is corrected and potassium can shift back into the cells (Brenner, 2003; Sherwin, 2004).

Calcium imbalances. There is a potential for calcium imbalances in PD. The PD solutions are available in concentrations of 7.0 mg/dL (1.75 mmol/L) and 5.0 mg/dL (1.25 mmol) of calcium. The latter solution is considered a low calcium prescription but in comparison with the serum ionized calcium is within the normal range. A risk of hypercalcemia is associated with higher calcium dialysate concentrations if there is no UF or if reabsorption occurs instead of fluid removal (Burkart & Piraino, 2001); however, increased fluid removal as occurs with 2.5% and 4.25% can result in enhanced calcium removal. For individuals who develop hypercalcemia secondary to the use of prescribed calcium-containing phosphate binders, a lower calcium dialysate can be used. This approach allows the continuation of medications beneficial for treatment of renal osteodystrophy while reducing the risks of hypercalcemia.

Complications Associated with Nutritional Status

Wang, Bernardini, Piriano, and Fried (2003) used albumin as a marker and concluded that hypoalbuminemia at the initiation of PD was associated with a higher peritonitis rate and felt that further studies were warranted to investigate this relationship and its effect on clinical outcomes. Since malnutrition contributes to morbidity and mortality, collaboration with the dietitian is imperative in early and continued interventions to improve the nutritional status of individuals treated with PD. PD is efficient at removing waste products; however, the membrane does not discriminate between wastes and essential nutrients. As a result, an average of 0.5 grams of protein/L of effluent is removed daily but up to 10-20 g per day has been described (Prichard, 2001). Additionally, 2-3 g of amino acids may be removed daily. Oral supplements, IP amino acids, total potential nutrition (TPN), and percutaneous enterostomal gastrostomy (PEG) tubes have been prescribed as methods for maintaining intake in individuals who are unable to meet their caloric and protein needs. Although more common in the pediatric population, PEG feeding in adults on PD has been reported; however, the approach is associated with a higher rate of complications (Madane, Forden, Fein, Morrell, Grossman, 2000).

Infectious Complications

Minnaganti and Cunha (2001), in a review of infections associated with uremia and dialysis, cited that infections accounted for "12% to 22% of deaths among dialysis patients in the United States and Canada" (p. 385). PD catheter exit site infections are reviewed in Chapter 28. Piraino (1998) wrote that "peritonitis remains a serious complication with associated risks including technique failure, catheter loss, and death" (p. 1956). Historically, CAPD was associated with a high incidence of peritonitis in the range of one every 10 weeks (Gokal, 2000). With improvements in technique, the incidence has decreased dramatically, but peritonitis rates remain a measurement used in determining the success of PD.

The literature has been variable with respect to the frequency of peritonitis in APD compared to CAPD (Diaz-Buxo & Crawford, 2002; Huang, Hung, Yen, Wu, & Tsai, 2001; Okechukwu & Swartz, 2001; Rodriguez-Carmona, Perez Fontan, Garcia Falcon, Fernandez Rivera, & Valdes, 1999). In a review of 198 patients with 327 episodes of peritonitis over a 10-year period, Yishak, Bernardini, Fried and Piraino (2001) found that although the failure rate for treatment was twice as high in APD patients compared to CAPD, there was no significant difference in the development of peritonitis based on treatment modality.

Peritonitis is an inflammation of the peritoneal cavity, which is primarily caused by infection. A diagnosis of presumed peritonitis is made if any of the three following criteria are met: abdominal pain, cloudy fluid, or a positive culture report from the peritoneal effluent. Identification of microorganisms with an increased white cell count greater than 100/mm^3 and more than 50% neutrophils confirms the diagnosis. Normally, the peritoneal cavity contains leukocytes such as macrophages, lymphocytes, and mesothelial cells, but in inflammatory states, neutrophils are recruited that contribute to the change in effluent clarity (Faull, 2000). The cloudy fluid is more readily recognized in CAPD than APD, and this finding can affect the timing of interventions and expected outcomes from treatment.

The presentation of peritonitis may range from a picture of no abdominal pain to mild abdominal cramps and cloudy fluid to extreme abdominal pain with rebound abdominal tenderness (Piraino et al., 2005). Nausea, vomiting, diarrhea, hypotension, and fever can also occur. Fever and hypotension, however, are not common findings and are generally associated with a more severe peritonitis such as *S aureus* with a septic presentation. The signs and symptoms of peritonitis are associated with other conditions such as gastritis, cholecystitis, appendicitis, pancreatitis, and ischemic bowel (Bargman, 2000; Minnaganti & Cunha, 2001; Prischl, Wallner, Schauer, Balon, & Kramar, 1999); hence, although it is tempting to label abdominal pain in people on PD as peritonitis, it is important to consider other abdominal pathologies.

Another finding that can occur is a transient decrease in UF as a consequence of the inflammatory process on the peritoneal membrane. Solute clearance may increase leading to reabsorption of the glucose with loss of the osmotic gradient for water removal. Close attention to the target weight during this critical period will be required to determine the appropriate bag strengths for exchanges (Burrows & Prowant, 1998). Icodextrin can be used during peritonitis to support UF.

Causes of Peritonitis

In recording episodes of peritonitis, it is important to document the causative organisms, contributing factors, and antibiotic sensitivity patterns. People presenting with peritonitis will be physically unwell and will be experiencing a range of emotional stress including guilt for the development of the infection. They need to be questioned in a non-threatening, non-judgmental way about the possibility of contamination; they may feel traumatized by questions included in the clinical assessment directed at understanding the source of the infection. Questions concerning PD technique, however, may reveal "interesting" problem solving strategies that demonstrate a need for enhanced learning opportunities. For example, Tzamaloukas and Quintana (1990) reported a case of insufflation peritonitis in which an individual attempted to relieve obstruction in the peritoneal catheter by blowing into the lumen. While the assessment is required to determine learning needs, individuals with peritonitis should be informed if the infection is not a technique-related issue. Thus, peritonitis from an endogenous source such as diverticular disease is not related to poor technique. The reaffirmation that individuals are not responsible for the infection may decrease fears and self-doubt with respect to ability to continue PD.

Routes of transmission for microorganisms are classified as periluminal, transluminal, transmural, transvaginal, and hematogenous. Table 29-1 defines these routes and potential organisms related to infection. In addition to these routes, peritonitis may also be caused by environmental factors including water contaminants from showering or swimming, soil contaminants, and organisms normally associated with animals (Cooke, Kodjo, Clutterbuck, & Bamford, 2004; Flynn, Meislich, Kaiser, Polinsky, & Baluarte, 1996; Kanaan et al., 2002; Sivaraman, 1999; Vas & Oreopoulos, 2001).

Table 29-1
Classifications of Routes of Contamination and Associated Organisms

Route.	Definition	Example	Associated Organisms	% Of Total Infections
Transluminal	Through the catheter lumen	Direct contamination	S epidermidis Acinetobacter	30 – 40
Periluminal	Along the outer surface of the peritoneal catheter	Exit site infection, with spread along tunnel to cavity	S epidermidis S aureus Pseudomonas Yeast	20 - 30
Transmural	Across the wall of the bowel	Diarrheal episode/ bowel perforation, diverticulosis	Gram negative enteric organisms Anaerobes	25 – 30
Transvaginal	Across the vaginal wall	Vaginal-peritoneal Fistula	Yeast Strep. Bovis Lactobacillus	5-10
Hematogenous	Spread through blood	Post dental work	Streptococcus M tuberculosis	2 – 5

Note: Adapted from Brown (2002); Brunier (1995); Vargemezis & Thodis (2001); Vas & Oreopoulos (2001).

Gram-positive, gram-negative, fungi, and mycobacterium or a combination of these organisms can cause peritonitis. Touch contamination with organisms such as *S aureus* and *S epidermidis* are associated with breaks in technique. Vas and Oreopoulos (2001) note that the incubation period for peritonitis can range from 6 to 48 hours although it is difficult to be precise about the time frame. Another source of bacteria is biofilm resulting from microbacterial colonies present on the inner surface of the peritoneal catheter. These colonies can adapt over time and develop antibiotic resistance (Dasgupta & Larabie, 2001). Occasionally, an individual may present with signs and symptoms of peritonitis; however, the microbiological sample is negative for any organism. This is known as "sterile" or culture negative peritonitis and may be caused by a number of reasons, such as:

- individual receiving antibiotics for another purpose, masking presence of organisms
- sampling delayed
- inadequate sampling
- volume too small for sample
- inadequate dwell time prior to collection of sample
- problems with culture technique in laboratory

The International Society for Peritoneal Dialysis (ISPD) recommendations (Piraino et al., 2005) detail approaches to collection of samples. These have been summarized in Table 29-2. The guidelines further caution that samples for APD collection should be interpreted according to the percentage of polymorphonuclear cells, as the dwell time may be shorter and influence the total number of white cells. Although 2 hours is the recommended minimum dwell period for collection, up to 4 to 6 hours has been suggested to yield an accurate appropriate cell count (Keane et al., 2000; Vas & Oreopoulos, 2001).

Nomenclature of Peritonitis

A single presentation of peritonitis is referred to as an

Table 29-2
Recommended Practice for Collecting and Processing Peritoneal Effluent

Collect first cloudy sample

- If CAPD, send first cloudy bag
- If APD, use day dwell or if dry, need to instill 1 liter minimum for 1-2 hours; if at night and can tolerate, try to instill for 1-2 hours, longer dwell if preferable
- If doubt with first sample in terms of results, repeat culture with a dwell time of at least 2 hours

Send to laboratory for analysis prior to initiation of antibiotics

- Options to take to closest laboratory or provide blood culture bottles at home or to refrigerate until able to bring to laboratory

Laboratory handling

- Centrifuge 50 mL at 3000 g for 15 minutes
- Resuspend sediment in 3-5 mL of sterile saline
- Inject into solid culture media and blood culture medium
- If unable to centrifuge, effluent can be injected directly into blood culture medium

"episode." Table 29-3 summarizes the terms used to differentiate episodes. Defining the infection facilitates treatment options and enhances data collection on peritonitis for both quality control and research. The expectation for treatment is clinical improvement; thus, non-responsiveness or worsening symptoms require further investigations. Reasons for non-response include "tunnel infection, intra-abdominal abscess, slime layer colonization of the intra-abdominal portion of the catheter, and inadequate antibiotic dosing" (Piraino, 2003, p. 73). If the individual is not improving and has developed a refractory peritonitis,

Table 29-3
Definitions of Peritonitis Episodes

Recurrent - occurs within 4 weeks of completing therapy, with a different organism than original infection

Relapsing - occurs within 4 weeks of completing therapy, with the same organism as the original infection or with one sterile episode

Repeat - occurs in more than 4 weeks following completing therapy, with the same organism as the original infection

Refractory - failure to respond to therapy within 5 days of receiving the appropriate antibiotic for the infection

Catheter-related - associated with exit-site or tunnel infection, with same organism, or with one site, sterile

Note: Adapted from Brenner & Rector (2004); Keane et al. (2000); Piraino et al. (2005); and Vas & Oreopoulos (2001).

removal of the catheter is indicated (Piraino et al., 2005).

Changes in peritonitis rates. Historically, peritonitis was associated primarily with gram-positive organisms (Posen, 1989). A reduction in gram-positive peritonitis has occurred with innovations such as disconnect systems, "flush before fill," and mupirocin prophylaxis. As a result, greater attention is now given to gram-negative organisms (Dasgupta & Larabie, 2001; Keane et al., 2000; Piraino, Bernardini, Florio, & Fried, 2003). Kim et al. (2004), in a 10-year retrospective review of 1,015 individuals from 1992 to 2001, reported that the majority of microorganisms associated with peritonitis were gram-positive, but noted a similar trend of changing organisms with greater proportions of gram-negative and methicillin-resistant staphylococci observed.

Polymicrobial peritonitis. Polymicrobial peritonitis refers to more than one organism causing the infection. Multiple gram-negative organisms on culture are generally associated with a more serious prognosis than multiple gram-positive organisms (Piraino et al., 2005). Catastrophic events including appendicitis and diverticulitis with bowel perforation have been associated with the development of polymicrobial peritonitis (Fried & Piraino, 2000; Harwell et al., 1997; Kern, Newman, Cacho, Schulak, & Weiss, 2002). Kim and Korbet (2000) reported that polymicrobial peritonitis accounted for 6% to 8% of all episodes of peritonitis with gram-negative and/or fungi as the causative organism. They further elaborated that the source of infection was often unknown and was not necessarily linked to catastrophic events. Szeto and colleagues (2002), in their review of 140 cases of polymicrobial peritonitis from 1995 to 2001, agreed with this report. They postulated that in many infections, contamination of the peritoneal cavity by migration of gram-negative bacteria across the bowel wall was the source for the organisms. The treatment of polymicrobial peritonitis has included catheter removal although successful treatment without catheter replacement has also been described (Holley, Bernardini, & Piraino, 1992; Kiernan et al., 1995; Kim & Korbet, 2000; Szeto, Chow,

Wong, Leung, & Li, 2002). Szeto et al. noted that catheter removal in their reviewed cases was more likely with peritonitis caused by anaerobes, fungus, or *Pseudomonas* species. The ISPD recommendations (Piraino et al., 2005) also note that resolution of polymicrobial gram-positive peritonitis may respond to antibiotics without catheter removal unless the catheter itself is the infectious source. On the other hand, the ISPD recommendations suggest that catheter removal is more likely with polymicrobial gram-negative organisms (Piraino et al., 2005).

Fungal peritonitis. Fungal peritonitis can occur as a primary infection or acquired peritonitis after treatment of a bacterial infection, particularly in association with long-term antibiotic administration (Ramalanjaona, 2003; Vas & Oreopoulos, 2001). Yeasts and filamentous fungi such as *Candida, Torulopsis glabrata, Aspergillus,* and *Fusarium* have been identified in peritonitis (Piraino, 1998; Vas & Oreopoulos, 2001). Huang and associates (2000) identified risk factors for fungal peritonitis as the use of antibiotics and steroids, prior diagnosis of lupus, increased frequency of peritonitis, and hospitalization. As these organisms can grow into the wall of the catheter, thus evading antibiotics, it is recommended that catheters be removed as soon as possible a part of treatment of fungal peritonitis (Keane et al., 2000).

Mycobacterial peritonitis. Both tuberculous (TB) and non-TB mycobacteria such as *M. fortuitum, M. kansasii,* and *M. gordonae* have been identified as causative organisms in peritonitis (Keane et al., 2000). TB peritonitis is frequently related to reactivation of prior disease (Keane et al., 2000) while *M. gordonae* are environmental and found in soil, water, and non-pasteruerized milk (Essnau et al. in Asnis et al., 1996). The diagnosis of mycobacterium can be difficult as skin tests and acid-fast bacillus (AFB) smears are often negative (Asnis, Bresciani, & Bhat, 1996). Additionally, the presentation may be as a culture negative peritonitis in some individuals, as the organism takes time to grow in the culture medium (Leehey et al., 2001; Vas & Oreopoulos, 2001). Treatment, in most instances, consists of three pharmacologic agents including rifampicin, isoniazid, and pyrazinamide (Keane et al., 2000). Ethambutol is not recommended because of the high risk of ocular toxicity in people with renal failure (Lui et al., 2001; Piraino et al., 2005).

Recognition and diagnosis of peritonitis. In preparing people for self-care, the signs and symptoms of peritonitis as well as the importance of reporting breaks in technique should be incorporated into the teaching programs. It is recommended that protocols be developed to facilitate treatment when breaks in technique occur; these situations typically require antibiotic therapy (Piraino et al., 2005). The *Toronto Western Hospital Patient Manual Eighth* edition (2002) defines these breaks as either "dry" or "wet" contaminations. A dry contamination infers that the peritoneal catheter was clamped but that a portion of the system has been touched and requires changing prior to continuation of procedures. A wet contamination is defined as having a potential risk of bacterial entry into the cavity. This may occur following a touch contamination with subsequent infusion of dialysate into the peritoneal cavity or as a result of a tear in the tubing and subsequent leaking of fluid and may require prophylactic antibiotics.

In the event of cloudy effluent, it is imperative that the first cloudy bag is saved for microbiological (gram stain and C&S) and hematological (white cell count) analysis prior to antibiotics in order to minimize false-negative culture results. Early intervention can promote home management of peritonitis, but delays in recognition and intervention can result in a more difficult course with potential hospitalization. Gram stains vary in their ability to identify organisms, with a positive report cited as occurring in "9% to 40% of peritonitis episodes" (Keane et al., 2000, p. 398); thus, it is important to continue broad antibiotic coverage until the culture reports are complete. Gram stains are also useful in the early identification of yeast (Fried & Piraino, 2000; Keane et al., 2000). Effluent analysis is useful to monitor white cell counts as an indication of the therapeutic response. A sustained high level or initial decrease followed by increase can be related to poor response to antibiotics, incorrect dosing, wrong antibiotic, or the rupture of an abscess within the peritoneal cavity (Piraino, 2003). On the other hand, decreasing white cell counts and clinical improvement are associated with resolution of the peritonitis.

Treatment of Peritonitis

Treatment of peritonitis includes flushes, IP antibiotics, pain management, and psychological support for both the individual with infection and caregivers who may experience feelings of guilt and distress with the development of the infection. Treatment should be commenced immediately as delays can lead to a more complicated course (Okechukwu & Swartz, 2001).

One to three flushes of dialysate in and out without a dwell time have been used in the initial presentation of infection to reduce the bacterial count and relieve pain; however, since there is a theoretical possibility that host defense factors will be washed out with the organism, additional flushes are not recommended. If flushes are used, the prescribed volume is generally the same as the individual's dialysis prescription; however, if the pain is severe, a lesser volume may be used according to individual tolerance levels. The ISPD guidelines no longer include flushes as part of the standard protocol and hence, unit specific policies need to review local practices. Given that cultures require time to grow for identification, empiric coverage of peritonitis is commenced to ensure that the most common organisms will be covered. Thus, the ISPD guidelines recommend broad-spectrum coverage for both gram-positive and gram-negative organisms with IP drug administration. The IP route is effective in allowing high concentration of drug in the peritoneal cavity as well as being convenient, particularly in individuals who may have nausea and vomiting, and are unable to tolerate oral antibiotics (Manley & Bailie, 2002).

Gram-positive bacteria can be treated with a first generation cephalosporin such as cefazolin, and gram-negative ones can be treated with either a third generation cephalosporin such as ceftazidime or an aminoglycoside such as tobramycin. In order to preserve residual renal function in individuals with greater than 100 ml urine in 24 hours, cephalosporins are preferred to aminoglycosides, which are more nephrotoxic. IP administration of antibiotics can be delivered either in each bag or in a single daily dose.

Following final culture and sensitivity reports, the antibiotics can be adjusted for the specific organism and sensitivity. Treatment duration ranges from 14 days for organisms such as *S epidermidis* to 21 days for *S aureus* species and anaerobes, although individual units may elect to prescribe a differing duration of therapy. The ISPD (2005) has published updated recommendations for PD related infections, and these can serve as an excellent guideline for developing unit specific protocols (ISPD, 2005).

Since the ISPD revised guidelines were first published, there have been controversies regarding the choice of antibiotics. Zelenitsky, Ariano, and Harding (2004) reviewed the literature on residual renal function decline and otovestibular damage and suggested that due to limited analysis, the generally held belief that aminoglycosides were associated with more side effects than cephalosporins was unwarranted and, thus, aminoglycosides remain a suitable alternative. These authors also expressed concern with resistance in continued use of ceftazidime. Kavanagh, Prescott, and Mactier (2004) in 31/2-year review of peritonitis in Scotland noted that vancomycin has remained the antibiotic of choice for treating gram-positive organisms despite ISPD recommendations and have attributed this to the local antibiotic resistance patterns. It should be noted that the recommendations emphasized the need to review local peritonitis patterns, organisms, and sensitivities in developing unit-specific guidelines.

Additionally, the ISPD guidelines are based on CAPD, and concerns have been raised regarding the efficacy of IP antibiotics in APD due to higher clearance rates compared to CAPD. Manley and Bailie (2002) recommended a day dwell of at least 4 hours for antibiotic administration in APD. For individuals who cannot tolerate a day dwell due to back pain or existing hernias, a smaller volume of dialysate can be used to deliver the antibiotic.

Individuals may be taught to self-manage peritonitis at home both with early recognition and intervention; however, some individuals may require admission to hospital for supportive measures during the peritonitis. For mild peritonitis, people may be able to cope at home with support from the home PD unit; however, if the symptoms preclude the individual from managing the dialysis techniques safely, admission may be warranted. In the event of severe peritonitis in which stabilization and investigations are required, admission is also preferred. Measures of severity can include hemodynamic instability with sepsis, pain requiring analgesia, classification of organism (i.e., polymicrobial, yeast), and underlying etiology of the infection.

Oral antibiotics. Although the traditional route for antibiotic administration in the management of peritonitis has been IP, there is increased interest in the use of oral antibiotics. In a review Passadakis and Oreopoulos (2001) concluded that despite concerns about resistance with oral monotherapy, quinolones alone could be used as a first-line approach. A 78%-83% success rate using the oral route alone was reported and was considered approximately equal to IP combinations of aminoglycosides and first-generation cephalosporins. They noted that a combination of an oral quinolone and a single IP antibiotic was also an effective alternative approach. Goffin et al. (2004) studied oral ciprofloxacin and IP vancomycin over a 9-year period and concluded that this combination as first-line agents showed similar outcomes to standard IP antibiotic regimens. Yeung and associates (2004) also studied the use of oral ciprofloxacin for individuals on CCPD; they advocated the use of this agent in the setting of *E. coli* and *Klebsiella* species but found suboptimal drug concentrations against *P. aeruginosa*. The current ISPD guidelines (Piraino et al., 2005) state that quinolines "appear to be acceptable alternative to aminoglycosides for gram-negative coverage" and suggest a dose of levofloxacin of 300 mg daily or pefloxacin 400 mg daily but do not recommend oral agents for severe cases of peritonitis or for *S. aureus* (p. 115). Passadakis and Oreopoulos (2001), while optimistic about the option of oral antibiotics, cautioned that further comparative randomized studies are needed in order to determine the efficacy of oral medications in peritonitis treatment. Additionally, if there is uncertainty about the gastrointestinal absorption of medications (i.e., vomiting), the IP route is preferred.

Heparin. In order to prevent fibrin formation associated with the inflammatory response, to maintain patency of the catheter, and to reduce sequestration of bacterial colonies in fibrin, intraperitoneal heparin is recommended (Diaz-Buxo, 2005). Heparin 500 units/L is recommended by the ISPD (Piraino et al., 2005) for "extremely cloudy effluent" (p. 113) although unit specific practices may range from 500 to 1000 units of heparin/L (UHN Division of Nephrology, 2005).

PD catheter removal. Although individuals committed to PD may be hesitant to temporarily stop their PD and utilize HD, there are some circumstances that may require such a change; thus, they should be supported through this period. Piraino (2003) summarizes reasons for PD catheter removal as "persistent exit site/tunnel infection; exit site/tunnel infection with associated peritonitis, refractory peritonitis with failure to clear effluent by 4-5 days with appropriate antibiotics, persistently positive effluent cultures, recurrent peritonitis (with) two or more episodes of peritonitis with the same organisms within 1 month of stopping antibiotics, and fungal peritonitis" (p. 74). Organisms strongly associated with the need for early catheter removal include *Pseudomonas, Mycobacterium,* and fungal and polymicrobial infections (Keane et al., 2000; Nannini, Paphitou, & Ostrosky-Zeichner, 2003; Okechukwu & Swartz, 2001; Szeto et al., 2002). Failure to remove the catheter in these situations could lead to serious peritoneal membrane damage or death.

ISPD recommendations based on opinion are for replacement of the peritoneal catheter 2-3 weeks after removal of the infected catheter; however, the interval may be extended in the event of severe infection or organisms such as fungi or tuberculosis. There have been reports of simultaneous catheter removal and replacement when the peritonitis has been attributed to biofilm or tunnel infec-

Table 29-4
Calculating Episodes of Peritonitis

Rates

1. Number of infections by organisms over time, divided by dialysis years' time at risk, expressed as episodes per year

2. Months of PD at risk, divided by number of episodes, expressed as interval in months between episodes

Percentage

1. As percentage of patients over a time period free of peritonitis

Time at Risk

Time at risk = number of patients on PD for the entire month x number of days in month + number of days on PD for newly trained for month + number of days on PD for patients who left PD during month (transplanted, died, transferred out) = Total days divided by number of days in month = months at risk.

Month at risk divided by 12 = years at risk

Number of events divided by years at risk = rate per year

(To determine the interval of months between episodes, 12 divided by rate per year)

Note: Adapted from Bernardini (2004); Piraino et al. (2005).

tion. This approach is undertaken if there is evidence that the individual has responded to antibiotics and the effluent white blood cell count has normalized (Majkowski, & Mendley, 1997; Swartz, Messana, Reynolds, & Ranjit, 1991). Thus, the effluent must be clear at the time of simultaneous removal and reinsertion of the catheter. Additionally, the simultaneous procedure is not recommended for peritonitis caused by *pseudomonas* species, fungus, or mycobacterium or if there is an associated intraperitoneal abscess (Keane et al., 2000; Okechukwu & Swartz, 2001).

Vigilance. Monitoring of peritonitis rates is essential for a PD program in order to follow the incidence of infection and identify contributing factors. The data can then be used to modify procedures, adapt teaching and evaluation processes and further develop guidelines for interventions. Calculation methods for peritonitis rates are in Table 29-4. Various targets have been set for expected rates of peritonitis including one less than every 18 patient months (The Renal Association, 2002). Vas and Oreopoulos (2001) suggested that an acceptable peritonitis rate be in the range of one episode every 24 patient months although Vas (2002) noted that there are reports of one episode every 36 to 48 patient months.

In interpreting rates of infection, one must also consider the population and associated risk factors when developing quality improvement strategies. New units, in particular, may expect to see a higher incidence rate than established units until the expertise is developed. Regardless of the units' experience, dedication to systematic monitoring and adherence to approved guidelines will have an impact on outcomes for individuals on PD.

Edwards, Calissi, and Kappel (2001) described the use of a multidisciplinary critical pathway for the management of peritonitis in the home dialysis setting. Through clear delineation of responsibilities and recording of events, Edwards et al. (2001) believed that the development of this pathway augmented the training provided for individuals self-managing PD and enhanced communication between the care providers and care recipients. They also discussed the necessity of revising such documentation with changes in recommendations for management. Kim et al. (2004) stressed the role of nurses trained in PD in the decline of peritonitis rates in their unit; the authors also highlighted the value of patient education programs in reducing infection rates. Hall et al. (2004) demonstrated fewer exit site infections and reduced peritonitis when a program of enhanced training was compared with the standard approach. The mean training time was 29 hours for the enhanced group and 22.6 hours for the standard group. Thus, time spent in education and follow-up is crucial in the prevention and subsequent management of peritonitis.

Prevention of Peritonitis

Measures to prevent the occurrence of peritonitis are vital to the outcome of the technique. The Center for Disease Control (CDC) (2004) recommends hand washing with soap and water or an alcohol based hand rub before handling dressings while Piraino (1998), in summarizing studies on hand washing and contamination of connection sites, stressed the need to adhere to aseptic techniques including hand washing and drying.

Prophylactic antibiotic coverage for procedures is of major importance but often gets overlooked. Colucci, Scalamogna, and De Vecchi (2001), in a review of 424 episodes of peritonitis in 353 people over 10 years, described four episodes of peritonitis within 7 days of procedures associated with organs close to or in the peritoneal cavity, such as colonoscopy and liver, prostate, or endometrial biopsies. The authors recommended prophylactic antibiotic coverage for any of these procedures as well as for transplant nephrectomy or barium enemas. In addition, prophylaxis for dental work is recommended (Oreopoulos & Vas, 2001; Piraino, 1998, Piraino et al., 2005). It is important to note that dental work includes cleaning as well as invasive dental procedures.

In a comprehensive review of randomized controlled trials for prevention of peritonitis, Strippoli, Tong, Johnson, Schena, and Craig (2004) identified six studies with successful outcomes associated with prophylaxis: one study supported the use of mupirocin topically for nasal staphylococci carriers, four studies reduced post-operative peritonitis with use of perioperative IV antibiotics, and one study reduced *Candida* species peritonitis by the use of oral nystatin as an additive to peritonitis protocol recommendations. Prophylactic measures should be reviewed and incorporated into unit practice.

Adherence to technique is also vital for prevention of PD peritonitis, thus PD programs should incorporate a variety of teaching and learning strategies including demonstration and return demonstration as well as skill updating and retraining, as required. Assessment of abilities is essential and occasionally can be enhanced with assistance by occupational therapists and the selection of appropriate assistive devices. The entire multidisciplinary team can help to evaluate episodes of peritonitis. The nature of the organism often helps to determine the most likely cause of the infection. This may provide direction for the nurse regarding the most appropriate approach to prevent future episodes of infection.

Psychologically, the burden of self-care and "burn out" can lead to inadequate or poor adherence to technique. Troidle et al. (2003) found an association with depression and frequency of peritonitis and suggested that this was an avenue for further studies. Lew and Piraino (2005) also noted the relationship between outcomes and psychosocial factors including depression. This would support a therapeutic relationship between the nephrology nurses and individuals on PD, particularly as with home dialysis where there is less peer support than with in-center dialysis. Thus, the nurses are in an ideal position to assess physical, social and psychological factors that affect the overall status of individuals.

Ultrafiltration (UF) Failure

UF failure refers to the inability to remove fluid efficiently. This can be a transient effect as noted with peritonitis or may be permanent secondary to changes in the peritoneal membrane for various reasons including exposure to irritants, scarring post-surgical interventions, or peritonitis and loss of aquaporin I channels (Oreopoulos & Rao, 2001).

In assessing for UF failure, warning signals can include the increased requirement for hypertonic solutions to remove fluid and decreased effluent returns with previously effective patterns of bag strength selection. Approaches to management include the use of icodextrin solutions, diuretics if the individual has residual renal function, and dietary sodium and fluid restrictions. If appropriate, a shift in PD therapy may be required. For example if the PET demonstrates that the individual is a rapid transporter who has been managed on CAPD, a change to CCPD with shorter dwells may facilitate improved water removal. If, however, PD options have been tried and proven ineffective, transfer to HD may be imminent and steps should be taken to prepare both physically and emotionally for the transfer.

Encapsulating Peritoneal Sclerosis (EPS)

This rare but increasingly identified complication of PD has been reported under a number of names including peritoneal sclerosis, sclerotic obstructive peritonitis, calcific peritonitis, abdominal cocoon, and sclerosing peritonitis. Over time, the peritoneal membrane can become sclerosed leading to encapsulation of the small bowel in a cocoon-like web of membrane. This ultimately results in intermittent small bowel obstruction; however, large bowel obstruction has also been reported (Choi, Kim, Kim, Jin, & Choi, 2004).

Reported incidence rates have ranged from 0.54% to

2.2% (Afthentopoulos, Passadikis, Oreopoulos, & Bargman, 1998; Nakamoto, Kawaguchi, & Suzuki, 2002; Rigby & Hawley, 1998). Rigby and Hawley (1998) reported a mortality rate of 56% in 54 individuals identified with EPS in a review of 7,374 people from 1978 to 1994 in Australia. Although the incidence rate of this complication is low, the consequence is great, as there is a high mortality rate from malnutrition and sepsis (Pollock, 2003).

People with this condition may present with manifestations while still remaining on PD or after transfer to HD or renal transplantation. Vague abdominal pain and, occasionally, hemoperitoneum may be found in the early stages of EPS, but as time progresses, intermittent small bowel obstruction, abdominal pain ranging from mild to severe, nausea, vomiting, weight loss, and decreased UF with PD help establish the diagnosis. Yamamoto et al. (2002) found an association between high transport membrane characteristics and the development of EPS after cessation of long-term PD. This is not always the case, as not all individuals with EPS have high transport characteristics as a defining feature of the condition (Kawaguchi, Kawanishi, Mujais, Topley, & Oreopoulos, 2000). Pollock (2003) suggests these differences in transport may reflect varying stages of disease progression, thus it is important to compare characteristics over time.

Abdominal x-rays are generally not helpful in establishing the diagnosis unless prominent calcification is noted in combination with specific ultrasound and CT findings. Calcification can occur without EPS (Bargman, 2000). Fixed, dilated loops of bowel that are tethered to the membrane, a "sandwich appearance" to the membrane, and entrapped fluid may be found on ultrasound.

Findings on CT may include adherent dilated bowel loops, air fluid levels, thickening of the intestinal wall and peritoneal membrane, and loculated fluid collections (Stafford-Johnson, Wilson, Francis, & Swartz, 1998). It is important to remember that many people on long-term PD will develop thickening of the peritoneal membrane; thus, this finding alone does not indicate a diagnosis of EPS.

The composition of dialysate solutions has been implicated in the development of EPS including use of acetate-based solutions, low pH, hyperosmolarity, and presence of glucose degradation products. Additionally, instillation of disinfectant into the peritoneal cavity, inline filters on administration sets for trapping bacteria, frequent peritonitis with associated scarring of the membrane, and longer duration of dialysis have been associated with EPS (Pollock, 2003). Nakamoto et al. (2002), in a retrospective analysis of 11,549 patients in 157 centers in Japan between 1980 and 2000, reported on 256 individuals with EPS and noted that there was a 3.3 times higher incidence of peritonitis in the diagnosed individuals. These authors also found that EPS developed an average of 99.6 (range 10-168) months after initiation of CAPD.

Treatment of EPS. Reported treatments for EPS have included the use of immunosuppressives, tamoxifen, TPN, peritoneal lavage, and surgical intervention (Allaria, Giangrande, Gandini, & Pisoni, 1999; del Peso et al., 2003; Martins, Rodrigues, Cabrita, & Guimaraes, 1999; Yamamoto et al., 2002). Medications such as tamoxifen

and immunosuppressive agents including azathioprine, cyclosporine, sirolimus, and prednisone have been used; however, series reports provide a range of outcomes from no benefit to improvement (del Peso et al., 2003; Mori et al., 1997; Rajani, Smyth, Koffman, Abbs, & Goldsmith, 2002). Recent studies suggest that immunosuppressive therapy in the early stages of EPS may be more beneficial than in later stages (Dejagere et al., 2005; Kawanishi et al., 2004). Tamoxifen, an anti-estrogen, has been used in the treatment of breast cancer and retroperitoneal fibrosis (Evrenkaya et al., 2004). The drug's action in EPS is not clear although the drug may affect growth factors. While not treating EPS, TPN, an adjunct to therapy to counteract the associated malnutrition, has been used but is not without risks including infection and hepatic failure (Nauth et al., 2004; Spencer & Compher, 2003). Since the membrane may be more prone to adhere without peritoneal fluid in the cavity (Bargman, 2000), a suggestion has been to perform intermittent peritoneal lavage in high-risk individuals who are no longer on PD, but this does not eliminate the primary pathologic process (Moriishi et al., 2002; Nakayama et al., 2002). Early surgical interventions have been associated with a high mortality rate; however, Smith, Collins, Morris, and Teele (1997) reported success with two individuals through a surgical procedure to peel the membrane away from the intestines. Increasing success with surgical approaches, including enterolysis, have been described (Kawanishi, 2002; Kawanishi et al., 2004; Slim, Tohme, Yaghi, Honein, & Sayegh, 2005). Enterolysis is generally a very complex surgical procedure that involves carefully separating the bowel from the entire peritoneal membrane.

Individuals with EPS and their families require additional counseling and support given the poor prognosis associated with this condition. In the era of computer information, individuals seeking information may lose hope if reviewing the current literature detailing high mortality and should be advised of new findings in the field as they are reported in order to maintain hope. Regrets regarding the choice of dialysis modality may also arise and require honest communication to maintain a trust relationship with caregivers. While the prognosis is guarded, newer therapies are offering hope to individuals with this condition.

Psychological Impact of PD

While self-determination and control of treatment are considered important to the success of PD, there may be people who become fatigued with the daily routine of dialysis and opt to alter the routine. Bernardini and Piraino (1998) examined compliance of individuals in a prospective study and found that one third of the people did not do the ordered exchanges faithfully. As evidenced by an inventory of supplies during home visits, only 74% of prescribed exchanges were carried out, and that compliance was higher with APD than with CAPD. This could reflect fatigue with the procedure. Wu et al. (2004) concluded that health-related quality of life (HRQOL) measurements improve in the first year of dialysis for both HD and PD. Although, losses also occur, the authors could not conclude that PD provided a better quality of life than HD. They reported that people on PD could expect less pain, less problems with diet, and better functional capacity for work with this option. They may experience more concerns with sleep or sexual functioning than people on HD.

In a prospective cohort study, Rubin and colleagues (2004) found that people on PD rated the care received by the nephrology team higher than people on HD. In this study, the people "receiving PD were 1.5 times as likely to rate their dialysis care excellent overall than were patients receiving HD" (p. 700). In this survey, it was found that dialysis information and information for making the choice of dialysis were most highly valued by the respondents. Shimoyama et al. (2003), in a study of 26 people on CAPD and 34 family caregivers, found that success of coping with chronic illness was affected by changes in social role and mental health. These studies support the important role of nurses in offering support and continued connection with individuals on PD, as well as incorporating assessment of psychological well-being as part of the on going nursing care. Strategies can then be developed to alleviate the impact, such as support groups, home visits, clinic visits, counseling programs, and referrals to health care services.

Summary

Medical treatments include both benefits and risks. In undertaking PD, individuals are committing themselves to a life-support therapy; however, as can be seen by the review of complications, the treatment can add stressors to both the biological and psychological burden of illness. While health care professionals highlight the normalization of illness to allow life to continue, the reality is that even in the most stable individual on PD, complications may be experienced. The early identification and intervention is of utmost importance in maintaining trusting relationships and support to encourage the continuation of PD. Tan and Morad (2003) described the need for PD nurses who are motivated, highly skilled in communication and willing to seek challenges beyond the normal environment. In training, assessing, monitoring, and supporting individuals on PD, nurses have the opportunity to contribute not only to the overall program but also to individual outcomes for people receiving treatment. Further, by documenting the nursing approach and interventions for complications, the professional body of knowledge can be enhanced in the ongoing evolution of PD as a treatment option.

References

Afthentopoulos, I.E., Rao, P., Bhaskaran, S., & Oreopoulos, D.G. (1997). Does a large dialysate volume (2.5 litres) increase hernia formation in CAPD? (Abstract). *Peritoneal Dialysis International, 17*(S1), S55.

Afthentopoulos, I.E., Passadakis, P., Oreopoulos, D.G., & Bargman, J. (1998). Sclerosing peritonitis in continuous ambulatory peritoneal dialysis patients: One center's experience and review of the literature. *Advances in Renal Replacement Therapy, 5*(3), 157-167.

Akheel, S., Rattansingh, A., & Furtado, S.D. (2005). Current perspectives on the management of gastroparesis. *Journal of Postgraduate Medicine, 51*, 54-60.

Allaria, P.M., Giangrande, A., Gandini, E., & Pisoni, I.B. (1999). Continuous ambulatory peritoneal dialysis and sclerosing encapsulating peritonitis: Tamoxifen as a new therapeutic agent? *Journal of Nephrology, 12*(6), 395-397.

Ashgar, R., Woodrow, G., & Turney, J.H. (2000). A case of eosinophilic peritonitis treated with oral corticosteroids (Letter). *Peritoneal Dialysis International, 20*(5), 579-580.

Asnis, D.S., Bresciani, A.R., & Bhat, J.G. (1996). *Mycobacterium gordonae:* Unusual pathogen causing peritonitis in a patient on chronic ambulatory peritoneal dialysis. *Clinical Microbiology Newsletter, 18*(15), 116-118.

Bargman, J.M. (2000). Non-infectious complications of peritoneal dialysis. In R. Gokal, R. Khanna, R. Krediet, & K. Nolph (Eds.), *Textbook of peritoneal dialysis* (pp. 60-646). Dordrecht: Kluwer Academic Publishers.

Bargman, J.M. (2001). Mechanical complications of peritoneal dialysis. In J.T. Daugirdas, P.G. Blake, & T.S. Ing (Eds.), *Handbook of dialysis* (pp. 399-404). Philadelphia: Lippincott Williams & Wilkins.

Bargman, J. (2004). The law of diminishing returns: It is not always ultrafiltration failure. *Peritoneal Dialysis International, 24*(5), 419-421.

Bargman, J.M., Zent, R., Ellis, P., Auger, M., & Wilson, S. (1994). Diagnosis of lymphoma in a continuous ambulatory peritoneal dialysis patient by peritoneal fluid cytology. *American Journal of Kidney Diseases, 23*(5), 747-750.

Bernardini, J. (2004). Peritoneal dialysis: Myths, barriers and achieving optimum outcomes. *Nephrology Nursing Journal, 31*(5), 494-498.

Bernardini, J., & Piraino, B. (1998). Compliance in CAPD and CCPD patients as measured by supply inventories during home visits. *American Journal of Kidney Diseases, 31*(1), 101-107.

Brenner, B.M. (2003). *The kidney* (7th ed.). St. Louis: W.B. Saunders.

Brown, E.A. (2002). An opportune time to develop new strategies against repeat peritonitis in patients on peritoneal dialysis? *American Journal of Kidney Diseases, 39*(6), 1318-1320.

Brunier, G. (1995). Peritonitis in patients on peritoneal dialysis: A review of pathophysiology and treatment. *ANNA Journal, 22*(6), 575-585.

Burkart, J.M., & Piraino, B. (Eds.). (2001). Hypercalcemia in a peritoneal dialysis patient (Peritoneal Dialysis Case Forum). *Peritoneal Dialysis International, 21*(4), 420-427.

Burrows, L., & Prowant, B.F. (1998). Peritoneal dialysis. In J. Parker (Ed.), *Contemporary nephrology nursing* (pp. 605-659). Pitman, NJ: American Nephrology Nurses' Association.

Burrowes, J.D. (2004). Incorporating ethnic and cultural food preferences in the renal diet. *Advances in Renal Replacement Therapy, 11*(1), 97-104.

Cárdenas, A., & Chopra, S. (2002). Chylous ascites. *The American Journal of Gastroenterology, 97*(8), 1896-1900.

Carter, T.B., Garris, A.G., & Ullian, M.E. (1996). Rusty peritoneal dialysis fluid after intravenous administration of iron dextran. *American Journal of Kidney Diseases, 27*(1), 147-150.

Centers for Disease Control (CDC). (2004). Retrieved from www.cdc.gove/drugresistance/healthcare

Choi, J.H., Kim, J.H., Kim, J.J., Jin, S.Y., & Choi, D.L. (2004). Large bowel obstruction caused by sclerosing peritonitis: Contrast-enhanced CT findings. *The British Journal of Radiology, 77*, 344-346.

Chow, K.M., Szeto, C.C., & Li, P.K. (2003). Management options for hydrothorax complicating peritoneal dialysis. *Seminars in Dialysis, 16*(5), 389-394.

Colucci, P., Scalamogna, A., & De Vecchi, A. (2001). Peritonitis following surgical procedures in peritoneal dialysis (Letter). *Peritoneal Dialysis Bulletin, 21*(2), 198-200.

Cooke, F.J., Kodjo, A., Clutterbuck, E.J., & Bamford, K.B. (2004). A case of Pasteurella multocida peritoneal dialysis-associated peritonitis and a review of the literature. *International Journal of Infectious Diseases, 8*(3), 171-174.

Crabtree, J.H., & Fishman, A. (2005). A laparoscopic method for optimal peritoneal dialysis access. *American Surgeon, 71*(2), 135-143.

Currier, H. (1995). Chylous ascites: An unexpected complication that resembles peritonitis. *ANNA Journal, 22*(2), 157-159.

Dasgupta, M.K., & Larabie, M. (2001). Biofilms in peritoneal dialysis. *Peritoneal Dialysis International, 21*(S3), S213-S217.

Daugirdas, J.T., Leehey, D.J., Popli, S., Hoffman, W., Zayas, I., Gandhi, V.C., & Ng, T.S. (1987). Induction of peritoneal fluid eosinophilia and/or monocytosis by intraperitoneal air injection. *American Journal of Nephrology, 7*(2), 116-120.

Dejagere, T., Evenepoel, P., Claes, K., Kuypers, D., Maes, B., & Vanrentergham, Y. (2005). Acute-onset, steroid-sensitive, encapsulating peritoneal sclerosis in a renal transplant recipient. *American Journal of Kidney Diseases, 45*(2), E33-E37.

del Peso, G., Bajo, M.A., Gil, F., Aguilera, A., Ros, S., Costero, O., Castro, M.J., & Selgas, R. (2003). Clinical experience with tamoxifen in peritoneal fibrosing syndromes. *Advances in Peritoneal Dialysis, 19*, 32-35.

De Schoenmakere, G., Vanholder, R., Rottey, S., Duym, P., Lameire, N. (2001). Relationship between gastric emptying and clinical and biochemical factors in chronic hemodialysis patients. *Nephrology, Dialysis, Transplantation, 16*,1850-1855.

Diaz-Buxo, J.A. (2005). Clinical use of peritoneal dialysis. In A.R. Nissenson & R.N. Fine (Eds.), *Clinical dialysis* (4th ed.) (pp. 421-489). New York: McGraw-Hill.

Diaz-Buxo, J.A., & Crawford, T.L. (2002). Peritonitis in continuous cycling peritoneal dialysis. *Advances in Peritoneal Dialysis, 18*, 161-164.

Dorval, M., Legault, L., Lessard, F., & Roy, L. (2000). Practical aspects of the addition of sodium bicarbonate to peritoneal dialysate. *Peritoneal Dialysis International, 20*(6), 791-793.

Dozio, B., Scanziani, R., Rovere, G., Sangalli, L., Sacerdoti, S., & Surian, M. (2001). Hemoperitoneum in a continuous ambulatory peritoneal dialysis patient caused by a hepatocarcinoma treated with percutaneous embolization. *American Journal of Kidney Diseases, 38*(3), E11.

Edwards, M., Calissi, P.T., & Kappel, J.E. (2001). A critical pathway for outpatient treatment of CAPD peritonitis. *Peritoneal Dialysis Bulletin, 21*(1), 79-83.

Enia, G., Mallamaci, F., Benedetto, F.A., Panuccio, V., Parlongo, S., Cutrupi, S., Giacone, G., Cottini, E., Tripepi, G., Malatino, L.S., & Zoccali, C. (2001). Long-term CAPD patients are volume expanded and display more severe left ventricular hypertrophy than haemodialysis patients. *Nephrology Dialysis Transplantation, 16*, 1459-1464.

Enoch, C., Aslam, N., & Piraino, B. (2002). Intra-abdominal pressure, peritoneal dialysis exchange volume, and tolerance in APD. *Seminars in Dialysis, 15*(6), 403-406.

Evrenkaya, T.R., Atasoyu, E.M., Unver, S., Basekim, C., Baloglu, H., & Tulbek, M.Y. (2004). Corticosteroid and tamoxifen therapy in sclerosing encapsulating peritonitis in a patient on continuous ambulatory peritoneal dialysis. *Nephrology Dialysis Transplantation, 19*, 2423-2424.

Faull, R.J. (2000). Peritoneal defenses against infection: "Winning the battle but losing the war?" *Seminars in Dialysis, 13*(1), 47-53.

Flanigan, M., & Gokal, R. (2005). Peritoneal catheters and exit-site practices toward optimum peritoneal access: A review of current developments. *Peritoneal Dialysis International, 25*, 132-139.

Flynn, J.T., Meislich, D., Kaiser, B.A., Polinsky, M.S., & Baluarte, H.J. (1996). Fusarium peritonitis in a child on peritoneal dialysis: Case report and review of the literature. *Peritoneal Dialysis International, 16*(1), 52-57.

Fraley, D.S., Johnston, J.R., Bruns, F.J., Adler, S., & Segel, D.P. (1988). Rupture of ovarian cyst: Massive hemoperitoneum in continuous ambulatory peritoneal dialysis patients: Diagnosis and treatment. *American Journal of Kidney Diseases, 12*(1), 69-71.

Fried, L., & Piraino, B. (2000). Peritonitis. In R. Gokal, R. Khanna, R. Krediet, & K. Nolph (Eds.), *Textbook of peritoneal dialysis* (pp. 545-564). Dordrecht: Kluwer Academic Publishers.

Gagnon, R.F., & Daniels, E. (2004). The persisting pneumatoenteric recess and the infracardiac bursa: Possible role in the pathogenesis of right hydrothorax complicating peritoneal dialysis. *Advances in Peritoneal Dialysis, 20*, 132-136.

Goffin, E., Herbiet, L., Pouthier, D., Pochet, J.M., Lafontaine, J.J., Christophe, J.L., Gigi, J., & Vandercam, B. (2004). Vancomycin and ciprofloxacin: Systemic antibiotic administration for peritoneal dialysis-associated peritonitis. *Peritoneal Dialysis International, 24*(5), 433-439.

Gokal, R. (1999). Fluid management and cardiovascular outcome in peritoneal dialysis patients. *Seminars in Dialysis, 12*(2), 126-132.

Gokal, R. (2000). History of peritoneal dialysis. In R. Gokal, R. Khanna, R. Krediet, & K. Nolph (Ed.), *Textbook of peritoneal dialysis* (pp. 1-17). Dordrecht: Kluwer Academic Publishers.

Gokal, R., Alexander, S., Ash, S., Chen, T.W., Danielson, A., Holmes, et al. (1998). Peritoneal catheters and exit-site practices toward optimum peritoneal access: 1998 update. *Peritoneal Dialysis International, 18*(1), 11-33.

Greenberg, A., Bernardini, J., Piraino, B., Johnston, J.R., & Perlmutter, J.A. (1992). Hemoperitoneum complicating chronic peritoneal dialysis: Single-center experience and literature review. *American Journal of Kidney Diseases, 19*(3), 252-256.

Hall, G., Bogan, A., Dreis, S., Duffy, A., Green, S., Kelley, K., et al. (2004). New directions in peritoneal dialysis training. *Nephrology Nursing Journal, 31*(2), 149-154, 159-163.

Harnett, J.D., Gill, D., Corbett, L., Parfrey, P.S., & Gault, H. (1987). Recurrent hemoperitoneum in women receiving continuous ambulatory peritoneal dialysis. *Annals of Internal Medicine, 107*(3), 341-343.

Halstead, J.C., Lim, E., & Ritchie, A.J. (2002). Acute hydrothorax in CAPD. Early thoracoscopic (VATS) intervention allows return to peritoneal dialysis. *Nephron, 92*(3), 725-727.

Harwell, C.M., Newman, L.N., Cacho, C.P., Mulligan, D.C., Schulak, J.A., & Friedlander, M.A. (1997). Abdominal catastrophe: Visceral injury as a cause of peritonitis in patients treated by peritoneal dialysis. *Peritoneal Dialysis International, 17*(6), 586-594.

Hawkins, S.P., Homer, J.A., Murray, B.B., Voss, D.M., & van der Merwe, W.M. (2000). Modified computed tomography peritoneography: Clinical utility in continuous ambulatory peritoneal dialysis patients. *Australasian Radiology, 44*, 398-403.

Health Guide for the Perplexed. (2005). Inguinal hernias or the dangers of groin and allied "ruptures." Retrieved July 7, 2005, from www.broward.org/medical/mei00227.htm

Holley, J.L., Bernardini, J., & Piraino, B. (1992). Polymicrobial peritonitis in patients on continuous ambulatory peritoneal dialysis (Abstract). *American Journal of Kidney Diseases, 19*, 162-166.

Hou, S. (2001). Conception and pregnancy in peritoneal dialysis patients. *Peritoneal Dialysis International, 21*(S3), S290-S299.

Huang, C.H., Chen, H.S., Chen, Y.M., & Tsai, T.J. (1996). Fibroadhesive form of tuberculosis peritonitis: Chyloperitoneum in a patient undergoing automated peritoneal dialysis. *Nephron, 72*(4), 708-711.

Huang, J.W., Hung, K.Y., Wu, K.I.D., Peng, Y.S., Tsai, T.J., & Hsieh, B.S. (2000). Clinical features of and risk factors for fungal peritonitis in peritoneal dialysis. *Journal of the Formosan Medical Association, 99*(7) 544-548.

Huang, J.W., Hung, K.Y., Yen, C.J., Wu, J.D., & Tsai, T.J. (2001). Comparison of infectious complications in peritoneal dialysis patients using either a twin-bag system or automated peritoneal dialysis (comment). *Nephrology Dialysis Transplantation, 16*(9), 1957-1958.

Hubalewska, A., Stompor, T., Placzkiewicz, E., Staszczak, A., Huszno, B., Sulowicz, W., & Szybinski, Z. (2004). Evaluation of gastric emptying in patients with chronic renal failure on continuous ambulatory peritoneal dialysis using 99 mTc-solid meal. *Nuclear Medicine Review Central East Europe, 7*(1), 27-30.

Hughes, G.C., Ketchersid, T.L., Lenzen, J.M., & Lowe, J.E. (1999). Thoracic complications of peritoneal dialysis. *Annals of Thoracic Surgery, 67*(5), 1518-1522.

International Society for Peritoneal Dialysis (ISPD). (2005) International Society for Peritoneal Dialysis releases new peritonitis guidelines/recommendations. Retrieved July 21, 2005, at http://www.pdserve.com/pdserve/pdserve.nsf/Content/PDServe+Connection+Newsletter+-+Vol.+4%2C+No.4c%2C+2000

Jobson, V.W., & Adams, P.L. (1983). Endometrial carcinoma diagnosed by examination of peritoneal dialysate. *Obstetrics and Gynecology, 62*(2), 264-266.

Kanaan, N., Gavage, P., Janssens, M., Avesani, V., Gigi, J., & Goffin E. (2002). Pasterurella multocida in peritoneal dialysis: A rare cause of peritonitis associated with exposure to domestic cats. *Acta Clinical Belgium, 57*(5), 254-256.

Kanagasundaram, N.S., Macdougall, I.C., & Turney, J.H. (1998). Massive haemoperitoneum due to rupture of splenic infarct during CAPD. *Nephrology Dialysis Transplantation, 13*, 2380-2381.

Karahan, O.I., Taflkapan, H., Tokgöz, B., Coflkun, A., Utafl, C., & Güleç, M. (2002). Continuous ambulatory peritoneal dialysis: CT peritoneography findings and assessment of related clinical complications. *Acta Radiologica, 43*(2), 170-174.

Kavanagh, D., Prescott, G.J., & Mactier, R.A. (2004). Peritoneal dialysis-associated peritonitis in Scotland (1999-2002). *Nephrology Dialysis Transplantation, 19*(10), 2584-2591.

Kawaguchi, Y., Kawanishi, H., Mujais, S., Topley, N., & Oreopoulos, D.G. (2000). Encapsulating peritoneal sclerosis: definition, etiology, diagnosis, and treatment. *Peritoneal Dialysis International, 20*(S4), S43-S55.

Kawanishi, H. (2002). Treatment for encapsulating peritoneal sclerosis. *Advances in Peritoneal Dialysis, 18*, 139-143.

Kawanishi, H., Kawaguchi, Y., Fukui, H., Hara, S., Imada, A., Kubo, H., et al. for the Long-Term Peritoneal Dialysis Study Group. (2004). Encapsulating peritoneal sclerosis in Japan: A prospective, controlled, multicenter study. *American Journal of Kidney Diseases, 44*(4), 729-737.

Keane, W.F., Bailie, G.R., Boeschoten, E., Gokal, R., Golper, T.A., Holmes, C.J., et al. (2000). Adult peritoneal dialysis-related peritonitis treatment recommendations: 2000 update. *Peritoneal Dialysis International, 20*(4), 396-411.

Kern, E.O., Newman, L.N., Cacho, C.P., Schulak, J.A., & Weiss, M.F. (2002). Abdominal catastrophe revisited: The risk and outcome of enteric peritoneal contamination. *Peritoneal Dialysis International, 22*(3), 323-334.

Khandelwal, M., Kothari, J., Krishnan, M., Liakopoulos, V., Tziviskou, E., Sahu, K., et al. (2003a). Volume expansion and sodium balance in peritoneal dialysis patients. Part I: Recent concepts in pathogenesis. *Advances in Peritoneal Dialysis, 19*, 36-43.

Khandelwal, M., Kothari, J., Krishnan, M., Liakopoulos, V., Tziviskou, E., Sahu, K., et al. (2003b). Volume expansion and sodium balance in peritoneal dialysis patients. Part II: Newer insights in management. *Advances in Peritoneal Dialysis, 19*, 44-52.

Kiernan, L., Finkelstein, F.O., Kliger, A.S., Gorban-Brennan, N.L., Juergensen, P., & Mooraki, A. (1995). Outcome of polymicrobial peritonitis in continuous ambulatory peritoneal dialysis (Abstract). *American Journal of Kidney Diseases, 25*, 464-464.

Kim, G.C., & Korbet, S.M. (2000). Polymicrobial peritonitis in continuous ambulatory peritoneal dialysis patients. *American Journal of Kidney Diseases, 36*(5), 1000-1008.

Kim, D.J., Kang, W.H., Kim, H.Y., Lee, B.H., Kim, B., Lee, S.K., et al. (1999). The effect of dialysate dwell on gastric emptying time in patients on continuous ambulatory peritoneal dialysis. *Peritoneal Dialysis International, 19*(S2), S176-S178.

Kim, D.K., Yoo, T.H., Ryu, D.R., Xu, Z.G., Kim, H.J., Choi, K.H., et al. (2004). Changes in causative organisms and their antimicrobial susceptibility in CAPD peritonitis: A single center's experience over one decade. *Peritoneal Dialysis International, 24*(5), 424-432.

Konings, C.J.A.M., Kooman, J.P., van der Sande, F.M., & Leunissen, K.M.L. (2003). Fluid status in peritoneal dialysis: What's new? *Peritoneal Dialysis International, 23*(3), 284-290.

Lam, M.F., Lo, W.K., Chu, F.S.K., Li, F.K., Yip, T.P.S., Tse, K.C., et al. (2004). Retroperitoneal leakage as a cause of ultrafiltration failure. *Peritoneal Dialysis International, 24*(5), 466-470.

Leblanc, M., Ouimet, D., & Pichette, V. (2001). Dialysate leaks in peritoneal dialysis. *Seminars in Dialysis, 14*(1), 50-54.

Lee, M., & Donovan, J.F. (2002). Laparoscopic omentectomy for salvage of peritoneal dialysis catheters. *Journal of Endourology, 16*(4), 241-244.

Leehey, D.J., Gandhi, V.C., & Daugirdas, J.T. (2001). Peritonitis and exit site infection. In J.T. Daugirdas, P.G. Blake, & T.S. Ing (Eds.), *Handbook of dialysis* (pp. 373-398). Philadelphia: Lippincott, Williams, & Wilkins.

Levy, R.I., & Wenk, R.E. (2001). Chyloperitoneum in a peritoneal

dialysis patient. *American Journal of Kidney Diseases, 38*(3), E12.

Lew, S.Q., & Piraino, B. (2005). Quality of life and psychological issues in peritoneal dialysis patients. *Seminars in Dialysis, 18*(2), 119-123.

Lui, S.L., Tang, S., Li, F.K., Choy, B.Y., Chan, T.M., Lo, W.K., & Lai, K.N. (2001). Tuberculosis infection in Chinese patients undergoing continuous ambulatory peritoneal dialysis. *American Journal of Kidney Diseases, 38*(5), 1055-1060.

Lupo, A., Tarchini, R., Segoloni, G.P., Gentile, M.G., Cancarini, G., Fellin, G., et al. (1988). Abdominal hernias in CAPD patients: Incidence, risk factors, and outcome. *Advances in Continuous Ambulatory Peritoneal Dialysis, 4*, 107-109.

Maaz, D.E. (2004). Troubleshooting non-infectious peritoneal dialysis issues. *Nephrology Nursing Journal, 31*(5), 521-533.

Mactier, R.A., Sprosen, T.S., Gokal, R., Williams, P.F., Lindbergh, M., Naik, R.B., et al. (1998). Bicarbonate and bicarbonate/lactate peritoneal dialysis solutions for the treatment of infusion pain. *Kidney International, 53*(4), 1061-1067.

Madane, S.J., Forden, L., Fein, P., Morrell, A., & Grossman, I. (2000). Outcome of PEG feeding in patients on peritoneal dialysis with end stage renal disease (Abstract). *American Journal of Gastroenterology, 95*(9), 2634.

Majkowski, N.L., & Mendley, S.R. (1997). Simultaneous removal and replacement of infected peritoneal dialysis catheters. *American Journal of Kidney Diseases, 29*(5), 706-711.

Mak, S-K, Nyunt, K., Wong, P-N., Lo, K-Y., Tong, G.M.W., Tai, Y-P., & Wong, A.K.M. (2002). Long-term follow-up of thoracoscopic pleurodesis for hydrothorax complicating peritoneal dialysis. *Annals of Thoracic Surgery, 74*, 218-221.

Manley, H.J., & Bailie, G.R. (2002). Treatment of peritonitis in APD: pharmacokinetic principles. *Seminars in Dialysis, 15*(6), 418-421.

Martins, L.S.S., Rodrigues, A.S., Cabrita, A.N., & Guimaraes, S. (1999). Sclerosing encapsulating peritonitis: A case successfully treated with immunosuppression. *Peritoneal Dialysis International, 19*(5), 478-481.

McCray, S., & Parrish, C.R. (2004). When chyle leaks: Nutrition management options. *Practical Gastroenterology, 17*, 60-76.

Min, C.H., Park, J.H., Ahn, J.H., Kang, E.T., Yu, S.H., Ch, S.J., Park, E.S., Yoo, J.H., & Song, J.S. (1997). Dialysis-related amyloidosis (DRA) in a patient on CAPD presenting as haemoperitoneum with colon perforation. *Nephrology Dialysis Transplantation, 12*, 2761-2763.

Min, F., Tarlo, S.M., Bargman, J., Poonai, N., Richardson, R., & Oreopoulos, D. (2000). Prevalence and causes of cough in chronic dialysis patients: A comparison between hemodialysis and peritoneal dialysis patients. *Advances in Peritoneal Dialysis, 16*, 129-133.

Minnaganti, V.R., & Cunha, B.A. (2001). Infections associated with uremia and dialysis. *Infectious Disease Clinics of North America, 15*(2), 385-406.

Mital, S., Fried, L.F., & Piraino, B. (2004). Bleeding complications associated with peritoneal dialysis catheter insertion. *Peritoneal Dialysis International, 24*(5), 478-480.

Mori, Y. Matsuo, S., Sutoh, H., Toriyama, T., Kawahara, H., & Hotta, N. (1997). A case of a dialysis patient with sclerosing peritonitis successfully treated with corticosteroid therapy alone. *American Journal of Kidney Diseases, 30*(2), 275-278.

Moriishi, M., Kawanishi, H., Kawai, T., Takahashi, S., Hirai, T., Shishida, M., Watanabe, H., & Takahshi, N. (2002). Preservation of peritoneal catheter for prevention of encapsulating peritoneal sclerosis. *Advances in Peritoneal Dialysis, 18*, 149-153.

Nace, G., George, A., Jr., & Stone, W. (1985). Hemoperitoneum: A red flag in CAPD. *Peritoneal Dialysis Bulletin, 5*, 42-44.

Nakamoto, H., Kawaguchi, Y., & Suzuki, H. (2002). Encapsulating peritoneal sclerosis in patients undergoing continuous ambulatory peritoneal dialysis in Japan. *Advances in Peritoneal Dialysis, 18*, 119-123.

Nakamura, H., Kitazawa, K., Kato, K., Inada, Y., Kato, N. Takahashi, M., Uekusa, Mitsugu, A., & Sugisaki, T. (2004). Stercoral perforation of the sigmoid colon in a patient undergoing CAPD: Case report. *Peritoneal Dialysis International, 24*(4), 399-401.

Nakayama, M., Yamamoto, H., Ikeda, M., Hasegawa, T., Kato, N., Takahashi, H., et al. (2002). Risk factors and preventive measures for encapsulating peritoneal sclerosis – Jikei experience 2002. *Advances in Peritoneal Dialysis, 18,* 144-148.

Nannini, E.C., Paphitou, N.I., & Ostrosky-Zeichner, L. (2003). Peritonitis due to *Asperigillus* and zygomyctes in patients undergoing peritoneal dialysis: Report of 2 cases and review of the literature. *Diagnostic Microbiology and Infectious Disease, 46,* 49-54.

Nassberger,L. (1982). Left-sided pleural effusion secondary to continuous ambulatory peritoneal dialysis. *Acta Medica Scandinavica, 211*(3), 219-220.

Nauth, J., Chang, C.W., Mobarhan, S., Sparks, S., Borton, M., & Svoboda, S. (2004). A therapeutic approach to wean total parenteral nutrition in the management of short bowel syndrome: Three cases using nocturnal enteral rehydration. *Nutrition Reviews, 62*(5), 221-231.

Nephrology Pharmacy Associates (NPA). (2003). Medfacts: Information on drugs in kidney disease – Diabetic gastroparesis: The potential for newer therapies. Retrieved July 21, 2005, from www.nephrologypharmacy.com

Nicholson, M.L., Burton, P.R., Donnelly, P.K., Veitch, P.S., & Walls, J. (1991). The role of omentectomy in continuous ambulatory peritoneal dialysis. *Peritoneal Dialysis International, 11*(4), 330-332.

Nomoto, Y., Suga, T., Nakajima, K., Sakai, H., Osawa, G., Ota, K., Kawaguchi, Y., Sakai, T., Sakai, S., & Shibata, M. (1989). Acute hydrothorax in continuous ambulatory peritoneal dialysis – A collaborative study of 161 centers. *American Journal of Nephrology, 9*(5), 363-367.

Ogunc, G. (2001). Videolaparoscopy with omentopexy: A new technique to allow placement of a catheter for continuous ambulatory peritoneal dialysis. *Surgery Today, 31*(10), 942-944.

Ogunc, G., Tuncer, M., Ogunc, D., Yardimsever, M., & Ersoy, F. (2003). Laparoscopic omental fixation technique versus open surgical placement of peritoneal dialysis catheters. *Surgical Endoscopy, 17,* 1749–1755.

Oh, S.Y., Kim, H., Kang, J.M., Lim, S.H., Park, H.D., Jung, S.S., & Lee, K.B. (2004). Eosinophilic peritonitis in a patient with continuous ambulatory peritoneal dialysis (CAPD). *Korean Journal of Internal Medicine, 19*(2), 121-123.

Ohtani, H., Imai, H., Komatsuda, A., Wakui, H., & Miura, A.B. (2000) Hemoperitoneum due to acute cytomegalovirus infection in a patient receiving peritoneal dialysis. *American Journal of Kidney Diseases, 36*(6), E33.

Okechukwu, C.N., & Swartz, R.D. (2001). Peritoneal dialysis-associated peritonitis. *Current Treatment Options in Infectious Diseases, 3,* 367-378.

Oreopoulos, D.G., & Rao, P.S. (2001). Assessing peritoneal ultrafiltration, solute transport, and volume status. In J.T. Daugirdas, P.G. Blake, & T.S. Ing (Ed.), *Handbook of dialysis* (pp. 361-372). Philadelphia: Lippincott, Williams, & Wilkins.

Passadakis, P., & Oreopoulos, D.G. (2001). The case for oral treatment of peritonitis in continuous ambulatory peritoneal dialysis. *Advances in Peritoneal Dialysis, 17,* 180-190.

Patterson, R.B., Whelan, T.V., & Schwab, C.W. (1988). Insertion of peritoneal dialysis catheters: The lateral approach. *Southern Medical Journal, 81*(5), 577-579.

Perez Fontan, M.F., Pombo, F., Soto, A., Perez Fontan, F.J., & Rodriguez-Carmona, A. (1993). Chylous ascites associated with acute pancreatitis in a patient undergoing continuous ambulatory peritoneal dialysis. *Nephron, 63*(4), 458-461.

Piraino, B. (1998). Peritonitis as a complication of peritoneal dialysis (Review). *Journal of the American Society of Nephrology, 9*(10), 1956-1964.

Piraino, B. (2003). Peritoneal dialysis catheter replacement: "Save the patient and not the catheter." *Seminars in Dialysis, 16*(1), 72-75.

Piraino, B., Bailie, G.R., Bernadini, J., Boeschoten, E., Gupta, A., Holmes, C., et al. (2005). Peritoneal dialysis-related infections recommendations: 2005 update. *Peritoneal Dialysis International, 25,* 107-131.

Piraino, B., Bernardini, J., Florio L., & Fried L. (2003). Staphylococcus aureus prophylaxis and trends in gram-negative infections in peritoneal dialysis patients. *Peritoneal Dialysis International, 23*(5), 456-459.

Pollock, C.A. (2003). Bloody ascites in a patient after transfer from peritoneal dialysis to hemodialysis. *Seminars in Dialysis, 16*(5), 406-410.

Posen, G.A. (1989). Canadian peritonitis registry (Final Report: January 1987 – September 1989).

Prichard, S. (2001). Metabolic complications of peritoneal dialysis. In J.T. Daugirdas, P.G., Blake, T.S. Ing (Eds.), *Handbook of dialysis* (pp. 405-410). Philadelphia: Lippincott, Williams & Wilkins.

Prischl, F.C., Wallner, M., Schauer, W., Balon, R., & Kramar, R. (1999). An important differential diagnosis in CAPD patients with the sudden onset of fever, vomiting, abdominal pain, and cloudy dialysate. *Peritoneal Dialysis International, 19*(1), 81-84.

Rajani, R., Smyth, J., Koffman, G., Abbs, I., Goldsmith, D.J.A. (2002) Differential effect of sirolimus *vs.* prednisolone in the treatment of sclerosing encapsulating peritonitis. *Nephrology Dialysis Transplantation, 17,* 2278-2280.

Ramalanjaona, G (2003). Chronic renal failure in children. Retrieved July 8, 2005, from www.antibiotic-consult.com/secure/text-bookarticles/Primary_Care_Book/25.htm

Ray, S.W., Secrest, J., Ch'ien, A.P.Y., & Corey, R.S. (2002). Managing gastroesophageal reflux disease. *Nurse Practitioner, 27*(5), 36-55.

Reissman, P., Lyass, S., Shiloni, E., Rivkind, A., Berlatzky, Y. (1998). *European Journal of Surgery, 164*(9), 703-707.

Rinaldi, S., Sera, F., Verrina, E., Edefonti, A., Gianoglio, B., Perfumo, F., el al.; Italian Registry of Pediatric Chronic Peritoneal Dialysis. (2004). *Peritoneal Dialysis International, 24*(5), 481-486.

Rigby, R.J., & Hawley, C.M. (1998). Sclerosing peritonitis: The experience in Australia. *Nephrology Dialysis Transplantation, 13*(1), 154-159.

Rocklin, M.A., Quinn, M.J., & Teitelbaum, I. (2000). Cloudy dialysate as a presenting feature of superior vena cava syndrome. *Nephrology Dialysis Transplantation, 15,* 1455-1457.

Rocklin, M.A., & Teitelbaum, I. (2001). Noninfectious causes of cloudy peritoneal dialysate. *Seminars in Dialysis, 14*(1), 37-40.

Rodriguez-Carmona, A., Perez Fontan, M., Garcia Falcon, T., Fernandez Rivera, C., & Valdes F. (1999). A comparative analysis on the incidence of peritonitis and exit-site infection in CAPD and automated peritoneal dialysis. *Peritoneal Dialysis International, 19*(3), 253-258.

Rubin, H.R., Fink, N.E., Plantinga, L.C., Sadler, J.H., Kliger, A.S., & Powe, N.R. (2004). Patient ratings of dialysis care with peritoneal dialysis vs. hemodialysis. *Journal of American Medical Association, 291*(6), 697-703.

Rudnick, R.R., Coyle, J.F., Beck, L.H., & McCurdy, D.K. (1979). Acute massive hydrothorax complicating peritoneal dialysis, report of 2 cases and a review of the literature. *Clinical Nephrology, 12*(1), 38-44.

Schiff, H., Mücke, C., Sorodoc, J., & Brendel, C. (2000). Gastrointestinal transit of an indigestible solid in patients on CAPD. *Peritoneal Dialysis International, 20,* 787-789.

Schoonjans, R., Van Vlem, B., Vandamme, W., Van Vlierberghe, H., Van Heddeghem, N., Van Biesen, W., Mast, A., Sas, S., Vanholder, R., Lameire, N., & De Vos, M. (2002). Gastric emptying of solids in cirrhotic and peritoneal dialysis patients: Influence of peritoneal volume load. *European Journal of Gastroenterology & Hepatology, 14,* 395-398.

Schwenk, M.H., Charytan, C., & Spinowitz, B.S. (2002). Dialysate leaks. In A.R. Nissenson & R.N. Fine (Eds.), *Dialysis therapy* (3rd ed.) (p.271) Philadelphia: Hanley & Belfus, Inc.

Schwenk, M.H., Spinowitz, B.S., & Charytan, C. (2002). Hydrothorax and peritoneal dialysis. In A.R. Nissenson & R.N. Fine (Eds.), *Dialysis therapy* (3rd ed.) (pp. 272-274). Philadelphia: Hanley & Belfus, Inc.

Shay, S., Schreiber, M., & Richter, J. (1999). Compliance curves during peritoneal dialysate infusion are like a distensible tube and are similar at multiple UGI sites. *The American Journal of*

Gastroenterology, 94(4), 1034 –1041.

Sherwin, R. (2004). Diabetes mellitus. In L. Goldman, *Cecil textbook of medicine,* (22nd ed.) (p. 687). St. Louis: W.B. Saunders.

Shimoyama, S., Hirakawa, O., Yahiro, K., Mizumachi, T., Schreiner, A., & Kakuma, T. (2003). Health-related quality of life and caregiver burden among peritoneal dialysis patients and their family caregivers in Japan. *Peritoneal Dialysis International, 23*(2), S200-S205.

Singh, S., Vaidya, P., Dale, A., & Morgan, B. (1983). Massive hydrothorax complicating continuous ambulatory peritoneal dialysis. *Nephron, 34*(3), 168-172.

Sivaraman, P. (1999). Meliodosis presenting as peritoneal dialysis-related peritonitis: What about the flower pot? *Peritoneal Dialysis International, 19*(2), 184-185.

Slim, R., Tohme, C., Yaghi, C., Honein, K., & Sayegh, R. (2005). Sclerosing encapsulating peritonitis: A diagnostic dilemma. *Journal of the American College of Surgeons, 200*(6), 974-975.

Smith, L., Collins, J.F., Morris, M., & Teele, R.L. (1997). Sclerosing encapsulating peritonitis associated with continuous ambulatory peritoneal dialysis: Surgical management. *American Journal of Kidney Diseases, 29*(3), 456-460.

Spadaro, J.J., Thakur, V., & Nolph, K.D. (1982) Technetium-99m-labeled macroaggregated albumin in demonstration of trans-diaphragmatic leakage of dialysate in peritoneal dialysis. *American Journal of Nephrology, 2*(1), 36-38.

Spence, P., Mathews, R., Khanna, R., & Oreopoulos, D.G. (1985). Improved results with a paramedian technique for the insertion of peritoneal dialysis catheters. *Surgery, Gynecology, Obstetrics, 161,* 585.

Stafford-Johnson, D.B., Wilson, T.E., Francis, I.R., & Swartz, R. (1998). CT appearance of sclerosing peritonitis in patients on chronic ambulatory peritoneal dialysis. *Journal of Computer Assisted Tomography, 22*(2), 295-299.

Steiner, R.W. (2002). Abdominal catastrophes, peritoneal eosinophilia, and other unusual events in peritoneal dialysis patients. In A.R. Nissenson & R.N. Fine (Eds.), *Dialysis therapy* (3rd ed., pp. 263-268). Philadelphia: Hanley & Belfus, Inc.

Strid, H., Simren, M., Stotzer, P.O., Abrahamsson, H., & Bjornsson, E.S. (2004). Delay in gastric emptying in patients with chronic renal failure. *Scandanavian Journal of Gastroenterology, 39*(6), 516-520.

Strippoli, G.F.M., Tong, A., Johnson, D.A., Schena, F.P., & Craig, J.C. (2004). Antimicrobial agents to prevent peritonitis in peritoneal dialysis: A systematic review of randomized controlled trials. *American Journal of Kidney Diseases, 44*(4), 591-603.

Swartz, R., Messana, J., Reynolds, J., & Ranjit, U. (1991). Simultaneous catheter replacement and removal in refractory peritoneal dialysis infections. *Kidney International, 40,* 1160-1165.

Szeto, C.C., & Chow, K.M. (2004). Pathogenesis and management of hydrothorax complicating peritoneal dialysis. *Current Opinion in Pulmonary Medicine, 10,* 315-319.

Szeto, C.C., Chow, K.M., Wong, T.Y.H., Leung, C.B., & Li, P.K.T. (2002). Conservative management of polymicrobial peritonitis complicating peritoneal dialysis – a series of 140 consecutive cases. *The American Journal of Medicine, 113,* 728-733.

Szeto, C.C., Chow, K.M., Wong, T.Y.H., Leung, C.B., Wang, A.Y.M., Lui, S.F., & Li, P.K.T. (2002). Feasibility of resuming peritoneal dialysis after severe peritonitis and Tenckhoff catheter removal. *Journal of the American Society of Nephrology, 13*(4), 1040-1045.

Tan, P.C., & Morad, Z. (2003). Training of peritoneal dialysis nurses. *Peritoneal Dialysis International, 23*(S2), S206-S209.

The Renal Association – Standards and Audit Subcommittee of the Renal Association. (2002, August). Treatment of adults and children with renal failure: Standards and audit measures. Retrieved July 21, 2005, from www.renal.org

Tokgöz, B., Dogukan, A., Güven, M., Ünlühizard, K., Oyma, O., & Utas, C. (2003). Relationship between different body size indicators and hernia development in CAPD patients. *Clinical Nephrology, 50*(3), 183-186.

Toronto Western Hospital Patient's Manual. (2002). Retrieved from www.pdtw.org

Tranaeus, A. (2000). A long-term study of bicarbonate/lactate-based peritoneal dialysis solution – clinical benefits. The Lactate/Bicarbonate Study Group. *Peritoneal Dialysis International, 20*(5), 516-523.

Troidle, L., Watnick, S., Wuerth, D.B., Gorban-Brennan, A.S., Kliger, A., & Finkelstein, F.O. (2003). Depression and its association with peritonitis in CPD patients. *American Journal of Kidney Diseases, 42*(2), 350-354.

Tzamaloukas, A.H., & Quintana, E.J. (1990) Insufflation peritonitis in continuous ambulatory peritoneal dialysis. *Peritoneal Dialysis International, 10*(2), 184.

Tzamaloukas, A.H., Saddler, M.C., Murata, G.H., Malhotra, D., Sena, P., Simon, D., Hawkins, K.L., Morgan, K., Nevarez, M., Wood, B., Elledge, L., & Gibel, L.J. (1995). Symptomatic fluid retention in patients on continuous peritoneal dialysis. *Journal of the American Society of Nephrology, 6*(2), 198-206.

Tsunezuka, Y., Hatakeyama, S-I., Iwase, T., & Watanabe, G. (2001). Video-assisted thoracoscopic treatment for pleuroperitoneal communication in peritoneal dialysis. *European Journal of Cardio-Thoracic Surgery, 20,* 205-207.

UHN Division of Nephrology. (2005). *Housestaff/ACNP guidebook.* Toronto, Ontario: University Health Network. Retrieved July 31, 2005, from http://intranet.uhn.ca/pdf/frame.asp?Page=http:// 142.224.24.159/intradoc/groups/public/@neph/@public/documents/documents/uhnprod006478.pdf

Van Vlem, B.A., Schoonjans, R.S., Strujik, D.G., Verbanck, J.J., Vanholder, R.C., Van Biesen, W.V., et al. (2002). Influence of dialysate on gastric emptying time in peritoneal dialysis patients. *Peritoneal Dialysis International, 22*(1), 32-38.

Vargemezis, V., & Thodis, E. (2001). Prevention and management of peritonitis and exit-site infection in patients on continuous ambulatory peritoneal dialysis. *Nephrology Dialysis Transplantation, 16*(S6), 106-108.

Vas, S.I. (2002). Infections related to prosthetic materials in patients on chronic peritoneal dialysis. *Clinical Microbiology and Infection, 8*(11), 705-708.

Vas, S., & Oreopoulos, D.G. (2001). Infections in patients undergoing peritoneal dialysis (Review). *Infectious Disease Clinics of North America, 15*(3), 743-774.

Vlahakos, D., Rudders, R., Simon, G., & Canzanello, V.J. (1990). Lymphoma-mimicking peritonitis in a patient on continuous ambulatory peritoneal dialysis (CAPD). *Peritoneal Dialysis International, 10*(2), 165-167.

Wang, Q., Bernardini, J., Piraino, B., & Fried, L. (2003). Albumin at the start of peritoneal dialysis predicts the development of peritonitis. *American Journal of Kidney Diseases, 41*(3), 664-669.

Williams, P.F., & Foggensteiner, L. (2002). Sterile/allergic peritonitis with icodextrin in CAPD patients (Letter). *Peritoneal Dialysis International, 22*(1), 89-90.

Wright, M., Woodrow, G., O'Brien, S., King, N., Dye, L., Blundell, J., Brownjohn, A., & Turney, J. (2004). Polydipisa: A feature of peritoneal dialysis. *Nephrology Dialysis Transplantation, 19,* 1581-1586.

Wu, A.W., Fink, N.E., Marsh-Manzl, J.V.R., Meyer, K.B., Finkelstein, F.O., Chapman, M.M., & Powe, N.R. (2004). Changes in quality of life during hemodialysis and peritoneal dialysis treatment: Generic and disease specific. *Journal of American Society of Nephrology, 15,* 743-753.

Yamamoto, R., Nakayama, M., Hasegawa, T., Miwako, N., Yamamoto, H., Yokoyami, K., et al. (2002). High-transport membrane is a risk factor for encapsulating peritoneal sclerosis developing after long-term continuous ambulatory peritoneal dialysis treatment. *Advances in Peritoneal Dialysis, 18,* 131-134.

Yeung, S.M., Walker, S.E., Tailor, S.A.N., Awdishu, L., Tobe, S., & Yassa, T. (2004). Pharmacokinetics of oral ciprofloxacin in continuous cycling peritoneal dialysis. *Peritoneal Dialysis International, 24*(5), 447-453.

Yishak, A., Bernardini, J., Fried, L., & Piraino, B. (2001). The outcome of peritonitis in patients on automated peritoneal dialysis. *Advances in Peritoneal Dialysis, 17,* 205-208.

Zelenitsky, S., Ariano, R., & Harding, G. (2004). A reevaluation of empiric therapy for peritoneal dialysis-related peritonitis. *American Journal of Kidney Diseases, 44*(3), 559-561.

Additional Readings

Bernardini, J. (2004). Peritoneal dialysis: myths, barriers and achieving optimum outcomes. *Nephrology Nursing Journal, 31*(5), 494-498.

Crabtree, J.H., & Fishman, A. (2003). Selective performance of prophylactic omentopexy during laparoscopic implantation of peritoneal dialysis catheters. *Surgical Laparoscopy, Endoscopy & Percutaneous Techniques, 13*(3), 180-184.

Oreopoulos, D.G. (2001). Pathogenesis and management of complications of peritoneal dialysis. *Nephrology Dialysis Transplantation*, 16 (S6), 103-105.

- The key to the management of peritoneal dialysis complications is in prevention, identification, and early intervention. Maintaining confidence in the therapy will be integral to the outcome for individuals engaged in self-care practices.

- In considering an individual for PD, age, co-morbidities, medications, and learning capabilities should be taken into account in preparing for the treatment and minimizing risks associated with the catheter implantation and dialysis procedure.

- Non-infectious complications encompass those conditions related to increased abdominal pressure, effluent appearance, metabolism, including fluid and electrolyte imbalances, and malnutrition.

- Abdominal pain related to PD may result from a variety of causes, such as catheter position, presence or lack of fluid in the peritoneal cavity, or dialysis technique.

- Hemoperitoneum refers to the presence of blood in the PD effluent. While the appearance can be alarming, the presence of bloody effluent can be related to a range of factors from benign to serious ones.

- Cloudy effluent returns are generally considered to be infectious; however, it is important for nurses and patients to be aware of the exceptions. By having cloudy fluid analyzed for both cell constituents and infectious organisms, the reason for the alteration in clarity can be determined.

- Since malnutrition contributes to morbidity and mortality, collaboration with the dietician is imperative in early and continued interventions to improve the nutritional status of individuals treated with PD.

- Peritonitis is an inflammation of the peritoneal cavity, which is primarily caused by infection. A diagnosis of presumed peritonitis is made if any of the three following criteria are met: abdominal pain, cloudy fluid, or a positive culture report from the peritoneal effluent.

- Treatment of peritonitis includes flushes (optional), IP antibiotics, pain management, and psychological support for both the individual with infection and caregivers who may experience feelings of guilt and distress with the development of the infection.

- Measures to prevent the occurrence of peritonitis are vital to the outcome of the technique and include adherence to aseptic techniques including hand washing and drying and prophylactic antibiotic coverage.

- Studies support the important role of nurses in offering support and continued connection with individuals on PD, as well as incorporating assessment of psychological well-being as part of the on going nursing care.

ANNP629 **Preventing and Managing Complications of Peritoneal Dialysis**

Elizabeth Kelman, MEd, RN, CNeph(C)
Diane Watson, MSc, RN, CNeph(C)

Contemporary Nephrology Nursing: Principles and Practice contains 39 chapters of educational content. Individual learners may apply for continuing nursing education credit by reading a chapter and completing the Continuing Education Evaluation Form for that chapter. Learners may apply for continuing education credit for any or all chapters.

Please photocopy this page and return to ANNA.
COMPLETE THE FOLLOWING:

Name: _____

Address:_____

City:_____ State: _____ Zip: _____

E-mail: _____

Preferred telephone: ☐ Home ☐ Work: _____

State where licensed and license number (optional): _____

CE application fees are based upon the number of contact hours provided by the individual chapter. CE fees per contact hour for ANNA members are as follows: 1.0-1.9 - $15; 2.0-2.9 - $20; 3.0-3.9 - $25; 4.0 and higher - $30. Fees for nonmembers are $10 higher.

ANNA Member: ☐ Yes ☐ No Member # (if available) _____

☐ Checked Enclosed ☐ American Express ☐ Visa ☐ MasterCard

Total Amount Submitted: _____

Credit Card Number: _____ Exp. Date: _____

Name as it appears on the card: _____

CE Evaluation Form
To receive continuing education credit for individual study after reading the chapter
1. Photocopy this form. (You may also download this form from ANNA's Web site, **www.annanurse.org**.)
2. Mail the completed form with payment (check) or credit card information to American Nephrology Nurses' Association, East Holly Avenue, Box 56, Pitman, NJ 08071-0056.
3. You will receive your CE certificate from ANNA in 4 to 6 weeks.

Test returns must be postmarked by **December 31, 2010.**

CE Application Fee
ANNA Member $15.00
Nonmember $25.00

EVALUATION FORM

1. I verify that I have read this chapter and completed this education activity. Date: _____

_____
Signature

2. What would be different in your practice if you applied what you learned from this activity? *(Please use additional sheet of paper if necessary.)*

_____
_____
_____
_____
_____
_____
_____
_____
_____
_____
_____
_____

Evaluation	Strongly disagree				Strongly agree
3. The activity met the stated objectives.					
a. Describe the nursing interventions necessary to prevent and manage non-infectious complications of peritoneal dialysis.	1	2	3	4	5
b. Describe the nursing interventions necessary to prevent and manage infectious complications of peritoneal dialysis.	1	2	3	4	5
4. The content was current and relevant.	1	2	3	4	5
5. The content was presented clearly.	1	2	3	4	5
6. The content was covered adequately.	1	2	3	4	5
7. Rate your ability to apply the learning obtained from this activity to practice.	1	2	3	4	5

Comments _____

_____

8. Time required to read the chapter and complete this form: _____ minutes.

This educational activity has been provided by the American Nephrology Nurses' Association (ANNA) for 1.0 contact hour. ANNA is accredited as a provider of continuing nursing education (CNE) by the American Nurses Credentialing Center's Commission on Accreditation (ANCC-COA). ANNA is an approved provider of continuing education by the California Board of Registered Nursing, CEP 0910.

Transplantation

UNIT 8

Unit 8 Contents

Organ Donation: The Supply and the Issues

Marilyn Bartucci, MSN, RN, CS, CCTC

Chapter Contents

Marilyn Bartucci, MSN, RN, CS, CCTC

Organ transplantation has evolved from being a medical experiment to a major therapeutic intervention for selected patients with end stage organ disease. Many advances have been made in organ procurement and preservation, surgical technique, tissue typing and matching, understanding the immune mechanisms that lead to organ rejection, and the development of potent immunosuppressive drug regimens that effectively prevent and treat rejection. These have lead to excellent 1- and 5-year patient (see Table 30-1) and graft survival rates (see Table 30-2). The fundamental requirement for transplantation is the organ donor. Without the availability of donor organs, transplantation as a treatment option is severely limited. This chapter will focus on kidney donation and provide an overview of the supply and demand issues, the evolution of kidney donation including initiatives to increase donation, sources of donor organs, the procurement process, and strategies to maximize the use of available kidneys. The responsibilities of agencies involved in the procurement and allocation of donor organs are discussed and the resources available for more information about organ donation and transplantation are provided.

Overview of Solid Organ Transplantation

In 2003, there were 25,451 organ transplants performed in the United States (Organ Procurement and Transplant Network/Scientific Registry of Transplant Recipients [OPTN/SRTR], 2003) and 1,804 in Canada (Canadian Organ Replacement Registry [CORR], 2003) (see Table 30-3).

Despite ever-improving health care and new advances in medical technology, the number of Americans and Canadians with end stage renal disease (ESRD) continues to increase. Diabetes remains the leading cause of new cases (36% U.S., 32% Canada), followed by hypertension (27% U.S, 20.8% Canada) and glomerulonephritis (8% U.S., 13.5% Canada) (United States Renal Data System [USRDS], 2003; CORR, 2003). In 2001, there were 392,023 patients with ESRD in the United States and 287,494 (73%) receiving dialysis therapy (USRDS, 2003). The number of patients waiting for kidneys has continued to increase, while the number of kidney transplants performed each year has remained fairly constant. During 2002, there were 53,704 patients on the kidney waiting list, but only 14,523 kidney transplants were performed; 8,207 from deceased and 6,236 from living donors (OPTN/SRTR, 2003). The consequences of the imbalance between supply and demand are an exponential increase in the number of patients waiting for a kidney transplant, increased waiting times, and an increase in the number of patients who die on the waiting list. The U.S. kidney transplant waiting list grew steadily from 24,704 in 1993 to 53,704 in 2002 and on December 24, 2004, the number of patients on the kidney waiting list surpassed 60,000 (OPTN, 2004). In Canada the number of patients on the waiting list has increased 84% over the same time period (McAllister & Badovinac, 2003). The U.S. median waiting times have increased by approximately 1 year from 747 to 1,121 days and the mortality rates for patients on the waiting list have

Table 30-1
Unadjusted 1- and 5-Year Patient Survival by Organ

Organs Transplanted	1-Year Survival (%)	5-Year Survival (%)
Kidney		
Deceased donor	94.2	82.5
Living donor	97.6	90.5
Pancreas alone	98.6	79.2
Pancreas after kidney	95.3	76.6
Pancreas and kidney	94.7	84.0
Liver		
Deceased donor	85.7	72.1
Living donor	89.1	80.0
Intestine	79.1	47.4
Heart	85.6	72.0
Lung		
Deceased donor	78.9	45.1
Living donor	70.9	41.6
Heart and Lung	67.1	36.7

Note: Based on OPTN data as of December 24, 2004.
Unadjusted first-year survival percentage refers to patients transplanted during 1999-2001, while corresponding 5-year refers to patients transplanted during 1996-1999.

Table 30-2
Unadjusted 1- and 5-Year Graft Survival by Organ

Organs Transplanted	1-Year Survival (%)	5-Year Survival (%)
Kidney		
Deceased donor	88.4	65.5
Living donor	94.5	78.6
Pancreas alone	77.3	41.8
Pancreas after kidney	79.4	46.0
Pancreas-kidney (kidney)	92.0	74.2
Pancreas-kidney (pancreas)	85.1	69.8
Liver		
Deceased donor	80.7	64.4
Living donor	79.5	70.8
Intestine	71.8	33.3
Heart	85.3	70.6
Lung		
Deceased donor	78.2	43.6
Living donor	69.6	39.9
Heart-lung	67.0	37.8

Note: Based on OPTN data as of December 24, 2004.
Unadjusted first-year survival percentage refers to patients transplanted during 1999-2001, while corresponding 5-year refers to patients transplanted during 1996-1999.

Table 30-3
2003 Organ Transplants Performed in the United States and Canada by Organ Type

Organ	United States	Canada
Kidney	15,122	1,053
Heart	2,055	156
Liver	5,671	398
Intestine	116	4
Pancreas	1,373	27
Lung	1,085	117
Heart-Lung	29	-
Multi-organ	-	49
Total	25,451	1,804

Note: From Organ Procurement and Transplantation Network/Scientific Registry of Transplant Recipients (2003) and Canadian Organ Replacement Registry (2003).

Table 30-4
Summary of Patient Survival on Dialysis, Following Deceased Donor Kidney Transplant and Living Donor Kidney Transplant at 1, 2, 5, and 10 Years

Years	Dialysis	Deceased Donor Kidney Transplant	Living Donor Kidney Transplant
1 (2000-2001)	77.8%	93.7%	97.6%
2 (1999-2001)	62.9%	91.6%	96.4%
5 (1996-2001)	31.9%	80.6%	90.4%
10 (1991-2001)	9.0%	58.9%	77.8%

Note: From United States Renal Data System (2003). *USRDS 2003 Annual Data Report*. Bethesda, MD: National Institute of Diabetes and Digestive and Kidney Diseases, National Institutes of Health, DHHS.

more than doubled between 1993 and 2001; and in 2001 alone, 3,209 patients with ESRD died waiting for a kidney transplant (OPTN/SRTR, 2003).

Kidney transplantation is the renal replacement therapy of choice for many patients with ESRD because it offers the greatest potential for a longer, healthier, productive life (Molzahn, Northcott, & Dossetor, 1997; USRDS, 2003; Wolfe, et al, 1999). A comparison of patient survival on dialysis and following deceased and living donor kidney transplantation revealed lower survival on dialysis at 1, 2, 5, and 10 years compared to kidney transplantation, regardless of the donor source. The survival difference worsened between dialysis and transplant at each subsequent time point. By 10 years, dialysis survival was 9% compared to deceased and living donor kidney transplant survival at 58.9% and 77.8%, respectively (USRDS, 2003) (see Table 30-4). Wolfe, Ashby, Milford et al (1999) used the USRDS database to compute and compare "projected years of life" for primary deceased donor kidney recipients and age-matched dialysis patients waiting for a kidney transplant. The results indicated transplantation offers a distinct survival advantage over dialysis-based renal replacement therapies for all age groups. The survival advantage was most striking for younger patients and those with diabetes mellitus. For example, non-diabetic

patients age 20 to 39 years with a kidney transplant had 31 projected life years compared to 20 years for waiting list patients. Diabetics in the same age group with a kidney transplant had 25 versus 8 projected life years for waiting list patients.

Initiatives to Increase Organ Donation

With success comes greater demand and the shortage of transplantable organs is an ongoing and frustrating reality. Two key factors are responsible for the critical shortage in the United States. First, reliance on deceased, brain-dead donors can provide only a limited number of potential donors; it has been estimated that no more than 10,500 to 13,800 such donors are available each year (Sheehy et al., 2003). Second, the rate of consent for organ donation by the next of kin is approximately 50% (Sheehy et al., 2003; Siminoff & Mercer, 2001). Increases in the total number of organs procured have resulted largely from an expansion of the donor pool (e.g., use of non-traditional donors including donation after cardiac death and expanded criteria donors) and from improvements in procedures for referring and requesting organ donation. Improving consent is the most promising solution to increasing the number of donated and recovered organs in the future.

Legislative Initiatives

Improving consent rates has been the target of a series of legislative and regulatory efforts. Organ donation in the U.S. is regulated by the Uniform Anatomical Gift Act (UAGA), drafted by the National Conference of Commissioners on Uniform State Laws in 1968 and modified in 1987. This law recognized the rights of individuals to donate by means of an organ donor card or the next of kin to give consent for organ donation of a deceased family member. The UAGA established altruism and volunteerism as the bedrock of organ donation. However, voluntarism was ineffective even though it was encouraged by the passage of the UAGA.

In 1978, the Uniform Brain Death Act expanded the traditional (cardiopulmonary) definition of death to include brain death. In 1980, the Uniform Determination of Death Act legalized brain death, and in 1981 the Uniform Definition of Death Act was adopted by the President's Commission for the Study of Ethical Problems in Medicine and Biomedical and Behavioral Research. It stated an individual who has sustained either irreversible cessation of circulation and respiratory function or irreversible cessation of all functions of the entire brain, including the brain stem, is dead and determination of death must be made in accordance with accepted medical standards.

Some of the difficulties in initiating the organ procurement process are related to the definition and declaration of death. In the past, both medical and lay public agreed that the absence of a heart beat and respirations were acceptable criteria for a declaration of death. However, the advances in life support technology that enabled health care professionals to maintain respiration and circulation in individuals whose brain function is absent helped to create uncertainty about death. Even with the Uniform Determination of Death Act, many health care professionals were uncertain about implementing the criteria. People are strongly conditioned to view a breathing body with a beating heart as alive even when those functions continue as a result of life support systems.

In 1986, in an attempt to overcome the reluctance of health care professionals to ask grieving families for organ/tissue donation, all 50 states in the U.S. passed required request laws. These laws mandated that all families be given the opportunity to donate the organs/tissues of a loved one who died in a hospital, if the deceased met eligibility criteria. The premise of the law was that all families have the right to decide about donation. If this decision-making opportunity is not provided by health care professionals, then these professionals are, in a sense, making the decision for the family against donation. It was hoped a policy of required request would lead hospital personnel to consider the need for transplantable organs/tissues routinely and the burden of decision concerning donation was equitably allocated among all families whose relatives might serve as donors. It was hoped that a standardized policy would lessen the psychological burden on both health care professionals and family members at a time of great stress and emotional upheaval. Finally, it removed the chance that a family may not be offered this option to donate while preserving their right to refuse consent, because voluntary choice is the ethical foundation for organ/tissue donation.

Experience with this legislation showed as much as a 300% increase in the number of tissue donors but no significant increase in the number of organ donors. However, changes in other public health policies were occurring when these laws were implemented, and this may have clouded the issue. For example, laws about drunk driving were enacted and strictly enforced. In addition, mandatory seat belt laws, mandatory helmet laws, lowered speed limits, and improved ability to transport accident victims quickly to tertiary care centers through air transport decreased traffic fatalities. Some believe the fact that organ donation remained constant during this time provided some evidence that these laws had a small positive impact on the organ supply.

When required request laws were implemented, there were reports that a greater percentage of families said "no" to the request. Part of the difficulty in evaluating these claims was the incomplete, inconsistent data collected prior to the implementation of the laws compared to the more complete data that is currently collected. Certificates on every death were required. These certificates included information about whether or not the deceased met donor eligibility criteria and the family's response to the request for an anatomical gift. In addition, health care professionals formerly relied on voluntarism or carefully evaluated families, making the request of families they were certain would respond favorably. A careful selection process was used prior to required request. With the enactment of required request, all potential donor families were offered the opportunity to make an anatomical gift. Another criticism of the law was there was not enough preparation of health care professionals on how to identify potential donors and approach grieving families to implement the law effectively. For required request to have a positive impact on the supply of organs/tissues for transplantation, health care professionals had to have the necessary

knowledge to identify potential donors and the skills to enable them to communicate sensitively and effectively with grieving families.

Required referral or routine notification was enacted in 1998 requiring hospitals to notify the local organ procurement organization (OPO) about all deaths and imminent deaths, but the family would be approached about donation in collaboration with the OPO. Underlying this regulation was the premise that health professionals alone were not effectively communicating with families about donation. Like required request, this regulation has had little impact on increasing consent rates. Even with new regulations, altruism and voluntarism continue to be the cornerstones of organ procurement, along with a reliance on family consent.

Many European countries have presumed consent laws where it is assumed that every individual is an organ donor unless measures are undertaken by the individual to "opt out" of the system. Spain is one such country. Although families are still approached about donation, the nature of the conversation is to determine if the deceased had ever "opted out" as an organ donor, not to obtain consent. With this presumed consent approach, national consent rates are 80% (Miranda, Vilardell, & Grinyo, 2003). In addition, Spanish hospitals "own" the donation process by having a compensated staff physician who assumes primary responsibility for donation.

Recently in the United States, new legislative acts, referred to as "first-person consent laws," have made it possible for donation to take place using the donor's valid donor card, entry onto a donor registry, or driver's license indication without seeking consent of the legal next-of-kin. Like in Spain, families are approached to reaffirm the donor's actual intent, not to obtain consent. It has been demonstrated that families rarely oppose donation once informed about the deceased's wishes. Since this is a new initiative and not universal, it is too early to determine if first-person consent laws will significantly increase the number of deceased donors (OPTN/SRTR, 2003).

Public Education

Consent for organ donation by families of brain-dead patients has been the major obstacle to maximizing the number of solid organs available for transplant. Despite public opinion polls reporting 99% of Americans are aware of transplantation and over 75% are willing to donate, fewer than half give consent (Siminoff & Mercer, 2001). Legislative efforts have yet to close the gap between donor potential and organs procured.

Differences in willingness to donate have been observed among various cultural groups. African Americans, for example, represent 13% of the American population but make up 35% of the kidney transplant waiting lists and in the past, had high rates of denial of consent for organ donation. After completing focus group sessions in the District of Columbia, the five most common obstacles to organ donation were identified: 1) lack of transplant awareness; 2) religious myths and misperceptions; 3) medical distrust; 4) fear of premature death after signing a donor card; and 5) racism (Callender & Maddox, 2004). Similar issues were found in the Latino/Hispanic, Asian Pacific Islander, Alaskan Native, and Native American groups. The National Minority Organ Tissue Transplant Education Program (MOTTEP) was founded to plan and implement a minority education program. Four main strategies were used to increase donation including: (a) utilization of transplant recipients, donors, candidates and their families, and health professionals as effective messengers within the community; (b) delivery of a culturally sensitive message by ethnically similar messengers known in the community; (c) community involvement in planning and implementing educational activities; and (d) collaboration with religious, social, and civic organizations. The success of this educational effort is demonstrated by similar rates of organ donation per million in the white (42.8), African American (40.8), and Latino/Hispanics (40.2) populations (Callender & Maddox, 2004).

Although the specific standards and positions about organ donation vary both within and among various faiths and denominations, the major religious groups all support donation and transplantation. Many groups (e.g., Roman Catholics, Amish, Muslims, and Jews) view donation as an act of charity, fraternal love, and self-sacrifice. Hindus, Jehovah's Witnesses, and various Protestant groups express the belief that donation is a matter of individual conscience (UNOS, 1995).

The focus of public education is to emphasize the success of organ transplantation, dispel common myths about donation, encourage individuals to make a decision about organ donation and sign a donor card or join a donor registry if that is their wish. Also, public education emphasizes the need to discuss the decision with family members before a crisis occurs.

Health Professional Education

The organ procurement organizations have worked diligently to educate health professionals about brain death, who can be an organ/tissue donor, and how to make a referral to the organ procurement organization. Although the organ procurement coordinators prefer to make the request for donation, they review the process of making a request so health professionals will become more comfortable with the process and can begin laying the groundwork by helping the family understand the gravity of their loved one's condition.

Requests for organ donation must be carefully timed and sensitive to the needs of the family. The donation process is initiated only after the physician has communicated to the family the hopelessness of the clinical situation and the family has had time to assimilate this information. Once the family has been informed of their loved one's death, the organ procurement coordinator, either alone or with the physician and/or nurse, can offer the family the opportunity to donate organs/tissues. The discussion takes place in a comfortable, private area, conducive to the family's expression of grief. The success of the request usually reflects the attitude exhibited by the caregivers during this sensitive period. The request for donation is handled as a part of the natural support provided to a family at the time of a loved one's death. It is the death that is the most important event, not the donation. The family is approached, not to acquire organs, but to show compassion and offer assistance and support during their bereavement. It has been shown that initiating a request for

organ/tissue donation before the family has had time to assimilate the news of their loved one's death results in a high rate of denied consent. Separating the explanation of the certainty of death from the request for donation (decoupling) allows for a period of acceptance and results in higher consent rates.

The organ procurement team responds to commonly expressed family concerns such as pain experienced by the donor, payment, disfigurement of the body, funeral delays, and confidentiality. A brief explanation of brain death can allay fears related to pain during the organ/tissue donation surgery. The family is informed that all costs associated with the procurement of organs/tissues and care of the donor, including laboratory tests, operating room costs, surgeon fees, and intravenous fluids and medications are paid by the procurement agency. The family remains financially responsible for all health care costs incurred up to the pronouncement of death. Families are often concerned about whether donation interferes with an open-casket funeral. Assurance can be given that the donor will appear normal, and donation does not preclude use of an open casket. Funeral delays usually are not necessary unless procurement teams are traveling from various parts of the country. After procurement, the body is released to the funeral home. Gifts of organ and tissue donation are confidential. No one who receives a transplant is told the identity of the donor, and donor families are only told what organs were transplanted, general information about the recipients, and how the recipients are doing after transplantation.

Health care professionals often fear that asking grieving families for organ/tissue donation adds to the family's grief. Studies have consistently shown, however, that the strongest advocates of donation are donor families, who view donation as the highest form of charity, giving the ultimate gift, life, to another person (Bartucci, 1987).

Types of Donors

Organs for transplant can be obtained from deceased donors, both heart-beating and non- heart-beating, and living donors. Deceased, heart-beating donors are previously healthy individuals who have had an irreversible brain injury. The most common causes of injury are: 1) cerebral trauma (e.g. motor vehicle accident or gunshot wound), 2) intracerebral or subarachnoid hemorrhage (e.g. cerebral vascular accident or ruptured aneurysm, and 3) anoxic brain damage resulting from cardiac arrest.

Management of Heart-Beating Donors

Prior to the declaration of brain death, therapeutic modalities are employed to maximize neurologic recovery. Ventilation and intravenous fluid therapy are altered to reduce intracranial pressure. Systemic blood pressure is supported with vasopressors to maintain adequate cerebral perfusion pressure. The diagnosis of brain death is made by a physician who is independent of the transplant team and therefore free of conflict of interest. Clinically, the diagnosis requires irrefutable documentation of the irreversible absence of cerebral and brainstem function (see Table 30-5). Electroencephalograms and isotope or dye angiography can be used to support the diagnosis, but they are not mandato-

Table 30-5

Clinical Criteria for Diagnosis of Brain Death

Irreversibility
• No sedating, paralyzing, or toxic drugs
• No gross electrolyte or endocrine disturbances
• No profound hyperthermia

Absent Cerebral Function
• No seizures or posturing
• No response to pain in cranial nerve distribution; spinal reflexes may be present
• Absent brainstem function
• Apnea in response to acidosis or hypercarbia
• No papillary or corneal reflexes
• No oculocephalic or vestibular reflexes
• No tracheobronchial reflexes

ry. When brain death is declared and consent for organ donation is obtained from the next-of-kin, therapy changes to optimize organ function. At this point, the management of the donor becomes the responsibility of the organ procurement team.

The goals of donor management are to maintain organ perfusion and organ oxygenation. Organ perfusion is a function of intravascular volume, vascular resistance, and cardiac function. Failure to maintain and balance these three components will result in impaired tissue perfusion, cellular dysfunction, organ deterioration, and organ death. Organ donors often have conditions such as thoracic injuries, shock, pneumonia, atelectasis, and other clinical problems that may result in diminished oxygenation and ventilation. Delivery of oxygen is essential to the maintenance of viable organ function. See Table 30-6 for nursing diagnoses, expected outcomes, interventions, and rationale for organ donor management.

Procurement of Deceased Donor Kidneys

The kidneys are removed en bloc (remaining attached to the aorta and vena cava), flushed with a sterile, cold preservation solution (e.g., UW, Collins, or HTK-custodial), and preserved in the cold solution via static or pulsatile perfusion for transport to the recipient's transplant center. Kidneys can be preserved for up to 72 hours, but most surgeons prefer to transplant kidneys before the cold ischemia time (the time between initiation of organ preservation in the donor and revascularization in the recipient) reaches 24 hours. Experience has shown that longer preservation time is associated with delayed graft function (DGF) from acute tubular necrosis (ATN), resulting in the need for dialysis until the ATN resolves.

Non-Heart-Beating Donor

Patients declared dead by traditional cardiopulmonary criteria are another source of kidneys acceptable for transplantation. Before the institution of brain death criteria in the United States in 1968, these donors were the major source of transplantable kidneys. Problems of extended warm ischemia time (the time between asystole and infusion of cold organ preservation solution) leading to cell and tissue

damage limited their usefulness and prompted most centers to rely solely on brain dead, heart-beating donors. However, as the gap between supply and demand for solid organs widened, there was renewed interest in reassessing the use of organs from donation after cardiac death (DCD) donors since the potential to increase the donor pool was estimated to be 20%-25% (Daemen et al., 1996).

The Institute of Medicine studied the medical and ethical issues of non-heart-beating donors (NHBD) and recommended: 1) all OPOs should explore the option of non-heart-beating organ transplantation; 2) the decision to withdraw life-sustaining treatment be made prior to any discussion of organ and tissue donation; 3) observational studies of patients after cessation of cardiopulmonary function be undertaken; 4) the NHBD process focuses on the patient and family; 5) a consensus on NHBD practices be developed; 6) adequate resources needed to cover the cost of outreach, education, and any increased costs associated with the NHBD process; and 7) research be undertaken to evaluate the impact of NHBD on families, care providers, and the public.

Donation after cardiac death can either be controlled or uncontrolled. Candidates for DCD in the controlled situation have a severe neurological injury (e.g. intracranial hemorrhage, stroke, anoxia, trauma), do not meet criteria for brain death, but have no chance for meaningful recovery. The family and attending physician have made the decision to withdraw life-sustaining treatment. It is only after the decision is made by the family to discontinue life support that the option of donating the organs/tissues of their loved one is broached. Since the decision to donate organs is made by the family before death, there is time for discussion, reflection, and informed consent before initiating any invasive procedure. The time and place of death is controlled to minimize warm ischemia time and the potential for organ and tissue damage. The patient is taken to the operating room where the femoral artery and vein are cannulated in preparation for organ preservation. Ventilatory support is removed, and death is declared using cardiopulmonary criteria. The waiting surgical team infuses cold organ preservation solution in situ to minimize warm ischemia time and a median sternotomy and midline abdominal incision are used for organ removal.

In the uncontrolled situation, family consent is obtained after cardiopulmonary death has occurred. In this situation, obtaining consent for donation is difficult because the family does not have time to adjust to the news of their loved one's death before having to make a decision about organ donation. In situ organ preservation must be instituted immediately after asystole to minimize warm ischemia time and potential organ and tissue damage.

The concern regarding the use of DCD donors is the potential impact on transplant outcomes from extended warm ischemia time compared to brain dead, heart-beating donors, most importantly, long-term renal function. Two important papers were published in 2002 examining long-term renal function in recipients of DCD donor kidneys. Weber et al. (2002), in a single center study from the University of Zurich in Switzerland, compared outcomes of 122 kidney transplants from DCD donors to 122 kidney transplants from brain dead, heart-beating donors. The recip-

Table 30-6
Nursing Care Plan for the Organ Donor

Nursing Diagnosis: Decreased cardiac output related to central nervous system dysfunction (loss of vasomotor control), hypovolemia

Expected Patient Outcome	Nursing Interventions	Rationale
Normal cardiac output as evidenced by systolic blood pressure greater than 100 mm Hg, heart rate within normal limits, and central venous pressure greater than 10 cm H_2O or 7 mm Hg	• Monitor hourly heart rate and blood pressure • Maintain continuous electrocardiographic monitoring • Monitor hourly central venous or pulmonary artery pressures • Monitor hourly fluid intake and output • Administer intravenous fluids (e.g. crytalloids, colloids, or blood products) as ordered • Administer vasopressors (e.g. low-dose dopamine) as ordered and document changes in blood pressure after administration	Deceased organ donor's regulatory mechanisms are partially or severely compromised. Neurogenic vasodilatation common in brain death may exacerbate hemodynamic instability. An adequate output is essential for maintaining perfusion to organs/tissues. Vital signs and hemodynamic parameters are basic measures of cardiac output.

Nursing Diagnosis: Impaired tissue perfusion related to central nervous system dysfunction, hypovolemia

Expected Patient Outcome	Nursing Interventions	Rationale
Adequate tissue perfusion as evidenced by systolic blood pressure greater than 100 mm Hg, central venous pressure greater than 10 cm H_2O or 7 mm Hg, urine output greater than 2-3 ml/kg per hour, good quality peripheral pulses, absence of cyanosis, and normal blood pH, urea nitrogen, and creatinine	• Monitor hourly heart rate, blood pressure, central venous pressure, or pulmonary artery pressure • Monitor quality of peripheral pulses • Monitor skin temperature and color • Check capillary refilling in fingertips • Observe nail beds and lips for cyanosis • Obtain arterial blood gases as indicated • Obtain serum electrolytes, blood urea nitrogen, and creatinine • Administer vasopressors (e.g. low-dose dopamine) as ordered and document changes in blood pressure and urine output after administration	Sustaining organ and tissue perfusion is the primary challenge prior to organ recovery. Critical monitoring of basic physical assessment parameters provides insight into status of peripheral perfusion.

Nursing Diagnosis: Impaired gas exchange related to central nervous system dysfunction (loss of respiratory mechanics), neurogenic pulmonary edema, atelectasis, aspiration pneumonia

Expected Patient Outcome	Nursing Interventions	Rationale
Adequate gas exchange as evidenced by PaO_2 levels greater than 100 mm Hg, oxyhemoglobin saturation 95% or above, $Paco_2$ between 40 and 45 mm Hg, IMV rate between 12 and 16 breaths per minute, tidal volume 12 to 15 ml/kg, pH 7.35 to 7.45, hemoglobin 12% to 18% to maximize content of oxygen in arterial blood. Adequate ventilation as evidenced by normal breath sounds bilaterally on auscultation and equal bilateral chest wall movement with respiration	• Monitor mechanical ventilation • Auscultate breath sounds bilaterally • Obtain arterial blood gases every 4 to 6 hours and after ventilator changes • Observe tracheobronchial secretions for amount, color, consistency, and odor • Maintain patent airway with sterile suctioning to remove tracheobronchial secretions • Turn every 2 hours and administer chest physiotherapy	Deceased donors lack any ventilatory drive and must be mechanically ventilated. Physical assessment and blood gases provide insight into the adequacy of gas exchange. Turning, suctioning, and chest physiotherapy help mobilize secretions to avoid stasis.

Nursing Diagnosis: Risk for fluid volume deficit related to diabetes insipidus

Expected Patient Outcome	Nursing Interventions	Rationale
Adequate fluid and electrolyte balance as evidenced by stable vital signs, appropriate urine output, stable weight, and normal serum and urine electrolytes	• Monitor hourly fluid intake and output • Monitor daily weights • Monitor urine specific gravity every 2 hours • Monitor serum and urine electrolytes and osmolality • Administer intravenous maintenance and replacement fluids as ordered • Administer aqueous vasopressin as ordered and titrate dose to maintain urine output between 150 to 300 mL/hr	Brain-dead patients commonly develop an imbalance of pituitary secretion of antidiuretic hormone. Monitoring intake and output, urine specific gravity, and urine and serum osmolality best assess the patient's fluid status. Daily weights reveal subtle and dramatic shifts in body fluid. IV fluids need to be administered to replace heavy fluid losses in urine. Vasopressin replaces antidiuretic hormone effect and reduces fluid losses.

Table 30-6 (continued)
Nursing Care Plan for the Organ Donor

Nursing Diagnosis: Impaired thermoregulation related to central nervous system dysfunction (damage to hypothalamus)

Expected Patient Outcome	Nursing Interventions	Rationale
Adequate temperature control as evidenced by normal body temperature, 97° to 100° F.	• Monitor body temperature for hypothermia • Maintain room temperature at 75° F or above • Keep body surfaces well covered at all times • Restore normal body temperature with the use of heating blankets as indicated • Warm intravenous fluids before administration if hypothermia is present	Without adequate central regulation, the capacity for shivering thermogenesis is absent. Passive heat loss may lead to progressive hypothermia, which is known to adversely affect cellular metabolism, oxygen release, and cardiac function. Frequent monitoring is essential. Cooling or rewarming may be necessary.

Nursing Diagnosis: Risk for infection related to presence of indwelling catheters and an endotracheal tube

Expected Patient Outcome	Nursing Interventions	Rationale
Absence of infection as evidenced by clear urine, white blood count within normal limits, absence of fever, and absence of purulent secretions and wound drainage	• Careful hand washing • Obtain complete blood count with differential • Maintain aseptic care of indwelling Foley catheter, observing urine for cloudiness, sediment, and odor • Monitor wounds, incisions, and puncture sites for erythema and drainage • Culture secretions, urine, and blood as indicated • Administer antibiotics as ordered	General asepsis is the best preventive measure. Presence of infection is monitored through blood work, results of cultures, and status of all wounds, incisions, and drainage sites. Prophylactic antibiotics may be administered to prevent sepsis.

Nursing Diagnosis: Grieving related to imminent death or death of a loved one

Expected Patient Outcome	Nursing Interventions	Rationale
Completion of the first task of grieving as evidenced by family's ability to discuss feelings about loss of a loved one. Knowledge and understanding of the normal grief process as evidenced by the family's ability to identify thoughts, feelings, behaviors, and physical sensations they experience as a result of their loss. Support system(s) in place as evidenced by the presence of other family members, friends, clergy, or counselor to help the family begin to work through their grief.	• Assess and evaluate accuracy of family's perceptions of loved one's condition • Listen attentively and with empathy to accounts of circumstances leading to death • Encourage family to talk about loved one • Allow family to visit any time and participate in care if they so desire • Explain variety of thoughts, feelings, behaviors, and physical sensations family may experience as normal part of grieving • Evaluate support systems (e.g. other family members, friends, clergy) • Refer for bereavement therapy if appropriate • Reinforce altruism and benefit of gift of organ donation	Brain death is a difficult concept because heart still beats. Coping with traumatic losses is fostered by allowing family to relive and process the circumstances. This involves talking about the loved one's life and personal qualities. Quiet time at the bedside can facilitate movement through the grief process. Brief discussion of grief can help family understand the nature of physical and emotional responses. Support systems are an essential coping resource, and bereavement therapy may help the family cope with their loss. Organ donation is a gift of life from sudden death. This is a comfort to many survivors.

Note: From Bartucci, M.R. (1999). Management of persons with organ/tissue transplants. In W.J.Phipps, J.K. Sands & J.F. Marek (Eds), *Medical-surgical nursing concepts and clinical practice* (6th Edition, pp. 2223-2225). St. Louis: Mosby, Inc.

ients were matched for age, gender, number of transplants, and calendar period of transplantation. There was no difference in death-censored graft function at 5 and 10 years between groups in spite of a significantly higher incidence of DGF in the recipients of kidneys from DCD donors (23.8%) and heart-beating donors (4%; $p<0.001$). At 10 years, the death-censored rate of graft survival was 78.7% for kidneys from DCD donors and 76.7% for kidneys from brain-dead donors ($p=0.98$). Forty-six percent of donors were uncontrolled, following unsuccessful cardiac resuscitation.

Rudich et al. (2002), in an analysis of 98,698 adult deceased donor transplants registered in the USRDS between January 1993 and June 2000, found the 6-year death-censored graft survival comparable between DCD donors (73.2%) and brain-dead donors (72.5%; p=ns), despite nearly twice the incidence of delayed graft function in the DCD donors. These studies provide convincing evidence that DCD donors are an acceptable source of kidneys for transplantation. In 2002, organs were recovered from 191 DCD donors (185 kidneys, 22 pancreata, and 103 livers), accounting for 3% of the total deceased donors, a 13% increase from 2001 and a five-fold increase over the decade (OPTN/SRTR, 2003). Preliminary data from 2003 shows a continuation of this trend with a 30% increase in DCD donors over 2002. Eighty-five percent of these donors are Caucasian, male (64%), and 18-49 years of age (56%) (Rosendale, 2004).

Expanded Criteria Donor

Attempts to expand the pool of kidneys from deceased donors have led to liberalizing criteria to include donors who would not have been considered previously. Such donors, called expanded criteria donors (ECD), include older individuals (up to 70 years) and those with medical conditions or other factors believed to be associated with decreased graft survival (e.g., diabetes, hypertension, certain infections, high-risk social behaviors but negative HIV, some hemodynamic instability, some chemical imbalances, and increased organ preservation time). Sometimes, two kidneys are transplanted into one recipient from such donors in order to maximize the mass of functioning nephrons; this strategy has been employed in an effort to use organs that would previously have been discarded.

The UNOS registry database was used to compare the outcomes of 403 dual kidney transplants and 11,033 single kidney transplants performed between 1997 and 2000. Graft survival at 1 year was 7% lower in the dual kidney group. However, graft survival was comparable to single kidney transplants when donors in both groups were over 55 years of age (Bunnapradist, Gritsch, Peng, Jordan, & Cho, 2003). It has been estimated these ECD donors have the potential to add 25%-39% to the organ donor supply. A careful evaluation, including histologic assessment of the recovered kidneys, must be made before transplantation. If on wedge biopsy, more than 20% of glomeruli are found to be sclerosed, the functional prognosis of the graft is poor, and these kidneys would be discarded (Kendrick, Singer, Gritsch, & Rosenthal, 2005). In addition, careful long-term follow-up must be maintained to ensure patient and graft survival rates are comparable to recipients of standard criteria deceased donor kidneys. The decision to transplant a kidney from an EDC donor requires not only a thorough anatomic and physiologic evaluation of the kidney, but a similar evaluation of the specific recipient that includes age, comorbid conditions, and immunologic compatibility. Much effort has gone into minimizing cold ischemia time, limiting the list of potential ECD kidney recipients to speed their allocation, and identifying patients who would most benefit from receiving an ECD kidney.

ECD kidneys are defined by the OPTN as kidneys with a relative risk of graft loss of 1.7 or greater, based on a combination of donor characteristics including age, history of hypertension, death from cerebrovascular accident, and elevated serum creatinine (> 1.5 mg/dL) at the time of kidney recovery. Using this definition, ECD kidneys constituted 8% of deceased donor transplants in 1993 and 15% in 2002. ECD kidneys had lower graft survival rates than kidneys from standard criteria donors (SCD). The unadjusted 3-month, 1-year, 3-year, and 5-year graft survival rates were 90%, 81%, 67%, and 51% for recipients of ECD kidneys compared to 95%, 90%, 81%, and 68% for recipients of SCD kidneys (OPTN/SRTR, 2003). The most appropriate use of ECD donor kidneys continues to be debated. Stratta et al. (2004) retrospectively studied 90 recipients of adult deceased donor kidneys transplanted between October 2001 and February 2003 and compared outcomes of ECD and SCD kidney transplants. ECD kidneys were used by matching estimated renal function mass to recipient need and recipients were selected on the basis of older age, HLA-matching, low allosensitization, and low body mass index. Patient and kidney survival rates were similar between groups as were the initial and mean serum creatinine levels up to 18 months posttransplant.

Living Donor

With the shortage of deceased donors, longer waiting times, and evidence of a distinct survival advantage for transplant recipients over dialysis patients, there has been a rise in the number of living donors in the United States. As in 2001, the number of living donors (6,618) exceeded the number of deceased donors (6,182) in 2002. Living donors have been used in kidney transplant since 1954. Over the past decade (1993-2002), living donation has become much more common, with living donor kidney transplants increasing from 28% of the total kidney transplants performed in 1993 to 43% in 2002 (OPTN/SRTR, 2002). This increase has accounted for nearly all of the growth in kidney transplant activity during this time period. The availability of the laparoscopic donor nephrectomy has provided additional motivation for promoting living kidney donation because compared to the standard open nephrectomy, there is decreased hospital length of stay, decreased requirements for pain medication, more rapid return to normal activity and work, and decreased risk of major and minor complications for the donor (Jacobs, Cho, & Dunkin, 2000).

There are a number of advantages to living donation. Compared with deceased donors, living donors offer the following advantages: better patient and graft survival; permit transplantation to be performed electively when the recipient is in optimal condition; avoid or minimize the need for dialysis; reduce the complications of organ procurement and preservation and thereby reduce the incidence of DGF and nephrotoxicity from calcineurin inhibitors; permit immunologic conditioning and immunosuppression to begin before surgery; reduce the waiting period for transplantation; and perhaps improve rehabilitation.

Preemptive renal transplant is an alternative therapy for the initiation of dialysis when renal replacement therapy is medically necessary and there is a willing and medically suitable living donor. The morbidities associated with dialysis are avoided (e.g. vascular access-related problems, cardiac systolic dysfunction) and studies have demonstrated a distinct short-term and long-term patient and graft survival advantage for preemptive transplant recipients compared with recipients transplanted after dialysis initiation (Kasiske, Matas, Ellison, Gill, & Kausz, 2002; Mange & Weir, 2003; Mange, Joffe, & Feldman, 2001; Meier-Kreische et al., 2000). These survival advantages have persisted despite substantial improvements in immunosuppression since 1994. Preemptive renal transplant is most successful when patients can be evaluated with sufficient lead time. This means patients as well as

Table 30-7
Living Kidney Donors: Exclusion Criteria

Age < 18 years or > 65 years

Blood type incompatibility

Positive T-cell crossmatch with potential recipient

Hypertension (>140/90 or use of antihypertensive medications)

Diabetes (abnormal glucose tolerance test or glycohemoglobin)

Proteinuria (> 250 mg/24 hours)

History of kidney stones

Abnormal glomerular filtration rate (creatinine clearance < 80 mL/min)

Microscopic hematuria

Urologic abnormalities in donor kidneys

Significant medical illness (e.g. chronic lung disease, recent malignancy)

Infectious disease (e.g. hepatitis B or C, human immunodeficiency virus, syphilis)

Obesity (30% above ideal body weight)

History of thrombosis or thromboembolism

Psychosocial contraindications (e.g. substance abuse)

Note: From Bartucci, M.R., & Hricik, D.E., (2002). Kidney transplantation. In S.A. Cupples & L. Ohler (Eds.), *Solid organ transplantation: A handbook for primary health care providers* (p. 201). New York: Springer Publishing Company.

Table 30-8
Medical Assessment of Living Kidney Donors

- Blood type and histocompatibility testing to determine recipient has no preformed antibodies against the donor HLA antigens
- Thorough history and physical examination
- Chest X-ray with posterior/anterior and lateral views
- Electrocardiogram
- Complete blood count, chemistry panel, rapid plasma reagin, serologic studies for cytomegalovirus, human immunodeficiency virus, and hepatitis B and C
- 24-hour urine for total protein and creatinine clearance, urinalysis, and culture
- Pregnancy test in females of child-bearing age
- Intravenous pyelogram or computed tomography to document anatomy of kidneys, ureters, and bladder
- Renal arteriogram or magnetic resonance angiography to outline anatomy of renal vasculature

Note: From Bartucci, M.R., & Hricik, D.E., (2002). Kidney transplantation. In S.A. Cupples & L. Ohler (Eds.), *Solid organ transplantation: A handbook for primary health care providers*. New York: Springer Publishing Company.

physicians need to be educated about the detection of asymptomatic renal disease and the benefits of early referral to a nephrologist.

There are ethical concerns about living kidney donors: subjecting a healthy person to the potential complications of an operation, loss of income if the donor is the primary wage earner in the family, unknown outcome for the recipient, and guilt felt by the donor if the recipient dies (Spital, 1997; Caplan, 1993). These implications for the donor must be weighed against the hope that living donation offers to the person with ESRD who is supported by long-term dialysis therapy. Respect for patient autonomy permits the donor to assume risk if there is reasonable certainty that the donor is competent to make the decision; is willing to be a donor; is medically and psychosocially suitable; is informed of the risk and benefits to the donor; understands the benefits and alternative treatments available for the recipient; is free from coercion; and is truly autonomous. A psychosocial evaluation by a social worker, psychologist, or psychiatrist is an essential component of the living donor evaluation. Exclusion criteria for living donors are listed in Table 30-6. Tests included in the medical assessment of living donors are listed in Table 30-7.

While living blood relatives (parent, child, sibling, grandparent, aunt, uncle, or cousin) are still the most common source of living donors, the number of transplants performed with living unrelated donors have added to the pool of available kidneys. These donors are not blood relatives, but have an emotional relationship with the potential recipient (spouse, significant other, in-law, adoptive parent or child, or friend). Most recently, living donors involved in paired kidney and

indirect exchange programs and anonymous or "Good Samaritans" have added to the living donor pool.

Paired exchange occurs when two kidney donors are unable to donate to their intended recipient because of ABO blood type incompatibility or a positive T-cell crossmatch. In a simple exchange, donor 1 donates a kidney to recipient 2, and donor 2 donates to recipient 1, with whom there is ABO compatibility and a negative T-cell crossmatch. The pairs do not necessarily know each other before being matched by the transplant center, and the surgeries occur simultaneously.

Indirect exchange occurs when a living kidney donor is ABO incompatible with an intended recipient. The donor gives a kidney to a matched recipient on the waiting list for a deceased donor. The donor's intended recipient becomes a priority on the waiting list for the next available ABO compatible kidney. This allows an extra living donor transplant to occur.

Non-directed donation occurs when a living donor gives a kidney to a transplant center without knowing who the recipient will be. This individual is sometimes referred to as a "Good Samaritan" donor. After a thorough living donor evaluation, the transplant center assigns the organ to the most suitable recipient on the deceased donor waiting list using the UNOS allocation algorithm. A non-directed donor is motivated by altruism, as are most other donors.

Organ Procurement and Allocation in the United States

Organ Procurement Organizations

Organ procurement organizations (OPOs) are responsible for organ and tissue donation services across the United States. Each OPO has a contiguous geographic service area designated by the Federal Government for which they provide 24-hour assistance to evaluate potential donors, discuss the option of donation with next-of-kin and obtain consent, and assist with physical assessment and hemodynamic mon-

Figure 30-1
The Organ Procurement and Transplant Network (OPTN) and Scientific Registry of Transplant Recipients (SRTR)

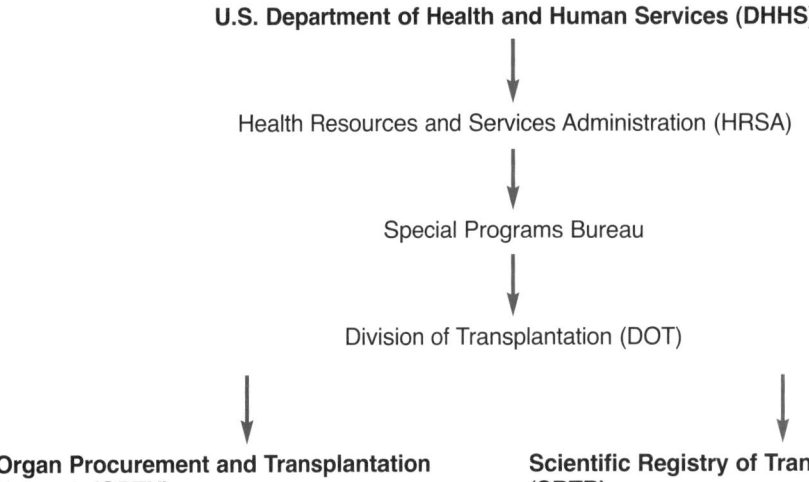

Note: From U.S. Department of Health and Human Services (2004). *Partnering with your transplant team: The patient's guide to transplantation* (p. 59). Rockville, MD: Health Resources and Services Administration, Special Programs Bureau, Division of Transplantation.

itoring to maintain organ function until surgical removal. They implement organ recovery and allocation of organs according to the policies set by the Organ Procurement and Transplantation Network/United Network for Organ Sharing. In addition, they provide follow-up bereavement support for donor families and information regarding the outcome of the donation. They also provide feedback to the donor hospitals regarding the transplant outcomes. There are 59 OPOs which provide deceased donor organs for the nation's 287 transplant centers. Fifty OPOs are independent (private, non-profit) and 9 are hospital-based (OPTN/SRTR, 2003).

United Network For Organ Sharing

UNOS is a tax-exempt, medical, scientific, and educational organization that has operated the national organ procurement and transplantation network (OPTN) under contract by the Division of Organ Transplantation of the Department of Health and Human Services since 1986 (see Figure 30-1). UNOS maintains a comprehensive database that includes information on every patient registered for an organ transplant since 1988 and follows each patient from listing to transplant or removal from the waiting list due to death or other reason. It is responsible for the equitable distribution of organs. The current allocation algorithm prioritizes the matching patients

in the local OPO service area, then regionally, then nationally. Policies for allocation consider medical status (heart, liver), blood type, HLA tissue type (kidney only), PRA (kidney only), donor weight (non-renal organs), and time waiting on the list. Additional points are given to children under age 18 (kidney only) because of the effect of uremia on skeletal growth, sexual maturation, cognitive performance, and psychosocial functioning, and to candidates who have previously donated a kidney. Other organ-specific allocation rules also exist. Zero HLA-mismatched kidney candidates are given national priority regardless of their geographic location or points accrued. Status 1 (medical urgency) liver registrants are also given priority within an OPTN/UNOS region over local candidates with less medical urgency. These allocation policies are continuously reviewed by the transplant community and the public and updated on the basis of advances in medical science.

Each time an organ is donated within an OPO service area, the allocation system matches the donor with the database of waiting transplant candidates. An ordered list is generated of all the potential recipients based on the algorithm for that organ system. Each organ is then offered by the OPO in sequence by communicating the donor's medical and social history to the medical professional (usually the transplant surgeon) at the transplant center where the patient is wait-listed.

The transplant center may accept or decline the organ on behalf of the transplant candidate, based on the medical professional's judgment of the medical status of the potential recipient at the time of the organ offer as well as the medical characteristics of the donor. Extrarenal organs are typically matched and allocated before the organs are recovered in order to limit cold ischemia time.

All transplant centers, organ procurement organizations, and tissue typing laboratories in the United States are members of UNOS. Those members who do not follow the policies set forth by UNOS will lose their Medicare funding. Because the waiting list became so long, minimum listing criteria were established to ensure only patients ready for transplant were on the list. A candidate for kidney transplant from a deceased donor is any patient undergoing renal replacement therapy who is deemed medically suitable for transplantation by a transplant team. Those patients not requiring renal replacement therapy must have a creatinine clearance 20 ml/minute.

Summary

As transplantation has become a major therapeutic intervention for selected patients with end stage organ disease, the demand for organs has far exceeded the supply and the disparity grows exponentially every year. Over the last decade, organ donation rates have plateaued. Living donation and the use of non-traditional donors has accounted for nearly all of the growth in transplant activity. There is ongoing analysis of outcomes in recipients of extended criteria donor organs to assure acceptable patient and graft survival rates as well as organ function. Consent for organ donation has been the major obstacle to maximizing the number of solid organs available for transplant, and legislative efforts have yet to close the gap between donor potential and organs procured.

References

Bartucci, M.R. (1987). Organ donation: A study of the donor family perspective. *Journal of Neuroscience Nursing, 19*(6), 305.

Bartucci, M.R. (1999). Management of persons with organ/tissue transplants. In W.J. Phipps, J.K. Sands, & J.F. Marek (Eds.), *Medical-surgical nursing concepts and clinical practice, Sixth Edition* (pp. 2219-2251). St. Louis: Mosby, Inc.

Bartucci, M.R., & Hricik, D.E. (2002). Kidney transplantation. In S.A. Cupples & L. Ohler (Eds.), *Solid organ transplantation: A handbook for primary health care providers* (pp. 189-222). New York: Springer Publishing Company.

Bunnapradist, S., Gritsch, H.A., Peng, A., Jordan, S.C. & Cho, Y.W. (2003). Dual kidneys from marginal adult donors as a source for cadaveric renal transplantation in the United States. *Journal of the American Society of Nephrology, 14*(4), 1031-1036.

Callender, C.O., & Maddox, G. (2004, November). Three decades of overcoming the African-American donation disparity. *Nephrology News & Issues,* pp. 39-40, 57.

Canadian Organ Replacement Register (CORR). (2003). Retrieved July 5, 2004 from http://www.cihi.ca

Caplan, A. (1993). Must I be my brother's keeper? Ethical issues in the use of living donors as sources of livers and other solid organs. *Transplantation Proceedings, 25,* 1997-2000.

Daemen, J.H.C., deWit, R.J., & Bronkhurst, M.W.G.A., et al. (1996). Non-heart-beating program contributes 40% of kidneys for transplantation. *Transplant Proceedings, 28,* 105.

Jacobs, S., Cho, E., & Dunkin, B. (2000). Laparoscopic donor nephrectomy: Current role in renal allograft procurement. *Urology, 55*(6), 807-811.

Kasiske, B.L., Matas, A.J. Ellison, M.D., Gill, J.S., & Kausz, A.T. (2002). Preemptive kidney transplantation; The advantage and the advan-

taged. *Journal of the American Society of Nephrology, 13,* 1358-1364.

Kendrick, E., Singer, J., Gritsch, H.A., & Rosenthal, J.T. (2005). Medical and surgical aspects of kidney donation. In G.M. Danovitch (Ed.), *Handbook of kidney transplantation* (Fourth Edition) (pp.135-168). Philadelphia: Lippincott, Williams & Wilkins.

Mange, K., Joffe, M.M., & Feldman, H.I. (2001). Effect of the use or nonuse of long-term dialysis on the subsequent survival of renal transplants from living donors. *New England Journal of Medicine, 8,* 726-731.

Mange. K.C., & Weir, M.R. (2003). Preemptive renal transplantation: Why not? *American Journal of Transplantation, 3*(11), 1336-1340.

McAllister, V.C., & Badovinac, K. (2003). Transplantation in Canada: Report of the Canadian Organ Replacement Register. *Transplant Proceedings, 35*(7), 2428-2430.

Meier-Kriesche, H-U., Port, F., & Ojo, A. et al. (2000). Effect of waiting time on renal transplant outcome. *Kidney International, 58,* 1311-1317.

Miranda, B., Vilardell, J., & Grinyo, J.M. (2003). Optimizing cadaveric organ procurement: The Catalan and Spanish experience. *American Journal of Transplantation, 3*(10), 1189-1196.

Molzahn, A.E., Northcott, H.C., & Dossetor, J.B. (1997). Perceptions of physicians, nurses, and patients regarding quality of life of patients with end stage renal disease. *ANNA Journal, 24,* 247-253.

Organ Procurement and Transplant Network/Scientific Registry of Transplant Recipients (OPTN/SRTR). (2003). Annual Report retrieved February 26, 2004 at http://www.optn.org/AR2003

Rosendale, J.D. (2004). Organ donation in the United States: 1988-2002. In J.M. Cecka & P.I. Terasaki (Eds.), *Clinical Transplants 2003* (pp. 65-76). Los Angeles: UCLA Immunogenetics Center.

Rudich, S.M., Kaplan, B., & Magee, J.C., et al. (2002). Renal transplanations performed using non-heart-beating organ donors: Going back to the future? *Transplantation, 74*(12), 1715-1720.

Sheehy, E., Conrad, S.L., Brigham, L.E., Weber, P., Eakin, M., Schkade, L., & Hunsicker, L. (2003). Estimating the number of potential donors in the United States. *New England Journal of Medicine, 349*(7), 667-674.

Siminoff, L.A. & Mercer, M.B. (2001). Public policy, public opinion, and consent for organ donation. *Cambridge Q Healthcare Ethics, 10,* 377-386

Spital, A. (1997). Ethical and policy issues in altruistic living and cadaveric organ donation. *Clinical Transplantation, 11,* 77-87.

Stratta, R.J., Rohr, M.S., & Sundberg, A.K. et al. (2004). Increased kidney transplantation utilizing expanded criteria deceased organ donors with results comparable to standard criteria donor transplant. *Annals of Surgery, 239*(5), 688-695.

United Network for Organ Sharing. (1995). *Organ and tissue donation: A reference guide for clergy.* Richmond, VA: Author.

United States Renal Data System (2003). *USRDS 2003 Annual Data Report.* Bethesda, MD: National Institute of Diabetes and Digestive Disorders and Kidney Diseases, National Institutes of Health, DHHS. Retrieved July 5, 2004 at http://www/usrds.org

Weber, M., Dindo, D., & Demartines, N., et al. (2002). Kidney transplantation from donors without a heart beat. *New England Journal of Medicine, 347*(4), 248- 255.

Wolfe, R.A., Ashby, V.B., & Milford, E.L. et al. (1999). Comparison of mortality in all patients on dialysis, patients on dialysis awaiting transplantation, and recipients of a first cadaveric transplant. *New England Journal of Medicine, 341*(23), 1725-1730.

- Organ transplantation is a successful therapeutic intervention for selected patients with end stage organ disease.

- The increasing success of organ transplantation has resulted in a disparity between the number of patients waiting for a transplant and the number of organs available from both deceased and living donors.

- The number of deceased donors has remained static over the last decade with only 50% of families giving consent for donation.

- Kidney transplantation is the renal replacement therapy of choice for patients with end stage renal disease because it offers the greatest potential for a longer, healthier, productive life.

- Deceased heart-beating donors are previously healthy individuals who have an irreversible brain injury and have no cerebral or brain stem function.

- Strategies to increase the number of available organs for transplantation include the use of non-heart-beating, expanded criteria, and living donors.

- Non-heart-beating donors are individuals who have a severe neurological injury, do not meet brain death criteria, have no chance for meaningful recovery, and the decision to discontinue life support has been made by the family and attending physician.

- Expanded criteria donors are over age 60 years or donors age 51-59 years with any two of the following additional risk factors: cerebrovascular death, hypertension, and serum creatinine above 1.5 mg/dl.

- The increase in living donors has accounted for nearly all of the growth in kidney transplant activity over the last decade.

- An ideal living donor is 18-65 years of age, blood type compatible with a negative T-cell crossmatch with the intended recipient, has normal kidney function, and has no obesity, diabetes, hypertension, urologic abnormalities, infectious disease, or significant medical illness.

- Organ procurement organizations are responsible for organ and tissue donation services across the United States including 24-hour assistance to evaluate potential donors, discuss the option of donation with next-of-kin and obtain consent, assist with hemodynamic monitoring to maintain organ function until surgical removal, and allocate organs according to policies set by the Organ Procurement and Transplantation Network and the United Network for Organ Sharing.

- The United Network for Organ Sharing is a non-profit organization responsible for maintaining the national waiting list for all organ transplant candidates and the computer system that matches donors with recipients, conducts national education and research initiatives, implements the process of developing national policies and collects donation and transplantation data from organ procurement organizations and transplant centers.

Organ Donation: The Supply and the Issues

Name of Resource	Brief Description	Where to Obtain Resource
Canadian Organ Replacement Register (CORR)	Records, analyzes, and reports on level of activity and outcomes of vital organ transplantation and renal dialysis activities in Canada	http://www.corr@cihi.ca
Coalition on Donation	Non-profit alliance of national organizations and local coalitions across United States, dedicated to inspiring all people to donate Life through organ and tissue donation	700 North 4th Street Richmond, VA 23219 Telephone: 804-782-4920 http://www.donatelife.net
Local Organ Procurement Organization (OPO)	OPOs serve as vital link between donor and recipient and are responsible for identification of donors and removal, preservation, and transportation of organs for transplantation. As resource to community, they provide public and professional education on critical need for organ donation. There are 59 OPOs across U.S.	Log on to http://www.optn.org/members/search.asp to identify local OPO and obtain contact telephone number
National Institutes of Diabetes and Digestive and Kidney Diseases (NIDDK)	Provides information about diseases of the kidneys and urologic system to people with kidney and urologic disorders and to their families, health care professionals, and public; answers inquiries, develops and distributes publications, and works closely with professional and patient organizations and Government agencies to coordinate resources about kidney and urologic diseases	National Kidney & Urologic Diseases Information Clearinghouse Office of Communications and Public Liaison NIDDK, National Institutes of Health Building 31, Room 9AO4 Center Drive MSC 2560 Bethesda, MD 20892-3580 Telephone: 301-654-4415 or 1-800-891-5390 http://www.niddk.nih.gov
National Minority Organ and Tissue Transplant Education Program (MOTTEP)	Provides educational programs to increase organ/tissue donation and promote healthier lifestyles to prevent diseases leading to need for transplantation in minority communities	Ambulatory Care Center 2041 Georgia Avenue, NW Suite 3100 Washington, DC 20060 Telephone: 1-800-393-2839 http://www.nationalmottep.org
North American Transplant Coordinators Organization (NATCO) Core Competencies For the Clinical Transplant Coordinator and the Procurement Transplant Coordinator	Provides core competencies for practitioners in field of clinical transplantation, organ and tissue procurement, and hospital development	P. O. Box 15384 Lenexa, KS 66285 Telephone: 913-492-3600 http://www.natco1.org
United Network for Organ Sharing (UNOS)	A nationwide umbrella for transplant community; non-profit organization that administers and maintains Nation's organ transplant waiting list; advances organ availability and transplantation by uniting and supporting its communities for benefit of patients through education, technology, and policy development	700 North 4th Street Richmond, VA 23219 Telephone: 804-782-4800 http://www.unos.org

Organ Donation: The Supply and the Issues

Name of Resource	Brief Description	Where to Obtain Resource
U.S. Department of Health and Human Services **Health Resources and Services Administration** **Special Programs Bureau** **Division of Transplantation**	Provides information and resources on organ donation and transplantation issues	5600 Fishers Lane, Room 16C-17 Rockville, MD 20857 Telephone: 301-443-7577 http://www.organdonor.gov
University Renal Research and Education Association (URREA) **Scientific Registry of Transplant Recipients (SRTR)**	A non-profit organization established for the purpose of conducting clinical and economic studies. It administers the Scientific Registry of Transplant Recipients (SRTR) under contract with the Health Resources and Services Administration of the U.S. Department of Health and Human Services	URREA SRTR 315 West Huron, Suite 260 Ann Arbor, MI 48103 Telephone: 734-665-4108 http://www.urrea.org http://www.ustransplant.org

ANNP630

Organ Donation: The Supply and the Issues

Marilyn Bartucci, MSN, RN, CS, CCTC

Contemporary Nephrology Nursing: Principles and Practice contains 39 chapters of educational content. Individual learners may apply for continuing nursing education credit by reading a chapter and completing the Continuing Education Evaluation Form for that chapter. Learners may apply for continuing education credit for any or all chapters.

Please photocopy this page and return to ANNA.
COMPLETE THE FOLLOWING:

Name: _____

Address:_____

City:_____ State: _____ Zip: _____

E-mail: _____

Preferred telephone: ☐ Home   ☐ Work: _____

State where licensed and license number (optional): _____

CE application fees are based upon the number of contact hours provided by the individual chapter. CE fees per contact hour for ANNA members are as follows: 1.0-1.9 - $15; 2.0-2.9 - $20; 3.0-3.9 - $25; 4.0 and higher - $30. Fees for nonmembers are $10 higher.

ANNA Member: ☐ Yes   ☐ No   Member # (if available) _____

☐ Checked Enclosed   ☐ American Express   ☐ Visa   ☐ MasterCard

Total Amount Submitted: _____

Credit Card Number: _____ Exp. Date: _____

Name as it appears on the card: _____

CE Evaluation Form
To receive continuing education credit for individual study after reading the chapter
1. Photocopy this form. (You may also download this form from ANNA's Web site, **www.annanurse.org.**)
2. Mail the completed form with payment (check) or credit card information to American Nephrology Nurses' Association, East Holly Avenue, Box 56, Pitman, NJ 08071-0056.
3. You will receive your CE certificate from ANNA in 4 to 6 weeks.

Test returns must be postmarked by **December 31, 2010.**

CE Application Fee
ANNA Member $15.00
Nonmember $25.00

EVALUATION FORM

1. I verify that I have read this chapter and completed this education activity. Date: _____

_____
Signature

2. What would be different in your practice if you applied what you learned from this activity? *(Please use additional sheet of paper if necessary.)*

_____
_____
_____
_____
_____
_____
_____
_____
_____
_____
_____
_____
_____

Evaluation	Strongly disagree				Strongly agree
3. The activity met the stated objectives.					
a. Give an overview of the initiatives being used to increase organ donation.	1	2	3	4	5
b. Discuss the types of donors that provide organs for transplantation.	1	2	3	4	5
c. Summarize the process for organ procurement and allocation in the United States.	1	2	3	4	5
4. The content was current and relevant.	1	2	3	4	5
5. The content was presented clearly.	1	2	3	4	5
6. The content was covered adequately.	1	2	3	4	5
7. Rate your ability to apply the learning obtained from this activity to practice.	1	2	3	4	5

Comments _____
_____

8. Time required to read the chapter and complete this form: _____ minutes.

This educational activity has been provided by the American Nephrology Nurses' Association (ANNA) for 1.5 contact hours. ANNA is accredited as a provider of continuing nursing education (CNE) by the American Nurses Credentialing Center's Commission on Accreditation (ANCC-COA). ANNA is an approved provider of continuing education by the California Board of Registered Nursing, CEP 0910.

Transplantation: The Procedure and Implications

Christine Mudge, MS, RN, PNPc/CNS, CNN, FAAN
Laurie Carlson, MSN, RN
Patricia Brennan, MSN, RN

Chapter Contents

Christine Mudge, MS, RN, PNPc/CNS, CNN, FAAN
Laurie Carlson, MSN, RN
Patricia Brennan, MSN, RN

Kidney Transplantation

Kidney transplantation has become the treatment option of choice for patients with end stage renal disease (ESRD). This is due to improved surgical techniques, improved immunosuppressive medications (see Chapter 32), opportunity for superior quality of life, and reduced cost (see Chapter 14) (Silkensen, 2000; Whiting, 2000). Overall, 1-year deceased (cadaveric) kidney transplant success rates are 89.4%, with 5-year success rates being 65%. For recipients of living donor kidneys, the success rates are 97% and 78%, respectively. Almost half of all kidney transplant recipients will be alive with a functioning graft 10 years after transplant (United Network for Organ Sharing [UNOS], 2001). Additional variables that impact patient and graft survival include primary disease and the general health of the recipient, race, immunosuppressive therapy, age, and compliance (Bresnahan et al., 2003; Foster et al., 2002; Vincenti, Jensik,

Filo, Miller, & Pirsch, 2002). Recipient and graft outcomes are further augmented by individualizing therapy and addressing each patient's risk profile (Vincenti, 2004).

The number of diseases that warrant renal transplantation is extensive (see Chapters 9 and 12). The more common causes of kidney disease leading to renal transplantation are outlined in Table 31-1 (Perryman & Stillerman, 1991). The type of renal support or replacement therapy an individual receives prior to kidney transplantation varies. Each situation must be carefully evaluated in collaboration with the patient and family and the transplant team. It is imperative that the nature and trajectory of ESRD and all treatment options be presented and discussed with the patient and family prior to instituting renal replacement therapy (see Chapter 13). This chapter will briefly review the kidney transplant surgical procedure and post-operative complications and management strategies.

Table 31-1
Disease Indications for Kidney Transplantation

Congenital Disorders	**Potential Irreversible Causes of Acute Renal Failure**
Aplastic	Cortical necrosis
Hypoplastic	Acute glomerulonephritis
Congenital nephrotic syndrome	Hemolytic uremic syndrome
Hereditary Nephropathies	Henoch-Schonlein syndrome
Polycystic kidney disease	Acute tubular necrosis
Alport's syndrome	**Inflammatory Disorders**
Medullary cystic disease	Chronic pyelonephritis
Familial nephritis	Membranoproliferative glomerulonephritis
Metabolic Disorders	Focal segmental glomerulosclerosis
Primary oxalosis (often combined kidney-liver transplant)	Hypocomplementemic nephritis
Nephrocalcinosis	Goodpasture's disease
Amyloidosis	Systemic lupus erythematous
Fabry's disease	Scleroderma
Cystinosis	Polyarteritis nodosum
Obstructive Uropathy	Wegener's disease
Congenital/acquired	**Tumors necessitating bilateral nephrectomy**
Reflux nephropathy	Renal carcinoma
Toxic nephropathies	Wilms's tumor
Lead nephropathy	Tuberous sclerosis
Analgesic nephropathy	**Other**
Trauma necessitating bilateral nephrectomy	Hypertensive nephrosclerosis
Renal Vascular Disease	Steroid resistant nephrotic syndrome
Renal artery occlusion	Multiple myeloma
Renal vein thrombosis	Macroglobulinemia
Renal infarct	

Kidney Transplant Surgical Procedure

Organs for kidney transplant are from two sources, living or deceased (cadaveric) donors. When compared to deceased organ transplants, living kidney transplants are often associated with improved graft survival, shorter waiting times, optimization of the recipient's general health, and reduced cost (Cohen & Galbraith, 2001; Vincenti, 2004). Although live donor renal transplants are increasing, they typically account for a minority of transplants performed (Cecka, 2000; UNOS, 2001). As a result, the number of individuals waiting for organ transplant increases every year. In response to the increased number of patients waiting, the transplant community has begun to utilize expanded donor criteria (ECD) in an effort to increase the deceased donor pool. ECD are those donors who, because of extremes of age or other clinical characteristics, are thought to produce allografts at risk for optimum function post-transplant (Whiting, 2000). Such donors might include those who are older than 55, diabetic, hypertensive or hypotensive, infected, or have abnormal organ function or a history of malignancy. Regardless of the donor source, the surgical procedure for the recipient is the same.

Donor Surgery

There are two approaches to the kidney donor surgical procedure, the open donor nephrectomy and the laparoscopic donor nephrectomy. Until recently, the open donor nephrectomy was the only surgical procedure known to accomplish living kidney donation. While effective, this surgery involves a large abdominal muscle incision, occasionally the removal of a rib from the donor, an extended hospital stay, and a prolonged recovery period. All of these factors have been historically considered disincentives to living kidney donation. Laparoscopic live donor nephrectomy was developed to decrease these disincentives to live donation (Ratner, Montgomery, & Kavoussi, 1998). With advances in laparoscopic surgery, this technique is becoming increasingly utilized, particularly for living kidney donors.

Open donor nephrectomy. In the conventional method, the donor is placed in a full lateral decubitus position by flexing the iliac crest and the ribs with the left or right flank anterior. The surgery uses a standard extraperitoneal flank approach with or without removal of the distal eleventh and twelfth ribs. The left side is usually preferred because it is technically easier and provides the kidney with a long vein, making the transplant procedure and ureteral anastomosis technically easier (Hanto & Simmons, 1987; Lind, Ijzermans, & Bonjer, 2002). The fascia is opened and the kidney mobilized to gain access to the renal vessels. The renal vessels, caval vein, and ureter are clamped and cut. It is imperative that during the dissection the blood supply to the ureter from the renal vessels is preserved. If indicated, *ex vivo* renal artery reconstruction is performed on a back table prior to transplant. In cases where there are multiple renal arteries, a Carrel patch may be used or the vessels implanted separately into the recipient's renal vessels (Salvatierra, 1987) (see Figure 31-1). With the dissection completed, the kidney is removed and flushed with an iced preservation solution (e.g., Euro-Collins). Flushing of the kidney is performed to remove

Figure 31-1
Vascular Techniques in Adults

Vascular anastomosis techniques in adults. A. end-to-end renal artery to external iliac artery anastomosis and renal vein to external iliac vein anastomosis; B. end-to-end artery to hypogastric artery anastomosis; C. a patch of aorta may be used for an anastomosis to the side of the external iliac artery for cadaver donors with multiple renal arteries; D. entire aorta used for two pediatric kidneys transplanted into an adult.

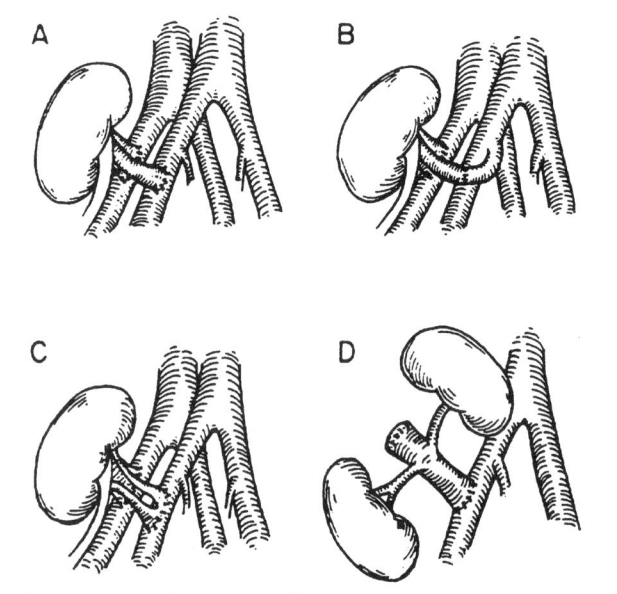

Note: Reprinted with permission from Hanto, D.W. & Simmons, R.L. (1987). Renal transplantation: Clinical considerations, *Radiologic Clinics of North America, 25*(2), 243.

blood products and reduce the core temperature of the kidney. The kidney is flushed until the venous effluent is clear and the kidney is discolored. The kidney then is placed in a sterile basin containing lactated Ringer's solution. The surgeon carefully examines and flushes the kidney before it is transported. Manipulation of the kidney should be minimized because it stimulates the nerves and can lead to vasospasm. Spasms can result in thrombosis, stenosis, and necrosis of the ureter, urinary leakage, and loss of graft (Diethelm, Barger, Whelchel, & Barber, 1987). The donor incision is closed. Living donors recover in the recovery room prior to returning to their room. The procedure takes approximately 4 to 6 hours. Open nephrectomy is a safe procedure for procuring donor kidneys in live donors, with reported mortality rates of 0.03% (Najarian, Chavers, McHugh, & Matas, 1992). In general, most deceased kidney donors undergo open donor nephrectomy.

Laparoscopic donor nephrectomy. Laparoscopic donor nephrectomy is a minimally invasive procedure. The patient is placed in a modified lateral decubitus position at 45 degrees, and the torso is allowed to rotate posteriorly to permit exposure to the lower midline (Kim, Ratner, & Kavoussi, 2000; Novotny, 2001). Three laparoscopic ports are placed under direct vision, one lateral to the rectus muscle between the umbilicus and iliac crest, one at the umbilicus, and one in the midline midway between the xiphoid and the umbilicus. The camera is positioned at the umbilical port. The surgery is performed through the other ports. It is often necessary to place a fourth port for the purpose of retraction. It is usually placed in the anterior axillary line at the level of the umbilicus (Fabrizio, Ratner, Montgomery, & Kavoussi, 1999; Novotny, 2001). Carbon dioxide is introduced into the abdominal cavity to mobilize the abdominal wall away from the organs and allow for more operating space. The kidney and ureter are dissected.

Typically, a right donor nephrectomy is performed to minimize serious potential vascular complications (Lind et al., 2002). The donor artery, vein, and ureter are carefully detached, and once the kidney is separated, it is removed through an incision just above the symphysis pubis. This incision does not go through the abdominal muscle wall. This procedure takes approximately 4 hours. Fabrizio et al. (1999), Novotny (2001), Philosophe et al. (1999), and Ratner et al. (1995) provide more complete descriptions of this procedure.

Several studies have shown that laparoscopic donor nephrectomy results in decreased post-operative morbidity, less pain, optimum cosmetic results, shorter hospital stay, and an earlier return to work (Cadeddu, Ratner, & Kavoussi, 2000; Kim et al., 2000; Novotny, 2001; Ratner et al., 1998). In addition, long-term recipient renal graft function of laparoscopic donor nephrectomy appears equal to that of open donor nephrectomy (Cadeddu et al., 2000; Kim et al., 2000; Novotny, 2001; Ratner et al., 1998). Laparoscopic surgery provides a significant benefit over traditional open surgery for kidney donation and is likely to become the "gold standard" for donor nephrectomy in the future (Handschein, Weber, Demartines, & Clavien, 2003).

Recipient Kidney Transplant Surgery

Kidney transplantation is a well-established surgical procedure. The kidney is typically transplanted extra-peritoneally into the recipient's iliac fossa (see Figure 31-2). The placement of the transplanted kidney in this location affords several advantages: close location of the graft to the vessels and bladder, enhanced ability to assess the graft post-operatively, and ease of accessibility in the event a biopsy or surgical intervention is necessary (Pattella & Weiskittel, 1991). An oblique incision is made from the midline symphysis pubis, curving laterally and superiorly to the iliac crest. The donor renal artery is anastomosed to either the recipient's external iliac artery, using an end-to-side technique, or to the recipient's hypogastric artery, using an end-to-end technique. Next, the donor renal vein is anastomosed to the recipient's external iliac vein. The final step is the anastomosis of the donor ureter into the recipient's bladder or into the ipsilateral native ureter as an ureterostomy. Situations that alter this standardized procedure include previous transplants, size mismatch between donor and recipient, pediatric recipients requiring an intraperitoneal placement of the kidney, and/or multiple donor renal arteries (see Figure 31-2). In some situations, such as severe polyuria or electrolyte wasting, polycystic kidney disease, uncontrollable hypertension, severe proteinuria, and recurrent pyelonephritis, recipient bilateral native nephrectomy is necessary (Benfield, 2003).

Figure 31-2
Kidney Transplant: The Right Lower Quadrant is the Usual Site for Kidney Transplantation

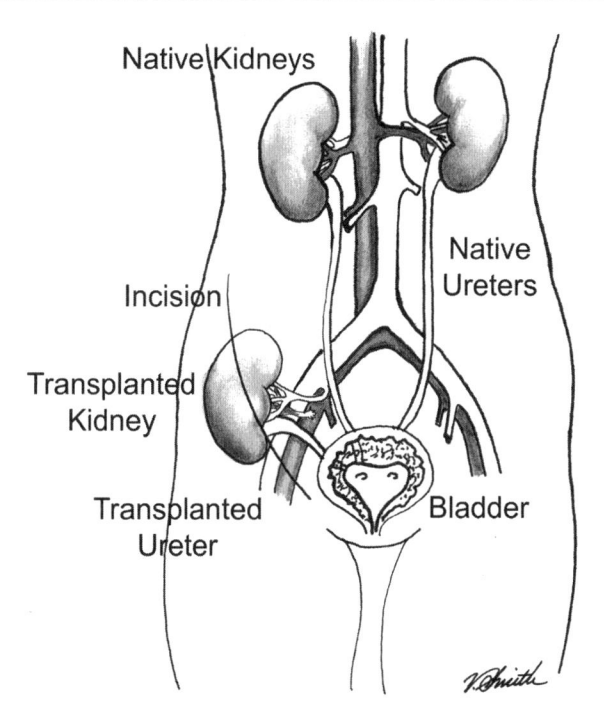

Note: This is an original drawing by Victoria Smith

Post-Operative Management and Nursing Care of the Kidney Transplant Recipient

During the post-operative period, patients must be encouraged to become active participants in their own care. Long-term post-transplant care is complex, requiring patients to have a relatively extensive knowledge of their health care management. Therefore, a comprehensive education program should be developed for every patient and family. Nursing care for the post-operative kidney transplant recipient can be challenging and rewarding. Although the care is very similar for any patient who has undergone major surgery, particular attention must be made to renal function and the pre-transplant long-term complications of uremia, the impact of immunosuppressive therapy, and the adjustment of the patient and family to the transplant process. Caring for the kidney transplant recipient and their family, therefore, mandates advanced nursing diagnosis and assessment skills, followed by prompt intervention.

Renal function. Assessment of renal function requires diligent monitoring of the color and character of urine flow rate, serum blood urea nitrogen (BUN), creatinine, electrolytes, and creatinine clearance. Renal function is confirmed by the immediate and continued formation of urine, an initial massive diuresis, a continual decline in serum BUN and creatinine, and the stabilization of electrolytes.

Delayed graft function (DGF) is the earliest marker of injury to the kidney that has an effect on long-term graft outcome. DGF is caused by both an ischemic phenomenon and immune factors (Shoskes, 2000). The major causes of

DGF are acute tubular necrosis, perfusion injury, hyperacute rejection, urological complications, endogenous donor renal disease (e.g., infection, tumors, renal diseases [IgA nephropathy, microvascular thrombosis]), and coexisting acute rejection (Sanfilippo, 1990).

Acute tubular necrosis (ATN) is the most likely cause of DGF early post-transplant. ATN occurs in approximately 10% – 30% of all patients after cadaveric transplantation and in less than 3% of those undergoing living-related renal transplantation. ATN is a reversible condition, lasting a few days to weeks. It is caused by changes in the donor kidney secondary to oxygen interruption during renal procurement, prolonged preservation time, or excessive handling during the surgery. Prolonged cold and warm ischemic times also contribute to ATN. Cold ischemia time is the length of time the kidney is preserved on ice from donor to recipient. With greater distance between donor and recipient (for example, from Boston to San Francisco), the cold ischemia time is likely to be longer. If the cold ischemia time is greater than 24 hours, there is an increased risk of ATN in the recipient. Warm ischemic time is the length of time between cessation of renal circulation to the achievement of adequate hypothermia in the donor organ. Vascular anastomosis takes approximately 20 to 30 minutes and, in some centers, is included in the warm ischemia time. Surgical complications related to the vascular anastomosis that can increase warm ischemia time include multiple renal arteries or hypovolemia.

There are two types of ATN, oliguric and non-oliguric. Oliguric ATN is the most common and is characterized by prolonged oliguria or anuria that can persist for several days to 2 months. Non-oliguric or high-output ATN is demonstrated by a normal or greater than normal urine output without adequate excretion of nitrogenous waste products. In both types of ATN, there is an elevation in BUN and serum creatinine with accompanying electrolyte disorders. A renal scan may be performed to evaluate the presence of ATN by assessing renal blood flow and excretion of a radioisotope. If ATN is present, there will be decreased uptake and excretion of the isotope. Renal biopsy will reveal tubular epithelial cell necrosis, mild edema, congestion, and inflammatory cell infiltration in the presence of ATN. If ATN is present, close judicious monitoring of fluids and electrolytes is necessary. Temporary dialysis may be needed and is often required in approximately 20% of deceased donor renal transplants in the early post-operative period (Garovoy, Stock, Bumgardner, Keith, & Linker, 1994). In general, gradual improvement in renal function can be observed over time.

Fluids and electrolytes. Monitoring of fluids and electrolytes is of paramount importance in determining renal function. The goal is to attain a euvolemic state and maintain renal perfusion. During the initial post-transplant period, there is large diuresis caused by a high osmotic load secondary to pre-transplant uremia, high glucose levels (due to steroid induced hyperglycemia, intravenous (IV) fluids, or diabetes), and volume overload from administration of intra-operative fluids. Adequate fluid replacement is given to match urine output, and diuretics are administered if necessary to secure continuing diuresis. Fluids are generally replaced with 0.45% normal saline with or without glucose. Inadequate fluid replacement can lead to oliguria and impaired renal function. Conversely, over-hydration can result in congestive heart failure or pulmonary edema, promote electrolyte disturbances, or contribute to hypertension. Therefore, it is imperative that the fluid status be closely monitored during the early post-transplant period. Typical assessment parameters include accurate daily weights, total intake and output, urine specific gravity, vital signs, and central venous pressure (CVP) measurement.

During the first 24 to 48 hours, intake and output are monitored every hour and in some centers every 30 minutes. All fluids (e.g., IV solutions, nasogastric secretions, urine, and infant's stool) are carefully measured to assure accurate balance. This is particularly important in children weighing less than 10 kilograms.

Blood clots are the most common cause of a diminishing urine output in the early post-operative period. If aseptic irrigation is unsuccessful in removing the clots, the catheter should be replaced after consulting with the surgeon. If urine volume is high, fluid administration is often increased to 30 ml plus urine output per hour. A CVP line may be placed to measure and titrate volume status more closely. CVP readings are usually kept between 6 mm and 12 mm Hg. Persistently low CVP readings may require additional fluid or albumin to ensure graft perfusion and maintenance of a euvolemic state. In addition, blood pressure should be maintained at greater than 110/70 mm Hg to insure adequate blood flow to the kidney.

Evaluation of the patient's volume status is facilitated by the assessment of skin turgor and mucous membranes for dehydration (assess infant fontanel; infants and children assess for tears), palpation and inspection of the extremities and sacral area for edema, and the inspection of the neck veins for distention (Perryman & Stillerman, 1991). The development of adventitious breath sounds, such as crackles, shortness of breath, and the presence of an S3 on cardiac evaluation are indicative of excess volume (Beckman, Schell, Calixto, & Sullivan, 1992).

Excess volume states are typically the result of intra-operative over-hydration to maintain renal perfusion or prevent ATN. Over-hydration is generally treated by administering diuretics (e.g., furosemide). In patients who do not respond to therapy, ATN must be suspected. In these patients, meticulous monitoring of fluid status is crucial. If the patient becomes over-hydrated, the physician is notified and further therapy is promptly instituted. Treatment often includes oxygen, nitroglycerin, and morphine sulfate as pre-cardiac load reducers. Morphine sulfate is utilized to relieve anxiety and relax airway smooth muscles, thus enhancing gas exchange and breathing (Beckman et al., 1992). If treatment is unsuccessful, emergent hemodialysis becomes necessary.

Dehydration can cause a reduction in renal perfusion and subsequent graft damage. Maintaining CVP levels above 4 mm Hg, systolic blood pressure greater than 110 mm Hg, and monitoring for adequate urine output are methods of ensuring renal perfusion.

Close monitoring of electrolytes is crucial with fluctuations in fluid status and varying degrees of renal function.

Table 31-2
Clinical Findings in Potassium Imbalance

System	Hypokalemia (< 3.5 mEq/L)	Hyperkalemia (> 5.5 mEq/L)
Cardiovascular	EKG changes: depressed ST segment, flat or inverted T wave, presence of a U wave, premature arterial or ventricular beats, progressing to paroxysmal atrial tachycardia, atrioventricular blocks, and ventricular tachycardia	EKG changes: spiked T waves, widened QRS complex, progressing to bradycardia, hypotension, loss of P waves, idioventricular pattern to systole, and cardiac arrest
Gastrointestinal	anorexia, nausea, vomiting, constipation, decreased bowel sounds	diarrhea, cramps, colic, increased bowel sounds
Muscle	weakness, flabby muscle	increased muscle irritability, increased tendon reflexes, muscle cramps
Central nervous system	lassitude, confusion	dizziness

Since electrolyte homeostasis is one of the kidneys' primary responsibilities (see Chapter 5), disruption in electrolyte balance is not an uncommon problem post-kidney transplant. The two most common imbalances are in potassium and glucose (see Table 31-2).

A normal potassium level is generally considered 3.5 to 5.5 mEq/L. Hyperkalemia or hypokalemia may develop post-kidney transplant. Hyperkalemia may be observed in the presence of ATN or acute rejection. In these situations, potassium is unable to be excreted by the damaged tubules and accumulates. Other factors that can cause hyperkalemia are administration of potassium, blood transfusions, and surgery, resulting in cell damage and the release of potassium ions. In addition, the initiation of one of the calcineurin inhibitors (cyclosporin or tacrolimus) may increase the risk of hyperkalemia (see Chapter 32). The presence of acidosis or hyperglycemia can contribute to hyperkalemia by creating ionic shifts. Hyperkalemia is initially treated with diuretics. However, if potassium levels are greater than 6.5 mEq/L, other forms of therapy should be implemented, such as dialysis or sodium polystyrene sulfonate (Kayexalate®) with sorbitol. Both hemodialysis and peritoneal dialysis effectively remove potassium. Kayexalate is an exchange ion that trades potassium ions for sodium ions in a ratio of 1:1 in the small bowel. Sorbitol is administered as an osmotic diarrhea agent to promote evacuation of the potassium from the intestines. A retention enema may be given to patients who have not progressed to oral feeds; however, in many centers, this is not recommended because of the pressure the enema can place on the surgical site.

Although many dialysis patients have developed a tolerance for elevated potassium levels, it is considered a medical emergency when potassium levels are greater than 6.5 mEq/L or when EKG changes are present. In these situations, administration of Kayexalate with sorbitol or emergency dialysis is usually performed. IV glucose, insulin, and bicarbonate may be employed, pending dialysis, to mobilize the potassium back into the cells. It must be remembered that the administration of glucose, insulin, and bicarbonate is only a temporary measure and that follow-up hemodialysis or Kayexalate with sorbitol is usually necessary. In severe emergencies, calcium gluconate may be ordered for its inotropic (improved contractility) effects on the heart. However, it must be remembered that calcium gluconate is contraindicated in patients taking digitalis. If hyperkalemia is an ongoing problem, dietary adjustment of potassium intake or additional medication is considered.

Hypokalemia (< 3.5 mEq/L) develops when potassium losses are greater than intake. In the early post-kidney transplant period, hypokalemia is usually the result of massive diuresis, excessive use of diuretics, large gastrointestinal losses, or lack of appropriate potassium replacement. The clinical manifestations and EKG changes caused by hypokalemia are outlined in Table 31-2.

Hypokalemia should be treated promptly to avoid EKG changes, particularly in patients receiving digitalis, which potentiates the effects of the drug. Treatment for hypokalemia requires cautious oral or IV potassium replacement with EKG monitoring and accurate measurement of gastrointestinal losses, which are high in potassium (e.g., nasogastric secretions, emesis, and stool [diarrhea]).

Nursing care for patients with an alteration in potassium levels focuses on prevention. This requires astute physical assessment, accurate measurement of gastrointestinal losses, EKG monitoring, and frequent evaluation of serum potassium levels. In the event that alterations in potassium develop, prompt intervention is mandated.

Hyperglycemia is a relatively common problem post-kidney transplant. It is typically characterized by a blood glucose level greater than 120 mg/dL. Hyperglycemia post-kidney transplant is often associated with the initial high doses of corticosteroids on glucose metabolism, use of tacrolimus, exacerbation of pre-existing diabetes mellitus, familial tendency toward diabetes, or the administration of large volumes of dextrose containing IV fluids. Patients with diabetes mellitus account for 25% of all patients with ESRD. Those who undergo renal transplantation require particularly close glucose monitoring and assessment for hyperglycemia. Risk factors for developing steroid-induced diabetes mellitus (SIDM) include a positive family history for diabetes, obesity, being over 40 years of age, and being female. The basic pathophysiology of SIDM is that corticosteroid therapy causes a decreased utilization of insulin by peripheral tissues. This results in prolonged hyperglycemia, causing a persistent stimulus for increased insulin secretion. Sustained hyperglycemia subsequently leads to a reduction in the number of insulin receptors sites, and the patient becomes "insulin resistant." In addition, hyperglycemia in these patients deprives cells of glucose because of the lack of available insulin. This leads to glycogenolysis in the liver, which further elevates serum glucose levels (see Chapters 11, 17, and 32).

Nursing care for patients at risk for SIDM includes close glucose monitoring by capillary glucose monitoring and serum levels and frequent physical assessment for clinical signs and symptoms of hyperglycemia. Common clinical manifestations of hyperglycemia include polydipsia, polyuria, glycosuria, weakness, fatigue, headache, blurred vision, nausea, vomiting, and abdominal cramps. Polyuria is the result of an osmotic diuresis caused by hyperglycemia, which can lead to dehydration. In the presence of a newly transplanted kidney, dehydration and decreased perfusion to the graft can result in graft damage. It is imperative, therefore, that meticulous fluid monitoring be adhered to in these patients.

Treatment of hyperglycemia is usually implemented when glucose levels are persistently elevated above 180 mg/dL. Short-acting regular insulin is used initially and adjusted as corticosteroids are tapered. Insulin needs are highly variable until steroid doses are stabilized. This mandates that the nurse provide close monitoring and evaluation of the patient's response to insulin administration during this time.

The onset of diabetes can be a very frightening and disturbing experience, and patients and their families may need additional support and education during this time. If hyperglycemic states do not resolve, it becomes necessary to instruct the patient and family in glucose monitoring and insulin injections prior to discharge from the hospital (see Chapter 11).

Patients with pre-existing Type 1 or 2 diabetes are usually controlled with continuous IV insulin infusion. The infusion rate is adjusted frequently based on glucose levels. Once the patient has stabilized, reinstitution of subcutaneous insulin or pump therapy can be considered. Most diabetic patients will need to re-assess their insulin needs post-transplant because of the alteration in glucose metabolism caused by prednisone and other medications they may be taking (see Chapter 32).

Urinary tract. Depending on the type of anastomosis, a urinary catheter is typically left in place for 2 to 5 days. The purpose of the catheter is to allow for close assessment of urinary flow, urine characteristics, and bladder decompression. Once the catheter has been removed, the patient is encouraged to void frequently to allow for continued monitoring of urine output, minimize pressure on the suture lines, and promote bladder healing.

Decreased urine flow may suggest ATN, rejection, a technical complication, decrease in circulating volume, or obstruction. Technical complications, such as a bladder leak, require prompt surgical intervention. If other clinical manifestations of hypovolemia are present, such as hypotension, a fluid bolus is often administered to improve renal perfusion and urine output.

Obstructive ureteral problems have many causes and may be as simple as a kink in the catheter. One of the major causes of catheter occlusion is blood clots. If the patient is passing large blood clots or has a decrease in urine output, it is often necessary to aseptically irrigate the catheter. Care must be taken during irrigation not to apply excess stress to the ureterocystostomy. This is particularly true in patients with exceptionally small bladders secondary to disuse and children, who naturally have smaller bladders. If clots are not removed, bladder distention, pain, and stress on the ureterocystostomy may develop. This may result in a leak at the site of the anastomosis. Occasionally, the surgeon will suture a stent to the end of the catheter passing through the ureter to prevent ureteral stenosis. The surgeon should always be notified prior to changing the catheter (Beckman et al., 1992).

Bladder spasms may develop, causing severe lower abdominal pain. Treatment includes belladonna and opium suppositories (B & O), oxybutynin chloride (Ditropan®), and propantheline bromide (Probanthine®). To allow for complete emptying of the bladder, treatment of bladder spasms should be stopped 24 hours before the catheter is removed. Urinary frequency after the catheter is removed can also be problematic for some patients. However, as the bladder stretches to accommodate larger urine volumes, urinary frequency generally resolves.

Cardiovascular. Nursing care with attention to the cardiovascular system post-kidney transplant requires frequent monitoring of the patient's blood pressure, vascular access for dialysis if present, and assessment of peripheral pulses.

Patients with ESRD often present with a number of cardiovascular disorders that need close monitoring post-transplant. These usually include hypertension, atherosclerosis, left ventricular hypertrophy and dysfunction, and/or a history of pericarditis or pericardial effusion (see Chapter 9). In order to secure optimum cardiovascular function post-transplant, blood pressure is frequently monitored. Hypertension post-transplant is most often related to pre-existing disease, volume overload, medications, or renal artery stenosis (RAS). It is generally treated with antihypertensive agents and diuretics. Hypertension caused by renal arterial stenosis generally requires surgical intervention. Hypotension can result from volume depletion or in response to medication (see Chapter 32). Hypotension subsequently leads to decreased renal perfusion, which can exacerbate ATN if present. A single hypotensive episode can also result in loss of the patient's arteriovenous (AV) vascular access, which can be detrimental in the event of graft failure. Frequent monitoring for a bruit and thrill and protection of the involved extremity by eliminating cuff pressures, blood draws, and IV line placements are important in maintaining the patient's vascular access.

During the surgical procedure, the kidney is anastomosed to the iliac vessels. Clots or thrombosis of these vessels can occur causing decreased perfusion to the affected extremity. Frequent assessment of femoral, popliteal, and pedal pulses will allow for early detection and prompt intervention of this problem.

Pulmonary. Prevention of pulmonary compromise is a major concern for the post-kidney transplant recipient. Smoking cessation prior to transplant is highly recommended. Causes of respiratory problems post-transplant include complications of pre-existing disease, pulmonary edema secondary to volume overload, atelectasis, and pulmonary infiltrates secondary to infection. Methods of ensuring sufficient oxygenation and maintenance of pulmonary function include adequate pain management to prevent splinting, early turning, coughing, deep breathing, ambulation, use of respiratory devices, and oxygen therapy if indicated. Periodic assessment of breath sounds, respiratory rate and effort, sputum, oxygen saturation, and patient color (e.g., ruddy, pale, cyanotic) can provide the nurse with the necessary information to assure adequate pulmonary function. If there is a change in pulmonary function, arterial blood gases and chest radiography will often be ordered to assess respiratory status. If pulmonary edema or infiltrates are observed on chest radiography, administration of diuretic medications (e.g., furosemide) and monitoring the patient's response are the first lines of therapy. In addition, if there is a change in the color and consistency of expectorated sputum, a sputum specimen for culture should be ordered and antibiotic therapy initiated if indicated.

Gastrointestinal. The gastrointestinal effects of surgery and general anesthesia secondary to kidney transplantation are similar to those of general abdominal surgery. Post-operative patients experience delayed gastric motility. Frequent assessment of the abdomen and knowledge of pre-transplant bowel patterns can be helpful. Abdominal assessment includes inspecting for abdominal distention; auscultating for the presence or absence of bowel sounds; palpating for tenderness; and monitoring for nausea, vomiting, diarrhea, constipation, and occult blood in the stool. Nausea and vomiting can develop for a variety of reasons, including anesthesia, medications, electrolyte disturbances, and dehydration. The cause should be addressed and treated appropriately. Antiemetics are often prescribed.

Constipation can occur as the result of antacids, analgesics, and/or decreased motility secondary to anesthesia. Increased mobility, dietary alterations, stool softeners, or changing medications from phosphate binders to histamine antagonists (e.g., ranitidine) are methods for minimizing constipation.

Diarrhea can develop as a result of immunosuppressant medication (e.g., mycophenolate mofetil; see Chapter 32), infection, or bleeding. If diarrhea persists, a complete stool work-up is performed, including culture, clostridium difficile, fecal leukocytes, and occult blood. Gastrointestinal bleeding may be related to corticosteroids or surgical stress. If active bleeding is present, endoscopy or colonoscopy with possible surgical intervention may be indicated. Clostridium difficile, one of the most common infections post-transplant, is typically treated for 7 to 10 days with antibiotics, usually oral Flagyl® or Vancomycin® (see Chapters 17 and 32).

Psychosocial considerations during the early post-operative period are often related to graft function, the relationship of the recipient to the living donor, and side effects of immunosuppressive therapy (see Chapter 32). With a successfully functioning graft and steroid administration, recipients often experience a general sense of well-being (Pattella & Weiskettel, 1991). The recipient may also have an improved self-esteem and body image (Thompson, McFarland, Hirsch, & Tucker, 1993). However, for patients who do not experience a successful transplant, the post-surgical period can be an extremely difficult time.

During the early post-transplant period, the recipient may express a wide range of emotional responses secondary to fear of rejection, conflict over the decision to undergo transplantation, incorporation of the graft into a sense of self, fear of assuming the characteristics of the donor, coping with feelings about the donor, family functioning, side effects of immunosuppression, pain, and financial worries. It is important that the nurse recognizes the recipient's concerns and provides appropriate support. In some situations, consultation with a social worker or financial counselor can be extremely helpful.

Early Complications Post-Kidney Transplantation

Early complications are those that occur during the first year post-kidney transplant. These complications are a result of the adverse side effects of immunosuppressive therapy discussed in detail in Chapter 32 and include rejection, infection, and technical problems related to the surgery. Surgical complications can further be classified as vascular, urologic, lymphatic, and wound management. The nurse can facilitate early and accurate diagnosis of complications by frequent and exact patient assessments. If complications do occur, appropriate nursing management, support, and education are implemented specific to the problem.

Rejection. Rejection continues to be one of the major problems in kidney transplantation. Although there is improvement in histocompatibility testing, immune modulating techniques, and the availability of new immunosuppressive therapy, many patients experience at least one rejection episode. There are four types of rejection: hyperacute, acute humoral antibody mediated, acute cellular, and chronic (Braun, 2003). A brief review of transplant immunology may assist the reader in understanding the concept of rejection. Mudge (1998), among others, provides an overview of transplant immunology that may be helpful (see Chapter 32).

Hyperacute rejection. Hyperacute rejection occurs minutes to 24 hours after transplantation. Clinical manifestations include an immediate and sharp decrease in renal function; pain over the allograft; and a swollen, mottled, cyanotic kidney with abrupt cessation of urine output. Hyperacute rejection is the result of pre-sensitization of the recipient to the donor's Class I human leukocyte antigens (HLA). The pathogenesis is an allograft-specific coagulopathy that is initiated by preformed anti-donor HLA antigens on the vascular endothelium and platelets. Fortunately, there has been a significant decrease in hyperacute rejection episodes because of more sensitive cross-matching techniques. Since the introduction of erythropoietin therapy in 1990 and the reduction of needed blood transfusions, there also has been a decrease in HLA panel reactive antibodies (PRA) in potential recipients (Braun, 2003).

Diagnosis of hyperacute rejection is made by evaluation of the patient's clinical manifestations (rising serum creatinine and blood urea nitrogen, decreased urine output, elec-

Table 31-3
Analysis of Diagnostic Studies in Renal Transplantation

Study	Goal	Interpretation
DTPA Radiology Study	Assess for blood flow to the allograft	*Normal* – presence of blood flow to the graft *Absence* – no blood flow; does not differentiate between ATN, rejection, or glomerular nephritis
Mag-3 Radiology Study	Assess for blood flow & extravasation of isotope indicating anastomotic leak	*Normal* – prompt uptake to the kidney with rapid clearance of the hippurate isotope from the kidney to the bladder and/or Foley catheter *ATN* – reduced isotope uptake with cortical retention *Cellular rejection* – initial changes show a reduction in excretion while later phases (days later) include a progressive reduction in uptake. A single scan can only be characterized as compatible with rejection but not diagnostic *Rejection-treatment phase* – the first response to treatment is one of improvement in excretion with subsequent improvement in uptake *Intrinsic parenchymal processes* – reduced uptake and excretion; the tubular luminal flow is fairly well preserved in contrast to the renal blood flow to the allograft
Renal Ultrasound	Evaluate the allograph for signs indicative of rejection: swelling, prominence of medullary pyramids, pelvic-infundibular wall thickening, resistive index (RI), and decreased sinus fat; may also be used to look for obstruction	*Normal* – no dilation to pelvis or ureters, may have small perinephritic fluid collections, normal sinus fat, and corticomedullary junction appearance and RI < 70% *Acute rejection* – swelling of allograft, reduced sinus fat (from compression), prominent medullary pyramids, pelvi-infundibular thickening, and RI > 70% (Note: These changes are seen when serum creatinine level is > 1 mg%.) *Obstruction* – dilated collecting structures (either intraureteral obstruction or periureteral obstruction secondary to lymphocele); changes are usually followed by anterograde pyelogram, IV pyelogram, or surgical intervention

trolyte abnormalities), renal scan that typically shows no uptake or excretion by the allograft (see Table 31-3), renal biopsy, and/or surgical exploration. Histological examination of the donor kidney demonstrates a diffuse intravascular coagulation in the glomerular capillaries and renal arterioles. There is initial antibody binding to the vascular endothelial cells, which activates complement and the coagulation cascade. This process results in polymorphonuclear leukocyte (PMN) chemotaxis and intravascular glomerular platelet deposition and thrombosis, which leads to congestion and edema, inflammatory injury to the renal vasculature and glomeruli with hemorrhage and necrosis, ischemic tubular injury, and frank cortical necrosis (Garovoy, Amend, Vincenti, & Feduska, 1987; Sanfilippo, 1990).

Absence of preformed HLA antibodies significantly reduces the risk of hyperacute rejection and humoral rejection episodes. Management and prognosis of hyperacute rejection is poor and transplant nephrectomy almost always necessary. Pre-transplant protocols have been reported, including plasma apheresis, that have shown some encouraging results in lowering recipients anti-donor HLA antibody titers (Montgomery et al., 2000; Schweizer et al., 1990).

Hyperacute rejection can cause emotional trauma for the patient and family. If there is a living donor, the loss of the graft may be even more devastating. Both the recipient and donor are forced to recover from a surgery that neither may feel benefited them. This may initiate feelings of failure, guilt, anger, or depression. It is not uncommon for these patients to feel neglected post-operatively (Ruse & Kottra-Buck, 1986). It is imperative that nurses assure that both receive support to deal with their loss.

Table 31-4
Differential Diagnosis for Allograft Dysfunction after Kidney Transplantation

Delayed Allograft Function

acute tubular necrosis
hyperacute rejection
acute rejection
perfusion injury during procurement
urological complications

Acute Dysfunction

acute rejection
calcineurin nephrotoxicity
drug reactions
infection
acute transplant glomerulopathy
malignant hypertension
ureteral or vascular complications
intravascular coagulopathy
recurrent disease

Chronic Dysfunction

chronic rejection
chronic calcineurin nephrotoxicity
chronic transplant glomerulopathy
arterio-nephrosclerosis
recurrent disease

Acute rejection. Acute rejection continues to be the most important cause of renal allograft dysfunction and the greatest obstacle to the success of kidney transplantation. It usually occurs 1 to 6 months post-transplant and has the potential to compromise long-term graft survival (Hariharan et al., 2000). A single episode of acute rejection during the first year post-transplant may be associated with a 50% reduction in renal allograft half life (Matas, Burk, DeVault, Monaco, & Pirsch, 1994). This is particularly noticeable in African-Americans, who demonstrate a 50% graft survival rate after acute rejection, as compared to 76% graft survival among Whites (Ojo et al., 1995).

Humoral antibody-mediated rejection. Humoral antibody-mediated rejection typically occurs 30 to 90 days post-kidney transplant. The incidence is approximately 10% in the first deceased donor transplant and 30% in repeat transplants, with 5% in mismatched living donor transplants, depending on the type of induction and ongoing immunosuppressive therapy (Braun, 2003). Clinically, there is a rapid rise in serum creatinine and BUN after initially good renal function. There may also be a decline in urine output and hypertension. Occasionally, there will be one of the following: fever, malaise, weight gain, and mild graft swelling and tenderness. Pathogenesis is based on the recipient's development of donor-reactive anti-HLA antibodies and possibly non-HLA antibodies. The differential diagnosis for a decline in renal function with similar abnormalities includes ATN, calcineurin nephrotoxicity, pre-renal azotemia, and obstruction (Garovoy et al., 1994) (see Table 31-4).

Detection of humoral antibody-mediated rejection is typically based on laboratory data, radiologic findings, and renal biopsy. Diagnosis of acute rejection can be facilitated by an ultrasound. Although not very sensitive, an ultrasound may demonstrate swelling of the kidney, blurring of corticomedullary junctions, and prominent pyramids in acute rejection. Magnetic resonance imaging (MRI), although expensive, may also be diagnostic and show loss of corticomedullary differentiation and swelling. In general, a renal biopsy is the "gold standard" for a definitive diagnosis to confirm kidney transplant rejection. Histologic examination of the graft is characterized by three cardinal diagnostic features: (a) morphologic evidence of acute tissue injury as exemplified by acute tubular injury, neutrophils, and/or mononuclear cells in the peritubular capillaries and/or glomeruli, and/or capillary thrombosis or intimal arteritis/fibrinoid necrosis/intramural or transmural inflammation in the arteries; (b) immunopathologic evidence for antibody action, exemplified by C4d and/or immunoglobulin in the peritubular capillaires, or immunoglobulin and complement in arterial fibrinoid necrosis; and (c) serologic evidence of circulating antibodies to donor HLA or other anti-donor endothelial antigens (Bohmig & Regele, 2003; Braun, 2003; Garovoy et al., 1987; Mauiyyedi & Colvin, 2002; Mauiyyedi et al., 2002; San Filippo, 1990).

Treatment of humoral antibody-mediated rejection is based mainly on anecdotal reporting, including apheresis, IV immunoglobin, Rituximab (antiCD 20 antibody), steroids, and other immunnosuppressive therapy (Bohmig & Regele, 2003). Although optimal treatment for mediated

rejection has yet to be established, depending on the transplant center, treatment is typically comprised of aggressive therapy with either a monoclonal antibody (OKT3) or polyclonal antibody (ATG); a course of apheresis, often with IV immunoglobulin (IVIG); and enhanced immunosuppression (e.g., conversion to tacrolimus and mycophenolate mofetil) (Montgomery et al., 2000; Pascual et al., 1998) (see Chapter 31). Acute humoral rejection occurs in approximately 20%–30% of acute rejection episodes. It has a poorer prognosis than cellular rejection and has been reported to be refractory to conventional immunosuppressive therapy (Herzenberg, Gill, Djurdjev, & Magil, 2002; Mauiyyedi & Colvin, 2002). It is important to note that treatment is often dependent on center protocols, degree of renal involvement, and the patient's response to therapy.

Acute cellular rejection. Acute cellular rejection usually occurs within the first 6 to12 months post-kidney transplant. The timing and severity are dependent on the type of immunosuppressive therapy, patient compliance, HLA compatibility between donor and recipient, and the recipient's innate immune response (Braun, 2003). Clinical manifestations include a gradual increase in serum creatinine and BUN, and increasing hypertension without a noticeable decline in urine output. The pathogenesis of acute cellular rejection involves delayed type hypersensitivity reaction and cytotoxic positive CD8 T-lymphocytes. A number of soluble mediators are also implicated, including cytokines, lymphokines, chemokines, vasoactive substances, and growth factors. Diagnosis is based on laboratory findings and renal biopsy. In otherwise stable transplants, subclinical acute cellular rejection may only be detected on protocol biopsies (Rush et al., 1998). Histologic findings in acute cellular rejection involve acute tubulitis, interstitial infiltration by positive CD4 and positive CD8 lymphocytes, monocytes, macrophages, B lymphocytes, and natural killer (NK) cells. Arteritis may also be present (Braun, 2003). Treatment typically includes steroids and conversion to tacrolimus and mycophenolate mofetil (or other enhanced immunosuppression). If arteritis is present, monoclonal or polyclonal antibody therapy may be employed. With the advent of newer and more potent immunosuppressant agents, the incidence of acute cellular rejection has declined significantly from 50% in the precyclosporine era to a current incidence of approximately 8%–15% (Braun, 2003; Vincenti, 2004).

Patients undergoing treatment for acute rejection must be closely monitored for drug side effects and episodes of infection. The additional immunosuppressive therapy used to treat acute rejection places the patient at an increased risk for infection. Frequent handwashing can help in preventing infection, and diligent physical assessment facilitates the detection of early manifestations of potential infection, promoting prompt intervention. Since high dose steroids are the most common treatment for acute rejection, it is imperative that the patient be monitored for gastric irritation by checking for occult blood in the stool, hyperglycemia, excessive fluid retention, and adjustment to temporary body image changes. Patients will often become cushingoid, gain weight, and develop acne. These side effects are particularly disturbing for adolescents, who should be monitored closely for compliance and provided with additional support. Nursing interventions for patients who are having a difficult time dealing with changes in their body image during rejection therapy include topical antibacterial medication to help control acne (e.g., benzyl peroxide), a nutritional consult to assist with appetite control and appropriate food choices, physical therapy or an exercise physiologist consult to increase activity level, and for young women different methods of applying their make-up. It is important to have an understanding of the patient's major concerns in order to appropriately develop an individualized plan of care. Rejection episodes are often an ideal opportunity to provide the patient and family with additional education and resources regarding transplantation. Patients should receive pre-transplant instruction regarding rejection to give them an understanding of signs and symptoms, course, and usual treatment. However, even those who have had instruction may feel shocked that they are undergoing a rejection episode (Ruse & Kottra-Buck, 1986). Responses to rejection are commonly a compilation of the rejection itself and the side effects of the drugs used to treat it. Emotional responses may include anger, depression, fear, withdrawal, or moodiness. During this time, it is important that the patient and family be provided with support. Transplant support groups can be very beneficial during rejection episodes.

Chronic rejection. Chronic rejection usually occurs months to years after kidney transplant (Braun, 2003). Chronic rejection has an insidious onset with a slow rise in serum creatinine, increasing proteinuria, and hypertension. It is typically unresponsive to an increase in immunosuppressive therapy and has a relentless downward trajectory in renal function. Clinical manifestations are highly variable depending on the degree of renal function. Initial presentation often includes proteinuria secondary to increasing glomerular permeability, an increasing serum BUN and creatinine, decreasing urine output, fluid retention, alteration in electrolytes, and an increase in renin production resulting in hypertension. It is widely accepted that the pathogenesis of chronic rejection includes immunologic and non-immunologic factors. Immunologic risk factors for chronic rejection include HLA mismatch, early rejection episodes, and late rejection episodes. In addition, those individuals, both children and adults, who experience one episode of acute rejection are at major risk for developing chronic rejection (Bradley, 2002; Samsonov & Briscoe, 2002; Seikaly 2004; Tejani & Sullivan, 2000). Non-immunologic risk factors include ischemia reperfusion injury, nephrotoxic drugs, viruses, hypertension, and hyperlipidemia (Basadonna et al., 1993; Bradley, 2002; Isoniemi et al., 1994; Matas et al., 1994; Samsonov & Briscoe, 2002; Seikaly, 2004; Tejani & Sullivan, 2000). Histologic findings in chronic rejection are characterized by interstitial fibrosis, tubular atrophy, intimal hyperplasia of the arterioles, glomerulosclerosis, and sometimes glomerulopathy. Over time, graft ischemia develops with subsequent loss of renal function (Braun, 2003; Garovoy et al., 1994; Isoniemi et al., 1994; Sanfilippo, 1990).

The host of alloantigenic independent factors involved in the histologic changes found in chronic rejection makes it difficult to differentiate. As a result, they have been included under the heading of "chronic allograft nephropathy" (CAN) or chronic allograft dysfunction. The histology of CAN is nonspecific and is characterized by fibrointimal thickening of the arteries, varying degrees of interstitial fibrosis, tubular atrophy, and a variety of glomerular changes (Braun, 2003; Braun & Yadlapalliet, 2002).

Renal biopsy is the most definitive method of diagnosing chronic rejection. Treatment of chronic rejection is generally conservative, focusing on graft preservation and delaying re-transplantation or dialysis. Management of chronic rejection is very similar to progressive ESRD, including medications, changes in diet, fluid restriction, monitoring of electrolytes, blood pressure control, anemia management, assistance in maintaining activity level, education, and support (see Chapter 12). In addition to education regarding medical management, patients and families will also need information regarding treatment options. For patients who have been previously dialyzed, assisting them in making the transition to dialysis is important. This will be highly variable, depending on how long it has been since they were last dialyzed. For those who have never been dialyzed, support and education are essential. These patients and families benefit from a support group and by speaking to other patients who are undergoing dialysis. They often require comprehensive instruction regarding ESRD and available treatment options (see Chapter 13). Many patients will want to be reconsidered for another transplant. For those patients interested in a second transplant, a complete evaluation to determine candidacy should be completed. As renal function deteriorates and renal replacement therapy becomes necessary, withdrawal of immunosuppressive therapy may be recommended. Transplant nephrectomy may be indicated for chronic symptoms, infection, or severe reflux nephropathy.

Infection

There are a number of risk factors that predispose the renal transplant recipient to infection. These include pre-existing uremia (see Chapter 11); underlying systemic disease such as diabetes, systemic lupus erythematosus (SLE), scleroderma, or malnutrition (see Chapter 9); or alterations in the host's defenses due to the transplant surgery and administration of immunosuppressive therapy (see Chapter 32). As a result of the surgery, the patient's first line of defense, the skin and mucous membranes, is broken. Further disruption is caused by invasive monitoring, urinary catheterization, central and peripheral IV access, and endotracheal intubation. Breakdown of primary defenses subjects the transplant recipient to infection. In addition, immunosuppressive therapy alters the body's secondary defense, the immune response, which augments the recipient's risk of infection. Disruption in the host's primary and secondary responses also predisposes the post-renal transplant recipient to infection. The most common indications for readmission to the hospital post-transplant are related to bacterial and viral infectious complications (Benfield, 2003) (see Table 31-5).

Urinary tract infections (UTIs). UTIs are the most common bacterial infections post-renal transplant (Anderson,

Table 31-5
Timetable for the Occurrence of Infection Posttransplant

Note: Reprinted with permission from Rubin, R. (1994) Infection in the organ transplant recipient (page 635). In R. Rubin & L. Young (Eds.), *Clinical approach to infection in the compromised host*, 3rd ed. New York: Plenum Publishing Corporation.

1986; Tolkoff-Rubin & Rubin, 1997). Risk factors include pre-transplant UTIs, polycystic disease, diabetes mellitus, post-operative bladder catheterization, immunosuppression, allograft trauma, and technical complications associated with ureteral anastomosis. UTIs after renal transplantation are attributed to urinary catheters, bladder atonicity, ureteral reflux, and obstructive abnormalities. The major sites of infection include the urethra (urethritis), bladder (cystitis), ureter (ureteritis), and the renal pelvis (pyelonephritis). The clinical manifestation of a UTI can vary between patients and site of infection. In general, clinical findings include fever; tachycardia; tachypnea; chills; supra-pubic or lower back pain; burning on urination; bladder spasms; frequency; urgency; hesitancy; incontinence; nocturia; hematuria; pyuria; cloudy, foul-smelling urine; nausea; and diarrhea (more common in infants). Diagnosis is based primarily on a urinalysis and urine for culture and sensitivity. The urinalysis will show large quantities of bacteria, pus, red blood cells (RBCs), white blood cells (WBCs), casts, and an increased urinary pH. A complete blood count (CBC) with differential may reveal an elevated WBC with a shift to the left. If bacteremia is suspected, blood cultures also should be obtained. Other diagnostic tests that may be employed are a computerized tomography (CT) scan or ultrasound to assess the status of the involved kidney for renal enlargement or abscesses in the renal tissue or structural abnormalities. Treatment usually includes systemic antibiotics (e.g., trimethoprim-sul-

famethoxazole, an aminoglycoside, or cephalosporin) and antibiotic bladder irrigations (if the catheter remains in place) for 14 to 21 days (Munoz, 2001). Fluid intake should be increased to 3,000 ml/day for adults to enhance flushing of the kidney and urinary tract. Prophylactic therapy may be necessary for recurrent infections. Follow-up cultures should always be performed to assure eradication of the infection. In addition to antibiotics, patients should be given analgesic and antipyretic medications to minimize their pain and lower their temperature.

The nurse can instruct the recipient to adhere to five preventative measures to minimize the risk of an UTI. First, empty bladder every 2 to 4 hours and drink at least two liters of fluid daily. Second, take showers rather than baths (no bubble baths), wash perianal area after every bowel movement, and do not use perfume in the genital area. Third, urinate before and after sexual activity, change tampons frequently, and seek prompt treatment for vaginal discharge. Fourth, avoid tight fitting pants and the use of chlorine bleach when laundering clothes. Fifth, adhere to antibiotic regime during an infectious episode or as prophylactic therapy.

Wound infections. Wound infections can be superficial or deep; those that extend into the perinephric space may result in a transplant nephrectomy. Less severe wound infections lead to prolonged healing and an extended hospital stay. Factors that contribute to the development of wound infections include hypovolemia, lack of oxygenation to the wound; obesity; diabetes mellitus; poor preoperative nutrition; and the pre-operative shave, which can lead to microscopic skin lesions where bacteria can colonize. In addition, immunosuppressive therapy also has an effect on delayed and altered wound healing. Clinical findings characteristic of wound infections are purulent drainage, pale tissue at the wound site with erythema around the edges, edema of surrounding tissue, fever, pain, nausea, and general malaise. Diagnosis is based on clinical manifestations and culture of the exudate or purulent drainage from the wound site. Obtaining an accurate culture can be difficult. It must be deep within the wound; superficial swabbing is generally not helpful and may reflect only skin pathogens. Management of wound infections involves systemic antibiotic therapy and meticulous wound management. Some infected wounds may require surgical debridement of necrotic tissue. Less severe wounds can be treated with irrigation and packing as ordered. Irrigation may be with normal saline, an antibiotic solution, or with a shower head. The latter is most helpful in enhancing wound healing by removing necrotic debris, as well as stimulating the surrounding circulation. Analgesic and antipyretic medications can be administered to minimize pain and reduce fever.

Vascular Complications

Renal artery thrombosis (RAT). RAT is an embolus completely blocking arterial flow to the kidney. RAT is an early complication post-renal transplant that results in graft infarction and failure. RAT typically occurs in 0.2%–1% of patients. It is generally the result of damage related to procurement, preservation, or transplantation; poor alignment of the intima during the anastomosis, especially when there is a disparity in vessel size; and excessive length of the vessels, particularly in an end-end anastomosis (Diethelm et al., 1987; Salvatierra, 1987). Clinical findings include sudden anuria, which may be the first clinical manifestation of RAT, suggesting a lack of blood supply to the graft. There is often accompanying tenderness over the graft and increasing edema of the thigh and leg on the side of the transplant. An elevated serum creatinine is also observed. Diagnosis of RAT should be suspected anytime there is a sudden decrease in urine output during the early post-operative period. Although other causes of acute renal failure are more likely, a missed diagnosis of RAT generally results in graft loss. Diagnosis is made by emergent renal scan, venogram with Doppler, or arteriogram of renal vessels demonstrating no flow to the graft. Management includes emergency exploration and revision of the vascular anastomosis. If the thrombosis cannot be corrected, transplant nephrectomy is often indicated.

Renal artery stenosis (RAS). RAS is a relatively frequent complication post-kidney transplant with an incidence of 1% to 23% being reported, depending on the definition of RAS and the frequency with which angiography is performed (Fervenza, Lafayette, Alfrey, & Petersen, 1998; Rengel et al., 1998; Wong et al., 1996). It is usually the result of vessel size mismatch at the site of the anastomosis; kinking or torsion of the renal artery; or intimal damage during procurement, preservation or transplantation. RAS is

manifested by "difficult to treat" hypertension secondary to hypoperfusion of the graft and stimulation of renin production. Thus, angiotensin-converting enzymes may exacerbate the effects of RAS. Other manifestations of RAS include decreased renal function, as demonstrated by an increasing serum BUN and creatinine, and an arterial bruit over the renal allograft or femoral artery close to the inguinal ligament. Diagnosis is based on Doppler examination and renal angiography, which is always performed when RAS is suspected (Fervenza et al., 1998). Renal angiography usually demonstrates poor concentrations of the radioisotope at the site of the stenosis with post-stenotic vessel dilatation. The renal angiogram is helpful in that it can also detect the status of the peripheral arteries. In the presence of multiple stenotic lesions, chronic rejection must be considered and renal biopsy should be performed. Treatment of RAS can be managed either medically or surgically by revascularization (Buturovic-Ponikvar, 2003). Percutaneous transluminal renal angioplasty and stenting is an alternative approach, with reports of favorable long-term follow-up (Fauchald et al., 1992; Merkus et al., 1993; Thomas, Riad, Johnson, & Cumberland, 1992). There are also reports of spontaneous regression of RAS (Chan, Ng, Ho, & Lau, 1985). Ongoing Doppler follow-up is recommended to assess the status of the stenotic area.

Renal vein thrombosis (RVT). RVT is the result of an embolus, usually in the renal vein and occasionally in the iliac vein. It is usually caused by an irregular intimal surface at the anastomosis site; intimal damage during procurement, preservation, or transplantation; and kinking or mechanical occlusion of the donor vein. Incidence is approximately 0.5%–6.2%, with graft thrombosis accounting for one third of all early graft failures (Bakir, Sluiter, Ploeg, van Son, & Tegzess, 1996; Patel, 2002). Clinical findings of RVT are characterized by proteinuria, hematuria, graft enlargement, and decreasing renal function. On occasion, iliac flow will be impaired, causing engorgement ipsilaterally on the affected side. Diagnosis of RVT is by venography. When venous thrombosis is suspected, there is no outflow of the radioisotope from the graft. Management focuses on early surgical intervention with vascular resection and re-anastomosis in order to facilitate graft preservation. Additional therapy may include the administration of systemic anticoagulation as soon as RVT is suspected. Nephrectomy may be indicated if damage is severe.

Graft rupture. Graft rupture is a very rare occurrence in kidney transplant recipients. Most occur within 2 to 3 weeks of surgery. Causes of graft rupture include swelling of the graft during an acute rejection crisis, renal biopsy, ischemic damage during procurement, urinary obstruction, emboli, lymphatic occlusion, or trauma. Rupture usually starts on the convex border of the kidney along the long axis. Clinical findings of graft rupture include pain and edema over the graft, abdominal swelling and tenderness, bleeding at incisional site, oliguria with declining renal function, hematuria, hypotension, tachycardia, cool and clammy skin, and changes in mental status. Care should be taken to monitor the patient closely to prevent vascular collapse secondary to blood loss and shock pending surgical intervention. Diagnosis is based on clinical manifestations.

It can be confirmed by ultrasonography, CT scan, or surgical exploration. Management mandates immediate surgical intervention. Depending on the extent of the damage, surgical repair of the renal capsule may be attempted. However, in most circumstances a transplant nephrectomy is the only treatment option.

Urological Complications

The incidence of urologic complications following kidney transplantation varies, depending on the complication. In general, urinary leaks are estimated at 9.2% and primary ureteric obstruction is estimated at 6.5%.

Urinary extravasation. Urinary extravasation (bladder leak) or fistula can be very problematic post-kidney transplant. Ureteral fistulas are one of the most serious post-kidney transplant complications. The most common cause of urinary extravasation or fistula is damage to the donor ureter. Damage usually occurs during the donor nephrectomy and results in injury to the donor ureteral blood supply, causing ischemic necrosis of the donor ureter. Insufficient closure of the cystotomy incision during transplant and pre-existing bladder abnormalities can contribute to inadequate bladder emptying and, subsequently, result in bladder leak. Patients at particular risk are insulin-dependent diabetics and those recipients with small contracted dysfunctional bladders previously requiring multiple urologic procedures, some with urinary diversion. Clinical findings are usually present within 5 weeks of transplant. The presenting signs and symptoms of a ureteral extravasation or fistula are pain and swelling over the graft, fever, elevation in serum BUN and creatinine levels, decreasing urine output, cutaneous urinary drainage over the surgical incision site, and possibly sepsis. Diagnosis is usually made by ultrasonography, revealing a periureteral fluid collection or hydronephrosis. A renal scan may demonstrate the isotope extravasating out of the ureter. In some cases, a cystogram may be necessary for diagnosis. Post-void scintophotographs are often included with the radioisotope renal scans to rule out small bladder extravasation that may not manifest itself until there is the increased intravesical pressure of voiding. Lower ureteral leaks can be diagnosed once the isotope has been evacuated by the bladder and is retained in an extravesical location.

Management strategies to prevent bladder extravasation include meticulous bladder anastomosis by the surgeon during the transplant procedure, decompression of the bladder with a Foley catheter, and the avoidance of bladder over-distention. It is a nursing responsibility to monitor for adequate urine output and the presence of clots, which may impede urinary drainage and contribute to bladder distention. If a leak does develop, the placement of a ureteral stent may be indicated or, in some circumstances, surgical reanastamosis may be required. Surgical reconstruction is totally dependent on the status of the ureter. If there is extensive necrosis of the ureter, alternate surgical approaches are necessary.

Ureteral obstruction. Ureteral obstruction is an uncommon complication early post-transplant. It usually occurs in 2%–10% of renal transplants (Berger & Diamond, 1998) and is generally due to a tight submucosal tunnel of the ureter into the bladder or torsion or the ureter. Late ureteral obstruction is more common and is the result of ureteral ischemia secondary to inadequate blood supply to the distal ureter. Lymphocele is often an extrinsic cause of ureteral obstruction. Other causes of ureteral obstruction include blood clots, strictures, ureteral torsion or compression, stones, infection, hematoma, spermatic cord obstruction, and periureteral fibrosis. Clinical findings of ureteral obstruction often present with a decrease in urine output, declining renal function as indicated by a rise in serum BUN and creatinine, local pain, and sepsis. Accompanying abdominal tenderness or pain and urinary leakage along the suture line may also be present. Diagnosis of ureteral obstruction is determined by ultrasonography, which typically demonstrates a marked narrowing at the stenotic or obstructed area and dilation of the ureter above the stenosis. Varying degrees of hydronephrosis may also be observed. A radioisotope renal scan can also be helpful, except in patients with only a mild obstruction. In severe ureteral obstruction, the presence of a large hilar defect in the graft and absence of radioisotope in the enlarged renal pelvis is diagnostic. Rejection can be differentiated from ureteral obstruction by the accumulation and stasis of the radioisotope in the enlarged renal pelvis. Management of ureteral obstruction often requires external drainage (Patel, 2002). However, a percutaneous stent may be placed anterograde or cystoscopically. The stent is left in place for a number of weeks prior to removal. It is not uncommon that the stenosis reoccurs with stent removal. Surgical intervention is often ultimately required. In the case of distal ureter pathology, reconstruction of the ureter and ureteroneocystostomy is often performed. If this procedure is not possible, the native ureter can be anastomosed to the donor ureter or renal pelvis. If there is inadequate ureter available, the bladder can be directly anastomosed to the renal pelvis. Particular attention must be paid to the latter type of anastomosis to minimize the risk of urinary tract infections to prevent transplant pyelonephritis.

Lymphatic Complications

Lymphoceles. Lymphoceles are a consequence of inadequate ligation of the lymphatics during renal transplantation. Lymphoceles are the collection of extraperitoneal fluid in the transplant fossa secondary to a leak of lymphatic fluid during the post-operative period. They typically develop 3 to 6 months post-transplant. The incidence of lymphoceles post-kidney transplant is reported to be 0.6% –18% (Amante & Kahan, 1994; Bischof et al., 1998). Clinical findings of a lymphocele vary, depending on their location. Small lympoceles may remain asymptomatic, but large lymphoceles usually cause deterioration in renal function and hydronephrosis because of compression on the ureter (Bischof et al., 1998). In general, clinical manifestations include a rising BUN and creatinine, decreasing urine output, mild lower abdominal discomfort on the affected side, and genital and/or ipsilateral edema of the extremity on the affected side. In extreme situations, the lymphocele may compress the transplanted ureter or iliac vein, causing bladder extravasation or extreme ipsilateral edema of the extremity on the affected side. Diagnosis of a lymphocele can be confirmed by ultrasonography or CT. A lymphatic fluid collection can be easily detected on ultrasound and depending on the location there may be an accompanying dilated ureter with or without hydronephrosis. Percutaneous aspiration for analysis can be helpful in an effort to differentiate it from urinomas, abscesses, and hematoma. Lymphocele fluid is typically comprised of BUN, creatinine, and electrolytes levels similar to those of the patient's plasma (Munoz, 2001). Management of a small non-obstructive asymptomatic lymphocele may include serial observation with ultrasonagraphy and monitoring of renal function. Symptomatic lymphoceles can be treated with external puncture and percutaneous drainage with varying success (Langle et al., 1990; Martin et al., 1996). Most lymphoceles require surgical intervention. The definitive treatment for non-infected lymphoceles is surgical fluid evacuation with the internal marsupialization of the lymphocele cavity into the peritoneal cavity to allow for subsequent drainage of the fluid (Boeckmann, Brauers, Wolff, Bongartz, & Jakse, 1996; Gonzalez, Duarte Novo, Gomez viega, Chantada Abal, & Alvarez Castelo, 1999). Infected lymphoceles should be managed with external drainage and appropriate antibiotic therapy (Munoz, 2001).

Long-Term Management Issues Following Kidney Transplant

Long-term management issues following kidney transplant can be categorized as kidney allograft dysfunction, problems related to immunosuppressive therapy, cardiovascular disease (CVD), hypertension, diabetes, hyperlipidemia, infections, malignancy, metabolic defects (e.g., bone disease), delayed growth and development in infants and children, problems related to sexuality and pregnancy, and psychosocial difficulties. This section will provide a brief overview of each of these management issues, with the exception of diabetes, which is discussed in Chapter 11, and problems related to immunosuppressive therapy, which are reviewed in Chapter 32.

Allograft dysfunction. Allograft dysfunction post-kidney transplant has been reported to be caused by chronic rejection, calcineurin nephrotoxicity, recurrent disease, RAS, and recurrent UTIs. In addition, non-compliance with immunosuppressive medications has been estimated to be between 5% and 43%, with variations in demographics and clinical variables (Didlake, Dreyfus, Kerman, Van Buren, & Kahan, 1988; Dunn et al., 1990; Rodriquez, Diaz, Colon, & Santiago-Delpin, 1991; Schweizer et al., 1990). Chronic rejection usually develops months to years after transplantation. It is clinically defined as a gradual but progressive impairment of renal allograft function in the absence of other specific causes. Risk factors predicting chronic rejection in renal transplant recipients have been reported to include elevated triglycerides, elevated low-density lipoprotein (LDL) cholesterol level, donor age, type and duration of immunosuppressive therapy, the incidence of at least one episode of acute rejection, previous infection, and the sum of histological changes taken over time as observed on biopsy (Basadonna et al., 1993; Isoniemi et

Table 31-6
Commonly Observed Recurrent Diseases after Renal Transplantation

Anti-Glomerular Basement Membrane (GBM) Disease
Cystinosis
Diabetic Nephropathy
Fabry Disease
Focal and Segmental Glomerular Sclerosis
Juxtamedullary Focal Glomerulosclerosis
Henoch-Schonlein Syndrome
Hemolytic Uremic Syndrome
IgA Nephropathy
Membranous Glomerulonephritis
Membranoproliferative Glomerulonephritis Types 1 and 2
Membranous Nephropathy
Primary Oxalosis
Rapidly Progressive Glomerulonephritis
Systemic Lupus Eryhtematosus

al., 1994; Matas et al., 1994). Typical histological changes occur in the renal vasculature, and treatment generally involves manipulation of immunosuppressive therapy. Other therapeutic methods that have been attempted include plasma exchange, dietary protein restriction, and antiplatelet agents.

The initial effect of cyclosporine (CSA) on renal structure and function is afferent arteriolar vasoconstriction. The drug may also cause more permanent changes such as arteriopathy, chronic arteriolar lesions that mimic nephrosclerosis, and interstitial and tubular fibrosis (see Chapter 32). Although reducing the dose is generally effective and may be associated with lower toxicity, there is an increased risk of rejection. In general, the majority of renal transplant recipients tolerate long-term cyclosporine therapy without progressively serious nephropathy (Burke et al., 1994)

Recurrent disease depends largely on the original disease and its natural history. Disorders that are known to have a high rate of reoccurrence after kidney transplantation are outlined in Table 31-6. Chadban (2001), Hariharan (2000), and Seikaly (2004) discuss management related to specific recurrent diseases post-kidney transplant.

RAS has been reported in approximately 12.4% of long-term post-kidney transplant patients (Buturovic-Ponikvar, 2003; Wong et al., 1996). However, since the presence of RAS is generally investigated only in patients with hypertension, these figures may grossly underestimate this complication. Management of RAS may require dilation and stenting of the stenosis or surgical resection and reanastomosis.

Recurrent UTIs also can cause renal dysfunction post-transplant and should be treated promptly to minimize the risk of septicemia. Patients with frequently occurring UTIs should be evaluated for obstruction in the ureteropelvic and ureterovesical junctions. A renal ultrasound or renal scan with furosemide stimulation usually will locate the obstruction if present. If severe, it may require placement of a percutaneous nephrostomy tube.

Cardiovascular disease (CVD). CVD represents the leading cause of death in patients with long-term functioning renal transplants and accounts for approximately 40%–50% of all deaths in this patient population (Briggs, 2001; Fellstrom, 2001; Ojo et al., 2000). Since diabetes mellitus and hypertension are the most frequently reported diseases leading to ESRD, it is not surprising that there is such a high incidence of CVD in this patient population. Specifically, hypertension and diabetes are known to accelerate atherosclerotic vascular lesions and undoubtedly contribute to the increased mortality and morbidity from myocardial infarction, transient ischemic attacks, and cerebrovascular accidents (CVA). Even in patients without a prior history of CVD, the incidence is reported to be 15.8% and up to 23% in adults post-kidney transplant (Kasiske, Guijarro, Massy, Wiederkehr, & Ma, 1996). Risk factors for CVD in patients post-kidney transplant include age (older patients are at great risk 49 ± 12 years), male, family history of CVD, diabetes, hypertension, pre-existing left ventricular hypertrophy, tobacco use, hyperlipidemia, hyperhomocysteinemia, hypertryglyceridemic, previous rejection episodes, cumulative doses of corticosteroids (Cohen & Galbraith, 2001; Kasiske et al., 1996; Kasiske, 1988; Kasiske & Klinger, 2000; Li et al., 1995; McLean, Hay, Woo, Padmanabhan, & Jardine, 2000; Stewart, Jardine, & Briggs, 2000).

With the high incidence of CVD post-kidney transplant, prevention and early treatment must be aggressive. Management measures include rigorous blood pressure and lipid control, weight loss and diet control, regular exercise, smoking cessation, diabetic control, prevention of rejection, and minimize daily steroid use to alternate day therapy when feasible (Cohen & Galbraith, 2001; Kiberd, 2002).

Hypertension. Hypertension is common in solid organ transplant recipients. It is estimated that 75%–85% of adults and 65%–75% of pediatric recipients will become hypertensive post-transplant (Kasiske et al., 2000). Several factors contribute to post-transplant hypertension, including pre-existing essential hypertension, allograft dysfunction, use of some immunosuppressive medications (e.g., calcineurin inhibitors and prednisone), RAS, remaining native kidneys causing increased renin and aldosterone levels, obesity, and diet (Rosenkranz & Mayer, 2000).

Blood pressure control is critical to prevent complications related to hypertension, particularly those associated with cardiovascular and atherosclerotic disease. In addition, hypertension is an important factor that may influence long-term graft survival. Hypertension is managed with a wide variety of available medications (see Chapters 9 and 12) and counseling regarding diet, exercise, and weight control. There are specific considerations when using antihypertensive medications in post-renal transplant recipients. For example, calcium channel blockers may reduce vasoconstriction, thus minimizing nephrotoxicity often caused by calcineurin inhibitors. Also, some antihypertensive medications in combination with routine post-transplant medications may either enhance or minimize the effects of the immunosuppressive agents. For example, some calcium channel blockers such as diltiazem and Verapamil® increase blood levels of calcineruin inhibitors and can potentially lead to over immunosuppression and nephrotoxicity. Loop diuretics may be helpful, but also can contribute to nephrotoxicity when given in conjunction with a calcineurin inhibitor. Although there are concerns regarding hyperkalemia and allograft dysfunction (in the presence of RAS), angiotensin-converting enzyme (ACE) inhibitors and angiotensin II receptor blockers may be considered optimum therapy for two reasons. First, they inhibit transforming growth factor (TGF) production and protect against calcineurin-inhibitor fibrosis. Secondly, they may have a protective effect by "hyperfiltering," the kidney having a favorable influence on chronic allograft nephropathy. Other antihypertensive therapies used in this patient population include centrally acting alpha agonist, beta-blockers, and vasodilators (Wong, 2000).

It is important in patients with refractory hypertension that renal renin levels be assessed and ultrasound be performed to rule-out RAS.

Hyperlipidemia. Hyperlipidemia is a common problem post-transplant and is estimated to affect over 60% of patients (Kasiske, 1998). Hyperlipidemia is characterized by increased total cholesterol (>200), excess LDL fraction, and increased triglycerides. Contributing factors to hyperlipidemia in this patient population include immunosuppressive medications (e.g., cyclosporine, prednisone, and sirolimus), obesity (body mass index [BMI] > 30), diet, genetic causes, hyperglycemia, lack of exercise, poor renal function, and proteinuria (McCune et al., 1998; Thorp et al., 2000). Hyperlipidemia contributes to CVD and chronic allograft nephropathy with additional risk of graft loss (Kasiske et al., 2000). Management of hyperlipidemia includes immunosuppressive therapy dose adjustments, change in diet, weight reduction, and regular exercise. If these measures are unsuccessful, drug treatment should be initiated. 3-hydroxy-3-methylglutaryl coenzyme A (HMG-CoA) reductase inhibitors (HMG CoA) have been safely and successfully used in transplant recipients. It is important to note that this class of medications may have additional immunosuppressive effects and decreases the risk of chronic rejection (Palinske, 2000).

Infections. Infections are common in transplant recipients, especially during the early post-transplant period, when the immune system is the most suppressed, and during treatment for rejection (see Table 31-5). Interestingly, renal transplant recipients have been associated with the lowest rate of infection in solid organ transplants (Kubak, Pegues, & Holt, 2001). Risk factors that contribute to infection in this patient population include those with poor renal function, recurrent treatment of rejection, higher levels of immunosuppression, leukopenia or pancytopenia, and/or post-splenectomy. These factors can alter the usual signs and symptoms of infection and delay diagnosis and treatment. It is imperative that the nurse always be aware of the patient's increased susceptibility to infection and take appropriate action, such as good handwashing. Because of the inherent risk of infection, prophylaxis for *Pneumocystis carinii*, cytomegalovirus (CMV), and oral candidiasis is routinely administered from the time of transplant to 1 month post-transplant or indefinitely post-transplant, depending on the center and specific patient considerations.

Lapsed time from transplant provides a model that may assist the provider in a timely and accurate diagnosis and, thus, more successful treatment (Rubin, 1994) (see Table 31-5). In general, most infections that develop post-transplant occur during three distinct time periods, the first month post-transplant, 1 to 6 months post-transplant, and later than 6 months post-transplant (Fishman & Rubin, 1998). Infections that occur during the first month include wound infections, UTIs, and pneumonia. UTIs are the most common infection in the transplant recipient, with an incidence of more than 30% in the first 3 months (Tolkoff-Rubin & Rubin, 1997). Prophylactic antibiotic therapy and close monitoring should be considered in patients with recurrent UTIs.

Infections are less common 1 to 6 months post-transplant. If an infection develops during this time frame, it is most likely an opportunistic infection such as CMV, *Cryptococcus*, and *Pneumocystis carinii* pneumonia. If one of these infections is present, there is an additional risk for other opportunistic infections to develop as well. It is also important to note that CMV infection can evolve in patients on prophylactic therapy. Six months post-transplant, infection and treatment of infection is much the same as the general population. However, in patients receiving large doses of immunosuppressive therapy, who have had recurrent episodes of rejection, or who are experiencing allograft dysfunction, the risk of an opportunistic infection is much higher.

Patients with chronic hepatitis B or C have an increased risk of morbidity and mortality related to liver disease post-transplant and should be monitored closely for cirrhosis, hepatocellular carcinoma, viral replication, and liver histology. Reduction in immunosuppressive therapy should be considered, if feasible. Antiviral therapy should be considered pre- and post-transplant, particularly with the advancement in newer treatment options (Van Thiel, Nadir, & Shah, 2002). Additional viral infections that regularly affect post-transplant recipients include herpes simplex type 1 and 2, *papillomavirus*, and, more recently, polyoma virus (Kazory & Ducloux, 2003; Yoshikawa, 2003).

Infections occurring more than 1 year post-transplant are expected to be similar to the general population and should be managed accordingly. Kidney transplant recipients on long-term immunosuppressive therapy should receive prophylaxis against infection. This is particularly true when undergoing dental procedures, surgery, or instrumentation of the gastrointestinal tract. In addition, daily prophylactic administration of penicillin (or erythromycin in penicillin sensitive patients) is recommended for splenectomized recipients. Prevention is central to the development of infection post-transplant. Any persistent fever or ongoing symptom, such as a cough, mandates evaluation. If possible, avoidance of unnecessarily high doses of immunosuppressive agents can assist in minimizing infectious episodes (see Chapter 31).

Mudge, Carlson, and Brennan (1998); Rubin (1994); and Silkensen (2000) are additional sources for a compre-

hensive review of infection post-transplant.

Malignancies. Malignancies remain a serious problem post-kidney transplant and following CVD and infection (Cohen & Galbraith, 2001; Lutz & Heemann, 2003). Basal-cell carcinoma of the skin and lips are the most common (Kasiske et al., 2000). Kaposi's sarcoma, carcinoma of the vulva and perineum, non-Hodgkin's lymphoma, squamous-cell carcinoma, hepatobiliary carcinoma, and carcinoma of the uterine cervix also have a higher incidence in transplant recipients than the general population (Penn, 2000).

Although typically not fatal, skin cancers are the most common malignancies after kidney transplantation (Dreno, 2003). Among the skin cancers, cutaneous pre-malignant and malignant epithelial lesions (carcinoma) are the most frequently observed in organ transplant recipients (Dreno, 2003; Ramsay, Fryer, Reece, Smith, & Harden, 2000). The incidence of skin cancer is reported to range between 10%–40% at 10 and 20 years post-transplant, with the incidence in Australians as high as 45%–70%, respectively (Goodman, Goldin, & Kuizon, 2000; Hartevelt, Bavinck, Kootte, Vermeer, & Vandenbroucke, 1990; Ramsay et al., 2000). The frequency of skin cancer in this population may be related to more intense sun exposure, skin type, and length of time after transplantation (Tessari, Barba, & Chieregato, 1999). High-dose immunosuppression, particularly multiple treatments with antilymphocyte preparations, augments the risk of malignancies, especially lymphoma (Kasiske, 2001; Suthanthiran & Strom, 1994). Immunosuppressive medications are also associated with a permissive effect on viral-related malignancies, particularly Epstein Barr Virus (EBV), that can subsequently lead to post-transplant lymphoproliferative disease (PTLD) and lymphoma particularly in children (Newstead, 2000).

Management of post-transplant malignancies varies and almost always includes a reduction in immunosuppressive therapy. Skin cancers are often easily detected and excised. Thus, all transplant patients should be routinely screened and referred to a dermatologist for any suspicious lesions (Reece, Harden, Smith, & Ramsay, 2002). The most significant factor in minimizing the risk of skin cancer is protection from sun exposure. Patients should be counseled to avoid excessive sun exposure, use sunscreen with SPF of 15 or higher, and wear protective clothing and hats (Wu & Orengo, 2001). Children, in particular, should be monitored for EBV and treated accordingly with an antiviral agent (e.g., ganciclovir) when they convert to being positive. Routine screening for breast, cervical, prostate, and colorectal cancers is the same as for the general population. In addition to conventional treatment of malignancies, reduction or cessation of immunosuppressive therapy is generally indicated.

Bone disorders. Bone disorders and alteration in mineral metabolism following renal transplantation are also common. These problems include hyperparathyroidism, osteomalacia, adynamic bone disease, and osteoporosis (Cueto-Manzano et al., 1999). Bone disorders are often the result of pre-transplant renal insufficiency (see Chapter 12) and immunosuppressive therapy (see Chapter 32). Osteoporosis can be observed in 60% of patients within 18 months of transplant (Kasiske et al., 2000). The causes of osteoporosis include corticosteriods, calcineurin inhibitors, hypogonadism, hyperparathyroidism, cigarette smoking, and poor calcium dietary intake (Kasiske et al., 2000; Lippuner, Casez, Horber, & Jaeger, 1998). Bone fractures are estimated at 5.7% in renal transplant recipients (Pichette et al., 1996). Monitoring of bone and mineral metabolism should include measurement of bone density, thyroid function tests, serum calcium, Vitamin D, parathyroid hormone, and testosterone levels. Treatment for osteoporosis and low bone mass starts early after transplant and should include calcium 1000–1500 mg/day, vitamin D 400–800 IU/day, weight bearing exercise, and avoidance of alcohol and tobacco. Biphosphates to prevent bone loss, hormone replacement therapy for women, and testosterone therapy for men have been suggested in specific patient populations (Cohen & Galbraith, 2001; Pichette et al., 1996). Patients with normal bone density should be monitored annually with DEXA scans.

Growth and development. Growth and development are often impaired in children at the time of transplant. Growth failure is usually due to chronic illness and organ failure secondary to nutritional, metabolic, and endocrine factors (Benfield, 2003). Theses changes are particularly significant in children with ESRD due to metabolic osteodystrophy and the coexistence of osteoporosis, hyperparathyroidism, osteomalacia, and ineffective utilization of growth hormone. In general, successful kidney transplantation corrects these changes and provides the child with an opportunity for normal growth and development, particularly with the use of subcutaneous growth hormone. Although growth and development post-kidney transplant is superior to dialysis, normal growth patterns are not always attained. Short stature and delay in the development of secondary sex characteristics can be difficult or even devastating for some children and teenagers. The use of growth hormone to maximize growth potential, as well as psychosocial support and education regarding strategies in managing altered body image, can facilitate coping and social adjustment, and minimize the risk of noncompliance.

Sexuality and pregnancy. Sexuality and pregnancy are concerns of most post-kidney transplant recipients. In general, fertility and reproductive function of both men and women return following transplantation. The possibility of conception emphasizes the need for counseling regarding contraception. Barrier methods of contraception are recommended for birth control and the prevention of sexually transmitted diseases.

There have been well over 7,000 pregnancies in renal transplant recipients (Armenti, Moritz, & Davison, 1998, 2003). However, pregnancies in transplant recipients are generally considered high risk and patients should be referred to an experienced high-risk obstetrician. In general, approximately 20% of babies born to renal transplant recipients are considered below normal gestational weight. Potential complications include pre-eclampsia, premature delivery, and decreased spontaneous delivery (Kasiske et al., 2000; Pesavento & Falkenhain, 1998). Pregnancy is usually discouraged the first 1 to 3 years post-transplant in order to ensure renal function and promote the outcome of a viable fetus. Because of the risks of potential graft loss, suggested guidelines for post-transplant pregnancy include average stable serum creatinine of < 2 mg/dL, normal blood pressure, maintenance of immunosuppressive therapy with close monitoring, adjustment of other medications as indicated, and waiting 1 to 3 years post-transplant (Cohen & Galbraith, 2001).

Psychosocial problems. Psychosocial problems following kidney transplantation range from anxiety and depression to exuberance and the feeling of having a new lease on life. These feeling may be the result of immunosuppressive therapy, alteration in family functioning, or reluctance to re-enter the work force. Individuals experience transplant differently, and their specific concerns must be taken into consideration to assist them in the transition.

Non-adherence is a major problem post-transplant, particularly among teenagers (Edwards, 1999). Non-compliance is the third leading cause of graft loss, and it is estimated that 20% of adult recipients will become non-compliant (De Geest et al., 1995; Gaston, Hudson, Ward, Jones, & Macon 1999). In general, risk factors for noncompliance include increased numbers of medications and medication side effects, depression, locus of control given over to others more powerful, unemployment, younger age, low socioeconomic status, and perceived amount of social and family support (Bunzel & Laederach-Hofmann, 2000; Kiley, Lam, & Pollak, 1993; Schweizer et al., 1990; Sketris, Waite, Grobler, West, & Gerus, 1994). It is the responsibility of nursing to work collaboratively with the transplant team and the patient and family to develop strategies to secure adherence to post-transplant routines and medications.

Pancreas Transplantation

Pancreas transplantation is a viable therapeutic option for insulin-dependent diabetes. The engraftment of a functioning endocrine pancreas into the insulin-dependent patient provides the optimal physiologic means of correcting altered metabolism. The goal of pancreas transplant is two-fold: to provide an insulin-independent lifestyle and to reverse the secondary complications associated with diabetes.

It has been very well established through the reporting of the Diabetes Control and Complications Trial Research Group (DCCT) in 1998 and 2000, respectively, that risks for long-term complications from Type I diabetes can be significantly minimized with the maintenance of normoglycemia. In concert with these reports, the successful development of less diabetogenic immunosuppressive agents, and the resurgence of interest in the previously stagnant islet cell transplantation field, the number of treatment options for the Type I diabetic patient abounds. What has yet to be determined are the short- and long-term outcomes of these various treatment modalities and, hence, the actual impact on the quality of life for the Type I diabetic patient.

Over the past decade, pursuing pancreas transplantation as a cure for diabetes has increased dramatically. The success rate (success defined as normoglycemia and insulin independence) is currently 80% at 3 years (Gruessner et al., 2001; Gruessner & Sutherland, 2002).

Figure 31-3
Islet Cell Infusion

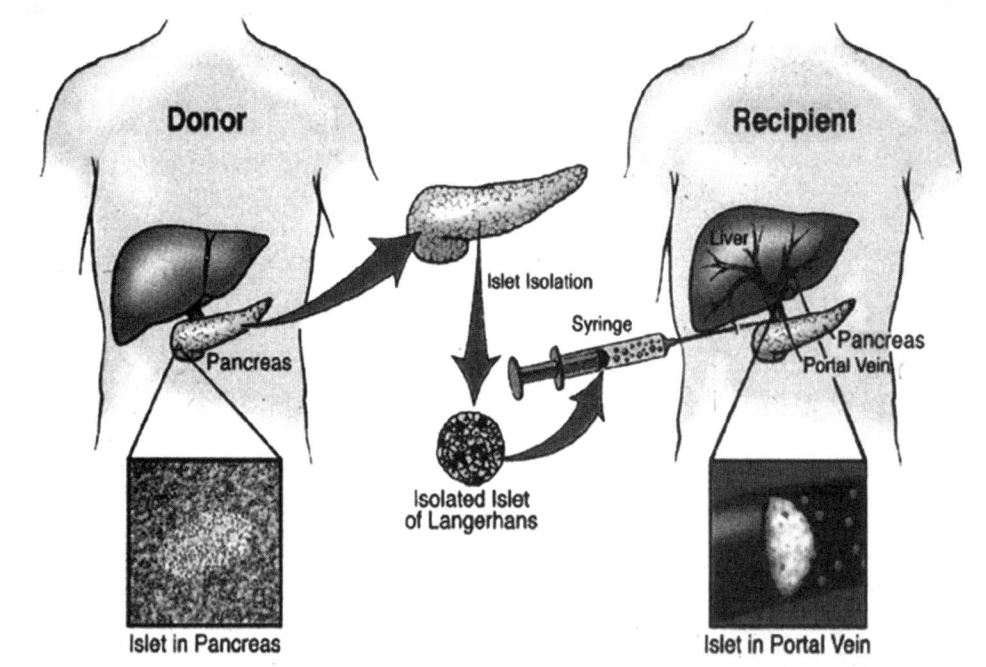

The 3-year graft survival for simultaneous kidney-pancreas transplant recipients is also estimated at 80%, as well as, for pancreas transplants performed after successful kidney transplant (Stock & Bluestone, 2004). It appears as though secondary complications of diabetes, such as diabetic nephropathy, are also halted (Fioretto, Steffes, Sutherland, Goetz, & Mauer, 1998). In addition, there are reported improvements in diabetic neuropathy and overall quality of life (Gross, Limwattananon, & Matthees, 1998; Navarro, Sutherland, & Kennedy, 1997).

With these promising results, researchers have been encouraged to pursue with great fervor the islet transplantation option for non-uremic diabetic patients (DeMayo, Elick, & Schanbacher, 1990). With the evolution of improved immunosuppressive therapy and the growing knowledge regarding appropriate islet cell mass, the prospect is that this less invasive procedure will prove to be a successful treatment modality for the diabetic patient.

Types of Pancreas Transplantation

Pancreas transplantation has taken several forms since its inception in the form of an animal model 35 years ago. There are three basic approaches to pancreatic transplantation: single or solitary pancreas transplant, islet cell transplantation, and combined kidney-pancreas transplant.

Solitary pancreas transplant. Solitary pancreas transplant or the transplantation of the pancreas alone had been attempted with limited success in the 1970s and early 1980s. Originally this procedure was considered to have significant immunologic risk due to the high incidence of rejection and graft loss. Due to the development of less diabetogenic immunosuppressive agents, solitary

pancreas transplant, following successful kidney transplantation, now enjoys the same 80% success rate at 3 years that has been demonstrated for the simultaneous kidney-pancreas transplant recipient. In addition to being an indication for the successful diabetic kidney transplant recipient to help maintain euglycemia, solitary pancreas transplant is becoming a more acceptable treatment modality for the pre-uremic Type I diabetic who suffers from significant problems with hypoglycemia or inability to control glucose levels resulting in life-threatening episodes requiring intervention. Despite the immunosuppressive advances that have made solitary pancreas a more successful treatment modality for this patient population, a very limited number of patients would qualify for such an extensive surgical procedure and involved immunosuppressive post-surgical protocol. As we begin to overcome the immunosuppressive barriers to solitary pancreas transplant with more effective and less toxic therapies, solitary pancreas transplant is still a treatment modality for only the most clinically robust patients. The re-emergence of the islet transplant procedure as a treatment modality for the unstable pre-uremic patient suffering from hypoglycemic unawareness and/or significant problems with hyperglycemia offers renewed hope to this select patient population.

Islet cell transplantation. Islet cell transplantation has been performed for over 25 years. However, until the breakthrough in 1999 at the University of Alberta, no one had consistently shown clinical states of insulin independence. The two significant changes this group brought to the field were the intraportal infusion (see Figure 31-3) of freshly isolated islets equaling 8,000-9,000 islet equivalents per kilogram and the use of effective immunosuppressive agents that are not toxic to the pancreatic islets (Stock & Bluestone, 2004). Islet cell transplantation involves the meticulous retrieval of cells from a deceased source. Retrieval and processing of islet cells remain a cumbersome and labor-intensive task. Once retrieved, the islets are injected into the recipient liver. The two main problems with islet cell transplantation remain the difficulty in islet cell isolation and the long-term viability of these cells (Sutherland et al., 1996; Zekorn et al., 1996). Islet cell transplant may become the procedure of choice if these two issues can be resolved. The advantages of avoiding a major surgical procedure would most certainly be desired. At the time of this publication, this particular type of beta cell replacement continues to be found in the context of a research study protocol. Current areas of research that continue to be explored in addition to islet cell transplantation are the use of islet cells from other animal models and islet cells from human fetal tissue (Dordevic et al., 1995; Farkas, Szasz, Lazar, Jr., Csanadi, & Lazar, 2002).

Combined kidney-pancreas transplantation. Combined kidney-pancreas transplantation is the simultaneous transplantation of a kidney and a pancreas from the same donor into a known Type 1 diabetic who also has renal failure. This procedure addresses the increasing number of diabetic patients who present with chronic renal failure.

Controversy still exists regarding whole versus segmental pancreas transplantation. Whole pancreas transplantation is the transplantation of the entire pancreas with or without a duodenal stump. Segmental pancreas transplantation usually involves the transplantation of only the body and tail of the pancreas. At this time it appears to remain physician preference as to which approach is taken.

The clinical future of pancreas transplantation is not completely clear. The trend toward islet cell transplantation continues to be pursued but will remain a possibility for only a select group of patients. With the increasing scarcity of deceased donors, living-related segmental pancreas transplantation may become a more viable option. However, the present procedure of choice is the combined cadaveric pancreas-kidney transplant for the Type I diabetic patient in renal failure and the solitary pancreas transplant for the pre-uremic Type I diabetic patient.

Pancreas Transplant Surgical Procedure

Pancreas transplant donors. Pancreas transplant donors are often simultaneous deceased kidney donors. Specifically, pancreatic donors are generally less than 50 years old without sepsis or pancreatic trauma. The donor's history must not include cancer, diabetes, chronic hypertension, or chronic alcoholism or IV drug abuse. Laboratory values are evaluated and the donor must have negative hepatitis and HIV serologies (Perkins et al., 1990). Alternatively, it appears as though the most optimal islet transplant donor is one with a higher BMI and increased donor age (Lakey et al., 1996). The point being that despite the scarcity of deceased donor organs, there appears to be very different selection criteria for donors required for solid organ transplant versus organs procured for islet iso-

Table 31-7
Pancreas Donor Selection For Islets and Pancreas

Whole Pancreas	Islets
HLA matching preferred	No HLA match
Donor age <45	Donor age > 15, <65
Absence of obesity	BMI >25%
Cold Ischemia <30 hrs	Cold Ischemia < 12 hrs

lation (see Table 31-7).

Regardless of the ultimate tissue usage, the entire pancreas is excised during the procurement. A button of the duodenum (the patch technique) or the intact duodenum (pancreaticoduodenal graft) is also recovered. Vascular components later used for anastomoses to the recipient include the portal vein and a Carrel patch of the aorta encompassing the celiac axis and superior mesenteric artery. Following procurement, the organ is flushed intra-arterially and preserved by cold storage using a variety of solutions.

Recipient surgery. Recipient surgery consists of one of three types of pancreas transplants: (a) islet cell transplants, (b) segmental or whole organ pancreatic transplants, and (c) simultaneous pancreas-kidney transplants. For purposes of this discussion, we will address combined pancreas-kidney transplant, whole pancreatic solitary pancreas transplant, and islet transplant infusion.

Combined pancreas-kidney transplant. In the combined pancreas-kidney transplant procedure, the pancreas is placed first intraperitoneally into the right iliac fossa. The arterial supply of the donor is anastomosed to the common iliac artery of the recipient. The venous drainage of the donor is anastomosed to the common iliac vein. Surgical anastomosis of the kidney follows and it is generally placed in the left iliac fossa.

Enzymal secretion and management of pancreatic transplantation has proved to be a technical challenge. Three types of exocrine drainage have been developed: ductal occlusion, enteric drainage, and urinary drainage. Ductal occlusion is performed by injecting a substance into the pancreatic duct, which hardens and occludes the duct (see Figure 31-4). Enteric drainage is accomplished by anastomosing the graft to a Roux-en-Y loop of the jejunum of the recipient (see Figure 31-5). Urinary diversion is accomplished by anastomosing the pancreas to the recipient's bladder by using a segment of the donor duodenum (see Figure 31-6).

There are advantages and potential complications to all three types of enteric drainage. The urinary drainage method has been the most common approach to enteric drainage. The advantage of this method is the ability to assess graft exocrine function by measuring urinary amylase levels. These levels have been shown to be early predictors of pancreas rejection (Sollinger et al., 1991). The drainage method is center and surgeon specific, often dependent on whether the pancreas transplant is performed concomitantly with a kidney transplant.

Figure 31-4
Injection of the Pancreatic Duct

Injection of the pancreatic duct to cause total duct occlusion and to suppress exocrine secretions.

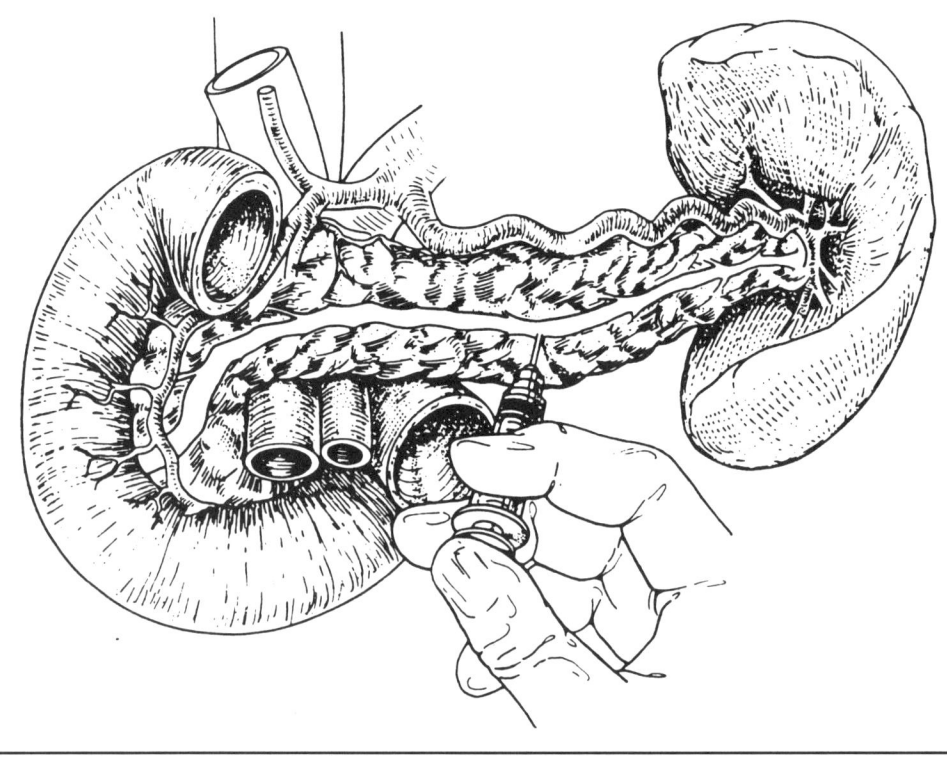

Note: From Groshek, M., & Smith, V. (1991). Pancreas transplantation. In M.K. Gaedeke Norris & M.A. House (Eds.), *Organ and tissue transplantation: Nursing care from procurement through rehabilitation.* Philadelphia: F.A. Davis, Figure 8.1, p. 157. Used with permission.

Solitary pancreas transplant. The solitary pancreas transplant procedure is accomplished using the above described anastomosing of the pancreas graft to the recipient's bladder by using a segment of the donor duodenum. Since there is no other marker to measure organ function with the solitary pancreas transplant patient, the urinary amylase levels described above function as surveillance markers for pancreatic function.

Islet transplant. The islet transplant procedure has been successful when performed via intraportal access through either a percutaneous transhepatic cannulation or via cannulation via direct exposure using a mini-laporatomy (Ryan et al., 2002; Shapiro, Ryan, & Lakey, 2001). Although other sites have been studied in the animal population, thus far the intraportal system has been the only one to manifest clinical success. The most significant complication post-infusion has been post-procedure bleeding requiring transfusions. Of other significance have been portal pressure elevations during the islet transplant infusion itself. This was a more common occurrence when non-purified islets were being used for transplant, most common during auto-islet transplantation. With the onset of purified islet transplant preparation, this complication is now much less common.

Pancreas Transplant Post-Operative Management and Nursing Care

Postoperative care of the pancreas-kidney transplant recipient is very similar to the care of the patient who receives only a kidney transplant (Trusler, 1991). The major considerations specific to pancreas transplantation are during the initial post-operative period.

The goal of the immediate post-operative period is to maintain hemodynamic stability and to prevent complications. If complications occur, early identification to allow for rapid treatment is optimal.

Institutional protocols will determine the place in which the recipient will recover from surgery. Most centers recover post-pancreas-kidney transplant recipients in the recovery room or the intensive care unit. Early extubation during recovery is routine, although supplemental oxygen may be required for a variable time following surgery. Invasive lines include: a central venous catheter, one or more peripheral lines, an indwelling urinary catheter, and several surgical drains.

The previous discussion of the post-kidney transplant recipient also applies to the post-pancreas-kidney transplant recipient. Post-operative management issues specific to the pancreas-kidney transplant patient include metabolic acidosis, urinary tract maintenance, pancreatitis, vascular patency, hemorrhage, rejection, and infection.

Figure 31-5

Pancreatico Enterostomy for Enteric Drainage of Pancreatic Exocrine Secretions

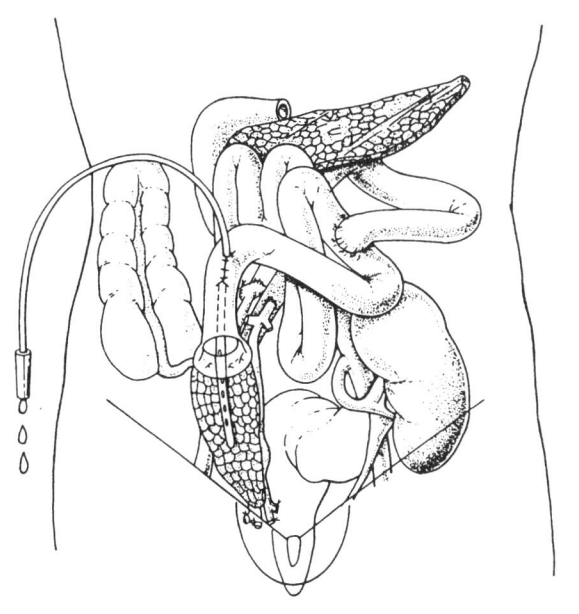

Note: From Groshek, G., & Smith, V. (1991). Pancreas transplantation. In M.K. Gaedeke Norris & M.A. House (Eds.), *Organ and tissue transplantation: Nursing care from procurement through rehabilitation.* Philadelphia: F.A. Davis, Figure 8.2, p. 158. Used with permission.

Metabolic acidosis. Metabolic acidosis is a frequent occurrence in the pancreas transplant patient whose exocrine drainage is done via urinary diversion. The cause is the loss of pancreatic electrolytes in the urine. In particular there is a significant loss of bicarbonate from the pancreas into the urine causing a systemic acidosis. If renal function becomes compromised there is an obligatory chloride retention augmenting the already present acidotic state. IV supplemental sodium bicarbonate may be required for a short period. In addition, it is not unusual that recipients will require oral supplementation of sodium bicarbonate later in their post-operative course (Willis & Post, 1990).

Nutritional status. Nutritional status may be an issue of concern for the pancreas transplant recipient. For the patient with significant problems with gastroparesis pretransplant, parenteral nutrition may be employed post-transplant; however, this is also a center-specific care issue. Generally, when normoglycemia is reached, problems with gastroparesis resolve. Each patient must be individually assessed to determine specific nutritional needs. In the case of the islet transplant recipient, many programs employ a low carbohydrate diet for the first several weeks to months following transplant in order to rest the newly infused islets. In addition, some centers continue with insulin infusions for a number of weeks post islet transplant to rest the newly infused islets.

Figure 31-6

Pancreaticoduodenocystomy for Urinary Drainage of Pancreatic Exocrine Secretions

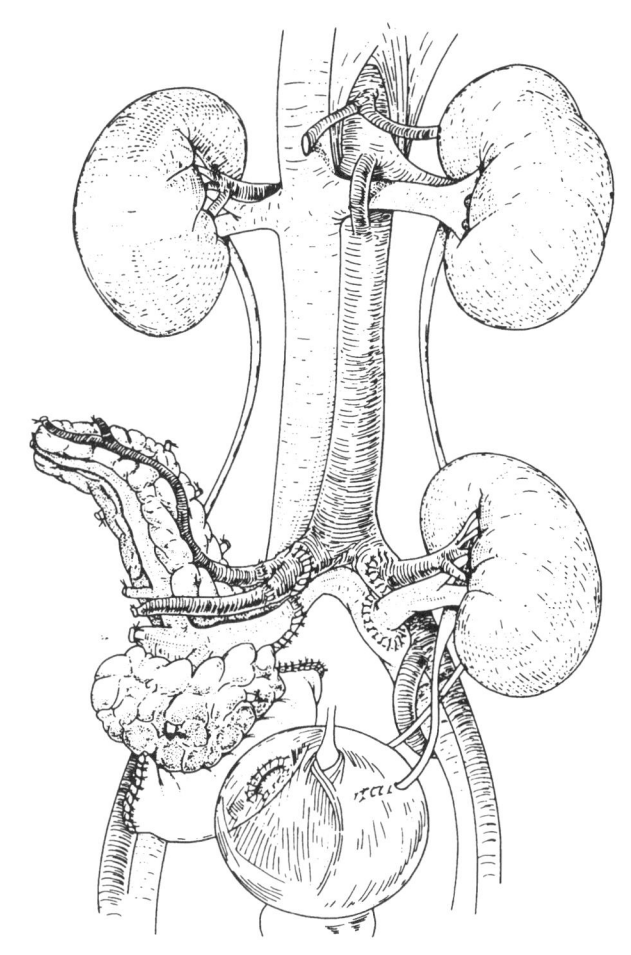

Note: From Groshek, M., & Smith, V. (1991). Pancreas transplantation. In M.K. Gaedeke Norris & M.A. House (Eds.), *Organ and tissue transplantation: Nursing care from procurement through rehabilitation.* Philadelphia: F.A. Davis, Figure 8.3, p. 159. Used with permission.

Urinary tract maintenance. Urinary tract maintenance is of the utmost importance during both the early and late post-operative periods. An indwelling Foley catheter is utilized to decompress and drain the bladder. Decompression of the bladder will promote healing of the suture line and bladder, and minimize the risk of anastomotic leaks. A urinary leak is diagnosed by a cystogram and may require long-term management with a Foley catheter or surgical repair.

Urinary reflux through the duodenal stump to the pancreas graft could also result from an inadequate drainage system. Clinically, urinary reflux produces a rise in serum amylase indicating pancreatitis.

Prompt irrigation of the Foley catheter is indicated with any decrease in urine output or suspicion of obstruction. Inability to re-establish an adequate drainage system by irrigating mandates that the Foley catheter be replaced immediately following consultation with the surgeon.

Graft pancreatitis. Graft pancreatitis is demonstrated by hyperamylasemia early or late during the post-operative period. Contributing factors include an inadequately drained urinary tract, damage to the pancreas during organ recovery, rejection, or trauma. Prompt identification of pancreatitis is crucial. Treatment includes administration of IV fluids, anticoagulation therapy to prevent thrombosis, and not allowing the patient to have anything by mouth (Willis & Post, 1990).

Vascular thrombosis. Vascular thrombosis continues to be of significant concern in the early post-operative period. Potential causes of thrombosis are mechanical obstruction, trauma to the pancreas during procurement, pancreatitis, thrombogenic effects of immunosuppressants, or microthrombi from the pancreas itself (Soon-Shiang, White, DeMayo, Koyle, & Danovitch, 1988). Graft thrombosis is manifested by hematuria, a sharp decrease in urine amylase with a simultaneous increase in serum glucose. Severe low abdominal pain is often reported by the patient. In addition, nuclear scans demonstrate lack of blood flow to the pancreas. Treatment is generally a total graft pancreatectomy (DeMayo et al., 1990). Careful monitoring of urinary amylase, serum glucose levels, and anticoagulation factors are all interventions utilized to monitor and prevent graft thrombosis. It has also been proposed that the avoidance of hypovolemia may assist in preventing vascular thrombosis post pancreas-kidney transplantation.

Hemorrhage. Hemorrhage post-operatively is associated with any type of surgery and must be monitored and assessed for frequently. Mild hematuria is common in the early post-operative period following pancreas-kidney transplantation. It is particularly common when the surgical approach for exocrine drainage is the urinary diversion. Persistent gross hematuria usually indicates an anastomotic leak at the duodenocystostomy site, ulcerations of the bladder, or duodenal cuff. Bladder irrigation is usually the initial intervention for hematuria. If the patient is receiving anticoagulation therapy it may need to be temporarily discontinued. Treatment of gross hematuria generally requires either surgical correction of the leak or medical/surgical treatment of the ulcerated duodenum (Willis & Post, 1990).

Rejection. Rejection is more difficult to diagnose in pancreas transplantation than other solid organ transplant and, thus, is a major cause of graft loss (Grundfest-Broniatowski, 1990). Pancreatic transplant rejection is also difficult to differentiate between other types of graft failure, such as vascular thrombosis, recurrent disease, and pancreatitis (Sollinger, Stratta, Kalayoglu, & Belzer, 1987). Clinical signs of rejection such as fever, ileus, and graft tenderness are often unreliable. A specific example is the elevation in transplant recipients' serum glucose levels, which may be a vague indicator of rejection. Unfortunately, serum glucose levels often remain normal until almost 90% of insulin-producing cells are destroyed. Another unreliable indicator is the elevation in serum amylase levels. The causes of high serum amylase levels vary and include preservation injury of the graft, pancreatitis, infection, and rejection.

Before the bladder drainage technique was instituted, it was difficult to monitor pancreas transplant rejection. As the use of the bladder drainage technique for exocrine drainage became more universally applied, graft survival rates improved. Graft survival improved because of the ability to identify and treat pancreas transplant rejection early based on urinary amylase levels. The bladder drainage technique allows for frequent monitoring of urinary amylase levels as an indicator of pancreas graft rejection. Immediately post-transplant a baseline urinary amylase level is obtained followed by close monitoring. The diagnosis of rejection can be made if there is a 25%–50% decrease in urine amylase from baseline (DeMayo et al., 1990). Other reliable predictors of pancreas graft rejection are a decrease in urinary bicarbonate and pH (Corry, 1987; Prieto, Sutherland, Fernandez-Cruz, Heil, Najarian, 1987).

Other methods that have been used to detect rejection post-pancreas transplantation include serum C-peptide levels, radionuclide imaging, open wedge or needle biopsy, and aspiration cytology (Grundfest-Broniatowski, 1990). A reversible increase in pancreatic graft size has been observed on CT scans during kidney transplant rejection (confirmed by biopsy) in combined pancreas-kidney transplants (Schaapherder et al., 1993). Biopsy of the transplanted pancreas can be performed through cystoscopy. Histological features that have demonstrated a high correlation with rejection include moderate to severe inflammation of the acinar tissue, acinar tissue loss and fibrosis, and vascular luminal narrowing (Nakhleh & Sutherland, 1992). Classification of pancreatic rejection has been suggested. Mild rejection would include endothelitis, and vasculitis would indicate severe rejection (Nakhleh & Sutherland, 1992). Cytologic features of acute rejection have been reported to include hypercellularity with lymphocyoturia, increased numbers of epithelial cells, and a positive staining for HLA-DR antigen.

A combined pancreas-kidney transplant from the same donor can be beneficial in terms of diagnosing rejection. In this situation the serum creatinine can be used as a reliable marker for detecting rejection and promptly instituting treatment (Sollinger et al., 1988). In combined pancreas-kidney transplantation, rejection is usually found in the kidney allograft first (Largiader, Baumgartner, Kolb, & Uhlschmid, 1983). Kidney rejection can occur independent of pancreas rejection; however, it is rare that the pancreas would reject independently. Early detection of kidney transplant rejection often precludes pancreas rejection. Generally, anti-rejection therapy is instituted immediately, thereby protecting the pancreas from an overwhelming rejection episode.

Infection. Infection, as with any other organ transplant patient, is a significant cause of morbidity in the pancreas transplant recipient. Astute nursing assessment for signs and symptoms of infection are crucial (see Table 31-5).

Long-Term Management of the Pancreas and Islet Transplant Recipient

Long-term management issues following solitary pancreas, simultaneous pancreas kidney, and islet transplantation are very similar to those previously outlined for the kidney transplant recipient. With the exception of those management issues related to high dose steroids, there are few differences. Long-term management issues can be cat-egorized as allograft dysfunction problems, problems with immunotherapy, hypertension, hyperlipidemia, infections, malignancy, problems related to sexuality and pregnancy, and psychosocial issues. Solitary pancreas, simultaneous kidney pancreas, and islet transplant patients are main-tained on similar immunotherapy post-transplant and, therefore, are susceptible to all the same risks associated with these drug regimes.

Graft loss involving pancreatic islet cells is ill under-stood at present. Many research studies are currently underway to assess the long-term outcomes of islet trans-plantation. Despite encouraging early successes both in Edmonton and elsewhere within the past several years, determining how long islets will be viable continues to be a challenge. Most patients require reinfusion of islets up to three times, increasing a patient's cumulative immunother-apy dose. This certainly adds further risk to the patient, specifically for malignancy and infection. Although it appears unlikely that islet patients will be rendered insulin independent with a single islet infusion and the need for some exogenous insulin may be required for a significant number of recipients, better glucose control with decreas-ing hypoglycemis episodes requiring intervention post-transplant seems to be the norm in this group. Hence, qual-ity of life may be improved with better control without complete insulin independence.

In addition to islet cell viability and longevity, the organ supply issue remains a significant problem for islet transplantation. This issue, although not unique to islet transplantation, is certainly more acute given the need for multiple donors in order for a patient to meet an outcome of improved glucose control or, optimally, insulin inde-pendence.

Liver Transplantation

Liver Transplant Surgical Procedure

Organs for liver transplantation come from two sources: living or deceased donors. There are a number of surgical approaches for the recipient undergoing liver transplantation, including reduced sized-grafts, split liver graft, living related left or right lobe liver transplant, auxil-iary liver transplant, and combined organ transplant (liver-kidney transplant).

Liver transplant donor. Liver transplant donor surgery, in general, is a very straightforward procedure. Donor liv-ers are matched to potential recipients based on blood type and body size. Although it is preferred that the donor and recipient be the same blood type, in cases of urgent need, ABO-incompatible donors have been used (Roberts, Forsmark, Lake, & Ascher, 1989). Donor and recipient weights within 20% of one another are generally consid-ered a likely match (Rosenthal, Podesta, Sher, & Makowka, 1994). If the donor liver is too large, it can result in pul-monary compromise, and if it is too small, there may be hepatic insufficiency or a mismatch in vessel size, which can lead to stenosis or thrombosis. However, with the advancement of surgical techniques in liver transplanta-

tion, this is not as much a limiting factor as in the past. With the advent of the paired or reduced-size graft, the surgeon is increasingly able to accommodate for variations in donor size. Generally, for hepatic donor procurement and to ensure stability of the donor's physiological condition, avoid prolonged warm ischemic time and rapidly remove the organs in the sequence agreed upon by the other trans-plant teams involved.

Surgical removal of the donor liver is performed through a mid-line incision. The major vessels around the liver are dissected, including the celiac trunk and branch-es, portal vein, and the inferior vena cava. The common bile duct is transected, with an attempt to maintain maxi-mum length of the duct for the recipient transplant opera-tion. Cool saline is flushed into the biliary tree via the gall bladder to remove stagnant bile and protect the biliary mucosa. The liver is then flushed in situ with cool heparinized lactated Ringer's to remove old blood, and then with University of Wisconsin (UW) solution for preser-vation. The suprahepatic cava is transected at the right atri-um and the infrahepatic cava just above the renal veins, preserving them for possible kidney transplantation. The portal vein is divided at the confluence of the splenic vein and superior mesenteric vein, and the abdominal aorta and hepatic artery excised to preserve the hepatic arterial sup-ply. The liver is packed in UW solution, stored on ice, and transported to the transplant center (Stock & Payne, 1990).

Recipient hepatectomy and transplant. Recipient hepatectomy and transplant are performed after the place-ment of multiple invasive lines. The recipient hepatectomy involves clamping the infrahepatic and suprahepatic inferi-or vena cava and dividing the portal vein. Venous return from the inferior vena cava is, thus, momentarily interrupt-ed, and the out-flow from the infrahepatic inferior vena cava and portal vein occluded. Decreased venous blood flow can lead to engorgement of all subdiaphragmatic ves-sels, causing an increase in portal hypertension and bowel congestion. Therefore, it is important to keep the time-frame of the anahepatic phase to a minimum (optimally less than 30 minutes). Some centers utilize a venovenous bypass system to minimize the risks during the anahepatic phase (Griffith et al., 1985). Other centers do not use it because of the risk of air embolism (Khoury, Mann, Porot, Abdul-Rasool, & Busuttil,, 1987).

Once the recipient's hepatectomy has been completed and homeostasis achieved, the donor liver anastomoses is initiated. There are five major anastomoses that are gener-ally completed in the following order: suprahepatic inferi-or vena cave, infraheptatic inferior vena cava, portal vein, hepatic artery, and biliary anastomosis. After the portal vein anastomosis is completed, the liver is reperfused. The liver is rewarmed and the hyperkalemic preservation solution vented through the anterior infrahepatic caval anastomosis. Stagnant splanchnic blood also is flushed. The reperfusion phase has been associated with electrolyte imbalances and coagulopathies (Stock & Payne, 1990).

There are two basic approaches to biliary reconstruc-tion, a choledochocholedochostomy or choledochoje-junostomy. A choledochocholedochostomy is an end-to-end anastomosis of the common bile ducts of the recipient and donor and is used whenever possible (see Figure 31-7). In the presence of biliary disease or a biliary duct-to-duct mismatch, a choledochojejunostomy is performed. This is an anastomosis of the donor bile duct to the recipient's jejunum, also referred to as a Roux-en-Y (see Figure 31-8).

Reduced sized-grafts. Reduced sized-grafts evolved to expand the donor pool primarily for pediatric patients (see Figure 31-9). This surgical technique was developed in response to the lack of available donors for infants and young children less than 2 years of age and has had good results. In reduced sized-grafts, the right posterior and anterior segments are resected, and the whole left liver with the vena cava is used (Emond, Whitington, & Broelsch, 1991; de Ville de Goyet et al., 1993).

Split liver transplantation. Split liver transplantation is a technique whereby the deceased donor liver is split between two recipients. The segmentation of liver anatomy allows the surgeon to perform this procedure, which has significant anatomical constraints and is substantially more complex than a reduced size graft. It requires two surgical teams and the allocation of structures is often not equal. Outcomes of split liver transplantation have been shown to be equivalent to whole organ transplants (Deshpande et al., 2002; McDiarmid, 2003).

Living-related liver transplantation (LRLTx). LRLTx evolved from the techniques applied during the reduced-size graft procedure. The impetus for developing LRLTx was the increasing number of children who were dying while on the waiting list (Broelsch et al., 1988). LRLTx is typically the donation of either the left lateral segment (segments 2 and 3) or the right lobe by a living-related donor (Belghiti & Kianmanesh, 2003; Broelsch et al., 1991). With increasing experience, LRLTx has become an accepted approach to liver transplantation for children (McDiarmid & Anand, 2002; Emond, 1993). Adult LRLTx has gained significant popularity over the last 5 years because the waiting list for deceased donors has grown at an exponential rate (Renz & Busuttil, 2000). The risk for donor mortality after right lobe donation is estimated to be 0.5%, and the risk for complications approximately 10%–20% (Humar, 2003). Patient and graft survival rates are slightly lower when compared to deceased donor transplants, which may be caused by the increased incidence of surgical complications. Biliary leaks are the main surgical complications for both donor and recipient (Broelsch et al., 2003; Humar, 2003). Although biliary complications may be more frequently observed in living donor transplants when compared to whole organ transplants, these usually do not impact on pediatric patient or graft survival (Egawa et al., 2001). Overall living-liver donors do exceptionally well post-donation, with 88% returning to pre-donation activities at 6 months and 100% at 1 year (Renz & Roberts, 2000).

Auxiliary liver transplantation. Auxiliary liver transplantation is a surgical procedure in which the liver graft is implanted without removing the native liver. It was originally introduced in 1972 to avoid the morbidity and mortality in total hepatectomy patients (Emond, 1993; Starzl et al., 1989a, b). Although this approach is rarely used, it may have a place in the future, particularly for those individuals with metabolic disorders.

Combined liver-kidney transplantation (LKTx). LKTx has been performed in patients with end stage hepato-renal disease and hepatorenal syndrome (Davis, Gonwa, & Wilkinson, 2002a). Outcomes for combined LKTx are influenced by the primary disease, severity of illness at the time of transplant, and location of the center performing the transplant. Liver transplantation has been reported to protect the kidney from rejection. Although early LKTx renal graft rejection rates are less than 10%, long -term protection of the kidney by the liver has not been established (Benedetti et al., 1996; Katznelson & Cecka, 1996; Lang et al., 2001; Larue et al., 1997). The surgical procedure is the same for single organ transplantation. In a combined transplant, the liver transplant surgery is performed before the kidney transplant. Post-operative management is the same for individual LKTx.

Liver Transplant Post-Operative Complications

The post-operative care and monitoring for complications of the liver transplant recipients is highly complex and requires a multidisciplinary approach and collaboration among team members (McGilvray & Greig, 2002). Liver transplant recipients are at risk for the same complications as any individual undergoing major abdominal surgery and organ transplantation. They also are at risk for the multiple side effects of immunosuppressive therapy and rejection and are at additional risk for infection (see Chapter 32). The complications of liver transplantation are briefly outlined.

Primary non-function (PNF). PNF is graft failure. It is clinically manifested by hepatic cytolysis, coagulopathy, altered synthetic function (e.g., decreased albumin and total protein, increasing prothrombin time and INR), lack of bile flow, high lactate levels, hyperkalemia, hypoglycemia, need for ventilatory support, hemodynamic instability, and often acute renal failure. In the presence of PNF, there is an initial elevation in serum transaminases, followed by a dramatic decrease and coinciding prolonged coagulation studies. These findings suggest hepatocyte death. Retransplantation is necessary for patient survival (Pokorny et al., 2000).

Hepatic allograft rejection. Hepatic allograft rejection has been classified by histological features, timing, response to therapy, and reversibility. The correlation between the histological severity of rejection and the degree of biochemical hepatic dysfunction has been poor. Therefore, liver biopsy and histology remain the "gold standard" for diagnosing alteration in hepatic graft function (Wiesner, Ludwig, van Hoek, & Krom, 1992). In addition, hepatic histology may enable rejection to be differentiated from viral hepatitis, bile duct obstruction, and other causes of hepatic dysfunction. The major targets of hepatic allograft rejection are the epithelial cells of the bile ducts and the endothelium of the hepatic arteries and veins. The hepatocytes appear to be less vulnerable.

Acute rejection post-liver transplant is generally a cell-mediated process that usually develops within 3 weeks to 3 months post-operatively (Goddard & Adams, 2002: McDiarmid & Anand, 2002). Clinical manifestations of acute cellular rejection may include fever, malaise, and/or fatigue. Laboratory manifestations include an elevation in

Figure 31-7
Choledochocholedochostomy

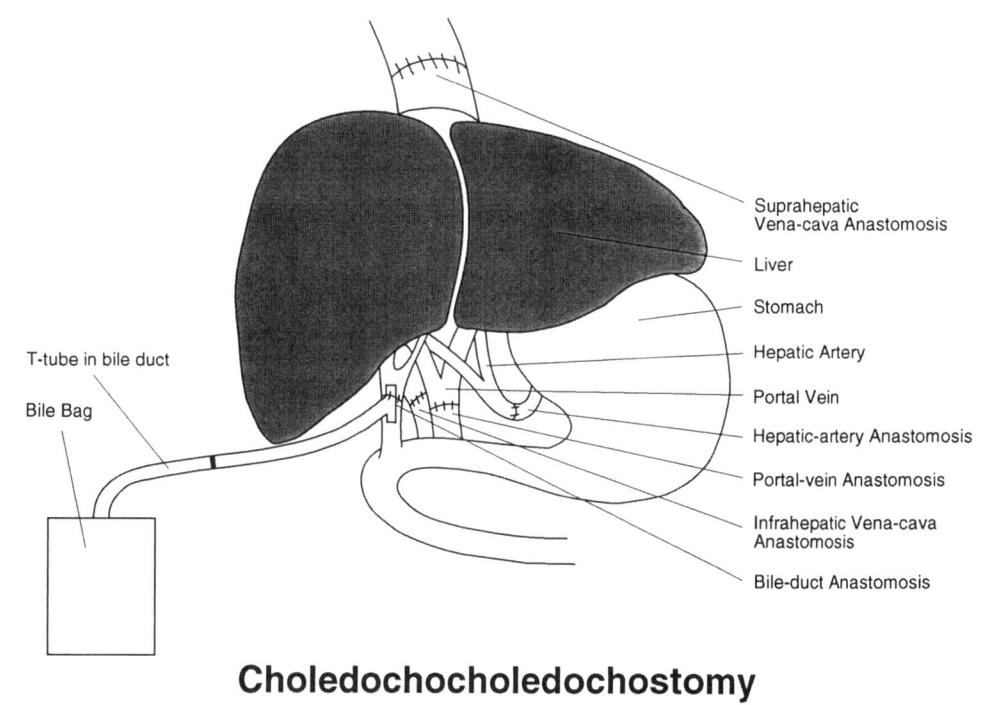

Suprahepatic
Vena-cava Anastomosis

Liver

Stomach

Hepatic Artery

Portal Vein

Hepatic-artery Anastomosis

Portal-vein Anastomosis

Infrahepatic Vena-cava
Anastomosis

Bile-duct Anastomosis

T-tube in bile duct

Bile Bag

Choledochocholedochostomy

Duct-to-Duct Biliary Anastomosis

Figure 31-8
Cholecochojejunostomy

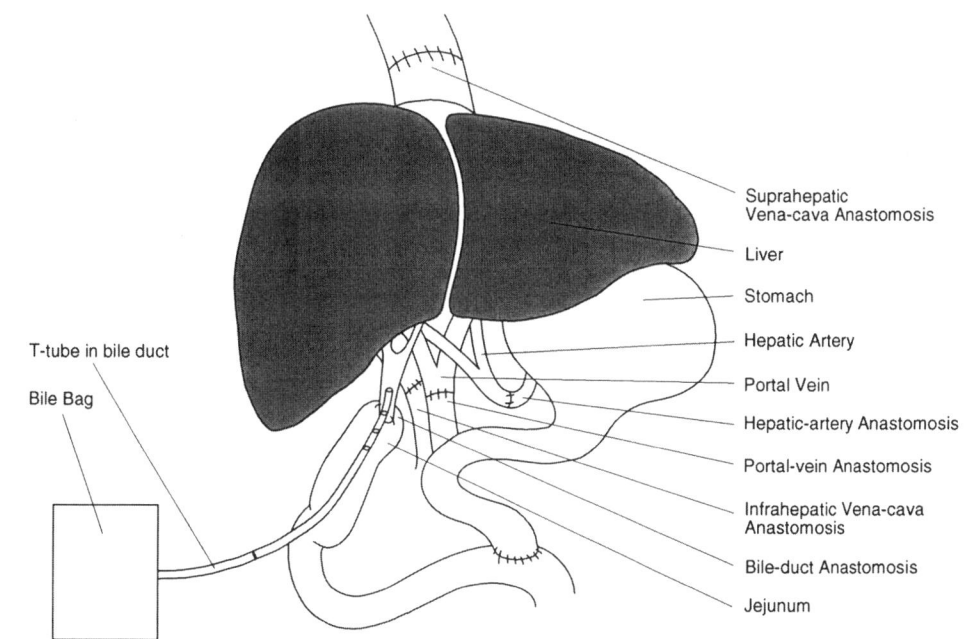

Suprahepatic
Vena-cava Anastomosis

Liver

Stomach

Hepatic Artery

Portal Vein

Hepatic-artery Anastomosis

Portal-vein Anastomosis

Infrahepatic Vena-cava
Anastomosis

Bile-duct Anastomosis

Jejunum

T-tube in bile duct

Bile Bag

Choledochojejunostomy (Roux "en" Y)

Figure 31-9
Surgical Anatomy for Reduced-Sized Liver Grafts

Review of the surgical anatomy that is the basis for reduced-sized grafts including living-related liver transplantation. A. total liver donor, with segments 2 and 3 being isolated for grafting. B. graft with interposition grafts used to extend the vessels. C. anastomosed liver graft with a Roux en Y jejunal limb.

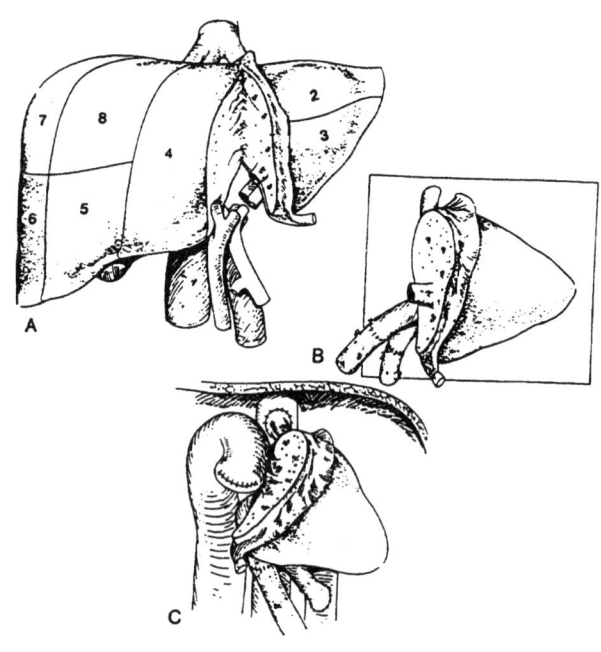

Note: Reprinted with permission from Emond, J. (1993). Clinical application of living-related liver transplantation. In J. Lake (Ed.), Advances in liver transplantation. *Gastroenterology Clinics of North America, 22*(2),

Table 31-8
Liver Laboratory Tests

Laboratory Tests	Normal Adult Values
AST/SGOT	7-39 U/L
ALT/SGPT	2-54 U/L
GGT	male 9-85 U/L female 6-58 U/L
Alkaline Phosphatase	41-133 U/L
Total Bilirubin	0.1-1.2 mg/dL
Direct Bilirubin	0.1 to 0.3 mg/dL
Indirect Bilirubin	0.2 to 0.8 mg/dL

hepatic transaminases (AST, ALT, GGT), alkaline phosphatase, and, in some situations, total bilirubin. Histological findings of acute hepatic rejection are portal or periportal inflammation, bile duct damage, and venous endothelitis (Snover, 1990). Rejection is treated differently

based on histolological findings, patient response to therapy, transplant center, and provider.

Chronic rejection post-liver transplantation is primarily a cell-mediated response that occurs in approximately 8% of patients. It is often diagnosed 6 weeks or more, post-liver transplant (Wiesner, Porayko, Lake, Batts, & Krom, 1993). It is defined as obliterative endarteritis with ischemic damage that may be accompanied by fibrosis, cirrhosis, and paucity of bile ducts ("vanishing bile duct syndrome") with cholestasis (Snover, 1990; Wiesner et al., 1992). Vanishing bile duct syndrome (VBDS) is characterized by loss of bile ducts in the absence of vascular rejection. Tacrolimus (Prograf®) has been used as rescue therapy for patients with chronic rejection and VBDS with a relatively favorable response (European FK506 Multicentre Liver Study Group, 1994; McDiarmid, Klintmalm, & Busuttil, 1993; Roberts et al., 1993). Chronic rejection seems to be increasingly unusual, which some investigators attribute to the increased use of tacrolimus in pediatric liver transplant recipients (Jain et al., 2001). Those patients who fail to respond to medical therapy typically require retransplantation.

Acute rejection typically develops early post-transplant and chronic rejection later. However, features of chronic rejection can develop early and acute rejection present late. Therefore, the differentiation between chronic and acute rejection is based primarily on histological findings.

Bleeding. Bleeding may develop the first few days postoperatively. Primary causes of early post-liver transplant bleeding include persistent coagulopathy, secondary to pre-existing splenomegaly with pancytopenia, poor hepatic function, or graft failure; collapse of one of the vascular anastomosis; or stress ulcers. Coagulopathies may be managed with a continuous infusion of fresh frozen plasma, platelet administration, and/or cryoprecipitated plasma. Recipients with poor graft function may require urgent retransplantation. Post-transplant bleeding may require re-exploration for possible hemorrhage and is generally performed in patients who present with normal coagulation parameters and compromised renal or pulmonary function (Stock & Payne, 1990).

Vascular complications. Vascular complications following liver transplantation typically include hepatic artery thrombosis (HAT), hepatic artery stenosis, portal vein thrombosis, and portal vein stenosis. HAT is the most common vascular complication post-transplant, with most cases occurring within the first 3 months. Predisposition for HAT includes anatomic problems, hypercoagulable state, rejection, prolonged ischemic time, and transplant for sclerosing cholangitis (Turka, 2001). It is typically diagnosed on Doppler ultrasound. If HAT develops early after transplantation, it generally presents with acute hepatic infarct manifested by a severe coagulopathy, hemodynamic instability, encephalopathy, hypoglycemia, hyperkalemia, renal impairment, and subsequent liver failure. HAT may also contribute to severe biliary complications (Bhattacharjya et al., 2001; Gunsar et al., 2003). Treatment of HAT is by surgical revascularization or retransplant (Denys et al., 2004). Retransplantation to prevent imminent death may be required in as many as 75% of patients (Turka, 2001).

Table 31-9
Manifestations of Liver Failure

Manifestation by System	Physiological Causes for the Manifestation
Constitutional fatigue, malaise, fever, anorexia, weight loss	progressive hepatic insufficiency, liver failure
Hepatic varies depending of disease (small retracted liver, enlarged cirrhotic liver (e.g., alcoholic cirrhosis)	fibrotic scaring
Cardiovascular portal hypertension dysrhythmias peripheral edema mild hypotension › left ventricular function	distorted hepatic architecture electrolyte imbalances altered hemodynamics hyperdynamic state
Dermatologic spider angiomata "stigmata" of cirrhosis palmar erythema jaundice xanthomas pruritus	unable to detoxify estrogens reduction in bilirubin excretion increased serum cholesterol increased serum bilirubin
Gastrointestinal abdominal discomfort/pain enlarged abdomen bleeding/hemorrhage fetor hepaticus nausea/vomiting/diarrhea	hepatic swelling, portal hypertension ascites; low albumin varices uncleared sulfur compounds decreased fat absorption
Hematological hypoalbuminemia, hypoprothrombinemia anemia leukopenia thrombocytopenia, ecchymoses	impaired protein synthesis decreased RBCs, hypersplenism hypersplenism impaired synthesis of clotting factors
Endocrine hypo/hyperglycemia gynecomastia, testicular atrophy, decreased libido	increased glucocorticoids, decreased glycogen increased estrogens; diuretic therapy
Neurological behavioral changes, reversed sleep/wake pattern, confusion, coma asterixis	hepatic encephalopathy
Pulmonary Dyspnea	elevated diaphragm secondary to ascites
Renal alteration in sodium/water balance hepatorenal syndrome	portal hypertension/ascites hepatic failure, cause unclear

Hepatic artery stenosis is less common and usually presents at the anastomotic site and can lead to hepatic ischemia and/or infarction. Proposed treatment involves surgical reanastomosis or percutaneous balloon dilatation (Abad et al., 1989; Denys et al., 2004).

Portal vein thrombosis is estimated to occur in 1.8% of cases post-liver transplant (Lerut et al., 1987). Contributing risk factors for portal vein thrombosis include pre-existing recannulized portal vein thrombosis, previous portacaval shunt, and an interposition vascular graft in the formation of portal vein anastomosis. Recipients of reduced size liver transplant grafts are at additional risk for portal vein complications (Hamady, Rela, & Sidhu,, 2002). Clinical presen-

tation is insidious and may include increasing ascites or portal hypertension with variceal bleeding. Diagnosis is based on hepatic ultrasonography or angiography (Friedewald, Molmenti, DeJong, & Hamper, 2003). If the diagnosis is made promptly, early surgical evacuation of the clot and reanastamosis with post-operative anticoagulation therapy may be successful. Treatment options have also included a combination of chemical thrombolysis and stent placement, and may require decompression of the splanchnic system through a splenorenal shunt or retransplantation (Bhattacharjya, Olliff, Bhattacharjya, Mirza, & McMaster, 2000).

Portal vein stenosis usually results from either a mis-

Table 31-10

Clinical Indications and Contraindications for Liver Transplantation

Clinical Indications	Contraindications

severe weakness and fatigue
intractable ascites
variceal hemorrhage
encephalopathy
intractable pruritus
recurrent cholangitis
spontaneous bacterial peritonitis
metabolic bone disease with fracture
intractable coagulopathy (PT > 5 seconds)
serum albumin < 2.5 g/dL
cholestasis, serum bilirubin > 10 mg/dL
hepatorenal syndrome
neurotoxicity
manifestation of certain metabolic disorders (e.g. glycogen storage disease)
	Absolute contradictions
	    AIDS with opportunistic infection
	    extrahepatic malignancy
	    inability to comply to immunosuppressive regime
	    active substance abuse
	    advanced cardiac or pulmonary disease
	    active infection
	    sepsis
	    documented anatomic anomalies precluding transplantation
	
	Relative contraindications
	    HIV seropositivity
	    acute renal failure
	    advanced malnutrition
	    primary hepatobiliary malignancy
	    portal vein thrombosis
	    previous side-to-side or end to side porta-caval shunt
	    chronic hepatitis B virus infection (HBsAg+)
	    chronic hepatitis C virus infection
	    psychosocial issues
	    lack of funding

Table 31-11

Disease Indications for Liver Transplantation

Indications	Contraindications
Cholestatic disorders Primary biliary cirrhosis Secondary biliary cirrhosis Primary sclerosing cholangitis Biliary atresia (extra & intra hepatic) Familial cholestatic syndromes Alagille's syndrome Bylers syndrome	**Fulminant hepatic failure** Viral hepatitis (A,B, C, B/delta) Drug induced (e.g. Acetaminophen) Toxins (e.g. amanita mushroom) Metabolic (e.g. Wilson's disease, Reye's syndrome, organic acidurias)
Hepatocellular disorders Chronic viral induced liver disease (hepatitis B, B/delta, C) Chronic drug induced liver disease Alcoholic liver disease Idiopathic autoimmune liver disease Cryptogenic cirrhosis Caroli's disease Angiosarcoma	**Metabolic liver disease** Alpha-1 antitrypsin deficiency Amyloidosis Wilson's disease Crigler-Najjar syndrome Erythropoietic protoporphyria Urea cycle deficiencies Glycogen storage disease Tyrosinemia Hemochromatosis Hereditary oxalosis Familial hypercholesterolemia Tyrosinemia Galactosemia
Hepatobiliary malignancy Hepatocellular carcinoma Hepatoblastoma	**Miscellaneous** TPN-induced cirrhosis Cystic fibrosis Congenital hepatic fibrosis
Vascular disease Budd-Chiari syndrome Veno-occlusive disease Hepatic vein occlusion	

match in the size of the donor-recipient's portal vein or a problem with the surgical technique. Balloon venoplasty with stent placement has been used to manage portal vein stenosis for over 15 years (Raby, Karani, Thomas, O'Grady, & Williams, 1991).

Pulmonary complications. Pulmonary complications seen frequently in the early post-operative liver transplant recipient include atelectasis and right pleural effusion. These problems result in poor ventilation and oxygenation, increasing the risk of pneumonia. Pulmonary complications are attributed to prolonged anesthesia, paralysis of the right diaphragm, ascites, a graft larger than the native liver pressing against the diaphragm, and pain. In addition, metabolic alkalosis and ascites can also interfere with proper ventilation and should be corrected. Vigorous pulmonary toilet, pain management, and early mobilization assist in reversing the effects of a pleural effusion and atelectasis, thus preventing pneumonia.

Renal insufficiency. Renal insufficiency is observed both pre-and post-transplant in patients undergoing liver transplantation. Pre-transplant disorders involving both the liver and kidney are extensive and impact on post-transplant patient and graft survival (Davis, Gonwa, & Wilkinson, 2002b). Post-transplant renal insufficiency in the presence of previously normal renal function may be due to massive hemorrhage and hypotension, hypovolemia, infection, calcineurin inhibitors, antibiotic therapy, or graft failure. Resuscitation with fluid, calculating appropriate antibiotic doses, and reducing intra-abdominal pressure through paracentesis can increase renal perfusion and preserve renal function.

Biliary complications. Biliary complications occur in 5%–15% of deceased liver transplant recipients. The incidence increases to 25% in recipients of reduced-size grafts. With the advent of right lobe living-related liver donors, the number of recipient biliary complications has also increased (Testa, Malago, Valentin-Gamazo, Lindell, & Broelsch, 2000). Biliary complications include bile leaks, strictures, and obstruction secondary to stones or biliary sludging caused by the shedding of the epithelial lining of the donor bile duct (Moser & Wall, 2001). Biliary leaks usually occur at the anastomosis within the first 3 weeks post-transplant. Bile leaks are often accompanied by peritoneal signs, acute abdominal pain, and fever. Since the hepatic artery delivers blood to the biliary system, it is important that HAT be ruled out as a potential cause of bile leaks. Doppler ultrasound of the hepatic artery or hepatic angiography can be used to determine hepatic artery patency (Friedewald et al., 2003). Management of biliary leaks includes antibiotic therapy, biloma drainage, and biliary drainage, which can often be performed in interventional radiology (Johnston, Gates, Reddy, Nickl, & Ranjan, 2000). In some cases, surgical intervention and revision of the biliary anastomosis may be necessary.

Biliary strictures can involve both the intrahepatic and extrahepatic biliary tree. Strictures are usually treated with balloon dilatation and stenting, either through endoscopy or a transhepatic approach (Denys et al., 2004; Friedewald et al., 2003). Although this is generally a successful treatment, it is not uncommon that these patients subsequently require retransplantation, particularly in situations where there are strictures secondary to HAT or biliary necrosis.

Recurrent disease. Recurrent disease is a major problem for patients with viral hepatitis or hepatic malignancies. In addition, patients with autoimmune hepatitis, primary biliary cirrhosis, and primary sclerosing cholangitis also have been observed to develop recurrent disease but rarely have significant clinical problems (Graziadei, 2002; Hubscher, 2001; Rosen, 2000).

The incidence of recurrent disease in patients with untreated hepatitis B pre-transplant is approximately 85%–95%. Individuals at highest risk are those who are hepatitis E antigen positive or demonstrate high serum levels of hepatitis B virus DNA, which is an indicator of high level viral replication (Davies et al., 1991; O'Grady et al., 1992). The use of combination prophylactic therapy employing hepatitis B immune globulin (HBIG) and lamivudine has been shown to reduce the overall rate of recurrent hepatitis B to 0%-10% (Lok, 2002). However, use of lamivudine prior to transplant has been associated with an increased risk for recurrent hepatitis B post-liver transplant due to drug resistance. Optimal dose and duration of therapy of HBIG in combination with lamivudine is not completely clear. Attention must be given to a cost-effective prophylactic regimen post transplant to prevent recurrent hepatitis B.

Hepatitis C (HCV) is the leading indication for liver transplant in adults and accounts for approximately 20%–30% of cases (McCaughan & Zekry, 2000). Recurrence after transplant is a major problem (Berenguer, 2002). The development of cirrhosis has been reported in 10% of patients with HCV at 5 years post-liver transplant (Feray et al., 1999). The 5-year survival rate for patients with HCV with cirrhosis has been reported to be 70% (Boker et al., 1997; Feray et al., 1999). Factors associated with a poorer prognosis include high pre-transplant viral load, co-existent hepatocellular carcinoma, older, non-White, high Child Pugh score at the time of transplant, genotype 1, and early/frequent rejection episodes (Charlton et al., 1998; McCaughan & Zekry, 2000). In addition, cumulative exposure to corticosteroids has been shown to be associated with increased mortality, higher levels of HCV viremia, and more severe histological recurrence. The development of steroid resistant rejection increases the risk of mortality in patients with HCV by greater than five fold. Before total bilirubin exceeds 3 mg/dl, pegylated interferon often in conjunction with ribavarin should be considered in recipients with histological recurrent HCV.

Conclusion

Transplantation is the treatment of choice for many people with end stage organ failure. It currently offers people with end stage organ failure the opportunity for a longer life of higher quality. The major challenges facing the future of transplantation are graft rejection and the shortage of donor organs. With continuing research on new immunosuppressive medications, fewer side effects are possible, as are even higher graft and patient survival rates.

References

Abad, J., Hidalgo, E.G., Cantarero, J.M., Parga, G., Fernandez, R., Gomez, M., et al. (1989). Hepatic artery anastomotic stenosis after transplantation: Treatment with percutaneous transluminal angioplasty. *Radiology, 171*, 661-662.

Amante, A.J., & Kahan, B.D. (1994). Technical complications of renal transplantation. *Surgery Clinics of North America, 74*, 1117-1131.

Armenti, V.T., Moritz, M.J., & Davison, J.M. (1998). Drug safety issues in pregnancy following transplantation and immunosuppression: Effects and outcomes. *Drug Safety, 19*, 219-232.

Armenti, V.T., Moritz, M.J., & Davison, J.M. (2003). Pregnancy in female pediatric solid organ transplant recipients. *Pediatric Clinics of North America, 50*, 1543-1560.

Anderson, R.U. (1986). Urinary tract infections in compromised hosts. *Urology Clinics of North America, 13*, 727-734.

Bakir, N., Sluiter, W.J., Ploeg, R.J., van Son, W.J., & Tegzess, A.M. (1996). Primary renal graft thrombosis. *Nephrology, Dialysis, Transplantation, 11*, 140-147.

Basadonna, J.P., Matas, A.J., Gillingham, K.J., Payne, W.D., Dunn, D.L., Sutherland, D.E.R., et al. (1993). Early versus acute renal allograft rejection impact on chronic rejection. *Transplantation, 55*, 993-995.

Beckman, N.J., Schell, H.M., Calixto, P.R., & Sullivan, M. (1992). Kidney transplantation: A therapy option. *AACN Clinical Issues in Critical Care Nursing, 3*, 370-384.

Belghiti, J., & Kianmanesh, R. (2003). Surgical techniques used in adult living donor liver transplantation. *Liver Transplantation, 9*(10 Suppl. 2), S29-S34.

Benedetti, E., Pirenne, J., Troppmann, C., Hakim, N., Moon, C., Gruessner, R.W., et al. (1996). Combined liver and kidney transplantation. *Transplant International, 9*, 486-491.

Benfield, M.R. (2003). Current status of kidney transplant: Update 2003. *Pediatric Clinics of North America, 50*, 1301-1334.

Berenguer, M. (2002). Natural history of recurrent hepatitis C. *Liver Transplantation, 8*(10 Suppl. 1), S14-S18.

Berger, P.M., & Diamond J.R. (1998). Ureteral obstruction as complication of renal transplant: A review. *Journal of Nephrology, 11*, 20-23.

Bhattacharjya, S., Gunson, B.K., Mirza, D.F., Mayer, D.A., Buckels, J.A., McMaster, P., et al. (2001). Delayed hepatic artery thrombosis in adult orthotopic liver transplantation: A 12-year experience. *Transplantation, 71*, 1592-1596.

Bhattacharjya, T., Olliff, S.P., Bhattacharjya, S., Mirza, D.F., & McMaster, P. (2000). Percutaneous portal vein thrombolysis and endovascular stent for management of posttransplant portal venous conduit thrombosis. *Transplantation, 69*, 2195-2198.

Bischof, G., Rockenschaub, S., Berlakovich, G., Langle, F., Muhlbacher, F., Fugger, R., et al. (1998). Management of lymphoceles after kidney transplantation. *Transplant International, 11*, 277-280.

Boeckmann, W., Brauers, A., Wolff, J.M., Bongartz, D., & Jakse, G. (1996). Laparoscopical marsupialization of symptomatic posttransplant lymphoceles. *Scandinavian Journal of Urology and Nephrology, 30*, 277-279.

Bohmig, G. & Regele, H. (2003). Diagnosis and treatment of antibody-mediated kidney allograft rejection. *Transplant International, 16*, 773-787.

Boker, K.H., Dalley, G., Bahr, M.J., Maschek, H., Tillmann, H.L., Trautwein, C., et al. (1997). Long-term outcome of hepatitis C virus infection after liver transplantation. *Hepatology, 25*, 203-210.

Bradley, B.A. (2002). Rejection and recipient age. *Transplant Immunology, 10*(2-3), 125-132.

Braun, W.E. (2003). Renal transplantation: Basic concepts and evolution of therapy. *Journal of Clinical Apheresis, 18*, 141-152.

Braun, W.E., & Yadlapalliet, N.G. (2002). The spectrum of long-term renal transplantation: Outcome, complications, and clinical studies. *Transplantation Review, 16*, 22-50.

Bresnahan, B.A., Cherikh, W.S. Cheng, Y., et al. (2003, May). *Short-term benefit of tacrolimus versus cyclosporine therapy after renal transplantation: An analysis of UNOS/OPTN database* [Abstract 1213]. Proceedings of the 2003 American Transplantation Congress, Washington, DC.

Briggs, J.D. (2001). Causes of death after renal transplantation. *Nephrology, Dialysis, Transplantation, 16*, 1545-1549.

Broelsch, C.E., Emond, J.C., Thistlethwaite, J.R., Whitington, P.F., Zucker, A.R., Baker, A.L., et al. (1988). Liver transplantation, including the concept of reduced-size liver transplants in children. *Annals of Surgery, 208*, 410-420.

Broelsch, C.E., Frilling, A., Testa, G., Cicinnati, V., Nadalin, S., Paul, A., et al. (2003). Early and late complications in the recipient of an adult living donor liver. *Liver Transplantation, 9*(10 Suppl. 2), S50-S53.

Broelsch, C.E., Whitington, P.F., Emond, J.C., Heffron, T.G., Thistlethwaite, J.R., Stevens, L., et al. (1991). Living transplantation of children from living related donors. *Annals of Surgery, 214*, 428-439.

Bunzel, B., & Laederach-Hofmann, K. (2000). Solid organ transplantation: Are there predictors for posttransplant non-compliance? A literature overview. *Transplantation, 70*, 711-716.

Burke, J.F., Jr., Pirsch, J.D., Ramos, E.L., Salomon, D.R., Stablein, D.M., Van Buren, D.H., et al. (1994). Long-term efficacy and safety of cyclosporine in renal-transplant recipients. *New England Journal of Medicine, 331*, 358-363.

Buturovic-Ponikvar, J. (2003). Renal transplant artery stenosis. *Nephrology, Dialysis, Transplantation, 18*(Suppl. 5), v74-v77.

Cadeddu, J.A., Ratner, L., & Kavoussi, L.R. (2000). Laparoscopic donor nephrectomy. *Seminars in Laparoscopic Surgery, 7*, 195-199.

Cecka, J.M. (2000). The UNOS scientific renal transplant registry—2000. *Clinical Transplants*, 1-18.

Chadban, S. (2001). Glomerulonephritis recurrence in the renal graft. *Journal of the American Society of Nephrology, 12*, 394-402.

Chan, Y.T., Ng, W.D., Ho, C.P., & Lau, W.C. (1985). Reversible stenosis of the renal artery following renal transplantation. *British Journal of Surgery, 72*, 454-455.

Charlton, M.R., Brandhagen, D., Wiesner, R.H., Gross, J.B., Jr., Detmer, J., Collins, M., et al. (1998). Hepatitis C virus infection in patients transplanted for cryptogenic cirrhosis: Red flag or red herring? *Transplantation, 65*, 73-76.

Cohen, D., & Galbraith, C. (2001). General health management and long-term care of the renal transplant recipient. *American Journal of Kidney Diseases, 38*(6 Suppl. 6), S10-S24.

Corry, R.J. (1987). University of Iowa experience in pancreatic transplantation. *Transplantation Proceedings, 19*(4 Suppl. 4), 37-39.

Cueto-Manzano, A.M., Konel, S., Hutchison, A.J., Crowley, V., France, V.W., Freemont, A.J., et al. (1999). Bone loss in long-term renal transplantation: Histopathology and densitometry analysis. *Kidney International, 55*, 2021-2029.

Davies, W.E., Portmann, B.C., O'Grady, J.G., Aldis, P.M., Chaggar, K., Alexander, G.J., et al. (1991). Hepatic histological findings after transplantation for chronic hepatitis B virus infection, including a unique pattern of fibrosing cholestatic hepatitis. *Hepatology, 13*, 150-157.

Davis, C. L., Gonwa, T. A., & Wilkinson, A. H. (2002a). Pathophysiology of renal disease associated with liver disorders: Implications for liver transplantation. Part I. *Liver Transplantation, 8*, 91-109.

Davis, C. L., Gonwa, T. A., & Wilkinson, A. H. (2002b). Identification of patients best suited for combined liver-kidney transplantation: Part II. *Liver Transplantation, 8*, 193-211.

De Geest, S., Borgermans, L., Gemoets, H., Abraham, I., Vlaminck, H., Evers, G., et al. (1995). Incidence, determinants, and consequences of subclinical noncompliance with immunosuppressive therapy in renal transplant recipients. *Transplantation, 59*, 340-347.

de Ville de Goyet, J., Hausleithner, V., Reding, R., Lerut, J., Janssen, M., & Otte, J.B. (1993). Impact of innovative techniques on the waiting list and results in pediatric liver transplantation. *Transplantation, 56*, 1130-1136.

DeMayo, E., Elick, B., & Schanbacher, B. (1990). Pancreas transplantation. In K.M. Sigardison-Door & L.M. Haggerty (Eds.), *Nursing care of the transplant recipient*. Philadelphia: W.B. Saunders.

Denys, A., Chevallier, P., Doenz, F., Qanadli, S. D., Sommacale, D.,

Gillet, M., et al. (2004). Interventional radiology in the management of complications after liver transplantation. *European Radiology, 14*, 431-439.

Deshpande, R.R., Bowles, M.J., Vilca-Melendez, H., Srinivasan, P., Girlanda, R., Dhawan, A., et al. (2002). Results of split liver transplantation in children. *Annals of Surgery, 236*, 248-253.

Didlake, R.H., Dreyfus, K., Kerman, R.H., Van Buren. C.T., & Kahan, B.D. (1988). Patient noncompliance: A major cause of late graft failure in cyclosporine-treated renal transplant recipients. *Transplantation, 59*, 340-347.

Diethelm, A.G., Barger, B.O., Whelchel, J.D., & Barber, W.H. (1987). Organ transplantation. In J.H. Davis (Ed.), *Clinical surgery*. St. Louis, MO: C.V. Mosby.

Dordevic, P.B., Lalia, N.M., Birkic, S., Jotic, A., Paunouc, I., Lalic, K. et al (1995). Human felt islet transplant in IDDM patients: An 8-year experience. *Transplant Proceedings, 27*(6), 31-45.

Dreno, B. (2003). Skin cancers after transplantation. *Nephrology, Dialysis, Transplantation, 18*, 1052-1058.

Dunn, J., Golden, D., Van Burne, D.T., Lewis, R.M., Lawen, J., & Kahan, B.D. (1990). Causes of graft loss beyond 2 years in the cyclosporine era. *Transplantation, 49*, 349-353.

Edwards, S.S. (1999). The "noncompliant" transplant patient: A persistent ethical dilemma. *Journal of Transplant Coordination, 9*, 202-208.

Egawa, H., Inomata, Y., Uemoto, S., Asonuma, K., Kiuchi, T., Fujita, S., et al. (2001). Biliary anastomotic complications in 400 living related liver transplantations. *World Journal of Surgery, 25*, 1300-1307.

Emond, J.C. (1993). Clinical application of living related liver transplantation. *Journal of Gastroenterology Clinics of North America, 22*, 301-315.

Emond, J.C., Whitington, P.F., & Broelsch, C. (1991). Overview of reduced size liver transplantation. *Clinical Transplantation, 5*, 168-173.

European FK506 Multicentre Liver Study Group. (1994). Reduced incidents of acute refractory acute and chronic rejection after liver transplantation with FK506 based immunosuppression. *Transplant Proceedings, 26*, 3260-3263.

Fabrizio, M.D., Ratner, L.E., Montgomery, R.A., & Kavoussi, L.R. (1999). Laparoscopic live donor nephrectomy. *Urologic Clinics of North America, 26*, 247-256.

Farkas, G., Szasz, Z., Lazar, G., Jr., Csanadi, J., & Lazar, G. (2002). Macrophage blockade induced by repeated gadolinium chloride injections saves human fetal islet xenografting in rats. *Transplantation Proceedings, 34*, 1460-1461.

Fauchald, P., Vatne, K., Paulsen, D., Brodahl, U., Sodal, G., Holdaas, H., et al. (1992). Long-term clinical results of percutaneous transluminal angioplasty in transplant renal artery stenosis. *Nephrology, Dialysis, Transplantation, 7*, 256-259.

Fellstrom, B. (2001). Risk factors for and management of posttransplantation cardiovascular disease. *BioDrugs, 15*, 261-278.

Feray, C., Caccamo, L., Alexander, G.J., Ducot, B., Gugenheim, J., Casanovas, T., et al. (1999). European collaborative study on factors influencing outcome after liver transplantation for hepatitis C. European Concerted Action on Viral Hepatitis (EUROHEP) Group. *Gastroenterology, 117*, 619-625.

Fervenza, F.C., Lafayette, R.A., Alfrey, E.J., & Petersen, J. (1998). Renal artery stenosis in kidney transplants. *American Journal of Kidney Diseases, 31*, 142-148.

Fioretto, P., Steffes, M.W., Sutherland, D.E., Goetz, F.C., & Mauer, M. (1998). Reversal of lesions of diabetic nephropathy after pancreas transplantation. *New England Journal of Medicine, 339*, 69-75.

Fishman, J.A., & Rubin, R.H. (1998). Infection in organ-transplant recipients. *New England Journal of Medicine, 338*, 1741-1751.

Foster, C.E., 3rd, Philosophe, B., Schweitzer, E.J., Colonna, J.O., Farney, A.C., Jarrell, B., et al. (2002). A decade of experience with renal transplantation in African-Americans. *Annals of Surgery, 236*, 794-804.

Friedewald, S.M., Molmenti, E.P., DeJong, M.R., & Hamper, U.M. (2003). Vascular and nonvascular complications of liver transplants: Sonographic evaluation and correlation with other imaging modalities and findings at surgery and pathology. *Ultrasound Quarterly, 19*(2), 71-85.

Garovoy, M.R., Amend, W.J.C., Vincenti, F., & Feduska, N.J. (1987). *Renal transplantation: The modern era.* New York: Gower Medical.

Garovoy, M.R., Stock, P., Bumgardner, G., Keith, F., & Linker, C. (1994). Clinical transplantation. In D.P. Stites, A.I. Terr, & T.G. Parslow (Eds.), *Basic and clinical immunology* (8th ed.). Norfolk, CT: Appleton & Lange.

Gaston, R.S., Hudson, S.L., Ward, M., Jones, P.L, & Macon, R. (1999). Late renal allograft loss: Non-compliance masquerading as chronic rejection. *Transplant Proceedings, 31*, S21-S23.

Goddard, S., & Adams, D.H. (2002). New approaches to immunosuppression in liver transplantation. *Journal of Gastroenterology and Hepatology, 17*, 116-126.

Gonzalez, M. M., Duarte Novo, J. E., Gomez viega, F., Chantada Abal, V., & Alvarez Castelo, L. (1999). Marsupialization via mini-laparotomy in the kidney transplant. *Archieves of Espanol Urology, 52*, 41-46.

Goodman, W.G., Goldin, J., & Kuizon, B.D. (2000). Coronary artery calcification in young adults with end stage renal disease who are undergoing dialysis. *New England Journal of Medicine, 342*, 1478-1483.

Graziadei, I.W. (2002). Recurrence of primary sclerosing cholangitis after liver transplantation. *Liver Transplantation, 8*(7), 575-581.

Griffith, B.P., Shaw, B.W., Jr., Hardesty, R.L., Iwatsuki, S., Bahnson, H.T., & Starzl, T.E. (1985). Veno-venous bypass without systemic anticoagulation for transplantation of the human liver. *Surgery, Gynecology and Obstetrics, 160*, 270-272.

Gross, C.R., Limwattananon, C., & Matthees, B.J. (1998). Quality of life after pancreas transplantation: A review. *Clinical Transplantation, 12*, 351-361.

Gruessner, A., & Sutherland, D. (2002). Pancreas transplant outcomes for United States (U.S.) and non-U.S. cases as reported to the United Network for Organ Sharing (UNOS) and the International Pancreas Transplant Registry (IPTS) as of October 2001.Richmond, VA: UNOS.

Gruessner, A.C., Sutherland, D.E., Dunn, D.L., Najarian, J.S., Humar, A., Kandaswamy, R., et al. (2001). Pancreas after kidney transplants in posturemeic patients with type I diabetes mellitus. *Journal of the American Society of Nephrology, 12*, 2490-2499.

Grundfest-Broniatowski, S. (1990). Pancreas transplantation: State of the art. *Cleveland Clinic Journal of Medicine, 57*, 564-570.

Gunsar, F., Rolando, N., Pastacaldi, S., Patch, D., Raimondo, M.L., Davidson, B., et al. (2003). Late hepatic artery thrombosis after orthotopic liver transplantation. *Liver Transplantation, 9*, 605-611.

Hamady, M., Rela, M., & Sidhu, P.S. (2002). Spontaneous resolution of a portal vein stenosis over a 21-month period in a "split-liver" transplant: Demonstration by colour Doppler ultrasound, catheter angiography and splenic pulp pressures. *European Radiology, 12*, 2280-2283.

Handschein, A.E., Weber, M., Demartines, N., & Clavien, P.A. (2003). Laparoscopic donor nephrectomy. *British Journal of Surgery, 90*, 1323-1332.

Hanto, D.W., & Simmons, R. (1987). Renal transplantation: Clinical considerations. *Radiologic Clinics of North America, 25*, 239-248.

Hariharan, S. (2000). Recurrent and de novo diseases after renal transplantation. *Seminars in Dialysis, 13*, 195-199.

Hariharan, S., Johnson, C.P., Bresnahan, B.A., Taranto, S.E., McIntosh, M.J., & Stablein, D. (2000). Improved graft survival after renal transplantation in the United States, 1988 to 1996. *New England Journal of Medicine, 342*, 605-612.

Hartevelt, M. M., Bavinck, J. N., Kootte, A. M., Vermeer, B. J., & Vandenbroucke, J. P. (1990). Incidence of skin cancer after renal transplantation in The Netherlands. *Transplantation, 49*, 506-509.

Herzenberg, A.M., Gill, J.S., Djurdjev, O., & Magil, A.B. (2002). C4d deposition in acute rejection: An independent long-term prognostic factor. *Journal of the American Society of Nephrology, 13*, 234-241.

Hubscher, S.G. (2001). Recurrent autoimmune hepatitis after liver transplantation; diagnostic criteria, risk factors, and outcome.

Liver Transplantation, 7(4), 285-291.

Humar, A. (2003). Donor and recipient outcomes after adult living donor liver transplantation. *Liver Transplantation, 9*(10 Suppl. 2), S42-S44.

Isoniemi, H., Nurminen, M., Tikkanen, M.J., von Willebrand, E., Krogerus, L., Ahonen, J., et al. (1994). Risk factors predicting chronic rejection of renal allografts. *Transplantation, 57*, 68-72.

Jain, A., Demetris, A.J., Kashyap, R., Blakomer, K., Ruppert, K., Khan, A., et al. (2001). Does tacrolimus offer virtual freedom from chronic rejection after primary liver transplantation? Risk and prognostic factors in 1,048 liver transplantations with a mean follow-up of 6 years. *Liver Transplantation, 7*, 623-630.

Johnston, T.D., Gates, R., Reddy, K.S., Nickl, N.J., & Ranjan, D. (2000). Nonoperative management of bile leaks following liver transplantation. *Clinical Transplantation, 14*(4 Pt. 2), 365-369.

Kasiske, B.L. (1988). Risk factors for accelerated atherosclerosis in renal transplant recipients. *American Journal of Medicine, 84*, 985-992.

Kasiske, B.L. (1998). Hyperlipidemia in patients with chronic renal disease. *American Journal of Kidney Diseases, 32*, S112-S119.

Kasiske, B.L. (2001). Long-term posttransplantation management and complications. In G.M. Danovitch (Ed.), *Handbook of kidney transplant* (3rd ed.) Philadelphia: Lippincott, Williams & Wilkins.

Kasiske, B.L., Guijarro, C., Massy, Z.A., Wiederkehr, M.R., & Ma, J.Z. (1996). Cardiovascular disease after renal transplantation. *Journal of the American Society of Nephrology, 7*, 158-165.

Kasiske, B.L. & Klinger, D. (2000). Cigarette smoking in renal transplant recipients. *Journal of American Society of Nephrology, 11*, 753-759.

Kasiske, B.L., Vazquex, M.A., Harmon, W.E., Brown, R.S., Danovitch, G.M., Gaston, R.S., et al. (2000). Recommendations for the outpatient surveillance of renal transplant recipients. *Journal of the American Society of Nephrology, 11*, S1-S86.

Katznelson, S., & Cecka, M. (1996) The liver neither protects the kidney from rejection nor improves kidney graft survival after combined liver and kidney transplantation from the same donor. *Transplantation, 61*, 1403-1405.

Kazory, A., & Ducloux, D. (2003). Renal transplantation and polyomavirus infection: Recent clinical facts and controversies. *Transplant Infectious Disease, 5*(2), 65-71.

Kiberd, B.A. (2002). Cardiovascular risk reduction in renal transplantation, strategies for success. *Minerva Urolology and Nephrology, 54*(2), 51-63.

Kiley, D.J., Lam, C.S., & Pollak, R. (1993). The study of treatment compliance following kidney transplantation. *Journal of Transplantation, 55*, 51-56.

Kim, F.J., Ratner, L.E., & Kavoussi, L.R. (2000). Renal transplantation: Laparoscopic live donor nephrectomy. *Urologic Clinics of North America, 27*, 777-785.

Khoury, G.F., Mann, M.E., Porot, M.J., Abdul-Rasool, I.H., & Busuttil, R.W. (1987). Air embolism associated with veno-venous bypass during orthotopic liver transplantation. *Anesthesiology, 67*, 848-851.

Kubak, B.M., Pegues, D.A., & Holt, C.D. (2001). Infections complications of kidney transplantation and their management. In G.M. Danovitch (Ed.), *Handbook of kidney transplantation* (3rd ed.), Philadelphia: Lippincott Williams & Wilkins.

Lakey, J.R., Warnock, G.L., Rajotte, R.V., Suarez-Alamazor, M.E., Ao, Z., Shapiro, A.M., et al. (1996). Variables in organ donors that affect the recovery of human islets of Langerhans. *Transplantation, 61*, 1047-1053.

Lang, M., Neumann, U., Kahl, A., Steinmuller, T., Settmacher, U., & Neuhaus, P. (2001). Long-term outcome of 27 patients after combined liver-kidney transplantation. *Transplantation Proceedings, 33*, 1440-1441.

Langle, F., Schurawitzki, H., Muhlbacher, F., Steininger, R., Watschinger, B., Derfler, K., et al. (1990). Treatment of lymphoceles following renal transplantation. *Transplantation Proceedings, 22*, 1420-1422.

Largiader, F., Baumgartner, D., Kolb, E., & Uhlschmid, G. (1983). Technique and results of combined pancreatic and renal allotransplantation in man. *Hormone and Metabolic Research, Supplement Series, 13*, 47-49.

Larue, J.R., Hiesse, C., Samuel, D., Blanchet, P., Goupy, C., Benoit, G., et al. (1997). Long-term results of combined kidney and liver transplantation at one center. *Transplantation Proceedings, 29*, 2365-2366.

Lerut, J., Tzakis, A.G., Bron, K., Gordon, R.D., Iwatsuki, S., Esquivel, C.O., et al. (1987). Complications of venous reconstruction in human orthotopic liver transplantation. *Annals of surgery, 205*, 404-414.

Li, P.K.T., Mak, T.W.L., Chan, T.H., Wang, A., Lam C.W.K., & Lai, K.N. (1995). Effect of fluvastatin on lipoprietn profiles in treating renal transplant recipients with dyslipoproteinemia. *Transplantation, 60*, 652-656

Lind, M.Y., Ijzermans, J.N., & Bonjer, H.J. (2002). Open versus laparoscopic donor nephrectomy in renal transplantation. *British Journal of Urology International, 89*, 162-168.

Lippuner, K. Casez, J.P., Horber, F.F., & Jaeger, P. (1998). Effects of deflazacort versus prednisone on bone mass, body composition, and lipid profile: A randomized double blind study in kidney transplant patients. *Journal of Clinical Endocrinology and Metabolism, 83*, 3795-3802.

Lok, A.S. (2002). Prevention of recurrent hepatitis B post-liver transplantation. *Liver Transplantation, 8*(10 Suppl. 1), S67-S73.

Lutz, J., & Heemann, U. (2003). Tumours after kidney transplantation. *Current Opinion in Urology,13*, 105-109.

Martin, X., Aboutaieb, R., Dawahra, M., Lagha, K., Garnier, J.L., Pangaud, C., et al. (1996). Treatment of lymphocele after kidney transplantation. *Progress in Urology, 6*, 260-263.

Matas, A. J., Burk, J.F, DeVault. G.A., Monaco, A., & Pirsch, J.D. (1994). Chronic rejection. *Journal of the American Society of Nephrology, 4*, S23-S29.

Matas, A.J., Gillingham, K.J., Payne, W.D., & Najarian, J.S. (1994). The impact of an acute rejection episode on long-term renal allograft survival (t1/2). *Transplantation, 57*, 857-859.

Mauiyyedi, S., & Colvin, R.B. (2002). Humoral rejection in kidney transplantation: New concepts in diagnosis and treatment. *Current Opinion in Nephrology and Hypertension, 11*, 609-618.

Mauiyyedi, S., Crespo, M., Collins, A.B., Schneeberger, E.E., Pascual, M.A., Saidman, S.L., et al. (2002). Acute humoral rejection in kidney transplantation: II. Morphology, immunopathology, and pathologic classification. *Journal of the American Society of Nephrology, 13*, 779-787.

McCaughan, G. W., & Zekry, A. (2000). Effects of immunosuppression and organ transplantation on the natural history and immunopathogenesis of hepatitis C virus infection. *Transplant Infectious Disease, 2*(4), 166-185.

McCune, T.R., Thacker, L.R., Peters, T.G., Mulloy, L. Rohr, M.S., Adams, P.A., et al. (1998). Effects of tacrolimus on hyperlipidemia after successful renal transplant: A Southeastern Organ Procurement Foundation multicenter clinical study. *Transplantation, 65*, 87-92.

McDiarmid, S.V. (2003). Current status of liver transplantation in children. *Pediatric Clinics of North America, 50*, 1335-1374.

McDiarmid, S., & Anand, R. (2002). SPLIT research group. Studies in pediatric liver transplantation: 2002 update. *Pediatric Transplantation, 6*, 34-56.

McDiarmid, S.V., Klintmalm, G.B., & Busuttil, R.D. (1993). FK506 conversion for intractable rejection of the liver allograph. *Transplant International, 6*, 305-312.

McGilvray, I.D., & Greig, P.D. (2002). Critical care of the liver transplant patient: An update. *Current Opinion in Critical Care, 8*, 178-182.

McLean, D., Hay, P., Woo, Y.M., Padmanabhan, N., & Jardine, A. G. (2000). Cardiovascular risk and renal transplantation: A mathematical model to explore future strategies. In M. Timio, V. Wizemann, & S. Venanzi (Eds.), *Cardionephrology 6*, Cosenza Editoriale Bios.

Merkus, J.W., Huysmans, F.T., Hoitsma, A.J., Buskens, F.G., Skotnicki, S.H., & Koene, R.A. (1993). Renal allograft artery stenosis: Results of medical treatment and intervention. A retrospective analysis. *Transplant International, 6*, 111-115.

Montgomery, R.A., Zachary, A.A., Racusen, L.C., Leffell, M.S., King, K.E., Burdick, J., et al. (2000). Plasmapheresis and intravenous immune globulin provides effective rescue therapy for refractory humoral rejection and allows kidneys to be successfully transplanted into cross-match-positive recipients. *Transplantation, 70,* 887-895.

Moser, M.A., & Wall, W.J. (2001). Management of biliary problems after liver transplantation. *Liver Transplantation, 7*(11 Suppl. 1), S46-S52.

Mudge, C. (1998). Immunology. In J. Parker (Ed.), *Contemporary nephrology nursing.* Pitman, NJ: American Nephrology Nurses Association.

Mudge, C., Carlson, L., & Brennan, P. (1998) Transplantation. In J. Parker (Ed.), *Contemporary nephrology nursing.* Pitman, NJ: American Nephrology Nurses Association.

Munoz, P. (2001). Management of urinary tract infections and lymphocele in renal transplant recipients. *Clinical Infectious Diseases, 33*(Suppl. 1), S53-S57.

Najarian, J.S., Chavers, B.M., McHugh, L.E., & Matas, A.J. (1992). 20 years or more of follow-up of living kidney donors. *Lancet, 340*(8823), 807-810.

Nakhleh, R.E., & Sutherland, D.E. (1992). Pancreas rejection. Significance of histopathologic findings with implications for classification of rejection. *American Journal of Surgical Pathology, 16,* 1098-1107.

Navarro, X., Sutherland, D.E., & Kennedy, W.R. (1997). Long-term effects of pancreatic transplantation on diabetic neuropathy. *Annals of Neurology, 42,* 727-736.

Newstead, C. G. (2000). Lymphoproliferative disease post-renal transplant. *Nephrology Dialysis and Transplantation,15,* 1913-1916.

Novotny, M.J. (2001). Laparoscopic live donor nephrectomy. *Urologic Clinics of North America, 28,* 127-135.

O'Grady, J.G., Smith, H.M., Davies, S.E., Daniels, H.M., Donaldson, P.T., Tan, K.C., et al. (1992). Hepatitis B virus reinfection after orthotopic liver transplantation: Serological and clinical implications. *Journal of Hepatology, 14,* 104-111.

Ojo, A.O., Hanson, J.A., Wolfe, R.A., Leichtman, A.B., Agodoa, L.Y., & Port, F.K. (2000). Long-term survival in renal transplant recipients with graft function. *Kidney International, 75,* 307-313.

Ojo, A.O., Port, F.K., Held, P.J., Wolfe, R.A., Turenne, M. N., Chung, E., et al. (1995). Inferior outcome of two-haplotype matched renal transplants in blacks: Role of early rejection. *Kidney International, 48,* 1592-1599.

Palinske, W. (2000) Immunomodulation: A new role for statins? *National Medicine, 6,* 1311-1322.

Pascual, M., Saidman, S., Tolkoff-Rubin, N., Williams, W.W., Mauiyyedi, S., Duan, J.M., et al. (1998). Plasma exchange and tacrolimus-mycophenolate rescue for acute humoral rejection in kidney transplantation. *Transplantation, 66,* 1460-1464.

Patel, C.S.U. (2002). Renal transplantation dysfunction: The role of interventional radiology. *Clinical Radiology, 57,* 772-783.

Pattella, P.S., & Weiskittel, P.D. (1991). Kidney transplantation. In M.K.G. Norris & M.A. House (Eds.), *Organ and tissue transplantation: Nursing care from procurement through rehabilitation.* Philadelphia: F.A. Davis.

Penn, I. (2000). Cancers in renal transplant recipients. *Advances in Renal Replacement Therapy, 7,* 147-156.

Perkins, J.D., Fromme, G.A., Nar, B.J., Southorn, P.A., Marsh, C.L., Munn, S.R., et al. (1990). Pancreas transplantation at Mayo: II. Operative and perioperative management. *Mayo Clinical Proceedings, 65,* 483-495.

Perryman, J.P., & Stillerman, P. (1991). Kidney transplantation. In S.L. Smith (Ed.), *Tissue and organ transplantation: Implications for professional nursing practice.* St. Louis, MO: C.V. Mosby.

Pesavento, T.E., & Falkenhain, M.E. (1998). Management of renal transplant patients. In A.K. Mandal & N.S. Nahman (Eds.), *Kidney disease in primary care.* New York: Williams and Wilkins.

Philosophe, B., Kuo, P.C., Schweitzer, E.J., Farney, A.C., Lim, J.W., Johnson, L.B., et al. (1999). Laparoscopic versus open donor nephrectomy: Comparing ureteral complications in the recipients and improving the laparoscopic technique. *Transplantation, 68,* 497-502.

Pichette, V., Bonnardeaux, A., Prudhomme, L., Gagne, M., Cardinal, J., & Quimet, D. (1996). Long-term bone loss in kidney transplant recipients: A cross-sectional and longitudinal study. *American Journal of Kidney Diseases, 28,* 105-114.

Pokorny, H., Gruenberger, T., Soliman, T., Rockenschaub, S., Langle,

F., & Steininger, R. (2000). Organ survival after primary dysfunction of liver grafts in clinical orthotopic liver transplantation. *Transplant International, 13*(Suppl. 1), S154-S157.

Prieto, M., Sutherland, D. E., Fernandez-Cruz, L., Heil, J., & Najarian, J. S. (1987). Experimental and clinical experience with urine amylase monitoring for early diagnosis of rejection in pancreas transplantation. *Transplantation, 43,* 73-79.

Raby, N., Karani, J., Thomas, S., O'Grady, J., & Williams, R. (1991). Stenoses of vascular anastomoses after hepatic transplantation: Treatment with balloon angioplasty. *American Journal of Roentgenology, 157,* 167-171.

Ramsay, H.M., Fryer, A.A., Reece, S., Smith, A.G., & Harden, P.N. (2000). Clinical risk factors associated with nonmelanoma skin cancer in renal transplant recipients. *American Journal of Kidney Diseases, 36,* 167-176.

Ratner, L.E., Ciseck, L.J., Moore, R.G., Cigarroa, F.G., Kaufman, H.S., & Kavoussi, L.R. (1995). Laparoscopic live donor nephrectomy. *Transplantation, 60,* 1047-1049.

Ratner, L.E., Montgomery, R.A., & Kavoussi, L.R. (1998). Living-donor nephrectomies: Laparoscopy and open techniques. *Archives of Surgery, 133,* 1253-1254.

Reece, S.M., Harden, P.N., Smith, A.G., & Ramsay, H.M. (2002). A model for nurse-led skin cancer surveillance following renal transplantation. *Nephrology Nursing Journal, 29,* 257-259, 267.

Rengel, M., Gomes-Da-Silva, G., Inchaustegui, L., Lampreave, J.L., Robledo, R., Echenagusia, A., et al. (1998). Renal artery stenosis after kidney transplantation: Diagnostic and therapeutic approach. *Kidney International, 68*(Suppl.), S99-S106.

Renz, J.F. & Busuttil, R.W. (2000). Adult-to-adult living donor liver transplantation: A critical analysis. *Seminars in Liver Disease, 20*(4), 411-424.

Renz, J.F. & Roberts, J.P. (2000). Long-term complications of living donor liver transplantation. *Liver Transplantation, 6*(6), S73-S76.

Roberts, J.P., Forsmark, C., Lake, J.R., & Ascher, N. (1989). Liver transplantation today. *Annual Reviews in Medicine, 400,* 287-303.

Roberts, J.P., Lake, J.R., Hebert, M., Nikolai, B., Ascher, N.L., & Ferrell, L.D. (1993). Reversal of chronic rejection after treatment failure with FK506 and RS61443. *Transplantation, 56,* 1021-1023.

Rodriquez, D., Diaz, M., Colon, A., & Santiago-Delpin, W.A. (1991). Psychosocial profile of non-compliant transplant recipients. *Transplant Proceedings, 23,* 1807-1809.

Rosen, H.R. (2000). Disease recurrence following liver transplantation. *Clinical Liver Diseases, 4*(3), 675-689.

Rosenkranz, A.R., & Mayer, G. (2000). Mechanisms of hypertension after renal transplantation. *Current Opinion in Urology,10*(2), 81-86.

Rosenthal, P., Podesta, L., Sher, A., & Makowka, L. (1994). Liver transplantation in children. *American Journal of Gastroenterology, 89,* 480-492.

Rubin, R. (1994). Infection in the organ transplant recipient. In R. Rubin & L. Young (Eds.), *Clinical approach to infection in the compromised host* (3rd ed.). New York: Plenum Publishing.

Ruse, L.A., & Kottra-Buck, C. (1986). Complications following renal transplantation. In C.J. Richards (Ed.), *Comprehensive nephrology nursing.* Boston: Little Brown.

Rush, D., Nickerson, P., Gough, J., McKenna, R., Grimm, P., Cheang, M., et al. (1998). Beneficial effects of treatment of early subclinical rejection: A randomized study. *Journal of the American Society of Nephrology, 9,* 2129-2134.

Ryan, E.A., Lakey, J.R., Rajotte, R.V., Korbutt, G.S., Kin, T., Imes, S., et al. (2002). Clinical outcomes and insulin secretion after islet transplantation with the Edmonton protocol. *Diabetes, 50,* 710-719.

Salvatierra, O. (1987). Renal transplantation. In J.F. Glenn (Ed.), *Urologic surgery* (3rd ed.). Philadelphia: J.B. Lippincott.

Samsonov, D., & Briscoe, D.M. (2002). Long-term care of pediatric renal transplant patients: From bench to bedside. *Current Opinion in Pediatrics, 14,* 205-210.

San Filippo, F. (1990). Renal transplantation. In G.E. Sale (Ed.), *A pathology of organ transplantation.* Boston: Butterworths.

Schaapherder, A.F., de Roos, A., Shaw, P.C., van der Woude, F.J., Lemkes, H.H., & Gooszen, H.G. (1993). The role of early baseline computed tomography in the interpretation of morphological changes after kidney-pancreas transplantation. *Transplant International, 6,* 270-276.

Schweizer, R.T., Rovelli, M., Palmer, D., Bossler, E., Hull, D., & Bartus, S. (1990). Noncompliance in organ transplant recipients. *Transplantation, 49,* 374-377.

Seikaly, M.G. (2004). Recurrence of primary disease in children after renal transplantation: An evidence-based update. *Pediatric Transplantation, 8,* 113-119.

Shapiro, A.M., Ryan, E.A., & Lakey, J.R. (2001). Pancreatic islet transplantation in the treatment of diabetes mellitus. *Best Practice & Research: Clinical Endocrinology & Metabolism, 15,* 241-264.

Shoskes, D.A. (2000). Non-immunologic renal allograft injury and delayed graft function: Clinical strategies for prevention and treatment. *Transplantation Proceedings, 32,* 766-768.

Silkensen, J.R. (2000). Long-term complications in renal transplantation. *Journal of the American Society of Nephrology, 11,* 582-588.

Sketris, I., Waite, N., Grobler, K., West, M., & Gerus, S. (1994). Factors affecting compliance with cyclosporine in adult renal transplant patients *Transplantation Proceedings, 26,* 2538-2541.

Snover, D.C. (1990). *The pathology of organ transplantation.* In G.E. Sale (Ed.), *The pathology of organ transplantation.* Burlington, MA: Butterworth-Heinemann.

Sollinger, H., Knechtle, S., Reed, A.D. Alessandro, A., Kalayogu, M., Bezer, F., et al. (1991). Experience with 100 consecutive simultaneous kidney-pancreas transplants with bladder drainage. *Annals of Surgery, 21,* 703-711.

Sollinger, H. W., Stratta, R.J., D'Alesandro, A.M., Kalayodu, M., Pirsch, J.D., & Belzer, F.D. (1988). Experience with simultaneous pancreas-kidney transplantation. *Annals of Surgery, 208,* 475-483.

Sollinger, H.W., Stratta, R.J., Kalayoglu, M., & Belzer, F.O. (1987). The University of Wisconsin experience in pancreas transplantation. *Transplantation Proceedings, 19,* 48-54.

Soon-Shiang, D., White, G., DeMayo, E., Koyle, M., & Danovitch, G. (1988). Mechanical obstruction of the portal vein as a cause of vascular thrombosis after pancreas transplantation in man. *Transplantation Proceedings, 20,* 399-402.

Starzl, T. E., Demetris, A. J., & Van Thiel, D. (1989a). Liver transplantation: Pt. 1. *New England Journal of Medicine, 321,* 1014-1022.

Starzl, T. E., Demetris, A. J., &Van Thiel, D. (1989b). Liver transplantation: Pt. 2. *New England Journal of Medicine, 321,* 1092-1099.

Stewart, G. Jardine, A.G., & Briggs, J.D. (2000). Ischaemic heart disease following renal transplantation. *Nephrology Dialysis and Transplantation, 15,* 269-277.

Stock, P.G., & Bluestone, J.A. (2004). Beta-cell replacement for type I diabetes. *Annual Review of Medicine, 55,* 133-156.

Stock, P.G., & Payne, W.D. (1990). Liver transplantation. *Critical Care Clinics, 6,* 911-926.

Suthanthiran, M., & Strom, T.B. (1994). Renal transplantation. *New England Journal of Medicine, 331,* 365-374.

Sutherland, D.E., Gores, P.E., Hering, B.J., Wahoff, D., McKeehen, D.A., & Gruessner, R.W. (1996). Islet transplant: An update. *Diabetes/Metabolism Review, 12,* 137-150.

Tejani, A., & Sullivan E. K. (2000). The impact of acute rejection on chronic rejection: A report of the North American Pediatric Renal Transplant Cooperative Study. *Pediatric Transplant, 4,* 107-111.

Tessari, G., Barba, A., & Chieregato, C. (1999). Risk factors for skin cancer in a group of renal transplant recipients. *Acta Dermato-Venereologica, 79,* 409-410.

Testa, G., Malago, M., Valentin-Gamazo, C., Lindell, G., & Broelsch, C.E. (2000). Biliary anastomosis in living related liver transplantation using the right liver lobe: Techniques and complications. *Liver Transplantation, 6,* 710-714.

Thomas, C.P., Riad, H., Johnson, B.F., & Cumberland, D.C. (1992). Percutaneous transluminal angioplasty in transplant renal arterial stenoses: A long-term follow-up. *Transplant International, 5,* 129-132.

Thompson, J.M., McFarland, J.K, Hirsch, J.E., & Tucker, S.M. (1993). *Mosby clinical nursing* (3rd ed.) St. Louis, MO: C.V. Mosby.

Thorp, M., DeMattos, A., Bennett, W., Barry, J., & Norman, D. (2000). The effect of conversion from cyclosporine to tacrolimus on gin-

gival hyperplasia, hirsutism and cholesterol. *Transplantation, 69,* 1218-1220.

Tolkoff-Rubin, N.E., & Rubin, R.H. (1997). Urinary tract infection in the immunocompromised host. Lessons from kidney transplantation and the AIDS epidemic. *Infectious Disease Clinics of North America, 11,* 707-717.

Trusler, L.A. (1991). Simultaneous kidney-pancreas transplantation. *ANNA Journal, 18,* 487-491.

Turka, N. (2001). *Primer on transplantation* (2nd ed.). Mt. Laurel, NJ: American Society of Transplantation.

United Network for Organ Sharing (UNOS). (2001). *2000 annual report of the U.S. Scientific Registry for transplant recipients and the organ procurement and transplantation network: Transplant data: 1990-1999.* Richmond, VA: Author.

Van Thiel, D., Nadir, A., & Shah, N. (2002). Hepatitis C virus and renal transplantation. *Transplantation Proceedings, 34*(6), 2433-2435.

Vincenti, F. (2004). A decade of progress in kidney transplantation. *Transplantation, 77*(9 Suppl.), S52-S61.

Vincenti, F., Jensik, S.C., Filo, R.S., Miller, J., & Pirsch, J. (2002). A long-term comparison of tacrolimus (FK506) and cyclosporine in kidney transplantation: Evidence for improved allograft survival at 5 years. *Transplantation, 73,* 775-782.

Whiting, J.F. (2000). Clinical and economic outcomes of the use of expanded criteria donors in renal transplantation. *Seminars in Dialysis, 13,* 316-319.

Wiesner, R.H., Ludwig, J., van Hoek, B., & Krom, R. A. (1992). Chronic hepatic allograph rejection: A review of ductopenic rejection and advantaging bio-duct syndrome. In L.C. Paul & K. Solez (Eds.), *Organ transplantation: Long-term results.* New York: Marcel Dekker.

Wiesner, R.H., Porayko, M.K., Lake, J.R., Batts, K.P., & Krom, R.A. (1993). Long-term management of liver transplant recipients. *Seminars in Gastrointestinal Disease, 4,* 151-164.

Willis, B.G., & Post, L.C. (1990). Pancreas transplantation. In S.L. Smith (Ed.), *Tissue and organ transplantation: Implications for professional nursing practice.* St. Louis, MO: C.V. Mosby.

Wong, K.S. (2000). Posttransplant hypertension. *Transplantation Proceedings, 32,* 1495-1496.

Wong, W., Fynn, S.P., Higgins, R.M., Walters, H., Evans, S., Deane, C., et al. (1996). Transplant renal artery stenosis in 77 patients — Does it have an immunological cause? *Transplantation, 61,* 215-219.

Wu, J.J., & Orengo, I.F. (2001). Squamous cell carcinoma in solid organ transplantation. *Dermatology Online Journal, 8*(2), 1-20.

Yoshikawa, T. (2003). Human herpes virus - 6 and -7 infections in transplantation. *Pediatric Transplantation, 7,* 11-17.

Zekorn, T.D., Horcher, A., Mellert, J., Siebers, U., Altug, T., Emre, A., et al. (1996). Biocompatibility and immunology in the encapsulation of islets of Langerhans (bioartificial pancreas). *International Journal of Artificial Organs, 19,* 251-257.

Additional Readings

Baumgartner, D., Largiader, F., Uhlschmid, G., & Briswanger, U. (1983). Rejection episodes in recipients of simultaneous pancreas and kidney transplantation. *Transplantation Proceedings, 15,* 1330-1331.

Lederer, S.R., Kluth-Pepper, B., & Schneeberger, H. (2001). Impact of humoral alloreactivity early after transplantation on the long-term survival of renal allografts. *Kidney International, 59,* 334-341.

Ratner, L.E., Montgomery, R.A., Maley, W.R., Cohen, C., Burdick, J., Chavin, K.D., et al. (2000). Laparoscopic live donor nephrectomy: The recipient. *Transplantation, 69,* 2319-2323.

Schweitzer, E.J., Wilson, J.S., Fernandez-Vina, M., Fox, M., Gutierrez, M., Wiland, A., et al. (2000). A high panel-reactive antibody rescue protocol for cross-match positive live donor kidney transplants. *Transplantation, 70,* 1531-1536.

- Kidney transplantation has become the treatment option of choice for patients with end stage renal disease (ESRD). Overall, 1-year deceased (cadaveric) kidney transplant success rates are 89.4%, with 5-year success rates being 65%. For recipients of living donor kidneys, the success rates are 97% and 78%, respectively.

- Organs for kidney transplant are from two sources, living or deceased (cadaveric) donors. Regardless of the donor source, the surgical procedure for the recipient is the same.

- There are two approaches to the kidney donor surgical procedure, the open donor nephrectomy and the laparoscopic donor nephrectomy.

- During the post-operative period, patients must be encouraged to become active participants in their own care. Long-term post-transplant care is complex, requiring patients to have a relatively extensive knowledge of their health care management.

- Pancreas transplantation is a viable therapeutic option for insulin-dependent diabetes. The engraftment of a functioning endocrine pancreas into the insulin-dependent patient provides the optimal physiologic means of correcting altered metabolism. The goal of pancreas transplant is two-fold: to provide an insulin-independent lifestyle and to reverse the secondary complications associated with diabetes.

- There are three basic approaches to pancreatic transplantation, single or solitary pancreas transplant, islet cell transplantation, and combined kidney-pancreas transplant.

- The major considerations specific to pancreas transplantation are during the initial post-operative period. The goal of the immediate post-operative period is to maintain hemodynamic stability and to prevent complications. If complications occur, early identification to allow for rapid treatment is optimal.

- Organs for liver transplantation come from two sources: living or deceased donors. There are a number of surgical approaches for the recipient undergoing liver transplantation, including reduced sized-grafts, split liver graft, living related left or right lobe liver transplant, auxiliary liver transplant, and combined organ transplant (liver-kidney transplant).

- The post-operative care and monitoring for complications of the liver transplant recipients is highly complex and requires a multidisciplinary approach and collaboration among team members (McGilvray & Greig, 2002). Liver transplant recipients are at risk for the same complications as any individual undergoing major abdominal surgery and organ transplantation. They also are at risk for the multiple side effects of immunosuppressive therapy and rejection and are at additional risk for infection.

ANNP631

Transplantation: The Procedure and Implications

Christine Mudge, MS, RN, PNPc/CNS, CNN, FAAN; Laurie Carlson, MSN, RN; and Patricia Brennan, MSN, RN

Contemporary Nephrology Nursing: Principles and Practice contains 39 chapters of educational content. Individual learners may apply for continuing nursing education credit by reading a chapter and completing the Continuing Education Evaluation Form for that chapter. Learners may apply for continuing education credit for any or all chapters.

Please photocopy this page and return to ANNA.
COMPLETE THE FOLLOWING:

Name: _____

Address:_____

City:_____ State: _____ Zip: _____

E-mail: _____

Preferred telephone: ☐ Home   ☐ Work: _____

State where licensed and license number (optional): _____

CE application fees are based upon the number of contact hours provided by the individual chapter. CE fees per contact hour for ANNA members are as follows: 1.0-1.9 - $15; 2.0-2.9 - $20; 3.0-3.9 - $25; 4.0 and higher - $30. Fees for nonmembers are $10 higher.

ANNA Member: ☐ Yes   ☐ No   Member # (if available) _____

☐ Checked Enclosed   ☐ American Express   ☐ Visa   ☐ MasterCard

Total Amount Submitted: _____

Credit Card Number: _____ Exp. Date: _____

Name as it appears on the card: _____

CE Evaluation Form
To receive continuing education credit for individual study after reading the chapter
1. Photocopy this form. (You may also download this form from ANNA's Web site, **www.annanurse.org.**)
2. Mail the completed form with payment (check) or credit card information to American Nephrology Nurses' Association, East Holly Avenue, Box 56, Pitman, NJ 08071-0056.
3. You will receive your CE certificate from ANNA in 4 to 6 weeks.

Test returns must be postmarked by **December 31, 2010.**

CE Application Fee
ANNA Member $30.00
Nonmember $40.00

EVALUATION FORM

1. I verify that I have read this chapter and completed this education activity. Date: _____

_____
Signature

2. What would be different in your practice if you applied what you learned from this activity? *(Please use additional sheet of paper if necessary.)*

_____
_____
_____
_____
_____
_____
_____
_____
_____
_____
_____
_____

Evaluation	Strongly disagree				Strongly agree
3. The activity met the stated objectives.					
a. Generate a plan of post-operative care for a patient having a kidney, pancreas, and/or liver transplant.	1	2	3	4	5
b. Contrast the nursing implications of the various post-operative complications possible with kidney transplantation.	1	2	3	4	5
c. Outline the long-term management necessary following a pancreas transplant.	1	2	3	4	5
d. Discuss the post-operative complications that are known to occur following a pancreas and liver transplant.	1	2	3	4	5
4. The content was current and relevant.	1	2	3	4	5
5. The content was presented clearly.	1	2	3	4	5
6. The content was covered adequately.	1	2	3	4	5
7. Rate your ability to apply the learning obtained from this activity to practice.	1	2	3	4	5

Comments _____
_____

8. Time required to read the chapter and complete this form: _____ minutes.

This educational activity has been provided by the American Nephrology Nurses' Association (ANNA) for 4.5 contact hours. ANNA is accredited as a provider of continuing nursing education (CNE) by the American Nurses Credentialing Center's Commission on Accreditation (ANCC-COA). ANNA is an approved provider of continuing education by the California Board of Registered Nursing, CEP 0910.

Pharmacotherapy of Transplantation

David Quan, PharmD

Chapter Contents

David Quan, PharmD

Functional deficits from end organ failure can be corrected by transplanting healthy organs from a cadaveric or live donor. Unless the recipient and donor are genetically identical, antigens on the donor organ will elicit an immunologic response by the host. This immunologic response, often referred to as rejection, if left untreated will lead to organ damage and ultimately graft loss. Drugs that suppress the immune system are given to the transplant recipient to prevent rejection of the transplanted organ.

Refinements in surgical technique and organ preservation have contributed to the success of solid organ transplantation. The development of immunosuppressive drugs have reduced the rates of acute rejection, and significantly increased graft and patient survival.

This chapter will focus on the pharmacotherapy of solid organ transplant recipients.

Immunology of Transplantation

The main function of the immune system is to discriminate self from non-self. The immune system protects the host from pathogens such as viruses, bacteria, and other organisms. The immune response first involves recognition of foreign material such as a pathogen, and then mounts an immune reaction to eliminate it. Allograft rejection is a natural response where the host immune system recognizes the transplanted organ as being non-self. Activation of the immune system causes a cytotoxic response resulting in organ damage.

The major histocompatibility complex (MHC) is a cluster of genes that controls the expression of human leukocyte antigens (HLA) on cells of the body. The HLA proteins are the primary antigens that aid the immune system in recognizing self from non-self.

T lymphocytes (T cells), B lymphocytes (B cells), natural killer (NK) cells, macrophages, and dendritic cells are the primary cellular components of the immune system. Macrophages engulf and destroy particles such as infectious organisms. In addition, macrophages interact with donor MHC molecules on the surface of the graft, processes them and presents (antigen presentation) to T cells for recognition. Binding via the T cell receptor (TCR), the T cells of the host will recognize the donor MHC molecules as foreign and initiate the rejection response. Helper T lymphocytes (T_H cells) release cytokines such as interleukin-2 (IL-2) and interferon-gamma (IFN-γ) to activate cytotoxic lymphocytes (T_C cells). Once activated, the T lymphocytes regulate the gene expression for IL-2 and IL-2 receptors. IL-2 stimulates T lymphocyte proliferation, and further recruitment and activation of other lymphocytes. In addition to IL-2, other cytokines such as IL-4 and IL-5 are involved with B lymphocyte activation. Production of IFN-γ and tumor necrosis factor-β (TNFβ) results in secondary macrophage activation. Activated T_C cells release inflammatory cytokines and lysozyme, which result in cell damage and allograft injury (Lake, Rossi, & Chodoff, 1997).

The types of grafts can be categorized in terms of the genetic disparity between the donor and recipient. Table 32-1 describes the nomenclature of different types of grafts in clinical transplantation.

Table 32-1
Graft Nomenclature

Type of graft	Description
*Allo*graft	From one person to another with different genetic makeup
*Auto*graft	Within the same person, from one part of the body to another (e.g. skin graft)
*Iso*graft	From one person to another with the same genetic makeup (e.g. identical twins)
*Xeno*graft	From one species to another species

Table 32-2
Types of Rejection

Type of rejection	Onset	Mediators
Hyperacute	Minutes to hours	Pre-formed anti-donor antibodies and complement
Accelerated	Days	Reactivation of sensitized T-lymphocytes
Acute	Days to weeks	Activation of T-lymphocytes
Chronic	Months to years	Unclear Antibodies, immune complexes, slow cellular reaction

The rejection response can be reduced if HLA histocompatibility tissue typing is performed. Serologic tests for the MHC class I (HLA-A, HLA-B, and HLA-C) and class II (HLA-DP, HLA-DQ and HLA-DR) antigens can be performed to match donor and recipient antigens. HLA matching of donor and recipients results in increased renal allograft survival (Takemoto, Terasaki, Cecka, Cho, & Gjertson, 1992). In renal transplant recipients, acute rejection is the most important predictor for chronic rejection. Chronic rejection has a detrimental effect on long-term graft survival, and is a leading cause of graft loss (Hariharan et al., 2000) (See Chapter 33 for further discussion of rejection). The type of rejection can be classified according to the time of onset after transplantation (Hutchinson, 1996). The types of rejection are summarized in Table 32-2.

The goal of immunosuppression is to control the immune response, while avoiding the complications of immunodeficiency, such as opportunistic infection and malignancy. Drugs that suppress the immune system can alter the immune response and decrease the risk of developing allograft rejection. The available immunosuppressive drugs used in solid organ transplantation are listed in Table 32-3.

Table 32-3
Available Immunosuppressive Drugs

Drug	Available Dosage Forms	Adult Dosing *	Administration
Antiproliferative Agents			
Azathioprine (Imuran)	50 mg tablets 100 mg/20 ml vials for injection	Initial dose: 3-5 mg/kg IV/PO QD Maintenance dose: 1-3 mg/kg/day	Take with food. Intravenous dose should be infused over 30-60 minutes.
Mycophenolate mofetil (CellCept)	250 mg capsules 500 mg tablets 200 mg/ml oral suspension 500 mg/20ml vials for injection	Renal: 1000 mg IV/PO BID Cardiac: 1500 mg IV/PO BID Hepatic: 1000 mg IV BID or 1500 mg PO BID Pediatric: 600 mg/m^2 PO BID	Intravenous dose should be administered over ≥ 2 hours. Take on an empty stomach. Patients with renal impairment (GFR <25 ml/min/1.73 m^2) should be carefully monitored for adverse events.
Mycophenolic acid (Myfortic)	180mg, 360 mg tablets	720 mg PO BID	Take on an empty stomach, or 1h before or 2h after meals. Do not crush, chew or cut tablets. Patients with renal impairment (GFR <25ml/min/1.73m^2) should be carefully monitored for adverse events.
Sirolimus (Rapamune)	1, 2 mg tablets 1 mg/ml oral solution (60ml bottle)	Initial dose: 6-15 mg Maintenance dose 2-5 mg PO QD	Oral solution should be refrigerated. Oral solution should be mixed with ≥ 2 oz. of water or orange juice in a glass or plastic container. Rinse container with ≥ 4 oz or water or orange juice and drink to ensure delivery of entire dose. Sirolimus should be given 4 hours *after* administration of cyclosporine.
Calcineurin inhibitors			
Cyclosporine (Sandimmune) Cyclosporine modified (Neoral, Gengraf)	Sandimmune: 25, 100 mg capsules 100 mg/ml oral solution (50ml bottle) 50 mg/5ml ampules for injection Neoral, Gengraf: 25, 100 mg capsules 100 mg/ml oral solution (50ml bottle)	Oral: 5-10 mg/kg/day Intravenous: 5-6 mg/kg/day (approximately 1/3 the oral dose)	Mix IV dose in 0.9% NS or D5W. Do not store in or infuse through PVC containing administration sets. Take dose in relation to meals consistently.
Tacrolimus (Prograf)	0.5, 1, 5 mg capsules 5 mg/1ml ampules for injection	Renal: 0.2 mg/kg/day (given as Q12h) Hepatic: 0.1-0.15 mg/kg/day (given as Q12h) Intravenous: 0.03-0.05 mg/kg/day as continuous infusion	Mix IV dose in 0.9% NS or D5W. Do not store in or infuse through PVC containing administration sets. Take dose in relation to meals consistently. Tacrolimus blood levels should be drawn just before the dose.

Table 32-3 (continued)
Available Immunosuppressive Drugs

Drug	Available Dosage Forms	Adult Dosing *	Administration
Antilymphocyte antibodies			
Antithymocyte globulin-equine (Atgam)	50 mg/5ml ampules for injection	Delay the onset of rejection: 15 mg/kg IV daily for up to 14 days Treatment of rejection: 10-15 mg/kg IV daily for up to 14 days	Mix in 0.45-0.9% NS or D5W 1/2 NS. Administer through 0.2 to 1 micron filter into a high-flow central vein. Infuse over at least 4 hours.
Antithymocyte globulin-rabbit (Thymoglobulin)	25 mg/5ml vials for injection	1.5 mg/kg IV daily for 7-14 days	Mix in 50-500 ml of 0.9% NS or D5W. Infuse through 0.22-micron filter. Infuse over at least 6 h for first dose, and 4h for subsequent doses. Administer into a high-flow vein.
Muromonab-CD3 (Orthoclone OKT3)	5 mg/5 ml ampules for injection	5 mg IV daily for 7-14 days	Dose should be drawn up into a syringe using a 0.2 or 0.22 micron low protein-binding filter. Give IV bolus (< 1 minute).
Interleukin-2 receptor antagonists			
Basiliximab (Simulect)	20 mg vials for injection	20 mg IV on day 0 and day 4 Pediatric (<35kg): 10 mg on day 4 & 4	May give as IV bolus. Mix in 50 ml of 0.9% normal saline or 5% dextrose water. Administer over 20-30 minutes. May give up to 2 h before surgery.
Daclizumab (Zenapax)	25 mg/5ml vials for injection	1 mg/kg IV on day 0, 14, 28, 42, & 56	Mix in 50 ml of 0.9% normal saline. Administer over 15 minutes. May give up to 24 h before surgery.
Corticosteroids			
Methylprednisolone (Medrol, SoluMedrol)	Medrol 2, 4, 8, 16, 32 mg tablets SoluMedrol 40, 125, 500, 1000 mg vials for injection	Taper will vary according to institutional immunosuppression protocols.	Intravenous methylprednisolone usually reserved for those unable to tolerate medications by the oral route. Infuse IV dose over several minutes. Large doses may be given in divided doses.
Prednisone (Deltasone, Orasone)	1, 2.5, 5, 10, 20, 50 mg tablets 1 mg/ml and 5 mg/ml oral solution	Taper will vary according to institutional immunosuppression protocols. Usual maintenance dose is 5 mg/day	Take with food to minimize GI upset. Large doses may be given in divided doses.

*Dose may vary according to transplant center specific immunosuppression protocols.

Table 32-4
Corticosteroid Equivalencies and Potencies

Glucocorticoid	Approximate equivalent dose (mg)	Relative antiinflammatory (glucocorticoid) potency	Relative mineralocorticoid potency
Hydrocortisone	25	1	2
Prednisone	5	4	1
Prednisolone	5	4	1
Methylprednisolone	4	5	0
Dexamethasone	0.75	20-30	0

Corticosteroids

The corticosteroids were the first immunosuppressive drugs used in solid organ transplantation, and remain a part of most immunosuppression regimens.

Pharmacology and Pharmacokinetics

Naturally occurring adrenocorticoid steroids possess both anti-inflammatory (glucocorticoid) and sodium-retaining (mineralocorticoid) activities. Hydrocortisone (cortisol) is typically used as replacement therapy for adrenocortical deficiency states (for example, "stress dose steroids"). Synthetic corticosteroids such as prednisone and prednisolone possess both glucocorticoid and mineralocorticoid activity. Other synthetic corticosteroids such as methylprednisolone and dexamethasone possess potent glucocorticoid activity, but are devoid of mineralocorticoid activity. These corticosteroids are used primarily for their anti-inflammatory effects. Table 32-4 summarizes the relative potencies of some of the commonly used corticosteroids (American Society of Health-System Pharmacists, 2004a).

Prednisone, prednisolone and methylprednisolone are the most commonly used corticosteroids in solid organ transplantation. The corticosteroids affect both cellular and humoral immunity. Corticosteroids block lymphocyte proliferation by inhibiting the synthesis of interleukin-1 (IL-1), IL-2 and IL-6 by macrophages and monocytes. The expression of TNF and IFN-γ is also inhibited. Corticosteroids also cause lympholysis by inducing apoptosis (programmed cell death) of immature T-lymphocytes. The corticosteroids have potent anti-inflammatory and nonspecific immunosuppressive effects on the immune system. While very effective, they are associated with many dose-related adverse effects. Acute adverse effects include psychosis, insomnia, and leukocytosis. Chronic adverse effects include hyperlipidemia, hypertension, edema, fat redistribution, osteopenia, and suppression of the adrenal axis. Please refer to Table 32-5 for a more complete list of adverse effects associated with corticosteroid use.

Dosing and Monitoring

The corticosteroids can be used to prevent or treat acute rejection. To prevent rejection, the first dose of intravenous methylprednisolone is often given intraoperatively, then tapered in a stepwise fashion to a usual maintenance dose of prednisone 5 mg/day (Woods et al., 1973). The dose and taper schedule will vary according to the type of organ(s) transplanted, concomitant medications and transplant center specific immunosuppression protocols. While corticosteroids are an integral part of many immunosuppression regimens, some transplant centers do not use corticosteroids at all (steroid avoidance) or taper the steroids off (steroid minimization) in select patient populations. Patients with osteopenia/osteoporosis or other endocrine disorders that may be exacerbated by the use of corticosteroids are potential candidates for these regimens.

High-dose intravenous methylprednisolone is often given for the treatment of acute rejection (Bell et al., 1971; Turcotte, Feduska, Carpenter, McDonald, & Bacon, 1972) (for example, 1 gram/day). The dose and duration will vary according to the type of organ(s) transplanted, severity of rejection, and transplant center-specific immunosuppression protocols. High-dose corticosteroids are effective in reversing acute rejection in greater than 80% of patients (Bell et al., 1971; Turcotte et al., 1972). For patients who do not respond to high-dose corticosteroids (steroid resistant rejection), treatment with an antilymphocyte antibody such as antithymocyte globulin or muromonab-CD3 may be necessary (refer to antilymphocyte antibody section).

Calcineurin Inhibitors

The calcineurin inhibitors (cyclosporine and tacrolimus) are the cornerstone of many immunosuppression regimens. Cyclosporine was isolated from a soil fungus in 1976, and found to have immunosuppressive activity (Borel, Feurer, Gubler, & Stahelin, 1976). Introduced into clinical practice in the early 1980s, cyclosporine revolutionized the field of transplantation by significantly reducing the incidence of acute allograft rejection and improving graft survival ("A randomized clinical trial of cyclosporine in cadaveric renal transplantation," 1983). While the calcineurin inhibitors are very effective in preventing acute rejection, they are not effective for the treatment of acute rejection.

Cyclosporine (Sandimmune®, Neoral®, Gengraf™)

Pharmacology and pharmacokinetics. Cyclosporine is a large cyclical peptide that binds to the intracellular protein, cyclophilin. The cyclosporine-cyclophilin complex inhibits calcineurin. Calcineurin is a serine phosphatase that is necessary for the transcription of the IL-2 gene. Inhibition of calcineurin leads to a decrease in the production and release of IL-2, resulting in selective inhibition of the activation and proliferation of T-lymphocytes.

Table 32- 5
Adverse Effects of Immunosuppressive Drugs

Calcineurin inhibitors: Cyclosporine

Nervous system	Gastrointestinal	Cardiovascular	Metabolic	Urogenital
Headache	Abdominal pain	Hypertension	Hyperkalemia	BUN increased
Paresthesia	Anorexia		Hyperlipidemia	Creatinine increased
Seizure	Diarrhea / vomiting		Hypomagnesemia	Renal dysfunction
Tremor	Gingival hyperplasia		LFT abnormalities	
	Hepatotoxicity			
	Nausea			
Dermatologic	**Hematologic**	**Other**		
Acne	Leukopenia	Edema		
Hirsutism	Lymphoma	Fever		
Pruritus		Opportunistic infections		
Rash		Malignancy		

Tacrolimus

Nervous system	Gastrointestinal	Cardiovascular	Metabolic	Urogenital
Headache	Diarrhea / vomiting	Hypertension	Hyperglycemia	BUN increased
Insomnia	Nausea	Myocardial hypertrophy	Hyperkalemia	Creatinine increased
Paresthesia	Anorexia		Hypomagnesemia	Renal dysfunction
Seizure			LFT abnormalities	
Tremor				
Dermatologic	**Hematologic**	**Other**		
Pruritus	Anemia	Abdominal pain		
Rash	Leukocytosis	Edema		
		Fever		
		Opportunistic infections		
		Malignancy		

Antiproliferative agents: Azathioprine

Hematologic	Gastrointestinal	Other		
Leukopenia	Diarrhea	Alopecia		
Thrombocytopenia	Hepatic veno-occlusive disease	Arthralgia / myalgia		
	Hepatotoxicity	Fever		
	Mucositis	Interstitial pneumonitis		
	Nausea / vomiting	Malignancy		
	Pancreatitis	Opportunistic infections		
		Rash		

Mycophenolate mofetil, mycophenolic acid

Hematologic	Gastrointestinal	Respiratory	Metabolic	Other
Anemia	Abdominal pain	Cough	Abnormal liver function tests	Anxiety
Leukopenia	Anorexia	Respiratory tract infections	Hypokalemia	Opportunistic infection
Neutropenia	Diarrhea	Sinusitis	Lactate dehydrogenase (elevated)	Rash
Thrombocytopenia	Dyspepsia			Sepsis
	Gastritis			Tachycardia
	Nausea / vomiting			Urinary tract infections
	Pancreatitis			Viral infections

Sirolimus

Hematologic	Metabolic	Dermatologic	Systemic	Other
Anemia	Hypercholesterolemia	Acne	Hypertension	Impaired wound healing
Leukopenia	Hypertriglyceridemia	Rash	Peripheral edema	Insomnia
Thrombocytopenia			Interstitial pneumonitis	Hepatic artery thrombosis
				Lymphocele formation
				Malignancy
				Opportunistic infections

Table 32- 5 (continued)
Adverse Effects of Immunosuppressive Drugs

Corticosteroids: **Methylprednisolone, prednisone**				
Neurologic Euphoria Hallucinations Insomnia Increased intracranial pressure Psychosis **Other** Cataracts Increased intraocular pressure Leukocytosis Opportunistic infection	**Gastrointestinal** Abdominal distension Gastritis Pancreatitis Peptic ulcer	**Musculoskeletal** Arthralgia Avascular necrosis of bone Muscle weakness Myopathy Osteopenia Osteoporosis Tendon rupture Vertebral compression fractures	**Cosmetic and Dermatologic** Acne Cushinoid syndrome Hirsutism Hyper- or hypopigmentation Fat redistribution "buffalo hump" Moon face Petechiae with ecchymoses Striae Sweating Thinning of skin	**Metabolic** Adrenal axis suppression Hyperglycemia Hyperlipidemia Impaired carbohydrate tolerance Impaired growth in children Impaired sexual maturation Impaired wound healing Increased appetite Menstrual irregularities Negative nitrogen balance Protein catabolism Sodium retention Water retention

Antilymphocyte antibodies: **Antithymocyte globulins**				
General Fever Chills Dizziness Hypersensitivity reactions Malaise Nausea Peripheral edema Pruritus	**Cardiovascular** Chest pain Hypertension Hypotension	**Hematologic** Leukopenia Serum sickness reaction Thrombocytopenia	**Others** Malignancy Phlebitis Opportunistic infections	

Muromonab-CD3				
Cytokine release syndrome Chills Diarrhea Dyspnea Fever Nausea Rigor Vomiting	**Central nervous system** Aseptic meningitis Dizziness Headache Tremor	**Cardiopulmonary** Chest pain Dyspnea Hypertension Hyperventilation Hypotension Tachycardia	**Hypersensitivity reactions** Anaphylactic reactions Angioedema Eosinophilia Immune complex deposition Serum sickness reaction Shock	**Other** Asthenia Edema Human antimouse antibody (HAMA) Malignancy Opportunistic infection Rash

Interleukin-2 receptor antagonists: **Basiliximab, Daclizumab**				
Hypersensitivity reactions	Injection site reactions	Gastrointestinal disorders	Opportunistic infections	

Cyclosporine is available in several formulations. The original formulation of cyclosporine (Sandimmune®) is formulated in olive oil, and requires bile for emulsification and absorption from the GI tract. Patients who have external biliary drainage, diarrhea, or cholestasis will have insufficient bile for absorption of cyclosporine from the GI tract. This can be overcome by giving the dose intravenously or refeeding bile with each dose of cyclosporine (Merion et al., 1989). The newer formulation, Neoral® is a microemulsion of cyclosporine, and other bioequivalent preparations (cyclosporine modified) are readily absorbed in the absence of bile. These newer formulations (Neoral® & Gengraf®) will be collectively referred to as cyclosporine modified, and the Sandimmune® formulation as cyclosporine. The cyclosporine-modified formulations are absorbed faster (shorter time to peak concentration), to a greater extent (greater area-under-the-concentration time curve and greater maximal concentration), and more consistently (decreased intrapatient and interpatient variability) than the original cyclosporine formulation (Kahan et al., 1994). Increased variability of cyclosporine pharmacokinetics is a risk factor for the development of rejection (Kahan, Welsh, & Rutzky, 1995). Because of the differences in the pharmacokinetic behavior between these formulations, they are not bioequivalent, and should not be used interchangeably. In addition, because of the pharmacokinetic limitations of the original formulation, it is no longer commonly used. Patients may be receiving Sandimmune® brand if they are on a stable regimen and wish to continue with this particular formulation. Most patients who are initiated on a cyclosporine-based regimen should be given a cyclosporine-modified formulation.

Cyclosporine is metabolized in the liver and GI tract via cytochrome P450-3A4 (CYP3A4). Cyclosporine is also a substrate for P-glycoprotein (PGP), the efflux pump found on the lumen of the intestines that drives drugs back into the intraluminal space, thus, decreasing absorption. There are many drugs that can interact with cyclosporine (see Table 32-6). The patient's medication list should be reviewed for potential drug interactions whenever new medications are prescribed.

Dosing and monitoring. Cyclosporine is used as part of an immunosuppression regimen, usually consisting of an antiproliferative agent (for example, mycophenolate, sirolimus, or azathioprine) and a corticosteroid to prevent rejection. The typical starting dose of cyclosporine or cyclosporine modified used to prevent allograft rejection is approximately 5 to 10 mg/kg/day given in divided doses twice a day (e.g. 2.5 to 5 mg/kg given every 12 hours).

An intravenous formulation of cyclosporine is available, but is infrequently used because most patients are able to tolerate medications by the oral route following transplantation. The dose is adjusted to achieve target cyclosporine whole blood concentrations of 150 to 400 ng/ml. This therapeutic range will depend on the type of cyclosporine assay used, as well as transplant center-specific immunosuppression protocols.

There are multiple ways of monitoring cyclosporine therapy. The most widely used method is to sample the trough (just before the dose) concentration. However, this method does not always correlate well with clinical outcomes such as acute rejection. Cyclosporine exposure, as measured by

Table 32-6
Drug Interactions with Cyclosporine, Tacrolimus, and Sirolimus

Drugs that inhibit cytochrome P450-3A4 and P-glycoprotein: (and increase cyclosporine/tacrolimus/sirolimus concentrations)	
Calcium channel blockers: Diltiazem, Nicardipine, Verapamil	*Antifungal agents:* Fluconazole, Itraconazole, Ketoconazole, Voriconazole
Antibiotics: Clarithromycin, Erythromycin	*HIV protease inhibitors:* Indinavir, Ritonavir
Others: Danazol, Grapefruits, grapefruit juice, Nefazodone	

Drugs that induce cytochrome P450-3A4 and P-glycoprotein: (and decrease cyclosporine/tacrolimus/sirolimus concentrations)	
Antibiotics: Rifabutin, Rifampin	*Anticonvulsants:* Carbamazepine, Phenobarbital, Phenytoin, Primidone
Others: St. John's Wort (Hypericum perforatum)	

* This is a partial list of drugs that can interact with cyclosporine, tacrolimus, or sirolimus.

the area-under-the concentration time curve (AUC_{0-12}) is a more sensitive method for predicting acute rejection. To determine the AUC_{0-12}, multiple blood samples must be taken during the 12-hour dosing interval, which is not only inconvenient, but also costly. Sparse sampling or abbreviated AUC algorithms are mathematical models that use a limited number of samples to estimate the AUC. Since most of the variability in absorption occurs in the first 4 hours after taking a dose of cyclosporine modified, the AUC_{0-4} is a sensitive marker for predicting acute rejection. The peak cyclosporine concentration at 2 hours (C_2 level) after administration of cyclosporine modified is an accurate marker for AUC_{0-4} and is correlated with improved outcomes such as decreased acute rejection (Levy et al., 2002a; Levy, Thervet, Lake, & Uchida, 2002b). To be within an acceptable margin of error, there is a 15-minute window before and after the 2-hour time point in which the sample can be taken. The precise timing of the sample dictates that this method of monitoring be undertaken in a controlled setting such as a hospital or transplant clinic.

Common dose-related adverse effects associated with cyclosporine therapy include renal dysfunction, neurotoxicity (headache, tremors, paresthesia and seizures) and hypertension. Other adverse effects include hyperlipidemia, gingival hyperplasia, hirsutism and opportunistic infections (see Table 32-5). Other drugs that are potentially nephrotoxic such as aminoglycosides (gentamicin, tobramycin), nonsteroidal anti-inflammatory agents (NSAIDS), and amphotericin B should be avoided in patients who are currently

Table 32-7
Tacrolimus Starting Dose and Target Levels

Type of patient	Initial oral dose*	Target whole blood trough concentration
Adult kidney transplant	0.2 mg/kg/day	month 1-3: 7-20 ng/ml month 4-12: 5-15 ng/ml
Adult liver transplant	0.1-0.15 mg/kg/day	month 1-12: 5-20 ng/ml
Pediatric liver transplant	0.15-0.2 mg/kg/day	month 1-12: 5-20 ng/ml

*In two divided doses, Q12h

receiving cyclosporine.

Neprotoxicity is a significant adverse effect of the calcineurin inhibitors, cyclosporine, and tacrolimus. The nephrotoxicity can be divided into acute and chronic effects. Acute nephrotoxicity typically manifests as a rise in the serum creatinine, hyperkalemia, and a decrease in urine output, particularly when cyclosporine or tacrolimus levels are above the normal therapeutic range (Olyaei, de Mattos, & Bennett, 1999). The calcineurin inhibitors acutely increase the renal vascular resistance, leading to a decrease in renal blood flow and glomerular filtration. Long-term calcineurin inhibitor use can result in cellular changes such as arteriolar hyalinosis, ischemic glomerulosclerosis, and interstitial fibrosis. Chronic allograft nephropathy is the result of incremental and cumulative damage to the nephrons, and is a leading cause of kidney transplant failure (Nankivell et al., 2003). Decreasing the cyclosporine or tacrolimus dose to target lower drug concentrations or the use of other nonnephrotoxic immunosuppressive drugs (e.g., sirolimus, basiliximab, daclizumab) are some ways of managing calcineurin inhibitor induced nephrotoxicity.

Tacrolimus (Prograf®)

Pharmacology and pharmacokinetics. Tacrolimus, previously known as FK506 is a macrolide antibiotic isolated from the soil bacterium, *Streptomyces tsukubaensis*, with immunosuppressive activity (Kino et al., 1987; Ochiai et al., 1987). Tacrolimus binds to the intracellular protein, FKBP-12. The tacrolimus-FKBP-12 complex inhibits calcineurin, resulting in decreased gene transcription of IL-2 and IFN-γ. The net effect is inhibition of T-lymphocyte activation and proliferation in a fashion similar to cyclosporine.

The first reported use of tacrolimus in humans was in 1989 for patients receiving an orthotopic liver transplant (Starzl et al., 1989). Tacrolimus has been shown to decrease the incidence of acute rejection in kidney, liver, heart, and lung transplantation (Griffith et al., 1994; Meiser et al., 1998; Miller, Mendez, Pirsch, & Jensik, 2000; Pirsch, Miller, Deierhoi, Vincenti, & Filo, 1997). Like cyclosporine, tacrolimus is metabolized by cytochrome P450-3A4, and is a substrate for PGP.

Dosing and monitoring. Tacrolimus is used in combination with corticosteroids to prevent allograft rejection. The starting dose of tacrolimus and target blood concentrations vary with the organ(s) transplanted, concomitant medica-

tions, and transplant center-specific immunosuppression protocols. Tacrolimus therapy is usually initiated at the doses listed in Table 32-7 and adjusted to achieve the desired target whole blood trough concentration. The target concentration may vary depending on the organ(s) transplanted, indication for transplantation (for example, autoimmune hepatitis vs. hepatitis C cirrhosis) as well as concomitant medications, medical conditions (e.g. renal dysfunction), and adverse effects. Many medications can interact with tacrolimus. Refer to Table 32-6 for a list of common drug-drug interactions with tacrolimus. Like cyclosporine, the use of other potentially nephrotoxic drugs such as the aminoglycosides, NSAIDS, and amphotericin B should be avoided. The most common adverse effects associated with tacrolimus include renal dysfunction, headaches, tremors, hypertension, hyperglycemia, and nausea (see Table 32-5).

Intravenous tacrolimus is available, and is usually reserved for patients unable to tolerate administration by the oral route. The initial dose of intravenous tacrolimus is approximately 0.03 to 0.5 mg/kg/day and is given as a continuous infusion. The intravenous formulation contains castor oil derivatives, which may result in anaphylactic reactions. The intravenous route of administration is infrequently used because most patients are usually able to tolerate medications by the oral route after transplant, and also because of an increased incidence of adverse effects with the intravenous preparation.

Antiproliferative Agents

The antiproliferative agents are a diverse group of drugs with a common mechanism of action. These drugs block the clonal expansion of lymphocytes in response to antigen stimulation. They are effective in preventing rejection, not for the treatment of rejection.

Azathioprine (Imuran®, Azasan®)

Pharmacology and pharmacokinetics. Azathioprine is a chemical analog of the naturally occurring purines, adenine, guanine, and hypoxanthine. Azathioprine is well absorbed following oral administration and is rapidly converted to the active form, 6-mercaptopurine (6-MP). 6-MP is a purine analog antimetabolite that interferes with nucleic acid metabolism, inhibiting RNA synthesis and ultimately cell division (American Society of Health-System Pharmacists, 2004b). Rapidly dividing cells such as T- and B-lymphocytes are very sensitive to the antiproliferative effects of azathioprine. Mercaptopurine is detoxified via the enzyme, xanthine oxidase, to 6-thiouric acid, which is excreted by the kidneys. Allopurinol, often used for the treatment of gout, is a potent inhibitor of xanthine oxidase. When allopurinol is given concomitantly with azathioprine, the pharmacologic effect and hematologic toxicities can be greatly magnified. Concurrent use of these two drugs should be avoided if possible. If it is necessary to use these two drugs together, one-third to one-fourth the dose of azathioprine should be used to minimize adverse effects.

Dosing and monitoring. Azathioprine is used as part of an immunosuppression regimen to prevent rejection. The typical starting dose of azathioprine is approximately 3-5 mg/kg/day beginning on the day of transplant (and in some cases 1-3 days before). An intravenous formulation of azathioprine is available, and is usually given at the same dose as the oral formulation. Reduction to a maintenance dose of 1-3 mg/kg/day is usually possible.

Myelosuppression is the most common dose-related adverse effect of azathioprine (Rossi, Schroeder, Hariharan, & First, 1993). Concomitant use of azathioprine with other myelosuppressive drugs such as trimethoprim/sulfamethoxazole (Septra®, Bactrim®), and angiotensin-converting enzyme inhibitors can potentiate leukopenia. Nonspecific cellular toxicities include alopecia, stomatitis, and esophagitis. Azathioprine also affects rapidly dividing cells in the gastrointestinal tract, resulting in nausea, vomiting, diarrhea, and abdominal cramping. Other adverse effects include hepatotoxicity, pancreatitis, myalgia, arthralgia, fever, and rash (see Table 32-5). There is an increased incidence of various types of skin cancers and lymphomas with long-term use of azathioprine.

Mycophenolate mofetil (CellCept®) and Mycophenolic acid (Myfortic®)

Pharmacology and pharmacokinetics. Mycophenolate mofetil (MMF) is an ester form of the active drug, mycophenolic acid (MPA). MMF is rapidly absorbed from the gastrointestinal tract and hydrolyzed to MPA. There is a secondary peak concentration of MPA probably the result of enterohepatic recirculation. MPA is metabolized to the inactive glucuronide (MPAG), which is excreted by the kidneys. In patients with severe renal dysfunction, MPAG can accumulate and be converted back to MPA. MPA selectively inhibits inosine monophosphate dehydrogenase (IMPDH), the key enzyme in the de novo pathway for purine biosynthesis. Inhibition of IMPDH by MPA blocks the synthesis of guanosine nucleotides necessary for the production of RNA and DNA. Rapidly dividing cells such as T- and B-lymphocytes are dependent on the de novo pathway for purine biosynthesis, and are particularly sensitive to the cytostatic effects of MPA. In addition, MPA also suppresses antibody formation by B-lymphocytes (Shaw et al., 1995). Mycophenolate mofetil has been shown to reduce the incidence of acute rejection in kidney, liver, and heart transplant recipients (Kobashigawa et al., 1998; Sollinger, 1995; Weisner Rabkin,& Klintmalm, 2001).

Mycophenolic acid (Myfortic®) is an enteric-coated formulation of MPA that is designed to release the drug in the small intestines. Mycophenolic acid 720 mg provides similar drug exposure as 1000 mg of mycophenolate mofetil, with similar efficacy and adverse effects (Salvadori et al., 2004).

Dosing and monitoring. Mycophenolate mofetil and mycophenolic acid are used as part of an immunosuppression regimen containing cyclosporine and a corticosteroid to prevent allograft rejection in renal, cardiac, and hepatic transplant recipients. The usual adult starting dose of mycophenolate mofetil is 1000 to 1500 mg orally twice a day. The usual dose of mycophenolic acid is 720 mg orally twice a day. The dose may be decreased due to adverse effects such as gastrointestinal intolerance, leukopenia, or thrombocytopenia. Other adverse effects include neutropenia, diarrhea, and viral infections (see Table 32-5). An intravenous preparation of mycophenolate mofetil is available, and is usually reserved for patients unable to tolerate administration by the oral route. Monitoring of MPA serum levels is not routinely performed. Aluminum and magnesium containing antacids will decrease the oral absorption of mycophenolate mofetil, and should not be administered at the same time. Bile acid binding resins such as cholestyramine can interfere with enterohepatic recirculation and decrease serum MPA levels.

Sirolimus (Rapamune®)

Pharmacology and pharmacokinetics. Sirolimus (previously known as rapamycin) is a macrolide antibiotic that was initially studied as an antifungal and antitumor agent, but was found to exhibit immunosuppressive effects (Sehgal, Baker, & Vezina, 1975; Sehgal, 2003).

Sirolimus binds to the same protein, FKBP-12, as tacrolimus. Instead of inhibiting calcineurin, the sirolimus-FKBP-12 complex inhibits the mammalian Target of Rapamycin (mTOR). Suppression of mTOR inhibits the IL-2 induced activation and proliferation of T-lymphocytes by preventing the progression from the G_1 to the S phase of the cell cycle (Saunders, Metcalfe, & Nicholson, 2001). Because sirolimus has a different mechanism of action (blocks the effects of IL-2) from that of the calcineurin inhibitors (blocks the production of IL-2), the combination act synergistically to prevent allograft rejection (Kahan et al., 1998).

Sirolimus is poorly absorbed from the gastrointestinal tract, and has a long elimination half-life of approximately 60 hours. Sirolimus is extensively metabolized in the liver and GI tract by cytochrome CYP3A4, and is a substrate for PGP. Many drugs are known to inhibit or induce the activity of CYP3A4 and PGP. Care should be exercised when starting a new drug known to inhibit or induce CYP3A4 or PGP. Please refer to Table 32-6 for a list of medications that may interact with sirolimus. Coadministration of cyclosporine, modified with sirolimus at the same time, results in increased sirolimus blood levels (see Dosing and Monitoring section) (Kaplan, Meier-Kriesche, Napoli, & Kahan, 1998).

Dosing and monitoring. Sirolimus is used to prevent allograft rejection as part of an immunosuppression regimen that contains cyclosporine and corticosteroids. Sirolimus has been shown to decrease the occurrence and severity of acute rejection in renal transplant recipients (Kahan, 2000; MacDonald, 2001). Sirolimus has also been shown to be effective in preventing acute rejection in liver, heart, and lung transplant recipients (Longoria et al., 1999; McAlister et al., 2000; Pham et al., 2002). In renal transplant recipients at low to moderate immunologic risk, sirolimus allows for cyclosporine to be withdrawn 2 to 4 months post-transplant, which can result in improved renal function and lower blood pressure (Johnson et al., 2001).

To rapidly achieve a therapeutic concentration, a loading dose of 6 to 15 mg (approximately 3 times the maintenance dose) can be given. A maintenance dose of 2 to 5 mg once a day is recommended for renal transplant recipients. For patients receiving cyclosporine as part of their immunosuppression regimen, it is recommended that sirolimus be given 4 hours after cyclosporine administration to minimize the effect of cyclosporine modified on increasing sirolimus blood levels. The target sirolimus trough level is 3 to 15 ng/ml in patients with an immunosuppression regimen using cyclosporine and sirolimus. The dose of sirolimus should be adjusted to achieve a target trough concentration within the range of 12 to 24 ng/ml in patients following withdrawal of cyclosporine (Rapamune [package insert], 2003). The combination of sirolimus with other immunosuppressive drugs and desired target concentrations will vary according to transplant center specific protocols.

Significant adverse effects associated with sirolimus include bone marrow suppression (leukopenia, thrombocytopenia), hyperlipidemia (hypercholesterolemia, hypertriglyceridemia), and impaired wound healing (see Table 32-5).

Antilymphocyte Antibodies

The antilymphocyte antibodies are potent immunosuppressive drugs that are typically reserved for the treatment of acute rejection or to prevent rejection in patients at high immunologic risk. Polyclonal antilymphocyte antibodies are nonspecific and can lead to significant side effects related to their reactivity against not only lymphocytes, but also nonwhite blood cells and other tissues. Unlike the polyclonal antilymphocyte antibodies preparations, monoclonal antilymphocyte antibodies are directed against specific targets on T-lymphocytes. In addition to specificity, monoclonal antibodies have high purity and reproducible biological activity.

Muromonab CD3 (Orthoclone OKT3®)

Pharmacology. Muromonab CD3 is a murine monoclonal antibody directed against the CD3 receptor on human T lymphocytes. Muromonab CD3 is an IgG immunoglobulin made by fusing mouse myeloma cells with splenic lymphocytes of mice immunized with a specific antigen. The resulting hybridoma possess the properties to produce an antibody to a specific epitope and the immortal nature of myeloma cells. This technique allows for large quantities of monoclonal antibodies to be produced. Muromonab CD3 was the first monoclonal antibody approved by the FDA for use in humans.

The CD3 receptor on T lymphocytes plays a key role in antigen recognition. Binding of muromonab CD3 to the CD3 receptor results in early activation followed by inhibition of T lymphocyte function. Muromonab CD3 blocks the generation and function of T lymphocytes. Following intravenous

administration, circulating CD3 positive cells are rapidly depleted within a matter of minutes. It is believed that the CD3 positive cells are opsonized and removed from circulation by the reticuloendothelial system in the liver and spleen. CD3 positive cells will slowly begin to reappear approximately 48 hours after discontinuing muromonab CD3 (Orthoclone OKT3 [package insert], 2003).

Dosing and monitoring. Muromonab CD3 can be used sequentially with other immunosuppressive drugs as part of an induction regimen to prevent rejection or to delay the addition of a calcineurin inhibitor such as cyclosporine (Norman et al., 1993; Opelz, 1995).

Muromonab CD3 is frequently used for the treatment of severe or steroid-resistant acute allograft rejection (Ortho Multicenter Transplant Study Group, 1985; Woodle et al., 1991). The recommended dose of muromonab CD3 for the treatment of acute allograft rejection is 5 mg as a daily intravenous bolus dose for 7 to 14 days. To decrease the severity of adverse effects, methylprednisolone, acetaminophen, and diphenhydramine can be given 1-4 hours prior to administration of muromonab CD3 (Chatenoud, Legendre, Ferran, Bach, & Kreis, 1991).

Periodic monitoring should be performed during therapy to ensure T-cell clearance (CD3 positive cells < 25 cells/mm^3) and/or plasma muromonab CD3 levels $\geq$ 800 ng/mL. Normalization of laboratory parameters, resolving of rejection on tissue biopsy, and return of organ function are clinical signs of efficacy. Since muromonab CD3 is an antibody derived from mice, it is immunogenic to humans. Approximately 50% of patients who receive a course of muromonab CD3 will develop IgG anti-OKT3 antibodies (human antimouse antibodies or HAMA). These neutralizing antibodies will decrease the effectiveness of muromonab CD3. Muromonab CD3 should not be given to patients with anti-mouse antibody titers in excess of 1:1000. Other antilymphocyte antibodies should be considered in this situation.

The early activation of T lymphocytes causes a release of cytokines (for example, TNF, IL-2, and IFN-γ), resulting in systemic manifestations collectively referred to as cytokine release syndrome (CRS) (Abramowicz et al., 1989; Thistlethwaite et al., 1988). CRS is typically associated with the first few doses and begins about 30 minutes after administration of muromonab CD3. The frequency and severity tends to diminish with subsequent doses. For the first few doses, emergency resuscitation equipment should be available and the patient be closely monitored for signs and symptoms of cytokine release syndrome. To decrease the risk of pulmonary edema, the patient should be assessed for signs of fluid overload prior to administration of muromonab CD3. Patients should have a clear chest radiograph and not weigh more than 3% above their minimum weight during the prior week (Orthoclone OKT3 [package insert], 2003). Muromonab-CD3 and the other antilymphocyte preparations increase the risk of cytomegalovirus infections and the development of lymphomas (Opelz & Dohler, 2004). Other adverse effects include headache, diarrhea, aseptic meningitis, and opportunistic infections (see Table 32-5).

Antithymocyte Globulin-Equine (Atgam®) and Antithymocyte Globulin-Rabbit (Thymoglobulin®)

Pharmacology. Antithymocyte globulin is gamma immune globulin (IgG) produced by immunizing horses or rabbits with human thymocytes (T lymphocytes). The animals produce antibodies against antigens expressed on the human T-lymphocytes. The antibodies are then collected and purified. The antithymocyte globulins suppress the immune response by depleting T-lymphocytes from circulation and modulating the T-lymphocyte activation, homing, and cytotoxic activities.

Antithymocyte globulins contain a mixture of antibodies that are specific for a number of surface markers, such as CD2, CD3, CD4, CD8, CD11a, CD25, etc., as well as some non-lymphoid cells (for example, erythrocytes, platelets) (Bonnefoy-Berard, Vincent, & Revillard, 1991; Rebellato, Gross, Verbanac, & Thomas, 1994). Within a day, there is a rapid depletion of circulating lymphocytes, the result of complement-mediated opsonization and lysis.

Dosing and monitoring. Antithymocyte globulin can be used as part of an induction regimen to delay or prevent acute rejection, or for the treatment of acute rejection (Brennan et al., 1999; Mariat et al., 1998). The decision to use induction therapy is based on the patient's medical needs and cost considerations. Induction therapy is usually reserved for patients at high immunologic risk of rejection (e.g., African-Americans, sensitized patients, retransplant recipients, or patients with delayed graft function [DGF]). Patients on corticosteroid-sparing or calcineurin inhibitor-sparing immunosuppression regimens can also be given induction therapy. The usual dose of antithymocyte globulin-rabbit (Thymoglobulin®) is 1 to 1.5 mg/kg administered daily for 7 to 14 days, while the dose of antithymocyte globulin-equine (Atgam®) is 10 to 30 mg/kg administered daily for 7 to 14 days. Corticosteroids, acetaminophen, and a histamine-1 blocker are usually given to minimize infusion-related adverse effects. Other drugs such as a calcineurin inhibitor and an antiproliferative agent are also given as part of the immunosuppression regimen. The dosing regimen will vary according to transplant center specific protocols. Fever, chills, rigors, opportunistic infections, malignancies, hypotension, and hypersensitivity reactions can occur with antithymocyte globulins (see Table 32-5). Severe thrombocytopenia and leukopenia may necessitate dose reduction.

Interleukin-2 (IL-2) Receptor Antagonists

The interleukin-2 receptor antagonist (IL-2Ra) is the newest class for drugs approved by the FDA for use in transplantation. The IL-2Ras are IgG monoclonal antibodies produced by recombinant DNA technology. The active binding portion (variable domain) of a mouse antibody directed against the alfa-subunit of the IL-2 receptor (Tac or CD25) is fused to the constant domain of a human IgG antibody. The rationale for combining a mouse antibody with a human antibody is to increase the length of time it remains in the body, and to decrease the antigenicity of the new molecule (Queen et al., 1989). Basiliximab and daclizumab are two IL-2 receptor antagonists currently available for the prevention of acute rejection.

Basiliximab (Simulect®) and Daclizumab (Zenapax®)

Pharmacology and pharmacokinetics. Basiliximab is a chimeric (70% human/30% murine), while daclizumab is a humanized (90% human/10% murine) monoclonal (IgG) antibody. Both basiliximab and daclizumab bind to the α-subunit of the interleukin-2 receptor found on the surface of activated T-lymphocytes. The highly specific binding of these drugs to the IL-2 receptor prevents IL-2 from binding to the receptor, thus preventing the IL-2 mediated activation of lymphocytes. Basiliximab exhibits a long elimination half-life of approximately 7 days. The duration of receptor blockage ranges from 36 to 59 days after administration of basiliximab (Simulect [package insert], 2002). Daclizumab also exhibits a long elimination half-life of approximately 20 days. At the recommended dosing regimen with daclizumab, the IL-2 receptor is blocked for up to 120 days (Zenapax [package insert], 2002). When used as part of an immunosuppression regimen, basiliximab and daclizumab have been shown to reduce the incidence of acute rejection in renal transplant recipients (Nashan et al., 1997; Vincenti et al., 1998).

Dosing and monitoring. Basiliximab or daclizumab are used as part of an immunosuppression regimen that contains cyclosporine and corticosteroids to prevent acute rejection. Basiliximab is given as a two-dose regimen of 20 mg each infused intravenously over 30 minutes. The first 20 mg dose is given 2 hours prior to transplant and the second dose is given on post-operative day 4. The standard dosing regimen of daclizumab consists of five 1 mg/kg doses given at 14-day intervals. The first dose can be given up to 24 hours prior to transplant. Each dose of daclizumab should be given as a short infusion over 15 minutes. The use of IL-2Ras in combination with other immunosuppressive drugs vary according to transplant center-specific protocols. Immunosuppression regimens of 2 doses of daclizumab have been used instead of 5 (Deierhoi, 2000).

Therapeutic blood level monitoring is not necessary for these drugs. Both basiliximab and daclizumab are generally well tolerated (see Table 32-5). Because these drugs contain part mouse antibody, hypersensitivity reactions such as anaphylaxis can occur. Patients should be monitored appropriately and have medications to treat hypersensitivity reactions readily available.

Other Medications

Opportunistic infections can cause significant morbidity and mortality in an immunocompromised patient. Antibiotics can be given for the treatment of an active infection or to prevent an infection (prophylaxis). Cytomegalovirus (CMV), herpes simplex virus (HSV), mucocutaneous candidiasis (thrush), and *pneumocystis carinii* pneumonia (PCP) are common opportunistic infections seen in solid organ transplant recipients. Antibiotic prophylaxis is usually given during the first few months following transplantation when immunosuppression is usually the most intense. Common antibiotics used in the transplant recipient are listed in Table 32-8. The antibiotic regimens will vary according to the organ(s) transplanted and transplant center-specific protocols.

Other medications include using aspirin to prevent arterial thrombosis and a proton pump inhibitor (PPI) or a hista-

Table 32-8
Other Medications Commonly Used in Transplantation

Drug:	Purpose:	Common dose:	Side effects:
Antivirals: Acyclovir (Zovirax) Ganciclovir (Cytovene) Valganciclovir (Valcyte)	Prevent cytomegalovirus (CMV), herpes simplex virus (HSV), varicella zoster virus (VZV) infections	Acyclovir 800 mg PO QID* Ganciclovir 1000 mg PO TID* Valganciclovir 900mg PO QD*	Acyclovir: Headache, crystaluria Ganciclovir/Valganciclovir: Leukopenia, thrombocytopenia
Antifungals: Clotrimazole (Mycelex) Fluconazole (Diflucan) Nystatin (Mycostatin, Nilstat)	Prevent mucocutaneous candidiasis (thrush)	Clotrimazole 10 mg QID-5x/day Fluconazole 100-200 mg PO QD* Nystatin 10 ml swish/swallow QID	Clotrimazole and fluconazole may inhibit the metabolism of cyclosporine, sirolimus, and tacrolimus
Trimethoprim/sulfamethoxazole (Bactrim, Septra) Dapsone Inhaled pentamidine (Nebupent)	Prevent *Pneumocystis carinii* pneumonia (PCP)	Trimethoprim/sulfamethoxazole: One single- or double-strength tablet PO every other day*. Dosing regimens may vary. Dapsone 50-100 mg PO QD Inhaled pentamidine 300 mg Q Month	Trimethoprim/sulfamethoxazole: Rash Leukopenia Thrombocytopenia Dapsone: Hemolytic anemia Inhaled pentamidine: Coughing
Aspirin	Prevent arterial (renal, pancreatic, hepatic) thrombosis	Aspirin 81 to 325 mg PO QD	Bleeding Stomach upset
Proton pump inhibitor: Lansoprazole (Prevacid) Omeprazole (Prilosec) Pantoprazole (Protonix) Rabeprazole (Aciphex) *H_2 blocker:* Famotidine (Pepcid) Ranitidine (Zantac)	Prevent stress gastritis	*Proton pump inhibitor:* Lansoprazole 15-30 mg/day Omeprazole 20-40 mg/day Pantoprazole 40 mg/day Rabeprazole 20 mg/day *H_2 blocker:* Famotidine 20-40 mg/day* Ranitidine 150-300 mg/day*	*Proton pump inhibitor:* Headache Diarrhea *H_2 blocker:* Cimetidine may inhibit the metabolism of cyclosporine, sirolimus, and tacrolimus

*Dose adjustment may be necessary in patients with renal dysfunction

mine-2 receptor antagonist (H2 blocker) to prevent stress gastritis. In addition, other medications may need to be initiated to manage other immunosuppressive drug-related adverse effects such as hypertension, diabetes, and hyperlipidemia. Opportunistic infections and other complications of transplantation are discussed in greater detail in Chapter 33, Preventing and Managing Complications.

Patients should be cautioned about self-medication with over-the-counter products. Many drugs are known to interact with immunosuppressive medications or may exacerbate other medical conditions. The patient should consult with a healthcare provider about the potential for any drug-drug or drug-disease interactions when starting a new medication. The use of herbal remedies or herbal products such as St. John's wort or echinacea should be avoided in this patient population (Barone, Gurley, Ketel, & Abul-Ezz, 2001; Breidenbach et al., 2000; Wilasrusmee et al., 2002). The use of immunosuppressive drugs may decrease the efficacy of vaccines. The use of live vaccines such as measles, mumps, rubella, oral polio, BCG, yellow fever, typhoid, and varicella should be avoided. Vaccination with a live vaccine can result in disseminated disease in immunosuppressed patients.

Clinical Use of Drugs

Immunosuppression has evolved from two-drug regimens (prednisone and azathioprine) in the early days of transplantation to the present with numerous complex regimens that allow for individualization of drug therapy based upon patient-specific conditions. The most commonly used immunosuppression combination in solid organ transplantation is a triple regimen, consisting of prednisone, an antiproliferative agent, and a calcineurin inhibitor. This combination maximizes immunosuppression, while allowing lower doses to be used in an attempt to minimize dose-related adverse effects (Simmons et al., 1985). Table 32-9 lists the typical medication regimen used in a post-transplant patient.

The choice of one drug over another may be influenced by the presence of other medical conditions. For example, an immunosuppression regimen that contains cyclosporine may be preferred over tacrolimus in a patient with a history of diabetes. If hyperglycemia develops in a patient due to tacrolimus, he or she can be converted over to a cyclosporine-based regimen (Butani & Makker, 2000; Pirsch et al., 1997). Similarly, a patient who develops hyperlipidemia on a cyclosporine-based regimen can be converted over to a tacrolimus-based regimen (Kohnle et al., 2000). Some immunosuppression regimens that use antibodies are aimed at avoidance of calcineurin inhibitors or corticosteroids in an effort to minimize nephrotoxicity and bone-related disorders respectively (Sarwal et al., 2001; Vincenti et al., 2001a; Vincenti et al., 2001b).

Monoclonal and polyclonal antibody preparations can be used as part of an "induction" immunosuppression regimen (that is, drugs that are prophylactically administered during the immediate post-transplant period to prevent acute rejection). Induction regimens are usually reserved for patients at high risk of rejection (for example, African-American, sensitized patients, retransplant recipients, and patients with delayed graft function), or in whom therapy with a calcineurin inhibitor will be delayed. The choice of a monoclonal versus polyclonal antibody, dose, other immunosuppressive drugs, and duration will vary according to transplant center-specific protocols. Following induction therapy, patients will be placed on a life-long maintenance regimen to prevent allograft rejection.

Drug Interactions

Many factors can influence the blood levels of various immunosuppressive drugs. Transplant recipients take multiple drugs to prevent allograft rejection and opportunistic infections. These patients often require other medications to treat underlying illnesses or concurrent medical conditions. Nurses can play a vital role in preventing medication-related adverse events by identifying drugs that may interact with transplant-related medications before administration to the patient. If a potential interaction is identified, the prescriber should be promptly notified, so an appropriate course of action can be taken. An alternative medication that will not interact with the immunosuppressive drugs should be first considered. If this is not feasible, then the blood concentration of the immunosuppressive drugs should be closely monitored and the dose adjusted to maintain levels within the desired therapeutic range. Often, clinicians will empirically

Table 32-9
Typical Post-Transplant Drug Regimen

Drug	Use
Tacrolimus	Anti-rejection
Mycophenolate mofetil	Anti-rejection
Prednisone	Anti-rejection
Acyclovir	CMV prophylaxis
Trimethoprim/sulfamethoxazole	PCP, UTI prophylaxis
Clotrimazole troches	Thrush prophylaxis
Omeprazole	Prevent stress ulcer

alter the dose of the medication in anticipation of a known drug-drug interaction. For example, the dose of tacrolimus should be decreased when therapy with fluconazole is started. Patients should also be instructed to check with their pharmacist or transplant clinic whenever a new medication is prescribed.

Delayed Graft Function

Delayed graft function (DGF), typically defined as the need for dialysis post-transplant, is associated with decreased graft survival (Shoskes & Cecka, 1998). The use of nephrotoxic drugs such as the calcineurin inhibitors, NSAIDS (such as ibuprofen), gentamicin, and amphotericin B should be avoided in this setting. Induction therapy with polyclonal or monoclonal antilymphocyte antibody (antithymocyte globulin, OKT3) can be used to delay the use of calcineurin inhibitors until renal function improves (Norman et al., 1993; Guttmann & Flemming, 1997). Interleukin-2 receptor antagonists such as basiliximab and daclizumab have also been used in this setting (Bumgardner, Ramos, Lin, & Vincenti, 2001; Gonwa et al., 2002).

Medication Compliance

Medication noncompliance is a complex problem and a major barrier to the success of solid organ transplantation. It has been reported that up to 55% of patients are not compliant with their medication regimen (Vasquez, Tanzi, Benedetti, & Pollak, 2003). Patient noncompliance is a major cause of chronic rejection and late allograft loss in renal transplant recipients (Didlake, Dreyfus, Kerman, Van Buren, & Kahan, 1988).

Noncompliance can range from skipping doses, stopping medications too soon, taking more or less than the amount prescribed, taking the doses erratically or at improper times, to not taking the medication at all. Factors that are associated with medication noncompliance include polypharmacy, a complex medication regimen, poor self-esteem, cultural beliefs, adolescent age, illiteracy, occurrence of adverse effects, fear, anxiety, the patient's perception of health beliefs, depression, and the lack of adequate financial or social support (Jindel, Joseph, Morris, Santella, & Baines, 2003; Loghman-Adham, 2003).

Patients and their caregivers should be educated during the transplant evaluation process about the need for life-long immunosuppression, common adverse effects, the importance of routine laboratory monitoring, and the costs associated with the transplant medications. Patients should be encouraged to attend a local support group to share their pre- and post-transplant experiences with others. In the post-transplant setting, the multidisciplinary transplant team plays a vital role in educating patients and their caregiver(s) about the proper way to take their medications, adherence to the medication schedule, and the importance of compliance with the medication regimen.

Some strategies that can help improve medication compliance include simplifying the medication regimen, using reminder systems such as medication schedules or medication boxes, minimizing financial impact to the patient, and offering support groups or mentoring programs.

Conclusion

The success of organ transplantation is dependent upon the use of drugs to suppress the recipient's immune response, while avoiding complications associated with immunodeficiency such as opportunistic infections and malignancies. Following organ transplantation, patients will require lifelong immunosuppression to prevent allograft rejection. The clinical use of immunosuppressive drugs is complex. Many of the immunosuppressive drugs have a narrow therapeutic range. Drug levels below this range are associated with allograft rejection, while drug levels above this range are associated with adverse effects. Other drugs and medical conditions may not only affect the disposition, but also the tolerability of immunosuppressive drugs. The cost associated with the acquisition of medications and drug monitoring can exceed $15,000 per year. Despite these enormous costs, renal transplantation has been shown to be more cost effective than long-term dialysis. It is imperative that health care practitioners taking care of transplant recipients be aware of the many issues surrounding transplant medications to ensure optimal patient outcomes.

References

A randomized clinical trial of cyclosporine in cadaveric renal transplantation. (1983). *New England Journal of Medicine, 309*(14), 809-815.

Abramowicz, D., Schandene, L., Goldman, M., Crusiaux, A., Vereerstraeten, P., & De Pauw, L., et al. (1989). Release of tumor necrosis factor, interleukin-2, and gamma-interferon in serum after injection of OKT3 monoclonal antibody in kidney transplant recipients. *Transplantation, 47*(4), 606-608.

American Society of Health-System Pharmacists. (2004a). Corticosteroids. In G.K. McEvoy (Ed.), *AHFS drug information 2004* (pp. 2886-2898). Bethesda, MD: Author.

American Society of Health-System Pharmacists. (2004b). Azathioprine. In G.K. McEvoy (Ed.), *AHFS drug information 2004* (pp. 3621-3624). Bethesda, MD: Author.

Barone, G.W., Gurley, B.J., Ketel, B.L., & Abul-Ezz, S.R. (2001). Herbal supplements: A potential for drug interactions in transplant recipients. *Transplantation, 71*(2), 239-241.

Bell, P.R., Briggs, J.D., Calman, K.C., Paton, A.M., Wood, R.F., & Macpherson, S.G., et al. (1971). Reversal of acute clinical and experimental organ rejection using large doses of intravenous prednisolone. *Lancet, 1*(7705), 876-880.

Bonnefoy-Berard, N., Vincent, C., & Revillard, J.P. (1991). Antibodies against functional leukocyte surface molecules in polyclonal anti-lymphocyte and antithymocyte globulins. *Transplantation, 51*(3), 669-673.

Borel, J.F., Feurer, C., Gubler, H.U., & Stahelin, H. (1976). Biological effects of cyclosporin A: A new antilymphocytic agent. *Agents Actions, 6*(4), 468-475.

Breidenbach, T., Kliem, V., Burg, M., Radermacher, J., Hoffmann, M.W., & Klempnauer, J. (2000). Profound drop of cyclosporin A whole blood trough levels caused by St. John's wort (Hypericum perforatum). *Transplantation, 69*(10), 2229-2230.

Brennan, D.C., Flavin, K., Lowell, J.A., Howard, T.K., Shenoy, S., & Burgess, S., et al. (1999). A randomized, double-blinded comparison of Thymoglobulin versus Atgam for induction immunosuppressive therapy in adult renal transplant recipients. *Transplantation, 67*(7), 1011-1018.

Bumgardner, G.L., Ramos, E., Lin, A., & Vincenti, F. (2001). Daclizumab (humanized anti-IL2Ralpha mAb) prophylaxis for prevention of acute rejection in renal transplant recipients with delayed graft function. *Transplantation, 72*(4), 642-647.

Butani, L., & Makker, S.P. (2000). Conversion from tacrolimus to neoral for postrenal transplant diabetes. *Pediatric Nephrology, 15*(3-4), 176-178.

Chatenoud, L., Legendre, C., Ferran, C., Bach, J.F., & Kreis, H. (1991). Corticosteroid inhibition of the OKT3-induced cytokine-related syndrome: Dosage and kinetics prerequisites. *Transplantation, 51*(2), 334-338.

Deierhoi, M. (2000). Two-dose daclizumab in cadaveric kidney transplant recipients [Abstract]. Transplantation, 69, S260.

Didlake, R.H., Dreyfus, K., Kerman, R.H., Van Buren, C.T., & Kahan, B.D. (1988). Patient noncompliance: a major cause of late graft failure in cyclosporine-treated renal transplants. *Transplant Proceedings, 20*(3 Suppl 3), 63-69.

Gonwa, T.A., Mai, M.L., Smith, L.B., Levy, M.F., Goldstein, R.M., & Klintmalm, G.B. (2002). Immunosuppression for delayed or slow graft function in primary cadaveric renal transplantation: use of low dose tacrolimus therapy with post-operative administration of anti-CD25 monoclonal antibody. *Clinical Transplantation, 16*(2), 144-149.

Griffith, B.P., Bando K., & Hardesty R.L., Armitage, J.M., Keenan, R.J., Pham, S.M. et al. (1994). A prospective randomized trial of FK506 versus cyclosporine after human pulmonary transplantation. *Transplantation, 57*, 848-852.

Guttmann, R.D., & Flemming, C. (1997). Sequential biological immunosuppression. Induction therapy with rabbit antithymocyte globulin. *Clinical Transplantation, 11*(3), 185-192.

Hariharan, S., Johnson, C.P., Bresnahan, B.A., Taranto, S.E., McIntosh, M.J., & Stablein, D. (2000). Improved graft survival after renal transplantation in the United States, 1988 to 1996. *New England Journal of Medicine, 342*(9), 605-612.

Hutchinson, I. (1996). Transplantation and rejection. In B.J. Roitt I, & Male D. (Ed.), Immunology (pp. 26.21-26.13). New York: Mosby.

Jindel, R.M., Joseph, J.T., Morris, M.C., Santella, R.N., & Baines, L.S. (2003). Noncompliance after kidney transplantation: A systematic review. *Transplantation Proceedings, 35*(8), 2868-2872.

Johnson, R.W., Kreis, H., Oberbauer, R., Brattstrom, C., Claesson, K., & Eris, J. (2001). Sirolimus allows early cyclosporine withdrawal in renal transplantation, resulting in improved renal function and lower blood pressure. *Transplantation, 72*(5), 777-786.

Kahan, B.D. (2000). Efficacy of sirolimus compared with azathioprine for reduction of acute renal allograft rejection: a randomized multicenter study. The Rapamune US Study Group. *Lancet, 356*(9225), 194-202.

Kahan, B.D., Dunn, J., Fitts, C., Van Buren, D., Wombolt, D., & Pollak, R., et al. (1994). The Neoral formulation: Improved correlation between cyclosporine trough levels and exposure in stable renal transplant recipients. *Transplantation Proceedings, 26*(5), 2940-2943.

Kahan, B.D., Podbielski, J., Napoli, K.L., Katz, S.M., Meier-Kriesche, H.U., & Van Buren, C.T. (1998). Immunosuppressive effects and safety of a sirolimus/cyclosporine combination regimen for renal transplantation. *Transplantation, 66*(8), 1040-1046.

Kahan, B.D., Welsh, M., & Rutzky, L.P. (1995). Challenges in cyclosporine therapy: The role of therapeutic monitoring by area under the curve monitoring. *Therapeutic Drug Monitoring 17*(6), 621-624.

Kaplan, B., Meier-Kriesche, H.U., Napoli, K.L., & Kahan, B.D. (1998). The effects of relative timing of sirolimus and cyclosporine microemulsion formulation coadministration on the pharmacokinetics of each agent. *Clinical Pharmacologic Therapy, 63*(1), 48-53.

Kino, T., Hatanaka, H., Miyata, S., Inamura, N., Nishiyama, M., & Yajima, T., et al. (1987). FK-506, a novel immunosuppressant isolated from a Streptomyces. II. Immunosuppressive effect of FK-506 in vitro. *Journal of Antibiotics (Tokyo), 40*(9), 1256-1265.

Kobashigawa J, Miller L, & Renlund D, et al. (1998). A randomized active-controlled trial of mycophenolate mofetil in heart transplant recipients. *Transplantation, 66*, 507-515.

Kohnle, M., Zimmermann, U., Lutkes, P., Albrecht, K.H., Philipp, T., & Heemann, U. (2000). Conversion from cyclosporine A to tacrolimus after kidney transplantation due to hyperlipidemia. *Transplantation International, 13* Suppl 1, S345-348.

Lake, K., Rossi S.J., & Chodoff L. (1997). Solid organ transplantation. In American Society of Health-Systems Pharmacists (Ed.), *Concepts in immunology and immunotherapeutics* (3rd ed.). Bethesda: American Society of Health-System Pharmacists.

Levy, G., Burra, P., Cavallari, A., Duvoux, C., Lake, J., & Mayer, A.D., et al. (2002a). Improved clinical outcomes for liver transplant recipients using cyclosporine monitoring based on 2-hr post-dose levels (C2). *Transplantation, 73*(6), 953-959.

Levy, G., Thervet, E., Lake, J., & Uchida, K. (2002b). Patient management by Neoral C(2) monitoring: An international consensus statement. *Transplantation, 73*(9 Suppl), S12-18.

Loghman-Adham, M. (2003). Medication noncompliance in patients with chronic disease: Issues in dialysis and renal transplantation. *American Journal of Managed Care, 9*(2), 155-171.

Longoria, J., Roberts, R.F., Marboe, C.C., Stouch, B.C., Starnes, V.A., & Barr, M.L. (1999). Sirolimus (rapamycin) potentiates cyclosporine in prevention of acute lung rejection. *Journal of Thoracic Cardiovascular Surgery, 117*(4), 714-718.

MacDonald, A.S. (2001). A worldwide, phase III, randomized, controlled, safety and efficacy study of a sirolimus/cyclosporine regimen for prevention of acute rejection in recipients of primary mismatched renal allografts. *Transplantation, 71*(2), 271-280.

Mariat, C., Alamartine, E., Diab, N., de Filippis, J.P., Laurent, B., & Berthoux, F. (1998). A randomized prospective study comparing low-dose OKT3 to low-dose ATG for the treatment of acute steroid-resistant rejection episodes in kidney transplant recipients. *Transplantation International, 11*(3), 231-236.

McAlister, V.C., Gao, Z., Peltekian, K., Domingues, J., Mahalati, K., & MacDonald, A.S. (2000). Sirolimus-tacrolimus combination immunosuppression. *Lancet, 355*, 376-377.

Meiser B.M., Uberfuhr P., & Fuchs A., Schmidt, D., Pfeiffer, M., Paulus, D., et al. (1998). Single-center randomized trial comparing tacrolimus (FK506) and cyclosporine in the prevention of acute myocardial rejection. *Journal of Heart Lung Transplant, 17*, 782-788.

Merion, R.M., Gorski, D.H., Burtch, G.D., Turcotte, J.G., Colletti, L.M., & Campbell, D.A., Jr. (1989). Bile refeeding after liver transplantation and avoidance of intravenous cyclosporine. *Surgery, 106*(4), 604-609, 610.

Miller, J., Mendez, R., Pirsch, J.D., & Jensik, S.C. (2000). Safety and efficacy of tacrolimus in combination with mycophenolate mofetil (MMF) in cadaveric renal transplant recipients. FK506/MMF Dose-Ranging Kidney Transplant Study Group. *Transplantation, 69*(5), 875-880.

Nankivell, B.J., Borrows, R.J., Fung, C.L., O'Connell, P.J., Allen, R.D., & Chapman, J.R. (2003). The natural history of chronic allograft nephropathy. *New England Journal of Medicine, 349*(24), 2326-2333.

Nashan, B., Moore, R., Amlot, P., Schmidt, A.G., Abeywickrama, K., & Soulillou, J.P. (1997). Randomized trial of basiliximab versus placebo for control of acute cellular rejection in renal allograft recipients. CHIB 201 International Study Group. *Lancet, 350*, 1193-1198.

Norman, D.J., Kahana, L., Stuart, F.P., Jr., Thistlethwaite, J.R., Jr., Shield, C.F., 3rd, & Monaco, A., et al. (1993). A randomized clinical trial of induction therapy with OKT3 in kidney transplantation. *Transplantation, 55*(1), 44-50.

Ochiai, T., Nakajima, K., Nagata, M., Suzuki, T., Asano, T., & Uematsu, T., et al. (1987). Effect of a new immunosuppressive agent, FK 506, on heterotopic cardiac allotransplantation in the rat. *Transplantation Proceedings, 19*(1 Pt 2), 1284-1286.

Olyaei, A.J., de Mattos, A.M., & Bennett, W.M. (1999). Immunosuppressant-induced nephropathy: Pathophysiology, incidence and management. *Drug Safety, 21*(6), 471-488.

Opelz, G. (1995). Efficacy of rejection prophylaxis with OKT3 in renal transplantation. Collaborative Transplant Study. *Transplantation, 60*(11), 1220-1224.

Opelz, G., & Dohler, B. (2004). Lymphomas after solid organ transplantation: a collaborative transplant study report. *American Journal of Transplantation, 4*(2), 222-230.

Ortho Multicenter Transplant Study Group. (1985). A randomized clinical trial of OKT3 monoclonal antibody for acute rejection of cadaveric renal transplants. *New England Journal of Medicine, 313*(6), 337-342.

Orthoclone OKT3 [package insert]. (2003). Raritan, NJ: Ortho Biotech Products, L.P.

Pham, S.M., Qi, X.S., Mallon, S.M., Kaplon, R.J., Bauerlein, E.J., & Katariya, K., et al. (2002). Sirolimus and tacrolimus in clinical cardiac transplantation. *Transplantation Proceedings, 34*(5), 1839-1842.

Pirsch, J.D., Miller, J., Deierhoi, M.H., Vincenti, F., & Filo, R.S. (1997). A comparison of tacrolimus (FK506) and cyclosporine for immunosuppression after cadaveric renal transplantation. FK506 Kidney Transplant Study Group. Transplantation, 63(7), 977-983.

Queen, C., Schneider, W.P., Selick, H.E., Payne, P.W., Landolfi, N.F., & Duncan, J.F., et al. (1989). A humanized antibody that binds to the interleukin 2 receptor. *Proceedings of the National Academy of Science, 86*(24), 10029-10033.

Rapamune. (2003). Package insert. Philadelphia, PA: Wyeth Laboratories; 2003.

Rebellato, L. M., Gross, U., Verbanac, K. M., & Thomas, J. M. (1994). A comprehensive definition of the major antibody specificities in polyclonal rabbit antithymocyte globulin. *Transplantation, 57*(5), 685-694.

Rossi, S.J., Schroeder, T.J., Hariharan, S., & First, M.R. (1993). Prevention and management of the adverse effects associated with immunosuppressive therapy. *Drug Safe, 9*(2), 104-131.

Salvadori, M., Holzer, H., de Mattos, A., Sollinger, H., Arns, W., & Oppenheimer, F., et al. (2004). Enteric-coated mycophenolate sodium is therapeutically equivalent to mycophenolate mofetil in de novo renal transplant patients. *American Journal of Transplantation, 4*(2), 231-236.

Sarwal, M.M., Yorgin, P.D., Alexander, S., Millan, M.T., Belson, A., & Belanger, N., et al. (2001). Promising early outcomes with a novel, complete steroid avoidance immunosuppression protocol in pediatric renal transplantation. *Transplantation, 72*(1), 13-21.

Saunders, R.N., Metcalfe, M.S., & Nicholson, M.L. (2001). Rapamycin in transplantation: A review of the evidence. *Kidney International, 59*(1), 3-16.

Sehgal, S.N. (2003). Sirolimus: Its discovery, biological properties, and mechanism of action. *Transplantation Proceedings, 35*(3 Suppl), S7-S14.

Sehgal, S.N., Baker, H., & Vezina, C. (1975). Rapamycin (AY-22,989): A new antifungal antibiotic. II. Fermentation, isolation and characterization. *Journal of Antibiotics (Tokyo), 28*(10), 727-732.

Shaw, L.M., Sollinger, H.W., Halloran, P., Morris, R.E., Yatscoff, R.W., & Ransom, J., et al. (1995). Mycophenolate mofetil: A report of the consensus panel. *Therapeutic Drug Monitor, 17*(6), 690-699.

Shoskes, D.A., & Cecka, J.M. (1998). Deleterious effects of delayed graft function in cadaveric renal transplant recipients independent of acute rejection. *Transplantation, 66*(12), 1697-1701.

Simmons, R.L., Canafax, D.M., Strand, M., Ascher, N.L., Payne, W.D., & Sutherland, D.E., et al. (1985). Management and prevention of cyclosporine nephrotoxicity after renal transplantation: Use of low doses of cyclosporine, azathioprine, and prednisone. *Transplantation Proceedings, 17*(4 Suppl 1), 266-275.

Simulect [package insert]. East Hanover, NJ: Novartis Pharmaceuticals Inc.; 2002.

Sollinger HW. (1995). Mycophenolate mofetil for the prevention of acute rejection in primary cadaveric renal allograft recipients. *Transplantation. 60*,225-232.

Starzl, T.E., Todo, S., Fung, J., Demetris, A.J., Venkataramman, R., & Jain, A. (1989). FK 506 for liver, kidney, and pancreas transplantation. *Lancet, 2*, 1000-1004.

Takemoto, S., Terasaki, P.I., Cecka, J.M., Cho, Y.W., & Gjertson, D.W. (1992). Survival of nationally shared, HLA-matched kidney transplants from cadaveric donors. The UNOS Scientific Renal Transplant Registry. *New England Journal of Medicine, 327*(12), 834-839.

Thistlethwaite, J.R., Jr., Stuart, J.K., Mayes, J.T., Gaber, A.O., Woodle, S., & Buckingham, M.R., et al. (1988). Complications and monitoring of OKT3 therapy. *American Journal of Kidney Diseases, 11*(2), 112-119.

Turcotte, J.G., Feduska, N.J., Carpenter, E.W., McDonald, F.D., & Bacon, G.E. (1972). Rejection crises in human renal transplant recipients: Control with high dose methylprednisolone therapy. *Archives of Surgery, 105*(2), 230-236.

Vasquez, E.M., Tanzi, M., Benedetti, E., & Pollak, R. (2003). Medication noncompliance after kidney transplantation. *American Journal of Health-Systems Pharmacy, 60*(3), 266-269.

Vincenti, F., Kirkman, R., Light, S., Bumgardner, G., Pescovitz, M., & Halloran, P., et al. (1998). Interleukin-2-receptor blockade with daclizumab to prevent acute rejection in renal transplantation. Daclizumab Triple Therapy Study Group. *New England Journal of Medicine, 338*(3), 161-165.

Vincenti, F., Monaco, A., Grinyo, J., Kinkhabwala, M., Neylan, J., & Roza, A., et al. (2001a). Rapid steroid withdrawal versus standard steroid therapy in patients treated with basiliximab, cyclosporine, and mycophenolate mofetil for the prevention of acute rejection in renal transplantation. *Transplantation Proceedings, 33*(1-2), 1011-1012.

Vincenti, F., Ramos, E., Brattstrom, C., Cho, S., Ekberg, H., & Grinyo, J., et al. (2001b). Multicenter trial exploring calcineurin inhibitors avoidance in renal transplantation. *Transplantation, 71*(9), 1282-1287.

Weisner R., Rabkin J., & Klintmalm G., McDiarmid, S., Langnas, A., Punch, J., et al.(2001). A randomized double-blind comparative study of mycophenolate mofetil and azathioprine in combination with cyclosporine and corticosteroids in primary liver transplant recipients. *Liver Transplantation, 7,* 442-450.

Wilasrusmee, C., Siddiqui, J., Bruch, D., Wilasrusmee, S., Kittur, S., & Kittur, D.S. (2002). In vitro immunomodulatory effects of herbal products. *American Surgery, 68*(10), 860-864.

Woodle, E.S., Thistlethwaite, J.R., Jr., Emond, J.C., Whitington, P.F., Black, D.D., & Aran, P.P., et al. (1991). OKT3 therapy for hepatic allograft rejection. Differential response in adults and children. *Transplantation, 51*(6), 1207-1212.

Woods, J.E., Anderson, C.F., DeWeerd, J.H., Johnson, W.J., Donadio, J.V., Jr., & Leary, F.J., et al. (1973). High-dosage intravenously administered methylprednisolone in renal transplantation. A preliminary report. *Journal of the American Medical Association, 223*(8), 896-899.

Zenapax [package insert]. (2002). Nutley, NJ: Roche Pharmaceuticals.

- The main function of the immune system is to discriminate self from non-self. The immune system protects the host from pathogens such as viruses, bacteria, and other organisms.

- The goal of immunosuppression is to control the immune response, while avoiding the complications of immunodeficiency, such as opportunistic infection and malignancy.

- Drugs that suppress the immune system can alter the immune response and decrease the risk of developing allograft rejection.

- The corticosteroids were the first immunosuppressive drugs used in solid organ transplantation, and remain a part of most immunosuppression regimens.

- Prednisone, prednisolone and methylprednisolone are the most commonly used corticosteroids in solid organ transplantation.

- The calcineurin inhibitors (cyclosporine and tacrolimus) are the cornerstone of many immunosuppression regimens.

- Introduced into clinical practice in the early 1980s, cyclosporine revolutionized the field of transplantation by significantly reducing the incidence of acute allograft rejection and improving graft survival.

- While the calcineurin inhibitors are very effective in preventing acute rejection, they are not effective for the treatment of acute rejection.

- The antiproliferative agents are a diverse group of drugs with a common mechanism of action. These drugs block the clonal expansion of lymphocytes in response to antigen stimulation.

- The antilymphocyte antibodies are potent immunosuppressive drugs that are typically reserved for the treatment of acute rejection or to prevent rejection in patients at high immunologic risk.

- The interleukin-2 receptor antagonist (IL-2Ra) is the newest class for drugs approved by the FDA for use in transplantation. The IL-2Ras are IgG monoclonal antibodies produced by recombinant DNA technology.

- Opportunistic infections can cause significant morbidity and mortality in an immunocompromised patient. Antibiotics can be given for the treatment of an active infection or to prevent an infection (prophylaxis).

- Immunosuppression has evolved from two-drug regimens (prednisone and azathioprine) in the early days of transplantation to the present with numerous complex regimens that allow for individualization of drug therapy based upon patient-specific conditions.

- The most commonly used immunosuppression combination in solid organ transplantation is a triple regimen, consisting of prednisone, an antiproliferative agent, and a calcineurin inhibitor.

- Many factors can influence the blood levels of various immunosuppressive drugs. Transplant recipients take multiple drugs to prevent allograft rejection and opportunistic infections.

- Nurses can play a vital role in preventing medication-related adverse events by identifying drugs that may interact with transplant-related medications before administration to the patient.

- Medication noncompliance is a complex problem and a major barrier to the success of solid organ transplantation. It has been reported that up to 55% of patients are not compliant with their medication regimen.

- Patient noncompliance is a major cause of chronic rejection and late allograft loss in renal transplant recipients .

Pharmacotherapy of Transplantation

Name of Resource	Brief Description	Where to Obtain Resource
American Journal of Transplantation	Web site for the American Journal of Transplantation.	www.blackwell-synergy.com/rd.asp?code=AJT&goto=journal
American Nephrology Nurses' Association	Web site for the American Nephrology Nurses' Association.	www.annanurse.org
American Society of Transplantation	Web site for the American Society of Transplantation.	www.a-s-t.org
Canadian Association of Nephrology Nurses and Technologists	Web site for the Canadian Association of Nurses and Technologists (CANNT).	www.cannt.ca
Coalition on Donation	Web site for the Coalition on Donation.	www.shareyourlife.org
Council of Nephrology Nurses and Technicians	Web site for the Council of Nephrology Nurses and Technicians.	www.kidney.org/professionals/CNNT
Medscape	Comprehensive news and information Web site. Has expert panel discussions and updates from recent professional meetings. Also offers continuing education units.	www.medscape.com/transplantationhome
National Kidney Foundation (NKF)	Web site for the National Kidney Foundation.	www.kidney.org
Nephrology Nursing Journal	Web site for the Nephrology Nursing Journal, the official journal of the American Nephrology Nurses' Association.	www.nephrologynursingjournal.net
North American Transplant Coordinators Organization (NATCO)	Web site for the North American Transplant Coordinators Organization.	www.natco1.org
Renal Physicians Association (RPA)	Web site for the Renal Physicians Association.	www.renalmd.org
Transplantation Journal Web site	Web site for the online journal, *Transplantation*.	www.transplantjournal.com
Transweb	A comprehensive Web site on many aspects of transplantation. Has a listing of local support groups.	www.transweb.org
United Network for Organ Sharing (UNOS)	Web site for United Network for Organ Sharing. Up-to-date information on transplant statistics. Searchable online database for transplant center-specific data.	www.unos.org

ANNP632   **Pharmacotherapy of Transplantation**

David Quan, PharmD

Contemporary Nephrology Nursing: Principles and Practice contains 39 chapters of educational content. Individual learners may apply for continuing nursing education credit by reading a chapter and completing the Continuing Education Evaluation Form for that chapter. Learners may apply for continuing education credit for any or all chapters.

Please photocopy this page and return to ANNA.
COMPLETE THE FOLLOWING:

Name: _____

Address: _____

City: _____ State: _____ Zip: _____

E-mail: _____

Preferred telephone: ☐ Home   ☐ Work: _____

State where licensed and license number (optional): _____

CE application fees are based upon the number of contact hours provided by the individual chapter. CE fees per contact hour for ANNA members are as follows: 1.0-1.9 - $15; 2.0-2.9 - $20; 3.0-3.9 - $25; 4.0 and higher - $30. Fees for nonmembers are $10 higher.

ANNA Member: ☐ Yes   ☐ No   Member # (if available) _____

☐ Checked Enclosed   ☐ American Express   ☐ Visa   ☐ MasterCard

Total Amount Submitted: _____

Credit Card Number: _____ Exp. Date: _____

Name as it appears on the card: _____

CE Evaluation Form
To receive continuing education credit for individual study after reading the chapter
1. Photocopy this form. (You may also download this form from ANNA's Web site, **www.annanurse.org.**)

2. Mail the completed form with payment (check) or credit card information to American Nephrology Nurses' Association, East Holly Avenue, Box 56, Pitman, NJ 08071-0056.

3. You will receive your CE certificate from ANNA in 4 to 6 weeks.

Test returns must be postmarked by **December 31, 2010.**

CE Application Fee
ANNA Member $15.00
Nonmember $25.00

EVALUATION FORM

1. I verify that I have read this chapter and completed this education activity. Date: _____

_____
Signature

2. What would be different in your practice if you applied what you learned from this activity? *(Please use additional sheet of paper if necessary.)*

_____
_____
_____
_____
_____
_____
_____
_____
_____
_____
_____
_____

Evaluation

	Strongly disagree				Strongly agree
3. The activity met the stated objectives.					
a. Relate the goal of immunosuppression to drugs used to achieve this state.	1	2	3	4	5
b. Compare steroids, calcineurin inhibitors, antiproliferative agents, antilymphocyte antibodies and interleukin-2 receptor antagonists as to uses and actions.	1	2	3	4	5
c. Describe the role of nurses in medication-related adverse events in patients on immunosuppressive agents.	1	2	3	4	5
4. The content was current and relevant.	1	2	3	4	5
5. The content was presented clearly.	1	2	3	4	5
6. The content was covered adequately.	1	2	3	4	5
7. Rate your ability to apply the learning obtained from this activity to practice.	1	2	3	4	5

Comments _____

_____

8. Time required to read the chapter and complete this form: _____ minutes.

This educational activity has been provided by the American Nephrology Nurses' Association (ANNA) for 1.5 contact hours. ANNA is accredited as a provider of continuing nursing education (CNE) by the American Nurses Credentialing Center's Commission on Accreditation (ANCC-COA). ANNA is an approved provider of continuing education by the California Board of Registered Nursing, CEP 0910.

Ethical, Legal, Public Policy and Legislative Issues

UNIT 9

Unit 9 Contents

Ethical Challenges in Nephrology Nursing

Rosalie Starzomski, PhD, RN

Chapter Contents

Ethical Challenges in Nephrology Nursing

Chapter 33

Rosalie Starzomski, PhD, RN

The rapid growth of knowledge in health care, the increasing use of technology for treating disease, and an aging population generate unprecedented opportunities and challenges in the delivery of health care. At the same time, this growth and expansion creates increasingly complex ethical challenges for health care professionals and the general public. As a result, ethics is an area in contemporary society that is receiving growing attention and is of interest not only to philosophers, but also to everyone involved in the development and provision of health care.

The role of ethics in health care is multifaceted. Every day in our health professional or citizen roles we are confronted with situations that require moral judgments and the ability to make ethical decisions. Nowhere is this more apparent than in nephrology nursing practice where, for example, decisions about selecting patients for treatment, as well as initiating, withdrawing, and withholding treatment are fraught with ethical concerns and questions about the fair and just allocation of limited resources. Although these dilemmas have been evident since the inception of dialysis and transplantation (Alexander, 1962), many of these issues are becoming more problematic as we face the challenges brought on by burgeoning technology, health care reform, and the shrinking resources available for health care delivery.

As nephrology nurses, we play an integral role in the provision of health care to people from a variety of ethnocultural backgrounds in settings such as hospitals, dialysis facilities, clinics, and the community. The pace of work is unrelenting with growing numbers of patients presenting with kidney disease and chronic kidney failure every year. The close relationships that develop between us and the persons for whom we provide care lead to many privileges and responsibilities as people allow us to enter their world and become aware of their choices, hopes, and fears.

Nephrology nurses have acquired knowledge about ethics and morality as a result of working in an environment where we are constantly called upon to make decisions based on our knowledge as well as our own values and beliefs. We identify ethical concerns related to social judgments, unnecessary suffering, incompetence, dehumanizing practices, and the demands of negotiating power relations, health care contexts, and resources (Redman, Hill, & Fry, 1997; Starzomski, 1998; Varcoe & Rodney, 2002; Varcoe et al., 2003). We make ethical decisions every day as we prioritize our time, determine patient assignments, interact with other health care professionals, and develop plans of care with patients and their families that are congruent with patient choices. Further, nephrology nurses, like nurses from other areas of practice, occupy a unique moral in-between position where they are answerable not only to patients but also to organizations (Storch, Rodney, & Starzomski, 2004; Varcoe & Rodney, 2002; Varcoe et al., 2003).

Consider the following situations that will be familiar to many readers:

- A 93-year-old man with kidney failure requires dialysis after 4 years of being managed in a chronic kidney failure clinic. His family wants him to begin dialysis, but the nurses are morally distressed about providing dialysis in this situation and wonder if doing so is acting in the best interest of the patient.
- A 29-year-old man with Type 1 diabetes receiving hemodialysis (HD) wishes to stop treatment because of his discomfort due to neuropathy and his decreasing quality of life. The dialysis team is deeply troubled by this request and wonders if the patient has the capacity to make such a decision.
- A nurse managing a continuous ambulatory peritoneal dialysis (CAPD) clinic is asked by a patient and his family members to accompany them to a local winery for a dinner and dance event to say thank you for all the care the nurse has given to the patient over the years. The nurse wonders whether doing so would constitute crossing professional boundaries.
- A 13-year-old Native American boy refuses to take his immunosuppressant medication post-transplant because he has learned from a traditional healer that he "no longer need to takes pills because they are poisoning his system." The transplant clinic staff are concerned that the boy is wasting a precious resource.
- Nurses on a transplant unit are aware, through a notice from administration, that the unit will be losing several nursing positions because of a lack of resources in the agency. The staff was not consulted about this decision and they are concerned that they will not be able to adequately care for their patients. They indicate that as advocates for their patients, they cannot accept this change.
- A 39-year-old woman calls an organ donation organization and indicates that she would like to be a kidney donor but wants to be able to direct her donation to a particular recipient.
- A 62-year-old South Asian man returns for follow-up in a transplant clinic where staff are aware he has purchased a kidney. The nursing staff are distressed that the patient has not "waited his turn on the transplant list," and they worry that he has disadvantaged a person in a third world country.

These scenarios challenge us in our practice, and they raise a myriad of ethical concerns. Although knowledge about ethics and ethical decision making are essential components of nephrology nursing practice, many of us feel unprepared to deal with ethical issues partly because we do not have the language to describe the ethical problems that we encounter daily in practice. Hence, if we are to make good ethical decisions, we must first understand the ethical foundations of our practice and develop ways to engage in decision making that will allow us to take an active role in discussing, planning, and implementing plans of care with patients, their families, and other team members. In this chapter, I provide information about ethics in nephrology nursing by outlining the ethical foundations necessary for practice. Although it is impossible to discuss all ethical issues that are problematic, I provide a framework in the chapter that can be used regardless of the issue. Throughout the chapter, many of the ethical challenges facing nephrology nurses today are highlighted, and resources are identified for further exploration of specific topic areas. Strategies that will assist nurses to uphold ethical standards are presented, and future directions in ethics and nephrology nursing are examined.

Moral Landscape: Ethical Foundations for Nephrology Nursing Practice

Ethics is the science or study of morals. The field of ethics is founded in the branch of human knowledge known as philosophy. The works of the influential ancient Greek philosophers, such as Socrates, Plato and Aristotle, established ethics as the "dispassionate and rational clarification and justification of the basic assumptions and beliefs that people hold about what is to be considered morally acceptable and morally unacceptable behavior" (Johnstone, 1999, p. 42). Ethics focuses critical reflection upon actions and events from the standpoint of right and wrong, good and evil, moral value and moral disvalue. In addition, ethics is concerned with policies, practices, duties, obligations, and rights; with fairness in the correction of wrongs (corrective justice); and with the fair distribution of benefits and burdens within society (distributive justice). Ethics is concerned with the resolution of moral disputes, controversies, and uncertainties (McDonald, Stevenson, & Cragg, 1992). Whereas the term ethics usually refers to the formal field of inquiry, morality usually refers to personal attributes and actions (Rodney, Burgess, McPherson, & Brown, 2004).

Ethics reflects what ought to occur in a given situation (Omery, 1989). Ethical issues (sometimes called problems or dilemmas) result from areas of concern that cannot be resolved solely through an appeal to empirical data and where there are conflicts of values as well as uncertainty about the amount or type of information needed to make decisions (Curtin, 1982).

Previously, the focus for ethics within health care was on biomedical ethics. Currently, health care ethics has evolved to a point where there is recognition that all health care professionals have ethical concerns and ethical responsibilities. The terms bioethics and health care ethics are used more frequently to clarify that it is not only medical practitioners but also all health professionals who must practice in an ethical manner (Roy, Williams, & Dickens, 1994). While bioethics and health care ethics have contributed to nursing ethics, nursing ethics is considered to be distinct from both and, in the last few decades, has been identified as a unique area of inquiry (Fry, 1989a,1989b; Rodney et al., 2002; Storch et al., 2002; Storch, 2004; Gibson, 1993).

Nursing organizations in North America have developed ethical standards that provide direction for nephrology nurses and articulate clearly our role as ethical practitioners and patient advocates. The American Nurses Association (ANA) proposed a tentative code of ethics in 1926 with several modifications made in subsequent years. The Canadian Nurses Association (CNA) adopted the International Council of Nurses (ICN) code as its first code of ethics in 1954 and developed its own code in 1980 with regular revisions occurring through the years.

Although it is difficult to determine when bioethics emerged as an important area in health care, it is thought to have occurred after Belding Scribner used a Teflon arteriovenous shunt for the continuous dialysis of Clyde Shields on March 9, 1960 (Jonsen, 1990). Following this major development, dialysis units, like the Northwest Kidney Center in Seattle, formed committees to decide which medically qualified patients would be chosen to receive dialysis in the few treatment slots available (Alexander, 1962; Fox & Swazey, 1992a). The Seattle group, called the God Squad by its critics, generated worldwide controversy since, up to that time, selection of patients for treatment with scarce resources was accomplished using an emergency triage system (developed in war-time and during natural disasters) where the sickest, treatable patients were given first priority for treatment (Jonsen, 1990). The Seattle committee, composed of middle and upper class members of the community, moved away from this method, and in the absence of any formal principles for selection, chose patients for treatment using criteria such as the likely success of the person on dialysis as well as criteria that rated the social worth of each potential candidate (Alexander, 1962; Jonsen, 1990; Fox & Swazey, 1992a). This selection process was described by Jonsen (1990) as using "some common sense maxims; younger rather than older patients, those with dependents rather than those without, the emotionally mature and stable, those with a record of public service and so on" (p. 46).

The story of the Seattle group illustrated one of the problems that brought bioethics to the forefront of nephrology. Because of a lack of resources, such as dialysis machines, trained personnel, and financial support, the issue of who should receive treatment, when all could not be treated, became a primary concern. The public attention given to the dialysis dilemma coupled with discussion about concerns arising out of unethical experimentation with human subjects (Beecher, 1966), stimulated scholarly reflection on these issues, thus contributing to the evolution of the field of bioethics (Jonsen, 1990).

Theoretical Landscape

What provides the basis for making ethical decisions? What guides our thinking and reasoning about ethical problems? In North America, we live in a pluralistic society composed of many ethnic communities, cultures, religions, and traditions, thus leading to different moral positions on many topics. Therefore, it is not possible to suggest that there is one universal ethic that all persons would agree upon, rather there are a variety of diverse perspectives that guide ethical decision making.

Several components are included when we think about the right course of action when confronted with an ethical concern, issue, or dilemma. In addition to considering our own values, beliefs, and attitudes, we can use ethical theory to provide direction for ethical decision making. Like all theory, ethical theory has not remained stagnant, rather it is constantly progressing as challenges to existing theories are made and new ideas are developed. The following brief review of theory development in health care ethics and nursing ethics will provide the background context for further discussion about ethical concerns in nephrology nursing and

Table 33-1
Ethical Theory Development

Ethical Period	Time
The Hippocratic Period	From the time of the Ancient Greek philosophers to the mid 1960s
The Period of Principlism	From the late 1960s to the 1980s
The Anti-Principlism Period Alternative Ethical Theories Proposed	From the 1980s to the present

Note: Adapted from Pellegrino, E. (1993).

provide direction for ethical decision making in the nephrology setting. In what follows, I endeavor to highlight the strengths and limitations of traditional approaches to health care ethics recognizing that because of space constraints, I do not do justice to the range of perspectives in this field or to the overlap among them.

Pellegrino (1993) views the development of ethical theory as comprising several distinct periods (see Table 33-1). Although focusing on biomedical ethics, Pellegrino's classification is useful in understanding the development of nursing ethics and health care ethics, as they parallel the development of biomedical ethics and share a similar history (Yeo, 1991).

The Hippocratic period. The first period described by Pellegrino is the interval in which the Hippocratic teachings, enhanced by contact with the Greek Stoics and religious traditions, formed the predominate ethic. During this period, ethical precepts such as obligations to do no harm, to do good, and to maintain confidentiality were evident in the Hippocratic Oath, an oath taken by physicians that provided direction for the practice of medicine. In addition, there were prohibitions in the Oath against abortion, euthanasia, and sexual relationships with patients. The physician was directed to follow the Oath, lead a life of virtue, and to act in conformity with the virtues of courage, temperance, and justice (Pellegrino, 1993, p. 1159).

The period of principlism. Principle-oriented ethical theory development began the second period of theory evolution in the mid 1960s when philosophical inquiry began to reshape the Hippocratic ethic (Pellegrino, 1993). Philosophers brought a variety of well-established moral traditions to health care ethics including two main ethical theories, teleological (consequentialist) and deontological theories. These theories lead to very different ways of examining ethical concerns.

Consequentialists (also called utilitarians) believe that the rightness or wrongness of an action is solely a function of the goodness or badness of the action's consequences. The whole of morality is reduced to one principle, that of utility, where actions are right if they maximize happiness. Proponents of utilitarianism believe that the end justifies the means. One major concern with this theory in contemporary practice is that it allows a person to do anything if it can be said that the act would produce the greatest net benefit for society as a whole. For example, if lying or killing someone would produce the greatest good for society, a utilitarian would suggest that the action should be carried out (Browne,

1994; Gibson, 1993; Mappes & Zembaty, 1991).

Deontological theory, such as that formulated by the philosopher Immanuel Kant, focuses on the nature of the act to be carried out and does not look merely at consequences. In Kant's theory, there are binding obligations or duties where an act is right if, and only if, it conforms to an overriding moral duty or obligation. Kant's central idea was always to treat people with respect and never solely as a means to an end. A concern with this theory is that there may be circumstances where the right thing to do may not conform to following a moral duty. For instance, Kant would say that one ought not to lie or to kill, however, what if lying would protect someone from harm or killing might protect one's child or occurred in self-defense? In these cases the theory does not provide clear direction (Browne, 1994; Mappes & Zembaty, 1991).

On their own, the theories described above were not sufficient to provide guidance for ethical decision making and action. As a result, a set of duties and principles was developed by Ross (1930/1988) and later modified by Beauchamp and Childress (1983) that included four principles seen as especially appropriate for biomedical ethics. These principles – autonomy, beneficence, nonmaleficence, and justice – were the cornerstone of the traditional approach to health care ethics and have become the "dominant way of doing ethics" (Pellegrino, 1993, p. 1159-1160) (see Table 33-2). The principles are viewed as codes of conduct that direct life and provide a basis for reasoning in ethics (Davis & Aroskar, 1991).

The first principle, autonomy, is defined as self-governance or self-rule by the individual who, at the same time, remains free from both controlling interferences by others and personal limitations that would prevent meaningful choices (Beauchamp, 1982; Beauchamp & Childress, 1989). Also known as respect for persons, autonomy directs us to see persons as worthy agents with a capacity for rational choice who are in control of their own bodies and lives.

Beneficence directs us to abstain from harming others and to help or benefit others, largely by preventing or removing possible harms. Non-maleficence is based on the Hippocratic Oath and is synonymous with the Latin phrase "primum non nocere" or "first do no harm." This principle directs us not to act in a manner that would harm an individual or society (Beauchamp, 1982; Beauchamp & Childress, 1989).

Justice is defined as fairness or providing persons with what they are entitled to or can legitimately claim.

Table 33-2
Traditional Principles of Bioethics

Principle	Definition
Autonomy	Individual self-governance or self-rule
Beneficence	Do good
Nonmaleficence	Do no harm
Justice	Treat people fairly

Distributive justice refers to just distribution of goods and services in society. This distribution is structured by various moral, legal, and cultural rules and principles that form the terms of cooperation for society (Beauchamp & Childress, 1989).

Justice can be viewed as a theory as well as a principle. Four major theories of justice include the utilitarian approach, Rawls' theory of justice as fairness (liberalism), the libertarian approach, and an egalitarian theory of justice.

Utilitarian theories reference the rightness or wrongness of actions or policies to the good or bad consequences they generate. Right acts and policies are those that achieve the greatest net good or happiness for the greatest net number (Buchanan, 1991).

Rawls' theory of justice is based on the idea that inequalities in the distribution of the primary goods of a society can be condoned only if these inequalities are to everyone's benefit, especially the least advantaged. His theory is based on three central principles: (a) the principle of greatest equal liberty, (b) the principle of equality of fair opportunity, and (c) the difference principle. With the principle of greatest equal liberty, Rawls contends that each person is to have an equal right to the most extensive system of equal basic liberties compatible with a similar system of liberty for all. In the principle of equality of opportunity, he suggests that offices and positions ought to be open to all and that people with similar skills and abilities ought to have equal access to offices and positions. Finally, in the difference principle, he proposes that social and economic institutions are to be arranged so as to benefit the maximally worst off (Rawls, 1971 as cited in Buchanan, 1991).

In a libertarian conception of justice, individuals have moral rights to life, liberty, and property that any just society must recognize and respect. From a libertarian perspective, coercion may only be used to prevent harm, theft, fraud, and to enforce contracts (Buchanan, 1991). Libertarian theorists suggest that attempts to force anyone to contribute any of his/her holdings for the welfare of others is a violation of property rights. However, libertarians do say that although justice does not require it, charity requires that those who seek aid are helped.

Egalitarians suggest that justice requires that social institutions work on the premise of moral equality where the life of everyone matters equally. Hence, similarities or equalities among individuals are emphasized. Distribution of health care ought to be carried out according to need with the provision of health care of the same extent and quality to everyone in society. The underlying aim of health care should be to meet equally the health care needs of all. Different treatment is justified only where the need is different or both needs cannot be met. Where these circumstances occur, then priority should be given to the greater need that can feasibly be met (Nielson, 1991).

Each of the theories of justice offers a theoretical basis for answering some fundamental questions concerning justice in health care, but none of them provides unambiguous answers to all of the questions. Each depends for its application upon many empirical premises that are not necessarily available (Buchanan, 1991).

The Anti-principlism period. The third period of ethical theory development, or anti-principle period, occurred when competing moral theories began to challenge the primacy of principles and when nurses began to question whether biomedical ethics was the ethical foundation for their practice (Fry, 1989a; 1989b). This period led to the contemporary era of ethical theory development. Pellegrino (1993) describes the current era as, "... one of crisis in which conceptual conflicts in ethics and the skepticism of moral philosophy challenge the very idea of a universal, normative ethic for medicine" (p. 1158). This same concern can be raised about health care ethics in general, where there is considerable discussion and tension among various ethical theorists.

The tension is particularly evident in the debate about the principle-oriented approach to ethics and the ethic of care. The principle-oriented approach to ethics is based on a lexical ordering and application of principles (such as autonomy, beneficence, nonmaleficence, and justice) (Veatch, 1991a). This ordering often occurs in a rational, objective, and impartial manner where the central issue is judging whether a person's actions are right or wrong (Cooper, 1991; Penticuff, 1991). In this cognitive approach, an action is considered morally right if it can be justified by a valid argument appealing to a valid moral principle as instituted in the social contract (Omery, 1989; Toulmin, 1981). Principle-oriented ethics is based on a model where reliance upon rules and principles is primary in moral action and justification (Cooper, 1991). Some proponents of a principle-oriented ethics generally believe that principles represent the moral truth and that there is a hierarchical ordering of principles where they are applied in a deductive, objective manner. In this ethic, there is a requirement of impartiality where the moral agent must not be influenced by personal feelings or special relationships to others. This requirement of universalizability implies that an action is right if any other person in a comparable situation ought to act in the same manner.

There has been considerable criticism, particularly in the nursing ethics literature, about the principle-based approach to ethics (Cooper, 1991; Penticuff, 1991), although some of this criticism may be related to how the principles have been used in practice rather than theoretical limitations in the principles themselves. For example, according to Rodney and colleagues (2004):

In the hands of busy clinicians, educators, and even ethicists, there has been a tendency to employ them [principles] in an a-contextual and reductionist manner. For instance, in applying the principle of autonomy to a dying patient's request not to have his family told of his prognosis, the discussion might quickly center around whether he was competent, informed, and unconstrained, with little exploration of the meaning behind his request, his understanding of his own and his family's grief processes, the values he held about his family's well-being, and so on. The principle of autonomy, with its rich theoretical traditions, can too easily be reduced to a binary equation (competent/incompetent; informed/ uninformed; constrained/unconstrained) if not handled with careful reflection and clinical insight (p. 67).

Critics have suggested that principle-oriented ethics is an "ethics of strangers" because of the detached way in which the theory is applied, and they have noted that there is a lack of consensus about the nature of fundamental ethical principles and that a hierarchical ordering of principles applied in a prescriptive, decontextualized manner is not practical in actual, complex ethical situations (Ackerman, 1983; Cooper, 1991). The approach has been criticized as actually representing a formula approach to ethics (Ackerman, 1983; Toulmin, 1981). Ackerman (1983) points out that principles may be more useful as heuristic devices or guidelines rather than absolutes. As a result of the criticism, there has been a move to explore other moral theories, several of which are described below.

There is growing interest in a return to contextual ethics in moral theory development. More interest is being expressed in virtue ethics and casuistry, two theories that arose in the first period of development described above (Jonsen, 1995; Pellegrino, 1993; Toulmin, 1981). The first of these, virtue ethics, describes a moral theory where the character of the moral agent is considered critical to ethical decision making. According to Pellegrino, virtue ethics cannot stand alone and should be anchored in some form of prior theory of right or wrong. He suggests that virtue ethics does not provide sufficient clear action for ethical decision making. Moreover, virtue ethics is prone to individual definitions of virtue or of the virtuous person (Pellegrino, 1993, p. 1161). However, Pellegrino believes that virtue ethics ought to be part of any ethical theory that becomes predominant in modern society.

Casuistry is based on case analysis where the decision maker looks for cases that are examples of principles then moves from these clear cases to more perplexing ones, ordering them by paradigm and analogy under a specific principle (Jonsen, 1990; Pellegrino, 1993, p. 1161). In casuistry, principles are valuable; however, they are not absolute. A criticism of casuistry stems from its development in the middle ages within Catholicism, where consensus was more easily obtained on certain principles. In a pluralistic, modern society, consensus is not always possible, thus, leaving casuistry as a method of case analysis rather than a guide to moral theory or practice (Arras, 1991; Pellegrino, 1993).

Further work in contextual ethics arose when theorists postulated that a theory conceptualized around the notion of care might actually be more useful in describing a nursing ethic than the justice-based model used in principle-oriented ethics. Historically, theories about moral development and moral reasoning had been strongly influenced by the work of psychologist Kohlberg and his Piagetian-based cog-

nitive theory of moral development (Blum, 1988). Gilligan (1982/1993) and Noddings (1984) challenged the field of moral psychology arguing that Kohlberg's singular focus on justice in his theory of moral development obscured another dimension of the moral concerns of individuals. Gilligan suggested that issues other than rights and fairness, the concerns of justice outlined in Kohlberg's model of moral development, helped to shape the way individuals frame moral conflict and choice. These included concerns about interdependence, maintaining connections and attachments among individuals, and assuring that someone not be excluded or hurt in the situation being examined (Fry, 1991). Gilligan described care as a "different voice" and not a voice lesser than Kohlberg's justice-based voice. She found that girls and women tended to approach ethical dilemmas in a contextualized, narrative way, looking for resolution in particular details of a problem situation. She identified this orientation in her research and called it an ethic of care. In contrast, boys and men seemed inclined to try to apply general abstract principles without attention to the unique circumstances of the case (Sherwin, 1992a). Gilligan described her theory as one way of changing the voice of the world by bringing women's voices into the open, thus starting a new conversation (1993).

In contrast to principle-oriented ethics, a care ethic has been described as a situational, intuitive process where the central issue is judging an action in terms of its web of relatedness (Fry, 1991). In this theory, moral concern deals with needs and responsibility as they evolve in a relationship (Cooper, 1991). Caring implies mutuality and reciprocity in relationships and is not unidirectional. An individual is considered moral when in a relationship with another and not because of a social contract as in the principled approach. The caring approach to ethics has been described as an ethic of "intimates" versus an ethic of "strangers" (Cooper, 1991; Fry, 1989a; 1989b; 1991; Penticuff, 1991).

There have been criticisms levied at those who suggest that caring is unique to women and to nursing, thereby excluding males and other health professionals (Gillon, 1992; Nelson, 1992; Starzomski, 1997). Gillon (1992) points out that Gilligan's theory describes a developmental process that involves a fundamental difference between men and women in their starting perspective on morality. He states, "... as she [Gilligan] points out in her last chapter, as men and women mature they increasingly come to appreciate the importance of both perspectives" (p. 172). Other critics have pointed out that the ethic of care may not provide direction at the macro level of health care because of its individualistic, relativistic, and relational underpinnings (Nelson, 1992). Finally, there are concerns that an ethic of care could lead to an impoverished self if individuals were required to care for all persons at all times (Fry, 1991; Nelson, 1992).

While principled ethics and contextual ethics are depicted in the literature as distinct theories, there are those who are proposing a principle-oriented ethic, woven with contextual features such as care and compassion and a focus on relationships. Bergum, Boyle, Briggs, and Dossetor (1993) have suggested that there should be a connection between the two processes of principled and contextual ethics where the focus is on the relationship itself – that space where health professionals and patients make connections. They state, "From the dialectic of close up and distant ethics comes synthesis, and this synthesis, in the narrative of our lives and those of our patients/clients, is what ethics is all about" (p. 1). Bergum (2004) further suggests that all relationships as experienced are moral since in every relationship individuals are enacting the question of what is the "right thing to do." Sherwin (1992a; 1992b; 1998) also considers the need for a broader and more contextualized understanding of health care ethics. For example, she calls for an alternative view of autonomy that she labels relational autonomy. Sherwin (1998) defines autonomy as "a capacity or skill that is developed (and constrained) by social circumstances. It is exercised within relationships and social structures that jointly help to shape the individual while also affecting others' responses to her efforts at autonomy" (p. 36).

Other work in nursing ethics describes the everyday relational context of nursing practice where trust and connectedness are paramount to making good ethical decisions (Hartrick Doane, 2002a, 2002b). Further, scholars studying nursing ethics are increasingly identifying contextual challenges where nurses are often constrained in their ability to practice ethically, for example, when nurses perceive they must ration their care in ways that interfere with their moral obligations in relationships with patients (Brown, Rodney, Pauly, Varcoe & Smye, 2004). Rodney, Pauly, and Burgess (2004) suggest that as part of expanding our thinking about alternative approaches to ethics, "we need to better understand and address the personal, social, and cultural aspects of health as well as the complex sociopolitical climates in which health care is delivered and in which resources for health are embedded" (p. 77).

Another area that is receiving attention in the development of ethical theory is the need to pay particular attention to cross-cultural issues, as there is considerable evidence to suggest that there is a lack of sensitivity to social and ethnocultural contexts in health care delivery. Coward and Ratanakul (1999) suggest that those of us practicing in Western health care are inclined to consider culture as being relevant only when we encounter people from "other" ethnic groups, forgetting that everyone comes from an ethnic background, and that as health care professionals we have our own disciplinary, specialty, and organizational cultures as well as our own background of personal, familial, and community values and beliefs. Culture is, of course, much more than ethnicity, and is not static but fluid and ever-changing and includes individualized as well as shared values and beliefs and encompasses notions of gender, race, and class (Anderson & Reimer Kirkham, 1998; Jecker, Carrese & Pearlman, 1995; Molzahn, Starzomski, McDonald, & O'Loughlin, 2004a, 2004b; Rodney, Pauly, et al., 2004).

In summary, the development of ethical theory over the centuries has been progressive, with a variety of approaches being proposed to determine how we should act when confronted with ethical concerns. The principles of bioethics have enabled health care professionals to find a method by which to engage in discourse about ethics. Current ethical theory development in nursing is moving away from the

Table 33-3
Levels of Professional Responsibility

Micro level - Individual Level
Meso Level - Institutional/Agency Level
Macro Level- Societal Level

application of principles as absolutes to consideration of the relationships among patients, their families, and the health professionals providing their care. In this latter scenario, principles are considered guidelines rather than universal absolutes with the personal, social, and cultural aspects of health and the sociopolitical climates in which health care is delivered becoming increasingly important.

Levels of Professional Responsibility

Meeting the ethical challenges confronting us in nephrology nursing, particularly as they are confounded by issues of resource allocation, requires us to think about our professional roles as they fit into three levels of involvement, as within each we have different levels of responsibilities (Rodney & Starzomski, 1994) (see Table 33-3). These three levels of involvement demand different types of decision making in order to arrive at ethically sound decisions. The first of these levels is the micro level. This is the level of individual professional responsibilities for patients and families under our care. At the micro level, we examine frameworks of ethical decision making for individual patients and their family members. The second level of responsibility is at the meso level or the level of institutional responsibilities for programs of care. Meso allocation is described as the division of a health care budget among various health care services. This decision making can be governmental, regional, or institutional. The third level is the macro level or the level of societal responsibilities for the health of the total population (Kluge, 1992; McDonald, 1993; Yeo & Donner, 1991). Macro allocation is most often described as the division of societal resources into various types of services to benefit the population (Rodney, Burgess, et al., 2004).

Throughout all levels of our involvement, we must keep in mind the need to foster the integrity of patient-professional relationships. Unique obligations befall health care professionals because their specialized judgment and skill is required for the good of patients. Given the trust that patients and family members place in professionals, fidelity is an important feature of professional/patient/family relationships (Beauchamp & Childress, 1989). Fidelity is based on trust and generates rules for promise-keeping structured around respect for autonomy.

One of the most difficult challenges facing us as we consider our roles in all three areas of professional responsibility is our ability to act in our individual patient's best interest, while at the same time involving ourselves in discussions about how resources are to be allocated in a just manner for the aggregate. In other words, how do we uphold our bedside covenant with patients to always act in their best interest (Pellegrino & Thomasma, 1988) and, at the same time, participate in decisions to allocate resources for groups of patients – decisions that may affect the care we are able to provide to individuals at the bedside?

Let us consider an illustration of these levels in nephrology nursing practice to help clarify how it is possible for nephrology nurses to be involved in micro, meso, and macro level decisions. Using the area of kidney transplantation as an illustration, at the micro level, we are concerned about how health care providers decide whether a transplant is in a particular patient's best interest. At the meso level, we are concerned about developing selection criteria for transplantation or deciding how much of an institutional budget should be used for transplantation compared to other programs. Furthermore, at the macro level, we are concerned about how much of the health care budget is to be used for transplantation in relation to other services (Rodney & Starzomski, 1994). At the macro level, we might also be called upon to advocate on behalf of all transplant patients if a particular service was threatened. If we do not get involved in progressive planning at the meso and macro level, we shall remain caught in a fundamental tension between our obligations to benefit individual clients and our obligations to benefit society (Fry, 1985; Kjellstrand, 1992).

Involving ourselves in meso and macro level activities does not mean that we have abandoned our patients at the micro level. On the contrary, by involvement in meso and macro level discussions, nephrology nurses may be in a better position to assure that activities at the micro level are carried out in the best interest of the patient. For example, in the late 1980s in Oregon, the state legislature determined there would be a budgetary shortfall in the funding of health services for Medicaid recipients (Klevit et al., 1991). The legislature decided, with little discussion and no public debate, to direct funds away from certain types of transplants in favor of prenatal and other forms of preventive and primary health care (Crawshaw, Garland, & Hines, 1989; Welch & Larson, 1988). There was extensive public outcry when two Oregon children in the Medicaid program were denied necessary transplants. The first child denied care was an infant with neuroblastoma whose family moved to Washington state and established Medicaid eligibility there in order to receive care for their son. The second case was a 7-year-old boy with leukemia who required a bone marrow transplant and reportedly died before his relatives could raise the money needed for him to receive necessary care. Extensive lobbying and political pressure from health care providers and citizens forced the state to rethink the decision and reinstate coverage for transplantation (Boisaubin, 1988; Welch & Larson, 1988). If health care providers had not lobbied for this change, they would have been unable to act in their patients' interest at the micro level since some patients would have been denied transplantation.

Making Ethical Decisions

An understanding of the development of health care ethics, ethical theory, levels of professional responsibility, and the role of the nephrology nurse as a moral agent provide the necessary knowledge to facilitate ethical decision making. With this foundation in place to provide direction for ethical decision making, how then do nephrology nurses make ethical decisions? In many cases, an ethical concern

surfaces when nurses feel concerned, anguished, or distressed about a particular situation. Awareness of the moral dimensions of a particular situation and consideration of the possibility of alternate courses of action are prerequisites to ethical deliberation. Ethical decision making is the application of various skills of ethical analysis and reasoning in an attempt to reach a well-grounded solution to an ethical problem or dilemma at times when value-based questions present difficulties in determining among options in the course of health care interactions (Benjamin & Curtis, 1986; Rodney et al., 2002). Ethical reasoning includes the need for thoughtful, critical thinking and an understanding of personal values when making ethical decisions. Ethical decision making focuses on determining what ought to occur in each situation and is an important part of each health care professional's ability to make good decisions about ethical concerns. Ethical decision making in modern health care settings is not the solitary activity of one team member but requires ongoing health care team communication and collaboration, remembering that the patient and family are integral team members, as well as nurses, physicians, technicians, social workers, dietitians, clergy, and other health professionals.

There are several frameworks that integrate various aspects of ethical theory to provide direction for decision making. Many of the models follow a process of rational deliberation similar to any decision making process. The model by MacDonald (2003), depicted in Table 33-4, is a comprehensive ethical decision-making framework that is based on care and compassion, where ethical principles are used as guidelines to assist in developing the best solution to a particular ethical concern or problem. This contextual approach to ethical decision making provides us with the ability to undertake a careful assessment of the patient's psychological and physiological status, personal wishes, cultural and spiritual beliefs, and overall quality of life, and to understand the patient in the context of his or her family and social environment. Like all frameworks it should function as a guide rather than a recipe, remembering that ethical decision making is a process that may vary depending on the circumstances of the case being considered. Ethical decision making is a process best done in a caring and compassionate environment. It will take time and may require more than one meeting with the patient, family, and team members. The goal is to arrive at a decision that best reflects what the patient would want if he or she were fully informed and well supported. Furthermore, it is essential to recognize that, because real cases are complex, it will not always be possible to obtain a perfect solution to an ethical problem. However, using a framework makes the process transparent to others and assures that key components have been considered.

In McDonald's framework the first step in decision making is identifying the problem and describing the case briefly with all the relevant facts and circumstances. At this stage it is important to clarify what decisions have to be made and by whom. In addition, it is necessary to know who needs to be involved in the decision, making certain to include the appropriate individuals in the discussion. Secondly, it is helpful to analyze the different alternatives that are practical and feasible given the circumstances of the case. Thirdly, it is

Table 33-4
An Ethical Decision-Making Framework for Individuals

A. Collect Information and Identify the Problem(s)
1. Identify what you know and what you don't know. Be prepared to add to/update your information throughout the decision-making process.
2. Gather as much information as possible on the patient's physical, psychological, social, ethno-cultural, and spiritual status, including changes over time. Seek input from the patient, family, friends, and other health care team members.
3. Investigate the patient's assessment of his or her own quality of life and wishes about the treatment/care decision(s) at hand. This includes determining the patient's competency. If the patient is not competent, look for an advance directive. Identify a proxy decision maker for patients who are not competent and seek evidence of the patient's prior expressed wishes. Regardless of the patient's competence (capacity), involve the patient as much as possible in all decisions affecting him or her.
4. Include a family assessment: their roles, relationships, and relevant "stories."
5. Identify the health care team members involved and circumstances affecting them.
6. Summarize the situation briefly but with all the relevant facts and circumstances. Try to get a sense of the patient's overall illness trajectory.
7. What decisions have to be made? By whom?

B. Specify Feasible Alternatives for Treatment and Care
1. Use your clinical expertise to identify a wide range and scope of alternatives.
2. Identify how various alternatives might be implemented (e.g., time trials).

C. Use Your Ethics Resources to Evaluate Alternatives
1. Principles/Concepts
   a. Autonomy: What does the patient want? How well has the patient been informed and/or supported? What explicit or implicit promises have been made to the patient?
   b. Non-maleficence: Will this harm the patient? Others?
   c. Beneficence: Will this benefit the patient? Others?
   d. Justice: Consider the interests of all those (including the patient) who have to be taken into account. Are biases about the patient or family affecting your decision making? Treat like situations alike.
   e. Fidelity: Are you fostering trust in patient/family/team relationships?
   f. Care: Will the patient and family be supported as they deal with loss, grief, and/or uncertainty? What about any moral distress of team members? What principles of palliative care can be incorporated in to the alternatives?
   g. Relational Autonomy: What relationships and social structures are affecting the various individuals involved in the situation? How can these relationships and social structures become more supportive of the patient, family members, and health care providers?
2. Standards
   a. Examine professional norms, standards and codes, legal precedents, and hospital policy.
3. Personal Judgments and Experiences
   a. Consider yours, your colleagues', and other members of the health care team.
4. Organized Procedures for Ethical Consultation
   a. Consider a formal case conference(s), an ethics committee meeting, or an ethics consultant.

D. Propose and Test Possible Resolutions
1. Select the best alternative(s), all things considered.
2. Perform a sensitivity analysis. Consider your choice(s) critically: Which factors would have to change to get you to alter your decision(s)?
3. Think about the effects of your choice(s) upon others' choices: Are you making it easier for others (health care providers, patients and their families, etc.) to act ethically?
4. Is this what a compassionate health care professional would do in a caring environment?
5. Formulate your choice(s) as a general maxim for all similar situations. Think of situations where it does not apply. Consider situations where it does apply.
6. Are you and the other decision makers still comfortable with your choice(s)? If you do not have consensus, revisit the process. Remember that you are not aiming at the perfect choice but the best possible choice.

Notes: Developed by Dr. Michael McDonald (1993-ongoing), W. Maurice Young Centre for Applied Ethics, University of British Columbia.
Adapted by Dr. P. Rodney and Dr. R. Starzomski (2003), University of Victoria School of Nursing & W. Maurice Young Centre for Applied Ethics, University of British Columbia
Versions of this framework are posted on the W. Maurice Young Centre for Applied Ethics Web page at www.ethics.ubc.ca

useful to consider various ethics resources to evaluate the alternatives that have been raised.

Within the framework, ethical principles are described, in addition to other ethics resources such as policies, professional norms, standards, codes of ethics, and legal precedents, that can provide valuable direction in deliberation about ethical problems. Contextual features of the case such as family relationships, past history, the illness experience, and spiritual and ethno-cultural considerations are critically important. All voices within the health care team must be heard, and the judgments of all team members need to be considered. There may be a need for an organized process for ethical discussion such as a case conference. Furthermore, an ethics committee or an ethics consultant can provide valuable advice and assistance with the case, if required.

After examining all the features of the case, a resolution to the problem can be proposed. How can we determine if we have made the best possible decision? One way is to perform a sensitivity analysis. We can consider critically the choice that was made – which factors would have to change to alter the decision? We can think about the effects of the choice made upon others' choices – is it easier or harder for relevant others such as health care providers, patients, and their families to act ethically? Furthermore, we can ask ourselves if this alternative is what a compassionate health care professional would do in a caring environment. Finally, the choice can be formulated as a general maxim (standard) for similar cases. It is useful to think about cases where it does or does not apply. The decision makers can then evaluate their level of comfort with the decision and implement the chosen alternative. If the decision makers are not comfortable with the decision, then it is essential to consider the factors that make them uncomfortable with the choice, with a view to coming up with a new general standard. This process is repeated until it appears that the best decision has been made in the time available. It is important to remember that the aim is not to develop the perfect choice, but a good choice.

Moral Climate: Ethical Issues in Nephrology Nursing

With this foundation for ethics in nephrology nursing and some resources for decision making, let us now move to an illustration of how to use this information in the context of some of the major ethical issues facing nephrology nurses. Some of the ethical concerns that nephrology practitioners encounter are representative of those that originated when dialysis and transplantation were in their infancy and are prototypical of ethical issues raised by high technology and life-sustaining treatments in health care. Others relate to concerns about workload, dehumanizing practices, unnecessary suffering, prolonging life, social judgment, and contextual constraints. Many of these everyday ethical issues often lead to moral distress for nurses if there are not leadership strategies in place to begin to address them in a systematic manner (Storch, Rodney, Pauly, Brown, & Starzomski, 2002).

In the early years of dialysis and transplantation, nephrology pioneer Belding Scribner identified several ethical issues that would be problematic in the future – patient selection, termination of treatment, suicidal patients, dying with dignity, and organ donor selection (Scribner, 1964). These concerns remain important today and, in some cases, have been joined by other issues, such as ensuring informed consent for treatment; deciding when to initiate, withhold, and withdraw treatment; advance care planning; end-of life decision making; and resource allocation concerns at the micro, meso, and macro levels of the system (Long, 1994; Moss, 1995, 1998, 2001a; 2001b; McCormick, 1993; Moss, Rettig, & Cassel, 1993; Neu, 1994; Pfettscher, 1993; 1996a; 1996b).

One of the most difficult issues in nephrology nursing is the increasing number of people requiring treatment for chronic renal failure and the diminishing resources available to care for them. More liberal treatment criteria, an aging population, and an increase in patients with conditions such as Type 2 diabetes are thought to play a major role in the increasing number of people requiring treatment. Although there are differences in how health care is funded in the United States (U.S.) and Canada, there are concerns in both systems about the ability to continue to fund end stage renal disease (ESRD) care in a manner that allows us to provide dialysis and transplantation for all who require these treatments (Balk, 1990; Glover & Moss, 1998; Mendez, Aswald, Dessouki, Cicciarelli, & Mendez, 1992; Moskop, 1987; Stiller, 1990).

It has been suggested that increasing kidney transplantation will resolve some of the concerns about the numbers of patients receiving expensive dialysis therapy. However, there are many unresolved ethical issues in the transplant realm

that remain problematic, and there are a variety of barriers to organ donation resulting in a chronic situation where the demand for organs exceeds the supply (Molzahn, Starzomski, & McCormick, 2003).

The important issues and questions arising in the transplant arena are manifested at the three levels of responsibility for health care. The community at large is faced with fundamental questions at the macro or societal level of the health care system about the level of resources to be allocated to life saving technology such as organ transplantation (Benjamin, 1992; Brooks, 1993; Turcotte, 1992, Veatch, 2000). Also at the macro level, a major worldwide organ shortage (Matesanz & Miranda, 2003) has raised questions about changing consent for human tissue by examining strategies for presumed consent (Andrews, 1992; Childress, 1992; Cohen, 1992; Menzel, 1992; Sadler, 1992; Veatch, 1991b; Youngner & Arnold, 1993), using fetal tissue for transplantation (Martin, 1992; Nelson, 1990), offering financial incentives for organ donation (Dickens, 1991; Evans, 1993), using marginal donors (Donnelly, Henderson, & Price, 1999), engaging in buying and selling organs (Guttmann & Guttmann, 1992; Kazim et al., 1992, Veatch, 2000), using anencephalic infant donors (Dickens, 1988; Roy et al., 1994), and considering the use of xenografts (transplanting from one species to another) as ways to solve the shortage of organs for human transplantation (Caplan, 1992; Rapaport, 1993; Reemtsma, 1992; Singer, 1992, Starzomski, 2004).

At the meso or institutional level of the health care system, questions are raised regarding the choice of the recipients for organ transplantation and how selection criteria should be developed (Kilner, 1988, 1990; Kluge, 1993; Seib, MacLeod, & Stiller, 1990). In addition, as transplant waiting lists grow, a question arises about the number of waiting lists on which a recipient should be listed. Another difficult question at the meso level arises when determining how decisions should be made about the proportion of an institutional budget devoted to transplantation compared to other programs (Balk, 1990).

Decisions at the micro level of the health care system are evident surrounding issues about how health care providers decide whether a transplant is in a given patient's best interest. For example, health care providers make decisions about removing kidneys from individual living donors to be transplanted into specific recipients (Hilton & Starzomski, 1994; Sells, 1992, Simmons, Marine, & Simmons, 1987). In addition, organs from unrelated and altruistic donors are being considered more frequently in transplant centers around the world (Author, 2002; Gohh, Morrissey, Madras, & Monaco, 2001; Siminoff & Leonard, 1999; Spital, 1992, 1993). Finally, there is the question of how many organs to which one individual is entitled (Evans, Manninen, Dong, & McLynne, 1993). Although this list is not exhaustive, it provides an overview of some of the most perplexing problems evident in transplantation today.

Concerns about the principles of autonomy and informed consent arise from the issues described above. Moreover, the critical principle of justice is embedded in many of these ethical issues about organ donation and transplantation, exposing deep tensions about the societal sense of what is true or just (Fox & Swazey, 1992a, 1992b; Jonsen,

1985, 1989; Kjellstrand & Dossetor, 1992). These situations raise a need for a collaborative approach among health care providers and the public to define and determine legitimate and just applications of organ transplantation technology (Fox & Swazey, 1992a, 1992b).

Case Analyses

The following cases, and the discussion that follows, highlight some of the ethical concerns and problems encountered by nephrology nurses and demonstrate how an ethical decision-making framework can be used to help resolve the problems.

Case 1 – To dialyze or not? Is that the question? Mr. T., an active 88-year-old man has been living in a private long-term care facility for the past 5 years. He is well liked by the staff and spends most of his time reading or playing cards. His health has been good for most of his life; however, at the age of 88 he was found to have a 4 cm abdominal aortic aneurysm that was considered by his surgeon too small to repair electively. The surgeon decided, with Mr. B., to continue to monitor the size of the aneurysm and consider surgery, if necessary, in the future.

One week ago, Mr. B. was found slumped over his bed by a nurse in the long-term care facility. He was unresponsive and an ambulance was called immediately. Mr. B. was taken to the emergency room (ER) of a large, tertiary care hospital. He arrested in the ambulance en route to the hospital and was resuscitated successfully by the ambulance attendants. In the ER it was confirmed that Mr. B.'s aneurysm had ruptured. He was rushed to the operating room, bumping two elective patients, and his aneurysm was repaired. In the operating room he was given 11 units of blood and then transferred to the intensive care unit (ICU). Mr. B. did not regain consciousness, and after 3 days, it was apparent that he was in acute renal failure. The nephrologist who saw Mr. B. recommended dialysis. As Mr. B had no relatives who could be involved in the decision, his surgeon decided that dialysis would be initiated.

Mr. B. was successfully removed from the ventilator, but after 3 weeks of dialysis treatment, he remained unconscious with no improvement in his kidney function. The nurses in the dialysis unit raised concerns about whether Mr. B. should be resuscitated if he arrested and, because of his poor prognosis, wondered whether dialysis should be continued. They were told that because the decision was made to initiate treatment by repairing his aneurysm, all must now be done to treat Mr. B. The dialysis unit nurses and social worker assigned to Mr. B. were upset about this decision and did not agree with the treatment plan. They spoke to nurses at the long-term care facility who knew Mr. B. very well, and these nurses stated that they believed Mr. B. would not want to be treated if he were aware of his condition. One nurse at the facility said that, in fact, Mr. B. would not have agreed to an aneurysm repair and was going to tell his surgeon this at his next appointment.

Because of the differences in opinion about how Mr. B. should be treated and the moral distress of the nurses caring for him, a team conference was called. Mr. B.'s family doctor and two nurses from the long-term care facility attended the conference as well as staff from the ICU, the cardiac sur-

geon, the social worker, two nurses from the dialysis unit, and the nephrologist.

Discussion. One of the major ethical concerns to be addressed by health care professionals in this case is whether treatment should be continued. Is Mr. B.'s best interest being considered given his prognosis and apparent wishes about surgical repair of his aneurysm (according to the nurses in the long-term care facility). Mr. B. is unable to speak for himself and has not left an advance directive or living will, nor does he have a relative or friend who could be named his surrogate decision maker. The dialysis unit nurses believe they are acting as Mr. B.'s advocates when raising the question of discontinuing dialysis, as they believe, after discussion with the nurses in the long-term care facility who have had a significant relationship with Mr. B. for many years, that he would not wish to continue the dialysis treatment.

Collecting more data about the case and examining the ethical principles outlined in the decision-making framework outlined earlier provide some guidance in this case. Mr. B. is unable to exercise his autonomy in his current state. The nephrologist believes that the dialysis treatment is providing some physiological benefit to Mr. B., is not harming him, and that his condition may improve. However, he is ambivalent about what course of action should now be taken since he has heard the information from the long term care nurses about Mr. B.'s wishes. The ICU physician believes Mr. B. may regain consciousness and be in a debilitated state, but at least he will be alive and then able to decide what treatment he wishes to have. The dialysis nurses disagree, stating that the pain and discomfort Mr. B. is currently experiencing in his weakened and debilitated state is burdensome and doing him harm. The nurses from the dialysis unit, long-term care facility, and ICU argue that the treatment is merely prolonging Mr. B.'s dying and not providing him with any real benefit. Mr. B.'s family physician, who has known him for several years, believes that Mr. B. would wish to discontinue treatment if he was unable to return to his former state and presses both the nephrologist and ICU physician for their realistic views about Mr. B.'s prognosis. When pressed, the ICU physician says he is certain that if Mr. B. does regain consciousness he would not return to his former level of health and would very likely have significant cognitive impairment. Traditional biomedical ethical approaches would have focused on Mr. B.'s consent to treatment and access to acute care resources. While these are important elements of the story, the traditional approach would have missed the ethically relevant problems of intra-and interdisciplinary team conflict.

When considering the principle of justice, the team believed that Mr. B. was entitled to be dialyzed and that when the outcome of a critically ill individual is uncertain then a trial of dialysis is appropriate. Considering the various theories of justice, they could see that all the theories would support Mr. B. receiving treatment. If, however, there was a question of limited resources, the utilitarian would say to provide care in the cases where there would be the greatest benefit. In other words, if a younger person who had a better prognosis and Mr. B. were competing for the same resource, then the person who would most benefit should receive the treatment. An individual operating from an egalitarian perspective would also consider examining who should receive the care if two individuals require it; however, different treatment would be justified only where the need was different or where both needs could not be met. Where these circumstances occur, then priority would be given to the greater need that could feasibly be met. In this institution, based on the resources available, treating Mr. B. is possible.

The dialysis unit nurses suggest that they are required to send a nurse to dialyze Mr. B. in the ICU, thus taking resources away from their own unit at a time when they are extremely busy. Their first concern is with the pain and suffering that Mr. B. is enduring and that his chances of recovery are very slim. They point out that the hospital policy with respect to withdrawing and withholding treatment states that there is no moral imperative to continue treatment if the treatment is futile. However, it is pointed out by another team member that futility is a very emotionally charged term and it is difficult to determine what it actually means.

The nephrologist volunteers that it is now very unlikely that Mr. B. will recover and that he has reviewed recent data from several studies where it is suggested that in cases like this the prognosis is very poor. In the end, the team agreed to continue treatment for another 2 days and consult with the hospital ethics committee to provide them with some guidance. In the interim, the surgeon and ICU physician agree to a "do not resuscitate" order, as they are convinced, based on resuscitation data from similar cases, that Mr. B. is not a candidate for resuscitation but should be allowed to die a natural death.

When reviewing the case with the ethics committee, the nurses once again suggest that Mr. B. be allowed to die with dignity and that continuing treatment would only prolong his suffering. The ethics committee helps the team review the facts of the case and the different alternatives. The ICU physician and the surgeon agree that because there has been no change in Mr. B.'s condition in the weeks he has been treated, continuing to dialyze him would only prolong his dying, and they agree that the treatment is medically futile. The team discusses whether they have made the right decision by coming to the conclusion that other caring and compassionate health professionals would make the same decision and determining that in similar cases, circumstances being the same, they would once again choose this option.

Following the case discussion, dialysis is discontinued. Mr. B. dies 2 days later without regaining consciousness.

The members of the team realize that the different values they held about death and dying, the absence of any relatives to speak for Mr. B. or a written advance directive, as well as their communication difficulties all made this case problematic. As a result of this case, the long-term care facility staff and the dialysis unit staff plan to develop and implement policies and programs to ensure that all patients are given the opportunity to discuss advance care planning. In addition, the members of the team in the agency began efforts and processes to improve their communication and decision making about ethical issues by instituting interdisciplinary ethics rounds that will be held twice a month where cases and concerns will be discussed. Moreover, they have committed to examining the outcome studies conducted about dialysis morbidity and mortality and, based on the data,

determining better selection criteria for treatment. They remain committed to ensuring patient choice in treatment decisions; however, they recognize the value of providing accurate data so people are able to make their decisions based on the best outcome information available. They recognize that to them the word "Team" means "together everyone achieves more."

Case 2 – Saying goodbye. Susan, a 29-year-old married nurse, developed ESRD as a result of diabetic nephropathy. She is legally blind, has severe peripheral neuropathy, and recently had a below the knee amputation because of a gangrenous foot. Susan has not worked for some time and, because of the complications of her diabetes, has been unable to have children, although she has had fertility treatments in the past. She is being followed in the Progressive Renal Insufficiency Clinic and wants to receive HD when her ESRD progresses to the point of requiring dialysis. There are no suitable living kidney donors who have come forward. Susan's husband is not considered a suitable donor because he also has diabetes. Susan is waiting for a transplant assessment to determine if she can be added to the transplant waiting list. She has told the nurses and her social worker that she sees this as her only hope.

Three weeks ago, Susan sustained a myocardial infarction (MI). She is currently in the cardiac ICU and will need quintuple bypass surgery as soon as her condition is stable enough. Because of her MI and the treatments she has received, Susan's renal failure has progressed, and she now requires dialysis. When this is discussed with Susan, she indicates that she does not want dialysis and wants to die peacefully. She says she is tired of treatments and surgeries. She describes how she watched one of her friends (who was also a diabetic) go through bypass surgery recently. Her friend died several days following surgery after experiencing a myriad of painful complications. Susan says that she would rather die of uremia than go through surgery and die, or worse, find out after surgery that she would not be a suitable transplant candidate. Susan's cardiac surgeon cannot say for certain whether Susan will survive the surgery and whether postoperatively her cardiac status will be stable enough for Susan to be a transplant candidate. He tells Susan she is considered an extremely high risk surgical candidate. Susan's husband and her parents do not believe that enough time has passed for Susan to make this decision. They want Susan to have dialysis and to think about her decision. Susan says she has thought of nothing else for the past few weeks. A psychologist who has been working with Susan for many years is convinced that Susan has sound decision-making capacity, she has reviewed all the alternatives, and that her decision should be respected. Some of the nephrology team members believe that Susan is making a bad decision and that she should start dialysis and then reconsider what she wishes to do.

Discussion. Several of the issues that emerge when people want to discontinue life-saving treatment are illustrated within this case. Family members and health care professionals often find it difficult to accept autonomous patient decisions partly because these decisions may conflict with their own values and wishes. There is, of course, the added concern of not wanting to lose a family member or friend who is loved dearly. When we examine the case, it is clear that Susan's family is having difficulty coping with the knowledge that she is dying. The family needs considerable emotional support to deal with this. Several of the health care team members believe Susan is refusing treatment that may improve her physical condition – albeit treatment that could potentially make her worse off than she is now. In the curative environment of dialysis and transplantation, professionals can be very uncomfortable when they are not able to provide a person with a treatment that will result in positive outcomes. In the pursuit of life, we may find it difficult to accept that people will die sometime and that our job may be to help them with a good death (Starzomski, 1994; Starzomski, 1997).

From Susan's perspective, no one can provide her with the information that she requires to assure her that she would have a better quality of life with the proposed treatments. Susan clearly articulates many of her concerns and has made her decision based on her individual circumstances and values. She has experienced many medical problems and claims she is tired of all the medical interventions. She is also aware (based on her friend's experience and what has been said to her by the cardiac surgeon) that the outcome of the cardiac surgery may not be positive. In considering the available information and determining the level of benefit she might receive, Susan is able to articulate her own choices and wishes. As an individual with decision-making capacity, Susan has the right to make choices about her own care. Some team members, attempting to act in a manner that they think would not cause Susan harm (in this case death), believe she should receive dialysis. They see her as a young individual who has much to live for and suggest that her life would be wasted if she were to stop dialysis. On the other hand, Susan believes the burdens of her treatment far outweigh the benefits. She believes that those who are not supporting her decision are acting in a paternalistic manner. There is a direct conflict between Susan's individual autonomy and the professional autonomy of the health care professionals who believe they are acting in accordance with the non-maleficence or the do no harm principle.

In this case, Susan needs the health care team to assist her and her family in preparation for her death. This is a task that some members of the team find particularly difficult. One way to help resolve the dilemmas that arise in this case is to encourage all team members (with Susan and her family being the pivotal part of that team) to discuss the issues in an open manner, using an ethical decision-making framework to help identify the problems, determine the alternatives, and arrive at a plan that would provide the necessary support and care for all involved. The solution here is not to consider treatment for the sake of others but to focus on what Susan wants and what she considers in her best interest, and to assist the family to cope with the reality that her condition is deteriorating and she is slowly dying.

What if the situation was different and Susan were not able to speak for herself? Clearly, there would be a variety of issues to consider, including whether Susan had a surrogate decision maker who could offer a substituted judgment (based on knowledge about what Susan would want through previous conversations with her or an explicit advance direc-

tive). In the absence of a named surrogate decision maker, a decision maker would be named who could provide a best interest judgment. There are a number of laws and regulations in the different jurisdictions governing informed consent, health care treatment decision making, and futility. As nephrology practitioners, we should be familiar with the laws and regulations that apply in our jurisdiction to assist us in making these difficult decisions.

Formal discussion about withholding or withdrawing treatment in dialysis and transplant units has been infrequent. In many situations, where death is imminent or where the potential outcome is extremely poor, there is great difficulty in shifting from a curative approach, to a palliative perspective, where palliative care principles can be applied and support provided, thus, giving people the option of dying with dignity (Starzomski, 1994). Some programs are moving in the direction of using palliative perspectives, incorporating discussion of advance directives, and developing guidelines for withdrawing and withholding treatments (Colvin & Hammes, 1991; Colvin, Myhre, Welch, & Hammes, 1993; Mendelsshon & Singer, 1994; Moss, 2001a; 2001b). However, there is still more to be done in many centers about systematically incorporating palliative care principles into programs of care. Most of the discussion about these areas occurs in an informal fashion in the coffee room or around the nursing station, where team members discuss their frustration about treatment decisions. Many programs are left with no clear direction about how to support individuals who are turned down for transplantation, choose not to be transplanted, elect not to start dialysis, or wish to discontinue the treatment. There are concerns about where, how, and by whom care is provided to the patient and family. In most cases, dialysis success is measured by patient survival through the treatment or, as in the case of transplantation, by patient survival and success of the graft, rather than on the overall quality of life for the individual (Starzomski, 1994).

How do we determine whether a treatment will in fact improve a patient's quality of life? There is agreement, in most situations, that practitioners are not obligated to offer and patients are not obligated to undergo treatments that are futile (Roy et al., 1994). But how do we determine futility – a heavily value-laden term? One way of ascertaining whether a treatment is futile or beneficial is by considering whether the proposed interventions will benefit the patient as a whole, or whether the treatment will become an additional burden that the person must bear as the dying process is prolonged (Starzomski, 1994).

Schneiderman, Jecker, and Jonsen (1990) believe futility has two distinct components, physiological effect and benefit. From their point of view, some treatments can be futile because they do not produce a desired physiological effect or the anticipated goal of treatment. Although this is a useful conceptualization, it is still difficult to apply in many cases because we do not have the outcome data with which to determine the potential physiological effect. What percentage of success is considered adequate to consider a treatment beneficial? Even with outcome data, each case must be evaluated in terms of the potential benefits as seen through the eyes of the patient. The patient must be the one, when presented with the information about the benefits and burdens of treatment, to make a choice based on his or her own individual interpretation of quality of life. Although some clinicians might suggest that this could lead to people asking for inappropriate care, it has been my experience in dealing with many hundreds of patients and families that there are very few who choose a treatment that has a potentially dismal outcome when the information about what is known is presented fairly and honestly, with the risks and benefits outlined accurately. Clearly, this information disclosure must occur in a supportive and caring environment where patients, families, and clinicians are working together in a collaborative manner (Starzomski, 1994, 2000).

Strategies to Enhance Ethical Decision Making

A variety of strategies, some of which have been mentioned briefly in the previous section, can enhance our ability to practice in an ethical manner. These strategies include team communication and collaboration, interdisciplinary education and rounds, use of resource persons for ethical decision-making assistance, research into the best methods to solve ethical problems, and greater public education and discussion about ethical issues.

Communication and Collaboration

Opportunities to be involved in ethical decision making at the bedside can serve to enhance the health care team contribution to the overall care of patients and their families. Special attention must be paid to comprehensive family assessment and consideration of the families' ethno-cultural beliefs and values. Use of resource people at the bedside, such as clinical nurse specialists, ethics consultants, and/or ethics committees can enhance overall ethical decision making by encouraging interdisciplinary team communication.

As the previous cases have illustrated, a vital component of making good decisions that are ethical in nature is having a well-developed health care team capable of working together and respecting each other's opinions, values, and responsibilities. Often, what have been thought of as ethical problems are confounded by problems with team conflict and communication. Finding solutions to the ethical challenges faced at the micro and meso levels of the health care system will require that we expand our thinking about teamwork and look at strategies that will lead to improved team collaboration (Rodney & Starzomski, 1994; Storch, 2004; Storch et al., 2004). Research shows that interdisciplinary collaboration requires mutual respect and can lead to developing common goals and positive patient outcomes (Baggs, 1993; Baggs, Ryan, Phelps, Richeson, Johnson, 1992; Mariano, 1989; Mitchell, Armstrong, Simpson, & Lentz, 1989). It is important that collaborative practice models, as opposed to vertical decision making models, be used in health care settings to promote optimal team work leading to the best possible patient care (Rodney & Starzomski, 1993, Storch et al., 2004).

When caring for people who are undergoing life-prolonging treatment, nurses must exercise moral judgment and use ethical decision-making approaches. There is considerable research suggesting that when nurses are constrained in their ability to practice morally they experience moral distress. Moral distress results when persons know what ought to be done, but they are unable to translate their moral choices into moral action (Jameton, 1984; Wilkinson, 1989). Thus, moral distress can occur when nurses are not included in decision making or when an institution or agency lacks appropriate processes or mechanisms for or actually constrains moral action (Rodney & Starzomski, 1993; Storch et al., 2004; Yarling & McElmurry, 1986).

In nephrology, we have valued teamwork since the inception of dialysis and transplantation. Indeed, the treatments have been improved and modified by nurses, physicians, and other professionals working together to provide the best care possible to people living with kidney disease. It is imperative that we continue to foster excellent team communication and collaboration to prevent nurses from becoming morally distressed and, at the same time, promote optimal patient care.

Ethics at the Bedside

Ethics rounds and discussions (including retrospective case discussions) are a means of operationalizing ethical decision making on an ongoing basis, at the same time encouraging participation and communication among all team members. Using a format similar to clinical rounds, ethics rounds can be educational in nature and/or may assist in clinical decisions. The rounds may be conducted by nurses or may be interdisciplinary. The cases reviewed may be actual cases in progress, past cases, or hypothetical cases. These rounds are an excellent way for interdisciplinary teams to work together improving communication and collaboration (Rodney & Starzomski, 1993). In many situations, it is useful to have an ethics interest group where issues can be discussed and new ideas and developments in the field of ethics explored. These can be nephrology specific or combined with other programs, depending on the needs of the individuals involved. Nurses need to have time to stop and reflect on their practice and have dialogue with nurse leaders about areas, for example, such as how to change the practice setting so that patient care is optimized.

Ethics Education

In order to value interdisciplinary decision making and to make good ethical decisions, more work needs to be done educating health professionals about ways to work together. In traditional educational settings, most professionals are socialized in the traditions and values of their own discipline. This does not always lead to a sense of understanding of what the issues are for members of other disciplines. There is not always a sense of the course of action that will lead to the most favorable outcome for the patient. Studies indicate that nurses and physicians, for instance, approach patients with what are quite often divergent philosophical stances (Campbell-Heider & Pollock, 1987; Grundstein-Amado, 1992; Stein, Watts, & Howell, 1990). This suggests the need for dialogue among nurses, physicians, and other team members during professional educational preparation so that the various members of the interdisciplinary team can appreciate each other's points of view (Rodney & Starzomski, 1993).

Interdisciplinary ethics education at the undergraduate and graduate level could do much to enhance understanding of values, beliefs, and responsibilities of the various health care team members. This understanding and respect can then be transferred to the clinical settings where the students will eventually be working together. Teaching team members about health care ethics and business and professional ethics should lead to better team communication since health care professionals will be able to articulate their own issues and concerns more effectively and understand the position of other team members. Finally, continuing education in the form of inservices and other educational offerings can assist team members to more effectively deal with ethical issues and situations as they arise in clinical practice (Rodney & Starzomski, 1993, Storch et al., 2002; Storch, 2004).

Ethics Consultation

Although ethical decision making should take place at the bedside, there are often times when consultation, advice, and guidance from resources such as ethics committees and consultants may be of value. Ethics committees are an effective resource to help team members with ethical decision making. Ethics committees are usually composed of an interdisciplinary group of physicians, nurses, administrators, clergy, ethicists, community members, and lawyers. However, past research shows that nurses are not always represented on these committees, or do not access them, often because they are unaware they exist (Storch & Griener, 1992). This situation requires change as nurses are an extremely valuable resource for ethics committees and are often in need of the assistance a committee could provide.

Most sources agree that institutional ethics committees have several roles including education, case consultation, and policy formulation (Blake, 1992; Storch & Griener, 1992; Storch, Griener, Marshall, & Olinek, 1990). Ethics committees can play a major role in disseminating information throughout the agency and acting as an educational resource. In addition, they are able to develop policies around topics, such as informed consent, resuscitation, and withdrawing and withholding treatment, that help provide guidance for ethical practice.

In many situations, ethics committees can provide consultation around individual cases and dilemmas. Sometimes this occurs with a few members of the committee or occasionally with the whole committee. In certain situations, ethics consultants are available in agencies to provide assistance with case consultation, education, and research. With proper institutional support, ethics committees and ethics consultants are invaluable in helping to develop healthy moral environments in hospitals and in the community.

Research

As we move into the future it is clear that activities within the health care system (including dialysis and transplantation) are undergoing considerable scrutiny, with emphasis on the need for all citizens to use resources in a responsible manner. More research needs to be conducted about the effects of the various reforms to the health care system. Furthermore, more research is required to determine what systems need to be in place to ensure that nurses are able to practice in an ethical manner.

Public and Health Care Provider Dialogue about Resource Allocation

One of the challenges for allocating resources efficiently in the health care sector is combining expert knowledge about the effectiveness of health care treatments and the structure and financing of the system with information about the values, preferences, and local circumstances of communities (Hurley, Birch, & Eyles, 1992). Stated another way, although health care providers possess expert knowledge about the expected effectiveness of health care in improving health status, individuals are the best judges of how these improvements affect their overall well-being. Therefore, there must be a partnership between the providers of care and consumers so that all voices are heard in the debate about how resources ought to be allocated for health care. We must give great attention to including those who are most at risk, as well as those who may not have the resources and energy to be involved in the process (Starzomski, 1997). More public debate is needed as the health care systems of both the U.S. and Canada continue to undergo reform. The process of opening up public discourse about resource allocation is a positive move. It is crucial that we become involved proactively in planning at the agency level as well as in the community and on the political scene. We must take initiative in discovering effective ways to maximize use of resources, while at the same time meeting the health care needs of persons with chronic renal failure and their families (McDonald, 1993). In the context of the discussion about resource allocation, several important ideas are useful to keep in mind:
- There must be full consultation, including public consultation and debate.
- The policies and their underlying principles should be open for all to see and compare with rival approaches.
- Everyone similarly situated should be similarly treated.
- Allocation decisions should be made on the best evidence available.
- Disparities in things such as wealth, social position, age, or responsibility for one's condition must not make a significant difference to the quality of health care one receives (Vancouver Coastal Health Corporate Ethics Committee, 2005).

Moral Horizons: Future Directions

The amazing success of the treatment of chronic renal failure has been the catalyst for an incredible array of ethical problems and issues. These ethical concerns will not go away. As we solve current problems, new ones will emerge. It is essential, therefore, that we develop a theoretical foundation and a method for ethical decision making that can be used by nephrology nurses regardless of the concern that is being discussed. Hence, my major goal in this chapter has been to provide a foundation and process for making ethical decisions that can be used by nephrology nurses wherever they practice.

Ethical theory is being developed constantly and can be thought of as work in progress. In order to make good ethical decisions, we must understand the evolution and application of ethical theory, and the role theory has, in helping us to make good ethical decisions.

As nephrology nurses, we have unique and pivotal roles at the micro level of the health care system as advocates for people with chronic renal failure and their families. Furthermore, we must also expand our thinking to include these individuals in the context of the society in which they live. In other words, we must be involved in ethical decision making at the meso and macro levels of the system.

If we are to make good ethical decisions, then we need to understand and emphasize the importance of team communication and collaboration, remembering that the patient is the central member of the team. Nurses need to continue to strive for better collaborative methods of delivering care in our nephrology programs. Emphasis should be placed on the need to encourage more open, public discussion about resource allocation for health care to ensure that all societal voices are heard, values are respected, and the best decisions are made about the just allocation of health care resources.

At the macro level of the system we require a collaborative approach to health care as we work together with consumers and governments to improve the health status of all citizens. We need to move beyond rhetoric to a place where there is true collaboration and consultation among these three groups as we strive to open moral space for continued societal ethical discourse (Rodney & Starzomski, 1994; Starzomski, 1997).

In the future, allocation of resources, selection of patients for treatment, and issues around withdrawing and withholding treatment will continue to require our ability to make ethical decisions. The shortage of human organs for transplantation will continue to push us to consider alternative sources for organs. Ethical concerns related to prenatal diagnosis of disease and gene therapy are not far off in nephrology as major strides are made in the identification of genes that cause specific types of kidney pathology such as polycystic kidney disease. Stem cell and cloning research may lead to regeneration of organs, and xenotransplantation may become a clinical reality. Nanotechnology may be used to diagnose and repair damaged tissues and organs. As we move in these new directions in nephrology, we must be ever vigilant, ensuring that the ethical concerns arising with each new type of treatment are adequately addressed to make certain that patients and their families receive the safe, high quality care they require. As nurses, we must always remember that we have a covenant with our patients and should always act in their best interest (Pellegrino & Thomasma, 1988). This is the pivotal requirement of caring, ethical nephrology nursing practice.

There are no simple answers to the complex challenges confronting us in nephrology. As we continue to move forward in this millennium, we must work together using thoughtful, critical, ethical decision making. Alternatives and solutions will emerge as we think about what it means to do good in nephrology nursing practice.

References

Ackerman, T. (1983). Experimentalism in bioethics research. *Journal of Medicine & Philosophy, 8*(2), 169-170.

Alexander, S. (1962, November 9). They decide who lives, who dies: Medical miracle puts a burden on a small committee. *Life,* 102-108; 111.

Anderson, J., & Reimer Kirkham, S. (1998). Constructing nation: The gendering and racializing of the Canadian health care system. In V. Strong-Boag, S. Grace, A. Eisenberg, & J. Anderson (Eds.), *Painting the maple: Essays on race, gender, and the construction of Canada* (pp. 242-261). Vancouver: UBC Press.

Andrews, L. (1992). The body as property: Some philosophical reflections - A response to J.F. Childress. *Transplantation Proceedings, 24*(5), 2149-2151.

Arras, J. (1991). Getting down to cases: The revival of casuistry in bioethics. *The Journal of Medicine and Philosophy, 16,* 29-51.

Author. (2002). The non-directed live-kidney donor: Ethical considerations and practice guidelines: A national conference report. *Transplantation, 74*(4), 582-589.

Baggs, J. (1993). Collaborative interdisciplinary bioethical decision making in intensive care units. *Nursing Outlook, 41*(3), 108-112.

Baggs, J., Ryan, S., Phelps, C., Richeson, J., & Johnson, J. (1992). The association between interdisciplinary collaboration and patient outcomes in a medical intensive care unit. *Heart & Lung, 21*(1), 18-24.

Balk, R. (1990). Should transplantation be part of a health care system? *Canadian Medical Association Journal, 36,* 1129-1132.

Beauchamp, T. (1982). Ethical theory and bioethics. In T. Beauchamp & L. Walters (Eds.), *Contemporary issues in bioethics* (2nd. ed.) (pp. 1-43). California: Wadsworth.

Beauchamp, T., & Childress, J. (1983). *Principles of biomedical ethics.* New York: Oxford University Press.

Beauchamp, T., & Childress, J. (1989). *Principles of biomedical ethics* (3rd. ed.). New York: Oxford University Press.

Beecher, H. (1966). Ethics and clinical research. *New England Journal of Medicine, 274*(24), 1354-1360.

Benjamin, M. (1992). Supply and demand for transplantable organs: The ethical perspective. *Transplantation Proceedings, 24*(5), 2139.

Benjamin, M., & Curtis, J. (1986). *Ethics in nursing* (2nd. ed.). New York: Oxford University Press.

Bergum, V. (2004). Relational ethics in nursing. In J. Storch, P. Rodney, & R. Starzomski (Eds.), *Toward a moral horizon: Nursing ethics for leadership and practice* (pp. 485-503). Don Mills, ON: Pearson Education Canada.

Bergum, V., Boyle, R., Briggs, M., & Dossetor, J. (1993). *Principle-based and relational ethics: Both essential features of bioethics theory and analysis.* Paper presented at The Canadian Bioethics Meeting, Montreal, Quebec.

Blake, D. (1992). The hospital ethics committee - Health care's moral conscience or white elephant? *Hastings Center Report, 22*(11), 6-11.

Blum, L.A. (1988). Gilligan and Kohlberg: Implications for moral theory. *Ethics, 98,* 472-491.

Boisaubin, E. (1988). Charity, the media, and limited medical resources. *JAMA, 259*(9), 1375-1376.

Brooks, J. (1993). The heart of the matter: Dalton Camp and his controversial transplant. *Canadian Medical Association Journal, 149*(7), 996-1002.

Brown, H., Rodney, P., Pauly, B., Varcoe, C., & Smye, V. (2004). Working the landscape: Nursing ethics. In J. Storch, P. Rodney, & R. Starzomski (Eds.). *Toward a moral horizon: Nursing ethics for leadership and practice* (pp. 126-153). Don Mills, ON: Pearson Education Canada.

Browne, A. (1994). *Ethics handout - Bridging the professions: An interdisciplinary course in health care ethics.* Vancouver, BC: University of British Columbia

Buchanan, A. (1991). Justice: A philosophical review. In T. Mappes & J. Zembaty (Eds.), *Biomedical ethics* (pp. 552-562). Toronto: McGraw-Hill, Inc.

Campbell-Heider, N., & Pollock, D. (1987). Barriers to physician-nurse collegiality: An anthropological perspective. *Social Science & Medicine, 25*(5), 421-425.

Caplan, A. (1992). Is xenografting morally wrong? *Transplantation Proceedings, 24*(2), 722-727.

Childress, J. (1992). The body as property: Some philosophical reflections. *Transplantation Proceedings, 24*(5), 2143-2148.

Cohen, C. (1992). The case for presumed consent to transplant human organs after death. *Transplantation Proceedings, 24*(5), 2168-2172.

Colvin, E., & Hammes, B. (1991). If I only knew: A patient education program on advance directives. *ANNA Journal, 18*(6), 557-560.

Colvin, E., Myhre, M., Welch, J., & Hammes, B. (1993). Moving beyond the Patient Self-determination Act: Educating patients to be autonomous. *ANNA Journal, 20*(5), 564-569.

Cooper, M. (1991). Principle-oriented ethics and the ethics of care: A creative tension. *Advances in Nursing Science, 14*(2), 22-31.

Coward, H., & Ratanakul, P. (Eds.). (1999). *A cross-cultural dialogue on health care ethics.* Waterloo, ON: Wilfred Laurier University Press.

Crawshaw, R., Garland, M., & Hines, B. (1989). Organ transplants: A search for health policy at the state level. *Western Journal of Medicine, 150*(1), 361-363.

Curtin, L. (1982). Human problems: Human beings. In L. Curtin & M.J. Flaherty (Eds.), *Nursing ethics: Theories and pragmatics* (pp. 37-42). Bowie, Maryland: Robert J. Brady.

Davis, A., & Aroskar, M. (1991). *Ethical dilemmas and nursing practice.* Toronto: Appleton & Lange.

Dickens, B. (1988). The anencephalic organ donor and the law. *Transplantation/Implantation Today, 5,* 42-46.

Dickens, B. (1991). WHO guiding principles on human organ transplantation. *Transplantation/Implantation Today, 8,* 12-18.

Donnelly, P., Henderson, R., & Price, D. (1999). Professional attitudes to bioethical issues ration the supply of "marginal living donor" kidneys for transplantation. *Transplantation Proceedings, 31*(1-2), 1349-1351.

Evans, R.W. (1993). Organ procurement and the role of financial incentives. *JAMA, 269*(24), 3113-3118.

Evans, R.W., Manninen, D., Dong, F., & McLynne, D. (1993). Is retransplantation cost-effective? *Transplantation Proceedings, 25*(1), 1694-1696.

Fox, R., & Swazey, J. (1992a). *Spare parts - Organ replacement in American society.* New York: Oxford University Press.

Fox, R., & Swazey, J. (1992b). *Leaving the field.* Hastings Center Report, 22(5), 9-15.

Fry, S. (1985). Individual vs. aggregate good: Ethical tension in nursing practice. *International Journal of Nursing Studies, 22*(4), 303-310.

Fry, S. (1989a). Toward a theory of nursing ethics. *Advances in Nursing Science, 11*(4), 9-22.

Fry, S. (1989b). The role of caring in a theory of nursing ethics. *Hypatia: A Journal of Feminist Philosophy, 4*(2), 88-103.

Fry, S. (1991). A theory of caring: Pitfalls and promises. In D. Gaut & M. Leininger (Eds.), *Caring: The compassionate healer* (pp. 161-172). New York: The National League for Nursing.

Gibson, C. (1993). Underpinnings of ethical reasoning in nursing. *Journal of Advanced Nursing, 18,* 2003-2007.

Gilligan, C. (1982/1993). *In a different voice: Psychological theory and women's development.* Cambridge: Harvard University Press.

Gillon, R. (1992). Caring, men and women, nurses and doctors, and health care ethics. *Journal of Medicine & Philosophy, 18*(4), 171-172.

Glover, J., & Moss A. (1998). Rationing dialysis in the United States: Possible implications of capitated systems. *Advances in Renal Replacement Therapy, 5*(4), 341-349.

Gohh, R., Morrissey, P., Madras, P., & Monaco, A. (2001). Controversies in organ donation: The altruistic living donor. *Nephrology, Dialysis, and Transplantation, 16,* 619-621.

Grundstein-Amado, R. (1992). Differences in ethical decision-making processes among nurses and doctors. *Journal of Advanced Nursing, 17*(2), 129-137.

Guttmann, A., & Guttmann, R. (1992). Sale of kidneys for transplantation: Attitudes of the health-care profession and the public. *Transplantation Proceedings, 24*(5), 2108-2109.

Hartrick Doane, G. (2002a). In the spirit of creativity: The learning and teaching of ethics in nursing. *Journal of Advanced Nursing, 39*(96), 521-528.

Hartrick Doane, G. (2002b). Am I still ethical? The socially-mediated process of nurses' moral identity. *Nursing Ethics, 9*(6), 623-635.

Hilton, A., & Starzomski, R. (1994). Family decision making about living related kidney donation. *ANNA Journal, 21*(6), 346-354; 381.

Hurley, J., Birch, S., & Eyles, J. (1992). *Information, efficiency, and decentralization within health care systems.* (CHEPA Working Paper # 92-21). Hamilton, ON, Canada: McMaster University.

Jameton, A. (1984). *Nursing practice: The ethical issues.* Englewood, NJ: Prentice-Hall.

Jecker, N., Carrese, J., & Pearlman, R. (1995). Caring for patients in cross-cultural settings. *Hastings Center Report, 25*(1), 6-14.

Johnstone, M.J. (1999). *Bioethics: A nursing perspective* (3rd ed.). Sydney: Harcourt Australia.

Jonsen, A. (1985). Organ transplants and the principle of fairness. *Law, Medicine, & Health Care, 13*(1), 37-39.

Jonsen, A. (1989). Ethical issues in organ transplantation. In R.M. Veatch (Ed.), *Medical ethics.* Boston: Jones and Bartlett Publishers.

Jonsen, A. (1990). *The new medicine and the old ethics.* Cambridge, Massachusetts: Harvard University Press.

Jonsen, A. (1995). Casuistry: An alternative or complement to principles? *Kennedy Institute of Ethics Journal, 5*(3), 237-251.

Kazim, E., Al-Rukaimi, H., Fernandez, S., Raizada, S., Mustafa, M., & Huda, N. (1992). Buying a kidney: The easy way out? *Transplantation Proceedings, 24*(5), 2112-2113.

Kilner, J. (1988). Selecting patients when resources are limited: A study of U.S. medical directors of kidney dialysis and transplantation facilities. *American Journal of Public Health, 78*(2), 144-147.

Kilner, J. (1990). *Who lives? Who dies? - Ethical criteria in patient selection.* New Haven: Yale University Press.

Kjellstrand, C. (1992). Disguising unjust rationing by calling it futile therapy. *The Bioethics Bulletin, 4*(2), 1-3.

Kjellstrand, C., & Dossetor, J. (1992). *Ethical problems in dialysis and transplantation.* Boston: Kluwer Academic Publishers.

Klevit, H., Bates, A., Castanares, T., Kirk, E., Sipes-Metzler, P., & Wopat, R. (1991). Prioritization of health care services: A progress report by the Oregon health services commission. *Archives of Internal Medicine, 151*(5), 912-916.

Kluge, E. (1992). *Biomedical ethics in a Canadian context.* Scarborough, Ontario: Prentice-Hall Canada Inc.

Kluge, E. (1993). Age and organ transplantation. *Canadian Medical Association Journal, 149*(7), 1003.

Long, R. (1994). Advance directives, informed consent, and the future of the ESRD program. *Contemporary Dialysis & Nephrology, 15*(5), 16-17; 21; 34.

Mappes, T., & Zembaty, J. (Eds.). (1991). *Biomedical ethics.* Toronto: McGraw-Hill, Inc.

Mariano, C. (1989). The case for interdisciplinary collaboration. *Nursing Outlook, 37*(8), 285-288.

Martin, D. (1992). Fetal tissue transplantation research: A Canadian analysis. *Health Law in Canada, 13*(1), 132-141.

Matesanz, R., & Miranda, B. (2003). International figures on organ donation and transplantation. *Transplant Newsletter, 9*(1), 1-43.

McDonald, M. (1993, May 7). Bio-ethical perspectives on health care cost containment. Resource allocation workshop handout, Calgary, Alberta.

McDonald, M., Stevenson, J.T., & Cragg, W. (1992). *Finding a balance of values: An ethical assessment of Ontario Hydro's demand/supply plan.* Unpublished report to the Aboriginal Research Coalition of Ontario.

MacDonald, M. (2003). *A framework for ethical decision-making: Version 6.0.* W. Maurice Young Centre for Applied Ethics, University of British Columbia. Retrieved from www.ethics.ubc.ca/mcdonald/decisions.html

Mendelsshon, D., & Singer, P. (1994). Advance directives in dialysis. *Advances in Renal Replacement Therapy, 1*(3), 240-250.

Mendez, R., Aswald, S., Dessouki, J., Cicciarelli, J., & Mendez, R. (1992). Costs and financing of kidney transplantation in the United States. *Transplantation Proceedings, 24*(5), 2127-2128.

Menzel, P. (1992). The moral duty to contribute and its implications for organ procurement policy. *Transplantation Proceedings, 24*(5), 2175-2178.

Mitchell, P., Armstrong, S., Simpson, T., & Lentz, M. (1989). American Association of Critical-Care Nurses Demonstration Project: Profile of excellence in critical care nursing. *Heart & Lung, 18*(3), 219-237.

Molzahn, A., Starzomski, R., & McCormick, J. (2003). The supply of organs for transplantation: Issues and challenges. *Nephrology Nursing Journal, 30*(1), 17-28.

Molzahn, A., Starzomski, R., MacDonald, M., & O'Loughlin, C. (2004a). Aboriginal beliefs about organ donation: Coast Salish viewpoints. *Canadian Journal of Nursing Research, 36*(4), 110-128.

Molzahn, A., Starzomski, R., MacDonald, M., & O'Loughlin, C. (2004b). Chinese Canadian beliefs toward organ donation. *Qualitative Health Research, 15*(1), 82-98.

Moss, A. (1995). To use dialysis appropriately: The emerging consensus on patient selection guidelines. *Advances in Renal Replacement Therapy, 2*(2), 175-183.

Moss, A. (1998). "At least we do not feel guilty:" Managing conflict with families over dialysis discontinuation. *American Journal of Kidney Disease, 31*(5), 868-883.

Moss, A. (2001a). New guideline describes nephrology community consensus on withholding and withdrawing dialysis. Recommendations regarding withdrawing dialysis. 2. *Nephrology News Issues, 15*(12), 58-61.

Moss, A. (2001b). Shared decision making in dialysis: A new clinical practice guideline to assist with dialysis-related ethics consultations. *Journal of Clinical Ethics, 12*(4), 406-414.

Moss, A., Rettig, R., & Cassel, C. (1993). A proposal for patient acceptance to and withdrawal from dialysis: A follow-up to the IOM report. *ANNA Journal, 20*(5), 557-561.

Moskop, J. (1987). The moral limits to federal funding for kidney disease. *Hastings Center Report, 17*(2), 11-15.

Nelson, H. (1992). Against caring. *The Journal of Clinical Ethics, 3*(1), 8-15.

Nelson, R. (1990). A policy concerning the therapeutic use of human fetal tissue in transplantation. *Western Journal of Medicine, 152*(4), 447-448.

Neu, S. (1994). Stopping chronic dialysis – The debate on a hot issue continues. *Contemporary Dialysis & Nephrology, 15*(5), 12-13.

Nielson, S. (1991). Autonomy, equality, and a just health care system. In T. Mappes & J. Zembaty. *Biomedical ethics* (pp. 562-567). Toronto: McGraw-Hill, Inc.

Noddings, N. (1984). *An ethic of caring. In caring: A feminine approach to ethics and moral education* (pp. 79-103). Berkeley, CA: University of California Press.

Omery, A. (1989). Values, moral reasoning, and ethics. *Nursing Clinics of North America, 24*(2), 499-506.

Pellegrino, E. (1993). The metamorphosis of medical ethics. *JAMA, 269*(9), 1158-1162.

Pellegrino, E., & Thomasma, D. (1988). *For the patient's good: The restoration of beneficence in health care.* London: Oxford Press Ltd.

Penticuff, J. (1991). Conceptual issues in nursing ethics research. *Journal of Medicine & Philosophy, 16*(3), 235-258.

Pfettscher, S. (1993). Bioethics in nephrology: Definitions and practices. *ANNA Journal, 20*(5), 543-547.

Pfettscher, S. (1996a). Dealing with difficult situations: Nephrology nurses, euthanasia, and assisted suicide. *ANNA Journal, 23*(5), 524-525.

Pfettscher S. (1996b). Dealing with difficult situations: When conflict arises regarding a patient's advanced directive and a physician's order. *ANNA Journal, 23*(2), 244-245.

Rapaport, F. (1993). Alternative sources of clinically transplantable vital organs. *Transplantation Proceedings, 25*(1), 42-44.

Redman, B., Hill, M., & Fry, S. (1997). Ethical conflicts reported by certified nephrology nurses (CNNs) practicing in dialysis settings. *ANNA Journal, 24*(1), 23-31; 32-33.

Reemtsma, K. (1992). Xenografts. *Transplantation Proceedings, 24*(5), 2225.

Rodney, P., & Starzomski, R. (1993). Constraints on the moral agency of nurses. *The Canadian Nurse, 89*(9), 23-26.

Rodney, P., & Starzomski, R. (1994). Responding to ethical challenges. *Nursing BC, 26*(2), 10-13.

Rodney, P., Varcoe, C., Storch, J., McPherson, G., Mahoney, K., Brown, H., Pauly, B., Hartrick Doane, G., & Starzomski, R. (2002). Navigating toward a moral horizon: A multi-site qualitative study of nurses' enactment of ethical practice. *Canadian Journal of Nursing Research, 34*(3), 75-102.

Rodney, P., Pauly, B., & Burgess, M. (2004). Our theoretical landscape: Complementary approaches to health care ethics. In J. Storch, P. Rodney, & R. Starzomski (Eds.). *Toward a moral horizon: Nursing ethics for leadership and practice* (pp. 77- 97). Don Mills, ON: Pearson Education Canada.

Rodney, P., Burgess, M., McPherson, G., & Brown, H. (2004). Our theoretical landscape: A brief history of health care ethics. In J. Storch, P. Rodney, & R. Starzomski (Eds.). *Toward a moral horizon: Nursing ethics for leadership and practice* (pp. 56-76). Don Mills, ON: Pearson Education Canada.

Ross, W. (1930/1988). *The right and the good.* Indianapolis: Hackett Publishing Co.

Roy, D., Williams, J., & Dickens, B. (1994). *Bioethics in Canada.* Scarborough: Prentice Hall Canada Inc.

Sadler, B. (1992). Presumed consent to organ transplantation: A different perspective. *Transplantation Proceedings, 24*(5), 2173-2174.

Schneiderman, L., Jecker, N., & Jonsen, A. (1990). Medical futility: Its meanings and ethical implications. *Annals of Internal Medicine, 112*(12), 949-954.

Scribner, B. (1964). Ethical problems of using artificial organs to sustain human life. *ASAIO Proceedings,* 209-212.

Seib, D., MacLeod, M., & Stiller, C. (1990). A step beyond: New limits in selection criteria. *Transplantation/Implantation Today, 7,* 47-51.

Sells, R. (1992). Some ethical issues in organ retrieval, 1982 to 1992. *Transplantation Proceedings, 24*(6), 2401-2403.

Sherwin, S. (1992a). Feminist and medical ethics: Two different approaches to contextual ethics. In H. Holmes & L. Purdy (Eds.), *Feminist perspectives in medical ethics* (pp. 17-31). Bloomington, IN: Indiana University Press.

Sherwin, S. (1992b). *No longer patient: Feminist ethics and health care.* Philadelphia: Temple University Press.

Sherwin, S. (1998). A relational approach to autonomy in health care. In S. Sherwin (Ed.), *The politics of women's health: Exploring agency and autonomy* (pp. 19-47). Philadelphia: Temple University Press.

Simmons, R., Marine, S., & Simmons, R. (1987). *Gift of life: The effect of organ transplantation on individual, family, and societal dynamics.* New Brunswick: Transaction Books.

Singer, P. (1992). Xenotransplantation and speciesism. *Transplantation Proceedings, 24*(2), 728-732.

Siminoff, L., & Leonard, M. (1999). Financial incentives: Alternatives to the altruistic model of organ donation. *Journal of Transplant Coordination, 9*(4), 250-256.

Spital, A. (1992). Unrelated living donors: Should they be used? *Transplantation Proceedings, 24*(5), 2215-2217.

Spital, A. (1993). Living organ donation is still ethically acceptable. *Archives of Internal Medicine, 153*(4), 529.

Starzomski, R. (1994). Ethical issues in palliative care: The case of dialysis and organ transplantation. *Journal of Palliative Care, 10*(3), 27-33.

Starzomski, R. (1997). *Resource allocation for solid organ transplantation: Toward public and health care provider dialogue.* Unpublished doctoral dissertation, University of British Columbia, Vancouver, Canada.

Starzomski, R. (1998). Ethics in nephrology nursing. In J. Parker (Ed.). *Nephrology nursing - A comprehensive textbook* (pp. 83-109). Pitman, NJ: American Nephrology Nurses Association.

Starzomski, R. (2000). Ethical issues: To dialyze or not? Is that the question? *CANNT Journal, 10*(4), 45-46.

Starzomski, R. (2004). The biotechnology revolution - A brave new world? The ethical challenges of xenotransplantation. In J. Storch, P. Rodney, & R. Starzomski (Eds.). *Toward a moral horizon: Nursing ethics for leadership and practice* (pp. 314-338). Don Mills, ON: Pearson Education Canada.

Stein, L., Watts, D., & Howell, T. (1990). The doctor-nurse game revisited. *New England Journal of Medicine, 322*(8), 546-549.

Stiller, C. (1990). Health care funding and transplantation in Canada. *Transplantation Proceedings, 22*(3), 980-981.

Storch, J. (2004). Nursing ethics: A developing moral terrain. In J. Storch, P. Rodney, & R. Starzomski (Eds.). *Toward a moral horizon: Nursing ethics for leadership and practice* (pp.1-16). Don Mills, ON: Pearson Education Canada.

Storch, J., & Griener, G. (1992). Ethics committees in Canadian hospitals: Report of the 1990 pilot study. *Healthcare Management Forum, 5*(11), 19-26.

Storch, J., Griener, G., Marshall, D., & Olinek, B. (1990). Ethics committees in Canadian hospitals: Report of the 1989 survey. *Healthcare Management Forum, 3*(4), 3-8.

Storch, J., Rodney, P., Pauly, B., Brown, H., & Starzomski, R. (2002). Listening to nurses' moral voices: Building a quality health care environment. *Canadian Journal of Nursing Leadership, 15*(4), 7-16.

Storch, J., Rodney, P., & Starzomski, R. (Eds.). (2004). *Toward a moral horizon: Nursing ethics for leadership and practice.* Don Mills, ON: Pearson Education Canada.

Toulmin, S. (1981). The tyranny of principles. *Hastings Center Report, 11*, 31-39.

Turcotte, J. (1992). Supply, demand, and ethics of organ procurement: The medical perspective. *Transplantation Proceedings, 24*(5), 2140-2142.

Vancouver Coastal Health Corporate Ethics Committee. (2005). How to make allocation decisions: A theory and test questions. *Healthcare Management Forum, 18*(1), 32-33.

Varcoe, C., & Rodney, P. (2002). Constrained agency: The social structure of nurses work. In B. Bolaria & H. Dickinson (Eds.), *Health, illness, and health care in Canada* (3rd ed.) (pp. 102-128). Toronto: Nelson.

Varcoe, C., Hartrick Doane, G., Pauly, B., Rodney, P., Storch, J., Mahoney, K., McPherson, G., Brown, H., & Starzomski, R. (2003). Ethical practice in nursing - Working the in-betweens. *Journal of Advanced Nursing, 45*(3), 316-325.

Veatch, R. (1991a). *The patient-physician relation: The patient as partner - Part 2.* Indianapolis: Indiana University Press.

Veatch, R. (1991b). Routine inquiry about organ donation – An alternative to presumed consent. *New England Journal of Medicine, 325*(17), 1246-1249.

Veatch R. (2000). *Transplantation ethics.* Washington, DC: Georgetown University Press.

Welch, G., & Larson, E. (1988). Dealing with limited resources – The Oregon decision to curtail funding for organ transplantation. *The New England Journal of Medicine, 319*(3), 171-173.

Wilkinson, J. (1989). Moral distress: A labor and delivery nurse's experience. *JOGNN, 18*(6), 513-519.

Yarling, R., & McElmurry, B. (1986). The moral foundation of nursing. *Advances in Nursing Science, 8*(2), 63-73.

Yeo, M. (1991). *Concepts & cases in nursing ethics.* Peterborough, Ontario: Broadview Press.

Yeo, M., & Donner, M. (1991). Justice. In M. Yeo (Ed.), *Concepts & cases in nursing ethics* (pp. 177-183). Peterborough, Ontario: Broadview Press.

Youngner, S., & Arnold, R. (1993). Ethical, psychosocial, and public policy implications of procuring organs from non-heart beating cadaver donors. *JAMA, 269*(21), 2769-2774.

Chapter Highlights

- The role of ethics in health care is multifaceted. Every day in our health professional or citizen roles we are confronted with situations that require moral judgments and the ability to make ethical decisions. Nowhere is this more apparent than in nephrology nursing practice where, for example, decisions about selecting patients for treatment, as well as initiating, withdrawing, and withholding treatment are fraught with ethical concerns and questions about the fair and just allocation of limited resources.

- Ethical theory is being developed constantly and can be thought of as work in progress. In order to make good ethical decisions, we must understand the evolution and application of ethical theory, and the role theory has, in helping us to make good ethical decisions.

- Pellegrino (1993) views the development of ethical theory as comprising several distinct periods: the Hippocratic Period, the Period of Principlism, and the Anti-Principlism Period. This classification is useful in understanding the development of nursing ethics and health care ethics, as they parallel the development of biomedical ethics and share a similar history (Yeo, 1991).

- Another area that is receiving attention in the development of ethical theory is the need to pay particular attention to cross-cultural issues, as there is considerable evidence to suggest that there is a lack of sensitivity to social and ethno-cultural contexts in health care delivery.

- An understanding of the development of health care ethics, ethical theory, levels of professional responsibility, and the role of the nephrology nurse as a moral agent provide the necessary knowledge to facilitate ethical decision making.

- Meeting the ethical challenges confronting us in nephrology nursing requires us to think about our professional roles as they fit into three levels of involvement: micro level, meso level, and macro level.

- One of the most difficult issues in nephrology nursing is the increasing number of people requiring treatment for chronic renal failure and the diminishing resources available to care for them.

- If we are to make good ethical decisions, then we need to understand and emphasize the importance of team communication and collaboration, remembering that the patient is the central member of the team.

- Ethics rounds and discussions (including retrospective case discussions) are a means of operationalizing ethical decision making on an ongoing basis, at the same time encouraging participation and communication among all team members.

- It is essential that we develop a theoretical foundation and a method for ethical decision making that can be used by nephrology nurses regardless of the concern that is being discussed.

ANNP633

Ethical Challenges in Nephrology Nursing

Rosalie Starzomski, PhD, RN

Contemporary Nephrology Nursing: Principles and Practice contains 39 chapters of educational content. Individual learners may apply for continuing nursing education credit by reading a chapter and completing the Continuing Education Evaluation Form for that chapter. Learners may apply for continuing education credit for any or all chapters.

Please photocopy this page and return to ANNA.
COMPLETE THE FOLLOWING:

Name: _____

Address: _____

City: _____ State: _____ Zip: _____

E-mail: _____

Preferred telephone: ☐ Home   ☐ Work: _____

State where licensed and license number (optional): _____

CE application fees are based upon the number of contact hours provided by the individual chapter. CE fees per contact hour for ANNA members are as follows: 1.0-1.9 - $15; 2.0-2.9 - $20; 3.0-3.9 - $25; 4.0 and higher - $30. Fees for nonmembers are $10 higher.

ANNA Member: ☐ Yes   ☐ No   Member # (if available) _____

☐ Checked Enclosed   ☐ American Express   ☐ Visa   ☐ MasterCard

Total Amount Submitted: _____

Credit Card Number: _____ Exp. Date: _____

Name as it appears on the card: _____

CE Evaluation Form
To receive continuing education credit for individual study after reading the chapter
1. Photocopy this form. (You may also download this form from ANNA's Web site, **www.annanurse.org.**)
2. Mail the completed form with payment (check) or credit card information to American Nephrology Nurses' Association, East Holly Avenue, Box 56, Pitman, NJ 08071-0056.
3. You will receive your CE certificate from ANNA in 4 to 6 weeks.

Test returns must be postmarked by **December 31, 2010.**

CE Application Fee
ANNA Member $25.00
Nonmember $35.00

EVALUATION FORM

1. I verify that I have read this chapter and completed this education activity. Date: _____

_____
Signature

2. What would be different in your practice if you applied what you learned from this activity? *(Please use additional sheet of paper if necessary.)*

_____

_____

_____

_____

_____

_____

_____

_____

_____

_____

_____

Evaluation	Strongly disagree				Strongly agree
3. The activity met the stated objectives.					
a. Discuss the foundations from which ethical issues are/can be addressed in nephrology nursing practice.	1	2	3	4	5
b. Devise strategies to enhance ethical decision-making in nephrology nursing.	1	2	3	4	5
c. Support personal ideas about the future ethical issues that will arise in nephrology nursing.	1	2	3	4	5
4. The content was current and relevant.	1	2	3	4	5
5. The content was presented clearly.	1	2	3	4	5
6. The content was covered adequately.	1	2	3	4	5
7. Rate your ability to apply the learning obtained from this activity to practice.	1	2	3	4	5

Comments _____

_____

8. Time required to read the chapter and complete this form: _____ minutes.

This educational activity has been provided by the American Nephrology Nurses' Association (ANNA) for 3.3 contact hours. ANNA is accredited as a provider of continuing nursing education (CNE) by the American Nurses Credentialing Center's Commission on Accreditation (ANCC-COA). ANNA is an approved provider of continuing education by the California Board of Registered Nursing, CEP 0910.

Medical Information and Documentation

Mary Rau-Foster, MBA, BS, JD, RN

Chapter Contents

Medical Information and Documentation

Chapter 34

Mary Rau-Foster, MBA, BS, JD, RN

The acquisition, documentation, utilization, and preservation of medical information are at the backbone of quality patient care. As well, full and timely reimbursement or payment is linked to accurate documentation of services provided. Of paramount importance to the complete and proper delivery of needed services is appropriate and timely written and verbal communication by and between members of the health care team. Appropriate and proper documentation of observations, assessments and actions can effectively aid in the defense of a medical negligence lawsuit. Failure to view and respect medical records as legal business documents, and to maintain them in a manner and style that will allow for easy access and use when needed, could harm an organization.

Privacy of Medical Information

During the course of treatment, patients share private details of their lives with physicians and other health care providers. No information is more sensitive or potentially more stigmatizing than personal health information and records. The disclosure of personal identifiable health care information can profoundly impact people's lives. It may affect decisions on whether they are hired or fired, whether they can secure business licenses and life insurance, and whether they are permitted to drive cars. Other secondary uses of the information, such as the use of genetic tests results for employment and insurance purposes, have the potential to harm the health care patient if the information is disclosed for unauthorized purposes. These facts accentuate the need for strong legal safeguards.

Patients trust their health care providers to respect their privacy, maintain the confidentiality of their health information, protect the integrity of the information, and assure its availability for their continuing care (Rhodes & Brandt, 2003).

For that reason, this information must be protected and maintained with the understanding that patients have a right to privacy and to have some control over the release of that information. Unauthorized disclosure, use, or communication of medical information is unlawful, unethical and a violation of a patients rights. Recent legislation and regulations have been enacted to provide for safeguards that will protect information shared by patients with health care providers in the course of treatment.

Communication of a medical history by the patient to the health care professional lays the foundation for the care of that patient. Without a level of trust and expectation that the information will be used to provide that care and will be protected from those without a legitimate need to know that information, the patients may withhold critical information that could affect the quality and outcome of care (Rhodes & Brandt, 2003). To that end, there must be policies, procedures, and practices established by the nephrology providers that will serve to address and protect the patient's privacy.

Confidentiality of medical information and records is regulated through various federal, state, and local statutes, ordinances, regulations, and case law. In addition, private accreditation standards, internal policies of facilities, and ethical guidelines of professional organizations also govern the confidentiality of information.

Healthcare Information Portability and Accountability Act (HIPAA): Federal Legislation

In 1996, important federal legislation, the Healthcare Information Portability and Accountability Act (HIPAA), was passed. HIPAA was introduced to improve Medicare and Medicaid patients' insurance program portability. Prior to the issuance of the HIPAA privacy rule, federal laws did not address the confidentiality of health care information collected and maintained by the private sector (doctors, hospitals, health plans, health insurers, and other health care-related entities).

Protecting the Privacy of Patients' Health Information

To address patient privacy and as part of HIPAA, Congress directed the Department of Health and Human Services (HHS) to issue patient privacy protection standards, including provisions designed to encourage electronic transactions and to create mandatory new safeguards to protect the security and confidentiality of health information. The final regulation covers health plans, health care clearinghouses, and those health care providers who electronically conduct certain financial and administrative transactions (e.g., enrollment, billing, and eligibility verification).

On April 14, 2003, the Federal privacy standards took effect for most health care providers. The provisions of the final rule generally apply equally to private sector and public sector covered entities. The purpose of the standards is to protect patients' medical records and other health information provided to health plans, doctors, hospitals, and other health care providers. HHS developed the standards with the intent that patients be provided with access to their medical records and have more control over how their personal health information is used and disclosed. These standards provide a uniform, federal privacy protections but do not impact state laws that provide additional protections to patient.

Patient Protections

The specific effect of the regulations is to limit the use of patients' personal medical information. They also protect medical records and other individually identifiable paper, electronic, or orally communicated health information. The standards, which includes the following, should be used to develop facility policies and procedures.

Access to medical records. Patients generally should be able to see and obtain copies of their medical records and request corrections if they identify errors and mistakes. An exception this standard might be if the physician determines for clearly stated reasons that disclosure to the patient is likely to have an adverse effect. The health care providers generally should provide access to these records within 30 days and may charge patients for the cost of copying and sending the records.

Notice of privacy practices. Providers must provide notice to their patients as to how their personal medical information might be used. They must also be notified of their rights under the new privacy regulation. Patients generally will be asked to sign, initial, or otherwise acknowledge that they received this notice.

Limits on use of personal medical information. The privacy rule sets limits on how providers may use individually identifiable health information. To promote the best quality care for patients, the rule does not restrict the ability of doctors, nurses, and other providers to share information needed to treat their patients. In other situations, though, personal health information generally may not be used for purposes unrelated to health care, and providers may use or share only the minimum amount of protected information needed for a particular purpose.

Prohibition on marketing. The final privacy rule sets new restrictions and limits on the use of patient information for purposes of marketing facilities services. The patients' specific authorization must be obtained before disclosing his or her information for marketing. At the same time, the rule permits doctors and other covered entities to communicate freely with patients about treatment options and other health-related information, including disease-management programs.

Confidential communications. Under the privacy rule, patients can request that providers take reasonable steps to ensure that their communications with the patient are confidential.

Complaints. Consumers may file a formal complaint regarding the privacy practices of a covered health plan or provider directly to the covered provider or health plan or to HHS' Office for Civil Rights (OCR), which is responsible for investigating complaints and enforcing the privacy regulation. When appropriate, OCR can impose civil monetary penalties up to $100 per violation and up to $25,000 per year for each requirement or prohibition violated for any violations of the privacy rule provisions. Potential criminal violations of the law are referred to the U.S. Department of Justice for further investigation and appropriate action. Criminal penalties apply for certain actions such as knowingly obtaining protected health information in violation of the law. Criminal penalties can range up to $50,000 and 1 year in prison for certain offenses; up to $100,000 and as much as 5 years in prison if the offenses are committed under "false pretenses;" and up to $250,000 and up to 10 years in prison if the offenses are committed with the intent to sell, transfer, or use protected health information for commercial advantage, personal gain, or malicious harm.

Written privacy procedures. The rule requires covered entities to have written privacy procedures, including a description of staff members who are permitted to have access to protected information, how it will be used, and when it may be disclosed. Providers must take steps to ensure that any business associates who have access to protected information agree to the same limitations on the use and disclosure of that information.

Employee training and designation of a privacy officer. Covered entities must train their employees in their privacy procedures and must designate an individual to be responsible for ensuring that the procedures are followed.

Public responsibilities. In limited circumstances, the final rule permits – but does not require – covered entities to continue certain existing disclosures of health information for specific public responsibilities. These permitted disclosures include: emergency circumstances; identification of the body of a deceased person or the cause of death; public health needs; research that involves limited data or has been independently approved by an Institutional Review Board or privacy board; oversight of the health care system; judicial and administrative proceedings; limited law enforcement activities; and activities related to national defense and security. The privacy rule generally establishes new safeguards and limits on these disclosures. Where no other law requires disclosures in these situations, covered entities may continue to use their professional judgment to decide whether to make such disclosures based on their own policies and ethical principles.

Medical Information Documentation

Documentation: Purpose and Methods

It takes a team of nephrology professionals (physicians, nurses, social workers, dietitians, patient care technicians, and others) to assess, analyze, plan for, and provide quality care and treatment to the nephrology patient. Each member of the team relies upon the observations, assessment, and expertise of the other team members in the endeavor to provide quality care and services to the patient.

It is important for all nephrology professionals to fully comprehend the necessity for complete, accurate written documentation. Accurate, accessible, and shareable health information is a well-accepted prerequisite of the provision of good health care, and documentation is an essential part of nursing practice and an important component in the care of the nephrology patient.

Documentation of care provided to the nephrology patient is of paramount importance but remains a challenge because the time constraints. The value of documentation cannot be minimized in the busy patient care environment. Quality patient care must go hand in hand with appropriate documentation of that care. Inadequate documentation can adversely affect patient care, reimbursement, care planning, and the ability to defend oneself in a medical malpractice or negligence claim.

Purposes of Documentation

Documentation serves many important purposes, including the following: (a) as an indicator of the nursing process, (b) as a communication tool by and between the team members caring for that patient, (c) as a permanent record of the events surrounding the care of the patient and the patient's response to the care, (d) for quality assurance purposes, (e) for reimbursement purposes, (f) for corporate compliance plan purposes, and (g) to provide a legal defense in the event of a medical malpractice or negligence claim.

The nursing process. All members of the nephrology team play important roles in the care of the patient. However, the nephrology nurse takes a lead role in the primary and day-to-day assessment and care of the patient. The most effective approach to patient care is a nursing process,

a problem-solving approach, and systematic method for implementing an individualized plan of care for the patient (Moreau et al., 2002). The systematic method includes the following steps:
1. assessment
2. nursing diagnosis
3. outcome identification
4. planning
5. implementation
6. evaluation (Moreau et al., 2002)

A nurse's duty includes performing an assessment regarding the health status of the patient and developing, implementing, and evaluating an appropriate plan of care. The nursing intervention required to stabilize the patient should be appropriate to the situation. Nurses cannot guarantee positive outcomes, but they can be judged on how reasonable and prudent their actions are under certain circumstances (Blair, 2003). Nurses are obligated to know and conform to laws, rules, and regulations at the federal, state, and local levels. When nurses accept patient assignments, they are accountable, legally and ethically, for the provision of safe care and the outcome of the care rendered.

An important element of the nursing process is decision-making about nursing interventions. Nurses must make assessments and decisions based upon subjective and objective data. Subjective data is derived from information relayed by patient, such as comments, history, and quotes obtained from patients and objective data arises from physical signs and laboratory data. The nephrology nurse may find it necessary to interpret this information as part of the assessment process as a prelude to making patient care decisions.

Decision making involves reviewing data and comparing it to appropriate standards or baselines to determine what problems, if any, exist. The goals and techniques of the quality control program must reflect the criteria found in the standards (Richards & Rathbun, 1982). The source of the standards includes legally imposed duties, those imposed by professional organizations, and facility-created rules, policies, and procedures. Detailed protocols must be developed to ensure compliance with the standards and there should be documentation in the medical record that demonstrates compliance with the standards and protocols.

Documentation of the nursing process. Each step of the nursing process requires documentation, especially the rationale behind the nurse's treatment decisions. Nursing documentation coupled with an outcomes management approach identifying pathway interventions and variances can provide an all-encompassing patient care documentation system (Windle, 1994).

Documentation as communication tool. The data gained from the nephrology professional's observations may alter the course of a patient's treatment and medical care. The failure to communicate those observations to the rest of the team members can impact the ability of the rest of the team to effectively assess and care for the patient. The medical record serves as one forum for communication by and between the team members.

Permanent record of events. A dialysis patient's condition and needs may change from one month to the next and, as such, may require the intervention of one or more mem-

bers of the nephrology team. Documentation in the medical record provides for a permanent record of what was done for the patient and why, the events surrounding the care of the patient, and the patient's response to the care. If a nephrology professional observes an event, situation, or patient condition but fails to report or to document the observations and treatment, there is no permanent record of what occurred and, therefore, an inability of the other team members to be aware of, appreciate, and respond to that information.

Documentation for quality assurance purposes. The records will be subject to review by representatives from many different agencies and representatives of regulatory bodies and used to evaluate the care provided by nephrology facility staff.

The surveyors will review the medical records to evaluate the quality of patient care and to ensure that the dialysis facility is complying with certain regulations as may be reflected in the medical records. The surveyor will also look at the records to see if there is evidence that the facility has implemented and is following its own policies and procedures and that they are in compliance with the regulations.

When a patient files a complaint with the state surveyors or the End Stage Renal Disease (ESRD) Network, a representative may review the medical records. The patient's complaints may relate to a quality of care issue to inappropriate treatment by the staff. That patient's records and those of other patients may be scrutinized to determine if the patient's complaint has some merit and if the quality of care being delivered to the patient(s) is at an adequate or substandard level.

The failure of the dialysis facility and staff to follow the Medicare regulations, including quality assurance and patient care issues, and the refusal to bring the unit into compliance with those regulations can result in a revocation of the Medicare certification. Medicare termination actions arise either from a provider's failure to comply with the Medicare Conditions of Participation (42 C.F.R. Part 482) or with other provisions of the Medicare law. This means that the nephrology facility will no longer be able to bill and receive funding from Medicare. Since many dialysis patients are covered through Medicare, this failure could result in the temporary or permanent closure of a dialysis facility.

Documentation for reimbursement purposes. Documentation can help ensure proper reimbursement by third parties. It must meet regulatory standards to justify billings and to ensure appropriate reimbursement for services and treatments. Payment may not be made unless the services are "reasonable and medically necessary." Medicare, Medicaid, and other third-party payors often disallow charges for treatments, equipment, supplies, and medication if documentation is inconsistent, inadequate, or absent. For example, the Center for Medicare and Medicaid Services (CMS) dictates that a patient's hematocrit must be at or below a specified level before reimbursement for the drug Epoetin alfa is provided. Inadequate documentation of the hematocrit level may result in denial of reimbursement. Although an isolated incident probably has only a minor impact on a facility's budget, several episodes can significantly affect financial status.

The facility's billing department bills for treatments, medications, and services rendered. In order to submit a request for payment, the billing representative must first review the records and prepare the bill according the Medicaid, Medicare, or third party insurance payor's procedure. This includes selecting a pre-established code based upon the services rendered or medication provided and billing using that code. These reimbursing entities require that a clean claim, one that can be processed without obtaining additional information from the provider, be submitted for payment. One of the Medicare standards is that claims submitted for reimbursement shall accurately represent services actually rendered, shall be supported by sufficient documentation, and shall be in conformity with applicable coverage criteria for reimbursement. The standard further states that the claims should be submitted only when appropriate documentation supports the claim and only when such documentation is maintained, appropriately organized in a legible form, and available for audit and review.

A lack of supporting documentation, missing signatures, invalid codes, and misinterpreted abbreviations are some of the most common coding errors (Jacob, 2001). Ascertaining what those errors are and educating one's staff on proper coding and documentation methods can result in fewer denied claims and improved financial reimbursement. Incomplete or incorrect identifying information can delay the processing of a claim. Such claims may have to be returned by the intermediary for re-submission (Medicare, n.d., chap. III, section 312).

Documentation for corporate compliance purposes. Every health care facility must have a corporate compliance plan to help prevent the submission of erroneous claims and to aide in combating fraudulent conduct. Federal and state laws and regulations prohibit health care providers from engaging in certain practices that are considered to be fraudulent or abusive of the reimbursement system and/or the services rendered to the patients covered under this program. Among the general prohibition categories are two areas that relate to provision of services such as dialysis. Two of the prohibitions, billing for unnecessary services and providing substandard care, require good documentation so as to disprove such allegations, presuming that the services were necessary and the care was in keeping with the standard of care.

Documentation as a defense tool. To provide a legal defense in the event of a medical malpractice or negligence claim, the nephrology staff member must be able to show that he or she acted or reacted in a reasonable manner. Failing to provide written documentation has made many medical malpractice or negligence lawsuits very difficult, if not impossible, to defend. The frequently repeated adage, "If it was not written, it was not done!" is a warning worth heeding. This statement simply means that to a lawyer, judge, or juror, your undocumented and uncorroborated memory of events may be of little value.

The written word is permanent whereas one's memory can be fleeting or grow fuzzy with time. Since most lawsuits are not tried for several years after an event has occurred, the written word has more credibility than one's memory. Jurors also have a tendency to believe information that is written at the time of the event, before there is any expectation or anticipation of a lawsuit; it has a greater ring of truth.

Medical Records as Legal Documents

Nephrology professionals have often been advised that medical records are considered legal documents and should be accorded the respect of any legal document. The medical record has status as a legal document because it is designated and recognized by the courts as a business record as long as it meets the established criteria.

The medical records are admissible in court as business records as exceptions to the hearsay rule. The exception to this rule allows the medical record to be introduced into evidence without requiring that each person who made entries to the record be called to testify about their entries, asked which entries they made, why they made them, and what information they based these entries upon. This would be a cumbersome and time-consuming task. When submitted to the court as evidence by a lawyer, the custodian of the medical records may be required to authenticate them as business records.

As an exception to the hearsay rule and to be deemed a business record, the medical record must meet four basic tests: (a) that the record be made in the regular course of the business; (b) that the entry in the record be made by an employee or representative of that business who had personal knowledge of the act, event, or condition that is being recorded in the record; (c) that the record be made at or near the time that the recorded act, event, or condition occurred, or reasonably soon thereafter; and (d) that the records be kept in a consistent manner, according to a set procedure.

Made in the regular or ordinary course of business. The policies and procedures of most, if not all facilities, require that patient assessment and care be documented in the medical record and specify when, how, by whom, and under what circumstances the entries be made. This requirement meets the first burden under the business record exception rule. The information in the record must pertain to the provision of medical care or to legal matters, such as guardianship status, that are necessary to the rendering of medical care. Information that does not meet the criteria should not be entered into the record.

Personal knowledge. The person making the entry into the medical record must be the one who has personal knowledge of the event being documented. An exception to this rule is if the person making the entry receives the information directly from the person who has personal knowledge of that event. For example, a patient care technician reports an event to a nurse who would document the information in the medical record. The notation would include the name and title of the person reporting the information and what was communicated to the nurse.

Timely entry. The record must be made at or near the time that the recorded act, event, or condition occurred, or reasonably soon thereafter. While the law does not specify a time limit, the test to measure what is considered timely is the test of reasonableness. What is considered reasonable will change as the circumstances also change.

Making notations on the patient's chart as soon as possible after an event has occurred helps ensure accurate information. It is dangerous to rely on your memory when the brain is attempting to receive, analyze, and file thousands of bits of information in a short period of time. Timely notations in the patient record are perceived as more accurate because they were made before a lawsuit was anticipated.

In the dialysis setting, it is easier to record pertinent information on the flow sheet at the time it is obtained. Flow sheets should be readily accessible to the staff member when checking the equipment and assessing the patient. The time noted must be accurate and the source of the time must be consistent, therefore all facility clocks and employee watches should be consistent. For example, if staff members use their own watches rather than a wall clock when making assessments or entering data on a patient, significant time discrepancies can occur. Time can vary by as much as several minutes. Such discrepancies may not be inconsequential. If a patient is found to have suffered a cardiac arrest, a variation of a few minutes has great significance. Discrepancies in the patient record are "fodder" for the plaintiff's attorney. Once a case reaches court, much time and attention are paid to the exact timing and response to the event.

Proper maintenance. The records must be kept in a consistent manner according to a set procedure. Each facility's policy and procedure should delineate how and in what manner records are maintained and stored.

Medical Records: Maintenance, Storage, Release and Destruction of Records

The established standards for Medicare-approved providers (as stipulated in the Medicare Conditions for Participation) are specific as to what is required of a dialysis facility in terms of creation, retention, preservation of medical records, and documentation requirements. Failure to comply with these conditions can subject the facility to exclusion from the Medicare program. The conditions and standards which are found in the Code of Federal Regulations (§ 405.2139) p149-150 are as follows:

§405.2139 – Condition: Medical records. "A dialysis facility maintains complete medical records on all patients (including self-dialysis patients within the self-dialysis unit and home dialysis patients whose care is under the supervision of the facility) in accordance with accepted professional standards and practices." The medical records must be complete and with accurate documentation, readily available, and systematically organized to facilitate the compilation and retrieval of information. A member of the facility's staff is designated to serve as supervisor of medical records services, and ensures that all records are properly documented, completed, and preserved.

(a) Standard: Medical record. Each patient's medical record contains sufficient information to identify the patient clearly, to justify the diagnosis and treatment, and to document the results accurately. All medical records contain the following general categories of information: Documented evidence of assessment of the needs of the patient, whether the patient is treated with a reprocessed hemodialyzer, the establishment of an appropriate plan of treatment, and the care and services provided (see §405.2137[a] and [b]); evidence that the patient was informed of the results of the assessment described in §405.2138(a)(5); identification and social data; signed consent forms; referral information with authentication of diagnosis; medical and nursing history of patient; report(s) of physician examination(s); diagnostic and therapeutic orders; observations and progress notes; reports of treatments and clinical findings; reports of laboratory and other diagnostic tests and procedures; and discharge summary including final diagnosis and prognosis.

(b) Standard: Protection of medical record information. The ESRD facility safeguards medical record information against loss, destruction, or unauthorized use. The ESRD facility has written policies and procedures which govern the use and release of information contained in medical records. Written consent of the patient or of an authorized person acting in behalf of the patient is required for release of information not provided by law. Medical records are made available under stipulation of confidentiality, for inspection by authorized agents of the Secretary, as required for administration of the ESRD program under Medicare.

(c) Standard: Medical records supervisor. A member of the ESRD facility's staff is designated to serve as supervisor of the facility's medical records service. The functions of the medical records supervisor include, but are not limited to, the following: ensuring that the records are documented, completed, and maintained in accordance with accepted professional standards and practices; safeguarding the confidentiality of the records in accordance with established policy and legal requirements; ensuring that the records contain pertinent medical information and are filed for easy retrieval. When necessary, consultation is secured from a qualified medical record practitioner.

(d) Standard: Completion of medical records and centralization of clinical information. Current medical records and those of discharged patients are completed promptly. All clinical information pertaining to a patient is centralized in the patient's medical record. Provision is made for collecting and including in the medical record medical information generated by self-dialysis patients. Entries concerning the daily dialysis process may either be completed by staff or by trained self-dialysis patients, trained home dialysis patients, or trained assistants and then countersigned by staff.

(e) Standard: Retention and preservation of records. Medical records are retained for a period of time not less than that determined by the State statute governing records retention or statute of limitations; or in the absence of a State statute, 5 years from the date of discharge; or, in the case of a minor, 3 years after the patient becomes of age under State law, whichever is longest.

(f) Standard: Location and facilities. The facility maintains adequate facilities, equipment, and space, conveniently located, to provide efficient processing of medical records (e.g., reviewing, filing, and prompt retrieval) and statistical medical information (e.g., required abstracts, reports, etc.).

(g) Standard: Transfer of medical information. The facility provides for the interchange of medical and other information necessary or useful in the care and treatment of patients transferred between treating facilities, or in determining whether such patients can otherwise be adequately cared for in either of such facilities" (42CFR405.2139, 2001, pp.146-147).

§405.2180 – Termination of Medicare coverage. "(a) Except as provided in §405.2181, failure of a supplier of ESRD services to meet one or more of the conditions for coverage set forth in this subpart U will result in termination of

Medicare coverage of the services furnished by that supplier."

"If termination of coverage is based on failure to meet any of the other conditions specified in this subpart, coverage will not be reinstated until CMS finds that the reason for termination has been removed and there is reasonable assurance that it will not recur" (p. 154).

Medical Negligence and Malpractice

In the event of an adverse occurrence, a patient has the right to pursue legal action against a health care professional for damages allegedly arising out of that professional's negligent act or omission. The burden of proving a claim of medical malpractice or negligence rests with the plaintiff (the patient or the person who is authorized by law to pursue legal action) by and through the lawyer retained to represent him or her. The law requires that the plaintiff show evidence of how the defendant (the health care professional) was negligent. The sources that are used to prove the case of medical malpractice or negligence include: medical records, interviews with witnesses, and sworn testimony of parties to the legal action.

One of the first steps that the plaintiff's lawyer takes in a medical malpractice or negligence case is to request a complete copy of the patient's medical records. He or she and an expert will review the records to ascertain what happened and to theorize as to why it happened. The attorney already knows what injury or illness that the patient suffered but now searches for evidence of negligent acts or omissions. The attorney has the luxury of comparing the outcome with the actions taken and criticizing the nephrology professional's actions. Attorneys and experts arrive at conclusions based on what they glean from the patient record and from the information obtained from interviews of the testimony of witnesses. They look at the end results of a medical procedure, examination, or treatment and decide whether the health care professional's actions were appropriate, timely, sufficient, and in keeping with the standard of care. Because they have the luxury of knowing the outcome, there is often an attempt to second-guess a decision to act (or not act).

The patient record should reflect the event, the judgment (i.e., the evaluation of the event), and the action taken. A nephrology professional should never record an event without interpreting its significance and noting the action taken. In a courtroom situation, the professional is often asked, "What did you do and why?"

The law requires that a person act in a reasonable manner, but the definition of "reasonable" is dependent upon the specific circumstances. The notations in the patient record should include an adequate description and a reflection of the nephrology professional's thought process regarding the circumstances and the actions taken (or not taken), as were appropriate under the conditions described. The notation should indicate the professional's judgment as he or she responds to the situation in the analysis, plan of action, implementation, and evaluation of the procedure or treatment rendered. If the outcome is less than desirable, the nephrology professional will then be better able to defend his or her actions (Rau-Foster, 1992).

Elements of Medical Malpractice or Negligence

The burden of proving the allegations of medical malpractice or negligence rests with the plaintiff's attorney. There are five elements of a negligent action which must be proven: (a) that there is a duty to comply with the standard of care, (b) that there is a failure to comply with the standard of care, (c) that the failure to comply with the standard of care is the direct and proximate cause of injury or illness, (d) that it was foreseeable that the failure to comply could result in injury or illness, and (5) that there was actual injury or illness (Health Law Center, 1975). The following are examples and explanations of the elements of medical malpractice or negligence:

There is a duty to comply with the standard of care. *Explanation.* What standard of conduct must be met by the health care professional to satisfy the duty owed to the patient? What steps must the nephrology professional take to protect and ensure that the patient is dialyzed in a safe manner?

Standard of care. The dialysis staff member shall conduct a pre-dialysis assessment of the dialysis machine in accordance with the facilities policies and procedures, including testing the following alarms: blood leak; arterial pressure; venous pressure; conductivity; ultrafiltration; high, air and foam detector; power failure; blood pump.

Act or omission. The dialysis staff member fails to checks all machine alarms and perform all pre-dialysis checks on the machine and dialyzer.

Documentation considerations and issues. The flow sheet should list each pre-dialysis assessment task with adequate space to enter the information. The person performing the checks should enter the information immediately upon performing the checks and his or her identification should be readily apparent on the flow sheet.

There is a failure to comply with the standard of care. *Explanation:* By error or omission, the health care professional fails to ensure that the patient's safety is protected in accordance with the standards promulgated by the profession.

Act or omission. Failure to test the air and foam detector alarm.

Documentation. The dialysis professional should not only perform the checks but also immediately document the results of the observations in the appropriate section of the dialysis flow sheet.

The failure to comply with the standard of care is the proximate (direct) cause of the patient's injury or illness. *Explanation.* The act or omission did, in fact, directly result in injury or illness to the patient. There are no other intervening forces that could have caused the problem.

Act or omission. The failure to check the air and foam detection alarm prevented the detection of air in the bloodlines and as a result air entered into the patient's circulatory system.

Documentation. The person performing the machine checks failed to check the alarms and to document that it was done.

It was foreseeable that the failure to comply with the standard of care could result in harm to the patient. *Explanation:* Removing and returning blood through tubing that is compressed by a blood pump subjects the tubing to damage and introduction of air into the bloodlines. If the air is not trapped into one of the two blood chambers, the air can enter the patient's body. Air in the blood stream can be incompatible with life and if the patient is not promptly treated can result in death. Since an air embolus is a recognized hazard of the procedure, for the patient's safety and well-being, the air detection alarm must be checked to ensure that it is working.

The patient sustained actual injury or illness. *Explanation:* The patient received air resulting in an air embolus and, ultimately, death.

Medical Records as Evidence in a Medical Malpractice or Negligence Case

The medical record can be a very effective defense tool for a malpractice or negligence case or claim. In the event of a lawsuit, experts will review the medical records at the request of the plaintiff and defense lawyers. The purpose of the review is to determine what, if any, negligent act or omission occurred that harmed the patient, how it occurred, who caused the injury, and whether that injury was in violation of the standard of care. The focus of the review will be on:

1. What happened?
2. Why did it happen?
3. What were the contributing factors?
4. What, if anything, was done? What was the staff member's thought process as evidenced by the act or omission?
5. What was not done? If a decision was made not to act, what was the reason for the decision and was it reasonable under the circumstances?
6. What was the outcome?
7. Was the patient injured as a result of any act or omission?
8. What was done wrong and by whom?

A Sample Scenario

The following example demonstrates how an assessment of the medical records might proceed in terms of determining negligence:

Mr. Doe is a 56-year-old man who has been on dialysis for 4 years. He is not always compliant with his medication and treatment prescriptions. He has numerous health problems, including hypertension and cardiac problems. On July 5, 1995, he comes to Dapper Dan's dialysis facility for treatment. He waits in the waiting room for about 20 minutes before he is brought back to the treatment area. He is ambulatory and requires some assistance. His pre-dialysis assessment is done, and his dialysis treatment is initiated. Approximately 1 1/2 hours into his treatment, the staff noticed that Mr. Doe was unresponsive and not breathing. All cardio-pulmonary resuscitative efforts are unsuccessful, and Mr. Doe is pronounced dead at the hospital emergency room. An autopsy was not done but the cause of death was listed as cardiac failure. The family sues for wrongful death.

The following are but a few of the questions that will be asked of any nephrology licensed and unlicensed staff members. They should be answered based on information documented in the medical record.

1. Was Mr. Doe's condition sufficiently stable so that he could be safely dialyzed on that date?
2. Was a proper pre-assessment done? By whom? What was included in the assessment? Did the assessment meet the standard of care?
3. Was he properly monitored during dialysis? By whom? How was he monitored? Did the staff member follow the monitoring policy and procedure?
4. Was the patient's condition stable during his dialysis treatment? How do we know? Who was evaluating the patient? How do we know?
5. Considering his cardiac and medical condition, should he have been monitored more frequently? By whom? If he should have been monitored more often, why wasn't he?
6. Was his dialysis machine in proper working order? How do we know? Who checked it? How do we know?
7. At what point should he have been noted to be unresponsive and in an arrest situation? Did the staff discover it in a timely manner? How do we know?
8. Did the staff respond to the situation in an appropriate manner? How do we know? What exactly did they do, who did it, and when? How do we know?
9. What emergency treatment was rendered? How do we know? Was it sufficient and appropriate? Who provided it? How do we know?
10. Did the clinic have complete and up-to-date policies and procedures in place? Were they followed at all times by all staff members involved in the care and treatment of this patient? How do we know? (Foster Seminars, 1998)

Documentation Specifics

The elements of good documentation include entries that are: contemporaneous, complete, concise, comprehensive, clear and correct and credible. These are the same criteria that the medical records must meet to be considered legal business records.

Elements of Effective Documentation

Contemporaneous – The information should be promptly recorded. There should be no procrastination or delay in making the entry into the chart. Information not entered into the record in a timely manner is most likely to be forgotten and omitted or recorded incorrectly, neither of which is acceptable. This helps ensure accurate information and improves the credibility in the juror's minds.

For example, someone fails to manually take the patient's blood pressure or to record it in the record and at a later point in time information, which may or may not have been perfectly recalled, is entered into the record. This information will lack credibility because its accuracy will be questioned.

Complete – The entries should be complete. Documentation should reflect a total picture of what occurred before, during, and after the treatment process. A complete dialysis patient record should reflect the total picture of what occurred before, during, and after the dialysis treatment process.

Pre-dialysis. The pre-dialysis phase includes information about the patient's condition, status, and complaints before beginning dialysis on a particular day. If the patient experienced a respiratory or cardiac arrest during treatment, this pre-dialysis information would play a vital role when there is a legal question as to whether the decision to initiate dialysis on that particular day was the right one. The question might be asked, "Given the patient's condition on that date and at that time, was it proper and appropriate to dialyze the patient in an outpatient dialysis setting?"

Documentation of a patient's comments or complaints about problems on non-dialysis days should be used to identify and evaluate the effects of treatment and medical prescriptions and, if applicable, the ways patients are contributing to their own health problems. This information should also alert other health care team members to the patient's needs. For example, if a patient indicates an inability to comply with dietary or medical requirements, the nurse's communication of this problem to the dietitian and social worker can trigger an investigation of the patient's financial status. Can the patient afford to purchase needed medications? Is the patient selecting foods incompatible with the diet prescription because prohibited food is cheaper or more readily available? The dietitian and social worker are also responsible for communicating their findings and recommendations to the other team members. This communication should be in writing to ensure that all team members are alerted to the patient's needs and to document the findings and rationale for the plan of action (which may be needed in the future to defend against allegations of negligence).

The dialysis equipment should be checked and the results recorded on the dialysis flow sheet before beginning treatment. There is substantial risk associated with mechanically removing blood, treating it, and returning it to the body. Even without negligence, the process can result in injury or death.

Dialysis equipment has mechanical safeguards to reduce risk and to diminish the severity of injury if the risk becomes a reality. However, not all risks can be mechanically eliminated. The manufacturer issues guidelines to follow in preparing, maintaining, inspecting, and using equipment. These procedures must be followed and documented. The patient's safety and well-being depend on the health care provider's compliance with these recommendations. Both the ability to determine the cause(s) of patient injury and the ability to provide a defense depend on written documentation.

During dialysis. Patient response is a major component of documentation during this phase, noting in the patient record the treatment procedure and the patient's response to medications and fluids administered. Nurses can use this information to evaluate whether the goals of the care plan have been met. A court can use the same documentation to determine whether the patient received adequate and reasonable care.

The second major component of documentation during dialysis is frequent evaluation of equipment. Such assessments are necessary because equipment can fail or malfunction at any time without adequate warning. The status of the safety alarms must be observed and recorded throughout the treatment. (The sloppy practice of disarming alarms and other safety features of the dialysis machine has resulted in patient injury and even death.) Not only is frequent monitoring and documentation of alarm status a standard of care for nephrology nurses, but the failure to perform these procedures may result in personal legal liability.

Post-dialysis. The patient's condition should be observed and described in the patient record following each dialysis treatment. This assessment can alert the health care professional to possible complications. If the patient seems to be in stable condition, a description of what constitutes "stable" should be noted. The phrase "the patient was stable at the time of discharge" may not stand up to scrutiny by a plaintiff's attorney. If the patient collapses, bleeds, or dies on the way home after dialysis, the person who made the assessment will be asked and must be able to define the term "stable" and what criteria were used to reach that conclusion.

The patient record should reflect the patient's condition at time of discharge. Factual documentation of the observation made becomes valuable if it is necessary to provide a defense against allegations of negligence. Unfortunately, many dialysis patients must drive themselves home against medical advice after treatment. In one recent lawsuit involving such a case, the patient struck another car after leaving the facility. When he was sued, he claimed that the dialysis staff should not have allowed him to drive home because he was not in stable condition. The only protection against claims of negligence in such a situation is documentation.

An example of an appropriate discharge note is:

"Patient was noted to be ambulating without difficulty or requiring assistance. Patient stated, 'I feel fine.' Voiced no complaints of weakness. The access site, which required the holding of pressure for an extra 5 minutes following the removal of the needles, was noted to be free of any bleeding at the time of discharge. Patient and her husband were instructed to apply pressure and to go to the emergency room if the access begins to bleed again. Patient and husband voiced their understanding."

Concise. Unnecessary duplication of information in the record should be avoided. An effective documentation system will reduce the need for unnecessary duplication of information in the record.

Comprehensive. Documentation should include all of the pertinent information. Proper documentation tells a very important story about the patient. It gives indication of his or her condition, what treatment was rendered (and if none was rendered, why not), and the patient's response to the treatment. This story also reflects your observations and thought process. It should describe what you did (or did not do) and why. The documentation should include enough information to allow the re-creation of the chain of events that led to the intervention, a description of the intervention, and a detailed report of the outcome of the intervention (Richards & Rathbun, 1982).

The following questions will help to assess the adequacy of documentation:
1. Does the information flow logically?
2. Are there any information gaps?
3. Are there abnormal test results without explanatory documentation?
4. Is there conflicting documentation in the patient record?
5. Are any required reports missing?

Clear. A description of the patient assessment, treatment, and response to treatment should be clearly understandable. The lack of standardized terms and nursing language can result in confusion, errors in patient assessment and care, and can be a threat to patient safety. A use of standardized and facility approved terms and abbreviations can effectively eliminate confusion and improve communication among the nephrology team members.

Correct. All information in the medical record must be correct. Incorrect information such as errors in patient's name or other information can have a negative impact on the overall perception of the credibility of person making the entry.

Credible. What accounts for credible entries made in the medical record? They are factual, legible, objective, timely, and respectable.

Factual. Describe what was seen, heard, and stated by the patient and/ or to the patient. Effective documentation includes answering the what, when, where, how, why, and who questions.

Legible. Write legibly. If the records and notations are sloppy, there will be a presumption that the care and treatment of the patient was also sloppy.

Objective. No judgmental or critical statements nor guesses should be included in the medical record. Unprofessional statements may lead to the presumption that the care and attention paid to the patient was substandard.

Timely. Don't delay documentation.

Respectable. Documentation must be respectable and respected for the role it can play in a successful defense to allegations in a lawsuit.

Documentation Tips

The following are suggestions for maintaining good documentation:

- Use only abbreviations that are standard in the industry and approved by your facility.
- Use only black or blue ink pens. (Other colors may not photo copy very well.)
- Write legibly. A jury may interpret illegible and or sloppy handwriting as being indicative of inadequate care or an attempt to hide or cover-up damaging information. If you cannot write legibly, print legibly.
- Spell all words correctly. Misspelled words can result in misinterpretation by others.
- Use only facility approved chart material. Never use notepaper; post it notes, scratch paper, or chart materials from or with another institution's name.
- Every page of the medical record or dialysis flow sheet must contain the following: (a) the patient's first and last name and middle initial (if there is another patient with the same or similar name), (b) the date including the year, and (c) the name of the person making an entry into the record. If the staff member uses his or her initials on the flow sheet, there must also be a notation on that same sheet indicating the name and initials being used.
- Charting should be completed in a sequential order. There should be no blanks or empty spaces in the narrative charting and each entry should be timed, signed, and include the title of the person making the entry.
- The timing of your record entry is important: Remember that documentation of an event that is made as soon as possible after an event has more credibility with a jury than one that is delayed.

- Make the entry as soon as possible after you have performed the task or made the observation.
- DO NOT make an entry in anticipation that you will do something.
- The entry should reflect that which you have already done and, therefore, use only the present or past tenses.
- Failure to chart medications or other treatments may be interpreted by another that the medication or treatment was not given. This can result in duplication of medication administration, treatments performed, or vital signs being unnecessarily repeated.
- No staff member should make an entry for or sign another person's name to a medical record documentation. On those rare occasions when it is necessary to do so, let the record clearly reflect that you are making an entry for another person. Include the reason why and the fact the notation is made on behalf of that person. Include the date and time you are making the entry and include the date (and time if known) that the absent staff member states that he or she performed the task.
- If you make a mistake in an entry on the medical record (which includes the nephrology flow sheets), the corrections or additions to the medical record must be made in a legally acceptable manner: (a) draw a line through the incorrect entry; (b) above the line, print the word "error" and include your initials and the date; (c) enter the correct information that corrects the error and sign you name; (d) do not use whiteout or correction tape!
- Do not alter or destroy any record. In some states any alteration or destruction of records is considered a misdemeanor crime.

What Should Be Charted?

- Observations of the patient (including vital signs).
- Responses by the patient to treatments, intravenous (IV) fluids, and medications (especially those that are not routinely administered as part of the treatment process).
- Observation of the patient's condition, pre, during, and post dialysis treatment.
- Patient education (information provided to the patient) and in what form that information was provided. (Was it verbal information only or did it also include written materials or audio or videotape education?). Also include how the patient responded and what his or her response was.
- Patient's refusal of treatment, medications, or to follow the facility's policies and procedures. (Include the reason that the patient gives for his or her refusal.)
- Physician visits, examinations, and treatments.
- Any abnormalities such as bruises, bleeding, wounds, or drainage. (Include information about the location, color, viscosity of the fluid, odor, and the amount of the drainage.)
- Any abnormalities or changes in vital signs or physical condition. Include information as to what you did about these noted changes and whom you notified about them. Also make notation of the patient's response to any treatments used to correct or improve his or her condition.

How Should Notations in the Chart Be Made?

- All information should be objective, factual, correct, and clearly documented.
- State your observations in terms of your senses:
  - What you saw (the patient convulsing)
  - What you heard (the gasping for breath)
  - What you felt (the skin was clammy)
  - What you smelled (the odor from the drainage)
- If you did not observe it or cannot factually validate, use "appears" language.
- Before using any "catch-all" phrases, ask yourself what real meaning those terms have. Also, be aware of how phrases can sound to those outside of the medical profession (i.e., jurors and judges):

  Improper: "Patient was found dead." ("Found" implies that you were nowhere around. Where were you? Was the patient left alone?)

  Proper: "Upon observation, patient was noted to be without a blood pressure, pulse, or respiration. I started CPR immediately."

  Improper: "Patient came here drunk as usual." (You don't like him much do you? So, therefore, you probably did not take good care of him.)

  Proper: "Patient was noted again today to have the presence of a strong smelling odor to his breath. His speech was slurred and his gait was unsteady. He has been observed to be in the same or similar conditions on many previous occasions."

  Improper: "Patient had no complaints." (Does that mean that you didn't hear any or that you didn't ask him? Or was it because he was comatose or dead and could not complain?)

  Proper: "Patient voices no complaints today…. or… patient states he is feeling well today."

All medical records are legal documents and should not be altered, changed, or destroyed. If a medical record becomes contaminated with blood, it is permissible to re-copy the information onto a clean record. However, the original record should be maintained in a plastic cover. The copied record should clearly indicate that it is a duplicate and why the chart had to be charted again on a new sheet. It should also indicate where the original document is kept (i.e., in the back of the chart or in the patient's previous medical records folder).

Documentation by Non-licensed Personnel

In many states, non-licensed personnel are permitted to document in the patient record (and particularly dialysis flow sheets) after undergoing a thorough training process. A countersignature by a registered nurse may be required to demonstrate supervision. By signing, the nurse is not necessarily attesting to the accuracy of assessments (e.g., vital signs) or the performance of the task by the non-licensed personnel, but is indicating that the entry was reviewed. The nurse is responsible for taking action if review of the documentation indicates that it is necessary. If the accuracy or validity of the information is questionable, the nurse has a duty to investigate the notation.

Issues Related to Documentation of Patient Termination

One of the most difficult situations that the nephrology team members face is the decision to terminate the relationship with a patient because of behavioral issues. When it become necessary for a facility to terminate the relationship with a patient, it is important to not only consider the steps in the Patient Termination Action and Documentation Checklist (see Table 34-1), but to answer the questions in the documentation process.

Improving Documentation

Too often, documentation is perceived as one more unrealistic requirement placed on an already overburdened professional. Over many decades, various methods of recording information in the medical record have been fashioned with a goal to simplify and improve the process. Such methods include narrative charting, problem-oriented charting, focus charting, charting by exception, SOAP (subjective, objective, assessment and planning), and SOAPIER (subjective, objective, assessment, planning, implementation, evaluation and revision) (Guido, Heaton, Leone, Rodano, & Swiggum, 1999). There are positive and negative aspects to each system. One such negative aspect is the failure of these methods to include an interdisciplinary approach to patient care.

More often than not, there was duplication of information or recording of information by other members of the interdisciplinary team that was not read or appreciated by the other team members. Health care focus topics replaced nursing diagnoses and served as a common thread to coordinate documentation of patient care. The many benefits identified thus far include daily interdisciplinary patient assessments and interventions documented on a single form, less time spent documenting, a handwritten system that provides for easy computerization in the future, a logical format for quick identification of patient status and changes related to a particular health care focus, and a format that facilitates future revision as prompted by ongoing evaluations (Scoates, Fishman, & McAdam, 1996).

Evaluation of Current Charting and Documentation Systems

Every facility should evaluate their documentation and medical records system. An effective evaluation method will ask and answer the following questions:
1. What works?
2. What does not?
3. What needs to change and how long will it take?
4. Will the new system be cost effective?
5. How will changing the system affect other members of the health care team?
6. How will the change impact the facility billing office?
7. How will you handle resistance to proposed changes? (Moreau et al., 2002)

The corrective action plan for documentation and medical record improvements will require valuable resources (time, people, money, systems, and equipment). The use of those resources to improve a system can reap future benefits and can actually pay for itself through decrease in waste, improvement in ability to store and retrieve and use information, and can decrease the financial impact that denied claims has on a facility.

Motivating Staff to Document: Why Does Documentation Continue to Remain a Problem?

In a profession and health care field where there is increased pressure to do more with less, shortcuts may be taken to meet the demands. The nephrology professional may argue that it is more important to provide patient care than to spend time documenting that care. However, there are several reasons why nephrology staff members are not properly documenting in the patient record: (a) they may think that they are doing it, (b) they may not know how or understand the purpose or proper methods of documentation, (c) there may be no perceived reward for doing so or consequences for non-compliance, and finally (d) they may think that their documentation methods and efforts are sufficient.

How to Improve Employee Compliance

Employee documentation efforts and compliance can be improved. Surveying the employees to find out what the obstacles are to effective documentation efforts is a good beginning. Acting upon the information to correct and improve upon documentation practices is imperative if a permanent improvement in the process is to be achieved. There are several primary and corrective methods that can be used to establish and maintain good documentation practices.

Training and education. Licensed personnel have undergone, as part of their training and education, classes in documentation. The unlicensed personnel who may be charting on the dialysis flow sheet will have to undergo training and education in the importance and proper methods of documentation. Regardless of prior training, all members of the health care team may require intermittent retraining to reinforce the need to and appropriate methods of documentation.

Time management techniques. Often the lack of organizational and time management skills will result in poor documentation. Ensuring that the nephrology team members have the tools, the time, and the time management training for performance of their jobs, including documentation in the medical record, may decrease the perception that there is no time to document.

Peer audits. A vital part of an effective documentation compliance program is implementing a method to monitor the nephrology staff's documentation efforts. One effective evaluation and correction method is the peer review or self-audit method. The peer-review or self-audit is not only a cost-effective way to protect against fraud and abuse, but they are also valuable educational tools for staff members to improve their coding and documentation skills. Auditing the patient record helps ensure that legal requirements have been met and that there are no omissions, inconsistencies, or gaps. The auditing process can be an efficient and simple one if procedures are properly defined. The report of the findings must be discussed in staff meetings, and the problems addressed and corrected in a timely manner.

Several staff members should share responsibility for the audits. Such sharing can serve as a useful motivational tool – having each staff member assess the patient record can be an

Table 34-1
Patient Termination Action and Documentation Checklist

Why is the patient being terminated?

Is the termination due to a violation of the facility policy, procedures, rules, or regulations by the patient? If so, what are they?

Have other patients been affected by the patient's actions? If so, how?

Have other patients been allowed to exhibit this type of behavior without corrective action being taken?

Have staff members been affected by the patient's actions? If so, how?

Is the problem behavior ongoing? Is it recent? How recent?

Was the patient aware of the policy, procedure, rules, or regulations? If so, how was he or she made aware of them?

Does the patient have the mental capacity to understand his or her actions and their consequences? If so, how was this determined?

What are the contributing factors for the patient's problematic behavior?

Were the concerns addressed with the patient? If so, when, how, where, by whom?

What was the patient's response?

Did the patient's problematic behavior change? If so, how?

What does the patient perceive as the problem? What does he or she perceive to be the contributing factors?

Were these concerns investigated and addressed? If so, by whom, when, how, and what were the results?

Did the patient receive one-on-one counseling? If so, when, where, by whom, and what were the results? If not, why not?

Did the patient participate in a group counseling session? If so, when, where, who was present, and what was the outcome? If not, why not?

Was a behavioral contract entered into with the patient? If so, when and what was the outcome? If not, why not?

Is the patient's family aware of the problems with the patient? If so, what was their response? If not, why not?

Has the patient been evaluated by a psychologist or psychiatrist? If so, what was the outcome? If not, what not?

What other steps could be taken prior to termination of the relationship?

Has the ESRD Network been advised of this situation? If so, when, how, and by whom? What was the response of the network?

Note: From Rau-Foster (1999), pp. 14-20.

incentive for all of them to be more proficient in their own documentation. For auditing to be effective, staff members must be held accountable for any inadequacies in documentation. It may be necessary to provide frequent inservice programs on documentation and to remind and motivate the staff that it is their duty to practice good documentation. If a staff member continues to be delinquent in or fails to comply with the documentation protocol, corrective action may be necessary and appropriate.

Enforce compliance. One way to enforce compliance by acknowledging appreciation for the staff member's compliance with good documentation practices and policies. In addition, immediate and appropriate corrective action must be taken for incidences of non-compliance. If education and retraining fails to correct the documentation errors and omissions, disciplinary action should be implemented. Not only should immediate corrective action be undertaken, but the employee's annual performance review should include an evaluation of compliance with documentation policies and procedures.

Create a culture of expectation. The staff member will look to, and be influenced by, what he or she perceives is of importance to and mandated by the management (and therefore facility) under the umbrella of the corporate culture.

Future of Medical Information Documentation and Records

The documentation methods and records retention practices continue to change. The use of computers, an increasing requirement that medical information be readily retrievable, and the need for better medical record storage systems are driving the recording and storing technology. These needs have led to Electronic Medical Records systems (EMR). The EMRs are being used by some health care facilities, and others are still utilizing paper records or a hybrid of paper and EMR systems. The Internet and Intranet have increased the possibility that information can be stored, accessed, and shared in a timely manner. While there are continued concerns regarding the security of electronic records, the ability to provide better patient care because of the ready access to the patient records will drive the change from paper to electronic records.

Personal digital assistants (PDAs) are one of the many useful and available pieces of technology that makes the health care professional's job, patient care planning, execution, and recording easier and more efficient. One health care organization, the Visiting Nurses Association (VNA) in California, recognized a need to improve the documentation and care process. The VNA issued to each of its nurses, a PDA that is specially programmed with in-depth clinical information and easy-to-use electronic nursing forms (Palm One, 2001). The staff response and enthusiasm has been very positive, as their tasks have been made easier.

Conclusion

A patient's medical information is a very important component in the planning and execution of quality care by the nephrology team members. Making a written record of the treatment provided to the patient does take time. However, not only is it a legal and regulatory requirement, it is also part of the nephrology professional's job. Documentation is not something that can be glossed over or dismissed as time consuming. It should be done not only because it is expected but also because as a professional it is part of the professional responsibility to the patient. This information must be protected, properly recorded, shared with members of the nephrology team, and stored. The nephrology facility must

have policies and procedures that are current and enforced. This will not only facilitate the delivery of quality patient care but will ensure that the facility is in compliance with the reimbursement guidelines and meets regulations and standards. Further, the documentation can also be used as a defense tool in a medical malpractice claim. To improve the nephrology team members' compliance with good documentation practices and standards, they must receive training and be held accountable for failure to comply with the facility's policies and procedures. The facility must be consistent in its enforcement of required practices.

References

Blair, P.D. (2003). Solid standards guard against malpractice. *Nursing Management, 34*(7), 10.

Code of Federal Regulations. (2001). *42 CFR 405.2139,* pp. 149-150. Washington, DC: Federal Government.

Code of Federal Regulations (2001) *42 CFR 405.2180,* p. 154 Washington, DC: Federal Government.

Code of Federal Regulations. (2001). *42 CFR. Part 482.* Washington, DC: Federal Government.

Guido, G.W., Heaton, M., Leone, C., Rodano, G.W., & Swiggum, R. (1999). *Surefire documentation.* St. Louis: Mosby, Inc.

Health Law Center. (1975) *Nursing and the law* (2nd ed.). Rockville, MD: Aspen Systems Corporation.

Jacob, J. (2001, July 2). Common coding errors can cost your practice. *American Medical News, 44,* 1.

Medicare. (n.d.). *In Medicare renal dialysis facility manual (pp. 3-4.1)* Baltimore: U.S. Government.

Moreau, D., Stockslager, J.L., Duksta, C., Eggenberger, T., Follin, S.A., Haworth, K., et al. (Ed.). (2002). *Charting made incredibly easy* (2nd ed.). Philadelphia: Lippincott, Williams & Wilkins.

Palm One. (2001, May). In PDAs: *The wave of the future.* Retrieved February 2, 2004, from www.palmblvd.com/articles/2001/5/2001-5-10-Nurses-Using-PDAs_print.html

Rau-Foster, M. (1992). Documentation: Priority or routine? *Nephrology Nursing, 2*(1).

Rau-Foster, M. (Producer). (1998). *Documentation in the dialysis clinic* [Video based training program]. Brentwood, TN: Foster Seminars.

Rau-Foster, M. (1999). *Dealing with challenging dialysis patient situations.* Brentwood, TN: FSC Publishing.

Rhodes, H., & Brandt, M.D. (2003, November). In *AHIMA practice brief: Protecting patient information after a facility closure.* Retrieved February 2, 2004, from www.ahima.org

Richards, E.P., & Rathbun, K.C. (1982). *Medical risk management: Preventative legal strategies for health care providers.* Retrieved January 25, 2004, from http://biotech.law.edu/Books/aspen/Aspen.html 1982

Scoates, G. H., Fishman, M., & McAdam, B. (1996). Health care focus documentation. *Nursing Management, 27*(8), 30.

Windle, P.E. (1994). Critical pathways: An integrated documentation tool. *Nursing Management, 1,* 25.

- The acquisition, documentation, utilization, and preservation of medical information are at the backbone of quality patient care. Failure to recognize medical records as legal business documents could harm an organization.

- Confidentiality of medical information and records is regulated through various federal, state, and local statutes, ordinances, regulations, and case law. In addition, private accreditation standards, internal policies of facilities, and ethical guidelines of professional organizations also govern the confidentiality of information.

- To address patient privacy Congress directed the Department of Health and Human Services (HHS) to issue patient privacy protection standards to protect the security and confidentiality of health information.

- Nephrology professionals must comprehend the necessity for complete, accurate written documentation. Accurate, accessible, and shareable health information is a well-accepted prerequisite of the provision of good health care, and documentation is an essential part of nursing practice and an important component in the care of the nephrology patient.

- Documentation serves many important purposes, including (a) an indicator of the nursing process, (b) a communication tool by and between the team members caring for that patient, (c) a permanent record of the events surrounding the care of the patient and the patient's response to the care, (d) for quality assurance purposes, (e) for reimbursement purposes, (f) for corporate compliance plan purposes, and (g) to provide a legal defense in the event of a medical malpractice or negligence claim.

- Nephrology professionals have often been advised that medical records are considered legal documents and should be accorded the respect of any legal document.

- Patients have the right to pursue legal action against a health care professional for damages allegedly arising out of that professional's negligent act or omission. The burden of proving a claim of medical malpractice or negligence rests with the plaintiff (the patient or the person who is authorized by law to pursue legal action) by and through the lawyer retained to represent him or her. The sources that are used to prove the case of medical malpractice or negligence include: medical records, interviews with witnesses, and sworn testimony of parties to the legal action.

- The elements of good documentation include entries that are: contemporaneous, complete, concise, comprehensive, clear, correct, and credible. These are the same criteria that the medical records must meet to be considered legal business records.

- Employee documentation efforts and compliance can be improved. Identifying obstacles to effective documentation and acting upon the information to correct and improve upon documentation practices is imperative.

- The documentation methods and records retention practices continue to change. The use of computers, an increasing requirement that medical information be readily retrievable, and the need for better medical record storage systems are driving the recording and storing technology.

ANNP634

Medical Information and Documentation

Mary Rau-Foster, MBA, BS, JD, RN

Contemporary Nephrology Nursing: Principles and Practice contains 39 chapters of educational content. Individual learners may apply for continuing nursing education credit by reading a chapter and completing the Continuing Education Evaluation Form for that chapter. Learners may apply for continuing education credit for any or all chapters.

Please photocopy this page and return to ANNA.
COMPLETE THE FOLLOWING:

Name: _____

Address:_____

City:_____State: _____Zip: _____

E-mail: _____

Preferred telephone: ☐ Home   ☐ Work: _____

State where licensed and license number (optional): _____

CE application fees are based upon the number of contact hours provided by the individual chapter. CE fees per contact hour for ANNA members are as follows: 1.0-1.9 - $15; 2.0-2.9 - $20; 3.0-3.9 - $25; 4.0 and higher - $30. Fees for nonmembers are $10 higher.

ANNA Member: ☐ Yes   ☐ No   Member # (if available) _____

☐ Checked Enclosed   ☐ American Express   ☐ Visa   ☐ MasterCard

Total Amount Submitted: _____

Credit Card Number: _____   Exp. Date: _____

Name as it appears on the card: _____

CE Evaluation Form
To receive continuing education credit for individual study after reading the chapter
1. Photocopy this form. (You may also download this form from ANNA's Web site, **www.annanurse.org**.)
2. Mail the completed form with payment (check) or credit card information to American Nephrology Nurses' Association, East Holly Avenue, Box 56, Pitman, NJ 08071-0056.
3. You will receive your CE certificate from ANNA in 4 to 6 weeks.

Test returns must be postmarked by **December 31, 2010.**

CE Application Fee
ANNA Member $20.00
Nonmember $30.00

EVALUATION FORM

1. I verify that I have read this chapter and completed this education activity. Date: _____

_____
Signature

2. What would be different in your practice if you applied what you learned from this activity? *(Please use additional sheet of paper if necessary.)*

_____

_____

_____

_____

_____

_____

_____

_____

_____

_____

_____

_____

Evaluation	Strongly disagree				Strongly agree
3. The activity met the stated objectives.					
a. Describe the guidelines and implications of maintaining patient privacy.	1	2	3	4	5
b. Summarize the documentation necessary to increase legal and ethical safety.	1	2	3	4	5
c. Itemize methods that can be used to improve documentation of patient care.	1	2	3	4	5
4. The content was current and relevant.	1	2	3	4	5
5. The content was presented clearly.	1	2	3	4	5
6. The content was covered adequately.	1	2	3	4	5
7. Rate your ability to apply the learning obtained from this activity to practice.	1	2	3	4	5

Comments _____

_____

8. Time required to read the chapter and complete this form: _____ minutes.

This educational activity has been provided by the American Nephrology Nurses' Association (ANNA) for 2.7 contact hours. ANNA is accredited as a provider of continuing nursing education (CNE) by the American Nurses Credentialing Center's Commission on Accreditation (ANCC-COA). ANNA is an approved provider of continuing education by the California Board of Registered Nursing, CEP 0910.

Public Policy Issues and Legislative Process

Kathleen Smith, BS, RN, CNN

Chapter Contents

Kathleen Smith, BS, RN, CNN

We live in interesting times. In just over 3 decades we have seen the birth of the Medicare End Stage Renal Disease (ESRD) program, which has provided access to lifesaving therapy to over 1.5 million people with chronic kidney disease (CKD) and has given hope to individuals who would otherwise face certain death. The enactment of that program provided a guarantee of federal payment for dialysis and transplantation, and coupled with private insurance coverage that followed, an industry was spawned that has expanded access to renal replacement therapy (RRT) to all those in need. Fixed dialysis reimbursement throughout the history of the program has led to efficiencies in care delivery, technological improvements, industry consolidation, and vertical integration in a number of provider companies and has affected the mix of registered nurses in staffing patterns. Medicare coverage for immunosuppressive drugs was the program's first foray into coverage of outpatient medications. In the late 1990s, quality was defined through the National Kidney Foundation (NKF) Dialysis Outcomes Quality Initiative (DOQI).

The ESRD program is a story of access, cost, and quality, the three policy issue areas related to health care. While separate and distinct, these areas are inextricably linked. Access was created with the passage of legislation and today refers more to beneficiaries' access to quality care than to treatment itself. Cost quickly became an issue due to the growing number of beneficiaries and continues to be dealt with in legislation that addresses coverage and regulations that determine payment policy for those covered items and services. Quality has moved far beyond the basic structure- and process-oriented conditions of participation or coverage in the Medicare program and is now defined and measured in terms of clinical outcomes.

For nurses working in nephrology, the ESRD program exists because a bill was introduced, responding to a recognized need in communities that was brought to the attention of legislators, and that was supported by the medical and scientific community of the time. As the largest group of health care professionals caring for individuals with CKD, the responsibility of nurses to continue the tradition and advocate for the future health of the ESRD program should be clear.

These are years of rapid change in health care. Nurses face many challenges and have many opportunities to participate in and influence the formation of health policy. Nurse citizens can become very effective in their lobbying efforts, whether on the federal, state, or local level, when they are visible and armed with information about the issues, key players, the processes, and their belief in what nursing can contribute to the health care system.

The purpose of this chapter is to introduce nephrology nurses to some of the current policy issues related to the ESRD program. In addition, the legislative process and the importance of its role in the development of public policy are addressed.

Contemporary Issues in the ESRD Program

Access Issues

The Medicare Beneficiary Improvement and Protection Act (BIPA) of 2000 required the General Accounting Office (now known as the Government Accountability Office) to study the access of Medicare beneficiaries to dialysis services (Pub. L. No. 106-554, App. F, § 422(d), 114 Stat. 2763, 2763A-517). The study was to determine whether there was a sufficient supply of facilities and whether Medicare payment levels were appropriate to ensure continued access to such services and to improvements in access and quality of care that could result in the increased use of long nightly and short daily hemodialysis modalities. The report, entitled "Medicare Dialysis Facilities: Beneficiary Access Stable and Problems in Payment System Being Addressed," found that patient access to care appeared to be adequate, although there is less access to home dialysis (General Accounting Office, 2004). They also noted that the reimbursement system was in need of change.

A draft recommendation that the Centers for Medicare and Medicaid Services (CMS) - the agency in the Department of Health and Human Services (DHHS) responsible for managing the two federal programs - redesign the prospective payment system to bundle the costs of services, including separately billable drugs, into one payment amount was not included in the final report since CMS does not believe it has authority to make such a change under current law. CMS noted that the Medicare Prescription Drug, Improvement, and Modernization Act of 2003 (MMA) requires the Secretary of DHHS to report to Congress by October 1, 2005, on the elements and features necessary in the design and implementation of a broader case-mix adjusted prospective payment system and is also required to conduct a 3-year demonstration project beginning January 1, 2006, that uses such a payment system (Pub. L. No. 108-173, § 623, 117 Stat. 2066, 2312-17).

The American Nephrology Nurses' Association (ANNA) nominated two nurses to serve on the Advisory Board to this demonstration project, and one of them, Bonnie Bacon Greenspan, BS, RN, MBA, was selected. In addition, since payment drives practice, nurses working in facilities that participate in the demonstration will experience first hand the changes that occur under the new payment system. ANNA will share the unique perspective of its members with those who will be evaluating the demonstration project.

Future access to care is another matter that looms on the horizon, given the projections that the ESRD population is expected to reach 650,000 by 2010 (Xue, 2001) and that by 2030 there could be over 2 million individuals on treatment for CKD (United States Renal Data System [USRDS], 2003). A number of current federal public health initiatives related to obesity and diabetes are, in part, targeting the long-term effects of those conditions on kidney function and, if successful, may lead to some reduction in this projection.

Access to nephrology professionals, nephrologists, and registered nurses is a related concern. The Renal Physicians Association and the American Society of Nephrology have begun to examine nephrologist workforce needs into 2010 and have expressed concern that demand may exceed supply under a number of assumptions. Can any future shortfall in nephrologists be met through the use of advanced practice nephrology nurses? Given the current nursing shortage and the aging of the nursing workforce, this may not be the solution. The average age of a registered nurse (RN) in 2000 was 45, and less than 10% of RNs were under age 30 according to the 2002 National Sample Survey of Registered Nurses, conducted by the Division of Nursing in the Health Resources and Services Administration (HRSA) of DHHS (http://bhpr.hrsa.gov/healthworkforce/reports/rnsurvey/rnss1.htm). Obviously, these workforce issues raise concerns about patient access to quality care by experienced nephrology clinicians.

On the state level, where nursing practice is regulated, nurses have faced legislative that address to establish nurse-patient ratios (primarily in hospital settings), mandatory overtime, the scope of practice for licensed practical nurses, and delegation authority to unlicensed personnel, to name a few. Specific to the dialysis setting, a number of states have taken action since the 1990s to regulate dialysis technicians or to deal with them specifically within the scope of RN and LPN delegation authority (O'Keefe, 2005). It is expected that such state-level activity will continue into the future and that nurses will need to educate state nurses associations, state boards of nursing, legislators, and other groups about their specific clinical practice areas and how these various attempts to protect citizens can be meaningfully applied, primarily in dialysis treatment settings.

With the aging of the population and the incidence of CKD later in life, there exists a potential access problem for the institutionalized elderly who require dialysis. The median age at which patients begin treatment for ESRD was 65 in 2003. Patients over age 75 made up one quarter of the new ESRD patients in 2003 (USRDS, 2005). In March and July 2004, CMS issued guidance (www.cms.hhs.gov/medicaid/survey-cert/sc0424.pdf and www.cms.hhs.gov/medicaid/survey-cert/sc0437.pdf, respectively) to dialysis facility and long-term care facility state surveyors that appears to change the Agency's view of these individuals as "home" dialysis patients and, instead, portrays them as patients of a dialysis facility requiring experienced licensed ESRD nurses on site in the nursing facility overseeing the dialysis and responsible for the care delivered. This is a major departure from the historical handling of such beneficiaries, and there will continue to be policy development and clarification on this subject, some of which may pose barriers to effective care delivery. Nurses will have to advocate for policies that meet the needs of this vulnerable subset of CKD patients.

Cost Issues

As documented by the USRDS and the CMS Annual Facility Survey, the rate of existing ESRD cases has increased each year since 1980, though the rate of increase

has been slowing since the early 1990s. Based on the most current data, over 452,000 patients were being treated for ESRD as of the end of 2003, nearly 325,000 of them on dialysis (USRDS, 2005). Prevalent patient rates continued to rise in 2003. More than 102,000 new patients started ESRD treatment in that same year, an adjusted incidence rate of 341 per million population (pmp).

The increase in the number of patients remains the driving force behind the overall growth in ESRD program expenditures. Changes in Medicare expenditures per patient year can arise from a number of causes, such as changes in the actual care that is given to ESRD patients, changes in the types of patients who are being treated (older, more diabetics, etc.), changes in prices paid by Medicare for specific services, and changes in Medicare billing practices.

Total spending in the United States for ESRD in 2003 from all sources was over $27 billion, an 6.8% increase over 2002; Medicare ESRD spending totaled $18 billion. Medicare spending per patient year 2003 was: ESRD total - $54,904; hemodialysis (HD) - $64,614; peritoneal dialysis (PD) - $43,384; transplant - $22,142 (excludes cost of organ procurement). On a per-patient-per-year basis, the cost increased over 2% between 2002 and 2003. This continued growth is related primarily to increases in the use of injectable medications such as epoetin, Vitamin D analogues, and iron preparations (USRDS, 2005).

The ESRD program covers less than 1% of all Medicare beneficiaries, but in 2002 it consumed nearly 7% of the Medicare budget. Clearly, a disproportionate share of Medicare expenditures is spent on Medicare ESRD beneficiaries. ESRD beneficiaries cost an average of at least 5 times more than beneficiaries in other categories: $6,211 is spent per aged beneficiary (> 65 years of age), $4,751 per disabled beneficiary (non-ESRD), and $34,709 per ESRD beneficiary. Average Medicare spending per beneficiary is $6,301. (Medicare Payment Advisory Commission [MedPAC], 2005).

This disproportionate spending will keep the ESRD program under the close scrutiny of legislators and CMS personnel, and alternative payment mechanisms, such as an expanded bundle of services included in the composite rate payment for dialysis, will continue to be explored. Nurses will have to be diligent in evaluating the impact and effectiveness such alternatives are likely to have on their workplaces and on patient care delivery and outcomes, and in sharing that evaluation with policymakers.

Quality Issues

Policy actions to ensure health care quality have been far less frequent or significant than actions to increase access to care or to decrease health care costs, making it the least visible aspect of the cost-access-quality policy triangle (Wakefield, 2002). This began to change in 1996 when President Clinton established the Presidential Advisory Commission on Consumer Protection and Quality in the Health Care Industry. This 32-member body was charged with making recommendations to the President on how to preserve and improve quality in the health care system.

Building on that work, in 1999 the Institute of

Medicine (IOM) Committee on Quality of Health Care in America released a highly-publicized report, *To Err is Human – Building a Safer Health System* (www.iom.edu). It suggested that as many as 95,000 people die annually in U.S. hospitals due to health care errors. In spring 2001, the same IOM committee released its final report, *Crossing the Quality Chasm: A New Health System for the 21st Century*, which made recommendations for achieving fundamental quality improvements in health care. Many of the recommendations addressed issues relevant to nursing, such as licensure and scope of practice; other recommendations related to changing reimbursement patterns were applicable to the nephrology setting.

Specifically, the 2001 report noted that current payment methods do not lend themselves to an environment of improved quality of care because there is little incentive to address overuse and misuse of services. To address these inherent flaws, the report advocated that providers able to demonstrate improved patient outcomes be properly rewarded for doing so.

In its March 2004 Report to the Congress, the MedPAC recommended that the Congress establish a quality incentive payment policy for physicians and facilities providing outpatient dialysis services (MedPAC, 2004). The Commission rightly pointed out that the outpatient dialysis sector is a ready environment for tying quality measures to payment in that (a) outcome measures are available that are evidence based, developed by third parties, and agreed-upon by the majority of providers; (b) CMS can collect provider-specific information without excessive burden on providers; (c) measures can be adjusted for case mix so providers are not discouraged from taking riskier or more complex patients; and (d) many providers can still improve upon some of the measures. However, MedPAC supported funding the quality payment by setting aside a small proportion (2%) of physicians' and facilities' payments as a means to motivate investment in better care.

Following the report, Sen. Max Baucus (D-MT), ranking Democrat on the powerful Senate Finance Committee, which has jurisdiction over Medicare, introduced legislation (S.2562, http://thomas.loc.gov) that, among other things, would have implemented the MedPAC and IOM recommendation. ANNA did not support the legislation because it was felt that the current dialysis composite rate was not sufficient for most providers to be reduced by the proposed 2% without putting access and quality care at risk. This legislation died with the close of the 108th Congress at the end of 2004, but similar legislation is expected to be introduced in the future.

The heightened interest in health policies that promote quality and protect consumers is likely to continue, and nurses have expertise to bring to this critical aspect of the policy debate.

Coming Together Around Access, Cost, and Quality

In 2003, the members of the kidney care community formed an alliance, Kidney Care Partners (KCP), a coalition that includes patient advocates, health care professionals, providers, and suppliers, united in a mission, individually and collectively, to ensure that CKD patients receive opti-

mal care and are able to live meaningful lives, that dialysis care is readily accessible to all those in need, and that research and development leads to enhanced therapies and innovative products (www.kidneycarepartners.com).

KCP was the first broad-based renal community stakeholder group in the history of the ESRD Program. ANNA was one of the first organizations to join KCP and has played an active role in the coalition's efforts since that time. The major initiative for 2003 was to have an annual update to the composite rate included in the Medicare prescription drug legislation, which seemed destined to move through the Congress that year.

Unsuccessful in that attempt, in 2004 the KCP member organizations prepared a more extensive agenda, this time adding other issues of access, cost, and quality in their legislative agenda. After months of defining and negotiating the elements, KCP was successful in getting the ESRD Modernization Act of 2004 introduced in both the House of Representatives and the Senate (H.R. 4927and S. 2614, respectively) to address their identified concerns (http://thomas.loc.gov).

These bills did not advance in 2004, as there was no Medicare legislation that year given the passage of the landmark Medicare prescription drug legislation the year before. They "died" with the close of the 108th Congress at the end of 2004.

Undaunted and committed to its goals, KCP was successful in getting legislation, the Kidney Care Quality and Improvement Act (H.R. 1298 and S. 635), reintroduced in 2005 (http://thomas.loc.gov). This legislation, like its predecessor, called on Congress to (a) establish an annual update framework for the ESRD composite rate, (b) create public and patient education initiatives to increase awareness about CKD, (c) provide Medicare coverage for CKD education services for Medicare-eligible patients, (d) improve the home dialysis benefit, (e) align the incentives for reimbursement for vascular access surgery with the stated clinical goal to promote creation of native fistulae, (f) establish a demonstration project to test outcomes-based ESRD reimbursement systems, and (g) evaluate the effect of the 2003 physician reimbursement changes for nephrologists.

In recent years, nephrology nurses have played a major role in educating local, state, and federal legislators about dialysis and transplantation by inviting them to visit their workplaces as part of ANNA's ESRD Education initiative. With the support of their employers and working with other professional colleagues, nurses have been the central figures in increasing the awareness and understanding of policymakers and their staff about CKD and the ESRD program.

The Importance of Action

It has been said that for a democracy to function successfully, its citizens must be willing to participate in their government. The First Amendment of our Constitution, adopted in 1791, guarantees us the freedom of speech, the right to assemble, and the right to petition the government. Therefore, speaking with policymakers to make our interests known and our concerns heard is a key component of our democratic government.

Participation in government takes many forms. The single most important activity of citizens in a successful democracy is exercising the right to vote. This implies an understanding of the issues and the potential impact brought about by election of the candidates. Other activities in which citizens may involve themselves include participating in campaigns, participating in organizations that promote or oppose certain legislative issues, contacting legislators about issues, and providing testimony at hearings. Citizens can even be involved in helping to originate and encourage the passage of specific legislation.

Much of nurses' professional lives will continue to be influenced by legislation at both the state and national levels. For this reason, it is imperative that nurses take on these responsibilities of citizenship. For example, the nurse practice act in each state controls nursing education and practice. These laws can be eliminated, amended, or totally rewritten in the legislative process. In addition, any law that involves not only health care but also general education and social issues may well have an impact on nursing, sometimes only because they affect the patient populations with which nurses work. On the national level, previous or existing legislation such as Medicare, Social Security, welfare reform, insurance reform, health professions' education programs, public health service programs, promotion of managed care, health research funding, and labor relations all affect nursing practice.

Keeping in mind that nursing is a predominantly female profession and that women only obtained the right to vote in 1924, it becomes easy to understand that nursing is barely out if its infancy in terms of developing its full potential in this area. Nurses still have a tendency to underestimate their strength in influencing legislation. But over the years there has also been increasing recognition that nurses must become involved in legislative issues. The consequences of nonparticipation are that someone else influences legislative decisions on health care in which nurses should have played a major role or that nursing issues are overlooked altogether. For example, nurses were not involved in the drafting of Medicare legislation, which, when enacted in 1965, did not include any reimbursement mechanisms for nurses.

In recent years, a number of nurses have successfully run for local, state, and national offices. Eddie Bernice Johnson (D-TX) was the first RN elected to Congress, although this did not occur until 1992. There are two other nurse members of the 109th Congress: Lois Capps (D-CA), a registered nurse, and Carolyn McCarthy (D-NY), a licensed practical nurse.

Since the advent of the 18-year-old vote, nursing students have become increasingly active in legislative affairs, and their impact has been felt often. For example, they have been influential in the passage of state child-abuse legislation, and they have been effective in providing testimony on federal funding for nursing education.

While nurses are becoming more sophisticated in the legislative process, they have not yet reached the full potential of their influence as individuals, as members of a profession that numbers nearly 3 million, and as members of other "power" groups. This is in part due to a lack of knowledge of the process itself and the resultant lack of understanding of the ways they can make their power felt and when they should take action.

Structure of the Federal Government

The three branches of the United States government include the executive, the judicial, and the legislative branches. Each branch has specific roles and functions, and each participates in a system of checks and balances that is provided by the due process of law in a democratic government.

Executive Branch

Included in the executive branch are the office of the president and the vice president and the federal departments and agencies. The duties of the executive branch include recommending legislation, such as President Clinton's sweeping health care reform proposal, the Health Security Act of 1993; administering laws; and signing or vetoing legislation. Current executive branch policy is usually presented to a joint session of Congress and to the nation by the president in the State of the Union address each January. Within the executive branch of government, responsibility for health policy lies with the DHHS. The Medicare and Medicaid programs are managed within DHHS by the CMS (formerly the Health Care Financing Administration – name changed in 2001).

Judicial Branch

The judicial branch of the government, the court system, has as its chief function the interpretation of laws and sometimes the changing of laws within its jurisdiction. One of the checks and balances in our system of government gives Congress the authority to supersede an unpopular Supreme Court decision by enacting new legislation. This has often been talked about in relation to the 1973 Roe vs. Wade abortion decision, but to date, the Supreme Court's ruling remains intact.

Legislative Branch

The legislative branch of government consists of the Congress, and its primary responsibility is to make laws. It is called the "heart of the government" because of its responsibility to listen and respond to the needs of the people. Our federal legislature is bicameral, meaning it has two chambers, the House of Representatives and the Senate. While the House has the constitutional responsibility to originate legislation that deals with raising revenue and spending it, sole authority rests in the Senate to approve the ratification of treaties, nominations by the president, and federal circuit court and Supreme Court nominations.

How a Bill Becomes Law

Nurses have long been involved in the drafting of policy and the procedures to carry them out within their employer organizations. National health policy is crafted in much the same way. At the federal level, however, such policies are written in the form of laws passed by the Congress (see Figure 35-1). The procedures for carrying out these laws are expressed in federal regulations and published in the Federal Register.

Figure 35-1
The Path of Legislation

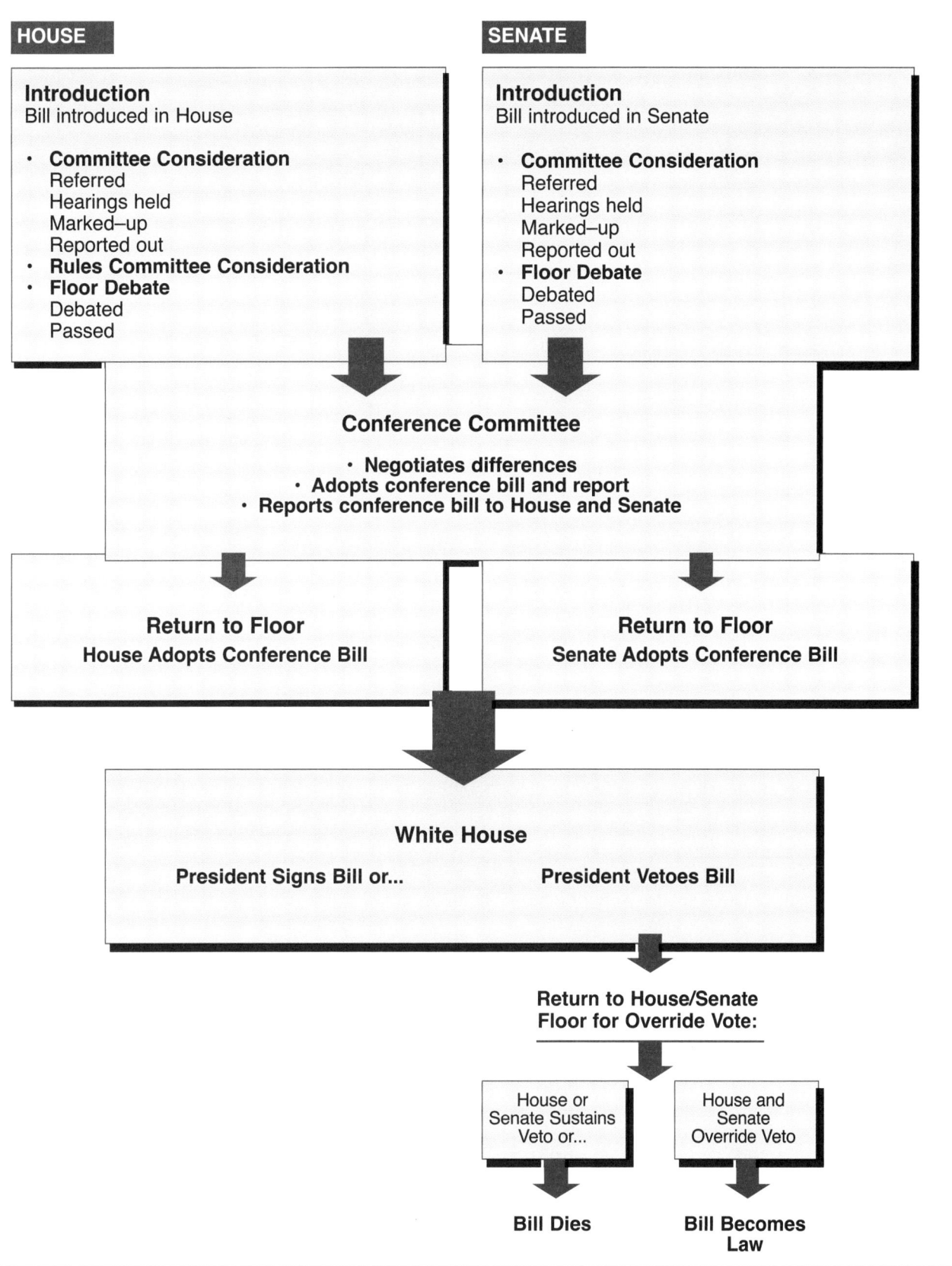

Figure 35-2
How Many Bills Become Law?

**Percentage of Bills Introduced That Became Law
In the 103rd Congress**

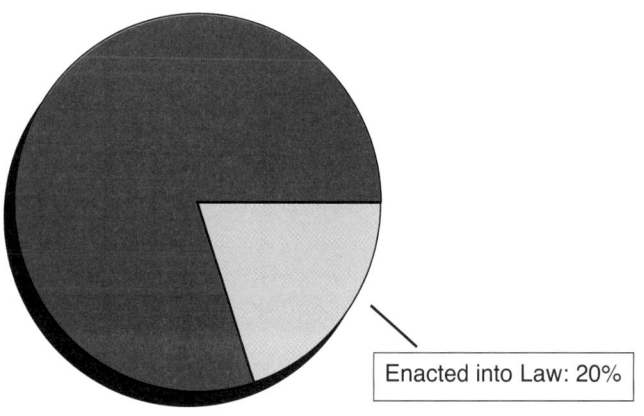

Enacted into Law: 20%

A bill faces difficult odds in winding its way through the House and Senate. Typically, in a 2-year session of Congress, some 10,000 bills are introduced. Less than 500 of them become law (see Figure 35-2). The only measures assured of passage are those that provide annual funds that keep the government operating, and sometimes they aren't passed on schedule. Otherwise, it takes strong White House support or the support of a substantial number of lawmakers for a bill to survive.

A bill can be introduced in either house of Congress, or it can be introduced in both houses simultaneously. Anyone can initiate a bill. It is a citizen's demand for action and it can originate from an individual who takes his ideas to a legislator, or it can originate within and be put forth by a special interest group, such as the KCP example stated earlier in this chapter. Obviously, the larger and more politically active the group is, the better chance they have of being heard. If there are a number of such groups representing even more citizens (that is, voters) with an interest in the issue, they may come together as a coalition in support of or in opposition to a legislative proposal and have even more clout.

In addition to individuals and special interest groups, some common originators of bills are a governmental administrator, agency, or department; a delegation of citizens in a legislator's district; a legislative committee; or a legislator. Many more citizens involve themselves in responding to legislation that has already been introduced than are involved in the initial introduction of a bill.

Committee Structure

Much of the work of Congress occurs in the House and Senate committees, each with jurisdiction over certain areas of law. Committees are further divided into subcommittees. Virtually all bills are sent to these panels after introduction, and many die there as a result of inaction.

The two major committees in the Senate that have

jurisdiction over health care and that oversee the activities of the DHHS are the Finance Committee and its Subcommittee on Health, with jurisdiction over Medicare and Medicaid; and the Health, Education, Labor, and Pension Committee, which authorizes programs under the Public Health Service Act, including federal funding of nursing education and research, National Institutes of Health programs, and the Centers for Disease Control and Prevention, to name a few.

In the House of Representatives there are also two major committees that are primarily responsible for health issues. The Energy and Commerce Committee, Subcommittee on Health, among other things, authorizes the programs under the Public Health Service Act, has jurisdiction over Medicaid, and shares jurisdiction for Medicare Parts B, C, and D with the Ways and Means Committee, Subcommittee on Health. The latter has exclusive jurisdiction over Part A (hospital insurance).

In both houses, the Appropriations Committees, Subcommittees on Labor, Health and Human Services, and Education, are responsible for yearly appropriations for health items in the federal budget, except the entitlement programs (like Medicare or Medicaid). Other committees in both houses, such as the Budget Committees, affect health care issues in their work.

Subcommittee Work

Once a committee takes up a bill, it usually holds public hearings. At this time, the members of the committee hear testimony from the bill's sponsors, expert witnesses, administration officials, and interest groups. Written testimony can be submitted for the record by a group or individual that is not asked to participate at the hearing.

The next step in the process is for the bill to go to "markup," which is a committee session during which the legislators go over the proposal line by line and vote on amendments, or changes. The committee then considers the bill. The outcome is either to approve the bill (report it out to the full committee) with or without amendments, some of which can change the nature of the bill completely; to "kill" or stop action on the bill; or to draft a new bill to accomplish the same goal but in a different manner.

The subcommittee to which a bill is referred is the first place where its fate can be influenced. If the bill is never put on the committee agenda or is not approved, it will generally not proceed further. The chairman, always a member of the majority party in that chamber, has the power to keep the bill off the agenda or to introduce it early or at a favorable time.

To get the desired action, which may be any of the above, interested persons/groups begin their legislative action at this point. All members of the subcommittee, especially the chairman, are important targets for the individuals or organizations interested in the outcome of the legislation. Individual members of these organizations whose legislators sit on the subcommittee may be asked to contact their legislator because of the influential position he or she has over the fate of the legislation at this point. Letters, phone calls, fax messages, e-mails, and personal contacts are used to reach the chairman and other committee members.

Committee Work

The same process outlined for subcommittees takes place at the full committee level, the next step in the legislative process for a bill that is reported out of the subcommittee. Opportunity for citizen/organization action occurs in the same way, focusing this time on the chairman and members of the full committee.

A bill that survives committee action can then be scheduled for action "on the floor," meaning the total membership of the body. Under certain circumstances, amendments may be proposed at this stage and are approved or rejected by the majority of those assembled.

House and Senate Action

In the House, most bills approved by committee proceed to the Rules Committee to determine how the bill will be handled on the House floor, how much time will be allotted for debate, and whether amendments will be permitted. The Majority Leader, who is chosen by the majority party, decides whether or when to call-up a bill for action. Members are given a limited amount of time to speak for or against the measure. Most issues are dealt with in a few hours.

In the Senate, bills approved by committees go directly to the calendar and are taken up whenever the Majority Leader of that body decides to call them. There are fewer limits on debate in the Senate than in the House, and rules allow members to speak twice for as long as they want on any issue before the Senate.

In light of this, to speed action on a bill, the Majority Leader may seek "unanimous consent" to vote at a certain time. If a member objects to this, a motion to limit debate (and therefore prevent a bill's opponents from "filibustering") may be offered. The procedure, called cloture, requires 60 affirmative votes. This is often difficult to obtain on closely divided issues. The Majority Leader rarely proceeds on an issue that he wants to succeed until he is assured of at least 60 votes.

The Voting Process

Roll-call votes in the House are cast electronically, each member using a plastic card and inserting it in terminals located throughout the chamber. The Senate still votes by voice; each Senator replies "aye" or "nay" as the roll is called. After a bill passes one chamber, it is sent to the other for a complete repetition of the process it went through in the first chamber.

Conference Committee

If the bill passed by the House and the one passed by the Senate on the same subject are not the same or if the bill has been amended by the second chamber after passing the first and the first chamber does not agree with the amendments, the bill is sent to a conference committee.

This committee consists of an equal number of members of each chamber, the "conferees," and usually includes members from the committees that originally handled the bills. Once the members of the conference committee are named by the leadership, opportunity for citizen action begins again.

The conference committee attempts to work out a compromise that will be accepted by both houses. Sometimes, however, the conferees are not able to arrive at a compromise and the bill dies, but usually an agreement is reached. The conference report issued by the committee when it achieves a compromise is sent to both chambers for vote. The compromise bill must be approved by each chamber before it is sent to the White House for action by the President.

Presidential Action

After passing both chambers, a passed bill goes to the President. If he approves it or fails to take action within 10 days, the bill becomes law. If Congress is not in session and the President does not sign the bill within the Constitutionally allotted 10 days, it does not become law. This is known as a "pocket veto." The President may veto the bill outright and return it to the chamber of origin. A two-thirds affirmative vote in both chambers is necessary to override the veto. Voting on a veto is often along party lines.

With such a complicated system of checks and balances provided by the due process of law in a democratic government such as the United States, often accompanied by extreme political pressure from within the government and the external influence of individuals and special interests, it is easy to understand why it is so difficult and time-consuming to translate an idea for legislation into law. This was the intention of our Founding Fathers, who envisioned a minimal role for the federal government and a more primary role for the states, as they created a true representative government.

Federal Budget Process

In early February each year, the president is required to submit his budget request to the Congress. This document represents a year of work by agency officials who channel their budget requests up to the cabinet level and through the Office of Management and Budget. It is their responsibility to reconcile the requests with the president's programs. Within 6 weeks after receiving the president's proposed budget, all standing House and Senate committees submit their views and estimates of expenditures for the coming year for programs under their jurisdiction to their respective budget committees. The House and Senate budget committees set economic priorities and make spending recommendations to the appropriations and tax committees.

Each spring Congress is required to pass a budget resolution that limits the level of funds that appropriations committees can approve. The resolution establishes a number of things, including targets for and ceilings on total federal spending and budget authority, targets for appropriations and other forms of spending in the budget, and a floor on total revenues. Once approved by Congress, the resolution serves as a guide to the appropriations and other spending committees on the amount of funding available for programs within their jurisdiction.

The annual congressional budget cycle is composed of three main processes: authorization, appropriations, and budget resolution. An authorization bill is a prerequisite for an appropriation bill. Passed through the process described above, authorizing legislation specifies the substance of federal programs and the agency that will implement them, and establishes program policies and the program's budget limit. A program may be authorized annually or less frequently. Renewal or modification of such programs is known as reauthorization. Responsibility for authorizing most health care programs rests with the committees of jurisdiction, which were previously mentioned.

Once an authorization bill is enacted, meaning a program is authorized under the law, Congress must pass yearly appropriation bills to determine the actual amount of funds that will be available for the authorized program. The appropriations process also determines how much funding each department or agency receives for a specific fiscal year. If zero funds are appropriated, the program is essentially dead for that fiscal year.

Within the House and Senate appropriations committees there are 13 subcommittees, one of which, the subcommittee on Labor, Health, and Human Services and Education, appropriates funds for most health programs. Because the Constitution requires all revenue measures to originate in the House of Representatives, it initiates all appropriations and taxation bills. Therefore, the House Appropriations Committee plays a major role in crafting spending bills. Interest groups and agencies appeal to the Senate Appropriations Committee when they disagree with the funding decisions made in the House.

As the federal fiscal year begins on October 1, it is expected that all appropriations bills for the new fiscal year will be enacted by that date. When this is not the case, to avoid a shutdown of the federal government, a Continuing Resolution may be passed by Congress that permits federal agencies to continue to operate at their current funding level until their regular appropriations bills are enacted.

Federal Regulatory Process

Action on a bill does not end with its passage. Laws are usually written very generally, as too much specificity makes them quickly obsolete. After a law is passed, it is sent to the particular federal agency that is responsible for writing the rules (also called regulations) which implement the law. These rules are as important as the law itself; they have the force of law and they spell out the specifics of how it will be carried out (see Table 35-1).

It is possible to influence policy at this point also and to strengthen or weaken the intent of the law. The opportunity to contribute to the development of regulations is available to interested organizations, which may make recommendations for individual appointments on advisory committees or offer informal participation and cooperation. Individuals and groups can also provide comment on proposed rules which are routinely published in the Federal Register (www.gpoaccess.gov/fr). ANNA has such a relationship with the CMS and is often called upon to educate key personnel by taking them on visits to dialysis facilities and transplant units.

Table 35-1
Steps in the Regulatory Process

1. Legislature passes law.
2. Law signed into law by Chief Executive (president or governor).
3. Public has opportunity to provide information to agency.
4. Executive branch agency drafts regulations to implement law.
5. Draft regulation published for public comment period.
6. Agency reviews public comments, may alter draft based on comments, and publishes final regulations.
7. Regulations have the weight of the law they are based upon.
8. Regulations should express the intent of the legislature when passing the underlying legislation and cannot exceed the scope of the statute.

Setting the Stage for Legislative Action

Influencing legislation cannot occur unless there is clear understanding of how our government works, how a bill becomes law, and how the legislative branch of government interacts with the executive and judicial branches. The congressional leadership is of critical importance; they are elected by their colleagues, they guide bills through the legislative process, and they act as chief advocates for the legislative agendas of their parties.

Most legislators are elected on platforms, either their own or their party's, and on promises for action that they make to their constituents. These platforms set their goals, the fulfillment of which comes with successful passage of appropriate legislation. However, they must also vote on other legislation to the satisfaction of their constituents. Most legislators want to be reelected to the same or higher office; many of their actions while in office reflect this desire.

As mentioned previously, during each 2-year Congress, lawmakers wade through thousands of bills, many of them on very intricate issues, only a small fraction of which are enacted into law. Obviously, not all of the bills introduced are brought to a vote, and certainly not all are of interest to nurses, but legislators need information on at least those bills that are of importance to their interests and constituents. On a typical workday, members of Congress scurry between committee hearings and meetings and sessions in the House or Senate chamber while trying to squeeze in meetings with constituents, lobbyists, and visiting dignitaries.

To help cope with their expanded workload, lawmakers have grown increasingly dependent on their staffs, a diverse group of lawyers, accountants, clerks, and others who act as secretaries, aides, assistants, schedulers, researchers, and policy analysts. In short, they keep the legislative machinery informed. These individuals review the issues and summarize background information on key bills and brief the legislators on the issues. They are very influential in that the legislators generally use this information to decide how they will vote. These staff members get information from numerous sources; organization representatives, individuals, and lobbyists usually become acquainted and maintain good relationships with them, providing information about the issues with which the legislator must deal. When nurses are not involved in this process, they find that the legislator may have received information about nursing that is either inaccurate, incomplete, obsolete, or skewed in another group's favor.

Placement on committees, where most preliminary action on bills takes place, is a measure of the influence a legislator has. Committee appointments are made by party leaders in each chamber of the Congress, that is, House and Senate. Committee chairmanships are particularly powerful positions; the chairmen are usually members of the majority party with seniority in their respective chambers. Some committees are more prestigious than others and are sought after eagerly. It is extremely important for citizens to know the committees on which their legislators sit because the action of committees affects the future of bills.

Congress is usually slow to act on controversial issues. The majority of lawmakers want to avoid the forefront of change for many reasons, including the wide diversity in political views that exists, regional interests, and general political caution. Congress seems more comfortable following trends than creating them, such that it often takes a groundswell of public pressure or a national crisis to shape consensus.

As a rule, the Senate is less reactive than the House, primarily because the senators are elected only every 6 years as opposed to House members who must be re-elected every 2 years. Also, House members are much closer to their constituents geographically as there is one Congressional representative for about 600,000 citizens. This is very different from the Senate, where there are two senators from each state, regardless of size. This structure, purposefully designed by our Founding Fathers, makes the Senate less compelled to react immediately to issues.

The Process of Lobbying

The increasing complexity of public issues has forced lawmakers to rely heavily on the expertise and opinions of professional and trade associations, as well as business, labor, and industry groups. Such expertise is provided by lobbyists, who are paid representatives of businesses and interest groups, many of which, depending on the size and contribution power of their constituencies, wield considerable power in legislative bodies.

It is important to remember that individual citizens can also "lobby" for or against legislation. Although there is certain mysticism about the process of lobbying, it is quite simply an attempt to legitimately influence legislators to promote or suppress proposed legislation.

Influencing the lawmaking process involves educating the legislators and staff members who decide what issues to consider in a given congressional year and who vote on those issues as they move through the legislative process. This process of influencing, or lobbying, is nothing more than educating, marketing, and selling. These are not foreign concepts to nurses who spend their days educating patients and colleagues, marketing ideas to physicians to get appropriate orders written, and selling good health

habits or practices to patients. There is no special skill set required of nurses who decide they want or need to involve themselves in the legislative process.

There are numerous ways in which lobbyists attempt to influence legislators. Much is done on the basis of direct contact in personal meetings and semi-social gatherings. Lobbyists provide information to the legislators and their staff, and introduce resource people to them. They are also valuable in that they keep their interest group informed about any pertinent legislation and aid the group in effective action.

Nurses and Political Action

From the foregoing, it can be seen that nurses and nursing students are major stakeholders in legislation. Whether acting as individuals or as part of groups, such as the American Nurses Association (ANA) and ANNA, they can make an impact on the political scene.

Learning to effectively communicate with legislators is essential to achieving positive results. While legislators want, and often need, to hear from their constituents, their time is limited. Carefully planned and organized contacts are usually the most effective means of communication.

One way that individuals 'lobby" is through membership in a professional association that establishes a legislative agenda and works as a group, and in coalitions with other like groups, to advance the agenda. For nurses, supporting these organizations with dues and making their opinions heard through various available mechanisms are some ways of indirectly influencing the legislative process.

However, to effectively influence a specific piece of legislation, multiple lobbying strategies need to be employed. ANNA's Board of Directors typically prepares a letter outlining the association's official position with regard to a specific piece of legislation in which it is interested. The letter is distributed to all members of the subcommittee or full committee to which the measure has been referred.

However, the individual members of those committees are more strongly influenced by what their own constituents tell them about a bill than they are by any other factors. This is where individual citizens become critical to the process and to their specialty association's ability to truly influence legislation. At this point, more direct lobbying techniques are necessary, such as communicating with legislators. ANNA members are notified, usually via the Internet, of those issues that are of interest to the association. ANNA's official position and its letter are posted, and sample letters are posted with E-mail links so the membership can send the letters directly to their legislators. In addition to E-mail, it is sometimes appropriate to mail letters and make phone calls and/or personal visits.

Becoming Knowledgeable

A number of ways exist for nurses to become more knowledgeable in matters of legislation. The ANA and its constituent state groups take a very active role in legislation, as does the National Student Nurses' Association (NSNA). A number of specialty nursing organizations devote significant resources to get involved in the legislative issues that affect their membership and its specific patient population. The major legislative activities of the nursing associations are discussed in the local chapters of these organizations. In addition, members are kept informed about legislation through the written materials of organizations. All major nursing journals routinely report key national legislative efforts and even those on the state level that have particular significance.

Another way for nurses to become more informed is by reading the newspaper. Feature articles, news stories, and editorials may not cover narrow pieces of legislation of special interest to nurses, such as reauthorization of the Nurse Education Act or funding for the National Institute for Nursing Research, but broader bills will be reported on, such as changes in the Medicare and Medicaid programs and welfare reform. Some newspapers list the major bills in the state legislature and in Congress, the action taken on those bills, and their current status. The votes of legislators on particular bills are also occasionally reported. This information enables readers to follow the path of a bill and to see how their legislators vote in general. The League of Women Voters and other political action groups can also be a source of such information.

One of the first pieces of information that nurses need to familiarize themselves with is the names of their own legislators. The easiest way is to use the Internet. For the House of Representatives, go to www.house.gov, and for the Senate, visit www.senate.gov. Otherwise, the information can be found at the local post office, city or county clerk's office, or libraries. A local or state League of Women Voters branch is also a good source, as is the district and state nurses' association. The state nurses' associations are usually headquartered in the state capital. Registration and voting are, of course, important, since voters are more influential than their nonvoter counterparts.

Preparing for Contact

Prior to contacting legislators, it is important to do some preparation on the issue at hand and on your legislators. With regard to the latter, make sure you are aware of your legislators' party affiliations and whether they have an interest in or any prior knowledge about the issue in question.

Legislators' local offices can be contacted, and are usually listed in the blue pages of the telephone book and through the Web sites mentioned above. Simply tell the staff what the issue is and ask if the legislator has taken a position on it or not. To call legislative offices in Washington, dial (202) 224-3121 for the Senate information operator and (202) 225-3121 for the House operator. Callers will be connected directly to their legislator's office, and operators will provide the direct phone number for future reference. This is still the most effective way to contact a legislator when time is of the essence, such as when an important issue is about to be voted upon.

Communicating by Letter

While this section focuses on writing a letter to a Congressional representative, it applies as well to writing state assembly representatives, city council members, the governor, the mayor, or even the President of the United States. The essentials of developing a letter to influence a policy maker are the same regardless of the intended recipient.

For members of Congress, letters can be mailed or sent via facsimile to the legislator's office. This is especially helpful if time is critical, and fax numbers are available from the legislators' offices.

The inside address and salutation should look like this:

The Honorable Full Name
United States Senate
Washington, DC 20510
Dear Senator _____:
or
The Honorable Full Name
U.S. House of Representatives
Washington, DC 20515
Dear Representative _____:
or
Dear Congressman/Congresswoman _____:

The writer should identify himself or herself immediately in the opening paragraph as (a) a constituent by indicating residence; (b) as a health care professional, including any relevant information that may be helpful, such as place of employment and the nature of work done, the patient population affected, etc.; and (c) as a member of a large group or coalition, such as ANNA or state nurses' association, which suggests strength in numbers. It may be important at times, however, to differentiate between issues that are of personal interest from those of any associations you belong to. Sufficient background should be provided to establish the writer as knowledgeable and credible in the specific area or issue of interest. At the end of the paragraph, state the issue and the purpose for writing.

General Guidelines

In terms of discussing the issues, there are several rules of thumb:

Rule #1. Be specific. Use the actual bill number if you know it. Share your position on the issue and why you have come to that position. Ask for your legislator's position on this issue. If you can, include information on the local impact of a specific proposal. Tell the member what you want done; for example, do you want the member to co-sponsor the bill to add support to it, do you want to urge hearings on the matter, or do you want a particular vote? Look for the member to make a commitment and ask for a response.

Rule #2. Be succinct. Legislators and their staff have very little time, and long letters and documents will not be read. Limit letters to one page and focus on one issue per letter. Pare down support material to a concise fact sheet, double-spaced, with bullets and good statistics and information that can easily be seen "at a glance;" such material will be kept and referred to as necessary.

Rule #3. Be positive. If you recognize a problem, suggest a solution, or if you think a particular bill is the wrong approach, explain what you think a better approach would be.

Rule #4. Be persistent. One contact probably will not be enough. Call the office a week or so after you have sent a letter to ask if it was received and to discuss it further with the appropriate staff member. (The staff members are assigned different types of issues. Typically, you will want to speak to the legislative assistant [LA] for health.) Ask for an appointment to discuss it with the legislator when he or she is in town. Keep the heat on!

Rule #5. Be courteous. It is not wise to threaten any kind of action if you don't get what you want from the legislator. If a vote is contrary to your position, let the member know politely how you feel.

Rule #6. Maintain contact. This need not be time-consuming and is important in relationship building. Send a note of thanks for a specific vote or for some activity that was held locally. Such behavior makes asking for something later a lot easier.

Rule #7. Report back. Let your organizations know what you have done. If you receive a reply letter from your member that indicates support, the association leadership can use that letter in Washington to ensure that support. Sometimes members say they cannot support a measure because they haven't heard from their constituents. Knowing that letters were sent and having copies of them can be very helpful.

Rule #8. Remember your manners. Always thank your legislator for time spent in a meeting or on the phone, or for a vote on your issue.

In closing the letter, establish yourself as a source of information and offer your assistance as a resource for more information. Prepare to be called if your issue becomes a hot topic. Invite the member or the staff to your workplace if that would help illustrate your point.

In terms of the form your letter takes, typed personal letters are acceptable and more commonplace with the predominance of personal computers, but handwritten letters are also acceptable. Many Members of Congress feel that handwritten letters are the only way to ensure that a personal letter is, in fact, personal. The next best thing would be to print the letter on personal stationery.

It cannot be stressed enough how much your letter counts! Sometimes specific letters are read by the members on the floor of the House or Senate; some letters are shared with colleagues if they illustrate a point particularly well. Members are told every day how much correspondence came in to both the district and Washington offices on a particular topic. Your voice will be heard. Don't forget to spread the word to others with whom you work or network. Urge them to write as well.

The Personal Visit

Personal visits with legislators and staff members are a very effective means of grassroots lobbying. It is generally wise to be on time and to stick to the agreed-upon time frame, to be friendly and polite, to greet the legislator with a firm handshake, and to keep the visit short. As with letter writing, it is important to identify yourself as a nurse and to offer to be a resource in the area of health care with which you are most familiar. Also, identify early in the meeting the purpose of your visit. Present the facts in an orderly man-

ner, be succinct, and avoid jargon or too many statistics.

It is thoughtful to comment on any of the legislator's bills or votes of which you approve and it is appropriate to ask if the legislator has taken a position on the issue you are there to discuss. Most of the guidelines for letter writing are also applicable to personal visits, including telling the legislator or staff member what you want the legislator to do and asking when you might have an answer on the legislator's position on your issue. If you are asked a question you cannot answer, do not lie; simply promise to get the information and provide it to them at a later date. This is one way to establish yourself as a reliable source of information that could improve your access to your legislator in the future.

At the end of the meeting, establish agreement on when you should follow-up and with whom, and then do so. Leave a one- or two-page fact sheet that summarizes the issue and your position and one that includes the name and phone number of a contact person if there should be a need for further information. Leave behind your business card as well. Remember the value of saying thank you and follow-up after the meeting with a letter thanking the legislator or staff member. Take this opportunity to reiterate your position, and include any information requested during the meeting.

Telephone Calls

Telephone calls are best for obtaining information. Lobbying calls should be kept very short. When making the call, ask for the legislative assistant who handles health issues, since this person can give you the best indication of the member's position on the issue. If you do not know your legislator's Washington office telephone number, call the Capitol switchboard at (202) 225-3121 (House) or (202) 224-3121 (Senate) and ask to be connected.

ANNA's Involvement in Legislative Arena

ANNA began its involvement in the legislative and regulatory arenas under the leadership and direction of Nancy Sharp during her tenure on the Board of the Directors and as the association's president in 1981-1982. The association established a Government Relations Committee to formally begin its journey into these arenas.

1980s Activities

When it was still known as the American Association of Nephrology Nurses and Technicians (AANNT), the association's first Legislative Policy Statement appeared in November 1983 (see Appendix E). It was a bold and visionary statement that addressed topics such as open physician staffing in dialysis facilities, the use of advanced practice nurses with reimbursement for their services under Medicare, elimination of certificate of need, and support for cost containment efforts in the ESRD program. This marked the first time the association had taken a public position on these issues. Many of the tenets, such as support for efforts to increase organ donation and the development of national standards and guidelines for the reprocessing of disposables and for water treatment safety, remain appropriate well into the 1990s (see Appendix D).

It is interesting to note that the early 1983 document supported concepts such as access, quality, cost effectiveness, along with issues of patient responsibility, data collection and reporting, and research. It even called for coverage of immunosuppressive drugs under Medicare. Given the contents of this document, it is clear that ANNA's Government Relations Committee was off to a very strong start.

Some of the early committee activities included two Head Nurse Surveys (one in 1984 and one in 1987) to evaluate the impact of the ESRD prospective payment regulations/reductions in reimbursement on the delivery of care in dialysis facilities.

In 1983 and 1984, the committee was very involved with then-Congressman Albert Gore and his staff as they were beginning to research the issues involved in organ transplantation. These activities resulted in the passage of the National Organ Transplant Act and the establishment of the Division of Organ Transplantation in the Health Resources and Services Administration of the Public Health Service, the Organ Procurement and Transplantation Network, and the Scientific Registry. Over the years, the committee has provided written and oral testimony to major House and Senate committees on such as topics as reuse, organ transplantation, the composite rate, and immunosuppressive drug coverage, and has responded to all proposed regulations that would affect the ESRD program.

In 1985 the association took a major step and hired a part-time legislative consultant. Years later, this became a half-time position, further demonstrating ANNA's commitment in this area.

Although the appointment of the state legislative representatives began during 1986-1987, it was during 1988-1989 that the State Legislative Representative Program was established to provide ANNA with a grassroots lobbying network and to provide the committee with information about state legislative activities. A Legislative Handbook was published and distributed for use by these state representatives, and the committee was reorganized with its members — regional advisors — coordinating the legislative activities within their regions. In 1993, the number of regional advisors was increased to two, with a legislative representative in almost every ANNA chapter.

1990s Activities

In 1990-1991, the Government Relations Committee became the Legislative Committee, and its first meeting was held in Washington, DC. During the following year, the first Legislative Workshop for 50 ANNA chapter Legislative Representatives was held in Washington, a chapter-level continuing education program was developed entitled "Influencing the Legislative Process," the legislative handbook was revised, and four reading packets were distributed to chapter Legislative Representatives.

In 1992-1993, to further increase grassroots participation in the legislative process, a section for Legislative Representatives was added to the ANNA Chapter Officer Orientation Manual, and the number of Legislative Representatives continued to grow. The Second Legislative Workshop was held in March 1994 in Washington, DC, with nearly 50 Legislative Representatives in attendance lobbying their elected officials on Capitol Hill.

2000 Activities

The committee became more formally entrenched in the Association's structure with the Regional Legislative Advisors becoming part of the Regional Executive Committees. Efforts focused on growing the base of State Directors and chapter Legislative Representatives.

ESRD Education Day, which became ESRD Education Week in 2005, was launched in 2003 along with the ESRD Briefing Book for State and Federal Policymakers, which was designed for use when hosting policymakers at dialysis facilities. Legislative Workshops were held in 2002 and 2004, the latter being held in conjunction with the annual symposium in Washington, DC. Nearly 300 nurses visited their Members of Congress on Capitol Hill as part of that event.

During these years, ANNA began taking members of Congress and their staff, as well as other government officials and representatives from CMS, on tours of dialysis and transplant units so they could better understand the policy issues of the day. Because the issues were expanding in scope, the Committee was renamed in 2004 as the Health Policy Committee.

One of the objectives of this committee has been to encourage more nurses to learn about and to incorporate legislative activity and public policy information into their professional activities. To that end, the committee and the legislative consultants have kept the membership informed through numerous articles in both the *ANNA Update* and the *Nephrology Nursing Journal* (formerly *ANNA Journal*), publishing the Legislative Agenda and Legislative Policy Statement each year after they are revised (see Appendix F) and sharing all formal letters, testimonies, and responses to proposed regulations in these publications. Since 1985, the year of the first Nurse in Washington Internship, ANNA members have participated in the planning of the event, have served as faculty, and have supported it with their attendance.

ANNA continues to stay involved with other nephrology organizations, specifically including the KCP coalition, as it anticipates the impact of various health care reform measures. Work continues in lobbying for appropriate reimbursement for dialysis and funding levels for the National Institute for Nursing Research and the Nurse Education Act. Collaboration continues with CMS and the ESRD Networks in support of quality initiatives in the ESRD program.

ANNA's Board of Directors, Health Policy Committee, and legislative consultant continually monitor and respond to issues affecting nursing, Medicare, and the ESRD program, providing information to policymakers on Capitol Hill, regulatory agencies, and those who influence policy decisions on various government boards and commissions. This is done based on ANNA's Legislative Agenda, which is updated and approved by the Board of Directors each year. The legislative agenda is to a large extent based on the association's Long-Range Strategic Plan.

Summary

As nursing activist Peggy Chinn has said, "For the remainder of this century, the most worthy goal that nurses can select is that of arousing their passion for a kind of political activism that will make a difference in their own lives and in the life of society." Let that continue to be a goal for nurses in the 21st century as well.

References

Committee on Quality of Health Care in America, Institute of Medicine (IOM). (1999). *To err is human: Building a safer health system.* Washington, DC: National Academy Press.

Committee on Quality of Health Care in America, Institute of Medicine (IOM). (2001). *Crossing the quality chasm: A new system for the 21st century.* Washington, DC: National Academy Press.

General Accounting Office. (2004). *Medicare dialysis facilities: Beneficiary access stable and problems in payment system being addressed* (GAO-04-450). Washington, DC: Author.

Medicare Payment Advisory Commission (MedPAC). (2004). *Report to the Congress: Medicare payment policy.* Washington, DC: Author.

Medicare Payment Advisory Commission (MedPAC). (2005). *A data book: Healthcare spending and the Medicare program.* Washington, DC: Author.

O'Keefe, C. (2005). State laws and regulations specific to dialysis: An overview. *Nephrology Nursing Journal, 32*(1), 31-37.

United States Renal Data System (USRDS). (2003). *USRDS 2003 Annual Data Report: Atlas of End-Stage Renal Disease in the United States.* Bethesda, MD: National Institutes of Health, National Institute of Diabetes and Digestive and Kidney Diseases.

United States Renal Data System (USRDS). (2005). *USRDS 2005 Annual Data Report: Altas of End-Stage Renal Disease in the United States.* Bethesda, MD: National Institutes of Health, National Institute of Diabetes and Digestive and Kidney Diseases.

Wakefield, M., et al. (2002). Contemporary issues in government. *Policy & politics in nursing and health care* (4th ed.). St. Louis, MO: Mosby.

Xue, J.L., et al. (2001). Forecast of the number of patients with end-stage renal disease in the United States to the year 2010. *Journal of the American Society of Nephrology, 12*, 2753-2758.

Additional Readings

American Nephrology Nurses' Association (ANNA). (1996). *ANNA legislative handbook.* Pitman, NJ: Author.

American Nephrology Nurses' Association (ANNA). (2004). *ESRD briefing book for state and federal policymakers* (2nd Ed.). Pitman, NJ: Author.

Smith, K. (1994). ANNA's involvement in legislative arena targets all levels of government. In *ANNA: Celebrating 25 years of service to the nephrology community* (p. 20). Pitman, NJ: ANNA.

U.S. Department of Health and Human Services (USDHHS), Health Resources and Services Administration, Bureau of Health Professions, Division of Nursing. (2002). *The registered nurse population, national sample survey of registered nurses-March 2000.* Rockville, MD: Health Resources and Services Administration.

- In just over 3 decades we have seen the birth of the Medicare End Stage Renal Disease (ESRD) program, which has provided access to lifesaving therapy to over 1.5 million people with chronic kidney disease (CKD) and has given hope to individuals who would otherwise face certain death.

- The Renal Physicians Association and the American Society of Nephrology have begun to examine nephrologist workforce needs into 2010 and have expressed concern that demand may exceed supply under a number of assumptions.

- The average age of a registered nurse (RN) in 2000 was 45, and less than 10% of RNs were under age 30 according to the 2002 National Sample Survey of Registered Nurses.

- In 1999 the Institute of Medicine (IOM) Committee on Quality of Health Care in America released a highly-publicized report, *To Err is Human – Building a Safer Health System,* which suggested that as many as 95,000 people die annually in U.S. hospitals due to health care errors.

- In spring 2001, IOM released its final report, *Crossing the Quality Chasm: A New Health System for the 21st Century,* which made recommendations for achieving fundamental quality improvements in health care.

- In 2003, the members of the kidney care community formed an alliance, Kidney Care Partners (KCP), a coalition that includes patient advocates, health care professionals, providers, and suppliers, united in a mission, individually and collectively, to ensure that CKD patients receive optimal care and are able to live meaningful lives, that dialysis care is readily accessible to all those in need, and that research and development leads to enhanced therapies and innovative products

- Much of nurses' professional lives will continue to be influenced by legislation at both the state and national levels. For this reason, it is imperative that nurses take on these responsibilities of citizenship.

- The three branches of the United States government include the executive, the judicial, and the legislative branches. Each branch has specific roles and functions, and each participates in a system of checks and balances that is provided by the due process of law in a democratic government.

- Nurses have long been involved in the drafting of policy and the procedures to carry them out within their employer organizations. National health policy is crafted in much the same way. At the federal level, however, such policies are written in the form of laws passed by the Congress (see Figure 35-1). The procedures for carrying out these laws are expressed in federal regulations and published in the Federal Register.

- Each year the president is required to submit his budget request to the Congress. This document represents a year of work by agency officials who channel their budget requests up to the cabinet level and through the Office of Management and Budget.

- Action on a bill does not end with its passage. Laws are usually written very generally, as too much specificity makes them quickly obsolete. After a law is passed, it is sent to the particular federal agency that is responsible for writing the regulations to implement the law. These regulations are as important as the law itself; they have the force of law and they spell out the specifics of how it will be carried out.

- The increasing complexity of public issues has forced lawmakers to rely heavily on the expertise and opinions of professional and trade associations, as well as business, labor, and industry groups. Such expertise is provided by lobbyists, who are paid representatives of businesses and interest groups, many of which, depending on the size and contribution power of their constituencies, wield considerable power in legislative bodies.

- A number of ways exist for nurses to become more knowledgeable in matters of legislation. The ANA and its constituent state groups take a very active role in legislation, as does the National Student Nurses' Association (NSNA). A number of specialty nursing organizations devote significant resources to get involved in the legislative issues that affect their membership and its specific patient population.

- ANNA began its involvement in the legislative and regulatory arenas under the leadership and direction of Nancy Sharp during her tenure on the Board of the Directors and as the association's president in 1981-1982. The association established a Government Relations Committee to formally begin its journey into these arenas.

ANNP635

Public Policy Issues and Legislative Process

Kathleen Smith, BS, RN, CNN

Contemporary Nephrology Nursing: Principles and Practice contains 39 chapters of educational content. Individual learners may apply for continuing nursing education credit by reading a chapter and completing the Continuing Education Evaluation Form for that chapter. Learners may apply for continuing education credit for any or all chapters.

Please photocopy this page and return to ANNA.
COMPLETE THE FOLLOWING:

Name: _____

Address:_____

City:_____ State: _____ Zip: _____

E-mail: _____

Preferred telephone: ☐ Home   ☐ Work: _____

State where licensed and license number (optional): _____

CE application fees are based upon the number of contact hours provided by the individual chapter. CE fees per contact hour for ANNA members are as follows: 1.0-1.9 - $15; 2.0-2.9 - $20; 3.0-3.9 - $25; 4.0 and higher - $30. Fees for nonmembers are $10 higher.

ANNA Member: ☐ Yes   ☐ No   Member # (if available) _____

☐ Checked Enclosed   ☐ American Express   ☐ Visa   ☐ MasterCard

Total Amount Submitted: _____

Credit Card Number: _____ Exp. Date: _____

Name as it appears on the card: _____

CE Evaluation Form
To receive continuing education credit for individual study after reading the chapter
1. Photocopy this form. (You may also download this form from ANNA's Web site, **www.annanurse.org**.)
2. Mail the completed form with payment (check) or credit card information to American Nephrology Nurses' Association, East Holly Avenue, Box 56, Pitman, NJ 08071-0056.
3. You will receive your CE certificate from ANNA in 4 to 6 weeks.

Test returns must be postmarked by **December 31, 2010.**

> **CE Application Fee**
> ANNA Member $20.00
> Nonmember $30.00

EVALUATION FORM

1. I verify that I have read this chapter and completed this education activity. Date: _____

_____
Signature

2. What would be different in your practice if you applied what you learned from this activity? *(Please use additional sheet of paper if necessary.)*

_____

_____

_____

_____

_____

_____

_____

_____

_____

_____

_____

_____

_____

Evaluation	Strongly disagree				Strongly agree
3. The activity met the stated objectives.					
a. Describe how the legislative, budgetary, and regulatory processes in the Federal government impact the issues faced in ESRD.	1	2	3	4	5
b. Outline methods nephrology nurses could use to become knowledgeable about the Federal government's processes that impact their practice.	1	2	3	4	5
c. Describe ANNA's involvement over the last 25+ years in the legislative arena.	1	2	3	4	5
4. The content was current and relevant.	1	2	3	4	5
5. The content was presented clearly.	1	2	3	4	5
6. The content was covered adequately.	1	2	3	4	5
7. Rate your ability to apply the learning obtained from this activity to practice.	1	2	3	4	5

Comments _____

_____

8. Time required to read the chapter and complete this form: _____ minutes.

> *This educational activity has been provided by the American Nephrology Nurses' Association (ANNA) for 2.6 contact hours. ANNA is accredited as a provider of continuing nursing education (CNE) by the American Nurses Credentialing Center's Commission on Accreditation (ANCC-COA). ANNA is an approved provider of continuing education by the California Board of Registered Nursing, CEP 0910.*

The Federal End Stage Renal Disease (ESRD) Program

Janel Parker, MSN, RN, CNN
Gail S. Wick, BSN, RN, CNN

CHAPTER 36

Chapter Contents

The Federal End Stage Renal Disease (ESRD) Program | Chapter 36

Janel Parker, MSN, RN, CNN
Gail S. Wick, BSN, RN, CNN

The End Stage Renal Disease (ESRD) Program is the only federal program that entitles people of all ages to Medicare coverage on the basis of their diagnosis. Any American who is either eligible for Social Security or is the dependent of someone who is eligible, is entitled to Medicare coverage for most, and occasionally all, of the costs of their treatment regardless of age, race or sex.

In the Social Security Amendments of 1972 (HR-1, Title XVIII), Public Law No. 92-603, Congress created this authorization to Medicare in support of persons with the diagnosis of chronic renal failure who were eligible for benefits under Social Security, and for the spouses or dependent children of these persons. These Medicare benefits, effective on July 1, 1973, provided access to dialysis treatments, kidney transplantation, and inpatient and outpatient care from physicians as well as renal treatment centers.

Since its inception, more than 1.3 million patients have received either dialysis or transplantation through financial support of the Medicare ESRD Program. Total enrollment for beneficiaries requiring dialysis or transplantation was approximately 16,000 in 1974 for a program cost of approximately $229 million (General Accounting Office [GAO], 2000a). By December 2002 almost 300,000 persons were enrolled (MedPAC, 2004a) at a cost of over $15 billion (GAO, 2003). The dialysis patient population alone is projected to increase to greater than 520,000 by 2010 based on an assumed 7% growth rate (GAO, 2003) and to quadruple by 2030. Forecast for total program costs in 2010 is $28 billion (GAO, 2003). The purpose of this chapter is to present an overview of the legislative and regulatory histories of the ESRD Program and a discussion of ESRD programs and issues that affect ESRD entitlements.

On an individual level, the ESRD program has been and remains important to the hundreds of thousands of individuals and their loved ones whose lives have been impacted by it. A broader perspective on its impact must recognize that the existence of a federal program spurred the further development of kidney disease treatment in this country, and influenced the rest of the world.

Genesis of the Medicare ESRD Program

The roots of the ESRD program date back to the 1960s and the development of two forms of treatment for ESRD, hemodialysis and transplantation. Prior to this time, treatment for people suffering from this disease was not possible, and the diagnosis of ESRD was in effect a "death sentence."

During the 1950s, it became possible to transplant kidneys between genetically non-identical donors and recipients (Levinsky, 1993; Plough, 1986). In the early 1960s, the first patient was initiated on chronic dialysis therapy (Scribner, 1990). With these advances in science, the federal government began to engage in a number of public policy efforts before creating the ESRD Program. The first facility for long-term dialysis, the Seattle Artificial Kidney Center located at Swedish Hospital in Seattle, was established in 1962 as part of a 2-year trial program to test the clinical and economic feasibility of chronic dialysis therapy (Albers, 1989). In 1963, the Veterans' Administration announced the establishment of dialysis centers in its hospitals throughout the country. The National Institutes of Health (NIH) began to fund kidney research in 1965, and the Public Health Service (PHS) supported a small number of dialysis centers as part of federally funded demonstration projects (Iglehart, 1993). With these exceptions, no systematic methodology had been established in the 1960s to fund dialysis and transplantation services.

In the early 1960s, renal failure was claiming 100,000 victims in the United States annually (Scribner, 1990), but there were not enough dialysis machines available to meet the demand. It is estimated that treatment costs were $15,000 per year (Scribner, 1990). Often a small number of patients were accepted into the few maintenance programs in existence based on social criteria. The social criteria included age (adults less than 45 years old were preferred), emotional stability and maturity, and the potential for return to a useful and productive role in society (Murray, Tu, Albers, Burnell, & Scribner, 1962; Schupak & Merrill, 1965). The psychiatric criteria used were criticized for mixing psychosocial evaluation with moral judgment (Abram, 1972).

The membership of these early selection committees reflected the demographic features of the medical profession and the values of the middle class, rather than those of the population of potential beneficiaries. In 1967, well-educated White men with stable marriages were represented among those chosen to receive treatment (Evans, Blagg, & Bryan, 1981), while today more members of minorities, women, and persons with less education are represented in the ESRD population.

In 1966, the President's Bureau of the Budget established an expert committee, under the chairmanship of Dr. Carl Gottschalk, to analyze the public policy issues related to ESRD. The following year, the committee concluded that dialysis and transplantation were established therapies for chronic renal failure and that the institution of a nationally funded clinical program was justified (Committee on Chronic Kidney Disease, 1967). This report is considered to have been most instrumental in the subsequent establishment of a federal policy for ESRD (Plough, 1986).

After the report was issued, the idea of a federal program for ESRD simmered in the Congress until December 1971. At that time, Arkansas Representative Wilbur D. Mills brought the idea forward by formally proposing the formation of such a program in the House of Representatives. This action followed 1 month after a patient underwent hemodialysis on the floor of the House of Representatives during a hearing of the House Ways and Means Committee, which Rep. Mills chaired.

History of the ESRD Program

Every year, thousands of bills are introduced in Congress, but only a few hundred pass the Senate and the House of Representatives and are signed into law by the President of the United States. Legislation authorizes the Center for Medicare and Medicaid Services (CMS), formerly the Health Care Financing Administration (HCFA), as the agency with administrative responsibility to formulate and oversee regulations that implement the public laws governing the Medicare ESRD Program. The regulatory process is a two-step procedure including a notice of proposed rule making (NPRM) and final regulations or rules. A NPRM is a text of the proposed regulation, history of the issue, description of the impact, and other related issues announced in the *Federal Register*. The public is invited to comment on the NPRM when specific instructions and deadlines are followed. Consideration is given to all comments in issuance of final regulations. Final regulations or rules include a statement of purpose and the basis for the regulation. All final regulations are published at least 30 days prior to the effective date (Bocchino & Burrows-Hudson, 1995).

Although the appropriate House or Senate committees never formally considered the legislation, Indiana Senator Vance Hartke successfully attached the measure as a floor amendment to the Social Security Amendments of 1972 after only 30 minutes of discussion. This amendment was adopted in the context of a broader provision of legislation that extended Medicare coverage to the disabled regardless of age.

On October 30, 1972, President Richard Nixon signed into law P.L. 92-603. Section 2991 of that law altered Title XVIII of the Social Security Act, declaring that chronic renal disease constitutes a disability. As a result, those suffering from ESRD would be covered for medical costs in the same ways as all other disabled individuals under Title XVIII. It is estimated that between 92% and 93% of the U.S. population is covered for treatment for ESRD through this entitlement. These Medicare benefits, effective on July 1, 1973, continue to provide access to dialysis treatments, kidney transplantation, and inpatient and outpatient care from physicians as well as renal treatment centers.

The growing cost of the ESRD Program has made it an increasingly visible part of the Medicare program. The cost to Medicare of maintaining a patient on chronic dialysis was an average of $52,000 in 2001, with all ESRD beneficiaries accounting for 6% of all Medicare spending (MedPAC, 2004b). These figures do not include additional costs for co-payments and deductibles not covered by Medicare.

The national expenditures for the ESRD Program have been much higher than initial estimates, which predicted expenditures of about $250 million by the end of 1977. Annual expenditures were $229 million in 1974, and had risen to over $15 billion by 2001 (GAO report, 2003). Part of the increase in cost is due to inflation; the cost per treatment of dialysis has actually fallen in constant dollars from 1974 to the present. The growth in the number of beneficiaries, which has far outpaced initial expectations, accounts for much of the cost of the program.

Congress and the CMS, the agency within the Department of Health and Human Services (DHHS) responsible for the management of the Medicare program, have periodically addressed various aspects of the ESRD Program. This action has resulted from the progressive increase in expenditures of the program in an increasingly constrained Medicare system and allegations in various reports that the quality of care of dialysis patients is not satisfactory (GAO, 2000b; GAO 2003).

Significant Legislative and Regulatory History of the ESRD Program

Social Security Amendments of 1972

Legislative activity. Public Law 92-603 extended Medicare benefits to patients suffering with chronic renal failure. Section 2991 created the ESRD Program. Effective date for Medicare coverage was July 1, 1973.

Regulatory action. Following enactment of P.L. 92-603, interim regulations implementing the law were published in the *Federal Register* on June 29, 1973, titled *Interim Conditions of Participation and Payment Rates for Dialysis and Transplant Services.* Additional regulations were published on April 22, 1975, making minor modifications to and republication of the initial interim regulations concerning coverage of services. A NPRM, published July 1, 1975, specified the "conditions of coverage" that facilities would be required to meet to qualify for Medicare reimbursement. It also included health and safety requirements of providers and directed the organization of the ESRD Network system. A Final Rule was published on June 3, 1976, that finalized the conditions of coverage for ESRD providers/suppliers.

ESRD Program Amendments of 1978

Legislative activity. On June 13, 1978, P.L. 95292 was enacted, amending the Social Security Act by including several new provisions for the ESRD Program to encourage home dialysis and transplantation.

Financial incentives were used to promote the use of lower cost, medically-appropriate self-dialysis (primarily home dialysis) as an incentive to the more costly incenter dialysis and to eliminate some of the existing financial disincentives to transplantation. The law provided for early Medicare entitlement for patients beginning self-dialysis or transplantation during the first 3 months following the initiation of chronic dialysis treatment. (Normally, Medicare entitlement begins 3 months *after* initiating treatment for chronic dialysis.)

The law also provided for the implementation of a prospective reimbursement method for dialysis payment, with incentives to assure more cost-effective delivery of services to patients dialyzing in facilities or at home. Medicare transplant benefits were extended from 12 to 36 months; that is, an individual with a functioning transplant would remain covered by Medicare under the ESRD benefit for 36 months posttransplant. The amendments included a mandate to develop a long-range national objective with respect to the most effective use of resources for treating renal disease and clarified the scope and responsibilities of the ESRD Networks.

In terms of background, Medicare's payment policy for outpatient dialysis services from 1973 to 1983 reimbursed independent renal facilities on a reasonable *charge* basis and hospital-based facilities on a reasonable *cost* basis, for both incenter and home dialysis services. Under the Interim Regulations, effective July 1, 1973, reimbursement for outpatient dialysis services was limited by a screen or payment ceiling of $138 per treatment (*Federal Register*, 1973). Home dialysis was paid for separately, and facilities managing home patients were reimbursed on a reasonable *cost* basis. Although home dialysis was the most economical modality in terms of overall program cost, it was simultaneously the least lucrative for facilities and physicians.

Congressional hearings on the ESRD Program were held in 1976, prompted by the rapid growth of ESRD expenditures and a concurrent decline in the proportion of patients treated by home dialysis (Rettig, 1980). These led to the ESRD Program Amendments of 1978.

Regulatory action. A final rule published on September 28, 1978, implemented the early entitlement to ESRD benefits for patients entering a program of self-dialysis training or transplantation. Another final rule, published October 19, 1978, defined self-dialysis services, training and facilities, and revised the minimal utilization rates and rate provisions for self-dialysis services. On October 19,1979, the final rule provided target rate reimbursement for facilities providing home dialysis services, equipment, and support services; developed incentives to allow providers to retain the difference between actual costs and the target rate reimbursement level; and encouraged more cost-effective services.

OBRA 1981

Legislative activity. The ESRD provisions in Section 2145 of the Omnibus Budget Reconciliation Act (OBRA) of 1981 (P.L. 97-35) again directed the Secretary of the DHHS to establish a prospective reimbursement system for outpatient dialysis to promote home dialysis, and revised physician payment to provide an incentive for home dialysis. To reduce the financial burden of the ESRD Program on total Medicare expenditures, the provisions also modified Medicare, making it the secondary payer to other private insurances for the first 12 months of Medicare entitlement.

Regulatory action. A NPRM published on February 12, 1982, with a subsequent final rule published on May 11, 1983, established the prospective composite rate payment system for dialysis in fulfillment of the requirements imposed by the ESRD Program Amendments of 1978 and the ESRD provisions of OBRA 1981. These regulations established a per-treatment payment rate adjusted for geographic wage differences, with slightly separate rates for hospital-based and independent dialysis facilities. The average composite rate for an independent facility was $123 per treatment, down from an average of $138 per treatment in the 1970s. The regulations also included a process for dialysis facilities to obtain an exception to the composite rate based on atypical patient mix, extraordinary circumstances, education costs, or designation as an isolated

essential facility. Physician payment was modified to a single monthly prospective capitation payment (MCP) that was inclusive of all routine medical care provided to ESRD beneficiaries.

For the first time, payments for home and center dialysis treatments were consolidated into a single base composite rate. Since providers would be reimbursed at the same per-treatment rate whether the patient dialyzed incenter or at home, the composite rate was intended to be an incentive to encourage dialysis providers to promote home dialysis among their patient populations.

Also, pursuant to the 1981 legislation, a final rule published on April 5, 1983, and effective May 5 of that same year, specified that Medicare would become the secondary payer for the first 12 months of Medicare entitlement for ESRD beneficiaries who are also covered under employer group health insurance.

National Organ Transplant Act of 1984

Legislative activity. The National Organ Transplant Act (P.L. 98-507) authorized the creation of the National Task Force on Organ Transplantation. It also amended the Public Health Service Act to address the acquisition and distribution of whole organs (including kidneys) through the Organ Procurement and Transplantation Network (OPTN) (Rettig & Levinsky, 1991). Kidney transplantation was covered by Medicare as a treatment for chronic renal failure as stated in the Social Security Amendments of 1972. Under these provisions, Medicare reimburses for organ procurement, the transplant surgical procedure, and related physician fees.

Regulatory action. A NPRM was published on July 31, 1987, with a subsequent final rule on March 1, 1988, that identified the conditions of coverage for the approval of organ procurement organizations (OPOs) for participation in the Medicare and Medicaid programs, and specified that there could be only one OPO for a defined service area. These regulations strengthened the OPOs by establishing the criteria by which they would be certified. The regulations required that each hospital participating in the Medicare/Medicaid programs must have written protocols for the identification of potential organ or tissue donors. They also required transplant providers to be members of and abide by the rules of the OPTN.

Congressional Omnibus Budget Reconciliation Act (COBRA) 1985

Legislative activity. In COBRA 1985 (P.L. 99272, Section 9214), Congress directed the Secretary of the DHHS to consolidate the 32 existing ESRD Networks into not less than 14 networks. The law also disallowed the merger of ESRD Networks to other organizations (Bocchino & Burrows-Hudson, 1995).

Regulatory action. A final rule was published on August 26, 1986, that delineated 14 Network areas and identified the criteria used to determine these areas.

OBRA 1986

Legislative activity. OBRA 1986 authorized the Secretary of DHHS to set the composite rate for dialysis

Figure 36-1
The ESRD Networks

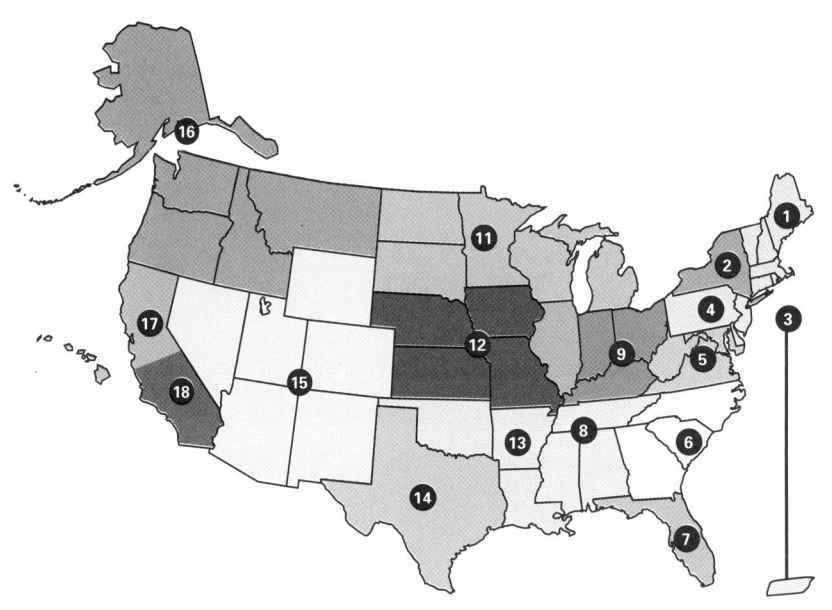

services provided between October 1, 1986, and October 1, 1988, at a level equal to that in effect as of May 13, 1986, reduced by $2.00. It further reduced the composite rate by an additional $.50 to finance the ESRD Networks.

OBRA 1986 also required a study to evaluate the effects of the payment reductions on access and quality of care. HCFA contracted with the Urban Institute in Washington, DC, to conduct the study. The report, *Review of the Impact of the Reduction of the Composite Rate for Renal Dialysis on Access and Quality of Care*, submitted in December 1987, concluded that reductions in the payment rates had made no impact on access to dialysis treatments and no deleterious effect on the quality of care provided (Bocchino & Burrows-Hudson, 1995).

OBRA 1986 established the U.S. Renal Data System (USRDS), a national ESRD registry to assemble and analyze data on the ESRD Program. The USRDS originated from discussions involving the renal community, Congress, and the National Institute of Diabetes and Digestive and Kidney Diseases (NIDDK) at the National Institutes of Health (NIH). Data are reported to the USRDS by Network organizations, transplant centers, and all other sources collecting information on ESRD patients. The registry was to:

- Prepare an annual ESRD report to Congress;
- Identify the economic impact, cost-effectiveness, and medical efficacy of alternative modalities of treatment;
- Evaluate the most appropriate allocation of resources for the treatment and research into the causes of chronic renal failure;
- Determine patient mortality and morbidity rates, and trends in such rates, and other indices of quality of care; and
- Conduct other analyses to assist the Congress in evaluating the ESRD Program.

The establishment of USRDS represented a major commitment by the NIH to kidney disease and related epidemiologic research. Since its inception, the USRDS has made a substantial contribution to the renal community by allowing researchers and clinicians to use its published data to explore a variety of unanswered questions regarding the care of ESRD patients (Rettig & Levinsky, 1991).

The 1986 legislation further modified and reorganized the ESRD Networks. OBRA 1986 required a reorganization of the Networks to establish not less than 17 Networks; this was later increased to 18 (see Figure 36-1). The legislation also defined the responsibilities of the Network organization as follows: (a) establishment of a medical review board to conduct onsite reviews and report on facilities and providers utilizing criteria and standards related to the appropriateness of patient care established by the Network organization; (b) review of medical records that fail to meet approved standards with local facility personnel and opportunities for the facility for discussion, written comment, the development of a Corrective Action Plan, specific educational activities, or sanctions; and, (c) data collection for annual census, population estimates, and population characteristics to be incorporated in the USRDS annual reports.

Payment was authorized for 1 year of immunosuppressive medications on an outpatient basis following transplantation. (This authorization was mainly in response to the high cost of cyclosporine.) The legislation also required standards and conditions for the safe and effective reuse of dialyzers and required organ procurement protocols as a requirement for hospitals and organizations involved in procuring organs for transplantation.

Regulatory action. On April 9, 1987, a NPRM outlined the revised 18 Network area designations; these were then published in a final rule on October 2 of that same year. Also in the April 9 notice, alternate sanctions were identified for suppliers of ESRD services and the requirement for such suppliers to participate in the activities and pursue the goals of the ESRD Networks was stated. These became effective October 19, 1988. In an October 1, 1987 final rule, the standards for the reuse of hemodialyzers, filters, and other dialysis supplies were published.

OBRA 1987

Legislative activity. OBRA 1987 (P.L. 100-203) required the Secretary of DHHS to direct a study of the Medicare ESRD Program by the National Academy of Sciences, Institute of Medicine (IOM). The study would examine the following issues:
- major epidemiologic and demographic changes in the ESRD patient population that may affect access to treatment, quality of care, or the resource requirements of the program;
- access to treatment by individuals with chronic renal failure, whether eligible for Medicare benefits or not;
- quality of care provided to ESRD beneficiaries, as measured by clinical indicators, functional status of patients, and patient satisfaction;
- effect of reimbursement on quality of care, and;
- adequacy of existing data systems to monitor these matters on a continuing basis (P.L. 100203, Section 4036d).

The final report, entitled *Kidney Failure and the Federal Government*, was edited by Rettig and Levinsky and published by National Academy Press in 1991. The authors published a "special report" entitled *The Medicare End Stage Renal Disease Program: A Report from the Institute of Medicine* in the *New England Journal of Medicine* (see Vol. 324, pp. 1143-1148, April 18, 1991, issue). The report, discussed later, set the stage for ESRD program going forward.

OBRA 1989

Legislative activity. The ESRD provisions of OBRA 1989 (P.L. 101-239) maintained the existing base composite rate for both hospital-based and independent dialysis facilities, including incenter and home dialysis patients, as those established in 1983 (and reduced by $2 in 1986) until October 1, 1990.

OBRA 1989 addressed the Method II form of reimbursement for home dialysis equipment and supplies and stipulated certain restrictions on Method II suppliers. It limited that reimbursement to the median national composite rate, with an exception for continuous cycling peritoneal dialysis (CCPD), which was set at 130% of the median national composite rate.

The Method II provisions in this legislation were largely in response to controversy surrounding Home Intensive Care, Inc. (HIC), a supplier of dialysis equipment and supplies to home patients. HIC saw the advantages to patients of the Method II billing methodology, as this rate was sufficient enough to allow the company to provide staff assistants to dialyze patients in their homes who would otherwise not have been able to do so (Rettig & Levinsky, 1991). Prior to this legislation, in February 1989, HCFA published

a NPRM attempting to reduce Method II reimbursement to the composite rate level through an inherent reasonableness ruling. This resulted in court action, which necessitated the inclusion of these provisions in the OBRA 1989 legislation.

OBRA 1989 reallocated funds for the 18 ESRD Network organizations to "report on facilities and providers that are not providing appropriate care" and "conduct onsite reviews of facilities and providers... utilizing standards of care established by the Network organization" (OBRA 1986). In addition, the legislation extended the provisions that applied to Peer Review Organizations (PROs) regarding protection of their liability for medical review to ESRD Networks. Following their reorganization, Networks existed in administrative oblivion until the issue of liability was resolved. The Networks now follow CMS quality assurance efforts (Rettig & Levinsky, 1991).

OBRA 1989 required the Secretary of DHHS to submit a report on the methodology and rationale used to establish a Medicare payment rate for erythropoietin. Recombinant human erythropoietin (EPO) was the first recombinant DNA-based biological for use in clinical practice. In June 1989, the Food and Drug Administration (FDA) approved EPO (Amgen, Inc.'s Epogen or Epoetin-alfa) for treatment of anemia in dialysis patients (FDA, 1989). HCFA responded immediately with a decision to provide coverage and an interim reimbursement policy (HCFA, 1989).

The interim rule was published on June 12, 1989, and specified that EPO for dialysis patients be paid for by an add-on amount to the ESRD facility composite rate (set nationally by HCFA). Reimbursement was initially set at $40 per administration of EPO for doses up to 10,000 units; an additional $30 was reimbursed if the patient required greater than 10,000 units per dose. The rule required certain documentation to be provided for payment.

The payment for EPO was not incorporated into the composite rate because all patients were not expected to receive it, nor were all patients expected to receive the same dose. Only the cost of the medication itself was recognized for reimbursement. Supplies, nursing care, medication administration, and laboratory services were absorbed by the facilities (Rettig & Levinsky, 1991).

In another interim rule published in November 1989, EPO was covered "incident to" a physician's service for patients on home dialysis. The rule specified that the EPO must be furnished in a non-facility setting (i.e., outpatient dialysis clinic or physician's office). In these cases, it was to be reimbursed at cost plus an administrative fee (to be deemed reasonable by local Medicare carrier).

Regulatory action. A NPRM published on December 26, 1990, and a final rule published on November 17, 1992, carried out the provisions of OBRA 1989 related to Method II reimbursement.

OBRA 1990

Legislative activity. OBRA 1990 was enacted as P.L. 101-508. It extended and expanded waivers for social health maintenance organizations (SHMOs). SHMOs consolidated the acute and chronic care delivery systems and managed care across a full range of services (acute care, post acute care, and expanded community care). Four innovative projects, created to refine methodologies and benefit design, were approved and, in addition, four existing SHMO sites were extended (Bocchino & Burrows-Hudson, 1995).

The President's budget for fiscal year 1991 (FY91), submitted to Congress in January 1990, recommended extending the secondary-payer provision from 12 to 18 months if the patient is covered by both Medicare and employer group health insurance. Congress adopted the provision in OBRA 1990 to become effective on February 1, 1991. Several organizations in the renal community supported this provision because: (a) providers generally received higher reimbursement from private insurers than they did from Medicare, (b) private insurers have a limited ability to track expenditures for ESRD patients in their claims processing systems, or (c) private payers were more reasonable payers than Medicare (Bocchino & Burrows-Hudson, 1995; Rettig & Levinsky, 1991).

In 1990, the GAO examined options to provide home dialysis aides for some dialysis patients. Some accepted "hardship case" criteria were patients who were confined to a bed or wheelchair, those unable to transfer without assistance or with no available transportation to the dialysis center, or those at risk while traveling (GAO, 1990). Several legislative proposals to implement payment for home partners resulted in Congress authorizing, in OBRA 1990 (Section 4202), a 3-year demonstration project to evaluate the safety and cost-effectiveness of staff-assisted home dialysis.

OBRA 1990 directed the Prospective Payment Assessment Commission (ProPAC) to study "the costs, services, and profit associated with dialysis treatment modalities," to recommend the method of payment for the facility component of outpatient dialysis services for fiscal year 1993, and the methodology for updating payments in subsequent years. (ProPAC was a federal commission that was responsible to advise Congress and the Secretary of DHHS on the Medicare Prospective Payment System [PPS].)

Section 4201(c) of OBRA 1990 made two changes in the EPO policy. Self-administration of EPO by competent home dialysis patients who do not require medical supervision became effective on July 1, 1991, and the payment for EPO administered to patients became $11 per 1,000 units.

Regulatory action. An interim rule published on September 4, 1991, and a subsequent final rule published on January 10, 1994, addressed the Medicare coverage of EPO used by competent home patients. The rule revised the conditions of coverage for these services furnished to ESRD beneficiaries to include patient selection; assessment of the patient's ability to administer the drug and the patient's compliance; the physician-supervised plan of care, including training to give the injection; monitoring of the drug's effectiveness; and the patient's ability to assess side effects.

Transplant Amendments Act of 1990

Legislative activity. Transplant Amendments Act of 1990 (P.L. 101-616) reauthorized the National Organ Transplant Act of 1984 for 3 years. In this legislation,

Congress expanded the authority of the Health Resources and Services Agency (HRSA) within DHHS to make grants related to organ procurement and factors affecting access, outcomes, and organ donation to nonprofit private organizations other than OPOs. OPOs shifted from being hospital-based to being independent entities, and multiple OPOs in a single statistical metropolitan area (SMA) were consolidated to assure "sufficient size, maximum effectiveness, and equitable distribution of organs." The minimum qualifications of the OPTN contractor, the composition of the OPTN Board of Directors, and the responsibilities of the OPTN were changed. The Secretary of DHHS was required to establish criteria to assure that an OPO meets target effectiveness regarding the number of organs procured each year.

The Transplant Amendments Act of 1990 called for a study by the GAO to determine the extent to which the procurement and allocation of organs had been equitable, efficient, and effective; the difficulties that were encountered in the procurement and allocation of organs; and the effect of state required-request laws.

Regulatory action. A NPRM published on June 21, 1991, and an interim final rule published on September 8, 1994, addressed the conditions of coverage for OPOs. The rules set the eligibility requirements and procedures for OPOs to receive Medicare and Medicaid reimbursement, clarified certification and designation, and redefined OPO service area. To obtain first time designation as an OPO, an organization must demonstrate that its service area has the potential to produce 50 donors or comprises an entire state; must procure a minimum of 24 donors per calendar year over a 2-year period; and maintain an average ratio of three organs per donor. The performance standards to evaluate OPO effectiveness became more quantitative on January 1, 1996.

In addition, the regulations specified that HCFA approval would be necessary for change of OPO ownership or service area; that OPOs must have a system in place for the equitable allocation of organs; and that OPOs must ensure that tests are done on all donors for the presence of communicable diseases, including AIDS.

Regulatory action. A NPRM, published on September 8, 1984, addressed the operation of the OPTN. The rules put forth the guidelines for OPTN functions, membership, and the governing board; addressed federal oversight of the allocation of organs to ensure fairness and equity; stated compliance requirements for participation in Medicare and Medicaid; and established minimum requirements to improve the outcome of transplantation and minimize the waste of donated organs.

OBRA 1993

Legislative activity. The ESRD provisions of OBRA 1993 (P.L. 103-66) extended coverage of immunosuppressive drug therapy from 12 months to 36 months. The extension period was phased in to reduce the impact on the federal budget. Effective in 1995, immunosuppressive drug therapy was covered for 18 months; during 1996, reimbursement was extended to 24 months; and during 1997, immunosuppressive drug therapy was extended to 30 months. As of 1997, the benefits were extended to 36 months (MedPAC, 2004a).

OBRA 1993 included physician self-referral limitations. Effective January 1, 1995, physicians were barred from referring patients for designated health services to any business entity with which that physician has a financial relationship if payment is to be made by Medicare or Medicaid. Eleven designated health services were specified as applicable for the self-referral ban. Such dialysis-related services included bone densitometry or other non-routine tests, durable medical equipment, parental and enteral nutrients, equipment and supplies, outpatient prescription drugs, and inpatient hospital services.

In OBRA 1993, Congress reduced payment for EPO to $10 per 1,000 units from $11 (OBRA 1990). In addition, self-administration of EPO was reimbursed for all dialysis patients and no longer limited to just those patients who dialyze at home.

The SHMO (OBRA 1990) waivers were extended under OBRA 1993 for 2 years, and one new site was authorized for an ESRD capitation demonstration project.

Medicare Amendments of 1993 and 1994

Legislative activity. These Medicare amendments were legislated as the Social Security Act Amendments of 1994 (P.L. 103-432). Known as technical amendments, they amended and corrected sections of OBRA 1986-1990 and 1993. Some of the provisions related to the ESRD Program included the following:

1. Conditions were defined under which a hospital could have an agreement with an OPO other than its designated OPO, including the waiver process and the criteria for granting waivers;
2. Eligibility criteria were defined for the staff-assisted home dialysis demonstration project and clarified that an individual could be a resident of a nursing facility and/or a skilled nursing facility; and
3. The extended coverage of immunosuppressive drug therapy was clarified to achieve budget neutrality and prevent gaps in coverage.

Balanced Budget Act of 1997

Legislative activity. The Balanced Budget Act (BBA) of 1997 (P.L. 105-33), signed by President Bill Clinton in August 1997, made sweeping changes to Medicare and contained many important provisions. It included several provisions specific to ESRD. The Act extended Medicare Secondary Payer coverage from 18 to 30 months, thus increasing the number of dialysis patients with a private payer as their primary source of insurance. HCFA was directed to develop and implement a method to measure and report the quality of renal dialysis services provided under the Medicare program. The Secretary of HHS was also told to audit cost reports of each dialysis provider at least once every 2 years beginning in 1996. The Act mandated that a "withhold" be applied to dialysis treatments received by Medicare managed care organization (MCOs) to fund the ESRD networks. Additionally, effective July 1, 1998, Section 4432 (b) (5) (D) expanded section 1861 (h) (7) of the Act to include coverage of services that are gen-

erally provided by skilled nursing facilities (SNF) or by others under arrangements with them made by the SNF. Dialysis services (which until then were specifically coverable as extended care services only when directly provided by either the SNF itself or its transfer agreement hospital) would also become coverable when provided under an arrangement between the SNF and a freestanding dialysis facility. While this makes dialysis coverable as a Part A SNF service, the SNF also has the option to unbundle the dialysis service altogether. If the SNF elects this latter option, dialysis services that meet the Part B dialysis benefit coverage requirements can be furnished and billed directly by an outside dialysis supplier without having to make an "arrangement" with the SNF in which the SNF does the Medicare billing. Specific criteria are listed in the Act for Part B consideration.

Regulatory action. A final rule published on August 15, 1997, specified the criteria HCFA uses to determine if a facility that furnishes dialysis services to Medicare patients with ESRD qualifies for a higher payment under an exception to its prospectively determined payment rate and the procedures that HCFA uses to evaluate ESRD payment exception requests. The regulations also revised the way HCFA computes acquisition costs for organs that are transplanted into Medicare beneficiaries.

Interim final rules for Medicare+Choice published on June 26, 1998, explained and implemented the provisions outlined in the BBA of 1997. The rule became effective on July 27, 1998, and it governs the operation of Medicare+Choice even though it is an interim final rule.

Balanced Budget Refinement Act of 1999

Legislative activity. The Balanced Budget Refinement Act of 1999 (P.L. 106-113) contained many important provisions such as establishment of the Medicare+Choice (M+C) Program, establishment of numerous demonstration projects, and Medigap protections. Several important ESRD provisions were also included. The 3.6% increase in the composite rate authorized by the bill represented only the second time in the history of the Medicare ESRD program that an increase in the composite rate had been granted. A 1.2% increase was effective on January 1, 2000, followed by a 2.4% increase effective January 1, 2001. Another major ESRD provision was one that extended Medicare coverage for immunosuppressive medications for aged and disabled beneficiaries whose 36-month coverage had not yet expired. This brought the total coverage to 44 months.

Regulatory action. The final rule for Prospective Payment System and Consolidated Billing for Skilled Nursing Facilities was published on July 30, 1999. This rule responded to comments submitted by the public to the May 12, 1998 interim final that implemented provisions in section 4432 of the BBA of 1997 regarding Medicare payment for SNF services.

Beneficiary Improvement and Protection Act (BIPA) of 2000

Legislative activity. The BIPA of 2000 (P.L. 106-554) was enacted on December 21, 2000. The Act required CMS to develop a full bundled payment system and an ESRD market basket payment formulation. It also provides for nutritional counseling to patients with chronic kidney disease (CKD).

Section 605 of the Act provides for revision of payment rates for ESRD patients enrolled in the M+C program. Section 620 allows ESRD beneficiaries to enroll in another M+C plan if their plan terminates its contract with HCFA. The provision applies to terminations occurring on or after the date of BIPA's enactment and retroactively to terminations on or after December 31, 1998.

Additionally, the Act provides a significant improvement in Medicare coverage for immunosuppressive medications required by transplant recipients as well as providing for two consecutive annual increases in composite rate for dialysis providers. While the legislation covered the same categories of transplant patients, it eliminated a time limit to coverage and extended lifetime coverage to them. Additionally, it did not limit benefits to transplants that were performed after a specified date as in the case of Balanced Budget Refinement Act of 1999. Included are all transplant recipients whose transplant was initially covered by Medicare or those who receive a transplant in the future and who meet age or disability requirements - are 65 or over or receive Social Security Disability Income (SSDI). The effective date of coverage was December 21, 2000, when the bill was signed by President Bill Clinton, but was implemented April 1, 2001.

Medicare Prescription Drug, Improvement, and Modernization Act of 2003

Legislative activity. President George W. Bush signed Public Law 108-173, known as the Medicare Prescription Drug, Improvement, and Modernization Act of 2003 into law on December 8, 2003. This legislation enacts the most far-reaching changes to the Medicare program since its creation in 1965 and will have major impact for the ESRD program for years to come.

From a reimbursement perspective, no change to the composite rate or drug reimbursement occurred in 2004, but a 1.6% composite rate increase was earmarked for January 2005. Beginning in 2005, the composite rate payment will be augmented by the difference between Medicare's payments and providers' acquisition costs for injectable drugs (i.e., the spread), and this augmented payment will be adjusted for patient case mix. Additionally, facilities will be paid the acquisition cost for dialysis injectable drugs. Beginning in 2006, annual updates will occur based on the growth in drug spending. The prohibition on dialysis facility exceptions to the composite rate (BIPA 422) was made inapplicable to pediatric facilities with 50% or more patients under age 18.

Other ESRD provisions include the requirement that by October 2005 the secretary is to submit a report to the Congress on a fully bundled dialysis prospective payment system. Dialysis-related drugs, including EPO, as well as laboratory services are to be rolled into an expanded composite rate. Additionally, the bill authorizes the development of a new 3-year demonstration project to begin in 2006 that will test a fully bundled, case-mix adjusted dialysis payment system. Facilities that participate in the

demonstration project will receive an additional 1.6% composite rate increase (Sharp, 2004). The Secretary must also create an Advisory Board to provide advice and recommendations with respect to the establishment and operation of the demonstration project.

The first report by the Office of the Inspector General DHHS mandated in the Act was released in May 2004. The purpose of the study was to determine the difference between the Medicare payment amount for separately billable end stage disease drugs and the acquisition costs of these drugs for facilities. The study also estimated the rate of growth of facilities' expenditures for these drugs. Overall, the study found that acquisition cost of the 10 drugs studied were less than the Medicare reimbursement with large discrepancies between large provider costs and facilities not owned or managed by the four largest providers (average 22% less versus 14%, respectively). When weighted by 2002 average sales prices (ASPS) for the drugs under review, ASP was, on average, 17% below the Medicare reimbursement amount. Medicare reimbursement for separately billable drugs is projected to rise by 11% ($216 million) between calendar years 2003 and 2005 (Office of Inspector General, 2004).

Regulatory action. In a November 7, 2003 Final Physician Fee Schedule Rule, CMS describes the background, rationale, and payment policies associated with the new MCP codes for physician payment. Questions and answers on the ESRD MCP G-Codes were released by CMS on December 22, 2003.

Organ Donation and Recovery Act of 2004

Legislative activity. The Organ Donation and Recovery Act of 2004 (P.L. 108-216) contains several key ESRD-related provisions. It establishes a federal grant program to provide assistance to living donors for travel and related expenses as well as incidental non-medical expenses incurred by individuals providing living organ donations. The legislation also grants money to states for programs designed to increase the number of organ donations (e.g., organ donor awareness, public education and outreach activities). The Secretary of HHS is required to establish a public education program to increase awareness about organ donation and the need for organs and to support development and dissemination of educational materials to inform health care professionals. Studies to evaluate the long-term effects associated with living organ donations are also authorized by the act. Finally, the Secretary of HHS is required to submit a report to Congress on the ethical implications of organ donation. Financial incentives designed to increase non-living donation is one example. The bill is designed to address the growing issue of over 85,000 patients awaiting kidney transplants as of April 2004 with only a little over 14,000 transplants performed each year.

Miscellaneous Regulatory Activity and Events Impacting the ESRD Program

Transplant. A final rule published on August 11, 1978, authorized temporary approval of renal transplantation centers for pediatric hospitals and allowed for Medicare approval and reimbursement for transplant facilities without the required minimal utilization for number of kidney transplants performed.

Dialysis. A NPRM published on January 15, 1981, specified the conditions of coverage for training-only dialysis facilities and provided limited approval of special purpose dialysis facilities on a time-limited basis for vacation and emergency purposes.

Dialysis. A NPRM published on July 17, 1988, declared the reuse of hemodialysis blood tubing to be subject to regulation by the FDA under the authority of the Medical Device Amendments of 1976. Blood tubing manufacturers were required to submit reuse protocols to the FDA for approval.

Dialysis and transplantation. A NPRM was published on May 30, 1989, addressing the occupational exposure to and transmission of bloodborne pathogens. The final rule was published on December 6, 1991, and became effective March 6, 1992. These regulations defined employer requirements to protect health care workers and members of other occupations who had exposure to blood and potential bloodborne pathogens through their employment. These regulations required that Hepatitis B vaccination be made available to all employees who have occupational exposure one or more times per month.

Dialysis. A NPRM published on January 6, 1994, revised the definition of ESRD and clarified the resumption of entitlement for individuals who return to a regular course of dialysis treatments after one course is ended and if a second transplant occurs after a beneficiary loses eligibility due to the 3-year rule.

Dialysis. A NPRM published on February 14, 1994, revised the guidelines on the reuse of hemodialysis filters (dialyzers) and addressed the standards for the quality of water used in dialysis. The 1993 Association for the Advancement of Medical Instrumentation (AAMI) guidelines on *Recommended Practice for Reuse of Hemodialyzers* were incorporated by reference in these regulations.

Dialysis. A NPRM published on June 17, 1997, addressed the updating and revising of HCFA's policy on coverage of ambulance services, including such services for ESRD beneficiaries. The current regulation limits ambulance transportation for ESRD beneficiaries living at home to the nearest hospital-based dialysis facility only. The proposed rule adds a provision that would cover medically necessary ambulance services for an ESRD beneficiary living at home to the nearest dialysis facility capable of furnishing the necessary dialysis services without regard to whether that facility is hospital-based.

Dialysis. A NPRM published on August 26, 1994, with a final rule published on August 15, 1997, specified the criteria the HCFA uses to determine if a facility that furnishes dialysis services to Medicare patients with ESRD qualifies for a payment rate higher than the prospectively determined payment rate, and the procedures the HCFA uses to evaluate ESRD payment exception requests. It also addressed and revised the way the HCFA computes acquisition costs for organs that are transplanted into Medicare beneficiaries.

Dialysis. The Health Insurance Portability and Accountability Act of 1996 forbids providers of dialysis services to furnish items or services for free or for a cost other than fair market value.

Dialysis. In February 1997, the HCFA issued a policy called the Hematocrit Monitoring Audit (HMA) that instructed Medicare contractors to monitor the hematocrit levels of ESRD patients receiving EPO. The policy provided for pre-payment review of EPO claims and denial of claims when the 90-day average hematocrit level exceeded 36.5%. The result was significant decreases in hematocrits in 1998. The HMA was retracted by the HCFA in July 1998, and the retraction was subsequently reconfirmed in August 2000 (Program Memorandum [PM] AB-00-76), July 2002 (PM AB-02-100), and September 2003 (PM AB-03-138).

Dialysis. On January 18, 2001, final rules for *Occupational Exposure to Bloodborne Pathogens; Needlestick and Other Sharps Injuries* were published by the Occupational Safety and Health Administration (OSHA). OSHA revised the bloodborne pathogens standard in conformance with the requirements set forth in the Needstick Safety and Prevention Act, P.L. 106-430, of 2000. The Act directs OSHA to revise the bloodborne pathogens standard to include new examples in the definition of engineering controls along with two definitions, "sharps with engineered sharps injury protections" and "needleless systems." It also required that exposure control plans reflect how employers implement new development in control technology; employers solicit input from employees responsible for direct patient care in the identification, evaluation, and selection of engineering and work practice controls; and certain employers establish and maintain a log of percutaneous injuries from contaminated sharps. The effective date was April 18, 2001.

The Continuance of the Medicare ESRD Program

Setting the Stage for the Future

The IOM, in response to a request by Congress (OBRA 1987, Section 4036d, P.L. No. 100-203), conducted a study of the Medicare ESRD Program. An IOM expert committee conducted the study. The individuals brought expertise to the study from internal medicine, nursing, nephrology, geriatrics, transplant surgery, economics, epidemiology, ethics, the social sciences, social work, and the perspective of a dialysis patient.

The committee submitted a report to Congress and the Secretary of the DHHS. It was published as *Kidney Failure and the Federal Government* by the National Academy Press, Washington, DC, in 1991. The objectives set forth for the Medicare ESRD program and recommendations based on the objectives set forth in the IOM report have had a profound impact on the ESRD Program throughout the 1990s and into the twenty-first century.

The IOM committee endorsed four objectives for Medicare ESRD program:
1. Guarantee access to treatment for all in which it is medically appropriate;
2. Provide care of high quality that achieves desirable health outcomes consistent with patient health status

and current professional knowledge;

3. Develop policies that steadily improve patient well-being and patient outcomes; and,

4. Manage the ESRD program prudently at the lowest cost compatible with adequate care.

Based on the four objectives set forth in the IOM report, numerous recommendations were made that have had a profound impact on the structure, process, and focus of the program. Highlights of the recommendations include:

- Medicare eligibility should be extended to all U.S. citizens and resident aliens.
- Congress should eliminate the 3-year Medicare eligibility limit for successful transplant patients and, thereby, authorize a lifetime entitlement comparable to that of dialysis patients.
- Coverage for payment of immunosuppressive medications for kidney transplant patients should be made coterminous with the period of entitlement.
- Donation of kidneys should receive high priority.
- Patients and clinicians in adult and pediatric nephrology and bioethicists should develop flexible guidelines for evaluating patients for whom the burdens of renal replacement therapy may substantially outweigh the benefits. Guidelines should be developed specifically for children and should describe the role of the parents in the decision making process.
- Nephrologists and other clinicians should discuss with all ESRD patients, their wishes about dialysis, cardiopulmonary resuscitation, and other life-sustaining treatments and encourage documented advance directives.
- ESRD clinicians should be encouraged to participate in continuing education in medical ethics and health law. Specialists in the medical ethics of renal disease should be available to educate clinicians, train members of the ethics committee, and to do research on ethical issues in dialysis and transplantation.
- Assess the shift of providers from not-for-profit to for-profit providers and the implications for access and quality.
- Eliminate CON as applied to dialysis facilities, recognizing that this is a state government rather than federal government action.
- Follow general Medicare payment policies in setting dialysis payment policies: update the rate, yearly; rebase the rate only when the HCFA rebases the other parts of Medicare governed by the PPS; ultimately, rebasing outpatient dialysis reimbursement from efficacy and quality studies that determine the components needed for appropriate dialysis care. An expert advisory body should be formed to periodically review the services that Medicare should reimburse; and ProPac, consistent with its charge to examine Medicare outpatient as well as inpatient reimbursement, should periodically review ESRD payment policy.
- Adopt certain reimbursement policies: evaluate the justification for the rate differential between hospital-based and independent facilities, especially in terms of patient complexity, and retain or eliminate the differential based on that analysis; establish a separate rate for hospital back-up units that treat both inpatients and outpatients that provide support to independent units in the care of complex outpatient cases; establish a separate rate for ESRD pediatric patients; and evaluate the need for a separate rate for rural facilities.
- HCFA should review the MCP regarding its exclusion from the Medicare Fee Schedule and the impact of this policy on the quality of care provided.
- The Medicare ESRD state survey system should be improved by HCFA to develop uniform training and certification requirements for surveyors and integrating the state survey system with other ESRD quality assurance (QA) efforts.
- HCFA's QA oversight of ESRD providers could be exercised by coordination within the CMS of all relevant bureaus (Health Standards and Quality Bureau [HSQB], Bureau of Policy Development, and Office of Research and Demonstrations), linking existing data bases to provide a systematic examination of the relation between cost of treatment and the quality of care, and integrate the ESRD networks and state surveys in a coherent national QA strategy; adequate financial support should be provided to facilities for QA activities by incorporating facility QA costs in reimbursement for both dialysis and transplantation; evaluate all policies, including reimbursement policies for their quality impacts on patients; establish an advisory group of nephrology professionals and experts in QA to design and develop ESRD-specific QA systems; support the regional and national data systems necessary for an effective QA system, and support a continuing program of ESRD QA research.
- A strong ESRD data acquisition and analysis capability should be maintained by HCFA.
- The USRDS should be authorized to conduct research linking epidemiologic and economic data on the ESRD patient population, and the special studies approach should be exploited to its full potential.
- The Secretary of the DHHS should take all steps necessary to fully implement all functions of the National ESRD Registry called for in OBRA 1986 within the next 2 years.
- The Renal Data System should be continued another 5 years when the current USRDS contract expires and the contract renegotiated at that time.
- NIDDK should expand its support for basic research that has the promise to prevent or to reduce the progression of kidney disease that leads to chronic renal failure.
- Clinical research on dialysis, supported by NIDDK or HCFA, should be resumed.
- Epidemiologic research should be supported to identify risk factors for renal failure and its clinical outcomes, the value of various interventions to prevent and treat chronic renal failure, and factors influencing access to care. Special attention should be given to racial and ethnic differences in the incidence and causes of renal failure and in transplantation (access, outcomes, and organ donation).

Table 36-1
NKF-DOQI Project Goals

Process Objectives	Outcome Objectives
• Develop and promulgate outcome goals for patients with chronic renal failure.	• Improve patient survival.
• Provide a road map on how to improve outcomes for these patients.	• Reduce patient morbidity.
• Facilitate adoption and use of practice guidelines within the renal community.	• Increase efficiency of care.
• Establish a mechanism for evaluating compliance with such standards of care.	• Improve quality of life for ESRD patients.

• Health services research should be supported to determine which components of medical care lead to better outcomes and to identify and validate quality measures for structure, process, and outcomes.

Review of legislation and regulations since the release of the report confirm that a number of the recommendations have come to fruition. Additionally, major strides have been made in data collection and reporting as well as demonstrated improvement in the quality of care. Examples are included below.

National Kidney Foundation-Dialysis Outcomes Quality Initiative (NKF-DOQI)

The advent of DOQI, now called K-DOQI for Kidney Dialysis Outcome Quality Initiative, was March 1995, with final guidelines on the original four topics issued in 1998. The K-DOQI project started as a joint renal community effort organized by the NKF and supported by Amgen, Inc. This initiative has built on and complements the work accomplished by other organizations and professionals in improving quality of care in dialysis. The NKF-KDOQI project represents an unprecedented effort to develop evidence-based clinical practice guidelines for patients with chronic renal failure, and most providers have embraced the K-DOQI recommendations for provision of care.

The purpose of the K-DOQI is to develop clinical practice guidelines (see Table 36-1). The original clinical practice guidelines developed were in the areas of vascular access, adequacy of dialysis, and anemia management. Another group of guidelines focusing on nutrition was later added, followed by guidelines on lipid management and treatment of bone disease. The implementation of the K-DOQI guidelines with the goal of increasing life expectancy and improving overall health and quality of life for the 290,000 people in the U.S. on chronic dialysis therapy (MedPAC, 2004b, combined with other quality-focused efforts by the renal community and CMS, has resulted in impressive increases in quality outcomes in recent years (CMS, 2003).

The areas selected for practice guidelines development are based on criteria that include: a high degree of variability in practice; high level of controversy or uncertainty; significant benefits or risks associated with the practice in question; significant number of patients affected; availability of sufficient information; and lack of contemporary practice guidelines.

The ESRD Clinical Performance Measures (CPM) Project

The ESRD CPM Project began in 1998 as a result of a directive in section 4558 (b) of the BBA of 1997 to CMS to develop and implement a method to measure and report the quality of renal dialysis services provided under the Medicare program (CMS, 2003). CMS funded the development of CPMs based on the National Kidney Foundation (NKF) K-DOQI Clinical Practice Guidelines. Sixteen CPMs were developed for quality improvement purposes in the areas of adequacy of hemodialysis and peritoneal dialysis, anemia management, and vascular access management. The CPMs are similar to the initial core indicators, the predecessor to the CPMs with the addition of measures for assessing a patient's vascular access. The CPM Project (also called the Core Indicator Project from 1994 to 1998) is designed to assess and identify opportunities to improve the care of patients with ESRD; the purpose is to provide comparative data to assist dialysis providers in improving patient care and outcomes. Since 1994 the project has documented continued improvements, particularly in the areas of adequacy of dialysis and anemia management. Data for hemodialysis patients are collected during a period of October to December and reported the following year while data for peritoneal dialysis patients are collected October to March. To facilitate quality improvement efforts, each report compares findings of the current study with those of previous studies and identifies opportunities to improve care for dialysis patients (CMS, 2003).

National Vascular Access Improvement Initiative (NVAII)

Vascular access is a major quality issue in ESRD. As a result, CMS identified vascular access as a significant quality improvement focus for ESRD Networks starting in July 2003. CMS has contracted with the Institute for Healthcare Improvement (IHI) to assist CMS, the ESRD Networks, and the renal community to develop a program to increase the likelihood that as many patients as possible will receive a fistula and that appropriate access monitoring and intervention will occur with a goal of minimizing the occurrence of vascular access complications. Working collaboratively with the renal community, consensus on the goals and structure of the project to avoid unnecessary burdens on the providers has been reached. As of 2004, a major national initiative is underway (CMS, 2004).

CPMs for Dialysis Facilities

Building on the experiences of the dialysis corporations, January 2000, the OIG conducted a comprehensive review of quality control and QA programs at some of the largest national dialysis chains [OE 01-99-00052]. The report found that "the corporations rely heavily on facility-specific clinical performance measures and have gained considerable experience on how to use them effectively to improve the quality of care they deliver (Office of Inspector General, 2002).

CROWN

CROWN, Consolidated Renal Operations in a Web-enabled Network, is a cooperative effort between CMS and the ESRD Networks that began in 2002. It is designed to improve the quality of ESRD information; to replace outdated, unsupported technology; to reduce errors and inconsistencies in ESRD data; to simplify ESRD systems; and to support electronic data collection at the information source, in a secure, integrated environment. The goal is simplified sharing of accurate data between dialysis facilities and CMS and the Networks (CMS, 2003).

Core Data Set

In 2003 CMS began a project to develop recommendations, with input from the renal community, for the elements of a data set that will be provided by dialysis facilities to fulfill all CMS and ESRD Network data needs. Reduction in the data-reporting burden on individual dialysis facilities without limiting the amount or quality of data provided is the major goal of the project. As in other data-related projects, CMS is cooperating with large dialysis provider organizations to have the data transmitted from the corporate offices and to ensure integrity of the data.

Dialysis Facility Reports

CMS funds the production of Dialysis Facility Reports that are based primarily on Medicare patient data. The reports provide each facility with information about itself. CMS's goal is to assist facility staff in quality of care improvement efforts. Each facility is given an opportunity by CMS to review its report and submit comments. The reports and any comments submitted by the facilities are then shared with the appropriate state survey agency to assist them in their survey activities.

Dialysis Facility Compare Web Site

Another initiative that focuses on quality data is the Dialysis Facility Compare (DFC) Web Site. The DFC Web site debut was on www.medicare.gov in January of 2001. It allows Medicare beneficiaries to search for and compare dialysis facilities geographically and contains facility-specific information such as location, ownership, types of services offered, etc., and clinical outcome data on the facility's patients. Annually, CMS provides facilities with an advanced preview of their quality measures and an opportunity to provide comments on their measures prior to the information being released to the public.

In-Center Hemodialysis Patient Perspective on Care Survey (ICH-CAHPS®)

In June 2000 the Office of Inspector General's office issued a report that included a recommendation that CMS require dialysis facilities to monitor patient satisfaction and develop a common instrument that facilities and others could use. CMS, in partnership with the Agency for Healthcare Research and Quality, is developing a standardized CAHPS patient experience of care survey for ESRD patients, focusing on hemodialysis patients in chronic dialysis centers. The survey is called *In-center Hemodialysis CAHPS® (ICH CAHPS)*. On August 25, 2003, a Federal Register Notice was published soliciting dialysis consumer experience of care/satisfaction measures or instructions. Recommendations for administration protocols and sampling methodologies were also solicited.

GAO Reports

In spite of great strides in quality outcomes over recent years, the GAO released two reports critical of the renal community and its quality of patient care as well as the oversight of the ESRD program by CMS. The first report entitled *Medicare Quality of Care: Oversight of Kidney Dialysis Facilities Needs Improvement,* a report to the Special Committee on Aging, was released in June 2000. *Dialysis Facilities: Problems Remain in Ensuring Compliance with Medicare Quality Standards*, a report to the chairman, Committee on Finance, was released in October 2003.

Medicare Quality of Care: Oversight of Kidney Dialysis Facilities Needs Improvement (June 2000). The June 2000 report focused on determining the extent to which onsite inspections of dialysis facilities are performed and problems identified as well as whether an effective process exists to ensure that dialysis facilities correct problems. It also explored the steps taken to use available monitoring resources as effectively as possible.

Recommendations were based on two conclusions. One conclusion was that only 11% of the dialysis facilities eligible for recertification in 1999 were surveyed in that year, compared to 52% in 1993. The second was that 15% of the surveyed facilities had deficiencies severe enough, if uncorrected, to warrant terminating their participation in Medicare.

The GAO recommended that the Administrator of CMS take the following actions:
- develop procedures on how and when to use CMS's existing authority to impose partial or complete payment reductions for ESRD facilities.
- establish procedures to facilitate better and more routine cooperation and information sharing between ESRD Networks and state survey agencies, particularly in targeting facilities for on-site surveys.

- evaluate the results of CMS's project for using clinical outcome data to select facilities for onsite review before it recommends that states use such data as a key factor in the selection process. A central component of the evaluation should be determining the extent to which the data are sufficient to predict which facilities have a higher likelihood of not complying with Medicare's conditions of participation (GAO, 2000b).

Dialysis Facilities: Problems Remain in Ensuring Compliance with Medicare Quality Standards (October 2003)

This follow-up report to the 2000 report had the same overall focus as the earlier report but used actual state survey data. A number of conclusions came out of the study. The GAO felt that a number of facilities studied did not achieve the minimum patient outcomes specified in clinical practice guidelines for a significant proportion of their patients. Examples were contained within the report. It was felt that, although ESRD survey activity had increased after the 2000 report, many states failed to meet the survey frequency goals set. The report also noted that facilities that corrected identified problems did not necessarily stay in compliance over time. As many as one in seven facilities surveyed from 1998 to 2002 had problems sufficiently severe (one or more condition-level deficiencies) to initiate the process of terminating the facility from the Medicare program. Examples were provided in the report.

At the conclusion of the report a number of actions and recommendations were made to strengthen oversight of ESRD facilities. They were as follows (GAO, 2003):
- establish a goal for state agencies to reduce the time between surveys for facilities with condition-level deficiencies
- publish facilities' survey results on its DFC Web site
- strongly encourage states to assign ESRD inspections to a designated subset of surveyors who specialize in conducting ESRD surveys
- make ESRD training courses more available to state surveyors, which may include increasing the number of classes and slots available as well as varying class location
- amend CMS's regulations to require that networks share facility-specific data with state agencies on a routine basis
- ensure that regional offices both adequately monitor state performance and provide state agencies ongoing assistance on policy and technical issues through regularly scheduled contacts with state surveyors.

Future Considerations for the ESRD Program

Predictions are that the ESRD patient population will double by 2010 and quadruple by 2030. Co-morbidities such as diabetes and hypertension that result in ESRD are on the rise while, to date, efforts at early detection and prevention have largely failed and education initiatives are often hit or miss, largely failing to reach susceptible populations. As of 2004, the ESRD program was underfunded, with providers losing an average of $13 per treatment for each Medicare patient, while labor and technology costs rose (Kidney Care Partners [KCP], 2004).

Going forward, because opportunities continue to exist to improve all aspects of quality, particularly nutrition, vascular access management, and bone disease management (MedPAC, 2004b; CMS, 2003), focus on quality improvement will continue and standards will rise. In addition to quality, there will a major focus on patient education, access to care, and patient safety. CKD will receive significant attention in an attempt to limit new cases of ESRD. Efforts by Congress, CMS, and the renal community to satisfy the four objectives for the Medicare ESRD Program established in 1991 (IOM, 1991) will progress as in the past. Yet, providers, regardless of commitment to quality, will continue to struggle to balance economic restrictions with allocation of resources to drive quality indicators upward. This will be the case until reimbursement catches up with costs.

The ESRD program will not continue as in the past. Change is not optional and changes in reimbursement and some form of ESRD Medicare Modernization are predicted to occur. Payment incentives that reward quality are likely. Inevitably, the questions "How should providers be rewarded?", "Will additional funding be required?", "Which quality measures should be used?", and "How will we keep other quality initiatives moving forward?" (MedPAC, 2004b) will be heavily debated and eventually resolved. MedPAC predicts that rewards will likely be based on improving care and exceeding national averages (MedPAC, 2004b). To achieve this, continued collaboration between CMS and providers will be key to success.

Summary

The ESRD program, while successful in the past, faces many significant challenges in the future. A successful future will depend on the active and passionate involvement of all those interested in ESRD and the care of its victims. Grassroots efforts to influence votes for key ESRD legislation as well as relentless focus on educating the public as well as public officials will be critical.

Who better than nephrology nurses to play key roles in molding the future of the program? Nephrology nurses have participated in the development of the clinical, legislative, and regulatory management of the ESRD Program since its inception. We will be instrumental in shaping the future through positive change in public policy so that our patients survive and thrive. We will need to adapt our expanding roles in delivering care to the patient with renal disease and to successfully advocate for fair and reasonable public policies. Will we rise to the challenge? No doubt. We can and we will.

References and Readings

Abram, H.S. (1972). Psychological dilemmas of medical progress. *Psychiatry Medicine, 3,* 51-58.

Albers, J. (1989). Reflections on the first dialysis nurse training program. *ANNA Journal, 16*(3), 230-231.

Bocchino, C., & Burrows-Hudson, S. (1995). Other salient issues related to ESRD and its treatment. In L.E. Lancaster (Ed.), *Core curriculum for nephrology nursing* (3rd edition) (pp. 423-446). Pitman, NJ: American Nephrology Nurses' Association.

Center for Medicare and Medicaid Services (CMS). (2003). *2003 Annual Report ESRD Clinical Performance Measures Project.* DHHS. Washington, DC: Author. [Also available on www.cms.hhs.gov/

esrd/l.asp]

Center for Medicare and Medicaid Services (CMS). (2004). *Fistula first brochure.* DHHS. Washington, DC: Author.

Committee on Chronic Kidney Disease. (1967). *Report of the Committee on Chronic Kidney Disease* (GPO Publication No. 933-491). Washington, DC: GPO.

Continuous quality improvement: HCFA plans important new patient-specific data collection initiative to improve CQI at the dialysis facility level. (1997). *Contemporary Dialysis & Nephrology, 18*(7), 17, 28.

Evans, R.W., Blagg, C.R., & Bryan, F.A. Jr. (1981). Implications for health care policy: A social and demographic profile of hemodialysis patients in the U.S. *Journal of the American Medical Association, 245,* 487-491.

Federal Register. (1973, June 19). No. 38, 17210. Washington, DC.

Food and Drug Administration. (FDA). (1989). *Summary basis of approval: Drug license name: Epoetin alfa.* Washington, DC: Author.

General Accounting Office (GAO). (1990). *Medicare: Options to provide home dialysis aides* (GAO/HRD-90-153). Washington, DC: Author.

General Accounting Office (GAO). (June 23, 2000a). *Letter to John Grassley.* Washington, DC: Author.

General Accounting Office (GAO). (2000b). *Medicare quality of care: Oversight of kidney dialysis facilities needs improvement.* Washington, DC: Author.

General Accounting Office (GAO). (2003). *Dialysis facilities: Problems remain in ensuring compliance with Medicare quality standards.* Washington, DC: Author.

Health Care Financing Administration (HCFA). (1989). Reimbursement for ESRD and transplant services. In *Medicare provider reimbursement manual: Transmittal No. 11.* Baltimore, MD: Author.

Iglehart, J.K. (1993). The American health care system: The end stage renal disease program. *New England Journal of Medicine, 328*(5), 367.

Kidney Care Partners (2003). Kidney Care Partner brochure. Washington, DC.

Kidney Care Partners (2003). Letter to the Honorable Charles E. Grassley. Washington, DC, October 6, 2003.

Kidney Care Partners (KCP). (2004, June 14). *Caring for patients with kidney failure: A briefing.* Washington, DC: KCP.

Kidney waiting list statistics are announced. (1997). *Contemporary Dialysis & Nephrology, 18*(5), 8.

Klahr, S. (1990). Rationing of health care and the end stage renal disease program. *American Journal of Kidney Disease, 16*(4), 392-395.

Levinsky, N.G. (1993). The organization of medical care: Lessons from the Medicare end stage renal disease program. *New England Journal of Medicine, 329*(19), 1395-1399.

MedPAC (2004a). *Report to the Congress: Medicare payment policy.* Washington, DC: Author

MedPAC (2004b). *Report to the Congress: New approaches in Medicare.* Washington, DC: Author.

Murray, J.S, Tu, W.H., Albers, J.B., Burnell, J.M., & Scribner, B.H. (1962). A community hemodialysis center for the treatment of chronic uremia. Transcript, *American Society for Artificial and Internal Organs, 8,* 315-320.

Office of Inspector General. (2004). *Medicare reimbursement for existing ESRD drugs* (OE1-03-04-00120). Washington, DC: Author.

Office of Inspector General. (Jan 2002). *Clinical performance measures for dialysis facilities: Building on the experiences of the dialysis corporations.* Washington, DC: Author.

Plough, A.L. (1986). *Borrowed time.* Philadelphia: Temple University Press.

Price, C. (1996a). President-Elect's message: Now is the time to get prepared for DOQI. *ANNA Update, 26*(1), 4, 6.

Price, C. (1996b). President's message: DOQI guidelines to be released to the renal community. *ANNA Update, 26*(6), 3.

ProPAC approves 2.8% increase in the composite rate. (1997). *Dialysis & Transplantation, 26*(3), 124.

Rettig, R.A. (1980). The politics of health cost containment: End stage renal disease (Editorial). *Bulletin of the New York Academy of Medicine, 56,* 115-138.

Rettig, R., & Levinsky, N.(Eds.).(1991). *Kidney failure and the federal government/Committee for the study of the Medicare ESRD program, Division of Health Care Services, Institute of Medicine.* Washington, DC: National Academy Press.

Scribner, B. (1990). A personalized history of chronic hemodialysis. *American Journal of Kidney Diseases, XVI*(6), 512.

Schupak, E., & Merrill, J.P. (1965). Experience with long-term intermittent hemodialysis. *Annals of Internal Medicine, 62,* 509-518.

Sharp, N. (2004). The Medicare bill and ESRD provisions in 2003. *ANNA Update, 34*(1), 13.

Smith, K. (1996). Representatives from the transplant community convene in Washington. *ANNA Update, 26*(5), 8.

Statement of principles on managed care and the ESRD population. (1997). *ANNA Update, 27*(3), 28.

United States Renal Data System (USRDS). (1990). *Annual report. National Institute of Diabetes and Digestive and Kidney Diseases.* Bethesda, MD: Author.

United States Renal Data System (USRDS). (2003). *Annual Report. National Institute of Diabetes and Digestive and Kidney Diseases.* Bethesda, MD: Author.

- In the Social Security Amendments of 1972 (HR-1, Title XVIII), P.L. 92603, Congress created authorization to Medicare in support of persons with the diagnosis of chronic renal failure who were eligible for benefits under Social Security and for the spouses or dependent children of these persons.

- The membership of the early selection committees reflected the demographic features of the medical profession and middle class values rather than those of the population of potential beneficiaries.

- In the 1960s and 1970s, the cost of health care represented a much lower percentage of the gross national product (GNP) than it does today; therefore, to deny life-saving treatment to Americans exclusively because of financial cost was given only cursory consideration.

- Legislation authorizes the HCFA as the agency with administrative responsibility to formulate regulations that implement the public laws governing the Medicare ESRD program.

- A national ESRD registry to assemble and analyze data, known as the United USRDS, was established by the Secretary of the DHHS as directed by Congress. The USRDS originated from discussions involving the renal community, Congress, and the NIDDK.

- The IOM committee submitted a report to Congress and the Secretary of the DHHS and the report was published in 1991 as Kidney Failure and the Federal Government through the National Academy Press, Washington, DC. The objectives for the Medicare ESRD Program and recommendations based on the objectives set forth in the IOM report had a profound impact on the ESRD Program for years to come (Klahr, 1990).

- The NKF-DOQI project represents an unprecedented effort to develop evidence-based clinical practice guidelines for patients with chronic renal failure.

- As the patient population has continued to increase, a greater number of geriatric patients, high-risk patients with co-morbid conditions, and minorities, which usually require more consideration of socio-economic problems, have entered the program.

ANNP636

The Federal End Stage Renal Disease (ESRD) Program

Janel Parker, MSN, RN, CNN, and Gail S. Wick, BSN, RN, CNN

Contemporary Nephrology Nursing: Principles and Practice contains 39 chapters of educational content. Individual learners may apply for continuing nursing education credit by reading a chapter and completing the Continuing Education Evaluation Form for that chapter. Learners may apply for continuing education credit for any or all chapters.

Please photocopy this page and return to ANNA.
COMPLETE THE FOLLOWING:

Name: _____

Address:_____

City:_____State: _____Zip: _____

E-mail: _____

Preferred telephone: ☐ Home   ☐ Work: _____

State where licensed and license number (optional): _____

CE application fees are based upon the number of contact hours provided by the individual chapter. CE fees per contact hour for ANNA members are as follows: 1.0-1.9 - $15; 2.0-2.9 - $20; 3.0-3.9 - $25; 4.0 and higher - $30. Fees for nonmembers are $10 higher.

ANNA Member: ☐ Yes   ☐ No   Member # (if available) _____

☐ Checked Enclosed   ☐ American Express   ☐ Visa   ☐ MasterCard

Total Amount Submitted: _____

Credit Card Number: _____ Exp. Date: _____

Name as it appears on the card: _____

CE Evaluation Form
To receive continuing education credit for individual study after reading the chapter
1. Photocopy this form. (You may also download this form from ANNA's Web site, **www.annanurse.org.**)
2. Mail the completed form with payment (check) or credit card information to American Nephrology Nurses' Association, East Holly Avenue, Box 56, Pitman, NJ 08071-0056.
3. You will receive your CE certificate from ANNA in 4 to 6 weeks.

Test returns must be postmarked by **December 31, 2010.**

CE Application Fee
ANNA Member $20.00
Nonmember $30.00

EVALUATION FORM

1. I verify that I have read this chapter and completed this education activity. Date: _____

   _____
   Signature

2. What would be different in your practice if you applied what you learned from this activity? *(Please use additional sheet of paper if necessary.)*

   _____
   _____
   _____
   _____
   _____
   _____
   _____
   _____
   _____
   _____
   _____
   _____
   _____
   _____
   _____

Evaluation	Strongly disagree				Strongly agree
3. The activity met the stated objectives.					
a. Outline the history of the ESRD program.	1	2	3	4	5
b. Discuss current initiatives and measures of compliance.	1	2	3	4	5
c. Project a future for the ESRD program in the United States.	1	2	3	4	5
4. The content was current and relevant.	1	2	3	4	5
5. The content was presented clearly.	1	2	3	4	5
6. The content was covered adequately.	1	2	3	4	5
7. Rate your ability to apply the learning obtained from this activity to practice.	1	2	3	4	5

Comments _____

_____

8. Time required to read the chapter and complete this form: _____ minutes.

This educational activity has been provided by the American Nephrology Nurses' Association (ANNA) for 2.7 contact hours. ANNA is accredited as a provider of continuing nursing education (CNE) by the American Nurses Credentialing Center's Commission on Accreditation (ANCC-COA). ANNA is an approved provider of continuing education by the California Board of Registered Nursing, CEP 0910.

Nephrology Nursing: A Global Perspective
Nicola Thomas, MA, BSc (Hons), RN

Chapter Contents

Nicola Thomas, MA, BSc (Hons), RN

This chapter provides the reader with an overview of nephrology nursing in a global context, encompassing topical issues in nephrology in Europe, Japan, Singapore, and Australia. The epidemiology of renal disease in these countries will be compared and contrasted, and the challenges of working in nephrology care across the world will be explored. The chapter will conclude with a discussion on improving renal care in developing countries and will also describe the work of the Renal Disaster Relief Task Force.

Epidemiology of Renal Disease World-Wide

Around the world, the incidence and prevalence of renal disease are increasing. Incidence of disease may be defined as the number of cases newly arising in a population during a specified period, divided by the size of the population at risk, whereas prevalence can be defined as the number of cases observed either at a particular time (point prevalence) or during a given time period (period prevalence) (Vetter & Mathews, 1999).

Causes of end stage renal disease (ESRD) throughout the world are similar to those in the United States (U.S.). The main underlying renal diseases in all countries usually include diabetes mellitus and glomerulonephritis, however variations can be seen among the European nations. In some countries, such as Finland, the rates of diabetes mellitus are very high, with the incidence of Type I (insulin-dependent) diabetes mellitus among children aged 14 years or under being the highest in the world and with an increase in incidence of approximately 3% per year (Rytkonen, Ranta, Tuomilehto, & Karvonen, 2001).

Treatment rates also vary among European countries (European Renal Association - European Dialysis and Transplant Association [ERA-EDTA], 2004), and in some countries, such as the UK, 29% of patients on dialysis have peritoneal dialysis, compared with only 9% in Austria (ERA-EDTA, 2004). In most countries in Western Europe, the number of new patients awaiting transplantation is increasing while transplant rates remain static. All these data will be explored in more detail later in the chapter.

Data from the Fresenius Medical Care dialysis network

structure, where 120 countries with established dialysis programs were identified, showed that at the end of 2001, 58% of the dialysis population worldwide was treated in just five countries: USA, Japan, Germany, Brazil, and Italy (Moeller, Gioberge, & Brown, 2002). These five countries accounted for < 12% of the world population. The next 10 countries ranked by size of their dialysis population accounted for 21% of the global dialysis patient population while representing 29% of the world population. The remaining 21% of global dialysis patients were treated in more than 100 different countries representing 50% of the world population. Table 37-1 shows the population, prevalence, and number of dialysis patients in different parts of the world.

Epidemiology of Renal Disease in Europe – The Role of the Registries

The epidemiology of renal replacement therapy (RRT) for ESRD varies considerably worldwide, but until recently it had been difficult to estimate and compare trends in the incidence of renal disease by age, gender, and cause in Europe. The ERA-EDTA Registry is a European Registry collecting data on RRT via the national and regional registries in Europe. It analyses these data and distributes the resulting information through registry reports presented at the annual ERA-EDTA congress and through publications in nephrology journals. The ERA-EDTA Registry is funded by the ERA-EDTA. Since June 2000, the Registry office is housed in the Department of Medical Informatics in the Academic Medical Center in Amsterdam, The Netherlands.

The most recently published results from the European Registry (Stengel et al., 2003) included data from nine countries participating in the ERA-EDTA registry: Austria, Belgium, Denmark, Finland, Greece, The Netherlands, Norway, Spain, and UK (Scotland). The adjusted incidence rate of RRT increased from 79.4 per million population (pmp) in 1990-1991 to 117.1 pmp in 1998-1999 (i.e., 4%-8% each year). This increase did not flatten out at the end of the decade, except in The Netherlands, and was greater in men than women, 5.2% versus 4.0% per year. The incidence of ESRD due to diabetes, hypertension, and renal vascular disease nearly doubled over 10 years; in 1998-

Table 37-1

Population, Prevalence, and Number of Dialysis Patients in Europe, Africa, Japan, and North America in 2001

Region	Population (million)	Prevalence of end stage renal disease (ESRD)	Number of dialysis patients (thousands)
European Union	380	790	196
Total Europe	804	490	269
Africa	833	55	43
Japan	127	1830	220
North America	311	1400	304

Note: Adapted from Moeller et al. (2002).

Figure 37-1
Number of Patients Accepted in the UK for RRT Between 1980 and 2001

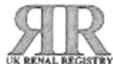

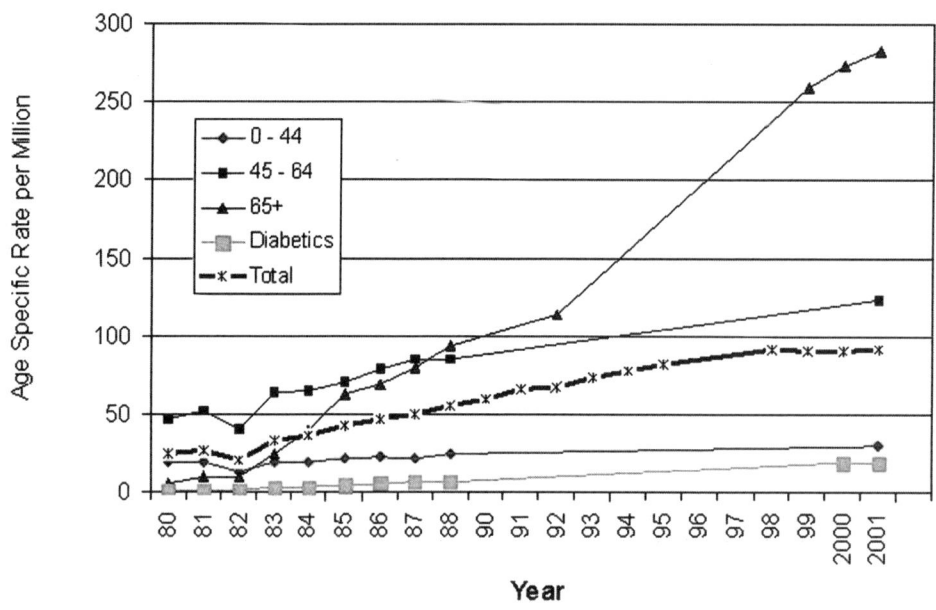

Notes: From U.K. Renal Registry (2003). Used with permission.

1999, it varied between countries from 10.2 to 39.3 pmp for diabetes, from 5.8 to 21.0 for hypertension, and from 1.0 to 15.5 for renal vascular disease.

It can be concluded that the requirement for RRT in Europe continues to rise but at various rates in the European countries studied. This results from increasing differences in the number of older people and, to a lesser extent, in the incidence of diabetes, hypertension, and renal vascular disease.

Epidemiology of Renal Disease in the United Kingdom (UK)

The UK Renal Registry provides a focus for the collection and analysis of standardized data relating to the incidence, clinical management, and outcome of renal disease. It, thus, acts as a source of comparative data for audit/benchmarking, planning, clinical governance, and research. The UK Renal Registry monitors indicators of the quality as well as quantity of care, with the aim of improving the standard of care. There is currently a concentration on data concerning RRT, including transplantation. At a later date there will be an extension to other forms of treatment for renal disease.

It has been suggested that the UK lags behind other European countries in the number of patients being offered RRT. In 2001, the UK Kidney Alliance (an umbrella body representing all organizations involved in renal services) suggested that acceptance rates for RRT in the UK were rising, but there remained geographical inequalities. There were some areas in the UK that did not have autonomous renal services or satellite dialysis units; therefore, both hospital and community-based services need to be expanded

to enable patients to have a choice of treatment.

The annual acceptance of new patients in the UK in 2002 was 93.2 pmp for adults and 1.7 pmp for children (UK Renal Registry, 2003). Although the acceptance rate is low compared with some parts of Europe, the number of patients on dialysis continues to rise in line with other countries. There are a number of reasons why UK rates are lower, including poor awareness among family doctors of the available dialysis facilities for older people, and also to some extent, the limited financial resources available. Under the National Health Service in the UK, dialysis services are free at the point of delivery, so any patient is able to have dialysis regardless of income or level of health care insurance. Figure 37-1 shows the number of patients accepted in the UK for RRT between 1980 and 2001.

Diabetic nephropathy as a cause of renal failure, seen in 18% of new patients, is not increasing and remains lower than in the U.S. and much of Europe.

The annual growth in the number of those receiving RRT is 7%, largely occurring for hemodialysis (HD). Of prevalent patients, 46.6% are transplanted, 37.1% are on HD, and 16.3% receive peritoneal dialysis (PD). PD is more common in the young, especially in those with diabetes, and the percentage of patients on PD is one of the highest in Europe. The number on RRT in the UK is predicted to rise for 20 years until a steady state position is reached.

Much of the rise in demand will occur even if there is no increase in the current acceptance rate. This growth will occur disproportionately in the older people treated by HD. The most realistic figures are over 45,000 patients (900 pmp), or a 4.5% average annual increase over the decade (Roderick et al., 2003).

Renal Replacement Therapies (RRT) in Europe

The Dialysis Outcomes and Practice Patterns Study (DOPPS) is a prospective, observational study designed to evaluate practice patterns in random samples of HD facilities and patients across three continents. Participating countries include France, Germany, Italy, Spain, and the UK (Euro-DOPPS), Japan, and the U.S. DOPPS data collection has used the same questionnaires and protocols across all participating countries to assess components of dialysis therapy and outcomes.

Hecking et al. (2004) described dialysis prescription, adherence, and nutrition among the Euro-DOPPS countries. In each Euro-DOPPS country, patients were selected randomly from 20-21 representative facilities. Among the five countries, mean delivered dose as measured by normalized urea clearance (Kt/V) varied from 1.28 to 1.50 and was accompanied by differences in dialysis prescription components, including blood flow rates, treatment times, and dialyzer membrane and flux characteristics. By country, a nearly two-fold difference was observed in indicators of patient adherence and management (skipping and shortening dialysis, hyperkalaemia, hyperphosphataemia, and high inter-dialytic weight gain), demonstrating clear differences in the management of HD patients across Euro-DOPPS. It is difficult to explain why these differences occur, but ways in which patients are educated about their illness and how far they are encouraged to take control of their illness may be some of the reasons.

In another DOPPS publication (Rayner et al., 2004) there was comparison made between mortality and hospitalization rates in random samples of patients on HD in the same five European countries. Results showed that hospitalization for cardiovascular disease was highest in France and Germany (0.40 and 0.43 hospitalizations per patient year, respectively) and lowest in the UK (0.19), although cardiovascular comorbidity was similar in the UK and France. Hospitalization rates for vascular access-related infection ranged from 0.01 hospitalizations per patient year in Italy to 0.08 in the UK, consistent with the higher dialysis catheter use in the UK (25%) versus Italy (5%). Differences in hospitalization rates across countries did not match differences in mortality rates, while causes of hospitalization differed substantially by country. The authors concluded that there was a need for further examination of whether hospital services are under-utilized in some settings for certain types of patient co-morbidity.

Comparisons have also been made between the European and U.S. outcomes on dialysis. Lameire (2002) explored some of the factors that may contribute and suggested that a higher co-morbidity of incident and prevalent patients on RRT, different vascular access policies with less use of arterio-venous fistulae (AVF), shorter dialysis times, and higher re-use of dialysis membranes in the U.S. may, among other factors, explain the higher mortality in the U.S. compared to Europe and Japan. Data from the DOPPS showed another variable may be to blame – serum albumin.

Port et al. (2004), for the DOPPS, estimated the percentage of patients who were managed outside published HD guidelines (K/DOQI and European Best Practice Guidelines for HD). Guidelines on dialysis dose, phosphate control, anemia, serum albumin, interdialytic weight gain, and use of catheters for vascular access were used, and the associated mortality risk was calculated. The authors estimated the number of life years that could be gained from adherence to these guidelines in the U.S. HD population for a 5-year projected period. Of the practices examined, the highest relative risk of mortality was associated with having albumin < 3.5 g/dl (relative risk = 1.38, $p < 0.0001$); 20.5% of the patients in the study fell outside the target range. The authors concluded that the magnitude of potential savings in life years should encourage greater adherence to guidelines and practices, as these are significantly associated with better survival.

In another DOPPS study (Rayner et al., 2003), data were analyzed from a random sample ($N = 3674$) of patients at the time of initiating HD, hemofiltration, or hemodiafiltration, in 309 units in five European countries, Japan and the U.S. There were large variations in the proportion of patients who commenced HD via an AVF, AV graft (AVG), or central venous catheter – 83% of patients in Germany commenced dialysis with an AVF, while only 15% did in the U.S. Median time to first cannulation also varied greatly between countries: Japan and Italy (25 and 27 days), Germany (42 days), Spain and France (80 and 86 days), UK and U.S. (96 and 98 days). Cannulation less than 14 days after creation was associated with a 2.1-fold increased risk of subsequent fistula failure ($P = 0.006$) compared with fistulae cannulated after 14 days. The authors concluded that significant differences in clinical practice currently exist between countries regarding the creation of AVF prior to starting HD and the timing of initial cannulation. As cannulation within 14 days of creation is associated with reduced long-term fistula survival, fistulae should ideally be left to mature for at least 14 days before first cannulation.

Different types of vascular access use across Europe have been observed in a recent EDTNA/ERCA survey (Elseviers et al., 2004). The European Practice Database (EPD) found that as the first choice for vascular access, AVF were mainly used in each of the participating countries. In northern England, the use of catheters was high (around 20% of all vascular access), whereas the use of AVGs was limited in Italy, the Czech Republic, and North England.

The Challenges of Renal Nursing in Europe

As in the U.S., there are increased numbers of patients who are older and more dependent and who require dialysis and transplantation. There are static transplantation rates in some countries. There are also decreased numbers of specialist nephrology nurses, so in some countries, such as the UK, many nurses are recruited from overseas.

It was considered by Ashwanden (2004) that as the population of the UK is an ageing one, this affects the number of young people applying to train as nurses as well as increases those who will be retiring. There is much literature exploring the explanations for the nursing crisis, although financial rewards and nursing perceived by young people to be a "low status job" compared with other diplomate/graduate careers seem to be the main reasons. Buchan and Sochalski (2004) provide a discussion on the policy context of the rise in the international mobility and migration of nurses. They conclude that policy options to manage nurse migration must include improving working conditions in both source and destination countries, instituting multilateral agreements to manage the flow more effectively, and developing compensation arrangements between source and destination countries (Buchan & Sochalski, 2004).

Nephrology nursing is an exciting and dynamic speciality, where the patients and their families and all the multi-disciplinary team work together to improve the quality and quantity of life, but there are still problems to be overcome. This section will now discuss the current trends in European renal care and will explore some of the initiatives that are aiming to overcome the challenges of increasing numbers of people requiring dialysis and transplantation. This section will conclude with an overview of the work of the European Dialysis and Transplant Nurses Association/European Renal Care Association (EDTNA/ERCA).

Prevention of Renal Disease

As in the U.S., there is a shift in focus in nephrology from only dialysis and transplantation to prevention of renal disease and collaboration with primary care practitioners. As well as the challenge of renal disease prevention, there is the problem of late referral. Jungers (2002) stated that up to 40% of patients suffering from chronic renal insufficiency (CRI) begin RRT less than 6 months after being referred to a renal unit, without having benefited from early nephrological care in the pre-dialysis period. Jungers (2002) goes on to state that late referral should not be considered only from the narrow point of view of its immediate or short-term effects resulting from lack of preparation to dialysis. A more pertinent concept is to consider the duration of pre-dialysis regular nephrological care and its consequences in the long-term on the length and quality of life of patients on dialysis.

It could be argued that nephrology nurses are well equipped to provide a much needed link role between primary and tertiary care in managing those with renal disease in the community. Across Europe there is much discussion about the role of renal physicians and nurses in prevention of renal disease, especially in control and management of diabetes mellitus and hypertension. In the UK, there have been recent publications on the management of renal disease in type II diabetes (National Institute for Clinical Excellence [NICE], 2002a), and a new contract for family doctors (British Medical Association [BMA], 2003) includes targets for blood pressure control, prescription of angiotensin-converting enzyme inhibitors (ACEIs), and microalbuminuria and creatinine testing.

An ongoing study into prevention and management of diabetic nephropathy (Thomas, 2004) involves collaboration between a renal nurse and six family doctor practices. Although the focus of the study is to see how far patient-centered education can influence the control of the parameters that lead to deterioration of renal function, the researcher has found that visiting and advising primary care teams can improve prescription of ACEIs for patients with microalbuminuria and can also improve referral rates for those with raised serum creatinine.

The trend is for renal care teams to focus on chronic kidney disease prevention, and nephrology nurses are well placed to advise their nursing colleagues in primary care and educate the patients who may be at risk.

Dialysis Trends

This section will explore a type of HD that is attracting renewed interest across Europe – home HD. In the 1980s, home HD was considered a superior therapy to unit-based dialysis, and decline in the 1990s was related to demographic, social, psychological, and financial factors as well as to competition with PD.

Piccoli and colleagues (2002) and other authors have published favorable results from their home HD programs and describe the most attractive feature for patients as being the individualized tailoring of dialysis schedules to work and family commitments. It is usual to have back-up support from nurses who can assist in case of short-term problems, while the main training center ensures follow-up for long-term clinical and logistic problems, such as technical/water supply difficulties. Piccoli et al. (2002) describe how dialysis schedules and controls are flexible and tailored; the range of dialysis time is between 1.20 -5 hours with 2-6 sessions per week; 8 patients were on thrice-weekly dialysis, and 7 on daily dialysis.

In the UK in 2002, the need for increased home dialysis provision was appraised by the NICE (2002b), which recommended that all suitable patients should be offered the choice between home HD and HD in a hospital/satellite. The report recommended that patients suitable for home HD would be those who:

- have the ability and motivation to learn to carry out the process and the commitment to maintain treatment
- are stable on dialysis
- are free of complications and significant concomitant disease that would render home HD unsuitable or unsafe
- have good functioning vascular access
- have a caregiver who has (or caregivers who have) also made an informed decision to assist with HD unless the individual is able to manage on his or her own
- have suitable space and facilities or an area that could be adapted within their home environment.

Home HD can give the flexibility that is often missing with unit-based dialysis, and although at first can be daunting for the patient and family, the benefits of the therapy often outweigh the disadvantages.

In some countries such as the UK, home dialysis therapy is funded as any other dialysis therapy, and patients are not required to pay any additional costs. However, in Belgium, where home HD is popular, costs are only reimbursed for three sessions per week (approximately 230 euros per session), which is less than for in-center HD. Patients in some centers in Belgium also have daily home dialysis,

Table 37-2
Number of Renal Transplants in Europe in 2003

Country	Number of renal transplants in 2003	Number of patients on waiting list
Austria[1]	372	774
Belgium and Luxembourg[1]	443	872
Germany[1]	2111	9479
Spain[2]	2032	
The Netherlands[1]	406	1182
United Kingdom[3]	1683 = 1245 (cadaver) + 438 (living)	5072

Notes: [1] From www.eurotransplant.org; [2] From www.donacion.organos.ua.es/ont;
[3] from www.uktransplant.org.uk

which means that the centers (not the patients) have to cover the costs for the additional sessions. In Belgium, the center also reimburses the patients if they dialyze at home for increased consumption of water and power.

Donor Transplant Initiatives

Many countries in Europe are experiencing a static transplantation rate. The number of transplants per year and the number of patients awaiting kidney transplants in 2003 are shown in Table 37-2.

In some parts of Europe, living donation and non-heart beating donation programs are promoted to improve transplantation rates. In Spain, there is a very successful program that began in 1989 with the creation of the National Transplant Organization (ONT). This program involved heavy investment and continues to give outstanding results (Matesanz, Miranda, Felipe, & Naya, 1996). The Spanish explored the identification of potential donors, the legal framework surrounding certification of death and consent, education and information, and the organization of recipient registration and organ allocation. Transplant coordinators were placed in every hospital, and the donation rate rose to 33.6 pmp within 10 years. A second initiative increased investment in neurosurgical facilities, which increased the number of potential donors available. A third step involved investing in public and health care worker education about the benefits of increasing cadaver donation. An opt-out law was introduced, but in practice, the consent of families is always sought. Clearly this change in practice has implications for nephrology nurses, many of whom have to increase their scope of practice to encompass organ donation and transplantation.

An opt-out system presumes consent unless the individual has specifically registered as unwilling to donate. Next-of-kin are still contacted. Belgium introduced an opt-out system in 1982, and the number of donors increased. Germany and Italy introduced it in 1997 and 2000, respectively. France was forced to modify its opt-out law in 1996 after adverse publicity, and since then donation rates have improved.

A European Association for Renal Professionals

The EDTNA/ERCA is an association of individual members. The members of the association are professionals working in the field of renal care and are drawn from a number of European states and other countries worldwide. At the end of 2003, the association had more than 5,000 members in more than 76 countries, with increasing membership from the countries of Central and Eastern Europe. The challenge of working with so many countries and languages cannot be underestimated.

European Research

The EDTNA/ERCA established the Research Board to promote research and provide opportunities for EDTNA/ERCA members to learn about research and take part in multi-center research projects organized through the Collaborative Research Program (CRP) and the European Practice Data Base (EPD).

The CRP offers members of the association an easy way to get involved in renal research. The first collaborative research project topic was vascular access, where 103 centers treating a total of 13,800 chronic HD patients were studied. Full reports on this project were published by Van Waeleghem, Elseviers, and Lindley (2000) and Elseviers et al. (2003). Vascular access recommendations (Van Waeleghem, Elseviers, & De Vos, 2004) have recently been published as a result of this initial study.

The EDTNA/ERCA survey of the provision of dietary advice in renal care was the second project organized through the CRP. Results from this study had an impact on the publication of the *EDTNA/ERCA European Guidelines for the Nutritional Care of Adult Renal Patients* (EDTNA/ERCA, 2004) (see www.edtna-erca.org).

The EDTNA/ERCA survey of the treatment of water for dialysis was the fourth project organized through the CRP. Data were collected from 69 HD facilities in 14 countries. Water quality in European dialysis units is mainly self-regulated. The majority of centers aimed to meet the requirements of the European Pharmacopoeia, but only 50% carried out tests to check compliance. The survey indicated that guidelines for water treatment were urgently needed,

Figure 37-2
Number of Centers in the European Practice Database 2002-2003

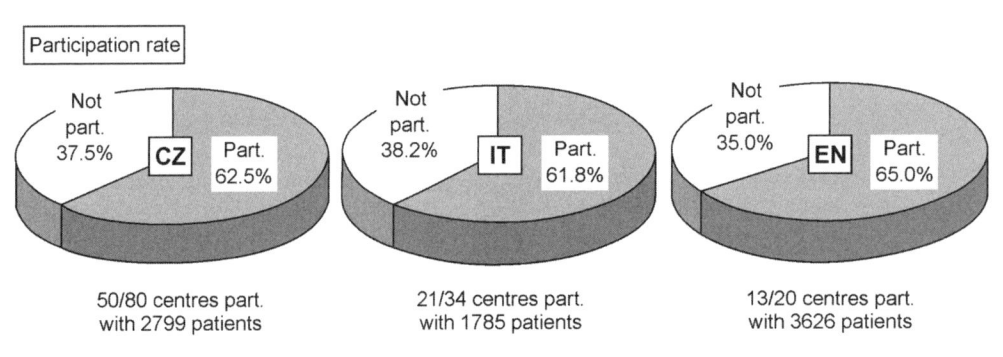

and the EDTNA/ERCA guidelines on the control and monitoring of microbiological contamination in water for dialysis were developed and are now available on the EDTNA/ERCA Web site (www.edtna-erca.org).

A study into the epidemiology and management of Hepatitis C Virus (HCV) aimed to investigate the management of hepatitis C in European HD centers, to measure the prevalence and incidence of HCV in the European countries, and to examine the association between clinical practice and seroconversion. The project is now in its third year and first results (Lindley et al., 2001) and policy recommendations (Zampieron et al., 2004) have been published.

European Practice Database (EPD)

The EDTNA/ERCA hopes to increase the research, which is comparing and contrasting practice across Europe, through the introduction of an EPD, which was piloted in the UK, Italy, and the Czech Republic. The number of centers in the pilot study is shown in Figure 37-2. Other countries (Greece, Belgium, Scotland, Norway) have joined the study in the second year.

The EPD project collects data on professional daily practice and outcome from dialysis centers of selected European countries aiming to audit local practice and to map routine practice in nephrology throughout Europe.

Data collection was performed using a center-based questionnaire translated in the appropriate languages of the participating countries. Basic information on routine daily practice was collected together with more detailed information on specific topics. The study covered all renal care disciplines and representatives of the EDTNA/ERCA Interest Groups participated in the development of specific questions for renal technicians, dietitians, social workers, pediatric renal care, and transplantation. Data collection was focused on center information not on individual patients.

Only results of the pilot phase of the project are available at present (Elseviers et al., 2004; Lindley et al., 2004; Pancírová, Kraciková, Lopot, De Vos, & Elseviers, 2004), but in the future it is hoped that the EPD will identify areas where the Research Board and the Special Interest Groups of the association identify differences in practice and the possible need for development of evidence-based European clinical guidelines.

Nephrology Education in Europe

The education board (EB) of the association has published a European framework for the *Professional Portfolio* (Thomas, 2003), the *European Basic Core Curriculum in Nephrology Nursing*, the *European Post-Basic Core Curriculum in Nephrology Nursing* (Thomas, Küntzle, & McCann, 2004), and has developed a European accreditation program for post-registration nephrology nursing courses (Hurst, Thomas, Sedgewick, & Reichardt, 2003). Basic education is undergraduate education, while post-basic or post-registration education is usually undertaken when nurses wish to specialize in a specific area of nursing, such as nephrology.

European Basic and Post-Basic Core Curricula in Nephrology Nursing

In the mid-1990s it was identified that renal nursing was not necessarily recognized as a specialty that required specific post-registration education. Because of this, the *European Core Curriculum for Post-Basic Nephrology Nursing* (now in its second edition) (Thomas, et al., 2004) was developed. The publication of this curriculum provided the impetus for some countries to develop nationally recognized post-registration courses, which meant that nurses did not have to repeat dialysis training when moving between one renal unit and another. In Germany for example, prior to 1996 there were no nationally recognized renal nursing courses. Some hospitals in Germany offered training courses, but these were often very different in terms of their scope, content, and course delivery mechanisms. However, in 1996 the Head Organization of German hospitals brought in broad guidelines for renal nurse education to harmonize education and training provision on a national level. The publication of the *EDTNA/ERCA Curriculum* in 1995 provided some impetus to this change in course recognition.

In 2000, it was recognized that a curriculum for pre-registration nursing students (*Basic Core Curriculum* [BCC]) and those working with renal patients in general wards was necessary to complement the already successful post-registration curriculum. The BCC has been written to provide an educational guide to teachers and educators who are providing education in nephrology nursing care.

The BCC is available on the EDTNA/ERCA Web site (in seven languages) and can be downloaded freely. It is available at www.edtna-erca.org.

A European Accreditation Program for Post-Registration Nephrology Nursing Courses

EDTNA/ERCA has recently started accrediting post-basic renal nursing courses that are running across Europe. The aim is to demonstrate that certain schools are running good quality courses based on the *European Post-Basic Core Curriculum in Nephrology Nursing*. As not all countries have regulatory bodies or have courses that are validated by universities, it was also hoped that course accreditation by the association could also encourage free movement of nurses across differing countries in Europe.

A pilot project began in 1997 and a list of 100 quality criteria within stated categories was devised. If the criteria were successfully achieved, it would demonstrate that a school provided excellent learning and teaching opportunities for students undertaking post-basic courses. A software package was developed allowing applicants to apply for accreditation electronically. At the end of the pilot project, the accreditation program had developed three stages:
- Completion of quality questionnaire
- Submission of evidence
- Possible visit by peer reviewer

A number of schools have been successfully approved during the last 3 years including schools from Germany, the UK, Portugal, and Finland. Further details are available on the EDTNA/ERCA Web site at www.edtna-erca.org

In this chapter, I will now discuss nephrology care outside Europe and will describe topical issues in the countries of Singapore, Japan, and Australia.

Nephrology Care in Singapore

Singapore is unusual in that the National Kidney Foundation in Singapore (NKFS) provides subsidized dialysis care to approximately 70% of the country's total ESRD population, based entirely on charitable donations.

Ramirez, Hsu, and McClellan (2003) have described how an exponential increase in prevalent dialysis patients receiving care through the NKF chronic dialysis program, and with the anticipated epidemic rise in patients with ESRD, an accelerated comprehensive strategy for the prevention of renal disease and its associated chronic diseases was developed. The NKFS's public health plan, which incorporates primary, secondary, and tertiary approaches to the prevention of chronic kidney disease includes: screening populations at risk for the development and progression of renal disease, the documentation of existing standards of care for chronic diseases associated with renal disease, and the institution of disease management programs that facilitate the systematic management of patients with chronic diseases that lead to ESRD.

Ramirez et al. (2003) described how longitudinal follow-up of the participating population is being performed in order to provide benchmarks for improvement and to determine future directions of the program. Such long-term monitoring also will facilitate the establishment of its efficacy in improving clinical outcomes, reducing the cost of care, and delaying the development and progression of chronic kidney disease.

Blake (2002) identifies that there are almost 30,000 patients maintained on PD in Asia, representing about 8% of all Asian dialysis patients. The largest numbers of PD patients are in Japan and China, but the highest PD penetration is in Hong Kong, Korea, and Singapore. There are excellent rates of both patient and technique survival in the richer Asian countries, such as Singapore, and Blake (2002) concludes that the healthier baseline health status in South East Asian patients, in particular, contributes to their impressive outcomes. The approach to both clearance and ultrafiltration is less aggressive in Asian countries than in the West (Blake, 2002).

Nephrology Care in Japan

The dialysis population of Japan in 2001 was 219,183 patients, up 6.3% over the year before. This equals 1721.9 dialysis patients pmp. The mean age of patients beginning dialysis was 64.2 years. The mean age of the overall dialysis population was 61.6 years, which was also a higher age than the year before. Among dialysis patients, the primary disease was diabetic nephropathy in 38.1% of patients, slightly down from 39.1% the previous year. Chronic glomerulonephritis was the primary disease in 32.4% of cases, a decrease from 34.7% the previous year. All these data were taken from a survey carried out by the Japanese Society for Dialysis Therapy (Patient Registration Committee, 2004).

While there are very high numbers of patients on HD, Japan has traditionally not had high numbers of patients who have received renal transplants. Nakahara et al. (2001) found that the percentage of patients seeking transplants declined from 61% in 1992 to 19.2% in 1999. The reasons given for not seeking transplants were the improvements of physical condition and resultant quality of life (QOL) due to progress in dialysis therapy, upgraded social welfare support, uncertainties of transplant medicine, loss of expectations due to limited availability of transplant kidneys, and aging of patients. In Japan, organ donation has not been widely accepted because of concerns about brain death and also because of Shinto beliefs regarding need for a whole body to go on to the next world. Legislation was passed in June 1997 that allowed organ donations from some brain-dead donors but the law is restrictive, and organ transplants in Japan are still limited (Kita et al., 2000).

Nephrology Care in Australia and New Zealand

In Australia, 1,855 new patients commenced treatment in 2002, a rate of 94 pmp per year. This was a decrease of 3% from 2001 and the first decrease since 1986. In New Zealand, the number of new patients entering renal failure programs was 453, a rate of 115 pmp. This was also a decrease (the first decrease since 1993) of 3% from the previous year (Australia and New Zealand Dialysis and Transplant Registry [ANZDATA], 2003)

The challenge of late referral is the same as in other countries world-wide with 26% of all new patients in Australia and 27% in New Zealand in 2003 referred late to nephrological care (i.e., less than 3 months before first dialysis).

In Australia, glomerulonephritis and diabetic nephropathy were the most common causes of ESRD (both 26%), followed by hypertension (16%), polycystic kidney disease (6%), and reflux and analgesic nephropathy (both 4%). In New Zealand, diabetic nephropathy (45%) was the most common cause of ESRD followed by glomerulonephritis (23%) and hypertension (9%). Type II diabetes (non insulin and insulin requiring) represented 92% of diabetic nephropathy (ANZDATA, 2003).

In Australia, the number of patients on the transplant waiting list in March of 2003 was 1,710, with 23% of the 7,300 patients dialyzing, compared to 25% last year. The 602 transplant operations performed in 2002 represented an increase of 11% compared to 2001 (540 operations). This was a transplant rate of 31 pmp compared to 28 per million in 2001. The living donor transplant rate was 38% (228 grafts) in 2002, compared to 39% (212 grafts) in 2001.

In New Zealand, of the 1,616 patients dialyzing in March 2003, 320 (20%) of the patients were on the transplant waiting list. The number of transplant operations (117) performed in 2002 represents a transplant rate of 30 per million (an increase of 6% from 2001). In relation to the source of organ donations, living donors made up 41% of all operations compared to 39% in 2001.

An interesting aspect of the data from the ANZDATA Registry is the current incidence, treatment, and outcomes of ESRD among indigenous groups in Australia and New Zealand. ESRD rates among indigenous groups in Australia and New Zealand exceeded non-indigenous rates up to eightfold in 2003 (MacDonald & Russ, 2003a) The median age of indigenous patients with ESRD was younger (51 vs. 60 years; $P < 0.0001$), and there was an excess of co-morbidities, particularly diabetes.

The incidence of ESRD did not differ in persons aged 0-14 years. In adults, Maori/Pacific Island people had similar rates of ESRD, a little more than half those of indigenous Australians except in persons aged 65 years and over in whom the rates were nearly equal, but 2-10 times the rates in "other" New Zealanders and non-indigenous Australians. It can be concluded that the incidence and pattern of treated ESRD differs quantitatively and qualitatively between Maori/Pacific Island people and other New Zealanders, and indigenous and non-indigenous Australians (Stewart, McCredie, & McDonald, 2004).

There also appear to be inequalities among access to renal transplantation. Cass et al. (2003) examined whether disparities in transplant rates between indigenous and non-indigenous Australians were due to a lower rate of acceptance onto the waiting list and/or a lower rate of moving from the list to transplantation. Indigenous patients had a lower transplantation rate (adjusted indigenous: non-indigenous rate ratio 0.32). They had both a lower rate of acceptance onto the waiting list and a lower rate of moving from the list to transplantation. The disparities were not explained by differences in age, sex, co-morbidities, or cause of renal disease. It was concluded that indigenous Australians face barriers to acceptance onto the waiting list and to moving from the list to transplantation. Further research is needed to identify the causes, which could facilitate strategies to improve equity in transplantation (Cass et al., 2003).

In summary, rates of ESRD among indigenous people in Australia and New Zealand are considerably higher than the non-indigenous population. The average age at the start of RRT for indigenous patients is approximately 10 years less than non-indigenous people. Among those starting RRT, rates of diabetic nephropathy are higher among indigenous patients, reflecting higher rates of diabetes. The increased burden of illness extends to coronary artery disease and chronic lung disease, which are present at rates 1.5 to 2 times non-indigenous rates.

Overall mortality outcomes are poorer for indigenous patients overall and for each RRT modality. These outcomes are not simply due to increased frequency of co-morbid illness – for indigenous people receiving dialysis treatment the mortality rate adjusted for age and gender is around one and one half times the non-indigenous rate. These data are consistent with studies showing increased rates of markers of early renal disease (in particular, albuminuria) between both Australian and New Zealand indigenous groups and reflect a broader health profile marked by high rates of diabetes, cardiovascular disease, and chronic lung disease. The authors conclude that addressing these issues is a major challenge for health care providers in these regions (McDonald & Russ, 2003).

World Foundation for Renal Care (WFRC)

There are major challenges throughout the world in caring for minority populations and for those who live in developing countries. Areas in the world where renal care is developing, such as some of the countries of Central and Eastern Europe and Africa, are in need of education and support from countries that have experience of dialysis and transplantation. The World Foundation for Renal Care (WFRC) has developed one such program.

The WFRC is a not-for-profit foundation committed to providing education to health care workers caring for patients with renal disease in emerging countries. The mission of the WFRC is to teach and share collective knowledge and expertise in the prevention, care, and treatment of renal diseases in countries that have established renal services. For more than 20 years, nursing leaders from the major nephrology nursing organizations around the world have conducted meetings to share and learn of clinical practices and professional concerns. But as access to renal care has expanded in emerging countries, training needs have grown and major educational support is now needed in each country.

The WFRC believes in a multidisciplinary approach to care, and teaching teams often consists of nurses, physicians, nutritionists, technicians, and others as dictated by a mutually agreed upon curriculum. The WFRC cooperates with colleagues in developing countries to assess educational needs related to RRT and also, when appropriate, assist in the development of screening and prevention programs.

WFRC activities are funded through educational grants and charitable donations, and all teachers volunteer their time. In order to better accomplish its mission, the WFRC has formed partnerships with the Commission for the Global Advancement of Nephrology (COMGAN) of the

International Society of Nephrology (ISN) and the International Federation of Kidney Foundations (IFKF). COMGAN's mission is to promote and provide basic nephrology education in emerging countries where the IFKF goal is to support the growth and development of kidney foundations around the world.

Teaching Tours

The WFRC addresses the educational needs of renal health care workers by sending teams of teachers to areas of the world where RRTs are being initiated.
The WFRC teaching teams:
- teach basic principles of RRTs
- train selected staff to teach others
- provide training materials for local teachers
- establish mentoring relationships
- provide follow-up from seminars and teaching visits

Previous teaching tours have included Russia and the Baltic States in 1995, where a multi-disciplinary team representing the ISN and the WFRC visited dialysis units and delivered lecture programs in Moscow, Petersburg, Estonia, and Lithuania. In 1997, the WFRC once again cooperated with the ISN in the planning and implementation of a combined tour to Russia and Turkey. To date, the WFRC has reached over 2,000 renal care workers in evolving countries, and the WFRC is currently assisting in the development of the Nephrology Nurses' Association of Peru, which has come to fruition after 4 years of continuing WFRC support. The WFRC team consisted of a multidisciplinary and multinational group of highly experienced renal care professionals who were able to bring the benefit of their long and valuable experience to colleagues who are hungry for knowledge and information.

No one group can meet all the needs in developing countries for education and treatment that the current world-wide epidemic of renal disease requires, but a growing coalition of interested groups stands ready to help.

International Disaster Relief

Following the devastating earthquake in Armenia in 1988, the ISN established the Renal Disaster Relief Task Force (RDRTF). Major earthquakes are followed by a substantial incidence of crush syndrome and pigment-induced acute renal failures (ARF), which can be fatal if dialysis is not available.

The primary challenge in these situations is organizational if complex therapeutic options need to be offered to a large number of victims. The ISN/ARF Commission has three different Task Forces for Renal Disaster Relief: one in North America, one in South America, and one in Europe (including Middle East and North Africa).

The European Task Force, through the Organization of Paramedical Personnel of Dialysis and Transplantation (ORPADT) centers in Belgium, the EDTNA/ERCA, and the Technicians Organization (DTV), has recruited volunteers to leave for the disaster area and offer their help, if necessary.

Besides the nephrology team (nurses, technicians, and doctors), other partners are involved. The first partner in this organization is Medecins Sans Frontieres (MSF) Belgium ("Doctors without Borders") who takes care of the general organization and logistic help. The second partner consists of a group of different important dialysis companies who take care of the necessary material supplies (dialysis machines, membranes, bloodlines, etc.). Other partners are the Pharmacy of the University Hospital of Ghent and, via MSF, the Belgian Airforce for the transport of goods.

One major earthquake where the RDRTF was involved was following the Marmara earthquake in Turkey in 1999. Here, in conjunction with MSF, a team landed at Istanbul Airport less than 22 hours after the disaster, and logistic and material support and manpower were provided over a period of approximately 1 month. Specific attention was paid to the choice of the RRT, the transport of victims and materials, the implementation of preventive re-hydration, and the problem of chronic renal failure patients dialyzed in the damaged area (Vanholder, Sever, De Smet, Erek, & Lameire, 2001). The RDRTF was also involved in providing assistance following earthquakes in Iran in December 2003 and in Northern Pakistan in October 2005.

Conclusion

This chapter has provided the reader with an overview of nephrology nursing in a global context. The challenges of renal care appear to be similar throughout the world namely, shifting the focus to prevention of renal disease, caring for an increased ageing and dependent population, improving transplantation rates, and enabling health professionals to have access to continuing professional development.

References

Ashwanden, C. (2004). Caring for staff in renal care. In N. Thomas (Ed.) *Advanced renal care.* (pp. 231-249). Oxford: Blackwells.

Australia and New Zealand Dialysis and Transplant Registry (ANZDATA). (2003). *Annual report.* Retrieved from www.anzdata.org.au

Blake, P.G. (2002). Peritoneal dialysis in Asia: An external perspective. *Peritoneal Dialysis International, 22*(2), 258-264.

British Medical Association (BMA). (2003). *New GMS contract: Investing in general practice.* Retrieved from the BMA at www.bma.org.uk

Buchan, J., & Sochalski, J. (2004). The migration of nurses: Trends and policies. *Bulletin World Health Organisation, 82*(8), 587-594.

Cass, A., Cunningham, J., Snelling, P., Wang, Z., & Hoy, W. (2003). Renal transplantation for indigenous Australians: Identifying the barriers to equitable access. *Ethnicity and Health 8*(2),111-119.

European Renal Association/European Dialysis and Transplant Association (ERA-EDTA) Registry. (2004). *ERA-EDTA registry 2002 annual report.* Amsterdam, The Netherlands: Academic Medical Center.

Elseviers, M.M., De Vos, J.Y., Pancírová, J., Zampieron, A., Lindley, E., Green, D., & Harrington, M. (2004). European Practice Database: Comparative results of the year 1 pilot project. *EDTNA/ERCA Journal, 30*(2), 64-70.

Elseviers, M.M., Van Waeleghem, J.P., & Lindley, E., for the Research Board of the EDTNA/ERCA. (2003). Management of vascular access in Europe: Part 2 – A multicenter study of related complications. *EDTNA/ERCA Journal, 29*(1), 45-50.

Hecking, E., Bragg-Gresham, J.L., Rayner, H.C., Pisoni, R.L., Andreucci V.E., Combe C., et al. (2004). Hemodialysis prescription, adherence, and nutritional indicators in five European countries: Results from the Dialysis Outcomes and Practice Patterns Study (DOPPS). *Nephrology Dialysis Transplantation, 19*(1), 100-107.

Hurst, J., Thomas, N., Sedgewick, J., & Reichardt, M. (2003). Accreditation of post-basic nephrology courses within the EDTNA/ERCA. *EDTNA/ERCA Journal, 29*(4), 181-184.

Jungers, P. (2002). Late referral: Loss of chance for the patient, loss of money for society. *Nephrology Dialysis Transplantation, 17*(3), 371-375.

Kita, Y., Aranami, Y., Aranami, Y., Nomura, Y., Johnson, K., Wakabayashi, T., et al. (2000). Japanese organ transplant law: A historical perspective. *Progress in Transplantation, 10*(2),106-108.

Lameire, N. (2002). Management of the hemodialysis patient: A European perspective. *Blood Purification, 20*(1), 93-102.

Lindley, E., Elseviers, M., Moll, R., Jadoul, M., Jayesekera, H., Zampieron, A., et al. (2001). Epidemiology and management of hepatitis C in hemodialysis patients: An informal multidisciplinary review. *EDTNA /ERCA Journal, 27*(3),156-162.

Lindley, E., Pancírová, J., Kracikova, J., Lopot, F., Green, D., Harrington, M., et al. (2004). Management of renal anaemia: Comparison of practice in the Czech Republic and Northern England. *EDTNA/ERCA Journal, 30*(2), 75-83.

Matesanz, R., Miranda, B., Felipe, C., & Naya, M.T. (1996). Continuous improvement in organ donation. The Spanish experience. *Transplantation, 61*(7), 1119-1121.

McDonald, S.P., & Russ, G.R. (2003). Current incidence, treatment patterns, and outcome of end stage renal disease among indigenous groups in Australia and New Zealand. *Nephrology (Carlton), 8*(1), 42-48.

Moeller, S., Gioberge, S., & Brown, G. (2002). ESRD patients in 2001: Global overview of patients, treatment modalities, and development trends. *Nephrology Dialysis Transplantation, 17*(12), 2071-2076.

Nakahara, N., Nakatani, T., Takemoto, Y., & Kishimoto, T. (2001). Japanese patients not seeking kidney transplants. *EDTNA/ERCA Journal, 27*(2), 92-96.

National Institute for Clinical Excellence (NICE). (2002a) *Guideline: Management of type 2 diabetes - Renal disease, prevention, and early management (Guideline F).* Retrieved from www.nice.org.uk

National Institute for Clinical Excellence (NICE). (2002b). *Guidance on home compared with hospital hemodialysis for patients with end stage renal failure,* London: NHS Executive, Technology Guidance 48. Retrieved from www.nice.org.uk

Pancírová, J., Kracikova, J., Lopot, F., De Vos, J.Y., & Elseviers, M.M. (2004). European practice database in the Czech Republic. *EDTNA/ERCA Journal, 30*(2), 71-74.

Patient Registration Committee, Japanese Society for Dialysis Therapy (2004). An overview of regular dialysis treatment in Japan (as of 31 December 2001). *Therapeutic Apheresis and Dialysis, 8*(1), 3-32.

Piccoli, G.B., Bermond, F., Mezza, E., Quaglia, M., Pacitti, A., Jeantet, A., et al. (2002). Home hemodialysis. Revival of a superior dialysis treatment. *Nephron, 92*(2), 324-332.

Port, F.K., Pisoni, R.L., Bragg-Gresham, J.L., Satayathum, S.S., Young, E.W., Wolfe, R.A., et al. (2004). DOPPS estimates of patient life years attributable to modifiable hemodialysis practices in the United States. *Blood Purification, 22*(1), 175-180.

Ramirez, S.P., Hsu, S.I., & McClellan, W. (2003). Taking a public health approach to the prevention of end stage renal disease: The NKF Singapore Program. *Kidney International, 83*(Suppl.), S61-S65.

Rayner, H.C., Pisoni, R.L., Bommer, J., Canaud, B., Hecking, E., Locatelli, F., et al. (2004). Mortality and hospitalization in hemodialysis patients in five European countries: Results from the Dialysis Outcomes and Practice Patterns Study (DOPPS). *Nephrology Dialysis Transplantation, 19*(1), 108-120.

Rayner, H.C., Pisoni, R.L., Gillespie, B.W., Goodkin, D.A., Akiba, T., Akizawa, T., et al. (2003). Creation, cannulation, and survival of arteriovenous fistulae: Data from the Dialysis Outcomes and Practice Patterns Study (DOPPS). *Kidney International, 63*(1), 323-330.

Rytkonen, M., Ranta, J., Tuomilehto, J., & Karvonen, M. (SPAT Study Group) (2001). The Finnish Childhood Diabetes Registry Group. Bayesian analysis of geographical variation in the incidence of Type I diabetes in Finland. *Diabetologia, 44*(Suppl. 3), B37-B44.

Roderick, P., Davies, R., Jones, C., Feest, T., Smith, S., & Farrington. K. (2003). Predicting future demand in England, a simulation model of renal replacement therapy. In United Kingdom Renal Registry, *Fifth annual report of the UK renal registry* (p. 65-83). Bristol: UK Renal Registry.

Stengel, B., Billon, S., Van Dijk, P.C., Jager, K.J., Dekker, F.W., Simpson, K., et al. (2003). Trends in the incidence of renal replacement therapy for end stage renal disease in Europe, 1990-1999. *Nephrology Dialysis Transplant, 18*(9), 1824-1833.

Stewart, J.H., McCredie, M.R., & McDonald, S.P. (2004). The incidence of treated end stage renal disease in New Zealand Maori and Pacific Island people and in indigenous Australians. *Nephrology Dialysis Transplantation, 19*(3), 678-685.

Thomas, N. (2003). Using and developing your EDTNA/ERCA professional portfolio. *EDTNA/ERCA Journal, 29*(4), 172-173, 177.

Thomas, N. (2004). Collaboration between hospital and primary care can improve the management of diabetic nephropathy, *British Journal of Diabetes and Vascular Disease, 4*(3), 202-204.

Thomas, N., Küntzle, W., & McCann, M. (Eds.) (2004). *European core curriculum for a post-basic course in nephrology nursing* (2nd ed.). European Dialysis and Transplant Nurses Association/ European Renal Care Association (*EDTNA/ERCA*).

UK Renal Registry (2003). *Fifth annual report of the UK renal registry.* Bristol, UK: UK Renal Registry.

Vanholder, R., Sever, M.S., De Smet, M., Erek, E. & Lameire, N. (2001). Intervention of the Renal Disaster Relief Task Force in the 1999 Marmara, Turkey earthquake. *Kidney International, 59*(2), 783-791.

Van Waeleghem, J.P., Elseviers, M.M., & De Vos, J.Y.(2004). EDTNA/ERCA vascular access recommendations for nephrology nurses. *EDTNA/ERCA Journal, 30*(2), 97-105.

Van Waeleghem, J.P., Elseviers, M.M., & Lindley, E.J. (2000). Management of vascular access in Europe Part I: A study of center-based policies. *EDTNA/ERCA Journal, 26*(4), 28-33.

Vetter, N., & Matthews, I. (Eds.) (1999). *Epidemiology and public health.* London: Churchill Livingstone.

Zampieron, A., Jayasekera, H., Elseviers, M.M., Lindley, E., DeVos, J.Y., Visser, R., et al. (2004). European study on epidemiology and management of hepatitis C in the haemodialysis population. Part 1: Center Policy. *EDTNA/ERCA Journal, 30*(2), 84-90.

Additional Readings

Elseviers, M., & Van Waeleghem, J.P. (2003). Complications of vascular access: Results of a European multi center study of the EDTNA/ERCA Research Board. *EDTNA/ERCA Journal, 29*(3),163-167.

Lindley, L., Lopot, F., Harrington, M., & Elseviers, M. (2000). Treatment of water for dialysis: A European survey. *EDTNA/ERCA Journal, 26*(4), 22-27.

McDonald, S.P., & Russ, G.R. (2003a). Burden of end stage renal disease among indigenous peoples in Australia and New Zealand. *Kidney International, 83*(Suppl.), S123-S127.

Sever, M.S., Erek, E., Vanholder, R., Kalkan, A., Guney, N., Usta, N., et al. (2004). Features of chronic hemodialysis practice after the Marmara earthquake. *Journal American Society of Nephrology, 15*(4), 1071-1076.

Thomas, N. (Ed.). (2004). *Advanced renal care.* Oxford: Blackwells.

Thomas, N. (Ed.). (2002). *Renal nursing* (2nd ed.). Edinburgh: Ballière Tindall.

Vijt, D., Castro, M.J., Endall, G., Elseviers, M.M., & Lindley, E. (2004). Post insertion catheter care in peritoneal dialysis (PD) centers across Europe: Complication rate and individual patients' outcome. *EDTNA/ERCA Journal, 30* (2), 91-96.

Vijt, D., Castro, M.J., Endall, G., Elseviers, M.M., & Lindley, E. (2004). Post insertion catheter care in Peritoneal Dialysis (PD) centers across Europe: Results of the PI project of the Research Board. *EDTNA/ERCA Journal, 30*(1), 42-47.

- Around the world, the incidence and prevalence of renal disease are increasing. The main causes of ESRD are similar to those of the United States (U.S.) and include diabetes mellitus and glomerulonephritis.

- The epidemiology of renal replacement therapy (RRT) for end stage renal disease (ESRD) varies considerably worldwide, but until recently it had been difficult to estimate and compare trends in the incidence of renal disease by age, gender, and cause in Europe.

- The ERA-EDTA Registry is a European Registry collecting data on RRT via the national and regional registries in Europe. It analyses these data and distributes the resulting information through registry reports presented at the annual ERA-EDTA congress and through publications in nephrology journals.

- The UK Renal Registry provides a focus for the collection and analysis of standardized data relating to the incidence, clinical management, and outcome of renal disease.

- The Dialysis Outcomes and Practice Patterns Study (DOPPS) is a prospective, observational study designed to evaluate practice patterns in random samples of HD facilities and patients across three continents. Participating countries include France, Germany, Italy, Spain, and the UK (Euro-DOPPS), Japan, and the U.S.

- Challenges of renal nursing in Europe are similar to those of the U.S. as there are increased numbers of patients who are older and more dependent and who require dialysis and transplantation. There are static transplantation rates in some countries. There are also decreased numbers of specialist nephrology nurses.

- EDTNA/ERCA is an association of 5,000 professionals from more than 76 countries working in the field of renal care with increasing membership from the countries of Central and Eastern Europe.

- Singapore is unusual in that the National Kidney Foundation in Singapore (NKFS) provides subsidized dialysis care to approximately 70% of the country's total end stage renal disease (ESRD) population, based entirely on charitable donations.

- While there are very high numbers of patients on HD, Japan has traditionally not had high numbers of patients who have received renal transplants. The reasons given include the improvements of physical condition and resultant quality of life (QOL), upgraded social welfare support, uncertainties of transplant medicine, loss of expectations due to limited availability of transplant kidneys, and aging of patients. In addition, organ donation has not been widely accepted in Japan because of concerns about brain death and because of Shinto beliefs regarding need for a whole body to go on to the next world.

- The WFRC is a not-for-profit foundation committed to providing education to health care workers caring for patients with renal disease in emerging countries. The mission of the WFRC is to teach and share collective knowledge and expertise in the prevention, care, and treatment of renal diseases in countries that have established renal services.

- The challenges of renal care appear to be similar throughout the world namely, shifting the focus to prevention of renal disease, caring for an increased ageing and dependent population, improving transplantation rates, and enabling health professionals to have access to continuing professional development.

ANNP637

Nephrology Nursing: A Global Perspective

Nicola Thomas, MA, BSc (Hons), RN

Contemporary Nephrology Nursing: Principles and Practice contains 39 chapters of educational content. Individual learners may apply for continuing nursing education credit by reading a chapter and completing the Continuing Education Evaluation Form for that chapter. Learners may apply for continuing education credit for any or all chapters.

Please photocopy this page and return to ANNA.
COMPLETE THE FOLLOWING:

Name: _____

Address:_____

City:_____ State: _____ Zip: _____

E-mail: _____

Preferred telephone: ☐ Home   ☐ Work: _____

State where licensed and license number (optional): _____

CE application fees are based upon the number of contact hours provided by the individual chapter. CE fees per contact hour for ANNA members are as follows: 1.0-1.9 - $15; 2.0-2.9 - $20; 3.0-3.9 - $25; 4.0 and higher - $30. Fees for nonmembers are $10 higher.

ANNA Member: ☐ Yes   ☐ No   Member # (if available) _____

☐ Checked Enclosed   ☐ American Express   ☐ Visa   ☐ MasterCard

Total Amount Submitted: _____

Credit Card Number: _____ Exp. Date: _____

Name as it appears on the card: _____

CE Evaluation Form
To receive continuing education credit for individual study after reading the chapter
1. Photocopy this form. (You may also download this form from ANNA's Web site, **www.annanurse.org.**)
2. Mail the completed form with payment (check) or credit card information to American Nephrology Nurses' Association, East Holly Avenue, Box 56, Pitman, NJ 08071-0056.
3. You will receive your CE certificate from ANNA in 4 to 6 weeks.

Test returns must be postmarked by **December 31, 2010.**

CE Application Fee
ANNA Member $15.00
Nonmember $25.00

EVALUATION FORM

1. I verify that I have read this chapter and completed this education activity. Date: _____

_____
Signature

2. What would be different in your practice if you applied what you learned from this activity? *(Please use additional sheet of paper if necessary.)*

_____
_____
_____
_____
_____
_____
_____
_____
_____
_____
_____
_____

	Strongly disagree				Strongly agree
Evaluation					
3. The activity met the stated objectives.					
a. Summarize the epidemiology of renal disease in selected countries around the world.	1	2	3	4	5
b. Discuss the challenges of renal nursing in Europe.	1	2	3	4	5
c. Describe the World Foundation of Renal Care.	1	2	3	4	5
4. The content was current and relevant.	1	2	3	4	5
5. The content was presented clearly.	1	2	3	4	5
6. The content was covered adequately.	1	2	3	4	5
7. Rate your ability to apply the learning obtained from this activity to practice.	1	2	3	4	5

Comments _____
_____

8. Time required to read the chapter and complete this form: _____ minutes.

This educational activity has been provided by the American Nephrology Nurses' Association (ANNA) for 1.0 contact hour. ANNA is accredited as a provider of continuing nursing education (CNE) by the American Nurses Credentialing Center's Commission on Accreditation (ANCC-COA). ANNA is an approved provider of continuing education by the California Board of Registered Nursing, CEP 0910.

Communication and Collaboration

Unit 10 Contents

Relating to Teaching and Learning

Janice McCormick, PhD, RN

C H A P T E R 38

Chapter Contents

Janice McCormick, PhD, RN

Patient education has long been considered one of the most important roles of the nurse. In fact, Florence Nightingale considered health teaching to be an essential aspect of nursing practice (Sanford, 2000). The educational role remains a core nursing and societal value today. For example, it is enshrined as an essential aspect of nursing practice in national, provincial, and/or state boards of nursing, as well as in nursing associations throughout much of the industrialized world. Furthermore, patient education is part of nursing's social mandate, and nurses have an ethical and legal duty to provide necessary teaching to patients and families. In addition, as this chapter will illustrate, the demand for nurses to provide education to patients and families will likely increase significantly over the next decade due to changes in health care delivery that began in the 1990s and is expected to continue into the foreseeable future. These changes will require that nurses have skills to assess clients' learning needs, and to plan, deliver, and evaluate learning outcomes in a timely and accurate manner.

Demand for Patient Education

The educator's role is becoming more important due, in part, to changes in health care delivery over the past two decades. Families, who already manage an estimated 80% of all health care needs and problems (Bastable, 2003), are increasingly expected to assume personal responsibility for their own health maintenance and health promotion (Brez & Taylor, 1997). Moreover, these shifts in responsibility have been accelerated by changes in hospital practices (such as same-day surgery and shorter hospital stays). Patients are being discharged from hospitals with a variety of medical and nursing needs that must be met by each patient's support system – usually female members of the patient's family (Anderson & Elfert, 1989; Polaschek, 2003). This can include everything from giving medications and changing dressings to performing peritoneal dialysis. This "expanded family care role" requires health care consumers to become more knowledgeable about the patient's condition and treatment, so they can provide the necessary care in the home. Nurses, who have traditionally performed this teaching role for patients and families, can expect the demand for this kind of teaching to increase. To meet these needs for health education, nurses will need to continue to develop their knowledge, skills, and expertise in providing education for patients and families.

The aging population in North America and Europe is another issue affecting the demand for patient education. This is particularly evident in the dialysis population because renal failure is predominately a disease of older people (Canadian Organ Retrieval Register [CORR], 2002; United States Renal Data System [USRDS], 2000). While certainly able and even keen to learn, older adults have some special needs that must be addressed in order to maximize their learning.

A Complex Medical Regimen

A significant factor in the growing demand for patient education is the fact that the educator's role in nephrology nursing practice is so extensive. Patients receiving renal replacement therapy have an especially complex medical regimen, involving multiple lifestyle changes that affect virtually every aspect of their lives. These lifestyle changes include diet and fluid restrictions, numerous medications to be taken several times each day, and often a long-term commitment to dialysis. Studies show that complex medical regimens and those requiring extensive lifestyle changes over an extended period increase the probability of errors or failure to adhere to one or more aspects of the regimen (Richards, 2003). These studies raise concerns that over time, patients on dialysis will not follow all aspects of their medical regimens, and that their health and even safety will be negatively affected. The intense preoccupation of many health care professionals with the issue of compliance creates an atmosphere that can be detrimental to patients who are labeled non-compliant, and this can interfere with the relationship between the nurse-teacher and the patient.

Rethinking Compliance

The topic of compliance is one that has generated an enormous amount of attention in the professional literature of physicians, nurses, pharmacists, dieticians, and others such as medical sociologists and anthropologists. Playle and Keeley (1998) observed that this body of literature has expanded rapidly over the past 30 to 35 years. In fact, they claim that over 4,000 papers and articles on compliance and non-compliance were published in English alone during the 1990s. The majority of these studies focused on links between specific variables and compliance, including demographic features of the patient population, characteristics of the regimen, diagnoses, types and number of medications, and satisfaction with the professional-patient relationship. Despite this prolific outpouring of research, according to Trostle (1988), the findings of these studies have been largely inconclusive. Furthermore, there are problems with the reliability of the methods used to assess non-compliance with medications. Issues of compliance and non-compliance in the nephrology setting are often perplexing, and a lot of nursing time and energy is taken up with a seemingly endless cycle of teaching patients about the regimen, monitoring patients for evidence of non-compliance, attempting to find reasons for non-compliance, reviewing the rationale for the regimen with patients, and reinforcing the need for adherence. Partly because of the complexity and pervasiveness of the renal regimen, perfect adherence to all requirements is probably very rare. Not only is the work of enforcing compliance a wasted effort, it is often misguided. This issue has the potential to be extremely detrimental to the establishment of an egalitarian relationship with the patient and can interfere with a therapeutic nurse-patient relationship. Labeling the patient as "non-compliant" and entering the cycle of monitoring, confronting, and "benevolent coercing" can potentially seriously impair the establishment of trust that is essential for relational practice (Scheid-Cooke, cited in Playle & Keeley, 1998).

As Richards (2003) notes, the term *compliance* has a manipulative or authoritative undertone that constructs the health care professional as the authority and the patient as submissive or obedient to authority. In response to critiques about the notion of compliance, many authors have substituted the term *adherence,* claiming it reflects the patient's commitment to following the prescribed regimen and implies a consensual agreement between patient and health care professional. However, this change is only semantic because expectations for the patient's behavior have not changed. One of the most often quoted definitions of compliance is from Haynes (1979), who states that compliance is "the extent to which the patient's behavior (in terms of taking medications, following diets, or executing other lifestyle changes) coincides with medical or health care advice" (p. 2). Fletcher (cited in Playle & Keeley, 1998), suggests that compliance means "patients doing what the health care professional wants them to do," and that the language used highlights the power relationship between health care professionals and patients. The power to label the patient as non-compliant remains the professional's prerogative. Moreover, as several researchers have pointed out, the language used to describe patients who fail to comply tends to blame patients. Playle and Keeley (1998) charge that compliance is an ideology of health care professionals, who see non-compliance as irrational and deviant. This perspective denies the legitimacy of patient choice. Discourses of non-compliance, in this view, are generated to maintain professional power and control (Playle & Keeley, 1998).

There does appear to be a change in thinking about compliance. In the past decade, articles and papers published on compliance have shifted from the earlier focus on the problem of non-compliance and ways of promoting greater compliance to the medical regimen to a tendency for scholars to take a critical stance toward the idea of compliance (Chater, 1999; Conrad, 1987; Edel, 1985; Thorne, 1990; Trostle, 1988; Wuest, 1993). For example, Thorne (1990) examined compliance from the perspective of chronically ill patients. It was discovered by interviewing patients that these patients made serious, reasoned choices to follow or reject specific aspects of their regimens, and that these choice were not irrational acts. Based on their understanding of their own body's needs and responses, patients attempted to control symptoms and side effects to achieve personal goals or outcomes for themselves. Thorne (1990) concluded that "non-compliance is a conscious and reasoned decision not to adhere to professional advice" (p. 63). In another study of patients' perspectives on compliance, Roberson (1992) noted that patients and health professionals have different definitions of compliance. "Patients define compliance in terms of their goals for their health and seek treatment approaches which are manageable, livable, and in their view, effective" (Roberson, 1992, p. 7). In contrast, many health care professionals continue to see the medical regimen as a non-negotiable prescription.

The critique of compliance suggests that a preferred approach to non-compliance is one that moves away from confrontation and coercion toward a relational approach that respects patients' rights to choose for themselves, recognizes the complexity of patients' lives, and acknowledges the multiple meanings of non-compliance for patients and families. Such an approach would help establish or maintain the relationship between the patient and nurse. Regardless of what choices the patient makes in terms of following the regimen, the nurse is responsible for ensuring that the patient receives instruction regarding management of the medical regimen. As Dukes Hess (1996) observed, "At the level of compliance, doing good means intervening to create conditions that make it *possible* for the client to comply" (p. 25). For the nurse-teacher, this means teaching patients appropriate self-care measures, which will allow patients to choose to meet their needs by providing self-care for those aspects of the regimen to which they want or need to adhere. A case study is presented to illustrate several key aspects of patient education in the nephrology setting (see Figure 38-1).

Life on Dialysis

Dialysis and transplantation are high technology settings where patients and families are thrust into an unfamiliar and sometimes frightening technological environment. The complexity of the medical regimen means that patients are suddenly expected to make radical changes in virtually every aspect of their lives. Besides needing dialysis three times a week, patients must take multiple medications several times a day, learn how to balance their complex diet and fluid restrictions, and may also have to cope with repeated medical or surgical procedures. Most, if not all, of these changes involve a learning process for the patient and family. Added to this is the life or death nature of the treatment they are undergoing, and it is easy to understand how frightening and stressful starting dialysis can be for the patient and for family members. Most patients feel overwhelmed at first and wonder how they will ever learn all the information they are expected to know. Many worry that they will never adapt to this radically altered lifestyle. The nature of these stresses and patients' adaptations plays a pivotal role in nurses' planning for health education teaching.

A case study is included in this chapter for two reasons: first, to highlight the importance of patients' personal biographies in all phases of the learning process, and second, to affirm the importance of the nurse-patient relationship to patient care and patient education. The relationships that patients and nurses form together are the basis for everything that will unfold over the time they spend together. A relational ethic stands in sharp contrast to practices rooted in behaviorism. Hartrick (1997) has criticized the dominance of behaviorism in nursing practice, arguing that the continued supremacy of the medical/technical *paradigm* has perpetuated the underlying mechanistic assumptions of that paradigm in aspects of nursing practice that are poorly suited to these assumptions. In particular, behavioral communication skills are taught to students as an approach for interpersonal nursing practice.

Although all indications point to an intensification of the demands on nurses to deliver increasingly sophisticated patient education, it is not just the *amount* of patient teaching that will distinguish patient education in the future, but also the *kind* of patient education that will challenge nephrology nurses as they map the course of future patient education. Nurses will be asked to re-think the theoretical frameworks they use to conceptualize and deliver patient education rather than simply doing more of the same things they have done in the past. The theoretical framework for patient education that nurses are most likely familiar with is not the framework most consistent with the nursing paradigm.

Patient Education as Relational Practice

The theoretical framework of behaviorism has underpinned patient education and nearly all educational work for most of the last century. Behaviorism, a predominant worldview in the medical/technological fields and in nursing practice, is a poor fit with the nursing *paradigm*, and should be rejected in favor of a model based on relational practice (Hartrick, 1997; Hartrick Doane, 2002). Behaviorism can be characterized as a belief that behavior is determined by principles of human conduct based on negative or positive reinforcements (Schwandt, 1997). It ignores the individual's cognitive and attitudinal changes in favor of observable behaviors. Further, it is a perspective that defines human learning and psychological functioning only in terms of observable changes in specific behaviors (Flew, 1984). In fact, metaphysical behaviorism goes as far as claiming that there is no such thing as consciousness because it cannot be proven behaviorally. This exclusive focus on the behavioral aspects of patients' lives as the sole criterion for learning is inconsistent with nursing's holistic worldview, making behaviorism a poor choice to guide patient teaching. Although behaviorism is still widely used in educational settings (including nursing education) it is increasingly being challenged and rejected. According to the philosopher Charles Taylor (1991), this behavioural approach so dominates thinking and institutions that technological solutions are sought even when something very different is required.

Some nurses (Paterson & Zderad, 1976) have criticized behaviorism for years, noting that it is inconsistent with nursing's caring focus. Bevis (1988) declared that behaviorist learning models lend themselves to training, not to education. She claimed that regardless of the theory of teaching and learning being used, when behavioral objectives are used as the sole guides for selecting and devising learning activities and content, and when they are the sole source of evaluation of learning, the *de facto* learning theory is behaviorism. An alternative to behaviorism in patient education is an approach based on nurses' relational capacities and *intersubjectivity*.

Hartrick's Model of Relational Practice

One such framework comes from Hartrick (1997), who critiques behaviorism and proposes an alternative model for nursing practice based on the principles of "relational capacities." Because nurses have relied almost exclusively on mechanistic models of human relationships that are based on behaviorist views, Hartrick (1997) developed an alternative model based on principles of human relating. The purpose of this new model is to establish an alternative to behaviorism that recognizes the importance of human caring and nursing practices aimed at establishing, maintaining, and nurturing relational capacities. In her model, Hartrick identified five relational capacities:

Figure 38-1
Case Study

Feeling numb with fear, Isobel opened the door to the Renal Unit, and then quickly put her hand into her pocket so her daughter, Cathy, wouldn't see how it was shaking. The nurses asked Cathy to remain in the waiting room until they had started the dialysis treatment for her mother. Isobel would like to have had Cathy in the room with her, but she didn't say anything – they must have a good reason for asking Cathy to stay outside, she thought. Isobel suddenly felt very sad and struggled to fight back her tears. If only she didn't feel so alone – This feeling of loneliness was something Isobel had been struggling with for the past 18 months since her husband, Fred, passed away. Isobel sat down on the edge of the recliner chair she was offered and cautiously looked around the room. She sighed. Here she was in the very place she had been dreading for months. She had tried to delay starting dialysis for as long as she could, but she knew that she could no longer function like this – she was so tired all the time – She hadn't read much of the patient information she had been given. She had tried to read the pamphlets she had been given, struggling to pay attention because she knew it was important. But every time she tried to read, the words seemed to fade or go out of focus, and after 10 minutes or so, she was too tired to continue. Because of this, she had only a vague idea of what was going to happen today. She fought the waves of anxiety that were once again threatening to wash over her. In a few minutes, a young woman greeted her by name and introduced herself as Kara. Kara said that she would be Isobel's primary nurse. Kara was friendly and welcoming, but Isobel's anxiety was increasing. With a growing sense of panic, she realized that she didn't know what 'primary nurse' meant. By now she could see the other patients sitting down beside machines, some being attended by the nurses. Suddenly realizing that the long red tubes she was looking at contained patients' blood, Isobel felt dizzy and thought she was going to faint. Noticing Isobel's pale face, Kara helped her to lean forward with her head over her knees until the dizziness passed.

After taking Isobel's vital signs and weighing her, Kara initiated dialysis via Isobel's temporary venous catheter, explaining what she was doing as she worked, and casually asking Isobel questions: How was she feeling today? Was she having any problems the nurses should know about? Where did she live? Did she have a family? What kinds of medications was she taking? How old was she? Did she have any questions? After she had initiated the dialysis treatment, Kara sat down and began to explain to Isobel what was happening – how the dialysis machine worked, what Isobel would need to do to follow her medical regimen at home, and how she would need to take her medications. Isobel tried to pay attention, but the explanations didn't make any sense to her. She had felt this sense of confusion for several weeks now – almost as if she were far away from the person talking. She understood the words, but couldn't make sense of the meaning. Kara was so kind, and Isobel knew Kara was trying to help her, so she just smiled and nodded, and didn't ask any questions. After 20 minutes, Isobel could no longer fight off her pervasive fatigue and nodded off to sleep right in the middle of Kara's instructions. Later, when dialysis was completed, Isobel was embarrassed that she might have offended Kara by falling asleep. She worried that she was too old to learn the things she would need to know to be on dialysis. "After all," Isobel thought, "I am going to be 80 in less than three months."

---

1. *Initiative, authenticity, and responsiveness.* These intertwined capacities involve active concern for and about others. The focus is on being present with another person and responding authentically to the expression of the other's feelings and thoughts.

2. *Mutuality and synchrony.* Mutuality refers to the acknowledgment and sharing of both commonalities and differences between people in interaction, whereas synchrony involves congruence between the internal rhythms and external actions of individuals (for example, mutuality and synchrony acknowledge the importance of rhythms of both dialogue and silence).

3. *Complexity and ambiguity.* Honoring complexity and ambiguity involves the recognition that complexity and ambiguity are intrinsic aspects of any interaction; to expand our capacity to recognize and live with complexity and ambiguity, we need to expand our capacity to trust, to be curious, to be comfortable with silence and not knowing, and learn to let go of the need for certainty and control.

4. *Intentionality in relating.* According to Hartrick (1997, p. 526), "Intentionality involves a clear and expressed congruence between espoused values and values-in-use (that is, the values one is drawing on to make decisions). Intentionality encompasses a) uncovering the values and beliefs that direct relational being/knowing/doing, and b) exercising choice in regard to following, expanding and/or transforming those values and beliefs." Hartrick's overall intent is to help people understand and clarify the meaning of their health, illness, and healing experiences, and to foster choice and a realization of one's own power.

5. *Re-imagining.* Re-imagining refers to the complex web of interconnections human beings form with each other and is an acknowledgment of the fact that human beings are interdependent, interrelating, and interconnected. We are constantly influenced by our interactions with others, and also affect the people with whom we interact. People are relational by nature, and relational practices are purposeful activities nurses carry out to create, maintain, and nurture these interconnections.

Continuing Dominance of the Behavioral Paradigm

Nevertheless, behavioral objectives continue to be widely used in educational settings. Many educators are attracted to the precision with which these objectives can be stated and the apparent ease of evaluating learning, at least for those objectives that can be stated in behavioral terms. However, other educators have criticized behavioral objectives, claiming that learning is reduced to mechanistic behaviors that fail to capture the diversity of learning experiences. Further, they note that behavioral objectives are unable to capture the more intricate cognitive processes that are not readily observable and measurable (Bastable, 2003). Most seriously for relational practice, preparing instructional objectives in advance means patients are being asked to work toward the nurse's or institution's goals, not the patient's own goals. In order for patients to commit to an educational plan, they must be able to see how the plan addresses goals

that are important to them. In creating educational plans, nurses need not only to help patients achieve their own meaningful goals; they need to understand something about learning theories so they can design learning approaches that work with patients' own learning styles.

Learning Theories

Learning theories were introduced into nursing primarily from educational psychologists, Gestalt theorists, and change theorists (for example, Kurt Lewin) (Knox, 2002). Learning theories explain how knowledge and skills are assimilated by the learner, and suggest effective ways to present material. Reflecting a time when the nursing profession actively introduced theories from other disciplines, chiefly psychology and sociology, these "borrowed" theories imported more than just those theories nurses applied to patient care situations. Embedded in these theories are underlying philosophical worldviews that reflect a particular way of seeing the world and our relationships with others. In order to appreciate the implications of the paradigm underlying the learning approach being used, it is necessary to understand the assumptions that underpin each paradigm. These include assumptions about how people learn, human nature, and the goals of learning. Unfortunately, there is no agreement on what the major learning approaches are. For example, Bastable (2003) reviews five major learning theories (behaviorist, cognitive, social learning, psychodynamic, and humanistic), but claims that only three of these are commonly used in patient education and health care practice (behaviorist, cognitive, and social learning theories). A more helpful and simpler distinction was drawn by Reese and Overton (1970), who divided learning theories into two major paradigms based on the underlying assumptions: the mechanistic paradigm and the organismic paradigm.

Mechanistic Learning Paradigm

The mechanistic paradigm, typified by behaviorism and behavioral learning objectives, represents the universe as a machine (orderly, predictable, and controllable). Behaviorism has been a dominant force in educational research and practice for most of the 20th century, and has had a significant influence on learning theory. Arising from mainstream psychology, behaviorism focuses mainly on what can be directly observed. Behaviorists measure the success of learning on direct evidence of a change in behavior of the learner. According to the mechanistic viewpoint, natural laws govern all natural phenomena, and therefore the scientific method is deemed appropriate for the study of human behavior. Human behavior is seen as reactive and passive. Forces external to the individual are responsible for initiating changes in behavior. Behaviorist theories describe the relationship between measurable stimuli and the behavioral responses elicited (sometimes referred to as S-R learning, or stimulus-response learning). Behaviorists believe that for learning to take place, objective and observable changes in behavior must occur (Knox, 2002).

In order to influence the direction of these changes, teachers in the behavioral paradigm prepare *behavioral objectives* that detail exactly what behaviors the learner must demonstrate. An essential criterion is that the change must be observable to the evaluator. Mager (1962), one of the first to identify the essential characteristics of behavioral instructional objectives, deemed that three steps were necessary to create a good behavioral objective:

Step 1: Specify performance. The instructor must identify the behavior that will be accepted as evidence that the learner has achieved the objective.

Step 2: Specify the conditions under which the behavior must occur (often stated as the resources the learner will be given while carrying out the behavioral objective).

Step 3: Specify the criteria of acceptable performance. This can be done by describing the level at which the learner must perform the behavior. For example, in the nephrology setting, a behavioral objective for Isobel by the end of her educational program might be:"Given a list of her own 9 medications, Isobel will identify the correct dosage and time for all 9 of her medications". Note that the conditions under which Isobel is to carry out the objective are stated: she is given a list (i.e., she doesn't have to memorize and recall all her medications), and the level of performance is given: she must know 9 out of the 9 medication dosages and time of day they should be taken.

Organismic Learning Paradigm

In contrast, the organismic model, exemplified by cognitive learning theories, perceives the universe as a unitary, interactive, developing entity with humans as the active source of behavior. Learning is defined as a process that creates a change in the individual, but this change does not have to be behavioral; it may be a change in insight, motivation, perceptions, mental associations, behavior, or a combination of these (Knox, 2002). Whereas behaviorists ignore the internal dynamics of learning and focus on the behavioral manifestations that signal learning, cognitive theorists stress the internal changes that occur in the learner. The key to learning for cognitive learning theorists involves changing the learner's internal perceptions, cognitions, and ways of processing and structuring information. Learning, according to adherents of cognitive learning theory, is viewed as an active process largely directed by the individual. It involves perceiving and interpreting information, and based on what is already known, reorganizing knowledge into new insights or understanding (Braungart & Braungart, 2003). I propose that the mechanistic model and behaviorism are inappropriate for nursing, and that they are inconsistent with the nursing paradigm of holism. Consequently, behaviorism should be rejected in favor of a relational approach.

Relational Practice as a Foundation for Interpersonal Nursing Practice

As far back as the 1960s, nursing theorists had begun to challenge the dominant models of nursing practice, rejecting the behaviorism then rampant in education, nursing, and many other fields, in favor of an approach based on interpersonal relationships, communication, caring, and humanism. For example, Paterson and Zderad (1976) drew on Buber's notion of "I – Thou" communication (Buber, 1958) in conceptualizing the relationship between nurse and patient. In this type of communication, the 'other' is perceived not as an object, but as subject. When the other is viewed as object,

an "I – It" relation exists. According to Buber (1958), this results in establishing distance between the self and the other. When nurses make movement toward patients by recognizing the patients' independent being, they move to establish a relationship – signaling a willingness to open themselves up to patients in an authentic relationship. This process makes effective communication between people possible. This relationship is characterized by authenticity, genuine communication, and acceptance of differences. Effective, genuine communication is the cornerstone of relational practice, an approach that can provide the basis for a transformative nurse-patient relationship.

Relational implies the complex web of interconnected relationships that characterize human interactions. When people interact, they become an integral part of each other's context, and mutually shape each other's perceptions, behaviors, and environment (Hartrick Doane & Varcoe, 2005). In recent years, there has been a growing body of literature on relational practice and relational capacities in a variety of fields including nursing (Hartrick, 1997; Hartrick Doane, 2002; Hartrick Doane & Varcoe, 2005), education (Noddings, 2003), ethics (MacDonald, 2002; Storch, Rodney, & Starzomski, 2004), and theology (Faust, 1998), among others. The approaches advocated in this literature reject the mechanistic models and interventions based on a behaviorist worldview, with its dehumanizing and instrumental approach that distances nurses from patients. Relational approaches acknowledge the reality that human beings are interdependent, interrelating, and interconnected. These assumptions stand in stark contrast to liberal political discourses, the predominant, if not always acknowledged, ideology in most Western industrialized countries.

Liberal Individualism in Contrast to Relational Practice

In contrast to a relational approach, the defining feature of liberalism is individualism (Browne, 2001). In her critique of liberal ideology, Browne noted that the cult of individualism constructs people as rational, self-sufficient, autonomous beings who can be considered independently of their context or environment. A relational perspective recognizes that people are interdependent and relational beings. Everything we do or say has an effect on others, and/or on the environment. In turn, we are affected by what others say and do. The importance of relationships in nursing practice and patient education was reinforced in the findings from two studies carried out in dialysis settings. In the first study, on the nature of dilemmas for nurses working in a dialysis unit, Wellard (1992) found that most of the dilemmas nurses experienced arose from conflicts in relationships with other people in the work environment, engendering stress, frustration, and job dissatisfaction. In the second study, 240 nurses and technicians from 307 randomly selected U.S. dialysis facilities were surveyed about specific domains of job satisfaction. Both the nurses and the technicians associated higher job satisfaction with their ability to engage in "desirable patient care practices." Two of these "desirable practices" were cited in the report: 1) being able to attend to patients' psychosocial needs and 2) being able to meet patients' educational needs (Perumal & Sehgal, 2003). These findings underscore the significance of relationships between people working together in a health care setting, and also suggest that health care professionals feel a sense of satisfaction when they are able to enact their professional practice roles and provide patients with the education they know patients need.

The pervasiveness of individualism shapes our consciousness in ways of which we may not be aware. Over time, we slip into ways of thinking that are familiar and comfortable (the status quo). We 'buy into' the rhetoric of liberal individualism without questioning it. It may come as a shock to realize that some of our most familiar and essential social concepts are not 'real'. Take, for example, 'society' and 'culture'. We speak about these two concepts as if they represented real entities, that is, something we can point to and say "that is society" or "this is culture." But society and culture do not exist outside of the ways we think or speak about them. What we think of as the social, organizational, or cultural environment in a particular unit of the hospital, for instance, is the cumulative effect of all of the interactions that take place within that context. The culture of the unit is, in other words, a daily performance enacted by all people who play roles in that setting (patients and families, health care professionals, supervisors, visitors, etc.). That is not to say that the effects of such interactions are not real in their consequences; this daily performance powerfully shapes how we interact in a work setting, affecting how satisfied we feel about the work we do, and ultimately molding our ways of thinking and reacting in that setting. Because unit culture doesn't exist "out there" but is constructed daily in what we say and do, the ways we interact with each other (nurses, patients, families, physicians, porters, lab staff, social workers, housekeepers, visitors, and all other health care professionals) are responsible for the unit or institutional culture. As such, all people interacting in a particular setting affect the culture by what they choose to say and do.

Every time we resist gossip and negative labels for patients, family members, nurses, or other health care workers; every time we consider the patient's lived experience and how these experiences might be shaping the ways patients and families react in a situation; every time we reach out to comfort, support, or make time to teach a patient and/or family member something they need to know to provide care for their loved ones; we create space for new ways of being-in-the-world for ourselves and all those around us. A relational way of thinking acknowledges the myriad ways we are interconnected and interrelating with others, influencing others at the same time we are being influenced. Moreover, it is a foundation for patient education that can be beneficial not only for patients and their families, but also for the educator (Noddings, 2003). There is evidence that the development of a positive relationship between the nurse-teacher and patients improves learning (Faust, 1998). Faust asserts that "effective teaching has more to do with the quality of the relationship and the process of learning than it has to do with content and static truth" (p. 467). He notes that a relational teaching model offers caring contexts where participation, growth, transformation, and insights occur for both teacher and learner. This can be especially advantageous for the elderly, as the nurse who has developed a close relationship with the patient is better able to assess readiness to learn, learning style, and to know what challenges the patient might have in learning. Because the elderly now constitute the fastest growing segment of the renal population, it is important to examine the special needs of the elderly in patient education.

Teaching Older Adults

Reflecting trends in the larger population, where those over 85 years of age comprise the fastest growing segment of the population, older adults are the fastest growing segment of the hemodialysis population as well (Chauhan, 2004; USRDS, 2000). According to Erikson (1963), the age ranges and developmental stages of these people are: middle adulthood (40 to 65 years – developmental stage: generativity vs. self-absorption and stagnation) or older adulthood (65 years and older – developmental stage: ego integrity vs. despair).

On the positive side, older people are in the 'formal operations' developmental stage where cognitive ability remains steady. Many in this stage of life possess a lifetime of experiences, skills, and resources that they bring to this new challenge. Physiological studies support the existence of two types of intelligence: crystallized intelligence and fluid intelligence. *Crystallized intelligence* is the knowledge individuals have gathered over a lifetime of experiences (for example, general knowledge, understanding, and being able to evaluate experience and social interactions, and numeric reasoning). This type of intelligence can improve with age and experience, unless there is dementia. *Fluid intelligence*, on the other hand, involves abstract thinking and reasoning ability; this kind of intelligence tends to decline with age, resulting in older people needing more time to process information, especially in making the connection between actions and results (Bastable & Rinwalske, 2003). A second consequence of the decline in fluid intelligence is a decrease in short-term memory, although long-term memory is unaffected. Although older adults may have slower processing time, they continue to do as well as younger people on IQ tests if they are given enough time to respond. There is also a diminishing of the senses: taste, vision, hearing, smell, and touch are all affected. It is important to remember that these findings are for people experiencing a 'normal' aging process; when older adults are also coping with ESRD, cognitive effects are more complex, and there are likely to be more problems with learning, memory, and the time needed to process information.

Returning to the case study, we note that Kara makes positive moves toward establishing a relationship with Isobel, setting the tone for their relationship. Kara welcomes Isobel and begins her treatment efficiently. She then makes sure she involves Isobel in conversation, finding out more about her so that she can begin to know her better – this is, after all, the beginning of her relationship with Isobel who is going to be her primary patient. Kara hopes that if Isobel has a better understanding of the way the machine works, her anxiety will decrease, and she will be more relaxed during dialysis. All of these intents are positive, but a number of the approaches Kara used are problematic. First, from a relational perspective, it would have been better to allow Isobel the option of having Cathy in the unit with her when she was starting dialysis for the first time. In a frightening situation, it might have been calming for Isobel to have a familiar face and the presence of a family member to reassure her. Because Isobel is still grieving the loss of her husband, she needs a familiar and loved presence around her to help her cope with all the changes she is experiencing at this time. Second, although Kara's desire to reduce Isobel's anxiety by explaining how the machine works is commendable, there are several reasons why the timing of her efforts was less than optimal. For example, despite the fact that patients are a 'captive audience' during the hours they are being dialyzed, there are compelling reasons for *not* scheduling patient education during these times. Almost all patients experience a variety of physical, emotional, and cognitive impairments resulting from their chronic renal failure and/or the dialysis treatment. These hemodynamic and physiologic changes have been shown to have a detrimental effect on patients' ability to learn.

Factors Affecting Learning in Patients with End Stage Renal Failure

The case study contains themes that will be familiar to many nephrology nurses: the growing numbers elderly patients, particularly women, receiving renal replacement therapy (Chauhan, 2004; USRDS, 2000); the difficulty finding an appropriate time and setting to carry out patient teaching; scarce resources for patient education (Turner, Wellard, & Bethune, 1999); and dealing with individual patient characteristics, symptoms, or side effects that can interfere with learning. Fatigue and problems concentrating figure prominently in this list of symptoms that can interfere with learning in patients with ESRD. Furthermore, there is evidence that these cognitive effects are exacerbated by dialysis (Smith & Winslow, 1990). These issues are explored in greater detail in the next section, and the research evidence is examined. The issues raised in the vignette underscore the importance of patient teaching in the nephrology setting and also flag some of the problematic issues surrounding patient education in a busy clinical unit.

Pathophysiological and Hemodynamic Effects of Hemodialysis

One of the insidious effects of the long slide into ESRD is something that doesn't show up on lab results: a slowing of cognitive responses that result in a decreased ability to concentrate, drowsiness (especially during dialysis), mental confusion (Levine, 1991), and mental fatigue (Heiwe, Clyne, & Dahlgren, 2003). There are conflicting opinions about the causes of this cognitive impairment. Some researchers point to uremic encephalopathy and uremic toxins (Bosch & Schlebusch, 1991; Evers, Tepel, Obladen, Suhr, Husstedt, Grotmeyer et al., 1998); and others have suggested anemia (Macdougal, 1998) as possible reasons for the cognitive deficits patients face. Anecdotally, patients have long complained about their lack of energy, fatigue, inability to concentrate, and paradoxically, difficulty getting to sleep or staying asleep through the night. These symptoms, particularly the extent of the mental and physical fatigue nephrology patients experience, have been confirmed by Heiwe, Clyne, & Dahlgren (2003) in a study designed to examine the impact of renal failure on the daily lives of patients. It has long been suspected that hemodialysis may temporarily cre-

ate conditions that make cognitive function more difficult. Certainly patients have expressed the opinion that they feel mentally fatigued and unable to think quickly or clearly during dialysis. Smith and Winslow (1990) were able to confirm that the hemodialysis treatment slows cognitive processes and temporarily exacerbates the degree of cognitive impairment patients experience. These researchers administered the Number Connection Test (NCT) to a group of 29 hemodialysis patients who volunteered to participate in their study. The NCT is a simple paper and pencil test consisting of 25 circles numbered in nonconsecutive order from 1 to 25. Patients were asked connect the numbers in consecutive order as quickly as they could. The score was the number of seconds taken to complete the task. The test was administered twice to each of the 29 volunteers: one hour before dialysis and one hour into the dialysis run. Patients required significantly more time to complete the test – an average of 17.16 seconds longer – during hemodialysis than before their treatments ($t = 3.29$, $p = .0027$). These results confirm what has been reported anecdotally: that patients experience cognitive slowing during dialysis. These findings support a policy of not planning patient education sessions during patients' hemodialysis treatment time.

This presents a dilemma for nephrology nurses; if teaching can't be provided during the hours when the patient is dialyzing, when can it be done? Because patients already spend many hours every week dialyzing or being seen by specialists, they are, understandably, unwilling to come to the hospital or clinic on their non-dialysis days. Brundage (1990) suggests some alternatives to face-to-face instruction, such as the use of written information for patients to study at home, with testing of knowledge by phone, telephone calls to provide teaching on non-dialysis days, content provided via instructional videos, audiotaped educational sessions, or posters demonstrating specific aspects of patient care. Nephrology nurses could use their imaginations to create easy-to-use instructional aids using photographs, photocopies of flow charts, or other instructional information to design individualized materials that patients and/or family members could access at times when they feel ready to learn and that are convenient for them.

Changing Demographics

Returning once again to the case study, experienced nephrology nurses will recognize many familiar patterns in the scenario presented in the case study. This case study was chosen because Isobel represents an increasingly common phenomenon in nephrology settings: the elderly patient beginning dialysis, particularly elderly female patients, although men on dialysis still outnumber women (Chauhan, 2004; USRDS, 2000). This older patient population may present some learning challenges of which nephrology nurses should be aware. Many patients on renal replacement therapy experience difficulty concentrating (Levine, 1991), and older patients may also have some problems with hearing and/or vision, which can interfere with their learning. Moreover, patients who are approaching 80 years of age, as Isobel is, were educated in the 1920s and 1930s, and reading skills can be lost over time through lack of practice (Jackson, Davis, Murphy, Bairnsfather, & George, 1994).

Furthermore, many older adults have not had extensive education. Citing U.S. statistics, Bastable (2003) claims that one-third of the elderly have only an eighth grade education, and 45% have less than a high school education. These statistics have implications for reading levels and literacy in this population.

Literacy

The extent of low literacy and illiteracy in North America is significant. An estimated 25 to 30% of North American adults (and about 40% of Americans over the age of 65) are considered to be functionally illiterate (Davidhizar & Brownson, 1999). This is a serious health issue as almost half (43%) of people who have low literacy live in poverty (Bastable, 2003). Despite the well-documented extent of illiteracy, health care professionals continue to rely heavily on print-based media for patient education (Brez & Taylor, 1997). Available research suggests that the reading level of much of these materials is beyond the capability of the groups for which it is intended (Conlin & Schumann, 2002; Davidhizar & Brownson, 1999) including much of the health care information available on the Internet (Sopczyk, 2003). In one study, researchers found that the reading levels of surgical consent forms were between 10.82 to 15.45 grade levels (Conlin & Schumann, 2002). Most printed education materials are written above the eighth grade level, with the average grade level falling between the 10th and 12th grades (Bastable, 2003). Research on reading levels and literacy has consistently shown that the reading levels of health care information should be no more than the eighth grade level; the mean literacy level is at or below the eighth grade, and studies show that people read two-to-four grade levels below their reported level of formal education (Bastable, 2003) (see Table 38-1 for a sample readability formula).

Compounding the generally low level of educational attainment of many elderly people is the fact that literacy demands have increased dramatically since the 1930s. Fain (1994, p. 52) claims that, "To be literate 100 years ago meant that people could read and write their own names. Today, being literate means that one is able to learn new skills, think critically, problem-solve, and apply general knowledge to various situations."Furthermore, reading and writing are only two of many expectations for literacy in the 21st century. Numeracy, or the ability to read and interpret numbers, is a skill that many seniors may not possess beyond simple arithmetic. As hospitals and clinics increasingly move to online information and educational programs, computer literacy is another area that is fast becoming an expectation for all adults to possess. Those unable to "surf the net" – to be able to go online to retrieve information from the World Wide Web – will fall behind and be at a disadvantage in their search for health care information. Nurses should be aware of the kinds of information being posted on Web sites in their institutions and monitor patients' abilities to access this information. Elderly people, even those who use computers for email, may lack advanced skills for navigating and problem solving in this medium.

The level of illiteracy or low literacy in the North America population has been termed "a silent epidemic," reflecting the large numbers of people affected. As such, it is

Table 38-1
How to Use the SMOG Readability Formula

1. Count 10 consecutive sentences near the beginning, 10 consecutive sentences near the middle, and 10 consecutive sentences near the end of the selection to be assessed. A sentence is any independent unit of thought punctuated by a period, question mark, or exclamation point. If a sentence has a colon or semi-colon, consider each part as a separate sentence.

2. From the 30 randomly selected sentences, count the words containing three or more syllables (these are polysyllabic words), including repetitions. Abbreviated words should be read aloud to determine their syllable count (for example, Sept. = September = three syllables). Letters or numerals in a string beginning or ending with a space or punctuation mark should be counted if, when read aloud in context, at least three syllables can be distinguished. Do not count words ending in –ed or –es if the ending makes the word have a third syllable. Hyphenated words are counted as one word. Proper nouns should be counted.

3. Approximate the reading grade level by: *first*, calculating the nearest perfect square root of the number of words with three or more syllables, and *second*, adding a constant of 3 to the square root. For example, if the total number of polysyllabic words in the 30 sentences was 53, the nearest perfect square would be 49. The square root of 49 is 7. Adding the constant of 3 makes the reading level of this sample the tenth grade. (Hint: Using a calculator with a square root function, simply enter the total number of words with three or more syllables, press the square root sign, and use the whole number that appears to the left of the decimal place as the nearest square root [disregard the numbers to the right of the decimal point]. This is the nearest square root. Add 3 to this number for the reading grade level).

very likely that a percentage of the patients that nurses are attempting to teach will struggle with reading to some degree. It is important in planning educational sessions not to assume that the patients can read and write. Older patients are more likely to have "test anxiety" and to resist attempts to formally test their reading ability; however, there are ways to predict which patients have a severe reading problem. For example, if the patient resists reading the materials he is given, says he will read it later, or says he has forgotten his glasses at home or that they are broken, he may be avoiding the task so he will not have to admit that he does not know how to read. Most people who are illiterate are embarrassed by this. In addition, people who cannot read or those who read poorly are usually very sensitive about it and will go to great lengths to hide it if they can. Although it would be ideal to do formal testing of the reading level of patients being taught so that appropriate learning materials could be used, it is important not to create undue anxiety in patients. Because formal testing may trigger test anxiety, the test may negatively influence the results. If testing is done, Brez and Taylor (1997) recommend that privacy and confidentiality be assured and communicated to the patient, and that testing be carried out by trained professionals. They also suggest that all patients, particularly those with low literacy skills, be offered a wide range of learning options developed for low reading

Table 38-2
Steps in the Teaching and Learning Relationship

1. The basis for the teaching and learning process is the establishment of open and honest communication, and a therapeutic nurse-patient relationship based on dialogue, appropriate self-disclosure, and thoughtful self-reflection.

2. Identify the *learning goals* and *learning objectives*. Ideally, this is a mutual process. Negotiate patient goals and objectives. In order for the patient to be invested in the process of working toward the goals, patients need to participate in identifying personal, meaningful goals. The nurse-teacher has a moral obligation to include teaching that enables patients and/or their family members to learn how to provide necessary self-care, prevent harm, and maintain a level of functioning acceptable to the patients.

3. Assess patient's readiness to learn, preferred learning style, current knowledge base, educational level, reading level, knowledge gaps, and physical, emotional, cultural, or psychological barriers to learning.

4. Select a variety of teaching strategies to present content, maximizing the patient's preferred learning style, and using active strategies to promote learning.

5. Note patient's responses, which goals and objectives are attained and which are not. Keep dialogue open to help determine what needs to be changed.

6. Evaluate progress toward each of the goals and objectives.

7. Revise goals and objectives as necessary and renegotiate goals as earlier ones are achieved. At all stages the patient should feel comfortable to disagree, suggest other goals, ask for more time, or ask for a time out.

levels and allow patients to select the materials that best suit their needs. This would avoid the risk of exposing patients with low literacy to embarrassment and subsequent stigmatization (Brez & Taylor, 1997). Learning materials could include audio-visual presentations or audio-taped information to augment other instructions and/or use non-print based teaching materials. If this is not possible, use the lowest reading level you can find or create, and see if the patient can read it. When people are sick, they prefer easy-to-read materials, even if their reading abilities are normally high. These statistics underscore the importance of carrying out a good assessment of the patient at the beginning of the educational process (see Table 38-2).

Patient Learning Assessment

The patient assessment should include an appraisal of the patient's physical and psychosocial needs, motivation to learn, readiness to learn, reading level, level of formal education, barriers to learning, current knowledge base, knowledge gaps, and an assessment of learning strengths and challenges. Assess the presence and extent of any problems or limitations with vision, hearing, movement or balance, as well as the presence of any diagnoses that might interfere with the patient's ability to learn (such as organic brain syndrome, Alzheimer's disease, receptive aphasia, or others).

The patient's preferred learning style is a determination of what senses he prefers for learning and how he learns best (for example, visual, aural, and kinetic). There are formal learning style instruments that can be used (Bastable, 2003), but the nurse-teacher can simply talk to the patient and ask questions about how he prefers to learn, and/or observe him in the teaching situation. The nurse-teacher might decide to do formal testing of reading to determine the patient's reading level if low literacy or illiteracy is suspected.

Learning Goals

It is important that nurses not approach all patients with the same predetermined learning goals, for example, using a pre-established set of goals and objectives in a patient education manual. The patient must have input into the learning goals and be able to work toward meaningful goals that are important to the patient and family. Ideally, it is only *after* such an assessment that learning goals can be identified and agreed upon, and teaching can be started. Learning goals divide the learning tasks into manageable portions designed to encourage the patient's progress toward her or his goals.

Planning Learning for Older Adults or Those with Low Literacy Skills

There are several things the nurse educator can do to maximize learning in older patients and/or those with low literacy.

1. Consistent with the relational focus of this chapter, the first task of the educator is to begin to create a positive, supportive relationship with the patient and family as the base for patient education and all other aspects of the patient's care over the course of illness and treatment.

2. Focus on the patient's strengths and demonstrate your confidence in his ability to learn what he needs to know in order to succeed.

3. Use the smallest amount of information possible to accomplish the negotiated goals. Particularly for patients who are in their early days of adapting to dialysis, pare information down to essentials and prioritize learning goals. Make sure that you do not impose the learning goals. People are more committed when working toward goals they are invested in and that are meaningful for them.

4. Make points of information as vivid and explicit as possible. Use simple terms and everyday language. For example, rather than saying "NPO," say "Nothing by Mouth" to avoid misunderstanding. Patients may not admit they don't know what NPO means. Remember to provide concrete examples whenever possible.

5. Teach one step at a time. Organize teaching in 'chunks' of related information, and give enough time for practice, asking and answering questions, and giving positive feedback.

6. Use multiple teaching methods and tools requiring fewer literacy skills. Oral instruction contains cues such as tone of voice, gestures, and expression that are lacking in print materials. These can help comprehension of the material, but remember to use everyday language and avoid medical jargon.

Table 38-3
Patient Learning Assessment

The patient assessment should include an appraisal of the patient's physical and psychosocial needs, motivation to learn, readiness to learn, reading level, level of formal education, barriers to learning, current knowledge base, knowledge gaps, and an assessment of learning strengths and challenges. Assess the presence and extent of any problems or limitations with vision, hearing, movement, or balance, as well as the presence of any diagnoses that might interfere with the patient's ability to learn (organic brain syndrome, Alzheimer's disease, receptive aphasia, or others). The patient's preferred learning style is a determination of what senses he prefers for learning and how he learns best (for example, visual, aural, kinetic). There are formal learning style instruments that can be used (Bastable 2003), but the nurse-teacher can simply talk to the patient and ask questions about how he prefers to learn, and/or observe him in the teaching situation. The nurse-teacher should attempt to do formal testing of reading if low literacy or illiteracy is suspected.

It is important that nurses not approach all patients with the same predetermined learning goals, for example, using a pre-established set of goals and objectives in a patient education manual. The patient must have input into the learning goals and be able to work toward meaningful goals that are important to him and his family. Ideally, it is only *after* such an assessment that learning goals can be identified and agreed upon, and teaching started.

7. Allow patients the chance to restate information in their own words and to demonstrate any procedures being taught. This can reinforce learning and also reveal any gaps or errors in understanding. Avoid asking questions that require a "yes" or "no" answer. Rather than asking him if he understands something, ask for specific feedback instead. Many people will simply say "yes" when asked if they understand.
8. Keep motivation high. People with low literacy may already feel like failures and need to know that the nurse is enthusiastic about the progress they are making and their chances for succeeding at the task. Use praise and encouragement.
9. Build in coordination of procedures. Use *tailoring* and *cuing*. *Tailoring* refers to coordinating patients' regimens into their daily schedules rather than having them change their daily routines to accommodate the regimen. *Cuing* focuses on using prompts and reminders to help people learn habits, such as placing medications in locations that remind patients to take medications at particular times of the day, or checking off medications as they are taken.
10. Use repetition to reinforce information. Repeating information using different words at intervals helps learning (see Tables 38-3 and 38-4).

Barriers to Teaching
Barriers to teaching are factors in the environment that can interfere with learning or with the teaching experience. Patient educators should examine these and prepare to eliminate or minimize them. The barriers include:

Table 38-4
Steps in the Process of Patient Education

1. Establish a relationship. The relationship the nurse-teacher forms with the patient is crucial to the teaching and learning process. When patients are treated with respect, consulted about their ideas and preferences in establishing the learning plan, including mutual goal setting and are involved in creating this plan, they are more invested in the outcomes and more willing to work on achieving the goals.
2. There are parallels between the nursing process and the teaching and learning process. It is essential that nurses begin with a thorough assessment of the learning strengths and challenges of the patient, and this learning assessment should be completed as soon as possible.
3. This process includes assessing the patient's preferred learning style, readiness to learn, existing knowledge base, level of education attained, reading level, and barriers to learning (physiological, psychological, language, cultural, or motivational problems) that affect learning.
4. The nurse-teacher and patient work together to negotiate a learning plan with goals and objectives important to the patient (and/or family) as well as goals relevant to learning essential knowledge to enable the patient to follow the medical regimen.
5. Based on the learning style assessment, the nurse-teacher selects a variety of learning tools and approaches to maximize learning. Research demonstrates that using a variety of learning approaches can increase learning.
6. The nurse-teacher selects learning activities that engage the patient actively rather than passively in the learning experience. The patient should be encouraged to restate principles or information in his or her own words, provide a return demonstration, or express other active learning strategies that allow the patient to manipulate ideas, concepts, and equipment. Active strategies have been found to facilitate learning.
7. It is important for the nurse-teacher to create an environment conducive to learning to bring about the 'teachable moment' rather than just waiting for it to happen (for example, by removing or reducing barriers to learning; promoting comfort and feelings of psychological, cultural, or emotional safety; and ensuring physiological aberrations are eliminated or minimized). The tenets of relational practice suggest that motivation to learn can be fostered when nurses have formed a strong and trusting relationship with patients and/or family members, and patients are working toward meaningful goals they participated in creating.
8. Evaluate teaching effectiveness. What progress toward the identified goals was the patient able to achieve? What problems were encountered? It is essential that teaching effectiveness be evaluated and documented. Teaching goals should be communicated to all staff so teaching can be reinforced and the teaching plan can be followed.
9. Document Teaching Process. All teaching efforts should be documented appropriately. Include negotiated goals, content areas, patient responses, problems, and attempts to address barriers, patient attainment of learning goals, and renegotiated goals.

- Real or perceived time restraints.
- Confusion about where the responsibility for education lies.
- Lack of communication among members of the health care team.
- Failure of employers to hold employees responsible for education.
- Failure of employers to provide adequate resources for teaching.
- Lack of continuity in the teaching and learning process.
- Attitudes and values that fail to recognize the importance of patient education.

Enhancing Patient Learning

Research shows that when a variety of teaching approaches are used, learning is enhanced. For example, when written materials at an appropriate reading level are given to patients along with verbal reinforcement, learning is facilitated. The following are ways to prepare learning materials that can be understood by the majority of patients:

- Decide with the patient what information is needed to meet the patient's learning needs.
- Select the best method (written, visual, demonstration, models, verbal, or a combination of these) to present the information.
- Organize the material in a logical sequence starting with the most important point first.
- Summarize the point again at the end.
- If information is of equal importance, start with the more general information and progress to the specific information.
- Use short words and sentences.
- Use the active voice – "You."
- Limit sentences to one main idea and support information per sentence.
- Open each paragraph with the main point or idea you want to get across.
- Write at the eighth grade level or lower.
- Print size should be at least 14 point.
- Use double or triple spacing.
- Don't clutter the information on the page; remember to leave empty "white space."
- Use illustrations, diagrams, or other visual or verbal cues to enhance learning.
- Build in time for reflection, questions, review, and giving positive feedback on performance.
- Pilot the materials before using them on patient populations.

Recommendations for Nurse Preparation in Patient Education

The gaps in formal nursing education programs noted at the beginning of the chapter remain an area of concern. With the demands on nurses for patient and family teaching likely to continue increasing in the future, nurses must have or obtain the skills to meet these needs. Clearly, if the nursing profession is to attain leadership in patient education, nursing educators must take seriously their responsibility to ensure that nurses are given a solid background in educational theory including principles of teaching and learning, knowledge

of learning theories, teaching strategies, presentation of educational materials, and evaluation of learning. Curricula in both undergraduate and graduate education should reflect the increasingly important role of patient education in practice to prepare nurses for excellence in education. In addition, individual nurse-teachers must engage in self study as well as take advantage of continuing educational opportunities to further develop their knowledge and skills in patient education. These issues must be addressed if nurses are to provide vital teaching for patients and families.

Summary

Patient education is a key nursing role, and it is an aspect of the social mandate of nursing. Nurses are legally and morally obligated to provide teaching that will enable patients to acquire the knowledge and skills they need to follow their medical regimen, prevent errors that could endanger their safety, and promote their health and well-being. At the same time, it is important for nurses to be aware of the fact that patients and families may have good reasons for deciding not to follow some aspects of the prescribed medical regimen. Patients are usually overwhelmed when beginning dialysis, which can negatively affect their ability to learn. Factors such as advanced age, lack of social support, dementia, or other physiological factors can also interfere with optimal learning. Evidence suggests that the educational role will continue to grow in importance, particularly in nephrology nursing practice.

Behavioral approaches, critiqued for being incompatible with nursing's holistic paradigm, are increasingly being replaced with relational approaches, which are founded on the importance of the relationship between the patient and nurse.

References

Alspach, J.G. (2000). *Preceptor handbook* (2nd ed.). Aliso Vieho, CA: American Association of Critical Care Nurses.

Anderson, J.M., & Elfert, H. (1989). Managing chronic illness in the family: Women as caretakers. *Journal of Advanced Nursing, 14,* 735-743.

Bastable, S.B. (2003). *Nurse as educator: Principles of teaching and learning for nursing practice* (2nd ed.). Sudbury, MA: Jones and Bartlett.

Bastable, S.B., & Rinwalske, M.A. (2003). Developmental stages of the learner. In S.B. Bastable (Ed.), *Nurse as educator: Principles of teaching and learning for nursing practice* (pp. 119-159). Boston: Jones and Bartlett.

Bevis, E.O. (1988). New directions for a new age. *Curriculum revolution: Mandate for change.* New York: National League for Nursing.

Bosch, B., & Schlebusch, L. (1991). Neuropsychological deficits associated with uraemic encephalopathy: A report of 5 patients. *South African Medical Journal, 79,* 560-562.

Braungart, M.M., & Braungart, R.G. (2003). Applying learning theories to healthcare practice. In S.B. Bastable (Ed.), *Nurse as educator: Principles of teaching and learning for nursing practice* (2nd ed.) (pp. 45-71). Boston: Jones and Bartlett.

Brez, S. M., & Taylor, M. (1997). Assessing literacy for patient teaching: Perspectives of adults with low literacy skills. *Journal of Advanced Nursing, 25,* 1040-1047.

Browne, A.J. (2001). The influence for liberal political ideology on nursing science. *Nursing Inquiry, 8*(2), 118-129.

Brundage, D. (1990). Research critique: Cognitive changes in chronic renal patients during hemodialysis. *ANNA Journal, 17*(4), 287.

Buber, M. (1958). *I and thou.* New York: Scribner.

Canadian Organ Replacement Registry (CORR). (2002). *Preliminary statistics on renal failure and solid organ transplantation in Canada: Data from 1981 - 2000.* Ottawa, ON: Canadian Institute for Health Information.

Chater, K. (1999). Risk and representation: Older people and noncompliance. *Nursing Inquiry, 6,* 132-138.

Chauhan, T. (2004). End-stage renal disease patients up nearly 19%. *Canadian Medical Association Journal, 170*(7), 1087.

Conlin, K.K., & Schumann, L. (2002). Literacy in the health care system: A study on open heart surgery patients. *Journal of the American Academy of Nurse Practitioners, 14*(1), 38-42.

Conrad, P. (1987). The noncompliant patient in search of autonomy. *Hastings Center Report, 17*(4), 15-17.

Davidhizar, R.E., & Brownson, K. (1999). Literacy, cultural diversity, and client education. *Health Care Manager, 18*(1), 39-47.

Dukes Hess, J.D. (1996). The ethics of compliance: A dialectic. *Advances in Nursing Science, 19*(1), 18-27.

Edel, M.K. (1985). Noncompliance: An appropriate nursing diagnosis? *Nursing Outlook, 33*(4), 183-185.

Erikson, E.H. (1963). *Childhood and society* (2nd ed.). New York: Norton.

Evers, S., Tepel, M., Obladen, M., Suhr, B., Husstedt, I., Grotmeyer, K., et al. (1998). Influence of end-stage renal failure and hemodialysis on event-related potentials. *Clinical Neurophysiology, 15,* 58-63.

Fain, J.A. (1994). Assessing nutrition education in clients with weak literacy skills. *Nurse Practitioner Forum, 5*(1), 52-55.

Faust, W. (1998). A model for effective adult and adolescent education in a relational mode. *Religious Education, 93*(4), 467-476.

Flew, A. (1984). *A dictionary of philosophy* (2nd ed.). London, UK: Macmillan.

Hartrick, G. (1997). Relational capacity: The foundation for interpersonal nursing practice. *Journal of Advanced Nursing, 26,* 523-528.

Hartrick Doane, G. (2002). Beyond behavioral skills to human-involved processes: Relational nursing practice and interpretive pedagogy. *Journal of Nursing Education, 41*(9), 400-404.

Hartrick Doane, G., & Varcoe, C. (2005). *Family nursing as relational inquiry – Developing health promoting practice.* Philadelphia: Lippincott, Williams & Wilkins.

Heiwe, S., Clyne, N., & Dahlgren, M.A. (2003). Living with chronic renal failure: Patient's experiences of their physical and functional capacity. *Physiotherapy Research International, 8*(4), 167-177.

Haynes, R.B. (1979). Introduction. In R.B. Haynes, D.L. Sackett, & D.W. Taylor (Eds.), *Compliance in health care* (pp. 1-10). Baltimore: Johns Hopkins Press.

Jackson, R.H., Davis, T.C., Murphy, P., Bairnsfather, L.E., & George, R.B. (1994). Reading deficiencies in older patients. *American Journal of the Medical Sciences, 308*(2), 79-82.

Knox, D. (2002). Learning theories. In M. McEwen & E.M. Wills (Eds.), *Theoretical basis for nursing* (pp. 321-344). Philadelphia: Lippincott, Williams, & Wilkins.

Levine, D.Z. (Ed.). (1991). *Care of the renal patient* (2nd ed.). Philadelphia: Saunders.

Luker, K., & Caress, S.L. (1989). Rethinking patient education. *Journal of Advanced Nursing, 14,* 711-718.

Macdonald, G. (2002). Transformative unlearning: Safety, discernment and communities of learning. *Nursing Inquiry, 9*(3), 170-178.

MacDonald, C. (2002). Nurse autonomy as relational. *Nursing Ethics, 9*(2), 194-201.

Macdougal, I. (1998). Quality of life and anemia: The nephrology experience. *Seminars in Oncology, 25,* 39-42.

Mager, R.F. (1962). *Preparing instructional objectives.* Belmont, CA: Fearon.

McEwen, M., & Wills, E.M. (Eds.). (2002). *Theoretical basis for nursing.* Philadelphia: Lippincott, Williams, & Wilkins.

Noddings, N. (2003). Is teaching a practice? *Journal of Philosophy of Education, 37*(2), 241-251.

Paterson, J.G., & Zderad, L.T. (1976). *Humanistic nursing.* New York: Wiley.

Perumal, S., & Sehgal, A.R. (2003). Job satisfaction and patient care practices of hemodialysis nurses and technicians. *Nephrology Nursing Journal, 30*(5), 523-528.

Playle, J., & Keeley, P. (1998). Non-compliance and professional power. *Journal of Advanced Nursing, 27,* 304-311.

Polaschek, N. (2003). The experience of living on dialysis: A literature review. *Nephrology Nursing Journal, 30*(3), 303-313.

Rankin, S.H., & Stallings, K.D. (2001). *Patient education: Principles and practices* (4th ed.). Philadelphia: Lippincott.

Reese, H.W., & Overton, W.F. (1970). Models of development and theories of development. In L.R. Goulet & P.B. Baltes (Eds.), *Life-span developmental psychology* (pp. 115-145). New York: Academic Press.

Richards, E. (2003). Motivation, compliance, and health behaviors of the learner. In S.B. Bastable (Ed.), *Nurse as educator: Principles of teaching and learning for nursing practice* (2nd ed.) (pp. 161-187). Boston: Jones and Bartlett.

Roberson, M. (1992). The meaning of compliance: Patients' perspectives. *Qualitative Health Research, 2*(1), 7-26.

Sanford, R.C. (2000). Caring through relation and dialogue: A nursing perspective for patient education. *Advances in Nursing Science, 22*(3), 1-15.

Schwandt, T.A. (1997). *Qualitative inquiry: A dictionary of terms.* Thousand Oaks, CA: Sage.

Smith, B.C., & Winslow, E.H. (1990). Cognitive changes in chronic renal patients during hemodialysis. *ANNA Journal, 17*(4), 283-286.

Sopczyk, D.L. (2003). Technology in education. In S.B. Bastable (Ed.), *Nurse as educator: Principles of teaching and learning for nursing practice* (2nd ed.) (pp. 427-463). Boston: Jones and Bartlett.

Storch, J.L., Rodney, P., & Starzomski, R. (Eds.). (2004). *Toward a moral horizon: Nursing ethics for leadership and practice.* Toronto: Prentice Hall.

Taylor, C. (1991). *The malaise of modernity.* Concord, ON: Anansi.

Thorne, S.E. (1990). Constructive noncompliance in chronic illness. *Holistic Nursing Practice, 5*(1), 62-69.

Trostle, J.A. (1988). Medical compliance as an ideology. *Social Science & Medicine, 27*(12), 1299-1308.

Turner, D., Wellard, S., & Bethune, E. (1999). Registered nurses' perceptions of teaching: Constraints to the teaching moment. *International Journal of Nursing Practice, 5,* 14-20.

USRDS. (2000). *Annual data report: Atlas of end-stage renal disease in the United States.* Bethesda, MD: National Institutes of Health, Diabetes, Digestive, and Kidney Diseases.

Wellard, S. (1992). The nature of dilemmas in dialysis nurse practice. *Journal of Advanced Nursing, 17,* 951-958.

Wuest, J. (1993). Removing the shackles: A feminist critique of noncompliance. *Nursing Outlook, 41*(5), 217-224.

- The educator's role is becoming more important due, in part, to changes in health care delivery over the past two decades. Families, who already manage an estimated 80% of all health care needs and problems (Bastable, 2003), are increasingly expected to assume personal responsibility for their own health maintenance and health promotion (Brez & Taylor, 1997).

- A significant factor in the growing demand for patient education is the fact that the educator's role in nephrology nursing practice is so extensive. Patients receiving renal replacement therapy have an especially complex medical regimen, involving multiple lifestyle changes that affect virtually every aspect of their lives.

- Dialysis and transplantation are high technology settings where patients and families are thrust into an unfamiliar and sometimes frightening technological environment. The complexity of the medical regimen means that patients are suddenly expected to make radical changes in virtually every aspect of their lives.

- The theoretical framework of behaviorism has underpinned patient education and nearly all educational work for most of the last century. Behaviorism, a predominant worldview in the medical/technological fields and in nursing practice, is a poor fit with the nursing paradigm, and should be rejected in favor of a model based on relational practice (Hartrick, 1997; Hartrick Doane, 2002).

- Because nurses have relied almost exclusively on mechanistic models of human relationships that are based on behaviorist views, Hartrick (1997) developed an alternative model based on principles of human relating. This new model established an alternative to behaviorism that recognizes the importance of human caring and nursing practices aimed at establishing, maintaining, and nurturing relational capacities.

- Learning theories explain how knowledge and skills are assimilated by the learner, and suggest effective ways to present material. Reflecting a time when the nursing profession actively introduced theories from other disciplines, chiefly psychology and sociology, these "borrowed" theories imported more than just those theories nurses applied to patient care situations.

- As far back as the 1960s, nursing theorists had begun to challenge the dominant models of nursing practice, rejecting the behaviorism then rampant in education, nursing, and many other fields, in favor of an approach based on interpersonal relationships, communication, caring, and humanism.

- One of the insidious effects of the long slide into ESRD is something that doesn't show up on lab results: a slowing of cognitive responses that result in a decreased ability to concentrate, drowsiness (especially during dialysis), mental confusion (Levine, 1991), and mental fatigue (Heiwe, Clyne, & Dahlgren, 2003).

- The extent of low literacy and illiteracy in North America is significant. An estimated 25 to 30% of North American adults (and about 40% of Americans over the age of 65) are considered to be functionally illiterate (Davidhizar & Brownson, 1999). This is a serious health issue as almost half (43%) of people who have low literacy live in poverty (Bastable, 2003).

- It is important that nurses not approach all patients with the same predetermined learning goals, for example, using a pre-established set of goals and objectives in a patient education manual. The patient must have input into the learning goals and be able to work toward meaningful goals that are important to the patient and family.

- Research shows that when a variety of teaching approaches are used, learning is enhanced. For example, when written materials at an appropriate reading level are given to patients along with verbal reinforcement, learning is facilitated.

- Clearly, if the nursing profession is to attain leadership in patient education, nursing educators must take seriously their responsibility to ensure that nurses are given a solid background in educational theory including principles of teaching and learning, knowledge of learning theories, teaching strategies, presentation of educational materials, and evaluation of learning.

- Patient education is a key nursing role, and it is an aspect of the social mandate of nursing. Nurses are legally and morally obligated to provide teaching that will enable patients to acquire the knowledge and skills they need to follow their medical regimen, prevent errors that could endanger their safety, and promote their health and well-being.

Behaviorism: Behaviorism, a theory that underpins the dominant medical/technical paradigm, postulates that psychological functioning is definable in terms of observed behavioral data (Flew, 1984). It can be characterized as a belief that behavior is determined in law-like ways by invariant principles of human conduct based on negative or positive reinforcements (Schwandt, 1997). For example, metaphysical behaviorism, one type of behaviorism, claims that there is no such thing as consciousness (Schwandt, 1997). Behaviorism is also the predominant worldview underpinning much of nursing practice. It is a realist position that rejects the individual's representations of events in favor of observable behaviors.

Behaviorist Learning Theory: This is one of several major learning theories. According to behaviorists, the focus for learning is mainly on what is directly observable, and learning is viewed as the product of the stimulus conditions (S) and the responses (R) that follow (sometimes termed the S-R model of learning). Much of behaviorist learning is based on respondent conditioning (classical or Pavlovian conditioning) and operant conditioning (reinforcement to bring about specific behaviors). Behaviorists view learning as a relatively simple process, as they ignore what goes on inside the individual and focus on observable behavior change (Bastable, 2003).

Cognitive Learning Theory: Cognitive Learning Theories perceive the universe as a unitary, interactive, developing entity with humans as the active source of behavior. Learning is defined as a process that creates a change in the individual, but this change does not have to be behavioral; it may be realized in terms of insight, motivation, perceptions, mental associations, behavior, or a combination of these (Knox, 2002).

Whereas behaviorists ignore the internal dynamics of learning, focusing instead on the behavioral manifestations that signal learning in the behavioral paradigm, cognitive theorists stress the internal changes that occur in the learner. The key to learning, in this view, involves changing the learner's internal perceptions, cognitions, and ways of processing and structuring information. Learning, according to adherents of cognitive learning theory, is viewed as an active process largely directed by the individual. It involves perceiving and interpreting information, and based on what the individual already knows, reorganizing knowledge into new insights or understanding (Braungart & Braungart, 2003).

De facto: Existing by fact (not necessarily by choice or right).

Determinism and Reductionism: Determinism is a way of thinking that assumes everything is caused by something in a predictable way. More specifically, determinism describes any theory that explains the world in a few narrowly defined factors to the exclusion of all others. Reductionism is the belief that human behavior can be reduced to or interpreted in terms of that of lower animals. For example, Pavlov with dogs, and Skinner with rats have used lower animals to illustrate instinctive behavioral patterns that can, by analogy, be correlated with some aspects of human behavior.

Intersubjectivity: This means "occurring between or among (or accessible to) two or more separate individuals" (Schwandt, 1997, p. 74). Although people make meaning through interpreting their experiences, these are known only to the individual. It is through dialogue that we create and maintain the basis for intersubjective or shared meanings.

Learning: Learning is defined as a relatively permanent change in mental processing, emotional functioning, and/or behavior as a result of experience. It is the lifelong, dynamic process by which individuals acquire new knowledge or skills and alter their thoughts, feelings, attitudes, and actions (Bastable, 2003).

Learning Assessment: This is a process of determining the learning strengths and challenges of the individual. It includes assessing factors known to affect learning, for example, the educational level attained and reading ability, diagnosing any physical and/or physiological problems known to affect ability to learn (such as hearing or visual problems, cognitive deficits due to organic brain syndrome or Alzheimer's disease), and identifying the existing knowledge base, preferred learning style, motivation to learn, and personal learning goals.

Learning Goal: A learning goal is "the final outcome of what is achieved at the end of the teaching and learning process. Goals are global and broad in nature; they serve as long-term targets for both the learner and the teacher" (Bastable, 2003, p. 321).

Learning Objective: An objective is a specific, single, intended, short-term outcome. These should be achievable at the conclusion of one teaching session or within a few days. There may need to be smaller subject-objectives in order for the patient to be able to work toward a larger goal.

Learning Theory: A learning theory is a coherent framework and set of integrated constructs and principles that describe, explain, or predict how people learn (Bastable, 2003).

Literacy: The ability of adults to read, understand, and interpret information written at the eighth grade level or above. Literacy is an umbrella term used to describe socially required and expected reading and writing abilities. It represents the relative ability of persons to use printed and written material commonly encountered in daily life (Bastable, 2003).

Obstacles to Learning: These include the following. 1) The stress of acute and chronic illness, anxiety, sensory deficits, and low literacy. Illness alone seldom acts as an impediment to learning, and may even act as an impetus for seeking the advice of a health care professional. 2) The negative influence of the hospital environment itself and social isolation. 3) Lack of time to learn due to rapid patient discharge from care. 4) Personal characteristics of the learner such as readiness to learn, motivation, and learning style. 5) The extent and complexity of the learning needed. 6) Lack of support or positive reinforcement from significant others. 7) Denial of learning needs. 8) The inconvenience, complexity, inaccessibility, fragmentation, and dehumanization of the health care system (Bastable, 2003).

Paradigm: A paradigm refers to a type of cognitive framework – an exemplar or set of shared solutions or approaches to substantive problems or issues in a particular discipline. Another sense of paradigm is that of a "disciplinary matrix," which includes the commitments, beliefs, values, methods, and outlooks held by members of a discipline (Schwandt, 1997). It is a particular way of viewing a discipline generally shared by members of that discipline (for example, what is important, how one goes about the practice and research of the discipline). Note: there may be two or more paradigms in any single discipline. Adherents will hold to their own paradigm perspective and carry out research and practice within their own paradigms until the competing paradigm(s) are disproved, or another paradigm arises to replace the existing paradigm.

Patient Teaching: Luker and Caress (1989) distinguish between patient teaching and patient education. Patient teaching "implies a didactic information giving approach;" patient education "implies something more comprehensive for which specialist skills are required" (p. 714).

Patient Education: In this chapter, the term patient education refers to a process of providing patients and/or their families with relevant information, knowledge, and/or skills training to enable them to achieve meaningful personal life goals and to control distressing symptoms. Patients may choose to use the knowledge gained to follow therapeutic regimens, or to attain, maintain, or regain a higher level of health functioning.

Patient teaching: Refers to activities of nurses that increase knowledge and understanding of specific information such as activities of self-care (Rankin & Stallings, 2001).

Readability: Measures of the reading difficulty level of a given sample of printed text. There are several commonly used tests for estimating readability (examples of some of the more common readability tests are: Cloze Procedure, Flesch Formula, Fog Formula, SMOG Formula, Fry Formula, and the Spache Grade Level Score). Most of these tests measure the level of reading difficulty of representative samples of educational print material by calculating a combination of the number of words with three or more syllables, or the number of words in each sentence or a representative sample of text. These formulas are not designed as writing guides, so their use does not guarantee writing good style. The procedure for using the SMOG Readability formula is included in this chapter as an example of how such formulas are used to calculate the reading grade level. Nurses preparing printed instructions for adult patients and their families should aim for no more than the eighth grade level; when people are ill or experiencing unstable health, the reading level should be lower or other methods of instruction should be used such as demonstration, audiotapes, or visual media including short films, photographs, or posters.

Readiness to Learn: Evidence of motivation at a particular time (Alspach, 2000). The time when the learner is receptive to learning, and is willing and able to participate in the learning process; that is, prepared or willing to learn (Bastable, 2003). People may signal their readiness by asking questions, showing interest, or closely watching when the nurse carries out a procedure or provides care, or by requesting information on particular topics. The nurse can also promote readiness by addressing barriers that might be limiting the patient's ability to learn, cueing the patient toward meaningful aspects of his care, and providing information relevant to the patient (based on the patient's identified learning goals).

Realist/Realism: A doctrine that proposes that there are real objects that exist independently of our knowledge of their existence (that is, a real world exists "out there" independently of anyone experiencing it). Scientific realism is the view that theories refer to real features of the world (Schwandt, 1997).

Rapid Estimate of Adult Literacy in Medicine (REALM): A reading skills test to measure a patient's ability to read medical and health-related vocabulary.

Relational Practice: The term *relational* describes the complex, interconnected nature of human life, the world, and nursing practice. A relational approach to nursing practice requires a view of the world through a relational lens where one examines how people, situations, contexts, and processes are integrally connected and shaping each other. A relational approach takes into account the interconnectedness of people and their world (Hartrick Doane & Varcoe, 2005).

Test of Functional Health Literacy in Adults (TOFHLA): An instrument for measuring patients' literacy level by using actual hospital materials, such as prescription labels, appointment slips, and informed consent forms (Bastable, 2003). This is also available in a Spanish version.

Teachable Moment: The time when the learner is most receptive to learning; nurses can maximize learning by assessing the patient's readiness to learn, and helping to create or foster the conditions to bring about the teachable moment (for example, by removing or reducing barriers to learning; promoting comfort and feelings of psychological, cultural, or emotional safety; and ensuring physiological aberrations are eliminated or minimized). The tenets of relational practice suggest that motivation to learn can be fostered when nurses have formed a strong and trusting relationship with patients and/or family members, and patients are working toward meaningful goals they participated in creating.

Unlearning: This is an educational concept first introduced by psychologists and change theorists. In order for people to change their present attitudes, practices, and beliefs, old ways of thinking and being need to be "unlearned" (especially when the old knowledge contradicts new evidence) in order to allow new evidence to inform decisions and learning to occur. This is not an automatic event. For example, presented with new evidence or practice guidelines that support a change in care practices, nurses must engage in a process of unlearning before they can effectively incorporate the new practices. In the same manner, patients and families may have to engage in an unlearning process before they can change their ideas and begin to adopt new information and ways of thinking. Unlearning is seen as essential to the process of creativity and is important in anti-racist, anti-sexist, antiviolence, and anti-discriminatory teaching practice. It is often characterized by powerful feelings as people move through a process of disequilibrium, denial/resistance, and eventual reconstruction as they unlearn knowledge, beliefs, or attitudes that had formed a familiar way of viewing the world (Macdonald, 2002). Patient educators may need to actively assist patients to unlearn past knowledge before they can move forward to learn new information.

ANNP638

Relating to Teaching and Learning

Janice McCormick, PhD, RN

Contemporary Nephrology Nursing: Principles and Practice contains 39 chapters of educational content. Individual learners may apply for continuing nursing education credit by reading a chapter and completing the Continuing Education Evaluation Form for that chapter. Learners may apply for continuing education credit for any or all chapters.

Please photocopy this page and return to ANNA.
COMPLETE THE FOLLOWING:

Name: _____

Address:_____

City:_____ State: _____ Zip: _____

E-mail: _____

Preferred telephone: ☐ Home   ☐ Work: _____

State where licensed and license number (optional): _____

CE application fees are based upon the number of contact hours provided by the individual chapter. CE fees per contact hour for ANNA members are as follows: 1.0-1.9 - $15; 2.0-2.9 - $20; 3.0-3.9 - $25; 4.0 and higher - $30. Fees for nonmembers are $10 higher.

ANNA Member: ☐ Yes   ☐ No   Member # (if available) _____

☐ Checked Enclosed   ☐ American Express   ☐ Visa   ☐ MasterCard

Total Amount Submitted: _____

Credit Card Number: _____ Exp. Date: _____

Name as it appears on the card: _____

CE Evaluation Form

To receive continuing education credit for individual study after reading the chapter

1. Photocopy this form. (You may also download this form from ANNA's Web site, **www.annanurse.org.**)

2. Mail the completed form with payment (check) or credit card information to American Nephrology Nurses' Association, East Holly Avenue, Box 56, Pitman, NJ 08071-0056.

3. You will receive your CE certificate from ANNA in 4 to 6 weeks.

Test returns must be postmarked by **December 31, 2010.**

> **CE Application Fee**
> ANNA Member $20.00
> Nonmember $30.00

EVALUATION FORM

1. I verify that I have read this chapter and completed this education activity. Date: _____

_____
Signature

2. What would be different in your practice if you applied what you learned from this activity? *(Please use additional sheet of paper if necessary.)*

_____

_____

_____

_____

_____

_____

_____

_____

_____

_____

_____

_____

Evaluation	Strongly disagree				Strongly agree
3. The activity met the stated objectives.					
a. Compare various learning/education theories used in adult education.	1	2	3	4	5
b. Discuss the factors that must be considered when planning education for people with ESRD.	1	2	3	4	5
c. Generate a plan of education for a patient newly diagnosed with ESRD.	1	2	3	4	5
4. The content was current and relevant.	1	2	3	4	5
5. The content was presented clearly.	1	2	3	4	5
6. The content was covered adequately.	1	2	3	4	5
7. Rate your ability to apply the learning obtained from this activity to practice.	1	2	3	4	5

Comments _____

_____

8. Time required to read the chapter and complete this form: _____ minutes.

This educational activity has been provided by the American Nephrology Nurses' Association (ANNA) for 2.1 contact hours. ANNA is accredited as a provider of continuing nursing education (CNE) by the American Nurses Credentialing Center's Commission on Accreditation (ANCC-COA). ANNA is an approved provider of continuing education by the California Board of Registered Nursing, CEP 0910.

Informatics and the Electronic Age

Francis Lau, PhD

Chapter Contents

Francis Lau, PhD

Over the past 10 years, there has been a dramatic increase in the use of computers in just about every facet of our lives and in society as a whole. This social phenomenon has had a significant impact within the health setting in terms of how health services are being delivered. Consumers have access to a vast amount of health information from the Internet, and health professionals need to adapt their day-to-day practice routines to cope with the increasingly computerized workplace. While the adoption of computers in the banking and airline industries has been readily accepted and is now mostly taken for granted, the use of computers by health professionals, especially nurses, to support patient care is still considered to be a major challenge at the present time.

Through earlier implementation of computer systems mostly in the hospital setting, a number of lessons have been learned as to how one should introduce these systems into the workplace. For instance, we have learned that we cannot treat the computer as a 'blackbox' and label non-adapters as being 'resistant to change.' In fact, experience has shown that the use of computers in the health setting involves a web of legislative, organizational, human, practice, system and performance issues that are highly complex and interrelated. In spite of what is known, the efforts to increase the utilization of computers within the health setting continue to be hampered by the lack of health professionals who are informatics-savvy and able to act as champions among their peers to promote the use of these systems in their local practice settings.

The purpose of this chapter is to present an overview of the field of health informatics and its relevance to nephrology nursing within a North American context. The chapter begins with a brief introduction of health informatics as an interdisciplinary field of study. Several key concepts in health informatics are then described to provide a coherent foundation to help one make sense of the role of computer systems (broadly referred to as health information systems, or HIS) within the health setting. Examples of different types of HIS that are used in practice, education and research settings are included to illustrate how health informatics can help support the work of health professionals and nephrology nurses. The chapter ends by highlighting a set of key issues in health informatics that are particularly relevant for all health professionals.

Introduction to Health Informatics

Computer technology has changed the way that health care services are delivered and how we deal with our personal health. Whether we are making a visit to the health clinic for a regular check-up, being admitted to the hospital for a surgical procedure, or filling a prescription at the local pharmacy, we will come across a computer, either directly or indirectly. For example, our visit to the clinic or admission to the hospital is most likely arranged through a computerized scheduling system; the details of our medical history, clinical assessments and interventions are likely maintained in an electronic chart; information about our prescriptions is kept in an online pharmacy database. In some rural communities, telehealth (such as videoconference) is used as an alternative to provide specialized health services, such as psychiatric consultation, that are not feasible otherwise.

Increasingly, we are using the Internet to access health information to help with our understanding and decision making of personal health-related matters. Some of us with particular ailments take part in online support groups and chat lines through the Internet to share information and offer support to one other. This is particularly the case for people with chronic illnesses such as renal disease where online support groups and personalized health information are available through different non-profit and advocacy organizations. We are also beginning to see selected health advice being provided online by health professionals through the use of computer technology.

In this section we provide a brief introduction of health informatics as a contemporary field of study. This includes giving a practical definition of health informatics, outlining the major areas of study, and how it is relevant to nephrology nursing.

Defining the Field

Broadly speaking, health informatics is an applied field of study concerned with the use of information and communications technology (ICT) to support the communication of health information and the delivery of health services. Health informatics is highly interdisciplinary in nature, drawing on a wide range of theories, methods and techniques from the fields of health service administration, psychology, computer science, organization studies, information science, operations research, and human communication. The term, medical informatics, is also used, particularly in the United States, reflecting its historical roots from the field of medicine. On the other hand, the term health informatics has gained popularity over the years as it is thought to go beyond 'medicine' in terms of disease and treatment to cover the broader concept of health and health service delivery. Other informatics-related terms still in use today that are aimed at specific disciplines include nursing informatics, dental informatics, public health informatics, and recently, bioinformatics, which pertains to the manipulation of genetic information.

Health informatics is also seen as both a scientific and an engineering discipline. The science agenda involves the need to understand the theories, principles, structures, methods, and processes involved with the use of health information, and the underlying ICT infrastructure to support health service delivery. For instance, how should patient information be classified and structured in order to enhance communication and decision-making? The engineering agenda includes the design and implementation of health information systems (HIS) to support service delivery in specific organizational settings. Of particular interests are the design of an appropriate user interface when constructing these systems, the implementation of common technical standards to enable the exchange of health information collected from different sources, and the protection of this information from improper disclosure and use.

Major Areas of Study

The study of health informatics can span the entire spectrum of health, ranging from the computer-based medical record for individual patients to the provision of nationwide health surveillance systems for selected populations as a whole. While achieving mastery in all of these areas is nearly impossible, it is important for health professionals to acquire a basic level of competency so they can interact effectively with the health information systems in their workplace. The need to build capacity in health informatics among health professionals is urgent, as the trend for computerization within the health sector is expected to continue in the foreseeable future. A practical scheme in organizing the major areas of health informatics study for health professionals should cover: health information; health information systems; information and communications technology; health information methods; and telehealth. These major areas of study are briefly outlined below and summarized in Table 39-1. Areas that are relevant to nephrology nursing are described in more detail in this chapter.

Health information. There are many types of health information ranging from an individual's health record, to aggregate health status and health service statistics, to research and lay health literature. The means by which this information is generated, collected, organized, stored, accessed, interpreted and used is of particular relevance to health professionals, policy makers, researchers, consumers and the public. To facilitate common understandings and ease of communication, such information as one's health record needs to be codified according to some international standards. Also of importance is the way in which this information should be protected to ensure privacy, confidentiality and security. For health literature, the main issue has to do the means by which it is produced and synthesized to ensure accuracy and credibility.

Health information systems. There are many types of health information system (HIS) applications used to support the delivery of health services and the communication of health information. Examples of traditional HIS used in hospital settings include the admission-transfer-discharge, order entry and results reporting, and laboratory, imaging and pharmacy systems. More contemporary examples are the community-based information systems, chronic disease management systems, and the electronic health record (EHR). Those that are aimed at individuals, such as consumers, include electronic health literature databases offered by commercial publishers, advocacy groups, and research organizations over the Web. Regardless of the type of system involved, the key aspect is the process by which the HIS is introduced into the organization. Often it involves the use of formal systems planning, design, implementation, and evaluation methodologies. Another aspect is the manner by which the change brought on by computerization is managed in the organization and community, which can be a highly politicized, arduous, and lengthy process.

Table 39-1
Major Areas of Study in Health Informatics

Health Information	The organization, processing and communication of data, facts or interpretations on a health issue or an individual's health condition
Health Information System	The planning, design, implementation, use and evaluation of computer applications that support health service delivery and access to health literature
Information and Communications Technology	The computer hardware, software and communication networks used to support health service delivery and access to health literature
Health Information Methods	The methods, tools and techniques used to analyze and interpret health information and literature to facilitate decision making
Telehealth	The use of communications technology to support healthcare delivery, patient/staff education and administration provided at a distance

Information and communications technology. The rapid technological advances over the last 10 years alone have led to the proliferation of different approaches to deploying ICT within the health sector. The widespread adoption of the Internet, broadband networks, and the World Wide Web has fundamentally changed the ways health organizations, communities, and individuals are interconnected with each other. The introduction of mobile devices such as tablet computers and personal digital assistants (PDAs) has also stimulated new ways of capturing and delivering health information at the point of contact. For health professionals, the challenges are to keep abreast of such technological advances and to integrate ICT into the workplace and their work practices in ways that are appropriate, respectful, and effective.

Health information methods. Different methods are used to analyze and make sense of the health information collected. These methods range from such techniques as odds likelihood ratio for clinical decision making at the individual level, to logistics management of the health services within an organization, to case-mix analysis at an aggregate level to compare the severity of the patient cases across organizations. For published literature, the techniques of critical appraisal and systematic review are used to determine its validity and relevance. Generally these methods are drawn from the disciplines of management science, epidemiology, biostatistics, and health services research. Also included are analytic techniques used to make sense of qualitative data such as thematic analysis of interview transcripts and written reports.

Telehealth. The use of ICT to communicate health information and deliver health services over a distance has become an important aspect of the health service delivery

Figure 39-1

Organizing Framework for Health Information Systems. Based on Androwich et al. (2003), p53.

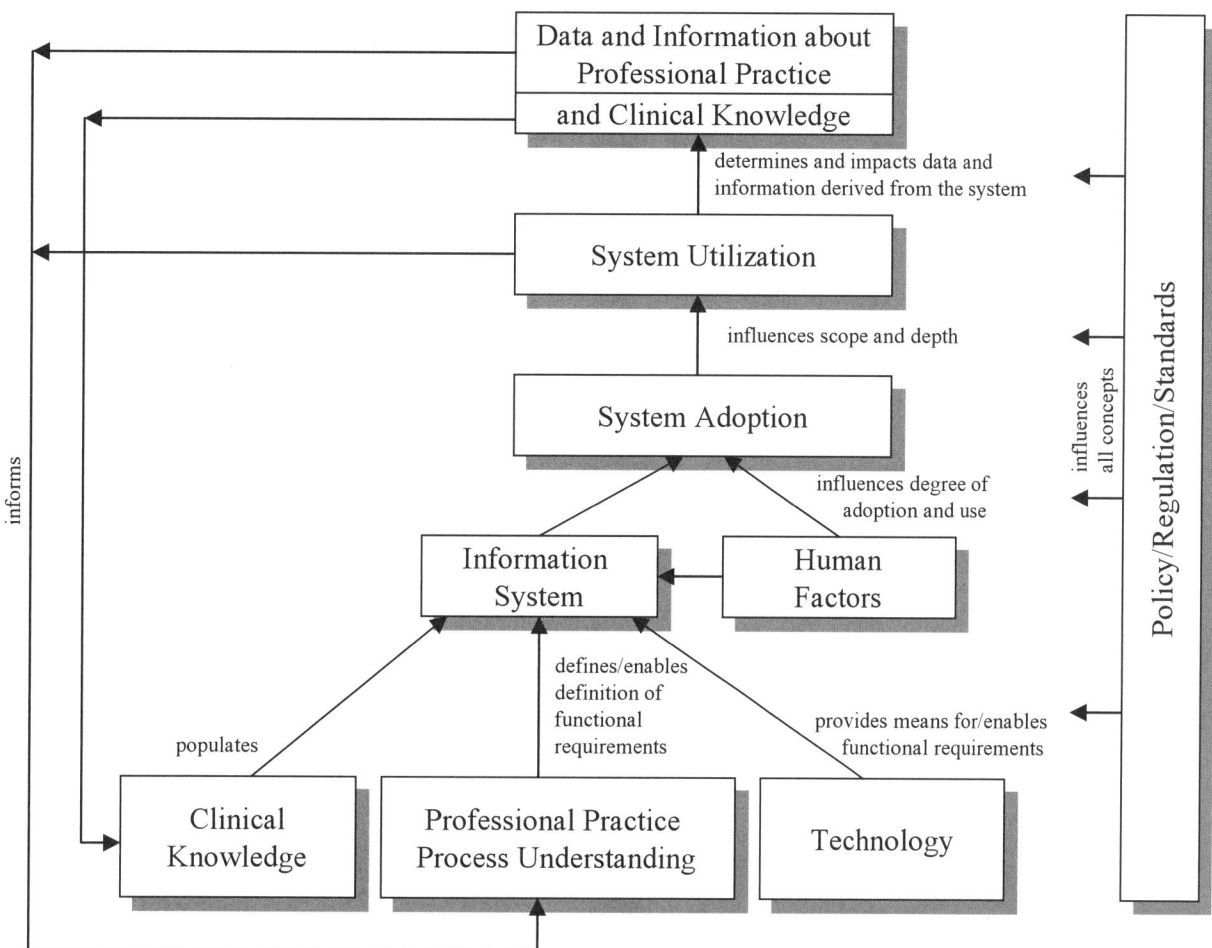

system given its vast geographic boundary. Over the years, telehealth has expanded from its initial scope of remote physician consultation to include a wide range of health-related activities such as telecare to provide direct care to patients at home, tele-education to support continuing professional development, and teleconference for administrative meetings among staff. To be successful in use of telehealth, there are different issues that should be considered, such as the readiness of the organization to offer telehealth, the jurisdiction and range of services to be provided, the methods to measure its cost-effectiveness, and plans to ensure its sustainability over time.

Relevance to Nephrology Nursing

Health informatics is relevant to nephrology nursing in many respects. First, there is a vast amount of health information that has to be collected, managed, and interpreted when caring for individuals with renal disorders, especially given the chronic nature of the disease. Second, HIS is becoming an integral part of health organizations in their

effort to manage the health information and services being delivered. Third, recent advances in ICT have led to an increased ability to deliver health services in the community and home settings through telehealth. Given these trends, it is essential for the nephrology nurse to acquire a basic level of informatics competency in order to interact with these changes effectively. Such competency should include a basic understanding of health informatics as an applied field of study, and how it can be used to enhance nephrology nursing practice. To do so, this chapter will provide a relevant set of health informatics concepts, HIS applications, and emerging issues considered important to nephrology nursing.

Concepts in Health Informatics

In the early days, computers were seen as a blackbox, much like a telephone, that could greatly improve the productivity of the workplace when implemented according to technical specifications. Over the years, learning from many costly failures and mistaken assumptions, we have come to realize the design and implementation of this so-called blackbox computer are much more complicated, especially within the health setting. In fact, we have learned that the HIS is really an artifact representing the policies, rules, and procedures that govern how professional work is performed at a given point in time within a health organization. Adoption is dependent on whether this system can support the work practices and information needs of its users - the health professionals.

Also, the functionality of the system and its ongoing utilization by the users will evolve over time as they adapt to each other. The more rigid the system, in terms of not being able to accommodate changes, the more its users would devise 'workaround routines' to bypass the system, that eventually will defeat its original intent.

In this section, health informatics concepts are described that are relevant to understanding the work practices of health professionals. These include an organizing framework for understanding the role of HIS within nursing practice; the process of introducing HIS into the organization; standardizing nursing vocabulary; and the evolution from telehealth to telenursing and how it impacts nursing as a profession.

A Framework for Understanding Health Information Systems

Androwich et al. (2003), of the American Medical Informatics Association and the American Nurses Association, have recently presented an organizing framework with a more holistic view of clinical information systems with an emphasis on nursing. This organizing framework has been broadened from clinical to health information systems, and an adapted version of the framework is included in Figure 39-1. When contemplating the planning, design, implementation, use, and evaluation of health information systems, it is important for us to refer to the concepts outlined in this framework in order to ensure a holistic view of these systems taking into account their underlying organizational and social contexts. The key concepts in this framework are described below.

Policy, regulation and standards. These provide the context for the overall health service delivery environment, which has a major influence on the organization and behavior of the HIS, as well as the resulting professional practice such as those in nursing.

Professional practice process understanding. These represent the specific activities performed by the health professionals as part of their scope of practice. Such practice standards, such as those for nursing, are usually defined by the respective professional and licensing bodies, which greatly influence the design of the HIS and their adoption and use.

Clinical knowledge. This represents the body of formal understanding, concepts, expertise and experience that define the field such as nursing. The means by which this knowledge is represented and used in HIS can greatly impact the scope of professional practice.

Technology. This refers to the ICT used to deploy the HIS within the organization. It includes all of the hardware, software, and databases required to operate the HIS, as

well as the underlying computer network infrastructures to provide the connectivity between systems.

Information systems. These refer to the HIS applications designed according to the functional requirements by which health professionals would interact with these systems as users to support their work.

Human factors. These are characteristics of the users and their perception toward the HIS, which can influence the extent to which the HIS is adopted and used over time.

System adoption. These refers to the extent that users have accepted the HIS as part of their professional scope of practice.

System utilization. This refers to the extent to which the users have incorporated the HIS into their day-to-day work routines as part of their professional practice.

Data and information on professional practice. Data generated from HIS at both the individual (e.g., patient data) and aggregate (e.g., statistics) levels can lead to better understanding of one's professional practice, performance, and effectiveness. In turn, this can further advance the clinical knowledge base of the discipline.

Process of Introducing HIS

The introduction of HIS into the health organization involves the process of systems planning, design, implementation, and evaluation. The extent to which these processes are formalized and applied depends on the type of system desired, the expertise available, and the overall readiness of the organization involved. The type of system refers to the complexity of the functions to be computerized and the extent to which the system is to be deployed within the organization. For instance, a patient care order system that is to be used 7 days a week by clinical staff throughout the hospital will require a more formal process for its deployment than a standalone application used only by the administrative department to analyze the pattern of service utilization for a particular program. The expertise available within the organization often influences the type of process used, as each process has its own set of assumptions, principles, techniques, and tools. The overall readiness of the organization refers to such factors as management commitment to change, staff attitudes toward computerization, technical infrastructure already in place, and resource availability to deploy the system. An overview of the system planning, design, implementation, and evaluation processes used to introduce HIS into the health organization are given below.

HIS planning. This starts with gaining an understanding of the overall mandate, vision, and objectives of the organization, and the strategy and tactics used to reach the ideal stage. The health information and service gaps, needs, and priorities that exist within the organization are then identified, and the types of HIS investment that can best support the transitions into this ideal stage are proposed. To ensure organizational buy-in at all levels, the HIS planning process should involve as many stakeholders as possible, ranging from frontline staff to department managers to senior executives. The planning focus should be sufficiently broad to include the service, information, and technical dimensions across the entire organization and how well they integrate with each other. The resulting HIS plan should serve as the master blueprint to guide the deployment of the proposed systems to improve the performance of the entire organization.

HIS design. This involves the methodical analysis of the information and service needs for the organization, and the detailed definition of the functional requirements in terms of what the HIS is expected to do. Once the requirements of the proposed HIS are defined, one has to decide whether to buy or build the system. This decision often depends on the availability and cost of commercial HIS on the market, the extent to which these HIS meet the requirements, and the culture within the organization regarding buying versus building systems. Increasingly, health organizations are turning to commercial vendors for packaged HIS solutions. As such, it is critical to accurately define the functions to be included in the proposed system, and to be thorough when negotiating the HIS contract with the vendor. For organizations that wish to build their own HIS, care should be taken to ensure there is sufficient in-house expertise for applications development, project management, and technical support.

HIS implementation. This refers to the process of deploying the HIS within the organization. It involves installing the HIS application and the underlying ICT components such as the hardware, software, databases, and telecommunication networks. Also included are the preparation and provision of user training, help-desk and technical support tasks during initial deployment, and ongoing operation of the HIS. In terms of user training, it is preferable to offer the sessions shortly before going 'live' with the HIS. This allows the users to apply what they have just learned on the new system. Aside from training users to navigate through the HIS interfaces, an effort should be made to help users make sense of the system to ascertain why computerized functions are there, and how they fit with or require change to fit with existing work practices. During HIS implementation, frequent communication among staff, management, and the implementation team is essential to ensure that everyone is up-to-date with all of the changes that are taking place (Lorenzi, 1997).

HIS evaluation. This is a critical but often-neglected step in determining the impact of the system once it has been deployed within the organization. There are many approaches to evaluating the impacts of HIS, ranging from controlled trials on the effects of clinical decision support systems (Hunt et al., 1998), to the use of mixed qualitative and quantitative methods to examine the effects of HIS across settings (Kaplan et al., 2001). Kaplan (1997) has proposed a 4C framework for evaluating the impacts of HIS that focuses on context, communication, care, and control issues. Context refers to the characteristics of the environment within which the HIS functions. Communication relates to how the pattern of information exchange may be changed as a result of computerization. Care relates to how the provision of health services may be changed as a result of the HIS. Control deals with how the organizational structure and power relationships between the various health professional groups, such as physicians and nurses, may change due to the new system. Regardless of the approach-

es, there are simply not enough evaluation studies done to date on the impacts of HIS in different health settings.

Standardizing the Vocabulary to Support Nursing Practice

Nursing care is an integral and vital part of the health service delivery system. Therefore, it is important to document the nursing care being provided to accurately reflect the degree of its contribution to the overall patient care processes and outcomes. As this documentation is also a legal record of care provision for the patient, it must be done in a consistent manner using a common vocabulary to facilitate understanding and comparison across systems, sites, and settings. Over the years, different approaches have been developed to document nursing care and outcomes. While substantial progress has been made in the classification of nursing practice, many challenges still remain to put these concepts into practice. In the following section, a review of different classification systems developed to support nursing practice is provided, the Omaha System is summarized as an illustration of one such system, and implementation issues to be considered by health organizations wishing to codify their nursing practice are identified.

Nursing classification systems. These are vocabulary schemes used to describe and categorize nursing practice in codified forms. Such schemes are intended to facilitate effective documentation and communication of the planned and actual nursing practice among nurses and with other health professionals. The nursing practice data collected can also be analyzed to identify the type of nursing care provided and the outcomes related to the provided care. Such classification is also a necessary step to capture nursing data in electronic form. Over the years, different classification systems have been developed for coding nursing diagnoses, interventions, and outcomes (Henry et al., 2000). These systems include the North American Nursing Diagnosis Association (NANDA), the Nursing Interventions Classification (NIC), the Nursing Outcomes Classification (NOC), the Omaha System, and the Home Health Care Classification (HHCC). Currently there are 167 nursing diagnoses in NANDA, 514 nursing interventions in NIC, and 330 outcomes classified into 6 domains and 24 classes within NOC. The Omaha System and HHCC each cover a comprehensive set of codes on nursing diagnoses, interventions, and outcomes. For example, the HHCC has 176 diagnoses, 197 interventions, and 3 qualifiers for the diagnoses to predict the outcome.

The Omaha System. The Omaha system is described here with a sample case to illustrate how nursing practice can be codified in a systematic manner (Omaha System, 2004). Within the Omaha System, there are 3 components that describe nursing practice: the problem classification scheme, intervention scheme, and problem rating scale for outcomes. These components are summarized in Table 39-2. By using these components together, one can describe the client needs, services provided, and their outcomes. The codification of this sample case is published on the Omaha System website by Ann Merrill of the University of Oklahoma College of Nursing. This case describes a nurse visiting a 70-year-old male living alone in a low-income apartment with a complaint of right arm pain from a fall in the bathroom 2 nights previously. The patient expressed pain, hugged his right arm to his body, and grimaced when asked to flex and extend his arm. His forearm and elbow were bruised and swollen without disfigurement of the joint. During discussion, it became apparent the patient was unsure about the cause of his pain but took aspirin that did not help. The nurse suggested additional ways to decrease pain and to make an appointment with the doctor, and also taught him symptoms of impaired circulation that should be reported immediately to the doctor should they developed. Partial codification of this case is shown in Table 39-3. For additional detail regarding this patient's living condition and fear of being evicted, see the rest of this case on the Omaha Web site under Case Study #2.

Implementation considerations. Issues that should be considered when selecting a classification system to codify nursing practice in an organization are: the type of information needed, its compatibility with the HIS already in place, and the resources required for its deployment. First, the information need will differ depending on the type of facility involved, such as an acute care hospital versus the home setting. For instance, the HHCC System has care components that are specific for home health nursing practice. Also the purpose of why the information is being collected should be made explicit in order to determine the appropriate classification system needed. Second, the HIS solutions already in use within the organization should be reviewed to ensure compatibility of the systems in terms of the technology and the vocabulary used. Increasingly, organizations are moving toward interdisciplinary care and integrated HIS in their setting that require the classification system to capture interdisciplinary and discipline-specific data as part of an integrated HIS. Third, the effort required to deploy a nursing classification system is substantial in terms of resources, leadership, time commitment, and organizational readiness. Once implemented, ongoing maintenance of the classification system is required to keep the vocabulary up to date. In 2000, the International Council of Nurses (ICN) established a formal International Classification for Nursing Practice (ICNP®) Programme to simulate the research, development, and implementation of a common nursing terminology scheme to ensure nursing practice data can be captured accurately as part of the HIS. At the present time, much work is still needed to harmonize the different nursing classification systems available and implement these systems as part of the HIS for use in different clinical settings.

From Telehealth to Telenursing

The Office for the Advancement of Telehealth (2001) in the United States defines telehealth as "the use of electronic information and telecommunications technologies to support long-distance clinical health care, patient and professional health-related education, public health, and health administration." The type of technology can range from the telephone to specialized videoconference equipment to the desktop computer. The type of communication channel can range from the regular phone line to integrated service data network (ISDN) to high-speed Internet.

Table 39-2
The Components of the Omaha System

Component	Detail of Scheme
Problem classification scheme	Level-1 with 4 Domains: Environmental, Psychosocial, Physiological, Behavioral Level-2 with 40 Terms: Client Problems, Needs/Strengths, Nursing Diagnoses Level-3 with 2 Sets of Modifiers: Deficit/Impairment/Actual, Potential, Health Promotion Individual or Family Level-4 with Signs and Symptoms
Intervention scheme	Level-1 with 4 Categories: Teaching/Guidance/Counselling, Treatment/Procedures, Surveillance, Case Management Level-2 with 62 Targets of Action 02 bladder care, 04 bonding, etc. Level-3 with Client-specific Information From nurses or other professionals
Problem rating scale for outcomes scheme	3 five-point Likert Scales Knowledge - Level no, minimal, basic, adequate, superior Behavior - Appropriateness not, rarely, inconsistently, usually, consistently Status – Signs and Symptoms extreme, severe, moderate, minimal, no

Table 39-3.
A Partial Sample Case of a Patient Fall

Component	Detail of Scheme
Problem classification	Modifiers: individual, actual Sign/Symptoms: 01 expresses pain/discomfort 02 compensated movement/guarding 03 facial grimaces
Problem Rating Scale Outcomes	Knowledge: 2 minimal knowledge Behavior: 2 rarely appropriate Status: 3 moderate signs/symptoms
Intervention	Category-1:teaching/guidance/counselling 1 anatomy/physiology discussed basis and cause of pain 44 medical/dental care described pain management technique 50 signs/symptoms of pain instructed reasons for pain & pattern of improvement in symptoms Category-2:treatments and procedures 6 other: applied sling to elbow joint Category-3:case management 31 medical/dental care encouraged client to visit physician

Telehealth practice has evolved from its early days in the form of telemedicine focused primarily on clinical consultation by physicians to now including a spectrum of health service deliveries, continuing professional education, and administrative meeting functions. The need for expensive and specialized videoconferencing equipment is now being replaced with low cost Web-based conferencing hardware and software that can run on a desktop computer.

In 1997, the American Academy of Ambulatory Care Nurses (AAACN) published the first standards for nurses engaged in telehealth practice. In that same year, the National Council of State Boards of Nursing issued a position paper that defines telenursing as "the practice of nursing over distance using telecommunications technology." Currently, the AAACN offers a Telehealth Nursing Practice Core Course that covers telephone triage, telehealth communication principles and techniques, telehealth patient care guidelines, and practical solutions to telenursing issues and legal concerns. There is also an active AAACN special interest group that addresses professional issues and educational needs of nurses engaged in telephone practice.

In this section, the types of telehealth in practice are described, the major issues are outlined, and a general framework of principles on telehealth nursing practice is provided.

Types of telehealth. The telehealth applications seen in North America (Swanson 1999) include teleconsultation such as telemedicine, telepsychiatry and teleradiology; education and training in different health disciplines through telelearning and telementoring; transfer of health information for health professionals and patients; and nursing telepractice. In teleconsultation, one can access health care expertise that is not available locally. The use of videoconferencing in teleconsultation, supplemented by radiological images as needed, allows better provider-client interactions through observable visual cues. Increasingly telehealth is used to provide on-site education and training of health professionals through real-time virtual large group lectures and case discussions, and one-on-one mentoring in specific clinical issues. The transfer of health information through direct online access via the Internet has provided citizens, patients, and health professionals, especially nurses, with up-to-date information on a variety of subject areas, with a caveat that the credibility of some of this information is questionable and should be used with caution. Telenursing is a more recent phenomenon that involves such tasks performed by nurses as communicating laboratory test results to clients, telephone triage for those with immediate concerns, follow-up for recently discharged clients, providing ongoing care and information for clients regarding chronic diseases such as diabetes, and monitoring home care clients via telephone or videoconferencing (Greenberg, 2003). Whatever the nature of the telehealth practice may be, the nurse charged with this responsibility should be adequately trained to manage the planning, setup, and delivery of the telehealth encounter effectively, including the use of the technology in an appropriate and competent manner.

Major issues in telehealth. The key telehealth issues include security and privacy of the telehealth encounter, regulation of telehealth practice, organizational readiness to implement telehealth, and the need for ongoing telehealth evaluation. Specifically, effort must be made to protect the security and privacy of the telehealth encounter in terms of access to the telehealth facility, informed consent, transmission of the client-provider interaction, documentation, and record-keeping. The regulation of telehealth practice is necessary to ensure compliance with established professional practice standards. In terms of organizational readiness, several factors must be considered, which include demonstrated need, technology availability, management commitment, and staff competency. To be credible, telehealth must be subject to rigorous evaluation to determine its quality, accessibility, cost, and acceptability in different organizational settings.

A framework of principles. The Canadian Nurses Association (CNA) proposed a set of guiding principles for nursing telepractice in Canada in 2001 (CNA, 2001). These principles are to ensure that the nursing telepractice (or telenursing) being provided is safe, competent, and ethical. The framework has six principles: nurse-client relationships; competencies; locus of accountability; security, confidentiality and privacy; informed consent and client choice; and professional practice environments. Nurse-client relationships in telenursing should be established through the nursing process of client assessment, planning, implementation, evaluation, and documentation. Competencies are critical for a nurse engaged in telenursing since the benefit of face-to-face interaction with the client does not exist. These include strong clinical/nursing knowledge and skills, an understanding of the psychosocial, spiritual and cultural needs and preferences of the client, and the appropriateness of the technology being used. Locus of accountability suggests the nurse engaged in telenursing is governed by the professional standards and legislation where he/she is located regardless of where the client is located. Security, confidentiality, and privacy policy must be in place to protect the client record and client-nurse interactions in telenursing. Informed consent and client choice suggest the client should be informed about the choices regarding nursing telenursing and the rights to other methods of care. Professional practice environments refer to the need for an environment that fosters professional practice to achieve quality care and client outcomes, and where telenursing can be provided safely, competently, and ethically.

Health Informatics in Practice

In this section, we provide five examples of health informatics in practice that are relevant to the nephrology nurse. The first example is the Veterans Health Administration (VHA) information systems in the United States and how they are changing the fundamental nature of health care delivery at VHA. The second example is telephone triage as illustrated by the BC NurseLine and Blue Cross call-line support systems that have emerged in recent years in North America. The third is the End Stage Renal Disease Networks and its use of information and technology to manage patients with chronic kidney disease in the

United States. The fourth is telehealth in renal care such as TELENEPHRO in New Brunswick, Canada and MyCareTeam from the Georgetown University Medical Center of the United States. The last example is on kidney disease registries such as the Canadian Organ Transplant Register and the U.S. Renal Data System that track renal dialysis and organ transplantation activities, practices and trends in Canada and the United States, respectively.

VHA Information Systems

The U.S. Veterans Health Administration (VHA) is one of the largest publicly funded health care system in the world with over 160 medical centers, 850 ambulatory care and outpatient clinics, and 300 long-term care facilities, counselling centers and home care programs serving 5 million patients each year. Until the mid-1990s, the VHA operated primarily as a hospital system providing medical and surgical services, and specialized in mental health care, spinal cord injuries, and long-term care through independently operated facilities. Then in 1996, major structural reform through the Veterans Health Care Eligibility Reform Act transformed VHA into a health care system with 21 geographically defined Veterans Integrated Service Networks, shifting care from hospital to ambulatory care facilities and home services (Perlin et al., 2004). The key guiding principles behind this structural transformation are based on six value domains of effectiveness by which VHA links quality to cost through a set of input and output performance measures. Five of these value domains are focused on outputs, including: technical quality of care, access to services, patient functional status, patient satisfaction, and community health. When measured against the financial resources as the input, the ratios of these input-output parameters become the sixth value domain of system cost-effectiveness. To ensure accountability, VHA has established an annual performance contract with the Office of Management and Budget based on the concept of evidence-based quality management and improvement.

The development of hospital computer systems at VHA began in the 1980s, which has since evolved over the years to become what is now known as VistA or the Veterans Information Systems and Technology Architecture (Hynes et al., 2004). VistA provides a standardized information technology framework to support the day-to-day operation of its network of 1,300 VHA facilities and affiliate organizations (e.g., academic medical centers). VistA has over 100 clinical, administrative, and financial applications, including such examples as admission-discharge-transfer, laboratory, remote order entry, radiology, dietetics, computerized patient record system (CPRS), imaging, pharmacy, home-based primary care, safety incident surveillance tracking, equipment request, integrated billing, and voluntary timekeeping. Health care providers can access these VistA applications via a common graphical user interface of the CPRS at any VHA facilities.

Currently, the CPRS is used by over 100,000 health care providers in all of the VHA facilities and medical centers nationwide. The CPRS allows the viewing of up-to-date patient information, including demographics, problem list, medications, allergies, laboratory results, hospitalization and outpatient clinic history, and medical images such as documents, x-rays, and photographs. This information is displayed immediately when the patient is selected in the CPRS, thus allowing the provider to review and update the patient's current medical record and place orders for medications, x-rays, laboratory tests, nursing care, diets, and consults, etc. in real-time electronically from different care sites. The CPRS is organized in such a way that it directly supports clinical decision making by the health care providers. These decision support features include real-time order checking for possible problems, automatic notification for clinically significant patient events, patient posting for alerts on warnings, adverse reactions and advance directives, and clinical reminders for preventive care.

The latest health information systems development efforts at VHA include the introduction of HealtheVet, My HealtheVet, and patient-centered care coordination (Perlin et al., 2004). In HealtheVet, aggregate registration, management, financial and provider data from VHA and non-VHA sources are collected and stored in a longitudinal database repository for research and population analyses. The My HealtheVet is a secure Web portal that provides patients with direct Internet access to their personal health record, online health assessment tools, instructions for prescription refills and appointment booking, and evidence-based consumer health information. In patient-centered care coordination, the VHA approach is to use technology to enable patients to manage their own chronic disease and health conditions at home. Through My HealtheVet, a patient can record his own physiologic measurements such as blood pressure and daily weight from home for review by the care coordinator at the local VHA facility. Any changes to the patient's condition that exceed the critical thresholds may trigger a home visit or a call by the coordinator to visit the clinic. A recent pilot program in Florida based on this care coordination approach has demonstrated improved satisfaction and health status for patients enrolled in the program. Another example is the use of daily telephone service with voice and/or text queries to aging veterans to assess their health status, medication compliance, and symptoms. Such approaches allow VHA patients to maintain their functional independence and social roles within the community in which they reside.

Telephone Triage and e-Health

BC NurseLine (2004) is an example of telenursing being offered in Canada. It is a 24-hour toll-free telephone service that is accessible 7 days a week to all residents in British Columbia (B.C.). The service is also available for those who are deaf or hearing impaired, and translation into 130 languages is available upon request. BC NurseLine is considered a form of tele-homecare where ICT is used to transfer data and information to assist in medical diagnosis, treatment and consultation between a client at home and health professionals from a health care organization. This example illustrates how the nurse can play a pivotal role in the delivery of health services and information through the use of a telephone triage call center and monitoring system.

BC NurseLine is staffed by registered nurses who are specially trained to provide confidential health information and advice on the telephone. The nurses answer questions about various health issues, provide information on treatment options, explain tests and procedures, advise on when to see a health professional, and point to health resources that exist in the caller's community. For assessment and symptom information, the nurses access a system called the *HealthWise KnowledgeBase*, which they use to triage the caller's question based on information provided and make appropriate recommendation regarding treatment and advice. This *HealthWise KnowledgeBase* resource is also accessible to the public online at www.bchealthguide.org.

Calls to BC NurseLine are documented and tracked in order to assist in future operations planning. The demographics about the caller and details of each call are recorded in a system known as the Call Manager. To ensure confidentiality, the caller's personal information is protected under the Freedom of Information and Protection of Privacy Act. The Minister of Health Services visited the NurseLine centre during the Nurses' Week Celebration in May of 2004 and reported that since its introduction, BC NurseLine had handled more than 500,000 calls. In 22,000 of the calls, the nurses identified an urgent need that required immediate medical attention, either through family doctors or emergency services. In 25,000 of the calls, the caller who believed they need 911 attention received advice that made them comfortable in choosing a less urgent level of service; 40,000 times, the call resolved the health issue, thus avoiding the need to visit the doctor, go to the emergency, or call 911. According to TCM TeleCare that manages this service, the BC NurseLine currently receives about 900 calls a day, and is being expanded to include a Pharmacist Referral Service.

BC NurseLine is just one component of the BC HealthGuide program in British Columbia that is aimed at providing an integrated self-care program where citizens have 24/7 access to credible information and advice wherever they live and when needed. The three other components of this program are the BCHealthGuideOnLine Website with over 3,000 health topics, tests, procedures and related resources, a 400-page BCHealthGuide on health concerns, tips and remedies, and a series of one-page fact sheets called *BCHealthFiles* on various health and safety issues. This program has the endorsement of the BC Medical Association, College of Family Physicians, College of Pharmacists of BC, and the Registered Nurses Association of BC.

In the United States, there are similar call-line services that provide health information and advice over the telephone. For example, the Blue Cross/Blue Shield of Florida ("Blue Cross") has a contracted health information call-line vendor that provides 24-hour/7-day telephone service to its members. This nursing call-line offers members information on their particular disease and treatment conditions. In addition, the call is linked to specific disease management protocols enabling Blue Cross to identify at-risk members for possible case management if needed. Recently, Blue Cross introduced e-Medicine via the Web as a way for its members to communicate with their physician offices for non-urgent care needs. Using the e-Medicine tools, mem-

bers can schedule appointments, receive normal laboratory results, request prescription renewals and refills, and consult with their physician on non-urgent health issues. Blue Cross also offers chronic disease management programs for diabetes, asthma, and congestive heart failure where members can sign up voluntarily to better manage their condition through online information and support. An educational website called Dialog Center is available 24 hours a day and 7 days a week with evidence-based information on clinical tests, medications, and treatment options. Members can speak privately on the telephone or online with health care professionals regarding their condition. The intent of these programs is to help individuals to take an active role in managing their own health, leading to improved outcomes.

Telehealth in Renal Care

TELENEPHRO (Robichaud 2001) is a telehealth program for nephrology that began in May of 1998 at the Beauséjour Hospital Corporation (BHC 2002) in Moncton, New Brunswick (NB), Canada. The program started as a pilot telehealth project under the Health Transition Fund Initiatives from Health Canada of the Federal Government. The project was implemented by a multidisciplinary BHC team in collaboration with Health Canada's Indian and Inuit Health Services Branch, and the NB Department of Health and Community Services. The objectives of TELENEPHRO are to improve the quality of life of renal dialysis patients; increase access to specialized services not available locally; maintain best possible dialysis care while coping with increasing demand for such services; reduce morbidity; and provide distance education to health professionals, renal patients, and their families.

TELENEPHRO links three remote sites and home-based patients across NB to bring specialist expertise to patients and health professionals where they reside. The three sites are the Regional Hospital Centre in Bathurst, located 150 miles north east of the BHC; a satellite centre for hemodialysis in Miramichi in Eastern NB; and the Big Cove Health Centre on an Aboriginal reserve in Eastern NB. TELENEPHRO uses ICT to link patients undergoing dialysis treatment at home or a satellite dialysis centre with specialists via telediagnosis, teleconsultation, teleradiology, and distance education. At the Bathurst Regional Hospital Centre, there is a dialysis unit staffed by nurses and medical internists. TELENEPHRO allows consultation between the internists and nephrologists; enables case conference with the health care team; and provides education sessions for health professionals, patients and their families. The Miramichi satellite centre handles six patients at a time under the supervision of nurses who can communicate with the nephrologists through videoconference for consultation. At the Big Cove Health Centre, a distance learning program on renal health is offered to those with high blood pressure or diabetes who are at risk in developing a renal disease.

The ICT used in TELENEPHRO includes a radiology image transferring system, a dialysis data management system, a videoconferencing system, and a clinical data transmission system, which are all interconnected over a high speed telecommunications network reserved for health care institutions throughout NB called the Wellness Network. The radiology imaging system allows nephrologists to view such images as chest x-rays and condition of fistulae of renal patients, while the dialysis data management system captures the patient's vital signs, weight loss, and length of session from the hemodialysis machine during dialysis. The videoconference system is a portable machine that allows the use of peripherals such as a digital stethoscope and headphone, and can store images in a database for subsequent comparison and review. The clinical data transmission system stores all data on the patient in a central database, which includes laboratory test results, pharmacy records, hemodialysis session data, and patient examination notes.

The TELENEPHRO program was evaluated in 2001 for its clinical efficacy, service quality, cost effectiveness, impact on patient health, participant satisfaction, and transferability to other settings. Qualitative and quantitative data were collected over 9 months through questionnaires, interviews, observations and a focus group. The findings show that the efficacy of the program for training, consultation, diagnosis, and dialysis treatment was rated very positively at 84% in terms of the clearness of the image, the connection, and equipment reliability. The quality of service was rated positive and satisfactory by those who responded. The cost savings were in reduced patient travel expenses. There was an improvement in the quality of dialysis treatments and some blood results for patients at the satellite units. Patients were 100% satisfied with the care received, and nephrologists were satisfied with the experience. For transferability, TELENEPHRO has since been used as a model in the implementation of other satellite centers in NB and Quebec.

In the United States, a Web-based system called MyCareTeam has been developed and piloted by researchers from the Georgetown University Medical Center to help patients manage peritoneal dialysis (PD) at home (Levine et al., 2000). The MyCareTeam Web site contains the patient's personal health record such as PD parameters and clinical data, laboratory results, appointment reminders, and PD prescriptions. Dialysis data from each session are automatically captured by the PD device and sent to a central database over the Internet. The Web site also include online self-monitoring tools, educational resources, and email communication ability with the hemodialysis care team. Thus far, feedback from the PD patients and care team have been positive in terms of automated data capture and online monitoring during the PD sessions.

End Stage Renal Disease Networks

The End Stage Renal Disease (ESRD) Networks Program is a national network of 18 organizations contracted by the Centers for Medicare & Medicaid services (CMS) to provide care for people with end stage renal disease in the United States. These Network organizations serve as liaisons between the federal government and ESRD service providers. Each Network can cover one or more states depending on the number of ESRD beneficiaries in

the given area. The responsibilities of these ESRD Networks are to oversee the quality of renal care being provided, collect performance data needed to manage the national Medicare ESRD program, and offer technical assistance to ESRD providers and patients within the designated geographic areas. In 2002, the ESRD program had close to 300,000 patients and 4,500 providers in its Networks. According to the 2003 Annual Report of the ESRD Networks, the four broad goals that govern the day-to-day activities of these Networks are: (1) improve the quality of care and quality of life for ESRD beneficiaries; (2) improve data validity, reliability, and reporting among ESRD facilities; (3) establish and improve partnerships and cooperative activities; and (4) support the marketing, deployment, and maintenance of CMS approved software applications.

The CMS and ESRD Networks have developed an integrated information system called the Consolidated Renal Operation in a Web-enabled Network (CROWN). CROWN has three key components: the Vital Information System to Improve Outcomes in Nephrology (VISION); the ESRD Standard Information Management System (SIMS); and the Renal Management Information System (REMIS). VISION is used by ESRD providers to store and transmit their local patient and facility data to their ESRD Network to be incorporated into SIMS through a secure Internet connection. SIMS is used by the ESRD Network to manage and report patient and facility-specific information. REMIS is used by CMS and the ESRD Networks in program oversight, including Medicare coverage and status, dialysis and transplant activities, and Medicare utilization of ESRD patients and their Medicare providers. Collectively these information systems provide the foundation by which the CMS and ESRD Networks can manage their ESRD programs, engage in quality improvement (QI) initiatives, and position their organizations strategically to ensure the ongoing provision of quality care to ESRD patients.

One recent QI initiative involving all the ESRD Networks is Fistula First, the National Vascular Access Improvement Initiative (NVAII) aimed at significantly increasing the use of arteriovenous fistulae (AVF) for hemodialysis access. NVAII is in response to the goals recommended by the National Kidney Foundation's Dialysis Outcomes Quality Initiative to increase the AVF rates from their current 29% to 50% or greater for incident patients and 31% to at least 40% for prevalent patients undergoing hemodialysis. To achieve these goals, the ESRD Networks partnered with the Institute for Healthcare Improvement (2005) to create a QI program to improve vascular access using the Plan-Do-Study-Act (PDSA) model. This program is guided by a set of clinical and organizational change recommendations such as to: incorporate vascular access into facility-based QI process; facilitate timely referral to nephrologists and early AVF evaluation by surgeons; place AVF in patients with catheters where feasible and secondary AVF in patients with AV grafts; provide cannulation training; and establish processes for monitoring and maintenance to ensure adequate access function. To be successful, this initiative requires accurate and timely patient and facility information to be collected and analyzed as quantifiable process and outcome measures on the improvement. Examples of process measures are investigations into non-AVF access as part of QI in the facility, and specification of AVF-only in referral to nephrologists and surgeons. Examples of outcome measures are fistula use and placement rates within the facility.

The Forum of ESRD Networks is a non-profit organization that advocates on behalf of all of the ESRD Networks and coordinates projects and activities of interest to its members. The Forum's Board of Directors (2005) has recently developed a strategic plan 2004-2007 document to provide a shared vision and future directions for the Networks. According to this plan, the envisioned future is for the Forum to be the recognized leader in chronic kidney disease (CKD) quality improvement, information management, and accountability. The specific strategies proposed to achieve the goals are: quality CKD care; support to networks and providers; information infrastructure; policy influence; and organizational effectiveness. Central to these strategies are the establishment of a comprehensive information systems framework that support the ongoing collection, analysis and reporting of accurate, complete and timely performance measures for the Networks. For example, in quality CKD care, up-to-date facility specific QI reports are needed to ensure high quality, safe and consistent care is being provided to patients. Similarly, the support to networks and providers can be improved through ongoing comparison of routinely collected patient and facility data on their relative performance. The establishment of a robust technology infrastructure where information can be easily accessible is key to improving the quality and availability of information for management. Such infrastructure can also increase the instances where policy makers seek information from the Forum as part of their policy development.

Kidney Disease Registries

In the United States, there is a national database system called the U.S. Renal Data System (USRDS) that is used to collect, analyze, and distribute information on ESRD in the country. The USRDS is funded by the National Institute of Diabetes and Digestive and Kidney Diseases (NIDDK) and the Centers for Medicare & Medicaid Services (CMS). The USRDS is administered through a coordinating center with the Minneapolis Medical Research Foundation, which works closely with members of the CMS, the United Network for Organ Sharing (UNOS), and the ESRD Networks. The goals of USRDS are to: characterize the ESRD population and describe its prevalence, incidence, mortality and disease rates; study relationships among ESRD patient demographics, treatment modalities and morbidity; identify new areas for renal research; and provide data to support ESRD research (USRDS, 2005). The USRDS database is a rich data resource with detailed profiles on ESRD patients and facilities, selected ESRD cohorts, claims, comorbidities and transplants that can be made available to researchers, health care organizations and the public.

UNOS is a non-profit organization created in the 1980s to coordinate the nation's organ transplantation system (UNOS, 2005). The Organ Procurement and Transplantation Network (OPTN) is a public-private part-

nership administered by UNOS to link health care professionals working in the donation and transplantation system with the intent to increase organ sharing and supply of donated organs in the country. Through OPTN, UNOS has developed an Internet-based network called UNet[SM] for registering patients for transplants, match donated organs to waiting patients, and manage transplant data for patients before and after their transplantation. The collected data are available at the center, state, regional and national levels, and are used by the government, researchers, organ transplant and procurement programs, and the public to track organ donation and transplantation in the country.

According to the highlights of the latest USRDS Annual Data Report (USRDS 2004): "Since 1993, hospital admission rates have dropped by 3% for hemodialysis and peritoneal dialysis patients who have been on therapy for less than 3 years, and are down 8% for transplant patients of similar vintage. For prevalent hemodialysis, peritoneal dialysis, and transplant patients on their modality less than 3 years, adjusted mortality rates have fallen. For hemodialysis patients of old vintage, rates have increased since 1994. Transitional costs from pre- to post-ESRD are considerable, with costs in the month of initiation, averaging $15,000 for Medicare patients and almost $25,000 for patients in employer group health plans. The greatest portion of costs is associated with hospitalizations" (USRDS, 2004). The 2004 OPTN/SRTR Annual Report has reported that: "Annual number of new wait-listed registrants under the age of 50 has remained fairly stable since 1994, but the number of new registrants aged 50 to 64 has doubled, and the number of new registrants over 64 has tripled during the past decade. In contrast to the steep increase in the number of candidates, there was only a 2.3% increase in the total number of kidney transplants performed in 2003; the fraction of kidney transplants from living donors remained constant at 44%. The transplant of ECD kidneys has increased steadily over the past decade, from 11% of kidney transplant in 1994 to 16% in 2003 (ECD kidney refers to expanded criteria donor age >60 or 50-60 with 2 of 3 conditions pre-donation serum creatinine < 1.5 mg/dL, stroke as cause of death, or hypertension). ECD kidneys made up 20% of all recovered kidneys and 16% of all transplants performed, compared with 15% in the prior year. Unadjusted graft survival for recipients of ECD transplants was 80% at one year and 51% at five years, compared to 91% and 69% for recipients of non-ECD transplants. For living donor recipients, results have been better than for non-ECD deceased donor transplants, with one and five-year unadjusted graft survival rates of 95% and 79%."

The Canadian Organ Replacement Register (CORR) is a national database that tracks vital organ transplantation and renal dialysis activities, outcomes, and trends in Canada. The purpose of this database is to: collect data on end stage organ failure and organ transplantation; provide national statistics on end stage organ failure for comparative analyses and research; increase availability of dialysis and transplantation data to facilitate better treatment decisions; provide a feedback mechanism to health care facilities in terms of quality assurance for treatment and a national standard for comparison; provide statistics on trends for the health care industry in the planning and delivery of renal treatment and transplant programs and services. CORR is managed by the Canadian Institute for Health Information (CIHI). Other CORR members and supporters are the Canadian Society of Nephrology, the Canadian Society of Transplantation, the Canadian Association of Nephrology Nurses and Technicians, the Canadian Association of Transplantation, and the Kidney Foundation of Canada.

CORR data are routinely collected from participating hospital and satellite dialysis centers, organ transplant centers,, and organ procurement organizations across Canada. The data collected consist of patient-specific disease, treatment, and outcome data on those receiving renal replacement therapy, and aggregate organ transplantation-related data. The patient specific data include demographics, risk factors, follow-up, and graft failures. The transplantation data include the number, type, and outcome of vital organ transplants, number of living and cadaveric organ donors, and number of patients on the transplant waiting list. The data series available are 1981-2001 for dialysis and kidney transplantation, and 1992-2001 for extra renal transplantation and organ donation. The CORR outputs include annual statistical reports, specific ad-hoc reports, selected data sets and Web-based interactive queries available to hospital administrators, health professionals, government officials, researchers, and the public.

The 2001 CORR Report on Renal Dialysis and Transplantation published on the CIHI (2001) website provides statistics on the activities, outcomes and trends for dialysis, organ donation, and transplantation during 1981-1999. According to the report, by the end of 1999, there were 23,601 patients on renal replacement therapy (RRT), which included 9,679 patients with a functioning kidney transplant and 13,922 patients on dialysis. Seventy-six percent of renal dialysis patients were on hemodialysis and 24% on peritoneal dialysis. There were 4,342 new RRT patients in 1999. The most common risk factors were hypertension, cardiovascular disease and diabetes. The proportion of new patients who were diabetic increased from 15% in 1981 to 32% in 1999. By the end of 1999, there were 4,793 diabetics receiving RRT for end stage renal disease. The survival rates for diabetic patients were lower than nondiabetic patients at 52% for 3-year and 34% for 5-year survival, versus 65% and 53%, respectively. In 1999 there were 1,663 single organ transplants in Canada, including 1,011 kidneys. Eighty-four percent of transplant recipients were between 18 and 64 years old, with males being the majority at 61%. As of September 30, 2000, there were 3,573 patients waiting for an organ transplant in Canada, with 79% being a kidney transplant. Organ donation has remained static over the years, with 421 cadaveric organ donors in 1999, representing 13.8 donors per million population.

Key Issues in Health Informatics

In this final section, a number of key issues in health informatics are discussed in terms of how they influence nursing practice. These issues cover the need and responsi-

bility to protect an individual's health information in the digital age, the plea for health professionals to acquire a basic level of health informatics competency as part of their initial/ongoing training, and the recognition of nursing informatics as an academic discipline. These issues are described below.

Protection of Health Information

The privacy of individuals, the respect for privacy, and trust are fundamental principles in a professional relationship. The proliferation of computer-based health information systems, the increasing variety of personal health information (e.g., genome) that is being captured, and the myriad of potential users of this information are challenging our existing assumptions of privacy and ways by which such information is protected from inappropriate use. These issues are particularly relevant to the nursing profession since it demands an increased level of awareness of the need to protect one's personal health information, and the translation of this awareness to become part of the nursing practice standards. The ways by which privacy, confidentiality, and security are addressed at the legislative, policy, and practical levels are briefly reviewed here.

In United States, the protection of health information for patients is guided by the Health Insurance Portability and Accountability Act (HIPPA) that was introduced in 1996 by the U.S. Congress but is just now being actively implemented in health care facilities across the country (Erlen, 2004). The HIPPA regulations are designed to protect patient's rights to privacy and their control in the disclosure of their personal health information. Increasingly, this information is being stored in computers and transmitted electronically over communication networks, telephones, emails, and facsimiles. As such, there need to be safeguards in place for those handling this information to ensure its proper disclosure and use. The HIPPA Privacy Rule, developed by the Department of Health and Human Services, sets the national standards for protection of health information and defines the circumstances for disclosure and use of this information. HIPPA applies to all health care agencies that provide patient care, bill for that care, and pay for the care received. Therefore, health care professional, nonprofessional, and volunteer staff who handle health information within these agencies must comply with HIPPA.

The American Nurses Association (ANA) wrote a position statement on privacy and confidentiality in light of the advances in technology. It emphasizes the protection of privacy and confidentiality as a way of maintaining trust with patients. The principles adopted by ANA are that:
1. The use and disclosure of identifiable health information should be restricted.
2. Patients have the right to access and amend their own information to ensure accuracy and make informed decisions.
3. Patients should receive written notice on how their health records are used and disclosed.
4. Informed consent from patients is required for use and disclosure of their information unless one's life is in danger, there is a threat to the public, or required by law;

5. Appropriate safeguards should be developed and implemented on proper use, disclosure, and storage of personal health information;

6. Privacy protection legislations and regulations should not impede public health and health care research efforts.

7. Enforceable remedies are needed for violations of privacy protection.

8. Federal legislations should provide a base to protection of privacy and confidentiality and not pre-empt other legislations that offer greater protection (ANA, 2005).

In practical terms, patients now have to sign a consent form upon their first encounter with the health care agency and are given a written notice explaining how their information is being protected, disclosed, and used. No information can be revealed about the patient unless it is used for treatment, billing and health care operation purposes within the facility. Patients can authorize and restrict who can access their medical records. They also have the right to access, review and make copies of their records. For the health care agency, privacy and security policies and procedures need to be established to ensure the organization is compliant with HIPAA. For example, there needs to be a designated privacy officer who oversees privacy and compliance matters within the organization, and privacy training should be mandatory for all new and continuing staff. For nurses, protection of patients' privacy and confidentiality is already inherent in professional ethical standards. Nevertheless, the rising prevalence of computer technology and electronic patient records increases the need for nurses to be aware of the changing technology and adopt good privacy practices on a day-to-day basis. For instance, not sharing computer login IDs, regular password changes, phoning ahead before faxing documents, shredding of duplicate records, and maintaining patient confidentiality are just a few examples of simple, yet effective practices to protect patient privacy.

Privacy impact assessment (PIA) has emerged in recent years as a popular method for examining the extent that the health information is being protected within an organization. Health professionals should become familiar with PIA as it is an excellent way to learn about the issues involved. The PIA is intended to address such questions as: What is the type of information being collected? What is the purpose for collecting this information? Who collects and uses the information? How is consent obtained? What security is in place to safeguard the information? What privacy training is provided to staff? What legislative authority, policies and procedures are involved? How is the professional relationship affected? What justifications are used to deal with exceptions? By addressing these questions in a proactive and systematic manner, one can become more accountable and be reassured that the rights of individuals and their personal information are being protected according to commonly accepted standards.

Health Informatics Competency

According to Canada Health Infoway Inc., a nonprofit private corporation created in 2001 to accelerate the deployment of electronic health records in Canada, there will be a steady increase in the number of health information systems being implemented across the country over the next 5 to 10 years. At the same time, many aspects of professional practice of physicians, nurses, and pharmacists alike will be transformed in fundamental ways with the deployment of these systems in clinical settings. Therefore, it is critical for health professionals to move beyond being merely computer literate to becoming competent in health informatics to embrace the ever-expanding digital age. This competency may be acquired through practical experience or formal education depending on the work environment and personal career aspirations. The increased use of health information systems in practice will generate new demands for health professionals to assume leadership roles within their organizations as the health informatics specialists. Opportunities are also available to join private firms engaged in commercial health information systems and consulting services, or to move into an academic career in health informatics education and research.

As described in the beginning of this chapter, health informatics is an interdisciplinary field spanning the domains of computer science, organizational studies, psychology, information science, health service administration, operations research, and human communication. It is impossible to be knowledgeable in all of these domains, but acquiring expertise in selected areas of health informatics will enhance professional practice. The required level of competency will vary depending on the expected role of the individuals involved. For instance, some health professionals may take on the role of being internal expert resources through the practical experience they have gained from the health information systems implemented in their department. Others may choose to work in the Information Systems Department as application and information analysts based on their health care experience supplemented with some formal informatics training. Health professionals have also pursued careers in the private sector with health information system vendors as client support analysts and account managers. A few will aspire to obtain advanced training to become specialists in health informatics research and education in academic settings.

Unlike the established health professions such as physicians and nurses in Canada that require certification or licensing prior to entering practice, there is no such regulation in place for health informaticians at present. This means that anyone with computer or related training can seek employment to work on health information systems in health organizations. This approach is becoming increasingly unsatisfactory, especially when implementing clinical information systems in a complex teaching hospital or community clinic where an understanding of the health care environment is essential. This understanding can only be acquired by those who already have a health care background or individuals with formal health informatics education. Recently, the United Kingdom has introduced a professional designation called the Certified Health Information Professionals, while in the United States, the American Health Information Management Association has introduced the designation of Health Information Systems

Professionals. While these designations are not requirements for entry to practice in health informatics, they are intended to move toward a basic level of competency to be considered for employment in health care organizations.

Nursing Informatics as a Subspecialty

Nursing informatics is considered a subspecialty within the broader field of health informatics. The Canadian Nurses Association (2001) defines nursing informatics as the application of computer science and information science to nursing. In particular, nursing informatics "promotes the generation, management and processing of relevant data in order to use information and develop knowledge that supports nursing in all practice domains." One view of nursing informatics is that it covers four interrelated nursing domains: clinical practice, education, administration, and research. Within each of these domains, the emphasis is on the appropriate use of health information and the supporting computer technology to achieve the goals involved. For instance, nursing informatics plays an important role in enhancing clinical practice in terms of defining, capturing, and using the nursing component of the electronic health record. In education, telehealth as a key aspect of nursing informatics is used to provide ongoing professional development for nurses. In administration, nursing informatics can provide the methods and tools such as workload measurement to improve the management of nursing practice. In research, nursing informatics can be an area of study in terms of the different types of health information systems involved.

An example of nursing informatics (NI) in practice is the NI-team that is part of the Nursing Department at the University Health Network (UHN) in the city of Toronto, Canada. The UHN website (UHN, 2004) includes a capsular summary of the NI team that is summarized here. At UHN, nursing informatics is defined as a discipline that "integrates nursing science, computer science, and information science to manage and communicate data, information and knowledge in nursing practice." The role of the NI team at UHN is to incorporate nursing information and knowledge needs into the health information systems being implemented to ensure they are consistent with the UHN professional nursing practice model. According to the UHN Nursing Department, the priorities of the NI-team are to provide the data and information that nurses need, implement computer-based tools to support nursing practice, and to integrate the ICT being deployed with the nursing workflow.

In the United States there are a number of organizations that offer nursing informatics education and training at different levels of competency (Gassert, 2000). For instance, the American Medical Informatics Association (AMIA) has a Nursing Informatics Working Group that offers workshops and seminars as part of AMIA's annual conferences. Rutgers University offers an annual spring conference that includes a nursing informatics stream. The Duke University School of Nursing offers a masters degree and post-masters certificate in nursing informatics. The masters degree has both full-time and part-time options, and can be taken mostly online with a 3-5 day on-campus

session each semester. The College of Nursing at the University of Utah offers a PhD in nursing with specialization in informatics.

Despite the plethora of NI education programs, there are common themes that define the NI as a distinct subdiscipline within nursing. An education think tank was held in 2004 by the AMIA-NI Working Group to refine the NI curricula across programs. A consensus emerged in that there are four major constructs that should be considered as part of a NI curriculum: data-information-knowledge, decision support, knowledge representation, and human computer interaction. These constructs are situated within a context bound by cultural, economic, and social physical aspects of the internal and external health care environment. The key informatics practice for nursing are information management, database management, systems, and project management (AMIA:NI-WG 2004).

Summary

Over the years, health informatics has emerged to become one of the most important fields of study, one that can change the nature of professional practice in fundamental ways. The field covers a spectrum of theories, methods, and applications around health information and ICT that provide the foundations and means necessary to redesign the patterns of professional work practices, especially those of the nurses. Examples include the electronic health record, telehealth and technology-enabled self-care that are key components of a well-functioning health care delivery system. Some of the evolving areas that are particularly important for nurses are nursing vocabulary, telehealth nursing practice, integrated information systems, and health informatics competency. For the nephrology nurse, the use of ICT in renal care, dialysis, and organ transplantation are further examples of where health informatics plays an important role in nephrology nursing practice.

References

American Medical Informatics Association, Nursing Informatics Working Group (2004). *Educational think tank report.*

American Nurses Association (2005). Privacy and confidentiality. *ANA Position Statements – Ethics and Human Rights.* Pending review and update 2005. http://www.ana.org/readroom/position/ethics/Etprivcy.htm; last accessed Mar 26, 2005.

Androwich, I.M., Bickford, C.J., Button, P.S., Hunter, K.M., Murphy, J., & Sensmeier, J. (2003). *Clinical information systems: A framework for reaching the vision.* American Nurses Publishing, Washington, DC.

BC NurseLine. *The BC healthguide program.* URL: http://www.bchealthguide.org/kbnurseline.stm. Last accessed May 27, 2004.

Beausejour Hospital Corporation (2002). *Telemedicine in nephrology.* URL: http://www.beausejour-nb.ca/templates/CHB/Chb1882d.html. Last accessed May 25, 2004.

Canadian Nurses Association. (2001, September). What is nursing informatics and why is it so important? *Nursing Now: Issues and Trends in Canadian Nursing.*

Canadian Nurses Association. (2001, November). *The role of the nurse in telepractice.* Position statement. Ottawa, Canada: Author.

Canadian Nurses Association (2003a). International classification for nursing practice: Documenting nursing care and client outcomes. *Nursing now: Issues and trends in Canadian Nursing,* 14, January.

Canadian Institute for Health Information (2001). Canadian organ replacement register. URL: http://secure.cihi.ca/cihiweb/dispPage.jsp?cw_page=services_corr_e. Last accessed May 27, 2004.

Erlen, J. A. (2004). HIPPA – Clinical and ethical considerations for nurses. *Orthopaedic Nursing, 23*(6), 410-413.

Forum of ESRD Networks. (2003, November). *Summary report of the ESRD Networks Annual Report.* Washington, DC: Author.

Forum of ESRD Networks. (2005, March 15). *The Forum of ESRD Networks' strategic plan 2004-2007* Accessed at http://www.esrdnetworks.org/strategicplan.htm.

French, C.G., Belitsky, P., & Lawen, J.G. Progress in renal transplantation. *Canadian Journal of Urology, 7*(3), 1030-7.

Gassert, C.A. (2000). Academic preparation in nursing informatics. In Ball, M.J., Hannah, J.J, Newbold, S.K., & Douglas, J.V. (eds). *Nursing informatics: Where caring and technology meet.* (3rd ed.). Springer-Verlag, NY.

Greenberg, M.E. (2003, January/February). Telehealth nursing practice SIG adopts teleterms. *AAACN Viewpoint.*

Kaplan, B., Brennan, P.F., Dowling, A.F., Friedman, C.P., & Peel, V. (2001). Toward an informatics research agenda: Key people and organizational issues. *JAMIA, 8*(3), 235-241.

Kaplan, B. (1997). Addressing organizational issues into the evaluation of medical systems. *JAMIA 4*(2), 94-101.

Henry, S.B., Warren, J.J., Lange, L., & Button, P. (2002). A review of major nursing vocabularies and the extent to which they have the characteristics required for implementation in computer-based systems. *JAMIA, 5*(4), 321-328.

Hunt, D. (1998). Effects of computer-based clinical decision support systems on physician performance and patient outcomes: A systematic review. *Journal of American Medical Association, 280*(5), 1339-1346.

Hynes, D.M., Perrin, R.A., Rappaport, S., Stevens, J.M., & Demakis, J.G. (2004). Informatics resources to support health care quality improvement in the Veterans Health Administration. *JAMIA, 11*(5), 344-350.

Institute for Healthcare Improvement. (2005, March 15). *End stage renal disease.* Accessed at http://www.ihi.org/IHI/Topics/ESRD/.

Levine, B.A., Alaoui, A., Hu, M. J., Winchester, J., & Mun, S.K. (2000). MyCareTeam Internet Site for home peritoneal dialysis patients.

Telemedicine Initiative Symposium Videos. Telemedicine and Telecommunications: Options for the New Century. National Library of Medicine March 13-14, 2001.

Lorenzi, N.M., Riley, R.T., & Blyth, A.J. Antecedents of the people and organizational aspects of medical informatics: Review of the literature. *JAMIA, 4*(2), 79-93.

National Council of State Boards of Nursing. (1997). *Telenursing: A challenge to regulation. National Council Position Paper 1997.* Accessed via URL: http://www.ncsbn.org/resources/complimentary_ncsbn_telenursing.asp

Office for Advancement of Telehealth. (2001). *2001 report to Congress on telemedicine.* Accessed via URL: http://telehealth.hrsa.gov/pubs/report2001/intro.htm#overview

Omaha System. (2004, May 22). The Omaha System: http://www.omahasystem.org; case study 2 by Merrill A of University of Oklahoma College of Nursing.

Perlin, J.B., Kolodner, R.M., & Roswell, R.H. (2004). The Veterans Health Administration: Quality, value, accountability, and information as transforming strategies for patient-centered care. *American Journal of Managed Care, 10*(11), 828-836.

Robichaud, S. (2001). Nephrology: The challenges of long distance care. *INFO NURSING.* December p.6-8.

Swanson, B. (1999). Introduction to telehealth. URL: http://telehealth.org.au/discussion_papers/intro_tele.html. Last accessed May 25, 2004

UHN Nursing Informatics. (2004). URL: http://www.uhn.ca/programs/nursing/site/about_nursing/index.asp. Last accessed June 2, 2004.

United Network for Organ Sharing. (UNOS). (2005, March 25). http://www.unos.org/

United States Renal Data System. (2004). 2004 USRDS annual data report, Précis. Washington, DC: Author.

United States Renal Data System. (USRDS). (2005, March 25). *About the USRDS.* Accessed at http://www.usrds.org/about.htm

U.S. Organ Procurement and Transplant Network and Scientific Registry of Transplant Recipients. (OPTN/SRTR). (2005, March 25). 2004 OPTN/SRTR Annual Report: Chapter 1 Trends and Results for Organ Donation and Transplantation in the United States, 2004 (page 6). Accessed at http://www.optn.org/AR2004/

- Through earlier implementation of computer systems mostly in hospital settings, a number of lessons have been learned as to how one should introduce these systems into the workplace. For instance, we have learned that we cannot treat the computer as a 'blackbox' and label non-adapters as being 'resistant to change'.

- Health informatics is highly interdisciplinary in nature, drawing on a wide range of theories, methods and techniques from the fields of health service administration, psychology, computer science, organization studies, information science, operations research, and human communication

- Androwich et al. (2003) have recently presented an organizing framework with a more holistic view of clinical information systems with an emphasis on nursing. This organizing framework has been broadened from clinical to health information systems, and includes an adapted version of the framework in Figure 39-1.

- The introduction of HIS into the health organization involves the process of systems planning, design, implementation, and evaluation. The extent to which these processes are formalized and applied depends on the type of system desired, the expertise available, and the overall readiness of the organization involved.

- Nursing care is an integral and vital part of the health service delivery system. Therefore, it is important to document the nursing care being provided to accurately reflect the degree of its contribution to the overall patient care processes and outcomes. As this documentation is also a legal record of care provision for the patient, it must be done in a consistent manner using a common vocabulary to facilitate understanding and comparison across systems, sites, and settings.

- The Office for the Advancement of Telehealth (2001) in the United States defines telehealth as "the use of electronic information and telecommunications technologies to support long-distance clinical health care, patient and professional health-related education, public health, and health administration." The type of technology can range from the telephone to specialized video-conference equipment to the desktop computer.

- The development of hospital computer systems at VHA began in the 1980s, which has since evolved over the years to become what is now known as VistA or the Veterans Information Systems and Technology Architecture (Hynes et al., 2004). VistA provides a standardized information technology framework to support the day-to-day operation of its network of 1,300 VHA facilities and affiliate organizations

- BC NurseLine (2004) is an example of telenursing being offered in Canada. It is a 24-hour toll-free telephone service that is accessible 7 days a week to all residents in British Columbia (B.C.). The service is also available for those who are deaf or hearing impaired, and translation into 130 languages is available upon request.

- The CMS and ESRD Networks have developed an integrated information system called the Consolidated Renal Operation in a Web-enabled Network (CROWN). CROWN has three key components: the Vital Information System to Improve Outcomes in Nephrology (VISION); The ESRD Standard Information Management System (SIMS); and the Renal Management Information System (REMIS).

- The privacy of individuals, the respect for privacy, and trust are fundamental principles in a professional relationship. The proliferation of computer-based health information systems, the increasing variety of personal health information that is being captured, and the myriad of potential users of this information are challenging our existing assumptions of privacy and ways by which such information is protected from inappropriate use.

- In the United States there are a number of organizations that offer nursing informatics education and training at different levels of competency (Gassert, 2000). For instance, the American Medical Informatics Association (AMIA) has a Nursing Informatics Working Group that offers workshops and seminars as part of AMIA's annual conferences. Rutgers University offers an annual spring conference that includes a nursing informatics stream. The Duke University School of Nursing offers a masters degree and post-masters certificate in nursing informatics.

ANNP639   **Informatics and the Electronic Age**

Francis Lau, PhD

Contemporary Nephrology Nursing: Principles and Practice contains 39 chapters of educational content. Individual learners may apply for continuing nursing education credit by reading a chapter and completing the Continuing Education Evaluation Form for that chapter. Learners may apply for continuing education credit for any or all chapters.

Please photocopy this page and return to ANNA.
COMPLETE THE FOLLOWING:

Name: _____

Address:_____

City:_____ State: _____ Zip: _____

E-mail: _____

Preferred telephone: ☐ Home   ☐ Work: _____

State where licensed and license number (optional): _____

CE application fees are based upon the number of contact hours provided by the individual chapter. CE fees per contact hour for ANNA members are as follows: 1.0-1.9 - $15; 2.0-2.9 - $20; 3.0-3.9 - $25; 4.0 and higher - $30. Fees for nonmembers are $10 higher.

ANNA Member: ☐ Yes   ☐ No   Member # (if available) _____

☐ Checked Enclosed   ☐ American Express   ☐ Visa   ☐ MasterCard

Total Amount Submitted: _____

Credit Card Number: _____ Exp. Date: _____

Name as it appears on the card: _____

CE Evaluation Form
To receive continuing education credit for individual study after reading the chapter
1. Photocopy this form. (You may also download this form from ANNA's Web site, **www.annanurse.org**.)
2. Mail the completed form with payment (check) or credit card information to American Nephrology Nurses' Association, East Holly Avenue, Box 56, Pitman, NJ 08071-0056.
3. You will receive your CE certificate from ANNA in 4 to 6 weeks.

Test returns must be postmarked by **December 31, 2010.**

CE Application Fee
ANNA Member $20.00
Nonmember $30.00

EVALUATION FORM

1. I verify that I have read this chapter and completed this education activity. Date: _____

_____
Signature

2. What would be different in your practice if you applied what you learned from this activity? *(Please use additional sheet of paper if necessary.)*

_____
_____
_____
_____
_____
_____
_____
_____
_____
_____
_____

Evaluation	Strongly disagree				Strongly agree
3. The activity met the stated objectives.					
a. Relate the increasing use of information and communications technology to the impact on nephrology nursing.	1	2	3	4	5
b. Compare informatics systems used in various health care settings.	1	2	3	4	5
c. Summarize the key issues in health care related to the use of communication technology.	1	2	3	4	5
4. The content was current and relevant.	1	2	3	4	5
5. The content was presented clearly.	1	2	3	4	5
6. The content was covered adequately.	1	2	3	4	5
7. Rate your ability to apply the learning obtained from this activity to practice.	1	2	3	4	5

Comments _____

_____

8. Time required to read the chapter and complete this form: _____ minutes.

This educational activity has been provided by the American Nephrology Nurses' Association (ANNA) for 2.5 contact hours. ANNA is accredited as a provider of continuing nursing education (CNE) by the American Nurses Credentialing Center's Commission on Accreditation (ANCC-COA). ANNA is an approved provider of continuing education by the California Board of Registered Nursing, CEP 0910.

Appendices

Problem & Clinical Manifestations	Nursing Intervention	Rationale
Hypervolemia Laboratory findings • Decreased hematocrit • Decreased urine specific gravity • Edema • Weight gain • Hypertension • Hypotension (if there is a decrease in EABV) • S3 gallop • Pulmonary rales • Pleural effusion • Cough • Ascites • Hepatic congestion • Elevated jugular venous pressure • Peripheral edema • Periorbital edema	Identify patients at risk for the development of hypervolemia.	All patients with compromised renal function are at risk. Close observation of these patients can help prevent acute complications.
	Weigh the patient daily or more often if indicated.	A rapid weight gain usually reflects fluid retention.
	Monitor 24-hour fluid intake and urine output. Also assess urine for presence of abnormal sediment.	As the GFR decreases the kidney loses the ability to excrete fluid and concentrate urine (see Table 13-2)..
	Maintain accurate records of intake and output (I&O). Compare findings. • Administer prescribed IV medications in the smallest amount of fluid possible. • Distribute the oral intake evenly throughout 24 hours. • Maintain the prescribed fluid restriction and sodium restriction. • Plan fluid intake schedule with the patient.	I&O records are important in evaluating the fluid status; however, weight is the *most accurate* indicator of volume status.
	Monitor BP and pulse in lying, sitting, and/or standing positions (if possible). Wait approximately 5 minutes between each reading. Note the rate and rhythm of the pulse. Monitor hemodynamic parameters if applicable, including CVP and PCWP.	Hypervolemia is frequently accompanied by an increase in BP and P, elevations of central venous, and pulmonary capillary wedge pressures. However, hypotension and a decrease in CVP and PCWP and an increase in P may be seen in patients with volume excess accompanied by a decreased EABV.
	Assess the neck veins with the patient sitting at a 45-degree angle. Measure the vertical distance in centimeters between the level of venous pulsation and sternal angle. An elevation of 3 cm or more is consistent with volume overload.	Intravascular fluid volume excess is associated with venous congestion and engorged neck veins. In fluid volume excess associated with decreased EABV, the neck veins may be "flat," even in the supine position.
	Monitor the heart sounds. Note the rate, rhythm, and presence of an S3.	The onset of an S3 is associated with heart failure and is an important clinical finding.
	Monitor the respiratory status. Assess the respiratory rate, characteristics of the respirations, and breath sounds. Note the quantity and character of sputum.	Tachypnea may be associated with fluid volume excess. The presence of crackles and wheezes indicates pulmonary congestion. Fluid can also accumulate in the pleural cavity and cause pain on respiration and decreased breath sounds over the area.
	Note periorbital, pedal, pretibial, and sacral areas for edema. If ascitic fluid is also accumulating, measure the circumference of the abdomen. Check tissue turgor. Provide meticulous skin care to prevent breakdown.	Edema is usually first noted in dependent areas.
	Administer prescribed medications including diuretics and dopamine. Monitor patients on dialysis and CRRT closely.	A diuretic may be prescribed to assist in fluid elimination. In ARF, dopamine may be used to increase renal blood flow and enhance diuresis
	Monitor the serum and urinary sodium, serum osmolality, fractional excretion of sodium, and hematocrit.	A patient with fluid retention may have a "dilution hyponatremia" and a drop in serum osmolality and hematocrit directly related to the excess fluid. Urinary electrolytes are important in the evaluation of tubular function.
	Consult with the physician about any changes that may indicate a deterioration of renal and/or cardiovascular function.	The following are reported promptly: • Weight gain greater than 5 lbs. in 24 hours • Development of wheezes and crackles or decreased breath sounds • Development of S3 • Sudden decrease in urine output

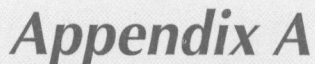
Problem & Clinical Manifestations	Nursing Intervention	Rationale
Hypervolemia (continued)	Encourage compliance with low-sodium diet. Educate patient regarding foods to avoid and fluid restriction.	Sodium promotes fluid retention.
	Provide psychologic support to the patient and family.	Fluid retention can precipitate anxiety and cause changes in body image.
Hypovolemia Laboratory Findings • Increased hematocrit • Increased BUN • Increased urine specific gravity • Weight loss • Hypotension • Thirst • Tachycardia • Decreased jugular venous pressure • Poor skin turgor • Dry skin and mucous membranes • Fatigue • Fever	Identify patients at risk.	Volume loss can be seen in early CRF and during the diuretic phase of ARF. Patients receiving diuretics are also at risk.
	Monitor weight daily or more often if indicated. Assess for volume losses from vomiting, diarrhea, drainage, etc.	Weight will assist in identifying insensible fluid losses.
	Monitor the blood pressure and pulse using the same procedure outlined under "Hypervolemia."	Orthostatic changes increase as volume decreases. Hypotension is usually seen in volume depletion.
	Assess for signs of hypovolemia: dry skin, decreased skin turgor, dry mucous membranes, sunken eyeballs, flat neck veins. Provide good skin care and oral hygiene.	Fluid volume deficit depletes intravascular, interstitial, and intracellular volume stores.
	Monitor laboratory studies, including hematocrit, sodium, BUN, creatinine, BUN: creatinine ratio, and urinary electrolytes. Consult with the physician about significant findings.	In hypovolemia, the hematocrit may increase. Depending on other factors, serum sodium levels are variable. The BUN may increase disproportionately to serum creatinine (normal ratio 10:1).
	Administer prescribed fluids, either orally or intravenously, or by both routes. • Monitor 24 hour intake and output	If nausea and vomiting are not present, the best way to replace fluids is orally. If fluids and electrolytes need to be replaced rapidly, the intravenous route is used.
	Provide psychologic support and education to the patient and family.	The patient and family are frequently anxious about the patient's current and future health status. They need to be instructed to increase fluid intake in situations where losses may increase.
Hyponatremia Laboratory Values • Serum Na+ < 135 mEq/L Gastrointestinal • Anorexia • Nausea • Vomiting Neurologic • Confusion, apprehension, anxiety • Stupor • Seizures • Coma • Weakness • Muscle cramps	Monitor serum Na+ levels. Assist in preventing hyponatremia. • Use normal saline instead of distilled water for irrigations • Avoid tap water enemas in bowel management • Replace fluid losses with fluid similar in composition • Monitor renal sodium losses • Monitor volume status closely	ARF and CRF patients may develop hyponatremia depending on urinary sodium loss and free water intake. Also free water can easily be absorbed during enemas and irrigations. Hyponatremia can occur with normal, increased, or decreased volume.
	Assess patient for signs and symptoms of hyponatremia. Monitor serum Na+ levels.	Signs and symptoms develop because of increased water content in brain and nerve cells.
	Assist with treatment which may include: • Water restriction • PO and IV sodium replacement • Discontinuing diuretic	Goal of treatment is to restore normal serum Na+ and osmolality.
	Monitor the neurologic status of the patient closely during treatment.	Rapid correction of hyponatremia can cause shrinkage of brain tissue resulting in severe neurologic signs and symptoms.
	Teach patient the importance of compliance with fluid restriction.	Excess water intake is a common cause of chronic hyponatremia in the CRF patient.

Problem & Clinical Manifestations	Nursing Intervention	Rationale
Hypernatremia Laboratory Findings • Serum Na+ >146 mEq/L General • Fever • Dry mucous membranes • Thirst • Flushed skin Neurologic • Lethargy • Altered mental status • Seizures Renal • Oliguria	Identify patients at risk and prevent problems if possible. Administer appropriate amounts of water. Monitor volume status closely. Identify sources of free water loss. Monitor serum and urinary sodium levels and serum osmolality and urine specific gravity. Monitor patient for manifestations hypernatremia Monitor correction of volume status. Follow: • Vital signs • Neurologic status • Muscle strength Educate patient and family regarding sodium restriction.	Most commonly occurs in patients with limited access to water. Hypernatremia can occur in hyper-, hypo-, or euvolemic status. Hypernatremia depletes ICF volume and leads to severe neurologic abnormalities. Volume replacement and/or diuretics may be used in an effort to restore normal osmolality. Rapid correction of osmolality may lead to cerebral edema, seizures, and death. Dialysis can assist in correcting hypernatremia. Usual diet is 2g Na+/day. Renal failure patients should not use salt substitute as these contain potassium.
Hypokalemia Laboratory Values • Serum K+ < 3.5 mEq/L • Alkalosis Neurologic • Confusion • Depression Cardiovascular • Hypotension • Increased sensitivity to digitalis • Arrhythmias • ECG changes Skeletal-Muscular • Weakness • Cramps • Paralysis Gastrointestinal • Anorexia • Vomiting • Diarrhea	Monitor serum K+ levels. Assess patient for signs and symptoms of hypokalemia. Assess renal and non-renal causes of potassium loss. Administer potassium supplements, monitoring potassium levels carefully. If possible, encourage intake of high K+ foods such as fruits and vegetables. • Monitor for GI irritation if using oral K+ supplementation. • Administer IV K+ slowly—monitor for phlebitis. Monitor patients who are receiving digitalis closely. Elevate K+ content of dialysate if indicated.	In renal insufficiency, significant potassium can be lost in the urine if the patient is on diuretics. Patients can also lose potassium via the GI tract, skin, or wound drainage. Patients on CAPD receiving insulin in the fluid may become hypokalemic since insulin facilitates movement of K+ into the cells. Patients in renal failure are at high risk for developing hyperkalemia. Patients on dialysis who are receiving digitalis may require an increased K+ concentration in the bath to prevent manifestations of digitalis toxicity. In renal failure, potassium excretion decreases placing patients at high risk for the development of hyperkalemia.
Hyperkalemia Laboratory Values • Serum K+ > 5.5 mEq/L • Acidosis Neuromuscular • Weakness • Paresthesias • Muscle cramps • Flaccid paralysis Cardiac • EGG changes • Cardiac arrest Gastrointestinal • Nausea • Vomiting • Abdominal pain • Ileus	Monitor serum K+ levels. Report elevations to physician. Assess patient for signs and symptoms of hyperkalemia. Administer treatment for hyperkalemia • Potassium restriction, kayexelate administration, diuretics, dialysis. • Administration of glucose and insulin or sodium bicarbonate. • Administration of calcium salts. Educate patient and family regarding K+ dietary restriction, importance of dialysis and severe, life-threatening complications of hyperkalemia. Monitor serum Ca++ levels.	Hyperkalemia increases the resting membrane potential and causes increased neuronal excitability. Treatment for hyperkalemia may include these interventions which: • Reduce body K+ content • Shift K+ into cells • Antagonize the effects of hyperkalemia on the heart muscle Diet compliance and regular dialysis treatments can prevent hyperkalemia.

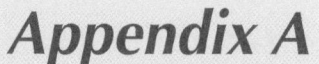
Problem & Clinical Manifestations	Nursing Intervention	Rationale
Hypocalcemia Laboratory Values • Serum Ca^{++} < 8.5 mg/dl Neuromuscular • Circumoral and acral paresthesias • Skeletal muscle cramps • Muscle cramps • Chvostek's/Trousseau's sign • Laryngeal stridor • Tetany • Weakness • Fatigue • Seizures Cardiovascular • Hypotension • ECG changes • Cardiac arrhythmias • Cardiac arrest Other (chronic) • Rickets • Osteomalacia • Cataracts • Dry Skin • Dental Caries	Assess patient for signs and symptoms of hypocalcemia. • Monitor albumin levels • Monitor serum pH Prevent hypocalcemia. • Administration of oral or IV Ca^{++} supplements and vitamin D as required. • Monitor patients carefully if on digitalis or if hypomagnesemia or hypokalemia are present. • Instruct patient in importance of keeping phosphate levels within normal limits.	Patients in renal failure have decreased intestinal absorption of Ca^{++} because of decrease Vitamin D levels. Hypocalcemia causes partial depolarization of neurons and increases neuromuscular excitability. Correct Ca^{++} level for albumin level and pH level. • A decrease of 1 g/dl in albumin is associated with an increase in serum Ca^{++} of 0.8 mg/dl. • A drop in pH of 0.1 units results in a reciprocal rise in ionized Ca^{++} of 0.1 mEq/L. Calcium and Vitamin D supplement are given as therapy. High phosphate levels promote the formation of calcium/phosphate complexes which precipitate out of solution and decrease ionized calcium.
Hypercalcemia Laboratory Values • Serum Ca^{++} > 10.5 mg/dl Neuromuscular • Personality changes • Acute psychosis • Weakness • Lethargy • Confusion and coma Cardiovascular • Hypertension • Shortening of the QT interval Gastrointestinal • Anorexia, nausea, vomiting • Constipation Renal • Polyuria • Nephrolithiasis Skeletal • Bone pain • Pathologic fractures Metabolic • Metastatic calcifications	Monitor serum Ca^{++} levels. Monitor patient for signs and symptoms of hypercalcemia. • Monitor albumin levels • Monitor serum pH Monitor serum phosphate levels closely. Follow calcium and phosphate product Administer appropriate therapy. A. In ARF or insufficiency • Saline and diuretics (if renal function permits) • Pamedronate - 30 mg over 4 to 6 hours • Calcitonin • Mithramycin B. In CRF or insufficiency • Withdrawal of Ca^{++} supplements and vitamin D therapy • Dialysis • Mithramycin • Surgical removal of parathyroid tissues	Major causes of hypercalcemia in ARF are bone destruction secondary to malignancy or release of Ca^{++} intracellular stores from injury or catabolism. In CRF, hypercalcemia is most often seen with calcium administration or Vitamin D therapy and secondary hyperparathyroidism. Hypercalcemia causes decreased neuronal excitability. When calcium $\times$ phosphate > 70, metastatic calcification can occur. • enhances renal excretion of Ca^{++} • reduces osteoclastic activity • inhibits PTH activity • slows bone resorption • decreases intestinal absorption of Ca^{++} • removes ionized Ca^{++}
Hypophosphatemia Laboratory Values • Serum PO_4 < 2.5 mg/dl in adults and 4.5 mg/dl in children	Monitor serum PO_4 levels.	Although hyperphosphatemia is more common in the renal failure patient, hypophosphatemia can occur with malabsorption syndrome and other abnormalities causing shifts of PO_4 into cells. Hypophosphatemia can also develop during TPN administration or when excess phosphate binders are given.

Problem & Clinical Manifestations	Nursing Intervention	Rationale
Neuromuscular • Encephalopathy • Parenthesis • Hyporeflexia • Seizures • Weakness Gastrointestinal • Anorexia • Dysphagia Hematologic • Impaired oxygen binding capacity • Hemolysis • Impaired leukocyte function • Impaired platelet function	Monitor patient for signs and symptoms of hypophosphatemia. Replace phosphate • IV supplementation may be necessary for severe causes. • Dietary supplement, such as milk • Oral phosphate supplement • Neutraphos Instruct RF patients in appropriate use of phosphate binders.	Symptoms are caused by decreased ATP synthesis in most cells and decreased 2, 3 DPG synthesis in red blood cells. Excessive use of phosphate binders is a cause of hypophosphatemia in CRF patients.
Hyperphosphatemia Laboratory Values • Serum PO_4 > 4.5 mg/dl • Associated with a decrease in serum Ca^{++} Metabolic • Metastatic calcification • Secondary hyperparathyroidism Renal • Deteriorating renal function Gastrointestinal • Abdominal cramps • Nausea • Diarrhea Neurological • Muscular cramps • Flaccid paralysis • Increased reflexes	Monitor serum PO_4 and Ca^{++} levels. Monitor patient for signs and symptoms of hyperphosphatemia. Administer treatment which may include: • Dietary restriction of phosphate • Phosphate binders are best given with meals • Aluminum antacids • Calcium carbonate • Calcium acetate • Dialysis Prevent hyperphosphatemia • Educate patient and family regarding dietary restrictions, use of phosphate binders, and long-term consequences of hyperphosphatemia • Never give RF patients phosphate-soda enemas	As renal function declines, phosphate excretion decreases. When the Ca^{++} x PO_4 is greater than 70, there is a drop in serum ionized calcium because of the formation and precipitation of calcium phosphate complexes. These interventions decrease intestinal absorption of PO_4. Use aluminum antacids only for initial control. Effective in removing limited amounts of phosphate.
Hypomagnesemia Laboratory Values • Serum Mg^{++} < 1.7 mg/dl (1.4 mEq/L) Neuromuscular • Personality changes • Tremors • Asterixis • Myoclonus • Seizures • (+) Trousseau's or Chvostek's sign Cardiovascular • Ventricular tachycardia • Increased risk of digitalis toxicity • Cardiac arrest	Monitor serum Mg^{++} levels. Monitor patient for signs and symptoms of hypomagnesemia. Treatment includes oral, IM, or IV Mg^{++} supplementation.	Hypomagnesemia usually occurs in malnourished dialysis patients or those receiving TPN. Hypomagnesemia increases release of acetylcholine at neuromuscular junctions which increases neuromuscular irritability.
Hypermagnesemia Laboratory Values • Serum Mg^{++} > 2.6 mg/dl (2.1 mEq/L) Neuromuscular • Lethargy • Confusion • Respiratory paralysis • Hyporeflexia	Monitor serum Mg^{++} levels. Assess patient for signs and symptoms of hypermagnesemia.	In the RF patient, hypermagnesemia is usually caused by intake of magnesium containing laxatives, enemas, or antacids. Hypermagnesemia decreases the release of acetylcholine at the neuromuscular junction, which causes decreased neuromuscular excitability.

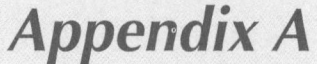
Problem & Clinical Manifestations	Nursing Intervention	Rationale
Hypermagnesemia (continued) Cardiovascular • Hypotension • Arrhythmias • Bradycardia • Arrest • EKG abnormalities (tall T-waves) Gastrointestinal • Nausea • Vomiting	Treatment is to discontinue magnesium containing compounds. Hemodialysis or peritoneal dialysis are also effective in removing magnesium. Administer prescribed medications • Calcium gluconate • IV insulin and glucose Instruct patient to avoid use of magnesium containing medications such as in some multivitamins, antacids, enemas, and laxatives.	Magnesium is in many antacids. • Calcium is a magnesium antagonist. • Promotes movement of magnesium into the cells.
Metabolic Acidosis Laboratory Values • Serum pH • Serum HCO3- Respiratory • Hyperventilation Neurological • Headache • Lethargy • Coma Gastrointestinal • Anorexia • Nausea and vomiting • Diarrhea Cardiac • Arrest • Dysrhythmias	Monitor arterial blood gases and serum HCO_3^- levels. Monitor patient for signs and symptoms of metabolic acidosis. Treatment includes: • Reduction of dietary protein • Supplemental sodium bicarbonate - oral or IV • Dialysis Educate patient regarding the importance of protein restriction.	As functional renal mass declines, the kidney is unable to excrete hydrogen and ammonium ions. Changes in serum pH alter cellular functioning. • Decreased acid loads of sulfates • Increase bicarbonate load • Removes H^+ and adds buffers
Metabolic Alkalosis Laboratory Values • Serum pH • Serum HCO3 Respiratory • Hypoventilation Neuromuscular • Confusion • Tetany • Convulsions Gastrointestinal • Nausea • Vomiting • Diarrhea	Monitor arterial blood gases and serum HCO_3^- levels. • Assess for sources of H^+ loss, vomiting, NG suction • Assess for bicarbonate load, i.e. antacids Monitor patient for signs and symptoms of metabolic alkalosis. Treatment includes correction of cause. Dialysis can assist in correcting the abnormality.	Metabolic alkalosis is uncommon in renal failure patients. However, it may occur as a result of vomiting, nasogastic suctioning, or when diuretics are used.

Expected Outcomes

1. Balanced intake and output with maintenance of patient volume states within established parameters.

2. Physical findings indicate optimum volume, electrolyte, and acid-base status as evidenced by:
   A. Normal vital signs (including hemodynamic parameters, if indicated)
   B. Good skin turgor without edema
   C. No signs and symptoms of electrolyte/acid-base balance alterations

3. Laboratory values are within normal limits. If abnormalities develop, they are promptly identified and treated.

4. Patient and family understand the importance of compliance with fluid and dietary prescription.

5. Patient and family understand the nature and use of medications used to treat fluid, electrolyte, and acid-base alterations.

Problem & Clinical Manifestations	Nursing Intervention	Rationale
Glucose Intolerance Laboratory Values • Elevated glucose levels in some patients. (However, fasting serum glucose levels are usually normal in non-diabetic hemodialysis patients. In patients on CAPD, fasting levels rarely exceed 160 mg/dl).	Monitor blood glucose levels—periodic fasting levels may be indicated. Assess insulin requirements of diabetic patients. Prevent hypoglycemia after dialysis. • Adequate oral intake prior to dialysis • Dialysate glucose bath of 200 mg/dl Consult with dietitian to plan appropriate diet. • Develop a dietary plan that will fit in with patient's lifestyle • Teach patient to incorporate diet into lifestyle	Urine testing is inaccurate in RF patients. Patients in renal failure have resistance to the peripheral utilization of insulin. However, there is also decreased excretion and metabolism of insulin. Thus, insulin dependent diabetics may require decreased doses of insulin. These patients may also have a blunted response to hypoglycemia. Although carbohydrate excess may contribute to hyperglycemia and development of obesity, patients need adequate caloric intake to prevent catabolism.
Abnormal Protein Metabolism Laboratory Values • Low serum albumin • Low serum transferrin • Low serum complements • Elevated BUN General • Weight loss • Muscle wasting	Monitor weight and anthropometric measurements. Monitor appropriate laboratory values - albumin, transferrin, and BUN. Consult dietitian and nutritional support team to conduct a nutritional assessment. Instruct patient to eat high biologic value protein foods. Provide patients with adequate protein intake: • Oral, enteral, or parenteral feedings Monitor patient for GI problems which might interfere with eating, appetite - diarrhea, abdomen distention, cramping. Provide adequate dialysis or CRRT. • Monitor KT/V and PCR Educate patient and family regarding the importance of appropriate protein intake	Patients in ARF and CRF have altered protein metabolism which places them at high risk for development of a protein wasting state. Nutritional assessment and history is important in determining nutrient needs. Protein foods of high biologic value such as meats and eggs provide essential amino acid. Adequate nutrition may help improve outcome of patient in ARF. On-going nutritional assessment is important to prevent catabolism and muscle wasting It is important to provide adequate removal of metabolic wastes in order to decrease uremic symptoms.
Abnormal Lipid Metabolism Laboratory Values • Elevated triglyceride levels > 200 mg/dl • Normal or slightly elevated serum cholesterol	Monitor cholesterol and triglyceride level. Consult dietitian and/or nutritional support team. Administer prescribed medications • Monitor liver function tests. • Avoid medications known to elevate lipid levels especially beta-blockers. Encourage patient to exercise. Assess patient for other risk factors which could accelerate arteriosclerosis. • Hypertension • Obesity • Smoking • Stress	Hypertryglyceridemia is believed to be caused by a deficiency of lipoprotein lipase. Lowering dietary intake of fats and carbohydrates can help in decreasing triglyceride levels but may be very difficult in view of other dietary restrictions. As cardiovascular disease is a major cause of death in the CRF patient, some physicians may prescribe antilipemic medications. Exercise can assist in decrease in triglyceride levels.
Endocrine Disorders Hypothyroidism • Hoarseness • Goiter • Weight gain • Dry skin • Cold intolerance	Assess CRF patient for signs and symptoms of endocrine-related disorders • Glucose intolerance • Hypertension (renin-dependent) • Hyperparathyroidism • Decreased gonadal function • Hypothyroidism	CRF patients have a variety of endocrine abnormalities related to changes in the synthesis, secretion, and metabolism of various hormone. Some endocrine abnormalities have been described in ARF patients, but these problems generally resolve after recovery of renal function.

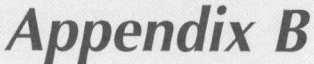

Problem & Clinical Manifestations	Nursing Intervention	Rationale

Endocrine Disorders (continued)
 	
Decreased gonadal function - male
• Atrophic testes
• Decreased sperm count and mobility
• Impotence
• Decreased libido
• Gynecomastia
• Galactorrhea
• Sluggishness
 	
Decreased gonadal function - female
• Amenorrhea
• Dysmenorrhea
• Decreased libido
• Galactorrhea
 	
Glucose intolerance
 	
Hypertension
 	
Hyperparathyroidism
	Monitor T_3, T_4, and TSH levels.
	• Assess patient for signs and symptoms of hypothyroidism
	• Administer thyroid supplements if needed
	
	Assess sexual functioning.
	A thorough history and physical is essential in work-up of sexual dysfunction.
	• Monitor appropriate laboratory values
	  FSH
	  Testosterone
	  Prolactin
	
	Patient and partner should receive sexual counseling to explore alternative methods of sexual satisfaction if impotence is not treatable.
	
	Provide emotional support for patient and partner.
	
	Administer prescribed medications
	• Bromocryptine
	• Testosterone
	• Zinc
	• Erythropoietin
		There is an increase in incidence of hypothyroidism in CRF patient. T_3 and T_4 levels are usually normal, but TSH levels are reliable in diagnosing hypothyroidism.
		Propylthiouracil (thyroid supplement) has increased half life in RF.
		
		Sexual problems are wide spread in dialysis patients. It is important to rule out vascular insufficiency and autonomic neuropathy.
		
		Dialysis patients endure a wide variety of emotional stresses.
		
		Correction of anemia with erythropoietin may improve sexual functioning.
		
		Hyperprolactinemia can be treated with bromocriptine. Zinc supplements have been reported to increase plasma testosterone levels.

Expected Outcomes

1. Patient's dry weight is appropriate for age, height, weight, and body frame.

2. Caloric intake is appropriate for energy demands and for the prevention of acceleration of catabolism.

3. Glucose levels are normal in non-diabetic dialysis patients. Glucose levels of diabetic patients are within established parameters.

4. Anthropometric measurements are appropriate for patient's size.

5. Laboratory values used to assess nutrition as status are at optimal levels.

6. Endocrine-related disorders are identified and treated appropriately.

7. Patients will express satisfaction regarding their sexuality.

Problem & Clinical Manifestations	Nursing Intervention	Rationale
Neurologic Manifestations Central • Headache • Lassitude • Apathy • Drowsiness • Insomnia • Emotional lability • Memory deficits • Somnolence • Confusion • Coma • Seizures • Sleep disturbances • Asterixis	Educate patient and family regarding neurologic effects of uremia and provide emotional support. Assess patient's ability to think and reason. Baseline cognitive function testing may be helpful in planning care. Allow patient adequate time to think about and respond to discussion. Conduct patient teaching according to patient's level of readiness. Provide frequent reinforcement. Observe for changes in general neurological status. • Perform baseline neurological exam and assessment of premorbid personality • Exam should be repeated as indicated Assess for other causes of CNS deficits: • Alcoholism • Drug abuse • B_{12}/folate deficiency Monitor patient for signs and symptoms of disequilibrium syndrome during dialysis. • Encephalopathy • Seizures • Headache • Blurred vision • Muscle cramps Assess sleep patterns. Instruct patient in sleep hygiene. • Retire and awaken at regular times • Have a relaxation period before going to bed • Avoid long day-time naps • Get at least one-half hour of sunlight within 30 minutes of out-of-bed time	The patient and family may become anxious regarding memory or behavioral changes. The psychosocial stresses associated with renal failure can aggravate neurologic symptoms. Cognitive abilities are decreased in uremia. The patient may require additional time to process information. Metabolism of drugs is altered in renal failure. Patients may respond to stress with drug abuse. Sodium modeling can help prevent this complication. Sleep disturbances can increase fatigue and worsen cognitive deficits. Sleep thrives on the "routine."
Peripheral • Paresthesias • Dysthesias • Decreased tendon reflexes • Muscle twitching • Restless leg syndrome • Gait abnormalities • Asterixis • Hearing loss • Facial asymmetry	Perform complete assessment of peripheral nervous system including cranial nerves. Maintain optimal fluid, electrolyte, and acid-base balance. Provide vitamin supplements. Restless leg syndrome may cause great discomfort and interfere with sleep. Educate patient regarding prevention of trauma to extremities: • properly fitting shoes • thermal precautions	Assessment may also include nerve conduction studies. Auditory studies may be indicated if hearing loss develops. Cranial nerve abnormalities can also occur. Metabolic abnormalities can aggravate peripheral neuropathies. Pyridoxine and B_{12} deficiencies can cause peripheral neuropathies. Benzodiazepines, opiates, and L-dopa can be used to treat this condition. Although tricyclics are frequently used to treat peripheral neuropathies, they can *worsen* leg movements at night. Trauma can lead to infection and possible loss of limb
Autonomic • Orthostatic hypotension • Depressed cough reflex • Decreased sweating	Assess patient for orthostasis. Take blood pressure and pulse in sitting and standing position. Use of TED stockings may help prevent orthostatic hypotension.	ANS abnormalities occur in renal failure, particularly in diabetic patients. Stockings help increase venous return to the heart.

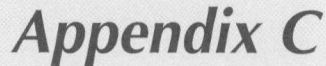
Expected Outcomes

1. Neurologic complications which occur are promptly recognized, evaluated, and treated.

2. Patient's comfort and safety is maintained.

3. Patient is maintained in optimum metabolic state.

4. Patient and family will understand the neurologic manifestations of the uremic syndrome.

Problem & Clinical Manifestations	Nursing Intervention	Rationale
Cardiovascular Manifestations • Hypertension • Congestive heart failure • Cardiac arrhythmias pericarditis • Cardiac tamponade • Accelerated atherosclerosis	Monitor BP, P, and weight. Instruct patient to take hypertensive medications.	Most hypertension is volume dependent but may also be related to excess production of renin.
	Monitor fluid and electrolyte status. Auscultate heart sounds for rate, rhythm, gallops, and murmurs. • Observe for distended neck veins • Palpate for enlarged liver • Check PMI placement	Fluid and electrolyte disturbances can cause changes in heart rate and rhythm. In addition, gallops (S_3 and S_4) may occur in congestive heart failure and hypertension. Murmurs develop with anemia, placement of vascular access.
	Assess for symptoms of pericarditis including tachycardia, ECG changes, pericardial friction rub (heard best when the patient is setting up and leaning forward), fever, and leukocytoses.	Pericarditis frequently occurs in uremic patients and may indicate the need for more aggressive dialysis. Pain of pericarditis is aggravated by movement, breathing, coughing, and lying down. The pain is relieved by sitting up and leaning forward.
	Monitor patient for signs and symptoms of effusion and tamponade i.e., paradox in the BP, distended neck veins, engorged liver, hypotension, displaced PMI, tachycardia, and enlarged heart on physical examination, CXR, and/or echocardiogram.	Effusion is the collection of fluid in the pericardial sac. Cardiac tamponade is a medical and/or surgical emergency
	Assess for signs and symptoms of atherosclerosis: • angina • decreased peripheral pulses • claudication	Accelerated atherosclerosis in CRF may be related to abnormalities in glucose and lipid metabolism.
	Educate patient and family regarding cardiac complications associated with renal failure and the roles that diet, medications, and dialysis play in their prevention. Educate patient regarding cardiac risk factor reduction.	

Expected Outcomes

1. Blood pressure is within normal limits.

2. Adequate cardiac output is maintained as evidenced by:
   A. stable vital signs
   B. ability to maintain consistent activity level
   C. strong peripheral pulses

3. Cardiac complications are promptly recognized, assessed, and treated.

4. Patient and family understand possible cardiac complications of uremia and can verbalize appropriate information regarding diet, medications, and signs and symptoms to report.

Problem & Clinical Manifestations	Nursing Intervention	Rationale
Respiratory Manifestations • Kussmaul's respiration • Pulmonary edema • Pneumonitis • Increased susceptibility to infections	Monitor respiratory rate and rhythm. Auscultate lung fields for: a. decreased breath sounds b. rales c. rhonchi d. pleural friction rub Monitor character and amount of sputum. Follow arterial blood gases and CXR as indicated. Instruct patient to avoid those with respiratory infections. Ensure patient receives appropriate vaccinations.	Respiratory rate may increase in compensation for metabolic acidosis. Rales and rhonchi develop in pulmonary edema. Decreased breath sounds occur with pleural effusion. Pleural friction rub is a sign of pleuritis. Pulmonary infections are characterized by increased, tenacious sputum production. Respiratory compromise may cause decreased oxygenation. Patients in renal failure have increased susceptibility to infection. Vaccination against the influenza virus is recommended annually. Pneumococcal vaccination is given according to antibody response.

Expected Outcomes

1. Respiratory rate less than 24/min. without dyspnea.
2. Absence of adventitious breath sounds.
3. Normal pO_2 and pCO_2 within limits of existing pathology.
4. Normal CXR.
5. Negative sputum culture.

Problem & Clinical Manifestations	Nursing Intervention	Rationale
Hematologic Manifestations Anemia • Fatigue • Decreased appetite • Increased angina • Cold intolerance • Hypotension • Reduced exercise tolerance • Dyspnea on exertion • Pallor • Tachycardia Increased bleeding tendency • Petechiae • Ecchymosis • Epistaxis • Hematochezia	Monitor hematocrit, iron studies, and bleeding time. Administer recombinant human erythropoietin (r-HuEPO) as ordered. Administer oral and/or IV iron and folate supplements as ordered. Keep iron saturation > 20%. Monitor patient for blood loss. • Check stool for occult blood • Bleeding from skin and mucous membranes • Bleeding from access or around IV lines Protect patient from trauma. Instruct patient in ways to prevent bleeding and bruising, i.e., avoid trauma, vigorous nose blowing, constipation, injury to gums during tooth brushing. • Administer appropriate medications if uncontrolled bleeding occurs.	Anemia develops in RF secondary to erythropoietin deficiency. Bleeding time is the most reliable test to evaluate bleeding tendency. r-HuEPO causes an increase in hematocrit within 8 to 12 weeks. Adequate iron and vitamin stores are necessary for RBC production. Platelet count may be only slightly ¬ but they do not function normally in uremic environment. • Cryoprecipitate, DDAVP, and estrogens may help control uremic bleeding. Dialysis also can improve bleeding time.

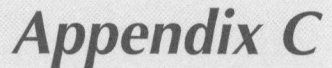
Problem & Clinical Manifestations	Nursing Intervention	Rationale
Hematologic Manifestations (continued) Impaired leukocyte function • Increased susceptibility to infections • Lymphopenia • Suppression of cellular and humoral immunity	Avoid penetration of skin/mucous membrane barriers. • Discontinue IV lines if possible • Avoid urinary catheter • Monitor WBC Teach patient good oral hygiene and skin care. Assess patient for viral, fungal, and parasitic infections.	Uremic patients have impaired leukocyte function. Infections are the major cause of death in ARF.

Expected Outcomes

1. Hematocrit is maintained at optimal level for patient (30%-35%).
2. Iron saturation is ≥ 20%.
3. Folate levels are within normal limits.
4. Blood losses are kept to a minimum.
5. Patient and family are knowledgeable regarding ways to prevent infection and bleeding.
6. Appropriate actions are taken to prevent infection.

Problem & Clinical Manifestations	Nursing Intervention	Rationale
Dermatologic Manifestations • Pruritus • Dry skin • Skin color changes • Pallor • Nail changes • Uremic Frost	Asses skin for dryness, signs of scratching, poor turgor, and changes in color. Consult dermatologist if necessary. Avoid use of drying soaps and use lanolin-based soaps. After bathing, patient should apply emollient while still wet and then pat dry. Instruct patient and family in good skin care. Advise patient to keep nails short and to avoid scratching. Explain nature of skin changes in renal failure. Instruct patient in control of phosphorus and calcium. Administer medications or treatments as ordered. • Diphenhydramine • Oral charcoal • UV light Assess nail for changes and signs of fungal infection.	Pruritus is a frequently described problem in acute chronic real failure. Possible causes indicate urochrome and metabolic waste retention, deposition of calcium phosphate crystals in skin, hyperparathyroidism, and histamine release. Applying emollient while wet helps seal moisture in skin. Trimmed nails can aid in preventing skin trauma from scratching. See Appendix B. • antihistamine • may bind with toxic substances in GI tract Nail changes do not occur in all uremic patients. Patients are susceptible to cutaneous infection.

Expected Outcomes

1. Patient's skin will remain intact and free from infections.
2. Patient will verbalize understanding of the dermatologic changes which occur in renal failure and importance of good skin and nail care.

Problem & Clinical Manifestations	Nursing Intervention	Rationale
Gastrointestinal Manifestations • Unpleasant taste in mouth • Gingival hyperplasia • Caries • Stomatitis • Anorexia • Nausea • Vomiting • Constipation • Diarrhea • Gastritis • Duodenitis • Colitis	Assess oral status. Examine gums, tongue, and mucous membranes. Assess for alterations in taste. To alleviate dry mouth, patient can be instructed to: • brush teeth frequency • chew gum • suck on hard candy • maintain daily fluid allotment	Oral membranes become pale. Metallic taste, halitosis, and stomatitis are caused by high urea concentration. Fluid losses can reduce salivary flow and cause dry mouth.

Problem & Clinical Manifestations	Nursing Intervention	Rationale
Gastrointestinal Manifestations (continued)	Teach patient the importance of good oral hygiene or perform oral care for patient. Instruct patient to have regular dental check-ups every 3-6 months. Dental prophylaxis is recommended for invasive procedures: • Penicillin V or K 1 gm 1 hour prior to procedure then 500 mg every 6 hours for 2 days. • Erythromycin - 1 gm 1 hour prior to procedure then 500 mg every 6 hours for 2 days. Assess patient for nausea, vomiting, anorexia and abdomen for pain, tenderness, distention and bowel sounds. • Plan food so that it is appealing • Small, frequent feedings may decrease nausea • Antiemetics can be used in small doses • Metaclopromide can enhance gastric emptying Assess patient for constipation/diarrhea • Stool softeners and bulk laxatives can be used to establish normal bowel habits. • Avoid excessive use of harsh laxatives • Saline enemas can provide relief • Diphenoxlate hydrochloride can be used to treat diarrhea. Periodically, check stools for occult blood. • Prophylactic use of antacids and H_2 blockers can help prevent ulcer formation in the ARF/CRF patient Educate patient and family in the gastrointestinal	Good oral hygiene habits and regular dental check-ups can help prevent morbidity. Gastropathy is related to high levels of urea. As renal function deteriorates, GI symptoms may worsen. Constipation may be due to decreased gastric motility and is a side effect of aluminum-based phosphate binders. Never administer a phosphate-soda enema to a renal failure patient as it will increase serum phosphate. Ulcerative lesions and platelet dysfunction predispose the renal failure patient to GI bleeding.

Expected Outcomes

1. Patient will maintain a good program of oral hygiene.
2. Patient will establish a desired bowel elimination pattern.
3. Gastrointestinal complications will be prevented. If problems develop they will be promptly recognized and treated.
4. Patient and family will verbalize an understanding of the GI manifestations of uremia and know how to best manage them.

Problem & Clinical Manifestations	Nursing Intervention	Rationale
Skeletalmuscular Manifestations Renal osteodystrophy • Bone pain • Pathological fractures • Metastatic calcifications	Monitor serum phosphate and calcium and the calcium phosphate product (calcium $\times$ phosphate) • Instruct patient and family in dietary phosphate restriction Administer phosphate binders with meals. Calcium binders should be used instead of aluminum binders if calcium phosphate product is less than 70 to prevent aluminum toxicity. • Assess patient for constipation Administer calcium supplements and Vitamin D therapy as indicated. Evaluate response to therapy. Follow PTH, alkaline phosphatase, aluminum levels in addition to bone biopsy results and hand and clavicle films.	As functional renal mass decreases, normal calcium and phosphate balance are disturbed. Hypocalcemia develops secondary to reduced Vitamin D levels. Hyperphosphatemia occurs from reduced renal phosphate excretion. The calcium phosphate product should stay below 70 to prevent metastatic calcifications. Phosphate binders bind with phosphate in the GI tract. Vitamin D (calcitriol) enhances intestinal absorption of calcium and suppress PTH secretion. Calcium and Vitamin D therapy should not be given if hyperphosphatemia is present as metastatic calcifications will occur. Elevated PTH and alkaline phosphatase levels are consistent with hyperparathyroidism. A bone biopsy will assist in diagnosing the presence and type of renal bone disease.

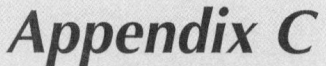

Problem & Clinical Manifestations	Nursing Intervention	Rationale
Skeletalmuscular Manifestations (continued)	Assess patient's ability to ambulate, range of motion, muscle strength, coordination, and bone pain. • Assess patient's environment for potential hazards. • Assess for soft tissues calcification • Joint pain • Pruritus • Conjunctivitis	These symptoms are associated with hyperparathyroidism. Changes in gait and muscle strength predispose patient to injuries.
	Educate patient and family regarding: • Manifestations of renal osteodystrophy. • Signs and symptoms to report to health care team. • Methods to minimize disability and enhance current mobility.	Calcium phosphate complexes can be deposited in soft tissues.

Expected Outcomes
1. Phosphate, calcium, PTH, aluminum, and alkaline phosphatase levels will remain within established parameters.
2. Patient will remain free of disability related to renal osteodystrophy.
3. Patient and family will verbalize an understanding of the importance of phosphate control in the prevention of renal osteodystrophy.

Preamble

ANNA is a national organization of registered nurses practicing in nephrology, transplantation, and related therapies, who are involved in the supervision and delivery of care to adults and children undergoing treatment for kidney disease and other disease processes that require replacement therapies. ANNA supports the multidisciplinary approach to health care and believes that registered nurses must be major participants in the planning, delivery, and evaluation of that care.

As a professional organization, ANNA has the obligation to set and update standards of patient care, educate practitioners, stimulate research and disseminate findings, promote interdisciplinary communication and cooperation, and address issues that may impact the practice of nephrology nursing.

This Health Policy Statement represents the ANNA viewpoint on major public policy issues relevant to the treatment of individuals with kidney disease and the practice of professional nephrology nursing. This document is provided to give the Association direction as legislative and regulatory issues are addressed on local, state and national levels. This document has been developed based on review of the issues and input from ANNA members, officers and committee chairpersons. The ANNA Board of Directors has approved the final document. This document is reviewed by the ANNA Health Policy Committee, Health Policy Consultants, and the Board of Directors when indicated.

Nursing

ANNA is committed to assuring and protecting access to professional nursing care delivered by highly educated, well-trained, and experienced registered nurses for individuals with kidney disease or other disease processes that require replacement therapies.

ANNA believes that registered nurses experienced in dialytic therapy must be present for the direct supervision of patient care activities and personnel during dialysis treatments.

ANNA believes that a registered nurse must be actively involved in determining staffing requirements in facilities providing care to patients with kidney disease, and that these requirements should be based on an assessment of patient acuity.

ANNA believes that care of patients with kidney disease is provided effectively and responsibly by registered nurses. Further, the use of advanced practice registered nurses in the management of patients with kidney disease can result in high quality care delivered at a lower cost, benefiting the health care delivery system in general, and the ESRD program in particular. ANNA supports the recognition of compensation for advanced practice registered nurses by all payers.

The Association believes that a sound education program is necessary to develop, maintain, and augment clinical and technical competence. ANNA believes that all licensed patient care personnel must complete a standard-ized nephrology education program reflecting the ANNA Standards of Clinical Practice for Nephrology Nursing.

ANNA endorses the certification of qualified nephrology nurses as defined by the Nephrology Nursing Certification Commission and continuing certification to refine the knowledge of nurses providing care to individuals in all stages and types of kidney disease across the life span.

ANNA supports the development of a standard national program of education and training for unlicensed personnel who provide direct care to individuals undergoing dialysis. ANNA believes such education and training is ideally done in a formal setting, with standardized competency testing upon completion of the program, and with continuing education requirements.

ANNA opposes the licensing of assistive personnel and supports the least restrictive approach to the regulation of such personnel, such as registration of individuals who meet specific educational or experiential requirements and who have demonstrated some level of competence. The Association supports the use of the term "certification" to designate voluntary private sector programs that attest to the competency of individual health professions and occupational groups.

ANNA supports a nurse's right to refuse to perform an act or take an assignment that in the nurse's judgment is not safe or is not within that nurse's skill, experience, qualifications or capability.

In accordance with our commitment to compassionate end-of-life care, ANNA believes that nurses should not participate in assisted suicide or active euthanasia and that such acts are in direct violation of the American Nurses Association (ANA) Code for Nurses with Interpretive Statements and the ethical traditions of the profession. (ANA, 2001) ANNA supports the ANA statement which asserts that, "Nurses individually and collectively have an obligation to provide comprehensive and compassionate end-of-life care which includes the promotion of comfort and the relief of pain and, at times, foregoing life-sustaining treatment." ANNA acknowledges that refusal to participate in assisted suicide or euthanasia does not constitute abandonment of patients.

ANNA believes that nephrology nurses should continue to advocate for health care environments that provide humane and dignified patient-centered care. The Association supports continued dialogue on end-of-life issues and appropriate decision-making related to withdrawal of treatment. ANNA has endorsed the *Clinical Practice Guideline on Shared Decision-Making in the Appropriate Initiation and Withdrawal from Dialysis* (February 2000), published by the Renal Physicians Association and the American Society of Nephrology.

ANNA supports the promotion of nursing's role in patient advocacy without fear of retribution or repercussions by providers.

ANNA believes personnel must be protected from occupational and environmental health hazards related to dialytic therapy and that standards for safety and protective measures should be developed, identified and implemented.

ANNA believes that any efforts to detect or test for substance abuse or communicable diseases must be consistent with good medical practice and shall not violate the individual's civil rights.

ANNA supports the promotion of the nurse's role in health policy advocacy through educational efforts, grassroots lobbying and activities that will promote the health of individuals with kidney disease or other disease processes that require replacement therapies.

ANNA supports the inclusion of registered nurses at the policy-making level and on all boards, commissions, expert panels, task forces and other groups setting policies and standards that affect nursing practice, the Medicare ESRD program, and its beneficiaries.

ANNA supports the efforts to resolve the current nursing shortage, especially as related to ESRD facilities.

ANNA continues to support the utilization of Advanced Practice Nurses (APNs) in all areas of nephrology.

ANNA supports grants to state Boards of Nursing to implement multistate licensure for health professionals through expansion of state compact process.

ANNA supports improved provision of and access to telehealth services, both distance learning for professionals and patients as well as treatment and home monitoring of chronic diseases in both Medicare and Medicaid.

Elements of Care

ANNA believes the practice of nephrology nursing is directed toward assessing and treating the health needs of individuals and their families who are experiencing the real or threatened impact of compromised kidney function, acute or chronic kidney disease, or other organ system failure states. This practice includes a commitment to help each individual and his/her significant others achieve an optimal level of functioning. Toward this end, nephrology nurses must establish high standards of patient care that are routinely updated.

ANNA believes that appropriate, quality treatment must be available to all individuals with kidney disease and other disease processes that require replacement therapies. ANNA supports providing these individuals with complete and accurate information about all alternative forms of therapy, including the associated risks and benefits, without regard for their cost. The Association believes that these individuals and families must be encouraged and allowed to be active participants in this decision-making process.

ANNA supports legislation promoting prevention and management of chronic kidney disease, including early diagnosis, education and creation of native fistulae for dialysis.

In order to achieve the goal of optimal rehabilitation, ANNA believes individuals must assume as much responsibility for their overall care as their physical and mental limits allow. ANNA supports all home and self-dialysis modalities, with training and supervision of persons choosing

these modalities under the direction of a qualified registered nurse. Additionally, ANNA supports research into barriers to home dialysis as a means to eliminating such barriers as the number of patients requiring dialysis in the next two decades is expected to more than double.

ANNA supports dialysis payment reform that would allow flexibility for the provision of daily or more frequent dialysis, and any other safe and effective emerging treatment modalities for chronic kidney disease, including incentives for patient self-management.

ANNA believes that all individuals must be protected from the possible threat of communicable diseases related to dialysis, transplantation, and other extracorporeal therapies, and that access to testing for such diseases should be available to all patients. ANNA endorses the vaccination of all patients against Hepatitis B, pneumonia, and influenza.

Transplantation

ANNA supports public and private sector efforts that promote organ donation and increase transplantation. The Association believes this can be accomplished by:
• Continued support for educational programs for the public and for health professionals concerning the lack of available donor organs and the appropriate identification of potential donors.
• Continued support for the federally funded OPTN.
• Implementation of uniform state codes and laws regarding organ donation, procurement, and transplantation:
  - Amend the Anatomical Gift Act to support that a desire to donate expressed in any form (a donor card, driver's license check-off, placement of name on a registry, or verbal statement) cannot be revoked by the next of kin, and to prohibit approach of families when there is evidence that the individual did not want to donate.
  - Amend the Anatomical Gift Act to facilitate Medical Examiner/ Coroner consent for 'John Doe' donations following a diligent search for identification and legal next of kin.
  - Add organ/tissue donation language in any existing or future legislation related to advance directives, living wills and durable powers of attorney.
  - Support of state registries for persons wishing to donate organs at the time of their deaths and federal funding for these registries.
• Continued federal support of transplant activities including medical research and coverage of immunosuppressive drug therapy and legislative initiatives to extend immunosuppressive drug coverage for the life of the transplanted organ(s).
• Education of insurers and other payers regarding the success and cost effectiveness of organ transplantation to their members in order to prevent actual or perceived barriers to transplantation.
• Removal of financial disincentives to live organ donation including funding for transportation and lost income.
• Studies to review the ethical implications of proposals to increase living non-related donation that may dispropor-

tionately affect certain populations.
• Support for research into the use of financial incentives for deceased donors as a mechanism to increase organ donation.

ANNA opposes coercive behavior in the solicitation of organs for transplantation and living donation when the donor's decision is based primarily on financial gain.

ESRD Program Management

ANNA is concerned that outdated payment policies negatively affect kidney patients' access to care and can lead to compromise in the quality of care delivered. ANNA supports ESRD payment reforms that will allow delivery of care that is consistent with both the standards of professional nephrology nursing established by ANNA, and the clinical practice guidelines established by the NKF-Kidney Dialysis Outcomes Quality Initiative.

ANNA believes that patients with progressive chronic kidney disease should have access to education and support services and clinical care that may improve their kidney function, delay the progression of their disease, or improve their health status and readiness for the initiation of end stage renal disease therapies.

ANNA supports amending Title XIX of the Social Security Act (Medicaid) to include dialysis as a mandatory service in state Medicaid programs.

ANNA believes that oversight of ESRD facilities should be an ongoing, collaborative effort by the Centers for Medicare and Medicaid Services (CMS) and its contractors, including state agencies and renal Network organizations. Members of the on-site survey team should be knowledgeable about the various aspects of the delivery of care to individuals with kidney disease. Assessment to assure that safe and effective care and treatment are delivered to all individuals must be included in the monitoring process.

Managed Care and Commercial Health Plans and the ESRD Population

Each health plan must develop a process to ensure access of members diagnosed with chronic kidney disease or end-stage renal disease to relevant specialists.

Each health plan must develop a protocol for screening their members for specific indications of kidney disease and early referral of those members to nephrologists for evaluation.

Each health plan must have a mechanism for providing its members who are children or adolescents with access to a pediatric nephrologist in the geographic area of coverage. If none is available, the plan's guidelines for care delivery to children or adolescents with kidney disease must be developed by a committee that includes a pediatric nephrologist.

Each health plan must have a mechanism for providing members with end-stage renal disease with access to dialysis and transplant providers that are geographically accessible, whose outcomes and waiting times are known to meet acceptable national standards and averages, and who are able to provide all forms of dialytic therapy currently available, including peritoneal dialysis, home dialysis, and a dialysis schedule that conforms with the members' employment or other rehabilitation needs.

Each health plan must develop mechanisms for rapid response from nephrology personnel when a referral request is received from a plan member with kidney disease.

Each health plan must involve nephrologists, nephrology nurses, renal social workers and renal nutritionists in the development of guidelines for care delivery for members with chronic kidney disease or end-stage renal disease.

Each health plan must have an ongoing education program for those members who have been diagnosed with chronic kidney disease or who are at risk for developing kidney disease, e.g. those with diabetes, hypertension, and hereditary diseases. This program is, ideally, managed by experienced nephrology nurses or, in their absence, other experienced nephrology professionals.

Each health plan must develop literature specific to the end-stage renal disease population that outlines the limits and extent of coverage to that population, including co-payments for dialysis treatments and associated therapies.

Each health plan must develop mechanisms to ensure the inclusion of members with end-stage renal disease in the ESRD Network programs and the United States Renal Data System (USRDS) database.

Each health plan must conduct periodic evaluations of all contractors (e.g. dialysis facilities and transplant programs) providing care to members with end-stage renal disease.

Each health plan must provide coverage for dialysis services for members who travel outside the health plan's normal coverage area.

Each health plan must provide coverage for immunosuppressive agents for all transplant recipients for the duration of the transplant.

No health plan may discriminate in any way against a member on the basis of a diagnosis of end-stage renal disease.

Adopted by the American Nephrology Nurses'
Association
Board of Directors
Revised and Reaffirmed: April 2005

Index

Note: *t*= table; *f*= figure

Index

Atgam (antithymocyte globulins-equine), 775*t*, 778*t*, 783

Atherosclerosis
- in chronic kidney disease, 251–252
- in end stage renal disease, 318–319, 318*t*

ATP, for acute renal failure, 216*t*

Atrial natriuretic factor. *See* Atrial natriuretic peptide

Atrial natriuretic hormone. *See* Atrial natriuretic peptide

Atrial natriuretic peptide (ANP)
- for acute renal failure, 216*t*
- renal hemodynamics and, 88
- sodium reabsorption and, 113

Atrial oncotic pressure, 112

Atriopeptin. *See* Atrial natriuretic peptide

Auditory system, renal-related information, 183*t*

Australia, nephrology nursing care in, 877–878

Autograft, 773*t*

Automated peritoneal dialysis (APD)
- cyclers for, 649
- historical aspects, 33–34
- peritonitis in, 696

Autonomic nervous system disturbances, in ESRD, 317–318

Autonomy, 362, 799, 805–806

Autoregulation mechanism (ARM), 85–86

Autosomal dominant disease, 165

Autosomal dominant polycystic kidney disease (ADPKD)
- genetic factors in, 170
- nephrectomy specimen, 150, 150*f*
- with PKD1 progression, 150

Autosomal recessive disease, 164–165

Autosomal recessive polycystic kidney disease (ARPKD), 150, 170

Autosome, 161*t*, 162

AV bridge grafts, for vascular access
- advantages of, 566
- assessment, 568
- cannulation technique, 568–569
- complications, 567–568, 567*f*, 569*t*
- disadvantages of, 566
- patient education, 569
- percent recirculation determination, 567, 569*t*
- placement, 566–567, 567*f*

AVF. *See* Arteriovenous fistula

Azathioprine (Imuran®; Azasan®)
- adverse effects, 777*t*
- dosage/administration, 774*t*, 781
- for kidney transplants, 35–36
- monitoring, 781
- pharmacology/pharmacokinetics, 780–781

Azotemia. *See* Prerenal failure

B

Bacillus-Calmette-Guerin vaccine (BCG vaccine), 440–441

Back filtration, 532, 533*f*

BACTEC system, 444

Bacteria
- antimicrobial-resistant, 422–427, 425*t*, 426*t*
- carriers, asymptomatic, 421–422
- causing peritonitis, 696–697, 697*t*
- colonization, 421
- infections, in hemodialysis unit, 421–442
  - antimicrobial-resistant bacteria and, 422–427, 425*t*, 426*t*

culture and follow-up, 424–426, 426*t*, 427*t*
- prevention of transmission, 422
- transmission, 421–422

Baker, Mary, 42*t*

Balanced Budget Act of 1997, 859

Balanced Budget Refinement Act of 1999, 859

Bartter syndrome, 164, 168*t*

Basiliximab (Simulect), 775*t*, 778*t*, 783

BCG vaccine (Bacillus-Calmette-Guerin vaccine), 440–441

BC NurseLine, 912–913

Bednar, Barbara, 44*t*

Behaviorism
- continuing dominance of, 890
- definition of, 900
- patient education and, 889

Behaviorist learning theory, 900

Beneficence, 362, 799

Beneficiary Improvement and Protection Act (BIPA), 859–860

Bereavement, 365

Berk, Hendrik, 31

Berk Enamel Company, 31

Bernbeck, Lois, 39*t*–40*t*

Beta$_2$-adrenergic agonists, for hyperkalemia in CKD, 412–413

Beta-adrenergic blockers
- for hypertension, in chronic kidney disease, 258–260, 258*t*
- use in renal insufficiency, 405

Bicarbonate
- anion gap and, 123
- buffering system, 102–103, 102*t*, 103*t*
- in dialysate, 542*t*, 543, 548
- generation, 104–105, 104*f*
- in peritoneal dialysis solutions, 646–647
- reabsorption, 97, 103–104, 103*f*, 104*f*

Bicitra, 475

Biddle, Geri, 42*t*–43*t*

Biguanides, for diabetes with kidney disease, 298*t*, 299

Bile-binding resins, use in renal insufficiency, 406

Biliary system complications, post-liver transplantation, 761

Bilirubin, in urine, 191*t*

Bilirubin tests, 758*t*

Bills, legislative process for, 838, 839*f*, 840–841

Bioavailability of drugs, 398

Bioimpedence spectroscopy, 583

Bioinformatics, 174

Biological wastes, from hemodialysis unit, 438

BIPA (Beneficiary Improvement and Protection Act), 859–860

Bladder
- capacity, 76
- distention, 186
- leakage, post-kidney transplantation, 745
- perforation, from PD catheter insertion, 670
- spasms, post-transplant, 738

Bleeding
- gastrointestinal
  - in acute renal failure, 222–223, 222*f*
  - in end stage renal disease, 321, 321*f*
- into peritoneal cavity, from PD catheter insertion, 670
- post-liver transplant, 758

Bleeding time in uremia, pharmacologic reduction of, 221, 221*t*

Blood analyses, diagnostic, 186–189, 187*t*, 188*t*

Bloodborne pathogens, occupational exposure, 861

Blood circuit for hemodialysis, intradialytic monitoring, 552–553

Blood clots, post-transplant urine output and, 736

Blood flow
- to liver, drug metabolism and, 397–398, 398*t*
- peritoneal, 637
- rate calculations for CRRT, 225, 225*t*
- renal, 81, 81*f*
  - pressure changes and, 85–86
  - renin-angiotensin mechanism and, 86–87, 86*f*

Bloodlines, hemodialyzer, 552, 594

Blood pressure
- classification, 249*t*, 250
- estimated dry weight and, 583
- high. *See* Hypertension
- management, for diabetes with kidney disease, 299–300
- mean arterial, 85

Blood urea nitrogen (BUN)
- normal range, 187, 187*t*
- in prerenal failure, 206
- in renal dysfunction, 187*t*
- for renal function assessment, 186, 187

Blood volume
- by age, 464, 464*t*
- depletion during hemodialysis, 588
- monitoring, during hemodialysis, 591–592

Bocchino, Carmella, 41*t*

Body temperature, during hemodialysis, 588

Body weight. *See* Weight, body

Bone disorders
- in chronic kidney disease, 250–251, 263*t*
- in end stage renal disease, 321–322
- post-kidney transplant, 748–749

Bone turnover, calcitriol and, 97

Borel, Jean-Francois, 36

Bostock, John, 30

Bowman, William, 30

Bowman's capsule, 78, 82

Bowman's space, 78

Bowman's space colloid osmotic pressure, 84, 84*f*, 85

Bowman's space hydrostatic pressure, 84, 84*f*, 85

Bradykinin
- synthesis of, 87
- type A dialyzer reactions and, 598

Brain death criteria, for organ donors, 718–719, 719*t*

Brennan, Dawn, 42*t*

Bright, Richard, 30

Bright's disease, 30, 36

Budget process, of federal government, 841–842

Buffer pairs, 102, 102*t*

Buffers
- in peritoneal dialysis solutions, 646–647
- physiological systems, 102, 102*t*
  - extracellular, 102–103, 103*t*
  - intracellular, 102–103, 103*t*

Bulk forming agents, for chronic kidney disease, 407

Static venous pressure, for vascular access monitoring, 573–574

Statins (HMG-CoA reductase inhibitors), 406

Steal syndrome, of AV bridge graft, 568

Stem cell research, 174

Stenosis, central venous catheter, 571

Sterilization methods
in hemodialysis unit, 437–438
for hemodialyzers, 539

Steroid-induced diabetes mellitus (SIDM), 737–738

Steroid resistant nephrotic syndrome, genetic factors in, 168*t*

Stool softeners, for chronic kidney disease, 407–408

Storage tanks, for water treatment system, 547

Streptokinase, for PD catheter obstruction, 676

Streptomycin, for tuberculosis, 446*t*, 447*t*

Stress
physical responses to, 334
psychological responses to, 334

Stressors
of aging, 508
family
kidney transplant-related, 333
peritoneal dialysis related, 332

Subclavian vein
central venous catheter placement, 570
occlusion, 561, 562*f*

Subcutaneous port devices, for vascular access, 572–573

Sulfonylureas, for diabetes with kidney disease, 298*t*, 299

Sulfur crystals, in urine sediment, 192, 193*t*

Supplemental Security Income (SSI), assistance, for families of pediatric CKD patients, 478–479

Support
private assistance, for families of pediatric CKD patients, 479
in promoting health/quality of life, 350

Support groups, for elderly, 512

Susceptibility genetic testing, 173

Swan-neck Missouri peritoneal catheters, 666–667, 666*f*, 669

Swan-neck peritoneal catheters, 665–666, 665*f*

Swartz formula, 189, 189*t*

Sympathetic nervous system
in hemorrhage control, 88, 89*f*
renin-angiotensin mechanism and, 86, 86*f*, 87

Symptom Assessment Index, 279

Symptom Interpretation Model, 278

Symptom Management Model, 278–279

Symptoms. *See also specific symptoms*
assessment tools, 279–280
associated pathological conditions, 181*t*
goals of, 277
management, 277–286
of fatigue, 280–282
of pruritus, 282–284
of thirst, 284–286
models of, 277–279
quality of life and, 349
renal related, by body system, 183*t*–184*t*

Symptom Self-Care Response Model, 278

Synchrony, 890

Synthetic dialyzer membranes, 537*t*, 538

Systemic lupus erythematosis, genetic factors in, 168*t*, 170–171

T

TAC (time-averaged concentration), 608

Tacrolimus (Prograf®)
adverse effects, 777*t*
dosage/administration, 774*t*
dosing/monitoring, 780, 780*t*
pharmacology/pharmacokinetics, 780

Tactile sensation, age-related changes, 504–505

TAD (time-averaged deviation), 608

Tamm-Horsfall mucoprotein, 190

Taste, sense of, age-related changes, 504

Teachable moment, 901

Teacher, nephrology nurse as, 21

Teaching
barriers to, 896–897
elderly, instructional systems design model for, 518–519, 518*t*
older adults, 892–893

Team approach, for advance care planning, 363–364

Telehealth
e-health, 912–913
health informatics and, 906–907, 906*t*
major issues, 911
nurses in, 910–911
in renal care, 913–914
telephone triage, 912–913
types of, 911

TELENEPHRO program, 913–914

Telephone triage, 912–913

Telomere, 162, 162*t*

Tenckhoff, Henry, 34

Tenckhoff catheters
coiled, curled or spiral, 664*f*, 665
development of, 34
for peritoneal dialysis for children, 469, 470*t*
single-cuff, 664–665, 665*f*
straight, 664–665, 664*f*

Test of Functional Health Literacy in Adults (TOFHLA), 901

Tetany, hypocalcemic, 130, 134*f*

T-fluted peritoneal catheter, 667–668, 668*f*

Therapeutic environment, for pediatric chronic kidney disease, 475–476

Therapeutic plasma exchange (TPE)
cascade or secondary plasma filtration, 231–232, 231*f*
complications, 233–234
continuous flow centrifugation, 230, 230*f*
equipment/supplies, 232–233, 232*t*
historical aspects, 228–229, 229*f*
intermittent flow centrifugation, 229–230, 229*f*
intraprocedural monitoring, 233–234
membrane plasma separators, 230–231, 231*f*
nursing literature on, 234–235
postprocedural care, 234
pretreatment nursing assessment, 232
research, 234–235
vascular access, 232, 232*t*
vs. hemodialysis, 232–234, 232*t*

Thermoregulation impairment in organ donor, nursing interventions for, 721*t*

Thiazide diuretics, for renal insufficiency, 402–403

Thiazolidinediones, for diabetes with kidney disease, 298*t*, 299

Thirst
assessment, 284–285
definition of, 284
etiologies of, 285
interventions for, 285–286

Three-pore model, of peritoneal membrane transport, 638–639

Thrombolytics, for PD catheter obstruction, 676

Thrombosis
of arteriovenous fisutula, 564–565, 565*t*
of AV bridge grafts, for vascular access, 567, 569*t*
central venous catheter, 570–571, 571*f*

Thrombotic thrombocytopenic purpura/hemolytic uremia syndrome (TTP/HUS), 149, 149*t*

Thymoglobulin (antithymocyte globulins-rabbit), 775*t*, 778*t*, 783

Thyroid hormone abnormalities, in end stage renal disease, 315*t*

Tidal drain volume, 643

Tidal fill volume, 643

Tidal volume peritoneal dialysis (TVPD), 643–644

Time-averaged concentration (TAC), 608

Time-averaged deviation (TAD), 608

Timeline representations stage, of CSM, 58

Time management techniques, 829

Time of day, nursing interventions for elderly and, 510

Title XVIII of Social Security Act, 854

T lymphocytes, transplant rejection and, 773

TMP (transmembrane pressure), 532, 589

TMP monitors, 544

Toenails, care practices, for diabetics, 304

TOFHLA (Test of Functional Health Literacy in Adults), 901

Toronto Western Hospital Type 2 peritoneal catheter, 666, 666*f*, 669

Total body fluid, 123, 123*t*

Total protein, urinary, 190, 192*t*

TPE. *See* Therapeutic plasma exchange

Transcellular fluid volume, 123, 123*t*

Transcription, 162, 162*t*, 165*f*

Transducer protector (TP), 541

Transitional epithelial cells, in urine sediment, 193*t*

Translation, genetic, 162, 162*t*, 165*f*

Transmembrane pressure (TMP), 532, 589

Transplant Amendments Act of 1990, 858

Transplantation
allocation of organs, 723–724, 724*t*
dietary restrictions, for children, 474
kidney. *See* Kidney transplantation
liver. *See* Liver transplantation
nephrology nursing specialty and, 9
overview, 715–716, 715*t*, 716*t*
pancreatic. *See* Pancreas transplantation
pharmacology of, 773–786
pharmacotherapy, resources, 790
prevalence rates, 715–716, 716*t*
procurement of organs, 723–724, 724*t*
quality of life and, 348
survival rates, 715–716, 715*t*

Treatment adherence
in chronic illness, 63
chronic kidney disease, 492–493

Treatment beliefs, Common-Sense Model of Self-Regulation of Health and Illness and, 64–65

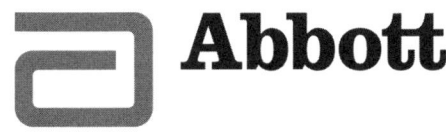

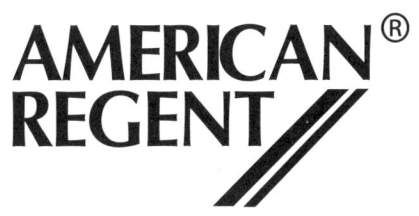

Abbott
200 Abbott Park Road
Department RA20
Abbott Park, IL 60064-6227
Telephone: 847-937-6100
Web site: www.abbott.com

Abbott is a global, broad-based health care company devoted to the discovery, development, and manufacture of pharmaceuticals, nutritionals and medical products, including devices and diagnostics. The company employs approximately 55,000 people and markets its products in more than 130 countries.

American Regent, Inc.
PO Box 9001
One Luitpold Drive
Shirley, NY   11967
Telephone: 800-645-1706 or 631-924-4000
Web site: www.americanregent.com
                      www.venofer.com

American Regent, "Your IV Iron Company," is proud to be the manufacturer and distributor of Venofer® (iron sucrose injection, USP), the #1 prescribed IV iron in the U.S.[1] Venofer® is available in 100mg/5mL single dose vials (preservative free). Venofer® is covered nationally by CMS/Medicare and has been assigned a permanent national HCPCS Code "J1756" for hemodialysis services.

American Regent continues its commitment to the renal community with quality services provided by a highly trained and knowledgeable field sales force and a clinical support team of nephrology specialists focused on issues impacting pre-dialysis, hemodialysis, and peritoneal dialysis patients. Some of these services include: Facility-Based In-Services and CE Presentations, Facility-Based Iron Utilization Reviews, Patient Education Programs, Professional Speakers Bureau, Patient Assistance Program, a Reimbursement Hotline, a Resource Center for Clinical Inquiries, and Regional Iron and Anemia Workshops. For additional information, visit our websites at www.americanregent.com and www.venofer.com.

[1] Based on IMS Health, National Sales Perspectives™ - 3rd Quarter 2005 Results – Total Sales Volume ($) and units (100 mg equivalents).

AMGEN®

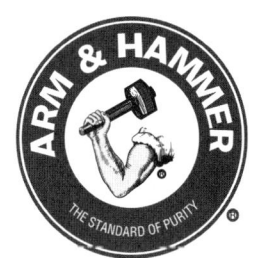

Amgen Inc.
Amgen Center
One Amgen Center Drive
Thousand Oaks, CA   91320
Telephone: 800-8AMGEN8 (800-826-4368)
Web site: www.amgen.com

Amgen, the world's largest biotechnology company, is a leader in bringing innovative treatment to nephrology patients. Amgen research and product development programs aim to help patients in four critical areas: metabolism/nephrology, oncology, inflammation and bone diseases and neurology. Two prominent erythropoietic agents discovered by Amgen include EPOGEN® (Epoetin alfa), the recombinant replacement for natural erythropoietin, and Aranesp® (darbepoetin alfa), for the treatment of anemia associated with chronic kidney disease. Amgen's first small molecule drug, Sensipar® (cinacalcet HCl) is a first-in-class calcimimetic agent, indicated for the treatment of secondary hyperparathyroidism in patients with chronic kidney disease on dialysis. Sensipar® is also indicated for the treatment of hypercalcemia in patients with parathyroid carcinoma.

Church & Dwight Co., Inc.
Performance Products Group
469 North Harrison Street
Princeton, NJ   08543
Telephone: 800-221-0453
Web site: www.ahperformance.com

Church & Dwight Co., Inc. is the maker of pure ARM & HAMMER® brand hemodialysis grade sodium bicarbonate, developed specifically for kidney dialysis. This outstanding product is available through our 'Partners in Quality Care,' a unique alliance between Church & Dwight and the nation's leaders in dialysis chemicals and equipment. Through this alliance, we provide our partners with resources for dialysis professionals and their patients. These resources add value to our product as well as enhance the roles dialysis professionals play in their facilities.

Among the resources are original educational materials such as the popular patient pamphlets, *A Guide to Managing Fluid Intake* and *A Guide to Taking Control of Your Life on Dialysis*. Debuting in early 2006 is *Hemodialysis Step by Step*, a take-home companion to the very well-received flip-chart presentation of the same name, used in clinics by dialysis staff with new hemodialysis patients. All three pamphlets are available in both English and Spanish.

Partners in Quality Care is a dynamic program that combines the very finest sodium bicarbonate with valuable information to promote better patient outcomes and compassionate patient care.

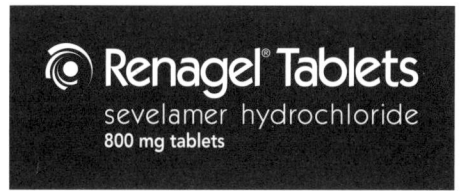

GAMBRO. Renal Products

Gambro Renal Products
10810 West Collins Avenue
Lakewood, CO   80215
Telephone: 800-525-2623 or 303-232-6800
Web site: www.usa-gambro.com

Gambro Renal Products (GRP) is a worldwide leader in intensive care therapies and dialysis technology and services that enable our customers to provide exceptional patient care. Our approach to superior dialysis treatment focuses on The Loop®, a holistic approach built around superior products, technology, delivery processes and people. The Loop provides a complete solution for physicians, administrators, clinicians and patients that improve dialysis treatment, while facilitating better patient outcomes and reducing lifecycle costs.

GRP's mission isn't to simply stay ahead of the curve. Instead, we're dedicated to creating it. We've been a leader in renal product development for over 40 years, and first to market with many innovations, including the first computerized dialysis machine. We also introduced the BiCart® cartridge, a dry bicarbonate concentrate cartridge that's become a world standard.

GRP also offers a full range of renal and intensive care services that give customers easy access to our expertise in logistics, clinical management, administration and education.

GRP is in the market for one simple reason: to help customers provide better care for their patients. We do this by offering solutions that improve treatment quality and efficiency, while allowing healthcare providers to focus on one thing—delivering the best patient care.

Gambro Renal Products. A better way to better care.

Genzyme Corporation
500 Kendall Street
Cambridge, MA   02142
Telephone: 800-932-3135
Web site: www.genzyme.com

One of the world's leading biotechnology companies, Genzyme is dedicated to making a major positive impact on the lives of people with serious diseases. Founded in 1981, Genzyme has grown from a small start-up to a diversified enterprise with more than 8,000 employees in locations spanning the globe and 2004 revenues of $2.2 billion. With many established products and services helping patients in more than 80 countries, Genzyme is a leader in the effort to develop and apply the most advanced technologies in the life sciences. The company's products and services are focused on rare inherited disorders, kidney disease, orthopaedics, cancer, transplant and immune diseases, and diagnostic testing. Genzyme's commitment to innovation continues today with a substantial development program focused on these fields as well as heart disease and other areas of unmet medical need.

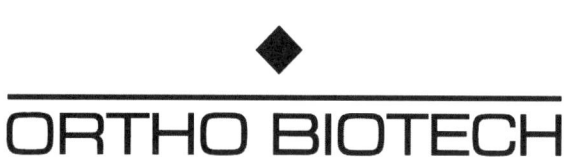

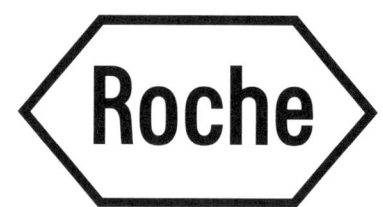

Ortho Biotech Products, L.P.
430 Route 22 East
Bridgewater, NJ 08807
Telephone: 908-541-4000
Web site: www.orthobiotech.com

In 1990, Ortho Biotech Products, L.P. was established in Raritan, NJ. Since that time, Ortho Biotech and its worldwide affiliates have earned a global reputation for researching, manufacturing, and marketing innovative healthcare products that enhance the quality of patients' lives. Ortho Biotech, located in Bridgewater, NJ, is an established market leader in Epoetin alfa therapy for anemia management.

Roche
340 Kingsland Street
Nutley, NJ   07110-1199
Telephone: 973-235-5000
Web site: http://www.rocheusa.com

Hoffmann-La Roche Inc. (Roche), based in Nutley, NJ, is the U.S. prescription drug unit of the Roche Group, a leading research-based health care enterprise that ranks among the world's leaders in pharmaceuticals and diagnostics. Roche discovers, develops, manufactures and markets numerous important prescription drugs that enhance people's health, well-being and quality of life. Among the company's areas of therapeutic interest are: dermatology; genitourinary disease; infectious diseases, including influenza; inflammation, including arthritis; metabolic diseases, including obesity and diabetes; neurology; oncology; osteoporosis; transplantation; vascular diseases; and virology, including HIV/AIDS and hepatitis C.

For more information on the Roche pharmaceuticals business in the United States, visit the company's web site at: http://www.rocheusa.com.

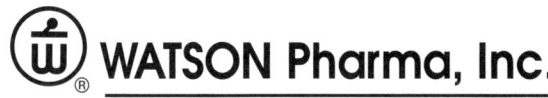

A Subsidiary of Watson Pharmaceuticals, Inc.

Watson Pharma, Inc.
A Subsidiary of Watson Pharmaceuticals, Inc.
360 Mount Kemble Avenue
Morristown, NJ   07962
Telephone: 973-355-8300
Web site: www.watsonpharm.com

Watson Nephrology offers specialty products for patients with kidney disease, including injectable iron therapies and vitamin formulations. We also provide support for nephrology professionals in hospitals and dialysis centers through iron reimbursement assistance, product information hotlines, and anemia management education programs. Watson Nephrology has enjoyed a long-standing relationship with healthcare providers and we are proud to continue working together for the benefit of hemodialysis patients. Watson Nephrology is a division of Watson Pharmaceuticals, Inc., a leading specialty pharmaceutical company that develops, manufactures, markets, sells, and distributes branded and generic pharmaceutical products.

AP® BIOLOGY EQUATIONS AND FORMULAS

Statistical Analysis and Probability

Mean (*See pages 12, 20*)

$$\bar{x} = \frac{1}{n}\sum_{i=1}^{n} x_i$$

Mode = value that occurs most frequently in a data set (*See pages 12, 21*)

Median = middle value that separates the greater and lesser halves of a data set (*See pages 12, 20*)

Mean = sum of all data points divided by number of data points (*See pages 12, 20*)

Range = value obtained by subtracting the smallest observation (sample minimum) from the greatest (sample maximum) (*See page 22*)

Standard Error of the Mean (*See page 24*)

$$SE_{\bar{x}} = \frac{s}{\sqrt{n}}$$

Standard Deviation (*See pages 22–24, 28*)

$$s = \sqrt{\frac{\sum\left(x_i - \bar{x}^2\right)}{n-1}}$$

Chi-Square (*See pages 374–376, 388–389*)

$$\chi^2 = \sum \frac{(o-e)^2}{e}$$

$\bar{x}$ = sample mean

n = sample size

s = sample standard deviation (i.e., the sample-based estimate of the standard deviation of the population)

o = observed results

e = expected results

$\sum$ = sum of all

Degrees of freedom are equal to the number of distinct possible outcomes minus one.

Chi-Square Table (*See page 375*)

P-value	Degrees of Freedom							
	1	2	3	4	5	6	7	8
0.05	3.84	5.99	7.81	9.49	11.07	12.59	14.07	15.51
0.01	6.63	9.21	11.34	13.28	15.09	16.81	18.48	20.09

Laws of Probability (*See pages 372–373, 386–388*)

If A and B are mutually exclusive, then:

$$P(A \text{ or } B) = P(A) + P(B)$$

If A and B are independent, then:

$$P(A \text{ and } B) = P(A) \times P(B)$$

Hardy–Weinberg Equations (*See pages 607–611*)

$$p^2 + 2pq + q^2 = 1$$
$$p + q = 1$$

p = frequency of allele 1 in a population

q = frequency of allele 2 in a population

Metric Prefixes

Factor	Prefix	Symbol
10^9	giga	G
10^6	mega	M
10^3	kilo	k
10^{-1}	deci	d
10^{-2}	centi	c
10^{-3}	milli	m
10^{-6}	micro	μ
10^{-9}	nano	n
10^{-12}	pico	p

Rate and Growth

Rate (*See page 198*)

$$\frac{dY}{dt}$$

Population Growth (*See pages 755–757, 774*)

$$\frac{dN}{dt} = B - D$$

Metric Conversions and Prefixes

Measurement	Unit and Abbreviation	Metric Equivalent	English-to-Metric Conversion Factor	Metric-to-English Conversion Factor
Area	1 square centimeter (cm^2)	= 100 square millimeters	1 square inch = 6.4516 cm^2	1 cm^2 = 0.155 square Inch
	1 square meter (m^2)	= 10,000 square centimeters	1 square foot = 0.0929 m^2	1 m^2 = 10.764 square feet
			1 square yard = 0.8361 m^2	1 m^2 = 1.196 square yards
	1 hectare (ha)	= 10,000 square meters (m^2)	1 acre = 0.405 ha	1 ha = 2.47 acres
Mass	1 microgram (µg)	= 10^{-6} gram		
	1 milligram (mg)	= 10^{-3} gram		1 mg = approx. 0.015 grain
	1 gram (g)	= 1000 milligrams	1 ounce = 28.35 g	1 g = 15.432 grains
				1 g = 0.0353 ounce
	1 kilogram (kg)	= 1000 grams	1 pound = 0.4536 kg	1 kg = 2.205 pounds
	1 metric ton (t)	= 1000 kilograms	1 ton = 0.907 t	1 t = 1.103 tons
Length	1 angstrom (Å)	= 10^{-10} meter (10^{-4} µm)		
	1 nanometer (nm) (formerly millimicron, mµ)	= 10^{-9} meter (10^{-3} µm)		
	1 micrometer (µm) (formerly micron, µ)	= 10^{-6} meter (10^{-3} mm)		
	1 millimeter (mm)	= 0.001 (10^{-3}) meter		1 mm = 0.039 inch
	1 centimeter (cm)	= 0.01 (10^{-2}) meter		1 cm = 0.3894 inch
	1 meter (m)	= 100 (10^{-2})	1 foot = 0.305 m	1 m = 39.37 inches
			1 yard = 0.914 m	1 m = 3.28 feet
				1 m = 1.09 yards
	1 kilometer (km)	= 1000 (10^3) meters	1 mile = 1.61 km	1 km = 0.62 mile
Volume (solids)	1 cubic millimeter (mm^3)	= 10^{-3} cubic centimeter = 10^{-9} cubic meter		
	1 cubic centimeter (cm^3 or cc)	= 10^{-6} cubic meter	1 cubic inch = 16.387 cm^3	1 cm^3 = 0.061 cubic inch
	1 cubic meter (m^3)	= 1,000,000 cubic centimeters	1 cubic foot = 0.0283 m^3	1 m^3 = 35.315 cubic feet
			1 cubic yard = 0.7646 m^3	1 m^3 = 1.308 cubic yards
Volume (liquids and gases)	1 microliter (µL or µl)	= 10^{-6} liter (10^{-3} milliliter)		
	1 milliliter (mL or ml)	= 10^{-3} liter = 1 cubic centimeter	1 teaspoon = approx. 5 mL	1 mL = approx. 15–16 drops (gtt.)
			1 fluid ounce = 29.57 mL	1 mL = approx. $\frac{1}{4}$ teaspoon
			1 pint = 473 mL	1 mL = 0.034 fluid ounce
			1 quart = 946 mL	
	1 liter (L or l)	= 1000 milliliters	1 quart = 0.946 L	1 L = 1.057 quarts
			1 gallon = 3.785 L	1 L = 0.264 gallon
	1 kiloliter (kL or kl)	= 1000 liters		1 kL = 264.17 gallons
Pressure	1 pascal (Pa)	= 1 newton/m^2 (N/m^2)	1 bar = 1 × 10^5 Pa	1 Pa = 1 × 10^{-5} bar
	1 kilopascal (kPa)	= 1000 pascals	1 bar = 100 kPa	1 kPa = 0.01 bar
	1 megapascal (MPa)	= 1000 kilopascals	1 bar = 0.1 MPa	1 MPa = 10 bars
Time	1 second (s or sec)	= $\frac{1}{60}$ minute		
	1 millisecond (ms or msec)	= 10^{-3} second		
Temperature	Degrees Celsius (°C) (0 K [Kelvin] = −273.15°C)	°F = $\frac{9}{5}$°C + 32	°C = $\frac{9}{5}$°C + 32	

Metric Prefixes

10^{-15} = femto (f)

10^{-12} = pico (p)

10^{-9} = nano (n)

10^{-6} = micro (µ)

10^{-3} = milli (m)

10^{-2} = centi (c)

10^3 = kilo (k)

10^6 = mega (M)

10^9 = giga (G)